evolve

To access your Student Resources, visit:

http://evolve.elsevier.com/BerryKohn

Evolve Student Resources for *Berry & Kohn's Operating Room Technique,*
11th Edition, offer the following features:

Student Resources

- **Student Activities**
  Review activities, including crossword and word search puzzles, Perfect Picture
  activities, sequencing exercises, and more

- **Tips for the Scrub Person and the Circulating Nurse**
  Highlight "pearls of wisdom" for scrub persons and circulating nurses that the
  author has been collecting for years

- **Geriatric Laboratory Values in the Normal Aging Process Appendix**

- **Glossary**
  Comprehensive list of key terms and definitions

- **Content Updates**
  Written by the textbook author to fill you in on the latest research findings, drug
  information, and much more

- **Perioperative Flash Cards**
  Incorporate images from the book to help you learn concepts such as positioning,
  dissection, incisions, and sutures

- **Key Term Flash Cards**
  A great study tool for mastering complex terminology

- **WebLinks**
  Regularly updated

Using a patient roller
Safety Pointers:
Moving a patient between two surfaces requires someone at both sides of the beds, someone at the foot, and someone at the head. The person at the head calls the count of 1-2-3 to initiate movement of the patient.

Zones of sterility of sterile attire
Safety Pointers:
Preventing contamination of sterile attire creates an environment of infection prevention and patient protection.

The level of the sterile field
Safety Pointers:
The level of the sterile field begins with the surgical site on the patient's body. The level is influenced by the height of OR bed and the position of the patient.

Seated team and level of sterile field
Safety Pointers:
When the team is seated for a procedure, the level of the sterile field changes. When one person sits, all members sit.

Pouring solutions onto sterile field
Safety Pointers:
The nonsterile circulating nurse pours solutions into containers on the sterile field without splashing or contaminating the sterile field. The bottle lip is considered contaminated once the solution has been poured and may not be recapped for sterile use.

Establishing a sterile field
Safety Pointers:
The sterile person drapes a small unsterile table with a sterile cover by opening the cover towards self first and away from self without reaching over the sterile surface. Never hover over a sterile field.

Sterile persons passing one another in the sterile field
Safety Pointers:
Sterile persons pass face-to-face or back-to-back. Never turn the back toward a sterile field.

Appropriate attire in the restricted area
Safety Pointers:
Basic appropriate attire in the OR includes: scrub suit, hair cover, and mask. If there is danger of a splash then eyewear is worn. A sterile gown and gloves are donned if entering the sterile field.

Removing contaminated gown
Safety Pointers:
The gown is peeled off and turned inside out, away from the body. The gloves are removed last using a glove-to-glove and skin-to-skin technique. Do not get contamination on the scrub suit during the removal process.

Passing a ring-handled instrument
Safety Pointers:
The sterile person holds the ringed instrument by the boxlocks as it is placed into the waiting hand of the sterile surgeon or first assistant.

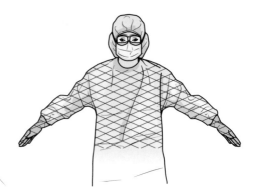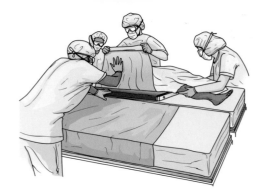

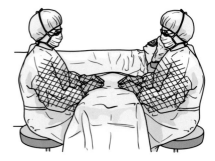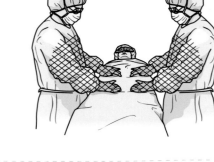

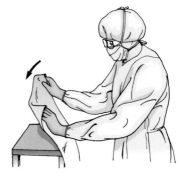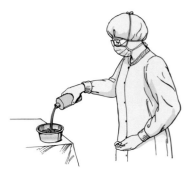

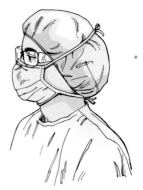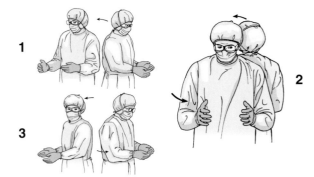

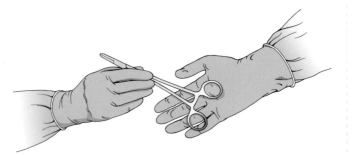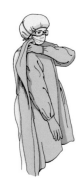

Tie on a passer
Safety Pointers:
The end of the free tie is positioned in the tip of a tonsil clamp or monihan clamp for use in the field.

Passing an item to the sterile field
Safety Pointers:
A nonsterile person can open and offer a sterile item to the sterile person without flipping it to the field. The sterile person touches only the sterile item to remove it from the packaging.

Flipping an item to the sterile field
Safety Pointers:
A nonsterile person can deliver an item to the sterile field using aseptic technique by opening the packet from one end and carefully flipping the item onto the table. Care is taken not to touch the item as its transferred and not to contaminate the sterile field during the transfer.

Overbed table attachment
Safety Pointers:
Care is taken to pad the axilla and avoid pressure on the patient's skin from the upright posts.

Position for tucked arms
Safety Pointers:
The arm is placed along side of the patient's body, and the draw sheet is secured with an arm protector.

Protection of the patient's arms when using table mounted equipment
Safety Pointers:
Care is taken not to cause compression of the brachial plexus by letting the patient's arms rest against an immobile surface such as a table mounted frame.

Armboard positioning
Safety Pointers:
The arms should not be abducted more than 90 degrees or the brachial plexus can be injured.

Lateral positioning frame
Safety Pointers:
Care is taken to pad the axilla and avoid pressure on the breasts and genitalia.

Andrews frame
Safety Pointers:
Kneeling position for spinal surgery requires the patient to be prone with the abdomen dependent. The arms are circumducted in diver's posture. Breasts, genitalia, and ears are protected. Secure with posterior board and boot straps.

Wilson frame
Safety Pointers:
The patient is prone over an arched frame with the abdomen dependent. The arms are circumducted into diver's posture. Breasts, genitalia, and ears are protected. Secure with leg straps over large muscle groups.

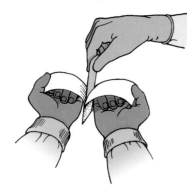
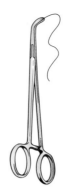
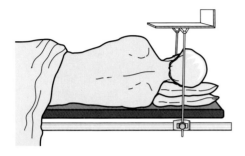
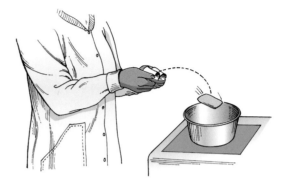
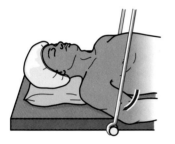
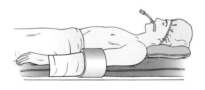
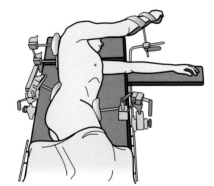

Correct
positioning

90 degrees

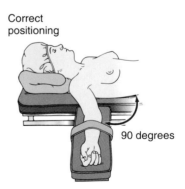
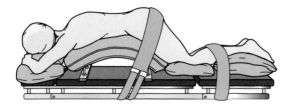
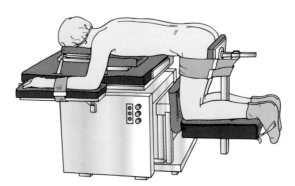

Using sling stirrups
Safety Pointers:
Care is taken to prevent a crush injury to the patient's hands in OR bed flex points. The legs should not come in contact with the upright posts of the stirrups. Injury to the peroneal nerve can cause footdrop.

Horseshoe headrest
Safety Pointers:
The horseshoe headrest is attached to the Mayfield frame. Care is taken to avoid pressure on the eyes or ears. Most horseshoe headrests are made of gel material.

Mayfield headrest
Safety Pointers:
Sterile pins are used to secure the patient's head in the Mayfield frame for head or cervical surgery.

Supine position
Safety Pointers:
Patient is face-up with arms tucked in at sides or positioned on armboards. Safety belt is over the thighs. A small pillow is under the knees and ankles as needed to relieve pressure to the lower back. The feet should not extend beyond the foot of the bed.

Frog-legged
Safety Pointers:
Care is taken not to permit stress on the externally rotated hip joint. Legs are secured in position for cardiothoracic or genitourinary procedures.

Trendelenburg's position
Safety Pointers:
The patient is positioned in a head down position. Care is taken to prevent shifting cephalad. Supine patients can have the footplate lowered to counter-balance the positioning. Intracranial pressure is increased. Abdominal organs shift cephalad to enhance visualization of pelvic organs.

Reverse Trendelenburg's position
Safety Pointers:
The patient is positioned feet down to shift organs caudad. Padding under the shoulders can hyperextend head and neck for anterior neck incisions. A padded footboard is used to prevent the patient from shifting toward the foot of operating bed.

Modified semi-Fowler's with shoulder free
Safety Pointers:
The patient is seated with the affected shoulder free. The head is secured and the eyes are protected.

Modified semi-Fowler's position: Beach chair
Safety Pointers:
The patient is partially seated in a beach chair pose. Note pressure points on buttocks. Small pillow is under the knees to relieve sacral pressure. Hands are placed across abdomen. Tucking the arms may cause the fingers to catch in the hinge of the operating bed.

Lithotomy position
Safety Pointers:
Two persons position the patient's legs into and out of the lithotomy position to prevent a rapid shift of blood pressure in the patient, to prevent sacral stretch, and to prevent injury in the caregiver. The patient's buttocks are positioned at the edge of OR bed. Strap is not placed over the abdomen to prevent an increase in pressure.

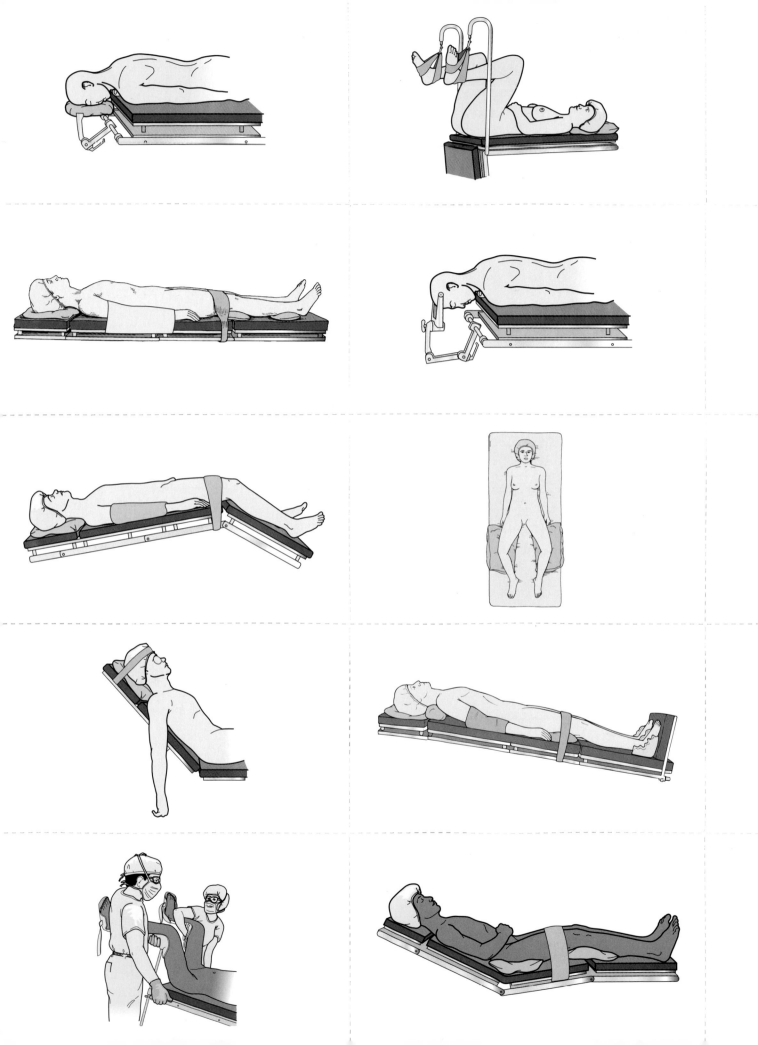

Prone position
Safety Pointers:
The patient is anesthetized on the transport cart. A minimum of 4 people are used to roll the patient face down on the OR bed. Arms are circumducted into diver position, axillary rolls are placed from shoulder to iliac crest, dorsum of feet are padded, and safety belt is across calves to prevent flexion. Thigh strap can be used.

Kraske (Jacknife) position
Safety Pointers:
The patient is anesthetized on the transport cart. A minimum of 4 people are used to roll the patient face down on the OR bed. Arms are circumducted into diver position, axillary rolls are placed from shoulder to iliac crest, dorsum of feet are padded, and safety belt is across calves. Thigh strap can be used. OR bed is flexed.

Left lateral
Safety Pointers:
The patient is positioned on a flat bed on the left side with both legs slightly flexed. Bottom axilla is padded, padding is placed between the knees, and the trunk is supported by pillows to prevent rolling.

Lateral positioning of cervical spine
Safety Pointers:
Care is taken to keep the cervical spine in alignment. Acute flexure can cause injury to cervical spine, discs, or vertebral arteries.

Right kidney position
Safety Pointers:
The patient is positioned on the left side with both legs slightly flexed. Bottom axilla is padded, padding is placed between the knees, and the trunk is supported by pillows to prevent rolling. The OR bed is flexed to elevate the right kidney, hence the name is for the target organ position when the OR bed is flexed.

Abdominal skin preparation
Safety Pointers:
The antiseptic skin cleansing is performed in a circular direction beginning at the incision site and extending toward the edges. A fresh sponge is used for each pass. The umbilicus is cleansed with a saturated cotton swab before the skin is prepped so the debris is not spread over the abdominal surface.

Chest and breast skin preparation
Safety Pointers:
The antiseptic skin cleansing is performed in a circular direction beginning at the incision site and extending toward the edges. All or part of the arm on the affected side will be prepped.A fresh sponge is used for each pass.

Perineal skin preparation
Safety Pointers:
The legs and abdomen are cleansed from the groin outward. The vagina is prepped next and the anus is cleansed last. The perineal prep is performed before a combined abdominal prep using a separate prep kit. This prevents perineal splashing to a clean abdomen. The abdomen is prepped last using a separate prep kit.

Hip skin preparation
Safety Pointers:
The skin is cleansed starting at the incision and working outward using a fresh sponge for each pass.

Limb skin preparation
Safety Pointers:
The limb is elevated by a limb holder or separate person wearing gloves. The skin is cleansed in a circumferential motion beginning at the distal part. A fresh sponge is used for each pass

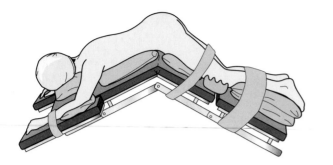

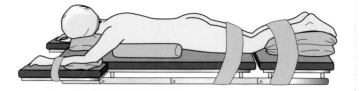

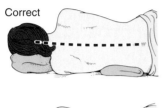

Correct

Incorrect

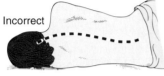

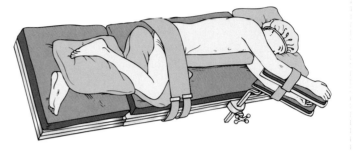

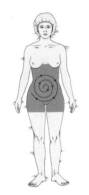

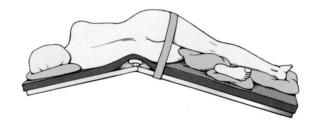

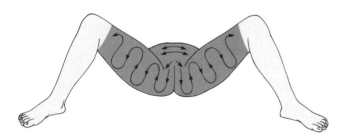

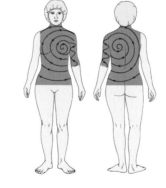

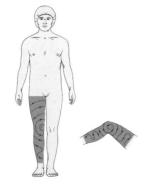

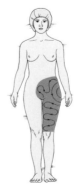

BERRY & KOHN'S

OPERATING ROOM TECHNIQUE

ELEVENTH EDITION

Nancymarie Phillips, RN, BSN, BA, MEd, RNFA, CNOR
Doctoral Candidate
Program Director, Perioperative Education
Perioperative and PeriAnesthesia Nursing
Registered Nurse First Assistants
Surgical Technology
Anesthesia Technology
Lakeland Community College,
Kirtland, Ohio

with 580 illustrations

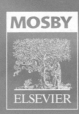

MOSBY

ELSEVIER

MOSBY
ELSEVIER

11830 Westline Industrial Drive
St. Louis, Missouri 63146

BERRY & KOHN'S OPERATING ROOM TECHNIQUE   ISBN: 978-0-323-04483-7
11th edition

Previous editions copyrighted 1955, 1960, 1966, 1972, 1978, 1986, 1991, 1996, 2000, 2003

ISBN: 978-0-323-04483-7

Acquisitions Editor: Kristin Geen
Developmental Editor: Lauren Lake
Managing Editor: Tamara Myers
Publishing Services Manager: Jeff Patterson
Design Direction: Jyotika Shroff

Printed in China

Last digit is the print number: 9 8 7 6 5 4 3

To

My Dad

Gilbert Dexter Howard, Jr.

He taught me to be brave and walk the walk.

Consultants

RUTH BAKST, RN, RNFA, CNOR
Perioperative Educator
Parma Community Hospital
Parma, Ohio
Registered Nurse Midwife
Capetown, South Africa

MARTIN A. PHILLIPS III, RN, BSN, CNOR, LTC
United States Army Nurse Corps
Reserve Component, 256th Combat Support Hospital
Brookpark, Ohio
399th Combat Support Hospital
Iraq
Perioperative Nursing
Veterans' Administration Medical Center
Cleveland, Ohio

M. JANE RUA, RN, BSN, JD
Attorney at Law
Jeffries, Kube, Forrest, and Monteleone, LPA
Cleveland, Ohio

JENNIFER KAVRAN, RN, BSN, CNOR
Wright Surgery Center
University Suburban Health Center
South Euclid, OH
Clinical Instructor
Perioperative Nursing and Surgical Technology
Lakeland Community College
Kirtland, Ohio

NATALIE BRIGHT, RN, BSN, CNOR
Perioperative Educator
Cleveland Clinic Health Systems-East
Mayfield Heights, Ohio

CATHERINE HYDE, RN, RNFA, CNOR
Obstetrics and Gynecology
Lake Hospital Systems
Willoughby, Ohio

PATRICK BURNISTON, RN, RNFA, CST, CNOR
Orthopaedic Surgery
Cuyahoga Falls, Ohio

SAM SIGNORE, RN, RNFA, CNOR
Cardiothoracic Surgery
E.T. Robbins, MD and Associates
Baptist Memorial Hospital, Memphis
Methodist Hospital,
Germantown, Tennessee

STEVE SUPANIK, RN
Spinal Surgery
Cleveland Clinic Foundation
Cleveland, Ohio

MICHELE GOULD, RN, BSN, RNFA, CNOR
Cardiothoracic Surgery
Maple Falls, Washington

REGINA ELAM, CST
General Surgery
Cleveland Clinic Foundation
Cleveland, Ohio

JACKI LAUSIN, ST
Lake Hospital System
Willoughby, Ohio

BONNIE VENCHIARUTTI, CST
University Hospital Health System East
Chardon, Ohio

Reviewers

Christina L. Baumer, RN, PhD, M.Ed, CNOR, CHES
Lancaster, Pennsylvania

Patricia E. Chapek, RN, BA, CNOR
Cleveland, Ohio

Roberta E. Clark, RN, BS, MSHSA, CNOR
Jacksonville, Florida

Sherry D. Ferki, RN, MSN
Portsmouth, Virginia

John F. Hanlon Jr., CRNA, MSNA, ARNP
Lowell, Massachusetts

Caryn B. Humphrey, RN, BSN
Muncie, Indiana

Michael J. Kremer, DNSc, CRNA, FAAN
Chicago, Illinois

Sherry M. Lawrence, RN, MSN, CNOR, ONC
Mobile, Alabama

Natasha Leskovsek, RN, MBA, MPM, JD
Washington, DC

Janet Anne Milligan, ST, RN, CNOR
Twin Falls, Idaho

Janice A. Neil, RN, PhD
Greenville, North Carolina

Carolyn J. Ragsdale, CST, BS
Champaign, Illinois

Nancy H. Wright, RN, BS, CNOR
Birmingham, Alabama

Saundra L. Seidel, APN, BC, CUCNS, CNOR
Fayetteville, Arkansas

Sarah Reidunn Tvedt-Pool, RN, MS
Rochester, Minnesota

Mary Ann Wehmer, RN, MSN, CNOR
Evansville, Indiana

Derek Wood, RN, BC, MS
Greeley, Colorado

Preface to the Eleventh Edition

As I survey the current editions of other texts in this field, I see that *Berry & Kohn's Operating Room Technique* is often imitated, but never duplicated. The attention to detail, explanations, and up-to-the-minute content surpasses the others. This time-honored text has its roots in the operating room (OR) orientation manual created by Mary Louise Kohn in the late 1940s while working as an OR educator at University Hospitals of Cleveland, Ohio. Her impeccable notes were a source of interest to many OR supervisors and educators who wanted to standardize their teaching techniques in accordance with Mary Louise's orientation tool. Many observers requested copies of her writings, and eventually the cost of providing copies became prohibitive.

In 1951, at the request of her publisher and with the encouragement of her superiors, Mary Louise assembled her orientation material into a manuscript suitable for publication. She spent countless hours writing and revising material until the birth of her daughter. Her dedication to her family led her to seek assistance for this project from Edna Cornelia Berry, who became her willing partner and coauthor throughout the first four editions.

The first edition of *Introduction to Operating Room Technique* by Edna Cornelia Berry and Mary Louise Kohn was published in 1955. I was fortunate to have obtained a copy for my collection. The first edition was dedicated to *"those nurses who accept the tension and challenge of coordinated teamwork as they minister to the patient in the operating room."* The main emphasis was on intraoperative care of the patient. The first edition had the following goals:

- To explain the principles of sterile and aseptic technique
- To stress the necessity for their application in all surgical procedures
- To provide insight into the physiologic and psychologic impact of surgical intervention on each patient as a unique individual

Berry and Kohn's Operating Room Technique has been the perioperative text of choice for more than 55 years because it emphasizes the importance of the patient and his or her reliance on the perioperative caregiver. The name remains "Operating Room Technique" because that is how it has been commonly known and identified, although the text has a comprehensive perioperative focus. It would be a disservice to our patients to merely describe the intraoperative phase and not include preoperative and postoperative care.

Every new edition of this classic perioperative text has addressed changing roles, needs, and evolving technologies while maintaining the fundamental focus that still remains valid after 55 years—the care of the surgical patient. This edition of the text identifies the knowledge and skill needs of the caregiver and strives to incorporate components of patient care from preoperative, intraoperative, and postoperative practice areas. A systems approach is introduced to help organize patient care to minimize the risk for human error.

Berry & Kohn's Operating Room Technique is designed to meet the needs of educators, learners, caregivers in diverse disciplines, and managerial personnel who care for surgical or interventional patients in many types of environments. Knowing the "why" of patient care is as important as knowing the "how." Additionally, it is important to stress that outcomes must be evaluated to support evidence-based practice. This text is the book of choice for certification preparation in diverse disciplines and incorporates all elements of the core curricula specified by several accrediting and certifying bodies.

FEATURES OF THE ELEVENTH EDITION

- A focus on the physiologic, psychologic, and spiritual considerations of perioperative patients to provide guidelines and standards for planning and implementing safe comprehensive individualized care.
- The systems approach is used as a foundation to support solid evidence-based practice to establish patient care procedures in such a way that all team members can identify their roles in a cooperative spirit of safety and efficiency.
- In-depth discussion of patients with special needs related to age or health status considerations, with an emphasis on the development of a plan of care tailored to the unique care parameters of all patients.
- Discussion of perioperative patient care in inpatient, ambulatory, and alternative sites/location to highlight considerations based on the setting as well as the surgical procedure.
- Encouragement of the caregiver to identify and examine personal and professional development issues that influence the manner in which care is rendered.
- Emphasis on teamwork among perioperative caregivers to encourage cooperation in attaining positive patient care outcomes.
- Detailed information about the fundamentals of perioperative nursing and surgical technology roles. No other text provides step-by-step explanations for each basic technique. Pertinent historical perspectives are included in each section to provide information about the evolution of the topic being discussed.
- Building of knowledge in a logical sequence—from fundamental concepts to implementation during surgical intervention—to enable readers to apply theory to practice.
- Comprehensive coverage of a broad range of essential topics to provide a thorough understanding of funda-

mental principles and techniques and an understanding of their applications in various surgical procedures.

• Specific surgical procedures are described in each specialty chapter to assist the learner and caregiver in planning and delivering patient care in the perioperative environment. The use of tables to organize the activities of the circulating nurse and the scrub person in specialty Chapters 33 through 45 is a new concept in the systems approach.

NEW TO THE ELEVENTH EDITION

Educators, learners, and caregivers in both academic and clinical settings will find the 12-section arrangement user-friendly. The logical and sequential order of the subject matter will enable perioperative caregivers of all disciplines to review and sharpen their knowledge and skill levels. The carefully planned tables, boxes, and figures further clarify the textual content. Line drawings are used throughout the text for emphasis and photographs are used to display specific identifiable subjects. *The AORN Standards, Recommended Practices, and Guidelines* have been incorporated to reflect modern perioperative practice. Web addresses are added in the text as in past editions, where appropriate.

• Chapter objectives have been updated to focus attention on important content to be learned in each chapter.

• Chapter outlines have been added in an abbreviated form to precede and describe the content of each chapter.

• Terminology and key words have been updated and revised to reflect modern practice. The key words and definitions appear at the start of each chapter to direct the reader's attention to the main premise for the material.

• Each chapter has been updated and revised to reflect current evidence-based practice and knowledge.

• The use of computers as learning and clinical tools is included throughout the text. Internet search engines are described, and pertinent websites are incorporated throughout the specialty sections. The advantages and disadvantages of computerized documentation are expanded. The Elsevier *Evolve* website has learning and teaching aids to enhance the classroom experience and support assimilation of knowledge.

• Educational support materials, such as PowerPoint presentations and test banks created by Jennifer Kavran, RN, BSN, CNOR, that follow each chapter are available.

• Perioperative flashcards that depict positioning images in the 11th edition are available for the first time in any perioperative textbook.

• Preoperative, intraoperative, and postoperative patient care chapters are clearly delineated and expanded to emphasis continuity for perioperative and perianesthesia caregivers.

• The Patient: The Reason for Your Existence (Chapter 7) reflects the care of the patient with some of the most common conditions. Caring for the victims of crime is described for the first time.

• Ambulatory Surgery Centers and Alternative Surgical Locations (Chapter 11) has been renamed. Ambulatory surgery centers are still described here, but other locations are introduced. Reviewers suggested descriptions and introduction to several new places, such as interventional suites, delivery rooms, mobile military installations, and veterinary facilities.

• Microbiologic Considerations (Chapter 14) has been updated to include new information about prion deactivation technology and antibiotic therapy. Bioterrorism is described for the first time.

• Surgical Instrumentation (Chapter 19) has been expanded to include twice as many illustrations as in previous editions. Select specialty instruments can be found in the specialty chapters.

• Surgical Pharmacology (Chapter 23) has been updated to collectively identify categories of drugs and pharmacologic substances used in perioperative patient care.

• Coordinated Roles of the Scrub Person and the Circulating Nurse (Chapter 25) has been updated to include tables that can be used to establish a systems approach to error prevention. Counts and the multiple reasons for counting and being accountable are described in depth.

• Endoscopy and Robotic-Assisted Surgery (Chapter 32) includes the concept of the Eight Essentials for Endoscopy, which were described for the first time collectively in the 10th edition. This section has been expanded to include robotics and the future of surgical practice.

• Spinal Surgery (Chapter 38) has been added. This chapter was developed to reflect modern practices that collectively incorporate neurologic and orthopedic disciplines for surgery of the spine.

• All illustrations and images are now in color. Many new illustrations and photos have been added to enhance the visual detail of basic perioperative principles and surgical anatomy.

• New boxes and tables serve to clarify and highlight information critical to perioperative practice.

ORGANIZATION

Section I describes education, learning, and professional issues. The correlation of theory and practice is integral to the success of patient care in the perioperative environment. Fundamental professional and personal attributes of the caregiver are examined, with an emphasis on objectivity in the development of the plan of care. Legal and ethical issues are discussed.

Section II delineates the roles of the members of the health care team as both direct and indirect caregivers. Non-physician first assistant roles and credentials are discussed in a separate chapter. Management of the perioperative patient care areas is described.

Section III provides in-depth information on patient assessment and the development of an individualized plan of care, with the patient viewed as a unique individual. Special needs are identified by health condition and age. Geriatric and pediatric chapters are included.

Section IV examines the physical plant of the perioperative environment—both hospital-based freestanding ambulatory facilities and alternative locations. Diagrams of conventional and nonconventional perioperative suite designs are included. Care of the perioperative environment, occupational hazards, and safety issues are examined in depth.

Section V explains microbiology and the importance of microbiologic control in the perioperative environment, with an emphasis on standard precautions. It delineates aseptic and sterile techniques as fundamental to intermediate aspects such as attire, scrubbing, gowning, and gloving. Separate chapters are provided regarding the sterilization and disinfection of surgical instrumentation and patient care supplies.

Section VI details the primary surgical instrumentation and equipment used during surgical procedures. The safe use of specialized surgical equipment is presented. Electricity is explained.

Section VII discusses preoperative patient care and includes the family/significant other in the plan of care. Diagnostic procedures and specimen handling are described.

Section VIII covers methods of anesthetic administration and the role of caregivers during this process. Physiologic patient responses and related potential perioperative complications are discussed in detail.

Section IX describes intraoperative patient care, including positioning, prepping, and draping. The interactive roles of the circulator and the scrub person are specified in Chapter 25. Economy of motion and the properties of physics are applied. Physiologic monitoring of the perioperative is described.

Section X focuses on the surgical site. Hemostasis and wound closure are discussed in detail. Wound assessment, dressing, and healing throughout the perioperative care period are described.

Section XI presents an expanded view of postoperative patient care. The postanesthesia care unit is explained. Prevention of patient complications is described. The death of a patient is discussed, and the importance of legal evidence is stressed.

Section XII covers the surgical specialties. Each chapter includes the historical development of the specialty. Salient surgical anatomy and procedures are described and illustrated in line drawings for clarity. Tables titled Tips for the Scrub Person and Tips for the Circulating Nurse are included for several common procedures.

Preface to the First Edition

The material in this text is the outgrowth of the coauthors' experience in the operating room—one as instructor of students, the other as head nurse with some responsibility for instructing and guiding students. It is an adaptation of the instructor's teaching outline for which there have been many requests.

The aim of the book is to facilitate the nurse's study of aseptic technique and care of the patient in the operating room. Although this text is intended primarily for the student, the authors hope it may prove useful to the graduate nurse as well.

Because it is assumed that the student has studied pathologic conditions necessitating surgical treatment, these conditions are not discussed. When applicable, and as a matter of emphasis, there is a reiteration of principles of sterile technique and safety factors for the patient. It is hoped this will aid in fixing the principles as patterns of thought and work.

Although operative routines vary in different hospitals, underlying principles are the same. Consequently, basic principles are stressed, and the authors have endeavored to keep the material as general as possible. Principles must be adapted to suit the situations found in individual hospitals. Specific linen, equipment, and procedures are mentioned merely to serve as a framework on which to demonstrate principles or as samples for points of departure. However, the specific examples mentioned are workable procedures that have evolved. They are kept as uncomplicated as possible for student teaching and for use in the practical situation.

Instruments for operations are not listed and few are mentioned because each hospital has its instrument lists, standardized for each case, to which students can refer.

Emphasis is placed on meeting the psychological as well as the physical needs of the surgical patient. An endeavor is made where possible to correlate briefly the preoperative and postoperative care with the operative procedure, to give the student a complete concept of patient care.

The frequent use of the imperative mood is for the purpose of brevity, organization, and emphasis. Questions and assignments in each chapter are to aid the student in reviewing the material, in recalling pertinent facts, and in applying the principles to his or her specific situation.

Obviously, if the student starts scrubbing for cases with an older nurse after the first day or two in the operating room and if operating-room theory is given concurrently with the practice, much of the material in this book will have been covered by individual instruction before class discussion.

The authors have attempted to maintain simplicity and brevity and to present a concise outline for preliminary study. They suggest that the student supplement this material by reference reading.

The authors wish to express their grateful appreciation and thanks to those people who by their interest and cooperation supported them:

To Miss Edythe Angell, supervisor of the Operating Rooms at University Hospitals of Cleveland, for helpful suggestions during the preparation of the manuscript and for reading, critically, the entire manuscript. We are gratefully indebted to her because we have learned from her much of what appears in this text.

To Miss Janet McMahon, Educational Director, School of Anesthesia, University Hospitals of Cleveland, for valuable assistance in preparing Chapter 21. Also, to Dr. Edward Depp, anesthesiologist, Euclid-Glenville Hospital, Cleveland, who offered suggestions on this chapter and reviewed it.

To Dr. C.C. Roe Jackson, of the faculty of Western Reserve University School of Medicine, for constructive criticism in reviewing Chapter 17. To Dr. Howard D. Kohn, also of the faculty, who has been most helpful in reading the manuscript and offering suggestions.

To Mrs. Geraldine Mink, librarian, for her assistance; to Mrs. Leona Peck for her patience in typing the manuscript and for her helpful suggestions; to Miss Ruth Elmenthaler and Miss Margaret Sanderson of the operating-room staff for their assistance in making the photographs; and to Mrs. Anita Rogoff for drawing the illustrations.

Edna Cornelia Berry
Mary Louise Kohn
Cleveland, Ohio

Acknowledgments

I want to thank so many people who have made this 11th edition possible. First, I want to thank all of the reviewers of the previous editions for their time in review and for their input to this 11th edition. The identified needs of this group provide the baselines for the growth and effectiveness of this work. The reviews were very detailed and appropriately critical.

I am so grateful to the many nurses from AORN's Membertalk and other listservs, and readers of previous editions who wrote to me or called requesting specialty topic coverage in this edition. I will do my best to meet these requests. I welcome feedback at all times and can be contacted via Lakeland Community College in Ohio or by either email address listed in the title page of this text.

I want to thank my assistant, Jacki Lausin, ST, for her help in compiling many tables and exhibits in this edition. Her help and input have been valuable and highly representative of the student population in our perioperative programs. Jacki is currently pursuing her associate degree in nursing at Lakeland Community College.

I want to thank my lab instructor, Regina Elam, CST for her patience and calm during this project. Her gentle style has helped so many beginners in the OR. Regina is employed at the Cleveland Clinic in General Surgery.

I want to thank my ongoing students in all disciplines (perioperative nursing, RNFA, and surgical technology) for asking hard questions and forcing me to step beyond the classroom and remain in the clinical site for answers to satisfy their needs. I see them as the future of patient care and the representatives of the high standards described in this text. It was because of them I won the 2006 AORN Perioperative Clinical Nursing Education Award and the 2006 Lakeland Community College Teaching Excellence Award.

I want to thank my perioperative nursing and surgical technologist colleagues for their professionalism and making the task of revision exciting and fresh. The instructors on my staff at Lakeland: Patty Chapek, RN, CNOR; Laurie Gronowski, BSN, RN; Caroline Vober, RN; Mike Hauser, RN; Steve Supanick, BS, RN; Linda Yoo, RN, BSN, CNOR; Regina Elam, CST; and Patrick Burniston, RN, BSN, RNFA, CST, CNOR, have contributed so much to the growth and the excellence of the students in all disciplines at the college and the clinical sites. I especially wish to thank Jennifer Kavran, RN, BSN, CNOR, for preparing the Instructor's Resource and PowerPoint presentations that accompany this text.

I want to thank Kristin Geen, Editor; Lauren Lake, Senior Developmental Editor; and Tamara Meyers, Managing Editor, Nursing Division, for their wonderful support and patience during the production of this edition. I was energized by their receptiveness to new ideas and was inspired to a new sense of creativity by their enthusiasm. It is great to have a team like this elicit rapid response in reviewers and to relay the information in a timely manner.

I want to mention my appreciation for the dean of Health and Science at Lakeland Community College, Deborah Hardy. As my immediate superior, she has supported me in ways that allow for the growth of my department at Lakeland and the growth and development of me as program director, author, doctoral student, and as a person. She has never turned down any idea for a new perioperative course or program. She is an inspiration as a forward-thinking academic woman.

I want to thank Mary Lou Kohn, RN, who trusted me with her wonderful creation. She is the epitome of the perioperative nurse we should strive to be. I put her foremost in mind before I commit any word to paper. I always ask myself, "How would Mary Lou describe this?" Or I think, "What would Mary Lou think about adding this?" I do this not only out of reverence for her trust, but because every time I see her to date, she continues to attend educational programs, she goes to the local AORN meetings at the Greater Cleveland Chapter, #3608, and she still exemplifies the highest standards of patient care despite being long retired. Mary Lou is a delightful human being and forever a perioperative nurse.

And last, but not least:

I want to thank my loving husband and best friend, Marty, who has been my greatest support and sounding board for all of my authorship projects and my doctoral work in the education of women. I am so fortunate to have a husband who is also a perioperative nurse educator with so much creativity and an unending sense of humor. He proofreads everything I write and helps with endless hours of research despite his obligations to his nurse educator position at work and being a lieutenant colonel in the Army Reserves Nurse Corps, 256th Combat Support Hospital. He is currently on duty in Iraq with the 399th CSH from Massachusetts. Marty is the greatest joy in my life and the best "Dog Father" to our "fur babies," Nina and Elliott, and our "feather babies," the six parakeets who sing from sunup to sundown.

Nancymarie Howard Phillips, 2006
nancymphillips@aol.com
nphillips@lakelandcc.edu

Contents

Chapter **1**

Perioperative Education

CHAPTER OBJECTIVES

After studying this chapter, the learner will be able to:
- Compare and contrast the art and science of surgery.
- Identify three characteristics of adult learners.
- Name five educational resources available for the learner.
- Define the difference between androgogy and pedagogy.
- Describe how adult learning principles apply to patient teaching.

CHAPTER OUTLINE

KEY TERMS AND DEFINITIONS

Androgogy   Teaching and learning processes for mature adult populations.

Behavior   Actions or conduct indicative of a mental state or predisposition influenced by emotions, feelings, beliefs, values, morals, and ethics.

Cognition   Process of knowing or perceiving, such as learning scientific principles and observing their application.

Competency   Creative application of knowledge, skills, and interpersonal abilities in fulfilling functions to provide safe, individualized patient care.

Critical thinking   The mental process by which an individual solves problems.

Disease   Failure of the body to counteract stimuli or stresses adequately, resulting in a disturbance in function or structure of any part, organ, or system of the body.

Knowledge   Organized body of factual information.

Learning style   Individualized methods used by the learner to understand and retain new information. These may be visual, auditory, tactile, sensory, or performance-oriented behaviors.

Mentoring   A nurturing, flexible relationship between a more experienced person and a lesser experienced person that involves trust, coaching, advice, guidance, and support. A sharing relationship guided by the needs of the less experienced person.

Objectives   Written in behavioral terms, statements that determine the expected outcomes of a behavior or process.

Pedagogy   Teaching and learning processes for immature and/or pediatric populations. A very directed style is used.

Perioperative   Total surgical experience that encompasses preoperative, intraoperative, and postoperative phases of patient care.

Preceptor   A person who observes, teaches, and evaluates a learner according to a prescribed format of training or orientation.

Psychomotor   Pertaining to physical demonstration of mental processes (i.e., applying cognitive learning).

Role model   A person who is admired and emulated for good practices in the clinical environment. The relationship between a role model and a learner can be strictly professional without personalized mentoring.

Skill   Application of knowledge into observable, measurable, and quantifiable performance.

Surgery   Branch of medicine that encompasses preoperative, intraoperative, and postoperative care of patients. The discipline of surgery is both an art and a science.

Surgical conscience   Awareness that develops from a knowledge base of the importance of strict adherence to principles of aseptic and sterile techniques.

Surgical procedure   Invasive incision into body tissues or a minimally invasive entrance into a body cavity for either therapeutic or diagnostic purposes during which protective reflexes or self-care abilities are potentially compromised.

SUPPLEMENTAL MATERIAL ON EVOLVE WEBSITE   *evolve*

http://evolve.elsevier.com/BerryKohn
- Content Updates
- Glossary
- Full Set of Perioperative Flash Cards
- Interactive Key Term Flash Cards
- Student Activities
- WebLinks

The main focus of this chapter is to establish the baseline or framework for an in-depth study of perioperative patient care and to support the educational process of the learner. Consideration is given to the perioperative educator, who may not have had a formal education in the teaching of adult learners. Both learners and educators should understand that the same learning and teaching principles apply to patient education. The key terms are commonly used terms that the learner should understand as the basis for learning about and participating in the science and art of surgery.

HISTORICAL BACKGROUND

Ancient Egyptian papyri chronicle the progress of medicine and surgery up to 1600 BC. Other influences on the historic development of surgery come from the Babylonian law—the Code of Hammurabi (1955-1913 BC). According to this law, if a patient died after a surgical procedure, retribution would be reflected on the surgeon in the form of amputation of his right hand. Ancient Persians had to perform successful procedures on three infidels before being pronounced as competent to practice surgery. Surgery was not considered a true medical discipline until the era of the physician Claudius Galen (AD 130-200), who is considered the father of experimental physiology. Despite his contributions, surgery remained a primitive practice and lacked a scientific base for the next 1200 years. Surgeons and barbers of thirteenth- and fourteenth-century England belonged to the same professional guild until 1540, when barbers agreed to confine their surgery practices to dentistry. These combined groups were dissolved in 1745, and by 1800 the Royal College of Surgeons of London was chartered.

Nineteenth-century authors describe the process of operating room education as a necessary element for the success of the surgical team. There were two different types of education, which targeted two different groups—the first group being the surgeons and their assistants, and the second group the surgical nurses. The early teams of that era recognized that the complexity of the surgical procedures was dynamic. The technical information considered current at any given time would be considered obsolete in a short time as methods and outcomes improved. The objectives for learning included gaining knowledge and skill that could be applied to the ever-changing surgical environment. The expectations of that era can be compared to the expectations of contemporary times for both groups of learners. Educators have a mission to prepare the learner with strong baselines of knowledge and skill that can be applied to surgical patient care.

THE ART AND SCIENCE OF SURGERY

Health is both a personal and an economic asset. Optimal health is the best physiologic and psychologic condition an individual can experience. Disease is the inability to adequately counteract physiologic stressors that cause disruption of the body's homeostasis. Additional influences, such as congenital anomalies, infection, or trauma, interfere with optimal human health and quality of life. As both a science and an art, surgery is the branch of medicine that comprises perioperative patient care encompassing such activities as preoperative preparation, intraoperative judgment and management, and postoperative care of patients. As a discipline, surgery combines physiologic management with an interventional aspect of treatment. The common indications for surgical intervention include correction of defects, alteration of form, restoration of function, diagnosis and/or treatment of diseases, and palliation. Table 1-1 describes some of the most common indications for surgery.

TABLE 1-1   Common Indications for Surgical Procedures

Indication for Surgical Procedure	Example
Incision	Open tissue or structure by sharp dissection
Excision	Remove tissue or structure by sharp dissection
Diagnostics	Biopsy tissue sample
Repair	Closing of a hernia
Removal	Foreign body
Reconstruction	Creation of a new breast
Palliation	Relief of obstruction
Aesthetics	Facelift
Harvest	Autologous skin graft
Procurement	Donor organ
Transplant	Placement of a donor organ
Bypass/shunt	Vascular rerouting
Drainage/evacuation	Incision of abscess
Stabilization	Repair of a fracture
Parturition	Cesarean section
Termination	Abortion of a pregnancy
Staging	Checking of cancer progression
Extraction	Removal of a tooth
Exploration	Invasive examination
Diversion	Creation of a stoma for urine

In the 1930s the English physician Lord Berkeley George Moynihan (1865-1936) said, "Surgery has been made safe for the patient; we must now make the patient safe for surgery." Surgical intervention is becoming a safer method of treating physiologic conditions. Most of the former contraindications to surgery that were related to patient age or condition have been eliminated because of better diagnostic methodologies and drug therapies. More individuals are now considered better candidates for surgery; however, each patient and each procedure are unique. Perioperative caregivers should not become complacent with routines but should always be prepared for the unexpected. Surgery cannot be considered completely safe all the time, and patient outcomes are not always predictable.

A surgical procedure may be invasive, minimally invasive, minimal access, or noninvasive. Any invasive or minimal access procedure enters the body either through an opening in the tissues or by a natural body orifice. Noninvasive procedures are frequently diagnostic and do not enter the body. Technology has elevated the practice of surgery to a more precise science that minimizes the "invasiveness" and enhances the functional aspects of the procedure. Recovery or postprocedure time decreases, and the patient is restored to functional capacity faster. Improvements in perioperative patient care technology are attributed to the following:

- Surgical specialization of surgeons and teams
- Sophisticated diagnostic and intraoperative imaging techniques
- Minimally invasive equipment and technology
- Ongoing research and technologic advancements

Surgical procedures are performed in hospitals, in surgeons' offices, or in freestanding surgical facilities. Many patients can safely have a surgical procedure as an outpatient and do not require an overnight stay at the facility. The types of surgical procedures performed on an outpatient basis are determined by the complexity of the procedure and the general health of the individual. Procedures performed on patients who remain overnight in the hospital vary according to the expertise of the surgeons, the health of the patient, and the availability of the equipment.

The purpose of this text is to provide a baseline for learning the professional and technical patient care knowledge and skill required to care for patients in the perioperative environment.

PERIOPERATIVE LEARNER

The learner in the perioperative environment may be a medical, nursing, or surgical technology student enrolled in a formal educational program, or the learner may be a newly hired orientee. Medical students have a surgical rotation that includes participation in surgical procedures. They learn some of the basic principles of surgical technology and sterile technique to ensure the safety and welfare of patients.

Some nursing schools offer basic exposure to perioperative nursing, either as part of the core curriculum or as an elective. After graduating from nursing school, the nurse needs further education before functioning as a perioperative professional. This education may take place in a postbasic/postgraduate perioperative nursing course offered by a community college or a hospital orientation program. Entry-level education for perioperative practice prepares nurses to be generalists. Basic perioperative nursing elective programs focus on the role of the perioperative nurse as both generalist circulator and scrub person. Specialization can follow a period in professional practice in a specific service. The perioperative nurse's role encompasses supervision of unlicensed personnel who scrub in surgery, such as surgical technologists and requires knowledge of practices and procedures performed under this title.

Surgical technology programs focus primarily on scrubbing in to prepare and maintain the surgical field and to handle instruments. Some surgical technology programs offer circulating experiences under the supervision of a registered nurse; however, the role of the circulator requires knowledge and skill not commonly covered in significant depth in shorter training programs. Most surgical technology programs provide scrub experiences in most specialties. After satisfactory completion of the program, many technologists are capable of functioning in the scrub role as a generalist or in some circumstances, a specialist. Advancing technology indicates the need for specialized competencies for all disciplines of perioperative patient care. Surgeons, perioperative nurses, and surgical technologists should continually strive to learn new procedures and technologies in a team-oriented environment.

Perioperative caregivers new to a particular practice setting should learn the specific performance standards and expectations of that institution. All personnel go through an orientation process to familiarize themselves with the philosophy, goals, policies, procedures, role expectations, and physical facilities specific to their institution. Departmental orientation is specific to the area in which the caregiver is employed.

Many graduates seek employment in the institutions where they performed clinical rotations. This is usually beneficial to the facility and the employee. Some students are hired into apprenticeships before graduation enabling them to work in the operating room (OR) in a limited capacity in anticipation of a permanent position. Schools that permit students to work while still in the education process should have a policy in place to delineate the student role from the employee role. The policy should be made known in writing to all clinical facilities hosting students and to students performing clinical rotations where apprenticeships are offered. The following are considerations in developing a policy for working students:

- Students may not work for compensation during official clinical hours.
- Students may not wear facility name or identification badges while performing clinical rotations as an agent of the school.
- Students may not wear school name or identification badges while performing work for compensation as an agent of the facility.
- Students may not take time off from classroom or clinical rotations to work for compensation.
- Students are not to be considered part of the clinical staff during clinical rotation hours.

All learners in the perioperative environment are adults and do not want to be treated as children. This concept applies whether the caregiver is experienced or a novice. Treating an adult learner in a pedagogic manner, as a child is treated, is counterproductive and becomes a barrier to learning. The learner can become resentful and unable to separate feelings of inexperience from feelings of inadequacy. Regardless of the level of learning required, the general characteristics of the adult learner (androgogic) as compared with the child learner (pedagogic) apply (Table 1-2). These concepts also should be applied to patient education programs.

Not everyone learns at the same speed or assimilates information in the same manner. Theoretic knowledge or a skill learned quickly by one individual may be difficult for another. Learning styles vary among individuals and are influenced by internal and external factors. Examples of learning style influences are listed in Box 1-1. Learning styles were described in the early 1990s by Howard Gardner at Harvard University. Understanding the differences in individual learners is the first step to imparting knowledge and skill. Seven learning skills identified by Gardner are summarized as follows:

1. Visual-spatial: Very environmentally aware. Learns well by observation, puzzles, graphics, and modeling.

TABLE 1-2	Characteristics of the Adult Learner as Compared with the Child Learner
Adult (Androgogy)	**Child (Pedagogy)**
Is self-directed	Is task oriented
Uses activities that follow transitions of maturity	Uses activities that follow stages of development
Uses intrinsic thought processes	Uses extrinsic thought processes
Uses problem-solving approach	Uses trial-and-error approach
Values self-esteem	Values self-esteem

2. Bodily kinesthetic: Keen sense of motion and hands-on sense. Communicates well by physical practice.
3. Musical: Learns well by listening and use of multimedia. Frequently learns better with music in the background.
4. Interpersonal: Group dynamics and study sessions work well for this learner.
5. Intrapersonal: Learns well through self-study and independence. Highly self-motivated and disciplined.
6. Linguistic: Very good with language and auditory skill. Learns effectively through lectures and explanation.
7. Logical-mathematical: Prefers to investigate and solve problems. Conceptual thinking precedes detailing with these learners.

Each facility should clearly define the role of the perioperative learner of each discipline. Activities of new perioperative nurses and surgical technology students are not the same. The perioperative nurse is involved with more direct patient care and decision making through physical assessment. The student surgical technologist is concerned primarily with preparing and maintaining the sterile field. Both disciplines of learners help prepare for, assist a qualified team member during, and clean up after surgical procedures, but they are not considered members of the staff complement. Learners are not expected to assume responsibilities for which they are not fully prepared. Only through continued study and experience can individuals qualify as team members in the perioperative environment.

The new perioperative nurse in a hospital orientation program, who will be functioning in interchangeable scrub and circulating roles, may learn the scrub role first in the learning sequence in order to learn the art of anticipation of surgeon and patient needs during a surgical procedure. This is the closest vantage point by which participation enables the perioperative nurse to be familiarized with the surgical process. An educator, preceptor, or other qualified staff member scrubs in as support and gradually allows the new perioperative nurse to take over more of the work in the sterile field. One of the primary behavioral objectives is to gain knowledge and skill in sterile technique. Performing the scrub role allows repetition of tasks performed within the sterile field and better prepares the perioperative nurse to supervise surgical technologists.

BOX 1-1   **Leaning Style Influences**

- Intelligence
- Attentiveness
- Cultural and ethnic background
- Educational preparation
- Motivation to learn
- Concentration and distractibility
- Personality characteristics
- Psychologic strengths or deficiencies
- Social skills, including communication skills
- Manual dexterity
- Physical senses
- Physical health
- Perceptual preferences and sensory partiality (e.g., visual vs. auditory)
- Environment

The second component of the perioperative nurse's learning sequence is the circulating role. A registered nurse preceptor is assigned to teach the new nurse the coordination of the scrub and circulating roles. Standard routines are taught under the supervision of an experienced perioperative nurse with comparable knowledge, skill, and educational preparation. Guidance and help from the clinical educator and other experienced staff members help the new perioperative nurse pull it all together. Surgeons and other staff members contribute to the learning process.

Personality traits, such as emotional maturity, social skills, and psychologic characteristics are continually assessed by the educator. A moody, easily angered, and negative person can be very difficult to deal with as a future team member. The learner who does not possess assertive skills for dealing with stressful events cannot function effectively in a team environment. Subjective responses to all activities should remain on a professional level if the team is to function efficiently. The perioperative nurse in training should be evaluated on a periodic basis to assess for increased competency levels.

PERIOPERATIVE EDUCATOR

Experience in the perioperative clinical setting should be planned and supervised by an experienced perioperative nurse educator. The term *educator* is used throughout this text to refer to the person responsible for planning, implementing, and evaluating the learner's experiences in the classroom and clinical perioperative setting. Other teaching personnel at the clinical site include perioperative nurse preceptors.

The educator should consider the effect on the learner who is seeing the perioperative environment for the first time. The operating room can appear cold, large, and overwhelming. A tour of the facility before beginning the program can help decrease the learner's anxiety.

A structured curriculum uses behavioral objectives, written guidelines, and relevant assignments for feedback to ensure that learning has occurred. Learner conferences are held at regular intervals to discuss procedures and progress. A sample outline for perioperative instruction is located online at www.nvo.com/delphipro/periopnursingclasses.

Didactic presentations should be incorporated into the teaching program to provide information concerning the theory and detail of all performed actions in the perioperative environment. Presentations should be offered by knowledgeable presenters who are well prepared to deliver the information to the group. If PowerPoint multimedia is used, the educator should be sure to use accurate and concise terminology when creating the slides. Handouts can be printed in several formats for distribution to the participants to use when following along with the talk or taking notes. Overloading each slide with wordiness and silly images causes confusion and wastes time. The key elements should be incorporated as a simple set of terms not to exceed six lines per slide that are explained verbally by the educator. Font style should be kept simple and the size should be readable at the back of the classroom. Avoid the use of all-capital letters. The slide color scheme and design can be selected as a template or customized per presentation. Colors such as blue and green are easier on

BOX 1-2	Performance Appraisal of the Scrub Role		
Evaluation	Meets Standard	Does Not Meet Standard	Comments
Wears OR attire properly: Dons personal protective gear Dons radiation badge as needed			
Performs housekeeping duties: Before first procedure of day Between procedures After last procedure of day			
Sterile supplies: Plans and gathers supplies Checks integrity of packages Checks sterility integrator Checks dates on perishables			
Places items on sterile surface: Opening wrapper(s) Peel packages Solution dispensing			
Scrubs for setup and procedure: Hand and arm scrubbing Hand hygiene with hand antiseptic			
Gowning: Gowns self correctly Gowns others			
Gloves: Closed method Open method Changes contaminated glove Gloves others			
Sterile setup: Drapes table and Mayo stand Positions items in the field			
Accountability: Labels solutions and drugs Reports amount of use Practices safety Maintains the sterile field			
Anticipates needs of surgeon: Coordinates with circulator Facilitates the first assistant Passes instrumentation			
Counts: Sponges Sharps Instruments			
Assembles instruments: Attaches knife blades on handles Loads or prepares suture Tests drills and devices Other			
Disassembles the table: Follows proper disposal of items Follows decontamination procedures			
Removes gown and gloves: Gown off first Glove-to-glove/skin-to-skin			

BOX 1-3	Performance Appraisal of the Circulating Nurse's Role		
Evaluation	Meets Standard	Does Not Meet Standard	Comments
Wears OR attire properly: Dons personal protective gear Dons radiation badge as needed			
Performs housekeeping duties: Before first procedure of day Between procedures After last procedure of day			
Sterile supplies: Plans and gathers supplies Checks integrity of packages Checks sterility integrator Checks dates on perishables			
Dispenses or transfers items to sterile surface as appropriate: Opens wrapper(s) and peel packs Opens closed container Solution dispensing Medication dispensing			
Validates implant parameters and documents in the lot log			
Practices aseptic technique: Dons and removes sterile or nonsterile gloves as appropriate for task Hand hygiene with hand antiseptic			
Gowning and gloving of others: Ties gowns for sterile team members Assists with contaminated glove removal Provides additional gowns and gloves as needed			
Accountability: Gathers and checks solutions and drugs for use on the field Documents amount of usage of drugs and solutions on the field Practices safety for the patient and team Monitors the sterile field and the members of the sterile team			
Anticipates needs of patient, anesthesia provider, surgeon, and other team members: Coordinates with the scrub person Obtains additional supplies and instrumentation as needed			
Provides safe and competent direct patient care: Patient advocate Patient identification Validates correct site protocol and time out procedures Patient assessment Supports psychosocial aspects of care Positioning and prepping as appropriate Monitoring physiologic and psychologic responses as appropriate Cares for specimens Patient teaching			

BOX 1-3	Performance Appraisal of the Circulating Nurse's Role—cont'd			
Evaluation	Meets Standard	Does Not Meet Standard	Comments
Counts: Sponges Sharps Instruments Documents any other item added to the field intraoperatively			
Attaches and activates surgical machinery and devices to the sterile field: Electrosurgery (ESU) cables, suction, power cords, and other peripheral equipment Activates, sets, and monitors peripheral equipment			
Supervises and manages the room: Plans and implements direct patient care using the nursing process Directs the activities of learners Communicates procedural progress to the control desk Communicates with family members Manages messages for the surgeon and first assistant Prevents inappropriate traffic through the room Documents procedural activities in patient record Computer literacy Manages patient charge items responsibly			

the eyes than reds, oranges, and bright yellows. Time should be planned between slides for questions or examples.

Positive reinforcement helps the learner build confidence and competence. The educator should not punish a learner for making honest errors during supervised learning. Degradation and damage to self-esteem are barriers to learning. The learner should not be put in a position to perform any function for which he or she has not had adequate training or guided practice. The educator should maintain a list of procedures in which the learner has participated and has demonstrated increasing levels of competence. Whether the learner is in a school-sponsored operating room education program or a departmental orientation program, the duration of the program should be sufficient to afford opportunities for adequate experience to facilitate success.

Check-off sheets can be used to track experiential progress during the education process. Box 1-2 shows an example of a basic check-off sheet for the evaluation of knowledge and skill in the scrub role. Box 1-3 shows an example of a basic check-off sheet for evaluation of knowledge and skill in the circulating nurse's role. This sheet can be modified to apply to specialties as needed. The Association of Surgical Technologists (AST) and the Association of periOperative Registered Nurses (AORN) have developed skills checklists, and these are available through the organizations.

Behavioral Objectives

The learner takes an active role in the teaching/learning process by helping identify behavioral objectives. Effective and organized educational experiences are identified and based on these objectives. The identified behavioral objectives are attained through critical-thinking exercises. Skill in questioning and encouragement in making discoveries allow the learner to use critical thinking as a learning tool.

Evaluation of the learner's progress is measured by how successfully the learner has met the behavioral objectives. Behavioral objectives are identified and written in behavioral terms and based on standards of expected performance and accepted standards of patient care. In 1956 Benjamin Bloom described the measurement of cognitive learning. He described six levels of learning, ranging from simple recall to advanced abstract thinking. Bloom's taxonomy provides a framework for structuring cognitive and affective learning. Therefore the concepts to be learned and the behavioral objectives to be met should form the foundation on which all perioperative caregivers build their practice. Each behavioral objective in Box 1-4 is measurable and is evaluated by performance standards.

Elements of Effective Instruction

The organization of the instructional material and the learning experience are further enhanced by the way the

---

BOX 1-4	Behavioral Objectives for Perioperative Caregivers

- To identify the role and responsibility of each team member
- To define current standard terminology associated with perioperative patient care through use of the perioperative nursing data set (PNDS)
- To compare and contrast knowledge of normal anatomy, physiology, and pathophysiology
- To discuss the interrelationships among physiologic, ethnocultural, and psychosocial factors that affect a patient and family's adaptation to the perioperative experience
- To identify the procedures necessary to prepare each patient as an individual for the intended surgical procedure
- To demonstrate the ability to select appropriate instrumentation, equipment, and supplies according to the individualized plan of care
- To apply the principles of sterilization, disinfection, and aseptic and sterile techniques in the preparation and use of all materials in the perioperative environment to prevent transmission of biologic contamination
- To identify the potential environmental hazards to the patient and team
- To demonstrate knowledge of the basic actions and uses of anesthetic agents, medications, fluid therapies, and electrolytes
- To demonstrate knowledge and skill during the surgical procedure by anticipating the needs of the patient and the team
- To discuss the principles of wound management
- To function as a team member by showing consideration for and cooperation with other perioperative caregivers
- To communicate effectively with personnel on other patient care divisions within the facility
- To develop the ability to perform safely and effectively during stressful situations

program is presented. The elements of effective instruction are summarized as follows:

- Set clear and concise behavioral objectives that are measurable in cognitive terminology that describes knowledge, comprehension, application, analysis, understanding, and evaluation.
- Establish a learning environment that is controlled by the educator.
- Provide variation in presenting material. Videotapes, DVDs, audiodiscs, and photographs can be alternated with lectures and hands-on practice. Handling instruments and supplies in a classroom is less intimidating than handling them in the perioperative environment for the first time.
- Encourage the exchange of questions and answers as an assessment tool. Learners often ask exactly what they need to know. The educator can determine areas of deficient knowledge.
- Reinforce learning. After a skill has been taught in a didactic manner, provide guided practice in the clinical laboratory before the task is actually performed in the perioperative environment. Provide positive support for desired behaviors. Self-assessment tools and performance evaluations provide feedback about the learner's progress.
- Summarize the learner's accomplishments at regular intervals. Reviewing daily activities helps reinforce the learning process by allowing the learner to associate the events of his or her experience with newly acquired knowledge.

The educator should work closely with the perioperative nurse manager. Classroom hours and clinical experience assignments are coordinated to provide the best experience for the learner. The nurse manager offers suggestions and coordination input for the benefit of the learner and staff members. The educator identifies areas of needed experience for the learner. An effort is made to confer and coordinate any changes in the program with all personnel in the department. The educator and the manager collaborate with the assigned preceptors as needed. These strategies foster a friendly and cooperative relationship among learners, educators, management, and preceptor staff.

All perioperative staff members indirectly assist in teaching the learners within the guidelines of the structured learning experience. The learners gain knowledge by observing and working with members of the entire team. Everyone should be familiar with the level of the learners, the behavioral objectives, and the teaching roles that staff members are expected to assume. Learners also should be responsible for updating the staff about needed experience and their current level of achievement.

Hospitals or facilities offering the clinical perioperative setting for educational programs have policies and procedures that are adaptations of national standards. All personnel, including faculty members and learners, are expected to adhere to their content.

LEARNING RESOURCES

Books, journals, videos, DVDs, slides, photographs, computers, and other audiovisual materials may supplement the lecture approach to perioperative education. Larger teaching institutions may have live closed-circuit television and interactive telecommunication systems that permit educators and learners to communicate from remote locations. Many audiovisual materials, such as videodiscs, audiotapes, and computer-assisted instruction, are self-contained units for self-study. A bibliography in a text such as this or at the conclusion of a journal article provides references to broaden the learner's database. Accessibility to current medical and scientific literature is without limit. Other sources include websites on the Internet and educational services that provide contact hours online.

The following are useful resources for acquiring and reinforcing knowledge:

1. Library and literature file. Books and current periodicals are available for the learner's reference in the medical library and learning centers at local colleges.
2. Educational literature and videotapes are available from surgical supply and instrument manufacturers. The literature that accompanies new equipment should be reviewed by all personnel who will be working with the item. Inservices usually are provided by clinical staff associated with the industry. The purchasing agent is a good source for these types of references.
3. Computer database information systems are available in most facilities or through personal Internet access providers for researching topics of interest for self-study or for supplementing classroom presentations. Web browsers such as Netscape Navigator, Microsoft's Internet Explorer, or Mozilla Firefox are used in searching the World Wide Web (WWW). Search engines on the Internet are valuable tools for finding special-

interest groups and professional medical associations. Several helpful search engines are listed in Box 1-5. Most health-related organizations have a website full of information for professionals and patients. AORN Online can be accessed at www.aorn.org. AST has a website (www.ast.org) that provides information about surgical technology. Terms associated with using the Internet and computer use are described in Box 1-6.

4. Specialty online news groups can be subscribed to through computerized online e-mail systems. Referred to as ListServe, these groups are communication tools for day-to-day discussions with others who have similar interests. They are available as daily e-mail entries or as a weekly digest. Perioperative nursing and nursing history ListServe lists are available for free subscription on the web. Table 1-3 describes how to sign up for the perioperative ListServe.

5. Literary databases are found on select websites and in most libraries. Examples of on-line literary databases include but are not limited to the following:
   a. Cumulative Index to Nursing and Allied Health Literature (CINAHL) is a widely used index for nursing and allied health. The database includes indexing by subject headings from virtually all English-language nursing journals and allied health literature from January 1983, with bimonthly updates.
   b. Medical Literature Analysis and Retrieval System Online (MEDLINE) is a computer-based reference system available at most libraries in the United States and Canada. Many websites on the Internet offer free MEDLINE access. Biomedical journals, including nursing journals, are referenced. The file contains references dating from 1966 at the National Library of Medicine (www.nih.gov).

BOX 1-5 | **Search Engines That Search Multiple Search Engines**

www.dogpile.com—Searches multiple search engines on general topics, and returns results organized according to each engine searched
www.google.com—Searches multiple search engines, but does not sort sites according to particular engines
www.cen.uiuc.edu/exploring.html—Internet jumpstation that enables the user to search multiple search engines, including maps, addresses, and directories

---

BOX 1-6 | **Terms Associated with Computer and Internet Use**

Address: Series of letters and/or numbers that enables the user to locate a specific website or e-mail directory; also known as *uniform resource locators (URLs).*

Adobe Acrobat .pdf file: A document, article, or file that is formatted for transfer and retrieval by use of proprietary software. A .pdf-formatted document retains its original appearance when opened by the Acrobat Reader software. Free sources for this program are located online at www.download.com.

Bookmark: Electronic marker selected by the user to record the address of a specific website for easy return.

Browser: Specialty software that enables the user to interact with or browse in websites. Examples include Firefox, Internet Explorer, and Netscape.

Cookie: An electronic notation placed in the user's computer hard drive that enables a website to recognize a return visitor to the site.

Download: Transfer of information over the Internet between computers or to a storage device such as a disk or flash drive.

E-mail: Communication between people over the Internet through a service provider such as America Online (AOL).

File transfer protocol (FTP): Method of retrieving files between computers.

Firewall: A computer program designed to deflect unwanted or uninvited downloads to the hard drive.

Flash drive: A removable storage device that connects to the USB (universal serial bus) port on the CPU (central processing unit) of the computer for the purpose of saving data or files. This device is small enough to fit on a key chain. Some flash drives have the capacity of several CD-ROMs.

Hypertext link: Location on a website that, when clicked with the left mouse button, connects the user to another page in the site or to another website entirely.

Hypertext markup language (HTML): Format for designing website pages.

Internet relay chat (IRC): Real-time discussion over the Internet through a service provider.

Internet service provider (ISP): Company that provides a method of gaining access to the Internet for e-mail and entry to the World Wide Web. Examples include America Online (AOL) and Netcom.

ListServe: Specialty communications through e-mail discussion group postings to a server. Messages between participants in a special-interest group are sent back and forth in response to topic threads.

Newsgroups: Discussion groups that post messages on electronic bulletin boards; can be accessed through an Internet service provider.

Search engine: Service sites available on the Internet that enable a person to leaf through multiple pages on multiple websites to collect specific information on a select topic. Examples include Google, Northern Light, Yahoo, AltaVista, Lycos, and Excite.

Thread: Specific topic line that is shared for several days through a newsgroup.

Virus: Harmful computer program that can enter a user's computer through a download or file transfer. Data can be destroyed or altered without the user being aware of the process. Care in downloading outside programs is recommended. Virus scanning software is commercially available to help protect computer systems. Updates are required periodically. Free virus scanning is available at www.housecalls.com.

Website: Place on the World Wide Web that features a specific topic of interest. It may consist of several website pages that can be accessed by clicking the left mouse button on a topic.

World Wide Web (WWW): Communication in text and graphic form that requires a computer, Internet service provider, and browser for access.

Zipped file: A large file that is compressed electronically for fast download. Can be opened to its full size by use of free unzipping software such as WinZip from www.download.com.

TABLE 1-3	How to Subscribe to Perioperative ListServe

Area on the E-mail Form	Type in This Information
Address line	periop-request@mailman1.u.washington.edu
Subject line	help

NOTE: Use e-mail to subscribe to the perioperative ListServe owned by Bob Baxter, RN, CNOR. After completion of the e-mail form, send it electronically like any other e-mail. Subscription confirmation should be received with 24 hours. You can reach the person managing the list at periop-owner@mailman1.u.washington.edu

c. Medscape (www.medscape.com) is a free article subscription service online. This site requires registration. The user selects an identification name and password. Many different specialty services are represented. A weekly digest is available at no charge and can be ordered for automatic delivery via e-mail.

6. Videotape and DVD library. The Hospital Satellite Network (HSN) is a telecommunication service provided to hospitals in which subscribers can view videotaped or digitally recorded programs transmitted by satellite. Video Journal provides a new videotape program to subscribers every 2 months. These sources of audiovisual programs are available for purchase or rental.

The array of health-related educational materials is endless. The Internet, which is accessible 24 hours a day, has opened many channels of information throughout the world. Many websites can be accessed in a multilingual mode, including Spanish, German, French, and Japanese. Some websites offer full-text articles that can be downloaded to a diskette or printed on a printer. Some of the articles are in .zip or .pdf format that requires WinZip or Adobe Acrobat Reader to open the file into a readable and/or printable document. WinZip and Acrobat Reader are free programs that can be downloaded and used repeatedly to open zipped or .pdf files. Websites such as www.download.com offer links to free file-opening software for download into your personal computer. These programs are frequently preloaded onto the hard drive of new computer models.

The advancement of computer technology has made computer equipment small enough to fit in a briefcase and economical enough for the average household to own one computer and possibly two. When researching scientific data on the Internet, it is advisable to review more than one website to support the accuracy of the information. Caution is advised regarding providing personal information such as credit card numbers over the Internet; security may be an issue.

APPLICATION OF THEORY TO PRACTICE

Learning is a process of discovery and mastery of skills. Performance-based learning to function competently in an area such as the perioperative environment should take place on three levels: cognitive, psychomotor, and affective. The learner should understand the scientific principles (cognitive learning) underlying the technical skills (psychomotor learning) and should appreciate the necessity of adhering to these principles (affective learning). In simpler terms, the learner should know why to do what (cognitive); how (psychomotor); and when, where, and by whom (affective). The learner should always have a rationale for each action. Learners and practicing perioperative caregivers should always know exactly why they are doing what they are doing—not just blindly perform tasks. This approach enables an intelligent modification of the plan of care in the event of an emergency or other untoward situation. In actual practice, this knowledge may be critical for patient safety and attainment of favorable outcomes.

Practice will give learners an opportunity to apply their knowledge of the basic sciences. Theory becomes meaningful and valuable only when put to practical use. Some knowledge is gained through observation, but skills are learned through actual hands-on experience in applying the theory learned in the classroom or self-study laboratory.

In the perioperative environment, the learner observes living anatomy; its alteration by congenital deformities, disease, or injury; and its restoration or reconstruction. Perioperative experience enables the learner to be a more understanding, observant, and efficient person. In close teamwork with surgeons and anesthesia providers, the nurse and the surgical technologist participate in vital resuscitative measures and learn to care for anesthetized, unconscious, and/or critically ill patients. Learning to function in life-threatening situations is critical to the patient's welfare. In addition, the learner discovers that emergencies such as cardiac arrest are more easily prevented than treated. By learning how theory applies to clinical practice, he or she gains valuable experience that is applicable to any nursing situation. The learner should strive to attain the following objectives:

• Appreciate what surgical intervention means to each patient.
• Recognize the importance of optimal physical and psychologic preoperative patient preparation.
• Validate the need for constant patient observation intraoperatively.
• Determine the cause of postoperative pain and/or complications.
• Differentiate between seemingly innocuous occurrences and situations that, if left unrecognized and allowed to progress, lead to injury of the patient or a team member or damage to departmental equipment.
• Cope with all situations in a calm, efficient manner, and think clearly and act quickly in an emergency.
• Attend to every detail, observe keenly, and anticipate the needs of the patient and team members.
• Determine the importance of aseptic and sterile techniques, and comprehensively and conscientiously apply knowledge to practice.
• Expect the unexpected. Situations or conditions can change at a moment's notice.

Above all, perioperative experience teaches that no surgical procedure is a minor event to the surgical patient!

The only predictable element in the perioperative environment is the potential for an unpredictable occurrence. For practical use, hospitals may classify surgical procedures as major or minor; however, in reality no such distinction exists. Every procedure has a deep personal meaning for each patient and his or her family, and the possibility of an unfavorable outcome can never be completely excluded. All perioperative procedures carry an element of inherent risk. A relatively safe procedure can rapidly become catastrophic, even fatal, if the patient:

- Is unknowingly allergic or sensitive to a chemical, substance, medication, or anesthetic drug
- Develops uncontrollable bleeding
- Has seizures
- Experiences cardiac arrest on the operating bed
- Goes into irreversible shock
- Succumbs to overwhelming postoperative infection

Although every precaution is taken to foresee and prevent adverse reactions, such reactions do occur on occasion. No matter how simple the procedure, an experienced, conscientious team member is always acutely aware of potential problems and gives undivided attention to the patient and procedure at all times.

During the learning experience, the learner will participate in or observe the preparation of supplies and equipment and learn their intended use. With practical experience, the learner will gain an appreciation for the precision of surgical instrumentation and equipment. Also, in helping to carry out a daily schedule of surgical procedures, the learner will become aware of the interdependence of the various departments within the facility and how they work together for the well-being of the patient. One of the most valuable learning experiences in the perioperative environment is the opportunity to see and become a part of real teamwork in action. Chapter 25 explores and explains the coordinated roles of the circulating nurse and the scrub person.

EXPECTED BEHAVIORS OF PERIOPERATIVE CAREGIVERS

Regardless of their respective roles, all perioperative caregivers are expected to be competent and humane. A patient's sense of security is grounded in how he or she perceives the behavior of the team as a whole. This leaves a lasting impression that patients associate with their experiences in the perioperative environment. The behavior of the team reveals self-confidence (or diffidence), interest (or indifference), proficiency (or ineptness), and authority (or indecision). In addition to possessing technical knowledge and skill, personnel should display appropriate personal attributes and communication skills that inspire confidence and trust in patients and other team members.

Personal Attributes

Personal attributes are manifest in the attitudes displayed by an individual while performing his or her duties. These inherent characteristics contribute to interrelatedness of the team and the final outcome for the patient. Although these concepts are intrinsic to the individual and are certainly open to interpretation, the main premise remains focused on providing safe and efficient patient care

through a team effort. Desirable personal attributes are listed in Table 1-4.

Communications

Communication is essential for exchanging information with another person. It is necessary for successful interpersonal relationships and serves to clarify actions. Communication is *proactive* when an idea or intent is relayed to another person and *reactive* when a response is received. Communication has taken place when the receiver interprets the message in the manner intended by the sender. Communication is effective only when the patient and caregivers understand one another. A key element is to demonstrate appropriate body language to match the spoken word.

Teamwork

A team is a group of two or more people who recognize common goals and coordinate their efforts to achieve them. Broadly defined, the health care team includes all personnel relating to the patient—those in direct patient contact, and those in other departments whose services are essential and contribute indirectly to patient care. Interdependence characterizes a team—without the other members, the goals cannot be met.

The team approach to patient care should be a coordinated effort that is performed with the cooperation of all caregivers. Team members should communicate and should

TABLE 1-4	Attributes Expected in a Perioperative Caregiver
Desirable Attribute	**Measurable Behaviors**
Empathy	Develop a sense of what the patient is feeling
Conscientiousness	No compromise in quality of care
Efficiency	Organized and properly prepared; time is not wasted duplicating steps
Sensitivity	Genuine caring and perceptiveness for the patient and the team
Open minded	Accepting of the ideas of others
Flexible and adaptable	Able to cope with changes in routine
Supportive	Nonjudgmental and sincere approach to relationships
Communicative	Exchanges information in a professional manner
Listens	Accepts and receives information in a professional manner
Even tempered	Hostility and anger have no place in the perioperative environment
Versatile	Knowledgeable and can troubleshoot
Analytic	Knowing how and why for each task
Creative	Able to innovate solutions
Sense of humor	Eases tension at appropriate times
Manual dexterity	Good eye-hand coordination
Stamina	Capable of standing for prolonged periods
Hygiene	Body odors cause discomfort for the team
Ethics	Strong sense of truth, honor, and goodness
Curiosity	Desire to know and learn new things

have a shared division of duties to perform specified tasks as a unified body. The failure of any one member to perform his or her role can have a serious effect on the success of the entire team. Performing as a team requires that each member exert an effort to attain the common goals competently and safely. The actions of each team member are important. No one individual can accomplish the goal without the cooperation of the rest of the team.

Pride in one's work and in the team as a whole leads to personal satisfaction. High morale is facilitated by adequate staff orientation, staff participation in departmental decision making and problem solving, the receipt of deserved praise, the opportunity for continuing education, and motivation to reach and practice at the highest potential.

The common goal of the perioperative team is the effective delivery of care in a safe, efficient, and timely manner. To function efficiently, team members must communicate effectively. Problems such as a break in aseptic or sterile technique must be identified and corrective actions taken. To fulfill expectations, team members must be aware of each other's needs for information. Efforts of other support services, such as radiology and pathology departments, must be coordinated with the needs of the surgeon.

Mutual respect is the foundation of teamwork. It is also a right. Respect is shown through collaboration, cooperation, and truthful communication. Verbal abuse, disruptive behavior, and harassment are out of place in the professional environment. Behavior that inhibits the performance of team members or threatens patient care should be factually documented and reported to superiors in the chain of command.

Teamwork requires the commitment and effort of team members to increase productivity, ensure quality performance, and participate in problem solving by communicating and cooperating with one another. A team approach is necessary for patient-centered care. Surgeons, assistants, anesthesia providers, patient care staff, and staff of supporting services should coordinate their efforts. Each discipline contributes to successful outcomes of surgical intervention by working together as team. Several factors contribute to these successful outcomes:

1. Interdepartmental communication is important for mutual cooperation, consideration, and efficient collaboration.
   a. Personnel on patient care divisions and physicians share pertinent information concerning patients. Collected data are documented, thereby protecting the patient, the patient care personnel, and the facility.
   b. Personnel work together in a congenial atmosphere with respect and appreciation for each other's unique skills and contributions. Team members benefit from the expertise of each other. Teamwork is at its finest in the perioperative environment.
   c. Personnel are considerate of each other and of the patient.
      (1) The surgeon should inform the team of any anticipated potential deviation from his or her regular routine for the scheduled procedure. An advance notice of changes can help avoid delays in obtaining needed equipment.
      (2) The perioperative team promotes a quiet atmosphere to ensure the surgeon's uninterrupted concentration. Interruptions during the procedure can cause the team to lose concentration and jeopardize the safety of the patient or team members.
      (3) The anesthesia provider and circulating nurse assist each other with certain procedures such as medication administration and intubation.
2. Adequate preparation and familiarity with the surgeon's preferences and the surgical procedure to be performed are fundamental to teamwork. If the perioperative staff members are unfamiliar with the routine and equipment, the patient or a team member may be at risk for injury. An adequately experienced and skilled team is essential for the effective performance of a safe, efficient procedure.
3. The patient has an unconditional right to the team's complete concentration and attention at all times. He or she is a unique individual who is completely dependent on the perioperative caregivers to work as a team.

Although the ideologic differences of personnel may at times be a source of conflict, the care of the patient should be a priority over personality differences. Complex procedures, busy surgery schedules, or shortages of personnel should not interfere with the delivery of efficient, individualized patient care.

Clinical Competence

On the basis of experience and performance, patient care personnel can be categorized as novice, competent, proficient, or expert. The novice lacks experience but is expected to perform to the best of his or her ability with assistance. Most employers provide a formal orientation program for new patient care personnel. During this orientation period, the necessary knowledge, skills, and abilities should be developed to perform at a level of basic competency. As experience is gained, proficiency expands from a minimal competency to an advanced level of expertise. Competent practice requires critical thinking skills and decision-making ability. Statements of clinical competency are established by professional organizations such as AORN and AST. These guidelines are published by each professional organization and made available to practitioners of all disciplines. Competencies are discussed in more detail in Chapter 2.

REALITIES OF CLINICAL PRACTICE

When a formal educational experience is completed, a learner or orientee is eager to apply his or her skills and knowledge in an employment setting. A transition from dependent learner to independent practitioner evolves over a period of time. The realities of the work environment and the emotional and ethical dilemmas of some situations are experienced as basic competencies are developed. It can take 6 months to 1 year to feel confident as a functioning perioperative team member. Many facilities require personnel to take calls for emergencies after business hours; therefore, the staff must be competent to fulfill this requirement independent of a preceptor.

Reality Shock

Reality is a sense of actuality, a feeling that this is what the real world is all about. Reality shock sets in as the transition takes place from being a beginning learner to becoming an employed graduate professional nurse or surgical technologist. The familiar educator and peer learners are not always present to give counsel, advice, and moral support. As professional caregivers attempt to adapt to new demands, they need to remember the following:

- Learning does not end with basic education. It is an ongoing process throughout the professional's career.
- Teaching at various levels is the responsibility of the entire team. New information is developed and shared by the group for the improvement of patient care practices.
- All caregivers were once novices (although some may have forgotten those novice days). They have experienced the feelings and frustrations of being the newest staff member. The experienced caregiver should try to remember these feelings and offer encouragement to new personnel.
- Patience is an asset while developing work habits and establishing working relationships. Expectations of self and of others should be realistic. Feelings of excitement and anticipation and the fear of failure or making mistakes are normal but should be expressed appropriately. Disruptive behavior distracts the attention of team from the patient.
- Applying the principles and techniques already learned will enable the caregiver to make sound judgments and appropriate decisions in the perioperative environment.
- It is important to ask questions and acknowledge not knowing how to do something. Seeking help promotes professional growth.

Everyone wants and needs to become an accepted member of both social and work groups. The entire perioperative team, including the surgeon and anesthesia provider, is both a social group and a work group. Ambivalent feelings may arise on entering these groups. The pleasures of functioning as a team member may be offset by uncertainty about the ability to perform well. Initial goals will be task and skill oriented as learning focuses on policies, procedures, and routines. Eventually insecurity will be replaced with self-confidence. The display of confidence will increase trust, respect, and recognition from others, as well as the personal satisfaction of accomplishment.

Dynamics of the Psychologic Climate

Learning to adapt to the variety of tasks and ever-changing demands in the perioperative environment is difficult. Some anxiety is normal, especially in situations in which feelings of insecurity are generated or a sense of intimidation pervades the environment. At times the demands of the job may seem to outweigh the personal resources of the caregiver. Confidence develops as skills are learned.

An understanding of expected performance is perhaps the most important element in the transition from novice to independent practitioner. Personnel in the perioperative environment play key roles in the beginner's development. There is a distinction between the roles of *preceptor, mentor* and *role model*. A *preceptor* works with orientees and learners according to a prescribed task-oriented lesson plan. The process offers minimal flexibility and little personalization for individual needs. A *mentor* has more experience with the personnel and the climate of the OR and can provide insight into the social atmosphere of the department. A mentor develops a relatively personalized relationship with less experienced orientees or learners and fosters a sense of nurturance for their growth and assimilation into the department. A beginner should look for a mentor to help bridge the gap between novice and proficient levels. Beginners should also look for *role models*—those experienced staff members who are emulated and respected for their clinical competence and pattern their emerging professional self after the behaviors of the role model. A personal relationship may not evolve with a role model in the same way as with a mentor.

The beginner should stick with the winners—those staff members who are reaping personal rewards and self-satisfaction from their work ethic. Their enthusiasm will be contagious and start the growth of an exciting career. The losers—staff members who have negative attitudes, complain, and do not make an effort to solve problems but instead create them—should be avoided.

Eustress versus Distress

Physical and emotional stresses are part of daily life. Stress is the nonspecific reaction of the body, physiologically and/or psychologically, to any demand. The demand may be pleasant or unpleasant, conscious or unconscious. The intensity of the stressor will dictate adaptation. An individual's perception of a situation will influence the reaction to it.

Stress is not only an essential part of life but also a useful stimulant. Positive stress, referred to as *eustress,* motivates an individual to be productive and efficient. It forces adaptation to the ever-present changes in the perioperative environment. The response should be quick (e.g., when a trauma victim arrives or a patient has a cardiac arrest). To expect the unexpected is part of perioperative patient care. Eustress fosters a sense of achievement, satisfaction, and self-confidence.

Stress that becomes overwhelming and uncomfortable is referred to as *distress*. In the perioperative environment, the behavior of others may be perceived as cause for distress. Policies, or a lack of them, can also be a source of distress if they are in conflict with the caregiver's expectations. Through adaptive mechanisms, the caregiver can cope with the tensions, conflicts, and demands of the perioperative environment in either a collaborative or a nonproductive manner. Even though perceived as distress, some conflict is necessary to stimulate a change in work methods and solve organizational problems. Sometimes it takes dissatisfaction with a situation to spark positive change and prevent stagnation.

Patient care personnel become distressed by the conduct of other team members. For example, it is uncomfortable to be harshly criticized by a surgeon in front of peers or patients. However, much that is said is not personally directed. Often the surgeon is reacting to his or her distress regarding unanticipated circumstances presented by the patient, team member, or equipment during the surgical procedure. The reactions of personnel will be influenced by their attitudes, mood, cultural and religious background, values and ethics, experiences, and concerns of the moment. Outbursts of anger are inappropriate in the operating room at any time. However, constant frustration and inner conflict create the distresses that can lead to job dissatisfaction. Behaviors that place patients or personnel at risk such as throwing objects should be reported to the nurse manager and documented.

Stress Reduction

Assertive behavior is a useful tool for conflict resolution. Shared professional communication can keep the tension in the environment at a minimum. The caregiver should keep his or her composure at all times and maintain a professional and assertive (not aggressive) attitude. Personal conflicts between team members should be dealt with privately.

Humor can be an effective method of reducing anxiety. It should be used appropriately to defuse tension. Laughing at oneself helps to preserve self-esteem while learning from the experience.

At the end of the work shift, the caregiver should evaluate the events of the day, the emotions evoked, and how they were handled. What was done effectively? What coping skills may be needed to improve or enhance positive attitudes in the work environment and in interpersonal relationships? Teamwork is essential in the perioperative environment, with every team member obligated to make a positive contribution.

Stress is a reality that need not create a sense of self-defeat. Regardless of the source of stress, the body responds and the physiologic and psychologic effects can be subtle or intense. The determination of whether a stressor is good or bad depends on an individual's perception of the circumstances. Any event that creates a feeling of impending danger also creates the perception of loss of control. A major factor in stress management is maintaining control, which can be accomplished by learning to tune in to the balance between the body and the mind. The caregiver can learn to be prepared for life's difficulties by understanding how the perception of stress can affect decision making, self-expression, and subsistence in the world.

Listening to the Body

The caregiver should develop a sense for how the body signals exhaustion, hunger, illness, and/or physical pain. The body is a sensory barometer of the environmental effects on the caregiver, and ignoring physical signals decreases the ability of the body to manage stress. Going without sleep or skipping meals creates physical stress that can be avoided. Sleep deprivation caused by long hours on call can be as dangerous as overuse of alcohol or using illegal drugs. The biologic need for sleep cannot be denied and is important for the health and safety of the individual and the others in the environment. Decision making, reaction times, memory, and generalized health are impaired by not getting enough rest. Regular sleep of at least 6 hours per day and rest periods, exercise, adequate dietary practices, and routine health checkups provide a sound basis for care of the body.

Maintaining the Mind

Mental relaxation can help the caregiver manage stress. Using meditation and mental imagery on a regular basis provides a break from stressful routines and allows the mind to fortify itself against the negative perceptions of a situation. Creating time to clear confusing thoughts and align productive thinking enables the body and the mind to support an emotional balance and a sense of well-being. This positive interaction can become an influence in a stressful situation and serve as an example to coworkers.

Bibliography

Alfaro-LeFevre R: Improving your ability to think critically, *Nurs Spectr* 2(3):25-29, 2001.
Durmer JS, Dinges DF: Neurocognitive consequences of sleep deprivation, *Semin Neurol* 25(1):117-129, 2005.
Gardner K: Maintaining a positive attitude when others don't, *Surg Serv Manag* 8(4):16-22, 2002.
Groah L: Mentoring: Designing the future, *Surg Serv Manag* 6(8):26-28, 2000.
Lewis JA, Kruckenberg KK: New roles for nurses, *Surg Serv Manag* 6(8):13-16, 2000.
Loving GL, Wilson JS: Infusing critical thinking into the nursing curriculum through faculty development, *Nurse Educ* 25(2):70-75, 2000.
Rosenstein AH, O'Daniel M: Disruptive behavior and clinical outcomes: Perceptions of nurses and physicians, *Nurs Manag* 36(1):18-28, 2005.
Smith AP: Partners at the bedside: The importance of nurse-physician relationships, *Nurs Econ* 22(3):161-164, 2004.
Watson V, Steiert MJ: Verbal abuse and violence: The quest for harmony in the OR, *Surg Serv Manag* 8(4):16-22, 2002.

Chapter 2

Foundations of Perioperative Patient Care Standards

CHAPTER OBJECTIVES

After studying this chapter, the learner will be able to:
- Discuss how standardization influences patient care.
- Describe two professional sources of patient care standards.
- List three main aspects of accountability.
- Identify the components of the nursing process.

CHAPTER OUTLINE

KEY TERMS AND DEFINITIONS

Accountability   Answering for performance of a service or task.
Accreditation   A method of professional evaluation and recognition of an institution for meeting educational, practice, and national standard parameters.
Advocacy   Active support of another person.
Benchmark   A point of reference that sets the evaluation point of activities.
Competency statement   A document based on empirical data that define expected and measurable clinical activities.
Domain   Set of knowledge that is specific and clearly identified.
Element   Smallest unit of data that is known and can be described and measured.
Guidance statement   A document based on empirical data that suggest processes for performance of clinical activities.
Guideline   A document or concept based on empirical data that guide clinical activities.

Licensure   Approval for practice granted by a governmental agency for a predetermined period of time, after which the approval process is repeated.
Nomenclature   A specialized set of terms.
Nursing diagnosis   Identification of patient problem, need, or health consideration, which may be actual or at risk; based on human response patterns according to NANDA International.
Nursing process   Organizational framework for planning patient care; this involves assessment, nursing diagnosis, outcome identification, planning, implementation, and evaluation of the plan.
Obligation   Duty or promise.
Outcome   The effect of an intervention.
PNDS   Perioperative nursing data elements. Standardized perioperative nursing language.
Position statement   A document that describes a particular belief.
Profession   Vocation in a specialty requiring specialized education and knowledge.
Recommended Practice   Activities believed to be the optimal level of professional practice that are achievable.
Responsibility   Social, moral, or legal duty.
Rights   Power or possession of privilege.
Standard   Authoritative statement that describes accountability, values, and priorities.
Taxonomy   An orderly classification based on interrelationships.

SUPPLEMENTAL MATERIAL ON EVOLVE WEBSITE — *evolve*

http://evolve.elsevier.com/BerryKohn
- Content Updates
- Glossary
- Full Set of Perioperative Flash Cards
- Interactive Key Term Flash Cards
- Student Activities
- WebLinks

This chapter establishes the basis for perioperative patient care. The opening section gives a glimpse of historic patient care and progresses to modern perioperative practice.

HISTORICAL BACKGROUND

Throughout history, practitioners of the healing arts have been both revered and feared. They have been depicted as magicians, holy men, and deities. As the population grew, so did the fascination with herbs and remedies. When a homemade concoction worked, it was considered divine intervention or magic; if it failed, it was considered evil. Without knowledge of the germ theory, mass epidemics that were not cured by local healers were considered suspect for demonic influence. Evil was thought to be the cause of all illness. During the Spanish Inquisition in the sixteenth century, a midwife who experienced complications with a complex childbirth was at risk for being accused of witchcraft or infant sacrifice. More female healers than male healers were accused and executed during this dark era of patient care.

Nonphysician patient care is credited to the Greek physician Hippocrates (460-377 BC), the "Father of Medicine." He instituted training for men who would administer the treatments and therapies prescribed by the physicians of the time. Although most care was rendered by family members, complex procedures were performed by these trained individuals. They were considered the first home caregivers. Aristotle (384-322 BC) was the son of a physician. He wrote *The Golden Cabinet of Secrets,* a collection of herbal remedies that included antispasmodics, astringents, sedatives, laxatives, and stimulants. This was a commonly used guide for medical care and was disseminated over the Middle East trade routes. Famous people such as Alexander the Great (356-323 BC), who was Aristotle's student, and Cleopatra (69-31 BC) used this herbal guide.

Traveling health care was started in the ninth and tenth centuries by military and religious groups, which consisted primarily of men. In 1050, 35 years before the first Crusade, a hospital for the ill was dedicated in Jerusalem by the Knight Hospitallers of Saint John. Originally intended to be a religious order, the knights learned military skills to protect civilians on pilgrimages to the Holy Land.

Churches ceased control of hospitals during the reformation of the eighteenth century. Free care associated with religious personnel was replaced with low-paid, uneducated workers. Most of the tasks were unpleasant and menial, and cleanliness was not a prime consideration. Hospitals became filthy dens of death. Low wages and abominable working conditions did not attract honest, educated people to the job. Those who could afford private treatment at home had a better chance of survival by avoiding cross-contamination with other patients.

John Howard (1726-1790), an English philanthropist and prison reformer, wrote a book titled *An Account of the Principal Lazarettos*[1] in Europe and Additional Remarks on the Present State of Prisons in Great Britain and Ireland (1777), which disclosed the deplorable conditions in hospitals and prisons. Many patients were treated worse than prisoners were. Personal possessions were stolen, and barbaric treatments resembled torture. Physicians wore bloody aprons during surgery and did not change or wash them between patients. Instruments were rarely even wiped clean between uses. Handwashing was considered unimportant. Decisions were made about treatments without consulting the patient or family. During that dark era of patient care, few people accepted responsibility for the adequate performance of duties, and quality assurance was not a consideration. Undesired outcomes of care were commonly blamed on divine punishment.

Early nineteenth-century patient care gave rise to the clear separation of medicine and nursing. The profession of nursing was validated by the first nursing theorist, Florence Nightingale (1820-1910) (Fig. 2-1). Her concepts included the identification of the nurse as a skilled worker under the direction of a physician, who was the architect of medical treatment. She demonstrated that the environment and cleanliness ultimately affected the patient. Perioperative patient care is grounded in the control of the environment and the cleanliness of the devices therein.

Florence Nightingale is credited with developing the environmental theory of patient care on which all perioperative patient care is based (Box 2-1). According to her theory, the caregiver is accountable for creating and maintaining the best possible environmental conditions to assist natural healing. She emphasized the need for prevention through education and teamwork. In her eyes, the team consisted of not only the caregivers but also the patient and family. She often approached her legislators with suggestions for bills and laws designed to protect patients and caregivers. Her numerous letters and writings chronicle her work.

Until Florence Nightingale established standards of patient care and nursing education, the practice was haphazard and performed mostly by uneducated, untrained individuals. Nightingale stated, "Prepare for the unexpected. Patience is often more effective than aggression. Timing is everything. Create effective systems for obtaining and distributing resources. Caring for the sick requires a holistic approach." Nightingale made this statement in her 1854 report to the British government as she prepared her nurses for service during the Crimean War in Turkey. Not everyone

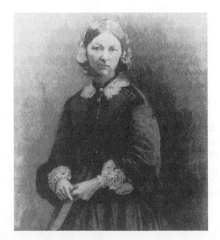

FIG. 2-1   Florence Nightingale, the first nursing theorist. (*Courtesy Florence Nightingale Museum Trust, London.*)

---

[1] A lazaretto is a place where people with contagious diseases, such as leprosy, are quarantined or housed.

BOX 2-1	Nightingale's Environmental Theory		
Physical Environment	**Psychologic Environment**		**Social Environment**
Sanitation	Communication		Mortality data
Ventilation	Advice		Prevention of disease
Lighting	Variety		Education of caregiver
Noise	Scientific knowledge base		Nursing as distinct from medicine
Odors	Creativity		Accountability
Temperature	Spirituality		Responsibility

had a family member to provide long-term care and all were commonly at the mercy of strangers. Box 2-2 lists several Internet addresses for further information on the history of patient care.

Both perioperative nurses and surgical technologists work toward a common objective—providing the safest possible care so that patients achieve favorable surgical outcomes. The perioperative nurse is responsible for the development of the patient-oriented plan of care, which is the creative application of the nursing process, scientific principles, judgment, skills, and professional competencies. Additional information about perioperative nursing can be found at www.aorn.org and surgical technology at www.ast.org.

SURGICAL CONSCIENCE

The key elements of perioperative practice are caring, conscience, discipline, and technique. Optimal patient care requires an inherent surgical conscience, selflessness, self-discipline, and the application of principles of asepsis and sterile technique. All are inseparably related.

The concept of a surgical conscience may be stated simply as a surgical Golden Rule: Do unto the patient as you would have others do unto you. The caregiver should consider each patient as himself or herself or as a loved one. Once an individual develops a surgical conscience, it remains inherent thereafter. Florence Nightingale summarized what is, in essence, its meaning when she said, "The nurse should keep a high sense of duty in her own mind, must aim at perfection in her care, and must be consistent always in herself."

A surgical conscience involves self-inspection coupled with moral obligation. Involving both scientific and intellectual honesty, it is self-regulation in practice according to a deep personal commitment to the highest values. It incorporates the caregiver's values and attitudes at a conscious level and monitors behavior and decision making in relation to those values. In short, a surgical conscience is

the inner voice for conscientious practice of aseptic and sterile techniques at all times. This conscientiousness applies to every activity and intervention, as well as to personal hygiene and health. An aseptic body image includes an awareness of body, hair, makeup, jewelry, fingernails, and attire. A team member with an infectious process, such as influenza, a cold, or an open skin lesion, clearly cannot work in the perioperative environment. Professional responsibility requires that patient safety is not compromised.

Correct practice of asepsis provides a foundation for development of a mature conscience—mastery of personal integrity and discipline. Development of this conscience incorporates knowledge of aseptic principles, perpetual attention to detail, and experience. All are facets of responsibility that involve trust. A surgical conscience does not permit a person to excuse an error but rather to admit and rectify one readily. It becomes so much an automatic part of the caregiver that he or she can see at a glance or instinctively know if a break in technique or violation of a principle has occurred. Conscience dictates that appropriate action be taken, whether the person is with others or is alone and unobserved. A surgical conscience therefore is the foundation for the practice of strict aseptic and sterile techniques. Practice according to that conscience results in pride in professional accomplishments, as well as an inner confidence that the patient is receiving the highest level of care.

A very important aspect in assisting the development of a surgical conscience in others is communication skill. A team member should not be criticized for an error; that person should be given credit for admitting the error and should be helped to correct the violation. Fear of criticism is the primary deterrent in admission of fault. No one should be reluctant to admit a frank or questionable break in technique. However, any individual unmotivated to carry out expected practices as close to perfection as possible has no place in the operating room (OR) suite.

PATIENT RIGHTS

As a consumer, the patient purchases services to fulfill health care needs and is entitled to certain rights. Access to health care is recognized as a right, not a privilege, of every human being.

Patient Advocacy

A patient advocate recognizes the patient's and the family's need for information and assistance in coping with the surgical experience, regardless of the setting. As an advocate,

BOX 2-2	Internet Sources of Nursing History

www.geocities.com/Athens/Forum/6011—Men in American nursing history
www4.umdnj.edu/camlbweb/blacknurses.html—Black nurses in history
www.aahn.org—American Association for the History of Nursing

the perioperative nurse can provide information discovered during patient assessment that identifies specific needs or health concerns that require action. Advance preparation can help the patient and family anticipate events. Assistance in coping acknowledges the anxieties and fears of the patient and family, regardless of how minimally invasive the procedure may seem. No procedure is minor to the patient! Each patient reacts differently. The patient senses some relief in knowing that the caregiver has taken the time to identify needs specific to his or her care. The patient advocate is a caregiver who does the following:

1. Establishes rapport with the patient, family, or significant others in a manner that conveys genuine concern and sincere caring
2. Encourages the patient and family or significant others to express feelings and to ask questions
3. Helps relieve anxiety and apprehension by providing factual information regarding what to expect
4. Helps the patient make informed decisions throughout the perioperative experience
5. Acts as a patient representative by communicating pertinent information to other team members
6. Oversees all activities throughout the perioperative experience to ensure the safety and welfare of the patient
7. Keeps the family informed of significant events throughout the perioperative experience
8. Protects the patient's rights by compliance with advance directives for care (living will, durable power of attorney, or both). Additional information about advance directives and durable power of attorney can be found in Chapter 3.

ACCOUNTABILITY

Accountability means answering to someone for an obligatory action. As both learners and caregivers, perioperative nurses and surgical technologists are accountable to the following:

- Patients receiving services
- Employer
- Educational institution providing learning experiences
- Profession or vocation to uphold established standards of practice
- Self and other team members

A lack of accountability for behavior in the perioperative environment may result in patient injury or dissatisfaction with care. Health care providers have a legal and moral obligation to identify and correct situations that threaten a patient's safety and well-being. Most incidents that could endanger the patient and lead to legal actions can be prevented. Prevention focuses on the responsible performance of duty and continual performance improvement. The provision of safe care of the patient also protects caregivers and the health care facility from liability. In addition, it upholds the reputation of the professions by maintaining the confidence of the consumer public. Failure of a caregiver to maintain accountability constitutes negligence. If negligence is established, any caregiver can be held liable for his or her own acts of omission or commission. Each person is responsible for his or her own negligent acts.

STANDARDIZATION OF PATIENT CARE
Importance of Standardization

Perioperative patient care personnel should be able to cope with all situations and to give patients the best of their skills and knowledge. Although the use of different techniques may achieve the same results, each hospital establishes policies and procedures for all personnel to follow based on standards, recommended practices, and guidelines that are developed by professional organizations and predicated on scientific research. These written policies, procedures, and guidelines help prevent confusion and foster coordination of activities. Uniformity and standardization of procedures help personnel develop skill and efficiency for the following reasons:

- The main purpose is to ensure the safety and welfare of the patient and personnel.
- It is easier for the perioperative educator and preceptors to teach learners consistent methods of patient care.
- Learning is easier if everyone performs procedures in the same way.
- Deviations show a need for evaluation of the procedures or the staff. Do the procedures need revision?
- Uniform procedures provide an efficient check during preparation for any surgical procedure.
- One person can take over for another at any time during the surgical procedure, if necessary, and know exactly where to find instruments and supplies.
- Routine procedures establish habits that increase speed in thought and action. Doing work in a certain way promotes a high level of proficiency.
- Knowing the standards allows intelligent decision making when a patient's condition requires modification of a routine.

Professional Sources of Standards

Standards of care are defined as those acts that a reasonably prudent person with comparable training and experience would perform under the same or similar circumstances. Professional standards delineate activities related to performance, performance improvement, continuing education, ethical behavior, responsibility, and accountability.

Standards established by regulatory agencies are governed by laws. Standards established by professional associations are voluntary. Standards of practice for perioperative patient care include professional and regulated standards. Several sources of perioperative patient care standards are identified in this list:

1. Standards of Perioperative Nursing. These standards, which originated as ANA standards of OR practice in 1975, were approved by ANA and by Association of periOperative Registered Nurses (AORN) and originally published in 1981. Reviews and revisions are done yearly as needed.

   These five sets of standards for an optimal level of perioperative nursing practice are published annually in *AORN Standards, Recommended Practices, and Guidelines*. The scaffold of the standards is premised in patient care quality and is primarily tri-fold—Structure, Process, and Outcome. These three components provide a means for the perioperative nurse to analyze and interpret care. Reviews and revisions are done yearly as needed.

a. Standards of Perioperative Administrative Nursing Practice. These are *structural* standards that provide a framework for establishing administrative and organizational practices in a variety of settings.

b. Standards of Perioperative Clinical Practice. These are *process* standards based on problem-solving techniques using principles and theories of biophysical and behavioral sciences. They describe how the nursing process is used in the perioperative setting. The *Perioperative Nursing Data Elements* (PNDS) provide a means to measure and collect performance improvement data.

c. Standards of Perioperative Professional Practice. These are *process* standards that describe a competent level of behavior for the professional role of the perioperative nurse. The activities relate to quality practice evaluation, continuing education, collegial relations, collaboration, ethical conduct, and use of resources, evidence-based research, and leadership.

d. Quality and Performance Improvement Standards for Perioperative Nursing. These are *process* standards to assist in the development of methods to measure, assess, and improve patient care.

e. Perioperative Patient Outcomes: Standards of Perioperative Care. These are *outcome* standards that reflect desired observable patient outcomes during preoperative, intraoperative, and postoperative phases of patient care. They focus on patient and family responses to intervention during surgical, diagnostic, or therapeutic intervention. Each outcome has a unique identifier in the PNDS.

2. The Operating Room Nurses Association of Canada (ORNAC, www.ornac.ca) has published Recommended Standards for Operating Room Nursing Practice and Quality Assurance Audit.

3. Association of Surgical Technologists Standards of Practice (AST, www.ast.org). These are process standards that provide guidelines for safe and effective patient care in appropriate preoperative, intraoperative, and postoperative practice settings. They include interpersonal skills, environmental safety, and application of principles of surgical technology.

4. Joint Commission on Accreditation of Healthcare Organizations (JCAHO) standards (www.jcaho.org). These standards, published in the *Accreditation Manual for Hospitals* are functional, performance-based standards that focus on actual clinical care provided directly to patients and on management of the health care organization providing services. They relate to efficiency, effectiveness, safety, and timeliness; to appropriateness, continuity, and availability of care; and to patient satisfaction. JCAHO evaluates compliance with these standards and reviews clinical outcomes of care provided as fundamental criteria for accreditation. Selective clinical indicators serve as outcome measurements for the processes of patient care. Additional information about error reporting and monitoring of patient care standards can be found in Chapter 3.

- JCAHO established National Patient Safety Goals in 2006
- Improve the accuracy of patient identification
- Improve the effectiveness between caregivers
- Improve the safety of using medications
- Reduce the risk of healthcare-associated infections
- Accurately and completely reconcile medications across the continuum of care

5. National Fire Protection Association (NFPA) standards (http://safety.science.tamu.edu/nfpa.html). These standards apply to environmental safety to reduce, to the extent possible, hazards to patients and personnel.

6. Association for the Advancement of Medical Instrumentation (AAMI) device standards (www.aami.org). These standards provide industry with reference documents on accepted levels of device safety and performance and test methods to determine conformance. AAMI standards have also been established for sterilization, electrical safety, and patient monitoring for health care providers in relation to evaluation, maintenance, and use of medical devices and instrumentation.

7. Clinically based risk-control standards. These standards are written by medical specialty groups and professional liability underwriters. They establish appropriate benchmarks of acceptable practices and outcomes specifically for controlling liability losses. They may be incorporated into the health care facility's risk management program.

Standards from Regulatory Bodies

The standards set by these organizations are enforceable by law:

1. Federal Medicare Act and all subsequent amendments to this Social Security Act (www.cms.hhs.gov). This legislation incorporates the provision that institutions participating in Medicare must maintain the level of patient care recognized as the norm. Specific requirements are included.

a. Health Insurance Portability and Accountability Act (HIPAA, www.cms.hhs.gov/hipaa). The Department of Health and Human Services (HHS) set national standards for electronic health care transactions and national identifiers for providers, health plans, and employers. It also addresses the security and privacy of health data. Many facilities require the employees to sign a confidentiality agreement upon hire.

2. American National Standards Institute (ANSI) standards (www.ansi.org). These standards concern exposures to toxic materials and safe use of equipment such as lasers.

3. U.S. Food and Drug Administration (FDA) performance standards (www.fda.gov). Federal Medical Device Amendments regulate the manufacture, labeling, sale, and use of implantable medical devices and many products used in or on patients. The FDA also controls treatment protocols for use of drugs. The manufacturer's lot number and product description of implanted devices should be attached to or included in the patient's chart.

4. Agency for Healthcare Research and Quality (AHRQ) clinical practice guidelines (www.ahcpr.gov). These standards include indicators for performance measurement. They are based on research and professional judgment regarding effectiveness and appropriateness of medical care, including safety, efficacy, and effectiveness of technology. This agency was created in provisions of the Consolidated Omnibus Budget Reconciliation Act of 1989. AORN has included perioperative interpretations of the AHRQ guidelines in the AORN *Standards, Recommended Practices, and Guidelines* publication.

5. Occupational Safety and Health Administration (OSHA) standards (www.osha.gov). These legally enforceable standards include permissible levels of toxic substances in the environment. Although explicitly developed to protect employees, patients receive secondary benefits from control of hazards in the environment.

Sources of Standardization Data within the Health Care Facility

Each patient care facility uses several sources from which to derive standardization data. Efficient use of time and resources is the end result. Establishing protocols and performance expectations that are specific to the needs of the facility benefits the patient, the caregiver, and the facility.

1. *Facility-specific patient care standards.* The patient care services department establishes standards for appropriate patient care based on the standards developed by the American Nurses Association (ANA). Optimal standards of nursing practice guide the provision of patient care throughout the institution. Written policies and procedures reflect these standards. Institutional standards are based on standards established at national levels by the JCAHO, AORN, ANA, and other nursing organizations and governmental agencies. Nurses should practice within the limitations of the nurse practice act of the state in which they are licensed and practice. Copies of facility-specific documents are available for review from the nursing or hospital administration.

2. *Hospital policy and procedure manual.* This manual contains basic and general administrative and patient care policies that apply to all hospital personnel. A copy is retained on each patient care unit and in all departments of the hospital.

3. *Safety plan manual.* The potential hazards and identifiable situations that may cause injury to a caregiver or patient are described in the manual provided by the hospital safety committee. Plans for fire or disaster drills and evacuation routes are outlined.

4. *Material safety data sheets (MSDS).* These detailed sheets describe chemicals used in the workplace and actions to take if they are spilled into the environment. Specific cleanup and disposal methods are outlined. Most facilities require a yearly review of the MSDS process. Individual MSDS sheets for specific chemicals is online at www.msds.com.

5. *Disaster plan manual.* This manual outlines the plans for both *internal* and *external* disasters. An internal disaster is an event that happens within the facility (e.g., an explosion, a fire) and requires employee assistance for control of the situation and evacuation of personnel and patients. An external disaster is an event that happens outside the confines of the facility (e.g., the World Trade Center terrorist actions of September 11, 2001). An external disaster could also be a natural phenomenon such as an earthquake or an accident (e.g., a train wreck). Both internal and external disasters require rapid activation of all services within the hospital. Personnel who are off duty will be called to the facility and will be assigned as needed.

6. *Infection control manual.* This manual contains the policies and procedures designed to minimize the risk of infection and control the spread of disease within the health care facility. It includes state, local, federal, and professional standards for the protection of the patient and the caregiver.

7. *Perioperative policy and procedure manual.* This manual, usually a hardcover ringed binder, contains the policies pertaining solely to the administration and operation of the perioperative environment. A copy is available for reference in the manager's office, at the control desk, or in both places. The primary purpose of the perioperative policy and procedure manual is to detail why and how procedures should be specifically performed within the perioperative environment. It includes both supportive activities and practices that involve direct perioperative patient care.

8. *Orientation manual.* This manual is designed to acquaint personnel with the environment, policies, and procedures specific to performance and the position descriptions of all personnel in the department.

9. *Instrument book.* The individual instruments and trays required for each surgical procedure are listed in a separate book that is kept in the instrument processing area. Photographs or catalog illustrations help instrumentation personnel identify the vast number of instruments and how they are compiled into sets.

10. *Surgeon's preference cards/case cart sheet.* A preference card is maintained for each surgical procedure that each surgeon performs. The surgeon's specific preferences and any variance from the procedures in the procedure book are noted on these cards. The cards are revised as procedures and personal preferences for new technology change. A set of these cards is kept readily available in a central file or in a computer under the surgeon's name, and they are pulled for each day's surgical procedures. In preparing for each surgical procedure, nurses and surgical technologists consult both these cards and the procedure book. A surgical central supply department may use these cards to pack a case cart for each individual procedure. Table 2-1 shows sample case cart sheet components incorporating the surgeon's preference card.

11. *Directories.* Alphabetic listings of the location of supplies and equipment are maintained for the instrument room, general workroom, sterile supply room, and general perioperative storage areas. Regardless of where the storage areas are located, personnel should know the location of supplies and equipment. Directories save time in trying to locate items.

TABLE 2-1	Sample Case Cart Sheet Components with Surgeon's Preferences*	

Surgeon:
  Dr. Jared
	Procedure:
	  Excision lipoma right anterior thigh
		Patient:
		  Martin Alexander

Gloves:
  Size 8
	Prep:
	  One-step iodophor
		Patient data: (e.g., age, sex, allergies)
		  26 years old, male, no allergies

Positioning:
  Supine
	Medications:
	  1% lidocaine plain
	  Sterile saline 1000 mL
		Drapes:
		  General custom pack
		  2 gowns

Instruments:
  Soft tissue set
	Suture:
	  3-0 Vicryl PS1
		Sponges:
		  2 packs Raytec

Special requests:
  Radio or CD player on low
	Disposable supplies:
	  None
		Notes:
		  Call family when procedure completed

*Components of computer-generated case cart procedure supply sheet. These sheets are generated at the time the procedure is scheduled using standardized surgeon's preference cards and patient-specific needs. Items listed under each heading are examples only.

RECOMMENDED PRACTICES

Recommended practices are optimum behavioral objectives for caregivers. They may not always be achievable, as standards are, because of limitations in a particular practice setting. Recommended practices state what ideally can be done.

AORN recommended practices for perioperative nursing concern aseptic techniques and technical aspects of nursing practice directed toward providing safety in the perioperative environment. They are based on principles of microbiology, scientific literature, validated research, and experts' opinions. Although compliance is voluntary, individual commitment, professional conscience, and the practice setting should guide perioperative caregivers in using these recommended practices. They represent what is believed to be an optimal level of practice and are intended to be achievable.

Guidelines and recommended practices of other agencies, including AAMI, the Centers for Disease Control and Prevention (CDC), the National Institute for Occupational Safety and Health (NIOSH), and the Environmental Protection Agency (EPA), also are used for environmental, patient, and personnel safety.

Policies and Procedures

Policies and procedures reflect variations in institutional environments and clinical situations. They are established to protect employees, learners, and patients. They establish the facility's standard of care. Policies should be consistent with regulatory and professional standards of practice. Procedures define scope, purposes, and instructions to be carried out and by whom. They should be clearly written, current, dated, and reviewed periodically. Although policies and procedures vary from one institution to another, they provide guidelines for patient care and safety in that specific physical facility. Learning and following policies and procedures are protective measures against potentially litigious actions.

Many facilities document in the employee's personnel file that policies and procedures have been reviewed during orientation to the employment setting. Employees may be asked to sign a notation verifying knowledge of a new or revised policy or procedure after its introduction. Some policies and procedures apply to all employees; others refer to a specific department. Because of the potential legal implications, adherence to all policies and procedures is mandatory. Personnel are evaluated on their ability to follow policy and perform procedures correctly. The following examples should be included in the perioperative department manual. These procedures are incorporated into discussions in subsequent chapters.

Identifying the Patient

When a patient enters the facility, a plastic identification wristband is put on the patient in the admitting area. Care is taken to place the wristband in a location that does not interfere with the surgical site. To verify accuracy, the patient should be asked to spell his or her name and pronounce it. The circulating nurse and anesthesia provider check the wristband with the patient and surgeon, the patient's chart, and the surgical schedule. The surgeon should visit with the patient before an anesthetic is administered. A parent, legal guardian, or individual with power of attorney can complete this identification process. JCAHO indicates that at least two methods should be employed to identify a patient as part of the patient safety goals.

Identifying the Surgical Site

The surgical site indicated by the consent form should be verified between the circulating nurse and the patient. Universal methods of surgical site verification include asking the patient to describe what he or she understands the planned procedure to be. If the procedure is to be performed on a particular side of the body, the patient should be asked to point to and clarify the site. The surgeon should mark the site with his or her initials in indelible ink that does not wash off during intraoperative skin preparation. Marking with an "X" is inappropriate and can be confusing if "X" is used to indicate the wrong side.

Before making the incision the entire team pauses for a "TIME OUT" as the surgical site listed on the consent form is read aloud. The entire team confirms that this is correct information. During this process the availability of the correct implants or special equipment is confirmed (Box 2-3).

The surgical site marking and identification process should be standardized within the facility and written into policy to avoid wrong-site procedures. The time out process

BOX 2-3	"Time Out" for Prevention of Wrong Site Surgery

- Correct patient?
- Correct position?
- Correct site?
- Correct procedure?
- Correct equipment?
- Correct images? (scans or radiographs in proper orientation)
- Correct implants? (as appropriate)

should be documented in the patient's record by the circulating nurse. More information can be found at www.aorn.org in the official statements section and on the JCAHO website at www.jcaho.org. JCAHO has described factors that contribute to wrong site, wrong patient, and wrong procedure surgery. They are as follows:

- Emergencies
- Morbid obesity
- Physical deformity
- Unusual equipment or setup of the OR
- Multiple surgeons
- Multiple procedures
- Unmarked patients
- Unverified patients
- No checklist
- No assessment
- Staffing issues
- Distractions
- Lack of information about the patient
- Organizational culture of the facility

Protecting Personal Property

Personnel in preoperative areas are responsible for removing valuables and prostheses before patients go to the OR. The circulating nurse is responsible for double-checking each patient and removing, as necessary, unnecessary items brought to the OR. Personal items such as religious medals, hearing aid(s), eyeglasses, dentures, and eye prostheses are commonly permitted to remain with the patient who is having local or regional anesthesia. The circulating nurse should inform the anesthesia provider and the surgeon of their presence and document them on the patient's chart. Artificial extremities, undergarments, wigs, hairpins, wristwatches, and rings should be removed. Jewelry could get lost, or a ring might become stuck on the patient's finger as a result of postoperative swelling. In addition to the danger of losing or damaging these items, some could cause pressure areas on the anesthetized patient's body.

Any item that is removed should be placed in a rigid container and labeled with the patient's name and number. The patient's personal property should not be wrapped in a paper or linen towel that could inadvertently be discarded in a trash receptacle or laundry hamper. The container may be retained by the circulating nurse during the surgical procedure and sent with the patient to the postoperative area. Alternatively, the circulating nurse may immediately ask a nursing assistant to return the container to the patient care unit. This person should obtain a receipt for the

patient's personal property from the person receiving it. The receipt is given to the circulating nurse to put in the patient's chart along with a notation of the transaction in the nurses' notes. Patients value their property. A caregiver can be held liable for loss or damage to a patient's personal property.

Observing the Patient

Unattended patients may fall from a stretcher or the OR bed. Falls are one of the most frequent causes of avoidable injuries. Side rails, restraints, and safety straps should be used to protect all patients, children as well as adults. A small child could reach and insert a tiny finger into an electrical socket. Patients should be observed at all times in the perioperative environment.

Positioning the Patient

Care is taken when moving all patients to and from the OR bed. The patient should be positioned to ensure adequate exposure of the surgical site for the surgeon but not compromise any body system. The anesthesia provider should determine the physiologic safety of the patient's body systems. Cardiopulmonary functioning should not be impaired. Adequate support of joints and limbs should be provided during movement into the desired position. Pressure areas should be adequately protected to prevent neurovascular damage. The plan of care should include appropriate numbers of personnel for safe patient movement. Patients who are incapable of assisting with physical motion require a minimum of four people to ensure a safe move from one surface to another. There should be at least one person on either side of the patient, one at the foot, and one at the head to monitor the patient's airway and physiologic response. The person guiding the patient's head should be the one who counts "one—two—three" to pace the synchronized movement from one surface to another.

The surgeon determines the appropriate surgical position in consultation with the anesthesia provider. The circulating nurse and first assistant help position the patient. A stretcher is kept nearby at all times if a patient is placed in a prone position or any position other than supine. In the event of an emergency, the patient will need to be placed in a supine position for treatment such as cardiopulmonary resuscitation (CPR).

Many patients receive a general anesthetic or heavy sedation and are therefore unconscious or not in control of their protective reflexes. Constant vigilance is essential to safeguard patients who are vulnerable and unable to protect themselves. Liability on the part of the team would be difficult to dispute. Everyone in the perioperative environment has a duty to monitor and protect the patient at all times without exception.

Aseptic and Sterile Techniques

Infection is a serious postoperative complication that may become life threatening for the patient. Perioperative patient care team members must know and apply the principles of aseptic and sterile techniques at all times. Established procedures for aseptic technique, sterilization, and disinfection should be followed meticulously. An emergency situation in which asepsis becomes a secondary concern is a rare occurrence. Asepsis should not be compromised for the sake of convenience of the caregiver. Each team member should consider how personal preferences for care of self or a loved one should be applied to the care of patients.

Postoperative wound infection can originate in the OR from a break in technique by any team member. Inappropriate reuse of disposable items may be indefensible, as can use of an unsterile endoscope introduced into a sterile body cavity. An unsterile scope can disrupt the mucous membrane and come into contact with the patient's vascular system. No area of the body is considered "dirty." Any area of the body is at risk when the vascular system is entered and should be worthy of sterile instrumentation. Microorganisms can be transferred via any access portal to the vascular system, including but not limited to the mouth, urethra, penis, vagina, rectum, and ear. Strict asepsis and sterile technique prevent many postperative complications. The following principle should be remembered: When in doubt about something's sterility, consider it unsterile, hence the phrase "When in doubt, throw it out."

Accountability of Accurate Counts

The primary responsibility for accounting for all sponges, sharps, and instruments before, during, and after every surgical procedure rests with the circulating nurse and scrub person. Laziness and a cavalier attitude surround the statement, "the incision is *too small* to lose anything." Don't ever be fooled by this. It can happen. There are several reasons to count and be accountable for items used in a surgical procedure.

1. Patients have been known to retain items from a surgical procedure regardless of the size or location of the surgical site. This is a serious safety breach that is not excusable.
2. Instruments are costly and should not "vanish into thin air." It is a shame that some hospitals x-ray all the trash and have metal detectors on the doors of the OR. Instruments stuck in washing machines cause damage to the mechanisms. Accountability significantly decreases this loss.
3. Many instruments have sharp tips or cutting surfaces. If an instrument is in the trash or laundry it can become a source of injury to unsuspecting housekeepers or laundry workers. Gloves worn for cleaning do not protect from sharp objects. This can result in prolonged illness and inability to work.

Any item put into the patient should be documented as part of the count and reconciled at the end of the procedure. The surgeon and first assistant facilitate the count of the items on the surgical field before closure; however, it is not their job to perform the actual counts. Because accountability for sponges, sharps, and instruments is recognized as essential to safe practice and the standard of care, omission of appropriate counts or a facility's lack of established procedures for counting and accountability could result in a serious threat of liability. There is no excuse for any retained foreign object if the systems for accountability are followed by the entire team.

The circulating nurse should document in writing the outcome of the final counts as correct or incorrect and any unusual incidents concerning them, including the need for a radiograph to look for a lost item. If a radiograph is taken, the name of the radiologist and his or her findings also should be documented. An incident report should be filed on all counts that remain unresolved. It is not necessary to indicate the actual number of sponges or needles used on the OR record. The documentation of correct or incorrect counts is sufficient. Any questionable count should be documented as resolved or unresolved and to whom the event was reported.

Facility policy and procedure should determine the disposition of any tally sheets used in the counting process. The tally sheets are merely worksheets and have no particular value to the permanent record. Some facilities use a wipe-off grease board to tally sponge, needle, and instrument counts. Additional information about the processes and rationale for counting and being accountable are described in Chapter 25.

Using Equipment

All instruments, equipment, and appliances should be used and tested according to the recommendations and instructions of the manufacturer. Safety devices such as personal protective attire or smoke evacuation apparatus should be employed as necessary. Electrical and laser equipment also should pass inspection by the biomedical engineering department and be tagged with a dated preventive maintenance sticker. Electrical equipment should be properly grounded to prevent electrical shock and burns. Equipment or devices that are known or suspected to be faulty are not used.

The facility should conduct appropriate training and competency reviews for all equipment used in patient care. Personnel who set up and operate facility-owned equipment may be found negligent if a patient is injured. Great care is critical to prevent injury when using all equipment in the perioperative environment. It is inappropriate to operate equipment or machinery for which the employee has had no training. All personnel should have adequate training on all equipment they are expected to operate during patient care in the OR. Records of such training should be on file within the department.

Preventing Skin Injury

Skin injury may be caused by an electrical or thermal device, chemical agent, sharp objects, or mechanical pressure. Pressure necrosis is possible after any procedure and especially after procedures lasting more than 2 hours. Patients who have been in holding areas or emergency departments may have pressure injury in process before arriving at the OR. The circulating nurse should assess the patient for skin injury.

A burn may occur from the use of a hot instrument taken directly out of the autoclave, such as a mouth gag or a large retractor. The scrub person should immerse a hot instrument in a basin of cool, sterile water before handing it to the surgeon. The hot item should not be placed in a damp towel and placed on the patient's skin; the heat from the item will transfer through the towel and cause a burn. Prolonged contact of even moderate temperatures can cause tissue damage. The patient under anesthesia has no protective reflexes to warn of an impending injury. Thermal injury can happen when any device or solution heated beyond 110° F (44° C) comes into contact with a patient's tissues.[2]

A patient may be burned during use of the electro-surgical unit (ESU). Inadequate skin contact or improper placement of the patient return electrode can cause a deep tissue burn that won't manifest immediately in the OR by a superficial reaction. Redness of the skin on removal of the patient return electrode may be caused by the adhesive rather than a burn. In a thermal injury, the deep tissue necroses and sloughs from the bottom up, leaving a full-thickness wound that may be insensate because of nerve damage. The tip of the ESU pencil, endoscopic instrument, or suction cautery probe remains hot after it is applied to tissues for hemostasis. Unintended burns may occur if the hot tip touches other body parts or if it is activated against a metal retractor or instrument. Use of a dry sponge against an activated tip causes ignition.

Alcohol and other flammable solutions such as some one-step prep chemicals can be ignited, causing flash fires if the solutions are pooled under the patient or allowed to saturate drapes, especially in the presence of oxygen. Vapors or oxygen can accumulate under drapes and ignite if exposed to the ESU pencil. A thermal burn also can occur from other types of electrical and laser equipment that is improperly used or maintained. The caregiver should be aware that the effects of some types of lasers on tissue are not readily visible until tissue necrosis takes place several days postoperatively.

Administering Drugs

Any drug that the surgeon uses in the surgical site, such as an antibiotic or local anesthetic, is recorded in the peri-operative note by the circulating nurse and surgeon. The drug is checked by a registered nurse and the scrub person before it is transferred to the sterile field. The sterile medication container and syringes (if used) are clearly labeled by the scrub person on the field. The scrub person frequently has more than one drug on the instrument table, and confusion could result if the drugs are not properly marked. Each is correctly labeled and administered appropriately. The scrub person repeats the name of the drug to the surgeon when passing it. Medications and medication handling are described in more detail in Chapters 23 and 25.

AORN has developed a medication toolkit for preventing medication errors. Contact AORN at www.aorn.org for more information about receiving this packet. Consider the "seven rights" of medication administration:
- Right patient
- Right drug
- Right dose
- Right reason
- Right time
- Right route
- Right documentation

Monitoring the Patient

The standard of care indicates that a registered nurse is responsible for monitoring the cardiac and respiratory status of a patient receiving local anesthetic, with or without intravenous (IV) conscious sedation, if an anesthesia provider is not present. The nurse is expected to interpret the monitoring equipment, assess the patient, and initiate interventions promptly if the patient has an untoward reaction. Policies and procedures are delineated by each facility for care of the patient receiving local anesthetic. The nurse who is monitoring the patient should not be assigned circulating duties that would distract attention from the patient. Patient monitoring is described in more detail in Chapter 27.

Preparing Specimens

With very few exceptions, tissue and objects removed from a patient are sent to the pathology department. The loss of a tissue biopsy specimen could necessitate a second surgical procedure to obtain another one. Incorrectly labeled specimens could result in a mistaken diagnosis, with possible critical implications for two patients. Also, the loss of a specimen could prevent determination of a diagnosis and subsequent initiation of definitive therapy. The pathology report becomes part of the patient's permanent record as added documentation of the diagnosis. Specimens from opposite sides of the body should be sent in separate marked containers.

Care for foreign bodies according to the policy of the facility. They may have legal significance and frequently are claimed by police, especially if the foreign body is a bullet or something implicated in a crime. These items are not to be left unattended at any time. A receipt from the person taking them protects personnel and the facility. Chain of custody is a serious issue.

Specimen handling can be hazardous for personnel. Best practices indicate that a sterile container and lid of the appropriate size on the sterile field is the safest way to prevent biologic exposure of other team members. The scrub person should contain the specimen completely before handing the container off to the circulating nurse, who is wearing protective gloves. Dropping a specimen into a cup being held by another is placing that person at risk for exposure. This is avoidable. Specific information about specimen preparation can be found in Chapter 22.

Patient Teaching

The patient and/or significant others need to be informed about treatment options and their roles in the process. The patient has the right to make decisions and to contribute to the development of the plan of care. The perioperative nurse can assist with preoperative teaching of deep-breathing exercises for postoperative recovery. Information should be provided verbally and in writing. The patient and/or significant others should respond appropriately in

---

[2] ECRI (formerly the Emergency Care Research Institute, www.ecri.org) is a nonprofit health services research agency. Its mission is to improve the safety, quality, and cost effectiveness of health care. It is widely recognized as one of the world's leading independent organizations committed to advancing the quality of health care.

such a way as to signify understanding of the information. This is particularly important for ambulatory surgery patients who will go home under the care of others. Patient teaching and demonstration of understanding should be documented in the chart. More information about patient teaching is located in Chapter 21.

PROFESSIONALISM

Professionals act responsibly in accord with their commitment to public trust and service. Simply stated, the word *profession* implies a combination and coordination of knowledge, skills, and ideals that are communicated through activities based in higher education. The following are characteristics of a profession:

- It defines its own purposes and code of ethics.
- It sets its own standards and conducts its own affairs; it is self-regulated and has autonomy.
- Through research, it identifies and develops its own body of knowledge unique to its role.
- It requires critical thinking skills in clinical judgment, as well as problem-solving and decision-making skills in the application of knowledge.
- It engages in self-evaluation and peer review to control and alter its practices and accountabilities.

PROFESSIONAL PERIOPERATIVE NURSING

Professional nursing is dedicated to the promotion of optimal health for all human beings in their various environments. AORN is the leading organization for perioperative nursing and sets the standard for professionalism. In the support of professional perioperative nursing in a wide variety of specialties, AORN has formed 23 specialty assemblies for specialized practice areas and professional interests. The specialty assemblies do not have regular meetings, but offer online and newsletter participation. Several times a year the specialty assemblies offer workshops. Assembly meetings are held at the annual AORN Congress. An abbreviated internal specialty assembly governance structure provides a chairman and other elected officials. A modest fee is charged for membership in each assembly. A perioperative nurse may belong to as many assemblies as desired. The specialty assemblies enforced, as of 2006, include the following:

1. Perioperative nursing informatics
2. Rural and small hospitals
3. RN first assistant
4. Minimally invasive and laser
5. Pediatric
6. Orthopedic
7. Ophthalmology
8. Neurosurgery
9. Leadership
10. Military/government nursing
11. Ambulatory surgery
12. Integrated health practices
13. Cardiothoracic
14. Educator/clinical nurse specialist
15. Business, industry, and consulting
16. Retired nurses
17. Advanced practice nurses
18. Endovascular
19. Central supply/sterile processing/materials management
20. General surgery/gynecology
21. Multicultural nursing
22. Plastic and reconstructive surgery
23. Trauma

Nursing in general is both a humanistic art and an applied science. The art of professional nursing practice involves nursing diagnoses and the treatment of human responses to health and illness in all patient care settings. The science behind the paradigm of nursing is based on theories about the nature of humankind, health, and disease. Nursing education prepares nurses to translate the art and science of nursing into relevant knowledge and skill. Professional nursing education is built on a solid base of general education in liberal arts, humanities, and natural and behavioral sciences. AORN Position Statements reflect that in the future minimal entry level into perioperative nursing should be the baccalaureate degree.

A wise physician once said that the physician's role is to cure sometimes, to relieve often, and to comfort always. The same can be said for the perioperative nurse, who is a registered nurse who embodies all that the words that "nurse" has traditionally meant to a patient—provider of safety and comfort, supporter, and confidante. The patient's safety and welfare are entrusted to the perioperative OR nurse from the moment of arrival in the perioperative environment until departure and the transfer of responsibility for care to another professional health care team member. The perioperative nurse is legally accountable for the delivery of care to patients in the perioperative environment, including interventions that assist the patient in a conscious or unconscious state. The primary emphasis of the nurse's responsibility is to the patient. The perioperative nurse identifies the physiologic, psychologic, and sociologic needs of the patient; develops and implements an individualized plan of care that coordinates interventions; and evaluates outcomes of the patient's perioperative experience. The nurse is accountable and responsible for delegated patient care.

Patient-Nurse Relationship

To practice in a technologically complex environment, perioperative nurses must be flexible and their skills must be diverse. Their roles incorporate both the technical and the behavioral components of professional nursing. Competent fulfillment of the perioperative nursing role is based on the knowledge and application of the principles of biologic, physiologic, behavioral, and social sciences. Perioperative nurses develop nursing diagnoses based on patients' problems, needs, and health status. This is essential information in the identification of expected outcomes and in the formulation of a perioperative plan of care.

The perioperative nurse shares a special humanized experience with the patient at a time of great stress and need in his or her life. This relationship encompasses feelings, attitudes, and behaviors, with mutual trust and understanding as vital components. Effective interaction encompasses concern for the unique personhood of both the patient and the nurse. The length of time spent with the patient is not as important as the quality of the interaction. The level of the interaction may directly affect the patient's perception of the delivery of care in the perioperative environment.

To achieve and maintain a viable cooperative relationship, the patient should be able to sense that the nurse unconditionally cares about his or her well-being. The nurse should remain aware that personal interaction is often predicated on culture, attitudes, beliefs, and experiences. Knowledge of the effect of care on the patient's outcome enhances the attainment of the desired result.

Perioperative nursing care is a specialized combination of individualized and standardized care. Individualized care, the art of nursing, demonstrates genuine concern for the patient as a person and is not purely technical. Standardized care, the science of nursing, is derived from a body of scientific knowledge that has been developed through research and clinical practice.

EVIDENCE-BASED PRACTICE

The medical model has used tradition or habit to determine the foundations of practice. In the 1980s medicine adopted an evidence-based framework premised in research as a foundation for patient care practices. Nursing has questioned the best methods for performing patient care and has sought confirmation of the rationale that supports nursing actions. The development of a systematic process involves research that yields evidence of best practices. The key elements involve obtaining and evaluating evidence and considerations for implementing newly established evidence in practice.

Caregivers should always question why they are doing a particular action and if it is truly effective. Behaviors should continually be evaluated for usefulness as opposed to ritualism. Many practices may no longer be necessary and are not supported by evidence. The following questions should be systematically reviewed when researching for evidence-based practice:

- Which practice area requires evidence?
- What comprises evidence?
- How can evidence be found?
- What is the value of individual increments of evidence?
- Can the increments of evidence be combined into a unit of practice?
- Can the unit of practice be implemented in patient care?

In order to set up a research project or a systematic review, the following should be well established:

- Who will make up the population to be studied?
- Which intervention will be studied?
- How does one intervention compare with another?
- Which outcomes are preferred?

NURSING PROCESS

Perioperative patient care requires developing a plan of care and identifying expected outcomes through the nursing process (Box 2-4). The nursing process is a systematic approach to nursing practice using problem-solving techniques. This six-part process provides a systematic foundation for assessing the patient, establishing a nursing diagnosis, identifying desired outcomes, planning interventions,

---

BOX 2-4	The Nursing Process

ASSESSMENT
- Identify the actual or potential problems, needs, and health status considerations through appraisal of the physiologic, psychosocial, objective, subjective, cultural, and ethnic data related to the patient as an individual. Assessment is based on functional health patterns.
- Document assessment data.

NURSING DIAGNOSIS
- Formulate prioritized actual or potential nursing diagnoses unique to the patient. Human response patterns guide the development of nursing diagnoses.

IDENTIFICATION OF OUTCOMES
- Develop measurable and attainable expected outcomes and mutual goals in collaboration with the patient, significant others, and other health care providers.
- Identify realistic time frames in which fulfillment may be accomplished.

PLANNING
- Establish and prioritize a working set of interventions for the actual problems, needs, and health status considerations.
- Establish a contingency plan for the potential problems, needs, and health status considerations that may become actual during the course of the perioperative experience.
- Include the patient's input for the construction of the individualized plan.
- Document the plan of care in a retrievable manner.

IMPLEMENTATION
- Share the plan with the perioperative team for continuity of care.
- Activate the interventions in a systematic order of priority.
- Discontinue any intervention that is ineffective.
- Document the implementation of the interventions and their effectiveness.

EVALUATION
- Determine the effectiveness of the plan as the expected outcomes and mutual goals are met.
- Reformulate the plan and implement new interventions as necessary.
- Document the effectiveness of the plan of care in an ongoing, systematic manner.

BOX 2-5	Human Response Patterns According to NANDA International

- Exchanging
- Communicating
- Relating
- Valuing
- Choosing
- Moving
- Perceiving
- Knowing
- Feeling

implementing care, and evaluating the success of the plan. Human response patterns to health and illness are key elements in establishing a nursing diagnosis (Box 2-5).

Integration of the Nursing Process into Perioperative Patient Care

The six components of the nursing process are integrated into the three phases of the patient's perioperative experience: the preoperative phase, the intraoperative phase, and the postoperative phase. Throughout the entire perioperative period, the patient is continually assessed, the plan of care is modified, implementation is effected, and the cycle is evaluated for the attainment of outcomes. The perioperative nurse is responsible for continually assessing the patient by observing and acknowledging parameters identified in Box 2-6. The system and the structure had been traditionally complex until specific data elements of perioperative patient care were clearly stated in a standardized manner.

AORN responded to this dilemma and has identified a Perioperative Patient Focused Model that consists of three primary areas of nursing concern: nursing diagnosis, nursing interventions, and patient outcomes (Fig. 2-2).

| BOX 2-6 | Assessment Parameters That Are Monitored Throughout Perioperative Care by the Circulating Nurse |

- Physiologic
- Medical diagnosis
- Surgical site and procedure
- Results of diagnostic studies
- Laboratory tests
- Review of systems
- Mobility, range of motion
- Prosthetics (internal or external)
- Sensory impairments
- Allergies
- Skin condition
- Nutritional and metabolic status
- Height and weight
- Vital signs
- Elimination pattern (e.g., continence)
- Sleep, rest, exercise patterns
- Medications
- Substance abuse
- Psychosocial
- Cognition (e.g., mental status)
- Cultural and religious beliefs
- Perception of procedure
- Expectations of care
- Knowledge base (e.g., informed consent)
- Readiness to learn
- Ability to understand and retain teaching
- Stress level (e.g., anxiety, fears)
- Coping mechanisms
- Support from family or significant others
- Attitude and motivation (e.g., health management)
- Affective responses (e.g., ability to express feelings)
- Speech characteristics (e.g., language)
- Nonverbal behavior

These areas are reflected in the model as domains that describe the perioperative patient's interaction with the health care system, in particular, surgery. The primary domains concerning perioperative nurses and their patients are patient safety, physiologic responses, behavioral responses: A, concerning the patient and the system and, B, concerning the nurse, ethics, and the patient's rights, and the health care system.[3]

---

[3] PNDS 2002 AORN.

FIG. 2-2   AORN Perioperative Patient Focused Model. The Perioperative Patient Focused Model consists of domains of nursing concern: nursing diagnoses, nursing interventions, and patient outcomes. These domains are in continual interaction with the health system encircling the focus of perioperative nursing practice: the patient.

Three of these domains—behavioral responses, patient safety, and physiologic responses—reflect phenomena of concern to perioperative nurses and are composed of the nursing diagnoses, interventions, and outcomes that surgical patients or their families experience. The fourth domain, the health system, is composed of the structural data elements and focuses on clinical processes and outcomes. Looking at the model, note the heavy line that indicates a differentiation between the health system and the patient. The model as a whole illustrates the dynamic nature of the perioperative patient experience and the nursing presence throughout that process. Working in a collaborative manner with other members of the health care team and the patient, the nurse establishes outcomes, identifies nursing diagnoses, and provides nursing care. The nurse intervenes within the context of the health care system to assist the patient to achieve the highest attainable health (physiologic, behavioral, and safety) outcomes throughout the perioperative experience.

(From AORN: Patient outcomes: standards of perioperative care. In AORN: Standards, recommended practices, and guidelines, Denver, 2001, The Association.)

Perioperative Nursing Data Set

AORN developed the perioperative-specific nursing vocabulary that defines and describes the perioperative patient's experiences from preadmission to discharge from care.[4] The standardized language of data elements identifies specific common components that are distinctly part of perioperative patient care.

A data element is the smallest unit of descriptive information available that retains its meaning. It allows the reader to conceptualize without added descriptors. The *Perioperative Nursing Data Set* (PNDS, 2nd edition) was published by AORN in 2002 and includes 74 perioperative nursing diagnoses, 133 perioperative nursing interventions, and 28 patient outcomes. The PNDS is described in four domains specific to the perioperative nursing process. These are as follows:

- Domain 1: (D1) Safety
- Domain 2: (D2) Physiologic responses
- Domain 3-A: (D3-A) Behavioral responses of patient and family: Knowledge
- Domain 3-B: (D3-B) Behavioral responses of patient and family: Rights and ethics
- Domain 4: (D4) Health system

The PNDS is important for capturing data in a systematic way that can be retrieved, measured, and evaluated by an information system. Box 2-7 lists examples of licensed perioperative software vendors that have incorporated the PNDS into their database for perioperative documentation. The standardized language has a letter and a number that are specific to the nursing activity it describes within the particular domain as described above. For example:

- X for nursing diagnosis
- I for nursing intervention
- O for outcomes

The PNDS was officially recognized by the American Nurses Association's Committee on Nursing Practice Information in 1999. The clinical relevance of the PNDS is specific to perioperative patient care and provides a standardized language to validate the value of the role of the professional perioperative nurse. The PNDS is clinically validated nursing language that is useful for clinical practice, education, and research. According to AORN, the advantages of PNDS usage include but are not limited to the following:

- Providing a framework to standardize documentation
- Providing a universal language for perioperative nursing practice and education
- Assisting in the measurement and evaluation of patient care outcomes
- Providing a foundation for perioperative nursing research and evaluation of patient outcomes
- Informing decisions about the relationship of staffing to patient outcomes
- Providing data about the contributions of nurses to patient outcomes in the perioperative arena
- Data can be gathered and tallied in a mechanized format.

---

[4] PNDS 2002 AORN brochure. For additional information, email pnds@aorn.org.

BOX 2-7   Examples of Perioperative Software Vendors That Have Incorporated the PNDS into Their Surgical Information Systems

Cerner Corporation, www.cerner.com
Deio, www.deiona.com
Epic Systems Corporation, www.epicsystems.com
GE Medical Systems Information Technologies, www.gemedicalsystems.com
McKessonHBOC, www.hboc.com
Mediware, www.mediware.com
PerSé Technologies, www.per-se.com
Picis Inc., www.picis.com
RES-Q Healthcare Systems, www.res-q.com
Surgical Information Systems (SIS), www.orsoftware.com
Unibased Systems Architecture, Inc. (USA), www.unibased.com

Sample documents using the PNDS are online at www.aorn.org/research/documentation.htm (Adobe Acrobat Reader, a free download, is required to read these documents). Consult AORN online at www.aorn.org/research/pnds.htm for additional information about obtaining a copy of the PNDS. Other nursing organizations with recognized forms of standardized language are listed online at www.nursingworld.org/nidsec/classlst.htm.

Preoperative Phase. The preoperative phase of the patient's surgical experience begins when the decision is made to undergo surgical intervention, and it ends when the patient is transferred to the OR bed. During this phase the perioperative nurse performs the assessment, determines the nursing diagnoses, identifies potential outcomes, and develops a plan of care. The nurse assesses the patient to identify any actual or potential physiologic, psychosocial, and spiritual needs, problems, or other health status considerations. In collaboration with the patient and/or significant others, the nurse then determines the nursing diagnoses and identifies the expected outcomes of the perioperative experience. The perioperative nurse plans, prioritizes, and initiates the patient care necessary for the attainment of the desired outcomes.

Intraoperative Phase. The intraoperative phase begins with placement of the patient on the OR bed and continues until the patient is admitted to a postprocedure or postoperative area. Implementation of the plan and evaluation of care continue during this phase. The perioperative nurse either personally carries out the plan of care or supervises others in carrying out the plan with skill, safety, efficiency, and effectiveness. Modification of the plan may be necessary during the procedure.

Postoperative Phase. The postoperative phase begins with admission of the patient to a postprocedure or postanesthesia area, which may be a postanesthesia care unit (PACU) or an intensive care unit (ICU). Patients admitted to the facility on an ambulatory 1-day-stay basis may return to the ambulatory unit. As indicated by his or her condition, the patient will transfer from the immediate post-operative patient care division for progressive stages of self-care on a surgical unit before being discharged from the hospital. The postoperative phase ends when the surgeon discontinues follow-up care. Evaluation, the sixth component of nursing process, is completed during this phase.

STANDARDS OF PERIOPERATIVE NURSING PRACTICE

A standard is an authoritative statement established and published by a profession and by which the performance of practice can be measured. The standards of nursing practice establish parameters and competency levels against which the practice of the profession may be compared.

The ANA Standards of Clinical Nursing Practice reflect the nursing process and state the interventions to be performed. These standards are a description of a competent level of practice common to all nurses and form the foundation of all decision making in the provision of care to all patients. The interpretive statements that accompany each standard provide definitions of terms along with the interventions and guidelines necessary to achieve these standards. Criteria for the achievement of each standard are also stated and remain consistent with current nursing practice.

Nursing practice is based on theory and is constantly evolving with the development of new technology and research. The standards are written in behavioral terms so nurses can measure to what degree each standard has been met.

The *Standards of Perioperative Clinical Practice*, originally published in 1981, were revised in 1992 by AORN. The nursing activities inherent in each standard are incorporated in the nursing process during the three phases of surgical care.

Standard I: Assessment

The perioperative nurse collects patient health data. Data collection is continual and ongoing. It may be gathered in the preoperative holding area, on the patient care unit, in the clinic, or by a telephone call to the patient at home. Information can be obtained from the patient's chart, by consultation with other members of the health care team (e.g., unit nurses, surgeon, anesthesia provider), through interviews with the patient and/or family or significant others, and by observation and physical assessment. Data collection is a progressive and orderly process of gathering meaningful information pertinent to the planned surgical intervention. It includes but is not limited to the following:

- Current medical diagnosis and therapy
- Diagnostic studies and laboratory test results
- Physical status and physiologic responses, including allergies and sensory or physical deficits
- Psychosocial status, including education level
- Spiritual needs, ethnic and cultural background, and lifestyle
- Previous responses to illness, hospitalization, and surgery
- Patient's understanding, perceptions, and expectations of the procedure

Pertinent data collected through physiologic and psychosocial assessment are documented. Box 2-6 lists the perioperative assessment parameters to be considered. The basic elements of a nursing assessment are described in the sections that follow.

- *Subjective data:* Include the patient's perceptions and expectations of the procedure and may be recorded in the form of a direct quote.
- *Objective data:* Include the nurse's observations of the patient and the interpretation of baseline data.

Physiologic Assessment. The perioperative nurse performs a physical assessment of the patient. Techniques include inspection/observation, auscultation, percussion, palpation, and olfaction. The assessment of major body systems establishes the baseline health status of the patient. It provides a basis for planning appropriate patient care and provides a database for postoperative evaluation.

The perioperative nurse should also be familiar with laboratory test norms so that critical deviations can be identified in all phases of perioperative care. Other important parameters for planning perioperative care include knowledge of allergies, skin integrity, sensory or physical limitations, prosthetic devices, nutritional/metabolic status, and chronic illness. The routine use of medications can affect or interact with anesthetic medications and postoperative recovery. A patient who smokes and who will have general anesthesia needs to be taught coughing and deep-breathing exercises. The patient who is dependent on alcohol or other drugs can suffer postoperative physiologic and psychologic manifestations of withdrawal. A chemically dependent person who is recovering from an addiction may refuse preoperative sedation and postoperative narcotics for pain.

Psychosocial Assessment. The perioperative nurse performs a psychosocial assessment. Illness makes a person vulnerable, and individuals vary in their ability to cope with stressful situations. Culture, religion, and socioeconomic factors have an effect on a patient's interpretation of illness and response to the interaction with the perioperative environment. Anticipatory apprehension, although normal to some degree, may diminish critical-thinking and decision-making abilities. Stress may initiate an exaggerated response of normal coping mechanisms for self-protection. Establishing a preoperative psychosocial baseline facilitates prompt recognition of maladaptation to a perioperative event.

Documentation. Pertinent information should be recorded in the patient's chart for use by the perioperative team. Data collection forms the baseline for ongoing care in the perioperative environment. Computer programs can be used to establish a computerized patient database. The nurse enters the data obtained from physiologic and psychosocial assessments through physical examination, interview, and observation. Use of the PNDS allows the nurse to use standardized terminology that in turn permits data collection about patient care. This is the foundation of evidence-based practice. A printed copy of the patient care plan is obtained for the patient's record. The nurse should review the printed copy and date and sign it for the permanent record.

Standard II: Diagnosis

The perioperative nurse analyzes the assessment data in determining the nursing diagnoses. Nursing diagnoses are conclusions based on analysis and interpretation of the human response patterns revealed by the assessment data. These are concise written statements about a patient's actual or potential problems, needs, or health status considerations amenable to nursing intervention.

A medical diagnosis defines problems on the basis of a patient's pathologic condition(s). NANDA International has developed a list of nursing diagnoses (www.nanda.org). This list, known as a *taxonomy*, classifies human response patterns and standardizes the nomenclature for describing them. It includes definitions and defining characteristics for each diagnosis. The PNDS has 74 nursing diagnoses specific to perioperative patients. A NANDA nursing diagnosis has three components:

1. *Defining characteristics.* Human responses to altered body processes and other contributing factors describe the acuity of an actual or potential health status deviation. The nurse identifies the characteristics for which nursing interventions can legally be used to maintain current health status or to reduce, eliminate, or prevent its alteration. These interventions are based on human response patterns:
   a. *Problem.* Any health care condition that requires diagnostic, therapeutic, or educational action. Problems can be active (requiring immediate action) or inactive (having been solved). Problem-oriented medical records are built on this premise. An ongoing list is maintained in a database and is used throughout the managed care environment.
   b. *Need.* A lack of something essential for the maintenance of health that may be met through the plan of care. Needs may be actual (in existence at the time of assessment) or potential (anticipated to become actual during the length of stay [e.g., deficient knowledge]). Many of these needs are met through the intervention component of the plan of care.
   c. *Health status considerations.* A personal habit, lifestyle, or influencing agent that if uncontrolled can lead to a decline in physiologic or psychologic well-being (e.g., occupational hazards, exposure to chemical agent or smoke, substance abuse).
2. *Signs (objective) and symptoms (subjective).* Data obtained during the assessment identify the defining characteristics of the patient's actual or potential health problems. The patient's functional health patterns are assessed (Box 2-8). Gordon has suggested that there are 11 functional health patterns that should be assessed. The domains include physiologic, psychologic, and sociologic aspects of observed behavior.
3. *Etiology/related factors.* The causes of problems may be related to physiologic, psychosocial, spiritual, environmental, or other factors contributing to the patient's health status. These causes define relevant risk factors to be considered in planning patient care.

BOX 2-8	Gordon's Functional Health Patterns of Observable Behaviors

- Health perception/health management
- Nutritional/metabolic
- Elimination
- Activity/exercise
- Sleep/rest
- Cognitive/perceptual
- Self-perception/self-concept
- Role/relationship
- Sexuality/reproductive
- Coping/stress tolerance
- Value/belief

Modified from Gordon M: *Manual of nursing diagnosis, 1997-1998*, St Louis, 1997, Mosby.

Documentation

Use of the PNDS terminology helps perioperative nurses establish standard communication when documenting nursing diagnoses. A common language facilitates continuity of patient care. The documentation of the nursing diagnosis is designated as the letter "X" with the corresponding nomenclature (terminology) and number from the PNDS list. Select random examples include:

- X1 Activity intolerance
- X35 Noncompliance
- X47 Disturbed sensory perception
- X63 Urinary retention
- X74 Chronic pain

Standard III: Outcome Identification

The perioperative nurse identifies expected outcomes unique to the patient. Each outcome can be affected by nursing care (also referred to as "nurse sensitive"[5]) and is specific to the individual, the family, and the community. The *Nursing Outcomes Classification* (NOC) taxonomy is built on five levels: domains, classes, outcomes, indicators, and measures.[6] The standardized terminology gives quantifiable language to the statement of outcomes and has numeric codes that can be used in nursing informatics systems. Each outcome is evidence based and was researched using qualitative and quantitative methods in 10 midwestern centers in the United States.

The nurse measures the patient's responses and uses a five-point Likert scale to tally the score. A numeric baseline range is documented and the numeric target outcome is identified. This method permits the use of the data in an information system and in empirical research. The 330 validated outcomes are closely linked and integral with 176 NANDA nursing diagnoses and can be used across the care continuum in all branches of nursing, including the perioperative care areas.

Expected perioperative outcomes are the desired and obtainable patient objectives after a surgical intervention. These outcomes occur within specified time frames and

---

[5] Terminology used in the *Nursing Outcomes Classification* (NOC) 3/e, 2004.
[6] NOC 3/e, 2004.

have specific criteria for evaluation as demonstrated in the 28 identified PNDS patient outcomes. They direct patient care to modify or maintain the patient's baseline functional physical capabilities and behavioral patterns. The patient's rights and preferences are the cornerstones for expected outcomes. They should be realistic, attainable, and consistent with medical regimen and patient outcome standards for perioperative nursing.

Documentation. The results of care should be documented in standardized language. Examples of PNDS outcomes are prefixed with the letter "O" and the nomenclature and number from the PNDS list. Select examples of PNDS documentation include the following:

- O30 The patient's neurologic status is consistent with or improved from baseline levels established preoperatively.
- O14 The patient's respiratory status is consistent with or improved from baseline levels established preoperatively.
- O13 The patient's fluid and electrolyte balance is consistent with or improved from baseline levels established preoperatively.

Standard IV: Planning

The perioperative nurse develops a plan of care that prescribes interventions to attain the expected outcomes. Based on the assessment data, nursing diagnoses, and identified expected outcomes, the perioperative nurse devises a plan of care. The plan should include a provision for all phases of patient care in the perioperative environment. Key concepts to consider in planning perioperative patient care include but are not limited to the following:

- Participation of the patient and/or significant others in formulation of the plan
- Medical diagnosis and effect of surgical intervention on the patient's physiology
- Psychosocial and spiritual needs of the patient and his or her significant others
- Environmental safety, comfort, and well-being
- Provision of supplies, equipment, and technical expertise
- Current best nursing practices

The plan of care should reflect current standards, facilitate the prescribed medical care, and work toward the attainment of desired outcomes. The scope of the plan is determined by assessment data. Any unusual data are considered for individualized patient care. Alternative options or interventions, not just routine procedures, are a necessary part of the plan. Regardless of format, the plan of care specifies the following:

- Patient care necessary to achieve expected outcomes
- Interventional priorities and sequence of care
- Availability of resources needed to implement the plan
- How, where, and by whom the care will be delivered
- Specific modifications for individualized aspects of care
- Methods for evaluating the effectiveness of the plan

Documentation. Standardized patient care plans may be developed for patient populations undergoing similar

procedures, with space provided to note any unique or unusual patient assessment data. These care plans can be organized on preprinted forms to include the usual nursing diagnoses and expected outcomes and may include, but are not limited to, the following:

- Patient will demonstrate understanding of the procedure.
- Patient will be injury-free.
- Patient will remain normothermic.
- Patient will be infection-free.
- Patient's skin will remain intact.
- Patient will remain physiologically stable.
- Patient will demonstrate psychologic comfort.
- Patient will return to normal activities of daily living.

The format of the record may include checklists and spaces for specific patient data. This record accompanies the patient throughout the perioperative environment and serves as a guide for the perioperative team. Use of a standardized language, such as the PNDS, is beneficial for precise communication. Dissemination of the plan to all personnel involved in providing care to the patient is essential for continuity of care. The plan is modified as indicated by ongoing evaluation data.

Standard V: Implementation

The perioperative nurse implements the direct and indirect interventions identified in the plan of care. A taxonomy of nursing interventions known as the *Nursing Intervention Classification* (NIC) is the basis for the standardization of terminology.[7] The NIC is linked to NANDA International and describes 514 evidence-based interventions that are grouped into 30 classes. The seven domains of the NIC are Physiological: basic, Physiological: complex, Behavioral, Safety, Family, Health, and Community. The standardized terminology of the NIC gives quantifiable language to the nursing interventions and has numeric codes that can be used in nursing informatics systems.

The plan of care is implemented throughout the perioperative care period by the entire team. Scientific principles provide the basis for patient care interventions that are consistent with the plan for continuity of patient care in the perioperative environment. They are performed with safety, skill, efficiency, and effectiveness.

The patient's welfare and individual needs are paramount in every facet of activity and must not be compromised. Seemingly routine details are significant. For example, taking a defective instrument out of circulation may prevent injury to the patient or team member. All preoperative preparations within the perioperative environment provide for the physical safety of the patient and team in an aseptic, controlled manner. The circulating nurse also provides emotional support to the patient before transfer to the OR bed and during induction of anesthesia.

This text focuses primarily on direct and indirect interventions that perioperative and perianesthesia nurses and surgical technologists perform to ensure achievement of expected patient outcomes. Implementation of safe and efficient patient care requires the application of technical

---

[7] *Nursing Intervention Classification* (NIC) 4/e, 2004.

and professional knowledge, sound clinical judgment, and a surgical conscience on the part of all team members. Nurses have a responsibility to monitor constantly the physical and psychologic responses of patients to care. They control environmental factors that affect outcomes of surgical intervention.

Documentation. All patient care interventions (both routine and individualized), observations of patient responses, and the resultant outcomes delineated in the patient care plan are documented as evidence of the care given. This written documentation becomes part of the patient's permanent record. The circulating nurse accountable for the patient's care is responsible for the documentation. The person completing the documentation should sign with a complete name and title. Interventions contributing to patient comfort and safety are identified. Activities other than direct patient care that are not recorded elsewhere and may affect patient outcomes are included (e.g., how tissue specimens were handled).

Writing nurses' notes or progress notes on the patient's chart or completing an accurate intraoperative observation checklist provides a profile of what has happened to the patient. The notes should contain what happened and why. Intraoperative records not only have legal value but also are valuable to the postoperative care team. The PNDS provides standardized language to describe 133 nursing interventions that are designated by the letter "I" and the nomenclature and number from the list. Select PNDS intervention examples include:

- I4 Administers care to wound site
- I5 Administers electrolyte therapy as prescribed
- I3 Administers care to invasive device sites
- I37 Evaluates for signs and symptoms of electrical injury
- I84 Manages specimen handling and disposition

Standard VI: Evaluation

The perioperative nurse evaluates the patient's progress toward the attainment of outcomes with an actual outcome statement as described in the PNDS. Evaluation is a continual process of reassessing the patient and his or her responses to implementation of the plan of care. Perioperative caregivers accommodate a variety of intense situations within a short time. The perioperative team is always on the alert for, and prepared to respond to, the unexpected. The flexibility of the team is manifest in the quick modifications to the plan of care during emergency situations.

All components of the nursing process are performed concurrently during the intraoperative phase as changes occur in the patient's internal and external environments. The patient is observed during the surgical procedure and evaluated for responses to all interventions.

Determination of patient responses and the realization of expected outcomes can be verified by direct observation of and/or conversation with the patient. The perioperative nurse observes the patient's responses to interventions during the immediate preoperative and intraoperative phases of care in the perioperative environment. The perioperative nurse may accompany the patient to the PACU or postprocedure area to determine the level of attainment of expected outcomes. Ideally, the perioperative nurse visits the patient postoperatively on the patient care division or phones an ambulatory patient at home within 24 to 48 hours after discharge.

Documentation

The patient's permanent record should reflect the ongoing evaluation of perioperative nursing care and its outcomes. This includes a comparison of expected outcomes to the degree of outcome attainment as determined by the patient's responses to nursing interventions. Documentation using a standardized language provides legal evidence of results of the plan of care and revisions to the plan after reassessment of the patient. Examples of PNDS in action include, but are not limited to, the following PNDS numbered nursing diagnoses and outcome statements:

- X30 Deficient knowledge—O31: Patient demonstrates knowledge of the expected responses to the procedure
- X50 Impaired skin integrity—O11: Patient has wound/tissue perfusion consistent with or improved from baseline levels established preoperatively
- X26 Hypothermia—O12: Patient is at or returning to normothermia at the conclusion of the immediate postoperative period
- X29 Risk for injury—O2: Patient is free from injury from extraneous objects

CLINICAL COMPETENCY OF THE PERIOPERATIVE NURSE

Using the framework of the nursing process, AORN published Competency Statements in Perioperative Nursing in 1986 and revised them in 1992. These broadly written statements of expected competencies can be used to develop position descriptions, to develop performance appraisals, and to organize orientation and staff development activities. They may serve as guidelines for the skills a nurse should reasonably expect to achieve to function as a perioperative nurse in the perioperative environment. These statements incorporate the many principles, procedures, and practices elaborated throughout this text for competent care of the surgical patient.

- Assess the physiologic health status of the patient.
- Assess the psychosocial health status of the patient and family.
- Formulate nursing diagnoses based on health status data.
- Establish the patient's expected outcomes based on nursing diagnoses.
- Develop a plan of care that identifies patient care interventions to achieve expected outcomes.
- Implement patient care interventions according to the plan of care.
- Evaluate the attainment of expected outcomes and effectiveness of patient care.
- Participate in patient and family teaching.
- Create and maintain a sterile field.
- Provide equipment and supplies based on patient needs.
- Perform sponge, sharps, and instrument counts.
- Administer drugs and solutions as prescribed.
- Physiologically monitor the patient during the surgical procedure and throughout the perioperative experience.

- Monitor and control the environment.
- Respect the patient's rights.
- Demonstrate accountability.

SCOPE OF PERIOPERATIVE NURSING PRACTICE

Perioperative nurses care for patients throughout the continuum of the perioperative intervention. The patient's needs are unique during this phase of care and require specific activities particular to the realm of perioperative nursing. The professional nurses render direct care or oversee the implementation of the plan of care through specialized activities that include but are not limited to the following:

- Educate staff and peers
- Emotionally support and reassure the patient and his or her family
- Serve as patient advocate
- Control environment
- Provide resources
- Maintain asepsis
- Monitor physiologic and psychologic status
- Manage aggregate patient needs
- Supervise ancillary personnel
- Validate and explore current and prospective practices
- Integrate and coordinate care across all disciplines
- Collaborate and consult

These activities are incorporated into the scope of perioperative practice by managers, educators, practitioners, and researchers. These practices take place in hospitals, clinics, educational facilities, physicians' offices, provider organizations, and industry.

SURGICAL TECHNOLOGY

The activities of registered professional nurses are supplemented and complemented by the services of allied technical health care personnel. The term *allied health care personnel* refers to individuals who have been trained in a health care–related science and have responsibility for the delivery of health care–related services but who are not graduates of schools of medicine, osteopathy, dentistry, podiatry, or nursing. Approximately two thirds of the health care workforce are designated as allied health professionals. Educational preparation may be offered in colleges, vocational-technical schools, hospital-based programs, or military service schools. Technologists, technicians, and therapists in more than 130 occupational categories work collaboratively with and under the direction of physicians and registered nurses.

The surgical technologist, or ST, is a member of the direct patient care team and works intraoperatively with the surgeon and anesthesia provider under the direction of the circulating nurse. This team is referred to as the perioperative team. The surgical technologist prepares instruments, supplies, and equipment to maintain a safe and therapeutic surgical environment for the patient. The surgical technologist performs specific techniques and functions designed to exclude pathogenic microorganisms from the surgical wound.

A surgical technologist completes a 9-month certificate to 2-year college degree intensive educational program. This program includes courses in anatomy and physi-ology, pathology, and microbiology as prerequisites to courses that involve the theory and application of technology during surgical procedures and for care of the perioperative environment. Other courses in the curriculum, such as pharmacology, help explain the underlying basis for the technical tasks to be performed. Courses in psychology, ethics, and interpersonal communication are fundamental to an appreciation of the humanities. According to the accrediting body's standards, a 9-month program should average 400 to 500 hours of didactic instruction and offer more than 500 hours of supervised clinical practice.

AST, NBSTSA (formerly LCC-ST), and ARC-ST have taken the position that an associate degree is the preferred educational level for entry into practice and that certification should be a condition of employment. This is documented in the 2005 combined meeting minutes and in the AST Recommended Standards of Practice.[8]

STANDARDS OF PRACTICE FOR SURGICAL TECHNOLOGISTS

AST has developed standards of practice that provide guidelines for the development of performance descriptions and performance evaluations. The quality of the surgical technologist's practice may be judged by these standards. The six authoritative statements that comprise the standards describe the scope of patient care and serve as a guide on which to base clinical practice.[9]

Standard I

Teamwork is essential for perioperative patient care and is contingent on interpersonal skills. Communication is critical to the positive attainment of expected outcomes of care. All team members should work together for the common good of the patient. For the benefit of the patient and the delivery of quality care, interpersonal skills are demonstrated in all interactions with the health care team, the patient and family, superiors, and peers. Personal integrity and surgical conscience are integrated into every aspect of professional behavior.

Standard II

Preoperative planning and preparation for surgical intervention are individualized to meet the needs of each patient and his or her surgeon. The surgical technologist collaborates with the professional registered nurse in the collection of data for use in the preparation of equipment and supplies needed for the surgical procedure. The implementation of patient care identified in the plan of care is performed under the supervision of a professional registered nurse.

Standard III

The preparation of the perioperative environment and all supplies and equipment will ensure environmental safety for patients and personnel. The application of the plan of

---

[8] AST, ARC-ST, and LCC-ST are located at 6 West Dry Creek Circle, Littleton, CO 80120.

[9] www.ast.org.

care includes wearing appropriate attire, anticipating the needs of the patient and perioperative team, maintaining a safe work area, observing aseptic technique, and following all policies and procedures of the institution.

Standard IV

Application of basic and current knowledge is necessary for a proficient performance of assigned functions. The surgical technologist should maintain a current knowledge base of procedures, equipment and supplies, emergency protocol for various situations, and changes in scientific technology pertinent to his or her performance description objectives. It is the responsibility of the surgical technologist to augment his or her knowledge base by studying recent literature, attending inservice and continuing education programs, and pursuing new learning experiences.

Standard V

Each patient's rights to privacy, dignity, safety, and comfort are respected and protected. Each member of the OR team has a moral and ethical duty to uphold strict observance of the patient's rights. The surgical technologist, like all members of the health care team, is expected to perform as a patient advocate in all situations. This is an accountability issue and should be part of each aspect of patient care.

Standard VI

Every patient is entitled to the same application of aseptic technique within the physical facilities. Implementation of the individualized plan of care for every patient includes the application of aseptic or sterile technique at all times by all members of the health care team. All patients are given the same dedication in their care.

CLINICAL COMPETENCY OF THE SURGICAL TECHNOLOGIST

The performance description developed by AST identifies performance objectives against which the surgical technologist may measure his or her level of competency. According to AST, the surgical technologist can aspire to three levels based on education, experience, and time in service. Each level requires the surgical technologist to be certified and employed in the operating room. The employment setting can be a clinic, private practice, or a facility, such as a hospital. These levels could be used to structure seniority, promotions, and salaries. The certified surgical technologist (CST) levels are as follows:

Level I CST

- Entry level as certified or a qualified applicant
- Graduated from an accredited program with a minimum of 125 cases in the scrub role
- Performs as first scrub in all assigned specialty cases

Level I Competencies

- Demonstrates knowledge and practice of basic patient care concepts
- Demonstrates the application of the principles of asepsis in a knowledgeable manner that provides for optimal patient care in the OR
- Demonstrates basic surgical case preparation skills

- Demonstrates the ability to perform in the role of first scrub on all basic surgical cases
- Demonstrates responsible behavior as a health care professional

Level II CST (Advanced)

- Current CST
- A minimum of 5 consecutive years of full-time employment
- Documentation of a minimum of 24 continuing education credits in a specialty area

Level II Competencies

- Demonstrates all competencies required for CST level I
- Demonstrates advanced knowledge and practice of patient care techniques
- Demonstrates advanced knowledge of aseptic and surgical technique
- Demonstrates advanced knowledge and practice of circulating skills and tasks
- Demonstrates knowledge related to OR emergency situations
- Demonstrates advanced organizational skills
- Demonstrates advanced knowledge in one or two specialty areas
- Demonstrates a professional attitude

Level III CST (Specialist)

- Current CST
- Associates degree in surgical technology or related field, or a minimum of 8 consecutive years of full-time employment
- Documentation of a minimum of 24 continuing education credits in a specialty or management area
- Documentation of a minimum of 20 continuing education credits in AST category 3 advanced practice

Level III Competencies

- Demonstrates all competencies required for CST level II
- Demonstrates superior knowledge and practice of patient care techniques
- Demonstrates superior knowledge of aseptic and surgical technique
- Demonstrates advanced knowledge and practice of circulating skills and tasks
- Demonstrates advanced knowledge related to OR emergency situations
- Demonstrates advanced organizational skills
- Demonstrates superior knowledge in one or two specialty areas
- Demonstrates a professional attitude
- Demonstrates leadership abilities

CONTINUAL PERFORMANCE EVALUATION AND IMPROVEMENT

Nursing research and experience have shown that quality cannot be ensured, only monitored and performance improved. JCAHO has adopted a definition of quality as "continual improvement" in patient care services to increase the probability of expected patient outcomes and to reduce the probability of undesired outcomes. Outcomes can be defined, monitored, and measured. Patient satisfaction is one outcome measurement that is critical in evaluating quality of performance. Satisfied patients are more cooperative and receptive to therapy and teaching.

Each patient deserves the best possible care. Without the structure provided by the nursing process, health care services would be fragmented and accountability for the quality of services rendered would be made difficult. Society demands the accountability of those who provide patient care services. Patients are protected by laws, standards, and recommended practices. Performance of care should comply with established policies and procedures of the hospital or ambulatory care facility and with professional standards of practice.

Performance Improvement Studies

Most studies are designed to measure compliance with current policies and procedures and to identify the need for change in practice guidelines or the need for education of staff. Both strengths and weaknesses in performance are identified. Ultimately the purpose is to correct deficiencies and deviations from expected standards. Important aspects that have an effect on the quality of patient care are identified, and a measurable indicator is established for each aspect. Data sources and methods of data collection should be appropriate for each indicator. Sample size and the frequency of data collection should be sufficient to identify trends or patterns in the delivery of care. A sample size of 5% of the monitored patient population selected for study or 25 patients or events, whichever is greater, is usually adequate to obtain reliable data.

Data are collected either concurrently or retrospectively and are organized for evaluation. A concurrent study begins with a current manifestation and links this effect to occurrences at the same time (i.e., is related to care in progress). This type of study focuses on a systematic series of actions that brings about an outcome. Through concurrent observation, the implementation component of the nursing process can be monitored during perioperative patient care to determine whether interventions are consistent with established standards for care and recommended practices. The interventions performed should protect the welfare and safety of the patient and should meet his or her identified physiologic and psychologic needs. The environment, including equipment or supplies used in the room, can also be evaluated at this time.

A retrospective study focuses on the end result of patient care or on a measurable change in the actual state of the patient's health as a result of care received. This evaluation of outcomes usually occurs through review of patient records. The study begins with a current manifestation and links this effect to some occurrence in the past (i.e., care previously given). Complications attributable to care in the perioperative environment may be identified (e.g., nerve palsy from poor positioning, infiltration of an IV infusion, postoperative wound infection). The source of these complications may be difficult to identify unless every detail of actual care given and any unusual occurrences are recorded in the patient's record. Accurate and complete documentation is therefore essential for meaningful retrospective studies.

Any method that systematically monitors and evaluates the quality of patient care can enable perioperative nurses and surgical technologists to take corrective action for improvement of performance. Quality improvement studies also assist in the coordination of plans for patient care with surgeons, improve communications with other departments, identify needs for revision of policies and procedures, and reassess equipment, personnel, and other aspects of patient care.

Benchmarking

Benchmarking is a term that is used to continually monitor progress of a competitor to discover methods for performance improvement and how to implement them. According to JCAHO, when processes within the same facility are measured against each other, this is referred to as *"internal benchmarking."* Measuring performance against an outside competitor is referred to as *"competitive benchmarking."* If another industry's activities are used as the comparison, the reference is then made to *"functional benchmarking."*

When practices are benchmarked, the current level of attainment is clearly identifiable and higher performance attributes can be viewed as the next step to work for.

Peer Review

Peer review differs from other quality improvement programs in that it looks at the strengths and weaknesses of an individual practitioner's performance rather than appraises the quality of care rendered by a group of professionals to a group of patients. An associate with the same role expectations and performance description examines and evaluates the clinical practice of a peer. The individual is evaluated by written standards of performance, and the review should offer constructive criticism of the performance observed. Through this framework, caregivers gain feedback for personal improvement or confirmation of personal achievement related to their effectiveness of professional, technical, and interpersonal skills in providing patient care.

Bibliography

Allen G: Maximizing nurses' advocacy role to improve patient outcomes, *AORN J* 71(5):1038-1050, 2000.

AORN (Association of periOperative Registered Nurses): *AORN standards, recommended practices, and guidelines,* Denver, 2005, The Association.

AORN (Association of periOperative Registered Nurses): *Perioperative nursing data set: the perioperative nursing vocabulary,* Denver, 2002, The Association.

Berger AM, Berger CR: Data mining as a tool for research and knowledge development in nursing, *Computers Inform Nurs* 22(3):123-131, 2004.

Beyea SC: Data fields for intraoperative records using the perioperative nursing data set, *AORN J* 73(5):952, 954, 2000.

Beyea SC: Perioperative data elements: interventions and outcomes, *AORN J* 71(2):344-352, 2000.

Beyea SC: Structural data elements: standardized terms and definitions, *AORN J* 71(3):541-549, 2000.

Collette CL: Understanding patients' needs is the foundation of perioperative nursing, *AORN J* 71(3):629-630, 2000.

Cunningham JH: Managing physician preferences collaboratively, *SSM* 6(11):16-21, 2000.

Dochterman JM, Bulechek GM: *Nursing interventions classification (NIC),* ed 4, St. Louis, 2004, Mosby.

Dock LL, Stewart IM: *A short history of nursing,* ed 2, New York, 1929, GP Putnam's Sons.

Ferguson L: External validity, generalizability, knowledge utilization, *J Nurs Scholar* 36(1):16-22, 2004.

Hewitt-Taylor J: Evidence-based practice, *Nurs Standard* 17(14-15): 47-55, 2002.

Keenan G et al: Toward collecting a standardized nursing data set across the continuum: case of adult care nurse practitioner setting, *Outcomes Manage* 7(3):113-120, 2003.

Kleinbeck SV, Dopp A: The perioperative nursing data set, *AORN J* 82(1):51-57, 2005.

Kleinbeck SV: Revising the perioperative nursing data set, *AORN J* 75(3):602-610, 2002.

Kleinbeck SV: Development of the perioperative nursing data set, *AORN J* 70(1):15-28, 1999.

Kleinpell R, Gawlinski A: Assessing outcomes in advanced practice nursing practice: The use of quality indicators and evidence-based practice, *AACN Clin Issues* 16(1):43-57, 2005.

Lipp A: The systematic review as evidence-based tool for the operating room, *AORN J* 81(6):1279-1287, 2005.

Lunny M et al: Feasibility of studying the effects of using NANDA, NIC, and NOC on nurses' power and children's outcomes, *Computers Inform Nurs* 22(6):316-325, 2004.

Mathews DE: Developing a perioperative peer performance appraisal system, *AORN J* 72(6):1039-1044, 1046, 2000.

Moorhead S, et al: *Nursing outcomes classification (NOC),* ed 3, St. Louis, 2004, Mosby.

Nightingale F: *Notes on nursing: what it is, and what it is not,* New York, 1969, Dover Publications.

Pape T: Boyer's model of scholarly nursing applied to professional development, *AORN J* 71(5):995-1003, 2000.

Rothrock JC, Smith DA: Selecting the perioperative patient focused model, *AORN J* 71(5):1030-1037, 2000.

Seifert PC: Registration, licensure, and accountability, *AORN J* 70(2):182-186, 1999.

Seifert PC: The perioperative nursing data set: power is knowledge, *AORN J* 70(1):8-11, 1999.

Legal, Regulatory, and Ethical Issues

KEY TERMS AND DEFINITIONS

Advance directive   Document that indicates wishes concerning health care and usually designates someone to make decisions if the patient is unable to do so for self.
Autonomy   Self-government or independence.
Causation   Action directly or indirectly causing an injury.
Consent   Voluntary, autonomous permission to proceed with an agreed-on course of action.
Damages   Compensation awarded to make restitution for an injury or a wrong.
Defendant   Person named as the object of a lawsuit.
Deposition   Statement given under oath that is a documentation of fact used in a court of law.
Iatrogenic   Injury or illness caused by professional intervention of a health care provider.
Indicator   A measured increment of performance, process, system, or outcome.
Liability   Legally responsible for personal actions.
Malpractice   Substandard delivery of care that results in harm.
Near miss   An event or situation that just by chance did not cause patient injury. A very close call.
Negligence   Careless performance of duty.

Plaintiff   Person who initiates a lawsuit.
Proximate cause   An act of commission or omission by one or more persons that caused a consequence to another.
Root cause analysis   The baseline reason for the occurrence of failure in a process or system.
Sentinel event   An unexpected occurrence that involves physiologic or psychologic injury or death. This occurrence signals the need for appropriate reporting and documentation, immediate investigation, and response.
Systems approach   A global attitude of improvement and safety that encompasses involvement of individuals and the organization at all levels. Adverse events are attributed not only to individuals but also failure of the interaction of the individual and the organization.
Tort   Wrong committed by one person against another; civil action.

Competent patient care is the best way to avoid a malpractice or negligence claim. Unfortunately, even under the best of circumstances, a patient may be injured and recover monetary damages as compensation. Understanding how a liability action starts and how it proceeds is important in the effort to avoid the many pitfalls that can lead to being named and successfully sued in a lawsuit.

Caregivers should consider that liability is not the only rationale behind competent care. The main focus should be the desired outcome for the patient and the exemplary delivery of care. Performing in a particular manner merely to avoid being sued is not an ethical practice.

HISTORICAL BACKGROUND

Hammurabi (1728-1686 BC) established one of the oldest known set of laws that included penalties for physicians/surgeons who did not cure, a schedule of acceptable fees, and organization for the delivery of medical treatment. Punishments were specified for infractions of the code. These 282 rules are inscribed on a large diorite stone in ancient Babylonian currently in a permanent display in the Louvre Museum *(Musée du Louvre)* in Paris, France. The Code of Hammurabi was considered unbreakable, even by a king or noblemen. The law could not be changed or altered because it was etched on the face of the stone. This is the origin of the phrase *carved or written in stone* as meaning unchangeable. More information about the Code of Hammurabi can be found at www.constitution.org/ime/hammurabi.htm.

The first recorded medical malpractice suit was tried in England in 1374. The first one in the United States occurred in 1794. Throughout the nineteenth century and the early part of the twentieth century, litigation against physicians was quite uncommon and rarely affected nurses. Malpractice suits began to increase markedly in the 1970s as an increasing number of people sought health care services and became aware of their humanitarian and consumer rights.

LEGAL ISSUES

Inherent in professional practice is the duty to safeguard the safety and rights of patients. The patient is at risk for harm during any surgical procedure. These factors also may present health care providers with ethical dilemmas that are complicated by legal issues. Respect for the patient's autonomy and the patient's right to make informed decisions about his or her own health care should be considered and balanced by the professional obligations of beneficence (the duty to benefit) and nonmaleficence (not to harm).

Any caregiver can be named in a lawsuit. Being named in a suit does not mean that you have been successfully sued and does not always means you are liable for anything. Attorneys frequently name everyone involved with the patient in the suit as part of the fact-finding process for building the lawsuit. When in doubt about personal competency for a new or unfamiliar procedure or piece of equipment, seek guidance from the clinical educator or immediate supervisor.

Regardless of who is in charge of the team, each team member is responsible for his or her own actions. When performing duties within the scope of practice and according to facility policy and procedure, the risk of being successfully sued in a malpractice or negligence suit is very limited. Honest mistakes can result in patient injury. If a suit is brought to court, a jury can evaluate a reasonable set of circumstances, facts, and testimony to render a verdict in favor of the caregiver. The plaintiff does not always win. If the verdict is found in favor of the plaintiff, the damages awarded may be for compensatory award. Many states have set limits on the amount of money that can be awarded by the court.

The quality of health care in this country is assessed through the outcome of services rendered. If the outcome is unacceptable, patients tend to take grievances to court. The severity of an injury usually determines whether a claim of merit will arise, but other contributing factors include a breakdown of rapport between the patient and the health care team members and unrealistic expectations about the outcome of care.

Causes for litigation lie in patients' and their families' belief that physicians and/or health care organizations have not provided appropriate diagnosis, treatment, or results. Although the physician is professionally responsible for patient care, other patient care personnel act as part of the health care team, carrying responsibility for their own actions. Medical and surgical sales personnel and suppliers of equipment and drugs also are indirectly involved in treatment and may be held responsible for product liability.

LIABILITY

To be liable is to be legally bound and responsible for personal actions that adversely affect another person. Every patient care provider should always carry out duties in accordance with standards and practice guidelines established by federal statutes, state practice acts, professional organizations, and regulatory agencies, as well as those that are common practice throughout the community. Deviation from these standards and practices that cause injury to a patient can result in liability for negligence or malpractice. For this type of civil suit to be successful for the plaintiff, he or she has to prove that negligent care or malpractice caused the injury.

Negligence is the failure to use the care or skills that any caregiver in the same or a similar situation would be expected to use. These acts of omission or commission that cause damage to a patient may give rise to tort action, which is a civil lawsuit.

Malpractice is any professional misconduct, unreasonable lack of skill or judgment, or illegal or immoral conduct. Malpractice and negligence claims usually are settled in a civil court; however, depending on the severity of the injury and the extent of the misconduct, they may be taken to criminal court. From the legal point of view of damages or fault, professional negligence usually is often synonymous with malpractice in a tort action. Factors contributing to a successful lawsuit on behalf of the plaintiff have been called the "four D's of malpractice":

1. Duty to deliver a standard of care directly proportional to the degree of specialty training received
2. Deviation from that duty by omission or commission
3. Direct causation of a personal injury or damage because of deviation of duty
4. Damages to a patient or personal property caused by the deviation from the standard of care

Statutory laws (laws by legislation) and common laws (laws based on court decisions) differ from state to state. Courts differ at times in their interpretation of laws. Any caregiver who is in some manner thought to be responsible for injury to a patient may be sued. The nurse manager or clinical educator responsible for assigning duties to this individual may be included in the suit if delegation and supervision are in question.

Caregivers, such as nurses, technologists, and technicians are considered employees of the health care facility. The facility is almost always named in the suit as being ultimately responsible for hiring, monitoring credentials, evaluating, and disciplining their employees.

The court may rule that a learner or an experienced practitioner is liable for his or her own acts. A learner may be held responsible for independent actions in proportion to the amount and type of instruction received and judged by the standard of other learners in training. An instructor can be named with the learner as partially liable.

Medical care and professional liability have become institutional problems. The primary cause of professional liability claims is iatrogenic medical injury—an injury or other adverse outcome sustained by a patient as a result of treatment. Many incidents in the perioperative environment have been causes for a lawsuit.

Liability Prevention for the Facility and the Team

Complex technologies, acuity of hospitalized patients' conditions, short-stay procedures, diverse roles of providers, inadequacy of staffing numbers, and other factors present challenges in managing risks of liability. Many surgeons restrict their practices to avoid patients who have complex diseases or who are at high risk of uncertain outcomes. Others practice defensive medicine, ordering tests principally to protect themselves against possible litigation. As lawyers have become increasingly sophisticated in representing injured patients, all health care providers need to take measures to protect themselves from litigation. A preventive strategy includes the following:

- Become active within the professional organizations associated with setting the standards for practice. Most organizations provide up-to-date education and resources for improvement of practice. Have a voice in shaping the future of the profession.
- Remain current with continuing education. Become certified, and maintain the credential.
- Establish positive rapport with patients. Patients are less likely to sue if they perceive that they were treated with respect, dignity, and sincere concern. Patients have the right to accurate information and good communication.
- Comply with the legal statutes of the state and standards of accrediting agencies, professional associations, and the health care facility policies.
- Adhere to the policies and procedures of the facility. Seek a position on the policy and procedure committee in order to have a say in the formation and revision of facility practices.
- Document assessments, interventions, and evaluations of patient care outcomes. Leave a paper trail that is easy to follow for the reconstruction of the event in question.
- Prevent injuries by adhering to policies and procedures. Shortcuts can be hazardous to the patient and team members.
- If an injury occurs, control further injury or damage by reporting problems and taking corrective action immediately.
- Maintain good communications with other team members.
- In addition to these strategies, the facility as the employer and the caregiver as the employee should take steps to avoid liability. The facility protects the patient, its personnel, and itself by maintaining safe and well-defined policies and procedures based on national standards and recommended practices.

Liability Insurance

Formerly it was thought that patients did not sue nurses and other patient care providers because they had no large assets. Unfortunately, this is no longer true. Increased autonomy increases the risk for liability. Perioperative nurses make independent nursing decisions based on their assessments, and they can carry out and/or delegate certain patient care interventions without a physician's order. No matter how careful the caregiver is, mistakes can happen. An unintentional wrong may cause injury to a patient. Most facilities carry insurance that covers incidents that result in harm to a patient when policies and procedures are followed; however, they may not cover the employee who fails to follow the established protocol. In some instances the facility's insurance may not adequately cover all of the expenses associated with a lawsuit, such as a private attorney and lost wages during suspensions and trial.

The caregiver who accidentally caused the injury may be named in the suit as an individual or as a codefendant. Carrying personal liability insurance protects against a possible discrepancy with the facility's insurance coverage and provides the employee with the opportunity for representation by a personal attorney. A professional liability policy can be individualized to meet the practice of the insured. The policy costs are tax deductible and the protection of personal assets and wages may well be worth the price of the coverage. Professional associations recommend individual professional liability insurance and frequently offer discounts to members.

Borrowed Servant Rule

In the past the surgeon was considered the captain of the ship in the perioperative environment and was liable for the negligent acts of servants. In the early 1940s and 1950s, courts held that this doctrine, based on the master–borrowed servant relationship, was applicable by the mere presence of the surgeon. Once having entered the operating room (OR), the surgeon was considered to have complete control over other team members. But courts now recognize that the surgeon does not have complete control over the acts of the perioperative patient care team at all times.

Each member of the team has significant performance autonomy. The surgeon usually is not held responsible when a perioperative caregiver fails to carry out a routine procedure as expected. Courts have decided that certain procedures do not need to be personally performed by the surgeon, such as counts or mixing medications on the sterile field. According to the borrowed servant rule, the surgeon is liable for acts of team members only when he or she has the right to control and supervise the way in which a perioperative caregiver performs the specific task. A good example of this is counting sponges, sharps, and instruments. The facility, not the surgeon, establishes the mechanism by which the employee team accounts for items used during a procedure. The surgeon does share some liability if he or she prohibits or prevents the team from accomplishing this task. If this is the case, the circulating nurse should clearly document the surgeon's refusal to permit counting in the medical record and report to the immediate supervisor.

Independent Contractor

The employer may be held responsible for employees under the master-servant rule. However, the current trend is to hold an individual responsible for his or her own acts under the principle of the independent contractor. For example, a private scrub person, biomedical technologist, or first assistant may contract with several surgeons to provide services on a fee-for-service basis. These individuals are not directly employed by the facility but are usually credentialed and given permission to work with the surgeon by the medical staff department. Some questions may arise concerning the level of responsibility of the facility for credentialing someone who is accused of substandard practice. The facility will be named in the suit initially but may be dropped at a later date.

In 2006, the Joint Commission on Accreditation of Healthcare Organizations (JCAHO) determined that the facility that permits independent contractors such as private first assistants, interns, residents, or other privately engaged personnel is responsible for specific standards associated with accountability. These standards are as follows:

- The contractor must be appropriately credentialed for the role.
- The contractor must be competent.
- The contractor must be providing care under the direct supervision of a licensed practitioner.
- The contractor may perform duties only within the scope of his or her intended role.
- The contractor must adhere to the policies and procedures of the facility.
- The contractor must be oriented to the facility's emergency evacuation procedures.
- The contractor must be current in immunizations and health screenings.
- The contractor must display appropriate identification at all times.
- The contractor must comply with all background checks, possibly including fingerprinting.

Doctrine of the Reasonable Man

A patient has the right to expect that all patient care personnel will use knowledge, skill, and judgment in performing duties that meet standards exercised by other reasonably prudent professionals involved in similar circumstances.

Whenever a mishap occurs in patient care, the cause of the event is compared to local and national standards of care. Experts are consulted by attorneys and the mishap is studied. The results should show whether the same event performed by someone else of the same or similar education and role would have had the same result under the same or similar circumstances. This is how the courts determine the reasonableness of a caregiver's actions. An example of this might be how drugs are administered. The average nurse in average circumstances would check and recheck to be sure the right patient gets the right drug. A careless nurse might omit checking the patient's ID and administer the wrong drug. This would be considered unreasonable and would be a source of liability.

Doctrine of *Res Ipsa Loquitur*

Translated from Latin, *res ipsa loquitur* means "the thing speaks for itself." Under this doctrine, the courts allow the patient's injury to stand as inference of negligence. The defendant has to prove that he or she did not act negligently. Before this doctrine can be applied, three conditions must exist:

1. The type of injury would not ordinarily occur without a negligent act.
2. The injury was caused by the conduct or instrumentality within the exclusive control of the person or persons being sued.
3. The injured person could not have contributed to negligence or voluntarily assumed risk.

This doctrine applies to injuries sustained by the patient while in the perioperative environment, such as a retained foreign object (e.g., sponge, towel, needle, other instrument), a fall, or a burn. The defendant must prove that a breach did not occur and that he or she was not negligent.

Doctrine of *Respondeat Superior*

An employer may be liable for an employee's negligent conduct under the *respondeat superior* master-servant employment relationship. This implies that the master will answer for the acts of a servant. If a patient is injured as a result of an employee's negligent act within the scope of that employment, the employer is responsible to the injured patient. The patient may name both the facility and the employee in a civil suit, but the employee may be dropped from the suit if he or she was following facility policy and procedure and acting within the appropriate scope of practice.

A facility may have outdated practiced or unsafe procedures. One example might be the labeling of drugs on the sterile field. Instead of requiring the name and dose of the drug to be written on the sterile container and the syringe, the facility may permit the scrub person to place the cap of the syringe into the medicine cup containing local anesthetic to signify the contents of both the syringe and cup. This is a practice that was in effect in some facilities up to a few years ago. It is clearly an unsafe practice to require a scrub person to manage drugs on the sterile field in this manner. The facility would be found liable for this action if it required the employee to perform at this unacceptable level.

Doctrine of Corporate Negligence

Under the corporate negligence doctrine, the facility may be liable not for the negligence of employees but for its own negligence in failing to ensure that an acceptable level of care is provided. The facility has a duty to provide services and is responsible for the following:

- Screening and verifying qualifications of all staff members, including medical staff, according to standards established by JCAHO
- Monitoring and reviewing performance and competency of staff members through established personnel appraisal and peer review procedures
- Maintaining a competent staff of physicians and other caregivers
- Revoking practice privileges of a physician and other caregivers when the administrators know or should have known that the individual is incompetent or impaired

Corporate negligence includes the use of personnel who are inadequately trained for the position they hold. The Alabama Supreme Court found HealthTrust, Inc. liable for permitting a surgical technologist to perform in the role of first assistant at Crestwood Hospital in 1997 (*Cantrell v. Crestwood*). The surgical technologist was holding a retractor during an open hip procedure on a pediatric patient and permanently injured the sciatic nerve. Her leg is disfigured, and she has undergone multiple failed surgeries to restore function. The surgeon was not found liable for the acts of the facility's employee.

Extension Doctrine

If the surgeon goes beyond the limits to which the patient consented, liability for assault and battery may be charged. This doctrine implies that the patient's explicit consent for a surgical procedure serves as an implicit consent for any or all procedures deemed necessary to cope with unpredictable situations that jeopardize the patient's health. By medical necessity and sound judgment, the surgeon may perform a different or an additional surgical procedure when unexpected conditions are encountered during the course of an authorized surgical procedure (e.g., finding an abscess near the target organ or finding a tumor extended into adjacent structures).

The surgeon may extend the surgical procedure to correct or remove any abnormal or pathologic condition under the extension doctrine. The court will determine whether the patient consented to a specific procedure or generally to surgical treatment of a health problem. The surgeon may not routinely remove the appendix or gallbladder during a tubal ligation.

Assault and Battery

In legal terms, assault is an unlawful threat to harm another physically. Battery is the carrying out of bodily harm, as by touching without authorization or consent. Lack of informed consent to perform a procedure is an important aspect of an assault-and-battery charge. Informed consent must be obtained by the physician and consent to perform a procedure must be given voluntarily with full understanding of implications by the patient. The purposes of a written, signed, and witnessed consent are to protect the surgeon, anesthesia provider, perioperative team members, and facility from claims of unauthorized procedures and to protect the patient from unsanctioned procedures. Consents are discussed in detail later in this chapter.

Invasion of Privacy

The patient's right to privacy exists by statutory or common law. The patient's chart, medical record, videotapes, radiographs, and photographs are considered confidential information for use by physicians and other health care personnel directly concerned with that patient's care. The patient should give written consent for videotaping or photographing his or her surgical procedure for medical education or research. The patient has the right to refuse photographic consent.

The patient has the right to expect that all communications and records pertaining to individualized care will be treated as confidential and will not be misused. This includes the right to privacy during interview, examination, and treatment. The surgery schedule bearing the names of the patients should not be posted in a location where the public or other patients can read it.

Some patients, such as celebrities, may request to be admitted with an alias. Care is taken when identifying these patients so that they will not be confused with other patients and receive the wrong procedure. Community hospitals may be admitting people from the surrounding neighborhood. The caregiver may be in a position to learn private information about a neighbor. Maintaining the confidentiality of patient information is imperative. Every health care worker has a moral obligation to hold in confidence any personal or family affairs learned from patients. Many facilities have implemented confidentiality agreements with all health care personnel on the premises. Schools for surgical personnel require students to sign confidentiality agreements before going to a clinical site. Figure 3-1 shows an example of a college confidentiality agreement.

Health Insurance Portability and Accountability Act (HIPAA)

HIPAA was published in the *Federal Register* in 2003 and the final rule took effect in April 2005. This act provides for confidentiality of health data involved in research or transmitted and stored by electronic or any other means. The release or disclosure of this protected health information (referred to as PHI) requires patient authorization. HIPAA covers far more than PHI—it covers fingerprints, voice prints, and photographic images.[1]

The Agency for Healthcare Research and Quality (AHRQ) reports on their morbidity and mortality website the case of an unmarried woman who was undergoing a D&C (dilation and curettage) because of a miscarriage.[2] The facility had closed-circuit TV cameras for security that were displayed at the control desk. A passerby saw the face of the woman and knew her procedure. The passerby gossiped to the neighborhood and caused great embarrassment for the patient.

Patients who are part of a criminal investigation have rights. Victims and perpetrators both have the right of privacy and should not have information provided to the news media or other people without express permission from the law enforcement agency in charge of the investi-

---

[1] www.hhs.gov/ocr/hipaa; Adobe Acrobat Reader is required to read the document of the HIPAA rule on the web.
[2] www.webmm.ahrq.gov; March 2004.

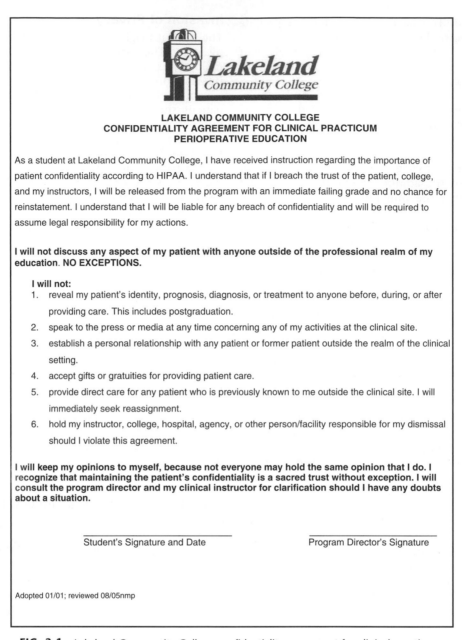

LAKELAND COMMUNITY COLLEGE
CONFIDENTIALITY AGREEMENT FOR CLINICAL PRACTICUM
PERIOPERATIVE EDUCATION

As a student at Lakeland Community College, I have received instruction regarding the importance of patient confidentiality according to HIPAA. I understand that if I breach the trust of the patient, college, and my instructors, I will be released from the program with an immediate failing grade and no chance for reinstatement. I understand that I will be liable for any breach of confidentiality and will be required to assume legal responsibility for my actions.

I will not discuss any aspect of my patient with anyone outside of the professional realm of my education. NO EXCEPTIONS.

I will not:
1. reveal my patient's identity, prognosis, diagnosis, or treatment to anyone before, during, or after providing care. This includes postgraduation.
2. speak to the press or media at any time concerning any of my activities at the clinical site.
3. establish a personal relationship with any patient or former patient outside the realm of the clinical setting.
4. accept gifts or gratuities for providing patient care.
5. provide direct care for any patient who is previously known to me outside the clinical site. I will immediately seek reassignment.
6. hold my instructor, college, hospital, agency, or other person/facility responsible for my dismissal should I violate this agreement.

I will keep my opinions to myself, because not everyone may hold the same opinion that I do. I recognize that maintaining the patient's confidentiality is a sacred trust without exception. I will consult the program director and my clinical instructor for clarification should I have any doubts about a situation.

_____   _____
Student's Signature and Date   Program Director's Signature

Adopted 01/01; reviewed 08/05nmp

FIG. 3-1   Lakeland Community College confidentiality agreement for clinical practicum.

gation. Information related to a crime discovered by health care personnel during the course of care should be reported to the immediate supervisor in charge, who should in turn arrange for the information to be relayed to the authorities as soon as possible. Personnel are advised not to promise secrecy to a suspected perpetrator who is a patient.

Abandonment

Abandonment consists of leaving the patient for any reason when the patient's condition is contingent on the presence of the caregiver. If the caregiver leaves the room knowing there is a potential need for care during his or her absence, even under the order of a physician, the caregiver is liable for his or her own actions.

In *Czubinsky v. Doctor's Hospital,* the surgeon ordered the circulating nurse to leave the room to help him start another procedure. During the circulating nurse's absence, the patient had a cardiac arrest. The only team members on hand were the anesthesia provider and the surgical technologist. At the trial, the circulating nurse admitted to knowing that it was wrong to leave the patient because of his condition but left because of the surgeon's insistence. The expert witness testified that the circulating nurse should not have been ordered away from the patient to work in another room. The court decided that if adequate help for resuscitation had been available in the OR during the patient's crisis, he would not have suffered permanent brain damage, which occurred because of this breach of duty. According to the court, the circulating nurse had a duty to remain with the patient.

If an event necessitates leaving a patient, it is important to transfer care to another caregiver of equal status and function. In uncontrollable circumstances, the perioperative manager should be consulted immediately. The patient must not be left unattended. No one, not even a physician, may release a caregiver from a responsibility to a patient. A child or disoriented patient left alone or unguarded in a holding area, for example, may sustain injury by an electric shock from a nearby outlet or by some other hazard within reach. The circulating nurse may be considered negligent by reason of abandonment for failure to monitor a patient in the OR. The circulating nurse should be in attendance during induction of and emergence from anesthesia and throughout the surgical procedure to assist as needed.

JCAHO AND SENTINEL EVENTS

Professional accountability requires professionals to monitor performance as it applies to patient outcomes. The identification of an undesired outcome may be the result of direct or indirect actions of the caregiver. Such an outcome is referred to as a *sentinel event*—an unexpected event that involves a risk for or the occurrence of death or serious physical or psychologic injury. Serious injury specifically includes loss of limb or function. The term *sentinel* was selected to represent the concept because the seriousness of the event requires immediate investigation and response. These events have a significant effect on patient outcomes; they should be evaluated for root cause, and a plan to prevent its occurrence should be prepared.

Root Cause Analysis

JCAHO developed and approved a list of sentinel events that should be voluntarily reported and other events that need not be reported (Box 3-1). The JCAHO publication *Conducting a Root Cause Analysis in Response to a Sentinel Event* has been made available to institutions as a guideline for investigating the causes of sentinel events. The objective is to improve the system that has permitted the error to occur. Guidelines include a fill-in-the-blank questionnaire to help track the cause of the event.

The guidelines suggested by JCAHO allow each facility flexibility in determining the root causes for events specific to the environment. Using flowcharts, the facility can identify one or more of these root causes. Each facility is encouraged but not required to report sentinel events to JCAHO. Other sources, such as the patient, a family member, or the media, may generate the report. If JCAHO becomes aware of an event, the facility is required to perform a root cause analysis and action plan or other approved protocol within 45 days of the event. A JCAHO glossary of sentinel event terminology can be viewed at www.jcaho.org.

Institutional Reporting of Sentinel Events

The Patient Safety and Quality Improvement Act of 2005[3] encourages a culture of safety in the health care system. JCAHO indicates that mistakes are minimized by designing systems that anticipate and possibly prevent human error.[4]

| BOX 3-1 | Reportable and Nonreportable Sentinel Events Identified by JCAHO |

REPORTABLE
- Any event that results in the loss of life or limb (e.g., death, paralysis, coma) associated with a medication error
- Suicide of a patient within 72 hours of being in an around-the-clock care setting
- Elopement or unauthorized departure of an individual from around-the-clock care facility that results in suicide or homicide or permanent loss of function
- Abduction from a care facility
- Rape
- Discharge of an infant to the wrong family
- Hemolytic transfusion reaction involving the administration of blood or blood products having major blood group incompatibilities
- Surgery on the wrong patient or the wrong body part
- Intrapartum maternal death related to the birth process
- A perinatal death unrelated to a congenital condition in an infant weighing more than 2500 g
- Assault, homicide, or other crime resulting in patient death or a major permanent loss of function
- A fall that results in death or major permanent loss of function as a direct result of the injuries sustained
- Hemolytic transfusion reaction involving incompatible blood
- A retained foreign object from surgery

NONREPORTABLE
- Any near miss
- Full return of limb or bodily function by discharge or within 2 weeks of the initial loss of function
- Medication errors that do not result in death or the permanent loss of function
- Any sentinel event that has not affected the recipient of care
- A death or injury that follows discharge against medical advice (AMA)
- Unsuccessful suicide attempts
- Unintentionally retained foreign body without permanent loss of function
- Minor hemolysis with no clinical sequelae

Data from www.aarc.org/sentinel_examples.html; also www.jacho.org/sentinel/se_pp.htm, June 2005.
JCAHO, Joint Commission on Accreditation of Healthcare Organizations.

Each procedure has inherent safety risks that are not always apparent. These tend to surface when systems thinking are not foremost in the procedure development process.

The 2005 act references data that show the incidence of reporting to be more accurate when done on a voluntary basis rather than when reporting is mandatory. Health care facilities have requested protection for reporting information because in order to rework the system the faults need to be known. This is the main way of studying problems and finding solutions for improved performance. Many states have adopted the National Quality Forum's (NQF) list of 27 adverse events as the foundation for mandatory adverse event reporting.[5] In 2004, Minnesota was the first

---

[3] This act is an amendment to Title IX of the Public Health Service Act.
[4] Institute of Medicine, *To err is human: building a safer health system,* Washington, D.C., 1999, National Academy Press, pp. 86-87.

[5] The full list of 27 adverse events as defined by the NQF is located on the Minnesota Department of Health's website: www.health.state.mn.us/patientsafety/adverse27events.html (Adobe Acrobat Reader is needed to view the two-page file).

state to adopt the 27 events as mandatory to report. In the first year of mandatory reporting, surgical adverse events were the highest reported of all the categories by early 2005. Other states have followed by implementing reporting systems and including additional categories of adverse events that are mandatory to report. For additional information about the NQF adverse event list, go to www.qualityforum.org.

CONSENT
General Consent

Most facilities require the patient or his or her legal guardian to sign a general consent form on admission. This form authorizes the attending physician and the staff to render standard day-to-day treatment or to perform generalized treatments and care as the physician deems advisable. This general consent is relied on only for activities performed in routine care. Physicians and nurses should be knowledgeable about the statements on the form used in their facility.

Each facility should have policies and procedures in place about the authorization of general consent. Many facilities require the patient or appropriate guardian to sign the general consent document in the admission department before admission to the facility. This is facilitated by the admissions clerk, who is a nonmedical person. This in no way equals informed consent. Box 3-2 compares content examples of general consent to treat versus informed consent.

Informed Consent

State statutes differ in their interpretation of the doctrine of informed consent, but all recognize the *physician's duty* to inform the patient of the risks, benefits, and alternatives of a procedure and to obtain consent before treatment. Failure to do so may be considered a breach of duty. **Informed consent is a process—not necessarily a mere document.** Explanations of the procedure, risks, benefits, and alternative therapy are made verbally to the patient's level of understanding. Some facilities have a special form that is used during this process. A surgeon or anesthesia provider may be held liable for negligence if the patient can prove failure to disclose significant information that would have influenced a reasonable person's decision to

consent. Informed consent is a protective act for the patient and the treating physician and should be documented appropriately. The circulating nurse, as patient advocate, should ensure that this process has taken place before permitting the patient to be transferred to the OR.

The anesthesia provider also has a responsibility to inform the patient of any potential for unfavorable reactions to any medication or anesthetic agent that may be given during the surgical procedure. The risks of anesthesia should be explained without causing the patient undue stress. If the surgeon intends or wants to perform a procedure not specified on the consent form, the circulating nurse has the responsibility to inform the surgeon and/or proper administrative authority of the discrepancy.

The surgeon may be approved by the U.S. Food and Drug Administration (FDA) as a clinical investigator or by the Department of Health and Human Services (HHS) as a researcher for the controlled experimental use of new drugs, chemical agents, or medical devices. Written consent based on an informed decision to participate in the research should be obtained from the patient before any investigational item, drug, or procedure begins. The surgeon completes an investigator's report that is returned to the supplier of the drug or device and eventually filed with the FDA (www.fda.gov). The patient is free to refuse or withdraw at any time from research carried out under the auspices of the HHS. All parties involved with the procedure are bound by HIPAA and the confidentiality implied therein. More information can be found on the HHS website (www.hhs.gov).

Informed Consent for a Surgical Procedure. According to the American College of Surgeons, a reasonable approach to informed consent should involve answering the following patient questions:
- What do you plan to do to me?
- Why do you want to do this procedure?
- Are there any alternatives to this plan?
- What things should I worry about?
- What are the greatest risks or the worst thing that could happen?

The patient has the right to waive an explanation of the nature and consequences of the procedure and has the right to refuse treatment. When a patient signs a consent

BOX 3-2 **Examples and Comparison of Consent Form Contents**	
General Consent to Treat	**Informed Consent**
Admission to facility	Name of patient and legal guardian as appropriate
Time and date admitted	Name of facility
Admissions clerk name	Specific procedures and who explained them
Mode of admission	Specific practitioners and their roles
Treating/admitting physician	Risks of the procedure
Person responsible for payment	Alternatives to treatment
Contact persons for emergency	Signatures: patient or legal guardian, surgeon(s), and the witness to the signatures
Basic care assumptions (such as dietary orders, activity orders, testing, examination by physician)	Date and time the process took place

Source: Centers for Medicare and Medicaid Services, 2005, pp. 161-162 (www.cms.hhs.gov; use A-0238 in search field).

agreement, consent is given only for the specific procedure indicated on the form. Additional procedures should be listed and signed separately—not added after the patient has already signed the form. Contents documented about informed consent should include but are not limited to the following:

- Who will be performing the procedure, including any residents, interns, or first assistants
- Each surgical procedure to be performed, including secondary procedures
- Any procedure for which an anesthetic is administered
- Procedures involving entrance into the body via an incision, puncture, or natural orifice
- Any hazardous therapy, such as irradiation or chemotherapy

Responsibility for Informed Consent Before a Surgical Procedure. The surgeon is responsible for obtaining informed consent from the patient, which should include the risks, benefits, and possible complications of all proposed surgical procedures. The explanation should include a discussion of the removal and disposition of body parts, the potential for disfigurement or disability, and what the patient may expect in the postoperative period. The preoperative discussion also should include advice to the patient regarding medications, diet, bathing, smoking, and other factors that might affect outcome and rehabilitation.

The surgeon has the ultimate responsibility for obtaining informed consent for the procedure and should document this activity in the appropriate place in the patient's permanent record. The patient or appropriate guardian may be required to sign this record in the presence of a witness. All consent documents become a permanent part of the patient's medical record and accompany him or her throughout the perioperative environment. When checking the patient's identity and chart on arrival in the OR, it is the duty of the circulating nurse and the anesthesia provider to be certain of the following:

- The appropriate consents are on the chart and are properly completed and signed.
- The information on the form is correct.

Validation of Consent

The patient should personally sign the consent unless he or she is a minor, is unconscious or mentally incompetent, or is in a life-threatening situation. The next of kin, legal guardian, or other authorized person should sign for these patients. The physician gives explanations to the parent of a minor or to the legal guardian of an incompetent adult.

A consent document should contain the patient's name in full, the surgeon's name, the specific procedure to be performed, the signatures of the patient and authorized witness(es), and the date of signatures. A signed consent is regarded as legally valid for as long as the patient still consents to the same procedure. Institutional policy may vary.

The patient giving consent for treatment should be of legal age and mentally competent. Except in life-threatening emergency situations, the patient should sign the consent form before premedication is given and before

going to the OR or other procedural/interventional area. This may be done in the surgeon's office, in the facility's admitting office, or on the patient care unit; it is done freely without coercion. If the patient is:

- A minor, a parent or legal guardian should sign.
- An emancipated minor, married, or independently earning a living, he or she may sign.
- A minor who is the parent of an infant or child who is having a procedure, he or she may sign for his or her own child.
- Illiterate, he or she may sign with an *X*, after which the witness writes, "Patient's mark." Because illiteracy implies the inability to read and write, the patient should indicate an understanding of a verbal explanation.
- Unconscious, a responsible relative or guardian should sign.
- Mentally incompetent, the legal guardian—who may be either an individual or an agency—should sign. A court order may be necessary to legalize the procedure in the absence of the legal guardian.
- An adult or an emancipated minor who is mentally incapacitated by alcohol or other chemical substance, the spouse or responsible relative of legal age may sign when the urgency of the procedure does not allow time for the patient to regain mental competence.

Consent documents vary. Policies related to informed consent are developed by the medical staff and governing body in accordance with legal requirements. All personnel involved in the care of patients should be familiar with these policies.

Witnessing a Consent. A witness verifies that the consent was signed without coercion after the surgeon explained the details of the procedure. The patient's or guardian's signature should be witnessed by one or more authorized people. The witnesses may be physicians, nurses, other facility employees, or family members as established by policy. Checking or witnessing the signature of the patient or other authorized person does not constitute validation of informed consent. The witness assumes no liability or responsibility for the patient's understanding. The witness signing a consent document attests only to the following:

- Identification of the patient or legal substitute
- Voluntary signature, without coercion
- Mental state of signatory (i.e., not coerced, sedated, or confused) at the time of signing

Consent in Emergency Situations. In a life-threatening emergency, the consent to treat and stabilize is not essential. Although every effort should be made to obtain consent, the patient's physical condition takes precedence over a procedure permit. The patient's state of consciousness may prevent him or her from verbalizing or signing a permit for treatment. Permission for a lifesaving procedure, especially for a minor, may be accepted from a legal guardian or responsible relative by telephone, fax, or other written communication. If it is obtained by telephone, two nurses should monitor the call and sign the form, which is signed later by the parent or legal guardian on arrival at the facility.

Right to Refuse a Surgical Procedure. The patient should reconcile the advantages and disadvantages of the surgical intervention. Each patient is entitled to receive sufficient information from which to intelligently base a decision regarding whether to proceed. The patient has the right to decide what will or will not be done to him or her. Only after making this decision is the patient asked to sign a written consent for a surgical procedure.

The patient has a right to withdraw written consent at any time before the surgical procedure. The surgeon is notified, and the patient is not taken into the OR. The circulating nurse documents the situation on the patient's record. The surgeon should explain the medical consequences of refusing the surgical procedure. If therapeutically valid, alternative methods of medical management should be offered. The surgical procedure is postponed until the patient makes a final decision. The procedure may be canceled.

The surgeon should document the patient's refusal for surgical treatment. For legal protection, the surgeon should also obtain from the patient, parent, or legal guardian a written refusal for the procedure or other treatment. The physician is required to inform the patient of the consequences of refusing diagnostic tests or therapeutic procedures.

Second Opinion. If the surgeon or patient has doubts about the necessity of a procedure, another opinion should be sought from a qualified specialist in the appropriate field of surgery. Consultation is a common and desirable part of good surgical practice. A second opinion may be required by third-party payers (i.e., insurance carriers) or managed care services. This is particularly indicated if the surgical procedure involves extended disability. Policy may require special consultation or consent for procedures resulting in reproductive sterilization or a pregnancy termination.

Advance Directives

The Patient Self-Determination Act enacted by the U.S. Congress in December 1991 ensures the patient the opportunity to participate in decision making before a procedure.[6] The law requires that patients be informed of their rights to make their own decisions regarding their health care. This act applies to hospitals, nursing homes, home health care agencies, hospice programs, and health maintenance organizations (HMOs). It does not apply to freestanding ambulatory or office settings.

Each patient has the right to determine the care received and to participate in the selection of delivery methods. The caregiver has the obligation to respect the patient's wishes regarding that care. This right extends to the issue of refusing treatment. Policies should be in place to provide for making patients aware of their right of self-determination.

The term *advance directive* encompasses durable power of attorney and living wills. The living will concept allows the patient to refuse treatment or nonessential measures to prolong life in a hopeless situation. A *durable power of attorney* document designates the person authorized to make decisions in the event that the patient is incapacitated. It allows the wishes of patients concerning their care needs to be met if they become impaired and cannot make decisions. The durable power of attorney does not apply to pediatric patients or to incompetent adults who are already under legal guardianship. These patients already have decision makers available to decide treatment options.

On admission to the facility, the patient is asked whether he or she has an advance directive or durable power of attorney. A federal regulation requires that the institution be aware of whether such a document exists and enact it in the event of impaired cognitive function of the patient. The perioperative team should be made aware of its existence. A copy, not the original, is placed in the patient's record. Advance directives may also indicate the patient's preferences concerning organ donation. The family is still asked for consent before any procurement occurs after the patient's death. In some states, the family has the right to refuse procurement regardless of the patient's last wishes.

DOCUMENTATION OF PERIOPERATIVE PATIENT CARE

Verbal communication between patients and health care providers does not constitute legal documentation of care. Entries in the record by nurses and physicians provide a history of the patient's clinical course and responses to treatment. The record serves to identify what was done. The broad assumption is that if something is not documented, it was not done. The record serves as a means of communication among providers for continuity of care. Policies and procedures should be in place for documentation. Each patient care facility is responsible for the following:

- Establishing, evaluating, and enforcing policies and procedures for patient care documentation
- Interpreting and outlining standards for care documentation in accordance with accreditation guidelines
- Protecting the privacy of patients by preventing unauthorized access and use of documented patient care data and reports
- Creating forms and charting formats for personnel to use in hard copy documentation
- Selecting protocol for computerized archives of patient care records and reports
- Providing a timely mechanism for retrieval of archived patient care records and reports for reference in a timely manner for routine or emergency care

All interactions with patients should be documented in the patient's chart in the appropriate format. Regardless of the format or the media used for the patient's record, all entries should be:

- Documented on the appropriate form (e.g., code sheet, perioperative record, medication sheet, progress note).
- Written legibly in ink without erasures. The charting procedure may be specific (e.g., all entries are to be made in black ink).
- Stated factually. Documentation of objective data and services rendered should be very specific.

[6] Patient Self-Determination Act, Public Law 101-508, *Federal Register* 57, March 6, 1992.

Observations and actions should be stated definitively, objectively, and concisely. Record what is seen, heard, felt, or smelled (i.e., the facts without judgment or opinion). Write quotes of the patient's subjective expression.

- Stated in understandable terminology. Abbreviations may be permissible only for very commonly accepted medical terms (e.g., T&A, D&C, TUR). Most institutions provide a standard list of their accepted medical abbreviations for charting purposes.
- Dated (month, day, year), including the time (AM/PM) the note is written and the time action was performed as appropriate for significant events or changes in the patient's condition. Late entries are documented as per facility policy.
- Signed with the full legal signature, title, and status of the writer, either in permanent ink or electronically.
- Corrected if an error is made. The date, time, and initials of the person making a correction should be noted next to the correction. A single line should be drawn through incorrect information without obliterating it (the mistake should not be scribbled out or erased), and the correct information should then be entered. Correction fluid is not acceptable. If an entire page must be recopied, the original is attached to the new copy and not destroyed.

Additional documentation in the patient's record should include the following:

- Execution of the physician's orders and the patient's responses
- Any teaching of the patient or family, including how he, she, or they indicated understanding
- Any unusual event, such as a fall, spontaneous change in condition, or injury
- All visitors, especially physicians
- Any notification of physicians or supervisors

The perioperative nurse should be alert to signs that a patient does not clearly understand what is going to happen as a result of surgical intervention. This should be documented and brought to the attention of the surgeon. Significant observations should be recorded in the chart. For example, if a patient verbally withdraws consent for a surgical procedure or expresses a fear of death in the OR, the perioperative nurse is responsible for communicating this information to the surgeon and anesthesia provider and for recording the patient's statement.

Benefits of Documentation to the Facility

There are many reasons for accurate documentation other than those for legal application. Some facilities use the data for strategic planning and growth of the organization. Benefits of accurate documentation to the facility include but are not limited to the following:

- Legal permanent record
- Billing and reimbursement
- Performance improvement (PI)
- Measurement of clinical pathways
- Budget and financial planning
- Staffing ratios
- Research protocol
- Utilization review

- Risk management
- Patient acuity and census

Standards and Methods for Documentation of Patient Care

The standards for patient care documentation are established by the American Nurses Association (ANA) and JCAHO. The national standard of care requires that patient care documentation reflect the application of the nursing process (assessment, nursing diagnosis, outcome identification, planning, intervention, and evaluation) during the entire length of stay, according to ANA and JCAHO. The use of the *Perioperative Nursing Data Set* (PNDS) is the method of choice for perioperative patient care documentation. The PNDS provides a standardized universal language for patient care documentation and is used by many surgical computer software manufacturers.

Charting Modalities. Many ways of recording patient care information have been used over the years. Changes in technology have created more methods of recording patient care. The following are examples:

- Narrative charting. Expository writing about significant events using third-person commentary, quotes, and standard abbreviations. Entries are sequential, timed, dated, and signed.
- Block charting. Short commentary on activity that resembles narrative charting covering a longer period of several hours or days. Entries are sequential, timed, dated, and signed. Some facilities use a checklist format.
- Focus charting. Specific documentation directed at a designated aspect of the patient's needs, status, or health considerations.
- Subjective-objective charting (subjective-objective assessment plan [SOAP]). Multidisciplinary approach to documenting care according to cues given by a patient with a specific set of signs and symptoms. This approach uses direct quotes and assessment data.
- Problem-oriented charting (problem-oriented medical record [POMR]). Approach using a problem list as the working element from which care is planned. Working from the list, patient priorities are investigated, diagnosed, treated, minimized, solved, or remain ongoing. As problems are solved, they are stricken from the list.
- Computer-generated charting. Use of standardized care plans formulated in the computer and modified for the individual patient. The computer time and date stamps the plan as it is printed for the hard copy record. This form of charting requires the caregiver's signature.
- Computer software programs, check-off forms, and flow sheets. Commonly used as shortcuts for record keeping. Unfortunately, it is easy to rely on the standardized data on these preprinted records and inadvertently omit potentially important individualized information.

Computerized Documentation. Many facilities have been using computers for patient admitting, billing, scheduling, and human resource information for several decades. Within the past 15 years, patient data have been recorded and stored electronically at the patient care unit level. Only a few personnel are permitted to access this information and must log on using employee identification and passwords to enter the computer system. Passwords are changed at routine intervals. Retrievable data recorded and accumulated in these electronic files include patient care information, laboratory results, surgical reports, admission and discharge summaries, and many highly sensitive details about a patient's financial status.

Nurses charged with the responsibility of accessing and contributing to computerized patient data should be aware that security and confidentiality must be protected. Failing to maintain the secrecy of passwords and failing to log off after use are common problems identified with unauthorized access. Some systems have a built-in log-off feature if the workstation is left idle for a prolonged period. If this happens, the user has to reenter the system by logging back on. Pros and cons of computerized documentation are listed in Box 3-3.

Perioperative Documentation. Specific care given in the perioperative environment should be documented on the patient's chart. Most facilities use a preprinted form with a standardized plan of care. Space is provided to add individualized patient needs and to document additional interventions. Data included in the record come from several patient care areas.

A checklist is commonly included with the chart to assist the circulating nurse to determine if all of the data are included on the chart. Expected outcomes should be

---

BOX 3-3 — Pros and Cons of Computerized Documentation

PROS
Terminology is standardized
Abbreviations are standardized
Useful for accumulation of data from many sources
Data retrieval is easier and efficient
Information is legible and in standard terminology
Uses standardized formats, flow charts, and graphs
Each entry and printing is time and date stamped
Can minimize error if physicians record orders online
Data can be transferred electronically between physician's office and care facility
Record updating is more timely and ongoing
Can save time, space, and resources
Easier to retrieve archived charts from previous admissions
Health care organizations with multiple remote sites can transfer patient data online

CONS
Can be confusing for inexperienced users
Failure to log off can leave system available to unauthorized use
Can be out of service for undetermined periods
Needs periodic maintenance and software updates
Backups of files are needed in case of failure
Paper records must be kept when system is down
Impersonal interaction between patient and caregivers
Preoutlined care plans are less individualized
Hardware and software can be costly to install
Potential for breach of security if files are transferred online

---

specified (e.g., the patient is free from injury). The circulating nurse should document specific activities performed to achieve the expected outcomes. The permanent perioperative record should include but not be limited to the following:

- Preoperative history, physical (H&P) examination, laboratory reports, consent form(s), and other documents in the chart per policy
- Patient identification and verification of the surgical site, intended surgical procedure, allergies, and nothing-by-mouth (NPO) status
- Significant intraoperative times, such as arrival in and departure from the OR, anesthesia start and finish, and incision and closure
- Patient's condition on transfer to and from the OR, as well as the method of transport to and from the OR, and by whom
- Level of consciousness or anxiety manifested by objective observation
- Patient position, and types of restraints and supports used for maintaining the patient's position on the OR bed and for protecting pressure areas, and by whom
- Personal property disposition, such as religious articles, hearing aid, spectacles, and dentures
- Skin condition and antimicrobials used for skin preparation, and by whom
- Intravenous (IV) site, time started, type of needle or cannula, solutions administered IV (including blood products), and by whom
- Medication types and amounts (including local anesthetic agents), irrigating solutions used and amounts, and by whom
- Tourniquet cuff location, pressure, inflation duration, identification of unit, and applied by whom
- Estimated blood loss and urinary output, as appropriate
- Sponge, sharps, and instrument counts as correct or incorrect. If inconclusive, state steps taken in remedy of the situation and notification steps taken
- Surgical procedure performed, location of the incision
- Specific equipment used (e.g., laser), electrosurgical unit (ESU), dispersive and monitoring electrode(s), and prosthetic devices implanted, if applicable, including the manufacturer and lot/serial number
- Specimens and cultures sent to the laboratory
- Site and types of drains, catheters, and packing as applicable
- Wound classification is documented at the end of the procedure when all risks for infection have been identified
- Type of dressing applied
- Any unusual event or complication, and action performed
- All personnel in the room and their roles, including physicians, visitors, sales personnel, students, and others as applicable

Incident Report

When an accident or unusual incident occurs involving a patient, employee, or property in the facility, the factual details should be reported to the nurse manager and documented according to institutional policy. Details should be objective, complete, and accurate. They should be written as statements of facts without interpretation or opinion. For example, it should be stated that the area of the patient's skin under the inactive dispersive electrode of the electrosurgical unit was mottled and red when the electrode was removed, rather than that the patient's skin appeared burned by the dispersive electrode. The details of equipment used, including the serial number or asset tag identification of the generator and the lot number of the electrode, should be included.

The action performed as a result of any adverse event should be described in detail. Any equipment in question should be removed from service and tagged as "out of order" for repair by the biomedical personnel of the facility. Any suspect device should be inspected and reapproved for use according to institutional policy before it is returned to service. All devices and their identifying wrappers suspected of being defective should be secured for inspection by the facility's risk management personnel.

Incident reports are completed per policy and retained by the risk management department. They should be reviewed as part of the overall institution and departmental quality improvement and risk management programs. Incident reports are considered work products and constitute privileged information. They may serve to refresh an individual's memory of events, however, for preparation of defense in a lawsuit. The fact that an incident report was completed should not be documented in the patient's permanent record. Examples of situations that require incident reporting are included in Box 3-4.

LEGAL ASPECTS OF DRUGS AND MEDICAL DEVICES

In 1906 the U.S. government enacted the Pure Food and Drug Act, with the U.S. Department of Agriculture as the enforcing agency, to ensure the introduction of safe and sanitary foods and drugs to the public. The Food, Drug, and Cosmetic Act of 1938 extended regulation to include cosmetics, drugs, and medical devices. The FDA, within the Department of Agriculture, became the enforcing agency with authority to implement a preclearance mechanism requiring drug manufacturers to provide evidence of safety

before a new drug could be sold. Sutures were classified as drugs.

The Kefauver-Harris Drug Amendments of 1962 added strength to the new drug clearance procedures. Drug manufacturers must prove to the FDA the effectiveness, as well as the safety, of drugs before making them commercially available. These amendments established a mechanism for clinical investigation to evaluate the efficacy of drugs. Depending on the nature of a drug, clinical studies often require several years before the FDA approves commercial sale of a product.

The Medical Device Amendments of 1976 gave the FDA regulatory control over medical devices. A medical device is defined as any instrument, apparatus, or other similar or related article, including any component, part, or accessory, promoted for a medical purpose that does not rely on chemical action to achieve its intended purpose. Under this definition, sutures were reclassified as devices. All of the wound closure materials discussed in this chapter are classified as devices.

In 1988 the FDA reclassified many devices, including surgical attire, masks, gloves, and drapes, for control under FDA regulations. Medical devices are classified and receive FDA approval before they are marketed. They are classified into one of three classifications:
- Class I devices are subject to general regulatory controls that ensure that they are as safe and effective as similar devices already being sold.
- Class II devices must establish safety and effectiveness performance standards for a new type of product.
- Class III devices are usually life-sustaining or life-supporting implants or external devices. The manufacturer must file for premarket approval before the device is tested clinically to substantiate effectiveness.

A mandatory device reporting regulation was put into effect in 1984. This regulation requires manufacturers and importers to report to the FDA any death or serious injury to a patient as a result of the malfunction of a medical device. Through the Safe Medical Devices Act of 1990, health care facilities are required to report directly to the FDA and to the manufacturer the probability that a device caused or contributed to a patient's death, serious injury, or serious illness. Additional requirements for tracking certain permanently implantable devices became effective in 1993. Manufacturers are responsible for tracking devices from the manufacturing facility through the chain of distribution (purchasers) to the end users (patients). Health care facilities that implant and explant (remove) these devices must submit reports to manufacturers promptly after devices are received, implanted, and/or explanted. The manufacturer must be able to provide to the FDA the following specific information:
1. Device
   a. Lot, batch, model, and serial numbers or other identification used by the manufacturer
   b. Date(s) of receipt or acquisition within the chain of distribution
   c. Name(s) of person(s) or supplier from whom the device was received
2. Patient
   a. Date of implantation

BOX 3-4	**Unusual Situations That Require an Incident Report**

- Falls or unexpectedly finding a patient, visitor, or other personnel lying on the floor
- Injury to patient, visitor, or other personnel
- Needlesticks
- Any fire or smoke event
- Possible theft or loss of an item
- Malfunctioning equipment
- Intruder or unauthorized personnel
- Medication error
- Medication reaction
- Lost sponge or instrument during a procedure (incorrect and unresolved count)
- Object retained within patient

b. Name, address, and telephone number of the recipient patient

c. Social Security number, if the patient's permission is obtained to release his or her Social Security number to the manufacturer

3. Physician(s) who prescribed, implanted, and/or explanted the device

4. End-of-life information about the device, as applicable

a. Date of explantation

b. Date of patient's death

c. Date the device was returned to the distributor or manufacturer

d. Date the device was permanently retired from use or disposed of

Also in 1993 the FDA began the voluntary MedWatch program to encourage physicians, nurses, pharmacists, and other health care professionals to report adverse events and defects or problems with regulated drugs and devices. The purpose of MedWatch is to provide a nationwide standardized system for reporting to the FDA any medical device or drug suspected of causing a patient's death, life-threatening injury or illness, disability, prolonged hospitalization, congenital anomaly, and/or experience that required intervention to prevent permanent health impairment.

FIG. 3-2 MedWatch reporting form. *(Courtesy U.S. Food and Drug Administration, Rockville, Md.)*

The FDA provides a MedWatch reporting form (Fig. 3-2). Examples of reportable problems include latex sensitivity, malfunction of drug infusion pumps, and failure of an alarm during malfunction of a ventilator. The MedWatch reporting forms are available for download online at http://origin.www.fda.gov/medwatch/getforms.htm.

Surgeons who implant or use medical devices, as well as nurses, surgical technologists, and others who handle them, must be adequately instructed in the proper care and handling of all devices to ensure patient safety. Most adverse events occur when devices are misused, are defective, or malfunction. However, an adverse patient reaction can occur when the device functions properly and is used

appropriately. The FDA is responsible for investigating a report of an adverse event or product problem and for taking corrective action.

ETHICAL ISSUES

Professions have codes of conduct and documents that include value statements derived from moral concepts. The Code of Ethics of the Association of Surgical Technologists (AST) (Box 3-5) provides guidance for surgical technologists. Nurses may refer to the International Code of Nursing Ethics and to a code established by their own professional association, such as the ANA Code for Nurses (Box 3-6) or the Code of Ethics for Nursing of the Canadian Nurses

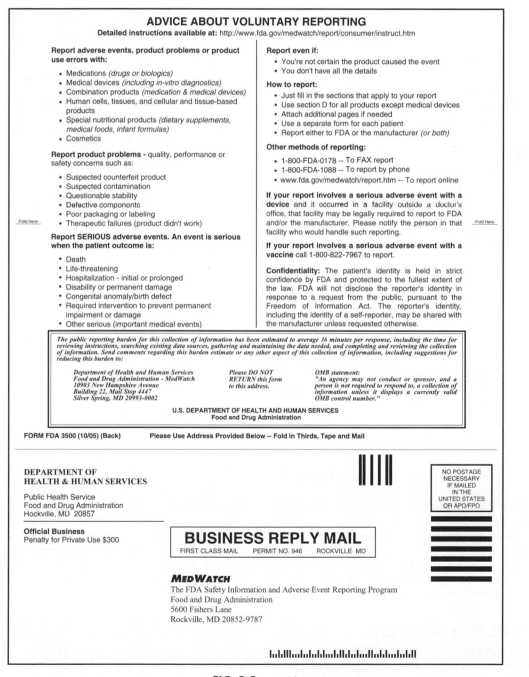

FIG. 3-2—cont'd

BOX 3-5	Code of Ethics: Association of Surgical Technologists

1. To maintain the highest standards of professional conduct and patient care
2. To hold in confidence, with respect to patient's beliefs, all personal matters
3. To respect and protect the patient's legal and moral right to quality patient care
4. To not knowingly cause injury or any injustice to those entrusted to our care
5. To work with fellow technologists and other professional health groups to promote harmony and unity for better patient care
6. To always follow the principles of asepsis
7. To maintain a high degree of efficiency through continuing education
8. To maintain and practice surgical technology willingly, with pride and dignity
9. To report any unethical conduct or practice to the proper authority
10. To adhere to the Code of Ethics at all times in relationship to all members of the health care team

Association of Surgical Technologists, 6 Dry Creek Circle, Littleton, CO 80120.

BOX 3-6	Code for Nurses: American Nurses Association (ANA)

1. The nurse provides services with respect for human dignity and the uniqueness of the patient, unrestricted by considerations of social or economic status, personal attributes, or the nature of health problems.
2. The nurse safeguards the client's right to privacy by judiciously protecting information of a confidential nature.
3. The nurse acts to safeguard the patient and the public when health care and safety are affected by incompetent, unethical, or illegal practice by any person.
4. The nurse assumes responsibility and accountability for individual nursing judgments and actions.
5. The nurse maintains competence in nursing.
6. The nurse exercises informed judgment and uses individual competency and qualifications as criteria in seeking consultation, accepting responsibilities, and delegating nursing activities.
7. The nurse participates in activities that contribute to the ongoing development of the profession's body of knowledge.
8. The nurse participates in the profession's efforts to implement and improve standards of nursing.
9. The nurse participates in the profession's efforts to establish and maintain conditions of employment conducive to high-quality patient care.
10. The nurse participates in the profession's effort to protect the public from misinformation and misrepresentation and to maintain the integrity of nursing.
11. The nurse collaborates with members of the health professions and other citizens in promoting community and national efforts to meet the health needs of the public.

From American Nurses Association: *Code for nurses with interpretive statements*, Washington, DC, 2001, The Association.

Association. In the statement of the nature and scope of nursing practice titled Nursing, a Social Policy Statement, developed by the ANA Congress of Practice in 1980, nurses committed to respect for human beings "unaltered by social, educational, economic, cultural, racial, religious or other specific attributes of human beings receiving care, including nature and duration of disease and illness." The ethics of a profession establish the role and scope of professional behavior and the nature of relationships with patients and colleagues.

Universal moral principles guide ethical decision making and activities in clinical practice (Box 3-7). These include the following:

- Values are operational beliefs an individual chooses as the basis for behavior. They may change over time. They may create conflicts when value systems are not compatible with the expectations of others. Values reflect ethics. Ethics refer to standards or principles of moral judgment and action. Ethics as a philosophy defines a systematic method of differentiating right from wrong within a specific belief system.
- Professional and societal codes and standards offer guidelines in this determination. Ethics and law are closely related. Legal doctrines often interpret ethical concepts.
- The Bill of Rights of the Constitution of the United States establishes individual rights based on moral principles that respect human worth and dignity. The courts have upheld the right to individual autonomy in making health care decisions, as evidenced by rulings about such issues as abortion, the right to die with dignity, and living wills.

BIOETHICAL SITUATIONS

An ethical dilemma arises in the work situation when the choice between two or more alternatives creates a conflict between an individual's value system and moral obligation to the patient, to the family or significant others, to the physician, or to the employer and coworkers. Conflicts can be between rights, duties, and responsibilities.

Both legal and ethical considerations can cause conflicts. Legally, a patient has the right to choose among treatment alternatives or the right to refuse treatment. Philosophically, the patient's preference may be different from that of the health care provider. The primary responsibility to the patient is to ensure delivery of safe care. This includes use of appropriate and available technology, but only if this is the patient's choice, with informed consent freely given, or is known to be the patient's wish. Conversely, the patient and the caregiver may be forced to face court-ordered procedures or treatments. This may impose the need to assist in a surgical intervention such as a cesarean section on a woman who has moral or religious objections to this form of treatment but who has been ordered by the court to have the procedure performed for the benefit of the unborn fetus.

This example is extreme, but the courts are constantly working to define the rights of the unborn. In the issue of viability versus possible death, the court usually supports measures necessary to sustain life. The caregiver who participates in a court-ordered procedure is protected by law, provided that the performance of his or her duties meets the standards of care.

Autonomy: Self-determination implies freedom of choice and ability to make decisions to determine one's own course of action. Decisions may be made in collaboration with others, based on reasonable and prudent information. Decisions should be acknowledged and respected by others.
Beneficence: Duty to help others seek balance between what is good to do and what might produce harm to another or self.
Nonmaleficence: Duty to do no harm.
Justice: Allocation of human, material, and technologic resources a person has a right to receive or claim (i.e., equality of care).
Veracity: Devotion to truthfulness (i.e., to give accurate information).
Fidelity: Quality of faithfulness, based on trust and honesty, that protects rights of individuals (e.g., dignity, privacy).
Confidentiality: Respect for privileged information received from another person with disclosure only to appropriate others.

Caregivers should decide for themselves the appropriate course of action when dealing with an ethical dilemma. By developing a personal philosophy and by understanding both professional and institutional philosophies, the caregiver may better answer many personal ethical questions such as the following:

- When does life begin?
- When does it end?
- What is my perception of quality of life between conception and death?
- What is my role in health care?
- What is my role as patient advocate?
- What are my moral rights in relation to my personal beliefs and values and those of others?
- Where are the dividing lines between a patient's personal rights to privacy and confidentiality and a legal or ethical duty of disclosure?

A few of the ethical dilemmas facing physicians and perioperative personnel are mentioned for personal consideration. It should also be noted that some of these issues are regulated by state statutes or federal court decisions. All caregivers should be familiar with statutes in the state in which they practice, particularly those regarding participation and the right to refrain on the basis of personal beliefs. The right to refuse to participate may be covered by a law but not at the expense of a patient's safety and welfare. The patient cannot be harmed by acts of commission or omission.

Reproductive Sterilization

Voluntary reproductive sterilization as a contraceptive method may be contrary to the moral, ethical, or religious beliefs of a caregiver. Consent is required to perform reproductive sterilization. Some facilities require consent from a patient's spouse.

Abortion

Legalized abortion allows for induced termination of pregnancy. In the 1973 decision of *Roe v. Wade*, the U.S. Supreme Court ruled that any licensed physician can terminate pregnancy during the first trimester with the woman's consent. During the second trimester, the Court requires a state statute that regulates abortion on the basis of preservation and protection of maternal health. During the third trimester, legal abortion should consider meaningful life for the fetus outside the womb and endangerment to the mother's life and health. By selective abortion, one or more fertilized ova may be aborted so that others may mature properly in a multiple pregnancy, which is perhaps a result of fertility drugs.

Although, by law, physicians may perform abortions in health care facilities, many people, individually and collectively, oppose abortion, believing that it is a form of active euthanasia because it takes the life of an innocent victim without consent.

In facilities where abortions and other reproductive procedures are performed, employees have the right to refrain from participation because of their moral, ethical, or religious beliefs except in an emergency that threatens the life of the mother. These beliefs should be made known to the employer in writing. Some states have a protective statute for employees and employers regulating good-faith efforts to accommodate employees' beliefs. In other states, laws protect an employee from being forced by an employer to assist in abortions.

Human Experimentation

Procedures still in developmental stages are performed in clinical research–oriented facilities with the patient's informed consent. Those willing to be pioneers in human experimentation have given or will give hope to many patients with poor prognoses. A caregiver should decide if he or she wants to participate in experimental surgery.

Fetal Tissue and Stem Cell Research

Experimentation with human tissues may be of moral concern to some individuals. The acquisition of the tissues may take place in the OR in the form of embryonic tissue, and the implantation may take place in the OR. Fetal tissue lacks lymphocytes that can cause graft-versus-host response. Advantages of fetal tissue include rapid proliferation of cells, quick reversal of the host's condition, and differentiation in response to cues of the host tissue. Studies have shown promise in the treatment of diabetes mellitus, Parkinson's disease, and certain blood disorders and that the fetal tissue used in the treatment of Parkinson's disease continues to proliferate and function for many years after transplant. Tissue from spontaneous abortion and ectopic pregnancy has generally undergone pathologic degradation and is not suitable for this use. The use of fetal tissue and organs is subject to state law.

HIV and Other Infections

The prevalence of human immunodeficiency virus (HIV) infection, with or without acquired immunodeficiency syndrome (AIDS), has created a catastrophic health problem with many inherent emotional issues. Unlike other communicable diseases, HIV infection is a fatal illness with no known cure at this time, although some drug therapies may slow its progression. Its mode of transmission and methods of prevention are known. Therefore personal biases and prejudices should not discriminate against the infected patient. However, underlying attitudes about homosexuality and IV drug abuse may subconsciously influence the care of such patients. Are these patients any different from patients with hemophilia or those who became infected through a contaminated blood transfusion? Should the infant with HIV be treated any differently than an infant with a congenital anomaly? Does the diagnosis make a difference to the health care provider and to the quality of care that the patient receives? Should it?

Knowing that HIV infection is transmitted by blood and body secretions, conscientious application of standard precautions for infection control should provide protection against occupational exposure to HIV, hepatitis, tuberculosis, and other communicable or resistant infections. The ANA Code for Nurses emphasizes that care is given regardless of the nature of health problems.

Other ethical questions concern screening and the reporting of test results versus confidentiality. Do the same considerations apply to team members as to patients? What constitutes valid reasons for restricting or terminating employment on the basis of health status? This question has broader implications than just the issue of being seropositive for HIV. No state mandates by law that a health care worker can refuse to provide care for a patient with HIV infection. Risks versus benefits to self, patients, and team members, plus potential litigation as a result of actions, should be evaluated in making ethical decisions. Confidentiality, privacy, and informed consent are human rights that should be protected, but the right to health care should be protected also.

Both AORN and AST have published statements encouraging health care facilities to provide policies and procedures to ensure the safety of patients and personnel. These organizations believe that providers have a right to know the HIV or other infectious status of patients but that caregivers do not have the right to discriminate against HIV-positive patients. They should follow the Centers for Disease Control and Prevention (CDC) guidelines in caring for all patients to prevent transmission of infection.

Quality of Life

Surgeons often must make critical decisions before or during surgical interventions regarding the quality of patients' lives after surgical procedures. Palliative procedures may relieve pain. Therapeutic procedures may be disfiguring. Life-support systems may sustain vital functions. Life-sustaining therapy may prolong the dying process. Many questions arise regarding care of terminally ill, severely debilitated or injured, and comatose patients. What will be the outcome in terms of mental or physical competence? When should cardiopulmonary resuscitation be initiated or discontinued? Physicians decide, but all team members are affected by the decisions.

Patients with advance directives have made many of these difficult decisions while in a lucid mental state. This saves the family or legal guardians the anguish of making the decision during times of duress. This helps provide some closure and a small sense of satisfaction that the loved one's wishes were known and followed.

Euthanasia

How is euthanasia defined? Is mercy killing ethical, legal, or justified? Does the patient, family or guardian, physicians, or courts have the right to decide to abandon heroic measures to sustain life? The patient who is aware of the options and whose decision-making capacity is intact has the right of self-determination. OR personnel develop the plan of care guided by an advance directive.

Euthanasia is derived from the Greek words meaning "good or merciful death." Both active euthanasia and passive euthanasia are intentional acts that cause death, but the methods are different. An act of direct intervention that causes death is active euthanasia. Withholding or withdrawing life-prolonging or life-sustaining measures is passive euthanasia. Death is caused by the underlying disease process, trauma, or physiologic dysfunction. This concept differs from physician-assisted suicide. Suicide involves the person causing his or her own demise.

The idea of euthanasia seems to violate traditional principles of medicine to preserve life, but our modern technologies can prolong life without preserving quality. Quality of life can be interpreted as life that has a meaningful value. Most human beings value having cognitive abilities, physical capabilities, or both, and living free of undue pain and suffering. This raises the ethical question of whether physicians should do what they technologically can do.

Right to Die

Courts have determined that patients have a constitutional right to privacy in choosing to die with dignity or a common law right to withhold consent and refuse treatment. A mentally competent adult older than the age of 18 years can execute a living will, an advance directive, directing physicians and other health care providers not to use extraordinary measures to prolong life. Most physicians designate "extraordinary" measures as those that are optional, such as mechanical respiration, hydration, nutrition, medication, or a combination of these, and that sustain life. If it is the expressed wish of the patient, the physician writes do-not-resuscitate (DNR) orders.

A living will relieves family members of decision making when the patient becomes terminally ill, incompetent, or comatose. No laws or court precedents deal specifically with the issue of DNR orders in the perioperative environment. Institutional policy should address this matter. Theoretically, a patient can attempt to sue for compensation for expenses under a negligence or battery charge. In general, courts are reluctant to hold health care workers liable for acts performed to maintain life. In *Anderson v. St. Francis,* defibrillation was performed despite a DNR order. The court found that sustaining life was not considered an injury and rejected the compensatory claim.

A patient who has a standing DNR order may require a procedure to decrease pain or palliate uncomfortable symptoms. Before going to the OR, the DNR order should be reaffirmed with the patient, guardian, or person who has durable power of attorney. The status of the DNR order must be clarified before the patient goes to the OR. In an emergency, if there is doubt about the validity of the DNR order or a question concerning reconsideration of the order, the caregiver should participate in resuscitation. If there is any question about the patient changing his or her mind, a second chance may not be an option during an emergency situation. If the patient or legal guardian is specifically clear about upholding the DNR order in the OR, the team has the responsibility to follow the patient's wishes. A caregiver who has a moral objection to upholding a DNR order may request reassignment through the nurse manager of the department.

The issue of discontinuation of life-sustaining measures becomes more difficult in a comatose, mentally incompetent patient who has not executed an advance directive. Family members, in consultation with physicians, may request DNR orders. Caregivers are obligated to follow DNR orders.

Organ Donation and Transplantation

As a result of the Uniform Anatomical Gift Act of 1968, many adults carry cards stating that at death they wish to donate their body organs or parts for transplantation, therapy, medical research, or education. Most states include this information on a driver's license. If this legal authority is not available, some states have a required request law. In the event of legally defined brain death, the caregivers are required by this law to ask the family if they wish to allow organ retrieval for transplantation.

Transplant surgeons rely on the perioperative patient care teams who procure donor organs, eyes, bone, and skin. Organ transplantation has complicated the issue of time of death. Perfusion of oxygenated blood through tissues must be sustained by artificial means during procurement of vital organs with functional viability. Brain death must be clearly established before procurement can proceed.

Legally, death has occurred when an individual has sustained either irreversible cessation of circulation, and respiratory functions or irreversible cessation of all functions of the entire brain, including the brainstem. Therefore the accepted definition of irreversible coma for potential donors includes unresponsiveness, no spontaneous movements of respiration, no reflexes, and a flat electroencephalogram.

When brain death is determined by two physicians who are not part of the transplant team, the donor will be taken to the OR with artificial support systems functioning to perfuse organs. Some caregivers have moral questions about assisting with removal of viable organs from seemingly living bodies. When the heart is removed, cardiopulmonary support is discontinued and the anesthesia personnel leave the room. This is a difficult time for the remaining team who may still have the assignment of procuring nonperfused tissues, such as skin, bone, or eyes.

Perioperative caregivers who believe that donation of organs and body parts is a gift of love find it easier and ethically acceptable to participate in procurement procedures. Family members of donors have been encouraged by surgical team members not to focus on their grief, but rather to focus on the gifts of life they are giving unselfishly to the recipients. This does not mean that the donor's family will not go through the grieving process. They will need support. Caregivers learn to cope with feelings associated with the procurement of donor organs in a manner similar to dealing with the sudden death of any patient in the perioperative environment.

Death and Dying

Intellectually, we know that death is inevitable. Death can be a difficult burden for caregivers to bear because our education, experience, and philosophy are dedicated to survival. Regardless of religious or cultural beliefs, death is a mystery, a passage from the known to the unknown. Perhaps partially for this reason, the death of a patient in the OR is an unsettling experience, especially if it is unexpected.

One of the most difficult aspects of a death in the OR for the team members is the period after the actual event. The surgeon goes to inform the family. The assistants and anesthesia provider leave the room. Often the perioperative team is left alone with the patient's body. The patient should be prepared so that the family can view the body in an area adjoining the perioperative environment, where they can have privacy in expressing their feelings. The perioperative nurse may be expected to accompany the family and to lend support during the viewing. A chaplain or other clergy should be called if desired by the family. Specific departmental policies should be developed to assist the caregiver with this difficult aspect of patient care. Coping strategies that can help team members may include the following:

- Realize that everyone involved is part of a team effort.
- Believe in a power greater than the skills of the team.
- Share feelings with others. It is helpful for perioperative patient care team members to talk with each other about what happened. Encourage each other to share feelings associated with the loss. Crying is acceptable behavior.
- Deal with the patient's death by identifying personally with the loss. Empathy is a positive emotion. Working through the grieving process brings a sense of closure to the relationship.
- Some facilities provide support groups to help staff members and bereaved families deal with death.
- Arrange a visit with the hospital chaplain or rabbi.

Bibliography

Agard A: Informed consent: Theory versus practice, *Natl Clin Pract Cardiovasc Med* 2(6):270, 2005.

AORN (Association of periOperative Registered Nurses): *AORN standards, recommended practices, and guidelines,* Denver, 2005, The Association.

Beya SC: Learning from sentinel event statistics, *AORN J* 80(2):315, 317-318, 2004.

Bogart JB et al: *Legal nurse consulting: principles and practice,* New York, 1998, CRC Press, Association of Legal Nurse Consultants.

Coyle G: Designing and implementing a close call reporting system, *Nurs Admin Quarter* 29(1):57-62, 2005.

Ebright P et al: Themes surrounding novice nurse near miss and adverse event situations, *J Nurs Admin* 34(1):531-538, 2004.

Edwards M, Moczygemba J: Reducing medical errors through better documentation, *Health Care Manage* 23(4):329-333, 2004.

Fortunato NM et al: *Nursing law in Ohio,* Eau Claire, WI, 1997, National Business Institute.

Institute of Medicine: *To err is human: building a safer health system,* Washington, DC, 2000, National Academy Press.

Joint Commission on Accreditation of Healthcare Organizations: *Health care at the crossroads: strategies for improving the medical liability system and preventing patient injury,* 2005, Washington D.C., The Organization.

Koski G et al: Cooperative research ethics review boards: a win-win solution? *IRB* 27(3):1-7, 2005.

Lantos J: In Practice: Ethics class, *Hastings Center Rep* 35(3):7, 2005.

McGraw KS: Should do-not-resuscitate orders be suspended during surgical procedures? *AORN J* 67(4):794-799, 1998.

Murphy EK: "Captain of the ship" doctrine continues to take on water, *AORN J* 74(4):525-526, 528, 2001.

Murphy EK: Intraoperative use of unlicensed assistive personnel, *AORN J* 68(4):678-681, 1998.

Wiessman JS et al: Error reporting and disclosure systems, *JAMA* 293(11):1359-1366, 2005.

Chapter 4

The Perioperative Patient Care Team and Professional Credentialing

CHAPTER OBJECTIVES

After studying this chapter, the learner will be able to:
- Define the concept of the sterile team.
- Define the concept of the nonsterile team.
- Describe the role of the circulating nurse.
- Describe the role of the scrub person.
- Describe the role of the first assistant.

CHAPTER OUTLINE

KEY TERMS AND DEFINITIONS

Anesthesia provider   Member of the nonsterile team who administers anesthetics during the surgical procedure; may be a physician (MD, DO), anesthesia assistant (AA), or a specially trained and certified registered nurse anesthetist (CRNA).

Certification   A method of professional evaluation and recognition of an individual for meeting educational, practice, and national standard parameters that range above minimal competency.

Circulating nurse   RN member of the nonsterile team who directs and coordinates the activities of the intraoperative environment during the surgical procedure. Role involves patient assessment, planning, and critical thinking skills.

Credentials   Validation of professional recognition, such as licensure or certification.

Delegation   A registered nurse or physician can assign and supervise tasks performed by a LPN/LVN, ST, or other UAP provided the tasks are not intended for a licensed individual's scope of practice and are within the capabilities of the person being assigned the tasks.

Licensure   Governmental regulation of approval to practice in a specific profession to provide specific services. Practicing without a license is illegal and punishable by law. Some license renewals include attainment of continued education in the profession.

Licensure is designed to ensure minimal competency of the licensee for the benefit of protecting the safety and welfare of the public. The laws that define the scope of practice governing a registered professional are called *practice acts*.

Nonsterile team   Intraoperative caregivers who provide direct care from the periphery of the sterile field and environment; do not wear sterile attire (i.e., radiology technician, anesthesia technologist).

Perianesthesia nurse   RN who renders care in the preoperative and postoperative environment. Member of the nonsterile team.

Registration   Establishing a record of name, address, and qualifications of a professional with a state authority. This does not establish stands of practice, does not require a certain entry level, and does not provide for continued competency verification or continued education.

Scrub person   Member of the sterile team who passes instruments and facilitates the surgical procedure. Is a surgical technologist (ST), registered nurse (RN), or licensed practical or vocational nurse (LPN/LVN).

Sterile team   Intraoperative caregivers who provide direct care within the sterile field; wear sterile attire. (i.e., surgeon, first assistant, scrub person).

Surgeon   Physician (e.g., MD, DO, DDS, DPM) who performs the surgical procedure.

Surgical assistant   Member of the sterile team who provides exposure and hemostasis during a surgical procedure. Is a physician, registered nurse first assistant (RNFA), surgical assistant (SA), physician assistant (PA), or certified surgical technologist specially trained and certified as a first assistant (CST/CFA).

SUPPLEMENTAL MATERIAL ON EVOLVE WEBSITE   *evolve*

http://evolve.elsevier.com/BerryKohn
- Content Updates
- Glossary
- Full Set of Perioperative Flash Cards
- Interactive Key Term Flash Cards
- Student Activities
- WebLinks

HISTORICAL BACKGROUND

Early surgical practitioners did not have qualified teams to rely on when a patient needed surgery. During the American Civil War (1861-1865), the Confederate Medical Departments of the Army and the Navy were staffed by medical officers, hospital stewards, matrons, nurses, and ward masters. The average regimental hospital worked out of two hospital tents, employing one or two surgeons, one steward, 10 nurses (all volunteers), and two cooks. The patient population during the war in the South consisted of 3 million sick and wounded. It was estimated that each of the 600,000 fighting forces fell ill or were wounded at least six times during the war, in addition to the 200,000 fatalities. The survival statistics were surprisingly good because most of the physicians and medical assistive personnel had little if any training for the roles they played.

Medical schools in the North offered a program of study that consisted of 5 months of lectures. Southern medical schools soon followed suit. The Medical College of Georgia set a new standard by increasing the study period to 9 months and employing eight professors. The increasing need for medical care sparked accelerated programs that addressed the eye as well as the ear of the learner. Lectures were supplanted by demonstrations of anatomic dissection. Medical graduates increased in number from 35 in 1850 to 133 in 1861 to meet the needs of war.

Training of nurses during the Civil War was sponsored by religious orders. They gave practical training to women who were considered "born nurses" or the "motherly type." Plain-looking, respectable women were asked to care for the sick and wounded. More than 2000 women responded to this call. The American Sisters of Charity, founded by Elizabeth Bayley Seton (1774-1821) in Emmitsburg, Maryland, and the American Sisters of Mercy, founded in Pittsburgh by Frances Warde (1810-1884), were two prominent Catholic orders that cared for both Northern and Southern soldiers on the battlefield and in military hospitals. The Sister-nurses were able to cross the battle lines with out a password because they were held in such high esteem. The soldiers called them "black caps." Spies for both sides of the American Civil War frequently dressed as nuns to gather military intelligence because they were able to move about freely without suspicion.

In the North, Dr. Elizabeth Blackwell (1821-1910), a friend of Florence Nightingale (1820-1910), supported formal training for nurses and tried to bring it into the formal hospital setting. Dr. Blackwell had founded a hospital for women and children in New York with her sister, Dr. Emily Blackwell, in 1859. Training schools were actually opened for the training of nurses in New England by Dr. Marie Zakrzewska. Still, most of the nurses available for war-time duty were wives, mothers, and sisters of the soldiers. During this time, Clara Barton (1821-1912), a New England schoolteacher, traveled to the front lines in 1861 to play a major role in the Civil War effort. She founded the American branch of the International Red Cross that was originated in 1863 by Jean Henri Dunant (1828-1910). More information about medicine and the American Civil War can be found at www.americancivilwar.com.

After the war, in 1872, Dr. Susan Dimock went to Kaiserswerth, Germany, to study the nursing education system set up by Florence Nightingale. She implemented the Nightingale teaching methods in the New England hospital and in 1873 graduated the first trained nurses in America, one of which was Linda Richards (considered the first trained nurse in America).

DEPENDENCE OF THE PATIENT ON THE QUALIFIED TEAM

The perioperative team works to promote the best interests of the patient every single minute. For the welfare and safety of the patient, the entire team must work efficiently as a functioning single unit. The members should be thoroughly familiar with procedures, setups, equipment, and policies and should be able to cope with the unpredictable. Their qualifications must be beyond reproach. They should have a high morale, mutual understanding, trust, cooperation, and consideration. Anyone who cannot function wholeheartedly as a qualified team member has no place in the operating room (OR).

All OR personnel should have the proven knowledge, skill, competency, and ability to perform at an optimal level at all times. The validation of clinical competence is an important aspect of providing safe patient care. Once each member of the team has passed the novice stage, other criteria demonstrate and document the knowledge and skills gained through experience and continuing education. Aligning professionally with local, state, and nationally recognized organizations that establish the standards of practice provides an opportunity for growth. Credentialing and certification may include completing a course of instruction or meeting certain criteria and passing an examination. Other measurements of competence include performance evaluations in a clinical setting.

CREDENTIALING OF QUALIFIED CAREGIVERS

Credentialing refers to the processes of accreditation, licensure, and certification of institutions, agencies, and individuals. These processes establish quality, identity, protection, and control for the competency-based education and performance of professional and allied technical health care personnel. Credentialing also protects the public from fraudulent practitioners.

Accreditation

An accrediting body of a voluntary organization evaluates and sanctions an educational program or an institution as meeting predetermined standards and/or essential criteria. The National League for Nursing (NLN) accredits schools of nursing. Surgical technology programs are accredited by the Commission on Accreditation of Allied Health Education Programs (CAAHEP) after a satisfactory review and recommendation by the Accreditation Review Committee on Education in Surgical Technology (ARC-ST).

The United States Government Department of Education has been accepted by the National Board of Surgical Technology and Surgical Assisting (NBSTSA) (formerly the Liaison Council on Certification for the Surgical Technologist (LCC-ST) as an accepted accrediting body after January 1, 2004, up to entrance May 1, 2006.[1] The Accrediting Bureau of Health Education Schools (ABHES) accredits many colleges and vocational settings in the United States. The Joint Commission on Accreditation of Healthcare Organizations (JCAHO) accredits hospitals and ambulatory care centers. Other professional organizations offer accreditation for special-interest groups.

Licensure and Registration

A license to practice is granted to professionals by a governmental agency, such as the state board of nursing or medicine. Licensure implies a certain amount of appropriate independence in actions. On completion of a formal academic education, nurses and physicians who successfully pass a state examination receive a license to practice in that state. To maintain this license, they must register with the state as required by law; hence the term *registered nurse.* Licensed practical/licensed vocational nurses (LPN/LVNs) also are licensed.

Most states grant a license by reciprocity or endorsement to applicants who wish to practice in their state but who took the examination in another state. Some states require licensure for some categories of allied health occupations, such as physical therapists.

Licensure is not offered on an indefinite basis. Applicants apply for renewal at specific time intervals determined by each state. Many states require proof of continuing education for nurses and physicians as a prerequisite for eligibility of relicensure.

Registration is a method of state regulation of practice parameters and designation for disciplinary action. Perioperative nurses are *registered* as well as *licensed.*

Certification

A nongovernmental private organization can award a credential that attests to level of knowledge above minimal competency of an individual who meets predetermined qualifications. Certification may be defined as documented validation of an individual's professional achievement of knowledge and skill in identified standards. To be certified is to demonstrate the attainment of more than minimal competency; it is a statement of certification-level knowledge. Certification for perioperative nurses and surgical technologists is voluntary, whereas licensure is mandatory for some disciplines.

Certification is usually granted for a limited time. To retain this credential, an individual must complete the recertification process established by the certifying body. For recertification, some certifying organizations require a specified number of clinical hours, continuing education contact hours, a written examination, or a combination of these in a portfolio format. Maintaining certification by going through this process demonstrates a high level of motivation and commitment.

Physicians, nurses, and allied health care personnel may be certified by their professional specialty association as being competent in knowledge and skills to practice. Applicants take an examination that tests knowledge in the area of specialization.

Some nursing associations grant recognition of professional achievement and competence in current practice. A perioperative nurse who has been in clinical perioperative practice for 24 months and who has successfully passed an examination is certified by the Competency & Credentialing Institute (CCI, www.cc-institute.org [formerly known as CBPN—Certification Board Perioperative Nursing]) as a *certified perioperative nurse,* which is designated as CNOR. Box 4-1 describes the required eligibility for CNOR certification and Table 4-1 describes the criteria for CNOR recertification. Several nursing specialty organizations, such as the National Association of Orthopaedic Nurses (NAON, www.orthonurse.org) and the American Society of Plastic Surgery Nurses (ASPSN, www.aspsn.org), offer certification examinations through their certifying bodies as an additional credentialing tool.

PERIOPERATIVE PATIENT CARE TEAM

At no other time during the health care experience will the patient be so well attended as in the perioperative care period. Preoperatively, the perianesthesia nurse performs the preoperative assessment and the patient has the opportunity to ask questions of the personnel administering the anesthetic. In the OR, the patient is surrounded by the surgeon, the surgical assistant, the scrub person, the anesthesia provider, and the circulating nurse. Postoperatively, the perianesthesia nurse cares for the patient until his or her physiologic status is stable. These individuals, each with specific functions to perform, form the perioperative patient care team. (More information is available at www.aspan.org; the role of the perianesthesia nurse is described in more detail in the postoperative section in Chapter 30.)

The perioperative patient care team is like a symphony orchestra, with each person an integral entity in unison and harmony with his or her colleagues to accomplish the expected outcomes.

U.S. Federal Medicare and Medicaid regulations Title 42, Public Health describe conditions for participation of individuals in surgical services departments. In Chapter IV, Part 482, Section 482.51, the regulation states that the OR must be supervised by an experienced registered nurse (RN) or doctor of medicine/doctor of osteopathy (MD/DO) and that the circulator must be an RN. It further states that an LPN/LVN and surgical technologists may serve as scrub nurses or assist with circulating duties under the supervision of the qualified RN.

The perioperative team is subdivided according to the functions of its members:

1. The nonsterile team
   a. Anesthesia provider
   b. Circulating nurse
   c. Perianesthesia nurse
   d. Others (e.g., students, sales representatives, laboratory or radiography personnel)
2. The sterile team
   a. Surgeon

---

[1] Department of Education accredits institutions offering predominantly allied health education. ABHES includes the accreditation of medical assistant, medical laboratory technician, and surgical technology programs within public and private institutions.

BOX 4-1 **CNOR-Eligibility Criteria**

- Licensed RN in state of practice and currently employed full or part time in administrative, teaching, research, or general staff capacity in perioperative nursing.
- Bachelor of science in nursing (BSN) not required for CNOR.
- Two years and 2400 hours of perioperative nursing experience.

Roles eligible for certification:
- Staff nurse
- Surgical services administrative nurse manager
- Surgical services nursing coordinator
- Assistant surgical services supervisor
- Surgical services director
- Surgical services information technology specialist
- Surgical services budget and finance manager
- Surgical services central processing manager
- Surgical services materials manager
- Surgical services quality assurance coordinator/auditor
- Surgical services head nurse
- Surgical services assistant head nurse
- Surgical services team leader
- Surgical services charge nurse
- Perioperative educator or staff development director (whether teaching registered nurses, student nurses, or surgical technologists)
- Private RN scrub nurse
- RN first assistant
- Perioperative administrative supervisor
- Medical-surgical instructor in perioperative nursing
- Perioperative clinical nurse specialist or nurse clinician
- Full-time student who meets applicant status requirements
- Perioperative nurse consultant
- Individual who handles the perioperative role in a noninvasive/invasive procedure setting, such as a radiology suite, a cardiac cath lab, an office surgery setting, or an endoscopy suite
- Clinical education consultant (who provides inservice programs to operating room staff)
- Case manager

Roles ineligible for certification
- Nurse anesthetist (eligible only if functioning as a perioperative nurse)
- PACU nurse or manager (eligible only if relieving in the operating room as needed or has responsibility for operating room/surgical services)
- Emergency department nurse
- OR labor and delivery nurse (eligible only if surgical procedures such as cesarean sections are done in delivery room)
- RN sales representative (eligible only if performing the role of perioperative nurse part time or the role of perioperative educator, i.e., providing inservice programs)
- Director or assistant director of nursing service (eligible only if directly responsible for the OR)
- RN hospital administrator/assistant administrator (eligible only if directly responsible for OR/surgical services)
- Nurse in surgical care or surgical rehabilitation units
- Intensive care unit (ICU) or coronary care unit nurse
- Infection control nurse/nurse epidemiologist (eligible only if directly responsible for OR/surgical services)
- Veterinary OR nurse
- Cardiopulmonary perfusionist (eligible only if performing the role of perioperative nurse)
- Nurse with inactive licensure and/or graduate nurse status

b. First assistant (second assistant if needed)
c. Scrub person

The team also may include biomedical technicians, specialty technicians, and others who may be needed to set up and operate specialized equipment or monitoring devices during the surgical procedure.

Sterile team members scrub their hands and arms, don a sterile gown and gloves, and enter the sterile field. The sterile field is the area of the OR that immediately surrounds and is specially prepared for the patient. To establish and maintain a sterile field, all items needed for the surgical procedure are sterile and handled in a sterile manner. Only sterile items and personnel dressed in sterile attire may enter the sterile field.

Nonsterile team members do not enter the sterile field; they function outside and around it. They assume responsibility for maintaining sterile and aseptic techniques during the surgical procedure. They handle supplies and equipment that are not considered sterile. Following the principles of aseptic technique, they keep the sterile team supplied, provide direct patient care, and handle situations that may arise during the perioperative care period.

NONSTERILE TEAM MEMBERS
Perianesthesia Team

The perianesthesia team consists of RNs and specially trained patient care assistants. Preoperatively, the RN assesses the patient and documents the findings. Any information that contributes to the care of the patient in the intraoperative area is communicated to the intraoperative team members. Some perianesthesia RNs specialize in the care of the patient before the surgical procedure and others specialize in the care of the patient postoperatively.

Anesthesia Provider

Anesthesia and surgery are two distinct but inseparable disciplines; they are two parts of one medical entity. Adequate communication between the surgeon and the anesthesia provider is the patient's greatest safeguard. The anesthesia provider is an indispensable member of the perioperative team. Functioning as a guardian of the patient throughout the entire care period, the anesthesia provider manages the patient's physiology using the principles of aseptic technique. Throughout this text the term *anesthesia provider* is used to refer to the person responsible for inducing and maintaining anesthesia at the required levels and managing untoward physiologic reactions throughout the surgical procedure. Medically delegated functions of an anesthetic nature are performed under the overall supervision of a responsible physician or in accordance with state regulations and individual written guidelines approved within the health care facility.

An anesthesiologist is an MD or DO, preferably certified by the American Board of Anesthesiology, who specializes in administering anesthetics to produce various states of anesthesia. To become eligible for certification, physicians complete a 2-year anesthesia residency program after successful completion of medical school. The term *anesthetist* refers to a qualified RN, anesthesiologist assistant (AA), dentist, or physician who administers anesthetics.

TABLE 4-1	CNOR Recertification	
Point System **300 Required to Recertify**	**Contact Hour Method** **125 Contact Hours in 5 Years**	**Examination for Recertification**

Continued education
• Limit 100 points
• 1 contact hour = 2 points
Academic credit hours for a degree
• Unlimited contact hours apply
• 1 semester credit = 15 contact hours
• 1 quarter credit = 10 contact hours
Teaching in a college or university
• Limit 60 points
• 1 course = 30 points
Presentation
• 30-60 minutes = 10 points (limit 50 points)
• 4-8 hours = 30 points (limit 90 points)
Publication
• Article = 25 points (limit 75 points)
• Book chapter = 40 points (limit 120 points)
• Entire book = 50 points (limit 50 points)
• Guest editor = 10 (limit 20 points)
• Book review = 5 (limit 15 points)
Service on a board or committee
• 20 points each (limit 60 points per year)
Cross-training into new area
• 30 points each (limit 90 points)
• Orientation to new hospital does not qualify
Precepting new employees or students
• 25 points each (limit 75)
Consult www.cc-institute.org for more
  information.
	As of 2006:
	• 75 contact hours must be directly
	  related to perioperative nursing
	• 65.2-contact-hour limit for
	  academic credit hours may be
	  applied
		• Discount for AORN members
		• Qualified perioperative nurses can test
		  during the second, third, and fourth quarters
		• If unsuccessful in the second quarter, the
		  exam can be retaken in the third or fourth
		  quarter if the appropriate deadline is met
		  for application
		• Unsuccessful candidates must wait until the
		  first quarter of the subsequent year to reapply
		  if the exam is not retaken by the fourth
		  quarter
		• Application must be made by the deadline
		  date for the testing window selected
		• Fees apply for each attempt at reexamination

An RN is required to have a minimum of a bachelor's degree in nursing or science for entrance into a school of nurse anesthesia. To become a certified registered nurse anesthetist (CRNA), a graduate of an accredited nurse anesthesia program (a minimum of 2 years) is required to have a master's degree in nursing and pass the certification examination of the Council on Certification of Nurse Anesthetists. Nurse anesthetists are recertified every 2 years.

An anesthesia assistant (AA) is a master's prepared non-physician, non-nurse anesthetist who administers anesthesia under the direction of an anesthesiologist. The AA's education consists of a baccalaureate in biologic science and 2 additional years of specialty training in biophysical science. (More information on the AA degree is available online at www.anesthetist.org.)

Some anesthesia providers prefer to specialize in one area, such as cardiothoracic or obstetric anesthesia. The latter involves the simultaneous care of two patients—the mother and the neonate. In some settings, anesthesia providers participate in teaching and research as well as in clinical practice.

Anesthesia providers are not confined to the perioperative environment, but this is their primary arena. In addition to providing anesthesia during surgical procedures, anesthesia providers oversee the postanesthesia care unit (PACU) until each patient has regained control of his or her vital reflexes. They also participate in the hospital's program of cardiopulmonary resuscitation as teachers and team members. They are consultants or managers for problems of acute and chronic respiratory insufficiency that require respiratory therapy, as well as for a variety of other fluid, electrolyte, and metabolic disturbances that require intravenous (IV) therapy. In the intensive care unit or emergency department, their advice may be sought regarding the total care of unconscious, critically ill, or injured patients with acute circulatory disorders or neurologic deficits. Anesthesia providers also are integral staff members of pain therapy clinics.

Circulating Nurse

The circulating nurse is a qualified RN. A qualified surgical technologist (ST) or LPN/LVN may assist with circulating duties under the supervision of the RN.[2] The circulating nurse is vital to the smooth flow of events before, during, and after the surgical procedure. Physical and psychological demands of the circulating nurse's role are described in Box 4-2.

The patient's medical record is required to identify who provided circulating duties. Patients undergoing a surgical intervention experience physical and psychosocial trauma.

---

[2] 42 CFR § 428.51: federal position on the RN circulator according to the Centers for Medicare and Medicaid Services.

BOX 4-2	Physical and Psychological Attributes of the Circulating Nurse's Role

1. Visual acuity with or without correction is critical to precise observation of the environment, patient, and team, and for reading small print. Protective eyewear is required at all times when in proximity to the surgical field or when at risk for a splash/aerosol exposure. Bright lights or dim lights are commonly used throughout the surgical procedure, and people with photosensitivity or susceptibility to light-mediated eye irritation will find the OR environment problematic. Visual accuracy is imperative.
2. Manual dexterity and accuracy of motion is required for fast action during emergencies. Inability to coordinate body motions could cause injury to the patient, team, or self. Physical ability to maneuver around the periphery of the sterile field without causing contamination or disruption of the surgical procedure is critical.
3. Eye-hand coordination is essential for safe and efficient delivery of sterile items to the field. Eye-hand coordination is imperative for the safety and preservation of the sterile field.
4. Ability to concentrate and remain alert during long procedures. Thinking on one's feet is a hallmark of the circulating nurse. Multitasking is essential because the coordination of the room, patient care, team, documentation, and anticipation demands clear thinking.
5. Ability to lift instrument trays of at least 20 pounds and assist with moving large incapacitated patients using proper body mechanics.
6. Auditory acuity in both ears with or without amplification is critical for hearing and understanding commands while machinery is running. Voices are kept low during surgery, especially when the patient is awake. Hearing correctly is imperative.
7. Ability to quickly anticipate and discern commands and needs of the team. Must be able to differentiate and prioritize the needs of the surgical team and the anesthesia provider efficiently and to be able to offer appropriate alternatives in extraordinary circumstances.
8. The ability to speak, understand, and document clearly using the English language is critical to safe patient care. Appropriate terminology and use of approved standard accepted abbreviations are essential to communication in the OR.
9. Communication is essential between the team, anesthesia provider, control desk, family waiting room, labs, and perianesthesia care areas. The circulating nurse coordinates pertinent information among all areas concerning the care of the perioperative patient.
10. The ability to remain calm and function quickly, safely, and precisely during an emergency. Must be able to make decisions and problem solve effectively without loss of emotional control.

BOX 4-3	Thirty-Four States That Require a Registered Nurse Circulator in the Operating Room

Alabama	Iowa	New York
Alaska	Kentucky	North Dakota
Arizona	Louisiana	Oklahoma
Arkansas	Maine	Oregon
California	Massachusetts	Pennsylvania
Colorado	Missouri	Rhode Island
Delaware	Montana	Tennessee
Florida	Nebraska	Texas
Georgia	Nevada	Utah
Hawaii	New Jersey	Wisconsin
Idaho	New Mexico	Wyoming
Indiana		

The surgeon is in charge at the operating bed, but he or she relies on the circulating nurse to monitor and coordinate all activities within the room and to manage the care required for each patient. The RN should be continuously knowledgeable about the status of the patient. To some extent, the circulating nurse controls the physical and emotional atmosphere in the room, which allows other team members to concentrate on tasks without distraction.

A qualified RN should be available at all times to respond to emergencies in the perioperative environment. "Immediately available" has been interpreted by nurse practice acts to imply that an RN can supervise an unspecified number of contiguous rooms but should be immediately available to assist in each of these rooms uninterrupted; he or she can leave a room for short periods but can return immediately to supervise or assist as needed. However, the regulations in 34 states specify that one RN circulate in each room (Box 4-3). The RN who is called to a room to manage a crisis is not "immediately available" to any other patient who may be in need. More than one crisis can happen at any given time. The circulating nurse would be abandoning one patient to tend to another. This is highly unsafe and places the nurse and the facility at risk for liability.

The circulating nurse is vital to the provision of care that includes, but is not limited to, the following:
1. Applying the nursing process to directing and coordinating all activities related to the care and support of the patient in the OR. Nursing diagnosis and decision-making skills are essential in assessing, planning, implementing, and evaluating the plan of care before, during, and after a surgical intervention. This is the professional perioperative role of the RN circulating nurse.
2. Creating and maintaining a safe and comfortable environment for the patient by implementing the principles of asepsis. The circulating nurse demonstrates a strong sense of surgical conscience. Any break in technique by anyone in the room should be recognized and corrected instantly. Although sterile technique is the responsibility of everyone in the room, the circulating nurse is on the alert to catch any breaks that others may not have seen. By stand-

They enter an alien environment removed from personal contact with family and friends, and their physical and psychological needs are great. At this critical time, patients need the professional judgment of others who function on their behalf, and these advocates should be within physical and social proximity at all times. The circulating nurse's role as the patient's advocate and protector is critical and extends throughout the entire perioperative environment.

ing farther away from the sterile field than others, the circulating nurse is better able to observe the entire field and the sterile team members.

3. Providing assistance to any member of the OR team in any manner for which the circulating nurse is qualified. This role requires current knowledge of the legal implications of surgical intervention. The circulating nurse knows the organization of the work and the relative importance of the factors involved in accomplishing it. An effective circulating nurse ensures that the sterile team is supplied with every item necessary to perform the surgical procedure efficiently. The circulating nurse must know all supplies, instruments, and equipment; be able to obtain them quickly; and guard against inadvertent hazards in their use and care. He or she must be competent to direct the scrub person.

4. Identifying any potential environmental danger or stressful situation involving the patient, other team members, or both. This role requires constant flexibility to meet the unexpected and to act in an efficient, rational manner at all times.

5. Maintaining the communication link between events and team members in the sterile field and people who are not in the OR but are concerned with the outcome of the surgical procedure. The latter includes the patient's family or significant others plus other personnel in the perioperative environment and in other departments of the hospital. The ability to recognize and effectively communicate situations involving the patient and/or other team members is a vital link in the continuity of patient care.

6. Directing the activities of all learners. The circulating nurse must have the supervisory capability and teaching skills necessary to ensure maintenance of a safe and therapeutic environment for the patient. Kindly given assistance builds up the learner's confidence. In this capacity the circulating nurse acts as a supervisor, adviser, and teacher.

STERILE TEAM MEMBERS

Surgeon

The surgeon must have the knowledge, skill, and judgment required to successfully perform the intended surgical procedure and any deviations necessitated by unforeseen difficulties. The American College of Surgeons (ACS) has stated the principles of patient care that dictate ethical surgical practice. Protection of the patient and quality care are preeminent in these principles. The surgeon's responsibilities include preoperative diagnosis and care, selection and performance of the surgical procedure, and postoperative management of care.

The care of many surgical patients is so complex that considerably more than technical skill is required of a surgeon. The surgeon cannot predict that a surgical procedure will be simple and uncomplicated. The surgeon must be prepared for the unexpected by having knowledge of the fundamentals of the basic sciences and by having the ability to apply this knowledge to the diagnosis and management of the patient before, during, and after surgical intervention. The surgeon assumes full responsibility for all medical acts of judgment and for the management of the surgical patient.

A surgeon is a licensed MD, DO, oral surgeon (doctor of dental surgery [DDS] or doctor of dental medicine [DMD]), or doctor of podiatric medicine (a podiatrist [DPM]) who is specially trained and qualified by knowledge and experience to perform surgical procedures. After earning a bachelor's degree, all physicians complete the equivalent of 4 years of medical school. To become a surgeon, a physician completes at least 2 years of general surgical residency training before completing additional years of postgraduate education in a surgical specialty. The surgical residency provides the physician with education and experience in the preoperative evaluation, intraoperative treatment, and postoperative care of patients. Consultation and supervision are available from faculty and attending surgeons.

By virtue of their postgraduate surgical education, most surgeons practice within a specific surgical specialty. Highly trained and qualified surgeons limit themselves to their specialty, except perhaps in emergency situations.

Qualification for surgical practice involves certification by a surgical specialty board approved by the American Board of Medical Specialists. Ten American specialty boards grant certification for surgical practice. All 10 boards governing the surgical specialties require at least 3 years of approved formal residency training, and most set the minimum at 4 or 5 years. Any physician who aspires to become a board-certified surgeon must meet these requirements.

Surgical procedures may be performed by physicians who do not meet the previously discussed criteria. These physicians include those who received an MD degree before 1968 and who have had surgical privileges for more than 5 years in a hospital approved by JCAHO, where most of their surgical practice is conducted; those who render surgical care in an emergency or in an area of limited population where a surgical specialist is not available; and those who by reason of education, training, and experience are eligible for but have not yet obtained certification.

A surgeon must become a member of the medical staff and be granted surgical privileges in each facility in which he or she wishes to practice. Standards for admission to staff membership and the retention of that membership are clearly delineated in the bylaws formulated by the medical staff and are approved by the governing body of the hospital. The credentials committee has the primary responsibility for thoroughly investigating not only the training of an applicant but also his or her integrity, technical competence, and professional judgment. In making its recommendations, this committee can limit a surgeon's privileges as it sees fit, which ensures that each surgeon performs only those services for which he or she has been deemed competent.

Patients are entitled to protection and the assurance that a surgeon's surgical privileges are limited to those for which he or she has been trained and competence has been demonstrated. The patient's choice of and confidence in a surgeon, as well as adherence to instructions and advice, are factors in the outcome of surgical intervention. A discerning patient will check the surgeon's qualifications before surgery.

A competent surgeon is a physician who realistically appreciates his or her own cognitive skills and personal characteristics and can intervene effectively in a patient's illness or injury. Appropriate clinical skills (e.g., data gathering, decision making, problem solving) and appropriate personal characteristics (e.g., humanistic concern, accountability, compassionate interpersonal behavior) are important attributes of a surgeon.

First Assistant

Under the direction of the surgeon, a qualified first assistant helps maintain visibility of the surgical site, control bleeding, close wounds, and apply dressings. The first assistant handles and manipulates tissues and uses instruments to provide hemostasis. The role of and need for a first assistant will vary with the type of procedure or surgical specialty, the condition of the patient, and the type of surgical facility. In determining this need, the characteristics of the surgical procedure should be evaluated: anticipated blood loss, anesthesia time for the patient, fatigue factors affecting the OR team, and the potential for complications. This role is critical to the well-being of the patient. Detailed information about the role and duties of the first assistant can be found in Chapter 5 of this text.

For many simple procedures, it is unreasonable to insist that a second surgeon assist a competent surgeon. Reimbursement is generally not provided for simple cases. The surgeon should evaluate all factors to determine his or her need for assistance during the surgical procedure and consider that some insurance providers do not reimburse for a physician first assistant. However, the assistance of another qualified surgeon is usually necessary for procedures requiring considerable judgment or technical skill and those requiring more than one sterile team. The hazards of a surgical procedure may depend more on the condition of the patient than on the complexity of the procedure itself. The surgeon should be able to provide rationale for his or her decision if challenged or if not in compliance with medical staff bylaws.

Scrub Person

The scrub person is a patient care staff member of the sterile team. The scrub role may be filled by an RN, LPN/LVN, or an ST. The term *scrub person* is used throughout this text to designate this role and to elaborate on the specific technical and behavioral functions of the individual performing on the sterile team in this capacity.

The scrub person should not simultaneously function the role of first or second assistant. Performing additional tasks takes the scrub person's attention away from the primary responsibilities. Holding retractors, for example, can cause permanent injury to a patient if inappropriately positioned, maintained in alignment, or placed in contact with electrocautery inadvertently.

The scrub person is responsible for establishing and maintaining the integrity, safety, and efficiency of the sterile field throughout the surgical procedure. Knowledge of and experience with aseptic and sterile techniques qualify the scrub person to prepare and arrange instruments and supplies and to facilitate the surgical procedure by providing the required sterile instruments and supplies. The scrub person must anticipate, plan for, and respond to the needs of the surgeon and other team members by constantly watching the sterile field. Manual dexterity and physical stamina are required. Other important assets include a stable temperament, an ability to work under pressure, a keen sense of responsibility, and a concern for accuracy in performing all duties. Box 4-4 describes the physical and psychological attributes required of the scrub person in the sterile scrub role.

Two scrub persons may join the team in teaching situations or during extremely complicated or hazardous surgical procedures. One scrub person may pass instruments and supplies to the surgeon while the other prepares the supplies. Two scrub persons should be assigned if two complete teams are working simultaneously.

An experienced preceptor may join the team to teach, guide, and assist the learner function as a scrub person. When unexpected, unusual, or emergency situations arise, specific instructions and guidance are received from the surgeon or RN. The ST provides services and assists with patient care under the supervision of an RN at all times.

BOX 4-4	**Physical and Psychological Attributes of the Scrub Person's Role**

1. Visual acuity with or without correction is critical to threading small needles and reading small print. Protective eyewear is required at all times when at the surgical field. Bright lights or dim lights are commonly used throughout the surgical procedure, and people with photosensitivity or susceptibility to light-mediated eye irritation will find the OR environment problematic. Visual accuracy is imperative.
2. Manual dexterity and accuracy of motion is required for fast action during emergencies. Inability to coordinate body motions could cause injury to the patient, team, or self. Manual dexterity is imperative.
3. Eye-hand coordination and alertness is essential for safe handling of instruments during surgery. Eye-hand coordination is imperative for the efficiency of the procedure.
4. Ability to delay nutritional intake for prolonged periods during long procedures.
5. Ability to stand in a confined space for prolonged periods.
6. Ability to lift instrument trays of at least 20 pounds and assist with moving large incapacitated patients using proper body mechanics.
7. Auditory acuity in both ears with or without amplification is critical for hearing and understanding commands while machinery is running. Voices are kept low during surgery, especially when the patient is awake. Hearing correctly is imperative.
8. Ability to quickly anticipate and discern commands and needs of the team. Must be able to differentiate between instruments and supplies efficiently and to be able to offer appropriate alternatives in extraordinary circumstances.
9. The ability to speak, understand, and document clearly using the English language is critical to safe patient care. Appropriate terminology and use of approved standard accepted abbreviations are essential to communication in the OR.
10. The ability to remain calm and function quickly, safely, and precisely during an emergency. Must be able to make decisions and problem solve effectively without loss of emotional control.

Some facilities permit RNs or STs privately employed by surgeons to come into the OR to perform the scrub role for their employers. These private scrub persons should adhere to all hospital policies and procedures and to approved written guidelines for the functions they may fulfill. They are not covered under the facility's liability insurance and should carry their own policy as independent contractors. There is no such thing as working under someone else's license such as a physician or a registered nurse. Each person is responsible for personal liability. Further discussion of independent practitioners can be found in Chapter 3.

Private scrub persons can create liability for the facility because the facility will be held liable by virtue of permitting them to work within the facility. They should not perform first assisting or be considered first assistants unless they are appropriately credentialed in the role. Several states have addressed who may and may not first assist in surgery.

STs who have completed an accredited surgical technology program and successfully pass an examination attesting to their theoretic knowledge are certified by the NBSTSA, the main certifying body for STs. These individuals become entitled to use the designator CST after their names. Although a fee is required, a discount is offered by the NBSTSA to members of the Association of Surgical Technologists (AST). Application for the certification exam may be made a soon as 30 days before graduation for the graduating class to apply as a group.

Certification for the CST is valid for 4 years, then must be renewed or it is considered lapsed. Eligibility for CST certification is described in Box 4-5. Renewal can be by either an examination or attainment of 60 continuing education credits. The NBSTSA voted in 2005 to request that AST remove the continuing education renewal requirement that specified categories one, two, and three for credits earned toward renewal of the CST or CFA credential. The NBSTSA believes that this change is necessary for alignment with widely accepted credential-renewal policy standards within the medical, nursing, and allied health professions.

The NBSTSA was concerned about the subjective criteria defining the individual categories and classification of each continuing education program. The emphasis will be placed on determining if credits were earned through a properly approved provider. (New versions of the continuing education forms are available for download from www.ast.org.)

BOX 4-5 | Eligibility for Certified Surgical Technologist (CST) Certification by Examination for Surgical Technologists

Currently or previously certified surgical technology
Graduate of a CAAHEP-accredited surgical technology program
Graduate of an ABHES from the U.S. Department of Health and Human Services. For additional information, visit www.abhes.org.
No minimum practice hour requirement (accredited programs have minimum case number ratings for new graduates)
(Consult www.nbstsa.org for additional information.)

Bibliography

AORN (Association of periOperative Registered Nurses): *Ambulatory surgery principles and practices,* ed 2, Denver, 2002, The Association.
AORN (Association of periOperative Registered Nurses): *Core curriculum for the RN first assistant,* ed 4, Denver, 2005, The Association.
AORN (Association of periOperative Registered Nurses): *Perioperative nursing data set,* ed 2, Denver, 2002, The Association.
AORN (Association of periOperative Registered Nurses): *Standards, recommended practices, and guidelines,* Denver, 2005, The Association.
Association of Surgical Technologists: *Core curriculum for surgical technology,* ed 5, Englewood, Colo, 2002, The Association.
Beyea SC: The ideal state for perioperative nursing, *AORN J* 73(5):897-901, 2001.
Cunningham HH: *Doctors in gray: The confederate medical service,* Baton Rouge, 1958, Louisiana State University Press.
Dock L, Stewart IM: *A short history of nursing,* ed 2, New York, 1929, GP Putnam's Sons.
Espin SL, Lingard LA: Time as a catalyst for tension in nurse-surgeon communication, *AORN J* 74(5):672-679, 2001.
Healy K: *Frances Warde: American founder of the Sisters of Mercy,* New York, 1973, The Seabury Press.
Hewitt J: A critical review of the arguments debating the role of the nurse advocate, *J Adv Nurs* 37(5):439-445, 2002.
Matson K: The critical "nurse" in the circulating nurse role, *AORN J* 73(5):971-975, 2001.
Murphy EK: Who can be called a nurse? *AORN J* 69(6):1238-1242, 1999.
Quinn DM: Schick L: *Perianesthesia nursing care core curriculum,* Philadelphia, 2004, Saunders.
Reeder JM: Patient safety, errors and mistakes, and perioperative nursing, *Semin Periop Nurs* 10(2):115-118, 2001.
Van Cleave C et al: Filling the void created by reductions in nurse staffing, *AORN J* 75(4):829-831, 833-834, 2002.
Weindorfer E, Larkin BG: A critical shortage of surgical technologists creates collaboration between rivals, *AORN J* 81(3):555-562, 2005.
Wood J: Scrub nurse practice: an ethical viewpoint, *Br J Periop Nurs* 12(2):64-67, 2002.

Chapter 5

The Surgical First Assistant

CHAPTER OBJECTIVES

After studying this chapter, the learner will be able to:
- Identify key components of the first assistant's knowledge and skill levels.
- List pertinent perioperative activities of the first assistant.
- Describe the patient care disciplines that with appropriate education function in the role of the first assistant.
- Discuss the legal implications of the first assistant role.

CHAPTER OUTLINE

KEY TERMS AND DEFINITIONS

Anastomosis   Creating a patent connection between two tubular structures by use of suture or specialized staples.

Buzzing a forceps   A method of applying the active electrode of a monopolar cautery against an instrument clamped to the patient's tissue for the purpose of spot hemostasis. The flat side of a metal cautery blade is placed in contact with a clamped instrument below the level of the operator's hand before activation of the current. The edge of a Teflon-coated cautery blade is placed against an instrument clamped to patient's tissue below the level of the operator's hand before activation of the current.

Cleavage lines   Tissue planes where the natural line of tissue growth permits dissection between areas that maintain anatomic structure.

Dissection   Separation of tissue planes by sharp or blunt means.

Dynamic tension   The stress on skin caused by underlying musculature, joints, and body motion.

Hemostasis   Preventing the loss of blood. Stopping the flow of blood.

Incise cut   Scalpel is used in a perpendicular position to slice tissue in a linear direction.

Langer's lines   Natural lines along skin caused by tension inherent in the structure of the dermal-epidermal layers.

Ligation   The act of tying or occluding an anatomic structure.

Palmed   Method of holding an instrument where the working end is nested in the palm of the hand of the assistant while the fingers remain free to grasp other items in the field. The working end can be presented and made functional by a rotation of the wrist. This method can be used for countertraction with some manual retractors.

Perpendicular   The intersection of surfaces at right angles. The scalpel is held perpendicular to the tissue during incision.

Press cut   Scalpel is pushed into the tissue rather than slid to incise. Press cutting can be a form of intentional puncture.

Raising a flap   Perpendicular countertraction is placed on superficial tissues as large areas are undermined by dissection. Care is taken not to disrupt vascularization of the elevated tissue.

Retraction   Displacement of structures by use of the hand or an instrument to expose the surgical site.

Scrape-cut   Scalpel is dragged laterally across tissues to separate cell layers rather than full tissue layers.

Skin tension   The turgor of the skin that is either static or dynamic. Tension factors largely in the final healing of the incision and the appearance of the scar.

Splitting   Separation of muscle tissue along the fascial layers. A form of blunt dissection.

Sponging   A method of providing exposure by removal of blood and fluid from the surgical site. The preferred way to sponge is to blot or pat the area so as not to remove biologic clots.

Static tension   The constant state of skin position over the framework of the body. Also known as Langer's lines.

Suction   Negative pressure used to clear the visual field of blood and body substances. Various styles of tips and tip protectors are used. On occasion, a rigid suction tip can be used to remove fluids and retract tissues simultaneously.

Surgical assistant   Member of the sterile team who provides exposure and hemostasis during a surgical procedure. A physician, RNFA, SA, PA, or CST specially trained and certified as a CFA.

Suture   (verb) The act of sewing tissues; (noun), a thread used for sewing tissue in surgery.

Thenar grip   Method of holding an instrument in which the ring handle is secured in the palm at the base of the thumb instead of placing the thumb through the ring. A small portion of the ring finger may be situated within the opposing ring of the handle.

Traction-countertraction   Displacement of a structure by pulling the tissue in an opposite direction to facilitate sharp or blunt dissection of tissue planes.

Transection   Cutting across natural anatomic lines. Can be done by sharp dissection or electrocoagulation.

Triangulation   Suturing three opposing points of a tubular structure so that the distance between two points can be approximated in a straight line.

Tripod grip   Holding an instrument or scissors in a steady position with the index finger on the box lock hinge and the thumb and ring finger partly in the ring handles for ease of release.

Undermining   Dissection of subsurface tissue planes. Care is taken not to devascularize upper layers of tissue.

HISTORICAL BACKGROUND

In the past, the first assistant to the surgeon ideally was a qualified surgeon or a resident in an accredited surgical education program. It was thought that the first assistant should be capable of assuming responsibility for performing the procedure for the primary surgeon under specific circumstances. The surgeon commonly requested the assistance of an associate physician with whom a surgical practice was shared and to whom part of the patient's care was delegated postoperatively. Complex surgical procedures required more than one surgical team and the services of a first assistant who was proficient in several surgical specialties.

Today in hospitals with accredited postgraduate surgical residency training programs, a surgical resident usually acts as the first assistant. The resident is given increasing responsibilities under supervision of the primary surgeon as he or she develops knowledge and skill. On completion of training, the resident is able to assume responsibility for continuity of surgical patient care. The staff surgeon in charge may delegate the performance of part of a surgical procedure to a resident, provided the surgeon is an active participant throughout the essential part of the operation. The patient should be informed and give consent if a resident will be responsible for surgical treatment.

In community and rural hospitals, surgical residents usually are not available to first-assist in surgery. Experienced professional nurses and other allied health care personnel have been trained to fulfill this role. Nonphysician first assistants are required to complete a formal educational program for first assisting according to their practice discipline. Whether nonphysician first assistants are employed by a surgeon or a health care facility, their practice privileges are based on verifiable credentials that attest to essential knowledge and skills. Legal issues associated with each role are defined by individual state law. Some states require licensure for first assistants.

The intent of the chapter is not to teach first-assisting behaviors but to acquaint the learner with the role and attributes of the professionally educated first assistant.

FIRST ASSISTANT'S KNOWLEDGE AND SKILL LEVEL
Surgical Anatomy and Physiology

The patient's body is a complex biosystem. Every surgical procedure interrupts multiple facets of a patient's anatomic structure and physiologic function. Lack of knowledge about each structure and its function could cause untoward disruption and injury. A single injury will affect many aspects of the patient's outcome and could progress to permanent disability or death. Anatomy and physiology are closely intertwined and should be considered as inseparable components of the whole person.

Knowledge of anatomic structures is critical to the first assistant. Tissue manipulation with instruments requires expert working knowledge of what is grossly seen and what is occluded from view. Improper retraction of tissue that has nervous and vascular structures contained within could cause complications such as neurologic dysfunction or vascular obstruction, resulting in thrombosis or embolization. Lack of this knowledge led to permanent damage to a child's sciatic nerve as documented by *Healthtrust v. Cantrell* in Alabama.[1] In this lawsuit, the surgical technologist, who was performing in the role of surgical first assistant, was unable to identify the location of the sciatic nerve and caused serious injury with a retractor. The surgical technologist stated that he knew how to use retractors and held them where the surgeon placed them. This is an unacceptable and unsafe practice.

The surgical first assistant must absolutely know all the ramifications of every action performed in the role and its effect on the patient's outcome. The actions of the surgical first assistant should reflect the ability to identify all of the normal and abnormal structures in the surgical site and make intelligent, informed decisions about patient safety. Each first assistant is responsible for personal liability. There is no such thing as "working under someone else's license" as commonly misinterpreted by some surgical staff members.

Pharmacology

Medications taken by the patient can cause complications in the perioperative environment. The first assistant should have a clear understanding of each drug the patient takes and its effect on the surgical procedure. Anticoagulants, for example, could cause intraoperative bleeding or postoperative hematoma. Other drugs such as birth control pills can predispose the patient to deep vein thrombosis, which in turn could lead to pulmonary embolism. Patients who take hypoglycemic medication may be predisposed to metabolic problems during the procedure and infections postoperatively. Knowledge of each drug's pharmacologic use and action can help prevent complications throughout the perioperative care period. The first assistant and the circulating nurse should collaborate concerning patient sensitivities and allergies.

Psychomotor Dexterity

Precise, purposeful movement at the sterile field is important for the maintenance of the sterile field and the protection of the patient and team. Many instruments used could cause puncture injury if mishandled, and the resultant contamination could cause transmission of a serious illness such as human immunodeficiency virus (HIV) or hepatitis B or C. Clumsiness can cause instruments to fall from the field to the floor, resulting in damaged equipment. Use of

[1] *Healthtrust v. Cantrell* (689 SO 2d 822 [Ala] 1997).

an item for a purpose other than its intended function can create liability for the facility if someone is harmed.

Efficiency is important to facilitate the procedure. The surgeon relies on the first assistant to help manipulate tissues with instrumentation in both open and endoscopic procedures. For open procedures, the surgical site is visually larger and requires the first assistant to be a "second set of eyes." The surgeon's attention may be focused on a particular organ system, and the first assistant helps by providing exposure and observing for problems in the periphery. For endoscopic procedures, the visual field is limited to the image on the video monitor. The first assistant needs a steady hand when using endoscopic instruments, because even the slightest motion can cause the entire surgical field to shift, placing the patient at risk for injury and causing nausea in team members who are viewing the video monitor. Extreme caution is exercised to prevent injury to tissue not in the direct visual field.

Procedure Knowledge and Techniques

The first assistant needs to know each step that will be encountered during the surgical procedure. It is important to anticipate and think in advance about each step to help the procedure move smoothly. The first assistant should have clear knowledge about not only the functional steps but also the indications for the procedure. Box 5-1 describes the most common indications for a surgical procedure.

When the surgeon incises tissue, the first assistant usually provides a clear field by retraction (traction or counter-traction), sponging, or suction. Some circumstances require the use of hemostatic actions, such as clamping, suturing, cauterizing, or application of some other pharmacologic preparation to stop bleeding.

The surgeon may request the first assistant to "buzz the forceps," which means placing the active electrode against a forceps that is holding patient tissue and delivering electrical current after the tip is in complete contact with the instrument (Fig. 5-1). The gloved hand holding the forceps should have as much contact with the instrument as possible before the current is delivered. This decreases the amount of current passing over the holder's hand and prevents concentration of electricity at a focal point on the hand. The current is delivered below the holder's hand and as close to the actual patient tissue as possible to minimize the risk of alternate current pathway. The forceps is not permitted to touch any other part of the patient's tissue or other instrumentation during this process or the patient will suffer burns to nontarget tissue.

Knowing how and when to perform each action is part of the knowledge base of the first assistant. Random clamping or cautery can cause serious tissue damage.

Surgical Site Management

Management of the surgical site is a crucial part of the successful outcome of the procedure for both physiologic and aesthetic reasons. Physiologically, a surgical site infection could be devastating to the health of the patient and be an incredible cost factor during the recovery period. Aesthetically, the closure is what the patient sees at the end of the procedure and how he or she judges the quality of care.

The first assistant commonly assists in closing the skin and applying dressings or supportive materials, such as casts. Improper technique of closure can lead to poor wound healing and unsightly scarring. Securing drains appropriately facilitates surgical site healing (Fig. 5-2).

BOX 5-1	Common Indications for a Surgical Procedure (with Examples)
Indication	**Example**
Diagnostic	Biopsy
Repair	Hernia
Removal	Hardware or foreign body
Reconstruction	Rebuild
Neoconstruction	Create
Palliation	Temporary relief
Aesthetic	Cosmetic
Harvest/procurement	Organ or graft
Transplant	Organ
Implant	To set in place
Bypass/shunt	Reroute vascular flow
Drainage/evacuation	Abscess
Parturition	Childbirth
Termination	Abortion
Stabilization	Fracture
Extraction	Teeth
Exploration	Open examination
Diversion	Colostomy

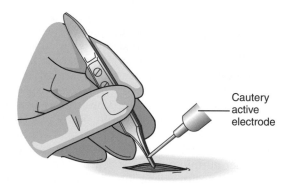

Cautery active electrode

FIG. 5-1 Buzzing the forceps. The active electrode tip is placed against the forceps to deliver current to a specific spot of bleeding.

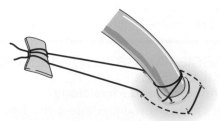

FIG. 5-2 The surgical drain should be secured with a suture.

WHAT DOES THE FIRST ASSISTANT DO?

Position, Prep, and Drape the Patient

The first assistant is frequently responsible for positioning the patient on the table after the anesthesia provider indicates it is safe to do so. In the absence of the first assistant, other members of the team may perform this function. Provision for safe exposure of the surgical site without compromising the physiology of the patient is the key to a successful procedure. Chapter 26 describes the processes for positioning, prepping, and draping the patient.

Handle Instrumentation

The role of the first assistant involves knowledge, skill, and dexterity in handling and using surgical instrumentation. A skilled first assistant can make the role look easy, but in fact his or her skill is reflected by precise action. Fumbling or struggling indicates lack of knowledge and skill in the role. The standard of care for the use of equipment or instrumentation in the role of first assistant includes the following:

- Knowledge of the equipment and instrumentation
- Knowledge of how and when to use the equipment and instrumentation
- Dexterity of holding and using basic instrumentation (Figs. 5-3, 5-4, 5-5, and 5-6)

- Skill in the use or operation of the equipment and machinery
- Knowledge of potential for injury to underlying and surrounding tissues

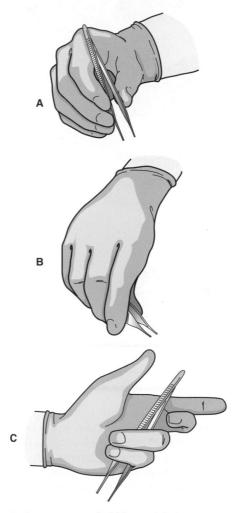

FIG. 5-4 **A,** Correct way to hold forceps. **B,** Incorrect way to hold forceps. **C,** Palming a forceps.

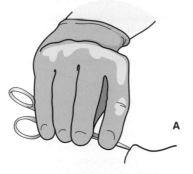
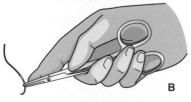
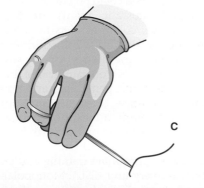

FIG. 5-3 **A,** Holding a needle holder correctly in dorsal view. **B,** Holding a needle holder correctly in palmar view. **C,** Incorrect way to hold a needle holder, with finger in.

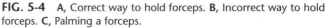
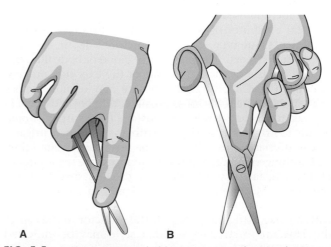

FIG. 5-5 **A,** Correct way to hold scissors, using the tripod grip showing dorsal hand view. **B,** Correct way to hold scissors with tripod grip showing the palmar hand view.

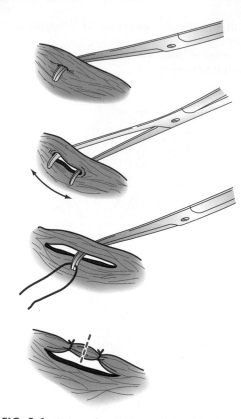

FIG. 5-6   Using a free tie to occlude a blood vessel.

Provide Exposure

Methods of providing exposure include use of rigid and flexible retractors, grasping instruments (e.g., clamps, forceps), Silastic bands (e.g., vessel loops), rubber drains (e.g., Penrose), umbilical tapes, Raytec sponges, laparotomy tapes, suture traction, plastic isolation bags (bowel bags), and suction, as well as by direct hand positioning. More recent technology includes the use of saline and carbon dioxide mister/blower to keep the field clear of blood during "off pump" cardiac bypass grafting. Care is taken not to introduce an air bolus into an open vessel.

The method used to provide exposure is carefully selected. Physical attributes of the patient are considered, such as body size, tissue type, adjacent structures, depth, and type of exposure needed. The presence of blood or body fluid can require the use of suction as part of the exposure process. Prolonged need for surgical exposure may require the use of a self-retaining retractor as possible. Whenever tissues are exposed to air for extended periods, the first assistant should be sure to irrigate the site lightly with an appropriate irrigant.

Use of manual retractors can be physically demanding, and prolonged use can contribute to repetitive stress injuries of the assistant's wrist and arm causing carpal tunnel syndrome. Most retractors are designed to be held in an ergonomic fashion and do not require the forces associated with a tense, struggling grasp. If the retractor in use causes the assistant to struggle, another style may be indicated for use.

Suction should be used with caution. Evacuation of fluids to clear the field of vision should be done in a manner that is not injurious to adjacent structures. The direct force of the vacuum against tissues can cause suction lesions that can become inflamed and necrose. Blind suctioning should be avoided because organs such as the spleen could be perforated and cause hemorrhage.

Provide Hemostasis

Prevention of active bleeding and blood loss is a major part of every surgical procedure. The surgeon takes great care to avoid vessels and organs during dissection, because blood and body fluids obscure vision in the surgical field and the loss of blood is a detriment to the patient. Unfortunately, some maneuvers during the procedure cause bleeding, and this bleeding must be cleared and controlled. The clearing of the field is part of the exposure process, but the control of bleeding and blood loss is referred to as hemostasis.

Methods and mechanisms of hemostasis are described in detail in Chapter 28, but a brief description is provided here for first assistant role description.

Hemostasis is provided by mechanical, chemical, or thermal means. The decision of which to use at a given point in a procedure requires significant knowledge and skill. Examples of each method include but are not limited to the following:

1. Manual hemostasis. Direct pressure over a part; indirect pressure adjacent to a part.
   a. Clip (metallic, plastic, temporary, permanent, absorbable)
   b. Suture (suture ligature, free tie) (see Fig. 5-6)
   c. Clamp and tie (hemostat: crushing or noncrushing) (Fig. 5-7)
   d. Tourniquet (Rummel vascular sliding occlusion, vessel loop, umbilical tape, Penrose drain, pneumatic tourniquet). Occlusion of the circulation should be held to the least amount of time possible to prevent tissue damage.
   e. Hand and/or fingers over area to create pressure. Directly hold or blot sponge over site. Do not wipe off the newly formed clot; doing so will cause bleeding to resume.
2. Chemical hemostasis. Agent is placed over localized bleeding surface to control active bleeding. Care is taken not to allow the material to be introduced into the systemic circulation. Hemostatic materials should not be permitted to contaminate blood salvage systems. The returned blood could potentially cause an embolus. Chemical hemostatic agents are topical (liquid, gelatin sponge, collagen fibers or sponge, cellulose, fibrin glue, or albumin). Epinephrine is commonly added to local anesthetics for its vasoconstrictive properties. (This is contraindicated in small distal vessels of the digits, penis, ears, and nose.)
3. Thermal hemostasis. Electrosurgical units or lasers are the most common means of thermal hemostasis. Safety is a critical factor in the use of such equipment. Personnel using thermal hemostatic devices should have appropriate training and credentials.
   a. Electrosurgery unit (ESU). Monopolar requires the use of return electrode on the patient. Active electrode can be touched directly to tissue or to a forceps holding a segment of tissue. Enhanced monopolar

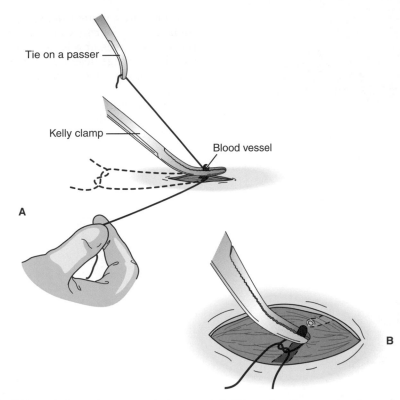

FIG. 5-7 **A,** Using a clamp to occlude a vessel. **B,** Using a free tie around a clamped vessel.

units may have argon beam (argon gas) coagulation properties that are useful for large bleeding surfaces. The tip of the argon beam coagulator is not touched directly to the bleeding surface because it can clog. The argon gas is nonflammable and is used to clear blood away as the current flows across the bleeding surface.

   b. Laser. Extreme caution is exercised at all times during laser use. Eyewear of the appropriate optical density is worn by everyone, including the patient. The environment should not support inadvertent injury by any stray laser light.

Handle Tissue

The first assistant should always be aware of each tissue type and the appropriate means by which to handle it. All tissue should be handled with care, using the fewest instruments possible. Knowledge of the instrumentation and its intended use is critical. Some instruments are considered crushing and should not be used to handle delicate lumens. Skin edges can be crushed by inappropriate grasping with a forceps (Fig. 5-8).

Dissection

The first assistant should be familiar with and skillful in methods of tissue dissection. Procurement of vascular conduit or preparing kidneys for transplant requires the first assistant to know sharp and blunt methods of separating tissue. Sharp methods require the use of a scalpel or scissors (Figs. 5-9 and 5-10). Blunt methods commonly use dull edges of instruments or a sponge-covered finger (Fig. 5-11).

Suture

The first assistant may be required to suture (Fig. 5-12) and cut suture (Fig. 5-13) during and at the end of the procedure. Suturing can entail the use of conventional suture material and needles, metallic or absorbable clips, staplers, wound tape strips, wound glue, wire, and other materials for joining tissue. Intraoperative suturing is performed for hemostasis, stabilization of a part, traction, or other tissue manipulation. At the end of the procedure the incision is closed by a closure method using one of the devices just mentioned.

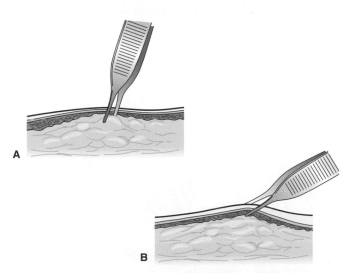

FIG. 5-8 **A,** Correct way to grasp subcutaneous tissue with forceps. **B,** Incorrect way to grasp tissue by crushing the dermis and epidermis in the jaws of the forceps.

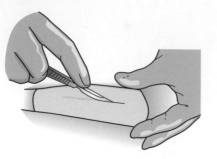

FIG. 5-9 Using a scalpel to create incision with right hand and exerting traction with the left.

Knot tying requires extensive practice and skill (Fig. 5-14). An insecure knot can lead to an obstructed view during the procedure if bleeding is not controlled and to postoperative hemorrhage leading to hematoma. Knot tying for conventional surgery is performed by one of the following methods:
- Two-handed tie (Fig. 5-15)
- Instrument tie (Fig. 5-16)
- One-handed tie (Fig. 5-17)

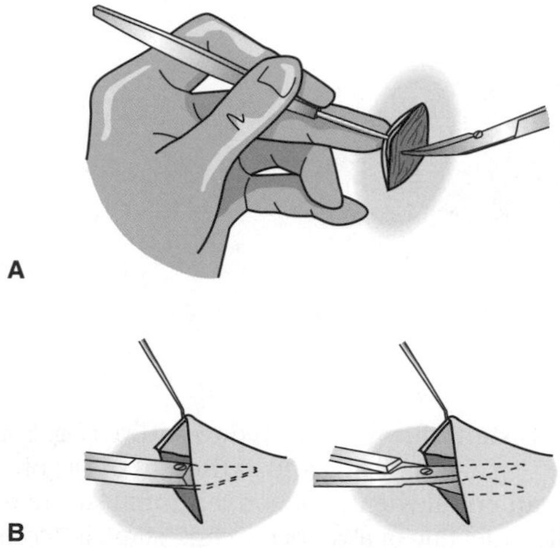

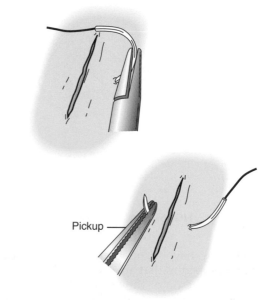

FIG. 5-12 Correct way to introduce the suture needle into the skin.

Pickup

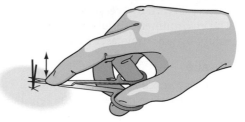

FIG. 5-10 Techniques for undermining the skin with scissors. **A,** Skin is peeled back over the left middle finger. Edge is held by delicate skin hook retractor. Scissors are used to nip at subcutaneous tissue. **B,** Closed scissors are placed under the skin at the incision line. **C,** Scissors are opened and spread to first bluntly dissect and separate tissues with the outer edge of blades. Sharp dissection can be used secondarily from within the pocket of dissection.

FIG. 5-13 Correct way to cut suture.

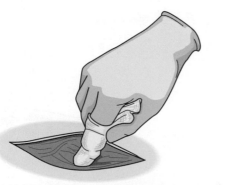

FIG. 5-11 Blunt dissection using a gauze sponge over the first finger.

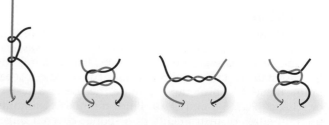

FIG. 5-14 Types of knots used in surgical procedures.

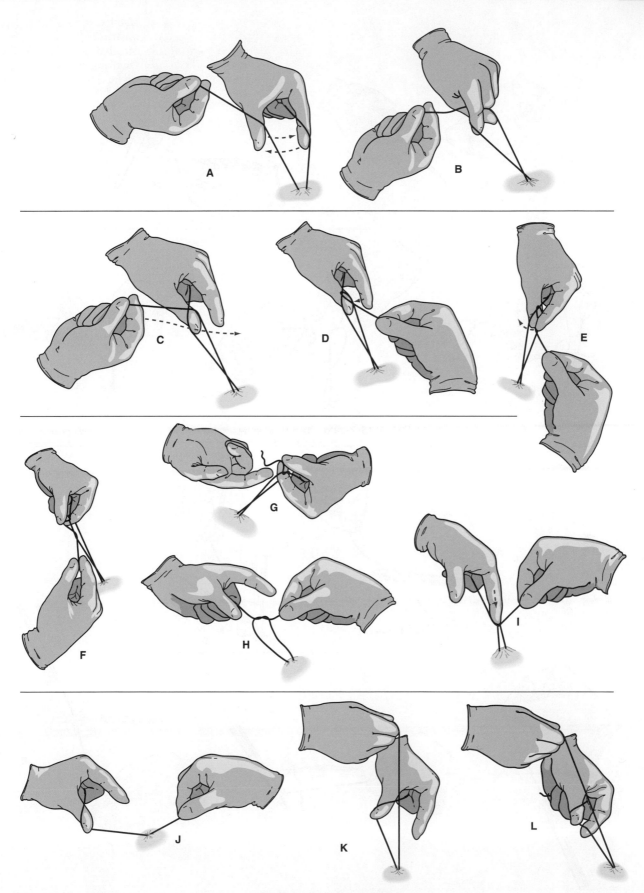

FIG. 5-15 Two-handed tie.

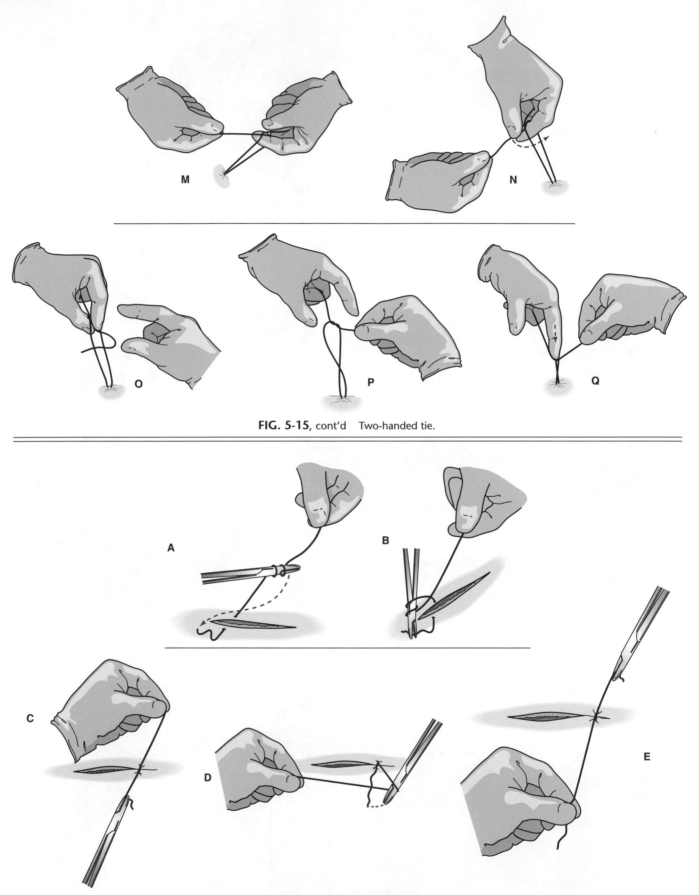

FIG. 5-15, cont'd   Two-handed tie.

FIG. 5-16   Instrument tie.

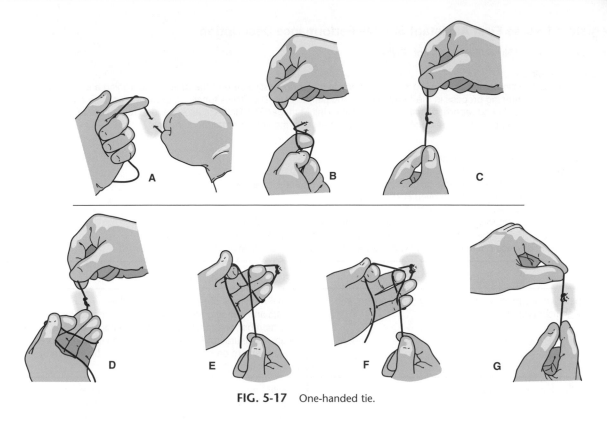

FIG. 5-17   One-handed tie.

Recognize Surgical Hazards

Surgical hazards are described in Chapter 13. The first assistant works with the surgeon and the rest of the team to provide a safe environment. Every step of the procedure requires diligence and care. The first assistant should be able to identify potential hazards and prevent them. Should an untoward event occur, the first assistant should know the steps to take to resume a safe environment. Primary hazards are biologic, physical, and chemical. Each hazard has a multitude of manifestations. Examples of hazards include but are not limited to the following:

- Biologic hazards. Exposure to contamination by both the patient and the team
- Physical hazards. Risk for needlestick injury, fire, tissue damage
- Chemical hazards. Medications, prep solution, sterilants

Respond Appropriately to Emergency Situations

The first assistant should be credentialed in cardiopulmonary resuscitation (CPR), preferably at the advanced cardiac life support (ACLS) level. The first assistant is a key member of the team during lifesaving procedures.

Patient Assessment

The assessment of the patient is an ongoing activity practiced by all the professionals rendering direct care. The advanced practice first assistant is master's prepared and has extensive education in physiology. Some states have granted prescriptive privileges to particular disciplines that participate in perioperative patient care. Orders written by first assistant personnel are cosigned by the surgeon or anesthesiologist; an exception is the nurse practitioner writing a prescription permitted under the authority of his or her own state.[2] Nurse practitioners have a number assigned by the U.S. Drug Enforcement Agency (DEA) that is to be included with the written prescription.

DISCIPLINES ASSOCIATED WITH FIRST-ASSISTING IN SURGERY

Registered Nurse First Assistant (RNFA)

A CNOR who has successfully completed a Competency & Credentialing Institute (CCI)–approved program based on the Core Curriculum for the Registered Nurse First Assistant of AORN (Association of periOperative Registered Nurses) may seek a position as an RNFA with a private surgeon, hospital, or clinic. The RNFA functions under the direct supervision of a surgeon. The RNFA functions solely as the first assistant and should not simultaneously perform the functions of a scrub nurse. A sample performance description is shown in Figure 5-18. The qualifications to function as a first assistant should include but are not limited to the following:

- Demonstrated competency in both scrub and circulating nurse roles for a minimum of 2 years
- Knowledge and skill in applying the principles of aseptic and sterile techniques to ensure infection control

---

[2] Byrne W: U.S. nurse practitioner prescribing law: a state-by-state summary, *Medscape Nurses* 4(2), 2002, Medscape.

Registered Nurse First Assistant Sample Performance Description

Job Title: Registered Nurse First Assistant (RNFA)

Purpose of Position:
Assist under the direction of the primary operating surgeon in the perioperative care of the patient undergoing a surgical experience. The RNFA uses the nursing process in the formulation of the plan of care. The RNFA functions within the policies and guidelines established by the facility and reports directly to the Surgical Unit Manager. The RNFA is an expanded role of the registered nurse and is accountable for exemplifying leadership and professionalism in the implementation of the role.

Qualifications:
1. Graduate of accredited school of nursing
2. Licensed to practice in the state of Ohio
3. Minimum of 24 months perioperative experience, both scrubbing and circulating
4. Satisfactory completion of CCI approved RNFA program
5. Certification in perioperative nursing (CNOR)
6. Certified in cardiopulmonary resuscitation, basic life-saver BCLS (CPR-ACLS preferred)
7. Accumulation of 125 contact hours of continuing education every 5 years to maintain CNOR status.
8. BSN and 2000 practice hours in role of RNFA if planning certification (CRNFA) credential with CCI.

Functions:	Satisfactory Performance:
1. Preoperative assessment and teaching of the patient and family (significant other)	1. RNFA reviews objective and subjective data. Is aware of lab results and pending tests. The assessment includes the patient as a member of a family unit and a member of society. RNFA is aware of cultural and personal influences in the interpretation of assessment data. RNFA communicates findings to the primary surgeon.
2. Formulation of nursing diagnoses	2. RNFA interprets the assessment data and plans care appropriate to the pending surgical procedure. RNFA collaborates with the primary surgeon and others to facilitate the pending surgical procedure and the attainment of favorable patient outcomes.
3. Recognizes potential hazards and initiates corrective action	3. RNFA is aware of the environment observing for potential sources of injury to self, team, and the patient. RNFA practices universal precautions at all times and is in observance of OSHA regulations.
4. Practices within the guidelines established by the state of Ohio	4. RNFA:
	a. Handles tissue
	b. Provides exposure
	c. Uses instrumentation
	d. Sutures
	e. Provides hemostasis
	f. Closes tissue and skin
	Prohibitions:
	a. May not perform the intended procedure
	b. May not perform the task of the surgeon
	c. Does not simultaneously function as scrub nurse

FIG. 5-18   Sample performance description for registered nurse first assistant.

5. Demonstrates intraoperative competency as an RNFA	5. Knowledge:
	a. Principles of asepsis and infection control
	b. Surgical anatomy and physiology
	c. Surgical procedures
	d. Recognizes hazards and effects safety measures
	Skill:
	a. Manual dexterity
	b. Suturing and ligating
	c. Providing hemostasis
	d. Exposing the surgical site
	e. Positioning, prepping, and draping
6. Continuous assessment of the patient during the intraoperative phase of the surgical experience	6. RNFA observes condition of patient and initiates emergency measures as needed.
7. Postoperative assessment, evaluation and teaching	7. RNFA accompanies the patient to the postoperative unit as needed and communicates with the patient and family (significant other) as designated by the primary surgeon. RNFA, in collaboration with the primary surgeon and others, evaluates the attainment of expected outcomes.
8. Communicates postoperative information as directed by primary surgeon	8. Writes orders as per policy for verbal orders with the co-signature of the primary surgeon.
9. Adheres to institutional policies and procedures reflecting attendance, registered nurse professional responsibility, standards of care, and communication through chain of command	9. Observes institutional policy and practices the art and science of registered nursing in the expanded role of the RNFA

FIG. 5-18, cont'd   Sample performance description for registered nurse first assistant.

- Knowledge of surgical anatomy, physiology, fluid and electrolyte balance, acid-base regulation, clinical pathology, and wound healing because these factors relate to surgical procedures
- Comprehension of risk factors and potential intraoperative complications and knowledge of actions to minimize them
- Technical skill and manual dexterity in handling tissue, providing exposure, using instruments and devices, providing hemostasis, tying sutures and knots, and applying dressings
- Ability to recognize safety hazards and initiate appropriate preventive and corrective actions
- Ability to perform cooperatively and effectively with other team members
- Ability to perform effectively in stressful and emergency situations
- CNOR is maintained. A minimum of 125 contact hours of continuing education is required, or the nurse can retake the CNOR examination
- Certification in cardiopulmonary resuscitation (basic cardiac life support or advanced life support preferred)
- Completion of formal CCI-approved RNFA program based on the *AORN Core Curriculum for the RN First Assistant*

Since 1995 the role of the RNFA is recognized in all states as being within the scope of nursing practice as an expanded role of the perioperative nurse. Credentialing as an RNFA is controlled by individual state boards of nursing.

Voluntary certification is attained by successfully passing a national examination. The CCI has developed a national certification examination for the eligible RNFA that includes the following requirements:
- Licensed as registered nurse (RN) in the United States
- Bachelor of science in nursing (BSN) or master of science in nursing (MSN) degree
- CNOR or certification in advanced practice nursing
- Completion of a CCI-approved RNFA program based on the AORN *Core Curriculum for the RNFA*
- 2000 hours of first-assisting experience during a period of 5 years. 500 hours must be within 2 years of taking the certification exam. Documentation of 2000 hours must be included with the application.

- 1400 hours must be in the intraoperative role; 600 hours may be in preoperative or postoperative settings.
- Documentation of clinical competency[3]

After meeting all requirements and successfully passing the certification examination, a certified RNFA may use the title certified registered nurse first assistant (CRNFA). The CRNFA may recertify every 5 years by contact hours or by examination. Eligibility for recertification includes maintenance of CNOR status and documentation of active clinical practice as an RNFA with continued clinical competency for the 2-year period preceding the recertification date. A combination of clinical practice hours or points and continued education can be used for recertification. Box 5-2 describes recertification through combined methods.

For ease of processing, the certifications for CNOR and CRNFA were merged in January 1998 to allow recertification at the same intervals. The requirement for the combination recertification is 200 contact hours every 5 years; 100 of these hours must be RNFA-specific. (More information is available at www.cc-institute.org.) Academic hours earned toward a baccalaureate or higher degree may be applied toward certification. Up to 62.5 academic-based contact hours can be applied toward recertification. The conversion formula for academic hours to contact hours is as follows:

- 1 semester hour equals 15 contact hours
- 1 quarter hour equals 10 contact hours

Certified Nurse Midwife

Certified nurse midwives (CNMs) are credentialed to provide perinatal care. The CNM is a master's prepared RN who has been licensed and credentialed by the state board of nursing in his or her practice locale. The scope of practice includes antenatal care, gynecologic care, parturition care, and postnatal care. The CNM works with female patients in wellness centers, preventive settings, and childbirth. Occasionally a pregnant patient will present with complications requiring cesarean delivery. Usually the CNM has been with the patient throughout labor and is present when the determination is made to perform a surgical delivery. The surgically trained CNM can shorten the interval wait for additional surgical staff to arrive by first assisting in the cesarean birth.

The CNM works collaboratively with an obstetrician who performs the surgical procedure. Most states permit the CNM who has had appropriate additional training to function in the role of first assistant in the cesarean procedure. Training includes surgical anatomy, procedure steps, suturing, and the safe use of surgical instruments. This does not qualify the CNM as a fully credentialed RNFA for all procedures—only those procedures associated with the female reproductive system during childbirth. Some CNMs are first-assisting during gynecologic procedures on nonpregnant patients. The CNM does not meet the requirements for certification as an RNFA unless an approved RNFA course has been completed. The CNM in the first

BOX 5-2	CRNFA Recertification Requires That the CNOR Credential Is Maintained

Clinical practice hours and contact hours. Half of the contact hours must be RNFA specific:

1000 clinical practice hours (at least 700 hours must be intraoperative care) and 200 contact hours

500 clinical practice hours (at least 350 hours must be intraoperative care) and 300 contact hours

Clinical practice hours and points:

1000 clinical practice hours (at least 700 hours must be intraoperative care) and 400 points

500 clinical practice hours (at least 350 hours must be intraoperative care) and 500 points

Recertification by examination:

1000 clinical practice hours to recertify by exam; 700 hours must be intraoperative care.

assistant role in the cesarean section provides continuity of care with his or her patient population.

This role is supported by the American College of Nurse-Midwives (ACNM), the American College of Obstetricians and Gynecologists (ACOG), and the American College of Surgeons (ACS). Some state boards of nursing prohibit the CNM from first assisting. They state that the CNM must also meet the same educational requirements as an RNFA to be permitted to first assist. (More information is available at www.acnm.org.)

Physician Assistant

The medical staff may approve privileges for an allied health care professional referred to as a physician assistant (PA) who is qualified by academic and clinical training to first-assist in the operating room (OR) and function in other areas of perioperative patient care. The extent of a PA's practice is defined by state law, facility policy, and preference of the employing physician. Prescription authority has been granted at various levels in 48 states.

Most students entering PA school have at least 4 years of health care experience and a minimum of a bachelor's degree.[4] Many PA programs are housed within medical schools, and their graduates are referred to as physician extenders. The first 2 years of the program are accomplished in the same classes with the medical students. The clinical component of their education includes 2000 clinical hours, and practice requirements include registration or licensure by the state wherein they practice. The role of the PA evolved in the late 1960s and now incorporates 134 accredited programs throughout the United States that incorporate 26 months of PA education.

Physician assistant is a generic term with two subcategories: the assistant to the primary care physician in the clinical area; and the first assistant to the surgeon. The PA who functions as a first assistant in surgery is required to have surgical training in addition to the baseline PA education. The surgical education process usually encompasses

---

[3] Jane Rothrock has described competencies for RNFAs in basic practice and advanced practice. Competency Assessment and Competence Acquisition: The advanced practice nurse as RN surgical first assistant, Medscape. Accessed April, 2005. www.medscape.com

[4] Navsaria D: *NPs and PAs: working with you, Medscape Med Students* 4(1), 2002, Medscape Portals, Inc. www.medscape.com

six semesters of clinical surgical experience. Eligibility for acceptance by the medical staff either as a PA or a surgical assistant (SA) is determined by the following criteria:

- Exercising critical thinking within areas of competence, with the physician member of the medical staff having the ultimate responsibility for patient care
- Participating directly in the management of patients under the supervision or direction of a member of the medical staff
- Documenting progress notes on patients' medical records and writing orders to the extent established by the medical staff
- Writing limited prescriptions in 47 states, Guam, and the District of Columbia. The educational requirement is a minimum of 78 credit hours in pharmacology.
- Performing direct patient care in conformity with applicable provisions of medical staff bylaws, which may include obtaining medical histories and performing physical examinations

The SA performs duties under the direct supervision of a surgeon, who maintains the direct responsibility for the patient. The assistant may perform tasks delegated by the surgeon for the care of patients in any setting for which the surgeon assumes responsibility. The SA education program has an intense intraoperative focus.

After completion of a formal Commission on Accreditation of Allied Health Education Programs/Accreditation Review Committee on Education for the Physician Assistant (CΛΛHEP/ARC-PA)–accredited academic program, the PA or SA should attain national certification by taking the Physician Assistant National Certifying Exam (PA-C). Recertification period is 6 years and includes a 100-hour continuing education requirement every 2 years. The medical staff bylaws delineate the practice privileges of the assistant within the hospital. Reimbursement for services is made to the PA's employer. Medicare reimburses at 85% of the physician's fee schedule for clinical care and 13.6% of the surgeon's fee for first assisting in surgery. The PA's reimbursement is paid directly to the employer whether it is a private physician practice or a hospital surgical department. More information is available at www.aapa.org. (Specific questions can be addressed by e-mail at aapa@aapa.org.)

Surgical Technologist

A certified surgical technologist (CST) may also be trained to first-assist in a program of study approved by the Association of Surgical Technologists (AST). An associate's degree should be the minimal entry-level requirement for CSTs who enter a postgraduate first-assisting program as described by the certifying and accrediting bodies for surgical technology. For CSTs with at least 2 years of first assisting experience during the previous 4 years, a national first-assisting certification examination is available from the National Board of Surgical Technology and Surgical Assisting (NBSTSA). After successfully passing this

examination, the CST first assistant may use the initials CST/CFA.

At the time of original certification as a CFA, the CST time period of the certification is adjusted to be of the same duration as the CFA portion of the certification. Both aspects of the certification will be adjusted for the same period of 6 years. Recertification as a CST/CFA is accomplished by providing documentation of practicing as a CST/CFA for 2 years of the 6-year certification period and by obtaining 100 continuing education credits in the categories defined by the NBSTSA. Another option is to document 2 years of practice as a first assistant within the 6-year period and take the certification examination again.

Several states have indicated that first assisting is not within the realm of the surgical technologist. The surgical technologist should not first-assist unless he or she has attended a formal training program. Holding retractors inappropriately can cause serious injury and should not be taken lightly. (More information is available at www.ast.org.)

Bibliography

American College of Nurse-Midwives: *The midwife as first assistant handbook*, Washington, DC, 2001, The Association.

Biggins J: The role of the RNSA in colorectal and general surgery, *Br J Periop Nurs* 12(6):222-226, 2002.

Edwards C, Keeley O: Competency-based learning for the surgical assistant, *Nurs Stand* 12(20):44-47, 1998.

Fazzino D: Integrating the independent RNFA into health care institutions, *SSM* 6(9):48-51, 2000.

Firlit BM et al: Registered nurse first assistant competencies, *AORN J* 76(4):671-679, 2002.

Franko FP: Providers of first assisting services, *AORN J* 79(6): 1311-1318, 2004.

Gavin M et al: Physician assistants: many general practitioners would welcome having physician assistants, *BMJ* 324(7339):735-736, 2002.

Grzybicki DM et al: The economic benefit for family and general medicine practices employing physician assistants, *Am J Manag Care* 8(7):613-620, 2002.

Homan T, Dunscombe A: Marketing the RN first assistant role, *AORN J* 72(2):234-240, 2000.

Huchinson L: The physician assistant: would the US model meet the needs of the NHS? *BMJ* 323(7323):1244-1247, 2001.

Ilton S: Perioperative nursing: the benefits of registered nurse first assistant practice, *Can Nurse* 98(6):22-27, 2002.

Mills AC, McSweeney M: Nurse practitioners and physician assistants revisited: Do their practice patterns differ in ambulatory care? *J Prof Nurs* 18(1):36-46, 2002.

Moes C, Thacher F: The midwife as first assistant for cesarean section, *J Midwifery Womens Health* 46(5):305-312, 2001.

Romig CL: AORN set for certified RN first assistant Medicare reimbursement in the new year, *AORN J* 71(2):414, 417-419, 2000.

Rothrock JC: *The RN first assistant: An expanded perioperative nursing role*, ed 3, Philadelphia, 1999, Lippincott.

Tanner J: First assistant activities, *Br J Periop Nurs* 11(4):172-178, 2001.

Vaiden RE et al: *Core curriculum for the RN first assistant*, ed 3, Denver, 2000, Association of periOperative Registered Nurses.

Wiley MJ: Is your practice staffed correctly? *Med Econ* 79(12):66-68, 73, 2002.

Chapter 6

Administration of Perioperative Patient Care Services

CHAPTER OBJECTIVES

After studying this chapter, the learner will be able to:
- Define the role of the perioperative management team.
- Describe the relationship between the perioperative environment and other patient care departments.
- Define the role of intradepartmental surgical services committees.
- Facilitate mediation in conflict resolution.

CHAPTER OUTLINE

KEY TERMS AND DEFINITIONS

Administrator   Person who directs or manages departmental affairs; may be a nurse or physician.

Capital budget   Monies for larger purchases that have lasting use implications for a time-defined period. Some items will depreciate over time and will need replacement as technologies change.

Committee   A group within the organization that is assembled to perform a specific task.

Evidence-based practice   A procedure or activity that is validated by scientific proof in a clinical setting.

Inservice education   Departmental programs designed to introduce or demonstrate equipment, techniques, or procedures used in perioperative patient care.

Learning organization   The functional group that includes all personnel involved with the facility. The organization needs to be able to learn from experience and the environment if it is to survive and grow. Stagnation and inflexibility are costly and a main cause of failure and financial loss.

Manager   Person who plans and executes directives passed down from administration.

Materials   Supplies, such as reusable or disposable goods, ordered and maintained in stock for departmental use in patient care.

Operational budget   Monies appropriated for the costs of doing day-to-day business.

Sacred cow   A practice that continues despite lack of scientific evidence or validation by evidence-based practice.

Systems thinking   A process by which the learning organization collectively examines practices and processes during the analysis of root causes. This mechanism examines long-term activity, not just one single change. It is a circular process of business and people skills.

HISTORICAL BACKGROUND

ESTABLISHING ADMINISTRATIVE ROLES

The perioperative patient care team surrounds the patient throughout the perioperative experience. This direct perioperative patient care team functions within the physical confines of the operating room (OR). This room is one part of the physical facilities that make up the total perioperative environment. Other areas in the perioperative environment include preadmission testing (PAT), the ambulatory services unit (ASU), and the postanesthesia care unit (PACU). Similarly, this team makes up only one part of the human activity directed toward the care of the surgical patient. Many other people function in an indirect relationship with the patient, contributing vital supporting services toward the common goal of ensuring a safe, comfortable, and effective perioperative environment.

The relationship and duties of perioperative staff members vary according to the size and extent of the physical facilities and the number of personnel employed. No person's job is insignificant. Each has important functions to perform, and each is responsible for assuming a part of the total workload.

The purpose of this chapter is to acquaint the perioperative staff with the role of the management team and the nature of the job they have to perform. This is not a "how-to" chapter on management, but a descriptive collection of structural and elemental components of the underpinnings of a surgical services department. This chapter could serve to create ideas or a conceptual framework for a new manager in the OR. Many article reviews and up-to-date notices for managers can be found at www.ssmonline.org. This is a leadership-based managerial website created by the Association of periOperative Registered Nurses (AORN), with a link that allows for email notification of updates. This keeps the manager informed of many new developments in the perioperative arena. (Other concerns for managers such as safety and efficiency can be explored at www.leapfroggroup.org, which offers many topics of interest to administrators, managers, and staff.)

Perioperative Administrative Personnel

Personnel should know the direction of the entire organizational effort as a prerequisite for their successful functioning. Administrative personnel interpret hospital and departmental philosophy, objectives, policies, and procedures to the perioperative staff. These terms are defined as follows:

1. Philosophy. Statement of beliefs regarding patient care and the nature of perioperative nursing that clarifies the overall responsibilities to be fulfilled.
2. Objectives. Statements of specific goals and purposes to be accomplished during the course of action and definitions of criteria for acceptable performance.
3. Policies. Specific authoritative statements of governing principles or actions, within the context of the philosophy and objectives, that assist in decision making by providing guidelines for action to be taken or, in some situations, for what is not to be done.

   a. Basic policies. Statements of the principles of administration and its approach to functioning. Examples include disallowing smoking by anyone on facility premises.
   b. General policies. Guidelines of the principles dealing with everyday situations that affect all personnel within the hospital. Examples include requiring all personnel, regardless of role, to be certified in cardiopulmonary resuscitation (CPR).
   c. Departmental policies. Guidelines structured to meet the needs of a specific work unit (e.g., OR policies). Examples include dress codes for specific areas.
4. Procedures. Statements of task- and skill-oriented actions to be taken in the implementation of policies.

Perioperative Nurse Manager

In most accredited facilities a registered nurse (RN) is responsible for administration and supervision of all perioperative patient care services. The perioperative environment is a business unit and high-cost center of the hospital. It should be managed as a business to manage costs and maintain effectiveness. Therefore the title and functions of the perioperative nurse manager reflect the extent and complexity of the administrative responsibilities.

In larger hospitals the perioperative nurse manager may hold some variation of the title of director of perioperative services or assistant vice president. Because of the magnitude of the administrative duties, actual supervision of personnel may be delegated to a line manager or charge nurse. In smaller hospitals where administrative responsibilities are not as time consuming, the perioperative nurse manager directly supervises personnel. In other situations one nurse may manage more than one clinical service, such as the OR, PACU, ASU, special procedures room, and/or central processing department. The term *manager* is used throughout this text to designate the perioperative nurse who is responsible for coordinating patient care and related support services of the department.

The perioperative nurse manager should have general knowledge of nursing theory and practice, specialized knowledge of OR technique and management, and knowledge of business and financial management. The manager should possess leadership skills to supervise and direct patient care within the perioperative environment according to established principles and professional standards. The main function of the manager is to provide leadership that promotes a cooperative team effort. To be a leader requires additional business skills and knowledge. These concern functions of management that include planning, organizing, staffing, directing, and controlling, plus the processes of problem solving, decision making, coordinating, and communicating.

The manager is responsible for the allocation and completion of work but does not do it all or make all of the decisions. Qualified personnel are employed, and they are delegated increasing responsibility as they develop competence in their work. The manager creates an organizational attitude that can function well in his or her absence.

The manager implements and enforces hospital and departmental policies and procedures. He or she also analyzes and evaluates continuously all patient care services rendered and, through participation in research, seeks to improve the quality of patient care given. The manager retains accountability for all related activities in the perioperative environment. The scope of this accountability includes the following:

- Provision of competent staff and supportive services adequately prepared to achieve quality patient care objectives
- Delegation of responsibilities to professional nurses and assignment of duties to other patient care personnel
- Responsibility for evaluating the performance of all departmental personnel and for assessing and continuously improving the quality of care and services
- Provision of educational opportunities to increase knowledge and skills of all personnel
- Coordination of administrative duties to ensure proper functioning of staff
- Provision and fiscal control of materials, supplies, and equipment
- Coordination of activities between the perioperative environment and other departments
- Creation of an atmosphere that fosters teamwork and provides job satisfaction for all staff members
- Identification of problems and resolution of them in a decisive, timely manner
- Initiation of data collection and analyses to develop effective systems and to monitor efficiency and productivity

Clinical Coordinator

An assistant nurse manager aids in administration and supervision of nursing service in the OR and is directly responsible to the perioperative nurse manager. This nurse acts as administrative head in the absence of the manager. The position usually does not exist in small hospitals. In large hospitals one or more clinical coordinators provide leadership to specific services and assist with the management of manpower and material resources.

Head Nurse or Charge Nurse

The head nurse or charge nurse functions in a line management position as a liaison between staff members and administrative personnel. In some hospitals the title of head nurse is given to the person whose position is comparable to that of a coordinator. In others, usually smaller hospitals, the perioperative nurse manager functions more or less in the capacity of a head nurse, so for simplicity, the term *head nurse* will be used to refer to this role.

In large hospitals with many surgical specialty services, a head nurse may be responsible for the administration and direct supervision of patient care in a particular specialty service, such as ophthalmology, neurosurgery, cardiovascular surgery, or urology. With this structure, several head nurses are in the department. These head nurses should have the technical proficiency required for the specialty service for which they are responsible and should have sufficient managerial ability to plan for and administer effectively the patient care activities.

The duties of the head nurse include, but are not limited to, the following:

- Planning for and supervising patient care activities within the OR suite or specific room(s) to which he or she is assigned
- Coordinating patient care activities with the surgeons and anesthesia providers
- Maintaining adequate supplies and equipment and providing for their economical use
- Observing the performance of all staff members and providing feedback
- Interpreting the policies and procedures adopted by the department and hospital administration
- Informing the perioperative manager of needs and problems arising in the department and assisting with problem solving
- Assisting with orientation of new staff members

Functions vary in different hospitals, but the position of head nurse, with its direct and continuous responsibility for both patients and staff, is an important one.

Perioperative Business Manager

Some hospitals employ a perioperative business manager, who sometimes has the title of unit manager. This person may report to the perioperative manager or directly to the hospital administrator. Lines of authority and responsibility between the business manager and the perioperative nurse manager should be clearly defined regardless of the organizational structure. The business manager directs the management of daily operational and indirect patient care functions in the perioperative environment.

Non-nursing administrative duties should include maintaining a clean, orderly, safe environment within the department for patients and personnel. This entails more than removing visible dust and dirt.

A safe environment is one that is free of contamination, electrical and fire hazards, and negligence. Formulation of procedures is necessary. Personnel should be trained. However, inspection and follow-up are equally important. The business manager coordinates these efforts with the supporting service departments: housekeeping, maintenance, laundry, and materials management.

A business manager may prepare and administrate the department budget. Doing so may include maintaining inventories and evaluating supplies and equipment. If the hospital does not employ a business manager, the nurse manager or coordinator assumes responsibility for these duties.

Advanced Practice Nurse

Within any organization a formal structure of authority and responsibility exists. However, the evolution of technology and the acute illnesses of patients have changed the focus of functions for many nurses within the hospital organization. With experience, an advanced practice nurse (APN) can manage patient care and direct the activities of others. This practitioner may hold the title of perioperative nurse clinician, clinical nurse specialist (CNS), or APN. Although the term *practitioner* is used to describe any or all of these advanced roles, differentiation is made within the profession on the basis of formal academic education to include master's degree preparation.

In general, minimum preparation for this expanded role is a baccalaureate degree in nursing (bachelor of science in nursing [BSN]). The CNS, however, in an advanced role, has been defined as a graduate of a master's degree program in nursing (master of science in nursing [MSN]), who is an expert in a clinical specialty, a role model for and consultant to professional nursing staff, and a teacher of patients and other personnel. He or she conducts research to validate nursing interventions. These skills can be used effectively for advanced practice in the perioperative environment. Many APNs are registered nurse first assistants (RNFAs), and those who have attained certification in this role are titled certified registered nurse first assistants (CRNFAs). Nurses in this role who have advanced nursing certification are not required to concurrently maintain a certified perioperative nurse (CNOR) status.

The APN is capable of exercising a high degree of discriminative judgment in planning, executing, and evaluating nursing care based on the assessed needs of patients having one or more common clinical manifestations. A practitioner may develop the plan of care for a group of orthopedic patients, for example. This plan is coordinated for each patient with the surgeon, other professional nurses, and allied health care personnel who assist in the performance of functions related to the plan.

Clinical nursing interventions are not necessarily performed by the practitioner. The APN decides which nursing interventions can be performed by others and which he or she personally should do. These decisions are based on personal interaction with each patient and knowledge of the clinical condition. The practitioner exercises a degree of autonomy and independence within the clinical setting. Some state boards of nursing have permitted select APNs to have minimal prescriptive powers.

Because a practitioner has advanced academic preparation in theoretic knowledge and clinical experience in a particular clinical patient care setting and is an expert in nursing situations in that setting, qualified clinical coordinators may function as practitioners. In this role they assist in planning the total care for each surgical patient, coordinating nursing and supportive services, and participating in the orientation, development, and evaluation of caregivers assigned to direct patient care functions in the perioperative environment.

APNs who assess individual patient needs through personal patient interviews and physical examinations and who plan for individualized care in the perioperative environment truly function as perioperative nurse practitioners. They make decisions relative to direct and indirect patient care in the perioperative environment, using specialized judgments and skills. Problem solving and decision making are the heart of professional management and professional leadership.

The practitioner may work solely or primarily with the surgeons in a specific surgical specialty. Some APNs work as independent contractors with a surgical group as a qualifier for APN certification. This concept of nursing specialization coincides with the specialization of surgeons. With practice and formal or informal study, nurses develop expertise in planning and implementing care for patients with similar surgical problems. Skills and knowledge become highly specialized. Surgeons in that particular specialty rely on these nurses to supervise the care of their patients and to direct less-experienced personnel on the perioperative team.

Perioperative Education Coordinator

Planned educational experiences are provided in the job setting to help staff members perform competently and knowledgeably. Most hospitals have a staff development department surgical services committee to plan, coordinate, and conduct educational and training programs.

An orientation program is planned for each new employee. All new personnel should become familiar with the philosophy, objectives, policies, and procedures of the hospital and patient care services. This general orientation program assists the new employee to adjust to the organization and environment. It is coordinated with an orientation to the duties in the unit to which the employee is assigned.

The inservice coordinator may be a member of the staff development department, administrative staff, or both. This person is responsible for planning, scheduling, and coordinating the orientation of new staff. This includes review of policies and procedures, performance description, and standards specific to the perioperative environment. Based on an assessment of individual skills, the new employee is given guidance and supervision for a period of weeks to months until basic competencies are adequate to function independently. Head nurses, preceptors, and other experienced staff members assist with the orientation of new personnel.

Inservice education programs should be planned to keep the perioperative staff up-to-date on new techniques, equipment, and patient care practices. Programs focusing on fire prevention, electrical hazards, security measures, and resuscitation training are important to ensure personnel and patient safety. Professional and technical programs designed to develop specialized job knowledge, skills, and/or attitudes affecting patient care are planned and presented. The inservice coordinator is responsible for assessing the educational needs of staff members collectively and individually and then for planning, scheduling, coordinating, and evaluating inservice programs. This individual may also conduct some sessions.

Staff development programs conducted on a continual basis enhance performance by maintaining job knowledge and clinical competence. Inservice programs may be supplemented by other appropriate continuing education programs held outside the health care facility or presented by qualified people representing industry.

Preceptor. The orientation process is facilitated by a one-to-one relationship between the new employee and an experienced staff member. The preceptor teaches, counsels, advises, and encourages the orientee until he or she can function independently. The preceptor is accountable for assessing the orientee's abilities, assigning activities accordingly, and assisting in carrying out duties safely. Learning needs can be assessed through interview, observation, and a skills checklist.

To ensure consistency in teaching, the preceptor coordinates development of appropriate and measurable behavioral objectives for the orientee with the inservice coordinator, management staff, or both. The preceptor should evaluate performance and offer constructive feedback to build the orientee's self-confidence. To be effective, the preceptor should have an interest in teaching and should have acquired the necessary skills and experience with adult learners.

INTERDEPARTMENTAL RELATIONSHIPS

The perioperative environment is one of many departments within the total hospital organization. To provide continuity in patient care, many departments coordinate their efforts through the administration of the formal organizational structure of the hospital.

Every hospital has a governing body that appoints a chief executive officer (CEO), usually with the title of hospital administrator, to provide appropriate physical resources and personnel to meet the needs of patients. Administrative lines of authority, responsibility, and accountability are defined to establish the working relationships among departments and personnel (Fig. 6-1).

A nurse executive, sometimes referred to as the vice president of patient care services or director of nursing services, reports to the hospital administrator. The perioperative nurse manager reports to the nurse executive if perioperative services are a division under management of the nursing service. In some facilities perioperative services are an independent unit not managed by the nursing service. The perioperative nurse manager then reports directly to the CEO, an assistant administrator, or the chief of one of the medical services. Through either channel of administration, many activities in the perioperative environment are coordinated with other patient care units and departments within the facility.

PATIENT CARE DEPARTMENTS
Patient Care Division

Patients come to the OR directly from a short-stay or in-house patient care unit, an outpatient ambulatory care area, or the emergency department (ED). Channels of communication should be kept open among perioperative personnel and patient care personnel in other units. Coordination of preoperative preparation and transportation of patients prevents downtime in the perioperative environment. Many facilities use a checklist system to ensure adequate preparation of surgical patients in a timely manner. An RN or licensed practical/vocational nurse (LPN/LVN) signs or initials each item accomplished. By the time the patient leaves for the patient care unit, all the preparations have been completed.

Emergency Department/Trauma Center

Victims of trauma and acutely ill patients often are seen initially in the hospital ED. Cardiopulmonary resuscitative and other equipment are available to initiate prompt triage and treatment. Minor injuries usually can be treated in the ED. Some patients must be scheduled for an emergency surgical procedure, however. These patients may arrive in the OR before the results of all diagnostic tests are confirmed. Therefore communication among OR, ED, laboratory, and radiology personnel is vital to the success of surgical inter-

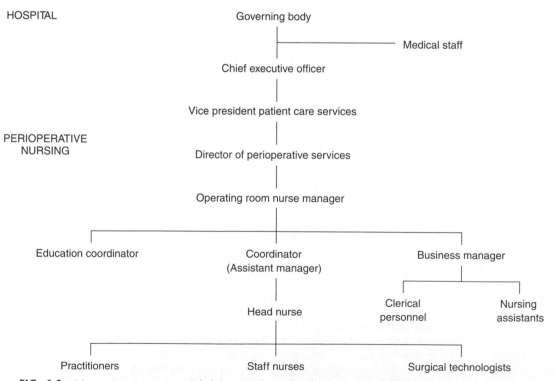

FIG. 6-1   Management structure. Administrative lines of authority, responsibility, and accountability are defined to establish working relationships among departments and personnel.

vention. OR personnel should be advised of the nature of the injury or illness to prepare all needed equipment and obtain supplies for the emergency surgical procedure.

Designated regional trauma centers should have teams of surgeons, anesthesia providers, and perioperative personnel who are immediately available in the hospital 24 hours a day. A trauma nurse coordinator is administratively responsible for all personnel and activities to ensure comprehensive trauma care.

Intensive Care Unit

Because surgery has become more specialized and complex, specialized patient care facilities where concentrated treatment can bring the patient to a satisfactory recovery have become a necessity. This care is provided in an intensive care unit (ICU), which is open 24 hours a day, 7 days a week. It is staffed by highly trained and specialized RNs. Critically ill patients who need constant care for several days are admitted directly from the OR, PACU, ED, or other patient care unit. Each bedside is equipped with therapeutic and monitoring equipment.

Depending on the size of the facility and its specialty services, more than one specially designed and equipped surgical intensive care unit (SICU) may be provided. One ICU may admit only cardiovascular surgical patients (coronary care unit [CCU]), another may admit only pediatric patients (pediatric intensive care unit [PICU]), and another may admit only neurologic patients (neurologic intensive care unit [NICU]). In addition to SICUs, most hospitals also have a unit for nonsurgical (medical) patients (medical intensive care unit [MICU]). The increased efficiency that these units afford serves the best interests of both the facility and the patient. They create the most effective use of personnel and equipment and lower morbidity and mortality rates.

Movements of patients to and from the SICUs should be closely coordinated with the anesthesia provider, the perioperative nurse, and the PACU personnel. If the surgeon or anesthesia provider anticipates that a patient will need intensive care postoperatively, a SICU bed is reserved at the same time the patient is scheduled for the surgical procedure. The appropriate SICU should be notified promptly when the surgeon determines that there is an unanticipated need for a bed. Sometimes the patient must wait in the OR or PACU for an available bed, and sometimes elective surgical procedures are postponed because sufficient SICU beds or staff is not available.

Obstetric Services

The obstetric unit is divided into three separate areas: labor and delivery (L&D), postpartum care, and newborn nursery. Most L&Ds are equipped and staffed for delivery by cesarean section (C-section). However, in other hospitals, patients scheduled for either elective or emergency C-section are brought to the OR. In addition to supplies needed for the surgical procedure, adequate resuscitative equipment must be available for the newborn. Some facilities require the OR personnel to be on call for all C-sections in both the OR and L&D.

L&Ds that staff for C-sections provide their own circulating and scrub nurses. These nurses are eligible for CNOR status. Many departments staff with their own RNFAs specific

to the role of assisting on C-sections. Certified nurse midwives serve in the first assistant capacity after appropriate training, but are not considered RNFAs unless they have completed a Competency & Credentialing Institute (CCI)–approved RNFA program.

PATIENT SERVICES DEPARTMENTS
Radiology and Nuclear Medicine Departments

Frequently, personnel from the radiology (x-ray) and nuclear medicine (radiation therapy) departments assist with diagnostic or therapeutic procedures in the OR. For some procedures it may be necessary for perioperative personnel to go to the radiology department to assist the surgeon during an interventional procedure requiring sterile technique. Whenever a diagnostic procedure or surgical procedure is scheduled that will require use of radiology equipment or a radioactive implant, all departments should be notified at least the day before. This facilitates the scheduling of personnel and workload in all departments. Provision for handling hazardous materials can be made.

Pharmacy

Many drugs are routinely stocked in the OR suite for the anesthesia providers' use, and some are kept for use by the surgeons during surgical procedures. These are obtained by requisition from the pharmacy. Narcotics are always kept under lock, and each dose is recorded as it is dispensed. A satellite pharmacy may be established in the surgical services department to dispense unit doses of medication on a per-case basis.

Pharmacists are resource people who convey drug information to physicians and nurses. They should be responsible for preparing all admixtures, but often the mixing of medications is done by RNs in the preoperative holding area, OR, PACU, and SICU to expedite administration. The pharmacist is responsible for quality control of drug product services throughout the hospital.

Blood Bank

All hospitals have a blood transfusion service or blood bank. This is a highly technical service for collecting, testing, processing, and distributing blood products. If the hospital does not have its own blood bank, blood may be supplied from a regional blood center. Written policies and procedures for blood transfusion services must conform to the standards of the American Association of Blood Banks. These include criteria for accepting blood donors, laboratory testing of donors' and recipients' blood, and preparing and administering blood products for therapeutic purposes. Blood banks dispense whole blood, plasma, packed cells, or platelets only as they are needed.

If in advance of an elective surgical procedure the surgeon anticipates that blood loss replacement may be necessary, the patient may have his or her own blood (autologous) drawn and stored in the blood bank for autotransfusion— a blood replacement procedure. Blood bank technicians also may participate on autotransfusion teams for collection of patients' blood intraoperatively and postoperatively.

If autologous blood is not available or additional units of donor blood (homologous) are needed, a sample of the patient's blood is sent to the blood bank for type and crossmatch. In emergency situations this sample may be sent from the ED or the OR. The units of blood products ordered by the surgeon or anesthesia provider are prepared and labeled with the patient's name and blood data. Suspected or recognized adverse reactions to blood transfusion must be documented on the patient's chart and reported to the blood bank.

Pathology Department

The pathologist, a physician who specializes in the cause and effect of disease, may be on call at a few minutes' notice to examine tissue while the patient is anesthetized. This enables the surgeon to proceed immediately with a definitive surgical procedure if malignant tumor cells are found, without subjecting the patient to a second surgical procedure at a later time.

A small laboratory may be located within the perioperative environment with equipment for microscopic tissue examination. This laboratory may be used for other tests and/or for taking photographs of tissue specimens removed from patients. Routinely, all tissue removed during a surgical procedure is sent to the pathology department for a minimum of gross examination.

Clinical Laboratory

Samples of blood, urine, or body fluids are taken to the clinical laboratory for analysis. Some analyses are routinely performed preoperatively. Others are done during a surgical procedure, such as blood gas analyses. Samples are obtained and immediately sent to the laboratory, or they may be obtained during a surgical procedure for analysis later, such as a culture to determine the cause of an infection.

Biologic testing of sterile supplies is done routinely. The perioperative environment may be biologically tested when a contamination problem is suspected. The bacteriologist, who specializes in the study of microorganisms, may come into the OR suite to collect samples for testing, or OR personnel may collect samples and send them to the laboratory. The results provide a method for evaluating the effectiveness of procedures and the degree of adherence to environmental standards.

DEPARTMENTAL SERVICE DIVISIONS
Medical Records Department

Clinical records include the admitting diagnosis, the patient's chief complaint, complete history and physical examination findings, the results of laboratory examinations, and the physicians' and nurses' care plans. Records should state the therapy employed, including surgical procedure(s), and include progress notes, consultation remarks, the patient's condition on discharge, or observations in case of death. A summary of the hospitalization experience should be complete. These records are signed by the physicians and nurses attending the patient.

The anesthesia record completed during the surgical procedure by the anesthesia provider also becomes part of the patient's record. The circulator should write pertinent remarks regarding the care rendered in the OR and the patient's response on the nurses' note sheet or the progress notes. Documentation is a responsibility of all professional team members implementing direct patient care.

Notes about the surgical procedure should be explicit, dictated promptly after completion of the procedure, and incorporated into the record of each surgical patient. For the surgeons' convenience, many hospitals have dictating machines or a phone hookup with the medical records department installed within the OR suite, usually located in the dressing room or lounge. Details of the preoperative and postoperative diagnosis and the surgical procedure itself may have medical and legal significance. It is the responsibility of the medical records department to transcribe the surgeon's dictation and to maintain the patient's chart after discharge from the hospital. The patient's chart may be put on microfilm for storage.

Environmental Services

Housekeeping functions are recognized as important preventive measures to eliminate microorganisms from the hospital environment. Each hospital establishes an environmental routine for its particular needs. Usually the environmental services personnel and perioperative personnel share housekeeping duties in the perioperative environment.

The amount of cleaning done by the perioperative personnel varies from one hospital to another. In many hospitals the members of the environmental services department terminally clean all furniture, flat surfaces, lights, and floors once a day at the end of the surgical schedule. In other facilities they also clean the furniture and floors before the schedule starts and between each surgical procedure throughout the day.

Whatever plan they follow, environmental services personnel should have a storage area within the OR suite in which to keep their equipment and supplies. Equipment used for cleaning in the OR is not taken outside the suite.

The director of environmental services and the perioperative nurse manager plan the division of work. Personnel in each department should understand their responsibilities. The perioperative nurse manager checks the work of the environmental personnel and keeps in touch with their director concerning their performance.

The director evaluates and chooses the proper solutions for effective cleaning, sets up a program and standard of performance for personnel, and sees that personnel are properly oriented and taught the appropriate procedures. This includes procedures for removal and disposal of trash and soiled laundry.

Using a checklist helps to cover all areas to be cleaned and inspected on a routine and preventive maintenance basis, whether it is daily, weekly, or monthly. Weekly or monthly cleaning routines include walls and ceilings, in addition to the daily cleaning schedule within the perioperative environment.

The director impresses on the personnel the importance of the work and the part they play in enabling the perioperative personnel to carry out aseptic technique. The environmental personnel function as members of the team when working with the scrub persons and circulators between surgical procedures.

Facilities Engineering

The facilities engineering department personnel work closely with the OR department by providing a preventive maintenance program. This includes routine monitoring of ventilation and heating, electrical and lighting systems, emergency warning systems, and water supply. Humidity is recorded every hour in the engineering department. All electrical equipment should be checked monthly by engineering department personnel. In addition, they regularly test the autonomous emergency power source and maintain a written record of inspection and performance.

The hospital water supply system should not be connected with other piping systems or with fixtures that could allow contamination of the water supply. The hot water supply and steam lines have temperature-control devices and filters regulated by the engineering department personnel. They are cleaned on a routine schedule, usually weekly, to prevent accumulation of mineral deposits.

Clinical Biomedical Engineering

Competent technical personnel should be available to every area of the hospital to ensure the safe operation of equipment. Nearly every surgical procedure uses some form of powered instrumentation. Because of the variety and complexity of the instrumentation currently in use, most hospitals have a clinical engineer and/or biomedical equipment technician on staff or available. This technical support group assists perioperative personnel in evaluating and selecting new equipment, installing and operating it, and maintaining it.

The clinical engineer is systems and applications oriented. This individual can compare different models and manufacturers' specifications and provide recommendations for purchase. The biomedical equipment technician is knowledgeable about the theory of operation, the underlying physiologic principles, and the practical, safe clinical applications of biomedical instrumentation. This individual can test, install, calibrate, inspect, service, and repair equipment. Every preventive service or repair is recorded in an instrument history file.

Materials Management

In an effort to control escalating health care costs, many hospitals belong to contract buying groups. This concept has changed the nature of the purchasing function and the management of supplies. The organizational administrative structure varies, but the basic functions of materials management are purchasing, processing, inventorying, maintaining proper function, and distributing supplies and equipment. Several departments are responsible for supplies.

Purchasing Department. The purchasing director coordinates the acquisition of supplies and equipment for the hospital. Standardization of products used throughout the hospital fosters quantity purchases, which provides leverage in negotiating prices with vendors. Items that are too expensive to stock in large quantities or that are used infrequently are ordered through the purchasing department as needed. In some hospitals this department is referred to as materials management.

Central Storeroom. The purchasing director or materials manager determines the supplies to be stocked for requisition by all of the departments of the hospital. Bulk inventories are received and warehoused in the central storeroom. Each department then requisitions supplies as needed, usually on a weekly basis.

Central Processing Department

One area of the hospital is designed specifically for processing, storing, and distributing supplies and equipment used in patient care. This department may be referred to as central service or central supply; central processing; supply, processing, and distribution; or materials management. The functional design and workflow patterns provide for separation of soiled and contaminated supplies from clean and sterile items. Supplies are replenished on the patient care units on a predetermined time schedule to maintain standard inventory levels. This may be done by central service using an exchange cart system (i.e., a cart of fresh supplies is exchanged for the one in use).

Control of patient charges for supplies also may be coordinated by central service. Inventory control is computerized in most hospitals. Bar code technology on individual packages may facilitate patient charges and inventory management.

Laundry Services

Many disposable, nonwoven fabrics are used. However, some woven fabrics are processed daily for use in the hospital, such as patient gowns, bedding, and towels. Hospitals that do not have laundry facilities as part of their physical plant use a commercial laundry service. An adequate inventory should be maintained for daily use. The manager of the laundry services assists in determining appropriate inventories and supervises the laundry processes. Reusable fabrics that must be sterilized before use are packaged and sterilized either in the central service or sterile processing department.

Human Resources Department

Careful selection of capable, highly motivated people contributes to efficiency and effectiveness. The human resources department helps to screen applicants with appropriate qualifications. Those seen as having potential for available positions are referred to the appropriate department head.

Potential employees are processed through human resources before an interview with the perioperative nurse manager is scheduled. The human resources department assists in hiring and terminating all employees. This department also provides resources for employee assistance and assists with progressive discipline.

COORDINATION THROUGH COMMITTEES

A committee is a group of people delegated to consider, investigate, take specific action on, and report on a matter of mutual concern or interest. Many activities within the facility are coordinated by multidisciplinary committees.

Each committee has a chairperson who conducts the flow of each meeting. A report or minutes that include an attendance roster should be generated to document the activities of the meetings. Each committee member has a special contribution to make in the progress in the work of the group. Each member has a voice in the final outcome charged to the group.

Committee members are usually allotted time during the workday to attend meetings. Other compensation should be made when meetings are scheduled at times when members are not scheduled to work.

Perioperative Committees

Surgical Services Committee. The surgical services committee is a committee of the medical staff that is vital to the management of the perioperative environment. One surgeon is appointed chief or director of the department of surgery. In teaching hospitals, a surgeon is appointed chief of each specialty service (e.g., chief of orthopedics). The anesthesia department also designates a director of that department. These individuals are responsible for professional practice and administrative activities within their respective departments. They should maintain continuing evaluation of the professional performance of all members of the medical staff who have been granted privileges in their specialty. They also serve as liaison representatives between the medical staff and the hospital administrators.

The chief of surgery, the chiefs or representatives of the specialty services, the chief of the anesthesia department, the perioperative nurse manager, the coordinator, and/or the OR business manager meet at regular intervals to review departmental activities. The hospital administrator and vice president of perioperative services also may be members of this committee or may be invited to attend meetings relevant to their concerns.

The surgical services committee formulates policies and procedures pertaining to use of facilities, a schedule of surgical procedures, and maintenance of a safe environment. Evaluation of techniques and selection of new products may require review of reports from other departments' surgical services committees in addition to those prepared by perioperative personnel.

Because this committee determines policies and procedures for efficient functioning within the OR suite, persistent problems are brought before the committee, where recommendations for corrective action are made. For example, if temperature and humidity controls are not being effectively monitored or maintained, the committee may recommend to the hospital administrators that procedures be reviewed and revised by the maintenance department or that new equipment be installed.

If surgeons are repeatedly late in arriving, thus delaying the surgical schedule, stronger policy may be indicated for the control and better use of facilities. If a new product is purchased, a new procedure may need to be written to specify its use and care.

Through data collection and a problem-solving approach to decision making, the surgical services committee seeks to improve the working relationships of all members of the OR team and the supportive services concerned with activities within the perioperative environment. Specific areas of concern for the surgical services committee include but are not limited to the following:

- Setting goals and objectives for the department
- Monitoring policies and procedures
- Planning for growth of services
- Interrelationships between patient care areas within the department and the facility

- Sanctions for noncompliance with policies and procedures
- Review of preparations for accreditation process
- Resolution of issues that interfere with the flow of the surgical services department

Policies and associated directives formulated and approved by the committee serve as guides for governing the actions of surgeons, anesthesia providers, and the patient care staff while in the perioperative environment. The perioperative nurse manager shares with the surgical services committee, hospital administrators, and nursing service the responsibility for clarification, implementation, and day-to-day enforcement of approved policies and procedures.

Operating Room Safety Committees

Radiation Safety Committee. The radiation safety committee reviews use of radiation exposure monitoring badges. This group sets policies and procedures for maintaining a safe environment where ionizing radiation is present. The committee may establish routines for periodic checking of lead aprons for intactness and for investigating reports of noncompliance with safety practices.

Laser Safety Committee. The laser safety committee establishes policies and procedures, standards, documentation systems, and credentialing criteria for the use of lasers in the health care facility. The laser safety committee also may be responsible for the development of training and continuing education programs for physicians, nurses, and surgical technologists. This may be a subcommittee of the surgical services committee. Members should include but are not limited to the chief of surgery, the chief of anesthesia, physician representatives from each surgical specialty using the laser, the perioperative nurse manager, laser nurse specialists, a biomedical technician, and a representative of administration.

This committee may delegate safety surveillance duties to a laser safety officer (LSO), who is responsible for identifying problems and safety concerns with the use of lasers. The LSO may be a physician, nurse, or specially trained laser technician. The LSO is given the authority to stop any laser procedure if safety is in question.

Infection Control Committee. The infection control committee investigates hospital-acquired (formerly referred to as nosocomial) infections (HAIs) and seeks to prevent or control them. Membership may vary but should include representatives of the medical staff, hospital administration, and nursing service and the epidemiologist or infection control coordinator. Representatives from other departments attend meetings when the agenda is relevant to their particular concerns.

The committee meets at least quarterly. Members form a defense against HAIs by reviewing environmental factors and by determining whether the hospital is providing a safe environment for patient care. They review all infection reports and investigate HAIs. Committee members also review policies and procedures and scrutinize the entire chain of asepsis in an effort to determine and then eliminate possible sources of infection.

This committee has the authority to approve changes necessary to eliminate any hazardous practices. Included in its jurisdiction is the education of personnel so that they can provide a high standard of patient care. A health care facility has a moral duty to provide a safe environment for its patients. The infection control committee aids the hospital in fulfilling this duty. Surveillance personnel assist in directing infection control policies, procedures, and practices.

Infection Control Coordinator. An infection surveillance, prevention, and control program uses the services of a key person and agent of the infection control committee—the infection control coordinator (ICC). Because this person is often an RN with special training in epidemiology, microbiology, statistics, and research methodology, he or she may be called an infection control nurse (ICN) or nurse epidemiologist.

The ICC monitors the environment for infections and works closely with the infection control committee. The ICC's duties are as follows:

1. Promptly investigating outbreaks of disease or infection above expected levels
2. Promptly identifying the origin and cause of outbreaks by epidemiologic study
3. Acquiring, correlating, analyzing, and evaluating surveillance data and bacterial colony counts. This includes gathering information to compute and classify specific wound infection rates for all invasive procedures. Rates should be entered in the infection control committee record and be available to the department of surgery.
4. Tracking factors that contribute to infection problems
5. Consulting with directors of critical areas, such as the OR. If an outbreak of postoperative infections occurs, the ICC confers with the OR nurse manager. They review the patients' intraoperative records to determine if the infected patients had the same procedure or same surgical team or were operated on in the same room. They review antiseptic agents used for skin preparation, antibiotics used for wound irrigation, and other commonalties in patient care. If a patient develops signs and symptoms of infection within the immediate postoperative period, a causative factor in the OR is suspect.
6. Coordinating educational programs for personnel who influence infection control. The ICC is a consultant to all hospital personnel and a liaison officer in disseminating information on infection control.
7. Assisting in employee health programs in regard to screening, immunizing, and monitoring the personal health of personnel
8. Assisting in development and implementation of improved patient care procedures
9. Comparing monthly statistics. A significant rise in the monthly reported surgical wound infection rate is cause for concern. Reports and data can be helpful in evaluating aseptic practices if they are brought to the attention of personnel.
10. Reporting appropriate diseases to public health authorities

11. Comparing products for effectiveness. The infection control committee approves disinfectants and antiseptics, for example, based on recommendations of the coordinator.
12. Obtaining information from surgeons about evidence of infection after discharge and conducting retrospective studies for statistical analysis

In short, the infection control coordinator identifies problems, collects data to find the causes, investigates solutions, and makes recommendations for appropriate hospital policies and procedures to prevent infections. In evaluating infection problems, the ICC attempts to find a common denominator. This often leads to the source of the problem. For example, an outbreak of postoperative respiratory infections would lead to investigation of the cleaning and sterilizing of anesthesia equipment and ventilators. Success of the control program depends in part on the information provided by a conscientious staff, including physicians.

Infection Control Program. An effective infection control program aims to reduce the incidence of infections and to control sources. Information collected through surveillance serves as a basis for corrective action. This information includes written records and reports of known or potential infections among patients and personnel. Guidelines and standards for infection control and surveillance are published by the Joint Commission on Accreditation of Healthcare Organizations (JCAHO) in the *Accreditation Manual for Hospitals* and by the Centers for Disease Control and Prevention (CDC). In general, these standards and guidelines include the following:

- Establishment of an effective hospital-wide program for surveillance, prevention, and control of infection
- Establishment of a multidisciplinary committee to oversee the program by reviewing surveillance reports and by approving policies, procedures, and actions to prevent and control infection
- Assignment of a qualified person(s) to be responsible for management of the infection surveillance, prevention, and control program
- Provision of written policies and procedures pertinent to infection surveillance, prevention, and control for all patient care departments and supporting services
- Provision of patient care support services that are adequately prepared to perform all required infection surveillance, prevention, and control functions

Surveillance. The CDC, an agency of the Department of Health and Human Services, is the third largest section of the U.S. Public Health Service. Functioning on both national and international levels, its activities are multifaceted. It carries out a national surveillance of disease incidence and a program, including health education, in prevention of communicable diseases.

Through liaison with state and local health departments, the CDC provides assistance and consultation to health care facilities for specific problem solving, analysis of surveillance data, or on-site investigation of serious outbreaks of infections. As part of its commitment to the prevention of HAIs, the CDC furnishes information on how to structure an infection control program.

Continuous Performance Improvement Committee. Members of the performance improvement committee include representatives of both clinical and administrative personnel. This committee monitors routine activities, evaluates clinical outcomes, reviews incident reports, and conducts problem-focused studies in an effort to identify practices deemed substandard.

Actual practices may be in violation of policy or not in compliance with accepted standards or governmental regulations. Noncompliance puts a hospital or ambulatory care facility at risk for legal liability. A productive and efficient committee will implement actions designed to eliminate real or potential problems, improve patient care, and reduce financial loss. Because of an emphasis on cost containment, use of facilities and risk management also may be concerns of this committee.

Many facilities employ a quality improvement coordinator and/or a risk manager to ensure implementation of committee decisions. The primary function of the person in this position is to assess actual practices and evaluate outcomes of patient care. The continuous performance improvement (CPI) coordinator may receive and respond to complaints about patient care or environmental hazards.

Each hospital department and patient care area may have its own quality improvement subcommittee. These unit-based committees monitor performance, identify ways to constructively solve competency problems, and seek opportunities for improvements in practices.

Other interdepartmental subcommittees may focus on specific activities or problems requiring input from several disciplines. Reports from these subcommittees are reviewed by the CPI coordinator. Mutual problems are shared with the hospital committee.

Ethics Committee. A multidisciplinary ethics committee should represent the hospital and the community it serves. Representatives include physicians, nurses, social workers, patient relations liaisons, clergy, lawyers, bioethicists, and laypersons from the community. Their primary purpose is to educate the staff and the community regarding moral principles and processes of ethical decision making in the face of diverse issues that arise in the care of critically and terminally ill patients. They provide consultation to professional staff, patients, and families. This committee recommends policies and guidelines on such issues as informed consent, research protocols, and advance directives.

Perioperative nurses and surgical technologists often are confronted with social, ethical, and legal decisions concerning genetic and reproductive biology, organ transplantation, and death with dignity. The ethics committee can provide a forum for discussion of these issues. Some hospitals have a nursing bioethics committee in addition to the hospital committee. These committees provide education and consultation and develop policies and procedures. They are not decision-making bodies. They do not get involved in disciplinary matters.

Hospital Safety Committee

Representatives from administration, the nursing service, the medical staff, the engineering and maintenance departments, environmental/housekeeping services, the dietary department, and the safety director form the nucleus of the hospital safety committee. This group writes policies and procedures designed to enhance safety within the hospital and on hospital grounds. They exchange information with the infection control and quality improvement committees and conduct hazard surveillance programs. They meet at least bimonthly to investigate and evaluate reported incidents. Action is taken when a hazardous condition exists that could result in personal injury or damage to equipment or facilities.

Disaster Planning Committee

Health care facilities should have an organized plan for caring for mass casualties if a major disaster occurs. External disasters happen outside of the health care facility, such as a terrorist attack, an airplane crash, or an event of nature (e.g., flood, Hurricane Katrina in 2005).

Internal disasters, such as a fire or an explosion, happen inside the health care facility. Planning by the intrahospital disaster committee includes consultation with local civil authorities and representatives of other medical agencies to establish an effective chain of command and to make appropriate jurisdictional provisions. This planning results in disaster-site triage to separate and distribute patients to ensure the most efficient use of available facilities and services.

Disaster drills are held at least twice a year to try out the plans developed by the committee, to seek to improve them, and to familiarize personnel with them. Plans for both types of disasters include the following:

- An information center within the hospital to facilitate a unified medical command and the movement of patients
- A receiving area for the injured. Severely wounded casualties are given emergency care according to their needs and are sent at once to the OR or to other units as indicated or transferred to another facility. Ambulatory patients may be treated in the ED for slight injuries and sent home or admitted to the hospital as indicated.
- Special disaster medical records or tags that accompany patients at all times
- A plan of organization of personnel. As soon as a hospital receives word of a disaster during the evening or night, several key people are called. These in turn telephone others previously assigned to them, and these call still others, until the full staff has been notified. If the disaster occurs during the day, the full staff is usually on duty, although any off-duty personnel may be called. Other departments are alerted and come on duty as needed; these include personnel for the blood bank, laboratory, pharmacy, materials management, radiology department, and patient care units, including the OR, PACU, and ICU. If disposable drape packs are not in use, it may be necessary to alert some laundry personnel. Some key maintenance personnel should be available, especially electricians.
- Written departmental instructions for personnel. For the perioperative staff these may include sign-in procedures, checklists of duties, and patient scheduling procedures.

Personnel must know where to report, what to do, and where extra supplies are kept in case of an emergency. Extra supplies are stored in reserve in sufficient quantities to fill possible needs for a minimum of 1 week.

SURGICAL SERVICES MANAGEMENT

Management of the surgical services department is key to the success of this high-cost center within the institution. Power and authority go hand-in-hand in the role of administrators and managers. Authority can be bestowed on a person in the role, but power is the ability to influence the outcome in a particular direction. The skillful and effective manager uses both of these attributes to maintain control over the activities and decision making of the department. Primary managerial activities will revolve around safe, efficient patient care, leadership, and budgetary concerns.

Administrative and Management Behaviors

Accreditation. Ongoing policy and procedure updates decrease the need for last-minute compliance documentation necessary for JCAHO. Most accreditation cycles are 3 years—ample time to establish and maintain an accreditation-responsible program. Some considerations for staying in readiness are the following:

- Set a routine schedule for reviewing and updating policies and procedures. Don't wait until a visit is anticipated to start trying to clean up outdated practices.
- Model each behavior in patient care after the desired outcome.
- Share information with the staff about the department's progress toward full compliance. Feature each stride with a report from the achievers during routine staff meetings.
- Keep a copy of the survey questions immediately available for the staff to review.
- Establish small groups to tackle small, manageable tasks. Collectively this will amount to a large improvement in participation. Tasks can be delegated to each service.
- Be sure the staff has all the necessary supplies, resources, and support to accomplish the mission.
- Present each item to be worked on in a positive attitude. Use the staff's natural talent and creativity.
- Pitch in and help whenever needed.
- Reward the accomplishments on an ongoing basis, not just for the moment.
- Remain current with modern practices. Dated or unfounded policies and procedures can undermine the authority of the manager in the eyes of the staff and physicians.

Leadership Qualifications and Competency. Leadership is difficult to define, but it is nonexistent without subordinate cooperation. The manager's style, capability, knowledge base, practice reputation, and experience help set the pace for the progress of the department. People skills are very important. Throughout the staff complement, some people will show informal leadership abilities that can be positive or negative. Some hallmarks of leadership competency include the following:

- Critical thinking skill
- Objectivity
- Using credible sources
- Planning ability
- Flexibility
- Creativity
- Self-control
- Negotiation skills

Informal leaders can be harmful if their influence directs the staff away from the main mission of the OR. Winning the support of informal leaders is a significant stride toward better cohesiveness for the staff. Informal leaders can be very disruptive when communications break down among the ranks.

Develop "systems thinking."[1] Each member of the team needs to identify personal strengths and his or her personal relationship with the organization that is working toward becoming a learning organization.

The main focus is continual improvement by tempering activities and behaviors of the individual in accordance to the needed productivity of the organization. Senge (1990) identified five constructs that are either group or individual relationships with the organization. The process cannot be paced with an exact timeline; however, it can be measured by improved productivity and personnel in a stable working relationship. The five constructs are simplistically paraphrased as follows:

- Personal mastery: clarify and deepen personal focus
- Mental models: identify the internal beliefs that cause us to act in a certain way
- Shared vision: working "on the same page" as the rest of the team. Sometimes this requires more commitment than compliance for growth of the vision. This is where some personnel will try to break away and do their own thing.
- Team learning: a coordinated group activity in which ideas are receptively expressed in an open dialog. No judgments are made as would happen in a discussion. Everyone is required to listen and not criticize the ideas of others in the group.
- Systems thinking: discover the root causes of events and fuses all the other four constructs together to effect long-range improvement

Systems thinking is a way to improve the quality of care and help set standards that can be expanded or contracted to meet the needs of the facility and the patient population. When the learning organization has a process of systems thinking in place, the emphasis is on the system, not the individual staff member. Error reduction in the OR can commonly be traced back to a flaw in a system that permitted something to go wrong, such as a retained sponge or a sharps injury. When a decent system is in place and followed by the group, the risk of error is minimized.

Leading by Example. The surgical services staff needs to have respect for the management team. Encouraging the staff to become professionally active and then joining them in professional activities can help cement a sense of pride in accomplishment.

---

[1] A series of five processes that integrates personal development, learning, group dynamics, and continuous improvement as described by Peter Senge in his 1990 book, *The Fifth Discipline*.

Nurse managers who have no clue about current practices are not only harmful to the organization but also less respected by the staff. Failure to keep up with the times makes the nurse manager appear unintelligent and uncaring, especially when the staff attends outside workshops for updates and are met with disdain by the manager. This is a common cause of losing staff to other, more progressive facilities.

Perioperative nurse mangers should be professionally involved and should be certified as CNORs and possibly certification as an administrator.

Although an academic degree is not always necessary, having one makes a statement of respect for education and personal growth. Support for line managers and staff who are pursuing degrees is an admirable trait in the management structure.

Rounding Up Those Sacred Cows.
Policies and procedures should have a firm foundation in scientific research and evidence-based practice. Practices that continue despite lack of scientific evidence are referred to as sacred cows. Managers lose much credibility and look ignorant when they enforce dated practices. The staff will respect the manager more when he or she can support the basis for best practice behaviors. Mechanically performing tasks without knowing why is a hazard to the patients and the staff. Excuses given by managers commonly include the following:

- "This is how we do it here."
- "This is how we have always done it."
- "We don't do it *that* way here" (in reference to the introduction of a newer, more modern approach).
- "The national standards are only voluntary, not mandatory."
- "This is how I was taught. That's good enough for my staff."
- "I did not know that the staff was doing that activity in that manner."
- "Because this is how I wanted it done."

Demanding that the staff perform procedures according to nonexistent rationale is time wasting and ridiculous. The manager looks incompetent when the staff is required to follow protocols that are not founded in evidence-based practice. Some areas for investigation concerning sacred cows in the OR include the following intraoperative behaviors:

- Requiring shoe covers and masks in all areas of the surgical suite
- Covergowns and lab coats are worn when leaving the OR
- Forbidding the use of nail polish, including fresh nail polish
- Skin preps as sterile procedures
- Surgical site hair removal
- Home-laundered versus facility-laundered scrubs
- Timed scrubs, counted brush stroke scrubs, and hand hygiene antisepsis
- Extent of between-case cleaning
- Excessive draping
- Setting time parameters on the sterility of items
- Covering tables
- Flash sterilization

Professional Involvement.
Managers should be members of their professional organizations and take part in the care and feeding of their profession. Managers should also be certified as a professional credential.

The administrative and management staff should be knowledgeable about current standards and trends in perioperative patient care. Offering to host professional meetings at the facility or holding open houses for new potential surgical services staff shows an interest in the departmental growth.

Meetings.
Most management personnel are required to attend and plan a multitude of meetings pertaining to the business of the department and the hospital as a whole. When planning daily activities, they should consider the need to attend these communication sessions. The manager should establish routine meetings within the surgical services department for the dissemination of information as appropriate and adhere to a set time parameter for the proceedings.

Some meetings require the attendance of people from other departments and need to be carefully planned. Offering to hold the meeting in a neutral location can help prevent disruptions by office phones and distractions.

The chairman or leader of a meeting should realize the importance of the meeting's beginning and ending on time. Complex topics should be interspersed with simpler group communications. Solicitation of agenda items from attendees in advance helps the chairman plan ahead and maintain the order of business with minimal digression.

Setting the Agenda.
Establishing a time period and content for each meeting is important. Personnel attending meetings should estimate the amount of time they will need to plan for attendance. The manager will need to plan release time for meeting attendees that does not interfere with the daily operation of the surgery department. A meeting agenda should have the following in its composition:

- Introductions of new personnel
- Short overview of discussion topics
- Old business
- New business
- Special topics
- Delegation of new tasks
- Exchange of information for the good of the group

Minutes of the Meeting.
Records of each meeting should be kept at a central location in the department. Personnel in process of patient care may not be able to attend formal staff meetings and need to keep informed about current events in the hospital and department. Secretarial staff or a designated team member should document pertinent facts for the record and verify the accuracy with members of the committee before the group meets for a session.

A loose-leaf notebook with meeting overviews can be maintained in a common area available to all departmental staff members. Copies of the minutes can be sent to appropriate people within the facility on a need-to-know basis. The minutes also serve to validate the activities transacted and any resolutions or expectations of future business.

Personnel Management

Motivation and Building a Unified Team. Staff meetings are useful forums for group exchange of ideas, reporting, and concerns. The manager should have regularly scheduled meetings with a formal agenda that has provision for staff input. Allowing the staff to have some ownership of the surgical services department encourages pride in group endeavors.

When the department consists of several areas with specific functions separate from the others, smaller personalized area meetings can be beneficial to work through items not of interest to the entire department. The PACU personnel may have different issues than the OR team. Collective meetings are useful for consolidating matters that are common to all the areas.

Staffing. Planning for adequate and appropriate staff to safely and efficiently provide patient care during the implementation of the surgical schedule is a complex task. Sometimes managers try to cut corners by stretching the staff numbers to bare-bones teams. It is important to remember that staff satisfaction and retention are not built on working them to a frazzle. Plans are necessary for break and lunch relief. Consideration should be given to assignments that are emotionally or extremely physically draining. Provision for the relief of an extremely stressed team member is reassuring to the entire staff that they will not be abandoned by management if the case becomes more complex or lengthy than originally planned.

Retention of staff is a cost-saving measure. The manger should think about the processes associated with hiring, orienting, and maintaining each person on roll. According to the 2004-2005 AORN National Committee on Education, the cost of replacing an experienced staff nurse ranges between $10,000 and $15,000. The cost of training a novice perioperative nurse from scratch ranges between $30,000 and $50,000. Some of the parameters for staffing with newly hired nurses include the following:

- Development or purchase of a perioperative nurse education program
- Recruitment costs
- Duration of orientation
- Preceptor costs
- Materials costs

The cost-effective means for retention is to look for what contributes to staff satisfaction. Giving the staff the opportunity to participate in staffing decisions such as "on call time" or mandatory overtime can help prevent staff burnout and resignations. Working the team to a frazzle is not the way to keep staff. Studies demonstrate overworked and exhausted staff frequently cause more surgical error and increase staff turnover.

Staffing decisions should not be made based solely on costs. Safety for the patient and the entire team should be foremost in the scheme of planning.

Delegation of Duties. When assigning a task to personnel within the department, the person receiving the instruction should be fully capable and knowledgeable in the action to be taken. The manager should consider appropriateness of roles and the assignment of duties according to the standards of care and in some instances the legality of the role. For example, some states have laws that indicate only a registered nurse may perform the role of circulator. Some states have laws that indicate who may or may not perform in the role of first assistant. Thought should be given to potential consequences of assigning staff to roles that are out of the scope of practice.

Clear instructions should be given, and feedback should be received indicating understanding. Recognition of a job well done should be freely given. Consequences for poor performance should be moderated appropriately. Competency of each employee should be validated on a regular basis and incompetent employees should brought up to speed or put on notice of progressive discipline.

Conflict Management. The operating room is a closed environment with a potentially fragile morale. When personnel work closely together for long periods, it is not uncommon for small disagreements to take place. The manager may need to intervene periodically. It is important to hear both sides of the disagreement before taking any action. Disruptive behavior should not be tolerated; instead, it should be managed with firmness and professionalism.

Lateral Violence. Conflicts should not be allowed to fulminate to overstated proportions. Use of the term *violence* indicates that there is/are victim(s). Abuse within the ranks is a form of violence and includes nonverbal innuendos, verbal confrontation, backstabbing, undermining behaviors, sabotage, and gossip.

Personnel have indicated that within their first 6 months they experienced some form of lateral violence.[2] Dissatisfaction among the staff leads to increased personnel turnover and is very costly to the facility. Compromise is a middle-of-the-road approach and should not favor one employee over another. Lateral violence is not a rite of passage in the perioperative environment. The manger needs to identify the problem in evolution in order to manage it. The staff should be held accountable for maintaining professional relationships and for preventing the "eating of one's young" as has been the case for many generations. The staff must not be permitted to "dish it out" or be forced to "take it in." The following is a list of behavioral signs that the staff is dissatisfied and is referred to as "red ink"[3] behavior to be investigated and managed:

- Excessive overtime and staff refusal to help out. Cases that run overtime are sometimes caused by staff not performing assigned tasks and failing to prepare appropriately for caseload. Foot-dragging.
- Low productivity. Turnover between cases is prolonged by staff coming back from breaks and lunch late. Work is unfinished or done poorly.
- Constant complaining. The manager needs to listen attentively to find the root cause.

---

[2] Discussion at the AORN managers conference in New Orleans, April, 2005. Martha Griffin. *Inter-Group Conflict: Lateral or Horizontal Violence.*

[3] Briles J: Zapping conflict in the health care workplace, *SSM* 9(6):27-31, 2003.

- High absenteeism and tardiness. These can be signs that morale is very low.
- Constant turnover of staff. Dissatisfied personnel will quit or transfer out when resolutions are not sought out or met.
- Temperaments flare up easily. Stress can result in acting-out behavior.

Downward Violence. Downward violence is any abusive behavior directed at lower-ranked individuals by higher-ranked individuals. This can be abuses by a manager to staff, from a surgeon to manager, or surgeon to staff. A study was done of OR abuses resulting in departmental transfers wherein 47% of transfer requests were sparked by management abuse toward staff.[4]

When the disagreement is with a surgeon, the automatic assumption of the staff is that they do not have a fighting chance to say their piece and that it won't matter what they say. This needs to be addressed as soon as possible after an incident.

Verbal abuse by surgeons is not acceptable under any circumstances regardless of the event, and can cause serious problems in the OR. A surgeon has no right to terrorize the staff. Sometimes bad behavior is a sign of incompetence and is an attempt to hide or smoke-screen personal insecurity. This is true of any person.

Throwing items or other physical displays by the surgeon in the OR are unsafe and should be subject of discipline at the level of the medical staff officers. Failure to attain resolution at that level warrants a report and meeting with the CEO of the facility. Care is taken to follow chain of command; however, the conscientious manager cannot knowingly allow staff or patient endangerment by a surgeon, regardless of his volume of revenue to the facility. It is hard to stand up for what is right and just, especially when one is standing alone. The staff will have a sense of respect for the manager who champions the cause of the department fairly and professionally.

Sometimes egos are factors, and a small disagreement gets blown out of proportion. The staff should be assured that many surgeon complaints are not meant on a personal level but, instead, are directed specifically at a situation. Personal attacks can cause anger initially but can cause grudges that last months, even years.

The manager, after hearing both sides, has the responsibility to mediate a truce but may have to involve the chief of surgery and the director of nursing service for the facility. Conflicts are very costly to the organization in many ways but primarily because of the following:

- Staff replacement costs either in orientation of new personnel or in the use of agency workers to fill gaps left in staffing
- Additional man-hours to complete the schedule at the end of the day; staff frequently take a sick day when feeling overwhelmed and depressed
- Refusal to stay overtime because of lack of loyalty
- Increased errors and carelessness
- Legal issues, such as suits for harassment

[4] Briles J, 2003.

- Poor productivity and low morale
- Lack of pride in the job can cause injury to the patient

What can the manager do about conflicts and/or verbal abuse? A few strategies can prove useful when facing this dilemma. Some ideas are as follows:

- The two people with the disagreement should have a face-to-face meeting away from the OR, perhaps in the manager's office.
- The manager should be present. Other support may include the chief of surgery, chief of staff, and the director of nursing service. If a physician representative is present, an additional nursing representative should also be present.
- Avoid blaming anyone. Remain objective, and maintain civil tones in all parties.
- Ask each party what would make the situation better on an individual level. Try to reach a compromise with this information.
- The surgeon should not have the right to demand an employee's resignation. Unfounded termination can result in a lawsuit against the facility, the manager, and the surgeon.
- Praise positive strides for a peaceful resolution. Be aware that some people are very overjoyed by being unhappy. Some people have a bad day every day.
- Assure both sides that you will all reach a satisfactory conclusion together.

Documentation. Records of performance reviews should be maintained in human resources and in the manager's file. Each employee should have a file that documents competency and practice attributes. Care is taken to document evaluations and anecdotal notes in professional terms because if a staff member files a grievance with higher administration or with a union, the records may be open to scrutiny. Inflammatory comments or slang references could be mistaken for inappropriate labeling of personnel and cause hard feelings.

The manger should evaluate personnel and have them do self-evaluations in preparation for a face-to-face discussion about performance and performance improvement goals. The contents of the documentation should be the framework for discussion. The staff member should be permitted to retain a copy of all performance evaluation for his or her personal records.

BUDGETING AND FINANCIAL RESPONSIBILITY

For the new nurse manager, preparing a budget for the first time can be very intimidating. Before beginning, meet with the facility finance personnel, business manager, and another nurse manager within the facility who may be willing to mentor this process. The materials manager can often shed light on the historical use of supplies, and the payroll department can provide information about salaries, performance reviews, and overtime. Computerized records can help with historical department activities and projection of future needs.

Reviewing previous copies of earlier budgets can be helpful. Most facilities have a specific fiscal year and begin the year with a budget overview meeting, at which time instructional packets are passed out. Computerized methods may include spreadsheets and graphs. Computer literacy is a must during this process.

After the initial budget is submitted and approved, plans should be under way to begin gathering information for the next fiscal year. Responsibility for the financial affairs of the department includes forecasting needs and growth. The budget, in itself, is a prime managerial planning tool, not an obstacle to progress.

Day-to-day financial management considerations may include several of the following budgetary factors:

- Engage the staff in budget dialog. Don't use the budget as a weapon or threat, but emphasize the ways the staff can safeguard against waste and promote loss prevention.
- Use the operational structure within the facility. Seek information and advice from other managers, department heads, and purchasing departments. Set up formal and informal meetings to monitor the financial climate of the institution.
- Cheapest materials may sometimes cost more in the long run. Establish evaluation groups for new products. Graph out the pros and cons of each item tried. Solicit input from other departments that might interface with the product.
- Encourage planning in ordering of stock. Keep a standard number of supplies on hand and discourage "squirreling away" of items by staff members. Discourage inventory accumulation in the individual operating rooms.
- Strive for standardization. Custom packs and routine basic supplies help in this process.
- Don't skimp on the education of the staff. The staff needs to know the products and trends associated with the procedures for which they are required to provide patient care. Have regularly scheduled inservices and have specialty leaders put on a small trade fair periodically. New machines and supplies can be introduced in an enjoyable atmosphere instead of "on the fly" when a new item is foisted on the team in the middle of a procedure.

Operational Budget

The operating budget directly reflects the department's revenues and expenses. Caseload and man-hours are the prime considerations during the development of the operational budget. If cases are increasing, so is the number of hours and possibly overtime by staff. One method of minimizing the overtime costs is to have staggered staffing shifts. A team that starts later in the day could be assigned to break and lunch relief for the early starting rooms. At the end of the day the late-start team could be available to finish rooms that are still running at the end of the shift. In some facilities, this decreases the need for a full second shift crew.

Most facilities provide a monthly departmental summary of expenditures that include line items such as the following:

- Noncapital purchases (usually less than $500)
- Charges for expenses such as laundry, preventive maintenance contracts, and repairs
- Supply and inventory charges (check the number and type of cases each month; are price increases expected?

Is there a purchasing contract with a distributor or a buying consortium?)
- Wages and salaries with benefits (holidays and vacation time is calculated; overtime may be projected and additional full time equivalents [FTEs] may be needed)
- Educational funds for continuing education, degree seeking courses, certification, and recertification

Each month the projected amount should be compared with the actual amount of each item. At first it can seem confusing, but with time this practice becomes second nature. Some vendors charge on a net 30-day basis, and the actual charges do not appear until 1 to 2 months after the fact. It is wise to always glance through 3 months at a time to compare and track charging trends. Keep a notebook for observations by the month. This will help to sort out confusing items. Jot down phone numbers and problematic issues as well as ongoing questions.

Keeping track of the facility's monthly census may provide some clues as to the accuracy of the figures and if they will be important for future budget preparation and identification of trends. As these data accumulate, they may demonstrate the need for a change in supplier. Keep good notes of positive and negative encounters with sales personnel. Always request a business card, and keep it on file for quick contact. A file should be started for each vendor used and notations made if they are associated with a hospital-wide buying contract.

A pocket computer or other portable electronic device is useful for tracking the budget and having portable information for meetings. The device can be synchronized and recharged with the desktop computer and the information can be kept current at all times. Some pocket computers have software that can be used for spreadsheets and document processing. It is important to password protect all devices in case of loss or theft. Some devices contain a cell phone.

Capital Budget

The capital budget is more concerned with improvements to the physical plant and purchases of large equipment. Patient care devices that are charged per use are considered capital equipment.

Surgeons frequently request equipment for the types of procedures they perform. Some surgeons have the opportunity to preview new equipment at seminars and conferences and bring the brochures to the manager for future trial use. Sometimes new equipment previewed at medical conferences is discounted to participants of the event. If special capital items are planned for future purchase it is useful for the manager to attend trade shows and medical conferences where these devices are displayed and demonstrated.

Keeping an ongoing list or file with information about specifications and cost is very useful at budget time when preparing requests for capital expenditures. Information that is useful in this process includes the following:

- Formal and generic name of the device
- Does the device require special hookups or storage?
- Who will use it?
- Who will educate the staff about its use?
- How frequently will it be used?
- Consumables necessary, such as disposable leads or parts

- What is the cost of its use to the facility and the patient?
- Is the use of the device reimbursable by third-party payer?
- Would renting the device be more cost effective than a purchase?
- Will this device become antiquated quickly?
- What is currently being used in its place?
- Vendor (include contact person, phone number, business card, and e-mail address; date this entry— sales force changes are common)
- If it is a new project or a replacement (one unit, or more?)
- If one is available for trial
- Why it should be purchased
- Costs (item, installation, preventive maintenance [PM] contract, tax, shipping, maintenance; get a secured price quote)
- Education or credentialing required to use it?
- Warranty and service information
- Delivery and turnaround time for repairs (loaner available?)
- Costs of basic repairs
- Is product support available during the phase-in process?

Outdated or poorly functioning machinery is replaced during this process. The American Hospital Association has prepared a "life expectancy" guideline for most types of devices used in patient care. This resource is valuable in establishing a replacement program for dated items. The manager should project needs and develop plans for growth or improvement for a 5-year cycle. Knowledge of current technology is a must to stay on top of new device knowledge. Some departments include anesthesia equipment with the OR and PACU capital budget.

NEW PRODUCT AND EQUIPMENT EVALUATION

The user of a product is best qualified to evaluate performance, safety, effectiveness, and efficiency. Before a decision is made to purchase or to standardize a particular item, a clinical evaluation should be conducted to solicit feedback from team members whose work will be affected by the product. This may involve the surgeons or anesthesia providers, as well as perioperative nurses and surgical technologists. Instruction should be provided on the correct use of the item before it is evaluated. Sales representatives may be permitted to assist in the trial of a product in the OR. Although not providing direct patient care, they offer suggestions and consult with the users during the product trial. Members of an interdisciplinary product selection committee might include:

- Pharmacist
- Nurse educator
- Biomedical staff
- Wound care team member
- Infection control nurse
- Occupational or physical therapist
- Nurse manager
- Nurses from the postsurgical areas

To be valid, feedback should be an objective evaluation of function, quality, and use. Does it meet a need? Does it solve a problem? Is it cost effective? Does it improve patient care? How does it compare with other brands? Several brands of the same product may be evaluated to select the most satisfactory one for the intended purpose and to standardize the inventory. Written evaluations are useful for the decision-making process after the trial period.

Many products are used only in the perioperative environment; some are used also in other patient care areas. Representatives from all user departments should assist the materials manager in selecting products. Most hospitals have a product evaluation committee for this purpose. A representative of the perioperative staff provides this committee with information regarding quality and effectiveness, based on feedback from user staff members.

Once a product has been purchased, the user assumes responsibility for its safety and its proper use for its intended purpose. Problems with medications or patient care items should be reported to the Food and Drug Administration (FDA) using the MedWatch system. The FDA tracks complaints and orchestrates recalls as appropriate (Fig. 3-1).

Working with Sales Representatives

Sales representatives are important sources of information and support. Each facility should have a policy in place that addresses who has the authority to work with the sales personnel and under what circumstances are they permitted in the department. The sales personnel should register at the main information desk in the lobby of the hospital and wear proper identification at all times. They should not cause any disruption or compromise patient privacy in any way.

AORN has established a position statement about sales representatives in the operating room that is useful for determining facility policies and procedures. Sales representatives should have a basic knowledge of sterile technique and should be able to enter the OR without disruption. AORN has developed a sales representative certification class to acquaint the sales force with the OR and its protocols. The following are some guidelines about working with sales representatives:

- The facility should have specific policies in place to govern the activities of sales representatives.
- Meetings are by appointment only. No meetings are to be scheduled with any of the staff without express permission from the manager.
- Physicians may not bring a sales representative into the department without going through proper channels.
- Facility security policies are followed at all times.
- The sales representative may not render direct patient care at any time. The patient should have the opportunity to give informed consent to the presence of sales personnel.
- Specialized and highly trained manufacturers' representatives may have indirect activities, such as calibration of pacemakers and defibrillators, as directed by the surgeon. These personnel should not be scrubbed in at any time.
- Only the products planned for the meeting will be presented.
- No fliers or materials are to be distributed without permission of the manager.

- Trial devices are brought in only by request and will be examined by the facility's biomedical department for safety.
- Disposable products for trial will have appropriate lot numbers for reporting problems or malfunctions.

Bibliography

AORN (Association of periOperative Registered Nurses): Standards of perioperative administrative practice. In *AORN standards, recommended practices, and guidelines,* Denver, CO, 2005, The Association.

AORN guidance statement: Safe on-call practices in perioperative practice settings, *AORN J* 81(5):1054-1057, 2005.

AORN guidance statement: Perioperative staffing, *AORN J* 81(5):1059-1066, 2005.

Briles J: Zapping conflict in the health care workplace, *SSM* 9(6):27-31, 2003.

Dexter F: How to design an effective surgical schedule, *Out-patient Surg* 11(3):17-23, 2001.

Dix K: Best practices for purchasing managers, *Infect Contr Today* 9(7):34-38, 2005.

Forsythe LL: Using an organizational culture analysis to design interventions for change, *AORN J* 81(6):1290-1302, 2005.

Gelinas LS: Defining the role of the nurse executive for the twenty-first century, *SSM* 6(1):34-37, 2000.

Hopper, WR: Surgeon's abusive behavior in the OR, *SSM* 9(6):46-48, 2003.

Hughes SJ: Analyzing the value of new technology, *SSM* 6(8):44-47, 2000.

Kerfoot KM: Surgical services in the new millennium, *SSM* 6(1):6-8, 2000.

Kondrat BK: Operating room nurse managers: competence and beyond, *AORN J* 73(6):1116, 1121-1124, 1126-1127, 1129-1130, 2001.

Maun C: Conflict management: What really works? *SSM* 6(6):37-40, 2000.

Northhouse PG: *Leadership: Theory and practice,* ed 3, Thousand Oaks, Calif, 2004, Sage.

Rearick T: A cost effective surgical infection control program, *SSM* 6(8):38-43, 2000.

Roark J: The materials management team: Uniting the key players in IC, OR, and purchasing, *Infect Contr Today* 9(1):22-23, 2005.

Rupert C, Kitzman S: The clinical voice in product selection and implementation, *SSM* 8(4):24-26, 2002.

Saver C: Staffing ratio trends: A survey of perioperative nurse managers, *AORN J* 81(5):1041-1044, 2005.

Seifert PC: Leaving the nineties behind, *SSM* 6(1):18-22, 2000.

Senge P: *The fifth discipline: The art and practice of the learning organization,* New York, 1990, Currency Doubleday.

Chapter **7**

The Patient: The Reason for Your Existence

CHAPTER OBJECTIVES

After studying this chapter, the learner will be able to:
- Describe Maslow's hierarchy of needs.
- Describe some characteristics of diversity in a patient population.
- List the key elements of a patient-centered approach.
- Describe how the patient may perceive care.

CHAPTER OUTLINE

KEY TERMS AND DEFINITIONS

Body mass index (BMI)   Calculation dividing body weight in kilograms by height in meters squared (kg/m^2).
Comorbidity   More than one disease entity in an individual.
Domestic violence   Abuse perpetrated in the home or living arrangement. Can be physical, psychological, verbal, or nonverbal.
Homeostasis   A balance of systems within a person that sustains life in a disease-free state.
Paradigm   Model used as a foundation for a conceptual framework.
Perception   Using the senses, cognition, and awareness to evaluate the collective stimuli of the environment.
Perpetrator   Person who is suspected of committing a crime against another person.
Polypharmacy   The use of multiple medications, either prescribed or self-administered.
Stress   Internal perception of and response to stimuli in a positive or negative manner.
Victim   Person who has been injured by the effects of the environment or suffered abuse by another person.

SUPPLEMENTAL MATERIAL ON EVOLVE WEBSITE   *evolve*

http://evolve.elsevier.com/BerryKohn
- Content Updates
- Glossary
- Full Set of Perioperative Flash Cards
- Interactive Key Term Flash Cards
- Student Activities
- WebLinks

HISTORICAL BACKGROUND

Patient care has changed throughout history. Patients have been treated by medicine men and women who were intrigued by birth, disease, and death. Primitive treatments consisted of driving away evil spirits with incantations, loud noise, and physical manipulation. Early medicine included trephining (drilling holes in the skull), ice cold baths, blood letting, purgatives and enemas, and herbal concoctions. Common belief was that the most effective treatment was the one that tasted the worst or contained the most foul ingredients.

Nursing as a career for women in patient care has its roots in mothering or nurturing. Males were involved with patient care in every era; however, the nurturing "mother-care" label was not assigned to them in the same regard. Two identified health care–related roles emerged as history unfolded—the medicine giver and the caretaker. Males commonly assumed the role of medicine giver and the women took on the role of caretaker. Initially these two roles were the same, but the tasks became separated and medicine and nursing emerged as powerful allies in patient care.

The traditional role of patient care encompassed care of adults and children in the sick bed, care during childbirth, care of the aged and infirm, care of the handicapped, and care at the end of life. Modern roles include health promotion, disease prevention, and supporting a sense of generalized well-being. Patient care became one of the first means for women to seek financial independence during the woman's movement based on skills they learned within their own households caring for families.

In 1922, medical texts by authors such as Morris King, MD, included sections for nurses regarding patient care. Much of the information was relayed in the same manner as environmental nursing theorist Florence Nightingale (1820-1910) directed in her classic text *Notes on Nursing: What It Is and What It Is Not*. Environmental influences included care of the sick room, attitudes and approaches of the caregiver, and housekeeping duties.

Directories of nurses and people providing patient care were available at pharmacies, physicians' offices, and hospital nursing departments. Patient care in the home setting was available at a moment's notice. Service and obedience to the physician were the most desired attributes. The usual salary for patient care was $4 to $5 per day.

An emphasis was placed on how the nurse or caregiver was expected to behave and look. A preference for single, plain-looking women between the ages of 25 and 30 years showed clear gender bias. A woman of this age in the late 19th and early 20th centuries may have passed her chances for making a marriage and was not likely to leave the profession to bear children and tend a family.

Early texts examined the psyche of the patient, illustrating an understanding of the need for clear communication in the effort to gain trust. Early authors suggested that speaking in normal tones and keeping extraneous noise to a minimum would promote rapid recovery and wellness. They also suggested that an explanation of necessary tasks and an avoidance of sudden, unexpected actions would foster cooperation during convalescence.

In 2005, President George W. Bush signed a bill into law[1] creating a role in health care facilities for trained counselors referred to as "patient navigators" to work with terminal or seriously ill patients. The purpose of the law is to test whether the patient navigators can help the patients overcome barriers such as economic, cultural, and geographic obstacles that block adequate and timely health care access.

THE PATIENT AS AN INDIVIDUAL

Patients are the reason for the existence of the health care team. They look to the perioperative team to fulfill their diverse needs during the preoperative, intraoperative, and postoperative phases of care (Fig. 7-1). The patient is always the center of attention—not just when under the operating room (OR) spotlight.

A patient may be defined as an individual recipient of health care services. Extremes of age (pediatric and geriatric) and comorbid disease entities require individualization of the plan of care. To meet a patient's requirements and expectations effectively, personnel should have knowledge of his or her needs, problems, and health considerations. From a perioperative perspective, it is important to understand the effect a surgical procedure has on a patient's lifestyle.

Characteristics that individualize patients include, but are not limited to, the following:
- They are worthwhile and unique individuals.
- They respond psychosocially on the basis of their personal values, beliefs, and ethnocultural background.
- They have the capacity to adapt to their internal as well as external environments.
- They have basic needs that must be met to maintain homeostasis.

---

[1] Patient Navigator Outreach and Chronic Disease Prevention Act, June 22, 2005. This bill provides funding for 5 years in the area of providing health care to the disadvantaged chronically ill. The bill was backed by the American Cancer Society, American Diabetes Association, and the National Association of Community Health Centers.

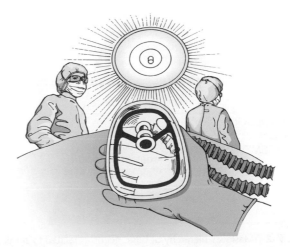

FIG. 7-1 The OR from the patient's perspective.

Homeostasis is a consistent internal environment maintained by the patient's adaptive capabilities, and it has a physiologic and a psychological component. From a physiologic aspect, the patient's body strives to maintain equilibrium within normal limits through control mechanisms located in the endocrine glands and in the reticular formation in the brainstem. This stability depends partly on the structural integrity of the body, the adequacy of its functions, and environmental influences.

Psychological homeostasis is based on emotional acceptance and a rational understanding of events that influence health and wellness. Fear and anxiety are common stressors that alter a patient's psychological response to the health care system.

Patients' Basic Needs

Needs are factors that must be controlled or redirected to restore altered function. Nursing diagnoses are based on knowledge and understanding of a patient's needs and how to fulfill them. The surgical patient faces a threat to the needs identified by humanistic psychologist and motivational theorist Abraham Maslow (1908-1970): physical, security, psychosocial, emotional, and spiritual.

Hierarchy of Needs. In following Maslow's concept of a motivational hierarchy of needs to set priorities for care (Fig. 7-2), the basic lower level (physiologic needs) essential for survival must be met first. Satisfaction of the higher level needs for safety and security, belonging and acceptance, self-esteem, and self-actualization can then be met. Health care personnel should be concerned with a total picture of the patient's needs and consider all of them.

In illness, needs can be influenced by factors such as location of the pathologic condition, type of surgical procedure, and effectiveness of therapy. Also, priorities may

change with changing situations. Preoperatively, anxiety and nutritional status are addressed. Intraoperatively, the team concentrates on the patient's physiologic needs for oxygen, circulation, and the prevention of shock and infection. Postoperatively, team members must prevent complications and encourage patient self-actualization. If the patient's needs are not met satisfactorily, undesirable consequences can occur.

Patients' Reactions to Illness

To meet a patient's needs, the health care team should be sensitive to his or her feelings about the illness. A patient's reactions influence his or her behaviors and the staff's behavioral responses. An understanding of the patient's basic methods of coping will be helpful to the caregiver in developing the plan of care (Table 7-1).

Behavior. Health and human behavior are interdependent and often age-dependent. Regardless of age, individuals with physiologic problems experience some emotional change that influences their behavior. Patients react to a new interpersonal environment according to their learned behavioral patterns. The following are basic facts about behavior:

- The perception of interaction within the environment creates individual differences in personality, behavior, and needs.
- A person's physical and psychosocial behavior is a response to stimuli in an attempt to maintain homeostasis.
- Behavior is complex. Behavioral acts have multiple causes in addition to a major precipitating one.
- A person functions on many levels simultaneously. Many factors determine an individual's response in a given situation.

Behavior should be evaluated in light of the person's specific situation and pertinent social forces such as family, culture, and environment. Patients respond to crises or personal threats in different ways. Some persons face suffering and surgical intervention with extreme courage, dignity, and fortitude. Others may revert to extreme fear or helplessness, even when faced with a relatively safe procedure.

Overt behavior is not necessarily consistent with one's feelings but often reflects them most accurately. Patients often express frustration and fear behaviorally in an effort to cope with environmental stimuli.

Adaptation. In 1984, theorist Sister Callista Roy proposed adaptation as a conceptual model for nursing. Any deviation from a person's normal daily pattern of living necessitates adaptation through innate or acquired defenses. Adaptation may involve physiologic or psychological changes. Her paradigm as it applies to perioperative patient care includes the following:

1. The patient takes in stimuli and processes the information to produce a response.
   a. Effective adaptation is exhibited by a favorable response.
   b. Ineffective adaptation is exhibited by unfavorable response.

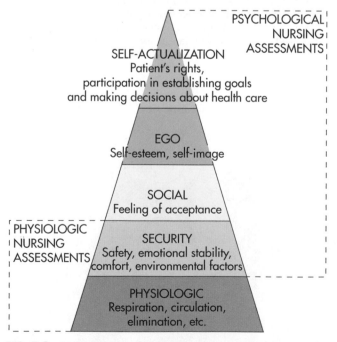

FIG. 7-2 Maslow's hierarchy of basic needs as related to surgical patients' needs during perioperative care.

TABLE 7-1	Common Coping Mechanisms		
Mechanism	**Meaning**	**Objective Assessment**	**Example**
Denial	Rejects responsibility; unable or unwilling to accept the truth	Stammers; may or may not make eye contact; seems to be making excuses	"I do not have lung cancer."
Displacement	Shifts blame to a weaker substitute	Is submissive to power figures, but critical and oppressive to subordinates	"My doctor never tells me anything. The lab must be wrong."
Identification	Acts like an admired hero or villain	Shows outward signs of indecisiveness and low self-esteem	"My sister and I both feel ill. We both have the same disease, I'll bet."
Projection	Attributes unacceptable behavior to others	Acts suspicious of others; assumes a defensive posture	"The cigarette manufacturer enticed me to smoke."
Rationalization	Justifies behavior with plausible statements	May be defensive or smug; trying to save face; can become hostile	"I became ill only because cancer runs in my family."
Reaction formation	Acts differently than he or she feels inside	Is confused; irrational; has mood swings; may seem overly conscientious and moral	"These are not tears of sadness; they are tears of joy because I will be dead soon."
Regression	Reverts back to a more primitive state of being	May assume closed, fetal position; has crossed arms and legs; looks downward, cries; has prolonged silences	"I want my mother."
Repression	Blocks unacceptable thoughts and feelings	Has a blank stare, a questioning look; no in-depth discussions	"I don't remember what my diagnosis is. Why am I here?"

2. The environment around and inside the patient is constantly changing. The patient responds either favorably or unfavorably to each change.
3. The health status of the patient integrates the whole person as he or she adapts to changes in internal and external forces.
4. The process of nursing is a science, and the application of patient care is an art.

Both the mind and the body must adapt successfully for the patient to recover. Adaptation requires energy, ingenuity, and persistence. The adaptive process includes physiologic or psychological changes that constitute an attempt to counteract stimuli so the individual can continue to function. If something interferes with this adaptation, the effects can be detrimental. Adaptation to illness includes the following three stages:

1. Transition from health: development of symptoms
2. Acceptance: coping and making decisions
3. Convalescence or resolution

Adaptation may be rapid or slow, depending on the nature of the stimuli and on the patient's culture, learned responses, and developmental needs. Adaptations may be sensory, motor, or sensorimotor. The extent of adjustment required is contingent on the type of illness, the magnitude of disability, and the patient's personality.

Stress. Stress can be defined as a physical, chemical, or emotional factor that causes tension, and it may be a factor in disease causation. It is the result of a perceived threat and is manifested by changes in physiologic and psychosocial behavior. Stress tolerance depends on the individual and on the stressor—its intensity, duration, and type (either localized or generalized, such as pain).

Stressful factors can originate from within the individual or from the external environment. Intrinsic factors, or those that originate within a patient, include the following:

- Hereditary or genetic factors, such as competency of the hormonal or enzymatic system.

- Nature of the illness or disease process. This may be influenced by nutritional or immunologic status.
- Severity of the illness or the presence of a stigma.
- Previous personal experiences with illness. Chronic illness has a disruptive effect on lifestyle.
- Age. Children feel threatened, whereas adolescents resent an interruption of activities and are painfully aware of body changes. Older people think about infirmity and death.
- Intellectual capacity. Misconceptions can lead to a knowledge deficit about the disease. Impaired cognitive function creates an inability to understand or comprehend.
- Disturbed sensorium. Hearing or sight loss intensifies a stressful experience.
- General state of personal well-being.

Extrinsic factors originate from external sources and include the following:

- Environment. The physical and social environment of the hospital is not the same as that of the home.
- Family role and status. Expectations and authoritative relationships affect lifestyle, attitudes, and communications.
- Economic or financial situation.
- Religion. Beliefs influence attitudes and values toward life, illness, and death. For example, Jehovah's Witnesses will not permit transfusion of whole blood or blood components. Orthodox Jews must follow dietary laws in any environment. The fatalistic attitudes derived from some religious beliefs give a person little control over his or her environment and can render a patient passive and apathetic.
- Cultural background, education, and social class. These factors are closely related to a patient's emotional responses and living habits. Significant cultural elements such as food habits; daily living patterns; hygiene; family organization; child care; and orientation to the past, present, and future should be

analyzed in relation to culture. An ethnic community is really a larger family. Roles taught by a cultural group influence the mores, beliefs, and social interactions of its members. Also, responses to pain may vary according to cultural or ethnic background. Some groups commonly show an exaggerated emotional response, whereas other groups believe it is more appropriate to conceal suffering and feelings.

- Social relationships. Family, significant others, and friends help satisfy the need for reassurance and provide a sense of being cared about.

Stress is both physiologic and psychological. It can adversely affect appetite and bodily functions such as digestion, metabolism, and fluid and electrolyte balance. The secretion of adrenocortical hormones delays wound healing and decreases resistance to infection. In addition, the patient's emotional needs come to the surface during times of markedly increased stress, which mobilizes defense mechanisms for fight or flight. The patient's ability to adapt depends in part on effective intervention.

Anticipatory apprehension, although normal to some degree, may diminish critical thinking and decision-making abilities and may initiate an exaggerated response. Patients feel vulnerable when threatened with the loss of body parts, bodily function, or life. The strangeness of the OR itself—its noises, odors, and equipment—represents an unfriendly environment.

Patients' Perceptions of Care

Studies have shown that a patient's perception is based on expectations of high-level care. The patient's belief system defines what he or she considers to be good care. Perceptions of caring behaviors vary according to the degree of illness, type of procedure, level of cognition, and setting. Most patients believe that proficient and efficient perioperative care includes assistance with pain control, warmth, comfort, and a safe environment. The caregiver is also perceived as a patient advocate and a communication link with the family and/or significant others.

Research has revealed that preoperatively a patient needs information about the surgical procedure, how it will be performed, and the type of anesthetic to be used. Intraoperatively, the patient assumes a passive role, entrusting his or her care to the perioperative team. Before administration of the anesthetic, the patient may be acutely aware of the surroundings and activities. Patients surveyed indicate that during this segment of intraoperative care they want to know what is happening as it takes place and desire reassurance from the circulator at his or her side. Patients expect the perioperative nurse to remain in physical proximity and act promptly in an emergency.

During and after the administration of the anesthetic, the patient places a strong sense of confidence in the team as a whole and has expectations of competence and efficiency. The professional nurse is considered a main source of protection during this period of vulnerability.

Postoperatively, the patient expects the perioperative nurse to monitor his or her condition closely and to provide pain relief as needed. In continuation of the passive role, the patient perceives the nurse as caring, protective, and efficient. Patients respond favorably to the following:

- Provision of privacy
- Sensitivity to the inconvenience of hospitalization
- Frequent family updates during the surgical procedure
- Attention to personal and special needs
- Acceptance of personal individuality
- Friendliness
- Accurate and understandable information about tests and treatments

Family/Significant Others

A discussion of the patient would not be complete without specific mention of the patient's family or of others significant in his or her life. Illness often creates an emotional and financial burden on the family. They may experience considerable anxiety over the outcomes of surgery, the feelings of isolation, and the disruption of lifestyle. Families' reaction to illness and perception of care is as individualized as the patient.

Families need preoperative instruction to prepare for the postoperative outcomes and rehabilitation. They also need to be kept informed of the patient's progress during the surgical procedure and recovery period. Time passes more slowly during waiting periods, and family members may fear something has gone wrong if the wait is longer than anticipated. Some family members may prefer to wait at home or at work. The surgeon should contact a spouse, family, or significant others when the surgical procedure is over. Discussions with anyone other than the patient concerning condition or personal information require the patient's permission as part of the Health Insurance Portability and Accountability Act (HIPAA) requirements concerning patient privacy.

THE PATIENT WITH INDIVIDUALIZED NEEDS

The debilitated, chronically ill, or age-extreme patient has an increased difficulty in combating the stress of surgery and anesthetic agents. Other problems or health considerations that predispose the patient to intraoperative or postoperative complications include substance abuse or other serious subclinical conditions not revealed during the preoperative assessment.

Preoperative diagnostic and laboratory studies assist in establishing diagnoses and in pinpointing areas of deficiency. Surgical intervention is often postponed until a physiologic situation is improved or controlled (e.g., high blood pressure is lowered; cardiac dysrhythmias are corrected). Preoperative therapy may be indicated to control diabetes, reduce obesity, or treat infection to decrease the risk of complications.

Patients of various ages and stages of development have different needs, and the ways of meeting these needs will vary. A family-centered approach to care is valuable. Family cooperation is essential for communication with, interpretation for, and assistance with patients, particularly geriatric patients.

The Patient with Sensory Impairment or Physical Challenge

Some patients come to the perioperative environment with conditions unrelated to the surgical problem. Sensory and physically challenged patients commonly have increased anxiety and require a highly individualized plan of care; these patients also have the potential for a problematic postoperative recovery.

Sensory Impairment. Communication is essential to assess adequately the needs of challenged patients and to care for them. Team members should know about and understand the patient's limitations. The patient has a right to know what will happen during the surgical experience and to participate in decisions about his or her care. The Rehabilitation Act of 1973 states that to receive federal funds, an agency "must provide, when necessary, appropriate auxiliary aids. . . to people with impaired sensory, manual or speaking skills to give them an equal opportunity to benefit from services." The complexities of each patient's situation should be evaluated and dealt with appropriately.

Language Barrier. A language barrier can be a complex challenge. Anxiety increases in proportion to one's inability to communicate in a stress-producing situation. The inability to understand or to express oneself verbally is frustrating, and the patient's behavior may reflect his or her feelings of inadequacy or insecurity. Nonverbal body language through eye contact, pleasant facial expressions, and a gentle touch can comfort the patient who speaks a different language. Every effort should be made to obtain an interpreter to assist the patient and the health care team; many hospitals use interpreters for the ethnic groups within the community.

Some patients are reluctant to share confidential medical information with a relative or friend. The interpreter should be trusted and accepted by the patient and should be sensitive to the needs of the surgeon and caregivers. The patient needs to be adequately informed before giving consent for a surgical procedure and must provide permission for release of information concerning the procedure.

Hearing Impairment/Deafness. Hearing impairment varies from inner ear conduction changes that occur during the aging process and affect the distinction of some high-frequency consonant sounds to congenital profound sensorineural deafness. Conductive or sensorineural deafness may result from disease or injury to the ear at any age. The degree of impairment will determine whether the patient communicates through sign language, has a hearing-assistive cochlear implant, has a hearing aid, and/or reads lips. Written information is always helpful, provided the patient is literate. Pictograms work well with most patients. An interpreter can assist with patients who use sign language.

The following steps should be observed when communicating with a patient who has a hearing impairment:
1. Make sure the room is quiet and well lit, with minimal distractions. Deaf patients may perceive extraneous sounds as buzzing or air-rushing. Deafness can be manifest in many degrees. Care is taken not to approach so quietly that the patient becomes startled.
2. Look directly at the patient. Speak clearly and slowly in a moderate tone of voice, with visible but not exaggerated lip movements. Facial expressions, touch, and body gestures can help communicate feelings and instructions.
3. Greet the patient without wearing a facemask and attract the patient's attention before speaking. Make eye contact.
4. Be sure the patient understands and responds appropriately to questions.
5. To help explain your actions, show the patient any equipment (e.g., a safety strap) before placing it on him or her.
6. Allow the patient to wear a hearing aid in the perioperative environment, if possible. Try to know what type of device the patient uses and how to adjust the controls if it should start humming during the procedure.

Visual Impairment/Blindness. Like deafness, blindness can be a part of the aging process or a congenital anomaly. Cataracts are a common cause of the loss of visual acuity; this condition may be inherited but is more often associated with aging. Vision is affected by the shape of the eye, other structural factors, and diseases and injuries.

Patients who are blind feel insecure in a strange environment; therefore, the following steps should be observed when communicating with them:
1. Address the patient by name in moderate tones and introduce yourself. Make some noise as you approach so as not to startle the patient.
2. Always speak to the patient before touching him or her. A gentle word followed by a gentle touch can be comforting.
3. To prevent a distressful reaction to unexpected noises or sensations, the patient should be told what is going to happen before any physical contact.
4. Guiding the patient's hand will help him or her feel secure, such as when being moved onto the operating bed.

A visually impaired patient should be permitted to wear eyeglasses in the perioperative environment as much as possible. If a general anesthetic is used, the glasses should be sent to the postanesthesia care unit (PACU) so they are available when the patient wakes up. Contact lenses must be removed before administration of a general anesthetic, because they may dry on the cornea or become dislodged.

Physical Challenge. Patients who are physically challenged require a highly individualized plan of care. Physical problems such as contractures or pressure sores may make it difficult to position the patient on the operating bed. Patients with spastic muscle motion as in cerebral palsy will require additional personnel around the operating bed for safety during transfer or the random body movement could cause the patient to fall. Creative supports and positioning aids are required, and additional assistance may be needed to move the patient safely. Exposure of the surgical site may be difficult to achieve.

Millions of people have some form of arthritis. Children with juvenile rheumatoid arthritis have many systemic problems as a result of the disease process, which continues into adulthood. The onset of this autoimmune disease can occur at any age and can result in stiffness, swelling, and deformity of the joints of the hands, feet, and neck; inflammation of blood vessels; and tissue damage to organ systems. Joints need solid but padded support. Long-term treatment with nonsteroidal antiinflammatory drugs (NSAIDs) or corticosteroid therapy may affect bleeding intraoperatively and wound healing postoperatively.

Paralyzed patients, such as those with spinal cord injury, are unable to move. Patients with lack of voluntary muscle control, such as with cerebral palsy, must be protected from falls or injuries during transport or transfer. These patients have decreased tactile sensitivity to heat and cold, so they must be protected from burns and hypothermia.

Impairment of Cognitive Function.
Communicating with patients who have impaired cognitive function is sometimes difficult. Cognitive functions are based on intelligence and the ability to think, learn, remember, and solve problems. Explanations about procedures and the environment may seem confusing and frightening to these patients. Verbal communication should be attempted at the patient's level of understanding and response. Simple phrases and soft vocal tones can be reassuring. Cooperation during the surgical procedure may be hard to attain, and preoperative sedation may be necessary.

The Patient with Alteration of Nutrition

Decreased intake and increased metabolic demands create nutritional problems in surgical patients. Drug therapy and procedure activities affect nutritional status; this should be considered when planning for a patient's nutritional needs. Table 7-2 describes the effects that certain drugs have on nutrition. The preoperative assessment may reveal risk factors associated with alterations of nutrition. Patients having procedures of the mouth, face, head, and neck may have mechanical difficulty taking adequate nutrition.

Malnutrition.
Malnutrition in the surgical patient is caused by an inadequate intake or use of calories and protein preoperatively and/or postoperatively. The discrepancy between the intake of essential nutrients and the body's demand for them creates a state of impaired functional ability and structural integrity. Surgical patients are commonly kept without food preoperatively for safe anesthetic administration and postoperatively to prevent nausea and vomiting. Patients who are undernourished have less than 70% to 80% of ideal body weight (IBW) and suffer greatly from the lack of caloric intake. As a result of malnutrition, the patient may experience the following:

1. Poor tolerance of anesthetic agents
   a. Decreased metabolism of chemicals by the liver
   b. Inadequate excretion of toxins by the kidneys
   c. Unstable vital signs
2. Altered wound healing potential
   a. Decreased protein synthesis postoperatively
   b. Increased protein wasting and breakdown of skeletal muscle after severe traumatic injury
   c. Negative nitrogen balance with a serum albumin less than 3 g/dL and blood urea nitrogen (BUN) less than 10 g/dL

TABLE 7-2	Drugs That Interfere with Nutritional Status
Drug	**Effect on Nutrition**
Aluminum hydroxide	Binds with other nutrients, causing phosphate malabsorption
Aminoglycosides	Reduce carbohydrate metabolism
Amphetamines	Suppress appetite, causing weight loss
Antacids	Alter gastrointestinal pH
Anticholinergics	Decrease gastrointestinal motility, causing malabsorption
Antihistamines	Stimulate appetite and can cause weight gain
Antihypertensives	Decrease gastrointestinal motility, causing malabsorption
Antineoplastics	Impair nutrient absorption
Antirheumatoids	Impair nutrient absorption
Benzodiazepines	Stimulate appetite, causing weight gain
Cathartics	Cause calcium and phosphate loss
Chloramphenicol	Inhibits protein binding
Cytotoxic agents	Suppress appetite, causing weight loss
Immunosuppressives	Suppress appetite, causing weight loss
Isoniazid	Causes pyridoxine deficiency
Neomycin	Interferes with bile acids, causing iron, sugar, and triglyceride malabsorption
Phenobarbital	Causes vitamin D deficiency
Phenothiazides	Stimulate appetite, causing weight gain
Phenytoin	Causes osteomalacia
Steroids	Deplete sodium
Tricyclic antidepressants	Stimulate appetite, causing weight gain

3. Decreased serum electrolytes associated with anorexia, bulimia, alcoholism, and other chronic metabolic disturbances
   a. Hypokalemia (low potassium level)
   b. Hypomagnesemia (low magnesium level)
   c. Hypocalcemia (low calcium level)
4. Increased susceptibility to infection from immunologic incompetence, with a total lymphocyte count less than 1500/mm^3
5. Sequential multisystem organ failure
   a. Dehydration
   b. Abnormalities in glucose regulation
   c. Abnormalities in clotting mechanisms
   d. Renal failure
   e. Cardiopulmonary failure
6. Increased risk of morbidity and mortality

Serum blood tests help determine nutritional status and include total proteins, albumin/globulin ratio, and BUN level. Body weight is also significant. The average adult patient needs a minimum of 1500 calories daily to prevent body protein catabolism. Hypermetabolic states can double that requirement to 3000 calories daily. If caloric intake is less than body requirements, protein is converted into carbohydrates for energy. Protein synthesis then becomes insufficient for restoration of body tissues. Box 7-1 describes conditions that place a patient at risk for protein deficiency and malnutrition.

Depleted reserves of essential elements must be replenished to replace tissue loss and expedite wound

BOX 7-1	Factors That Increase a Patient's Risk for Protein-Based Nutritional Deficit

- Chronic illness
- Acute illness
- Stress
- Metabolic disease
- Sensory impairment
- Unconsciousness
- Polypharmacy
- Depression
- Immobility
- Edentulousness

healing. Protein deficiency impairs collagen formation, thereby delaying the healing process. Water-soluble vitamins C and B complex are important for tissue repair and nervous system function. The fat-soluble vitamins A, D, E, and K are important for neurovascular activities. The patient's depleted nutritional status lowers host resistance by impairing lymphocyte and neutrophil production. A definite relationship has been demonstrated between hypoproteinemia and proliferative postoperative infection. Wound healing is impaired.

Metabolism. Metabolism is the phenomenon of synthesizing foodstuffs into complex elements and complex substances into simple ones in the production of energy. It involves two opposing phases:

1. Anabolism—the conversion of nutritive material into complex living matter; tissue construction
2. Catabolism, or destructive metabolism—breaking down or dissolution by the body of complex compounds, often with the release of energy

Metabolic disorders such as diabetes and the stress response of traumatic injury can complicate the outcome of a surgical intervention. Hormonal responses to physical stress involve both anabolic and catabolic effects on the body, with catabolism being the predominant effect. The degree of metabolic reaction may depend greatly on the body's reserve of labile protein. The patient's preoperative nutritional state, the type and extent of the surgical procedure, and the effect of the surgical procedure on the patient's ability to digest and absorb nutrients affect immediate postoperative metabolism.

Catabolic responses are augmented by preoperative fasting, cathartic preparation, adrenocortical responses to tissue trauma during the procedure, blood loss, and alterations in fluid and electrolyte balance. Patients with burns, traumatic injury, absorptive disorders, or toxemia need careful nutritional replacement, because they usually have a severe protein deficit. Hydration and renal function are closely observed and monitored in the perioperative environment.

Drugs also can have an adverse affect on metabolic balance. Broad-spectrum antibiotics limit a disease process, but in association with dietary inadequacy they can cause vitamin K deficiency in older patients by inhibiting the intestinal bacteria that produce that vitamin. Drug detoxification and/or excretion may be altered in patients with impaired kidney or liver function, leading to possible drug overdose.

Nutritional Supplements. Dietary management is used to correct metabolic and nutritional abnormalities before the surgical procedure. In some patients, special nutritional supplements are indicated to build up or compensate for a permanent metabolic handicap. Enteral feedings help maintain the integrity of the gastrointestinal mucosa. Successful therapy is indicated by weight gain, a rise in plasma albumin, and a positive nitrogen balance. A chemically defined elemental diet may be administered via the following routes:

- Oral intake
- Nasogastric tube for enteral nutrition
- Gastrostomy tube, with or without infusion pump for enteral nutrition
- Intravenous (IV) infusion of protein and dextrose through a peripheral vein for parenteral nutrition
- Central venous cannulation for hyperalimentation for parenteral nutrition

The Patient with Diabetes Mellitus

Diabetes mellitus is an endocrine disorder that affects glucose metabolism and the production of insulin in the beta cells of the pancreas. Insulin is a hormone that helps break down carbohydrates. If insulin is not produced in sufficient quantities or is of poor quality, carbohydrates are not metabolized and are excreted in the urine as glucose. Glucose molecules are large and damage the cellular structure of the renal tubules of the kidneys.

Usually genetic in origin, diabetes mellitus can be triggered in predisposed individuals by environmental stress. Management of the surgical patient with diabetes depends on the type and control of the disorder, which will be one of three types:

1. Type 1: insulin-dependent diabetes mellitus (IDDM). The pancreas produces little or no insulin, thus necessitating regular administration of insulin by injection. Onset may be at any age but usually occurs in juveniles (adolescents ages 12 to 16 years) and adults up to age 40 years.
2. Type 2: non–insulin-dependent diabetes mellitus (NIDDM). The pancreas produces varying amounts of insulin. Onset may be at any age but usually occurs after age 40 years in obese persons. Blood glucose levels are controlled by diet and the administration of oral antihyperglycemics.
3. Diabetes mellitus associated with other conditions or syndromes. Impaired glucose tolerance may be secondary to pancreatic or hormonal disease, drug or chemical toxicity, abnormal insulin receptors, or other genetic syndromes. The diabetes may be latent, asymptomatic, or borderline.

Stress caused by physical and emotional trauma, infection, or fever raises blood glucose levels and stimulates the pituitary and adrenal glands. The pituitary gland secretes adrenocorticotropic hormone (ACTH), which stimulates the production of glucocorticoids. These glucocorticoids in turn increase gluconeogenesis—the formation of glucose by the liver from noncarbohydrate sources. The resultant extra glucose enters the bloodstream. Coincidentally, the adrenal glands secrete epinephrine, which accelerates the conversion of glycogen in the liver to glucose and also raises the level of blood sugar. More insulin is needed to metabolize this additional blood sugar. The primary goal in controlling diabetes is to maintain a stable internal environment, thereby averting a metabolic crisis. Extreme care must be taken to prevent the following:

1. Hyperglycemia and ketonuria
   a. A rise in blood glucose and ketones can precipitate severe fluid loss, causing dehydration and hyperkalemia from the release of potassium from cells.
   b. Some medications (e.g., cortisone) increase the level of blood sugar and antagonize the effect of insulin.
2. Ketoacidosis and acetonuria
   a. These conditions are caused by insulin insufficiency from natural causes or from a reduced or omitted insulin dosage.
   b. These conditions may result in coma and ultimately death if allowed to progress untreated.
3. Hypoglycemia and hypoglycemic shock
   a. These conditions are caused by too much insulin.
   b. They are of faster onset than ketoacidosis.
   c. Hypoglycemia is especially dangerous. It can occur during major surgical procedures because of the omission or delay of oral intake.
   d. These conditions can cause brain damage and put stress on the cardiovascular system.

Prevention of these states depends on the following:
- Physician's treatment of choice for diabetes
- Severity and type of disorder
- Existence of complicating conditions
- Type of surgical procedure

The preoperative assessment of patients with the potential for impaired glucose metabolism includes laboratory testing for fasting and postprandial blood glucose levels, urinalysis, complete blood count, BUN, and serum electrolyte determinations. A chest radiograph study and electrocardiogram (ECG) also are advisable.

Common Complications of Diabetes Mellitus. The balance between caloric intake and glucose metabolism is disrupted during the perioperative experience. Patients with type 2 diabetes usually withstand a surgical intervention without crisis. Intraoperative metabolic control may be more difficult in patients with type 1 diabetes who have marked unpredictability and greater extremes in blood sugar levels. Lengthy major surgical procedures with extensive tissue trauma present the greatest challenge to regulation. Patients with diabetes are prone to the following:
- Dehydration and electrolyte imbalance
- Infection
- Inadequate circulation from neurovascular disease, causing deficient tissue perfusion (Fig. 7-3)
- Hypertension
- Hyperlipemia that affects both coronary and peripheral arteries. Peripheral edema can lead to gangrene.
- Delayed wound healing as a result of increased protein breakdown or compromised circulation. Glycogenesis,

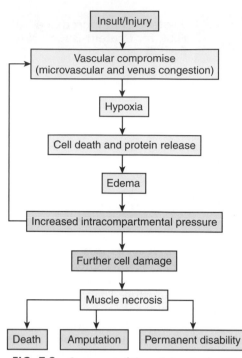

FIG. 7-3 Outcomes of tissue injury in the OR.

the breakdown of glycogen to glucose in the liver, diverts protein from tissue regeneration.
- Neuropathy or nervous system disorders, which causes motor and sensory deficit
- Nephropathy, which affects small blood vessels in the kidneys
- Retinopathy, which affects small vessels in eyes, and blindness
- Neuropathic musculoskeletal disease. Severe bone destruction may cause neuropathic fractures.
- Neurogenic bladder, which causes incontinence. Urinary tract infections are common.

Diabetes causes many bodily changes that increase in frequency with duration of the disease. Physiologic dysfunctions, as listed in Table 7-3, make a person with diabetes a potentially high-risk patient.

Special Considerations. Scheduling elective surgical procedures early in the day for patients with diabetes minimizes the period during which oral intake is restricted. Assessment of these patients can minimize potential risks:

1. Capillary blood should be tested preoperatively for fasting serum glucose. The results provide baseline data to assess postoperative control.
2. The preoperative insulin dose may be reduced or eliminated to guard against hypoglycemia or insulin shock during the surgical procedure.
3. Continuous IV access is vital throughout the surgical procedure in case of a metabolic problem. An infusion of dextrose in water may be started to begin administering the daily carbohydrate requirement before the patient comes to the OR.
   a. Optional methods of management for patients who are insulin dependent are determined by the severity of the disease, the preoperative control

TABLE 7-3	Physiologic Dysfunctions in High-Risk Patients with Diabetes and Obesity

Diabetes Mellitus	Obesity
INTEGUMENTARY SYSTEM	
Skin that may be dry, itchy	Hirsutism in women
Loss of fat from adipose tissue	Excess subcuticular fat
Injuries that heal slowly	Injuries that heal slowly
MUSCULOSKELETAL SYSTEM	
Neuropathic skeletal disease with bone destruction	Osteoarthritis
Leg pain, neuropathy	Chronic back pain
Muscular wasting	Strain on joints and ligaments
	Joint pain
	Diminished mobility
CARDIOVASCULAR SYSTEM	
Increased heart rate	Myocardial hypertrophy
Predisposition to coronary artery disease	High blood pressure
Predisposition to thrombophlebitis	Arteriosclerosis
Peripheral edema	Venous stasis
	Varicose veins
RESPIRATORY SYSTEM	
Predisposition to infection	Shortness of breath
	Decreased tidal volume
	Decreased lung expansion
RENAL SYSTEM	
Nephropathy	Vascular changes in kidneys
Increased excretion	Decreased intestinal mobility
Neurogenic bladder	Predisposition to liver and biliary disease
GASTROINTESTINAL SYSTEM	
Secretion of glucose by liver	
NEUROLOGIC SYSTEM	
Neuropathy	
Sensory impairment	
Retinopathy and blindness	
ENDOCRINE SYSTEM	
Poor or nonexistent insulin production	Predisposition to diabetes mellitus
Poor metabolic control	Pituitary abnormalities
Increased production of cortisol by adrenal glands under stress	Poor metabolic control
Electrolyte imbalance	Dysfunctional uterine bleeding

regimen, and the type of surgical procedure. Insulin may be added to the infusion or administered by subcutaneous injection. Amounts are determined by serum glucose levels.

b. Adequate hydration must be maintained because a rising blood glucose level upsets osmotic equilibrium. Electrolytes may be added to maintain metabolic status.

c. Fluid intake and output must be monitored to maintain hydration without fluid overload.

4. A metabolic crisis in an unconscious patient is difficult to detect without frequent blood tests. Therefore, during long surgical procedures, blood glucose levels are monitored for hyperglycemia or hypoglycemia. Glucometers accurately measure capillary blood glucose levels. Monitoring is necessary to ascertain the patient's requirements for insulin, glucose, or both.

5. Nasogastric suction may cause acidosis, dehydration, or electrolyte imbalance.

6. Antiembolic stockings are usually worn by the patient during the surgical procedure and postoperatively as a precaution against thrombophlebitis and thromboembolism. Some surgeons use sequential compression leg wraps to prevent deep vein thrombosis during long periods of immobility.

7. Skin integrity must be guarded to avoid breakdown.
   a. Strict aseptic and sterile techniques are extremely important to the infection-prone diabetic patient.
   b. To protect bony prominences and to prevent pressure sores, foam padding or a gel mattress should be placed on the operating bed for surgical procedures expected to take more than 2 hours.
   c. Hyposensitive tape is used to affix dressings.

The Obese Patient

Obesity is prevalent in our society. Obesity is referred to as morbid obesity when weight exceeds 100 pounds (45.4 kg) over the ideal weight. The patient's body mass index (BMI) exceeds 25 to greater than 30 kg/m^2. The term *morbid* is used to describe from 110% to greater than 120% of IBW and its serious effect on health and lifestyle. It may be of one of two origins:

1. Endocrine—usually associated with biliary, hepatic, or endocrine disease
2. Nonendocrine—commonly associated with excessive caloric intake

Common Complications of Obesity. Surgical patients who are 10% or more overweight have an increased incidence of morbidity and mortality caused by concomitant systemic diseases and physical problems. The degree of morbidity varies with the severity of the obese condition. The physiologic dysfunctions of obesity are listed in Table 7-3.

Obesity predisposes an individual to several conditions:

• Increased demand on the heart. Pulse rate, cardiac output, stroke volume, and blood volume increase to meet the metabolic demands of the adipose tissue (fat). Eventually this overload leads to myocardial hypertrophy (enlargement of the heart), and congestive heart failure may result. Coronary artery disease also is common.

• Hypertension (high blood pressure). Vascular changes in the kidneys are associated with hypertension and affect the elimination of protein wastes and the maintenance of fluid and electrolyte balance.

• Varicose veins and edema in the lower extremities. Poor venous return results from pressure on the pelvic veins and the vena cava. Venous stasis can ultimately contribute to thrombophlebitis and thromboembolism. Some surgeons use sequential compression leg wraps or antiembolic stockings to prevent deep vein thrombosis during long periods of immobility.

• Pulmonary function abnormalities. Hypoxemia, or inadequate oxygen in blood, may be associated with decreased tidal volume or poor gas exchange caused by excessive weight on the thoracic cavity. Patients who are obese are susceptible to postoperative pulmonary infection and pulmonary embolism.

- Respiratory compromise sleep apnea is common.
- Diseases of the digestive system, such as liver or gallbladder disease. Diverticulosis is not uncommon.
- Osteoarthritis. This condition may limit mobility of the spine and joints and may in fact contribute to excessive wear on joint cartilage.
- Diabetes mellitus. Type 2 diabetes.
- Malnutrition. Even though the obese patient is overweight, he or she may have a protein deficiency or other metabolic disturbance such as hyperlipidemia.

Special Considerations. The physical size of an obese patient presents problems for the OR and PACU teams. Safety precautions against injury to the patient and staff, falls, and burns must be emphasized. Problems include the following:

1. Transporting and lifting the patient. Size-appropriate wheelchairs and stretchers should be used. Mechanical patient lifters are desirable. If these are not available, extra people are needed to ensure safety in lifting.
   a. Stretchers and operating beds must be weight appropriate and stabilized. Most standard operating beds cannot support more than 300 to 350 pounds. The manufacturer's instructions should be consulted. Operating beds should be tagged with clearly visible weight restrictions. Larger weight loads can be borne by beds especially designed for obese patients.
   b. In moving the patient from the stretcher to the operating bed, the wheels should be locked and it should be suggested that the patient sit up. The back of the patient's gown should be untied, and the patient should be asked to feel for the side of the operating bed so that he or she does not move too far and fall over the opposite side. Additional personnel should stand at the opposite side of the bed to prevent falls.
   c. Safety belts should be long enough to provide secure limitation of unwanted mobility. When the patient is supine, the circulating nurse should place a small pillow under the patient's knees to relieve low back strain. The safety belt is placed over the thighs 2 to 3 inches above the knees. The circulating nurse should be able to slide one hand between the safety belt and the patient to ensure that no pressure is on the patient. A second safety belt may be needed for the lower legs if the patient's calves occupy the spaces closest to the edge of the bed because of the inability to close the legs when supine.
2. Keeping bodily exposure to a minimum as with all patients. Gowns are often small and obese patients may feel self-conscious.
3. Induction, intubation, and maintenance of anesthesia.
   a. On rare occasions, venous cutdown may be necessary to establish an IV line if peripheral veins are hard to access. Some anesthesia providers may use a central line for better venous access.
   b. Mobility of the cervical spine to hyperextend the neck for intubation may be limited. The anesthesia chapter of this text (Chapter 24) discusses neck and throat considerations for complex intubation. Some patients may require awake intubation.
   c. Inefficient respiratory muscles, poor lung/chest wall compliance, and/or increased intraabdominal pressure in the supine position reduce ventilation capability.
   d. Inefficient ventilation lowers the concentration of gases entering the alveoli of the lungs, which prolongs induction time.
   e. Continuous uptake by adipose tissue requires higher concentrations of anesthetic agents to maintain anesthesia. Drug dosages are calculated by body weight in kilograms (2.2 kg = 1 lb). The circulating nurse should double-check that the patient's weight is listed in kilograms on the chart for the anesthesia provider.
   f. The recovery period may be prolonged because adipose tissue retains fat-soluble agents and because the poor blood supply in this tissue eliminates agents slowly.
4. Positioning, prepping, and draping on the operating bed.
   a. Extra personnel may be necessary to assist with positioning.
   b. Massive tissue and pressure areas must be protected. Protuberances must be padded to prevent bruising and pressure injuries (Fig. 7-4). Tissue folds, breasts, and genitalia should not be compressed. Alternating pressure reduction surfaces such as gel pads should be used. Rolled blankets are not appropriate padding because once compressed, they do not disperse the body weight and become a source of localized pressure.
   c. Ventilation and circulation must be ensured.
   d. When an electrosurgical unit is used, the patient's dispersive electrode is applied on a flat, dry, smooth surface and is not surrounded by overlapping skinfolds, because tissue could be burned.
   e. An additional person may need to help hold the legs during Foley catheter insertion.
   f. More than one skin prep tray may be needed to accommodate large body habitus.
5. Increased operating time because of mechanics of the surgical procedure.
   a. In an open procedure, the accessibility of deep organs (e.g., gallbladder) may be a problem.
   b. Large instrumentation may contribute to surgical trauma and postoperative pain.
6. Thromboembolic complications, which may occur because of venous stasis; erythrocytosis, which increases the viscosity of the blood; and a decrease in fibrinolytic activity. Anticoagulants such as subcutaneous heparin may be given prophylactically.
7. Delayed healing because of poor vascularity of adipose tissue. Obese patients have an increased incidence of postoperative wound infection and disruption.

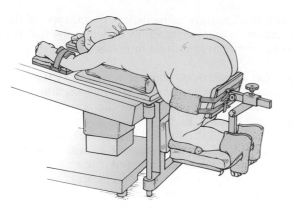

FIG. 7-4 Positioning an obsese patient for spinal surgery on an Andrews frame.

a. A sterile, closed drainage system is often used to drain accumulated fluid, thereby facilitating healing.
b. It is harder to eliminate "dead space" in wound closure.

THE PATIENT WITH CANCER

Oncology is the study of scientific control over neoplastic growth. It concerns the etiology, diagnosis, treatment, and rehabilitation of patients with known or potential neoplasms. A neoplasm is an atypical growth of abnormal cells or tissues that may be a benign or malignant tumor.

Both malignant and benign neoplasms consist of cells that divide and grow uncontrollably at varied rates. The stimulus for growth can be intrinsic (e.g., hormonal) or extrinsic (e.g., exposure to external elements). Neoplastic overgrowth or the invasion of surrounding tissue causes dysfunction and may eventually cause the death of the patient.

Cancer is a broad term that encompasses any malignant tissue change and is potentially curable. Treatment and prognosis are based on the type of cancer and the extent of the disease. Each type differs in its symptoms, behavior, and response to treatment.

The exact cause of cancer is unknown, but is the second leading cause of death in the United States. Cancerous tumors can be caused by exposure to chemical toxins, ionizing radiation, chronic tissue irritation, tobacco smoke, ultraviolet rays, viral invasion, and genetic predisposition. Studies have shown that immunosuppression may contribute to the incidence of cancer by altering biochemical metabolism and cellular enzyme production. Other research has shown that dietary influences, such as nitrates, salt-cured or smoked foods, and high-fat diets, may contribute to cancer in certain individuals.

Oncologists study the cause (epidemiology) of cancer, as well as the diagnosis, treatment, and rehabilitation of cancer patients. Moreover, patients are demanding that their surgeons give attention to the reconstruction of body image and rehabilitation to a useful life. Therefore the management of patients with cancer must be accomplished through the efforts of a multidisciplinary team of oncologic surgeons in conjunction with pathologists, radiation oncologists, pharmacists, immunologists, medical oncologists, and others. In addition to physical care, nurses in all patient care settings provide psychologic support for cancer patients and their families.

Cancer Risk Avoidance Behaviors

Patient education should include information about avoiding cancer-causing behaviors and how to minimize the risk for cancer. Behaviors to discuss include the following:

• Avoiding smoking and exposure to smoke. The Department of Health and Human Services reports that exposure to cigarette smoke is responsible for 83% of all cases of lung cancer. Each year more than 100,000 children 12 years of age and younger begin smoking, which leads to habitual use. Secondhand smoke, referred to as environmental tobacco smoke (ETS), has been implicated in the development of cancer in nonsmoking people who are exposed to smoke on a regular basis.
• Increasing dietary intake of fiber and low-fat foods. Antioxidants such as vitamins C and A may reduce an individual's risk for developing cancer. High-fat diets have been implicated in the development of breast, colon, and prostate cancers. According to reports of the American Cancer Society, 35% of cancer deaths are related to dietary causes and are possibly preventable. A desirable weight should be maintained, and obesity should be avoided. Excessive alcohol intake should also be avoided.
• Minimizing sun exposure, especially between the hours of 10:00 AM and 3:30 PM. Sun exposure has been shown to be the major cause of skin cancer, especially melanoma. Severe sunburn in childhood may be linked to the development of skin cancer later in life. Certain medications, such as tranquilizers, antidiabetic agents, diuretics, antiinflammatory agents, and antibiotics, can predispose an individual to sunburn. Certain cosmetic products, such as tretinoin (Retin-A) and alpha-hydroxy acid are extremely reactive to sunlight and can increase the risk of sunburn within 30 minutes of exposure. Tanning booths also can be hazardous to the skin.
• A waterproof sunscreen lotion with a sun protection factor (SPF) of at least 15 should be applied whenever sun exposure is likely. Sun-blocking products of SPF 30 to 45 are preferred and should provide protection from both ultraviolet A and ultraviolet B (UVA, UVB) rays. (UVA rays can increase the damage caused by UVB rays.) Sunscreen should be applied at least half an hour before going outdoors and reapplied every hour thereafter.
• Having regular checkups, especially yearly checkups after 40 years of age. Knowing the warning signs of cancer may promote prompt diagnosis and treatment. Signs to consider in young children include frequent swelling (lymphadenopathy) or bruising, unexplained headaches or fevers, dramatic weight loss or gain, and localized pain.
• Self-examining the skin, breast, and testes, which may reveal an early sign of cancer. These self-examinations should be performed monthly.

Extent of Disease

Carcinoma In Situ. In carcinoma in situ, normal cells are replaced by anaplastic cells but the growth disturbance of epithelial surfaces shows no behavioral evidence of invasion and metastasis. This cellular change is noted most often in stratified squamous and glandular epithelium. Carcinoma in situ is also referred to as intraepithelial or preinvasive cancer. Common sites for in situ carcinoma include the following:

- Uterine cervix
- Uterine endometrium
- Vagina
- Anus
- Penis
- Lip
- Buccal mucosa
- Bronchi
- Esophagus
- Eye
- Breast

Localized Cancer. Localized cancer is contained within the organ of its origin.

Regional Cancer. In regional cancer, the invaded area extends from the periphery of the organ or tissue of origin to include tumor cells in adjacent organs or tissues (e.g., the regional lymph nodes).

Metastatic Cancer. In metastatic cancer, the tumor extends by way of lymphatic or vascular channels to tissues or organs beyond the regional area.

Disseminated Cancer. In disseminated cancer, multiple foci of tumor cells are dispersed throughout the body.

Cancer Treatment Modalities

Cancer is a systemic disease. Therapy is curative if the disease process can be totally eradicated, but the success of therapy depends largely on early diagnosis. Tumors are classified to determine the most effective therapy. When a cure is not possible, palliative therapy relieves symptoms and improves quality of life but does not cure the disease.

Adjuvant Therapy. Surgical resection, endocrine therapy, radiation therapy, chemotherapy, immunotherapy, hyperthermia, or combinations of these procedures are used to treat cancer. The surgeon or oncologist determines the most appropriate therapy for each patient. When determining the most appropriate therapy, the following are considered:

- Type, site, and extent of tumor and whether lymph nodes are involved
- Type of surrounding normal tissue
- Age and general condition of the patient, including nutritional status and whether other diseases are present
- Whether curative or palliative therapy is possible

Before beginning therapy, a patient with cancer undergoes an extensive pretreatment workup. Each form of cancer therapy has certain advantages and limitations. Several factors affect a patient's response to treatment: host factors, clinical stage of malignancy, and type of therapy. The patient is followed carefully to determine the effectiveness of treatment at routine intervals.

Surgical Resection. Surgical resection is the modality of choice to remove solid tumors. The resection of a malignant tumor is, however, localized therapy for what may be a systemic disease. Each patient is evaluated and treated individually, and the surgical procedure is planned appropriately for the identified stage of disease. Depending on localization, regionalization, and dissemination of the tumor, the surgeon selects either a radical curative surgical procedure or a salvage palliative surgical procedure.

Surgical debulking, in which the tumor is partially removed, may be the procedure of choice for some types of surgically incurable malignant neoplasms. With surgical debulking, the intent is not to cure but to make subsequent therapy with irradiation, drugs, or other palliative measures more effective and thereby extend survival. In planning the surgical procedure, the surgeon considers the length of expected survival, the prognosis of surgical intervention, and the effect of concurrent diseases on the postoperative result.

Accessible primary tumors are often treated by excision. An extremely wide resection may be necessary to avoid recurrence of the tumor. The pathologist is able to make judgments about questionable margins by evaluating frozen sections while the surgical procedure is in progress. The pathologist's findings guide the surgeon during resection so that residual tumor is not left in the patient. The specimen is also tested after permanent section fixation in the pathology laboratory. Final results are available in 2 to 3 days. Additional discussion about cancer diagnostics is found in Chapter 22.

Many surgical procedures are performed for ablation of tumors by primary resection. In addition, a lymphadenectomy (removal of local lymph nodes) may be performed as a prophylactic measure to inhibit the metastatic spread of tumor cells via lymphatic channels. These nodes are tested to determine the extent of tumor cell spread. Other modalities of therapy may be administered preoperatively, intraoperatively, and/or postoperatively to reduce or prevent a recurrence or metastasis.

Considerations for Intraoperative Care

Malignant tumor cells can be disseminated by manipulation of tissue. Because of their altered nutritional and physiologic status, patients with cancer also may be highly susceptible to the complications of postoperative infection. To minimize these risks, the following specific precautions are taken in the surgical management of patients with cancer:

1. The skin over the site of a soft tissue tumor should be handled gently during hair removal and antisepsis. Vigorous scrubbing could dislodge underlying tumor cells; this is avoided by the use of "no-touch" techniques. With vascular tumors, manipulation during positioning or skin preparation could cause vascular complications such as emboli or hemorrhage. The no-touch technique means that the tumor is handled as little as possible during its removal.

2. Gowns, gloves, drapes, and instruments may be changed after a biopsy (e.g., a breast biopsy) before incision for a radical resection (e.g., a mastectomy). The tumor is deliberately incised to obtain a biopsy for diagnosis.

3. Instruments placed in direct contact with tumor cells may be discarded immediately after use. Even when the tumor appears to be localized, most cancers have disseminated to some degree. Therefore some surgeons prefer to use each instrument once and then discard it.

4. Some surgeons prefer to irrigate the surgical site with sterile water instead of sterile normal saline solution to cause the destruction of cancerous cells by crenation. This practice is common during mastectomy.

5. As a prophylactic measure, antibiotics are administered preoperatively, intraoperatively, and postoperatively to provide an adequate antibacterial level to prevent wound infection.

6. Time-honored precautions such as handling tissue gently, keeping blood loss to a minimum, and avoiding an unduly prolonged surgical procedure influence the outcome for the patient.

During a long surgical procedure, the circulating nurse conveys periodic messages to the patient's family members or significant others to reassure them that their loved one is receiving care from a concerned perioperative team.

Cancer Therapy

Patients may have many treatments of a varied nature before they come to the OR for resection. The team should have an understanding of the treatment regimen the patient is undergoing in conjunction with surgery. The following methodologies have many different types of effects on the patient's physiology and can alter response patterns during surgical intervention. Some of these treatments require combined chemical, radiation, and surgical procedures in order to be effective.

Endocrine Therapy. Tumors arising in organs that are usually under hormonal influence (e.g., breast, ovary, and uterus in female patients; prostate and testes in male patients) may be stimulated by hormones produced in the endocrine glands. Cellular metabolism is affected by the presence of specific hormone receptors in tumor cells: estrogen and/or progesterone in a female and androgens in a male.

Certain breast, endometrial, and prostatic cancers depend on sex hormones for growth and maintenance. Therefore the recurrence or spread of disease may be slowed by therapeutic hormonal manipulation. Endocrine manipulation does not cure, but it can control dissemination of the disease if the tumor progresses beyond the limits of effective surgical resection or radiation therapy.

Hormonal Receptor Site Studies. Identifying the hormonal dependence of the primary tumor through studies of the receptor site is a fairly reliable way of selecting patients who will benefit from preoperative or postoperative endocrine manipulation. After a positive diagnosis of cancer, either by a frozen section biopsy or by pathologic permanent sections, the surgeon will probably request a receptor site evaluation of a primary breast, uterine, or prostatic tumor. The tissue specimen removed by surgical resection should be sent fresh or in saline. It should not be placed in formalin preservative solution because doing so will alter the receptor cells enough to negate the hormonal study.

Endocrine Ablation. Since 1896, surgeons have described positive clinical responses in patients with metastatic breast cancer after treatment by endocrine ablation—the surgical removal of endocrine glands. If the surgeon plans to eliminate endocrine stimulation surgically in a patient with a known hormone-dependent tumor, all sources of the hormone should be ablated chemically, hormonally, or surgically.

- Bilateral adrenalectomy and oophorectomy. Both adrenal glands and/or ovaries may be resected to prevent the recurrence of endocrine-derived cancer. These may be removed as a one-stage surgical procedure (i.e., bilateral adrenalectomy/oophorectomy). If two separate surgical procedures are preferred, the bilateral oophorectomy precedes the bilateral adrenalectomy, except in menopausal women in whom only the latter surgical procedure may be indicated.

- Bilateral adrenalectomy and orchiectomy. After prostatectomy for advanced carcinoma of the prostate, both testes may be removed (i.e., bilateral orchiectomy) to eliminate androgens of testicular origin. Bilateral adrenalectomy also may be indicated.

- Hormonal therapy. Hormones administered orally or via injection can alter cell metabolism by changing the systemic hormonal environment of the body. For hormones to be effective, tumor cells must contain receptors. Hormones must bind to these receptors before they can exert an effect on cells.

- Antiestrogen therapy. Patients with medical contraindications to endocrine ablation may receive antiestrogen therapy. An estrogen antagonist deprives an estrogen-dependent tumor of the estrogen necessary for its growth. Nafoxidine and tamoxifen (Nolvadex) are synthetic nonsteroidal drugs that inhibit the normal intake of estrogen at estrogen receptor sites; they are taken orally.

- Corticosteroids. Prednisone, cortisone, hydrocortisone, or some other preparation of corticosteroids may be administered as an antiinflammatory agent along with the chemotherapeutic agents given to control disseminated disease.

Photodynamic (Laser) Therapy

For photodynamic therapy (also referred to as photoradiation), an argon tunable dye laser is used to destroy malignant cells by photochemical reaction. A photosensitive drug, either hematoporphyrin derivative (HPD) from cow's blood (Photofrin) or purified dihematoporphyrin ether, is absorbed by malignant and reticular endothelial cells.

The photosensitive drug is injected intravenously via venipuncture or Hickman catheter 24 to 48 hours before the photodynamic therapy and is taken up by cells to make them fluorescent and photosensitive. It remains longer in malignant cells than in normal cells before being excreted from the body. When exposed to light from an argon laser, the tunable rhodamine B dye laser produces a red beam of approximately 630 nm. Other dyes, such as dicyanomethylene, may produce different wavelengths. HPD in cells absorbs the laser light, which leads to a photochemical reaction that causes tissue-oxygen molecules to release cytotoxic singlet oxygen and destroy tumor cells. Depending on tumor site, the laser can be delivered interstitially, endoscopically, externally, or retrobulbarly.

Photodynamic therapy may be used to debulk tumors of the eye, head and neck, breast, esophagus, gastrointestinal tract, bronchus, and bladder. The tunable dye laser also may be used to diagnose tumor cells. The OR should be darkened or have shades to block outside daylight during the laser treatment. The patient is cautioned to avoid exposure to sunlight or other sources of ultraviolet light both after injection of the dye and postoperatively. Photosensitivity is the primary side effect of the dye and may last 4 to 6 weeks.

Radiation Therapy

Radiation is the emission of electromagnetic waves or atomic particles that result from the disintegration of nuclei of unstable or radioactive elements. The treatment of malignant disease with radiation may be referred to as radiation therapy, brachytherapy, or radiotherapy. Ionizing radiation is used for this type of therapy, which involves the use of high-voltage radiation and other radioactive elements to injure or destroy cells. Like surgical resection and photodynamic therapy, radiation therapy is localized therapy that is applicable for a limited number of specific tumors.

Ionizing Radiation. Ionization is the physical production of positive and negative ions capable of conducting electricity. Ionizing radiation is radiation with sufficient energy to disrupt the electronic balance of an atom. When disruption occurs in tissue cells or extracellular fluids, the effect can range from minor changes to profound disturbances. Radiation may come either from particles of the nuclei of disintegrating atoms or from electromagnetic waves that have no mass. Types of ionizing radiation include:

- Alpha particles. Alpha particles are relatively large particles that have a very slight penetrating power. They are stopped by a thin sheet of paper. They have dense ionization but can produce tremendous tissue destruction within a short distance.
- Beta particles. Beta particles are relatively small, are electrical, and travel with the speed of light. They have greater penetrating properties than do alpha particles. Their emissions cause tissue necrosis, and they produce ionization, which has destructive properties.
- Gamma rays and x-rays. Gamma rays and x-rays are electromagnetic radiations of short wavelength but high energy and are capable of completely penetrating the body. They affect tumor tissue more rapidly than normal tissue. These types of rays are stopped by a thick lead shield. Protons ranging in energy from 30 kilovolts (kV) to 35 million electron volts (eV) are available for the treatment of various cancers. Gamma rays are emitted spontaneously from the nucleus of an atom of a radioactive element.

Effects of Radiation on Cells

Cancer cells multiply out of normal body control; they are in a state of active, uncontrolled mitosis (the nuclear division of the cytoplasm and nucleus). Radiation affects the metabolic activity of cells. Cells in an active state of mitosis are most susceptible. Over time, gamma rays and x-rays cause a cessation of cell growth and a regression of the tumor mass. Cells die and are replaced by fibrous tissue.

The sensitivity of a tumor to radiation varies. Some tumors can be destroyed by a small amount of radiation, whereas others require a large amount. The sensitivity of the tumor cells is determined by the sensitivity of the normal cells from which the tumor cells are derived. The effects of radiation therapy also depend to a large extent on tissue oxygenation. As a tumor grows, the periphery is well oxygenated but the central portion becomes necrotic and poorly oxygenated. The number of cells killed by radiation therapy is directly related to the amount of tissue and oxygen within the tumor. Therefore the hypoxic effect is a factor in determining therapeutic dosage of radiation.

Radiation therefore cannot be limited solely to the area being treated. The danger of injuring normal surrounding tissue is a limiting factor in the dosage and selection of the most appropriate type of radiation therapy. A factor in dosage is the ratio of tumor tissue to the surrounding normal tissue. The dosage is computed in rads (roentgen-absorbed doses). A rad is the unit used to measure the absorbed dose of radiation. One rad is the amount of radiation required to deposit 100 ergs of energy per gram of tissue.

Radiophysics or instruments such as Geiger counters or scintillation probes are used to determine the dose of radiation delivered to a specific tissue site; the dose is measured by distance from the source and duration of exposure. Doses are measured in rads to determine whether the dosage is adequate for therapy but not so excessive that it would cause damage to normal tissues.

The penetration of radiation energy is calculated from the rate of decay or disintegration, known as half-life. Half-life is the time required for half of the radioactive element to disintegrate and to lose half of its activity through decay.

Sources of Radiation

Although the effects of the different types of radiation therapy are similar, their sources and applications do differ. Some sources are implanted into the body in direct contact with tumor tissue, whereas other sources use an external beam to pass the radiation through the body to the tumor.

- Radium. Radium is a radioactive metal. Mme. Marie Curie (1867-1934), a research chemist, and her husband, Pierre (1859-1906), a physicist, discovered and named this metal in 1898. Several years earlier, Mme. Curie had been given the task of finding out why pitchblende would record its image on a photographic plate. She and her husband knew this material emitted more radiation than would be justified by the known minerals contained in it. It took 6 years of painstaking, difficult work for the Curies to isolate radium as a pure element and to learn of its radioactive properties. Their research eventually led to the use of radium in the treatment of malignant tumors.

- Metallic radium is unstable in air. Radium chloride or bromide salts emit fluorescence and heat. One gram gives off 134 calories per hour. Alpha and beta particles and gamma rays are products of its disintegration. The half-life of radium is approximately 1620 years; half the remaining life is lost in another 1620 years, and so on. The final product is lead.
- Radon. Radon is a dense, radioactive gas liberated as the first by-product of the disintegration of radium. Mme. Curie discovered this gas and first named it emanation. Radon is collected by an intricate process in radiopaque glass or gold capillary tubing, and the seeds for implantation are then cut and sealed. The dosage is computed according to the hours of insertion into tissue. It is measured in millicurie-hours. The half-life of radon is 4 days; its total life is approximately 30 days.
- Radionuclides. A radionuclide is an element that has been bombarded with radioactive particles in a nuclear reactor. A radionuclide shows radioactive disintegration and emits alpha and beta particles or gamma rays. Radionuclides that emit beta particles and gamma rays are used primarily for treating malignant tumors. Therapeutic radionuclides also may be referred to as radiopharmaceuticals. Historically they were known as radioactive isotopes, or radioisotopes, and these terms are still found in the literature. Cesium, cobalt, iodine, iridium, and yttrium are the most commonly used elements for therapy.

Radionuclides are controlled by the Atomic Energy Commission and are released only to individuals trained and licensed to use them. Available in liquid or solid forms, they may be ingested orally, infused intravenously, instilled into a body cavity, injected or implanted into a tumor, or applied to the skin externally. The ionizing radiation emitted has an action on tissue similar to that of radium, but radionuclides differ from radium in the following ways:

The half-life of radionuclides is short. Radionuclides disintegrate at varying rates depending on their type. Each element has a specific half-life that varies from a few hours (e.g., the 6 hours of technetium-99) to the 8 days of iodine-131 or the 5.3 years of cobalt-60.

Irradiation with radionuclides does not spread so much into adjoining tissue; therefore a stronger dose can be used in a malignant tumor. Radiation is not absorbed by bone and other normal body tissues. It can be more easily shielded for safe handling. The surgeon and other personnel get less radiation exposure in placing or removing radionuclides.

As with exposure to radium and radon, exposure to radionuclides is always potentially dangerous. Radiation may treat cancer, but it can also cause a malignant neoplasm.

Implantation of Radiation Sources

All radiation sources for implantation are prepared in the desired therapeutic dosages by personnel in the nuclear medicine department. Many types of sources are used to deliver maximum radiation to the primary tumor. No single type is ideal for every tumor or anatomic site.

Interstitial Needles. Interstitial needles are hollow sheaths and are usually made of platinum or Monel metal. Radium salts or radionuclides are encased in platinum or platinum-iridium short units or cells, which in turn are sealed in the metal sheath of the needle for implantation into tumor tissue. A needle may contain one or several short units or cells of the radiation source, depending on the length of needle to be used. Needles vary in length from 10 to 60 mm, with a diameter of 1 to 2 mm. The choice of length depends on dosage and on the area involved. Dosage is measured in milligram-hours, which can be converted to rads.

The interstitial needles, which usually contain cesium-137, are implanted in tumors near the body surface or in tissue accessible enough to permit their use (e.g., vagina, cervix, tongue, mouth, neck). In certain patients, stereotactic techniques are used to implant needles for the irradiation of brain tumors.

In the OR these needles are inserted at the periphery of and within the tumor. One end of the needle is pointed, and the other end has an eye for a heavy (size 2) suture. Needles are threaded to prevent loss while in use and to aid in removal. After the surgeon inserts the needles, the ends of the sutures are tied or taped together and are taped to the skin in an adjoining area or secured to buttons. Depending on the anatomic site, a template may be used to position and secure the needles.

A template consists of two acrylic plates that are separated by rubber O-rings and held together with screws. The plates have holes for insertion of the interstitial needles. The template remains in place until the needles are removed. Depending on the planned dosage to the tumor bed, needles are usually left in place for 4 to 7 days.

Interstitial Seeds. Sealed radionuclide seeds may be implanted permanently or temporarily. Because they have a short half-life, gold seeds are permanently implanted, most commonly into the prostate, lungs, or pancreas. Seeds containing cesium-137, iridium-192, or iodine-125 implanted directly into tumor tissue are removed after the desired exposure.

Seeds are useful in body cavities, in localized areas, and in tumors that are not resectable because of their location near major vessels or the spinal cord. Because they are small, the seeds can be placed to fit a curved area without requiring immobilization. However, they may move about if there is much motion.

Radionuclide seeds are 7 mm or less in length, are 0.75 mm in diameter, and have a wall 0.3 mm thick. The length of the seed depends on the desired dosage. Seeds can be inserted with or without an invasive surgical procedure. They may be strung on a strand of suture material or placed in a hollow plastic tube with sealed ends. With a needle attached, the strand or tube is woven or pulled through the tumor. Seeds in a plastic tube may be inserted through a hollow needle, such as a catheter through a trocar. Empty tubes may be inserted in the OR and afterloaded (i.e., the seeds are put into the tube at a later time and place). A microprocessor-controlled machine that pulls wire attached to radioactive material through the tube may be used for remote afterloading.

Brachytherapy. The term *brachytherapy* comes from a Greek term meaning "short-range treatment." Tiny titanium cylinders that contain a radioactive isotope are implanted to deliver a dose of radiation from the inside out that kills cancer cells while sparing healthy tissue. Brachytherapy is performed for many types of cancers, including breast and prostate (Fig. 7-5). Brachytherapy, an internal application with sealed sources of radionuclides, has almost totally supplanted the use of radium and radon. For example, the gamma rays of cesium-137 have greater penetrating power than radium does.

Brachytherapy is useful for delivering higher cell-killing doses in shorter periods than conventional radiation treatments. The capsules are placed under ultrasound guidance. A rapid delivery system that uses a catheter with a balloon on the tip has been developed to treat breast cancer smaller than 3 cm. The catheter is placed into the breast tissue during tumor excision, and the balloon is expanded with water. Twice per day for 4 to 5 days a high-dose radiation pellet is placed inside the catheter to treat the tissue. When the treatment period is complete, the catheter and pellet are removed. Patient selection includes those with clear margins of the tumor and with fewer than three affected lymph nodes.

Intracavitary Capsules. A sealed capsule of radium, cesium-137, iodine-125, yttrium-192, or cobalt-60 may be placed into a body cavity or orifice. The capsule may be a single tube of radioactive pins fixed in a tandem loader or a group of individual capsules, each of which contains one radioactive pin. Commonly used to treat tumors in the cervix or endometrium of the uterus, a capsule is inserted via the vagina for treatment of the uterine body.

In a patient with cervical cancer, an instrument such as an Ernst applicator is used. A metal or plastic tube with radioactive pins is inserted in the uterus. Metal pins are used in conjunction with heat. The tube is attached to two vaginal ovoids, each of which contains a radioactive pin, that are placed in the cul-de-sac around the cervix. This type of application delivers the desired dosage in a pear-shaped volume of tissue, which includes the cervix, corpus, and tissue around the cervix but spares the bladder and rectum from high doses of radiation.

A blunt intracavitary applicator is used to position the parts. The applicator is held securely and remains fixed to ensure proper dosage to the tumor without injuring the normal surrounding structures. For stabilization, the surgeon may suture the applicator to the cervix; vaginal packing also is used. Two different methods of application are used for inserting the radiation source: afterloading techniques and preloading techniques.

Afterloading Techniques. Afterloading techniques afford the greatest safety for OR personnel. In the OR, a cold, unloaded, hollow plastic or metal applicator, such as the Fletcher afterloader, is inserted into or adjacent to the tissues that will receive radiation. After radiographic verification of correct placement, the radiation source is loaded into the applicator at the patient's bedside.

Preloading Techniques. Preloading techniques require insertion of the "hot" radiation capsule in the OR by the surgeon. OR personnel should not be permitted in the OR during this procedure. To deliver a uniform dose to the desired area, the surgeon inserts an adjustable device designed to hold the radiation source in proper position in the tissues (e.g., the Ernst applicator). The bladder and rectum are held away from the area with packs to avoid undesired irradiation. To calculate the necessary dosage, the surgeon uses radiographs of the pelvis to check the position of the radiation source and to measure its distance from critical sites.

All preparations for insertion are made by nursing team members before they leave the room. (They wait in the substerile room during insertion.) Preparations include setting the sterile table with vaginal packing, antibiotic cream for packing, radiopaque solutions for radiographic studies, and a basin of sterile water; placing the radiograph cassette on the operating bed and notifying the radiology technician; obtaining the radiation source; positioning the patient; and putting a radiation sheet on the patient's chart and a card on the stretcher.

Intracavitary Colloidal Suspensions. Sterile radioactive colloidal suspensions of gold or phosphorus are used as palliative therapy to limit the growth of metastatic tumors in the pleural or peritoneal cavities. Radioactive colloidal gold-198 is most commonly used; it has a half-life of 2.7 days. It may also be instilled within the bladder. The effect of these suspensions is caused by the emission of beta particles, which penetrate tissue so slightly that radioactivity is limited to the immediate area in which the colloidal suspension is placed. A trocar and cannula are introduced into the pleural or peritoneal cavity, and the colloidal suspension is injected through the cannula from a lead-shielded syringe. After use, these instruments are stored in a remote area until the decay of radioactivity is complete.

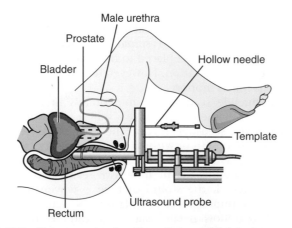

FIG. 7-5   Placement of radioactive cylinders for brachytherapy.

External Beam Radiation Therapy

Ionizing radiations of gamma rays or x-rays generated from machines are used externally to alter tumor cells within the body. This type of radiation therapy is noninvasive.

A maximum dose of radiation is concentrated on the malignant tumor below the skin, with a minimum dose to surrounding tissue. The angle of approach is changed a number of times during treatment to spread the amount of radiation to normal tissue over as wide an area as possible. Both orthovoltage equipment (low-voltage equipment that produces 200 to 500 kV) and megavoltage equipment (e.g., cobalt-60 beams and linear accelerators or betatrons) are used for external beam radiation therapy.

With some cancers, external radiation may be the only therapeutic modality used. It is difficult to determine the dosage of radiation that will provide the optimal cure with an acceptable balance of complications. With the advent of stereotactic techniques and the use of megavoltage equipment, intense rays can deliver cancer cell–killing doses without permanently injuring normal tissue and causing skin irritation. Even so, for many tumors most oncologists recommend a combination of radiation therapy and surgical resection; radiation therapy may be administered preoperatively and/or postoperatively or intraoperatively. External radiation therapy may also be combined with internal sources, such as intracavitary radiation capsules, to build up the dosage to large tumor areas.

Intraoperative Radiation Therapy. During a surgical procedure, a single high dose of radiation may be delivered directly to an intraabdominal or intrapelvic tumor or tumor bed to provide an additional palliative or localized means of control. Normal organs or tissues can be shielded from exposure. Radiation may also be used after resection of the bulk of the tumor.

An orthovoltage unit may be installed in a lead-lined OR for performing intraoperative radiation therapy. The sterile Lucite cone is placed directly over the tumor site. All team members leave the room during treatment. In some hospitals the patient is transported from the OR to the radiation therapy department. After exposure to a megavoltage electron beam, the wound may be closed in the treatment area or the patient may be returned to the OR for further surgery and/or wound closure. The open wound is covered with a sterile drape during transport, and sterile technique is used for closure.

Stereotactic Radiosurgery. Gamma knife technology was developed in Sweden in the early 1950s by surgeon Lars Leksell and Borje Larsson, PhD. They experimented with guiding devices and proton beams. Cobalt-60 was found to be most effective in the treatment of brain tumors and was selected as the energy source for the gamma knife. In 1975 the device was used to treat brain tumors in humans.

With stereotactic radiosurgery, fiberglass fixation pins are used to apply a base ring (the Leksell head frame) to the patient's head preoperatively. Two small rods are placed in the ear canals to stabilize the head frame during fixation. Care is taken not to injure the ear canal or tympanic membrane during this process. A calibrated ring is affixed to the frame to form X, Y, and Z coordinates to localize the brain lesion. The frame and ring sit within a larger helmet that aims the radiation at the tumor.

The gamma knife delivers highly concentrated doses of gamma rays to inoperable or deep-seated vascular malformations or brain tumors 1 to 10 cm^3 in size. The localized area is determined by precision stereotaxis. The neurosurgeon places the patient's head, with the Leksell head frame and localizing ring, into the collimator helmet so that the focusing channels direct 201 pinpointed cobalt-60 beams to the tumor. (The radiation sources are housed in a large spherical chamber that is housed within a special room.) The patient is placed on a sliding bed that accommodates and aligns with the helmet as it enters the spherical chamber. The gamma knife process lasts 3 to 4 hours. During the procedure, the patient is in video and voice communication with the perioperative team. All personnel leave the room during treatment because of the intensity of the radiation and its cumulative effects.

Safety Rules for Handling Radiation Sources

The cardinal factors of protection from radiation sources are distance, time, and shielding. For both personnel and patients, the following principles of radiation safety apply to handling all types of radioactive materials:

- The intensity of radiation varies inversely with the square of the distance from it (i.e., double the distance equals one quarter the intensity). Personnel should stay as far from the source as is feasible.
- Radiation sources (e.g., needles, seeds, capsules, suspensions) are prepared by personnel in the nuclear medicine department. Personnel prepare these sources behind a lead screen, and their hands are protected by lead-lined gloves, if possible, or special forceps during handling.
- Radiation sources are transported in a long-handled lead carrier so they are as close to the floor and as far away from the body of the transporter as possible. The lead carrier should be stored away from personnel and patient traffic areas while it is in the OR suite.
- When radiation sources are delivered to the OR, each needle, seed, or capsule is counted by the surgeon with the radiation therapist. This number is recorded.
- Glutaraldehyde solution is poured into the lead carrier to completely submerge the radiation sources. When ready to use, the radiation source is transported in the lead carrier into the OR. The needles, seeds, or capsules are removed from the lead container with sterile long-handled instruments and are rinsed thoroughly with sterile water.
- All radiation sources are handled with special long, ring-handled forceps from behind a lead protection shield. Radiation sources should never be touched with bare hands or gloves. Radiation sources are never handled with a crushing forceps because the seal of hollow containers can be broken. A groove-tipped forceps that is designed for this purpose is used.
- Radiation sources are handled as quickly as possible to limit the time that personnel are exposed to radiation.
- All radiation sources are accounted for before and after use, and any loss is immediately reported to the OR

nurse manager. Nothing should be removed from the room. To locate a lost radiation source, a radiation therapist or nuclear medicine department technician is called to bring a Geiger counter. A Geiger counter has a radiation-sensitive gauge with an indicator that moves and a sound that increases when near radioactive substances. A Hazmat team may be summoned.

- A radiation documentation sheet is completed and put in the patient's chart. The surgeon fills in the amount and exact time of insertion and the time the source is to be removed. Each nurse who cares for the patient on the unit signs this sheet just before going off duty, thereby passing responsibility for checking the patient and radiation source to the nurse who relieves. To check needles, the sutures attached to each needle are counted.
- The patient's bed and door to the room are conspicuously labeled with a radiation-in-use card or symbol (Fig. 7-6).
- The radiation source is removed by the surgeon at the exact time indicated so the patient will not be overexposed.
- Radiation is neither seen nor felt. Therefore the rules are carefully observed. Exposure is monitored and minimized.

Effects of Radiation Therapy on the Perioperative Patient

The patient may be undergoing several treatment modalities and may experience the specific tissue and systemic effects of each. The perioperative nurse should understand how radiation affects the patient and how it affects the attainment of desired outcomes. The plan of care should include consideration for the potential side effects of radiation therapy.

Chemotherapy

Either alone or in combination, a variety of chemotherapeutic agents is capable of providing measurable palliative remission or regression of primary and metastatic disease, with a decrease in the size of the tumor and no new metastases. In some instances a complete response, with the disappearance of all clinical evidence of the tumor, is achieved.

The trend is toward earlier and greater use of adjuvant chemotherapy. More than one agent may be administered to enhance the action of another cytotoxic or antigenic

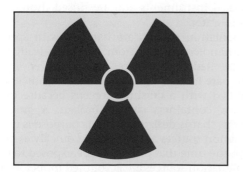

FIG. 7-6 Universal symbol for radiation.

substance. Adjuvant therapy is designed to maximize the benefits of each agent in the combination while avoiding overlapping toxicities. The following factors are important in determining the ability of tumor cells to respond to chemotherapy:

- Size and location of the tumor. The smaller the tumor, the easier it will be to reach cells. The mechanism for the passage of drugs into the brain differs from that for other body organs.
- Type of tumor. For example, cells of solid tumors in the lung, stomach, colon, and breast may be more resistant than cells in the lymphatic system.
- Combinations of adjuvant therapy. In select patients, chemotherapy may be used as an adjunct to all other types of therapy. Precise scheduling of dosages is necessary to attain effective results.
- Specific biochemical requirements of the tumor. Agents are selected according to the appropriateness of their structure and function. More than one agent is usually given.
- State of life cycle of the cancer cells. Cancer cells and normal cells go through the same life cycle phases. An understanding of this phenomenon is necessary for understanding chemotherapy.

Indications for Chemotherapy

Patients who are at risk for or who have systemic signs of advanced or disseminated disease (generally indicated by extranodal involvement) may be candidates for preoperative or postoperative chemotherapy.

Preoperative Chemotherapy. The objective of preoperative chemotherapy may be to shrink the tumor sufficiently to permit surgical resection. Adjuvant radiation therapy may be used in combination with chemotherapy to increase tumor regression and necrosis. Agents also may eliminate subclinical microscopic metastatic disease.

Postoperative Chemotherapy. Surgical resection followed by regional chemotherapy often can control local disease to keep a tumor in remission. Residual metastatic disease may be treated with systemic chemotherapy to cure the patient or to prolong life. Multiple doses may be given over a long period (several months to a year or more) to delay or eliminate recurrence of the tumor.

THE PATIENT WITH CHRONIC COMORBID DISEASE

Patients come to the OR for surgical procedures unrelated to a chronic cardiopulmonary or pulmonary disease. Even for unrelated surgeries the presence of these conditions may present a high risk for physiologic complications.

Cardiovascular Disease

The surgeon is particularly concerned about hemostasis and the potential for hemorrhage in a patient who is taking an anticoagulant medication. A patient who takes a daily dose of 81 mg of aspirin prophylactically may be instructed to discontinue its use for 2 weeks preoperatively. Anticoagulation is commonly prescribed for patients who have cardiac stents in place.

The anesthesia provider regulates the medications of patients who have an unstable blood pressure. Blood pressure is also monitored and maintained with appropriate medications in patients with a history of hypertension or hypotension. Tissue perfusion and oxygenation are critical to wound healing and depend on the circulatory status of the patient.

Pulmonary Disease

Any chronic condition that compromises pulmonary function presents a potential risk for a patient undergoing general inhalation anesthesia. Bronchoconstriction, edema, and excess mucus production cause uneven airway narrowing creating a ventilation-perfusion mismatch. Severe hypoxemia, an abnormal deficiency of oxygen in arterial blood, can trigger life-threatening dysrhythmias and respiratory failure.

Adequate ventilation is difficult in patients with asthma, chronic bronchitis, and pulmonary emphysema. Chronic obstructive pulmonary disease (COPD), which includes these conditions, is characterized by diminished inspiratory and expiratory capacity of the lungs. It is aggravated by cigarette smoking and air pollution. Smokers are advised to stop smoking at least 3 weeks preoperatively and are taught to use a spirometer postoperatively to clear respiratory secretions.

Deep-breathing and coughing exercises may be helpful postoperatively. Mechanical ventilation or intermittent positive pressure breathing (IPPB) apparatus may be necessary postoperatively to assist or control respiration. Patients who have trouble breathing are usually highly anxious and need emotional support.

The Patient with Induced or Acquired Immunosuppression

The immune system creates local barriers and inflammation to protect the body from invasion by pathogenic microorganisms and foreign bodies. Humoral and cell-mediated responses develop if these first-line defenses do not provide adequate protection. The humoral response produces antibodies to react with specific antigens. The cell-mediated response mobilizes tissue macrophages in the presence of a foreign body. Immunocompetence is he ability of the immune system to mobilize and deploy its antibodies and other responses to stimulation by an antigen. Immunocompetence may be threatened by a disease, a virus such as hepatitis B or HIV, or an immunosuppressive agent. Patients who are immunocompromised have a weakened or deficient immune response with a resultant decreased resistance to infection.

Immunosuppression. Immunosuppressive agents include corticosteroid hormones, which are given to prevent or reduce the inflammation caused by certain diseases. They are often prescribed for patients who have an autoimmune collagen disease (e.g., rheumatoid arthritis, systemic lupus erythematosus, scleroderma) or an autoimmune hemolytic disorder (e.g., idiopathic thrombocytopenic purpura or acquired hemolytic anemia). They also are given to patients with adrenal insufficiency, as well as after organ transplantation to combat rejection. Antineoplastic cytotoxic agents for chemotherapy and radiation therapy, which are used to reduce malignant tumor cells, also may cause immunosuppression.

Common Complications. The manifestations and clinical characteristics of the patient who is immunocompromised depend on the specific disease and the affected organ or system. For example, systemic lupus erythematosus can affect every organ system in the body. Adrenal insufficiency, as caused by Addison's disease, may be characterized by generalized systemic reaction. In contrast, organ transplantation or a malignant tumor may affect a single organ.

Special Considerations. Many patients who are immunocompromised have skin rashes or lesions, painful joints, poor nutrition, and/or generalized malaise. They need physical and emotional support throughout the perioperative care period. Aseptic and sterile techniques are important considerations for all surgical patients but are especially crucial for immunosuppressed and immunocompromised individuals, who are at high risk for developing a postoperative infection.

Acquired Immunodeficiency Syndrome. Patients with acquired immunodeficiency syndrome (AIDS) test positive for the human immunodeficiency virus (HIV) in serum and exhibit one or more signs and symptoms of an opportunistic disease, including pneumonia, fungal and/or parasitic infection(s), and malignant neoplasms. HIV can remain inactive and undetected in the body for many years before seroconverting and causing immunodeficient illness known as AIDS. During this time, no outward signs of HIV infection are noted, but it is possible for the patient to transmit the virus through blood, body fluids, or sexual contact.

Both males and females, including infants and children, may be HIV positive or diagnosed with AIDS. HIV was once thought to be transmitted only through homosexual behavior among men, IV drug use, or tainted blood transfusions. It is now known that the virus is also transmitted through heterosexual contact, and an infected mother may transmit the virus to her fetus.

The diagnosis of an HIV infection is confirmed by at least two separate tests. One positive test is not a conclusive diagnosis and is usually repeated for clarity. Initial testing with the enzyme-linked immunosorbent assay (ELISA) is performed to detect the presence of HIV antibodies in the blood. The diagnosis is confirmed with either the Western blot test or the indirect immunofluorescence assay.

If a patient tests seropositive for HIV infection, it does not mean that he or she has AIDS. HIV invades and destroys T lymphocytes. During this process the patient's immune system is disabled. The normal T lymphocyte level is 1000/mm^3; the severity of an HIV infection is measured by the level of T lymphocyte cells in the patient's blood. When the T cell level decreases to between 200 and 500/mm^3, the patient has seroconverted to an immunodeficient state and is considered to have AIDS.

There is no known cure for HIV infection or AIDS. Some medications are available to delay seroconversion in HIV infection and to prolong the life of a patient who has seroconverted to AIDS. Pharmacologic therapy may include broad-spectrum antibiotics, antivirals, antidiarrheals, vitamins, and antineoplastics.

Common Complications. A patient with HIV infection may complain of night sweats, unexplained fevers, dry cough, weakness, diarrhea, weight loss, and swollen lymph glands. A patient who has seroconverted to AIDS may have multiple opportunistic infections and malignancies concurrently and generalized poor health. Extreme muscle and tissue wasting is common.

Many patients with AIDS have multiple external and internal lesions. The skin may have open wounds with infectious exudate and/or large, swollen, purple lesions associated with Kaposi's sarcoma (a malignant multifocal neoplasm of reticuloendothelial cells that spreads in the skin and metastasizes to the lymph nodes and viscera). Large, painful masses of lymph tissue may be present in the neck, axilla, and groin. Mechanical obstruction caused by Kaposi lesions in the esophagus may prevent swallowing of food. Intestinal lesions may prevent the absorption of nutrients or cause bowel obstruction.

Constant anorexia, nausea, vomiting, and diarrhea may prevent adequate intake by mouth. Nutritional supplementation by hyperalimentation may be indicated to meet a patient's high caloric needs. Hyperalimentation is discussed in Chapter 23

AIDS causes the body to be susceptible to opportunistic infections because of the lowered resistance of the immune system. Opportunistic infections are caused by microorganisms that normally are nonpathogenic in a healthy individual. The mucous membranes of the mouth and genital areas may have herpes virus lesions or white patches of candidiasis, a yeastlike fungus. Neurologically, the patient may have recurrent episodes of cryptococcal meningitis or toxoplasmosis, causing persistent motor dysfunction and mental changes.

The patient with AIDS experiences a continual cycle of acute and chronic respiratory infections. *Pneumocystis jiroveci* pneumonia is the most common lung infection, followed by multiple-drug–resistant tuberculosis (MDR-TB). The patient may be in a perpetual state of respiratory distress. Central and peripheral cyanosis may be present. The respiratory effort expends high energy levels, causing the patient to deteriorate rapidly.

Special Considerations. Patients with AIDS may be in poor physical condition, depending on how the body systems have been affected. Most systems are eventually involved. The plan of perioperative care should incorporate the following considerations:

1. Moving the patient from the transport stretcher to the operating bed may require additional personnel for total lifting. The patient may not be able to move because of weakness or pain in the joints, muscle and tissue wasting, and superficial skin lesions.
2. Bony prominences and areas of decreased muscle mass and devascularized tissue must be protected throughout the positioning process and surgical procedure. Blankets, restraints, monitoring devices,

electrosurgical dispersive electrodes, drapes, instruments, and routine care devices may cause inadvertent harm to the patient despite the team's best efforts to protect the patient from injury.
3. IV line insertion, induction of anesthesia, and maintenance of the airway may be difficult. A suitable vein for infusion may be hard to identify because of former IV drug use or large areas of epidermal Kaposi's sarcoma. In extreme cases the only IV site may be a central venous catheter. Endotracheal intubation may be contraindicated because of potential hemorrhage from Kaposi lesions in the trachea. Placement of an esophageal stethoscope or rectal temperature probe may rupture other internal Kaposi lesions with the same result.
4. Postoperative wound healing is delayed or absent because of poor nutrition, decreased circulation, poor tissue integrity, and a continued immunodeficient condition.

Many patients with AIDS have been rejected by their families, especially if the virus was transmitted through a route not accepted or understood by family members. The diagnosis of AIDS may be the first time the family is made aware of the patient's alternative lifestyle. Psychological support systems may consist of a small circle of friends, who also may be infected with HIV or have AIDS. Preoperative consideration should be given to power of attorney, living will, and the potential for future do-not-resuscitate (DNR) status.

Continual counseling should be emphasized in the postoperative discharge plan to include provisions for physiological care and support. The patient, family, and significant others should be educated about the potential routes of transmission, such as exposure to blood and body fluids through sexual contact or shared IV needles. The virus is also potentially transmissible through shared razors, toothbrushes, and tweezers because of the possibility of blood contamination. Dishes and eating utensils are considered safe when washed in hot, soapy water, rinsed, and dried.

Education should include learning about physical activities that do not pose a risk of transmission, such as hugging, shaking hands, and sitting close.

Confidentiality is a concern because of the nature of the routes by which HIV can be transmitted. It is an issue of the patient's right to privacy. Testing for HIV is not a routine preadmission laboratory procedure. If a patient is tested, the results should be placed in the appropriate section of the patient's chart with other laboratory results, not displayed on the front of the chart. Reporting of the results should be governed by institutional policy and treated in the same manner as all patient confidentiality issues.

Dissemination of confidential patient information to inappropriate people is a breach of duty to the patient's privacy and may be subject to legal action. Physicians and nurses may face disciplinary action, such as license suspension or revocation by the boards of medicine or nursing, as indicated.

Perioperative patient care personnel should provide care to all patients with equal professionalism, compassion, empathy, and positive regard despite any personal feelings about a patient's lifestyle or disease entity. Nonjudgmental care is essential for the psychological wellness of patients with AIDS.

THE PATIENT WHO IS A VICTIM OF CRIME

Violent crime is prevalent in society. As health care professionals, we manage the care of the victims of crime and sometimes the accused perpetrator(s). Victims and perpetrators involved with the same incident may present to the same emergency department (ED) within moments of each other. Both are entitled to the same care and legal considerations, including privacy and basic tenets of respect.

The perpetrator is considered innocent until proven guilty in a court of law. Both patients have equal rights to patient advocacy, regardless of the circumstances of their injuries. All members of the health care team need to be in control and aware of subjective feelings and place personal biases and prejudices in proper perspective when caring for these individuals.

Crimes can involve drugs, domestic abuse, shootings, stabbings, gang violence, mugging, sexual assault, and hit-and-run motor vehicle accidents. Injuries can occur to bystanders at a crime scene, such as a robbery, drive-by shooting, or gang fight. All patients who arrive at the ED may provide potential forensic evidence for law enforcement officials and should be carefully processed according the facility policy.

On Arrival to the Emergency Department

Physical assessment is performed immediately on contact with the health care system by paramedics and continued on arrival to the facility by additional medical personnel. The level of consciousness is evaluated and the ABCs (airway, breathing, and circulation) are prioritized and stabilized. The first concern is to preserve life, followed closely by the concern to preserve the chain of evidence. Severely injured patients may need to bypass the ED and go directly to the OR.

Notation should be made of psychological affect. Many crimes are associated with drug abuse, and the administration of medications in the hospital could interact with drugs ingested on the street. The use of street drugs should be carefully ruled out by toxicology screens because they may alter baseline laboratory tests, interfere with lifesaving treatment, and potentiate anesthetics used during emergency surgery.

Unusual odors, such as chemicals, alcohol, gasoline, or other volatile substances should be investigated and documented. Chemicals can be hazardous in the OR, where fires can be triggered by electrosurgical devices in the presence of volatile materials.

Baseline vital signs, radiographs, scans, antibiotic prophylaxis, tetanus toxoid, pain control, and hemostasis are some of the prime concerns for stabilization. Facility spokespeople should handle all media interviews, and respect for patient privacy should be provided. Standard precautions are strictly followed at all times concerning all body substances.

Consent for treatment is required and should be obtained as soon as possible. This is important as the chain of evidence is constructed. The chain of evidence incorporates documentation of all material and observational findings associated with the victim, the suspected perpetrator, and the incident. An unconscious person is given full treatment regardless of consent status until family can be consulted.

Forensic Evidence in the Operating Room

Forensic evidence is critical for the reconstruction of events involved in a crime or suspected illegal activity. All forensic evidence is preserved according to institutional policy and procedure and is relinquished only to the appropriate authorities. The documentation of handling and disposition of evidence is referred to as a chain of evidence. This chain is maintained by requiring the signatures of everyone who comes into contact with forensic evidence. The goal is to attempt to validate that the evidence has not been tampered with before reaching the appropriate law enforcement agency.

Any potential evidence discovered during physical assessment should be carefully documented and secured until it can be turned over to appropriate law enforcement authorities. The Fourth Amendment to the Constitution of the United States provides equal protection against unreasonable search and seizure. Items found while intentionally searching a conscious patient without consent may be interpreted as unreasonable search and are potentially not admissible in court.

Illegal substances or weapons discovered during the routine course of assessment and that have not been obtained through unreasonable means may be used as evidence in some states. They are packaged dry and in an impervious container to prevent injury. Gloves are worn in handling evidence. Nothing is washed, wiped clean, or discarded. A clear chain of evidence is often difficult to maintain in a crisis, but every attempt is made to document the disposition of evidence and the location from which it was taken.

Assessment of the Crime Victim

Data collection begins with Emergency Medical Service (EMS) and police reports. If a patient with a suspicious injury, such as a gunshot or stab wound arrives at the ED by some other means, the police should be notified. Critical information about the injury includes where, when, and how the injury occurred and should be documented. Direct quotation of the patient's words is preferred. Differences between accounts of the incident by the patient and other observers should be carefully noted. Variance in reporting by a potential victim may mean that an accused perpetrator is innocent.

Patients, who are critically injured may be taken directly to the OR. The perioperative nurse should document physical injury patterning on the OR nurses' notes before evidence, such as bloody hand prints that are washed away during the skin preparation process. Most ORs have cameras or photographic staff available. Pictures of the injuries should be photographed in the lighting of the OR for clarity.

The patient may not be able to communicate vital information, such as when the last meal was eaten, if he or she has allergies, or if medications are taken on a routine basis for some condition. Family may not be available to give a medical or surgical history. It is critical to communicate to the team every detail discovered during the preparation of the patient for surgical intervention. Close observation for responses to treatment and physiologic clues is the key to providing safe care.

The patient's clothing may provide important information for the police and should be preserved intact if possible. This can be complex if the patient must come to the OR for lifesaving intervention. If clothing must be cut off, care should be taken to avoid cutting through bullet holes or stab wounds as possible. Keep in mind that the patient may have sharp objects in his or her clothing that could injury a caregiver. If possible, the patient should be placed on a separate bed sheet before clothing is removed and the fabric of the clothing should be cut along the seams. Hairs, carpet fibers, and other environmental information may be contained in folds of fabric and should be left with the clothing for the forensic examiners. The sheet forms a wrapper for the clothing before it is placed in an approved receptacle.

Clothing should not be placed in airtight containers or plastic bags because that may cause degradation of biologic matter. Paper bags may be used provided the bag has not been used before and the moisture of the clothing is not going to seep through the surface. Contamination of the outer aspect of the paper bag is a hazard to the examining teams and the law officials. Underclothes of sexual assault victims must be carefully preserved in the same manner. Storage and handling of these items should be well documented, and signatures are required when turned over to proper authorities. Some facilities provide tamper-proof evidence tape to seal the package and prevent altering of contents.

The patient's skin is observed for bruising, swelling, and open wounds. Characteristic marks, such as finger/hand-shaped injuries, tire marks, and repetitive patterning like stripes should be documented. The locations of the marks should be indicated on a human-like diagram in the patient's record. Whenever possible, the injuries should be photographed. This may require separate consent.

The study of ballistics is the scientific matching of a particular weapon to its projectile. As a bullet travels down the barrel of a gun it picks up characteristic markings. Removed bullets should be handled with care so the ballistic markings are not altered. Placing bullets or metallic evidence in a metal specimen basin could alter the longitudinal design of the identifying marks. Only plastic containers should be used. No solution should be added.

The presence of gunpowder and its distribution pattern around a bullet entrance wound on skin or clothing is important in determining muzzle-to-body distance. The closeness of the gun barrel determines the amount of skin damage on impact. Small-caliber bullet wounds have a smaller inverted entrance and larger everted exit points. Some bullets are designed to flatten on entry and may exit the body after traveling through several layers of soft tissue or organs. If contact is made with bony structures, the bullet may remain embedded in the body. Fragmentation bullets are designed to burst into tiny pieces as they enter the body, and may embolize. Close examination of the victim's back may reveal a gaping bullet exit wound or additional injuries initially unnoticed. Wounds should be copiously irrigated with sterile saline. Some surgeons will request antibiotic solution.

Absence of an exit wound may indicate the presence of a nonexploded fragmentation bullet. A retained malfunctioning fragmentation bullet could be deadly during an emergency surgical procedure. The explosive mechanism could inadvertently activate, causing injury to a member of the OR team.

Victims may present with obvious injuries, but may also have concealed damage. The initial assault may have been a gunshot or a stab wound, but incidental injury may include blunt trauma caused by falling to the ground. Some victims also have been beaten with fists or solid objects, causing damage to underlying organs and structures.

Crime victims are at high risk for misdiagnosis of secondary head injury or ruptured viscus. This may be further complicated if the victim is pregnant. Two patients may be affected: the mother and her unborn child. OB-GYN staff may need to be included in the surgical team.

Broken bones are misdiagnosed less frequently because of the use of routine radiography. The victim of a hit-and-run driver often suffers a fractured tibia and fibula at the height of the car's bumper. The measurement of the point of impact will enable investigators to determine if the vehicle was traveling at a constant rate of speed or braking at the time of the collision. Thorough head-to-toe assessment is followed by a complete review of all body systems. Every aspect of the physical exam and treatment becomes part of the evidence discovery process.

The Patient Who Is a Victim of Sexual Assault

Most patients who have been raped or sexually assaulted begin treatment in the ED. Severe injuries or multitrauma victims are frequently treated in the OR. Although frequently used, the term *rape* is a legal conclusion, not a medical diagnosis. Rape is a felony and one of the most underreported crimes—only 20% of all rapes are reported. Sexual offenses include marital rape, sexual battery, felonious sexual penetration, sexual imposition, and corruption of a minor. Sexual assault is the appropriate term for both male and female victims.

In reality, 1 of every 3 females will be sexually assaulted during her lifetime. Only 1 in 10 ever reports it. One of every 7 males will experience some form of sexual assault. More than 75% of the assailants are known to their victims.

The rape crisis center should be involved in every aspect of care for both sexes. Female rape trauma victims should always be examined by the gynecology staff, preferably female. Victims of sexual assault may fear examination or physical contact by members of a specific sex. Females may wish to have a female examiner. A male also may prefer a female examiner, especially if his assailant was male. This holds true of the OR team—the patient may have a sexual prejudice that needs to be respected. Sensitivity to the needs of the victim is important, and documentation and preservation of evidence should be maintained. Sexual assault is a crime of violence and power.

Physiologic and psychological stabilization is critical. Additional physical injuries, such as gunshot or stab wounds, may complicate care related to sexual assault. Medical history, such as current medications, immunizations, and allergies, should be assessed. Postassault douching, bathing, urination, or defecation may have altered evidence and are taken into consideration. Genital trauma should be closely evaluated.

Considerations for the Patient with Sexual Trauma

The psychological affect of a sexual assault victim can range from flat to hyperreactive. The victim should be approached with patience and understanding. Minors may be accompanied by their natural or court-appointed guardians. Quick, brisk moves by a caregiver can create undue emotional stress. The caregiver should always wear gloves to depersonalize touch and should allow the victim to guide his or her hands during the physical assessment to provide an element of self-control. Loss of control and violation increase the victim's anxiety. A calm demeanor can provide a sense of security for any victim of crime, but in particular, for a sexual assault victim. The OR should reflect a sense of stability and prevent nonessential noise.

Preoperative assessment of a female sexual assault victim should include past sexual, menstrual, and contraceptive history. The possibility of existing or resultant pregnancy should be considered. A blood test for beta human chorionic gonadotropin should be drawn. Hormonal pregnancy prophylaxis ("morning-after pill") may be used within 72 hours of the assault to induce menses and is 95% to 98% effective in preventing implantation of a fertilized ovum. Some women may desire the morning-after pill or abortion counseling at a later date. Approximately 1% of sexual assaults result in pregnancy.

During the examination, the victim's pubic hair should be combed into a clean white envelope. A few clippings of the victim's pubic hair and the comb should be sealed inside with the examiner's signature, date, and time on the outside. The assailant's hair may be present and is valuable as evidence. Examination with an ultraviolet Wood's lamp should be performed because prostatic secretions and seminal fluid appear fluorescent even when dried. Dried scrapings of blood and secretions from under fingernails and around genitalia should be saved in an appropriate container. Dried semen is sometimes used to verify an assailant's identity by blood type and DNA.

A colposcope with a green filter can be used to examine and photograph vaginal tears. The green filter is useful for identifying vascular structures as a direct contrast to reddened or bleeding tissue. Speculum, proctoscopic, and/or bimanual pelvic exams are performed using only sterile water as lubrication. Oral, vaginal, and/or anal mucosal smears, swabs, and washings should be fixed according to laboratory protocol. Commercial rape-evidence kits are available for the collection of specimens, preservation of evidence, and documentation of physical findings. Baseline blood tests for HIV, hepatitis B virus (HBV), hepatitis C virus (HCV), and syphilis should be performed with follow-up tests in 4 to 6 months. Cultures for gonococci also should be obtained. Antibiotic prophylaxis may be indicated.

The Patient Who Is a Victim of Domestic Violence

Victims of domestic violence may be male or female. Most are female and exhibit a common set of specific injuries. Many beatings go unreported because of fear of retaliation, low self-esteem, and embarrassment over enduring repeated abuse. Others claim they love the abuser and want to keep the family together. A battered woman may feel she deserved the beating and may avoid going to the ED unless she experiences symptoms she interprets as life-threatening.

Signs of physical abuse are commonly found around the face and head and consist of multiple abrasions, contusions, chipped teeth, fractured facial bones, epistaxis, and blackened eyes. Often the woman is pregnant for the first time, which is a common theme in 8% to 15% of gravid females suffering abusive treatment. Domestic violence occurs in all socioeconomic groups, but poverty and unemployment may precipitate the event.

The victim of domestic abuse may be afraid to report the event to the police. Emergency department personnel are not bound by law to report domestic violence. Emergency department nurses should completely and accurately document the event and if possible photograph the injuries with the patient's permission. Assure the victim that all information is confidential. Referral can be made to a battered women's shelter as necessary. Most shelters have a 24-hour crisis intervention

The Patient Who Is the Victim of Child Abuse

Children are the most helpless victims and more than 1000 die each year as a result of abuse or neglect. Of reported deaths, 60% are younger than 2 years of age. Child abuse can occur in any socioeconomic group and may take the form of psychological, physical, and sexual abuse. Other forms of victimization include neglect of physical, psychological, and medical needs. Infants and young children are unable to ask for help and are dependent on adults and health care workers to recognize abuse and neglect, treat them for it, and report it. Many injuries and illnesses are characteristic of abuse. However, many forms of abuse are discovered incidentally when a child is brought to the ED, clinic, or physician's office for an unrelated illness. OR personnel may discover signs of abuse when performing simple procedures such as myringotomy. Health care personnel should be educated to observe for unspoken signals from these helpless victims.

First signs of child abuse may be discovered while obtaining the child's history from the adult caretaker, parent, or guardian. Clues to look for include discrepancies about injury patterns, visits to multiple hospitals, lack of a consistent medical history, delays in seeking treatment, and visible evidence of old untreated injuries in various stages of healing. Observation of the child's affect can be misleading. Some children may be overcooperative with painful procedures or display extremes of affection.

A child who has known only abuse may show no response to the environment or fail to thrive. The abused child may cling to the abuser or exhibit avoidance behavior.

Response patterns can be unpredictable at times. Patient assessment should compare the developmental stage of the child to physical findings. Examples of discrepancies include long bone fractures in nonwalking infants or head injuries (whiplash-type) associated with violent shaking such as retinal and cerebral hemorrhage.

Violent shaking is a common form of abusive treatment between the ages of 6 weeks and 4 months during episodes of crying. Abusers may feel that shaking a crying infant is more acceptable than actually hitting. Crying may cease during the shaking because of brain edema, and the abuser may repeat the action because it made the baby stop crying. Clinical signs of trauma-induced brain injury are loss of consciousness, seizures, vomiting, and apnea. Brain injury also is caused by nutritional deficit and is manifest by personality change, learning disability, and diminished functional skill.

Visible injuries such as circumferential bruising around wrists or ankles from being held down are sometimes noted. Multiple clusters of similarly shaped discolored skin markings could indicate repeated strikes with a belt or stick. These are sometimes found to be in various stages of healing. Questionable burns may be found on soles of feet, backs of hands, or inside thighs. A scalded stocking pattern may be identified on a child who has been dipped in hot water. Children who accidentally burn themselves by grabbing hot objects usually have burns on the palms of the hands or irregular splash-shaped burns from pulling a pan off the stove. Venereal disease in a child is usually the result of sexual abuse.

Some conditions commonly mistaken for child abuse include dermatologic conditions, bone diseases, coagulation disorders, infections, skin discoloration (Mongolian spots), and folk healing remedies. Birthmarks can appear bluish and give the impression of bruising in various stages of healing. Some markings can be caused by clothing dyes or inks. Most of these markings can be removed with rubbing alcohol. Phytodermatosis is a skin discoloration that occurs when lime, lemon, celery, or herbal preparations are rubbed into the skin and exposed to sunlight. These phototoxic reactions can appear like hand marks if an adult was squeezing lemons or limes for summer beverages.

Folk remedies include coining, which involves rubbing a coin over an afflicted area. This sometimes causes striped bruises that resemble strap marks. To avoid erroneous reports of child abuse, the examiner should perform a careful history and physical, including appropriate laboratory studies. When in doubt, consult with a specialist, who can critically evaluate suspicious injury or illness.

Recognition of child abuse during physical assessment may not be instantly obvious. If the injury or illness does not match the explanation, the child may be a victim of abuse and the incident should be further investigated. In every state, a health care worker who suspects child abuse is mandated to report it to child welfare authorities.

Outcomes of Victimization

Regardless of the victim's age or social status, the postassault, postvictimization results can be devastating. Sequelae to victimization may include posttraumatic stress disorder (PTSD), augmented attention-deficit disorder with or without hyperactivity (ADD/ADHD), psychosis, depression, and continued feelings of victimization. Children may experience secondary enuresis and ecopresis as a form of regression and display inappropriate sexual behaviors toward adults or other children. Anger may be projected toward pets and smaller siblings in the form of cruelty and abuse. Abused children may grow up to become abusers. Nightmares are common in all ages. Coping mechanisms become distorted and conversion reactions can be confused with somatic complaints. Unfortunately, death is sometimes the final outcome of violent crime.

Prevention of violent crime is not always an option. Health care workers become aware of the event after the fact. Referral agencies are available to provide emergency shelter and temporary solace. Encouraging adult victims to report violent acts and follow through with prosecution is equally as important as treating physical injury. The victim who is fearful and unwilling to prosecute is at high risk for being victimized again. Minor victims are helpless and unable to report their injuries without help. Health care workers are required to report confirmed or suspected child abuse to proper authorities.

END-OF-LIFE CARE

Although perioperative patient care personnel are most often involved with patients who have a favorable prognosis, they also care for patients of all ages who have a catastrophic illness and are having surgery to palliate or relieve a specific problem. The procedure may be palliative rather than curative. Included in this category are patients with the following:

- Malignancies that result in severe debilitation and terminal illness
- Severe traumatic disabilities requiring lengthy hospitalization, such as after high spinal cord injury or extensive burns
- End-stage renal disease, or patients waiting for an organ transplant
- Patients with a DNR order

Maximum patient comfort and the relief of physiologic disturbances are primary concerns. All of these patients require highly individualized care. The manner in which patients are told the diagnosis and prognosis obviously has a great effect on their hope for recovery. Patients who have been thoroughly and considerately informed are easier to talk to, accept therapy more readily, and have greater trust in and communicate more openly with caregivers.

Each patient deals with such a diagnosis in his or her own way. Although it is not always so, many people consider the diagnosis of cancer a death warrant and react accordingly. To be supportive, the caregiver should mentally review Elisabeth Kübler-Ross's (1926-2004) stages of dying: denial, isolation, anger, bargaining, depression, and acceptance. (These stages do not always occur in this sequence.) Emphasis is placed on the present, with a focus on the patient's strengths and attributes and how best to use them. It is difficult to find hope when facing a radical, disfiguring procedure. Listening to the patient is particularly important.

DEATH OF A PATIENT IN THE OPERATING ROOM

Although it is an uncommon occurrence, a patient may die while on the operating bed or shortly after reaching the PACU or intensive care unit (ICU). When this happens, the perioperative manager should be notified immediately. Ideally, the family or significant others are informed by the surgeon or the surgeon's designee. It may be appropriate to have organ procurement personnel discuss organ donation with the family if death is imminent and to request permission to proceed with plans for potential organ procurement. If circumstances warrant, an autopsy may be necessary.

In the event of a high-profile accident or event, the facility's public relations personnel should be the contacts with the press or news media. Perioperative or perianesthesia personnel should not provide information about any patient to any person not authorized in the patient's care. A breech of confidentiality is a serious ethical consideration, and is especially contained in the event of a police investigation or medical malpractice suit.

Coroner's Cases

In some states the body of a patient who dies in the OR or does not awaken from general anesthesia automatically becomes the property of the coroner. Patients who die as a result of or in the commission of a crime become property of the coroner. Family consent for autopsy is not necessary in these situations. The coroner must give approval for organ procurement and has the right to overrule the wishes of the family.

Individual state law and institutional policy determine the postmortem care of the patient's body. For example, all drainage tubes, implants, and catheters may need to be left in place for removal and examination at autopsy. All medication vials and intravenous solution containers should remain with the body.

The body of a patient who dies under these circumstances is also considered the property of the coroner, but postmortem care is more complex. Critical medical-legal issues should be considered if the patient was a suspected victim or perpetrator of violence or was injured in a suspicious manner. All information about the patient's condition, personal effects and attire, and materials discovered during the surgical procedure are considered forensic evidence.

Postmortem Patient Care

A death may occur as a result of shock after extensive traumatic injuries, exsanguination after rupture of an aortic aneurysm, unsuccessful cardiopulmonary resuscitation after cardiac arrest, or other causes. The circulator's responsibilities after intraoperative death include the following:

1. Provide after-death care for the body as appropriate, or ensure that forensic protocol is followed before releasing the body to authorities or the morgue.
   a. Follow institutional policy and procedure.
   b. Be sure identification is correct.
   c. Place the patient supine in correct alignment with one pillow under the head. This will minimize pooling fluids in dependent tissue.
   d. Secure the patient's personal effects.
   e. Do not wash the body if it is considered part of forensic evidence.
2. Arrange for transportation of the body from the OR to the morgue, or release it to an appropriate authority.
   a. Release the body from the OR according to institutional policy and procedure.
   b. Avoid exposing other patients, visitors, and family to removal of the body.
   c. If the religious or cultural preference of a patient and/or family is known, an appropriate member of the clergy or a spiritual adviser may be consulted concerning after-death practices.
3. Complete the intraoperative chart and additional documentation as required by institutional policy.

Policy may allow the family to view a loved one before the body is transported to the morgue. The room in which the viewing takes place should be clean, presentable, and private. The perioperative nurse (or designee) should remain with the family and lend support. Parents may wish to hold a deceased child. Chairs and facial tissues should be available in the room. If forensics are involved, the nurse should not leave the patient's body unattended at any time.

Care is taken not to make statements to the family that sound cliché,[2] such as the following:

- "It was God's will" or "God has a plan."
- "Your loved one is in a better place now."
- "God needed an angel."
- "Everything happens for a reason."
- "Things will work out for the best."
- "Time will heal."
- "You have to be strong for your remaining loved ones."
- "Your loved one wouldn't want you to be sad."
- "At least your loved one is not in pain anymore."
- "You shouldn't be so sad. It is for the best."
- "At least your loved one lived a good life."

After a death in the OR, from whatever cause, team members should be given time to express their grief and deal with their feelings about the event. Tears and sadness are normal responses and should not be criticized. The team should be supportive of each other, including the surgeon and the anesthesia provider.

---

[2] www.elisabethkublerross.com.

Bibliography

Almagro P et al: Mortality after hospitalization for COPD, *Chest* 121(5): 1441-1448, 2002.
AORN (Association of periOperative Registered Nurses): *AORN standards, recommended practices, and guidelines,* Denver, 2005, The Association.
Beddhu S et al: The effects of comorbid conditions on the outcomes of patients undergoing peritoneal dialysis, *Am J Med* 112(9):696-701, 2002.
Dierker LC et al: Smoking and depression: An examination of the mechanisms of comorbidity, *Am J Psychiatry* 159(6):947-953, 2002.
Gunther M, Alligood MR: A discipline-specific determination of high quality nursing care, *J Adv Nurs* 38(4):353-359, 2002.

Huckleberry Y: Nutritional support and the surgical patient, *Am J Health System Pharm* 61(7):671-682, 2004.

Kells K: Ability of blind people to detect obstacles in unfamiliar environment, *J Nurs Scholarsh* 33(2):153-157, 2001.

Leksell JK et al: Power and perceived health in blind diabetic and nondiabetic individuals, *J Adv Nurs* 34(4):511-519, 2001.

Majasaari H et al: Patient's perceptions of emotional support and information provided to family members, *AORN J* 81(5):1030-1039, 2005.

McCahill LE et al: Indications and use of palliative surgery, *Ann Surg Oncol* 9(1):104-112, 2002.

Michard F, Teboul JL: Predicting fluid responsiveness in ICU patients, *Chest* 121(6):2000-2008, 2002.

Mouradan MS et al: How well are hypertension, hyperlipidemia, diabetes, and smoking managed after a stroke or transient ischemic attack? *Stroke* 33(6):1656-1659, 2002.

Nash T et al: Identifying cause for advancement to amputation in patients with diabetes, *Wounds* 17(2):32-36, 2005.

Plummer ES: Chronic complications, *RN* 64(5):34-40, 2001.

Shannon SE et al: Patients, nurse, and physicians have differing views on quality of critical care, *J Nurs Scholarsh* 34(2):173-179, 2002.

Valenti WM: The HIV specialist improves quality of care and outcomes, *AIDS Read* 12(5):202-205, 2002.

Wang JJ et al: Visual impairment, age-related cataract, and mortality, *Arch Ophthalmol* 119(8):1186-1190, 2001.

West SK et al: How does visual impairment affect performance on tasks of everyday life? *Arch Ophthalmol* 120(6):774-780, 2002.

Perioperative Pediatrics

KEY TERMS AND DEFINITIONS

Atresia   An interruption in the continuity of a tubular anatomic structure such as the trachea or esophagus.
Congenital physiologic   Condition that is present since birth.
Intussusception   Intestinal condition in which the bowel slides backward into itself, causing obstruction and pain.
Neonate   Newborn.
Puberty   Period of transition between childhood and adulthood when secondary sex characteristics develop. Commonly ages 8 to 13 for girls and ages 10 to 15 for boys.

The surgical problems peculiar to children from birth to postpuberty are not limited to any one area of the body or to any one surgical specialty. Malformations and diseases affect all body parts and therefore may require the skills of any of the surgical specialists. However, pediatric surgery is a specialty in itself and is not adult surgery scaled down to infant or child size. Indications for surgery include congenital anomalies, acquired disease processes, and trauma. Many of these conditions are treatable or curable by surgical intervention. (Additional information can be found at www.pedisurg.com.)

HISTORICAL BACKGROUND
INDICATIONS FOR SURGERY
Congenital Anomalies

A congenital anomaly is a deviation from normal structure or location in any organ or part of the body that is present from birth. It can alter function or appearance. Multiple anomalies may be present at birth. If an anomaly does not involve vital life functions, surgical intervention may be postponed until the results can be maximized and the risks of the surgical procedure are minimized by growth and development of body systems. If a newborn has a poor chance of survival without a surgical procedure, the risk is taken within hours or days after birth. Defects in the alimentary tract are the most common indication for an emergency surgical procedure during the newborn period, followed in frequency by cardiac and respiratory system defects. Mortality in the newborn is influenced by three uncontrollable factors: the multiplicity of anomalies, prematurity, and birthweight.

The presence of three or more physical congenital anomalies is referred to as the VACTERL association or syndrome:
   Vertebral defect, such as spina bifida or myelomeningocele
   Anal malformation, such as imperforate anus
   Cardiac anomaly, such as patent ductus arteriosus or ventricular and atrial septal defects
   Tracheoesophageal fistula
   Esophageal atresia
   Renal anomaly, such as horseshoe kidney and renal dysplasia
   Limb defect, such as short radius syndrome or syndactylism

Acquired Disease Processes

Among acquired disease processes, appendicitis is the most common surgically corrected childhood disease. Malignant tumors occur in infants and children but with minimal frequency when compared with occurrence rates for adults. Benign lesions are surgically excised, usually without further difficulty to the child.

Trauma

Accidental injury is the leading cause of death in children. The margin for error in diagnosis and treatment of a child is less than that for an adult with a similar injury. A child's blood volume is low compared with body size, and even a small loss of blood can be critical. Because the child's chest cavity is small, an abdominal or chest injury can be critical. Diagnosis is made quickly, and the patient is sent to the operating room (OR) if indicated. Examples of common injuries include blunt intestinal trauma caused by seat belt use on small children or head injuries caused by improper use of infant car seats. Other injuries, such as lacerations, fractures, or crushing injuries of hands and arms, may result in nerve, vessel, tendon, bone, and/or other soft tissue damage.

Skill is required in performing pediatric surgical procedures regardless of the indication for the procedure. Specialists in all fields develop these skills as a refinement of their specialties. Surgeons who perform pediatric surgery should have knowledge of the embryologic, psychological, physiologic, and pathologic problems peculiar to the newborn, infant, and child. Knowledge has advanced pediatric surgery through the following:

- Recognition of differences between pediatric patients and adults.
- Accurate diagnosis and earlier treatment. This facilitates a more favorable outcome, especially in the fetus and preterm neonate. Neonatology is a growing subspecialty of pediatrics.
- Understanding preoperative preparation of the patient and family.
- Availability of total parenteral nutrition (TPN) and other measures of supportive care for perioperative pediatric management.
- Advances in anesthesiology. These include new agents, perfection of techniques of administration, and an understanding of the responses of pediatric patients to anesthetic agents.
- Refinements in surgical procedures and instrumentation.
- Understanding of postoperative care. Larger facilities have neonatal and pediatric intensive care units.

CONSIDERATIONS IN PERIOPERATIVE PEDIATRICS

The nursing process is tailored to meet the unique needs of each pediatric patient. Assessment and nursing diagnosis are based on chronologic, psychological, and physiologic factors specific to each patient. The plan of care should reflect consideration for age and reflect interventions modified according to the child's developmental stage as identified in Table 8-1. Developmental theorists emphasize that although the child has reached a certain age or physical size, psycho-

logical growth is the key parameter by which communication is measured. Understanding individual differences enables the perioperative team to develop a positive rapport with the patient and family, which facilitates attainment of expected outcomes.

Not every patient of a particular age-group will meet standardized height and weight criteria; a child may be short or tall or thin or heavy for his or her age. Although norms have been established by age-groups, the plan of care should reflect consideration for individual differences. (Additional information about developmental theory and theorists in PowerPoint format can be found at www.coping.org.)

Chronologic Age

The chronologic age of the patient is a primary consideration in the development of the plan of care. An age-related baseline is a useful beginning for assessing pediatric patients effectively. No child will exactly meet all criteria in chronologic versus emotional age. Authors may vary in small time increments; however, no author can state that all children fit all templates exactly, because each is an individual. Terminology used to approximately categorize ages of pediatric patients includes the following:

1. Embryo: not compatible with life
2. Fetus: in utero after 3 months' gestation
3. Newborn infant, referred to as a neonate
   a. Potentially viable: gestational age more than 24 weeks; birthweight more than 500 g and capable of sustaining life outside the uterus (as defined by the World Health Organization)
   b. True preterm: gestational age less than 37 weeks; birthweight 2500 g or less
   c. Large preterm: gestational age less than 38 weeks; birthweight more than 2500 g
   d. Term neonate: gestational age 38 to 40 weeks; birthweight greater than 2500 g usually between 3402 and 3629 g (if less than 2500 g, the neonate is considered small for gestational age [SGA])
   e. Postterm: gestational age extended by more than 8 weeks
4. Neonatal period is first 28 days of extrauterine life
5. Infant: 28 days to 18 months
6. Toddler: 18 to 30 months
7. Preschool age: 2½ to 5 years
8. School age: 6 to 12 years
9. Adolescent: 13 through 18 years

PERIOPERATIVE ASSESSMENT OF THE PEDIATRIC PATIENT

Pediatric Psychosocial Assessment

Assessment of psychologic development is based on age-related criteria (see Table 8-1) but includes assessment of individual differences.[1,2] Comparison of established norms

---

[1]Additional Erikson definitions can be found at www.childdevelopmentinfo.com/development/erickson.shtml.
[2]Additional Piaget definitions can be found www.childdevelopmentinfo.com/development/piaget.shtml.

TABLE 8-1	Psychologic Developmental Stage Theories			
	Developmental Stage by Theorist			
Chronologic Age Ranges (Approximate)	Erikson	Piaget	Loevinger	Characteristics of Psychologic Development
Birth-18 months	Trust vs. mistrust	Sensorimotor	Presocial	Learns to view self as being separate from the environment; begins to develop the concept of hope; learns to develop attachments to others; is dependent on caregiver for warmth, security, nourishment, nurturing, and stimulation; begins to use sounds and short words to communicate ideas; may view hospitalization as abandonment
19 months-3 years	Autonomy vs. shame/doubt	Preoperational	Symbiotic	Develops a two-way relationship with primary caregiver; suffers separation anxiety when isolated from established relationships; has short trials of independence; personality becomes introverted or extroverted; establishes a sense of will; uses sentences for communication; has fear of immediate threats; does not project thoughts beyond the present situation
4-6 years	Initiative vs. guilt	Preoperational	Impulsive	Asserts a separate identity; begins to have fear of real and imagined situations; senses peer acceptance and/or rejection; is concerned about disfigurement; may act out feelings; believes that every action has a purpose, either reward or punishment; learns to be self-protective; fears death or nonexistence; death is not always understood as being permanent; develops short-term self-control; uses compound sentences to communicate; mimics terminology used by fantasy characters
7-11 years	Industry vs. inferiority	Concrete operational	Conformist	Imitates actions and attitudes of peers and heroes; is aware of the differences of others and identifies with a particular social group; fears loss of self-control; understands the world in moderate detail; prefers honest explanations and reassurance of safety; does not want to be treated like a baby; strives for competency in daily tasks; can distinguish between fact and fantasy; has a greater understanding of death and its permanence; wants to be accepted as an individual; communicates well verbally and with basic writing skill
12-16 years	Identity vs. role confusion	Formal operational	Self-aware, conscientious	May change opinion in response to stereotypes; develops close relationships; understands values, rules, and ideals; begins to feel more important as an individual; fears alienation; body image is extremely important; is capable of abstract thought and reasoning; has a sense of aesthetic beauty; can merge sensory information and logic to derive a conclusion; prefers privacy and confidentiality; may question authority; is aware of opposite sex; may explore sexual activity; dreams about future lifestyle; wants to prove self-worth; globally communicates verbally and in writing

TABLE 8-1	Psychologic Developmental Stage Theories—cont'd			
	Developmental Stage by Theorist			
Chronologic Age Ranges (Approximate)	**Erikson**	**Piaget**	**Loevinger**	**Characteristics of Psychologic Development**
17 years-adulthood	Intimacy vs. isolation	Formal operational	Individualistic	Becomes aware of and accepts the interdependence of mankind; may feel some hostility toward authority; sometimes torn between the desire to be totally independent and dependent; seeks companionship of opposite sex; may be sexually active; refines interpersonal skills; demands privacy and confidentiality; plans for independent lifestyle as approach; refines verbal and written communication skill

and assessment data is helpful in developing the plan of care. Environmental and parental influences can cause variance in affect, attitude, and social skills. Environmental influences on psychological development include ethnic, cultural, and socioeconomic factors. The age of the patient may indicate his or her level of involvement with the environment. For example, an infant may have exposure only to immediate family members for external stimuli but a preschool child may have daily experience with children in preschool and other children. Coping and social skills may be developed, depending on the child's developmental stage.

Parenting practices may directly influence the way the patient responds to caregivers and the perioperative environment. Pediatric patients respond differently in the presence of parents or guardians. Infants may be more cooperative if a parent is present. Conversely, an adolescent may want to demonstrate independence by asking the parent to leave the room. These actions may be completely opposite if the child has been abused or neglected. Lack of parental nurturing can cause a global deficit, including poor development of language and cognitive skills. Understanding the patient's level of psychological development can help the caregiver communicate more effectively with the pediatric patient throughout the perioperative experience. Interaction should be according to his or her individual developmental level regardless of chronologic age.

Pediatric Physical Assessment

The physiologic assessment of pediatric patients is compared with national averages when establishing baseline norms. Physiologic development is influenced by genetics, nutrition, health status, and environmental factors. The physical assessment may reveal conditions that can adversely affect the outcome of a surgical procedure. Comparison of the patient's age, size, and psychological development with established norms may enable the caregiver to assess for deficiencies in size or weight that may indicate a potential health problem. Unexplained marks or bruises may be signs of physical abuse.

A small, frail child may have a congenital cardiac deformity or a malabsorption syndrome. Abuse or neglect may be manifested as a nutritional deficit. An extremely thin, malnourished adolescent may be intentionally bulimic or anorexic in response to a psychological body image problem. An obese child may have an endocrine disease or a psychological disturbance that causes overeating. These issues are important considerations because most dosages of medications given to pediatric patients are based on body weight in kilograms. Absorption and metabolism of medication will be influenced by the same physiologic parameters that govern nutritional status.

Metabolism and Nutritional Considerations. Infants have relatively greater nutritional requirements than do adults for minimizing loss of body protein. The resting metabolic rate of an infant is two to three times that of an adult, resulting in rapid metabolic imbalances in infants. The potential for complications increases proportionately with the duration of fluid restriction, because infants are prone to hypovolemia and dehydration.

The neonate's body weight represents 70% to 80% fluid. Fluid weight is directly related to body fat content. Preterm infants have less body fat and consequently lose fluids easily. Other fluid losses are associated with urinary loss, gastrointestinal loss, insensible loss through respiration, and surgical loss by evaporation via the skin and drains. Fluid replacement for babies is calculated according to body weight as follows:

- Preterm: 120 to 50 mL/kg/24 hr
- Term neonates: 100 mL/kg/24 hr
- Infants more than 10 kg: 1050 mL/kg/24 hr

Procedures performed on infants and toddlers should have priority on the surgical schedule so that these patients can return to a normal fluid and feeding routine as quickly as possible.

Infants may be given regular formula or a varied diet up to 6 hours before anesthesia and clear liquids, usually dextrose in water, up to 2 hours before the surgical procedure. A satisfactory state of hydration is thus maintained, and milk curds are absent from the stomach. Infants may be breastfed up to 4 hours before the surgical procedure. Breast milk has less or no curd and empties faster from the stomach than does formula. Infants should not miss more than one or two feedings. Oral intake is resumed promptly after the infant recovers from anesthesia.

Toddlers and preschool children may be permitted clear liquids up to 2 to 4 hours preoperatively. Intake of clear oral fluids in small amounts decreases the level of gastric acid contents by stimulating gastric emptying and diminishes the hunger-deprivation response.

Children older than 5 years may have nothing by mouth (NPO) after midnight or 6 hours before induction of anesthesia. Exceptions may be necessary for children with fever, diabetes, or other special problems. For these children, clear liquids with supplemental glucose may be ordered to be given orally up to 2 hours preoperatively.

Older children may require slower progression of oral dietary intake postoperatively and are maintained with supplemental intravenous (IV) therapy that includes protein and vitamins. Vitamins K and C may be given to patients of any age-group.

Fluid and Electrolyte Balance Considerations. The newborn is not dehydrated and withstands major surgical procedures within the first 4 days of life without extensive fluid and electrolyte replacement. The renal system is easily overloaded by the administration of IV fluids. The newborn has a lower glomerular filtration rate and less efficient renal tubular function than does an adult. (Renal function improves during the first 2 months of life and approaches adult levels by age 2 years.) During the time of an average surgical procedure on a newborn, a total of 10 to 30 mL of fluid may be administered. Usually 5% dextrose in half-strength normal saline solution is infused.

Administration of excessive IV dextrose solution is avoided in infants younger than 1 year because they maintain lower glycogen stores. During physiologic stress, the patient easily becomes hyperglycemic. Hyperglycemia acts as an osmotic diuretic, causing increased urinary output and dilutional hyponatremia. The increased urine volume can be a false indicator of renal and hemodynamic status. Seizures and neurologic damage may result. Seizures may be clinically undetected while the infant is under general anesthesia because the pharmacologic agents act as anticonvulsants.

Infants have a relatively larger body surface area/body mass ratio than do adults. When they become dehydrated, which can occur rapidly, bodily functions are disturbed, as is the acid-base balance. Plasma proteins differ in concentration from those of an adult. Fluid and electrolyte replacements are necessary. In children older than 1 year, isotonic solutions, such as normal saline or Ringer's lactate, are given IV per kilogram of body weight.

Urinary output is directly related to body size and age. Neonates can concentrate 400 mOsm/L initially and 500 mOsm/L progressively over the first few days compared with 1200 mOsm/L in the average size adult. This concentration and excretion of the solute load results in 2 to 4 mL/kg/hr urinary output. Older children (toddlers and preschoolers) produce 1 to 2 mL/kg/hr of urine when adequately hydrated. Urine measurement in children is difficult to monitor without a Foley catheter.

The hemoglobin level is lowest at 2 to 3 months of age (Table 8-2). The blood volume of the average newborn is 250 mL—approximately 75 to 80 mL/kg of body weight (Table 8-3). Significant blood loss requires replacement. Blood is typed and crossmatched in readiness. Although blood loss is small in most cases, loss of 30 mL may represent 10% to 20% of circulating blood volume in an infant. The small margin of safety indicates the need for replacement of blood loss exceeding 10% of circulating blood volume. When replacement exceeds 50% of the estimated blood volume, sodium bicarbonate is infused to minimize metabolic acidosis.

Hypotension in an infant is not apparent until 50% of the circulating volume is lost. Hypotension is usually caused by myocardial depression from anesthetic agents, primarily inhalation anesthesia. The infant's myocardium has fewer contractile muscle fibers and more noncontractile connective tissue than is present in an older child or adult and therefore lacks myocardial force to maintain cardiac output. The cardiac output depends on the heart rate. Any decrease in heart rate directly affects blood pressure and body tissue perfusion.

IV infusions should be administered with the following precautions:

- Dehydration should be avoided. Therapy for metabolic acidosis, should it develop, is guided by measurement of pH, blood gases, and serum electrolytes.
- Blood volume loss should be measured as accurately as possible and promptly replaced. In an infant, rapid transfusion of blood may produce transient but severe metabolic acidosis because of citrate added as a preservative.
- IV fluids and blood should be infused through pediatric-size cannulated needles or catheters connected to drip chamber adapters and small solution containers. Umbilical vessels may be used for arterial or venous access in newborns less than 24 hours after birth. In extreme circumstances the umbilical vein can be accessed through a small infraumbilical incision and cannulated from inside the peritoneal cavity for rapid infusion. Scalp veins are used frequently on infants.

TABLE 8-2	Pediatric Hematologic Value Ranges			
Age	Hemoglobin (g/dL)	Hematocrit (%)	Leukocytes (mm^3)	Platelets (mm^3)
Cord blood	13.7-20.1	45-65	9000-30,000	350
2 weeks	13-20	42-46	5000-21,000	260
3 months	9.5-14.5	34-41	6000-18,000	250
6 months-6 years	10.5-14	33-42	6000-15,000	250
7-12 years	11-16	34-40	4500-13,500	250

TABLE 8-3	Pediatric Blood Volume
Age	Blood Volume (mL/kg)
Neonate	75 to 80
6 weeks-2 years	75
2 years-puberty	72

If venous access cannot be quickly established, intraosseous infusion may be indicated for fluid replacement (Fig. 8-1). A cutdown on an extremity vein, usually the saphenous vein, may be necessary for toddlers and older children. An extremity should be splinted to immobilize it. A 150- or 250-mL solution drip chamber, sometimes referred to as Burette, Buritrol, Metriset, or Soluset, is used to help avoid the danger of overhydration. This chamber is available in sizes ranging from 50 to 250 mL from manufacturers such as Abbott, Braun, and Baxter. Adapters are set for accurate control of the desired flow rate.

Body Temperature Considerations.
Temperature regulation is controlled in the anterior hypothalamus. Cooling causes vasoconstriction for the conservation of body heat. Extremes of cooling cause shivering in infants older than 3 months that generates body heat and increases metabolic needs, causing a 200% to 500% increase in oxygen consumption.[3]

Neonates (especially preterm), infants, and children have wider average body temperature variations than do adults. Infants younger than 3 months do not have a shiver response because of immature neurologic development. Body temperature in the newborn tends to range from as low as 97° to 100° F (36.1° to 37.7° C). Temperature begins to stabilize within this range 12 to 24 hours after birth if the environment is controlled. The relatively high rate of heat loss in propor-

tion to heat production in the infant results from an incompletely developed thermoregulatory mechanism and from a body fat/lean mass ratio with only a thin layer of subcutaneous brown fat for insulation.

Extensive extracorporeal circulation also causes rapid dissipation of heat from the body. A hypothermic newborn or infant metabolizes anesthetic agents more slowly and is susceptible to postoperative respiratory depression and delayed emergence from anesthesia. The first sign of significant hypothermia in a pediatric patient younger than 1 year is a heart rate less than 100 beats per minute, metabolic acidosis, hypoglycemia, hyperkalemia, elevated blood urea nitrogen (BUN), and oliguria.

Oxygen consumption is at a minimum when abdominal skin temperature is 97° F (36.1° C). A room temperature 5° F (15° C) cooler than that of abdominal skin produces a 50% increase in oxygen consumption, creating the hazard of acidosis. These factors account for the pediatric patient's susceptibility to environmental changes. The following can result in heat loss:

- Evaporation. When skin becomes wet, evaporative heat loss can occur. Excessive drapes can cause sweating. As sweat evaporates, it elicits a cooling effect.
- Radiation. When heat transfers from the body surface to the room atmosphere, radiation heat loss can result.
- Conduction. Placing the pediatric patient on a cold operating bed causes heat transfer from the patient's body to the surface of the bed.
- Convection. When air currents pass over skin, heat loss by convection results. Cold, wet diapers and blankets can cause heat loss by conduction.

Neonates, infants, and children are kept warm during the surgical procedure to minimize heat loss and to prevent hypothermia. Body temperature tends to decrease in the OR because of cooling from air-conditioning and open body cavities. Room temperature should be maintained as warm as 85° F (29.4° C). Continuous core body temperature monitoring should be performed (skin temperature sensors may be sufficient for short procedures). Other precautions should also be taken as follows:

- A hyperthermia blanket or water mattress may be placed on the operating bed and warmed before the infant or child is laid on it. It is covered with a double-thickness blanket. The temperature is maintained between 95° and 100° F (35° to 37.7° C) to prevent skin burns and elevation of body temperature above the normal range. Excessive hyperthermia can cause dehydration and convulsions in the anesthetized patient.
- A radiant heat lamp should be placed over the newborn to prevent heat loss through radiation. Warming lights with infrared bulbs may be used if a radiant warmer is not available. These lights should be about 27 inches (69 cm) from the infant to prevent burns; the distance should be measured. Plastic bubble wrap also provides insulation around the newborn to prevent heat loss by conduction but can cause heat loss by evaporation.
- Wrapping the head (except the face) and extremities in plastic, such as plastic wrap or Webril helps prevent heat loss in infants and small children. An aluminum warming suit or blanket may be used for toddlers and

---

[3]Akin A et al: Postoperative shivering in children with causative factors, *Pediatr Anesth* 15:1089-1093, 2005.

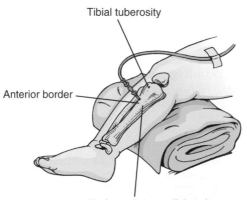

Tibial tuberosity

Anterior border

90 degrees to medial surface

FIG. 8-1   Intraosseous infusion into tibia. Insertion site for needle placement is in anterior midline 1 to 3 cm below tibial tuberosity. Note that needle is perpendicular to medial surface and that tubing is secured on thigh.

older children. Forced-air warming blankets also are effective in maintaining core temperature. Booties or socks can be helpful.

- Rectal, esophageal, axillary, or tympanic probes are used to measure core temperature. A probe placed into the rectum should not be inserted more than 1 inch (2 or 3 cm), because trauma to an infant through perforation of the rectum or colon can occur. Urinary catheters with thermistor probes may be useful if urinary catheterization is indicated. Tympanic temperature measurement can be inconsistent with measurements taken elsewhere in the body and should not be the only parameter by which determination of body temperature is made.[4]
- Drapes should permit some evaporative heat loss to maintain equalization of body temperature. An excessive number of drapes, which can retain heat and put a weight on the body, are avoided. Combinations of paper, plastic, and cloth drapes may cause excessive fluid loss through diaphoresis and absorption into the drapes.
- Solutions should be warm when applied to tissues to minimize heat loss by evaporation and conduction. The circulator should pour warm skin preparation solutions immediately before use. (Check the manufacturer's recommendations for warming solutions. Some iodine-based solutions become unstable when heated. The concentration of iodine increases when the fluid portion evaporates.) The scrub person moistens sponges in warm saline before handing them to the surgeon. Irrigant for urologic procedures should be warmed to body temperature except where contraindicated.
- Blood and IV solutions can be warmed before transfusion by running tubing through a blood and fluid warmer. Carbon dioxide (CO_2) for insufflation during laparoscopy can be warmed this way.
- Blankets should be warmed to place over the patient immediately after dressings are applied and drapes are removed. The patient should be kept covered whenever possible before and after the surgical procedure to prevent chilling from the air-conditioning.

Indicators of Thermoregulatory Status. Hyperthermia (i.e., core temperature of the body over 104° F [40° C]) during the surgical procedure can be caused by fever, dehydration, decrease in sweating from atropine administration, excessive drapes, and drugs that disturb temperature regulation, such as general anesthetics and barbiturates. If the patient is febrile preoperatively, the surgical procedure may be delayed to allow reduction in temperature and to permit fluid administration. If an immediate surgical procedure is necessary and fever persists, anesthesia is induced and external cooling is employed. IV fluids may be given at room temperature instead of warmed during administration.

Beginning signs of hypothermia include initial tachycardia and tachypnea as the body tries to compensate by circulating warmed blood throughout the body. As chilling progresses, the pediatric patient becomes bradycardic with shallow respirations because metabolic processes have slowed.

A sudden rise in temperature during the surgical procedure may indicate malignant hyperthermia. Immediate cooling with ice and cool fluids is necessary. More detailed information about malignant hyperthermia is described in Chapter 31.

Cardiopulmonary Status Considerations. The heart rate fluctuates widely among infants, toddlers, and preschool children and varies during activity and at rest (Table 8-4). Infants younger than 1 year tolerate a heart rate between 200 and 250 beats per minute without hemodynamic consequence. Heart rhythm disturbance is uncommon unless a cardiac anomaly is present. Cardiopulmonary complications manifest as respiratory compromise more frequently than as cardiac dysfunction. After age 5 years, cardiopulmonary response to stress resembles that of a young adult.

Cardiac and respiratory rates and sounds are continually monitored in all age-groups by precordial or esophageal stethoscopy. Blood pressure, vital signs, electrocardiogram (ECG), and other parameters as indicated also are monitored throughout the surgical procedure (see Table 8-4). A pulse oximeter can be placed on the palm of the hand or on the midfoot of a newborn or small infant. Smaller patients experience oxygen desaturation easily. A disadvantage of pulse oximetry is that it cannot detect instantaneous drops in oxygen saturation. It gives readouts of levels that have already occurred. Because of increased carboxyhemoglobin levels, it may be ineffective for patients who have had smoke inhalation or carbon monoxide poisoning. A pulse oximeter reading of 80% is clinically diagnostic of central cyanosis. Hypoxemia can cause bradycardia to decrease oxygen consumption of the myocardium.

Infants are particularly susceptible to respiratory obstruction because of their anatomic structure. They are primarily obligate nasal breathers. They have small nares, a relatively large tongue, lymphoid tissue present, and a small-diameter trachea, causing disproportionate narrowing of the airway. A cylindric thorax, poorly developed accessory respiratory muscles, and increased volume of abdominal contents limit diaphragmatic movement. The chest is more compliant and collapses easily.

Pediatric Infection Risk Considerations. Newborns and infants are susceptible to nosocomial infection. Many preterm infants who have respiratory distress and circulatory problems survive because of advances in perinatal medicine. This has increased the population of high-risk and debilitated infants with reduced humoral and cellular defenses to infection. Aseptic technique is essential in handling neonates and all other pediatric patients.

An elective surgical procedure should be delayed in the presence of respiratory infection because of the risk of airway obstruction. Intubation of inflamed tissues may cause laryngeal edema. Coryza, inflammation of mucous membranes of the nose, is often a sign of an infectious respiratory disease.

Frequent use of antibiotics may lead to antibiotic resistance in some microorganisms. Many types of antibiotics are used to treat infection; however, it is advised that

---

[4]Barclay L: Ear temperature poorly correlated with rectal temperature, *Lancet* 360:603-609, 2002.

TABLE 8-4	Pediatric Vital Sign Ranges			
Age	Heart Rate/Minute Awake	Heart Rate/Minute Asleep/at Rest	Respirations/Minute Asleep/at Rest	Blood Pressure Systolic* (mm Hg)
NEWBORN (2-3 kg)	100-180	80-160	30-60	60±10
INFANT				
1 month (4 kg)	110-150	70-120	26-34	80±16
6 months (7 kg)	115-130	80-180	24-50	89±29
1 year (10 kg)	100-150	70-120	22-30	96±30
TODDLER				
18-30 months (12-14 kg)	110-130	70-100	22-28	99±25
PRESCHOOL				
4 years (16-18 kg)	80-120	60-90	20-30	99±20
SCHOOL-AGE				
6-9 years (20-32 kg)	70-115	60-90	20-30	100±20
10 years (33 kg)	60-100	60-90	18-22	112±20
ADOLESCENT				
14 years (50 kg)	60-100	60-90	16-20	120±20

*www.emedicine.com.

Excerpted from the following references. Weights from the National Institute of Health (NIH) represent a combined estimate of weight for girls and boys. www.vh.org/pediatric/index.html; www.clinicalexam.com; www.cc.nih.gov/ccc/pedweb/pedsstaff/age.html; http://anesthesia.uihc.uiowa.edu

prevention by aseptic and sterile techniques is more beneficial to the patient.

Pediatric Pain Management Considerations.
Infants and children are sensitive to pain with the same intensity as adults. Their pain may be intense, but infants, toddlers, and preschool children are unable to describe its location and nature with specific terms, although they have some limited pain descriptive vocabulary around the age of 18 months.

Neonates and infants can be assessed for pain using physiologic parameters such as heart rate and oxygen saturation with facial expressions such as brow bulge, eye squeeze, and nasolabial furrow and body movements.

Another method of measuring pain is the FLACC Behavioral Pain Assessment Scale (Face, Legs, Activity, Cry, and Consolability) developed by nurses and physicians at C. S. Mott Children's Hospital at the University of Michigan Health System in Ann Arbor. The chart measures and scores five categories of behavior in pediatric patients ages 2 months to 7 years in relationship to pain (Table 8-5).

School-age children may refer pain to a part of the body not involved in the disease process. Figure 8-2 describes the Wong-Baker FACES Pain Rating Scale that can be used to determine the severity of pain experienced by a pediatric patient. Insecurity and fear in an older child may be more traumatic than the pain itself. Children should be observed for signs of pain (i.e., vocalizations, facial expressions, crying, body movements, physiologic parameters). Children also differ from adults in their response to pharmacologic agents; their tolerance to analgesic drugs is altered (Table 8-6).

Most pediatric medication errors occur because children vary significantly in body weight. The number of near-

TABLE 8-5	Pain Assessment in Pediatric Patients 2 Months to 7 Years Old: FLACC Behavioral Pain Assessment Scale		
	Scoring		
Categories	0	1	2
Face	No particular expression or smile	Occasional grimace or frown, withdrawn, disinterested	Frequent to constant quivering chin, clenched jaw
Legs	Normal position or relaxed	Uneasy, restless, tense	Kicking, or legs drawn up
Activity	Lying quietly, normal position moves easily	Squirming, shifting back and forth, tense	Arched, rigid or jerking
Cry	No cry (awake or asleep)	Moans or whimpers; occasional complaint	Crying steadily, screams or sobs, frequent complaints
Consolability	Content, relaxed	Reassured by occasional touching hugging or being talked to, distractible	Difficulty to console or comfort

Each of the five categories is scored from 0 to 2, resulting in a total score between 0 and 10.
The FLACC scale was developed by Sandra Merkel, MS, RN; Terri Voepel-Lewis, MS, RN; and Shobha Malviya, MD, at C.S. Mott Children's Hospital, University of Michigan Health System, Ann Arbor. Copyright © 2002, The Regents of the University of Michigan.

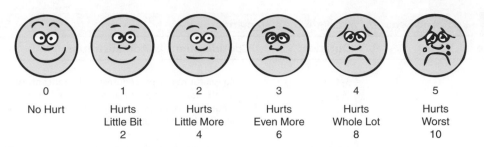

0	1	2	3	4	5
No Hurt	Hurts Little Bit	Hurts Little More	Hurts Even More	Hurts Whole Lot	Hurts Worst
	2	4	6	8	10

Original instructions:

Explain to the child that each face is for a person who feels happy because he has no pain (hurt) or sad because there is some or a lot of pain. **Face 0** is very happy because he doesn't hurt at all. **Face 1** hurts just a little bit. **Face 2** hurts a little more. **Face 3** hurts even more. **Face 4** hurts a whole lot, but **Face 5** hurts as much as you can imagine, although you don't have to be crying to feel this bad. Ask the child to choose the face that best describes own pain.

Rating scale is recommended for persons age 3 years and older.

Brief word instructions:

Point to each face using the words to describe the pain intensity. Ask the child to choose face that best describes own pain and record the appropriate number. *Note:* In a study of 148 children ages 4 to 5 years, there were no differences in pain scores when children used the original or brief word instructions. (In Wong D, Baker C: *Reference manual for the Wong-Baker FACES Pain Rating Scale*, Duarte, CA, 1998, City of Hope Pain/Palliative Care Pain Resource Center; also available on the website *www.elsevierhealth.com/WOW/*).

Wong-Baker FACES Pain Rating Scale:

Available at no charge from Purdue Pharma, L.P., One Stamford Forum., Stamford, CT 06901-3431; (800)733-1333 or (203) 588-5000, ext. 7314. Spanish and Portuguese translations by Ellen Johnsen; French translation by Thomas Angelo; Italian translation by Madeline Mitchko; Romanian translation by Bogdan R. Dinu; Bosniau translation by Barbara Bogomolov; Vietnamese translation by Yen B. Isle; Chinese translation by Hung-Shen Lin; Japanese translation from *After the announcement of cancer*, Tokyo, 1993, Iwanami Shoten, Pub; German translation from Wong DL: *Pediatric quick reference*, Berlin, Wiesbaden, 1997, Ullstein Mosby.

*This figure may be photocopied for clinical use.

FIG. 8-2 Wong-Baker FACES Pain Rating Scale.
(From Hockenberry MJ and others: Wong's nursing care of infants and children, *ed 8, St Louis, 2007, Mosby.)*

misses are nearly 7 times greater in children than in adults. Many errors are as high as 10 times the usual dose because of decimal placement mistakes in calculation. Considerations in pediatric medication should include the following:

- Children cannot determine and communicate their own responses to drugs with reliable precision.
- Parents frequently do not understand drug administration instructions.
- Data are minimal about pediatric responses to medication.
- Few clinical trials are used to support drug use for children, although the drugs are commonly used.
- Pediatric dosage forms and packaging are not available in all drugs used for children.
- Children have unpredictable disease states and organ responses to drugs.
- Reactions in children may not reflect the responses exhibited by adults.

Prevention of pediatric medication errors should include, but are not limited to, the following activities:

- Be sure the pediatric patient's weight is recorded in grams or kilograms (as appropriate for age and size) on the chart because weight-based dosages require accurate measurement for calculation.
- Do not abbreviate dosages or volumes.
- Clarify any questionable drug, dose, or route.

- Check for allergies. Observe the pediatric patient for new signs of allergy if a new medication is added to the regimen.
- When the drug is measured in decimals: be sure to use a zero at the left of the decimal to signify the fraction (e.g., 0.2 mg rather than .2 mg). Do not use a zero at the right of the decimal (e.g., 5 mg rather than 5.0 mg). Errors happen when someone does not see the decimal.
- Use generic names of drugs as a routine.
- Be sure to have clear signatures and contact numbers for the person prescribing the drug.
- Avoid verbal orders if possible.
- Know the medication and its actions before giving the drug.
- Know the medication delivery devices before using them (e.g., infusion pumps).

PREOPERATIVE PSYCHOLOGIC PREPARATION OF PEDIATRIC PATIENTS

The pediatric surgical patient should be considered as a whole person with individual physical and psychosocial needs assessed in relation to the natural stages of development. Equally important are the adjustment and attitude of the parents toward the child, the illness, and the surgical

TABLE 8-6	Pediatric Sedation and Pain Management	
Drug and Dosage	**Duration**	**Considerations in Administration**
ACETAMINOPHEN 10 mg/kg PO 20-25 mg/kg rectally	3-4 hours	Analgesia for minor procedures; antipyretic; absorption is delayed in infants, so dose should not be repeated for 6 hours; no effect on coagulopathy; no respiratory depression; may be combined with narcotic for major procedures
CODEINE 0.5-1 mg/kg IM or PO	3-4 hours	Moderate pain relief; not given IV; can be given with acetaminophen
DIAZEPAM 0.04-0.02 mg/kg IM or IV 0.12-0.8 mg/kg PO Not used for continuous infusion	1-3 hours 3-4 hours	Sedation and seizure control; can cause respiratory depression, jaundice, and vein irritation at IV site
FENTANYL 1-2 mcg/kg IM or IV Continuous infusion: 0.5-2 mcg/kg/hr PO lozenge is available	30-60 minutes	Excellent pain and anxiety relief; metabolized slowly in smaller children and infants; reversible with naloxone; short half-life; can cause respiratory depression, nausea, and vomiting; PO lozenge provides sedation but causes high incidence of preoperative nausea and vomiting
HYDROMORPHONE 1-4 mg per dose every 4 hours IM, IV, or PO	4-5 hours	Not used for infants and young children; used for adolescents; side effects include CNS and respiratory depression, hypotension, bradycardia, increased intracranial pressure, and peripheral vascular dilation
IBUPROFEN 5-10 mg/kg PO or rectally*	3-4 hours	Can cause gastrointestinal bleeding; may affect platelet aggregation
LORAZEPAM 0.1 mg/kg IV	6-8 hours	Long half-life; sedation and seizure control; can cause respiratory depression, nausea, vomiting, and vein irritation at IV site; used for adolescents
MEPERIDINE 1-1.5 mg/kg IM, IV, or subQ Can be given PO, but less effective	3-4 hours	Excellent pain relief; reversible with naloxone; can cause respiratory depression, suppression of intestinal motility, and hypotension; may cause nausea and vomiting; not used in increased intracranial pressure; poor sedation; not a good premedicant
MIDAZOLAM 0.1 mg/kg IV 0.08 mg/kg IM 0.5-0.75 mg/kg PO 0.3 mg/kg rectally in 5 mL normal saline Continuous infusion: 0.1 mg/kg/hr	30-60 minutes	Short half-life; may cause respiratory depression; excellent amnesic; sedation of choice for most pediatric patients
MORPHINE 0.1-0.2 mg/kg IM, IV, or subQ; not well absorbed PO; continuous infusion: 0.25-2 mg/kg/hr; average dose 0.06 mg/kg/hr	4-5 hours	Excellent pain relief; reversible with naloxone; can cause respiratory depression, suppression of intestinal motility, and hypotension; may cause nausea and vomiting; not a good premedicant
PENTOBARBITAL 2-4 mg/kg IM, PO, or rectally	3-4 hours	Causes sedation and hypnosis; short acting
SUFENTANIL 1-2 mcg/kg IV; nasal spray	1-2 hours	Is 10 times more potent than fentanyl; very short half-life

*Additional values can be found at www.virtual-anaesthesia-textbook.com/vat/peds.htm.
CNS, Central nervous system; *IM,* intramuscularly; *IV,* intravenously; *PO,* by mouth; *subQ,* subcutaneously.
Kyllonen M et al: Perioperative pharmacokinetics of ibuprofen after rectal administration, *Pediatr Anesth* 15(7):566, 2005.

experience. Parents' anxiety about the impending surgical procedure may be transferred to the child. Emotional support of the patient and the parents and teaching the patient and the parents are important aspects of preoperative preparation to help them cope.

When an event is threatening, the patient changes cognitive and behavioral responses to deal with the specific demands of the situation. Most adults face stress with more control when fear of the unknown is eliminated. Therefore, parents need to be informed of events that will occur and to be taught how to care for their child preoperatively and postoperatively. If children are informed of sensations to be experienced, cognitive control of the event may occur. Children do not differ from adults in this respect. However, understanding varies with age.

The following are general considerations:

1. Psychologically it may be better for both the infant and the parents if a congenital anomaly is corrected as soon after birth as possible. The infant younger than 1 year will not remember the experience. Parents will gain confidence in learning to cope with a residual deformity as the infant learns to compensate for it. Fear of body mutilation or punishment may be of paramount importance to a preschool or young school-age child.

   Children from 2 to 5 years of age have great sensitivity and a tenuous sense of reality. They live in a world of magic, monsters, and retribution, yet they are aggressive. School-age children have an enhanced sense of reality and value honesty and fairness. Their natural interest and curiosity aid communication. These children need reassurances and explanations in vocabulary compatible with their developmental level. Words should be chosen wisely. Negative connotations should be avoided, and the positive aspects should be stressed. The nurse should talk on the child's level about his or her interests and concerns.

   Anxiety in the school-age child may be stimulated by remembrance of a previous experience. Many children undergo two or more staged surgical procedures before the deformity of a congenital anomaly or traumatic injury is cosmetically reconstructed or functionally restored. Familiarity with the nursing staff reassures the child. Ideally, the same circulator who was present for the first surgical procedure should visit preoperatively and be with the child during subsequent surgical procedures.

   Fear of the unknown about general anesthesia may become exaggerated into extreme anxiety with fantasies of death. The school-age child and adolescent need facts and reassurances. General anesthesia should not be referred to as "putting you to sleep." The child may equate this phrase with the euthanasia of a former pet that never returned home. Instead, the nurse should say, "You will sleep for a little while," or "You will take a nap." Tell the child about the "nice nurses" who will be in the "wake-up room after your nap." Parents should be encouraged to also display confidence and cheerfulness to avoid transmitting anxiety.

   Parents should be honest with their child but maintain a confident manner. The perioperative nurse should do the same. However, a school-age child should not be given information not asked for; questions should be answered, and misunderstandings should be corrected. The nurse should be especially alert to silent, stoic, noncommunicative children, many of whom have difficult induction and emergence from anesthesia. Children who have lost a sibling or friend to death often fear hospitalization.

2. Some facilities hold parties or get-togethers for children and their parents before or after admission to explain routines and procedures before the surgical experience. At other facilities, personnel take children to the OR with their teddy bears so that they can see the different attire, lights, tables, anesthesia machine, and other equipment that might interest them. A child-size anesthesia mask becomes a toy that they are allowed to handle and place on the teddy bear. A clear plastic mask is less psychologically traumatic to a child than is an opaque, black rubber mask. An effective method of explaining procedures to children is to use the child's teddy bear and dress it as the child will look postoperatively. For example, a bandage is put on the bear if the child will have one postoperatively.

3. Separation from parent(s) or a trusted guardian is traumatic for infants older than 6 months, toddlers, and preschool children. Infants require cuddling and bonding. Toddlers are only reaching the autonomy stage when hospitalization forces them into passive behavior, and thus their separation anxiety is greatest. Young children may fear strangers. The parent's presence is necessary for the toddler, and the parent should be encouraged to stay with the hospitalized child as much as possible.

   The child should be permitted to bring a toy or other security object to the OR suite if a parent cannot be present. Many anesthesia providers encourage parents to accompany an infant or child to the OR and to stay through induction if they wish. The presence of a parent can significantly reduce anxiety and ease induction. Some facilities allow parents to accompany the child to the holding area but restrict entrance into the OR. Highly anxious parents who have difficulty coping with stress may cause an increase in the child's anxiety level.

4. Ambulatory surgery, if feasible, is an advantage, because the child enters the facility 1 to 2 hours before the surgical procedure and returns home after recovery from anesthesia. This minimizes the trauma of separation.

5. A preoperative visit by a perioperative nurse should be planned to get to know the child, confirm appropriate consents, and provide emotional support to the family. Parents should be taught to provide postoperative care, especially before and after an ambulatory procedure. Verbal instructions may be supplemented with a videotape or storybook to reinforce understanding for both the child and the parents.

6. The perioperative nurse should bring the patient to the OR in a crib or on an appropriate-size cart. Carrying him or her into the OR presents the risk for dropping or bumping the child. Each situation should be determined by the patient's need. Some facilities use toy wagons for child transport.

PEDIATRIC ANESTHESIA

Pediatric anesthesia has become increasingly specialized as the many variables in the management of infants and children have become better understood. The anesthesia provider recognizes and respects the small margin for error and the uniqueness of the physiology and responses to drugs of pediatric patients. For example, the high metabolic rate of children causes rapid oxygen consumption. Changes occur rapidly in infants and children.

Preoperative Assessment by the Anesthesia Provider

A preoperative visit by the anesthesia provider to establish rapport and assess the patient is also a vital part of preparation of the pediatric patient. This visit is made preferably with the parents present so that the child will consider the anesthesia provider a trustworthy and caring friend. During physical assessment, special attention is given to the heart, lungs, and upper airways. Loose teeth are noted. Possible difficulties are anticipated.

Preoperative care includes correction of dehydration, reduction of excessive fever, compensation for acidosis, and restoration of depleted blood volume. An American Society of Anesthesiologists (ASA) physical status classification is assigned to the pediatric patient. The patient's age, developmental stage, psychological characteristics, and history are considered to determine the patient's probable response to the anesthesia experience.

Premedication

Psychological preparation of the child older than 7 years can decrease the need for an anxiolytic (i.e., a sedative or minor tranquilizer to reduce anxiety). Crying greatly increases mucus in the respiratory tract. At the discretion of the anesthesia provider, premedication may be ordered to produce serenity. Some anesthesia providers prefer children to be well medicated; others favor minimal or no sedation. Infants younger than 1 year usually do not require premedication, but pacifiers with medication ports are commercially available for delivery of oral drugs. Premedication, which is tailored to the individual, varies considerably by age, weight, and health status. Preanesthetic sedation should allow the patient to be taken to the OR lightly asleep or drowsy and should facilitate induction of anesthesia without awakening the child. It should also provide some analgesia during the recovery period.

Timing of administration is extremely important. To be effective, drugs should be given at least 45 to 60 minutes before the surgical procedure. The circulator should check with the anesthesia provider and the surgeon before sending for the patient. If ample time is not available for the appropriate effect of premedication, the anesthesia provider may prefer to omit the medication to avoid precipitation of psychological trauma. Fast-acting drugs are available and may be useful for rapid sedation preoperatively. Narcotics, such as morphine and meperidine (Demerol), are rarely indicated for routine premedication in healthy pediatric patients.

No ideal premedicant exists, but the following drugs are commonly used (see also the comparison of sedatives in Table 8-6):

- Sufentanil (Sufenta) given nasally (i.e., sprayed onto the nasal mucosa) facilitates separation from parents by causing relaxation and drowsiness. The child becomes calm and cooperative.
- Fentanyl (Sublimaze) can be incorporated into a lozenge or a flavored hard candy mounted on a stick (i.e., an anesthetic lollipop). When the child licks the candy, the drug is absorbed into the bloodstream through the oral mucosa and produces sedation for 30 to 60 minutes.
- Diazepam (Valium), 0.04 to 0.02 mg/kg administered intramuscularly (IM) or 0.12 to 0.8 mg/kg given orally (PO), causes relaxation for 3 to 4 hours. This drug has very few cardiovascular side effects.
- Midazolam (Versed), 0.08 mg/kg administered IM 15 minutes before induction, greatly reduces anxiety. Oral preparations also work well. This drug is also good for intravenous conscious sedation (IVCS) during endoscopy. Doses range between 0.2 and 0.3 mg/kg IV. Cardiovascular stability is good, and ventilation is not depressed.
- Scopolamine, 0.006 mg/kg, may be added to an IM injection of midazolam for further sedation and amnesic effect.
- Atropine, 0.01 to 0.02 mg/kg, may be administered IM, IV, or subcutaneously (subQ) to inhibit secretions, especially in a child with a severe airway problem, or to counteract bradycardia. Cardiac effects last about 1 hour. Dosage is decreased to 0.004 mg/kg for infants less than 5 kg. It is not given in the presence of fever or glaucoma.
- Glycopyrrolate (Robinul), 0.004 to 0.01 mg/kg administered IM, lowers gastric acidity. It may be given as an alternative to atropine sulfate to reduce secretions. It is contraindicated in the presence of paralytic ileus, urinary tract obstruction, and glaucoma.

Anesthesia Equipment

Simple, lightweight anesthesia equipment is used. Disposable equipment is popular. Facemasks, designed for minimal dead space, are available to closely fit a child's relatively flat face. Nonrebreathing circuits provide less resistance and valves for fresh flow of gas at higher flow rates relative to a child's metabolism and ventilation. To avoid hypothermia, anesthetic gases are warmed and humidified. Neonates are especially at risk for fluctuations in temperature regulation.

Induction

Induction is facilitated by a quiet atmosphere, a soft voice, and a reassuring touch. A parent may be present if the policies of the facility permit. Children should be told what to expect without precipitating fear. The induction experience can be described as getting on a merry-go-round. Noises will seem louder. To avoid confusion, it is best for the child to listen to one person speak at this time. The circulator should remain at the patient's side, maintain a gentle touch, and be alert to the patient's needs and condition.

The following are considerations for anesthesia induction:
1. Restraints should be loose. Minimal pressure should be applied. If the patient is a newborn, infant, or toddler, restraint straps are omitted while the circulator holds the patient during induction. A toddler or preschool-age child is less frightened when holding on to someone's hands. Restraints can be applied after the patient is asleep.
2. A few drops of food extract of the child's choosing (e.g., mint, banana, strawberry) can be placed in the facemask. This makes the anesthetic gas more acceptable and gives the patient a sense of control. The scent

of anesthetic gas may be compared with the scent of special jet fuel used for airplanes or spaceships.

3. If the child is awake, crying, or struggling, apprehension during induction can be avoided by distraction and rapport. It is not easy to establish rapport with young children. If a parent is present, the child may be more cooperative. The child's cooperation may be solicited by counting out loud, singing the alphabet song, blowing up a balloon, taking a space trip or discussing a favorite plaything or television character. The facemask can be held slightly above the face, permitting anesthetic gas to flow by gravity, and lowered gently as the child becomes drowsy. Some anesthesia providers permit the child to hold the mask.

A child who has been crying may have somewhat edematous tissue in the nose and larynx. Secretions are frequently increased. Note that the parent, who may be present, is viewing his or her child's activities range from animated to lethargic. This gives the appearance of helplessness or death. The parent may feel emotional and shed tears. Reassurance should be given, and the parent should be escorted to the waiting area before intubation takes place.

4. Induction may be accompanied by regurgitation and aspiration of gastric contents in infants with pyloric stenosis, tracheoesophageal fistula, intestinal obstruction, or food in the stomach. The hazard is minimized by aspirating gastric contents with a sterile catheter before induction and leaving the tube in place for drainage during the surgical procedure. Rapid-sequence induction may also be used. This consists of thiopental sodium, muscle relaxant, and intubation with cricoid pressure (Sellick's maneuver) applied to close the esophagus and avoid silent regurgitation of food from the stomach. All trauma patients should be considered to have a full stomach.

Types of Induction

Inhalation. If asleep from premedication on arrival in the OR, the child can be anesthetized quickly. If the child is awake, induction may be initiated with inhalant anesthetic.

Nitrous oxide may increase peripheral vascular resistance if it is used to maintain general anesthesia for cardiovascular procedures. It may also increase the risk of air embolus because it combines with smaller air bubbles that may enter the system during repair of congenital heart defects. Potent inhalants are absorbed more rapidly in the presence of nitrous oxide and may cause myocardial depression and decrease cardiac output in very young children. Atropine may minimize this effect.

Rectal Induction. Given by enema, methohexital (Brevital), 15 mg/kg of 1% solution, produces sleep in 6 to 8 minutes and lasts 45 to 60 minutes. This is a painless method used in the presence of parents for preschoolers or toddlers. The parent may hold the child. It is a good method for short diagnostic procedures. The anesthesia provider remains with the patient. Once the child is asleep, the anesthesia state may be maintained with an inhalant. Gentle, assisted ventilation may be needed. This method is tolerated best in children younger than 3 years.

Intravenous Infusion. IV infusion is often preferred for patients older than 9 or 10 years. Induction with a small dose of barbiturate or ketamine is rapid. Studies have shown that IV induction causes less psychological trauma than do inhalant methods. A mixture of lidocaine and prilocaine in a cream base is commercially available for application to the site to decrease pain associated with venipuncture.

Care is taken if the child has a central line because infection or thrombosis may result. If the central line is used for anesthetic administration, all residual drug is flushed from the port so that none remains in the tubing after the procedure.

Ketamine, 1 to 2 mg/kg IV, is useful in a combative, burned, or hypovolemic patient. If given IM to a healthier child who weighs less than 10 kg, the usual dose is 5 to 10 mg/kg. The pharmacologic predictability of ketamine is a good reason for its use in pediatric sedation. Its onset takes place 1 to 2 minutes after IV administration and 5 minutes if given IM. Either way the duration of the dose is approximately 45 minutes. Low doses provide sedation and analgesia. Higher doses cause general anesthesia. Ketamine provides a moderate level of general anesthesia while maintaining blood pressure, breathing, and airway reflexes.[5] Ketamine offers a safer choice of anesthesia if the patient is a known or potential risk for malignant hyperthermia.

Epidural Block. A caudal epidural block may be used in combination with general anesthetic for orthopedic, abdominal, or thoracic procedures.

Intubation and Airway Placement. Airway obstruction in infants and children usually occurs early during anesthesia administration, especially if the child has been crying. When anesthesia deepens, oral airway insertion is essential after assisted ventilation with oxygen. Assisted or controlled ventilation reduces the labor of breathing and therefore reduces metabolism. Some anesthesia providers prefer the use of a laryngeal mask airway.

Intubation. Placement of an endotracheal tube in the trachea of a newborn or infant differs from placement in a child or adolescent. Regardless of age, the airway must remain patent. Sterile equipment and gentle manipulation to avoid soft tissue injury are essential for intubating and suctioning. Other considerations include the following:

- Endotracheal intubation is used by some anesthesia providers for all procedures in infants younger than 1 year. It is necessary for intraabdominal, intrathoracic, and neurosurgical procedures and for those in the head or neck areas, as well as for emergency procedures when contents of the stomach are uncertain. Intubation while the patient is awake may be used in neonates. A certain amount of jaw tightness (masseter muscle rigidity, trismus) is common in pediatric patients after the administration of succinylcholine, but this should be observed closely because it also may be a sign of malignant hyperthermia.

[5]Lin C, Durieux ME: Ketamine and kids, *Pediatr Anesth* 15:91-97, 2005.

TABLE 8-7	Recommended Endotracheal Tube Sizes
Age	Diameter (mm)
Preterm	2.5-3
Newborn	3
Newborn-6 months	3.5
6-12 months	3.5-4
12 months-2 years	4-4.5
3-4 years	4.5-5
5-6 years	5-5.5
7-8 years	5.5-6
9-10 years	6-6.5
11-12 years	6.5-7
13 years and older	7-7.5

- The size of the endotracheal tube is selected according to the width and length of the trachea (Table 8-7). Endotracheal tubes for children younger than 8 years are not cuffed. The uncuffed tube allows for a slight space around the exterior circumference and a wider internal diameter than a cuffed tube. Soft tissue at the narrowest level of the cricoid cartilage, located just below the vocal cords, forms a loose seal around the tube. The pediatric larynx sits more cephalad (higher) in the throat (C3 in a preterm infant and C4 in the average child compared with C5-6 in an adult).
- The nasotracheal tube may inadvertently dislodge adenoid tissue and carry it into the trachea.
- The head of a newborn or infant is elevated slightly and not hyperextended during placement of the endotracheal tube. A toddler also has a larger occiput and therefore needs little posterior extension of the head. A child with Down syndrome is predisposed to instability of the odontoid articulation at the first cervical vertebra (C1) and is at risk of dislocation if the head is placed in extreme hyperextension.
- A straight blade generally is used on the laryngoscope because the epiglottis must be raised to visualize the glottis during intubation (Fig. 8-3). An infant's epiglottis is long and stiff and projects posteriorly at an angle of 45 degrees above the glottis. The epiglottis of a toddler and a preschool child is short and easily traumatized.
- Intubation and suctioning are preceded and followed by oxygen administration. If the process of introducing the endotracheal tube takes longer than 30 seconds, the patient should be ventilated with 100% oxygen before additional attempts at intubation ensue.
- The length and diameter of the suction catheter should be considered when suctioning oropharyngeal secretions.

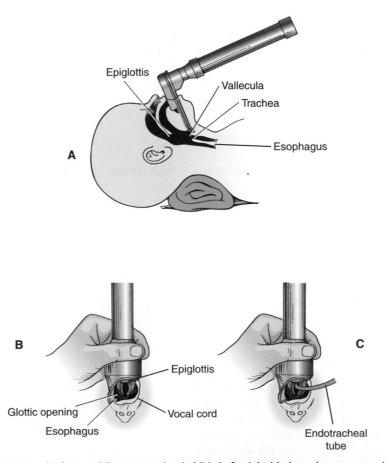

FIG. 8-3 Intubation of infant, toddler, or preschool child. **A,** Straight blade on laryngoscope is advanced to vallecula, space between base of tongue and epiglottis. **B,** Gentle elevation of tip of blade lifts epiglottis to visualize glottic opening between vocal cords. **C,** Endotracheal tube is advanced below blade into trachea.

An oversized catheter may perforate the oropharynx, trachea, bronchus, or esophagus.

- The newborn's head is maintained in a neutral position, midway between full extension and full flexion, while an endotracheal tube is in place. The tip of the tube should be positioned in the midtrachea. The average distance between the vocal cords and the carina, where the trachea separates into two branches, is only about 2 inches (4 to 5 cm) in a term neonate and much less in a preterm neonate. If the head shifts, the tube can shift, leading to inadequate oxygenation.

Anesthetic Agents and Maintenance

The following characteristics of anesthetic agents and maintenance of anesthesia are considered:

1. Topical agents are not often used because of the hazard of overdose. Local anesthetic cream (eutectic mixture of local anesthetics [EMLA]), may be used to start an IV access point with minimal risk of toxicity.

2. Inhalation anesthesia, especially with halothane or sevoflurane, is popular. Nitrous oxide–oxygen-halothane is frequently used in combination with IV agents. Halothane and succinylcholine are contraindicated if there is a family history of malignant hyperthermia, because they trigger the condition. Nitrous oxide is used with caution in patients with congenital cardiac defects, particularly in cyanotic conditions. Isoflurane (Forane) is irritating, necessitating slow and more difficult induction to prevent laryngospasm, but it offers the advantage of circulatory support. It is not useful in short procedures. Sevoflurane is less irritating to the airway and is comparable to halothane for induction. Emergence is smooth and rapid. Pain sensation may be immediate after arousal. Analgesia should be administered.

   Alveolar concentrations of inhaled anesthetics rise much more rapidly in pediatric patients than in adults because of relatively greater blood flow and smaller functional residual capacity. Children therefore have higher anesthetic requirements than do adults. To produce the same level of anesthesia, neonates require about 40% more halothane than do adults. Increased anesthetic requirement and more rapid induction can cause hypotension and reduced cardiac output in infants and children.

3. Ketamine provides sedation for preschool children during invasive diagnostic procedures. It is a short-acting general anesthetic for short procedures, such as burn debridement, tonsillectomy, or circumcision. Because it does not alter pharyngolaryngeal reflexes or skeletal tone, intubation is unnecessary. Cardiovascular and respiratory stimulation is minimal; ketamine may be useful in asthmatic and other poor-risk patients. It is contraindicated in the patient who has increased intracranial pressure. It is not advised for teenagers. Premedication with diazepam counteracts possible emergence delirium.

4. Local anesthesia is commonly used as a supplement to light general anesthesia. Long-acting agents, such as bupivacaine (Marcaine), prolong postoperative analgesia, thus reducing or eliminating the need for narcotics (Table 8-8). Epinephrine added to bupivacaine enhances its duration to a greater extent in children than in adults. Large doses of epinephrine may interact with halothane and cause dysrhythmias. Doses of epinephrine up to 10 mg/kg are considered safe.

5. Epidural anesthesia can be administered for sensory blockade intraoperatively. The epidural catheter may be left in place for prolonged postoperative analgesia. A continuous infusion of narcotics provides uninterrupted pain management, as administered to adults to attenuate postoperative stress response.

6. Narcotics are used in situations similar to adult indications. Nitrous oxide–narcotic-relaxant provides stable anesthesia for the very ill patient. Fentanyl has minimal cardiovascular effect.

7. The critically ill neonate does not tolerate anesthesia well. Adequate ventilation and oxygenation are vital, but care is taken to avoid oxygen toxicity with resultant retrolental fibroplasia; neovascularization of the retina can produce blindness. Neonates and preterm infants less than 34 weeks' gestational age and 1500 g or less body weight are at risk. Adequate blood-gas tension is ensured only by intraoperative invasive measurement.

8. Neuromuscular blockers are used judiciously. Infants younger than 1 year exhibit a lesser degree of blockade from succinylcholine than do older children. Bradycardia and an increase in intraocular tension are more conspicuous in infants. Response decreases with age. Dosage varies. A peripheral nerve stimulator should be used to assess blockade to avoid overdosage. Blockers seldom are required in infants because of their poorly developed abdominal musculature.

9. Consideration is given for postoperative analgesia. When halothane is reduced near the end of the surgical procedure, a narcotic may be given. Regional or local infiltration will also provide relief of pain (e.g., after circumcision or cleft lip repair).

Emergence and Extubation

Airway problems are the most common concern on emergence from anesthesia and immediately postoperatively. At the conclusion of the surgical procedure, the oropharynx is

TABLE 8-8	Local Anesthesia for Pediatric Patients
Agent	**Maximum Pediatric Dose**
Lidocaine	
Without epinephrine	4.5-5 mg/kg
With epinephrine (epinephrine should not exceed 10 mcg/kg)	7-10 mg/kg
Bupivacaine	3 mg/kg
Tetracaine	2 mg/kg
Procaine	15 mg/kg
Chloroprocaine	15 mg/kg
Cocaine	1 mg/kg

www.anesthesia-nursing.com/manual.html

suctioned. Some anesthesia providers also suction the stomach. All monitors are left in place until the patient is fully awake and extubated.

Reversal with a narcotic antagonist such as naloxone (Narcan) may be used to reverse narcosis but also has the effect of reversing analgesia. Pain sensation may result in restlessness. The usual dose is 0.01 to 0.1 mg/kg for infants and older children.

Extubation of an infant or child is preceded and followed by oxygen administration and performed either with the patient under deep anesthesia or on return of spontaneous respiration, because laryngospasm is possible between these periods. Heart and breath sounds are monitored after extubation. If spasm occurs, oxygen is given by positive pressure. Airway obstruction, aspiration, and hypothermia are hazards of the recovery period. Children, particularly in the 2- to 5-year age-group, may develop hoarseness and a croupy cough after removal of an endotracheal tube. Racemic epinephrine (Vaponefrin) provides relief; 0.5 mL of 2.25% diluted in 3 mL of sterile water can be delivered through a facemask and nebulizer. Constant observation after extubation is required.

The patient should not be taken from the OR with a body temperature less than 95° F (35° C). Below this crucial level, the risk for acidosis, hypoglycemia, bradycardia, hypotension, and apnea increases. This metabolic depression and delayed return of activity set the stage for possible sudden cardiac arrest. Dehydration and low humidity increase the viscosity of secretions. Pediatric patients require close observation for development of laryngeal edema, which is noted by croupy cough, sobbing inspiration, intercostal retraction, tachypnea, or tachycardia. Laryngeal edema greatly reduces the small diameter of the airway of an infant or toddler. Controlled humidity and oxygen are vital.

INTRAOPERATIVE PEDIATRIC PATIENT CARE CONSIDERATIONS

Basic principles of patient care and OR techniques used for adults apply to pediatric surgery; however, some additional considerations are required in the plan of care. The room should be warmed to 73° F (22.8° C) or slightly warmer before the pediatric patient is taken to the OR. Heat loss is a serious issue. A warmed blanket should be positioned on the OR bed as an undercover to prevent conduction of the child's body heat into the cooler mattress. A second warmed blanket should be placed over or around the child to prevent heat radiation into the room air.

To differentiate this specialty from care of adult patients, a few points specific to pediatric surgery are mentioned as follows:

1. Hair is not removed with a depilatory or shaved, except for cranial procedures and as ordered by the surgeon for an adolescent. All hair removed should be saved and given to the parents. Some parents feel their child's hair is a keepsake.

2. Diagnostic studies may be done in the OR with the patient under local anesthesia before induction of general anesthesia for an open surgical procedure. An infant may be swaddled on a padded (papoose) board to restrain him or her from moving while radiographs are taken and to permit easy change of position. A pacifier will help comfort and keep the infant quiet. Pacifiers with built-in medication chambers to deliver sedation are commercially available.

3. The patient is protected from injury. An infant or child should never be left alone anywhere in the perioperative environment. Preparation for induction should be made before the child's arrival.

   a. Guard against a fall from a crib or stretcher. Side rails should remain up at all times. An over-bed cage or mesh crib cover on a crib helps confine a toddler without restraint. Children are restrained at all times while on a stretcher or in a specially designed pediatric cart.

   b. Do not place a crib where the patient can reach an electrical outlet or near any article that can be picked up and cause injury.

   c. After the infant is asleep, pad wrists and ankles with several layers of sheet wadding (Webril). Restrain with Kerlix or Kling roller gauze, and pin straps to the sheet on the operating bed. Sheet wadding prevents possible abrasion of delicate skin by the restraint straps. Care is taken not to restrict circulation.

   d. Safety pins, open or closed, or other small objects are not left within reach of an infant or child.

4. Catheters as small as 8 French (Fr) are available for use as needed in newborns and infants. A plain-tip or whistle-tip catheter is used for a stomach tube. An indwelling Foley catheter with a 3-mL balloon may be used for urinary drainage. Small, calibrated drainage containers are connected to permit accurate determination of output.

5. Positioning principles are essentially the same as those described for adults. Figure 8-4 depicts ideas for positioning small infants. Correspondingly smaller towel rolls, pillows, gel pads, and beanbags are used to stabilize anesthetized infants and children. The size of the child or adolescent determines the appropriate supports to maintain the desired position. A small towel roll or stockinette-covered IV bag at each side of the body takes the weight of drapes off the small body of an infant or keeps the patient in a lateral position.

6. A disposable drape sheet without a fenestration is often advantageous: the surgeon can cut an opening of the desired size to expose the site of intended incision. Small towels and nonpiercing towel clips are used with a laparotomy sheet if self-adhering and disposable drapes are not available. A standard opening 3 × 5 inches (7.6 × 12.7 cm) in a pediatric laparotomy sheet is frequently too large for a newborn or infant. Part of the fenestration may be covered with a towel. Pediatric drapes are commercially available.

7. Blood loss on sponges is measured by weighing them while they are still wet. Blood loss on the drapes is estimated, and blood loss through suction is measured. The surgeon and anesthesia provider will determine if blood replacement is necessary, volume

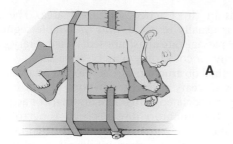

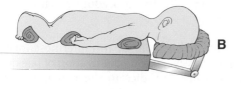

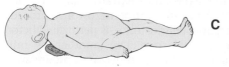

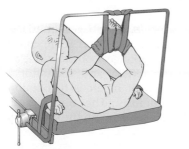

FIG. 8-4   Positioning of infant.
(From Fortunato N: Perioperative nursing series: Plastic and reconstructive surgery, *St Louis, 1998, Mosby.)*

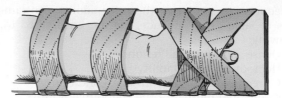

FIG. 8-5   Upper extremity restraint to splint elbow and hand of infant or toddler. Hand is pronated on armboard.

10. A stockinette pulled over dressings on an extremity protects them from becoming soiled and helps keep them in place. This can be changed easily as needed, leaving the dressings in place.

Instrumentation

Gentleness and precision in handling small structures and fragile tissues are essential. Basic or standard instrument sets, sutures, needles, and other items used for surgical procedures on adults are duplicated in miniature to take care of infants and children in each surgical specialty. The perioperative nurse and surgical technologist should be informed about their patient and then use good judgment in preparing supplies for pediatric surgery. The following principles apply:

- Size and weight are more critical factors than age in the selection of instruments, sutures, needles, and equipment.
- Small instruments are used on the delicate tissues of a newborn, infant, or small child.
- Hemostats should have fine points. A mosquito hemostat will clamp a superficial vessel but not a major artery.
- Noncrushing vascular clamps permit occlusion of major blood vessels. They also can be placed across the intestine of a newborn or infant rather than a large, heavy intestinal clamp.
- Lightweight instruments will not inhibit respiration. Instruments not in use on tissues are never laid on the patient, especially not on the chest. An instrument's weight could restrict respiration or circulation or cause bruises. Return instruments to the Mayo stand or instrument table immediately after use.
- Umbilical tape or vessel loops are used frequently to retract blood vessels and small structures, thereby giving the surgeon greater visibility in a small surgical site and eliminating the weight of retractors.
- Needle holders have fine-pointed jaws to hold small, delicate needles.
- Surgical procedure on an adolescent will require adult-size instruments.
- Scrub person closely watches the tissue being dissected and selects the instruments to hand to the surgeon accordingly.

COMMON SURGICAL PROCEDURES
General Surgery

Endoscopic Procedures. Gastroscopy, colonoscopy, and laparoscopy are performed for diagnosis of complaints of abdominal pain or symptoms of intestinal obstruction or inflammation. The indications for pediatric endoscopic

for volume, as it is lost. The measurements are calculated in grams. The calculation is 1 g equals 1 mL of blood. Discussion about weighing sponges is found in Chapter 31.

8. Adhesive tape is abrasive to tender skin and should be avoided when possible. A chemical wound cover like Nu Skin or collodion is adequate over a small incision with a subcuticular closure and is especially desirable under diapers unless dressings are needed to absorb drainage. Care is taken that clothing or the blanket does not touch this substance until it is dry. Skin-closure strips may be used instead of a chemical wound cover.

9. Dressings on the face or neck should be protected from vomitus and food particles, as well as from an infant's or toddler's hands. Elbows should be splinted when the patient potentially may disturb the incision, dressings, or a tube (Fig. 8-5). This is particularly important after eye surgery or cleft lip or palate surgery or when a tracheostomy tube is inserted.

procedures are similar to those for adults. Contraindications to laparoscopy include, but are not limited to, the following:

- Dense abdominal adhesions
- Hemodynamic instability
- Coagulopathy or hemorrhagic condition
- Congenital hernias of the abdominal wall
- Diaphragmatic hernia

Preparing the pediatric patient for laparoscopy should include (1) emptying the bladder by catheterization and (2) inserting a nasogastric tube. Small 0- and 30-degree telescopes are useful. Body size may indicate the use of specialized equipment for unconventional use, such as arthroscopic scopes because of shorter shafts and sheaths.

The potential for anomalous organ position should be considered when placing trocars and sheaths. The open method is preferred over the use of a Verres needle. CO_2 pressures should be kept low at around 8 to 10 mm Hg as tolerated until insufflation is complete. Although an open method is preferred for the primary trocar, sharp insertion of the secondary trocars may be performed under direct vision.

Potential for injury to nontarget organs is great. The bowel and adjacent organs are in close proximity and could inadvertently be injured by graspers or electrosurgical instruments. Small injuries can go unnoticed, resulting in subsequent postoperative bleeding.

Alimentary tract obstruction in a newborn or young infant is the most frequent cause for an emergency surgical procedure. The common sites of obstruction are in the esophagus, duodenum, ileum, colon, and anus. Atresia, an imperforation or closure of a normal opening, and stenosis, a constriction or narrowing, are the common causes of obstruction. Abnormal fistulae can develop between passages, such as in the tracheoesophageal area. The obstructive lesion is usually resected, and the viable segments of the visceral passages are anastomosed. A temporary gastrostomy, ileostomy, or colostomy may be necessary.

Intestinal obstruction can develop in infants and children months to years after the newborn period from a predisposing or associated congenital anomaly or acquired disease process. Inflammatory diseases such as necrotizing enterocolitis, ulcerative colitis, Meckel's diverticulum, or Crohn's disease, as well as other intestinal conditions such as Hirschsprung's disease or familial polyposis, require intestinal resection and anastomosis. An endorectal pullthrough may be the procedure of choice to preserve the rectum.

Biliary Atresia. A form of intrauterine cholangitis that results in progressive fibrotic obliteration of bile ducts, biliary atresia may cause jaundice in the newborn. If untreated, this condition can cause cirrhosis and death within the first year of life. Excision of extrahepatic ducts or hilar dissection with a hepatic portoenterostomy procedure, such as portal hepaticojejunostomy, is performed before the infant is 2 months old to relieve jaundice by improving bile drainage. If liver function becomes progressively impaired, liver transplantation may ultimately be necessary for survival (Fig. 8-6).

Esophageal Atresia. Esophageal atresia, with or without tracheoesophageal fistula, is an acute congenital anomaly characterized by esophageal obstruction, accumulation of secretions, gastric reflux, and respiratory complications (Fig. 8-7). The goal of repair is to obtain an end-to-end esophageal anastomosis. The timing and technique to accomplish this goal depend on the specific type of anomaly,

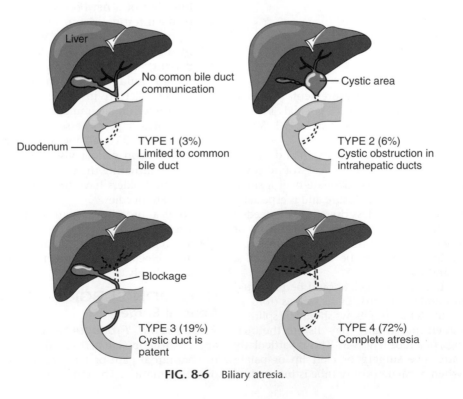

FIG. 8-6 Biliary atresia.

degree of prematurity, birthweight, and extent of other associated anomalies.

Repair may be either primary or staged. Gastrostomy (either open or endoscopic) is performed initially to establish a conduit for feeding the newborn less than 1200 g. Percutaneous placement of the gastrostomy tube (percutaneous endoscopic gastrostomy [PEG] tube) is commonly performed (Fig. 8-8).

Open repair includes division of the tracheoesophageal fistula, if present, and anastomosis of the esophageal pouches. Submucosal myotomies and lengthening of the upper pouch permit primary anastomosis to establish alimentary tract continuity. This may be delayed to allow the esophagus to grow as the infant grows so that the gap between the pouches shortens. A transthoracic or retrosternal interposition colon graft may be necessary for esophageal replacement if

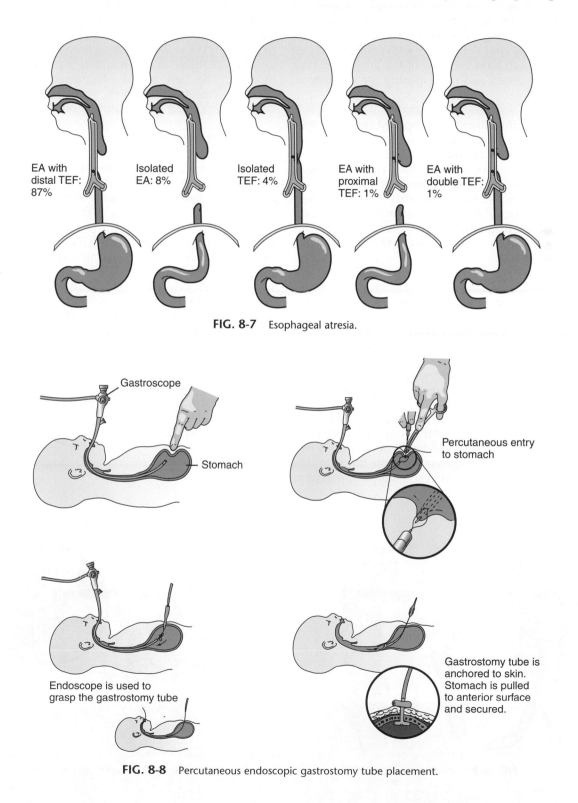

EA with distal TEF: 87%

Isolated EA: 8%

Isolated TEF: 4%

EA with proximal TEF: 1%

EA with double TEF: 1%

FIG. 8-7   Esophageal atresia.

Gastroscope

Stomach

Percutaneous entry to stomach

Endoscope is used to grasp the gastrostomy tube

Gastrostomy tube is anchored to skin. Stomach is pulled to anterior surface and secured.

FIG. 8-8   Percutaneous endoscopic gastrostomy tube placement.

the gap between the proximal and distal segments is too large for a primary esophageal anastomosis. Usually an extrapleural approach is used for these procedures.

Imperforate Anus. Anorectal malformation generally occurs during the 4th to 12th weeks of fetal development. The incidence of anal malformations is 1 in 4000 live births. More males have the condition than females. Imperforate anus (IA) is classified as high or low in relation to the levator muscles. Males have more high level IA incidence and manifest fistulas between the colon and bladder. Females may have more low level IA incidence with vestibular-vaginal fistulas but also can have a fusion of the anogenital tract referred to as a cloaca—a single opening for the urethra, rectum, and vagina.

If the anus remains closed (i.e., imperforate) during fetal development, the intestinal tract is opened surgically soon after birth. A posterior sagittal anorectoplasty or an abdominoperineal pullthrough procedure may be done for primary management with a temporary colostomy. Some children experience fecal incontinence or chronic constipation as they grow into their teens after repair procedures for high IA in infancy. Various secondary procedures are performed, most frequently an endorectal pullthrough procedure or gracilis muscle transplant for reconstruction of the rectal sphincter.

Intussusception. A portion of bowel slides into another segment and causes obstruction (Fig. 8-9). The most common site is the ileocolic junction. The motion is like a telescope. The bowel becomes inflamed, hemorrhagic, and necrotic. Most are diagnosed between 5 months and 1 year and incidence ranges from 1 to 4 in 1000 live births. This is the most common surgical emergency for children younger than 2 years and occurs primarily in the spring and fall months.

Theories about the cause include lingering viral infection that causes inflammation of the lymph glands (Peyer's patch) in the lumen of the bowel that develop hypertrophied adhesions. These adhesions cause the bowel to stick together during peristaltic motion stimulated by digestion.

Other theories indicate that when a baby is weaned from the bottle or breast and new foods are introduced into the diet, the digestive track has not yet adjusted to the change. Intussusception occurs in more males than females.

The symptoms range from intense pain to nausea and vomiting. A sausage-shape curve is sometimes apparent across the abdomen over the location of the intussusception. The baby may have bloody, jellylike stool.

Treatment can range from hydrostatic reduction with a barium enema to open laparotomy through a right lower quadrant incision. Some surgeons use oxygen as a gas enema to insufflate the colon and small bowel for intussusception less than 12 hours' duration and no signs of obstruction or bleeding. The flow rate is maintained around 2 L/min without exceeding 80 mm Hg pressure until fluoroscopy demonstrates small bowel insufflation.[6]

Pyloromyotomy. Pyloric stenosis is a congenital obstructive lesion in the pylorus of the stomach. The onset of symptoms usually occurs between the third and eighth weeks of life. The stenosis is relieved by modified pyloromyotomy also known as a Fredet-Ramstedt. After cutting through serosa, muscle layers of the pylorus are divided.

Herniorrhaphy. Herniorrhaphy (i.e., hernia repair) is the most frequently performed elective surgical procedure in infants and children by general surgeons. Of the four types of hernias seen in pediatric patients, indirect inguinal hernia is the most common; it occurs much more frequently in male patients than in female patients and appears during the first 10 years of life. Female patients who have an inguinal hernia also may have a prolapsed ovary in the hernial sac. Although they are frequently seen, most umbilical hernias do not require surgical intervention. Femoral hernias require surgical correction but are rarely acute problems in childhood. A hiatal hernia is a surgical emergency in the newborn if abdominal contents are in the chest, causing acute respiratory distress (Fig. 8-10). Diaphragmatic hernias

---

[6] home.coqui.net.

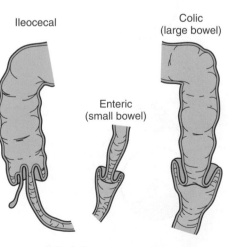

FIG. 8-9 Intussusception.

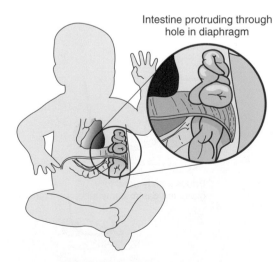

FIG. 8-10 Diaphragmatic hernia.

in infants and children are caused by congenital weakness in the fascia, abdominal wall, or diaphragm.

Omphalocele. Failure of abdominal viscera to become encapsulated within the peritoneal cavity during fetal development results in herniation through a midline defect in the abdominal wall at the base of the umbilicus (i.e., omphalocele) (Fig. 8-11). Contents in the omphalocele sac are surgically reduced back into the peritoneal cavity. The method of closure depends on the extent of the defect. Skin may be closed primarily if the defect is small. More commonly, primary closure of the abdominal wall is facilitated by vigorous stretching of the wall and emptying of intestinal contents from the sac. Closure is performed without undue tension. Synthetic mesh or sheeting may be used.

For large defects, closure of the abdominal wall usually is staged, with implantation of a silicone silo or expansion prosthesis to reduce intestines at the first stage, followed by removal of the device and abdominal wall closure at the second stage. Similar techniques are used for closure of gastroschisis, a full-thickness abdominal wall defect lateral to and separate from the umbilicus, with herniation of abdominal viscera.

Appendectomy. Appendicitis, an acute inflammation of the appendix, is the most common cause for an abdominal surgical procedure in the school-age child. Gangrene or rupture may occur before diagnosis or surgical intervention. A questionable diagnosis may be confirmed by laparoscopy. Appendectomy may be performed by laparoscopy or open laparotomy.

Splenectomy. Removal of the spleen may be indicated to correct hypersplenic disease, either congenital or acquired. Emergency splenectomy is necessary after rupture of the spleen, usually from blunt trauma. An attempt is made to salvage as much of the organ as possible to minimize future susceptibility to infection.

Bezoars. Intestinal obstruction can be caused by ingested matter that forms a foreign body that accumulates in the stomach and can extend into the small bowel. The foreign

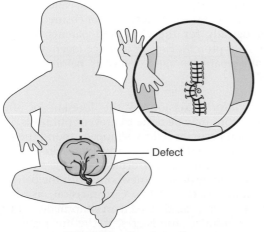

FIG. 8-11 Omphalocele.

body consists of hair *(tricho-)*, vegetable matter *(phyto-)*, or milk curd *(lacto-)* and is commonly associated with strange appetite compulsions (trichophagia) and emotional disturbances. Removal can be done endoscopically by hydrodissection or by open laparotomy. Shock-wave therapy is sometimes successful in fragmenting the bezoar mass for endoscopic removal.

Genitourology

Pediatric urology concerns itself basically with the diagnosis and treatment of infections and congenital anomalies within the genitourinary tract. Some type of anomaly of the genitourinary system may be found in 10% to 15% of newborns. Secondary infections are frequently associated with congenital anomalies; chronic diseases are frequently associated with infections. Pediatric and adolescent gynecology is discussed in Chapter 34. The following surgical procedures include those most commonly performed by pediatric urologists.

Cystoscopy. Diagnostic evaluation and therapeutic removal of obstructions within the structures of the genitourinary tract may be performed through an infant-size or child-size cystoscope. Cystoscopes from 9.5 through 16 Fr are used for infants and children. A size 3-Fr ureteral catheter can be introduced through the smallest-size cystoscope. Hypothermia can occur when the sterile water used to expand the bladder is cooler than body temperature.

Nephrectomy, Nephrostomy, or Pyeloureteroplasty. Hydronephrosis, congenital or acquired, may necessitate surgical intervention. Nephrectomy is indicated only if severe disease is unilateral, with a contralateral kidney capable of life-sustaining function. More conservative nephrostomy or pyeloureteroplasty is indicated for bilateral or moderate to mild kidney disease.

Wilms' Tumor. Wilms' tumor is a malignant, solid, renal tumor that develops rapidly in a child usually younger than 5 years. Nephrectomy is necessary to resect the tumor. If the adrenal gland is intimately connected to the tumor in the upper pole of the kidney, the gland is resected en bloc with the renal mass. Vascular extension of the tumor into the suprahepatic vena cava may necessitate a cardiopulmonary bypass to ligate all tumor vessels. Ipsilateral periaortic lymph node dissection often is performed to stage the extension of cancerous cells.

Neurogenic Bladder. Defective bladder function may be a result of a central nervous system lesion such as a myelomeningocele or spinal cord trauma. To preserve renal function and to achieve urinary continence in the presence of a neurogenic bladder, an enterocystoplasty may be performed. This procedure retains an intact urinary tract. An artificial urinary sphincter can be implanted to achieve dryness in the child who has sufficient dexterity to operate the pump.

Exstrophy of the Bladder. In exstrophy of the bladder, a congenital anomaly, the bladder herniates through the lower abdominal wall in the suprapubic region. Repair requires reconstruction of the lower abdominal wall and external genitalia. This can usually be accomplished in one surgical procedure on a female infant but requires two or more staged procedures on a male. A gastrocystoplasty may be the procedure of choice. If urinary continence cannot be established, urinary diversion through ureteral reimplantation may become necessary.

Ureteral Reimplantation. Repositioning the ureters (i.e., ureteral reimplantation) may be performed to correct either congenital or acquired total urinary incontinence or vesicoureteral reflux.

Incontinence causes parents to seek help for an infant or child. Incontinence is usually not caused by a single factor. The urologist plans the procedure on the basis of an accurate assessment of anatomic and physiologic causes. Creation of a tubularized trigonal muscle, when reconstructed into a new bladder neck, acts as a sphincter to maintain continence. With ureters in the normal position, this muscular tube in the bladder wall cannot be constructed. Therefore, the ureters are reimplanted superiorly into the bladder through a created tunnel. Care is taken that the ureters are not hooked or angled but follow a smooth curve into the bladder.

Vesicoureteral reflux is the most common reason for reimplanting ureters in pediatric patients. Chronic reflux, regurgitation of urine from the bladder into the ureters, can lead to pyelonephritis and hydronephrosis. Ureteral reimplantation may be required to prevent kidney damage. The objective of the surgical procedure is to position a segment of the ureters at a higher level within the bladder wall so that the level of urine is below the orifices and intravesical pressure prevents reflux.

When ureters cannot be reimplanted in the bladder, a urinary diversion procedure may be necessary. Ureters are usually anastomosed to a nonrefluxing colon conduit.

Urethral Repair. The external opening (meatus) of the urethra may be displaced at birth. Hypospadias is an anomaly in the male in which the urethra terminates on the underside of the penis or on the perineum (Fig. 8-12); in the female with hypospadias, the urethra opens into the vagina. With epispadias in the male, the urethra terminates on the dorsum of the penis; in the female, it terminates above the clitoris. Multistage procedures are usually necessary to correct these anomalies. The goal is to center the meatus at the tip of the glans penis of the male. This may be accomplished in a one-stage procedure by a transverse island flap derived from prepuce or by a vertical-incision/horizontal-closure technique for distal coronal or subglandular hypospa.dias. The female with meatal anomalies may need multistage procedures to approximate normal anatomic position. This procedure is usually performed between ages 1 and 4 years.

Orchiopexy. One or both testicles that failed to descend during fetal development can be brought into the scrotum and stabilized with a traction suture until healing takes place (Fig. 8-13). In the two-stage Torek operation, the testicle and supporting structures are dissected free from the inguinal region. An adequate length of spermatic vessels is released to permit the testicle to reach the scrotal sac. After

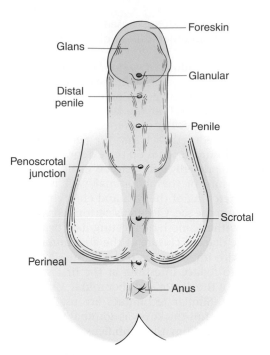

FIG. 8-12   Meatal opening in hypospadias.

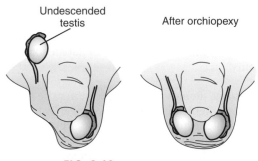

FIG. 8-13   Cryptorchidism.

it is pulled down through the scrotum, the testicle is sutured to fascia of the thigh. At the second-stage procedure, 2 to 3 months later, the testicle is freed from the fascia and embedded into the scrotum.

If one or both testicles are absent, silicone prostheses may be inserted into the scrotum for cosmetic appearance. Psychologically for the child and parents, undescended testicles (cryptorchidism) or absence (agenesis) of testicles is usually repaired at age 5 or 6 years, before the boy begins school.

Circumcision. Excision of the foreskin of the penis (circumcision) may be done to prevent phimosis, in which the foreskin becomes tightly wrapped around the tip of the glans penis, or to remove redundant foreskin. Circumcision is the most commonly performed pediatric surgical procedure. It should be done on newborns with the patient under local anesthesia (Fig. 8-14). Circumcision, as an elective procedure, is contraindicated if an abnormality of the glans penis or urethral meatus is present. Urethral repair generally uses the foreskin as graft tissue.

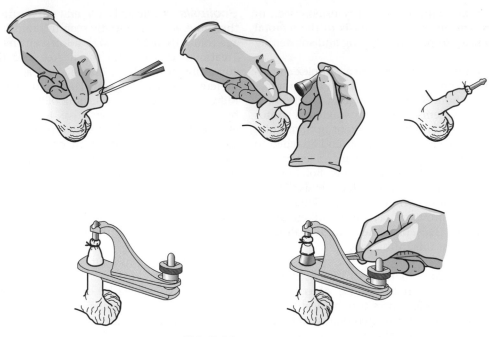

FIG. 8-14 Circumcision.

Orthopedic and Spinal Surgery

Pediatric orthopedic surgery is principally elective and reconstructive to correct deformities of the musculoskeletal system. These deformities may be congenital, idiopathic, pathologic, or traumatic. The extent the anomalies and functional disorders often involves prolonged immobilization and hospitalization. Many patients require a series of corrective procedures. Some of the conditions most commonly seen in the OR include those discussed in the following sections.

Fractures. Fractures that occur in infants and children generally are treated as they are in adults. Fixation devices are not well tolerated by children and often prevent uniting of the fracture. Closed reduction of long bone fractures is preferable.

Tendon Repair. Tendons may be lengthened, shortened, or transferred to correct congenital deformities of the hand or foot. Lacerated tendons are repaired to restore function. A tourniquet is used to control bleeding. The tourniquet cuff size should be appropriate for the size of the infant or child. Padding under the cuff is applied smoothly. Sheet wadding may be used under an infant cuff to protect delicate skin. The cuff should be tight but without restricting circulation before inflation. The time of inflation is closely watched to prevent ischemia. The surgeon may ask the circulator to release the pressure every 30 minutes on an infant or up to every 1 to 2 hours for an older child, depending on age. Tendon procedures are often lengthy.

Congenital Dislocated Hip. Displacement (dysplasia) of the femoral head from its normal position in the acetabulum can be present at birth, either unilaterally or bilaterally. If dysplasia is diagnosed early in infancy, closed reduction with immobilization usually corrects the dislocation without residual deformity (Fig. 8-15). If dysplasia is not diagnosed until after the child has begun to walk, open reduction of the hip with an osteotomy to stabilize the joint may be necessary.

Leg Length Discrepancies. The epiphyseal cartilaginous growth lines progressively close as the child matures. Bones lengthen from the activity of the epiphyses. The absolute physiologic criterion for completion of childhood is when this cartilage becomes a part of bone. A discrepancy in activity of an epiphyseal line may retard or overstimulate growth of a bone in one extremity and not in its contralateral counterpart. When this occurs in one femur, legs become unequal in length. The orthopedic surgeon may correct leg length discrepancies, usually in excess of 1 inch (2.5 cm), by epiphyseal arrest (i.e., stopping growth of the bone). This is done in the contralateral leg to let the shorter extremity catch up. The longer leg may be shortened by a closed intramedullary procedure. Under fluoroscopy, a reamer is inserted into the medullary canal of the femur through a small incision high on the hip. After the reamer widens the canal, a rotating saw is manipulated to cut a section from the bone. The bone ends are aligned and fixed with a flexible intramedullary rod.

Slipping of the upper femoral epiphysis causes displacement of the femoral head, which can occur as a result of

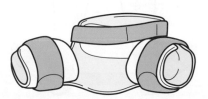

FIG. 8-15 Hip abduction splint for congenital dislocation of the hip.

traumatic injury or as a chronic disability usually seen in obese adolescents. Fusion of the epiphysis to the femoral neck may be necessary to prevent slipping and shortening of the leg.

Many limb deformities in children are a complex combination of angulation and shortening as a result of trauma, infection, metabolic bone disease, congenital deformity, and developmental problems. The Ilizarov external fixator technique provides an alternative treatment option. Thin, strong wires are transfixed through bones and attached to rings under tension. The rings, which encircle a leg or arm, are held firmly in place with threaded rods. Bolts on the rods are turned several times a day to pull cut ends of bone apart. Corticotomy, performed through a small skin incision after wires are inserted, preserves periosteal and endosteal blood supply to bone. This promotes rapid healing to regenerate new bone that fills in the gap.

Talipes Deformities. Combinations of various types of deformities of the foot, especially those of congenital origin, are referred to as talipes plus the medical term to describe whether the forefoot is inverted (varus) or everted (valgus) and whether the calcaneal tendon is shortened or lengthened.

Talipes Varus. Talipes varus, known as clubfoot, is the most common of the talipes deformities and may be unilateral or bilateral. The forefoot is inverted and rotated, accompanied by shortening of the calcaneal tendon and contracture of the plantar fascia. Conservative treatment by casting during infancy usually corrects a mild postural deformity before the infant bears weight on the foot (Fig. 8-16). A wedge cast with turnbuckles may be applied to an older child to allow gradual manipulation. If conservative treatment is unsuccessful, an open surgical procedure may be necessary.

Talipes Equinovarus. Talipes equinovarus, an idiopathic true clubfoot deformity, almost always requires surgical intervention for correction. In varying degrees, talipes equinovarus includes an incomplete dislocation (subluxation) of the talocalcaneonavicular joint with deformed talus and calcaneus bones, a shortened calcaneal tendon, and soft tissue contractures. As a result, the forefoot curls toward the heel (adduction, supination), the midfoot points downward (equinus), and the hindfoot turns inward (varus). The orthopedic surgeon uses a sequential-release approach to obtain maximum correction of all contractures and realigns bones in the ankle joint. Pins are inserted, and the extremity is put in a cast to maintain alignment of the foot and ankle.

Scoliosis. Scoliosis is a lateral curvature and rotation of the spine, most frequently seen in rapidly growing school-age (older than 10 years) or adolescent females (Fig. 8-17). Treatment depends on the degree and flexibility of the curvature, chronologic and skeletal age of the child, and preference of the surgeon. The child may be fitted with a Milwaukee brace (Fig. 8-18), immobilized in a cast, or stretched by traction. As an alternative to these techniques, an electrical device may be applied with an underarm brace to stimulate muscle contraction on the convex side of the curvature. If untreated at an early stage, scoliosis produces secondary changes in vertebral bodies and in the rib cage. Spinal fusion is ultimately performed if the curvature has become severe (50% or more) or must be stabilized after corrections. Government-mandated screening programs in schools have reduced the need for surgical correction in many children.

The following procedures may be used for correction of scoliosis:

1. A wedge body jacket or Minerva jacket may be applied. Turnbuckles may be incorporated. Turnbuckles are adjustable metal rods placed along the edges of the wedge of the cast. Gradual opening of the turnbuckles by the surgeon as tolerated by the patient corrects the lateral curvature of the spine.

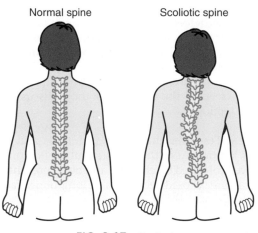

Normal spine   Scoliotic spine

FIG. 8-17   Scoliosis.

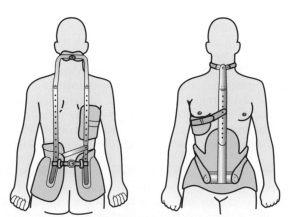

FIG. 8-18   Milwaukee brace for scoliosis.

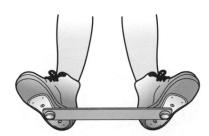

FIG. 8-16   Denis Browne splint for clubfoot deformity.

A Sayre sling, an appliance used for head traction, is sometimes used when applying a body jacket to correct slight scoliosis. Traction is obtained by means of pulleys and a rope suspended from the ceiling or an arm of the fracture table.

2. Halo traction is used to stretch the spine in some patients in whom the spine is too rigid to be straightened in a cast. A metal band is applied to the skull by means of four pins inserted into the cortex of the skull. A Steinmann pin is inserted into the distal end of each femur. A traction bow is put on each pin. Weights, usually equal, are put on the halo and Steinmann pins and gradually increased as tolerated. When radiographs show maximum correction, a spinal fusion is done. Traction may be continued until healing has taken place to the degree that there will be no loss of correction; a plaster jacket is then applied.

3. A Risser jacket is applied a few days preceding posterior spinal fusion to gain as much correction as possible. The orthopedic table is used. Traction is applied by a chin strap, similar to a Sayre sling, and countertraction is applied by a pelvic girdle. The spine is straightened as much as possible, and the body and head are encased in plaster.

Posterior spinal fusion may be performed as a two-stage procedure: vertebral body wedge resection at the first stage and insertion of Cotrel-Dubousset or Harrington rods (Fig. 8-19) with fusion at the second stage. Bone fragments removed during the first stage may be saved for the second-stage fusion or sent to the bone bank. Rods and hooks are stainless steel; appropriate instruments are required to insert them. Two rods are inserted—one on either side of the curvature. These rods are secured to the spine and force it into a more nearly normal position. Implanted on the outside of the vertebral column, the rods apply a longitudinal force on the spine. The spine is then fused.

The procedure may be done through a window in the Risser jacket, but usually the cast is bivalved and the patient lies in the anterior section. If the proce-

dure is done through a window, an electric cast cutter should be at hand to bivalve the cast if the patient has any respiratory difficulties. After the procedure, the bivalved posterior part is put in place and the jacket is fastened together by several rounds of plaster or by webbing straps with buckles. The patient is in the Risser jacket for a year. Progress is checked by radiographs.

4. Segmental spinal fixation with Luque rods may be the procedure of choice to stabilize the spine after fusion. Two L-shaped rods are placed next to the spinous processes and held by wires threaded under the lamina of each vertebra to be fused. Transverse traction internally on each vertebra stabilizes the spine without the need for a postoperative cast.

5. Anterior spinal fusion through a transthoracic approach is performed as a one-stage procedure to correct severe curvatures in patients who have malformed vertebral bodies. With Dwyer instruments, titanium staples are fitted over vertebral bodies on the convex side of the curve. Each staple is held in place by two titanium screws. A multistrand titanium cable, threaded through the heads of the screws, is tightened to compress the vertebrae and straighten the curve. Staples and screws are secured the full extent of the curvature. A plaster body jacket may be applied after the procedure to immobilize the back until the fusion is healed. The patient is then ambulatory.

Ophthalmology

Congenital Obstruction of the Nasolacrimal Duct. An obstruction, usually at the lower end of the nasolacrimal duct that enters the inferior meatus of the nose, often results in dilation and infection of the lacrimal sac. Treatment consists of passing a malleable probe from the lid punctum through the nasolacrimal passages to push out the obstructing plug of tissue.

Oculoplastic Procedures on the Eyelids. Congenital malformations such as ptosis (drooping of the upper or lower eyelid) are corrected by extraocular procedures. Ptosis repair is indicated when the levator is inadequate. In the levator resection procedure, which shortens the muscle and gives a more physiologic result, the levator muscle may be approached through the skin (Berke's method) or the conjunctiva (Iliff's method). A fascial sling procedure to support the lid consists of attaching the upper lid margin to the frontalis muscle. Materials used include autogenous fascia from the thigh, homograft fascia, or synthetic nonabsorbable suture material. The Fasanella-Servat operation is a simpler procedure for obtaining only a small amount of lid elevation.

Extraocular Muscle Procedures. Surgical procedures on extraocular muscles to correct strabismus or squint are the third most commonly performed pediatric procedures between ages 6 months and 6 years. The trend is to correct the congenital type during infancy and the acquired type in preschool years. Patterns of using two eyes together are more flexible and adaptable in a young child. These procedures on extraocular muscles are done to correct

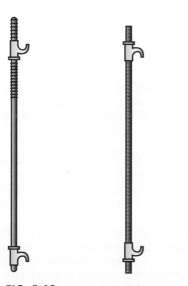
FIG. 8-19   Harrington rods.

muscle imbalance and promote coordination either by strengthening a weak muscle or by weakening an overactive one. The mechanical strength of a weak muscle can be increased by the following:

- Tucking. A tuck is sutured in the muscle to shorten it, thereby increasing its effective power.
- Advancement. The attachment point of the muscle is freed and reattached closer to the cornea, thereby increasing its leverage.
- Resection. Part of the muscle is removed to shorten it, and cut ends are sutured together.

An overactive muscle can be weakened by the following:

- Tenotomy. The point of attachment of the muscle is severed, and the muscle is dropped back, held by ligaments only.
- Recession. The muscle is detached from the eyeball and reattached farther back to decrease its action.
- Myotomy. The fibers of a section of the muscle are divided to diminish muscle action.
- Myectomy. A section of the muscle belly is excised.
- The Faden procedure. The muscle belly is sutured to the posterior sclera, thereby restricting muscle action considerably, producing a super-weakening effect.

Intraocular Procedures

Congenital Cataract Extraction. Under the operating microscope, with use of irrigation-aspiration and cutting instruments, the cataract and often the posterior capsule and a portion of the anterior vitreous are removed at one time. This procedure obtains a clear optical zone so that a contact lens can be fitted on the infant's eye within a few days postoperatively. The goal is to avoid intractable amblyopia (lazy eye) by correcting the defect during the first few weeks of life. An intraocular lens may be implanted. More commonly, epikeratophakia is performed to reshape the cornea.

Goniotomy. Although congenital glaucoma is rare, early surgical intervention is urgent to prevent blindness. Goniotomy is a microsurgical procedure that involves dividing a congenital layer of abnormal tissue covering the drainage angle of the anterior chamber. It is performed by use of a special operative contact lens placed on the eye that permits visualization of the angle. An incision is made through an opening in the contact lens.

Otorhinolaryngology

Myringotomy. Secretory otitis media is the most common chronic condition of childhood. Fluid accumulates in the middle ear from eustachian tube obstruction. This condition is corrected by myringotomy—an incision in the tympanic membrane (eardrum) for drainage (Fig. 8-20). Through aspiration of fluid and pus, pressure is released, pain is relieved, and hearing is restored and preserved. Myringotomy is done to prevent perforation of the eardrum and possible erosion of middle ear ossicles. When exudate is especially viscid, the patient has "glue ear" or mucoid otitis media.

Tympanostomy is commonly performed bilaterally in association with myringotomy. A self-cleaning, plastic pressure-equalizing tube is placed through an incision in

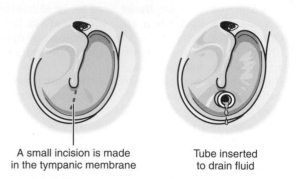

A small incision is made in the tympanic membrane

Tube inserted to drain fluid

FIG. 8-20   Myringotomy with perieustachian tube.

the tympanic membrane, bypassing the eustachian tube, to facilitate aeration of the middle ear space and to prevent reformation of serous otitis media. The tube usually extrudes spontaneously. Premature extrusion before normal eustachian tube function resumes may necessitate replacement of the tube.

Middle Ear Tympanoplasty. Congenital fused ossicles in the middle ear often are associated with stenosis or absence of an external auditory canal. Depending on the deformity, tympanoplasty may be performed with a temporalis fascia graft. If mobilization or ossiculoplasty is impossible, a total or partial ossicular prosthesis may be implanted to replace one or more ossicles. Congenital or acquired conductive deafness may be helped by tympanoplastic surgical techniques. Single-channel cochlear implants, approved for children, may be helpful for the profoundly deaf child.

Correction of Choanal Atresia. Newborns are obligate nose breathers and may die at birth if choanal atresia, congenital closure of nasal passages, is undiagnosed. They are unable to breathe and feed properly without an adequate nasal airway. Bone or fibrous tissue blocking the posterior choanae usually is excised via a transseptal approach to create an opening into the nasopharynx. A CO_2 laser may be used to develop appropriate apertures.

Adenoidectomy. Abnormally enlarged lymphoid tissue or infected adenoids can obstruct breathing. A child usually is at least 2 years old before having adenoid tissue in the nasopharynx removed, but adenoidectomy can be done at an earlier age. Removal of adenoids can positively influence the outcome of otitis media with effusion in childhood. Adenoidectomy is usually performed in conjunction with tonsillectomy.

Tonsillectomy. Tonsillectomy, the excision of hypertrophied or chronically infected tonsils, is not generally advised before the child is 3 years of age (Fig. 8-21). General anesthesia is used for patients up to about 14 years of age. Tonsillectomy and adenoidectomy frequently are performed together, appearing on the surgical schedule as T&A. Sterile technique is carried out throughout the procedure because the patient's vascular system is encountered. Precautions during the surgical procedure include control of bleeding and prevention of aspiration of blood or tissue.

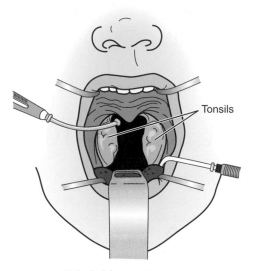

FIG. 8-21   Tonsillectomy.

Esophageal Dilation. Children, usually of preschool age, may ingest caustic agents that cause chemical burns of the mouth, lips, and pharynx and corrosive esophagitis. Long-term, gradual esophageal dilation with balloon catheters or bougies may be necessary to restore adequate oral intake of food after the acute phase of traumatic injury. When all attempts at dilation fail, the esophagus is replaced. The most satisfactory source of esophageal replacement is the colon.

Laryngeal Papillomas. Recurrent respiratory papillomatosis is localized in the larynx of children. Laryngeal papillomas are benign, wartlike lesions caused by the human papillomavirus. Hoarseness is an early symptom; airway obstruction is a later, life-threatening sign. Ablation with the CO_2 laser, manipulated through the operating microscope, preserves underlying laryngeal muscles and ligaments while vaporizing papillomas located on vocal cords. Laser ablation is not a cure; recurrence often necessitates repeated procedures to maintain a patent airway.

Tracheal or Laryngeal Stenosis. Some accidental injuries result in a narrowing (i.e., stenosis) of the trachea or larynx. Of greater concern are the injuries that result from therapy for respiratory problems, especially in newborns. Prolonged endotracheal intubation can lead to injury from tubes that are too large for the lumen, are too long, or move too much. These injuries may require balloon dilation and/or endoscopic resection of the stenotic area. Most infants then require an intraluminal stent to maintain patency of their airways.

In the presence of severe circumferential intraluminal scarring with involvement of the cartilages, surgical reconstruction becomes necessary. Laryngotracheoplasty widens the stenosed cartilaginous framework of the airway in the midline anteriorly and posteriorly and reconstructs the mucosal lining. Free or composite rib cartilage grafts are taken with mucosal tissue of the perichondrium for lining the airway. A stent assembly with a tracheostomy tube supports the reconstructed airway during healing. It can then be removed and the tracheostomy closed.

Tracheotomy. Tracheotomy, incision into the trachea and insertion of a tracheostomy tube, is advisable in cases of severe inflammatory glottic diseases, when endotracheal intubation would be required for longer than 72 hours, and when respiratory support is necessary for longer than 24 to 48 hours to treat respiratory problems. Appropriate sizes and types of tracheostomy tubes for infants and children should be available. Tubes that are too large, too rigid, or too long or that have an improper curve can produce ulceration and scarring at pressure points. Strictures that develop at the site of the tracheotomy may require resection to relieve airway obstruction after decannulation. Infants have a shorter neck and are prone to distal displacement of the tracheostomy tube from the intratracheal insertion point. Head motion will cause the tube to shift superiorly if it is not secured in position by ties.

Plastic and Reconstructive Surgery

With the exception of burns and other traumatic tissue injuries, most plastic and reconstructive surgery performed on infants and children is to correct congenital anomalies. The most common of these surgeries include those discussed in the following sections.

Cleft Lip. Lack of fusion of the soft tissues of the upper lip creates a cleft or fissure. The degree of cleft lips varies from simple notching of the lip to extension into the floor of the nose (Fig. 8-22). The cleft may be unilateral or bilateral. The number of procedures required for correction depends on the severity of the deformity. Some plastic surgeons do a primary cheiloplasty, closure of the cleft lip, within the first few days after birth to facilitate feeding and to minimize psychologic trauma of parents. Surgeons who prefer to wait until the infant is older follow the "rule of 10s": 10 weeks of age, 10 g of hemoglobin, 10 pounds of body weight. Regardless of preferred timing, infiltration of a local anesthetic agent with epinephrine is usually the anesthetic of choice.

To relieve tension on the incision postoperatively, a Logan bow (a small, curved metal frame) may be applied

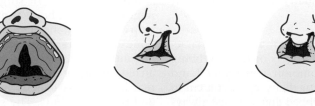

FIG. 8-22   Cleft lip and palate.

over the area of the incision and held in place by narrow adhesive strips to splint the lip. Skin closure strips may be used. Arm or elbow restraints are used to prevent the infant from removing the bow or strips and injuring the repaired lip. These restraints are applied in the OR.

Cleft Palate. Failure of tissues of the palate to fuse creates a fissure through the roof of the mouth. Palatal clefts may be a defect only in the soft palate or may extend through both hard and soft palates into the nose and include the alveolar ridge of the maxilla. Cleft palate is often associated with cleft lip; however, the two deformities are closed separately. Palatoplasty, closure of the soft palate, is done before speech begins, to avoid speech defects. A mouth gag is used during the surgical procedure to permit access to the palate without obstructing the airway. General anesthesia is administered via an endotracheal tube. This may be supplemented by infiltration of a local anesthetic agent. When epinephrine is used by the surgeon to minimize bleeding, the anesthesia provider is informed.

In patients with bilateral and, frequently, unilateral clefts, an additional surgical procedure is performed to elevate the tip of the nose and correct asymmetry before the child is 4 years of age.

Hemangioma. Hemangiomas are the most common of all human congenital anomalies. A hemangioma is a benign tumor (angioma) made up of blood vessels that may pigment or appear as a growth on the skin. All hemangiomas have abnormal patterns of hemodynamics, which is the effect of blood flow through tissues. Variations in vessel size distinguish the different types of these tumors. Argon or tunable dye laser or surgical excision in combination with a skin graft or pedicle flap repair is the treatment of choice for intradermal capillary hemangiomas (port-wine stain). Cryosurgery, surgical excision, or steroid therapy may be used for some other cavernous-type tumors.

Otoplasty. Abnormally small or absent external ears can be reconstructed in several surgical stages. An autogenous rib cartilage graft with the perichondrium intact or a silicone or a porous polyethylene prosthesis is used for the supporting framework to produce an anatomic contour. Usually necessitated by microtia, a congenital anomaly, reconstruction of the external ear can follow traumatic injury with loss of all or part of the pinna. Free flaps of temporoparietal fascia are used to secure a prosthesis or may be used to cover a carved cartilage armature for secondary reconstruction.

Otoplasty procedures to correct protruding or excessively large ears are performed more frequently than are procedures for microtia. These procedures often are done on preschool-age children, usually boys, to prevent psychological harm from teasing.

Syndactyly. Syndactyly is a congenital anomaly characterized by fusion of two or more fingers or toes. Webbing between fingers is the most common congenital hand deformity (Fig. 8-23). Tissue holding digits together is cut to separate fingers. Separation of webbed digits almost always requires skin grafts to achieve good functional results.

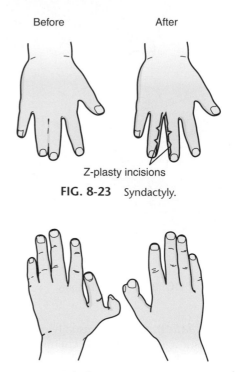

Before   After

Z-plasty incisions

FIG. 8-23   Syndactyly.

FIG. 8-24   Polydactyly.

Polydactyly. Polydactyly is a congenital anomaly characterized by the presence of more than the normal number of fingers or toes. A supernumerary digit may be alongside a thumb or little finger on one or both hands (Fig. 8-24). Extra digits on the feet are less common. Skin and tissue resemble a rudimentary digit. Some supernumerary digits contain bone, ligament, and tendon. Excision is recommended at an early age. If the excised digit contains rudimentary bone, multistage procedures may be required to enhance function of the remaining digits of the affected extremity.

Neurosurgery

Children of all ages sustain head injuries with hematomas that must be evacuated. Although brain tumors occur in children, the more frequently performed pediatric neurosurgical procedures are related to correction of congenital anomalies.

Craniosynostosis. If one or more of the suture lines in the skull, normally open in infancy (Fig. 8-25), fuses prematurely (craniosynostosis), the skull cannot expand during normal brain growth. A newborn with multiple-suture involvement may require surgical intervention because of increased intracranial pressure. Even fusion of a single suture puts a newborn at risk for altered cranial capacity and brain damage. The surgeon performs a craniectomy to remove the fused bone and to reopen the suture line(s). A strip of polyethylene or Silastic film may be inserted to cover bone edges on each side, or newly formed suture lines may be cauterized with Zenker's solution to prevent refusion. In an older infant or child, more extensive freeing of other bones may be necessary to achieve decompression of frontal lobes and orbital contents. The standard procedure takes up to 8 hours or more to perform.

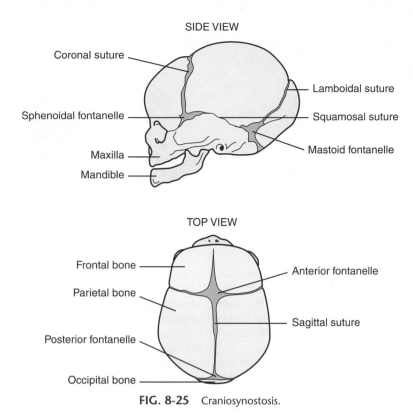

SIDE VIEW

Coronal suture
Lamboidal suture
Sphenoidal fontanelle
Squamosal suture
Maxilla
Mastoid fontanelle
Mandible

TOP VIEW

Frontal bone
Anterior fontanelle
Parietal bone
Sagittal suture
Posterior fontanelle
Occipital bone

FIG. 8-25   Craniosynostosis.

Craniofacial microsomia with severe facial asymmetry and the dysostosis of Apert's syndrome and Crouzon's disease also are associated with multiple skull and facial deformities. Craniofacial surgery, performed by a multidisciplinary team, involves repositioning and reshaping of skull and facial bones and a variety of soft tissue reconstructive techniques. Microplating systems may be used for rigid fixation of bones. The skull may provide a donor site without creating a deformity if bone grafts are required. Demineralized cadaver bone powder may be used to stimulate bone growth.

Endoscopic techniques have been developed in New York that enable the surgeon to separate the dura from the skull and snip away stenosed suture lines to free up the skull segments. The whole procedure takes less than 1 hour. The child then wears a skull-molding helmet for several months. Blood loss has been minimized, and the maximum hospital stay is 3 days. The endoscopic procedure is preferred for infants younger than 3 months; however, infants younger than 6 months can still be cared for using this method. The most commonly stenosed suture lines are the sagittal, coronal, metopic, and lambdoid. Older children are treated with the more extensive form of surgery, because they have more stenotic areas.

Encephalocele. Encephalocele is the herniation of brain and neural tissue through a defect in the skull. This is present at birth as a sac of tissue on the head. Usually these lesions can be removed 6 to 12 weeks after birth, unless the condition is complicated by hydrocephalus.

Hydrocephalus. Usually a congenital condition, hydrocephalus occurs when the passages between the ventricles are blocked and are dilated by accumulated cerebrospinal fluid. Failure of the absorptive mechanisms also can produce impairment in the normal circulation of cerebrospinal fluid, causing excess fluid to accumulate in the ventricles. Intracranial pressure thus created causes enlargement of the infant's head if the condition develops before fusion of cranial bones and often causes brain damage. Hydrocephalus may be diagnosed in utero by cephalocentesis, and a ventriculoamniotic shunt may be inserted to drain the ventricles. After birth, surgical treatment involves establishment of a mechanism for transporting excess fluid from the ventricles to maintain a close to normal intracranial pressure. This may be done by implantation of a shunt, which carries fluid from the lateral ventricle to the peritoneal cavity (ventriculoperitoneal shunt) or to the right atrium of the heart (ventriculoatrial shunt) (Fig. 8-26). Ventriculoatrial shunts are more commonly associated with infection, pleural effusion, and cardiac dysrhythmia. Other types of shunts are used, but less commonly, to bypass localized obstructions.

One end of the shunt catheter is put into the ventricle; the other end may connect to a one-way valve, which in turn is connected to the catheter that drains fluid distally from the head. An endoscopic technique may be used for catheter placement in the ventricle. Shunt malformation is usually caused by obstruction by the choroid plexus or debris. This complication can be reduced by positioning the shunt catheter tip opposite the foramen of Monro visually via a miniature fiberoptic pediatric neuroendoscope.

Catheters are made of silicone. An antithrombotic coating may be incorporated into the distal end. Some valves are regulated to open for drainage when predetermined pressure in the ventricle is reached. Other valves are designed as

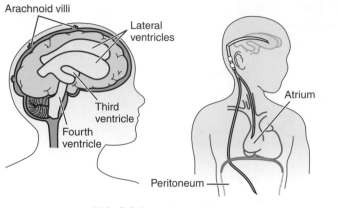

FIG. 8-26   Hydrocephalus.

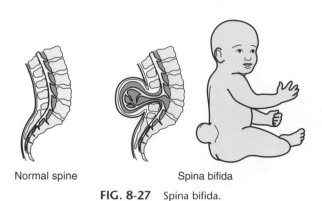

Normal spine   Spina bifida

FIG. 8-27   Spina bifida.

flushing devices to keep the distal catheter patent; the skin over the device is manually depressed to flush the system. For each patient the surgeon chooses the shunt mechanism that will be safest for the particular type of hydrocephalus being treated. Follow-up minor revisions are sometimes necessary, generally because of growth of the child.

As an alternative to a shunt procedure, a ventriculostomy can relieve intracranial pressure. A rigid neuroendoscope is introduced into the third ventricle. The contact fiber of a neodymium:yttrium-aluminum-garnet (Nd:YAG) laser, inserted through the scope, blanches and perforates the floor of the third ventricle at several points to establish circulation of cerebrospinal fluid into the subarachnoid space.

Myelomeningocele. A saclike protrusion may bulge through a defect in a portion of the vertebral column that failed to fuse in fetal development. If the nerves of the spinal cord remain within the vertebral column and only the meninges protrude into the sac, the congenital anomaly is a meningocele. However, if the sac also contains a portion of the spinal cord, it is a myelomeningocele, with associated permanent nerve damage. The degree of impairment depends on the level and extent of the defect. Clubfeet, dislocated hips, hydrocephalus, neurogenic bladder, paralysis, and other congenital disorders often accompany a myelomeningocele.

Each patient is evaluated and treated individually according to his or her needs. In general, it is best to delay the surgical procedure to repair a myelomeningocele until danger of development of hydrocephalus has passed or cerebrospinal fluid has been shunted. If the sac is covered with a thin membrane, meningitis (infection of meninges) is an imminent danger unless the defect is repaired soon after birth, usually within the first 48 hours, to close cutaneous, muscular, and dural defects.

Spina Bifida. Spina bifida, incomplete closure of the paired vertebral arches in the midline of the vertebral column, may occur without herniation of the meninges (Fig. 8-27).

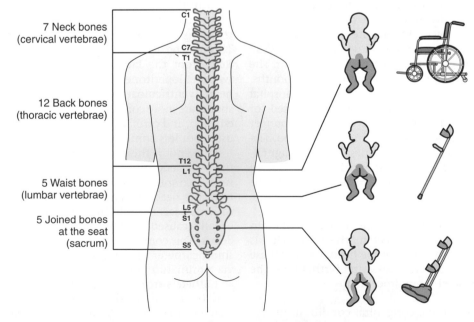

FIG. 8-28   Levels of spina bifida.

A spina bifida may be covered by intact skin and can occur at different levels of the spine (Fig. 8-28), causing various types of disability. Laminectomy may be indicated to repair the underlying defect.

Spastic Cerebral Palsy. Selective posterior rhizotomy can improve muscle tone and function of school-age children with spastic cerebral palsy. The procedure involves division of lumbar and sacral posterior nerve roots associated with an abnormal motor response as identified by nerve stimulation.

Thoracic Surgery

Aspiration of a foreign body can seriously compromise a child's respiratory status. Bronchoscopy with the child under general anesthesia may be necessary to remove the object. Bronchoscopy is also performed to diagnose tracheobronchial compression by an innominate artery, a vascular ring, or some other pathologic condition causing obstruction, stridor, or apnea. Thoracoscopy provides visualization of the chest wall and visceral pleura for diagnosis of diffuse or localized pulmonary disease. An intrathoracic biopsy can be obtained via a thoracoscope.

Pectus Excavatum. Pectus excavatum, a congenital malformation of the chest wall, is characterized by a pronounced funnel-shaped concave depression over the lower end of the sternum beginning at the angle of Lewis and extending to the xyphoid. Cardiopulmonary impairment can result from extreme pectus excavatum during the pubertal growth period. Children with moderate to severe forms have displacement of the heart and lung tissue, resulting in exercise intolerance and chest pain.

Minimally invasive procedures have been developed that require a curved metal bar to be slid under the ribs to elevate the sunken part (Fig. 8-29). No ribs or cartilage is removed. Thoracoscopic vision is used to guide the metal bar through two incisions made in the bilateral chest at the level of T4-5 interspace. The bar is secured to the ribs on each side to maintain the elevation of the deformity. Each bar is individually tailored to the recipient. The patient remains in

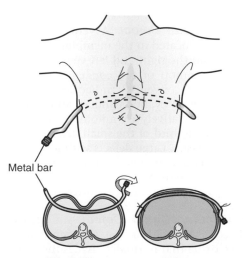

FIG. 8-29 Pectus excavatum.

Metal bar

the hospital for 2 to 3 days to monitor for complications and frequently has a thoracic epidural for pain management. The child can return to school within 2 weeks.

The Nuss procedure, developed in 1987 by Dr. Donald Nuss, is less complicated in younger children because the cartilage is softer and less calcified. Teens and young adults can have the procedure performed successfully, but their osseous tissue is less flexible. The bar is removed after 2 years as an outpatient procedure.

The deformity can be corrected during an open procedure by resecting lower intercostal cartilages and substernal ligaments to free up the sternum in a procedure referred to as the Ravitch repair. The sternum is elevated, and the cartilages are fitted to the sides of the sternum. Occasionally a pediatric patient will have transient postoperative brachial plexus injury caused by extremes of arm positioning during the procedure for the insertion of the bar and the camera.

Care is taken to try to avoid extreme positioning of the arm in abduction by suspending the arm rather than exceeding a 90-degree angle of shoulder-arm positioning. Risks of the Nuss procedure include bleeding, cardiac perforation, pericardial effusion, pneumothorax, and dysrhythmias.

Pectus Carinatum. Pectus carinatum is a protrusion of the breastbone. The cartilage buckles and causes pain. The condition progresses during periods of growth. The chest is rigid and stationary in a full inspiration position. Respiratory effort is compromised using the diaphragm and accessory muscles instead of the normal processes. Pulmonary function is diminished, and emphysema can develop. The problem may be genetically mediated and develops more commonly in males than in females. It increases in severity with age.

Pectus carinatum is seen in combination with some connective tissue disorders such as Marfan's syndrome or Ehlers-Danlos syndrome. Some have scoliosis and mitral valve prolapse. Other vascular disease is sometimes present.

In mild cases the patient wears a brace across the chest for 12 to 18 months. In moderate to severe cases, a transverse incision is made across the chest for an open correction. Bilateral wedges are removed from the ribs and excess cartilage over the sternum is removed to correct the condition. The perichondrium is left in place to grow over the excised area. The patient is required to remain hospitalized for several days. Outcomes are usually excellent.

Cardiovascular Surgery

Congenital cardiovascular defects are the result of abnormal embryologic development of the heart or major vessels. During fetal life, blood bypasses the lungs through the foramen ovale and the ductus arteriosus to the placenta. From the placenta, the blood bypasses the liver through the ductus venosus. The right ventricle pumps 66% of the circulation, and the left ventricle pumps 34%. At birth the pulmonary ventilation is established, and the increasing pressure causes increased left atrial force that in turn causes the foramen ovale to close. The right atrial pressure drops, causing the blood flow to reverse. The ductus arteriosus usually closes after 15 hours. Some neonates have a delay of 1 to 3 weeks for the complete closure of the ductus.

Most cardiovascular defects are diagnosed in infancy, often when symptoms of congestive heart failure develop within the first few days or months after birth. Corrective or palliative procedures are necessary to sustain or prolong the life of these infants. Many of these cardiovascular procedures are enhanced by or are made possible with the use of profound hypothermia and cardiopulmonary bypass. However, significant brain damage may be associated with a cardiovascular bypass in infants. Bypass perfusion time should not exceed 40 minutes between periods of temporary normal circulatory perfusion. Congenital defects in infants or children that are amenable to surgical intervention include the following:

Anomalous Venous Return. Failure of any one pulmonary vein or a combination of these veins to return blood to the left atrium precludes the full complement of oxygenated blood from entering the systemic circulation. The anomalous pulmonary vein or veins are transferred and anastomosed to the left atrium.

Coarctation of the Aorta. A coarctation is a narrowing or stricture in a vessel. This is one of the more common congenital cardiovascular defects, usually occurring in the aortic arch. It may cause hypertension in the upper extremities above the obstruction and hypotension in the lower extremities from slowed circulation below the coarctation. To correct the defect, the coarctation is resected and the aorta may be anastomosed end-to-end. An aortic patch graft may be necessary when the length of the coarctation prevents anastomosis. A subclavian flap angioplasty capable of growth in length and width, referred to as the Waldhausen procedure, is the surgical procedure of choice in infants.

Patent Ductus Arteriosus. During fetal life the ductus arteriosus carries blood from the pulmonary artery to the aorta to bypass the lungs. Normally this vessel closes in the first 24 hours after birth to prevent recirculation of arterial blood through the body. If closure does not occur, blood flow may be reversed by aortic pressure, causing respiratory distress (Fig. 8-30).

Signs of patent ductus arteriosus (PDA) include widening pulse pressure and a characteristic murmur. The incidence of PDA is 10% of all congenital cardiac defects and is usually diagnosed by 1 month of age. Surgical intervention is indicated, in lieu of prolonged ventilatory support, to prevent development of chronic pulmonary changes. The PDA can be clamped and ligated with ligating clips or suture in an open procedure or occluded using a transcatheter approach.

Septal Defects. An open heart procedure with cardiopulmonary bypass is necessary to close abnormal openings in the walls (septa) separating the chambers within the heart.

Atrial Septal Defect. An opening in the septum between the right and left atria may be sufficiently large to allow oxygenated blood to shunt from left to right and return to the lungs (Fig. 8-31). An atrial septal defect (ASD) can

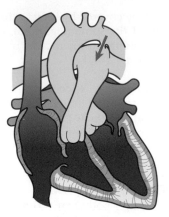

FIG. 8-30 Patent ductus arteriosus.

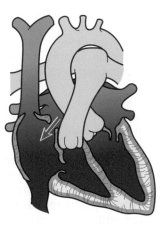

FIG. 8-31 Atrial septal defect.

increase pulmonary blood flow, with resultant pulmonary hypertension, if the defect is not closed. The incidence of ASD is 8% to 14% of all congenital heart defects and can remain asymptomatic until adulthood. Signs include acyanosis, thin body stature, and decreased tolerance to exercise. ASD is more common in females than in males (4:1). If the defect cannot be closed with sutures, a patch graft is inserted.

Ventricular Septal Defect. A ventricular septal defect (VSD) is usually located in the membranous portion of the septum between the right and left ventricles (Fig. 8-32). It is the most common of the congenital heart anomalies (25% to 30% of all congenital cardiac defects). Signs include alternation between cyanosis and acyanosis. Patients with small defects are relatively asymptomatic, and repair may be unnecessary. One third of the small defects spontaneously close by age 2 years. Large defects with left-to-right shunting of oxygenated blood back to the lungs, thus increasing pulmonary hypertension, become symptomatic by age 2 months. A patch graft may be required to close the defect.

Atrioventricular Canal Defect. An atrioventricular canal defect is present if the atrioventricular canal of connective tissue that normally divides the heart into four chambers has failed to develop. Deficiencies are present in

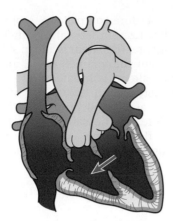

FIG. 8-32   Ventricular septal defect.

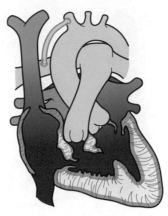

FIG. 8-34   Blalock-Taussig repair.

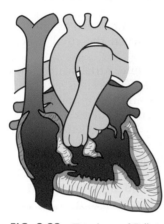

FIG. 8-33   Tetralogy of Fallot.

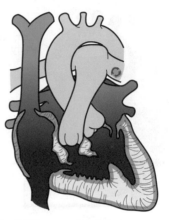

FIG. 8-35   Potts-Smith-Gibson repair.

the lower portion of the interatrial septum, upper portion of the interventricular septum, and tricuspid and mitral valves. The result is a large central canal that permits blood flow between any of the four chambers of the heart. A corrective procedure referred to as the Rastelli procedure involves repair of mitral and tricuspid valves and patch grafts to close septal defects. Creation of a competent mitral valve is of utmost importance to relieve pulmonary hypertension.

Tetralogy of Fallot. Tetralogy of Fallot is a combination of four defects (Fig. 8-33):
1. VSD (large)
2. Stenosis or atresia of the pulmonary valve and/or outflow tract into the pulmonary artery
3. Hypertrophy of the right ventricle
4. Dextroposition (displacement) of the aorta to the right so that it receives blood from both ventricles

Often referred to as "blue babies," infants with tetralogy of Fallot are cyanotic because insufficient oxygen circulates to body tissues. The incidence is 8% of all congenital cardiac defects and is commonly associated with Down syndrome. Total correction of the multiple anomalies is difficult. Assessment of the technical ease of correction is generally the dominant consideration. If cyanosis is severe, one of the following palliative shunt procedures may be performed during infancy to increase pulmonary blood flow:

- Blalock-Taussig procedure. The right subclavian artery is anastomosed, end-to-side, with the corresponding pulmonary artery (Fig. 8-34). Mixed arteriovenous blood from the aorta flows through the shunt to the pulmonary artery and into the lungs for oxygenation. A modification of this includes the use of a conduit graft, such as Gore-Tex.
- Potts-Smith-Gibson procedure. The descending aorta is anastomosed, side-to-side, with the left pulmonary artery (Fig. 8-35). The shunt enlarges as the child grows, but it is more difficult to reconstruct than a Blalock-Taussig shunt at a later time, when a corrective procedure is performed.
- Glenn procedure. The superior vena cava is anastomosed with the right pulmonary artery. Modern versions are bidirectional, allowing flow to the right and left pulmonary arteries.
- Waterston procedure. The ascending aorta is anastomosed with the right pulmonary artery (Fig. 8-36). The anastomosis is placed on the posterior aspect of the aorta to provide perfusion to both pulmonary arteries.

With cardiopulmonary bypass and hypothermia, the VSD is closed with a patch graft that also corrects the abnormal communication between the right ventricle and the aorta. Then the obstruction to pulmonary blood flow is relieved. This may include enlarging the pulmonary valve and/or

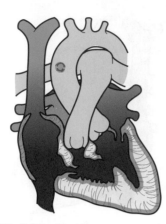

FIG. 8-36 The Waterston procedure.

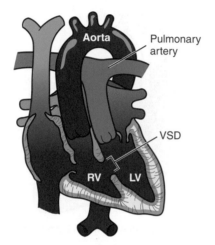

FIG. 8-37 Transposition of the great vessels.

widening the outflow tract. Resection of obstructing cardiac muscle may be necessary with insertion of a prosthetic outflow patch.

An aortic allograft containing the aortic valve with the septal leaflet of the mitral valve and the ascending aorta attached may be inserted. The septal leaflet of the mitral valve is used as a portion of the right ventricular outflow patch. All or part of the aortic valve and ascending aorta is used as a new conduit with the pulmonary artery or as a patch graft.

Transposition of the Great Vessels. In a transposition, the aorta arises from the right ventricle and the pulmonary artery arises from the left ventricle (Fig. 8-37). This creates essentially two separate circulatory systems—one systemic and the other pulmonary—but they are not interconnected as in normal anatomy. Life depends on the presence or creation of associated defects to permit exchange of blood between the two systems. The incidence of complete transposition of the great vessels is 10% of all cardiovascular defects. Males are affected more than females (2:1). A palliative procedure, such as one of the following, is performed in the newborn to improve oxygenation and sustain life until the infant grows enough to tolerate a corrective procedure:

- Rashkind procedure, or balloon septostomy. In the cardiac catheterization laboratory, under fluoroscopy, a balloon catheter (deflated) is advanced into the right atrium, through the foramen ovale, and into the left atrium. The balloon is inflated and pulled backward out of the left atrium across the atrial septum to enlarge the foramen ovale, thus creating an ASD.
- Park procedure. In the cardiac catheterization laboratory, under fluoroscopy, a catheter with a knife tip is passed through the right atrium to enlarge the opening of the foramen ovale.
- Blalock-Hanlon procedure. Atrial septectomy is done to create an ASD. A segment of the right atrium is excised.
- Pulmonary artery banding. The pulmonary artery is constricted in the presence of a large VSD to prevent irreversible pulmonary vascular obstructive changes from developing.

A corrective procedure, such as one of the following, is usually performed when the child is between 18 and 36 months of age:

- Mustard procedure. Atrial switch: An intraatrial baffle made of pericardial tissue is sutured between the pulmonary veins and the mitral valve and between the mitral and tricuspid valves. The baffle directs systemic venous return into the left ventricle and lungs and allows pulmonary venous return to enter the right ventricle and aorta.
- Senning procedure. Atrial switch: Flaps of the intraatrial septum and right atrial wall form new venous channels to divert pulmonary venous blood flow. Any atrial and/or septal defects are closed.
- Jantene procedure. Atrial switch: The aorta and pulmonary artery are anatomically switched (i.e., transposed). This procedure is useful in infants with a VSD or a large PDA in addition to transposition of the great arteries.

Tricuspid Atresia. The absence (atresia) of a tricuspid valve between the right atrium and ventricle prevents normal blood flow through the chambers of the heart. Blood flows through an ASD, into an enlarged left ventricle, and through a small rudimentary right ventricle to the pulmonary artery. Anastomosis of the superior vena cava with the right pulmonary artery or an aorticopulmonic artery shunt may be created as a palliative procedure to increase pulmonary blood flow in infancy. When the child is 3 or 4 years old, the corrective reconstructive Fontan procedure is performed. This procedure involves direct anastomosis of the pulmonary artery to the right atrium to create a connection between the pulmonary and systemic venous circulation.

Truncus Arteriosus. In truncus arteriosus a single great artery carries blood directly from the heart (with a large associated VSD) to the coronary, pulmonary, and systemic circulatory systems. A single tricuspid valve is present with two to six cusps. Initial palliative banding of the pulmonary arteries, as close to their origins off the truncus as possible, decreases pulmonary blood flow in an infant in congestive heart failure. At a later stage a corrective procedure can be performed to close the VSD and insert a conduit with an ascending aortic graft and aortic valve. Correction in infancy requires replacement of the conduit as the child grows. Incidence of this defect is 1% of all congenital cardiovascular defects.

Valvular Stenosis. Congenital aortic and/or pulmonary valve stenosis requires valvotomy, which is also referred to as the Brock procedure. An incision is made into the valve to open the narrowed or constrictive area obstructing blood flow.

Hypoplastic Left Heart Syndrome. Hypoplastic left heart syndrome is the most common cause of cardiac death in the first week of life. The left ventricle is severely under-developed (Fig. 8-38). The severity of the situation can vary according to the multitude of defects that can be present. The systemic perfusion of the aorta is entirely through a patent ductus arteriosus. The right ventricle is overloaded, and the patient is extremely dusky. The patient is in complete heart failure within 28 hours of life. The only real immediate treatment is cardiac transplant. Hearts available for neonatal transplant are few in number.

POSTOPERATIVE PEDIATRIC PATIENT CARE

The patient is taken to a postanesthesia care unit (PACU) for observation. Larger facilities have a PACU specifically designed to accommodate phase I and II pediatric patients. Parents are usually permitted in the pediatric PACU. The patient usually finds comfort in parental presence.

The PACU nurse receives the postanesthesia report from the anesthesia provider and a postprocedure report from the perioperative nurse. Vital signs are taken and include temperature, pulse, respirations, and blood pressure. The objective signs found in the head-to-toe assessment are compared with preoperative baseline values. Cardiac

monitoring and pulse oximetry are done. Physical assessment is performed and compared with other data obtained about the patient. Fluid intake and output are evaluated. The surgical site is inspected. Specific physician's orders pertaining to treatments and laboratory work are carried out.

The patient's recovery is evaluated at 5- to 15-minute intervals as the patient emerges from anesthesia to a more alert state. Each evaluation is documented in the patient's record per facility policy. The patient will be discharged from the PACU when reaching specific physiologic parameters according to departmental policy. The anesthesia provider is responsible for the patient in the PACU and is responsible for release criteria. The pediatric patient is never to be left unattended.

The parents are instructed in postoperative home care and are informed about signs and symptoms that should be reported to the physician. The instructions should be given verbally and in writing with the appropriate emergency phone consult numbers included. Directions for prescription medications such as antibiotics or analgesics should be explained to the parents by the PACU nurse. Pediatric patients who are of an age of reason and understanding should be addressed directly and given the opportunity to ask questions.

Within 24 to 48 hours after discharge, a postoperative phone call should be made as a follow-up to care. Pertinent information should be exchanged about the care of the patient and progress in recovery. The caller should be qualified to answer questions about the procedure and the recovery phase. Patient and family satisfaction should be evaluated. Some facilities ask the parent to call in during the evening hours to give an update to the PACU nurse.

Bibliography

Akin A, Esmaoglu A: Postoperative shivering in children and causative factors, *Pediatr Anesth* 15:1089-1093, 2005

American Academy of Pediatrics: *Prevention of medication errors in the pediatric inpatient setting,* Policy Statement, Grove City, IL, 2003.

Catlain A: Pediatric medical errors part 2: Case commentary, a source of tremendous loss, *Pediatr Nurs* 30(4):331-335, 2004.

Dowdell EB: Pediatric medical errors part 1: The case, *Pediatr Nurs* 30(4):328-330, 2004.

Fox ME et al: Positioning for the Nuss procedure: Avoiding brachial plexus injury, *Pediatr Anesth* 15:1067-1071, 2005.

Holland-Hall CM: Evaluation of the adolescent with chronic abdominal or pelvic pain, *J Pediatr Adolesc Gynecol* 17:23-27, 2004.

Inge TH et al: Reduced hospitalization cost for patients with pectus excavatum treated using minimally invasive surgery, *Surg Endosc* 17:1609-1613, 2003.

Kyllonen M et al: Perioperative pharmacokinetics of ibuprofen after rectal administration, *Pediatr Anesth* 15(7):566, 2005.

Mace SE et al: Clinical policy: Evidence-based approach to pharmacologic agents used in the pediatric sedation and analgesia in the emergency department, *Ann Emerg Med* 44(4):342-352, 2004.

van der Laan M et al: The role of laparoscopy in the management of childhood intussusception, *Surg Endosc* 15:373-376, 2001.

Vernon AH et al: Pediatric laparoscopic appendectomy for acute appendicitis, *Surg Endosc* 18:75-79, 2004.

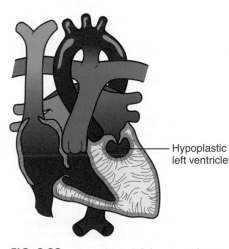

— Hypoplastic left ventricle

FIG. 8-38 Hypoplastic left heart syndrome.

Perioperative Geriatrics

KEY TERMS AND DEFINITIONS

Aged Social or legislative policies define aged as 65 years. Physiologic evaluation terms incorporate aged as 75 years.
Gerontology The study of aging and the elderly in all phases of life: sociologic, biologic, psychological, and physiologic.
Life cycle The span of time and events from birth to death.
Longevity The condition of living a prolonged life span.
Senile The state or process of aging. Derived from the Latin word *senex*, meaning "old man" or "old age." Aging takes place at all biologic levels.

HISTORICAL BACKGROUND

Traditionally the study of geriatrics did not contain a full realm of practices that included a specific study of surgical implications for the elderly. In some cultures, the elderly were not thought to be capable of leading productive lives as members of society. Historically, there were times when a person was considered at middle age at 35 years and at the end of life in their 40s or 50s. In 1901, the average life span was 49 years in the United States, but was increased to 65 years in 1940. As the average life span has increased the process of aging has become the center of scientific study concerning an ever-increasing life span, rich with continued contribution to society. Under ideal conditions a person could live past 100 years of age and possibly to 115.[1] As of 2005, the Centers for Disease Control and Prevention (CDC) indicate that the average life span is 77.6 years in the United States.

The oldest legitimately recorded person in modern times was a French woman named Jeanne Calmet who died at age 122 in 1997, although it is thought that some Asian people have lived past 150 years. Today, 1 in 10,000 people is 100 years of age.[2]

Women tend to live longer than men; however, this is equalizing because women are sharing many of the life shortening hazards such as smoking and risky occupations. Underdeveloped countries, such as some of the African nations, continue to have a low life expectancy ranging from 33 to 49 years of age.[3] Causes of death are related to health and below-poverty-level income.

The medical discipline of geriatrics is related to the clinical implications of the physiology of aging and the diagnosis and treatment of diseases that affect older adults. Gerontology is the comprehensive scientific study of all aspects of the aging process, including the physiologic, psychological, economic, and sociologic problems and considerations of the aging person. These factors are studied from the standpoint of the effect they have on the aging individual and the older population within society.

The Joint Commission on Accreditation of Healthcare Organizations (JCAHO) has identified the need for age-

---

[1] *Life span* is an idealized, species-specific biologic parameter that quantifies maximum attainable age under optimal environmental conditions. Historical anecdote suggests that human life span has remained constant at 110 to 115 years for at least the past 20 centuries according to the American Society of Anesthesiologists at www.asahq.org/clinical/geriatrics/geron.htm.
[2] Couzin J: How Much Can Human Life Span Be Extended? *Science* 309(5731): 83, 2005.
[3] http://en.wikipedia.org/wiki/List_of_countries_by_life_expectancy.

specific education. This chapter deals with the concept of the aging patient and the perioperative care of the surgical geriatric patient. The chapter contents are designed to meet the needs of preoperative, intraoperative, and postoperative care personnel. (An online textbook with additional information about geriatrics at www.geriatricsatyourfingertips.org is sponsored by the American Geriatrics Society and the John A. Hartford Foundation of New York City. Registration for use of this resource is required; however, there is no cost.)

PERSPECTIVES ON AGING

The process of aging is an orderly transformation of the body and mind that begins with birth and concludes with death. The term *geriatric* is taken from the Greek *yeros* (γερος), which means "old." People older than 65 years are often considered old or elderly. In actuality, a person with advanced age may maintain functional capabilities throughout his or her lifetime until adaptation to biologic, psychological, and/or social influences is no longer sufficient to sustain the independent activities of daily living. The main influences on the aging process are genetics, environment, and lifestyle.

Data about the changes that occur as the result of natural processes and environmental exposure are inconclusive because the only data available are those derived from comparisons among existing generations. The experiences and exposures of these generations have been vastly different and widely influenced by the period of the life span. No normal measurements are available on which to base the parameters of the aging process.

Life expectancy has increased steadily with major advancements in the study of disease processes, prevention, and treatment. The U.S. Department of Health and Human Services indicates that a person born in 1954 can expect to live to 68 years of age; a person born in 1988 can expect to live to 74 years of age. By the year 2030, 1 in every 10 people will be older than 85 years, with only 41% of the population younger than 35 years. The median age will be 40 years. This increase in life expectancy and decrease in mortality mean that the largest patient population will be geriatric patients—the fastest growing segment of the population.

As the life expectancy of the geriatric population increases, so does the incidence of comorbidity. Comorbidity is the existence of two or more disease processes in a single individual (e.g., coronary artery disease in a patient who has osteoporosis and may also be hypertensive and diabetic). It is the most common negative influence on the health status and functional ability of geriatric patients. A chronic condition affects recovery after surgical intervention, and many geriatric patients have multiple chronic or debilitating health problems. Comorbidity is also a major consideration in the attainment of expected outcomes; all medical diagnoses should be considered in the development of the plan of care.

Aging is viewed from many perspectives—some positive, some negative. The positive aspects involve respect for maturity and the wealth of knowledge gleaned from experiences. The negative aspects involve the debilitation, pervading weaknesses, and dependence that can occur during the closure of life. Philosophers tend to focus on the positive, inner peace derived from the wisdom acquired over many years. The view of aging adopted by an individual is based in part on the view of aging created by his or her cultural background. Geographic, financial, educational, and subjective influences shape the prototype of the older adult's place in society.

Cultural Considerations

Positive views of aging are found in many cultures that can trace their heritage back for many generations. Repetitious storytelling and historical accounts support the cultural growth of an individual from youth to old age. Many cultures appreciate, honor, and respect their older members for their experience and maturity. Growing old with dignity is not feared or deemed repulsive. A positive view of aging may be observed in an individual who is a first-generation immigrant to a new land, because he or she may not have assimilated the value systems of the new environment. The individual may have retained many time-honored beliefs of his or her country of origin; the values are held dear and are deeply ingrained.

Negative views of aging may be generated by cultures that are primarily youth oriented. Most members of these societies are second- and third-generation descendants of immigrants. They have developed value systems that do not reflect their country of origin. In a close community, values are supported within the belief structure of the group as a whole.

A culture is a set of structured social behaviors and personal beliefs that enable an individual to respond to social situations and relationships within a close community. The foundation of human relationships in a culture is more than ethnicity or race. Specific cultural practices such as dietary habits, lifestyle, and hygiene should be of concern to the perioperative nurse. For example, a patient's physical condition may be a direct result of a traditional activity such as fasting. A geriatric patient who has been fasting may appear dehydrated, malnourished, or confused. This should be considered before the patient undergoes a surgical procedure.

The psychological assessment may reflect a high risk for an alteration in self-image, because although patients may feel comfortable in their culture, they may have had a negative interaction with societal influences. For example, the media glorify young bodies and degrade the natural aging process, with advertisers using models that reflect the desirable aspects of youth and beauty. Cultural climate has a direct effect on the geriatric patient. The expected outcomes of the geriatric patient undergoing a surgical intervention will be influenced by his or her cultural views of aging and those of society as a whole.

Theories of Aging

Biologic, psychological, and ethnocultural factors influence the manner in which an individual ages. The extrinsic influences surrounding the physical and psychosocial components depend on the interaction of the person with the environment and his or her view of health and wellness. Many older people tend to optimistically overstate their actual health status and minimize or dismiss symptoms as age related. The intrinsic influences on the aging process are also interdependent, but to a less controllable degree. Certain inherited traits, such as pathologic conditions, are continued through the generations.

Each aged individual is unique. Perioperative nurses should understand the distinct aspects of each geriatric patient before developing a plan of care. Generic care plans do not address the specific problems, needs, and health considerations of the individual. Understanding the theories of the aging process enables the perioperative nurse to provide care throughout the surgical experience that will optimize the attainment of identified expected outcomes. The following theories explain aging as it is defined by science and research.

Wear-and-Tear Theory. The wear-and-tear theory suggests that the body loses its ability to keep pace with life processes. The sustenance of life suffers because the body begins to deteriorate in a natural, wearing-down process. The body continually tries to maintain homeostasis but degenerates over time because of cellular loss and destruction caused by interactions with the environment. During this process the body becomes increasingly vulnerable to injury and disease. If a disease state occurs, the body is less able to maintain normal homeostasis and even less able to tolerate the assault of illness. Eventually the body is unable to support life and ceases to function. Examples of wear and tear include but are not limited to the following:

- Prolonged exposure to the sun and other external sources can cause breakdown of the skin. Thinning of the skin makes bedridden or inactive people vulnerable to pressure sores.
- Turbulent blood flow in the areas of bifurcation of blood vessels may cause rupture if the vessels are weakened by arteriosclerosis.
- Abuse of chemical substances and alcohol can damage liver and brain cells. Nicotine is responsible for many effects of smoking. Although these effects are self-induced rather than the result of natural wear and tear, they do affect health status.

Genetic Mutation Theory. Deoxyribonucleic acid (DNA) has been a target for age-related changes, because it preserves the ongoing genetic message for cell replication and organism maintenance. DNA is a template, or coding mechanism, for the preservation of the life processes of cellular structures. Various agents damage DNA codes through physical, chemical, or biologic interactions. An alteration in the structure of DNA can cause an organism to change. This alteration can occur within the cell itself or be caused by a force in the environment. Mutated DNA cannot perform the processes necessary for normal cell activities. A cell containing wrongly coded DNA will continue to replicate itself in the wrong patterns. It will not return to normal.

In the aging process, DNA may mutate for a variety of reasons and will continue to produce the wrong type of cells during replication. For example, skin cells may be deficient in collagen or in the elastic properties associated with supple tissue. As a result, the skin replication process may yield drier, less elastic skin. This is characteristic of the skin of an older person. In certain circumstances, the mutated DNA could cause tumor production or other pathologic conditions, such as skin cancers.

Major organ systems affected by these changes are the central nervous system, the musculoskeletal system, and the cardiovascular system. Other systems affected include the gastrointestinal, genitourinary, endocrine, and integumentary. Essentially, all body systems change during the aging process.

Viral Theory. Researchers have approached the concept that viruses may invade human cells and remain inactive until the body loses its ability to suppress them. This theory is closely linked to the genetic mutation theory, because the virus can hide undetected in the DNA for many years. The replication process of the virus is similar to the replication of DNA. Some viruses are able to use genetic materials as a disguise to fool the body's immune system. The body does not recognize the virus as an invader or foreign substance.

The mechanism of viral activation is unknown but is very injurious to the body. Major targets include the endocrine, nervous, and immune systems. The incubation period may be several decades. Because there is no proof of the viral theory, a treatment or cure is unknown.

Environmental Theory. Exposure to natural and synthetic elements in the environment may accelerate the aging process. Although climate is often blamed for an increased rate of aging, studies indicate that the natural flow of the aging process is comparable among different geographic regions. Tropical climates are cited most often as areas of premature aging. Studies of tropical populations show that aging is not accelerated by the temperature, although mortality in these areas is affected by poor nutrition, parasites, and tropical diseases. Both tropical and desert groups tested did not show any mean blood pressure elevations diagnostic of hypertension, arteriosclerosis, or coronary artery disease between the ages of 20 and 83 years. The most astounding finding was the absence of angina pectoris and sudden heart attack deaths. This may be partly a result of a physically strenuous lifestyle and a diet that is low in animal fat.

Extremes of climate do not seem to accelerate the aging process. Studies involving Eskimo populations have shown that despite the difficult conditions of their lifestyles, blood pressure and cholesterol measurements do not vary significantly between the ages of 20 and 54 years. Mortality is affected by the harshness of the cold climate and the risk of physical injury or death associated with hunting and lifestyle practices. The CDC tables of life expectancy show longevity in colder climates.

Altitude has not been shown to accelerate the aging process. Studies performed among Peruvian Indians have shown stable blood pressures in a range lower than that of people living at sea level. Incidence of ischemic heart disease is very low at higher altitudes. In several documented communities of mountain-dwelling people, many residents were older than 100 years.

Ionizing radiation has been targeted as a cause of environmentally accelerated aging, but studies have not shown this to be true. Relevant evidence has shown that exposure to ionizing radiation does accelerate disease processes and pathologic conditions such as skin cancer, blood dyscrasias, and reproductive anomalies. Populations living in areas where nuclear tests frequently occurred have not shown signs of rapid aging when compared with control groups in nuclear-free areas. The most significant finding was an increase in leukemia and skin tumors.

Pollution causes many physiologic changes in the body. Chemicals in air, food, and water supplies have been shown to increase the incidence of health decline and disability. Exposure to pollutants throughout the life span dramatically shortens an individual's life expectancy through pathologic processes such as chronic lead poisoning and lung cancer.

Physical Factor Theory. Free radicals are being investigated as a potential cause of premature aging. Free radicals represent imbalances between the production and the elimination of unstable chemical compounds in the body. More research is needed to prove or disprove this theory.

Low-calorie diets do not alter the aging process in human beings. In populations studied for dietary habits, no increase in the life span is evident between control groups and groups who have a low-calorie intake. The most remarkable factor is the lack of increase in body weight after 30 years of age. A low-calorie diet may range between 1800 and 2500 kilocalories (kcal) per day depending on body size and gender. Notably, low-calorie diets are usually deficient in animal protein. Aged individuals who have low-calorie diets generally have lower blood pressure and lower serum cholesterol levels, with no significant change throughout the aging process. Subcutaneous fat deposits do not increase with age.

High-calorie diets that exceed 3200 kcal per day for men and 2200 kcal per day for women have the opposite effect on aging. An increase in caloric intake is accompanied by an increase in body mass that causes the individual to decrease body mobility. This is particularly evident in Euro-American populations, who often show a steady increase in weight up to the age of 60. Women in particular experience a thickening in fat deposits as they mature. Blood pressure and serum cholesterol levels steadily increase. The most significant elevations begin at age 50, with the development of coronary artery heart disease and atherosclerosis.

Animal fat content and excess calories are not the only considerations in the dietary aspect of aging and health. Vegetarians do not always follow a low-calorie pattern. They, too, can have a diet rich in fats, particularly if they consume saturated fats in the form of coconut oil. Salt is another consideration in the aging of the cardiovascular system. Diets high in sodium tend to increase circulating blood volume, thereby increasing systolic blood pressure. Studies have shown that an increase in systolic blood pressure significantly increases the risk of heart disease and stroke.

Exercise plays an important role in the health of the aging individual. Most populations studied have an exercise regimen linked to their activities of daily living. People in cultures characterized by many intrinsic diseases, parasites, malnutrition, poor hygiene, and harsh living conditions have remarkable physical fitness because of the amount of exercise they must perform to sustain life. People in affluent societies, in which the inhabitants are overfed and underexercised, do not enjoy good health in the same manner as the moderately fed and highly exercised residents of less-advantaged societies.

As the body ages, the endocrine system declines and the hormones responsible for the regulation of many interrelated body systems decrease in volume. Beta cells of the pancreas, thyroid, ovaries (in females), and testes (in males) exhibit less activity, which affects many other organ systems. For example:

- A decrease in estrogen production can increase the risk for osteoporosis and heart disease in women.
- A decrease in thyroid activity will decrease the basal metabolic rate and increase weight gain.
- A decrease in the efficiency of insulin production will decrease the efficiency of glucose metabolism.
- A decrease in testosterone production may decrease the libido in men.

Myths about Aging

Many misconceptions surround the process of aging. Myths, from the Greek *meethos* (μηθοζ), are stories created to explain the practices or beliefs of unknown origin regarding a person, place, or event. The creation of a myth about aging may be based on an isolated incident or a single observation and may not apply to all older adults.

Some myths have a small basis in fact, but most are unfounded and have a harmful effect on social policy and interpersonal relationships. Myths about the aging process may result in negative stereotypes, and a belief in negative stereotypes results in discrimination and improper treatment of the aging individual. Abnormal signs, symptoms, or behaviors exhibited by a geriatric patient usually indicate the presence of a pathologic process and should not be discounted as normal expectations of the aging process. The following are some of the negative myths about aging:

- *MYTH:* Older adults are senile. *TRUTH:* If mental processes decline, it is usually the result of a contributing factor such as stroke, carotid insufficiency, or Alzheimer's disease.
- *MYTH:* Older adults do not engage in sexual behavior. *TRUTH:* Sexual desire remains throughout the life span. Sexual activity may decline because of decreased physical mobility, circulatory impairment, or the unavailability of a partner. Self-gratification may be the only outlet.
- *MYTH:* Older adults always decline in health after a surgical procedure. *TRUTH:* The identification of problems, needs, and health considerations during the assessment phase of the nursing process decreases the probability of unmet expected outcomes.

Myths and stereotypes should not be allowed to influence the assessment of geriatric patients. Every aspect of the physical, psychosocial, and ethnocultural data should be assessed as unique to each individual and not as a generic group expectation. Reaching the age of 65 years does not instantly transform individuals into being old and debilitated. As people grow older, they may experience more developmental aging before they experience physical aging. Some people become frail as they age, but this is not true of everyone. Age alone does not make individuals less productive members of society. By the 21st century, limitations and disabilities may be decreased because of scientific advances and a better understanding of the aging process and health-promotion activities.

PERIOPERATIVE ASSESSMENT OF THE GERIATRIC PATIENT

The patient's ability to adapt to aging should be assessed by the perioperative nurse as part of the nursing process. With the exception of nursing diagnoses directly associated with the anticipated surgical procedure, specific nursing diagnoses should be associated with the patient's adaptation to the aging process. If positive adaptation has not been met, the risk is high for an augmentation of existing health conditions, such as a cardiovascular incident (e.g., stroke, myocardial infarction, hypertensive crisis). Comorbidity is a leading cause of death among older adults. More than 73% of all geriatric patients have more than one medical diagnosis capable of causing death. Therefore recognizing potential problems in the attainment of expected outcomes is as important as identifying actual problems.

Geriatric patients may present to the perioperative environment for urgent or emergent surgery because of the clinical signs and symptoms associated with a life-threatening illness. Common urgent problems include intestinal obstruction, ruptured diverticula, and orthopedic fractures. Vascular incidents such as ruptured aneurysm or bleeding from the gastrointestinal tract require immediate surgery. Sudden arterial occlusion that is unresponsive to chemical treatment is also considered emergent.

The postoperative phase of care is very important to the well-being of the geriatric patient. Maintaining or improving the preoperative level of wellness should be considered a primary expected outcome. A preoperative functional assessment is the foundation of the plan of care. Baseline parameters vary to a high degree among individuals, and all patients do not age at the same rate. Some patients are very young at 70 years of age, and some are very old. The difference should be assessed, and optimal outcomes should be identified for each geriatric patient. Influences on the level of functioning include physical ability, psychosocial support and resources, and environmental interactions.

Functional Assessment

Functional assessment can serve multiple purposes. In the preoperative phase, the plan of care includes the patient's unique differences, family involvement, resources, and level of independence. Many of these data are obtained by observation, interview, and lifestyle questionnaires. The information may be obtained from the patient, family, or significant others.

Many aspects of the patient's unique nature are easily discerned during the preoperative interview. Adequate time should be allowed for the interview (at least 30 minutes) so the patient has time to reflect and respond. Reaction time slows with age. The nurse should listen for subtle modifications or inconsistencies in the patient's information regarding health status. Sensory deficits should be considered, and the environment should be modified as needed during the interview. The nurse should establish rapport and have respect for the patient's dignity.

During the intraoperative phase, the functional assessment may allow for anticipation of needed supplies or additional help to accommodate the patient's needs. The patient's physical capabilities allow some independence in self-care. Patients tend to regress when they are not permitted to do things for themselves. A self-care deficit takes place when a patient feels the loss of independence while restrained on an operating bed. The freedom to assist with the transfer from the transport stretcher to the operating bed gives the patient a sense of participation in his or her own care. Maintaining a high level of self-esteem and value will enable the patient to prevent emotional regression or loss of control.

Activities of Daily Living. During the course of a normal day, an individual performs self-maintenance tasks and interacts with the environment. The ability to perform these activities of daily living (ADLs) is influenced by health status, emotions, mental clarity, and mobility. Limitations in performing these activities may be permanent or temporary, and many of the temporary limitations can be eliminated by medical or surgical treatment.

The perioperative nurse should assess the activity level of the geriatric patient. Advance preparations may need to be considered before the patient can undergo a surgical procedure. Because of identified physical limitations, special positioning or additional padding may be needed in combination with some form of communication assistance at the time the surgical procedure is performed. The functional baseline is the patient's capacity to perform self-care (e.g., feeding, bathing, toileting). Any deviation from the baseline assessment in the postoperative phase should be recorded and reported to the patient's physician.

Functional Activities. The activity patterns of geriatric patients reflect many aspects of their daily lives. Their ability to feed, bathe, and toilet themselves is one way to measure physical and psychological wellness. Basic daily activities such as grooming and dressing may be indicators of the level of the patient's involvement with his or her own care. The range of self-care activities depends on various factors, such as whether the patient is active and mobile enough to shop for food and prepare meals or is living in assisted housing where these services are provided. The ability to provide self-care should be assessed preoperatively to evaluate the outcome in the postoperative phase (i.e., resumption of activity level).

Functional Capacity. A basic assessment of physical strength and endurance will indicate whether the patient will be able to move from the transport stretcher to the operating bed. A patient who is weak or disabled by arthritis will need assistance or a total lift device. A patient who is visually impaired also may need assistance.

Communication through speech and hearing is vital to establishing the cognitive baseline. A hearing deficit or aphasia could be mistaken for a cognitive impairment. The patient who uses a hearing-assist device should be permitted to wear it to the operating room (OR) and, if possible, throughout the surgical procedure. It should be in place during emergence from anesthesia the patient can hear requests to deep breathe or move extremities.

The patient's sensory ability should be assessed. Tactile sensation dulls with age, and a patient's inability to feel external stimuli may lead to an inadvertent injury. Any sensory deficit, including a visual or hearing impairment, should be documented in the plan of care. The administration of a general anesthetic will alter the tactile assessment parameter during the intraoperative phase of care. As the patient emerges from anesthesia, the postanesthesia recovery nurses use the baseline assessment to measure the progress of the patient in the postoperative phase. Because of the interdependent aspects of the central nervous system with other vital physiologic systems, the evaluation of expected outcomes should include a sensory assessment.

Cognitive ability should also be assessed. The patient may be required to comprehend a command that is vital to the perioperative experience. A cognitive deficit may be of organic origin or result from a language barrier. Regardless of the reason, an inability to understand can cause anxiety for the patient and the caregiver. Alertness, short-term memory, capabilities to concentrate and problem solve, and motivation toward self-care are areas of cognition that influence the ability of the geriatric patient to adapt to illness and recovery. A patient who is cognitively impaired experiences disorientation and responds inappropriately to the environment. The impairment may be temporary but often is prolonged after anesthesia. Cognitive impairment also may be a permanent or chronic condition.

The patient's psychological state should be assessed preoperatively, because a change in mood or temperament may indicate an unexpected outcome caused by an injury or a physical problem resulting from the surgical procedure. Dementia, delirium, and emotional depression are common in older adults. Sudden withdrawal or a change in affect should be investigated promptly.

External Interactions. The manner in which an individual experiences illness depends on external forces and the number of barriers that may interfere with the attainment of outcomes. The nursing diagnoses may include Self-Care Deficit or Impaired Mobility. These diagnoses factor significantly in the postoperative phase and should be considered and placed in the plan of care. The reaction of the patient to either one of these nursing diagnoses will depend on his or her interactions with the external environment, the availability of resources, and the presence of barriers.

Resources. The level of independence exercised by the geriatric patient may depend on the resources available. The type of housing may depend on self-care ability and financial security. In developing the plan of care, the perioperative nurse should consider how the patient will meet his or her postoperative needs at home. Will help be available, or will arrangements for a visiting nurse or a family caregiver be needed? The patient's possible need for transportation to and from the surgeon's office for postoperative checkups should be considered.

Barriers. The type of housing may be a problem for the postoperative geriatric patient. If he or she lives alone in a multilevel dwelling, going up and down stairs may pose a significant problem. The location of the bathroom or kitchen may complicate the self-care process. Financial constraints may limit the number of home health care visits by an independent agency. The unavailability of family members may necessitate planning for institutionalization, which may be temporary but may become permanent.

Psychosocial Assessment

Gathering data about a geriatric patient should begin with the assessment of how this individual views other aged people and his or her own progression through the aging process. The assessment of a patient's self-concept may be an important indicator of a decline in the status of his or her psychological health. A patient's views of health and normative activity are influenced by his or her culture and affect the attainment of outcomes.

If the patient believes that older people are helpless, he or she may see the role of the aging process as one of helplessness. Although capable of many independent activities, this individual may adapt to an illness by becoming helpless. Even needing help temporarily may cause an older patient to believe that the condition is permanent. The perioperative nurse should be aware that the geriatric patient might experience a temporary period of helplessness. By establishing a functional baseline and stressing the temporary nature of postoperative recovery, the nurse can help the patient return to his or her routine.

The geriatric patient may feel rejected, unsupported, and worthless. Between 10% and 65% of geriatric patients experience depression and an alteration in self-image. The physical decline may be rapid when psychological well-being is threatened. The perioperative nurse should be aware that the geriatric patient who is depressed and lonely needs additional emotional support throughout the surgical experience.

The perioperative nurse should be aware of his or her own subjective views of aging and cultural attitudes and should not allow personal feelings to influence the assessment process. When assessing the geriatric patient, the nurse should consider the culture of origin, the cultural influence of the patient's current residence, and the patient's subjective perception of wellness and illness. Self-perception has a great influence on how well the geriatric patient adapts to aging. The nursing diagnoses should reflect the patient's adaptation because adaptation will affect the attainment of the expected outcomes. The perioperative plan of care should reflect the need for ongoing evaluation by postoperative caregivers.

Adaptation to the Aging Process. An individual should make many adjustments during the aging process.

The adaptation to aging is unique for each individual and is influenced by physical condition, psychological strengths and weaknesses, family and significant others, social support systems, financial resources, and functional ability. The geriatric patient develops a belief system about life expectations primarily on the basis of subjective feelings. If the patient is in decline, the outlook is usually negative, based on how he or she feels at a particular time. If the patient is feeling well and able-bodied, the outlook is usually positive, which helps delay the patient's fear of declining health outside the expected parameters of aging.

The prevention of decline not related to normative aging is a key factor in avoiding health deficits. The patient who can postpone health problems caused by factors that include avoidable health considerations—accidents, poor nutrition, inactivity, depression, and the effects of loneliness, smoking, substance abuse, and obesity—will enjoy a higher quality of life in the later years.

Self-Perception of Health. The patient's view of his or her health plays an important role in the actual health status. If the patient perceives health as important, preventive health maintenance should be a priority. The patient who feels well will perform the activities of daily living to the best of his or her ability. Minor interruptions in health status will not cause a major problem in the long-term prognosis of the patient's return to baseline parameters.

Physical Assessment

The physical assessment of the geriatric patient begins with general appearance. The perioperative nurse should first observe the patient from head to toe. The basic picture or image the patient creates can provide information about the health status. The patient should be assessed for posture, mobility, gait, rising or sitting, dexterity, body height and weight, body odors, psychological affect, communication, and comprehension of surroundings. The perioperative nurse should perform an assessment of the total patient by each body system. A summary of the physiologic changes associated with the normal aging process is provided in Table 9-1.

Any medications the patient takes on a routine or periodic basis should be listed on the chart, with their last dosages itemized. The patient should be encouraged to discuss all medications, including vitamins and topical ointments. Recreational drugs (e.g., street drugs, narcotics) should not be excluded from consideration just because the patient is older. Many medications can alter the results of bloodwork and the findings of the physical assessment. Drugs such as aspirin can alter blood tests for clotting times. Pain medications can alter sensorium.

Smoking and alcohol use are important to assess because they can affect many body systems. All assessment data should be recorded in the chart. The perioperative nurse should read the physician's medical history and physical examination report and review laboratory reports to discern the medical diagnoses (see Appendix A). Any additional abnormal findings should be reported to the surgeon and the anesthesia provider.

Integumentary System. Establishing a preoperative baseline for the condition of the skin will facilitate evaluation of the expected outcome (i.e., no injury to the skin as a result of surgical intervention). Assessment of the integumentary system includes the skin, fingernails and toenails, and all hair patterns of the body, face, and scalp. The nurse should ask the patient if any skin changes have taken place within the past several months. The skin is inspected for color, temperature, sensation, texture, turgor, thickness, and amount of subcutaneous tissue. The geriatric patient has a decreased number of sweat glands and an increased sensitivity to external temperature. The patient may complain of skin dryness, itching, and flaking.

The surface of the body should be inspected for sores, ulcers, and moles that have exhibited change over time. Broken or injured skin areas may indicate a pathologic condition such as skin cancer or diabetes. Skin rashes may indicate an allergy. Skin color can indicate liver disease or problems with other body systems (e.g., cardiovascular, respiratory). Bruises or abrasions may indicate a recent fall or possible elder abuse. Careful assessment of the body surface can reveal pertinent data about the patient's health status, but differentiating normal from abnormal skin conditions may be difficult. Skin is often wrinkled as a result of changes in connective tissue. Pigmentation and skin tags can be normal lesions in the aging process.

The nails and nailbeds of the fingers and toes should be observed for their presence or absence, texture, growth pattern, cleanliness, infection, and color. Clubbing and cyanosis of the fingertips and nailbeds may indicate cardiovascular disease. Extreme overgrowth and deformity of the toenails may indicate decreased circulation to the feet and legs. An accumulation of soil and debris under the nails may indicate an inability to wash properly. Twisted and gnarled digits may be painful to the touch, and this should be considered when planning positions for the surgical procedure (Fig. 9-1). The nurse should be aware that even the weight of the surgical drapes might create enough pressure to cause discomfort on the toenails.

Hair patterns on the scalp may show areas of thinning or loss. The nurse should note the condition of the hair, such as cleanliness, hair dye, and grooming. The condition of the hair may indicate the patient's level of interest or ability in performing self-care. A lack of care may be caused by inability or disinterest caused by depression. A patient with dementia may be unaware that the hair is dirty or uncombed.

Body hair patterns may be sparsely distributed in geriatric patients, with areas of thinning or absence. For

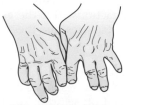

Rheumatoid arthritis   Hammertoes

FIG. 9-1 Deformities of the hands and feet.

TABLE 9-1	Physiologic Changes Associated with Normal Aging Processes in the Geriatric Patient

Age-Related Factors	Assessment Factors
INTEGUMENTARY SYSTEM	
Decreased subcutaneous fat, decreased turgor (elasticity)	Thin, dry skin, wrinkles
Diminished sweat glands, dulled tactile sensation	Poor thermoregulation, heat and cold sensitivity
Thickened connective tissue	Keratosis (patchy overgrowths of dermis), warts, skin tags (especially on face and neck)
Increased fat deposits over abdomen and hips	Poor excretion of fat-soluble drugs
Diminished capillary blood flow, reduced vascularity, capillary fragility	Pressure sores, delayed wound healing, purpura or lentigo (liver spots), bruises
Dry mucous membranes, decreased salivation and secretions	Dry mouth and vagina
MUSCULOSKELETAL SYSTEM	
Diminished protein synthesis in muscle cells, decreased muscle mass and tone	Muscle weakness, reduced strength, muscle wasting
Erosion of cartilage, thickened synovial fluid, fibrosed synovial membranes	Joint pain, swelling, stiffness, diminished range of motion
Diminished mobility, flexibility, and balance	Poor gait, poor posture, risk of falling
Increased porosity and demineralization of bone, thinning of intervertebral disks, decreased height	Ankylosing spondylosis, kyphosis, osteoporosis
RESPIRATORY SYSTEM	
Atrophied respiratory muscles, kyphosis or other postural changes, rib cage rigidity	Chest wall limitations
Reduced vital capacity	Dyspnea
Risk of pneumonia	Ineffective cough
CARDIOVASCULAR SYSTEM	
Decreased cardiac output and stroke volume	Chronic fatigue and dyspnea, orthostatic hypotension
Myocardial irritability and stiffness, decreased size of sinoatrial and atrioventricular nodes	Slow heart rate and circulation, dysrhythmias and murmurs
Increased vascular resistance, rigidity in arteries	Hypertension
Thickening and dilation of veins	Venous insufficiency, varicosities
Decline in renal blood flow	Edema in tissues
GASTROINTESTINAL SYSTEM	
Decreased esophageal peristalsis, slowed emptying of stomach	Indigestion, frequent antacid use
Diminished saliva production, which slows breakdown of carbohydrates; reduced gastric secretion of hydrochloric acid, which impairs absorption of vitamins and minerals; hepatic insufficiency, which affects absorption of fats	Malnutrition
Loss of perineal and anal sphincter tone	Diarrhea, fecal incontinence
Decreased intestinal peristalsis, loss of abdominal muscle turgor, reduced mucosal secretions in intestines	Constipation, frequent laxative use
ENDOCRINE SYSTEM	
Reduced hormonal activity, decreased physical activity	Slowed basal metabolic rate, subnormal temperature
Slowed release of insulin from pancreas	Impaired glucose metabolism
Reduced thyroid hormone production	Dry skin, temperature intolerance, poor appetite, lethargy, memory lapse
Disturbed fluid and electrolyte balance	Hydration status
GENITOURINARY SYSTEM	
Decreased renal blood flow, reduced number of glomeruli, reduced glomerular filtration rate, decreased excretory ability	Diminished renal function, risk of acid-base imbalance and drug toxicity
Loss of elasticity and muscle tone in ureters, bladder, and urethra	Urinary frequency, urgency, and nocturia
Decreased bladder muscle and sphincter tone, estrogen deficiency in female	Stress incontinence
Enlarged prostate in male	Urinary retention
Reduced testosterone, hypertrophied prostate, sclerosis of penile arteries and veins	Male: slow erection and ejaculation
Reduced estrogen; atrophied vulva, clitoris, and vagina	Female: sagging breasts, painful intercourse
NERVOUS SYSTEM	
Decreased number of brain cells, reduced cerebral blood flow, reduced oxygen supply to brain	Cognitive deficits: delirium, temporary state of confusion, forgetfulness, disorientation, irritability, and/or insomnia; dementia, a permanent state of cognitive impairment
Decreased neurons	Paresthesia, akinesia, diminished pain perception
Diminished neurotransmitters, decreased neurons	Tremors, head nodding, or other repetitive movements
Degeneration of myelin sheath, which lessens motor neuron conduction	Slowed reflexes and reaction time
Reduced sound transmission as eardrum thickens, decreased hair cells and neurons, reduced blood supply to cochlea	Auditory impairment
Weakened lens muscles, hardening of lens, flattening of cornea, reduced blood supply (which leads to macular deterioration), increased rigidity of iris, reduced pupil size	Visual impairment: decreased acuity, poor perception of light and color, poor peripheral vision

this reason, hair removal from the surgical site is not routinely indicated.

The extremities should be observed for the patterns of hair growth or its absence. The lower legs may not have much hair because of circulatory changes. The color of the legs should be observed at this time; duskiness and mottling may indicate a problem with arterial blood flow, whereas ruddiness may indicate a venous blood flow problem and possible deep vein thrombosis (DVT) risk. The shape, size, and equality of the lower legs should be checked for edema or ulceration. The condition of the extremities may have implications for positioning during the surgical procedure and may indicate the need for further systemic testing.

Musculoskeletal System. Assessment of the musculoskeletal system includes muscles, bones, posture, and gait. Muscle mass is usually decreased because muscle fibers atrophy, decrease in strength, and are fewer in number. Fibrous tissue replaces the lost mass. With less exercise and motion, muscle strength is compromised. Tendons become hardened, and range of motion decreases. Muscle cramps are common.

The patient may report a decrease in height. This is caused by demineralization of the bones, kyphosis, and narrowing of disk spaces in the vertebral column. The long bones do not decrease in length but become thin and brittle (osteoporosis), especially in older women; 78% of all patients older than 70 years have some degree of osteoporosis that is complicated by osteoarthritis (Fig. 9-2). Estrogen supplements after menopause may decrease the occurrence of brittle bones. However, fractures in the hips, vertebrae, wrists, and ends of long bones are common in older adults (Fig. 9-3).

Assistance with moving or total lifting may be necessary to help the geriatric patient move from the transport stretcher to the operating bed for the surgical procedure. The plan of care should include lifting help or devices and adequate positioning supplies. Care must be taken not to injure bony structures that may be weakened by osteoporosis.

Ankylosing spondylosis, a chronic inflammatory disease characterized by the fixation or fusion of a vertebral joint, often causes age-related postures. The body of the geriatric patient assumes an altered shape with an increased forward thoracic curvature (kyphosis) and a flattening of the lumbar curvature, particularly common in osteoporosis (Fig. 9-4). The patient may not be able to lie flat on the operating bed. Supine positioning may be painful unless the upper back and neck are supported. Fractures or subluxation of the cervical spine are possible if the ankylosed neck is allowed to fall back with the weight of the head. Twisting and forceful flexion can cause permanent damage to the vertebral column or contribute to rupture of the vertebral arteries.

Anteroposterior angles of the chest may be increased because of respiratory disease. Respiratory effort and chest excursion should be considered in planning positioning. In the preoperative assessment, the flexibility of the patient's spine and the presence of any deformity or associated disease should be noted. Flexion at the hip may be painful when the legs are maintained in a straight position. Placement of a safety belt over the thighs may exert counterpressure on the thighs, causing the legs to forcefully straighten against the flattened lumbar curvature. Modified positioning may include a small pillow under the knees and thighs to allow the age-related flexion angle of the hips to assume a natural position. Care in the place-

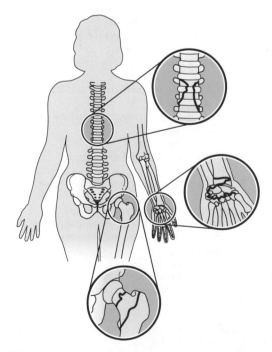

FIG. 9-2 Areas of the body commonly affected by osteoarthritis.

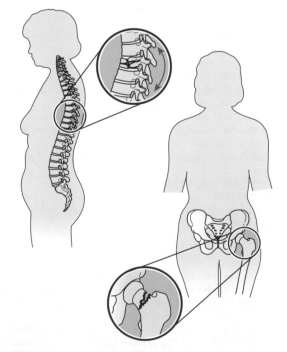

FIG. 9-3 Spontaneous fractures in the geriatric patient.

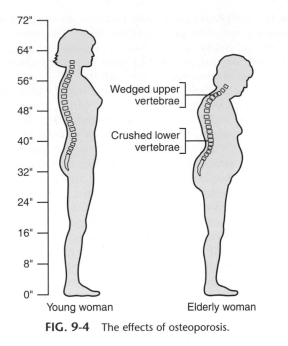

FIG. 9-4 The effects of osteoporosis.

ment of a safety belt or other restraint should include circulatory checks throughout the surgical procedure. The blankets should not exert pressure on the toenails, which can be painful.

The hands and feet may have painful deformities that should be considered when moving the patient to the operating bed and during positioning. Joints may be affected by arthritis, thickened synovium, and crystalloid formation in the synovial fluid. Patients may have osteoarthritis (Fig. 9-5) caused by the condition of cartilage degeneration, or they may have rheumatoid arthritis (Fig. 9-6) caused by the attack of the autoimmune system on joint lining. Either type of arthritis can cause pain on motion and positioning difficulties.

The patient may have a long history of taking non-steroidal antiinflammatory medications, corticosteroids, salicylates, and analgesics. The preoperative assessment should include an evaluation for the side effects associated with the long-term use of these medications. Gastrointestinal bleeding, prolonged clotting times, renal insufficiency, liver changes, loss of appetite, and alteration in mental status are common side effects that could adversely affect the desired outcomes of the surgical procedure.

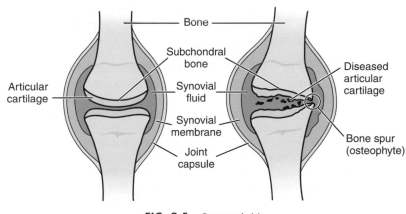

FIG. 9-5 Osteoarthritis.

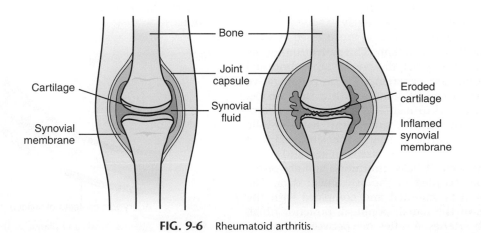

FIG. 9-6 Rheumatoid arthritis.

The patient's center of gravity is altered by multiple changes in body shape. Postural imbalance caused by impaired mobility is often the cause of falls that result in fractures. Some geriatric patients limit attempts at ambulation because they fear the possibility of falling. The risk of falls is further increased by complicating conditions such as sedation, electrolyte imbalance, impaired vision, and altered proprioception (muscular stimulation). Orthostatic hypotension contributes to the potential for falling when the geriatric patient rises from a sitting position and experiences a sudden drop in blood pressure. A fall may be symptomatic of a health problem or a systemic illness.

Cardiopulmonary System. Assessment of the lungs, heart, and circulation provides a good source of information about the general health condition of the patient. The cardiovascular and respiratory systems are closely interrelated. To assess the lungs, the nurse should ask the patient to describe how his or her breathing is affected by exertion. The nurse can assess difficulty or inefficiency in breathing by observing the patient's physical activity, respiratory effort, chest shape, and lip color. The nurse should palpate the trachea to determine if it is in midline. A deviation to the right or left may indicate the presence of a tumor. Tracheal position is an important consideration in the maintenance of an airway during a surgical procedure.

By listening to lung sounds with a stethoscope over the intercostal spaces, the nurse can refine the assessment to include specific sounds found in identified areas of each lobe. Percussion of the posterior chest wall tends to produce resonance except in very thin older adults, in whom tone is very hyperresonant. The normal sound is hollow and moderately loud, with a low pitch and long duration; the sound flattens over the rib bones. If the patient slumps forward and rounds the shoulders, the intercostal spaces widen for better percussion.

Establishing a preoperative respiratory system baseline is important. Intraoperative breathing difficulties may be avoided by adapting a position to accommodate the needs of the patient. Postoperative problems may be diagnosed and treated more efficiently if the patient's original respiratory condition has been assessed. Lung disease may affect the ability to clear secretions from the bronchial tree by coughing. Pneumonia is a common postoperative complication in geriatric patients. Coughing and deep-breathing exercises should be taught preoperatively.

The heart and systemic circulation are assessed as separate units and together as a system. The patient should be asked if dizziness, fainting, palpitations, or other abnormal subjective symptoms are experienced. The perioperative nurse should listen to heart sounds with a stethoscope. Dysrhythmias unrelated to heart disease are not uncommon in the geriatric patient, and many have systolic murmurs caused by aortic stenosis. The sinoatrial and atrioventricular nodes decrease in size with age, and signal interruption may occur. Clicks, murmurs, and abnormal sounds should be recorded in the assessment data. The apical pulse should be counted and compared with the peripheral pulses of the radial, popliteal, posterior tibial, and dorsalis pedis arteries. A difference between the apical

and the peripheral pulse may indicate an obstruction in a major artery. The jugular veins should be observed for distention. Veins in the lower extremities should be inspected for varicosities. Leg pain caused by circulatory impairment is common in older adults.

The carotid arteries should be auscultated with a stethoscope. Bruits and systolic murmurs, which are abnormal sounds, may indicate an evolving blockage (Fig. 9-7). Dizziness or cognitive impairment may be caused by carotid insufficiency. Care must be taken not to exert pressure over the carotid area, because manipulation of a plaque could cause an embolus to break loose and travel to the brain. Sudden changes in mental status during a surgical procedure performed with a local anesthetic could be the result of an arterial occlusion caused by a plaque embolus.

The geriatric patient usually has decreased or slowed circulation to all areas of the body. This should be considered while administering local anesthetics, because absorption of the medication will take longer and the effects will be delayed. The surgical site should be tested for the effects of the anesthetic before the incision is made. Vasoconstrictive additives, such as epinephrine, may have an exaggerated effect. Postoperative dressings should not be applied too tightly because healing is affected by circulatory efficiency.

Blood pressure should be assessed in the sitting and lying positions, and measured in both arms. Elevated systolic and diastolic blood pressures are a common finding in 40% of the geriatric patient population.

Assessment of laboratory blood values is important (see Appendix A). Anemia is common among older adults and is often overlooked as a potential cause of cerebral ischemia. Both men (21%) and women (34%) have slight normal decreases in hemoglobin and hematocrit levels because the blood-forming mechanisms lose efficiency with age. In men, the decrease in androgen production may cause a noticeable decrease in hemoglobin.

Extreme decreases in hemoglobin and hematocrit values are significant in the diagnosis of pathologic conditions in major organ systems, especially the gastrointestinal or genitourinary system. Anemic conditions also can be caused by a nutritional deficit. In the absence of any other confirmed pathologic condition, hemoglobin or hematocrit levels less than the lower limit of altitude-adjusted normal values (at sea level: hemoglobin 12 g/dL, hematocrit 35%) may signal anemia caused by malnutrition.

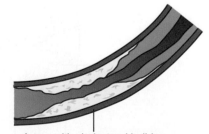

Artery with cholesterol buildup

FIG. 9-7   Atherosclerosis and plaque of the carotid artery.

The white blood cells do not decrease in number, but they do decrease in effectiveness. Inflammatory responses may be decreased or absent in the geriatric patient. This natural body response to injury may leave the patient more vulnerable to infection. The febrile response to infection may be diminished and therefore may not be a good indicator of a disease process. Older adults often have a subnormal baseline temperature.

Gastrointestinal System. Assessment of the gastrointestinal system should begin by observing for the visual signs of nutritional status, such as body weight, muscle wasting, bloating, and generalized weakness. Postoperative healing is profoundly affected by the ability of the cells to repair themselves. Both adequate nutrition and the ability to handle the necessary nutrients in the gastrointestinal system are essential for tissue restoration. Many socioeconomic, psychological, and physiologic factors influence the nutritional status of the geriatric patient. Living on a fixed income may limit the amount of nutritious food a patient can purchase. An adequate diet should include at least 1 g of protein per kilogram of desirable body weight, with an emphasis on a decreased number of calories. The average daily caloric intake of an older woman should range between 1280 and 1900 calories; for an older man the average daily caloric intake should range between 1530 and 2300 calories.

The perioperative nurse should keep in mind that actual caloric needs are unique for each patient and may vary in the presence of diabetes or other disease processes. A rapid weight gain or loss may indicate a serious pathologic condition and not an increase in body fat. Dietary control should focus on the quality, not the quantity, of food. Weight should be considered a vital sign in older adults and should be recorded in both pounds and kilograms because many medications are prescribed according to body weight in kilograms.

Psychologically the patient may feel that food does not taste right and may refuse to eat. Many psychological reasons for malnutrition are rooted in a physiologic cause. The geriatric patient's appetite may be decreased because there are fewer taste receptors in the mouth. The sense of smell may be diminished, or the patient's teeth may be in disrepair. Some patients are totally edentulous (toothless). The inability to taste, chew, and swallow discourages eating. Saliva production decreases and makes swallowing more difficult. Loose or missing teeth must be assessed because of the danger of aspirating a tooth during the surgical procedure.

The anesthesia mask may not seat well over an edentulous mouth. During the preoperative assessment, the perioperative nurse may find that a decreased ability to taste salty and sweet foods may cause the patient to increase the amount of salt and sugar in the diet. Increased salt intake may predispose the patient to congestive heart failure and fluid retention, and added sugar may cause an increase in unwanted body fat in proportion to muscle mass and difficult management of blood glucose.

The geriatric patient undergoing general anesthesia may receive stimulants and depressants; many of these are fat soluble. The fat-soluble drugs absorb faster but are excreted

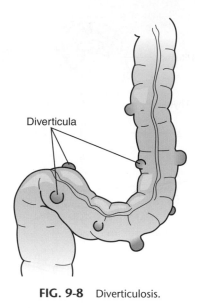

FIG. 9-8 Diverticulosis.

more slowly because of lower levels of intracellular fluid. Medications are unevenly distributed in the body, and the anticipated actions are unpredictable because fewer receptor sites react to the presence of the drug.

Digestion can be assessed by questioning the patient about food intake and the effects of the presence of food in the stomach. Older adults have decreased stomach motility, decreased gastric secretions, and slower stomach emptying time. The esophagus loses muscular tone and dilates slightly. Food may remain in the esophagus for longer periods. The perioperative nurse should ask the patient about the use of antacids and laxatives. Frequent use of antacids may indicate swallowing or stomach problems that should be investigated. Esophageal reflux in the presence of a hiatal hernia may need to be assessed preoperatively to prevent aspiration of gastric secretions. The inability to lie flat with food in the stomach may be the first symptom of a high-risk situation. Positioning and rapid-sequence induction of anesthesia may be considerations. Cricoid pressure (Sellick's maneuver) or awake intubation may be necessary to prevent aspiration.

The geriatric patient may use laxatives to maintain bowel regularity. Constipation is caused by decreased motility, lowered intake of bulk and fluids, and inactivity. Oil-based laxatives can lead to malabsorption of the fat-soluble vitamins A, D, E, and K, which further impairs nutritional and general health status. The absorption of nutrients is impaired naturally in older adults as a process of aging because intestinal blood flow is reduced and the absorptive cells lining the intestines are decreased. Diverticulosis and diverticulitis are common (Fig. 9-8). Fiber is an important dietary additive but should be used with caution because it can cause bowel obstruction or diarrhea. Diarrhea in the geriatric patient causes a serious threat to well-being because it may lead to dehydration.

The minimum oral fluid intake should be 1500 mL daily. Some geriatric patients have limited fluid intake. A patient may fear incontinence, have altered sensorium and cognition, be unable to drink fluids independently, or have

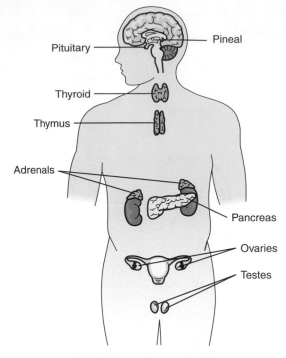

Pituitary

Pineal

Thyroid

Thymus

Adrenals

Pancreas

Ovaries

Testes

FIG. 9-9 Endocrine glands.

a decreased thirst sensation as part of the aging process. The serious nature of fluid balance in older adults is reflected in unstable electrolyte values and their direct effect on cardiac status. The perioperative nurse should perform a preoperative assessment of hydration. Signs of dehydration are dry tongue, sunken cheeks and eyes, severe loss of skin turgor, concentrated urine, and in some instances, mental confusion. Blood tests may show a urea level greater than 60 mg/dL. A geriatric patient who is dehydrated should receive preoperative intravenous fluids to prevent complications.

Endocrine System. The endocrine system interfaces with all major systems of the body. The assessment of endocrine functioning is complicated by the normal age-related changes in other body systems. The endocrine system consists of the thyroid gland; the parathyroid gland; the pancreas; the adrenal, pituitary, and pineal glands; and the ovaries or testes (Fig. 9-9).

Thyroid hormone production decreases by age 60 in men, whereas women experience decreased production by age 70. By 80 years of age, the thyroid gland reduces thyroid hormone production by 50%. The effects of this decreased production may be dry skin, memory lapse, temperature intolerance, lethargy, and appetite disturbance. Many signs and symptoms of thyroid disease may be confused with the normal aging process. Comorbidity may lead to abnormal laboratory test results in a patient with normal thyroid function.

Insulin is produced by the beta cells in the pancreas and affects the metabolism and storage of glucose. In healthy patients, glucose levels in the blood cause the pancreas to release insulin. The response of the pancreas

is slowed in older adults, and the release of insulin may not be triggered by the same stimulus. Many geriatric patients have diabetes mellitus with impaired glucose metabolism. Diabetes mellitus may be caused by deficient insulin production, insensitive insulin receptors, altered insulin release mechanisms, or inactivation of circulating insulin. An imbalance in blood glucose levels during the surgical procedure may predispose the patient to an unwanted outcome. Patients with diabetes mellitus often experience more postoperative infections and complications than do nondiabetic patients. Uncontrolled blood glucose metabolism has negative implications for all major body systems. Therefore, ongoing assessment is important to attain expected outcomes.

Genitourinary System. Assessment of the genitourinary system includes the bladder, urethra, ureters, kidneys, reproductive history, and genitalia. The first noticeable sign of a problem with the genitourinary system may be the odor of urine on clothing. The odor may be caused by lack of cleanliness but usually is from incontinence. More than 30% of the older population experience some form of urinary incontinence, but many are reluctant to discuss this problem and may try to avoid it. The problem may stem from stress incontinence, confusion, neurologic disorders, urinary tract infection, or immobility that prevents the patient from getting to the bathroom quickly.

The geriatric patient may fear loss of bladder control during the surgical procedure. Previous bladder or prostate gland surgery may predispose a patient to involuntary urine release. The perioperative nurse should include this situation in the plan of care. The problem may be minimized during the surgical procedure if the patient has an opportunity to empty the bladder preoperatively. The nursing diagnoses should reflect not only urinary incontinence but also the associated anxiety level of the patient.

Assessment of the genital area should include observation of the perineum for redness and excoriation. The bladder should be palpated with the patient in the supine position. The presence of a distended bladder after the patient has voided may indicate urinary retention with an overflow condition. This condition should be checked preoperatively before the patient is catheterized in the OR. The urethra could be inadvertently traumatized if an obstruction (e.g., tumor, enlarged prostate gland) is present.

The effectiveness of the kidneys decreases as the patient ages. By 50 years of age, renal blood flow and glomerular filtration rate decrease by as much as 50%. Although there may be no overt signs of a disease process, the perioperative nurse should be aware that the older patient is at increased risk for renal insufficiency and is highly susceptible to fluid overload, dehydration, or renal failure.

The perioperative nurse should make a baseline assessment of intake and output. During the surgical procedure, urinary output may be used to monitor the renal status of the patient. Renal impairment may delay the excretion of drugs by the kidneys and further complicate fluid balance. The urine should be assessed for color, concentration, the presence of particulate matter, and odor. Urinary output during the procedure should be at least 30 mL/hr; more

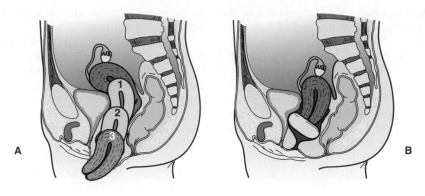

FIG. 9-10   **A,** Uterine prolapse. **B,** Donut pessary in place to correct uterine prolapse.

urine may be produced if the patient is taking diuretics or medications for blood pressure or cardiac control. Monitoring urinary output is difficult if the patient does not have an indwelling catheter or experiences urinary incontinence during the procedure. Postoperative care should include emptying the bladder to evaluate the expected outcome of adequate urinary output.

The reproductive assessment consists of the number of pregnancies a woman had during her childbearing years. Data about the method of birth should be included. Childbirth by cesarean section or a previous gynecologic surgery may indicate the possibility of pelvic adhesions that may be encountered if the planned surgical procedure includes entering the peritoneal cavity. Multiple vaginal births may cause uterine and bladder prolapse. The presence of a pessary[4] for uterine or bladder elevation should be noted (Fig. 9-10). The use of estrogen replacement therapy should be documented with the current dosage and the last doses taken. The possibility of osteoporosis and heart disease is greater in older women who have not had estrogen replacement after menopause.

The breasts of both male and female patients should be palpated for masses. The male patient may exhibit gynecomastia, which is an increase of breast tissue caused by decreased production of testosterone. Previous mammograms should be available if breast surgery is planned. Any hormonal therapy should be noted in the assessment. If a biopsy of the breast is performed, the specimen may be tested for estrogen receptor sites. The loss of fibrous breast tissue in the woman is normal. The main palpable finding will be the terminal milk ducts, which feel like strands or spindles. Masses are not a common finding and should be investigated.

Nulliparous women and those with a history of hormone replacement therapy (HRT) may be predisposed to breast cancer. Nipple discharge or retraction may indi-

cate a serious condition. The breasts of the elderly woman may be pendulous and flaccid. Prepping and draping may be slightly more difficult because of sagging skin and lack of muscle tone.

In males, size of the genitalia may be diminished. The penis may be smaller, and the testes descend lower into the scrotum because the rugae are decreased or absent. Pubic hair may be sparse, pale, and coarse. The ability to achieve an erection may be decreased or absent, and the ability to ejaculate may be diminished. Orgasm may still be possible without the presence of an erection. The prostate may be enlarged, and the incidence of prostatic cancer increases with age. The male geriatric patient may experience embarrassment during a prostate examination, and all efforts should be made to preserve his dignity.

Positioning for this examination may be difficult because of inflexible joints. The patient can be placed in a lateral, modified jackknife, or modified dorsal recumbent position. The presence of stool may hinder the palpation. For many prostate biopsies, transrectal ultrasound and needle aspiration are used. Rectal sphincter tone should be assessed in the patient who is undergoing a transrectal procedure. Anal tears, hemorrhoids, fissures, and defects in the musculature should be documented in the assessment data. Any stool present on the examiner's gloved finger should be tested for occult blood to establish the baseline; otherwise, postoperative bleeding could be wrongly assessed as a problem caused by the surgical procedure. Baseline data may help resolve the situation.

The female genitalia should be assessed both externally and internally. The patient should be placed supine in a modified lithotomy position. Spinal curvature or respiratory difficulty may prevent the patient from lying flat, and arthritic joints make lithotomy positioning painful. Care should be exercised not to create embarrassment during the examination. The vulvar area should be inspected. The mons and labia will appear smaller and looser because of the loss of subcutaneous fat pads and the decrease in estrogen production. Lesions and discolorations should be noted. The skin of the perineum may be shiny, atrophic, and dry. The prepuce and clitoris may be atrophied, but orgasm is still possible. The vaginal opening may appear small, dry, and inelastic. A previous history of hysterectomy or oophorectomy should be obtained. The absence of

---

[4]Pessaries are sometimes used to conservatively treat prolapsed pelvic organs. Some women use a pessary to minimize urinary incontinence. Patients are taught to remove the device for cleaning before bedtime and replace it in the morning. Pessaries are useful for the patient who cannot withstand a surgical procedure for prolapse, cystourethrocele, or rectocele.

the uterus or ovaries does not preclude examination of the vaginal vault. The anus should be inspected for tears, fissures, and hemorrhoids.

The internal assessment of the female genitalia includes a very gentle examination that involves insertion of a gloved, well-lubricated finger into the vagina. The vagina may feel shortened. The position of the bladder, rectum, and cervix should be ascertained. Protrusion of the bladder, rectum, or cervix may be present because the patient experiences a loss of muscle tone with age. The abdomen is palpated as the uterus is carefully elevated. The uterus atrophies as part of the aging process; enlargement is caused by disease. The endometrium will still respond to the stimulation of hormonal therapy, causing uterine bleeding. The adnexa are identified, and no masses should be palpable.

The use of a smaller, prewarmed, well-lubricated speculum is usually necessary for visualization of the cervix and for obtaining a Papanicolaou (Pap) smear. Pediatric instrumentation may be needed. The vaginal lining will look thin, smooth, dry, and atrophied. Care is essential to prevent trauma when fingers or instruments are inserted into the vagina. Discharge and foul odors are abnormal and should be reported. Vaginal bleeding is a sign of a pathologic condition in the older woman.

Sexuality in older adults is an often overlooked and ignored reality. The activity between geriatric sex partners may vary in performance, but sexual pleasure is not abandoned because of advancing age. Intercourse may not take place in the same way as when the partners were young, but sexual contact and mutual gratification remain pleasurable. Many geriatric patients have been forced to deny their sexuality because of the loss of their sex partner. Self-gratification may be practiced but is not openly discussed because of the personal nature of the act.

The subject of sexuality should be approached gently, without jokes or condemnation. Dislocations of total hip joint prosthetics can occur during sexual intercourse. A surgical procedure that may alter sexual habits can be devastating. Empathy is critical to the patient's adjustment to a change of lifestyle. Counseling may be necessary to assist the patient and the sex partner in expressing concerns. The perioperative nurse should be prepared to answer questions and listen to the patient as he or she expresses a sense of loss. When appropriate, the plan of care should reflect the nursing diagnosis of sexual dysfunction or ineffective sexuality patterns.

Nervous System. Assessment of the nervous system includes the brain, spinal cord, peripheral nerves, and sensory organs. The nervous system is uniquely interdependent with every system of the body. Age-related changes in the brain consist of a decreased number of neurons, a decreased rate of impulse transmission, an increased reflex response time, and a decreased brain mass.

The perioperative nurse should assess the geriatric patient and establish a baseline of neurologic function. Any deviation from baseline during the surgical procedure may indicate the presence of an additional or new pathologic condition involving the brain (e.g., stroke). Postoperatively, the ongoing assessment monitors the risk for a postprocedure deficit caused by medication or a pathologic condition.

The spinal cord and peripheral nerves are assessed together. During the functional assessment, the patient is observed ambulating, sitting, standing, maintaining posture, making intentional hand motions, and performing cooperative and purposeful actions such as writing. The perioperative nurse is able to observe for tremor, gait disturbance, shuffling of feet, unilateral weakness, or an alteration in mobility caused by a neurologic deficit. An assessment of the medications taken at home is important to determine the presence of transient nervous system side effects such as shaking and intention tremor. Smoking can cause a temporary decrease in cerebral blood flow, resulting in dizziness that may mimic a neurologic problem.

The sensory changes associated with aging involve decreased pressure and pain perception, difficulty differentiating between hot and cold, hearing loss, decreased visual acuity, and alterations in the senses of smell and taste and in spatial perception during locomotion. Preoperative assessment of tactile sensory conditions will enable the nurse to develop a plan of care that reflects the need for protection of bony pressure points and for caution during the use of heat- or cold-producing equipment such as a hypothermia/hyperthermia mattress.

If a patient has sensory impairments such as a visual disturbance, a hearing loss, or altered spatial perception, there is a high risk for injury caused by falls. Patients with cataracts may be sensitive to the glare from bright OR lights. Allowing the patient to wear hearing aids and eyeglasses to the OR helps the patient adapt to the surgical environment. Unexpected outcomes caused by sensory alteration can be prevented by developing a plan of care that considers the combined baseline abilities and sensory needs of the patient. For example, an assessment of hearing ability will dictate the need to facilitate communication.

INTRAOPERATIVE CONSIDERATIONS

Special precautions are indicated in caring for geriatric patients in the OR. The following factors should be considered:

• *Hypothermia.* Geriatric patients are at risk when their core body temperature falls below 96.8° F (36° C). A decreased basal metabolic rate, limited cardiovascular reserves, thinning of the skin, and reduced muscle mass affect the production and conservation of body heat. Measures must be taken to prevent inadvertent hypothermia caused by environmental factors. Precautionary measures include raising room temperature; using warm blankets and devices to circulate warmed air over body surfaces not included in the surgical site; warming anesthetic gases, solutions, and intravenous fluids; and covering the patient's head.

• *Positioning.* Patients should be lifted, not pulled, during transfer to and from the operating bed and during positioning on the operating bed. Skin is sensitive to abrasion because of decreased dermal thickness and turgor (elasticity). Joints may be stiff or painful because of calcification or degenerative osteoarthritis. Support of the back and neck prevents discomfort from osteoporosis, kyphosis, or rheumatoid arthritis. Padding and air supports protect pressure points and bony prominences. Circulation and respiration must not be further compromised. Decreased cardiac output, arteriosclerosis, venous stasis, reduced vital lung capacity, and reduced tissue oxygenation are characteristic changes in older adults.

- *Antiembolic measures.* Slow circulation and hypotension predispose older adults to thrombus formation and emboli. Antiembolic stockings or a sequential compression device on the legs helps decrease this risk.
- *Monitoring.* A decrease in renal circulation and excretory ability affects electrolyte balance and the excretion of drugs. Fluid and blood losses are not well tolerated, and hypovolemia can progress rapidly. Blood loss and urinary output must be monitored. Blood gases and electrolytes may need to be monitored, depending on the type of surgical procedure and the patient's preoperative condition. The reaction to any anesthetic agents and drugs is closely monitored in all patients. Fluctuations in cardiac rate and rhythm may portend an impending crisis.

Anesthesia Considerations

Geriatric patients present a special challenge to the anesthesia provider. Physiologic function gradually deteriorates with age but not in a predictable manner or progression. The aging process is not a disease but a fundamental biologic alteration. In geriatric patients, disease is superimposed on senescent changes. Elders are more prone to multiple organ system failure. Changes in the central nervous system produce effects on other body systems.

Characteristics of some older adults include memory loss and confusion (which are exaggerated in an institutional environment), malnutrition, anemia, osteoporosis, low blood volume, poor liver or renal function, arteriosclerosis, diminished autonomic tone and reflexes, instability of circulation, and diabetes. Reactivity to stimuli decreases with advancing years. These patients therefore experience an altered response to stress, which is exemplified by a high pain threshold. They are more susceptible to the action of all drugs. Abnormal sleeping and breathing patterns, with the production of apnea by hyperventilation, are accentuated by opioids. These phenomena translate to a need for lower doses of anesthetics and of opioids for analgesia; the minimum anesthetic concentration required declines progressively with advanced age.

In older adults, oxygen masks may be difficult to fit because of the loss of teeth and/or bony substance in the jaw. Induction may be prolonged and ventilation made difficult because of chronic obstructive pulmonary disease such as emphysema. With a rapid fall in blood pressure, patients are susceptible to hypoxia, stroke, renal failure, and the development of myocardial infarction. The problems of anesthetization are augmented because with geriatric patients, surgical procedures tend to be major and take longer; many procedures pertain to malignant tumors, with additional surgery necessary.

A decrease in muscle mass, including the myocardium, with a corresponding increase in body fat takes place in the aging process; most anesthetics are fat soluble. Cardiac output and pulmonary capacity also diminish with age, with a decline in maximal oxygen uptake. In addition, anesthetics may reduce oxygen to the heart, kidneys, and brain, and geriatric patients are prone to hypotension, hypothermia, cerebral edema, and hypoxemia postoperatively. These fundamental physiologic changes necessitate a reduction of anesthetic dosages in geriatric patients.

Surgical mortality is higher in older adults than in the general population, especially if the surgery is an emergency procedure, which does not allow sufficient time for a thorough preoperative evaluation and preparation. Complications related to the cardiovascular system and cerebral circulation often are followed by respiratory problems, aspiration, and infection. Surgical morbidity can be reduced, however, by skillful anesthesia management.

POSTOPERATIVE CONSIDERATIONS

The health status of geriatric patients is compromised by the interaction of drugs and anesthetics and by the surgical procedure itself. The following must be monitored postoperatively:

- Drug interactions. Tolerance may be poor, and detoxification is slow. Drugs metabolize slowly in the liver and are excreted slowly by the kidneys. Fat-soluble drugs have a prolonged duration because they are absorbed by body fat, which increases with aging. Many anesthetic agents are fat soluble and are myocardial and respiratory depressants. Narcotics and sedatives interact with anesthetics. Patients must be monitored for hypoxia because oxygenation to the heart, kidneys, and brain will be less efficient. General anesthetics and some drugs cause transient mental dysfunction.
- Aspiration. Older adults may have difficulty swallowing because of dry mucous membranes, reduced salivation, and reduced esophageal peristalsis. Coughing is less productive because of muscular atrophy in the chest and rigidity of the rib cage. Patients must be watched for aspiration.
- Infection. Respiratory, urinary, or gastrointestinal tract infections may develop as a result of immunodeficiency. Pneumonia can be fatal. Poor dental hygiene may be the source of systemic infection. Healing is further delayed if an infection develops in a wound already compromised by a reduced vascular supply. The fever associated with infection in younger patients may not be as obvious in geriatric patients. Elevation of white blood cell count may be a better indicator if the patient is not immunocompromised as the result of some other disease.

Geriatric patients require a thorough preoperative assessment, an experienced anesthesia provider, considerate and knowledgeable caregivers, meticulous aseptic and sterile techniques, and careful postoperative management. The patient and his or her family and/or significant others should be included in the development of the postoperative discharge plan. Planning should incorporate follow-up care with the surgeon.

Bibliography

Anonymous: Trends in aging—United States and world wide, *MMWR Morbid Mortal Wkly Rep* 52(6):101-114, 2003.

Bailes B: Perioperative care of the elderly surgical patient, *AORN J* 72(2):186-207, 2000.

Blanc S et al: Energy requirements in the eighth decade of life, *Am J Clin Nutr* 79(2):303-310, 2004.

Clarke A et al: Seeing the person behind the patient: Enhancing the care of older people using a biographical approach, *J Clin Nurs* 12(5):697-706, 2003.

Inaba K et al: Long-term outcomes of injury in the elderly, *J Trauma Injury Infect Crit Care* 54(3):486-491, 2003.

Jacobs DG: Special considerations in geriatric injury, *Curr Opin Crit Care* 9(6):535-539, 2003.

Kestleloot HE, Verbeke G: On the relationship between cardiovascular, cancer, and residual mortality rates with age, *Eur J Cardiovasc Prevention Rehab* 12(2):175-181, 2005.

Martin JH, Haynes LC: Depression, delirium, and dementia in the elderly patient, *AORN J* 72(2):209-217, 2000.

McIntosh L: The role of the nurse in the use of vaginal pessaries to treat pelvic organ prolapse and/or urinary incontinence: A literature review, *Urol Nurs* 25(1):41-48, 2005.

Mueller PS et al: Ethical issues in geriatrics: A guide for clinicians, *Mayo Clin Proc* 79(4):554-562, 2004.

Pisani MA et al: Under-recognition of preexisting cognitive impairment by physicians in older ICU patients, *Chest* 124(6): 2267-2274, 2003.

Rao SS: Prevention of falls in the elderly, *Am Fam Phys* 72(1):81-81, 2005.

Wachtel RE, Dexter F: Differentiating among hospitals performing physiologically complex operative procedures in the elderly, *Anesthesiology* 100(6):1552-1561, 2004.

Physical Facilities

CHAPTER OBJECTIVES

After studying this chapter, the learner will be able to:
- Identify specific areas within the surgical suite wherein attire and behaviors affect the manner of care delivery.
- Discuss how environmental layout contributes to aseptic technique.
- Describe methods of environmental controls that contribute to an aseptic environment.
- Describe the specialty rooms used for endoscopy, minimally invasive procedures, and urology

CHAPTER OUTLINE

KEY TERMS

Cesarean delivery   A specialized procedure that requires surgical intervention during the birth of a baby.

Endoscopic procedures   Surgical procedures that use natural body orifices or percutaneous techniques with fiberoptic lighting to employ cameras and long specialized instruments during tissue manipulation and invasive intervention (e.g., colonoscopy, bronchoscopy).

Interventional radiographic procedure   A specialized surgical procedure that permits the use of radiologic imaging during tissue manipulation and invasive intervention through small incisional portals.

Minimally invasive surgical (MIS) procedure   Surgical procedures that use small incisions and fiberoptic lighting to employ cameras and long specialized instruments during tissue manipulation and invasive intervention (i.e., laparoscopy or mediastinoscopy).

Operating room (OR)   A specialized room where the actual surgery takes place. This room is one part of the restricted area of surgical suite.

Sterile core   A special room within the suite where sterile supplies are stored for ease of use. This room is one part of the restricted area of surgical suite.

Substerile room   A room with a double sink that is separated from the operating room by a door and where select clean and contaminated activities take place during the process of the surgical procedure. Some substerile rooms have warming cabinets for solutions or blankets, a steam autoclave, and a STERIS unit. A disposal sink for contaminated fluids might be in here.

Suite   A collection of rooms that are used interactively during a surgical procedure wherein each room has a specific purpose (e.g., operating room, substerile room, scrub sink room, and sterile storage core).

SUPPLEMENTAL MATERIAL ON EVOLVE WEBSITE   *evolve*

http://evolve.elsevier.com/BerryKohn
- Content Updates
- Glossary
- Full Set of Perioperative Flash Cards
- Interactive Key Term Flash Cards
- Student Activities
- WebLinks

HISTORICAL BACKGROUND

Surgical procedures were not always performed within the confines of a formal hospital setting. The surgeon made house calls when summoned to see a patient. In the early 1900s, the surgical nurse was sent to prepare a suitable room with little traffic and ambient noise for the surgical procedure—usually the dining room, but occasionally the kitchen. Everything was removed from the room, especially carpets, drapes, pictures, and unnecessary furniture. The room was fumigated with sulfur dioxide for 12 hours if time allowed. This was accomplished by burning 3 pounds of sulfur in an iron pot for each 1000 cubic feet of air space. The windows and doors were sealed shut as much as possible. When the fumigation was complete, the walls and surfaces were scrubbed with 5% carbolic acid or hot soda solution. Von Esmarch described cleansing of wallpaper by a process that involved rubbing the surface with soft bread. He based this activity on personal experiments. If time did not permit the fumigation/scrubbing process, the room was to be penetrated with steam from a kettle.

Linen napkins and towels were boiled for 5 minutes in soda solution for use as sponges. The stove and oven were useful as sterilizers. Bricks were kept in the oven for use as warming devices for chilly patients. The kitchen or dining room table was padded for use as the operating bed and placed under the chandelier, with the head toward a north window. For privacy, fine white tissue paper was secured to the window using flour paste. Many surgeons had portable lamps for use in homes equipped with electricity. This was useful at night. White bed sheets were nailed to all of the walls as protective coverings.

The physical environment was of keen importance to the surgeon. The temperature of the room was to be maintained at 75° to 80° F and additional warming measures, such as heated blankets, hot water bottles, and heated bricks wrapped in flannel were used. In addition to preparing the environment, the nurse was required to have 10 gallons of hot sterile water and 10 gallons of cold sterile water ready for use. Her role included preparing sterile saline by boiling a large container of water and adding 2 teaspoons of table salt. The mixture was boiled for 30 minutes then filtered through cotton that has been baked to a brownish color into a sterile bottle. A cork was used to seal the opening. If the solution was to be kept for future use, the sealed bottle was boiled for 20 minutes for 3 consecutive days. This was believed to prevent spore generation.

At the conclusion of the surgical procedure the nurse was required to disassemble, boil, dry, and pack the surgeon's private instrumentation into his black bag. The room was returned to its original condition by removing the sheets from the walls and sending them out for laundering and restoring carpets and furniture to their usual position. The aim of the nurse was to leave the place as she found it.

PHYSICAL LAYOUT OF THE SURGICAL SUITE

Efficient use of the physical facilities is important. The design of the surgical suite offers a challenge to the planning team to optimize efficiency by creating realistic traffic and workflow patterns for patients, visitors, personnel, and supplies. The design also should allow for flexibility and future expansion and should control for environmental atmospheric regulation (Table 10-1). Architects consult surgeons, perioperative nurses, and surgical services administrative personnel before allocating space.

Construction or Renovation Planning and Design Team

The planning and design of the perioperative environment require a multidisciplinary team, which may include the following:
- Department director
- Nurse manager
- Physicians (surgeon, anesthesia provider)
- Senior perioperative nursing personnel
- Project manager (may be in-house personnel or a consultant)
- Information technologist
- Communications (e.g., telephone, intercom, emergency call) personnel
- Support services (e.g., laboratory, radiology) personnel
- Infection control personnel
- Architect
- Interior decorator

No one particular construction or renovation plan suits all hospitals; each is individually designed to meet projected specific future needs. The number of operating rooms, storage areas, and immediate perioperative patient care areas required depends on the following:
- Number, type, and length of the surgical procedures to be performed
- Type and distribution by specialties of the surgical staff and equipment for each

TABLE 10-1	Environmental Controls in the Surgical Suite		
Environmental Controls	**OR**	**Postanesthesia Care Unit**	**Storage Areas**
Temperature	68°-73° F (20°-22° C)	70°-75° F (21°-24° C)	68°-73° F (20°-22° C)
Humidity	30%-60%	30%-60%	30%-60%
Air exchanges per hour	15	6	4 (minimum)
Recirculated by room unit	No	No	No
Pressure related to adjacent areas	Positive	N/A	N/A
Exchanges with outdoor air per hour	3	2	N/A

Modified from American Institute of Architects Committee on Architecture for Health; US Department of Health and Human Services, *Guidelines for Construction and Equipment of Hospital and Medical Facilities*, Washington, DC, 2001, American Institute of Architects Press.

- Proportion of elective inpatient and emergency surgical procedures to ambulatory patient and minimally invasive procedures
- Scheduling policies related to the number of hours per day and days per week the suite will be in use and staffing needs
- Systems and procedures established for the efficient flow of patients, personnel, and supplies
- Consideration of volume changes and need for future expansion capabilities
- Technology to be implemented and plans for potential technology to be developed
- Safety of staff, patients, and other personnel during construction or renovation

Principles in Construction or Renovation Planning

The universal problem of environmental control to prevent wound infection exerts a great influence on the design of the surgical suite and the plans for construction or renovation. Buildings with surgical suites older than 30 years do not have the capability of supporting newer technology with renovation for space and technologic and electrical capabilities. Architects, administrators, and surgical suite designers follow several concepts in planning the physical layout and construction of a surgical suite:

1. Strategic planning
   a. Avoid as much inconvenience to facility personnel as possible.
   b. Include facility personnel in the planning phase as much as possible.
   c. Expedite completion as fast as possible without compromising safety of patients, staff, and construction personnel.
   d. Keep costs down by planning ahead. Do not substitute cheap materials for durable materials. They will only cost more to replace later. Always follow manufacturer's and blueprint specifications.
   e. Plan the project in steps, completing each area before starting the next.
   f. Minimize the ordering of supplies for patient use to only those items needed for immediate procedures. Inventory storage will be an issue as the project unfolds.
   g. Resolve replacement issues for current equipment in use. Sometimes it is financially better to buy units in a lot than to replace one at a time. Deals can be made regarding pricing when planning equipment for the new rooms. Better to install equipment from scratch than to add later at an added construction/installation cost.
   h. Plan for the closing of rooms without too much disruption if they are to be updated.
   i. Determine the balance of fixed equipment versus mobile equipment for use in several rooms.
   j. Determine the need for dedicated rooms such as for endoscopy, cystoscopy, minimally invasive procedures, interventional radiology, trauma, and cardiac procedures.
2. Plans for emergencies

   a. Power, communications, medical gases, vacuum system, waste gas scavenger, air-handlers, water, and sewage cannot be interrupted. A plan should be in place to counter any accidental cutting of lines by construction personnel. Legionella has grown in standing water lines during phases of construction.
   b. Protect monitoring equipment from interference from radiofrequencies caused by construction machines or devices.
   c. Plan for capability of construction work stoppage at a moment's notice if requested by a surgeon during a critical phase of surgery.
3. Exclusion of contamination from outside the suite with sensible traffic patterns to and from the suite
   a. Barrier must be in place between working operating rooms (ORs) and the portion of the suite under construction. Wood or drywall panels as temporary walls sealed over all edges with duct tape can keep dust from entering the suite. Plastic sheeting is not sturdy and can easily be punctured.
   b. Negative pressure must be maintained in halls with exhaust filtered to the outside of the building.
   c. Traffic patterns must be unobstructed for debris removal. Aspergillosis has been isolated in construction debris of older buildings. Toileting and hand-cleansing areas must be available to construction workers.
   d. Traffic patterns must be unobstructed for bringing in construction supplies and materials.
4. Separation of clean areas from contaminated areas within the suite during the building phase
   a. Patient traffic should be separated from construction traffic.
   b. Clean supplies are transferred in an area separate from construction supplies.
   c. Biologic decontamination and processing areas remain functional at all times.
5. Noise control
   a. Noise pollution should be kept at a minimum when surgical procedures are in process or the general patient population in the hospital is sleeping.
   b. Vibrations from powered equipment and jack-hammers can disrupt microscopic or other procedures.

Physical plant design and construction/renovation planning of a surgical suite should include detailed consideration for the activities of patients, caregivers, and environmental maintenance.

Type of Physical Plant Design

Most surgical suites are constructed according to a variation of one or more of four basic designs:

1. Central corridor, or hotel plan (Fig. 10-1)
2. Central core, or clean core plan with peripheral corridor (Fig. 10-2)
3. Combination central core and peripheral corridor, or racetrack plan (Fig. 10-3)
4. Grouping, or cluster plan with peripheral and central corridor (Fig. 10-4)

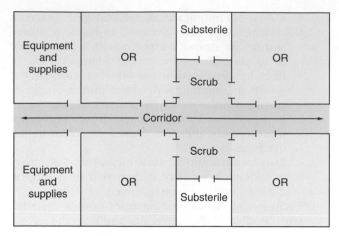

FIG. 10-1   Central corridor, hotel style.

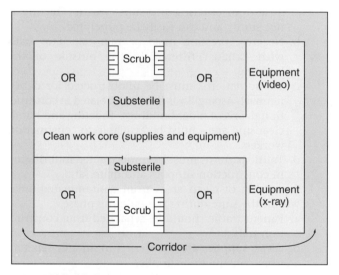

FIG. 10-2   Central core, peripheral corridor style.

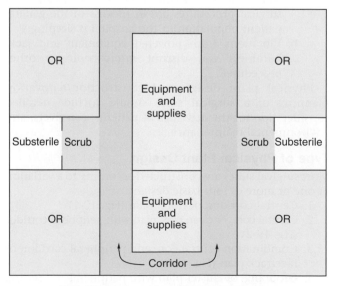

FIG. 10-3   Central corridor, racetrack style.

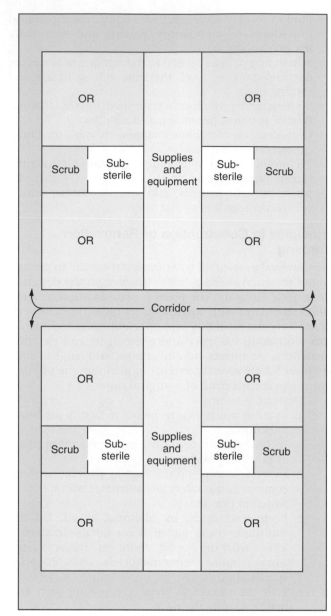

FIG. 10-4   Cluster combination, peripheral and central corridor style.

Each design has its advantages and disadvantages. Efficiency is affected if corridor distances are too long in proportion to other space, if illogical relationships exist between space and function, or if inadequate consideration was given to storage space, material handling, and personnel areas.

Location

The surgical suite is usually located in an area accessible to the critical care surgical patient areas and the supporting service departments, the central service or sterile processing department, the pathology department, and the radiology department. The size of the hospital is a determining factor because it is impossible to locate every desirable unit or department immediately adjacent to the surgical suite. A terminal location is necessary to prevent unrelated traffic from passing through the suite. A location on a top floor is not necessary for microbial control because all air is specially filtered to control dust. Traffic noises may be less evident above the ground floor. Artificial lighting is controllable, so the need for daylight is not a factor; in fact, it may be a distraction during the use of video equipment and other procedures requiring a darkened environment. Most surgical suites have solid walls without windows.

Space Allocation and Traffic Patterns

Space is allocated within the surgical suite to provide for the work to be done, with consideration given to the efficiency with which it can be accomplished. The surgical suite should be large enough to allow for correct technique yet small enough to minimize the movement of patients, personnel, and supplies. Provision must be made for traffic control. The type of design will predetermine traffic patterns. Everyone—staff, patients, and visitors—should follow the delineated patterns in appropriate attire. Signs should be posted that clearly indicate the attire and environmental controls required. The surgical suite is divided into three areas that are designated by the physical activities performed in each area.

Unrestricted Area. Street clothes are permitted. A corridor on the periphery accommodates traffic from outside, including patients. This area is isolated by doors from the main hospital corridor or elevators and from other areas of the surgical suite. It serves as an outside-to-inside access area (i.e., a transition zone). Traffic, although not limited, is monitored at a central location.

Semirestricted Area. Traffic is limited to properly attired, authorized personnel. Scrub suits and head coverings are required attire. This area includes peripheral support areas and access corridors to the ORs. The patient's hair is also covered.

Restricted Area. Masks are required to supplement OR attire where open sterile supplies or scrubbed personnel are located. Sterile procedures are carried out in the OR. The area also includes scrub sink areas and substerile rooms or clean core area(s) where unwrapped supplies are sterilized. Personnel entering this area for short periods, such as laboratory technicians, may wear clean surgical coveralls or jumpsuits to cover street clothes. Hair covering is worn and masks are donned as appropriate.

TRANSITION ZONES

Both patients and personnel enter the semirestricted and restricted areas of the surgical suite through a transition zone. This transition zone, inside the entrance to the surgical suite, separates the OR corridors from the rest of the facility.

Preoperative Check-in Unit

If a remote same-day procedure unit is not available for admission of patients who arrive shortly before a surgical procedure, facilities must be provided within the unrestricted area of the surgical suite for patients to change from street clothes into a gown. The area must ensure privacy. It may be compartmentalized with individual cubicles or be an open area with curtains. The decor should create a feeling of warmth and security. Lockers should be provided for safeguarding patients' clothes. Lavatory facilities must be available.

Preoperative Holding Area

A designated room or area should be available for patients to wait in the surgical suite; that area should shield them from potentially distressing sights and sounds. The corridor outside the OR is the least desirable area. The area should provide privacy. Individual cubicles are preferable to curtains. Hair removal and insertion of intravenous (IV) lines, indwelling urinary catheters, and gastric tubes may be done here. The anesthesia provider may insert invasive monitoring lines and give regional blocks. These procedures require good lighting. Each patient area is equipped with oxygen, suction, and devices for monitoring and cardiopulmonary resuscitation.

A nurses' station within the area provides for medication storage and preparation and for interdepartmental and intradepartmental communication. Computer access to patient information, such as laboratory reports, and to patient care documentation facilitates completion of patients' records, if necessary. Coordination with people managing the surgical schedule is essential to prevent delays.

Induction Room

Some hospitals have an induction room adjacent to each OR, where the patient waits and is prepared preoperatively before administration of anesthesia. Invasive IV lines are placed and/or regional anesthesia may be induced in this area. These are more common in larger facilities, where procedures such as open heart surgery or transplantation is performed.

Postanesthesia Care Unit

The postanesthesia care unit (PACU) may be outside the surgical suite, or it may be adjacent to the suite so that it may be incorporated into the unrestricted area with access from both the semirestricted area and an outside corridor. In the latter design, the PACU becomes a transition zone for the departure of patients.

Hospitals and ambulatory care facilities accommodate patients and their families. A designated waiting area must be provided for families. This is most conveniently located outside the surgical suite adjacent to the recovery area.

Dressing Rooms and Lounges

Dressing rooms must be provided for both men and women to change from street clothes into OR attire before entering the semirestricted area, and vice versa. Lockers are usually provided. Doors separate this area from lavatory facilities and adjacent lounges. Walls in the lounge areas should have an aesthetically pleasing color or combination of colors to foster a restful atmosphere. A window view of the outdoors is psychologically desirable. Dictating equipment and telephones should be available for surgeons in lounges or in an adjacent semirestricted area.

PERIPHERAL SUPPORT AREAS

Adequate space must be allocated to accommodate the needs of OR personnel and support services. The need for equipment, supply, and utility rooms and housekeeping determines support space requirements. Equipment and supply rooms should be decentralized, placing them near the appropriate ORs.

Central Control Desk

From a central control point, traffic in and out of the surgical suite may be observed. This area usually is within the unrestricted area. The clerk-receptionist is located at the control desk to coordinate communications. A pass-through window may be used to stop unauthorized people, to schedule surgical procedures with surgeons, or to receive drugs, blood, and various small supplies. A computerized pneumatic tube system within the hospital can speed the delivery of small items and paperwork, thus eliminating some courier services, such as from the pharmacy to the control desk. Tissue specimens or blood samples also can be sent to the laboratory through some tube systems.

Computers may be located in the control area. Automated information systems and computers assist in financial management, statistical recording and analysis, scheduling of patients and personnel, materials management, and other functions that evaluate the use of facilities. An integrated system interfaces with other hospital departments. It may have a modem or wireless Internet that allows surgeons to schedule surgical procedures directly from their offices.

Retrieval for review of patient records gives the perioperative nurse manager the opportunity to evaluate the patient care given and documented by nurses. Personnel records can be maintained. Other essential records can be stored in and retrieved from computer databases. The central processing unit for the OR computer system usually is located in or near the central administrative control area. A fax machine may be available for the electronic transfer of documents, records, and patient care orders between the OR and surgeons' offices.

Security systems usually can be monitored from the central administrative control area. Alarms are incorporated into electrical and piped-in systems to alert personnel to the location of a system failure. A centralized emergency call system facilitates summoning help. Narcotics are kept locked up and can be signed out only by appropriate personnel. Access to exchange areas, offices, and storage areas may be limited during evening and night hours and on weekends. Doors may be locked. Some hospitals use alarm systems, television surveillance, and/or electronic metal detection devices to control intruders and to prevent vandalism. Computers and records must be secured to protect patients' confidentiality.

Offices

Offices for the administrative patient care personnel and the anesthesia department should be located with access to both unrestricted and semirestricted areas. The staff members frequently need to confer with outside people and to be kept informed of activities within all areas of the suite.

Conference Room/Classroom

Ideally, a conference room or a classroom is located within the semirestricted area. This is used for patient care staff inservice educational programs and is used by the surgical staff for teaching. Closed-circuit television and/or video-cassettes may also be available for self-study. The departmental reference library may be housed here.

Support Services

The size of the health care facility and the types of services provided determine whether laboratory and radiology equipment is needed within the surgical suite.

Laboratory. A small laboratory where the pathologist can examine tissue specimens and perform frozen sections expedites the decisions that the surgeon must make during a surgical procedure when a diagnosis is questionable. A designated refrigerator for storing blood for transfusions also may be located in this room. Tissue specimens may be tested here by frozen section before they are delivered to the pathology department for permanent section.

Radiology Services. Special procedure rooms may be outfitted with radiologic and other imaging equipment for diagnostic and invasive radiologic procedures or insertion of catheters, pacemakers, and other devices. The walls of these rooms contain lead shields to confine radiation. A darkroom for processing radiographic films usually is available within the surgical suite for immediate processing of scout films or contrast dye studies of organ systems.

Work and Storage Areas

Clean and sterile supplies and equipment are separated from soiled items and trash. If the surgical suite has a clean core area, only clean or sterile items are stored there. Soiled items are taken to the decontamination area for processing before being stored, or they are taken to the disposal area. Work and storage areas are provided for handling all types of supplies and equipment, whether clean or contaminated.

Anesthesia Work and Storage Areas. Space must be provided for storing anesthesia equipment and supplies. Gas tanks are stored in a well-ventilated area separated from other supplies. Care is taken not to allow tanks or cylinders to be knocked over or damaged. They should stand upright in a secure, stable base for safety. Nondisposable items must be thoroughly decontaminated and cleaned after use in an area separate from sterile supplies. A separate workroom usually is provided for care and processing of anesthesia equipment. Dirty and clean supplies must be kept separated.

The storage area includes a secured space for drugs and anesthetic agents. Some facilities have drug-dispensing machines that require positive identification to obtain medications for patient use. Larger facilities have a pharmaceutical station where a pharmacist dispenses drugs on a per-case basis. Signatures are required for controlled substances. Unused drugs are returned to the pharmacist for accountability.

Housekeeping Storage Areas. Cleaning supplies and equipment need to be stored; the equipment used within the restricted area is kept separate from that used to clean the other areas. Therefore, more than one storage area may be provided for housekeeping purposes, depending on the design and size of the surgical suite. Sinks are provided, as well as shelves for supplies. Trash and soiled laundry receptacles should not be allowed to accumulate in the same room where clean supplies are kept; separate areas should be provided for these. Conveyors or designated elevators may be provided for prompt removal of bags of soiled laundry and trash from the suite.

Central Processing Area. Conveyors, dumbwaiters, or elevators connect the surgical suite with a central processing area on another floor of the hospital. If efficient material flow can be accomplished, support functions can be removed from the surgical suite. Effective communications and a reliable transportation system must be established. Some ORs send all of their instruments and supplies to the sterile processing department for cleaning, packaging, sterilizing, and storing. This system eliminates the need for some work and storage areas within the surgical suite, but exchange areas must be provided for carts. The movement of clean and sterile supplies must be kept separate from that of contaminated items and waste by means of space and traffic patterns.

Utility Room. Some hospitals use a closed-cart system and take contaminated instruments to a central area outside the surgical suite for cleanup. Some perform cleanup procedures in the substerile room. Many, by virtue of the limitations of the physical facilities, bring the instruments to a utility room. This room contains a washer-sterilizer, sinks, cabinets, and all necessary aids for cleaning. If the washer-sterilizer is a pass-through unit, it opens also into the general workroom, which eliminates the task of physically moving instruments from one room to another.

General Workroom. The general work area should be as centrally located in the surgical suite as possible to keep contamination to a minimum. The work area may be divided into a cleaning area and a preparation area. If instruments and equipment from the utility room are received from the pass-through washer-sterilizer into this room, an ultrasonic cleaner should be available here for cleaning instruments that the washer-sterilizer has not adequately cleaned. Otherwise, the ultrasonic cleaner may be in the utility room.

Instrument sets, basin sets, trays, and other supplies are wrapped for sterilization here. The preparation and sterilization of instrument trays and sets in a central room ensure control. This room also contains the stock supply of other items that are packaged for sterilization. The sterilizers that are used in this room may open also into the next room, the sterile supply room. This arrangement helps to eliminate the possibility of mixing sterile and nonsterile items.

Storage

Technology nearly tripled the need for storage space in the 1980s. Many older surgical suites have inadequate facilities for storage of sterile supplies, instruments, and bulky equipment. Storage space should fit logically into the design of the suite. Those responsible for calculating adequate storage space for instruments, sterile and unsterile supplies, and mobile equipment, such as special OR beds, specialty carts, and equipment, should consider the size of the entire surgical suite. The size of the entire suite is calculated into square

feet, and 50% of the total number of square footage of the department is added to serve as storage. This floor space does not include additional storage space needed for postanesthesia equipment. Using a case cart system may slightly decrease the amount of instrument space needed. Plans should include accommodation for the size of each type of case cart used and the numbers that will be in the suite at a given point in the daily surgical schedule.

Sterile Supply Room. Most hospitals keep a supply of sterile drapes, sponges, gloves, gowns, and other sterile items ready for use in a sterile supply room within the surgical suite. As many shelves as possible should be freestanding from the walls, which permits supplies to be put into one side and removed from the other; thus older packages are always used first. However, small items must be contained in boxes or bins to prevent them from falling to the floor. Inventory levels should be large enough to prevent running out of supplies, yet overstocking of sterile supplies should be avoided. Storage should be arranged to facilitate stock rotation.

The sterile storage area should be adjacent to or as close as possible to the sterilizing area if sterilizing is done in the surgical suite. Access to the sterile storage area should be limited; it should be separated from high-traffic areas. Humidity should be controlled at 30% to 60%, and temperature should be 68° to 75° F (20° to 24° C). Humidity in excess of 70% would cause concern for condensation within sterile packages and may permit microorganism transfer by capillary action. There should be positive pressure with a minimum of four fresh air exchanges per hour in the sterile storage area.[1]

Instrument Room. Most hospitals have a separate room or a section of the general workroom designated for storing nonsterile instruments. The instrument room contains cupboards in which all clean and decontaminated instruments are stored when not in use. Instruments usually are segregated on shelves according to surgical specialty services.

Sets of basic instruments are usually cleaned, assembled, and sterilized after each use. Special instruments such as intestinal clamps, kidney forceps, and bone instruments may be stored after cleaning and decontamination. Sets are then made up according to each specialty as needed.

Storage Room. Some large, portable equipment must also be stored in the surgical suite, readily accessible for use. A storage room for this equipment, such as the orthopedic table that may not be used daily, keeps equipment out of corridors when not in use. Lasers and video equipment can be damaged if inadvertently bumped by a passing stretcher in a corridor.

Scrub Room

An enclosed area for preoperative cleansing of hands and arms should be provided adjacent to each OR. Water spills on the floor are particularly hazardous if the scrub area is

[1]AAMI ST46: Good hospital practice: steam sterilization and sterility assurance, AAMI Standards and Recommended Practices Part I, 2000.

in a traffic corridor. An enclosed scrub room is a restricted area within the surgical suite. Paper towel dispensers and mirrors should be located in this area. Trash receptacles, limited to only those items used within this room, should be emptied several times per day. Some facilities have boxes of additional caps, masks, shoe covers, and eye protection in the event of biologic contamination requiring a change of these items during a procedure. The contaminated item should be discarded in the biohazardous trash bin in the OR after changing.

OPERATING ROOM

Each OR is a restricted area because of the need to maintain a controlled environment for sterile and aseptic techniques (Fig. 10-5).

Size

The size of individual ORs varies. In the interest of economy and flexibility, it is desirable to have all ORs the same size so that they can be used interchangeably to accommodate elective and emergency surgical procedures. Adequate size for a multipurpose procedure room for ambulatory surgery or endoscopy is at least 20 × 20 × 10 feet (6 × 6 × 3 m), or 400 square feet (approximately 37 m²) of clear floor space. Approximately 20 square feet of space should be planned between fixed cabinets and shelves on two opposing walls. Larger rooms for cardiac or other large procedures are 20 × 30 × 10 feet (600 square feet [approximately 60 m²]). Renovated rooms may be 360 square feet with 18 feet between the fixed shelving units.

A room may be designed for a specialty service if use by that service will be high. The room must accommodate equipment, such as lasers, microscopes, or video equipment, either fixed (permanently installed) or portable (movable). Portable equipment may require more floor space—a minimum of 22 × 22 × 10 feet (484 square feet [approximately 45 m²]). A specialized room, such as one equipped for cardiopulmonary bypass or trauma, may require as much as 600 square feet (approximately 60 m²) of useful space.

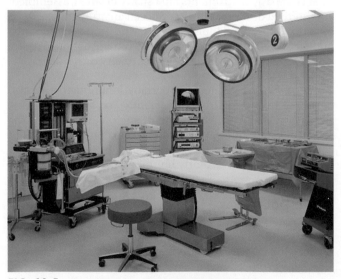

FIG. 10-5 Basic operating room. *(Courtesy Grey McVicar. In Lewis et al: Medical-surgical nursing: assessment and management of clinical problems, ed 7, St. Louis, 2007, Mosby.)*

Some rooms are designated for special procedures, such as gastrointestinal endoscopy, interventional radiologic studies, or the application of casts. Other rooms have adjacent areas used for specific purposes, such as visitor viewing galleries, or for installing special equipment, such as monitors.

Substerile Room

A group of two, three, or four ORs may be clustered around a central scrub area, work area, and a small substerile room. Only if the last-mentioned room is immediately adjacent to the OR and separated from the scrub area will it be considered the substerile room throughout this text.

A substerile room adjacent to the OR contains enclosed storage cupboards, a sink, steam sterilizer, a STERIS unit, and a warming cabinet. Although cleaning and sterilizing facilities are centralized, either inside or outside of the surgical suite, a substerile room with this equipment offers the following advantages:

- It saves time and steps. The circulating nurse can do emergency cleaning and sterilization of items here. This reduces waiting time for the surgeon, reduces anesthesia time for the patient, and saves steps for the circulating nurse. The circulating nurse, or scrub person if necessary, can lift sterile articles directly from the sterilizer onto the sterile instrument table without transporting them through a corridor or another area.
- It reduces the need for other personnel to obtain sterile instruments and allows the circulating nurse to stay within the room.
- It allows for better care of instruments and equipment that require special handling. Certain delicate or sensitive instruments or perhaps a surgeon's personally owned set usually are not sent out of the surgical suite. Only the personnel directly responsible for their use and care handle them; the circulating nurse and scrub person can clean them within the confines of the OR and this adjacent room.
- Rooms adjacent to orthopedic or cast rooms should have a sink with a plaster trap for disposal of casting solutions.
- The substerile room also usually contains a combination blanket and solution warmer, cabinets for storage, and perhaps a refrigerator for blood and medications. Empty sterile specimen containers and labels may be conveniently stored in this room. Slips for charges or other records may be kept here. Individual hospitals may find it convenient to keep other items in this room to allow the circulating nurse to remain in or immediately adjacent to the OR during the surgical procedure.

Doors

Doors should be 4 feet wide for ease in moving patients on carts and in beds. Ideally, sliding doors should be used exclusively in the OR. They eliminate the air currents caused by swinging doors. Microorganisms that have previously settled in the room are disturbed with each swing of the door. The microbial count is usually at its peak at the time of the skin incision, because this follows disturbance of air by gowning, draping, movement of personnel, and opening and closing of doors. During the surgical procedure, the microbial count rises every time doors swing open from either direction. Also, swinging doors may touch a sterile table or person. The risk of catching hands, equipment cords, or other supplies is increased. Doors should not swing out into the hallway.

Sliding doors should not recede into the wall like pocket styles, but should be of the surface-sliding type. Fire regulations mandate that sliding doors for ORs be of the type that can be swung open if necessary. Doors do not remain open either during or between surgical procedures. The room air circulation is higher pressure than in the halls to minimize the amount of dust and debris pulled in toward the sterile field. Closed doors decrease the mixing of air within the OR with that in the corridors, which may contain higher microbial counts. Air pressure in the room also is disrupted if the doors remain open.

When construction or renovation is in process, it is important to always keep the doors closed when not transporting patients. The air-handling systems are under a strain because of the disrupted processes and are further compromised when the airflow is allowed to equalize. This causes unstable temperature and humidity control. The desired temperature should be between 68° and 73° F (20° and 23° C), with a relative humidity of 30% to 60%. The risk for airborne contaminants is significantly increased.

Ventilation

The OR ventilation system must ensure a controlled supply of filtered air. Air changes and circulation provide fresh air and prevent accumulation of anesthetic gases in the room. Concentration of gases depends solely on the proportion of pure air entering the air system to the air being recirculated through the system. Fifteen air exchanges per hour with three exchanges of fresh air are recommended for operating rooms with recirculated air.[2] Some state building codes require 100% fresh air; others permit up to 80% recirculation of air. If air is recirculated, a gas scavenger system is mandatory to prevent the buildup of waste anesthetic gases. Various types of scavengers and evacuators are used to minimize air pollutants that are health risks for perioperative team members.

Ultraclean laminar airflow is installed in some ORs to provide up to 600 air exchanges per hour. This high-flow, unidirectional air-blowing system is housed in a wall or ceiling enclosure. The airflow can be vertical or horizontal. Staff should not pass between the airflow and the sterile field or the purpose for using ultraclean air is defeated.

Laminar airflow was first trialed during hip replacement surgery by Sir John Charnley in Great Britain in the 1950s. Charnley believed that if particulate could be removed from the air, the 7% infection rate could drop. His studies showed that the infection rate did fall to less than 2%. The value of this system in reducing airborne contamination is inconclusive because the rate continued to fall to less than 1% with changes in surgical dressing practices. Although the laminar system contributes to removing particulates, the improvements in sterile technique overall may have a larger effect on infection rate.

Other types of filtered air-delivery systems that have a high rate of airflow are as effective in controlling airborne contamination. Filtration through high-efficiency particulate air (HEPA) filters can be 99.7% efficient in removing particles that are larger than 0.3 mm. These microbial filters in ducts filter the air, practically eliminating all dust particles. The ventilating system in the surgical suite is separate from the hospital's general system and is to be cleaned, inspected, and maintained on a preventive maintenance (PM) schedule.

Positive air pressures (0.005 inch [0.013 cm] of water pressure) of 10% in each OR are greater than that in corridors, scrub areas, and substerile rooms. Positive pressure forces air from the room. The inlet is at the ceiling. Air leaves through the outlets at floor level. If the reverse is true, air is drawn into the room around the doors and through open doors. Microorganisms in the air can enter the room unless positive pressure is maintained. Closed doors maintain this environment and prevent equalization of air pressure. The recommended parameters include a dual filtration system with two filters in succession. The first filter should be at least 30% efficient, and the second filter should be at least 90%.

An air-conditioning system controls humidity. High relative humidity (weight of water vapor present) should be maintained between 30% and 60%. A relative humidity of not less than 50% to 55% is ideal. Moisture provides a relatively conductive medium, allowing static charge to leak to earth as fast as it is generated; sparks form more readily in atmospheres of low humidity.

Operating room temperature is maintained within a range of 68° to 73° F (20° to 23° C). A thermostat to control room temperature can be advantageous to meet patient needs; for example, the temperature can be increased to prevent hypothermia in pediatric, geriatric, or burn patients. Overmanipulation of controls can result in calibration problems. Controls should not be adjusted solely for the comfort of team members; patient normothermia is a strong consideration. Only the maintenance department can regulate temperature in some surgical suites.

Even with controls of humidity and temperature, air-conditioning units may be a source of microorganisms that come through the filters. The filters are changed at regular intervals. Ducts are cleaned by maintenance personnel on a regular schedule.

Floors

In the past, floors were conductive enough to dissipate static from equipment and personnel but not enough to endanger personnel from shock or cause explosions from flammable anesthetic gases. Conductivity is not a prime concern in OR design because explosive anesthetic gases are no longer used. The most common flooring used today is seamless polyvinyl chloride that is continued up the sides of the wall for 5 or 6 inches and welded into place. These materials should not degrade or stain with age and cleaning. Metal oxides can be incorporated to decrease the slipperiness of the surface when wet.

[2]American Institute of Architects Academy of Architecture for Health, Facilities Guidelines Institute, "General hospital" in *Guidelines for Design and Construction of Hospital and Health Care Facilities, 2001* (Dallas: Facilities Guidelines Institute, 2001) 72.

A variety of hard plastic, seamless materials are used for minor procedure room floors. The surface of all floors should not be porous but suitably hard for cleaning by the flooding, wet-vacuuming technique. Personnel fatigue may be related to the type of flooring, which can be too hard or too soft. Cushioned flooring is available. The floor should be slip-proof when wet because surgical hand cleansing causes splashes and spills around the scrub sink and into the OR, where the hands are dried.

Most of the glues and adhesives used in the installation of the flooring are malodorous and potentially toxic. During construction or renovation, care is taken to vent these fumes from the area. A minimum of 2 weeks may be needed to fully rid the area of the smell before it can be safely used for patient care.

Walls and Ceiling

Finishes of all surface materials should be hard, nonporous, fire-resistant, waterproof, stain-proof, seamless, nonreflective, and easy to clean. The ceiling should be a minimum of 10 feet (3 m) high and have seamless construction. The height of the ceiling will depend on the amount and types of ceiling-mounted equipment. The ceiling color should be white to reflect at least 90% of the light in even dispersion.

Walls should be a pastel color, with paneling made of hard vinyl materials that is easy to clean and maintain. Seams should be sealed by a silicone sealant. Laminated polyester or smooth, painted plaster provides a seamless wall; epoxy paint has a tendency to flake or chip. Dust and microorganisms can collect between tiles, because the mortar between them is not smooth. Most grout lines, including those made of latex, are porous enough to harbor microorganisms even after cleaning. Tiles can also crack and break. A material that is able to withstand considerable impact also may have some value in noise control. Stainless steel cuffs at collision corners help prevent damage.

Walls and ceilings often are used to mount devices, utilities, and equipment in an effort to reduce clutter on the floor. The ceilings should be reinforced with steel beams to support the load. In addition to the overhead operating light, the ceiling may be used for mounting an anesthesia service column, operating microscope, cryosurgery device, x-ray tube and image intensifier, electronic monitor, closed-circuit television monitor and camera, and a variety of hooks, poles, and tubes. Demands for ceiling-mounted equipment are diversified.

Suspended track mounts are not recommended because they engender fallout of dust-carrying microorganisms each time they are moved. If movable or track ceiling devices are installed, they should not be mounted directly over the operating bed but away from the center of the room and preferably recessed into the ceiling to minimize the possibility of dust accumulation and fallout.

Piped-In Gases, Computer Lines, and Electrical Systems

Vacuum for suction, anesthetic gas evacuation, compressed air, oxygen, and/or nitrous oxide may be piped into the OR. The outlets may be located on the wall or suspended from the ceiling in either a fixed, rotating orbiter or in a retractable column. The anesthesia provider needs at least two outlets

for oxygen and suction and one for nitrous oxide. To protect other rooms, the supply of oxygen and nitrous oxide to any room can be shut off at control panels in the corridor should trouble occur in a particular line. A panel light comes on, and a buzzer sounds in the room and in the maintenance department. The buzzer can be turned off, but the panel light stays on until the problem is corrected. The buzzer should be tested on a routine schedule.

Computer lines for monitors or personal computers (PCs) are commonly located adjacent to the anesthesia machine and the circulating nurse's writing desk. Additional lines may be attached to computers used in specialties such as neurosurgery, which uses immediate computed tomography (CT) scanning images during the intraoperative care period. Care is taken not to use the keyboard with soiled hands or soiled examination gloves. The keyboard should be of a design that permits adequate cleaning between patients.

Electrical outlets must meet the requirements of the equipment that will be used. Some machines require 220-volt power lines; others operate on 110 volts. Permanently mounted fixtures, such as a clock and radiograph view-boxes, can be recessed into walls and wired rather than plugged into outlets. Outlets suspended from the ceiling should have locking Hubble plugs to prevent accidental disconnection. Grounded wall outlets are used. Electrical cords that extend down the wall and/or across the floor are hazardous. Straight or curved ceiling-mounted tracks are satisfactory for bringing piped-in gases, vacuums, and electrical outlets close to the operating bed. They eliminate the hazard of tripping over cords, but insulation materials around electrical power sources from mobile ceiling-mounted tracks must be protected from repeated flexing to prevent cracks and damage to wires. Rigid or retractable ceiling service columns eliminate these hazards.

Multiple electrical outlets should be available from separate circuits. This minimizes the possibility of a blown fuse or a faulty circuit shutting off all electricity at a critical moment.

All personnel must be aware that the use of electricity introduces the hazards of electric shock, power failure, and fire. Faulty electrical equipment may cause a short circuit or the electrocution of patients or personnel. These hazards can be prevented by taking the following precautions:

1. Use only electrical equipment designed and approved for use in the OR. Equipment must have cords of adequate length and adequate current-carrying capacity to avoid overloading.
2. Test portable equipment immediately before use.
3. Discontinue use immediately if any malfunction takes place, and report any faulty electrical equipment.
4. If a ground fault buzzer sounds, unplug the last device engaged and remove it from service.

Fire safety systems are installed throughout the hospital. All personnel must know the fire rules. They must be familiar with the location of the alarm box and the use of fire extinguishers.

Lighting

General illumination is furnished by ceiling lights. Most room lights are white fluorescent but may be incandescent. Recessed lights do not collect dust. Lighting should be evenly distributed throughout the room without harsh shadows. The anesthesia provider must have sufficient light, at least 200 foot-candles, to adequately evaluate the patient's color. Intraoperatively, the lighting should not cause the organs to appear discolored.

To minimize eye fatigue, the ratio of intensity of general room lighting to that at the surgical site should not exceed 1:5, preferably 1:3. This contrast should be maintained in corridors and scrub areas, as well as in the room itself, so that the surgeon becomes accustomed to the light before entering the sterile field. Color and hue of the lights also should be consistent.

Illumination of the surgical site depends on the quality of light from an overhead spotlight source and the reflection from the drapes and tissues. Drapes should be blue, green, or gray to avoid eye fatigue. White, glistening tissues need less light than dull, dark tissues. Light must be of such quality that the pathologic conditions are recognizable. The overhead operating light must:

- Make an intense light, within a range of 2500 to 12,500 foot-candles (27,000 to 127,000 lux), into the incision without glare on the surface. It must give contrast to the depth and relationship of all anatomic structures. The light may be equipped with an intensity control. The surgeon will ask for more light when needed. A reserve light should be available.
- Provide a light pattern that has a diameter and focus appropriate for the size of the incision. An optical prism system has a fixed diameter and focus. Other types have adjustable controls mounted on the fixture. Most fixtures provide focused depth by refracting light to illuminate both the body cavity and the general operating field. The focal point is where illumination is greatest. It should not create a dark center at the surgical site. A 10- to 12-inch (25 to 30 cm) depth of focus allows the intensity to be relatively equal at both the surface and depth of the incision. To avoid glare, a circular field of 20 inches (50 cm) in diameter provides a 2-inch (5-cm) zone of maximum intensity in the center of the field with 20% intensity at the periphery.
- Be shadowless. Multiple light sources and/or reflectors decrease shadows. In some units the relationship is fixed; others have separately maneuverable sources to direct light beams from converging angles.
- Produce the blue-white color of daylight. Color quality of normal or diseased tissues is maintained within a spectral energy range of 3500° to 6700° Kelvin (K). Most surgeons prefer a color temperature of about 5000° K, which approximates the white light of a cloudless sky at noon.
- Be freely adjustable to any position or angle by either a vertical or horizontal range of motion. Most overhead operating lights are ceiling-mounted on mobile fixtures. Some have dual lights or dual tracks with sources on each track. These are designed for both lights to be used simultaneously to provide adequate intensity and minimize shadows in a single incision. Many fixtures are adapted so that the surgeon can direct the beam by manipulating sterile handles attached to the lamp or by remote control at the sterile field. Automatic positioning facilitates adjustment, and braking mechanisms

prevent drift (i.e., a movement away from the desired position). Fixtures should be manipulated as little as possible to minimize dispersion of dust over the sterile field. To obtain the best illumination in the shortest time, the first spotlight should be positioned at the surgical site, followed by the second. Ideally, the light can be maneuvered in a 360-degree rotation as needed, quickly and without effort. Smaller lights commonly are restricted because of wiring bundles.

- Produce a minimum of heat to prevent injuring and drying exposed tissues. Most overhead lights dissipate heat into the room, where it is cooled by the air-conditioning system. Halogen bulbs generate less heat than do other types. Lamps should produce less than 25,000 mW/cm^2 of radiant energy. If multiple light sources are used, collectively they must not exceed this limit at a single site. Beyond this range, the radiant energy produced by infrared rays changes to heat at or near the surface of exposed tissues. A filter globe absorbs some infrared and heat waves over the lightbulb or by an infrared cylindric absorption filter of a prism optical system.
- Be easily cleaned and maintained. Tracks recessed within the ceiling virtually eliminate dust accumulation. Suspension-mounted tracks or a centrally mounted fixture must have smooth surfaces that are easily accessible for cleaning. Lightbulbs should have a reasonably long life. Changing the bulb should not require additional tools because time may be an issue in a critical part of a surgical procedure. The bulb is usually too hot to touch with the bare hand. Many styles are available that contain several bulbs that provide backup light when one bulb burns out.

A supplemental surgical task light may be needed for a secondary surgical site, such as for the legs or arms during conduit procurement for cardiovascular procedures. Some hospitals have portable explosion-proof lights. These lights should have a wide base and should be tip-proof. Others have satellite units that are part of the overhead lighting fixture. These should be used only for secondary sites unless the manufacturer states that the additional intensity is within safe radiant energy levels when used in conjunction with the main light source. The use of multiple teams in complex multidisciplinary procedures requires adequate lighting for each operating surgeon.

A source of light from a circuit separate from the usual supply must be available for use in case of power failure. This may require a separate emergency spotlight. It is best if the operating light is equipped so that an automatic switch can be made to the emergency source of lighting when the usual power fails. Flashlights with fresh batteries should always be immediately available.

Some surgeons prefer to work in a darkened room with only stark illumination off the surgical site. This is particularly true of surgeons working with endoscopic instruments and the operating microscope. If the room has windows, light-proof shades may be drawn to darken the room when this equipment is in use. Because of the hazard of dust fallout from shades, the windows may have blinds contained between two panes of glass with a handle to open or close the louvers in rooms where this equipment is routinely used. Although the surgeon may prefer the room darkened, the circulating nurse or anesthesia provider must be able to see adequately to observe the patient's color and to monitor his or her condition. One spotlight can be aimed away from the field in the direction of the anesthesia provider. In some circumstances, the radiograph view-box can be turned on for additional illumination.

Some surgeons wear an adjustable headlight designed to focus a light beam on a specific area, usually in a recessed body cavity such as the nasopharynx. Fiberoptic headlights produce a cool light and reduce shadows. Both the surgeon and first assistant may wear a headlight. Alternatively, a light source that is an integral part of a sterile instrument, such as a lighted retractor or fiberoptic cable, may be used to illuminate deep cavities or tissues difficult to see with only the overhead operating light. Fiberoptic cables should not be permitted to become detached from the instrument and shine directly on the drape for a prolonged period, because a fire may ignite.

Radiograph View-Boxes

Radiograph view-boxes can be recessed into the wall. The viewing surface should accommodate a minimum of four standard-size films. The best location is in the line of vision of the surgeon standing at the operating bed. An additional view-box should be located near the anesthesia provider for review of chest films. It can also provide indirect illumination of the anesthesia machine or instrument table during procedures requiring a darkened room. Lights for view-boxes should be of high intensity. A film-holding basket should be planned within reach of each view-box station.

Many facilities have changed from plain film viewing to digital computer monitors. In this circumstance it is still useful to have lighted view-boxes available in the event old films are brought from the archives for comparison with the patient's new digital images.

Clocks

Two clocks should be in each OR. A standard clock for basic time observation should be visible from the field. A time-elapsed clock, which incorporates a warning signal, is useful for indicating that one or more predetermined periods of time have passed. This may be used during surgical procedures for total arterial occlusion, when using perfusion techniques or a pneumatic tourniquet, or during cardiac arrest. Start, stop, and reset buttons should be within reach of the anesthesia provider and the circulating nurse.

Cabinets or Carts

Each OR may be supplied with stationary cabinetry unless a cart system or pass-through entry is used. Supplies for the types of surgical procedures done in that room are stocked, or every OR may be stocked with a standard number and type of supplies. Having these basic supplies saves steps for the circulating nurse and helps eliminate traffic in and out of the OR. Glass shelves and sliding doors provide ease in finding and removing items. Many cabinets are made of stainless steel or hard plastic. Wire shelving minimizes dust accumulation. Cabinets should be easy to clean. One cabinet in the room may have a pegboard at the back to hang items,

such as table appliances. Gloves used in patient care should be removed when opening the cabinet and removing supplies.

Pass-through cabinets that circulate clean air through them while maintaining positive air room pressure allow transfer of supplies from outside the OR to inside it. They help ensure the rotation of supplies in storage or can be used only for passing supplies as needed from a clean center core. Some pass-through cabinets between the OR and a corridor accommodate supply carts directly from the sterile core, which are easily removable for restocking.

In lieu of or as an adjunct to cabinets, some hospitals stock carts with special sutures, instruments, drugs, and other items for some or all of the surgical specialties. The appropriate cart is brought to the room for a specific surgical procedure.

Furniture and Other Equipment

Stainless steel furniture is plain, durable, and easily cleaned. Each OR is equipped with the following:

- Operating bed with a mattress covered with an impervious surface, attachments for positioning the patient, and armboards.
- Instrument tables. These are commonly called "back tables," although they are actually at the side of the scrub person during the surgical procedure.
- Mayo stand. The Mayo stand is a frame with a removable rectangular stainless steel tray. The frame slides under the operating bed and over the sterile field. The tray serves to bring near the surgical field a supply of instruments that are used frequently during the surgical procedure.
- Small tables for gowns and gloves and/or the patient's skin preparation equipment and catheterization supplies.
- Ring stand for basin(s). This is optional because most ORs do not use splash basins.
- Anesthesia machine and table for anesthesia provider's equipment.
- Sitting stools and standing platforms.
- IV poles for IV solution bags.
- Suction canisters, preferably portable on a wheeled base.
- Laundry hamper frame.
- Kick buckets in wheeled bases. Commonly called "sponge buckets."
- Wastebasket.
- Writing surface. This may be a wall-mounted stainless steel desk or an area built into a cabinet for the circulating nurse to document in the records.
- Computer terminal station. This may be permanently affixed to a hardwired station or mobile wireless. The keyboard should be positioned so the circulating nurse can observe the sterile field. A scanning device may be incorporated for bar-coded drugs and supplies.

Communication Systems

A communication system is a vital link to summon routine or emergency assistance or to relay information to and from the OR team. Many surgical suites are equipped with telephones, intercoms, call-lights, video equipment, and computers. These communication systems may connect the OR with the clerk-receptionist's desk, the nurse manager's office, the holding area, the family waiting room, the PACU, the pathology and radiology departments, the blood bank, and the sterile processing department. These systems make instantaneous consultation possible through direct communication.

Voice Intercommunication System. Either monodirectional or bidirectional voice systems, via telephone or an intercommunication (intercom) system, are useful devices for the OR team but are potentially hazardous for the patient. Sounds are distorted to the patient in early stages of general anesthesia. Incoming calls over an intercom should not be permitted to disturb the patient at this time. Also, an awake patient should not receive traumatic information about a pathologic diagnosis (e.g., from a strange voice coming through an intercom speaker box after a biopsy has been performed). Installing any type of intercom equipment either in the adjacent substerile room or scrub area rather than in the OR helps eliminate sounds that could disturb both the patient and the surgeon.

Call-light System. In addition to or instead of a voice system, a call-light system can summon assistance from the anesthesia staff, pathologist, patient care staff, and housekeeping personnel. Activated in the OR by a foot- or hand-operated switch, a light alerts personnel at a central point in the suite or displays at several receiving points simultaneously.

Closed-Circuit Television. Television surveillance is an easy way for the nurse manager to keep abreast of activities in each OR. By means of a black-and-white or color video camera with a wide-angle lens mounted high in the corner of each OR, the manager may make rounds simply by switching from one room to another by pushing buttons at his or her desk and viewing a monitor in the office. Signs should be posted to indicate that video surveillance is in process.

More commonly, television monitors serve a number of useful purposes for the surgeon within the OR. They are widely used for teaching surgical techniques. This minimizes the number of visitors in the OR, which, in the interest of sterile technique, is advantageous. In addition, monitors provide a better view for more people to see the surgical procedure from a remote area or through a microscope or endoscope. They can also be used for record keeping and documentation for legal purposes for the surgeon. Video recording is possible for this purpose. If video recording is done while patients are in the rooms, each patient should have the opportunity to sign a permission form.

As an aid to diagnosis, an audiovisual hookup between the OR and the radiology department permits radiographs to be viewed on the television screen in the OR without having to be transported into the OR and mounted on view-boxes. With such a hookup, the surgeon gains the advantage of remote interpretive consultation when it is desired.

A two-way audiovisual system between the frozen-section laboratory and the OR enables the surgeon to examine the microscopic slide by video in consultation with the pathologist without leaving the operating bed. The pathologist can view the site of the pathologic lesion without entering the OR.

For these purposes the color television camera may be mounted over the operating bed in a number of ways. Usually it is attached to the stem of the operating light and outfitted with detachable sterilizable handles. An operating light with a television camera mounted in the center is available.

Video screens usually are adapted television sets and may be wall mounted or placed on floor stands that can be moved readily. All pieces of television equipment must be labeled to indicate that they comply with applicable electrical safety regulations for use in the OR. They also must be encased in nonporous materials that can be easily cleaned.

Computers. A computer terminal or PC in each OR affords access to information and allows data input by the circulating nurse. The type of hardware and software programs available dictates the capabilities of the automated information system. A keyboard, light pen, and/or bar-code scanner may be used for input. The computer processes and stores information for retrieval on the viewing monitor and by printout from a central processing unit. The system should be wireless for fast transmission of data and should require a password of each user in the system for security. The computer database helps the circulating nurse obtain and enter information that may include the following:

- Schedule, including the patient's name, surgeon, procedure, special or unusual equipment requirements, wound classification, whether procedure is elective or emergency
- Preoperative patient assessment data, nursing diagnoses, expected outcomes, and plan of care
- Results of laboratory and diagnostic tests
- Surgeon's preference card with capability to update
- Inventory of supplies and equipment provided and used
- Charges for direct patient billing
- Intraoperative nursing interventions
- Timing parameters, including anesthesia, procedure, and room turnover
- Incident reports
- Postoperative care in the PACU

The computer terminal may be mounted on the wall or placed on a shelf or a portable table or cart. The computer keyboard should be wireless so it can be moved so that the circulating nurse can see the patient and the activities of the OR team while electronically documenting intraoperative information into the record. The computerized patient information that is generated in the OR may interface with the hospital-wide computer system.

Monitoring Equipment

Monitors and computers are designed to keep the OR team aware of the physiologic functions of the patient throughout the surgical procedure and to record patient data. The anesthesia provider or a perioperative nurse uses monitoring devices as an added means to ensure safety for the patient during the surgical procedure.

SPECIAL PROCEDURE ROOMS

Certain procedures or outpatient treatments may indicate the need for rooms designed for a specific purpose, such as interventional radiology, endoscopy, or cystoscopy. These rooms are designed with equipment for performing the specific interventional procedures, including specialized radiologic and monitoring devices. A radiologist and several endoscopists should be consulted when planning these types of facilities.

Interventional Radiography Room

Endovascular stenting, balloon angioplasty, and other interventions requiring fluoroscopy can be performed in a room with fixed radiographic equipment and specialized radiographic beds (Fig. 10-6). The proximity to the OR is important in case of an emergency that necessitates an open procedure.

Cardiac catheterization may be performed within the surgical suite in a room equipped for fluoroscopy. Imaging screens are located near the head of the operating bed to allow the surgeon and the team to visualize the coronary arteries during the procedure. Monitors, suction, oxygen, and cardiopulmonary resuscitation equipment are available in this room for each cardiac catheterization procedure. The team must be alert for emergency situations, such as a perforated coronary artery, and be prepared for an emergency thoracotomy or transfer to an OR for an open procedure.

MIS Room (Minimally Invasive Surgery)

Some rooms are equipped for laparoscopic procedures. A dedicated MIS room has all the equipment for puncture endoscopy located on a large cart or a ceiling-mounted boom. The use of a boom in these rooms helps minimize the amount of equipment spread around the room by providing a central vertically organized placement of the machinery used for the procedure. Several TV monitors are located around the room for ergonomic viewing of the surgical field by the surgical team. The monitors can be attached to articulated arms on the main boom.

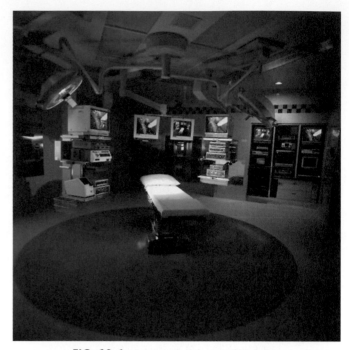

FIG. 10-6   Interventional operating room.

These rooms should have the capability of immediately converting to an open procedure in the event of an untoward event such as excessive bleeding.

Endoscopy Room. Many surgical suites have a designated room in which nonpuncture flexible or rigid endoscopic procedures, such as bronchoscopy, gastroscopy, sigmoidoscopy, or colonoscopy, are performed. Most are equipped for the use of lasers and electrosurgery. Some endoscopy rooms have radiographic and video capabilities. Some specialized equipment such as light sources can be permanently mounted from ceiling booms or orbiters and is not portable between rooms.

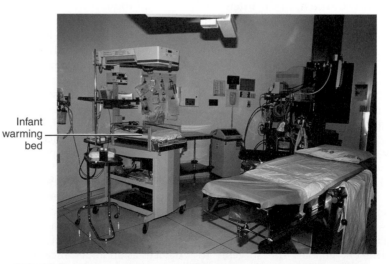

Infant warming bed

FIG. 10-7   Cesarean delivery room. *(Courtesy Michael S. Clement, M.D.)*

Cystoscopy Room. A cystoscopy room (cysto room) may be available for a urologic endoscopic examination or procedure. Ideally, the room should be 350 square feet with a minimum of 15 feet of clear space between fixed cabinets. Waste fluids are collected in special canisters and are disposed of like other biologically contaminated fluids. Older cystoscopy rooms may be equipped with special floor drains for the disposal of fluids during the procedure. Modern styles have eliminated this drain for infection control reasons.

A cysto room is also equipped with radiographic and fluoroscopy machines because many procedures require the use of radiopaque contrast media to visualize the kidneys, ureters, and bladder. Radiograph view-boxes should accommodate a minimum of four films simultaneously and may be situated near digital monitors. Imaging screens are located in the room to allow the urologist to visualize the urologic structures during fluoroscopy. Some urologists use ultrasonic equipment, lasers, and electrosurgery to perform minimally invasive procedures.

Cesarean Delivery Room. Most facilities that have obstetric departments will have a self contained operating room within the delivery suite (Fig. 10-7). This room is a restricted room with an attached substerile room and scrub sink area. The purpose of this room is to provide equipment and supplies in support of a surgical birth of the baby through the mother's abdomen (cesarean section) instead of a vaginal birth.

A few differences of the cesarean delivery room include resuscitation supplies and equipment for the newborn and a specialized warming bed that can be used to transport the baby to the special care nursery.

CONCLUSION

The surgical suite is a highly specialized area with distinct environmental controls for safety, cleanliness, and minimization of contamination. Personnel who work in the perioperative environment are required to know and understand the "hows and whys" of appropriate attire, what activities are safe, what environmental controls are in effect, and how to determine if the controls are effective. Environmental sanitation is described in Chapter 12 and environmental hazards are discussed in Chapter 13.

Bibliography

American Institute of Architects Committee on Architecture for Health in conjunction with Department of Health and Human Services: *Guidelines for construction and equipment of hospital and medical facilities,* Washington, DC, 1997, AIA Press.
AORN (Association of periOperative Registered Nurses): *AORN standards, recommended practices, and guidelines,* Denver, 2005, The Association.
Centers for Disease Control and Prevention: *Guidelines for prevention of surgical wound infection,* Atlanta, 1999, The Centers.
Chobin N: Construction in the sterile processing department, *SSM* 7(4):46-51, 2001.
Collins J: The team aspect of planning a new surgical services department, *SSM* 7(4):39-44, 2001.
Davis JL, Hollander SR: Construction project management, *SSM* 5(2):22-30, 1999.
Elledge JL: The surgery suite: Planning, design, and construction, *SSM* 7(4):11-20, 2001.
Fannin M: Domesticating birth in the hospital: Family-centered birth and the emergence of "homelike" birthing rooms, *Antipode* 35(3):513-535, 2003.
Friberg B: Ultraclean laminar airflow ORs, *AORN J* 67(4):841-851, 1998.
Haines RC, Brooks LR: Remodel or rebuild? *SSM* 5(2):32-35, 1999.
Illuminating Engineering Society of North America: RP-29 Lighting for hospitals and healthcare facilities, *SSM* 5(2):51-55, 1999.
Knepper B: Dirt and aspergillosis in surgical suite renovation: Planning a clean fight, *Infect Control Today* 6(1):26, 28, 2002.
McKee K: Surgeons speak out about surgical lights, *Outpatient Surg* 3(4):61-66, 2002.
Meltzer B: How to design a lap/endo suite, *Outpatient Surg* 3(3):18-26, 2002.
Osman C: Getting the OR ready, *Infect Control Today* 3(10):60-62, 1999.
Senn N: *A nurse's guide for the operating room,* ed 2, Chicago, 1905, Chicago Medical Book Co.
Stout G: Designing the ideal operating room, *Infect Control Today* 3(3):20-23, 1999.
Tydell PA: Nosocomial infection control during construction and renovation of healthcare facilities, *Infect Control Today* 6(6):47-49, 2002.
Warnshuis FC: Principles of surgical nursing, Philadelphia, 1918, Saunders.
Wetzel JC: Planning for effective OR design, *SSM* 7(4):21-25, 2001.

Chapter 11

Ambulatory Surgery Centers and Alternative Surgical Locations

CHAPTER OBJECTIVES

After studying this chapter, the learner will be able to:
- Compare the differences between hospital-based services and ambulatory surgery centers (ASCs).
- Distinguish between activities in fixed and mobile surgery locations.
- Describe key elements of human versus veterinary surgery.

CHAPTER OUTLINE

KEY TERMS AND DEFINITIONS

Ambulatory care   Care delivered to a patient who is not confined to bed or in need of formal admission to a facility for a prolonged period.

Deployment   A term that refers to sending one or more active duty soldiers forward into an area where medical war support is needed. Average length of stay is 3 days.

DEPMEDS   A system of mobile military hospital components that are assembled and dismantled close to the location of military activity.

Monitoring   Clinical observation of a patient's condition and vital signs through continuous interpretation of vital signs, activities, and responses.

PAT center   Area of a facility designated for patient assessment and preprocedural examination.

SUPPLEMENTAL MATERIAL ON EVOLVE WEBSITE

http://evolve.elsevier.com/BerryKohn
- Content Updates
- Glossary
- Full Set of Perioperative Flash Cards
- Interactive Key Term Flash Cards
- Student Activities
- WebLinks

HISTORICAL BACKGROUND

The concept of ambulatory surgery is not new; it can be traced back to Egypt in 3000 BC. Simple surgical procedures have been performed in physicians' offices for years. The first ambulatory surgery facility was opened in 1970 in Arizona. The concept gained widespread acceptance and was endorsed by the American Medical Association (AMA). Ambulatory surgery became acceptable for both local and general anesthesia with select patients, and in 1973 guidelines provided by the American Society of Anesthesiologists (ASA) strengthened the premise of same-day procedures.

For both patients and insurance providers, a cost savings is realized when the patient goes home after a short recovery period. Less invasive surgical procedures that allow for rapid return to function are well suited to ambulatory surgery. The number of surgical procedures performed as ambulatory or outpatient procedures increases each year.

Changes in minimally invasive technologies have been cost-effective, convenient, and efficient while remaining consistent with the same standards of care followed for hospitalized surgical patients. Patients have a right to expect comprehensive perioperative care from an ambulatory care facility. The risks, anxiety, and fears associated with a surgical procedure are not eliminated just because the setting is different or because advanced instrumentation is used.

AMBULATORY SURGICAL SETTING

Ambulatory surgery can be defined as surgical patient care performed under general, regional, or local anesthesia without overnight hospitalization. Some ASCs offer diagnostic testing and radiologic examinations, such as mammography.

Professional organizations with an ambulatory surgery focus are listed in Box 11-1. The following are organizations specifically for professional ambulatory surgical nurses:
- American Society of PeriAnesthesia Nurses (ASPAN)—www.aspan.org
- American Academy of Ambulatory Care Nurses (AAACN)—www.aaacn.org
- Association of periOperative Registered Nurses (AORN)—www.aorn.org

American Society of Anesthesiologists (ASA)—www.asahq.org

American Association for Accreditation of Ambulatory Surgery Facilities (AAAASF)—www.aaaasf.org

American Society of PeriAnesthesia Nurses (ASPAN)—www.aspan.org

Accreditation Association for Ambulatory Health Care (AAAHC)—www.aaahc.org

The Federated Ambulatory Surgery Association (FASA)—www.fasa.org

Joint Commission on Accreditation of Healthcare Organizations (JCAHO)—www.jcaho.org

Society for Ambulatory Anesthesia (SAMBA)—www.sambahq.org

American Academy of Ambulatory Care Nurses (AAACN)—www.aaacn.org

AORN has established a specialty assembly for nurses who practice in the ambulatory setting. A chairperson and council are selected by the assembly membership to serve 3-year terms. AORN's website has an ambulatory practice portal at www.aorn.org.

Ambulatory Surgery Programs

Various terms are used to describe ambulatory care facilities, including outpatient surgery, same-day surgical unit, day surgery, and ambulatory surgery center. Conceptually, an ambulatory facility has the following:

- Preprocedural testing and assessment area (PAT center)
- Admitting area
- Changing and dressing room with lockers and toilets
- Preoperative holding/preparation area
- Operating room (OR)
- Postanesthesia care unit (PACU) (or access to a PACU)
- Family waiting room

The decor of the ambulatory facility should be pleasing to enhance relaxation of the patient and family. Recliners are commonly available for postprocedure recovery. Many facilities have televisions with videocassette capability. Figure 11-1 depicts a sample floor plan showing the various areas within an ASC.

Priority patient parking areas should be conveniently located near the entrance to the facility, with parking spaces for disabled patients located nearest the entrance. Many hospital-based ASCs offer valet parking. The convenience of dropping off and picking up patients should be accommodated in the design of the facility. Studies have shown that this is a point of patient satisfaction. Space requirements for parking areas are determined by the number and types of surgical procedures to be performed.

The location of an ASC may vary. The Federated Ambulatory Surgery Association (FASA) indicates that a true ASC is not dependent on the main hospital and is physically independent in services, such as operating rooms, postprocedure care, and central service. ASCs are not designed to take emergency patients and typically employ fewer than 20 employees. Examples of outpatient surgery departments attached to hospitals include the following:

- Hospital-based dedicated unit. Patients come to a self-contained unit that is located within or attached to the hospital but physically separate from the inpatient OR suite.
- Hospital-based integrated unit. Ambulatory patients share the same OR suite and other hospital facilities with inpatients. The preoperative admission and holding area is shared. Ambulatory patients usually return to the same admission area for discharge after the procedure.
- Office-based center. Patients come to a physician's office that is equipped for surgery. Many private surgeons, dermatologists, periodontists, and podiatrists perform surgical procedures in their offices using a local anesthetic. This office-based center may accommodate one or more surgeons in the same specialty, or it may be a multiphysician, interdisciplinary clinic. Although these are not always attached to a hospital, they are not considered an ASC by FASA.
- Examples of ambulatory surgery centers by the definition of FASA are the following:
- Hospital-affiliated satellite surgery center. Patients come to an ambulatory surgery center that is owned and operated by a larger facility but geographically separate from it.
- Freestanding ambulatory surgery center. Patients come to a completely independent facility. Many of these facilities are owned and operated by physicians.

Accreditation of Ambulatory Facilities

The ASC should comply with standards set by the Accreditation Association for Ambulatory Health Care (AAAHC) (www.aaahc.org), the Joint Commission on Accreditation of Healthcare Organizations (JCAHO) (www.jcaho.org), American Association for the Accreditation of Ambulatory Surgery Facilities (AAAASF) (www.aaaasf.org), and the American Osteopathic Association (AOA) (www.osteopathic.org). These four patient advocacy and consumer groups advise patients to select facilities carefully and to look for accreditation and credentialing by professional and governmental agencies.

The 2006 Ambulatory Care and Office-Based Surgery National Patient Safety Goals includes the following:

- Improve the accuracy of patient identification: Use a minimum of two patient identifiers (excluding the patient's room number) when administering pharmacologic agents or blood, taking blood samples or specimens, or providing any treatments or procedures.
- Improve communications among caregivers: all verbal orders or results should be read back to the person delivering the information, standardize a list of all abbreviations, acronyms, and symbols that are not to be used within the organization, and improve the timeliness of information exchange between the reporter and receiver regarding test results and values. Standardize the hand-off report[1] of patient care between phases of care.

---

[1]Hand-off refers to the report given by the preoperative team to the intraoperative team and the intraoperative team to the postoperative team.

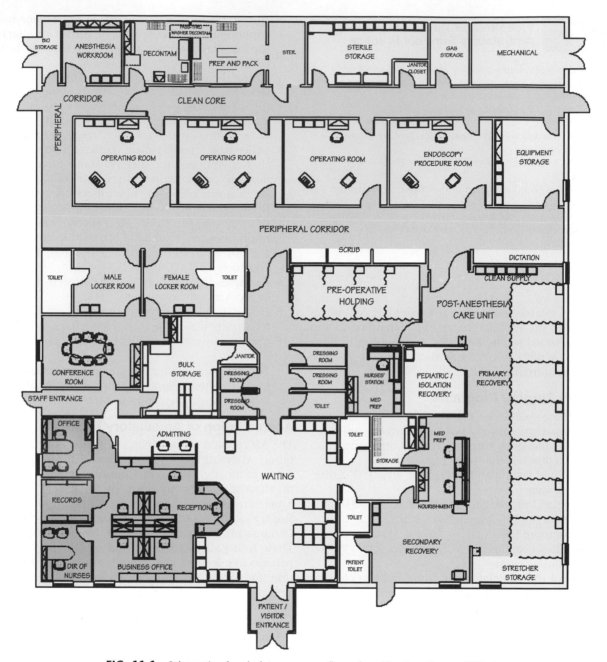

FIG. 11-1 Schematic of ambulatory surgery floor plan. *(Courtesy Herman Miller.)*

- Improve medication safety: Standardize the numbers and concentrations of drugs within the facility, identify sound-alike/look-alike medications and limit their use to prevent error, label all containers and delivery devices with the name and concentration of the drug,
- Reduce the risk of health care–related infections: Comply with Centers for Disease Control and Prevention (CDC) recommendations for hand hygiene, and all deaths or permanent injuries associated with health care–related infection will be treated as sentinel events.
- Identify and reconcile patient medications across the continuum of care: All home and hospital medications will be identified and relayed to all caregivers in the hand-off report.

- Reduce the risk of surgical fires: Staff education should include spark, fuel, and ignition sources including oxygen concentration under drapes as a source of surgical fire.

Licensure of ambulatory surgery centers is required in 43 states. Requirements for licensure are similar to those for accreditation. Inspection visits are scheduled on a routine basis. Ambulatory centers are highly regulated by governmental agencies. Approximately 85% of ambulatory surgery centers are approved for Medicare. Accreditation and credentialing of a facility can be attained by but is not limited to the following:

- Compliance with structural standards
- Establishment of policies and procedures that support competent standards of care

- Appropriate credentialing of personnel
- Emergency preparedness
- Appropriateness of procedures performed at the facility

Approximately 65% of all surgical procedures are performed on an ambulatory basis safely and without complications. Some smaller facilities limit the use of ambulatory surgery to procedures that can be performed with local or regional block anesthetics. Facilities with PACU capability allow surgeons to perform procedures with the patient under general anesthesia. Although procedures performed in an ambulatory care facility are usually of short duration (15 to 90 minutes), the appropriate selection and evaluation of patients are essential. Patient care and anesthesia management also are crucial factors in the experience of the ambulatory surgical patient. Some facilities are prohibited from performing complicated laparoscopy because of the risk for injury to the patient. (More information can be found at the Federated Ambulatory Surgery Association website at www.fasa.org.) Professional organizations that take part in setting the standards of care are listed in Box 11-2.

Patient Selection for Ambulatory Surgery

After a surgical procedure, patients may prefer to recuperate at home rather than in the hospital. These patients may be candidates for ambulatory surgery, depending on the nature and extent of the surgical procedure and on the patient's ability to follow instructions or to receive adequate care at home. Consideration is given to the duration and complexity of the surgical procedure, the risk of anesthesia, and the probability of postoperative complications.

BOX 11-2 | PTAC: Organizations Involved with JCAHO in the Development of Ambulatory Surgery Standards

American Academy of Family Physicians
American Academy of Pediatrics
American Association of Oral and Maxillofacial Surgeons
American College of Emergency Physicians
American College Health Association
American College of Physicians
American College of Surgeons
American Dental Association
American Hospital Association
American Medical Association
American Medical Group Association
American Nurses Association
American Podiatric Medical Association
American Society of Anesthesiologists
Association of periOperative Registered Nurses
Bureau of Primary Health Care
Centers for Medicare and Medicaid Services
Coalition of Rehabilitation Therapy Organizations
Department of Defense
Federal Bureau of Prisons/U.S. Department of Justice
Indian Health Service
North American Association for Ambulatory Urgent Care
Society for Ambulatory Anesthesiology

PTAC, Professional and Technical Ambulatory Committee; JCAHO, Joint Commission on Accreditation of Healthcare Organizations.

Patients are carefully screened before being considered safe candidates for ambulatory surgery. The following are some of the criteria considered:

1. General health status. Acceptable patients are in class I, II, or stable III of the physical status classification of the ASA. Patients are evaluated physically and emotionally to determine the possibility of complications during or after the surgical procedure. This evaluation includes a complete medical history, physical examination, and preanesthesia evaluation.
2. Results of preoperative tests. Patients may have tests on admission the morning of the surgical procedure, but preferably these tests are performed before the scheduled surgery date so the results can be evaluated. This prevents cancellation on the day of surgery if test results are unsatisfactory. Test results are placed on the chart that accompanies the patient to the OR. Preoperative tests may include the following:
   a. Complete blood count (CBC) and urinalysis (usually included in basic laboratory tests)
   b. Pregnancy test
   c. Multichemistry profile for higher-risk patients
   d. Chest radiograph (may be required if clinically indicated)
   e. Electrocardiogram (ECG) (may be required before general anesthesia for patients older than 35 years)
3. Willingness and psychological acceptance by patient and family. The patient should be willing and able to recuperate at home. Some patients lack adequate home care and may need other arrangements.

Each patient is individually assessed. Provision is made for competent care at home either by an agency or the patient's family. Compliance with preoperative and postoperative instructions by the patient and the availability of a responsible adult support person are essential. Other factors to consider when screening a patient for possible ambulatory surgery include the following:

- Recovery period. The surgeon should anticipate minimal or no postoperative complications. Patients in whom a prolonged period of nausea and vomiting is anticipated or in whom pain will not be relieved by oral analgesics are not ideal candidates for ambulatory surgery.
- Reimbursement sources. Most third-party payers prefer less-costly ambulatory surgery whenever a procedure can be safely performed in this setting. Patient safety and quality of care depend on patient screening and support systems.

Preoperative Patient Care

Written instructions for both preoperative and postoperative care are given to the patient by the surgeon during an office visit or by the nurse during a preadmission visit to the ambulatory care facility. These instructions describe the admission, preoperative, intraoperative, recovery, and discharge procedures, and they should be written in a language the patient can understand. To protect both the surgeon and the facility, the patient should sign for receipt of these instructions and should sign that informed consent has been given to the surgeon for the intended surgical procedure. Instructions should include the following:

1. Preoperative instructions
   a. Make an appointment for preadmission assessment and testing.
   b. Take nothing by mouth (NPO) after midnight (or other specified hour) before admission unless ordered to do so by the surgeon. This includes medications, unless ordered.
   c. Perform any necessary physical preparation such as bathing with antimicrobial soap as ordered.
   d. Arrive at the facility by ____ AM/PM. (Time will depend on the scheduled time for the surgical procedure. A minimal wait at the facility helps to reduce preoperative anxiety. Patients are usually admitted at least 1 hour before the scheduled time of their surgical procedure.) Figure 11-2 shows an ambulatory preoperative holding area.
   e. Notify the surgeon immediately of a change in physical condition, such as a cold or fever.
   f. Wear loose and comfortable clothing, leave jewelry and valuables at home, and remove makeup and nail polish. (This may include the removal of acrylic fingernails for some procedures if affixing the pulse oximeter to another location is not an option.)
2. Postoperative instructions
   a. Arrange for a responsible adult support person to take you home. (After some procedures, the patient may not be permitted to drive or leave unattended.)
   b. Do not ingest alcoholic beverages, drive a car, cook, or operate machinery for 24 hours if a sedative or general anesthetic has been administered.
   c. Delay important decision making until full recovery is attained.
   d. Take medications only as prescribed, and maintain as regular a diet as tolerated.
   e. Shower or bathe daily unless instructed otherwise. This helps to relieve muscle tension and discomfort and keeps the wound clean.
   f. Call the surgeon if postoperative problems arise.
   g. Report to the nearest emergency department if your condition deteriorates.
   h. Keep follow-up appointment with the surgeon.

The patient should be reminded that the postoperative information will be reinforced and possibly updated at the time of discharge. The patient's level of understanding of the preoperative instructions and planned procedure is assessed by a telephone call from the perioperative nurse to the patient the day before surgery; at this time, the scheduled date and arrival time are also verified. The patient should be reassured that he or she will be given a set of written instructions before discharge from the facility. The nurse should document patient instructions and responses in the record.

Intraoperative Patient Care

Intraoperatively, the same precautions are observed by all team members as for any surgical procedure. These include strict adherence to the principles of aseptic and sterile techniques and other OR routines. Consideration for patient privacy and avoidance of embarrassment are essential. The general layout of the operating room is similar to larger facilities, but on a smaller scale (Fig. 11-3).

The careful selection of patients, preoperative evaluation, and instructions help prevent complications from the anesthetic. Premedication, if given, is minimal. The surgical procedure should be less than 90 minutes in duration for general anesthesia and less than 3 hours for regional block. Local anesthesia or a regional block is preferable if appropriate. Spinal anesthesia is seldom used.

Cardiopulmonary resuscitation (CPR) equipment and nurses certified in CPR at a minimum level of basic cardiac life support (BCLS) should be available during the procedure (certification in advanced cardiac life support [ACLS] is preferred). Perioperative nurses specializing in the care of pediatric patients should have certification in pediatric advanced life support (PALS).

Patients who undergo general anesthesia or moderate sedation (formerly referred to as intravenous conscious sedation (IVCS)) are scheduled for surgery early in the day; this allows for a maximum recovery time. Rapidly dissipating agents are administered, and various combinations of agents and drugs are used. Drugs associated with prolonged recovery are avoided unless there is a specific indication for their use. Doses of IV agents, such as narcotics and barbiturates, may be reduced to avoid delayed emergence.

Technologic monitoring, including bispectral analysis (BIS monitoring), allows the anesthesia provider to administer minimal amounts of an agent based on the patient's level of consciousness and sensorium. Anesthetic techniques should provide adequate depth of anesthesia but with minimal cardiopulmonary changes and side effects. Indications for endotracheal intubation are the same as for inpatients.

The patient who is undergoing local anesthesia is monitored continuously for any reaction to the medications and/or a change in physiologic status. If an anesthesia provider is not in attendance, a qualified perioperative nurse should be assigned to monitor the patient for behavioral and physiologic changes. This nurse should have a basic knowledge of the function and use of monitoring equipment and should not be assigned other duties while monitoring the patient's condition.

The monitoring perioperative nurse measures and records the patient's vital signs before the injection of a local or regional block anesthetic or analgesic and every 15 minutes thereafter, monitors physiologic status according to written policy and procedure, and institutes emergency measures if an adverse reaction occurs. This nurse should be responsible for interpreting, identifying, and reporting abnormal readings to the surgeon. Additional functions of this nurse may include starting oxygen, administering IV therapy, or giving medications when clinically indicated. Suggested noninvasive intraoperative monitoring methods for patients undergoing local anesthesia are listed in Box 11-3.

BOX 11-3	**Noninvasive Monitoring Equipment Used for Patients under Local Anesthesia**

- Electrocardiograph
- Pulse oximeter
- Blood pressure apparatus

Ambulatory Surgery
Pre-Operative Holding

Pre-Operative Holding

Patients arriving for surgical procedures are held in this area until the appropriate operating room is ready.

Patients will change into hospital attire in dressing cubicles before entering the pre-operative holding area. An area should be available to store patients' clothing and personal belongings.

This area also may be called pre-anesthesia as patients may be given medications or intravenous fluids under close observation of the nursing staff.

A nurses control station and medication preparation area are often an integral part of this area.

Movable Modular Casework Applications

A pre-operative holding area can be planned using movable modular casework and may include

- Small workstation.

- Locker to hold patient care supplies.

- L cart, procedure/supply cart, or rail-hung C frame storage unit placed near each stretcher.

- Procedure/supply carts.

- Extra-deep modular shelving units.

- Sink unit.

- Med prep area.

Plan View of a Pre-Operative Holding Area

A pre-operative holding area will range in size from 350 to 800 square feet.

```
  8  linear feet work surface
  6  linear feet overhead storage
 40  filing inches
  1  locker for medications
  1  locker for IVs
  2  lockers for supplies
  1  C frame storage unit per bed
504  square feet
```

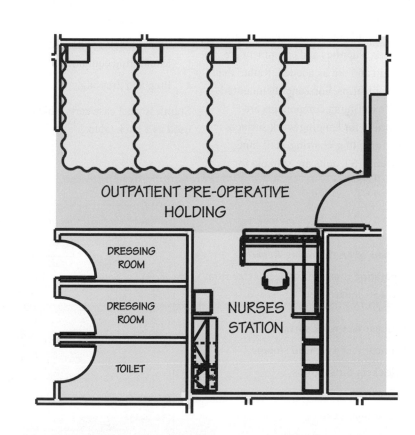

FIG. 11-2 Preoperative holding area. This area is used for patients preoperatively and can be used postoperatively. If a local anesthetic has been used, the patient returns directly from the operating room. If more complex anesthesia is used, the patient will return here after postanesthesia care unit discharge. *(Courtesy Herman Miller.)*

Scrub Area

Scrub areas are placed strategically outside operating rooms. Surgical scrub sinks are generally ceramic or stainless steel with foot or knee controls. It is helpful to place shelves above the sink to hold scrub brushes and masks.

Movable Modular Casework Applications

Depending on the design of the scrub area, scrub brushes and masks can be housed in modular shelving hung on rail, on wall strips above the sinks, or in rail-hung C frame storage units with drawers beside the sinks.

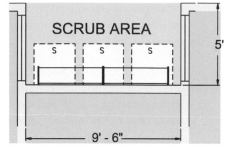

Plan View of a Scrub Area

  8 linear feet overhead storage (2 feet per sink)

50 square feet

Operating Room

An operating room is the area where surgical procedures are performed under strict sterile techniques.

For sanitization purposes, operating rooms should contain little or no built-in casework. Supplies and equipment are moved in and out as needed. Rather than using wall strips, horizontally mounted rail with rail-hung components are appropriate for hanging work surfaces for documenting/charting. Rail-hung shelves or CST units are suitable for overhead storage.

Movable Modular Casework Applications

An operating room can be planned using movable modular casework and may include

L carts or procedure/supply carts used for

- Anesthesia supplies and equipment.
- Suction and cautery equipment.
- Monitoring equipment.
- Prep and dressing.

Stainless steel case carts which can also be used as a back table.

Lockers used for

- General supply storage.
- Backup supplies.
- Specialty procedure carts.

Process tables used as

- Administrative/computer workstations.
- Back table for instruments.

Plan View of an Operating Room

An operating room will range in size from 300 to 450 square feet.

  4 linear feet work surface

  4 linear feet overhead storage

  3 lockers for supplies

  1 L cart

  1 anesthesia cart

     case carts as required

336 square feet

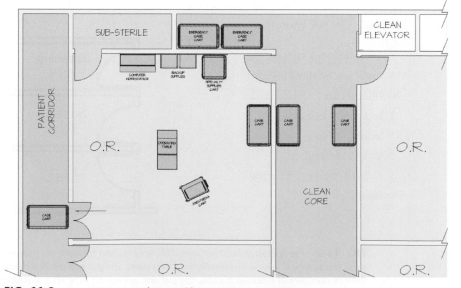

FIG. 11-3   Operating room layout. *(Courtesy Herman Miller.)*

The policies and procedures for monitoring patients undergoing local anesthesia should include patient risk criteria, the type of monitoring to be used, and interventions within the scope of nursing practice. All pertinent data and therapy are documented according to the policies of the facility.

The awake and alert patient needs to receive physical and emotional comfort throughout the surgical procedure. The field of vision may be small while the patient is draped, and tactile and other stimuli will come as a surprise if he or she is not forewarned. The patient should be told what is about to occur (e.g., "You will feel a needle sting"), what to expect (e.g., "You will have a burning sensation"), and what is expected of him or her (e.g., "Tell us if you feel pain"). The patient's questions should be answered truthfully and realistically. He or she should be reassured that appropriate amounts of the anesthetic will be administered as needed.

Conversation by team members should be appropriate and kept to a minimum. Hand signals between the surgeon and scrub person are more useful than a verbal request for instruments. However, the surgeon may request a No. 10 or 15 rather than a knife, or a Mayo or Metz rather than scissors. Strange noises should be explained to the patient (e.g., suction to remove an irrigating solution; the sound and odor of an electrosurgical unit [ESU]).

Background music of the patient's choice may help to relax and distract him or her. Headsets are one option for this purpose and help to block out other noises. Although headsets can distract the patient from the ambient room noise, they can also distract the patient from following necessary directions during the procedure; therefore cautious use is suggested. Traffic in and out of the room should be kept to a minimum. A sign should be placed on the door to indicate the type of anesthesia being used (e.g., "Patient awake, local anesthesia").

Postoperative Patient Care

Patients who have received a local anesthetic are returned to the ambulatory unit for a brief assessment and discharge. Patients who have undergone general anesthesia or IVCS or who need postoperative pain management are taken to the PACU for stabilization and observation (Fig. 11-4). Medications may be given intravenously in small dosages; oral medications may cause nausea and vomiting that may prolong the length of stay. Routine orders may be established by policy for these analgesics and antiemetics.

Consciousness, rational behavior, and ambulation do not imply full recovery. Blood pressure and pulse rate may return to the normal range while residual myocardial depression continues. Patients may lapse back into sleep or drowsiness as the drugs used for general anesthesia are metabolized. Patients are under observation at all times in the PACU. Although the Aldrete Scoring System (Table 11-1) is commonly used for establishing postoperative discharge criteria, this method should not be used to replace patient assessment data in determining suitability for discharge.

A hospital short-stay unit may provide postoperative care for observation and pain control for up to a 23-hour stay. When all discharge criteria are met, patients are discharged on written order of the anesthesia provider and/or surgeon

according to policy. Discharge is contingent on the patient's generalized condition. Vital signs are measured and compared with baseline, and the condition of the surgical site is documented. Patients who have questionable vital signs or an unstable physiology should be seen by a physician before discharge.

Patients are not allowed to drive home if a general or regional anesthetic has been administered. The patient should leave the facility via an appropriate mode of transportation and accompanied by a responsible adult. Select patients who have undergone local anesthesia without sedation may be permitted to drive home if an order is written by the surgeon. The means of the patient's discharge, regardless of transportation, should be documented.

Patient education is an essential element of ambulatory surgical care. Written discharge instructions are verbally reviewed with the patient and a responsible adult. The perioperative nurse should document how the patient or his or her representative signified understanding of the instruction. Some patients can verbalize or perform a return demonstration as confirmation. The patient is instructed when to arrange for a follow-up visit with the surgeon. Appropriate phone numbers for the surgeon, ambulatory center, and emergency help should be listed on the discharge instruction sheet. If problems occur after discharge, the patient is encouraged to contact the surgeon or ambulatory care facility.

Recovery Centers. Freestanding recovery care centers have been developed to accommodate a 24- to 48-hour uncomplicated postanesthesia recovery period. Although they occur infrequently, the most common reasons for admission to a freestanding recovery care center or hospital after ambulatory surgery are pain, nausea and vomiting, urinary retention, and concern for wound integrity. Several types of home/hotel-like facilities provide care for up to 72 hours after surgery. For select ambulatory surgery patients, arrangements for postoperative care can be made with a private home health agency.

Interfacility Transfer Management. If complications develop (e.g., adverse reactions to an anesthetic), the patient may need to be admitted to a hospital for intensive care monitoring. Therefore, freestanding ambulatory surgery centers and office-based centers need to have a patient transfer/admission agreement with a nearby hospital. The team in the room should notify the nurse in charge and arrange for transport. Smaller facilities use the emergency number 911 to request emergency medical services [EMS] personnel for the physical transport of the patient to the hospital. The doorways of office-based practices should be wide enough to accommodate the EMS stretcher. A registered nurse may be designated to travel with the patient. The plans for emergency transfer of a patient should be reviewed with the entire staff on a routine basis.

Follow-up Phone Calls. Most complications occur within the first 48 hours after surgery. Therefore, a registered nurse should call to check on the patient's progress and to reiterate postoperative instructions the following day or, at most, within 2 days of discharge. The nurse reminds the

Post-Anesthesia Care Unit (PACU/Recovery Room)

This area is adjacent to the operating room. Patients are brought to this area after surgery to recover from anesthesia and regain stable vital signs. After the patients are stable, they are moved to secondary recovery before being discharged.

The space is usually in an open area with patients separated with cubicle curtains. Those patients who need to be isolated are kept in a separate isolation recovery room. The isolation room also can be used for pediatric patients.

The layout of this space usually includes a nurses control station with a medication preparation area, a physicians' dictation area, an area for supplies and equipment, hand-washing sinks, and a patient toilet.

Movable Modular Casework Applications

Movable modular casework components appropriate for use in the post-anesthesia care unit include

- Nurses control station.

- L carts or rail-hung C frame storage units with drawers for supplies for each patient.

- Lockers for linen and medical supplies.

- Cantilevered sink units.

- Dictation area.

Plan View of a Post-Anesthesia Care Unit

A post-anesthesia care unit will range in size from 2000 to 4000 square feet.

26	linear feet work surface
18	linear feet overhead storage
80	filing inches
8	lockers for supplies
1	locker for medications
1	L cart for supplies
1	L cart for isolation cart
1	emergency cart
1	C frame storage unit per bed
	dictation area
2126	square feet

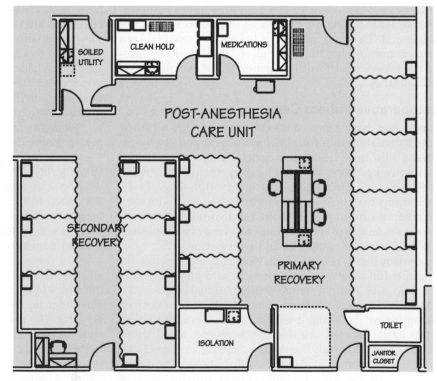

FIG. 11-4 Post-anesthesia care unit. *(Courtesy Herman Miller.)*

TABLE 11-1	Aldrete Postanesthesia Scoring System							
				Admit	15 min	30 min	45 min	60 min
Activity	Able to move voluntarily on command	4 Extremities		2	2	2	2	2
		2 Extremities		1	1	1	1	1
		0 Extremities		0	0	0	0	0
Respiration	Able to breathe deeply, cough freely			2	2	2	2	2
	Dyspnea or limited breathing			1	1	1	1	1
	Apnea			0	0	0	0	0
Circulation	BP + 20 of preanesthesia level			2	2	2	2	2
	BP + 20-50 of preanesthesia level			1	1	1	1	1
	BP + 50 of preanesthesia level			0	0	0	0	0
Consciousness	Fully awake			2	2	2	2	2
	Arousable on calling			1	1	1	1	1
	Not responding			0	0	0	0	0
O_2 saturation	Able to maintain O_2 saturation >92% on room air			2	2	2	2	2
	Needs O_2 inhalation to maintain O_2 saturation >90%			1	1	1	1	1
	O_2 saturation <90% even with O_2 supplementation			0	0	0	0	0

Modified from Aldrete A, Wright A: Revised Aldrete score for discharge, *Anesthesiol News* 18:17, 1992.
BP, Blood pressure.

patient to keep the follow-up appointment with the surgeon. Patients who plan to return to work within 1 or 2 days after surgery may be asked to phone the nurse themselves, because they may not be home when the nurse makes routine calls during the day. Patient satisfaction can be surveyed using this method of postoperative contact.

Documentation of Ambulatory Procedures

The development, implementation, and evaluation of the plan of care should be documented in the patient's medical record. Documentation should include but is not limited to the following:

1. Preoperative care
   a. Preanesthetic evaluation by the anesthesia provider if a general, regional, or local anesthetic with sedation is to be given
   b. Nursing assessment data, nursing diagnoses, expected outcomes, plan of care, and preoperative teaching by the perioperative nurse
   c. Medical history and physical examination
   d. Laboratory reports and results of other tests
   e. Informed consent for the surgical procedure
2. Intraoperative care
   a. Anesthetic and medications administered
   b. Vital signs and intraoperative monitoring data
   c. Intraoperative implementation of the plan of care
   d. Surgical procedure note by the surgeon
   e. Wound classification at the end of the procedure
   f. Any unexpected outcomes
3. Postoperative care
   a. Postanesthesia care, including monitoring of patient responses and medications
   b. Discharge instructions, including follow-up appointment with the surgeon and signs and symptoms

of potential complications that require immediate medical attention
   c. Radiology, pathology, and any other medical reports
   d. Physical and psychological status at the time of discharge
   e. Attainment of expected outcomes
   f. Mode of transport from the facility and destination, including relationship to the accompanying support person
4. Remote postoperative care
   a. Follow-up phone call within 24 to 48 hours to assess the patient's progress
   b. Follow-up phone call within 6 weeks to assess the patient's satisfaction with outcomes and services (for continuous quality improvement data)
   c. Patient follow-up with the surgeon

Most patients who receive ambulatory surgery are satisfied with their care. Studies have shown that if further surgery is indicated, most patients will choose to have the new procedure performed in an ambulatory setting. Fewer incidents of postoperative complications have been documented, as well as lower costs of treatment for the patient. Preoperative teaching is beneficial in helping patients attain the expected outcomes. Careful patient evaluation and planning can make the ambulatory surgery a successful and positive experience for the patient, family, significant others, and caregivers.

ALTERNATIVE SITES WHERE SURGERY IS PERFORMED

Mobile Army Military Hospital

Military medical personnel can be categorized as active duty or reserves. Several branches of military service personnel operate hospitals in the time of war. Colonel Michael DeBakey,

MD, was integral in the initial design of the Mobile Army Surgical Hospital (MASH) and received the Legion of Merit Award in the early 1940s. This section discusses the Army Nurse Corps and the activities associated with mobilization of a mobile surgical hospital in the second millennium. (Additional information can be found at www.armymedicine. army.mil/index.html.)

Active duty personnel can be stationed in their homeland or abroad for a particular tour of duty. Wherever they are located there are medical facilities for the care and health maintenance of the troops in times of peace and of war. Nurses and other supporting personnel provide care according to the same standards followed by health care personnel located in main hospitals in civilian locations. Nurses and other medical support personnel are deployed to the duty area in the same manner regardless of active duty or reservist status. Many surgical personnel are members of reserve units and could be called for active duty.

Reservists who are called to active duty for any augmentation or supporting role first go through mobilization activities to prepare for deployment. During the mobilization period, which can be several days or weeks, the soldiers are prepared for the specific area where they will be stationed for active duty. Activities include creating family care plans, immunization updates, physical examination, overview of geographic location, briefing on local native customs, and military-specific roles. Family care plan considerations are finalized by providing support for dependents and confirming childcare arrangements for single parents. During the Persian Gulf War, 16,337 single parents were called to active duty.

Nursing and medical support personnel are considered soldiers and are responsible for erecting their hospital and support structures for the deployment period (Fig. 11-5). Teams specially trained in setting up mobile medical facilities construct patient care wards, intensive care units, emergency triage tentage, supply areas, and operating rooms. Additional service structures, such as lab, radiology, and pharmacy are set up as well. All services are self-supporting, such as electricity, water supply, sanitation, food service, and communications.

Deployable medical systems (DEPMEDS) are essentially mobile hospital units (Fig. 11-6). One type, the combat support hospital (CSH) consists of special tents measuring 64 × 20 feet known as TEMPER tents, which are designed to be used in all climates (Fig. 11-7). They are used in combination with large rooms destined to be ORs or labs fashioned from fold-out steel box-rooms referred to as ISOs (Fig. 11-8). Some of the ISOs open out to create a protected environment double or triple its size. The operating room ISO is designed to provide a surgical setting for two patients at once (Fig. 11-9). Passages made of canvas, referred to

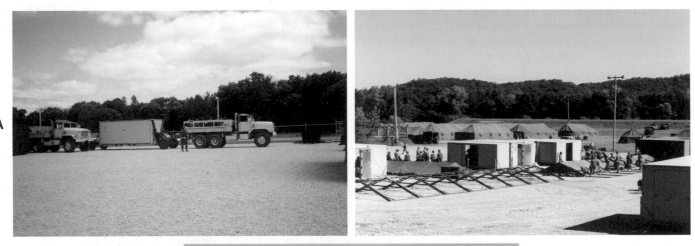

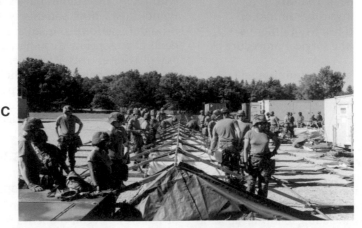

FIG. 11-5 **A,** Hospital being moved into position. **B,** Hospital under construction. **C,** Teamwork setup.

as vestibules, connect the TEMPER tents and ISOs to form the working environment of the hospital in a series of passages complete with climate control for all weather (Fig. 11-10).

The grounds on which the mobile DEPMEDS hospital is built are surveyed and cleared of hazards. Some dangers to look for are unexploded landmines, poisonous plants and animals, disease-carrying insects, and man-made booby traps. A specialized administrative team inspects the grounds and marks off each site for the layout to the exact inch. If the team miscalculates the plan, the TEMPERs and the ISOs will not line up correctly when the vestibules are attached. The integrity of each structure is inspected daily for stability in all types of weather.

In a hostile environment, the functionality of the hospital may depend on the maintenance of the physical plant. Security patrols continually monitor the perimeter of the area and diligently protect the hospital from sabotage by the enemy. Power generators and water supplies are prime targets for disabling the effectiveness of the mobile hospital's mission. The constant threat of chemical and/or biologic weapons is also a consideration. The personnel of the hospital must be prepared to dismantle the hospital and move to a new location in short notice.

Patient care in the mobile hospital is based on returning the soldier to duty as soon as possible. Studies have shown that soldiers who are separated from their units for prolonged

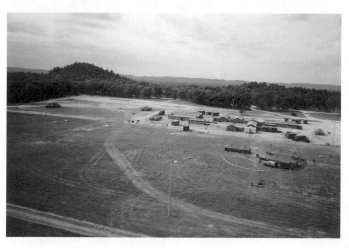

FIG. 11-6   Aerial view.

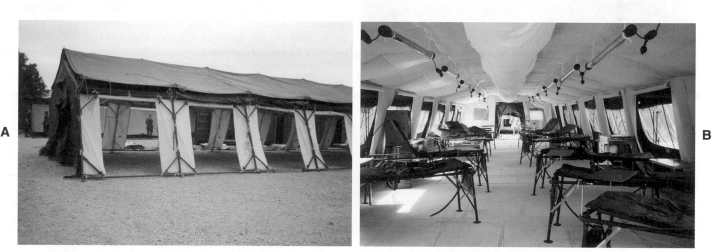

FIG. 11-7   **A,** TEMPER tent frame. **B,** TEMPER tent setup for patient care area.

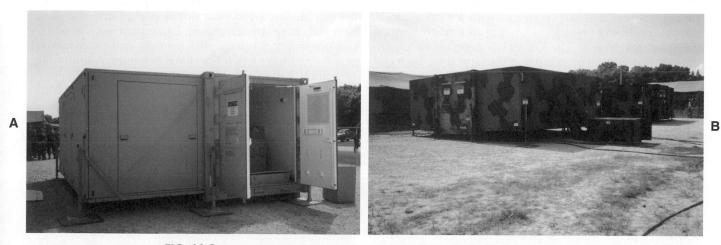

FIG. 11-8   **A,** Fold-out ISO with door open. **B,** Completed ISO setup from outside.

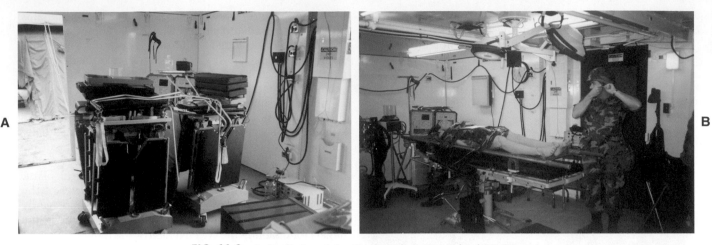

FIG. 11-9 **A**, Duplicate sets for the OR ISO. **B**, One side of OR ISO.

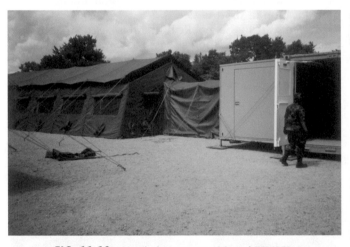

FIG. 11-10 Vestibule connects ISO and TEMPER.

periods due to war inflicted injury suffer increased duration of traumatic stress. A wounded soldier who can be saved with available resources is triaged and treated according the type of injury or injuries incurred.

Surgery in a Mobile Hospital Setting

Injured soldiers that can be treated with a surgical procedure are taken to a presurgical holding area, where they are stabilized for surgery. The OR ISO is designed to accommodate two surgical procedures at the same time. Each end of the room is set up with anesthesia equipment at the head of each OR bed. The ISO has two spotlights centered over the two OR beds that are aligned side by side. The surgical procedures are performed by two separate teams who maintain individual sterile fields for both patients. Postoperatively, the patients are taken to the postsurgical recovery area. The ISO is cleaned and set up for two more patients. The instrumentation is taken to an adjoining tent for cleaning and sterilization to prepare for subsequent surgical procedures. The processing area is referred to as CMS (central materiels service).

Each type of injury is carefully evaluated. Wounded soldiers, who require extraordinary surgical procedures and are not likely to survive, are transferred to an expectant ward where they receive comfort measures until they expire. This is extremely stressful to the nursing and medical staff, because in the civilian sector resources are frequently expended in the care of the hopeless, regardless of survivability. In a CSH environment, standard operating procedures mandate the type of care given to patients who are treated onsite, patients who are shipped out, and those who are beyond treatment.

Consideration is given to the injured enemy prisoners of war (EPW). A separate hospital facility is set up to accommodate EPW care. Security is very complex and additional training is required to manage patient care. Interpreters should be available. EPWs are allocated resources according to need per the Geneva Convention.

Service animals, such as mine-sniffing dogs may need surgical treatment. A separate surgical tent is set up for their care. Instrumentation and other sterile supplies are processed separately from items used in human care. A separate sterilizer may be set up for the sterilization of instruments used in animal surgery.[2]

The living quarters of the mobile hospital personnel consist mainly of tents capable of housing 20 or more people. During field training exercises smaller two-man tents are used to conserve space and expedite setup. Personal belongs are limited to what can be packed into two duffel bags and carried by one person. Equipment, such as protective masks, pistol belts, Kevlar helmets, and other survival gear leaves little room for personal belongings. Uniformity in attire is part of the unity of the group. Individuality is not stressed. The standard clothing is referred to as battle dress uniform (BDU).

The work day is 12 hours long. Every soldier is expected to perform the manual labor necessary to keep the hospital running 24 hours. Physical preparedness includes remaining strong through proper exercise and diet. A regular routine of workouts and running keeps the soldiers in condition.

[2]Vane E: Behind the scenes: Patient safety in the operating room and central material service during deployments, *Adv Patient Safety* (3), 2005.

Periodic physical testing (sit-ups, push-ups, and running 2 miles) is performed to assess each soldier's status. The intensity of the testing is determined by age and sex.

Stress of combat is unavoidable. Although nurses are healers, not warriors, they suffer the same levels of combat stress as fighting soldiers. The treatment for a nurse or other caregiver suffering from posttraumatic stress disorder (PTSD) is the same as that for a combat soldier. After a war, nurses suffering from PTSD may experience intense intrusive thought, such as flash-backs and may have many personal issues to resolve. Psychological counseling is usually indicated. Specific categories of military caregivers are designated for the psychological care and well-being of military personnel.

Much preparation goes into the readiness for war. Medical personnel learn the same soldiering skills as the fighting force in combination with remaining current in health care knowledge. In a CSH environment, the nurses and medical personnel must be prepared to defend the hospital in case of attack.

Veterinary Surgical Facilities

Animals have been the companions of humans since the beginning of time. They serve as a physical source of medication, food, and other by-products that we encounter every day. Service animals have a special place in our society because they are used to protect humans from harmful substances and items by their keen sense of smell, they serve as part of search and rescue teams, guides, transportation, and lately have served as diagnosticians by sensing seizures and sniffing cancer cells. Specialized facilities, such as veterinary clinics provide health services to this unique segment of society. Animal health insurance is becoming a popular concept for animal health care.

Scrub personnel are sometimes employed in a facility where investigational procedures are performed on animals or employed by veterinary clinics for the treatment of domestic animals. This specialized role requires knowledge in sterile and aseptic techniques, instrumentation, and modifications of positioning, prepping, and draping according to the size and body habitus of the veterinary patient.

The setting for performance of surgical procedures on animals should be treated with the same sterile and aseptic techniques as used for human surgery. The outcomes will directly reflect the care given by the absence of infection and freedom from other untoward injury. Microbial carriage of an animal undergoing a surgical procedure can be minimized by containment of contaminated fur, fins, and feathers with adequate cleansing and draping practices. Antiseptic preparations can reduce the microbial load of the skin in the same way they render human skin surgically clean.

Instrumentation is decontaminated and sterilized by the same methods as implements used in human care. Some hospitals have animal labs and clinics for research purposes within a separate section of the facility. Care is taken to isolate and process animal care instrumentation and supplies in a location that does not intermix with instruments and supplies intended for surgical procedures on humans. The risk for inadvertent transmission of infectious material, such as prions between species is significantly increased when instrumentation is mixed.

The physical plant is similar to ORs used for humans with the exception of specialized beds and positioners for extremely large animals such as horses or for small animals such as birds or rodents. Postanesthesia care areas for large standing animals, such as horses, should have padded walls and floors and minimal equipment to prevent an animal's self-inflicted injury.

Institutional animal care is accredited by the Association for Assessment and Accreditation of Laboratory Animal Care (AAALAC). Policies and procedures are specifically designed to meet the needs of animals in laboratory settings. Funding and grants for research commonly include provisions for the care and use of animal subjects. Humane treatment is stressed. Documentation of housing, bedding, feeding, and watering is required as part of the accreditation process.

Regulation of hazardous materials and infection control is required for the safety of human handlers and the welfare of the animals in their care. Waste disposal and sanitation is monitored. Animals involved in investigational studies are tagged for identification and sometimes quarantined as part of the study.

Bibliography

AORN (Association of periOperative Registered Nurses): *Ambulatory surgery: principles and practices,* Denver, 2002, The Association.

Beaver TM, Schenarts PJ: Battlefield surgery 2005, *Int J Surg* 3:171-175, 2005.

Bryant KJ: The federated ambulatory surgery association, *SSM* 6(2):15-17, 2000.

Franko FP: State laws and regulations for office-based surgery, *AORN J* 73(4):839-846, 2001.

Grevemeyer B: Infection control plan for the equine surgery suite, *Equine Vet* 17(3):266-274, 2005.

Hancox JG et al: Why are there differences in the perceived safety of office-based surgery? *Dermatol Surg* 30(11):1377-1379, 2004.

Iqbal Y, Taylor D: Megatrends: Four powerful forces that will shape the future of outpatient surgery, *Outpatient Surg* 3(3):28-33, 2002.

Kessler NW: The American Association of Ambulatory Surgery Centers, *SSM* 6(2):10-13, 2000.

King B, Jatoi I: The mobile army surgical hospital (MASH): A military and surgical legacy, *J National Med Assoc* 97(5):648-656, 2005.

Lancaster KA: Care of the pediatric patient in ambulatory surgery, *Nurs Clin North Am* 32(2):441-455, 1997.

Musinger C: Building an ambulatory surgery center, *SSM* 6(2):43-46, 2000.

National Center for Health Statistics: *Quarterly fact sheet: Monitoring health care in America, spotlight on ambulatory care in the US,* Hyattsville, Md, June 1997, US Department of Health and Human Services.

Pyrek KM: Preventing infections in the ambulatory surgery setting, *Infect Control Today* 6(8):38-42, 2002.

Quinn DM: *Ambulatory surgical nursing core curriculum,* Philadelphia, 1999, Saunders.

Vane E et al: Behind the scenes: Patient safety in the operating room and central material service during deployments, *Adv Patient Safety* 3:469-482, 2005.

Chapter 12

Care of the Perioperative Environment

CHAPTER OBJECTIVES

After studying this chapter, the learner will be able to:
- Describe how a room is prepared for the first case of the day.
- Describe how a room is cleaned and prepared between patients.
- Describe how a room is terminally cleaned at the end of the day.
- Discuss environmental responsibility.

CHAPTER OUTLINE

KEY TERMS AND DEFINITIONS

Between case "clean-up" Cleaning that takes place at the end of one case to prepare the environment for the next case of the day. Also referred to as "turnover."

Case cart system Computerized method of selecting and delivering instrument sets and supplies to the perioperative environment. Some models include provision for the return of instruments and contaminated items to the appropriate decontamination area.

Contamination Potentially pathogenic material that must be contained.

Custom packs Prepackaged disposable supplies standardized and assembled into packages and sterilized by the manufacturer or the distributor according to specific instructions and requests by a particular service at a facility.

Terminal cleaning Thorough cleaning and disinfection of the perioperative environment at the end of daily use.

Turnover Cleaning and preparation of the OR between cases for the next patient's arrival. Areas are cleaned according to level of need.

SUPPLEMENTAL MATERIAL ON EVOLVE WEBSITE *evolve*

http://evolve.elsevier.com/BerryKohn
- Content Updates
- Glossary
- Full Set of Perioperative Flash Cards
- Interactive Key Term Flash Cards
- Student Activities
- WebLinks

HISTORICAL BACKGROUND

The perioperative environment has changed many times throughout history. In ancient times, the healer, or shaman, came to the patient's dwelling to perform the healing arts. The family would gather around to chant and pray to great spirits, and amulets, or charms, were displayed. Mysticism and ceremony played a big part in the treatment. Surgical procedures, such as trephining (drilling holes in the head), or bloodletting were performed to purge evil. Medicinal herbs and hallucinogenic compounds often were used to dull the senses during the procedure, which was performed with crude knives and stone instruments. Knowledge of human anatomy and physiology was limited. Archeologic evidence has demonstrated that some of these patients survived the procedures.

Later eras were witness to procedures performed in the patient's home. Formal hospitals had not been established. Physicians would engage public nurses and family members to prepare the room in the home. In some circumstances the procedure was performed on the kitchen table using instruments taken directly from the physician's black bag. These implements had not been washed since the previous use. Most were merely wiped clean by the nurse. Gloves and other surgical attire were not worn. Procedures performed were limited to the pain tolerance of the patient. Intra-abdominal procedures were not performed, with the exception of cesarean sections for childbirth.

As anesthetic techniques improved and surgical procedures became somewhat safer, hospitals were the exclusive location of surgical suites. Hungarian obstetrician Ignaz Semmelweis (1816-1865) described the beginnings of the theory of infectious transfer between patients, and French bacteriologist Louis Pasteur (1822-1895) confirmed the existence of harmful microorganisms. This necessitated the need for a clean environment and clean practices.

STANDARDS FOR CLEANLINESS IN THE SURGICAL ENVIRONMENT

AORN has established standards and recommended practices for cleaning and maintaining optimal cleanliness in the perioperative environment. The recommendations include, but are not limited to, the following:
1. All patients are entitled to a clean environment for their surgical procedures.

2. Any contamination encountered during a surgical procedure should be contained and confined.
3. Between-case clean up should reestablish the cleanest environment possible for the next patient.
4. Procedure rooms and utility areas should be cleaned daily.
5. A schedule should be in place for routine cleaning of all areas and equipment in the surgical department.
6. All environmental sanitation processes should be defined by facility policy and procedure.

ESTABLISHING THE SURGICAL ENVIRONMENT

The duties of the scrub person and circulating nurse are many and varied as they prepare for the arrival of the patient in the operating room (OR). They are responsible for the cleanliness of the environment preoperatively, intraoperatively, and postoperatively so that the potential for contamination of the patient is kept to a minimum. They prepare and maintain the sterile field, work within it, and then break it down for terminal cleaning. These activities are performed in specific steps to minimize the risk of infection and maximize the use of time and supplies.

Preliminary Preparations

Preliminary preparations of the OR are completed by the circulating nurse and scrub person before each patient enters the OR. Assistance is provided by environmental service personnel. It is a cooperative effort. Clean, organized surroundings are part of total patient care. A visual inspection of the room and its contents should be performed by the team before bringing in supplies for a case. Basic room contents should include the OR bed, anesthesia machine and supplies, electrosurgical unit (ESU), instrument table, preparation (prep) table, Mayo stand, suction apparatus, and receptacles for trash and reusable woven fabrics (Fig. 12-1). Other tables and equipment are added as needed.

Before the First Surgical Procedure of the Day. The following housekeeping duties should be done before bringing supplies into the room for the first case of the day:
1. Remove unnecessary tables and equipment from the room. Arrange the appropriate furniture in an organized manner away from the traffic pattern.
2. Damp-dust (with a facility-approved disinfectant solution and lint-free cloth) the overhead operating light, furniture, flat surfaces, and all portable or mounted equipment. Start at higher surfaces, and work down to lower levels.
3. Damp-dust the tops and rims of the sterilizer and/or washer-sterilizer and the countertops in the substerile room adjacent to the OR.
4. Visually inspect the room for dirt and debris. The floor may need to be damp-mopped.

ROOM TURNOVER BETWEEN PATIENTS

Physical facilities influence the flow of supplies and equipment after the surgical procedure. However, basic principles of aseptic technique dictate the procedures to be carried out immediately after a surgical procedure is completed, to prepare the OR for the next patient. Every patient has the right to the same degree of safety in the environment. In addition, personnel working in surgical services should be protected. Some patients have known pathogenic microorganisms; others have unknown infectious organisms. Therefore, every patient should be considered a potential contaminant in the environment. Cleanup procedures should be rigidly followed to contain and confine contamination, known or unknown.

The routine cleanup procedure can be accomplished expeditiously by the circulating nurse and scrub person working cooperatively. While the circulating nurse assists with the outer layer of dressing and prepares the patient for transport from the OR, the scrub person begins to dismantle the sterile field before removing gown and gloves. All instruments, supplies, and equipment should be decontaminated, disinfected, terminally sterilized, or contained for disposal as appropriate before being handled by other personnel.

After a patient leaves the room, the immediate environment is cleaned and all surfaces are dried. Room cleanup between patients is directed at the prevention of cross-contamination. The cycle of contamination is from patient to environment and from environment to OR personnel and subsequent patients. Exposure to infectious waste is a hazard to everyone who encounters it. After each surgical procedure, the environment should be made safe for the next patient to follow in that room. Institutional policies and procedures for routine room cleanup should be designed to minimize the OR team's exposure to contamination during the cleaning process.

Room Turnover Activities by the Scrub Person

The patient should be thought of as the center, or focal point. The surrounding sterile field and all areas that have come in contact with blood or body fluids are considered contaminated. The primary principles of cleaning procedures are to confine and contain contamination and to physically remove microorganisms as quickly as possible. The sterile field is dismantled by the scrub person, who remains protected with the gown, gloves, a mask, protective eyewear, and a cap during the dismantling procedure. Contaminated supplies, instruments, and basins are prepared by the scrub person and sent to the processing department for terminal cleaning and sterilization.

The following are also activities/responsibilities of the scrub person:
1. Remain sterile until the patient leaves the room. Push the Mayo stand and instrument table away from the operating bed as soon as the intermediate layer of the dressing is applied. Do not contaminate the table or Mayo stand until the patient has actually left the room.
2. Check drapes for towel clips, instruments, and other items. Be sure that no equipment is discarded with disposable drapes or sent to the laundry with reusable woven fabric drapes. Roll drapes off the patient from head to foot to prevent airborne contamination; do not pull them off.

   Disposable drapes are placed in a biohazard plastic bag for disposal. Soiled drapes, whether disposable

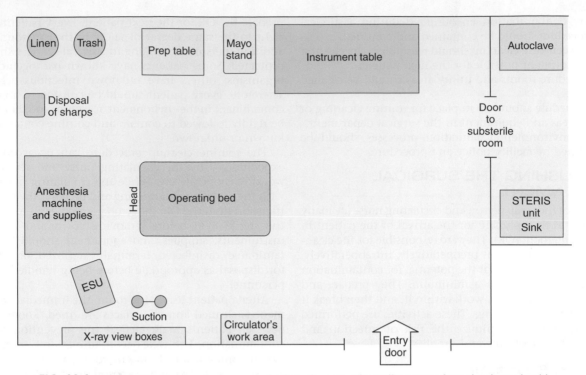

FIG. 12-1 Layout of basic operating room and substerile room. The traffic pattern from the doors should not interfere with the setup of the sterile tables or the transfer of the patient to the operating bed.

or reusable, should be handled as little as possible and with minimum agitation to prevent gross microbial contamination of air by dispersal of lint and debris.

3. Discard soiled sponges, other biologically contaminated waste, and disposable items in appropriate impervious biohazardous waste receptacles.
4. Discard unused sponges, nonwoven drapes, and other nonbloody disposable waste into the trash.
5. Dispose of sharp items safely. Special care should be taken in handling all knife blades, surgical needles, and needles used for injection or aspiration. Remove the tip from the electrosurgical handle (pencil). Place these items in an appropriate rigid, puncture-resistant container for safe disposal to prevent injury and potential risk of contamination.

The primary cause of accidental cuts and punctures to personnel, both within and outside of the OR, is disposal of surgical sharps at the end of the surgical procedure. Adherence to standardized systems designed specifically for safe handling and disposal of sharps prevents virtually all accidental cuts, punctures, and lacerations. Unused suture packets are discarded. Blades and needles should not be discarded loose in trash receptacles. These sharp items should be enclosed and secured for disposal in a sharps disposal container. A self-closing adhesive pad or box designed for this purpose is the safest device to use. A safe disposal procedure should be implemented and adhered to.

a. Remove knife blades from handles using a heavy hemostat; never use fingers. Using a needleholder causes the jaws of the instrument to become misaligned. Point the blade toward the table, away from the field and other people in the area so that if it breaks or slips, it will not fly across the room.

Do not put knife handles in an instrument tray with blades left on them. Other instruments designed for replaceable cutting blades, such as dermatomes, should have blades removed; thereafter they may be handled with other instruments.

Unloaded scalpel handles and other instruments with sharp tips or edges, such as scissors should be placed in a container separate from the other instruments so they can be easily identified by the processing personnel.

b. Place reusable surgical needles, either on a needle rack or loose, into a perforated stainless steel box to be disinfected, terminally cleaned, and sterilized with the instruments.
c. Dispose of burrs and drill bits in the same manner.
6. Remove blood, tissue, bone, and any other gross debris from instruments. All instruments, used and unused, must be cleaned, terminally sterilized, or undergo high-level disinfection before they are handled for definitive cleaning and sterilization and checked for proper functioning before reuse. Instruments should be presoaked and/or prerinsed before processing in a washer-sterilizer or decontaminator.

Any biologic material remaining on instruments is more difficult to remove after the instruments have been heat-sterilized because the material becomes baked on them. The biologic debris inhibits sterilization and disinfection processes.

7. Load the instrument-washing tray with heavy instruments in the bottom. All hinged instruments are fully opened to expose maximum surface area, including box locks. Instruments designed to be disassembled are taken apart. Carefully space instruments to prevent contact of sharp edges or points with other instruments. Concave surfaces should be turned down. Load the tray into the case cart for return to the processing department.

8. Put glass syringes, medicine glasses, and other glassware, including those used by the anesthesia provider, into a separate tray. Reusable syringe plungers are removed from the barrels. Discard disposable items in the trash without needles.

9. Suction detergent-disinfectant solution through the lumen of reusable suction tips. Thorough cleaning of the lumen is difficult to accomplish if biologic debris dries. Disposable suction tips and tubing are recommended and are discarded with other infectious waste.

10. Invert small basins and solution cups over the instruments. Basins and trays too large for the washer-sterilizer or standard instrument sterilizer are put into plastic bags for transport to the decontamination area. The Mayo tray may be included. Place these on the lower shelf of the case cart.

11. Dispose of solutions and suction bottle contents in a flushing hopper connected to a sanitary sewer. Wear personal protective equipment to protect from splashes. Disposable suction units simplify disposal. Commercial substances can be added to liquid in the disposable canister to solidify or gel contents for solid waste disposal. If disposable units are not used, decontaminate contents with disinfectant before hopper disposal.

    SafeCycle 40 (STERIS Corporation, Mentor, Ohio) is a fluid waste management system that collects and holds up to 40,000 mL of fluid and bloody waste. It uses wall suction connections, collects suctioned material, and automatically decontaminates and disposes of it in the processing area without the need for exposure of personnel to the contaminated fluid. The unit self-cleans using sealed canisters of disinfectant. The circulating nurse should disconnect wall suction units to avoid contamination of the internal wall outlet. Rinse the container, plunger, and lid. Reusable glass suction containers are sterilized along with basins and trays.

12. Discard all used disposable table drapes in a plastic bag with used disposable patient drapes. All reusable woven fabric drapes from open packs should be laundered to replace moisture lost to the fabric by sterilization. Unused along with used reusable woven fabric drapes should be sent to the laundry.

13. Remove the gown before removing gloves. The circulating nurse unfastens neck and back closures. Protect arms and scrub clothes from the contaminated outside of the gown. Grasp the right shoulder of the gown with your left hand, and in pulling the gown off your arm, turn the sleeve inside out. Turn the outside of the gown away from your body with a flexed elbow. Then grasp your other shoulder with the other hand and remove the gown entirely, pulling it off inside out. Discard the gown in a laundry hamper if it is reusable or in a trash receptacle if it is disposable.

14. To remove gloves, use glove-to-glove, then skin-to-skin technique to protect clean hands from the contaminated outside of gloves, which bear cells of the patient. Turn gloves inside out as they are removed to contain the biologic contamination, and then discard them into a trash receptacle. Wash hands after removing gloves.

15. Make sure the case cart is covered with an impervious drape or closed before it is returned to the processing area.

Room Turnover Activities by the Team

After the patient leaves, the environmental service personnel should be available to perform room cleaning. Regardless of which member of the team performs them, specific functions should be carried out to complete room cleanup. The following personnel and areas are considered contaminated during and after the surgical procedure:

- Members of the sterile team, until they have discarded their gowns, gloves, caps, masks, and shoe covers. These items remain in the contaminated area; scrub clothes are changed if they are wet or contaminated.
- All furniture, equipment, and the floor within and around the perimeter of the sterile field. If accidental spillage has occurred in other parts of the room, these areas are also considered contaminated.
- All anesthesia equipment
- Stretchers used to transport patients and patient moving devices. These should be cleaned after each patient use.

Clean, but not sterile examination gloves are worn to complete the room cleanup. The scrub person changes gloves after the sterile field is dismantled. Decontamination of the environment includes the following the following tasks:

- Furniture. Wash horizontal surfaces of all tables and equipment, including the anesthesia machine, with a disinfectant. Apply disinfectant from a squeeze-bottle dispenser, and wipe with a clean cloth or a disposable wipe that is changed frequently. Spray bottles can cause particles to become aerosolized and should be avoided. All surfaces of mattress, pads, and screw connections of the operating bed are included. Safety straps should be cleaned between patients. Velcro straps can be laundered according to the manufacturer's recommendations. Mobile furniture can be pushed through disinfectant solution used for floor care to clean casters.
- Overhead operating light. Wipe overhead light reflectors with a clean cloth that has been wetted with disinfectant solution specifically intended for this purpose. Commercial reflector cleaner prevents clouding of the surface that can cause dullness and glare. Lights and overhead tracks become contaminated quickly and present a possible hazard from fallout of microorganisms onto sterile surfaces or into wounds during surgical procedures. Clean these daily.
- Anesthesia equipment. Most masks and anesthesia tubing are disposable. Any reusable anesthesia masks

and tubing are cleaned and sterilized between patient uses. Some of this equipment can be steam-sterilized; if not, it may be sterilized by ethylene oxide gas and aerated before reuse. If this method is not available, items should be chemically sterilized according to the sterilant manufacturer's recommendations.

- Laryngoscope blades and handles should be disassembled, thoroughly cleaned, and disinfected according to Spaulding's classification of patient care items. Any parts that can tolerate a sterilization process should be terminally sterilized.[1] Noncritical items, such as blood pressure cuffs should be wiped clean with an approved disinfectant between patient uses.

- Laundry. After all cleaning procedures have been completed, discard cleaning cloths or put into a laundry bag if they are not disposable. When all reusable woven fabric items, used and unused, have been placed inside the laundry bag, close it securely. To help protect laundry personnel, an alginate bag that dissolves in hot water may be used as the primary laundry bag or as a liner within a cloth bag. Transport reusable woven fabrics soiled with blood or body fluids in leak-proof bags.

- Trash. Collect all trash in plastic or impervious bags, including disposable drapes and kick bucket and wastebasket liners. Bags should be sturdy to resist bursting or tearing during transport. Trash can be separated into infectious waste, noninfectious trash, and recyclable items. Separate receptacles should be available. Disposition of potentially infectious waste must comply with local, state, and/or federal regulations for contamination control measures. Use appropriately labeled and color-coded leak-proof bags for infectious waste, and use puncture-resistant containers for sharps.

- Floors. Clean a perimeter of 3 to 4 feet in circumference of the surgical field between cases. This perimeter expands in the direction of visible soilage. Hot water may hasten the biocidal action of the disinfectant agent but may also soften tile adhesive. Standing platforms are considered part of the floor and should be cleaned between cases.

- Fresh, clean mops are used with fresh Environmental Protection Agency (EPA)–registered disinfectant solution. The floor can be flooded with detergent-disinfectant solution. One mop is used to apply solution, and one is used to take up solution. Continually dipping and mopping spreads the biologic matter instead of removing it. After one-time use, remove mop heads and place in a laundry hamper with other contaminated reusable woven fabrics. Mop handles should be cleaned with disinfectant after use and stored in the housekeeping storage area until they are needed again. Use clean mops and disinfectant solution for each cleanup procedure.

- Walls. If walls are splashed with blood or organic debris during the surgical procedure, wash those areas. Otherwise, walls are not considered contaminated and need not be washed between surgical procedures.

Cart System Cleanup

All reusable instruments, basins, supplies, and equipment, including suction bottles, are put on or inside the case cart. The cart is covered or closed and taken to the central decontamination area outside surgical services for cleanup. A closed cart, especially if it has been used as the instrument table, is wiped with a disinfectant solution before it is taken out of the room. A cart with contaminated supplies should be removed from surgical services via the outer corridor if this is the design of the suite. If dumbwaiters or elevators are used, a separate one is provided for the contaminated cart. Clean and contaminated supplies are always kept separated.

The cart is designed to go through an automatic steam cart washer or a manual power wash for terminal cleaning after it is emptied and before it is restocked with clean and sterile supplies.

Getting the Room Ready for the Next Patient

The cleaning procedures described provide adequate decontamination and terminal sterilization after any surgical procedure. With a well-coordinated team, minimal turnover time between surgical procedures can be accomplished; in an average time of 10 to 15 minutes, the room will be ready for the next patient. The turnover time includes cleaning up after one procedure and setting up for the next procedure. Additional equipment brought into the room for the next patient should be damp-dusted before sterile supplies are opened.

Individual Patient Setups. Each patient has a right to individual supplies prepared just for him or her. Sterile supplies should not be opened until they are ready to be used. Tables should not be prepared and covered for use at a later time. The scrub person, working with an efficient circulating nurse, should have time to set up the instrument table immediately before each surgical procedure. There is no arbitrary life span of a setup table once it is open and prepared as a sterile field for a patient. The sterile table must be under surveillance at all times.

The practice of covering sterile setups is not in the best interest of the patient. Unless it is under constant surveillance, sterility of any setup cannot be guaranteed. Uncovering a sterile table is difficult and may compromise sterility. If a scheduled surgical procedure is delayed and a sterile setup has not been contaminated by the patient's presence in the room, the setup may remain open, under surveillance by someone in the room, with the doors closed. The setup should be used as close to the time of preparation as possible. Sterility is mainly event related, not time dependent.

If a patient is taken into the OR and for some reason the surgical procedure is canceled before the procedure has begun, the tables should be torn down and the room cleaned as if the surgical procedure had taken place. The setup is considered potentially contaminated and may not be saved for another patient. Disposable items may be useful for the clinical educator in the department during orientation and education sessions.

---

[1]AORN recommends that reusable laryngoscope handles have low-level disinfection after cleaning. Studies have shown that 40% to 50% of handles tested positive for blood residue.

DAILY TERMINAL CLEANING

In the Operating Room

At completion of the day's schedule, each OR, whether or not it was used that day, should be terminally cleaned. Additional and more rigorous cleaning is done in all areas already discussed for cleanup between surgical procedures. At the end of the day's schedule, the following routine should be followed:

- Furniture is thoroughly scrubbed, using mechanical friction in addition to chemical disinfection. Disinfectants are only adjuncts to good physical cleaning; "elbow grease" is probably the most important ingredient.
- Casters and wheels should be cleaned and kept free of suture ends and debris. Equipment is available that automatically washes stretchers, tables, and platforms and then steam-cleans and dries them within a matter of minutes.
- Equipment, such as ESUs and lasers, should be cleaned with care so as not to saturate surfaces to the degree that disinfectant solution runs into the mechanism, causing malfunction and requiring repairs.
- Ceiling- and wall-mounted fixtures and tracks are cleaned on all surfaces.
- Kick buckets, laundry hamper frames, and other waste receptacles are cleaned and disinfected; these items are sterilized when feasible.
- Floors are given a thorough wet-vacuum cleaning with wet-vacuum pickup used dry and then wet.
- Walls and ceilings should be checked for soil spots and cleaned as necessary.
- Cabinets and doors should be cleaned, especially around handles or push plates, where contamination is common.
- Air-intake grills, ducts, and filter covers should be cleaned.

Outside the Operating Room

- Countertops and sinks in the substerile room should be cleaned. The outer surface of the sterilizer, including the top, should be washed.
- Scrub sinks and spray heads on faucets should undergo thorough cleaning daily. A mild abrasive on sinks removes the oily film residue left by scrub antiseptics. Spray heads, faucet aerators, or sprinklers should be removed and disassembled, if possible, for thorough cleaning and sterilization of parts. Contaminated faucet aerators and sprinklers can transfer organisms directly to hands or items washed under them. Scrub sinks should not be used for routine cleaning purposes.
- Soap dispensers should be disassembled, cleaned, and terminally sterilized, if possible, before they are refilled with antiseptic solution. These dispensers can become reservoirs for microorganisms.
- Walls around scrub sinks should receive daily attention. Spray and splash from scrubbing cause buildup of antiseptic soap film around the sink. This film should be removed.
- Transportation and storage carts need to be cleaned, with specific attention given to wheels and casters.
- Cleaning equipment should be disassembled, cleaned, and dry before storage.

Weekly or Monthly Cleaning

A weekly or monthly cleaning routine is set up, in addition to the daily cleaning schedule, by the director of environmental/housekeeping services and the OR manager. Any routines for housekeeping are based on the physical construction of the department. However, if specific schedules are not established, some areas could be inadvertently missed. Areas to be considered are the following:

- *Walls.* Walls should be cleaned when they become visibly soiled. If they are painted or tiled with wide porous grouting, these factors should be considered in planning cleaning routines. Washing walls in the OR and throughout the suite once a week is reasonable, but less frequent time intervals for cleaning may be acceptable if spot disinfection is performed on a daily basis. This requires adequate continuous supervision.
- *Ceilings.* Ceilings may require regular special cleaning techniques because of mounted tracks and lighting fixtures. Specialized ceiling mounts for microscopes and booms for suspended equipment should be included in this plan. The types of fixtures are considered in planning cleaning routines.
- *Floors.* Floors throughout surgical services should be machine-scrubbed periodically to remove accumulated deposits and films. Conductive flooring should never be waxed. Rounded corners and edges facilitate cleaning.
- *Air-conditioning grills.* The exterior of air-conditioning grills should be vacuumed at least weekly. Additional cleaning is necessary when filters are checked and changed. Debris may be discharged into the room when the filter is changed. In-room air handlers are positive pressure. The filters should be changed on an off-shift or on the weekend. The room should be terminally cleaned after changing the filters.
- *Storage shelves.* Storage cabinets have been replaced in many OR suites by portable storage carts or pass-through shelving to a sterile core. Storage areas should be cleaned at least weekly or more often, if necessary, to control accumulation of dust, especially in sterile storage areas.
- *Sterilizers.* All types of sterilizers should be cleaned regularly and tested as recommended by the manufacturer.
- *Transfer zones.* Walls, ceilings, floors, air-conditioning grills, lockers, cabinets, and furniture should be cleaned on a regular schedule.

Environmental Responsibility

Many surgical supplies are recyclable. Recycling reduces not only air pollution and the amount of waste in landfills but also the amount of virgin resources consumed. Paper wrappers and many plastic items that are noninfectious, nonregulated trash can and should be recycled.[2] Recycling in the OR should be an integral part of the overall recycling

---

[2]AORN has a recommended practice that defines environmental responsibility as a set of practices performed by facility personnel that supports and promotes ecologic behaviors for future generations.

program of the health care facility. Consideration of recycling potential can be part of the evaluation process in selecting products.

The team should take care not to use more consumable product than necessary. Overfilling prep basins with chemical antiseptic solution and then disposing of it in the sanitary sewer exposes the environment to risk for resistant microorganisms and pollution.

Bibliography

AORN (Association of periOperative Registered Nurses): *AORN standards, recommended practices, and guidelines,* Denver, 2006, The Association.

Ellis K: Partners in clean, *Infect Control Today* 9(5):40-44, 2005.

Neil JA et al: Environmental surveillance in the operating room, *Infect Control Today* 82(1):43-49, 2005.

Pyrek KM: Follow standard precautions when handling soiled linens, *Infect Control Today* 6(3):12-14, 2002.

Seavey R: Environmental cleaning in the operating room, *Infect Control Today* 9(3):32-33, 2005.

Chapter 13

Potential Sources of Injury to the Caregiver and the Patient

KEY TERMS AND DEFINITIONS

Ionizing radiation Sufficient radiant energy to yield ions from the disintegration of the nuclei of unstable or radioactive elements. This radiation occurs naturally from cosmic rays, and these ions disrupt the electronic balance of atoms. Synthetic x-rays and nuclear power are capable of modifying molecules within body cells as they pass through tissue. They can be mutagenic (i.e., cause mutations of deoxyribonucleic acid [DNA]) in somatic body cells, predisposing a person to cancer, and in germ cells, predisposing a person to spontaneous abortion or congenital malformations.

Nonionizing radiation Radiant energy that does not produce ions but can produce hyperthermic conditions that are harmful to the skin and eyes. With the possible exception of ultraviolet rays, wavelengths from electromagnetic spectrum do not alter DNA in body cells.

HISTORICAL BACKGROUND

Historically, the operating room (OR) has been a place full of hazards for both the patient and the caregiver. The primary dangers include but are not limited to fire, chemical exposure to anesthetic agents, and direct exposure to biologic material.

Concern about fire and explosions caused by anesthetics and other flammable agents intensified in 1925 with the introduction of ethylene gas; the use of drop ether was already popular. In the following decade another highly flammable gas, cyclopropane, became popular. Proper ventilation systems and gas-scavenging systems for waste gases were either absent or highly inefficient. The potential hazard of static electricity causing combustion of flammable anesthetics has been minimized by elimination of the flammable agents. However, ignition from thermal devices continues to remain a fire hazard.

Special conductive shoes or conductive shoe covers were worn by personnel in the OR to minimize the risk of fire caused by a spark of static electricity. On entering the suite, each person was required to stand on a conductivity testing device near the entrance to the department. At one time, undergarments made from synthetic fibers were discouraged in the OR because they were considered a potential source of static.

ENVIRONMENTAL HAZARDS

The perioperative environment poses many hazards for both patients and personnel. The potential for physical injury from electric shock, burns, fire, explosion, exposure to bloodborne pathogens, and inhalation of toxic substances is ever present. Therefore, it is important that staff have knowledge of the hazards involved in equipment use, the causes of accidental injury, and the sources of health risks. Faulty equipment or improper usage increases the hazards of potential risk factors. The health care facility should be made as safe as possible.

Potential hazards should be identified and safe practices established. The facility's risk management personnel is charged with the responsibility of tracking issues of safety and potential injury. The recommendations that arise from these data are established to guide personnel in corrective actions. Patients and caregivers are never completely free from risks, but the risks can be minimized.

Safety refers to conditions that will not cause injury or harm to the employee, the patient, and other people in the health care facility. Safety goes hand in hand with knowledge, skill, and competency. Some equipment, such as lasers, radiographic equipment, and chemical sterilizers, can cause long-range injury if personnel are lax in safety and protective practices. The education and training of personnel are essential to create an awareness of the potential hazards. No one should be permitted to use equipment until properly instructed in its correct use and care.

Each caregiver should seek instruction when needed and follow the safety and control measures established by facility policies and procedures. Failure to use equipment and devices safely places both the caregiver and the patient at risk for injury.

Competency in using equipment should be tested periodically because technology changes frequently and the knowledge and skill associated with one piece of equipment may not apply to a newer model. In some instances the technology may become safer, but this is not always the case.

Classification of Hazards

Injuries can be caused by using faulty equipment, using equipment improperly, exposing oneself or others to toxic or irritating agents, or coming into contact with harmful agents. Hazards in the OR environment can be classified as follows:

- Physical, including back injury, fall, noise pollution, irradiation, electricity, and fire[1]
- Chemical, including anesthetic gases, toxic fumes from gases and liquids, cytotoxic drugs, and cleaning agents[2]
- Biologic, including the patient (as a host for or source of pathogenic microorganisms), infectious waste, cuts or needlestick injuries, surgical plume, and latex sensitivity[3]

Regulation of Hazards

Standards, guidelines, and recommended practices have been developed by many professional associations, such as the Association of periOperative Registered Nurses (AORN), and governmental agencies, such as the Department of Health and Human Services (HHS). The policies and procedures of the health care facility should be developed and enforced in compliance with local, state, and federal regulations. Other agencies include but are not limited to the following:

- The American Conference of Governmental Industrial Hygienists (ACGIH) (www.acgih.org) sets standards for threshold limits for exposure to toxic materials.
- The American National Standards Institute (ANSI) (www.ansi.org) sets standards to limit exposures to devices that emit light or sound, such as lasers, ultraviolet light, and nonionizing radiation.

- The National Fire Protection Association (NFPA) (www.nfpa.org) sets standards for electrical codes and fire safety.
- The Joint Commission on Accreditation of Healthcare Organizations (JCAHO) (www.jcaho.org) sets standards of patient care for accreditation.
- The Centers for Disease Control and Prevention (CDC) (www.cdc.gov) sets standards for infection control.
- The National Institute for Occupational Safety and Health (NIOSH) (www.cdc.gov/niosh) sets standards for ventilation systems and environmental protection in the workplace.
- The Environmental Protection Agency (EPA) (www.epa.gov) sets standards for the disposal of infectious and hazardous waste.
- The U.S. Food and Drug Administration (FDA) (www.fda.gov) sets standards and controls for the use of drugs, biologics, devices, and chemicals in patient care.
- The Center for Devices and Radiologic Health (CDRH) (www.fda.gov/cdrh) sets standards for the management and monitoring of radiation in patient care.
- The National Patient Safety Foundation (NPSF) (www.npsf.org) sets goals for patient safety in health care organizations.

In 1970 the Occupational Safety and Health Administration (OSHA) was created within the U.S. Department of Labor. Initially, OSHA adopted preexisting federal and national consensus standards and guidelines for environmental, patient, and personnel safety. Since its inception, OSHA has issued new standards and amended others, such as permissible exposure limits (PELs) to various occupational health and safety hazards. OSHA is authorized by law to enforce its standards, which may require employers to measure and monitor exposure to toxic or harmful agents, to notify employees of overexposure and provide medical consultation or care, and to maintain records of corrective actions. OSHA inspects health care facilities for compliance with standards. (More information can be found at www.osha.gov.)

The CDC oversees the activities of NIOSH. The research branch of NIOSH is the National Occupational Research Agenda (NORA).

PHYSICAL HAZARDS AND SAFEGUARDS

The architectural design of the perioperative environment affects its overall efficiency and productivity. The physical facility is designed to control traffic patterns, decrease contamination, facilitate the handling of equipment and supplies, and provide a comfortable working environment.

Environmental Factors

Several factors contribute to providing a safe, comfortable working environment: temperature control, ventilation, lighting, color, and noise. Temperature control should provide physical comfort (i.e., it should not be too warm or too cool).

The ventilating system in the perioperative environment usually evacuates odors fairly quickly by exchanging air 15 times per hour, with 3 exchanges of fresh air. The ventilating system should help remove toxic fumes and anesthetic gas waste that is not picked up by the scavenger system on the

---

[1]NIOSH publishes ergonomic safety information online at www.cdc.gov/niosh/topics/ergonomics.
[2]NIOSH publishes an online chemical hazards index as a .zip file at www.cdc.gov/niosh/npg.
[3]NIOSH publishes an online collection of strategies for health care workers and biologic exposure prevention at www.cdc.gov/niosh/topics/healthcare.

anesthesia machine. Perfume and other odors can cause headaches, nausea, or respiratory congestion in sensitive people. Heavy perfume can also have an annoying, lingering effect, and therefore people in the perioperative environment should avoid wearing it.

Lighting should be adequate, but excessive glare causes fatigue. Illumination is the product of the light and the reflectance of the target. A bright, highly polished mirror finish on an instrument tends to reflect light and can restrict vision. Satin- or dull-finished instruments eliminate glare and lessen eyestrain. These instruments are made with varying degrees of dullness depending on the manufacturer. Lightly tinted or polarized eyewear may save sterile team members from visual fatigue but should not distort the color of tissues. For drapes and walls, soft, cool colors, especially blues and greens, are less reflective than white. Drapes with blue, gray, or green tones help to reduce the contrast between most tissues and the surrounding field.

Although attention is given to ventilation, lighting, and color, less attention is given to the design of the OR in terms of auditory effects. Some facilities have piped-in music in waiting areas. Music can be stimulating for personnel and relaxing for patients who are awaiting surgery or undergoing a surgical procedure under local anesthesia. The selection of music should be appropriate for the intended listener. Music with a low volume, moderate rhythm, and bright tone can motivate muscular activity and increase levels of efficiency of OR personnel. However, this type of music would not be conducive to relaxation for the patient who is awaiting surgery. On the other hand, music can be a distraction and an annoyance, especially for the anesthesia provider, who may depend on auscultation when monitoring the patient. Music should be turned off at the request of the patient, surgeon, or anesthesia provider.

Extreme noise from drills, fan motors in equipment, and other sources can be annoying and potentially dangerous to patients and personnel. The noise can become intense enough to increase blood pressure and to provoke peripheral vasoconstriction, dilation of the pupils, and other subtle physiologic effects. It also can interfere with necessary communication and thereby provoke irritation. The EPA recommends that noise levels in hospitals not exceed 45 decibels during daytime hours.

The OR should be as quiet as possible except for the essential sounds of communication among team members directly concerned with the patient's care. Any necessary talking should be done in a low voice. Counts or requests for supplies should be done quietly or by hand signals. Conversation unrelated to the surgical procedure is out of place. Even during the deep stages of anesthesia, a patient may perceive and remember noise that occurs during the surgical procedure. This phenomenon is referred to as *anesthesia awareness.*

If a regional or local anesthetic is used, the patient can hear the conversation. Because patients interpret anything they hear in terms of themselves, all words should be guarded.

Major sources of noise in the OR involve paper, gloves, objects wheeled across the floor, instruments striking one another, monitors, and high-pitched power instruments, including suction. The scrub person should keep in mind the sources and the effects of this noise. The clattering of instruments should be avoided. Except while in actual use, suction tubing can be clamped or kinked to minimize noise. Paper wrappings should not be crushed. Monitors with audible signals should be placed as far away from the patient's ears as possible; continuous monitor beeps also can distract the surgeon and anesthesia provider. The circulating nurse should keep the doors to the OR closed to shut out the noise of the corridors, of water running in the scrub room, or of the sterilizer operating in the substerile room.

Working in a pleasantly quiet environment is less fatiguing, produces fewer psychological and physiologic adverse effects, and allows for greater efficiency on behalf of the patient.

Body Mechanics

Backache is a leading cause of work-related lost time, second only to upper respiratory infections. Standing for prolonged periods, often in an awkward position, is a common cause of low back pain. Tiring body motions or an awkward or strained body posture should be avoided. Weight bearing on only one foot causes additional strain. When the feet are placed together while standing, constant muscular effort is required by the thigh muscles to maintain an erect posture. In contrast, when the feet are apart, the ligaments of the hips and knees support the body with less effort. Therefore maintaining a wide stance while standing at the operating bed for prolonged periods will be less fatiguing for the scrub person.

While in a location to observe both the surgical procedure and the instrument table, the circulating nurse can stand with the upper and lower extremities in a resting position. In this standing position, the arms are clasped behind the back and the feet are in a wide stance.

Shoes should be considered for comfort and safety. Soft canvas or leather athletic shoes that tie or secure with Velcro provide adequate support for the foot. If running is required during an emergency, these shoes will be more secure than clog varieties with open backs. Soft shoes do not afford protection from dropped items.

The operating bed is adjusted to the best working height for the surgeon, which may not be the most comfortable position for the other members of the sterile team. Team members should be able to stand erect with their arms comfortably relaxed from the shoulders, without stooping, and they should not need to raise their hands above the level of their elbows for the majority of their work motions. Standing platforms (stepstools, referred to as steps) may be needed to elevate the scrub person and/or the assistant to a feasible working height. These platforms should be long enough and wide enough to allow a wide stance. A shorter surgeon can stand on steps to allow the team to have the operating bed at a comfortable working height.

Correct posture while in the sitting position is equally important. The back is strongest when it is straight. When seated, team members should sit well back in the chair or on the stool with the body straight from hips to neck. They should lean forward from the hips, not from the shoulders or waist. This position puts the least strain on muscles, ligaments, and internal organs. Before and after the surgical procedure, the circulating nurse and scrub person(s) should rest in a sitting position between periods of standing. If work is done in a sitting position, the stool or chair should be adjusted to the correct height for the working surface.

First assistants may develop carpal tunnel syndrome as a result of holding retractors in one position for prolonged periods. Carpal tunnel syndrome is a form of repetitive stress injury caused by tenosynovitis that places pressure on the median nerve of the hand. Consequently, the thumb, index, and ring fingers tingle and feel swollen. Self-retaining retractors help to relieve some of this strain.

Sprains and strains are common injuries sustained to the back, arms, or shoulders as a result of lifting patients or moving equipment. Several principles of body mechanics should be observed to minimize physical injury:

- Keep the body as close as possible to the person or equipment to be lifted or moved while maintaining a straight back.
- Lift with the large muscle groups of the legs and abdominal muscles, not the back.
- Bend the knees to get body weight under the load, and then straighten the legs to lift with the heels flat on the floor.
- Lift with a slow, even motion, keeping pressure off the lumbar (lower back) area.
- Push, do not pull, stretchers, tables, and heavy equipment on wheels or casters.
- Use large body muscles to maneuver the base of portable equipment such as laser equipment or microscopes.
- If standing for prolonged periods, stand in a wide stance with the heels apart so the ligaments of the hips and knees can support the body without effort.
- Distribute weight evenly on both feet, but shift the body occasionally during prolonged periods of stand-ing. Don't stiffen the legs at the knee. A slight flex is less stressful.
- Sit with the back straight from the hips to the neck, and lean forward from the hips.
- Align the head and neck with the body when standing or sitting, maintaining the lumbar curve.
- Change position, stretch, or walk around occasionally if possible.
- Pivot the entire body to avoid twisting at the waist.
- Bend forward with hip flexion and hand support.
- Avoid overhead reaching or overstretching; keep materials in the chest-to-knee range if possible; use steps as appropriate.

A lifting frame or Davis roller helps to relieve the potential strain of moving unconscious or obese patients (Fig. 13-1). Moving these patients alone can cause injury to the patient or the caregiver. Assistance is also needed to position patients on the operating bed. Physical therapy department personnel or the occupational health director can be a resource for teaching the patient care staff the proper techniques for lifting, bending, reaching, and pivoting.

Ionizing Radiation

Radiation cannot be seen or felt. Ionizing radiation produces positively and negatively charged particles that can change the electrical charge of some atoms and molecules in cells. These changes can alter enzymes, proteins, cell membranes, and genetic material. This can cause the death of cancer cells when radiation is used in therapeutic doses; however, exposure to radiation also can cause cancer, cataracts, bone marrow injury, burns, tissue necrosis, genetic mutations, spontaneous abortion, and congenital anomalies.

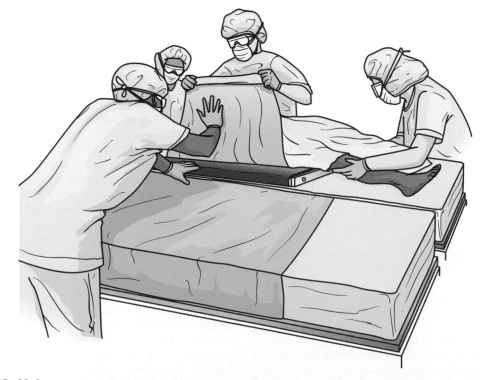

FIG. 13-1 Four surgical personnel using a patient roller correctly to move the patient from one surface to another.

Perioperative patient care personnel may assist with invasive radiographs. If personnel are unprotected, they are exposed to scatter radiation from the patient during intraoperative procedures when radiographs are taken or when fluoroscopes and image intensifiers are used. Team members are exposed also during the implantation or removal of radioactive elements. Patients exposed to radioactivity for therapeutic purposes or by accident may emit radiation.

Intraoperative radiographs may be taken during, but are not limited to, orthopedic procedures, urologic examinations, biliary tree visualization, angiography, or arteriography. The sterile team should be wearing lead protective garments under the sterile gown or should step behind a lead screen when the image is made. The radiograph cassette may need to be draped or encased in a sterile cover and the surgical incision may need to be protected with a sterile drape to prevent contamination by the radiograph machine. When a C-arm radiograph machine is used, a specialized sterile clear plastic tubular drape is slid over the entire machine (Fig. 13-2).

The effect of radiation is directly related to the amount and length of time of exposure. Exposure is cumulative, and because there is an extended latency period, the effects may not be evident for years. Therefore, constant vigilance for personal safety is essential to avoid excessive exposure to ionizing radiation. Protection implies understanding the basic terms and adhering to strict policies and procedures.

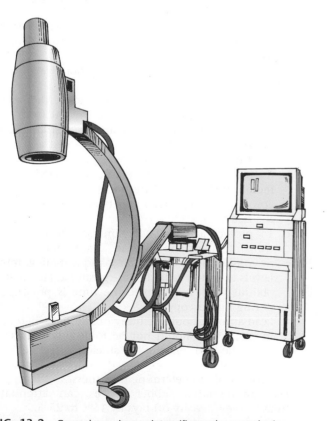

FIG. 13-2 C-arm keeps image intensifier and x-ray tube in alignment to amplify fluoroscopic optical image.

Safety Considerations in the Use of Ionizing Radiation. Because of the adverse and cumulative effects of ionizing radiation on body tissues, safety precautions are taken to protect patients and personnel from the potential hazards. Box 13-1 lists safe radiation exposure limits according to the area of the body. If protective precautions are used, OR personnel rarely, if ever, exceed these safe limits.

Patient Safety. A patient can be exposed to the primary beam of x-rays, the radioactivity of implants, and scatter radiation. Any exposure to radiation has biologic risks, and therefore the exposure should be as low as possible. To reduce the amount of radiation exposure, the following precautions should be taken:

1. The fluoroscope should be turned off when not in use. The patient is continuously exposed to radiation during fluoroscopy.
2. Every effort should be made to reconcile an incorrect sponge, sharps, or instrument count. A radiograph should be made only as a last resort to locate a missing item.
3. Body areas should be shielded from scatter radiation or the focused beam whenever possible. A lead shield can be positioned between the patient and radiation source if it will not interfere with the sterile field or visualization for the radiographic study. The shield is placed before the patient is draped. A shadow shield connected to the x-ray tube may be a preferable alternative if a lead shield cannot be used.
   a. Lymphatic tissue, the thyroid gland, and the bone marrow of the sternum are especially sensitive to radiation. Therefore a thyroid/sternal shield should be used during radiographs or fluoroscopy of the head, upper extremities, and chest.
   b. To protect the testes or ovaries, a gonadal shield should be used during radiographs or fluoroscopy of the hips and thighs.
   c. A lead shield should always be used to protect the fetus of a pregnant patient. Even low levels of scatter radiation may be harmful to the fetus. Therefore radiographs to the abdomen and pelvis are avoided, especially during the first trimester.

BOX 13-1	Permissible Doses of Radiation as Established by the National Council on Radiation Protection and Measurements

Permissible doses of radiation are based on units of an equivalent dose quantity that express all radiations on a common scale for the purpose of calculating their biologic effects. The maximum permissible doses per year for occupationally exposed people older than 18 years of age varies by body parts:
- Whole body, including blood-forming organs, bone marrow, and gonads: 5 rem, 50 mSv
- Lenses of eyes: 15 rem, 150 mSv
- Other organs and tissues: 50 rem, 500 mSv
- Fetus in utero: 0.5 rem, 5 mSv; no more than 50 mR, 0.5 mSv in any 1 month of gestation during pregnancy

Exposure should not exceed 100 mR, 1 mSv per week.

Intraoperative documentation should include the anatomic location of the direct radiographs or fluoroscopy, the type and location of radioactive implants, and shielding measures to protect the patient from scatter radiation.

Personnel Safety. Safety precautions should be taken to protect team members from the potential hazards of ionizing radiation. Three key factors must always be remembered: time, distance, and shielding.

Time. Overexposure and unnecessary exposure should be avoided in everyone, and especially in those of childbearing age. Changes may occur in the reproductive cells as a result of radiation, leading to potential genetic defects. The following precautions should be used to limit the length of exposure to radiation:

- Patient care personnel should rotate assignments on procedures that involve radiation.
- Staff members may request relief from exposure during pregnancy. If this is not possible, a pregnant staff member should leave the room or be adequately shielded when radiographs are performed or fluoroscopy is used.
- Radiation from an x-ray tube, fluoroscope, and image intensifier is present only as long as the machine is energized. These machines should be turned off when not in use.
- Radioactive elements should remain in lead-lined containers until ready for implantation. Trained personnel should handle the radioactive elements as quickly as possible and always with special forceps.
- A patient who has received radioactive substances for diagnostic studies may emit up to 2 millirads mR per hour. If possible, the surgical procedure should be delayed for at least 24 hours after the test.
- Personnel should limit the time spent in proximity to a patient who has had a diagnostic study with or an implantation of radioactive elements until disintegration reaches a low level.
- Body tissues and fluids removed from patients with radioactive emissions should be contained quickly.

Distance. Automatic or manual collimators, which confine the x-ray beam to the precise size of the radiograph or fluoroscopic screen, are required for all equipment. Most image intensifiers have a lead shield as part of the installation. A single-frame computerized recording device incorporated into the fluoroscopy system also helps reduce exposure. Fluoroscopy produces more scatter radiation than do direct x-ray beams. Personnel should distance themselves as far as possible from the source of radiation, as demonstrated by the following procedures:

- Unsterile team members who can safely do so should leave the room during each single radiograph exposure.
- Inanimate holding devices should be used to maintain the position of the radiograph and patient.
- Sterile team members and others who cannot leave room should stand 6 feet (2 m) or more from the patient, if possible, and out of the direct beam during exposure. Team members should remember the inverse square law of distance: double the distance equals one fourth the intensity.

- If possible, team members should stand behind or at a right angle to the beam on the side of the patient where the beam enters, not exits.
- Lateral or oblique radiographs increase scatter radiation. Positioning the beam in a plane vertical to the pelvis or thighs helps reduce scatter. For supine and upright radiographs, the beam should be directed at the floor or walls.

Shielding. Lead that is at least 0.5 mm thick offers the most effective protection against gamma rays and x-rays to halt and absorb radiation scatter. Alpha and beta particles do not require shielding. The following guidelines for shielding should be observed:

1. The walls of rooms with fixed radiation equipment are usually lined with lead. Gamma rays can penetrate lead to a depth of 12 inches (30.7 cm). X-rays can be stopped with lead or thick concrete.
2. Portable lead screens should be available.
   a. Sterile team members and others who cannot leave the room should stand behind a screen while radiographs are taken or while the patient is exposed to intraoperative radiation therapy. The screen(s) should be positioned behind a portable machine.
   b. When a lateral exposure is taken, the screen should be positioned behind the radiograph cassette to absorb rays that penetrate through or scatter from the cassette.
   c. People preparing radioactive implants that emit gamma rays should do so from behind a lead screen that is up to 12 inches (30.7 cm) thick. A sterile drape can be put over the screen so the scrub person or other sterile team member can stand behind the screen and reach around it.
3. Sterile and unsterile team members should wear lead aprons.
   a. The lead apron is worn under the sterile gown. Lead aprons that bear the total weight from the shoulders can cause fatigue and back strain. Lead protective attire can be worn like a vest and skirt to distribute the total lead weight.
   b. If the apron does not wrap around the body, team members should face the radiation source so the apron provides protection between the source and the body.
   c. To protect against beam and scatter radiation, team members should wear aprons during fluoroscopy and for lateral or oblique radiographs. Levels of scatter radiation are greater at lateral and oblique angles, and exposure time is prolonged during fluoroscopy.
   d. Lead aprons should be hung or laid flat when not in use. They should not be folded. Folding can crack the lead, making the shield ineffective. The aprons should be examined under radiographs periodically to determine intactness.
4. Lead-impregnated rubber gloves can attenuate (reduce the intensity of) rays by 15% to 25%.
   a. Sterile team members should wear sterile gloves over lead-impregnated gloves when the hands will

be in direct exposure (e.g., during fluoroscopy), when injecting radioactive dyes or elements, and while handling radioactive implants.
   b. If it is necessary to hold a cassette in position for a single radiograph exposure, lead gloves should be worn.
   c. Lead gloves may be supplied sterile or sterilized by the appropriate method for reuse. The rubber should allow adequate aeration to avoid skin irritation of the wearer.
5. Lead thyroid/sternal collars or shields should be worn during fluoroscopy and exposure to oblique-angle radiographs. Personnel within 6 feet (2 m) of the radiation source, including the anesthesia provider, risk exposure of the head and neck.
6. Leaded glasses may be worn to protect the eyes from cataract formation during fluoroscopy.

   Lead shields should be tested routinely by the radiology department every 6 months and whenever damage is suspected. Defects may not be visually detected.

Monitoring Radiation Exposure. All personnel exposed to ionizing radiation with any frequency or during prolonged procedures should wear a monitoring device. The purpose of the device is to measure the total rems of accumulated exposure. Therefore, the monitor is worn only by the person to whom it is issued and at all times of exposure for the designated period. Exposure data on the monitor are recorded for each individual either monthly or weekly, depending on the type of monitor.

Film badges are the most widely used monitors. These monitors contain small pieces of photographic film that are sensitive to different types of radiation: beta rays, gamma rays, and x-rays. Thermoluminescent badges and pocket dosimeters also are available. More than one monitor, of the same or a different type, may be worn.

Placement of the monitor is determined by which body parts are being monitored. The monitor should be worn consistently at the same area. A single monitor can be worn outside a lead apron at the level of the neck to measure exposure of head and neck, especially during fluoroscopy. Another monitor may be worn under the apron to measure exposure of the whole body and gonads.

Nonionizing Radiation

Radiant energy in the form of heat and/or light is emitted from radiowaves, microwaves, televisions, computers, radiant warmers, and light sources. For example, overhead operating lights produce heat. Fiberoptic light cables are cool, but the light transmitted is intense and can produce heat. Radiation from these sources is nonionizing (with the exception of ultraviolet lights, which can produce radiant energy in wavelengths and intensity sufficient to alter deoxyribonucleic acid [DNA] in cells, burn tissue, and damage the eyes). Nonionizing radiation does not accumulate in the body and therefore does not require monitoring. Nonionizing radiation per se is not hazardous when properly controlled.

Lasers, one form of nonionizing radiation, concentrate very-high-energy light beams within a small circumference to produce intense heat. (*Laser* is an acronym for light amplification by stimulated emission of radiation.) Laser equipment should be used in accordance with established regulatory standards and guidelines and the manufacturer's instructions for laser safety. Lasers can vaporize, cut, or coagulate tissues directly exposed to the beams. They can cause thermal burns from indirect exposure. Fire, explosion, eye and skin exposure, and laser plume (smoke) also are potential hazards for patients and personnel. Eyewear of the correct optical density is required and reflective surfaces should be covered. Safety measures should be taken.

Magnetic Energy

The first human testing of magnetic imaging took place in 1977. It took more than 5 hours to accomplish. Today this technology is becoming a diagnostic and interventional standard. Some larger facilities have interventional suites with high tech surgical equipment for real-time magnetic imaging during a surgical procedure that creates three-dimensional maps of the patient's body with radiowaves. Patients with implanted stainless steel clips and other components, such as older-style pacemakers can suffer injury in the presence of magnetic resonance imaging (MRI). Implanted clips may be attached to intracranial vessels or other structures that could be injured if exposed to extreme magnetic forces.

Patients with stimulator leads are at risk because the metal in the leads will become superheated, causing tissue injury. Examples of implanted stimulators include pacer wires, spinal or neurologic stimulators, and internal defibrillator wires.

No magnetic metal object can be used within the MRI environment. Items have been pulled from caregiver's pockets, including scissors. Instrument tables, IV poles, oxygen tanks, instrumentation, and OR furniture cannot be composed of any magnetic substance. Titanium or plastic is commonly used in this environment because it is inert and nonmagnetic.

Electricity

The appropriate use of electronic devices is a prime concern of health care providers and industry personnel who seek safer patient care. Underlying this concern is the rapidly expanding use of electronic equipment. The marketing and safety standards of medical electronic devices used in the perioperative environment are federally regulated. The standards and practices recommended by the Association for the Advancement of Medical Instrumentation (AAMI) are helpful to both manufacturers and users. Standards set by JCAHO also should be met for facility accreditation. Inadequately trained personnel or the malfunctions of devices such as electrosurgical units (ESUs), defibrillators, and radiograph machines are responsible for the fatalities and near-fatalities that occur.

Parameters of Electricity. Electricity is the flow of electrons along a path. It consists of three basic parameters: voltage, resistance, and current.

Voltage. Voltage forces electrons to move through material in one direction and causes current to flow. It is measured in volts. The greater the number of volts, the more direct the path of the current.

Resistance. Resistance is the measurement of opposition to the flow of electrons through material. It is measured in ohms. Electricity flows easily through conductors (e.g., metals, carbon, water); flow is minimized by insulators (e.g., rubber, plastic, glass) that prevent the flow of electricity. The resistance of the human body is more similar to a conductor than an insulator.

Current. Current is the rate of flow of electrons through a conductor. It is measured in amperes—the number of electrons passing a given point each second. Current flow is proportional to voltage and inversely proportional to resistance. Current may be one of two types:

1. Direct current (DC), as from a battery. This is a low-voltage current.
2. Alternating current (AC), as from a 110- or 220-volt line. This type of current has an alternating directional flow. AC is considered low voltage, but it is three times more powerful than low-voltage DC.

Grounding. The grounding of all electrical equipment is essential for safety and the prevention of stray current leakage. Grounding systems are designed to discharge any harmful electricity directly to the ground without including the patient in the circuit. This prevents the inadvertent passage of electric current through the patient, thereby preventing shock or burn.

ESUs are grounded. When using an ESU a return electrode is positioned on the patient to disperse the electrical energy and return it to the generator. The pad itself is not a ground, but a path for the current to return back to the machine.

Electrical power is supplied through two wires—hot and neutral—that transmit current to the three-wire outlets in the building. The third wire is the ground wire. When the cord from an electrical device is plugged into an outlet, the hot and neutral wires deliver the current. The ground wire is attached to a copper pipe that is driven into the ground at the point where power enters the building. An electrical connection to the ground provides a means for current to flow through the ground wire (or any other conductive surface) to the ground rather than going to the neutral wire. The copper ground wire is used to prevent the metal housings of electrical equipment from becoming electrically "hot." The ground wire within the three-wire power plug and cord connects the equipment (instrument) housing to the ground contact in the receptacle (wall outlet). This provides a constantly available return path for current to the electrical source.

When an instrument is grounded, leakage current returns through the ground wire to earth, causing no damage. However, if the ground path is absent or broken, leakage current will seek another path to ground. For example, if the insulation on wires is defective (e.g., broken or frayed cords or plugs), some current will leak or flow to other nearby conductors, such as the equipment housing. The same is true of endoscopic instrumentation with fractured insulation. The current will pass into the patient's tissues causing an inadvertent injury.

Equipotential Grounding System. Current flows between points only when a voltage difference exists between them.

Therefore electric shock can be minimized by eliminating voltage differences. One system designed to do this is the equipotential grounding system, which maintains an equal potential or voltage between all conductive surfaces near the patient. To achieve equipotential grounding, all exposed conductive surfaces within 6 feet (2 m) of the patient are electrically connected to a single point that is itself connected by a copper conductor to the ground tie point at the electrical distribution center serving the area. Consequently, all exposed metal surfaces are electrically tied together and to the ground.

Isolation Power System. Isolated power systems are used in hazardous locations such as ORs. An isolation transformer isolates the OR electrical circuits from grounded circuits in the power mains. Thus the isolated circuit does not include the ground in its pathway; the current seeks to flow only from one isolated line to the other. As a result, accidental grounding of people in contact with the hot wire does not cause current to flow through the individual.

A line isolation monitor checks the degree of isolation maintained by an isolated power system by continually measuring the resistance and capacitance between the two isolated lines and the ground. This measurement is called the hazard index. The monitor, a wall-mounted meter, has an alarm that is activated at the 2-milliampere level. This warning system indicates when inadvertent grounding of isolated circuits has occurred and alerts personnel to a dangerous situation. Because grounding can take place only when faulty equipment is plugged into ungrounded circuits, maximum safety is afforded by use of the isolation transformer. Ungrounded circuits fed through isolation transformers are required in OR and obstetric suites. Permanently installed overhead operating lights and receptacles in anesthetizing locations should be supplied by ungrounded electrical circuits.

The following steps should be taken in the event that the line isolation monitor alarm is activated during a surgical procedure:

1. Unplug the last piece of electrical equipment that was plugged into the power system.
2. Continue to unplug all equipment in the OR to identify the faulty equipment. A battery-operated backup system may be needed.
3. Close the OR until a biomedical engineer can check for current leakage.

Electric Shock. Electrocution occurs when an individual becomes the component that closes a circuit through which a lethal current may flow. Lethal levels may be attained by currents through the intact body via the skin or by currents applied directly to the heart. Electric shock occurs when a current is large enough to stimulate the nervous system or large muscle masses (e.g., when the body becomes the connecting link between two points of an electrical system that are at different potentials).

The physiologic effect of shock may range from a mere tingling sensation to tissue necrosis, ventricular fibrillation, or death. This effect is an electrical response of sensory cells, nerves, or muscles to electrical stimuli that originate either intrinsically (within the body) or extrinsically (outside the body). The severity of shock depends on the magnitude of the current flow and the path taken through the body. There are two types of shock: macroshock and microshock:

1. *Macroshock.* Macroshock occurs when current flows through a relatively large surface of skin. It usually results from inadvertent contact with moderately high voltage sources, expressed in milliamperes (1/1000 ampere). A current intensity of 1 to 5 milliamperes through the chest can cause severe burn at the point of contact. If the cardiac conduction system is involved, a current intensity of 50 to 100 milliamperes through the chest can cause ventricular fibrillation because the heartbeat is electrically controlled.

   Macroshock occurs through the trunk of the body, with the current following many paths; each path carries a fraction of the current. It may or may not be harmful, depending on how much current flows through a susceptible heart along its path. Common sources of macroshock are electrical wiring failures that allow skin contact with a live wire or surface at full voltage. The victim, instrument, or surface should never be touched with bare hands in a case of shock. The power supply should be disconnected, or an insulating material should be used to push the victim away from the source of electricity.

2. *Microshock.* Microshock occurs when current is applied to a very small contact area of skin. The development of medical techniques that permit the application of electrical impulses directly to the heart muscle has raised awareness of the extreme danger of microshock to an electrically sensitive patient. Cardiac microshock is a potential hazard of indwelling catheters filled with conductive fluid, probes inserted into the great vessels, and electrodes implanted around the heart. These devices multiply the potential for electrocution because they can be conductors of electricity.

   The external portion of a cardiac catheter generally consists of two parts: an inner conductor(s) of wires or conductive fluid and an outer insulating sheath. When there is a highly conductive pathway from outside the body to the great vessels and heart, small electric currents may cause ventricular fibrillation and cardiac arrest. When a shock has an internal route to the heart, it takes only one thousandth as much electricity to be fatal as when the shock is transmitted through the surface of the skin. Microshock occurs only if current from an exterior source flows through the cardiac catheter or conductor. Conductive intravascular catheters that disperse current at skin level diminish the risk of microshock. The most important precaution is to protect the exposed end of the cardiac conductor from contact with conductive surfaces, including the body. Rubber or plastic gloves should always be worn when handling the external end of a cardiac catheter or conductor.

Safeguards. Although the value of electronic devices is unquestionable, their use must not be allowed to cause electric shock or electrocution. Cardiac fibrillation and arrest may occur if a patient encounters an excess of accumulated small currents while connected to the ground through implanted electronic devices or by contact with other grounded objects, such as electrocardiograph (ECG) leads. Faulty electrical equipment may cause a short circuit or electric shock or can cause severe sparks that may be a source of ignition. The following safeguards should be used when working with electrical equipment:

- Particular care should be used when operating high-voltage equipment such as radiograph machines, ESUs, lasers, and electronic monitoring devices. These machines should be checked for frayed or broken power cords, properly functioning power switches, and grounding.
- Power cables should not be stretched taut or across traffic lanes.
- Liquids should never be placed on an electrical unit. A spill could cause an internal short circuit.
- Electrosurgical and laser units may interfere with the operation of other equipment. Therefore, they should be located on the operator's side of the table and as far as possible from the monitoring equipment. Preferably, these units are plugged into separate circuits to avoid overloading power lines. They should not be plugged into extension cords.
- Equipment should be properly grounded to prevent small extraneous current leaks.
- Machines should be turned off when plugging them into or unplugging them from the power receptacle and when attaching cords to the machine.
- Power cords should be unplugged by pulling on the plugs, never the cords; this prevents breakage of wires.
- All electrical equipment, including a surgeon's personal property, should be inspected by the biomedical engineering department before its initial use. Every piece must meet Underwriters Laboratories (UL) standards or other electrical safety requirements. All equipment should be inspected, preferably monthly but at least quarterly, and verified as safe for use. Equipment should be used according to the manufacturer's instructions.

Electrical and Thermal Burns. Monitors and all high-powered equipment are hazardous. Electrical energy is converted into thermal energy, and therefore the electricity supplied by a defective system may cause burns. The amount of heat produced depends on current density, contact time, and tissue resistance. As little as 300 milliamperes of current for 20 seconds can produce enough heat (113° F [45° C]) to burn intact skin. Current that is concentrated or has a high density at the point of contact can result in an electrical burn severe enough to require debridement.

Electrosurgical units generate high-frequency current. In these units, current flows to an active electrode that is used to cut or coagulate tissue. The patient is protected by using a dispersive electrode (also known as return electrode or Bovie pad). This provides the high-frequency current present at the active electrode with a low-current density pathway back to the generator. This is not the same as a ground. Proper connections from the dispersive electrode to the patient and to the unit are essential to prevent burns. Deep tissue burns can occur at the site of a dispersive electrode if it does not have adequate surface contact with skin or body tissue. Burns also can occur at the site of rings or other metal jewelry, ECG electrodes, or other low-resistance points from invasive monitor probes (e.g., temperature probes) if the current diverts to an alternate path.

Conductive surfaces should be capable of providing a return path for current other than through the operating bed or its attachments. If the return circuit of high-frequency equipment is faulty, the circuit may be completed through inadvertent contact with metal parts or attachments of the operating bed. If the pathway for the current is small, the current passing through the exposed area of skin contact will be relatively intense, causing a deep burn to the patient. For example, one such contact point may be the thigh touching the leg stirrup when the patient is in the lithotomy position.

Surface burns can occur when battery-operated equipment, such as a peripheral nerve stimulator, is used with external electrodes. Tetanic stimuli should be limited to 1 or 2 seconds. Handheld battery-operated cautery pencils can cause pinpoint burns when the tip remains hot after use. The heat from this tip can cause ignition to drapes or dry sponges.

Other potential sources of burns include malfunctioning controls on heat-generating devices that are in contact with the patient, such as radiofrequency diathermy or hypothermia/hyperthermia machines. Individual reactions to electrical hazards are influenced by factors such as the patient's nutritional state, the amount of body fat that acts as insulation, and the circulation in the body part in contact with the device.

Static Electricity. Static electricity consists of current of high voltage and low ampere. An electrostatic spark develops from friction and accumulates on physical objects. When two static-bearing objects come into contact, the one bearing the higher potential discharges to the one with the lower potential. Air is a nonconductor, but a high enough potential can overcome air resistance and jump the gap to a lower potential object. This causes an arc across air gaps, which are seen as spark(s) from the heat thus generated. These sparks can ignite flammable materials or gases.

Objects accumulate static in inverse proportion to their conductivity. A spark between two objects can occur only when an electrical path of good conductivity does not exist between them. Because earth has a zero potential, a charge is discharged to earth if it is brought into contact with earth directly or indirectly through a conductor. The aim is to provide adequate channels for the dissipation of static. Moderate conductivity has a tendency for the gradual spread of charge over both objects so they come to the same potential. The generation of static electricity cannot be prevented absolutely because its intrinsic origins are present at every interface. For static electricity to be a source of ignition, the following should be present:

- An effective means of static generation
- A means of accumulating the separate charges and maintaining a suitable difference of electrical potential
- A discharge of energy adequate to make a spark in an ignitable mixture

Fire and Explosion

Fire should be a matter of prime concern in the OR. Fires in an oxygen-enriched atmosphere (OEA) are fundamentally different in character from those occurring in normal atmosphere. The fire severity potential should be regarded as serious, with the potential for extensive damage and endangerment to lives of patients and personnel. The presence of flammable and combustible liquids, vapors, and gases in an OEA can result in the ultrarapid combustion of surrounding materials with explosive violence (Fig. 13-3).

Anesthesia providers have discontinued the use of highly flammable anesthetic agents (e.g., cyclopropane, ether) in favor of halogenated agents. These noncombustible agents are mixed with air, oxygen, or nitrous oxide. Although oxygen and nitrous oxide are nonflammable gases, they do support and accelerate combustion. A fire or explosion is the result of a combination of these factors:

- A flammable gas, vapor, or liquid (e.g., ethylene oxide, alcohol, ether, methane from the bowel, collodion). Dry sponges are flammable.
- A source of ignition (e.g., laser, electrosurgery)
- Oxygen (pure or in air with greater than 21% oxygen) or some other substance that provides oxygen, such as nitrous oxide gas. Oxygen can build up under the drapes and cause ignition when the cautery is used.

Safeguards. Standards of the NFPA and AAMI are evaluated by JCAHO to safeguard against fire and explosion in anesthetizing locations. Requirements are less stringent where only nonflammable inhalation agents are used. For example, nonconductive flooring and footwear are acceptable when a nonexplosive anesthetic is used. The factors that can cause fire should be controlled.

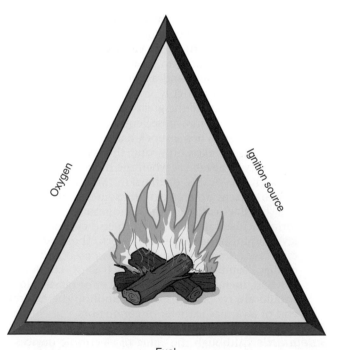

FIG. 13-3 Fire triangle.

Flammable Agents. Spontaneous combustion can occur when flammable agents are exposed to an ignition source in the presence of oxygen. The following are safeguards to prevent spontaneous combustion:

- Anesthesia machines, cylinders of compressed gas, and flammable liquid containers should be kept away from any source of heat and must not touch one another. A mixture of gases under high pressure is hazardous.
- Oil or grease is not used on oxygen valves or on parts of anesthesia machines. Oil or grease should not contact any cylinders, including those containing ethylene oxide, compressed air, or nitrogen.
- Flammable antiseptics containing alcohol and fat solvents are used with care for preoperative skin preparation before laser or electrosurgery. Vapors under drapes or pooled material on or around the skin can ignite if the prep solution is not completely dry before draping. Common pooling areas include the umbilicus and the sternal notch.
- Petroleum products used on the skin can ignite in the presence of ESU or laser. Water-soluble jelly can be used to coat eyebrows and lashes to render them less likely to ignite.
- Bowel gases (methane) are flammable. The rectum should be packed with a moist sponge before using ESU or laser near the perineum.
- Other flammables include collodion, benzoin, paraffin, and white wax (bone wax).

Ignition Sources. The minimum ignition temperatures of combustible materials in an OEA are lower than in air. The following list contains precautions to use when working with combustible materials:

1. Thermal devices and other heated objects can cause a fire or explosion.
   a. Precautions should be taken to prevent a laser beam, either directly or indirectly, from igniting drapes, sponges, and gowns or from melting an endotracheal tube. Place damp towels around the surgical site when using a carbon dioxide laser.
   b. Electrosurgical units should not be used on the neck, trachea, nasopharynx, and adjacent areas. Oxygen can cause a fire if the endotracheal tube is ignited or leaks into the field. Avoid using pieces of red rubber catheter as electrode insulation.
   c. Inadvertent activation of laser and electrosurgical units should be avoided. When not in use, handpieces should be placed in a holder on the sterile field, not left loose. Handpieces are hot after activation. Laser units should be on "stand-by" or turned off as appropriate.
   d. Beams from fiberoptic light carriers should not be directed onto a drape. Heat can build up until sufficient to produce burning or smoldering.
   e. Lights and sources of heat should be kept at least 4 feet (more than 1 m) away from the anesthesia machine and cylinders.
   f. Heat-generating equipment, such as the operating microscope and the projection lamp for fiberoptic lighting, must not be completely enclosed. Heat can build up under the covering.
   g. The hypothermia/hyperthermia machine should be at least 3 feet (1 m) away from the anesthesia machine, and both should be adequately grounded.
   h. Only approved photographic lighting equipment with suitable enclosures can be used. Strobe lamps are preferred.
   i. High-speed burrs and drills create extreme heat and can cause ignition.
2. An electrostatic (incendiary) spark can be an ignition source.
   a. The relative humidity (weight of water vapor present) in the perioperative environment should be maintained between 50% and 60%. Moisture provides a relatively conductive medium, therefore allowing static electricity to leak to earth as fast as it is generated. Sparks form more readily in low humidity.
   b. Explosion-proof electrical receptacles or locking Hubble plugs cannot be pulled apart accidentally. Grounding adapter plugs, multiple-outlet plugs, and extension cords are prohibited.
   c. Power cords should be rubber coated, and switches should be explosion-proof. Electrical equipment should be plugged into the power receptacle before the anesthetic is administered and before the power switch is turned on.
   d. Motion should be minimal in the area around the anesthesia equipment and the patient's head. Friction on the reservoir bag should be avoided. Team members should watch that drapes do not touch the bag or cover the anesthesia machine.
   e. Patients are covered with cotton blankets. Woolen or synthetic blankets are prone to producing static electricity.
   f. The hair of patients, personnel, and visitors is covered to avoid static discharge.
   g. Antistatic outer garments are worn. Hose and undergarments in close contact with the skin may be made of synthetic material.
   h. Antistatic liners in kick buckets are handled with caution.
   i. Metals should not make contact with a force sufficient to produce percussion sparks.
   j. Anesthesia is discontinued as soon as possible if the ground monitoring system indicates a warning. After completion of the surgical procedure, the room is not used until the electrical defect is corrected.

Fire Safety. All health care facilities have fire warning and safety systems. Staff members should be familiar with the location and operation of fire alarms and fire extinguishers as well as with evacuation routes and procedures. Fire drills should be scheduled routinely and should be part of competency testing. Personnel should know the uses of fire extinguishers, be able to distinguish among the three main classes of them, and how to operate them:

- Class A (pressurized water for combustibles such as paper, cloth, wood). A picture of a trash can or campfire may be on the side. The "A" is imprinted within a triangle.
- Class B (carbon dioxide or dry chemical to smother flammable liquids, oil, gas). A picture of a gas can may

be on the side. The "B" is imprinted inside a square. A number may precede the B. This number represents the distance in feet the spray will reach.

- Class C (halon [bromochlorodifluoromethane halogenated compressed gas] to smother an electrical or laser fire without leaving a residue on equipment). A picture of an electrical plug may appear on the side. The "C" is imprinted in a circle.

When a fire extinguisher is used, the mnemonic PASS may aid in remembering how to operate the device:

Pull the safety ring out of the handle.

Aim the nozzle.

Squeeze the handle.

Sweep the spray over the base of the fire.

If fire should occur in the OR during a surgical procedure, the first concern is for the safety of the patient and personnel. To prevent explosion, the burning article is removed immediately from the proximity of the oxygen source and the anesthesia machine or outlet of piped-in gases. The fire on the field is smothered with wet towels, and burning drapes are removed from the patient. The shut-off valves for piped-in gases are turned off, and electrical power cords are unplugged.

The mnemonic RACE may aid in preventing panic and should enable the team to act quickly in the event of fire anywhere within the perioperative environment:

Rescue anyone who is in immediate danger.

Activate the fire alarm.

Contain the fire if possible.

Evacuate the area.

The patient should be removed immediately from any danger and the fire should be extinguished in the room, if possible. The anesthetized patient is evacuated on the operating bed to a distant location on the same floor. Lateral evacuation is when the team movement from the fire is creating a distance from danger on the same floor. Anesthesia personnel should be assisted with life-support equipment, such as breathing bags (Ambu bag) and tubing. Keep in mind that oxygen will support the fire.

Pack the surgical site with saline-moistened lap tapes, and cover with a sterile towel or drape. Although attempts are made to prevent infection, this is a secondary thought to the loss of life. All fires, no matter how small must be reported to the facilities risk management department. Team members should refer to the departmental policy and procedure manual for evacuation and safety protocols specific to the facility.

Fires within the patient's body are usually small, but deadly. The most common type is an endotracheal fire. The cause is usually laser or ESU contact with a flammable endotracheal tube. In the event of an endotracheal fire, immediately withdraw the burning tube and pinch the nose and mouth shut to extinguish the fire (this removes the fuel and oxygen).[4] The anesthesia provider must immediately reintubate with a smaller, uncuffed tube and reoxygenate the patient. A cuffed tube would increase pressure on the damaged tissue.

---

[4]AORN Standards, Recommended Practices, and Guidelines, Fire Prevention in the Operating Room, 2005.

CHEMICAL HAZARDS AND SAFEGUARDS

Health care providers are exposed to many hazardous chemicals daily. The hazards of these chemicals include irritation of the eyes or mucous membranes, contact dermatitis or burns, toxicity that causes renal or liver disease, and exposure to carcinogens or mutagens. These or other effects may be immediate, delayed, or chronic. Hazardous chemicals in the workplace are controlled by government regulations, such as those of OSHA and EPA in the United States or those of the Control of Substances Hazardous to Health (COSHH) in Great Britain.

Chemicals should be labeled by the manufacturer with the identity of the agent(s) and appropriate warnings of hazards. The latter may be symbolic, that is, pictures added to words. Labels must not be removed or defaced. Employees should read the labels and understand procedures for safe handling and use. OSHA has incorporated right-to-know regulations in its standards. One part of this Hazard Communication Standard requires that employees have access to material safety data sheets (MSDSs) supplied by the manufacturer for each hazardous chemical in the workplace. An MSDS specifies the following:

- Composition and common names of the chemical
- Chemical and physical properties
- Known acute and chronic health effects, such as carcinogenic, mutagenic, or allergenic
- Exposure limits
- Protective measures
- Antidote or first-aid measures

OSHA standards are legally enforceable. Although not legally enforceable, NIOSH and ACGIH recommendations for exposure limits to hazardous gases and vapors in ambient air should be adopted for the safety of personnel.

Anesthetic Gases

Air-conditioning or ventilating systems help to prevent pockets of anesthetic gases in the OR, although concentrations around the anesthesia machine and the patient's head may not be remarkably reduced. Substantial amounts of gases can escape during surgical procedures. The patient's exhalations also can pollute the air in the OR and the postanesthesia care unit (PACU). Heavy gas can accumulate and channel along the floor as far as 50 feet (15 m). Confining agents by using a closed carbon dioxide absorption technique tends to restrict gases from getting into airstreams.

Waste anesthetic gases are gases and vapors that escape from the anesthesia machine and its hoses and connections; from around the facemask on the patient; and from the patient's expirations. Although not conclusive, data indicate that personnel may incur health hazards if chronically exposed to waste anesthetic gas. Stress, long working hours, and other unknown related factors may contribute to this occupational risk. Possible health hazards include the risk of spontaneous abortion, congenital abnormalities in the offspring of male and female personnel, cancer, and hepatic and renal disease. Significant behavioral changes have been observed and include decreased perception, cognition, and manual dexterity. Personnel also may complain of fatigue or headache.

Studies of the retention of anesthetic agents in anesthesia providers after the administration of clinical anesthesia have demonstrated traces of gas in expired air for varying lengths of time—from 7 hours after nitrous oxide administration to 64 hours after halothane administration. It has been shown that high doses of nitrous oxide block the metabolism of vitamin B_{12}. Chronic exposure to trace levels of nitrous oxide may also lead to neurologic problems or neuropathy.

Because millions of inhalation anesthetics are administered annually, a substantial number of OR staff are occupationally exposed to these gases. OSHA enforces the NIOSH recommendations that room air not be contaminated by more than 0.5 parts per million (ppm) of halogenated agents per hour when used in combination with nitrous oxide or by more than 2 ppm per hour when used alone. Nitrous oxide should be controlled to less than 25 ppm during an 8-hour time-weighted exposure.

The use of scavenging equipment and procedures is strongly recommended. Scavenging involves the removal of waste anesthetic gases, mainly by trapping them at the site of overflow on the breathing circuit; this is followed by disposal to the outside atmosphere, where the gases are safely diluted. The rate of removal of gases by the disposal system depends on the rate at which fresh air enters the OR and the patterns taken by air currents as they circulate through the room.

The proper use of scavenging equipment can reduce exposure to trace concentrations of gas by 90% to 95%. Personnel exposure should be reduced to the lowest practicable limits by reducing waste gas to the most technically feasible level. A waste-gas control program to ensure the continuing purity of environmental air includes the following measures:

1. Good work practices of anesthesia providers. The major source of waste gas in the OR is the intentional outflow of gases from the anesthesia breathing system. The quantity of gases discharged varies depending on the type of breathing system, the gas flow rate, and gas concentration.
2. Use of a well-designed, well-maintained scavenging system. Inexpensive, practical, and effective exhaust systems are available. The gas evacuation system should be attached to every anesthesia machine and ventilator to scavenge excess gases directly into a vacuum line with a minimum flow rate of 440 ppm.
3. Use of proper anesthesia technique:
   a. Different techniques of administration result in different exposure levels. Some leakage is uncontrollable.
   b. All components of the breathing system should fit well. Masks should fit facial contours to ensure a good seal. An oral or nasal airway may reduce the escape of gas from around the mask.
   c. Liquid halogenated agents should not be spilled. The gas flow should not be turned on until the mask is in place or the patient is intubated and the endotracheal tube is connected to the breathing circuit.
   d. Masks, tubing, reservoir bags, and endotracheal tubes should be inspected after each cleaning for leaks, holes, and abnormalities. Disposable equipment is preferable to recycled equipment.
4. Proper maintenance of anesthesia equipment through the following measures:
   a. Daily routine checking of anesthesia machines for leaks. NIOSH recommends that the total leak rate of each machine not exceed 100 mL/min at 30 cm of water pressure. Leaks can be detected with a gas analyzer or bubble test.
   b. Periodic preventive maintenance of all machines and fittings by a manufacturer's representative every 6 months, with in-house monitoring at least quarterly.
5. Maintenance of a high flow rate of fresh air into the air-conditioning system through engineering control procedures. A good ventilating system (preferably not a recirculating one) is also important in the PACU. The ventilation system should comply with the minimum requirements of 20 air changes per hour.
6. Use of an OR atmospheric monitoring program to record trace anesthetic levels and to determine the effectiveness of the previous measures. Specialized monitoring equipment, such as an infrared analyzer, is the only way to detect leaks. Dosimeters are available for each individual to wear to indicate exposure.

Sterilizing Agents

The chemical agents used to sterilize heat-sensitive items can be toxic or can vaporize to emit noxious fumes that are irritating to the eyes and nasal passages, even at low levels of exposure.

Ethylene Oxide. Ethylene oxide (EO) is used in a gaseous form for sterilization and is known to be a mutagen and carcinogen. The residual products can be toxic if there is direct contact with the skin or if the gas is inhaled. Exposure can cause dizziness, nausea, and vomiting. Ethylene glycol and ethylene chlorohydrin are by-products of a reaction with moisture, such as on the hands. All porous items sterilized with EO should be aerated to dissipate the gas. The PELs for EO are 5 ppm for a short-term exposure of 15 minutes and 1 ppm time-weighted average (TWA) over 8 hours.

Formaldehyde. Formaldehyde may be used in a gaseous or liquid form. The vapors are toxic to the respiratory tract. Formaldehyde is a potent allergen, mutagen, and carcinogen, and it can cause liver toxicity. The PEL is 1 ppm TWA (NIOSH recommendation) to 3 ppm TWA (OSHA standard) over 8 hours.

Glutaraldehyde. Glutaraldehyde is the least toxic of the three sterilizing agents, but the fumes from the liquid form may be irritating to the eyes, nose, and throat. Contact dermatitis and hives have been reported. The PEL is 0.2 ppm per exposure. Glutaraldehyde should be used only in a closed container and in a well-ventilated area. Protective eyewear should be worn. A dosimeter is available to determine the airborne concentration of fumes.

Disinfectants

Some of the disinfectants used to clean or decontaminate equipment and furniture can be irritating to the skin and eyes. Gloves and goggles should be worn when using these chemicals, and the agents should be used in proper dilution. The fumes from some agents can irritate the nasal passages. The following can cause gloves to degrade:

- Isopropyl alcohol
- Phenol
- Sodium hypochlorite
- Glutaraldehyde
- Hydrogen peroxide
- Quaternary amines
- Povidone iodine

Methyl Methacrylate

Commonly referred to as bone cement, methyl methacrylate is a mixture of liquid and powder polymers. It should be mixed at the sterile field just before use. The vapors released during mixing are irritating to the eyes and can damage soft contact lenses. The vapors are also irritating to the respiratory tract, and they can cause drowsiness.

Methyl methacrylate may be a mutagen, a carcinogen, or toxic to the liver. The liquid solvent can cause corneal burns if it splashes into the eyes. It also can diffuse through latex gloves to cause an allergic dermatitis; gloves that are impermeable to this solvent are available. A scavenging system should be used to collect the vapors during mixing and to exhaust it to the outside air or absorb it through activated charcoal. The PEL for methyl methacrylate has been established at 100 ppm TWA.

Drugs and Other Chemicals

Antineoplastic cytotoxic drugs used for chemotherapy can be hazardous, as can laser dyes and other pharmaceuticals. All chemical agents should be prepared and administered to minimize unnecessary exposures for both patients and personnel. Chemicals should be combined or mixed with diluents only when this is known to be a safe practice, as specified by the manufacturer.

Intraperitoneal chemotherapy can be administered in the OR during laparotomy. The surgeon can use the Coliseum technique where the chemical is introduced via a Tenckhoff catheter and a roller pump with a heat exchanger set at 111.2° F (44° C). The solution remains in the patient's abdomen for 90 minutes. The surgeon, wearing two sets of sterile gloves, continually manipulates the intraabdominal organs to evenly distribute the heated chemical as it continually circulates through the cavity and is removed through several abdominal drains. The air is continually filtered through activated charcoal and a smoke evacuator to protect the OR environment from aerosolization of the drug.

Safe Handling of Cytotoxic Agents

Antineoplastic cytotoxic agents have carcinogenic and mutagenic properties, and most can cause local and/or allergic reactions. Personnel should avoid inadvertent direct contact with skin or eyes, inhalation, and ingestion during handling.

Written precautions and procedures for handling, preparing, administering, and disposing of cytotoxic agents should be followed. Basic guidelines for the use of cytotoxic agents include the following:

1. Protect self from skin and respiratory contact. Preferably, prepare agents under a vertical laminar flow hood. Whether or not a containment hood is available, wear thick gloves, a mask, eye protection, and a gown.
2. Wash hands after handling cytotoxic agents and all items that have been in contact with them, including those used for administration.
3. Place all cytotoxic waste in sealed leak-proof bags or containers. Incineration is recommended for all materials used in preparing and administering cytotoxic agents.

BIOLOGIC HAZARDS AND SAFEGUARDS

The transmission of infection and disease within the health care facility is a concern of both consumers and providers. Biologic hazards do exist in the environment, and every effort should be made by health care providers to protect their patients and themselves. Standard precautions are a necessity (i.e., treating all body fluids and materials as infectious). Employers must ensure that the appropriate protective equipment is available and that employees are trained to wear and use it.

Surfaces such as door handles and computer keyboards have been found to harbor active vancomycin-resistant *Enterococcus* (VRE), methicillin-resistant Staphylococcus aureus (MRSA), and *Pseudomonas aeruginosa* (PSAE) for prolonged periods. Simple handwashing is becoming less effective in adequately removing these microorganisms. Antiseptic gel hand hygiene is recommended. Cleaning contaminated surfaces such as computer keyboards may be unreliable because these surfaces were not designed for exposure to disinfectant solutions. Some chemicals and solutions can damage the equipment.

Infectious Waste

Infectious medical waste is an environmental concern both within and outside the health care facility. The EPA defines infectious waste as waste containing pathogens with enough virulence and quantity that exposure to them could result in an infectious disease in a susceptible host. The disposal of potentially infectious waste generated in health care facilities is regulated by governmental mandates. Although regulated medical waste refers to the portion of waste that has the potential to transmit infectious disease, a uniform definition of what constitutes regulated medical waste has not been universally adopted. Factors that should be considered in deciding if something is infectious waste include the following:

- The presence of pathogenic organisms in sufficient numbers to be capable of causing infection in living beings. Many microorganisms are incapable of causing infection.
- The presence of a portal of entry into a susceptible host. A cut, needlestick, puncture wound, or skin lesion provides a portal of entry, but not all living beings are susceptible hosts to infectious diseases.

These two factors permit the regulation of medical waste that poses a risk to public health and the environment and creates aesthetic concerns for the public. Potentially infectious waste is considered to be blood and blood products, pathologic waste, microbiologic waste, and contaminated sharps. This includes items contaminated by blood, such as sponges, drapes, gowns, and gloves. These items should be segregated from general waste, such as wrappers.

Infectious waste is placed in leak-proof containers or bags strong enough to maintain integrity during transport, and these bags should be closed and either labeled or color-coded. For example, red bags may be used to differentiate infectious waste. Needles and sharps should be put in puncture-resistant containers. If the outside of the container is contaminated, double-bagging is necessary for safe handling during transport to the disposal area. Waste can be steam-sterilized or decontaminated with microwaves before compaction and disposal in a landfill, or it can be incinerated. Federal, state, and local regulations should be followed for disposal.

Biohazards

All patients are potential sources of infection. OSHA defines occupational exposure as reasonably anticipated skin, eye, mucous membrane, or parenteral contact with blood or other potentially infectious materials during the course of duty. This contact includes blood, tissues and organs, and all body fluids. Careful handling of and adequate protection from potentially contaminated equipment also are important. Handwashing is a must after every patient contact or glove removal. Personal exposure should be a concern of all team members.

To be in compliance with OSHA standards, every health care facility must develop a written exposure control plan that includes procedures for evaluating an incident and for determining when exposure has occurred. Engineering controls include safety devices or equipment designed to minimize or eliminate a biohazard. Likewise, restrictions or changes in work practices should ensure the safety of all patients and personnel in the environment. For example, food must not be stored in the same refrigerator as blood products or specimens. Eating and drinking are prohibited in areas where contact with blood or other potentially hazardous material is possible. Eating should never be allowed in the OR during a surgical procedure.

Bloodborne Disease. A penetrating injury (e.g., needlestick, cut) or a splash (e.g., into the eye, onto mucous membranes) with fluid contaminated with blood or body fluids must not be ignored. Hepatitis, human immunodeficiency virus (HIV), and other bloodborne pathogens can be transmitted through breaks in the skin or contact with mucous membranes. The hepatitis B vaccine is recommended for all high-risk health care workers.

If exposure to blood or body fluid occurs, the following procedures should be performed:
1. Stop activity immediately, and step back from the point of contamination.
2. Squeeze the skin around the needlestick or cut to expel blood and contaminants.
3. Cleanse the puncture site or flush the eye with cool water. Flush cut or puncture with alcohol or iodine preparation.
4. Report the incident according to facility policy and procedure and seek medical attention promptly.
5. Follow the particular protocol established by the facility for follow-up.

If a needlestick is involved, most facilities will draw a baseline blood sample from the patient and the injured caregiver. Periodic blood samples are drawn over a period of months to make sure results remain clear. Caregivers who have been contaminated by a high-risk patient or a patient known to have hepatitis B or to be positive for HIV should be treated with the appropriate drugs and followed by the employee health department. Additional information about postexposure prophylaxis and guidelines for treatment can be found at www.cdc.gov.[5]

Surgical Plume. Plume (surgical smoke) is generated by the thermal destruction of tissue or bone. Bloodborne pathogens, mutagens, carcinogens, and other toxic substances can be aerosolized by lasers, electrosurgery, and powered surgical instruments. Masks capable of filtering particles at least as small as 0.1 mm are recommended to prevent inhalation. Face shields, goggles, or eyeglasses with side shields should be worn to protect the eyes.

A smoke evacuator should be used to suction laser and electrosurgical plumes. The evacuator has a filtration system that incorporates a prefilter to trap particles, an ultralow penetrating air filter for particles in the 0.1-mm range, and a charcoal filter to absorb odor and hydrocarbons. The vacuum nozzle should be held close to the surgical site. Wall suction is not recommended for smoke evacuation because an inline filter is necessary to avoid clogging the system.

OR personnel can change the filters in some evacuators, whereas others require maintenance by a biomedical technician. Filters are contaminated with biohazardous material and should be disposed of in the same manner as items contaminated with blood and body fluids. Gloves, masks, and protective eyewear should be worn when changing filters because the connecting couplers have been contaminated with plume and the material may be released into the air when the connection is disengaged.

Reproductive Hazards

Male Reproductive Health Implications. Chemical, radiologic, and physical exposures can cause abnormalities in sperm numbers, shapes, and motility. The reaction experienced by an individual will depend on the agent, duration of exposure, and other health status considerations. Chemicals such as ethylene varieties can accumulate in the epididymis, seminal vesicles, or prostate, causing decreased sperm production and decreased ability to fertilize an ovum. Some chemicals can affect a man's ability to perform sexually either because of impotence or decreased libido. Chromosomal DNA can be affected, because sperm are produced every 72 days and are stored in the epididymis for 15 to 25 days, where they mature and begin to swim. These changes can cause fetal abnormality if fertilization takes place.

According to NORA, more than 1000 workplace chemicals can cause reproductive effects in animals. Many chemicals have never been tested and also may be implicated in birth defects. (More information is available at www.cdc.gov/niosh/malrepro.html.)

---

[5]CDC website update 2005: Guidelines for HIV prophylaxis after occupational exposure.

Female Reproductive Health Implications. Excessive exposure to ionizing radiation, waste anesthetic gases, and ethylene oxide during pregnancy may cause a spontaneous abortion or a congenital fetal anomaly. Pregnant employees may be more susceptible to fatigue from standing for prolonged periods, lifting heavy items, and eating and taking breaks at irregular intervals. Exposure to infectious diseases also is a hazard. The health care facility should have a policy for pregnant employees, which may include transferring a pregnant employee from a hazardous area such as the OR. For the safety of the fetus, assignments should limit exposures whenever possible. For example, a pregnant woman should not assist with the implantation of radioactive elements.

An employee who is pregnant is responsible for her own welfare and for the safety of her fetus. Immunizations should be current, especially for hepatitis B and rubella, and she should follow the safeguards described in this chapter to limit her exposures to the lowest possible levels. Ultimately, the employee should decide whether she wishes to continue working in the perioperative environment.

Latex Sensitivity/Allergy

Many items used in the OR, such as surgical gloves, catheters, drains, medication vial stoppers, tubing, anesthesia breathing circuits, endotracheal tubes, breathing bags, and syringe plungers, contain natural rubber latex (Table 13-1). Some

TABLE 13-1	Care of the Latex-Sensitive Patient		
Commonly Used Latex Products	Latex-Free Alternatives	Patient Teaching	Considerations
Anesthesia breathing circuit, endotracheal tube, Ambu breathing bag	Disposable plastic breathing circuits and endotracheal tubes	NA (not applicable)	Dispose of used equipment
Bite blocks for oral surgery	Dental rolls, rolled gauze squares, silicone blocks	NA	Avoid using counted radiopaque sponges
Catheters, enema tips, and drains	Silicone catheters and drains	Instruct patient to report irritation or discomfort in area of drain or catheter	Patients rarely have silicone sensitivity; check product for content in manufacturer's enclosed literature
Electrocardiogram (ECG) leads, dispersive electrodes, pulse oximeter leads	Nonlatex gel pads	Instruct patient to report irritation at application site	Patient may have sensitivity to conductive gel; may need to use water-soluble lubricant
Elastic bandages, antiembolism stockings	White cotton bandages	Instruct patient to report any sensory changes in bandaged part, such as tingling, pain, or loss of sensation	Nonelastic bandages or stockings may restrict movement and have less expansion properties; circulation may become impaired if applied too tightly
Elastic and adhesive tape	Plastic, paper, or silk tape	Instruct patient to report irritation around or under area of tape	Some patients have sensitivity to adhesive rather than tape backing
Elastic bands on surgical caps, shoe covers, urinary catheter leg bags, plastic pants, disposable diapers	Cloth towel or paper caps with ties to cover hair; cloth hook and loop leg bands, cloth diapers	Instruct patient to report irritation around hairline or leg(s)	Cloth diapers will not be impervious to leaks; cloth hook and loop bands may impair circulation to leg
Embolectomy catheters	Silicone catheters	NA	Check composition of entire catheter and balloon
Hypothermia/hyperthermia blanket, hot water bottle, heating pad, mattress cover	Disposable plastic warming blankets and pads	Instruct patient to report irritation or discomfort	Observe for temperature control of device to avoid skin injury
Latex gloves, finger cots	Plastic or other nonlatex gloves	Instruct patient that utility gloves used at home may contain latex	Use nonlatex sterile gloves; vinyl utility gloves for nonsterile activities
Positioning devices, such as egg crate–type, donuts, wedges, rolls	Rolled blankets and towels	NA	Roll blankets around larger objects, such as plastic water bags, for more height
Rubber shods	Silicone catheter or plastic tubes	NA	Should be radiopaque; plastic shods are not as pliable
Syringe plungers in plastic syringes	Glass syringes	Instruct patient that plungers in plastic syringes used for self-administered injectable medications contain latex	Air-powered autoinjector device or implantable medication dispensing mechanism are options at home
Tubing as on blood pressure cuffs and endoscopic insufflators	Disposable plastic tubing and cuff covers	NA	Wrap limb with cotton sheet wadding to avoid contact

synthetic products are referred to as latex but do not contain the protein that causes reaction. Natural rubber latex is manufactured from the milky sap *(Hevea brasiliensis)* obtained from rubber trees. A water-soluble protein in natural latex contains an antigen that can cause a fatal allergic response.

Two types of responses have been identified: local and systemic. Local reactions are less severe and occur when latex comes into contact with the skin, causing skin rash, itching, redness, and burning. A patient may have a systemic reaction when a latex product comes into contact with the mucous membranes, serosa, or peritoneum during a surgical procedure. This reaction is more severe, causing anaphylactic shock or death. The signs of severe anaphylaxis are hypotension, tachycardia, bronchospasm, and generalized erythema.

FDA studies have shown that 6% to 7% of direct patient care personnel and surgeons are sensitive to natural rubber latex. Health care personnel who are frequently exposed to latex products can become sensitized. Several items used in the OR contain latex but are not identified as having natural rubber latex as a content (e.g., the elastic bands on caps and shoe covers or mattress and pillow covers). The manufacturer should be consulted to determine whether a product in use contains latex and whether a latex-free substitute is available.

Latex proteins can contaminate the starch on prepowdered gloves, thus providing a potential route of airborne exposure to allergens during donning. Sterile surgical nonlatex gloves are available commercially but are more expensive. They should be used only when an allergy is confirmed or is highly suspected in the user or in a patient receiving care.

Testing procedures are available for the detection of a latex allergy. Testing all personnel and patients would be a costly endeavor, but testing people suspected of having a latex sensitivity should be considered. According to the CDC, 8% to 12% of all health care personnel are sensitive as compared with 1% to 6% of the general population. Patients should be asked preoperatively if they have a known sensitivity (i.e., a history of a reaction after handling a toy balloon or wearing rubber gloves). Children with spina bifida, people with constant latex exposure, and those with multiple allergies are known to be prone to latex allergy. Allergies to certain foods, such as avocados, potatoes, bananas, tomatoes, chestnuts, kiwifruit, and papaya, may be implicated in natural latex allergies per NIOSH.

RISK MANAGEMENT

The perioperative environment is a high-risk environment. The risks can be minimized by adhering to the many safeguards discussed in this chapter. An effective risk management program continually seeks to provide working conditions that will not jeopardize the health and safety of employees. Such a program has at least four key elements:
1. Administration
   a. Regulations, recommendations, guidelines, and laws should be enforced to prevent disastrous consequences of occupational hazards.
   b. Policies and procedures should be written, reviewed periodically, and updated as appropriate. All employees should have access to them.
   c. Protective attire and safety equipment should be made available to employees, as appropriate.
   d. Monitoring devices should be used in all hazardous locations as recommended by regulatory agencies.
   e. Employee health services should be provided for immunizations and in the event of injury.
2. Prevention
   a. Regular inservice programs should be conducted to keep employees informed about hazards and safeguards.
   b. Employees should be taught how to use and care for new equipment before it is put into service.
   c. Employees must know the location and use of emergency equipment, such as fire extinguishers and shut-off valves.
   d. Employees must wear protective attire, as appropriate.
   e. Routine preventive maintenance should be provided for all potentially hazardous equipment.
3. Correction
   a. Faulty or malfunctioning equipment should be taken out of service immediately.
   b. Any injury should be reported, with medical attention sought as soon as possible.
   c. Unsafe conditions should be reported.
4. Documentation
   a. Records of preemployment medical examinations and periodic examinations for the surveillance and early detection of disease should be maintained for each employee. These records should be retained in a permanent file after termination of employment in case there is a future health problem.
   b. At the time of employment, new employees may be given a letter explaining the occupational risks.
   c. Incident reports regarding injuries to personnel and patients should be filed with the administration of the facility.

The prevention of injuries is vital to maintaining a safe environment. It is everyone's responsibility.

Bibliography

Awan MS, Ahmed I: Endotracheal tube fire during tracheostomy: A case report, *Ear Nose Throat J* 81(2):90-92, 2002.
Bain EI: Assessing for occupational hazards, *Am J Nurs* 100(1):96, 2000.
Brisley T et al: Safe handling of cytotoxic chemotherapy: Implications for cancer nursing practice, *Austral J Cancer Nurs* 4(2):15-21, 2003.
Burm AG: Occupational hazards of inhalational anaesthetics, *Best Pract Res Clin Anaesthesiol* 17(1):147-161, 2003.
Converso A, Murphy C: Winning the battle against back injuries, *RN* 67(2):52-8, 47, 82, 2004.
Daane SP, Toth BA: Fire in the operating room: Principles and prevention, *Plastic Reconstruct Surg* 115(5):73-75, 2005.
ERCI: Sharps injuries in the operating room—A new focus for OSHA, *Operating Room Risk Manage* December, 2004.
Harstall R et al: Radiation exposure to the surgeon during fluoroscopically assisted percutaneous vertebroplasty, *Spine* 30(16):1893-1898, 2005.
Jackson SH, Cheung EC: Hepatitis B and hepatitis C: Occupational considerations for the anesthesiologist, *Anesthesiol Clin North Am* 22(3):357-377, 2004.
Johnston JN, Killion JB: Hazards in the radiology department, *Radiol Tech* 76(6):417-423, 2005.
Logan C: Risk management: Patient safety in the operating room: Fire safety and the perioperative nurse, *Dissector* 30(4):12-14, 2003.

Marenzi B: Hazards of smoke plume, *Dissector* 30(4):19-21, 2003.

McCarthy PM, Gaucher KA: Fire in the OR—Developing a fire safety plan, *AORN J* 79(3):588-597, 600, 2004.

Melzer HS et al: Gel-based surgical preparation resulting in an operating room fire: Case report, *J Neurosurg* 102(3):347-349, 2005.

Metules T: Latex-safe periop care, *RN 2003* 66(3):1-6, 2003.

Niedhammer I: How is sex considered in recent epidemiological publications on occupational risks? *Occup Environ Med* 57(8):521-527, 2000.

Trim JC: Raising awareness and reducing the risk of needlestick injuries, *Profess Nurse* 19(5): 259-61, 263-4, 2004.

Twomey CL: Latex allergy: current and future, *Emerg Med Services* 33(10):141-147, 2004.

Weiss ES et al: Prevalence of blood-borne pathogens in an urban, university-based general surgical practice, *Ann Surg* 241(5):803-807; discussion 807-809, 2005.

Chapter 14

Microbiologic Considerations

CHAPTER OBJECTIVES

After studying this chapter, the learner will be able to:
- Differentiate between microorganisms.
- Describe the natural lines of defense of the human body.
- Identify several favorable living characteristics of microorganisms.
- Describe how disease is spread.

CHAPTER OUTLINE

Historical Background, p. 232
Microorganisms: Nonpathogens Versus Pathogens, p. 232
Types of Pathogenic Microorganisms, p. 235
Antimicrobial Therapy, p. 246

KEY TERMS AND DEFINITIONS

Aerobe   Microorganism that requires air or the presence of oxygen for maintenance of life.

Anaerobe   Microorganism that grows best in an oxygen-free environment or one that cannot tolerate oxygen (e.g., *Clostridium* species that causes gas gangrene).

Antibiotics   Substances, natural or synthetic, that inhibit growth of or destroy microorganisms. Used as therapeutic agents against infectious diseases; some are selective for a specific organism; some are broad-spectrum antibiotics.

Antimicrobial agent   Chemical or pharmaceutical agent that destroys or inhibits growth of microorganisms.

Bioterrorism   Covert event involving introduction of microbial contamination and infection of humans or animals.

Cross-contamination   Transmission of microorganisms from patient to patient and from inanimate objects to patients and vice versa.

Epidemiology   Study of occurrence and distribution of disease; the sum of all factors controlling the presence or absence of a disease.

Florae   Bacteria and fungi normally inhabiting the body, resident or transient.

Infection   Invasion of the body by pathogenic microorganisms and the reaction of tissues to their presence and to toxins generated by the organisms.

- **Community-acquired infection** Infectious disease process that developed or was incubating before the patient entered the health care facility.
- **Nosocomial infection** Hospital-associated or acquired infection not present when the patient was admitted to the health care facility. Infection may occur at the surgical site or as a complication unrelated to the surgical site.
- **Superinfection** Secondary subsequent infection caused by a different microorganism that develops during or after antibiotic therapy.

Microorganisms   Living organisms, invisible to the naked eye, including bacteria, fungi, viruses, protozoa, yeasts, and molds.

Opportunists   Microorganisms that do not normally invade tissue but are capable of causing infection or disease if introduced into the body mechanically through injury, such as tetanus bacillus, or when resistance of the host may be lowered, as by human immunodeficiency virus (HIV) infection.

Pathogenic   Producing or capable of producing disease.

Sepsis   Severe toxic febrile state resulting from infection with pyogenic microorganisms, with or without associated septicemia. Septicemia is a clinical syndrome characterized by significant invasion into the bloodstream of microorganisms from a focus of infection in tissues. Microorganisms may multiply in the blood. Infection of bacterial origin carried through the bloodstream is sometimes referred to as bacteremia.

Standard precautions   Procedures followed to protect personnel from contact with blood and body fluids of all patients (formerly referred to as universal precautions).

SUPPLEMENTAL MATERIAL ON EVOLVE WEBSITE *evolve*

http://evolve.elsevier.com/BerryKohn
- Glossary
- Full Set of Perioperative Flash Cards
- Interactive Key Term Flash Cards
- Student Activities
- WebLinks

HISTORICAL BACKGROUND

Approximately five million types of microorganisms live in the Earth's many habitats. Each type of microorganism has specific features that distinguish it from the rest. The mechanism and rationale for grouping and categorizing microorganisms were originally described in 1763 by Swedish naturalist Carolus Linnaeus (1707-1778) and refined by French scientists Antoine Laurent de Jussieu (1748-1836) (plants) and Georges Leopold Cuvier (1769-1832) (animals). Contributions made by German biologist Ernst Haeckel (1834-1919) (bacteria) and American scientist Robert H. Whittaker (1924-1980) (fungi) further refined the study of microbiology.

As techniques and instrumentation became more refined, American biologist Herbert Copeland (1902-1968) (protozoa) reclassified all known microorganisms and segregated nucleated and nonnucleated microorganisms into separate kingdoms. Scientific classification of organisms currently identifies five kingdoms: animals, plants, fungi, Monera (bacteria), and Protista (algae, protozoa, and parasitic organisms). Similarities, physical structure, and relationships, as well as differences and independent life cycles, define how each microorganism is assigned to its kingdom. Further identification includes subdivisions within each group.

The study of microorganisms has led to many lifesaving advantages. Vaccines created from microbial activity have been developed to prevent many communicable diseases. The first of these was developed by Edward Jenner (1749-1823), an English physician. In 1796 he inoculated a child with a cowpox vaccine to prevent smallpox. Subsequently, vaccines and antitoxins have been developed to provide passive immunity against such infectious diseases as diphtheria, rubella, and poliomyelitis. Although many diseases have been nearly eradicated, these and other infectious diseases still occur, sometimes in epidemic proportions.

MICROORGANISMS: NONPATHOGENS VERSUS PATHOGENS

Specific numbers of microorganisms with plantlike or animal-like characteristics are considered nonpathogenic in the human if they are not transferred to a different location in the body. Nonpathogenic microorganisms do not pose a particular threat to health if they remain constant in microbial numbers. Natural resident florae can be found in the reproductive tract secretions, gastrointestinal tract, nasopharyngeal mucus, respiratory passages, and any superficial ductal opening, such as sweat and oil glands. Resident florae have specific roles in their natural location. Some resident florae of the large intestine aid in the synthesis of vitamin K, vitamin B_{12}, and folic acid but can cause an infection if they are relocated to a surgical incision.

The term *infection* is used when nonresident florae invade a susceptible area. The term *superinfection* is used when resident florae are out of balance and the increased number causes a pathogenic condition. If the count of microbial colonies increases above normal or the colonies grow in an area where they are not usually found, an infection results and the microorganisms are considered pathogenic. They can invade healthy tissue through some power of their own or can injure tissue by producing a toxin. Pathogenic microorganisms can cause sepsis—a severe toxic febrile state – or death.

In a healthy state, body fluids such as urine and cerebrospinal fluid do not normally contain microorganisms and are considered sterile. Other fluids that under normal circumstances do not contain microorganisms include blood, peritoneal fluid, synovial fluid, amniotic fluid, tears, semen, and breast milk. Because microorganisms are not visible on gross inspection, exposure to any body substance should be considered contaminated and treated accordingly.

Identification of Microorganisms

Microorganisms, with the exception of viruses, have intracellular deoxyribonucleic acid (DNA). The DNA is either enclosed in a nuclear membrane (eukaryotic) or loose in the cytoplasm (prokaryotic). Bacteria and blue-green algae are the only prokaryotic microorganisms. Bacteria remain in a primitive state unchanged by evolution. All other microorganisms are eukaryotic and have changed many times on an evolutionary scale.

Specimens and cultures of tissues or body fluids may be sent to the microbiology laboratory for identification. Treatment is prescribed according to the type of microorganism present in the body. The type of substance taken from the body for testing may be a clue as to the type of microorganism.

Accurate identification of the microorganism is critical to the selection of the appropriate therapy. Criteria used by laboratory personnel to identify the type of microorganism include the following:

* Cell morphology
* Mobility or motility
* Presence or absence of spores
* Native pigment
* Gram-stain reaction
* Growth factors (optimal growth conditions, speed of replication/reproduction, and how it grows in various media)
* How it colonizes
* Antibody detection in the host
* Metabolism and atmosphere requirements
* Biochemical activity (endotoxin or exotoxin)
* Sensitivity to exogenous chemicals or substances

Viability of Microorganisms

Any microorganism can become a pathogen when transferred from one place to another. Each type of microorganism has its own method of duplicating itself. Bacteria pass through four phases during their colonization/duplication/reproductive stage:

1. *Lag phase.* The microorganism adjusts to the new environment.
2. *Exponential (logarithmic, or log) growth phase.* This is characterized by a maximum and constant rate of multiplication. If conditions are favorable, *Escherichia coli (E. coli)* can double in 20 minutes. *Mycobacterium tuberculosis* (tubercle bacillus) may require 5 hours.

3. *Stationary phase.* The multiplication rate and death of microbes equalize and balance. This period can last several days.
4. *Death.* The rate of microbial death exceeds the rate of multiplication. A few living cells can linger for several days or months but not at the same level as the growth phase.

The rate of bacterial growth is depicted in Fig. 14-1. The population of microbes will double during the log phase at a predictable interval referred to as generation time or doubling time. Changes in temperature, moisture, illumination, nutrients, and pH can influence the rate at which any microbe passes through doubling time. If all favorable living conditions are met, the microbe can proliferate into disease state. Any change in the favorable conditions can alter the amount of time it takes for the microbe to pass through any one of the four phases. Box 14-1 describes the favorable living conditions associated with the proliferation of microorganisms.

The key element in preventing pathogenic disease is to understand the microorganism's mode of transmission, life cycle, and favorable living conditions. Interference with the viability, doubling, and survival of pathogenic microorganisms can minimize the risk of infection.

Three Lines of Defense

The human body is remarkable in its ability to protect itself by intact barriers, membranes, and bacteriostatic secretions. Three lines of defense are particularly important for prevention of disease.

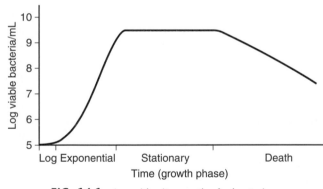

FIG. 14-1 Logarithmic growth of a bacterium.

BOX 14-1	**Favorable Living Conditions for Microorganisms**

Can live with oxygen (aerobic) or without oxygen (anaerobic); some require no special gaseous environment (facultative).
Can live with or without moisture; some can completely dry out and be reconstituted.
Can live with or without light; some like complete darkness.
Can live in a neutral or alkaline pH; most will die in an acidic environment.
Can live with or without warmth; some can grow in the freezer compartment of the refrigerator.
Can get nourishment from a living host or decayed matter; some can absorb nutrients from the environment of the host.

The first line of defense involves generalized good health and incorporates natural biochemical, mechanical, and anatomic protection through the following:
- *Skin.* Stratified epithelium contains sweat (sudoriferous) and oil (sebaceous) glands, which are bactericidal. Natural florae inhibit each other. The epithelium must remain intact to afford protection. Desquamation and low pH impede bacterial colonization.
- *Mucous membranes.* An effective barrier when intact, these line all natural body orifices except the ears, which secrete cerumen (earwax). Mucous membranes have bactericidal properties and a slightly acidic pH.
- *Reflexes.* Examples include vomiting, gagging, and blinking.
- *Sneeze.* Mucociliary escalator of the respiratory tree moves mucus and debris from the respiratory tract.
- *Genitourinary/reproductive tracts.* Immunoglobulin A (IgA), found in mucus, and enzymes are produced; these have a slightly acidic pH. Peristalsis is unidirectional.
- *Eyes.* Enzymes and IgA protect the conjunctiva and structures of the eye.
- *Cellular level.* Interferon is naturally formed in the cell to fight against viral attack.
- *Stomach acid.* Acid kills most pathogens.
- *Muscular closure of orifices.* Muscular closure provides a mechanical barrier against orifices such as the cervix and sphincters.

The second line of defense involves the collaborative effort of several body systems to prevent the proliferation of pathogenic microorganisms. These provide secondary protection if the microorganism breaks through the first line of defense. The second line of defense includes the following:
- *Inflammatory response.* This can be localized or systemic; biochemical, mechanical, and anatomic activities fight invading microorganisms and lay the groundwork for healing.
- *Antibody production.* Production is stimulated by the presence of an antigen. Some antibodies can be replicated for future exposures to the same microorganism.
- *Temperature elevation.* This can be localized or systemic. Some microorganisms are destroyed or repelled by heat.

The third line of defense can be acquired naturally or induced therapeutically. The third line of defense requires actual exposure to the pathogen in some form during which temporary or quasi-permanent resistance is attained. Methods include the following:
- *Passive immunity.* A "preformed" immunoglobulin (antibody) is introduced into the body. No memory for replication of the protective antibodies remains in the body.
- *Active immunity.* The body has the ability to develop a memory for production of antibodies in response to specific antigens. Live, dead, or attenuated microorganisms trigger the response. Some exposures require a booster injection to spark the memory and maintain immunity.

Pathogenic Invasion

Pathogenic microorganisms initially invade and aggregate in a body system or at a localized site, such as an abscess.

The proliferation of infectious material is easily supported by the warmth, chemical composition, moisture, and other components of the body. Local spread is supported by the surface of the wound, necrosis of tissue, diminished inflammatory response, and absence of anatomic barriers. Other pathways of infection include any body orifice, duct, or lumen of a broken vessel.

Veins are particularly vulnerable, because they are often associated with venous sinuses and have low pressure. The central nervous system (CNS) shares a similar risk for infection because the cerebrospinal fluid is under lowered pressure and has components that are rich in nutrients. As microbial colonies increase in number, infection may be carried through the body in the lymphatic system and may eventually become bloodborne. Major organ systems can become involved and can result in multisystem organ failure and death. Any body fluid or substance is a potential carrier of pathogens (Box 14-2).

According to the CDC, 14% to 16% of all health care-associated infections are surgical-site infections (SSI). Approximately 77% of surgical patients who die are reported to die of sepsis associated with these infections. SSI increases the length of stay and increases the cost of care.

Knowledge of how the cycle of infection works is the most important element of prevention. Considerations include but are not limited to the following:
- Identifying the reservoir of the pathogen
- Identifying the portal of exit of the pathogen from the reservoir
- Identifying how pathogens are transmitted
- Identifying the portal of entry into a susceptible host
- Identifying the invasion of the susceptible host

Infectious Processes in the Body

Clinically, infection is the product of the introduction, metabolic activities, and pathophysiologic effects of microorganisms in living tissue. It can develop in the surgical patient as a preoperative complication after an injury or as a postoperative complication.

A localized infection may begin at the surgical site between the fourth and eighth postoperative days. Infection, usually bacterial in origin, develops as a diffuse, inflammatory process, known as cellulitis, and is characterized by pain, redness, and swelling. This inflammatory response is the body's second line of defense directed toward localization and containment of the infecting organism after it has passed through the first line of defense. Red blood cells, leukocytes, and macrophages infiltrate the area, with pus formation (suppuration) often following. An abscess forms as a result of tissue liquefaction with pus formation, supported by bacterial proteolytic enzymes that break down protein and aid in the spread of infection. Fibrinolysin, for example, an enzyme produced by hemolytic streptococcus, may dissolve fibrin and delay surgical-site healing. The body attempts to wall off an abscess by means of a membrane that produces surrounding induration (hardened tissue) and heat. Localized pus should be drained promptly.

If localization is inadequate and does not contain the infectious process, spreading and extension occur, causing *regional infection*. Microorganisms and their metabolic products are carried from the primary invasion site into the lymphatic system, spreading along anatomic planes and causing lymphangitis. Failure of the lymph nodes to hold the infection results in uncontrolled cellulitis. Subsequently, regional and/or systemic infection may develop, characterized by chills, fever, and signs of toxicity. Septic emboli may enter the circulatory system from septic thrombophlebitis of regional veins communicating with local infections. These emboli and pathogenic microorganisms in the blood seed invasive infection and abscess formation in remote tissues.

Sepsis elevates the patient's metabolic rate 30% to 40% above average, imposing additional stress on the vital systems. For example, cardiac output is about 60% above normal resting value. The body's defenses and ability to meet the stress govern whether the infectious process progresses to systemic infection, or septic shock. Multiple infection sites, the presence of shock, and inappropriate antibiotic therapy result in a poor prognosis. Obviously, the key to avoiding infection is prevention, but if an infection begins, the next most important step is to identify the microorganism and treat it appropriately. More than one microorganism may be present; therefore, treatment is highly individualized. Diagnosis of systemic infection may include any two of the following:
- Temperature more than 38° C (100.4° F) or less than 36° C (96.8° F) (late sign)
- Heart rate more than 90 beats per minute (bpm)
- Respiratory rate more than 20 to 22 breaths per minute

BOX 14-2	**Body Fluids and Substances that May Transmit Pathogens**

Blood
Semen
Vaginal secretions
Breast milk
Feces
Urine
Cerebrospinal fluid
Unfixed tissue specimen
Synovial fluid
Vitreous humor
Aqueous humor
Saliva
Amniotic fluid
Tears
Nasal secretions
Respiratory secretions
Peritoneal fluid
Pericardial fluid
Plume from electrosurgery or laser
Irrigation solution
Carbon dioxide gas from deflation
Cerumen
Sebum
Smegma
Bile
Tissue
Any open wound
Any exudate or transudate

- White blood cell count more than 12,000/mm^3 or less than 4000/mm^3

Septic shock may include decreased urinary output (less than 30 ml/hr), altered mental state, and hypoxemia. The patient usually becomes very hypotensive (low blood pressure) and has signs of blood-clotting defects.

The ultimate resolution of infection depends on immunologic and inflammatory responses capable of overcoming the infectious process. This is associated with drainage and removal of foreign material, including debris of bacteria and cells, lysis (breakdown) of microorganisms, resorption of pus, and sloughing of necrotic tissue. Healing then ensues.

Who Is at Risk for Exposure?

Perioperative personnel who provide direct and indirect patient care are at risk for exposure to potentially harmful microorganisms. Wearing personal protective equipment (PPE), such as gowns, gloves, and eyewear with side shields, decreases the risk but does not eliminate it. The risk for exposure is proportionate to the proximity to the patient in the operating room (OR). The closer to the surgical field (source of blood and/or body substance), the higher the risk. The surgeon, assistants, and scrub persons have a higher risk by role and proximity. They share an increased incidence of needle-sticks and puncture wounds. The circulating nurse, environmental services personnel, and instrument processors are also at increased risk for body substance exposure because of specimen handling, cleaning processes, and other contaminants in the environment.

Exposure rates to blood and body substances for OR personnel have been reported as 10 per 100 procedures. Sharps were responsible for 3 of 100 exposures reported. Of glove tears reported, 93% were in single-gloved caregivers. Approximately 63% of glove tears in a single-gloved individual revealed a blood exposure. In 20% of double-gloved individuals who had a glove puncture, only 6% had evidence of inner-glove puncture. Double-gloving is not an assurance of avoiding puncture in the event of a needle-stick. In 74% of injuries with sharps, the injuries were self-inflicted by carelessness.

The patient is also at risk. If a needle-stick occurs, the needle may come into contact with the patient after penetrating the caregiver, thereby exposing the patient. Some patients have health conditions that predispose them to vulnerability for infection. Considerations related to higher risk include immunosuppression, an immature immune system (preterm and term infants), radiation therapy, burns, diabetes, nutritional depletion, smoking, chemotherapy for cancer, older patients, steroid use, sickle cell disease, alcoholism, liver and kidney disease, and pre-existing infection being treated with antibiotic therapy (superinfection/opportunistic infection may ensue).

Biofilm Formation

Biofilm forms when one or more species of bacteria and other microorganisms adhere to surfaces of all kinds of moist material–such as implantable metals, plastics, and tissue. The slimy material that binds the microorganisms to the surface of the device creates a barrier against antibiotic treatment that results in a persistent disease state. Biofilm infections can develop on medical devices implanted in the body such as catheters (tubes used to conduct fluids in or out of the body), artificial joints, and mechanical heart valves. The infection can be nearly impossible to eliminate and the affected implant must be explanted.

A biofilm infection may linger for months, years, or even a lifetime, regardless of the state of the patient's intact immune system. It may not cause the patient's death, though the infection can consume resources and financially drain the family. Research has shown that biofilm is a genetically-mediated process wherein bacteria exchange intercellular information that give rise to newly formed biofilm.

Persistent bacterial cells contain a gene *(HipA)* that codes for a toxic protein, which puts the cell into hibernation until the effects of a specific antibiotic have worn off. Antibiotics work only on growing, animated cells. When the antibiotic ceases to work the cells reanimate and repopulate the site. Deleting or deactivating the *HipA* gene could end the ongoing battle with biofilm.

Mandatory Reporting of Health Care–Acquired Infections (HAI)

The Healthcare Infection Control Practices Advisory Committee (HICPAC) of the Centers for Disease Control and Prevention (CDC) has published a document in 2005 on reporting health care–acquired infections (HAIs).[1] Infections to be reported include a wide range of patient-related infections that are traceable to health care intervention. Examples include but are not limited to the following:

- Indwelling catheter infections
- Surgical site infections (SSIs)
- Ventilator-associated pneumonia
- Central line infections
- Communicable diseases
- Septicemia

Methodology and surveillance activities are described by HICPAC in the recommendations to the CDC. The pros and cons include public reporting of infection rates, but a potential for misunderstanding by the general lay-population and misrepresentation of published data.

TYPES OF PATHOGENIC MICROORGANISMS

Infections may be caused by one or several combinations of microorganisms. In this chapter, each of the five main types of microorganisms is described according to structure, life cycle, and mode of transmission; examples of each type of microorganism are provided (Table 14-1).

Bacteria

Bacteria are essential to human life. We depend on many of their metabolic processes. Many antibiotics are derived from bacteria, such as erythromycin, chloramphenicol, and kanamycin. Some photosynthesizing types convert carbon dioxide to water and oxygen. More than 5000 species of bacteria have been named, and many more exist

---

[1]www.cdc.gov.

TABLE 14-1	Common Microorganisms in an Operating Room Environment	
Microorganism	**Usual Environment**	**Mode of Transmission**
Staphylococci	Skin, hair	Direct contact
	Upper respiratory tract	Airborne
Escherichia coli	Intestinal tract	Feces, urine
	Urinary tract	Direct contact
Streptococci	Oronasopharynx	Airborne
	Skin, perianal area	Direct contact
Mycobacterium	Respiratory tract	Airborne, droplet
tuberculosis	Urinary tract	Direct contact
Pseudomonas	Urinary tract	Direct contact
	Intestinal tract	Urine, feces
	Water	Water
Serratia marcescens	Urinary tract	Direct contact
	Respiratory tract	Water
Clostridium	Intestinal tract	Direct contact
Fungi	Dust, soil	Airborne
	Inanimate objects	Direct contact
Hepatitis virus	Blood	Bloodborne
	Body fluids	Direct contact

unidentified. Most of the morphologic differences in bacteria are found in metabolism, chemical composition, or resultant effect on the host. Unfortunately, many varieties of bacteria are pathogenic or are capable of becoming pathogenic (Fig. 14-2).

Bacteria can survive in diverse environments. For example, *Thermoplasma acidophilum* is found in the hot springs of Yellowstone Park and is capable of living in a 140° F

(60° C) environment with an acidic pH of 1 to 2. *Bacillus stearothermophilus* is used to test steam sterilizers because it can withstand temperatures up to 140° F (60° C). *Bacillus subtilus* is used to test dry heat and low temperature hydrogen peroxide sterilizers because it is destroyed at a lower temperature of 98.6° F (37° C).

Characteristics

1. *Structure.* Bacteria are microscopic, single-cell structures (1 to 10 mm). Two billion bacteria can be contained in a single drop of water. Bacteria have DNA but no formal nucleus (prokaryotic) and no membrane-bound organelles.
   a. Cocci are round. Examples include strains of *Staphylococcus* and *Streptococcus*. Diseases include impetigo and gonorrhea.
   b. Bacilli are rod shaped, and some can form spores. They are the most common types of bacteria. Examples include *Escherichia, Proteus,* and *Pseudomonas* species.
   c. Spirochetes are spiral shaped. Diseases include syphilis, leptospirosis, and Lyme disease.
   d. Pleomorphs can change shape from rod to round, making positive identification difficult. Diseases include mycoplasmal infection, typhus, rickettsial infection, chlamydia, psittacosis, and Rocky Mountain spotted fever. Rickettsia and chlamydia organisms must live in a host cell. They are intracellular parasites.
2. *Life cycle.* Bacteria can be aerobic, anaerobic, facultative, or microaerophilic. They can reproduce asexually by binary fission (split into equal halves). Some studies have shown that some genes may be transferred between bacterial species during viral infection (plasmid transfer).
3. *Transmission.* Infection is transmitted by direct contact or through animal or insect bites.

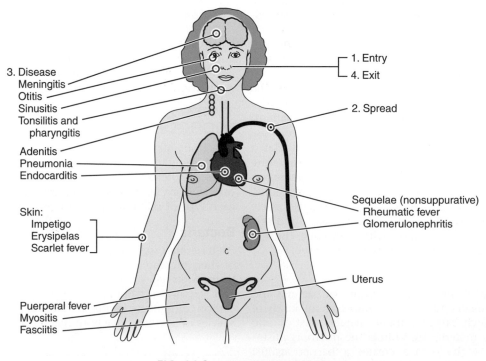

FIG. 14-2 *Streptococcus* infection.

4. *Encapsulation.* Some bacteria are encapsulated, which is a defense mechanism against phagocytic activity of leukocytes. These bacteria may be ingested by white blood cells, but instead of being killed and digested, they remain within the phagocyte for a time and are then extruded in a viable condition. The presence of a capsule is associated with virulence among pathogenic bacteria.

Differentiation of Bacterial Types. A universal way to determine the differences in bacteria is to stain the cell. Danish physician Christian Gram (1853-1938) developed a method of applying a solution of crystal violet and iodine (gentian violet) to the cell wall followed by exposure to 95% alcohol and acetone. Gram-positive bacteria retain a stain of dark purple-blue. Gram-negative bacteria retain only a stain of light pink after the rinsing process (Table 14-2). Gram stain is also used to identify nonbacterial substances such as trophocysts (helminth eggs) and larvae.

Endospores. Endospores are the resting, protective stage of about 150 species of gram-positive rod-shaped bacilli. Gram-negative bacilli do not form endospores. Select bacilli are capable of producing one endospore in response to an environmental threat, such as extreme heat or chemicals. When conditions suitable for bacterial growth are reestablished, the endospore reverts back to its original cellular structure for active vegetative growth and reproduction (Fig. 14-3).

In the vegetative or active growth state, spore-forming bacilli are no more difficult to kill than non–spore-forming bacteria. Most other microorganisms are killed easily by the processes of sterilization and disinfection, but bacterial spores are not. Examples of heat- and chemical-resistant spores include *Bacillus* and *Clostridium* species. Nonpathogenic varieties of the bacillus spore-forming microorganisms are used in sterilizers to test for efficacy (e.g., *Bacillus subtilus*). Other examples of potentially fatal diseases caused by spore-forming bacilli are anthrax, tetanus, gas gangrene, and botulism (Fig. 14-4).

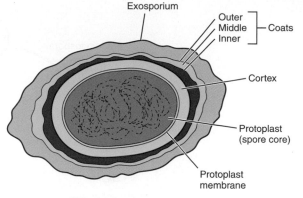

FIG. 14-3   Bacterial endospore.

Bacterial Toxicity. Pathogenic microorganisms produce substances that upon invasion adversely affect the host locally and/or systemically. Toxic substances affecting tissues, cells, and possibly enzyme systems diffuse from the microbial cells. The cellular substance of a wide variety of organisms is toxic also. In addition, harmful effects may be produced indirectly by activation of tissue enzymes by bacteria. Such toxic substances include the following:

1. *Exotoxins.* These classic bacterial toxins are the most potent toxins known. As little as 7 ounces (200 mL) of crystalline botulism type A toxin is said to be able to kill the world's entire population. Exotoxins appear to be proteins, are denatured by heat, and are destroyed by proteolytic enzymes, which break down protein. These bacteria are typically gram-positive and form spores. Examples of diseases are tuberculosis, clostridial infection, diphtheria, anthrax, and leprosy.

2. *Endotoxins.* These toxins are contained within the cell wall of bacteria and are released when the cell wall is broken. They are heat-stable and are not digested by proteolytic enzymes. On parenteral inoculation, they cause a rise in body temperature

TABLE 14-2	Bacterial Gram Stain Chart			
	Gram-positive Cocci	**Gram-negative Cocci**	**Gram-positive Rods**	**Gram-negative Rods**
Aerobic	Staphylococcus aureus	Neisseria gonorrhoeae	Listeria monocytogenes	Escherichia coli
	Staphylococcus epidermidis	Neisseria meningitidis	Bacillus anthracis	Klebsiella pneumoniae
	Streptococcus pneumonia	Moraxella catarrhalis	Cornyebacterium diphtheriae	Proteus mirabilis
	Streptococcus pyogenes			Serratia marcescens
	Streptococcus viridians			Pseudomonas aeruginosa
	Enterococcus faecalis			Enterobacter
	Enterococcus faecium			Haemophilus influenzae
				Legionella pneumophila
				Salmonella
				Shigella
				Brucella
				Bortadella
				Campylobacter
Anaerobic	Peptostreptococcus		Clostridium difficile	Bacteroides fragilis
	Peptococcus		Clostridium perfringin	Fusobacterium
			Clostridium tetani	
			Actinomyces	

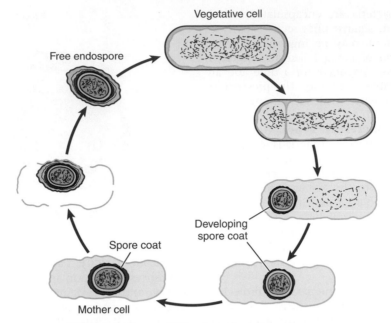

FIG. 14-4   Process of forming a bacterial endospore.

and are known as bacterial pyrogens. They increase capillary permeability with the resultant production of local hemorrhage. Endotoxins cause injury to body cells at the site of infection, but more important, they cause serious, often lethal, effects by dissemination and widespread injury to many tissues throughout the body. Endotoxic shock may occur in bacteremia caused by gram-negative bacteria. Examples of diseases are typhoid, shigellosis infection, and the plague. Microorganisms include *E. coli, Salmonella,* and *Pseudomonas.*

3. *Heterogeneous substances.* Microorganisms also form a variety of other heterogeneous (dissimilar) toxic substances, which may contribute to the disease process directly or facilitate the establishment of foci of infection. Toxins, which diffuse from the intact microbial cell, have the following various effects:

   a. Cytotoxic effect (leukocidin) destroys white blood cells (e.g., causing leukopenia, or reduction of the number of leukocytes below normal).

   b. Kinase effect interferes with the clotting mechanism of blood.

   c. Enzymatic effect causes bacterial hemolysins to dissolve red blood cells or fibrin, thereby inhibiting clot formation. Coagulase, an enzymatic substance of bacterial origin, is causally related to thrombus formation. Coagulase-positive *Staphylococcus, B. subtilis, E. coli,* and *Serratia marcescens* accelerate clotting of blood and induce intravascular clotting.

Toxic Shock Syndrome.   Toxic shock syndrome (TSS) is an acute condition caused by exotoxins secreted by strains of *Staphylococcus aureus.* The pathogen can invade any part of the body. TSS is characterized by fever over 102° F (38.9° C), hypotension, erythematous rash, and injury to multiple organ systems. Diagnosis is based on

the presence of abnormal clinical and laboratory findings. Prompt supportive treatment and antibiotic therapy are crucial. Desquamation, peeling of skin (usually from the palms of the hands and soles of the feet), occurs 1 to 2 weeks after onset.

Recovery is usually complete, but TSS is potentially fatal if untreated. It can originate from a surgical wound, burn, postpartum infection, or septic abortion infected or colonized with the implicated toxin. TSS can afflict any age-group of either sex (Fig. 14-5).

Septic Shock.   Septic shock is a state of widely disseminated infection, often borne in the bloodstream (i.e., septicemia). Early septic shock may begin with fever, restlessness, sudden unexplained hypotension, a cloudy sensorium, hypoxia, tachycardia, tachypnea, and/or oliguria. One or more of these signs and symptoms may be present. Toxic or metabolic by-products increase capillary permeability, permitting loss of circulating fluid into the interstitial fluid. Endotoxins released by bacteria promote vasodilation and hypotension.

Septic shock is most frequently produced by gram-negative bacteria. As shock progresses, the patient develops cold, clammy skin; sharply diminished urinary output; respiratory insufficiency; cardiac decompensation; disseminated intravascular coagulation (DIC); and metabolic acidosis. The high-risk category comprises patients with severe infection (e.g., peritonitis), trauma, burns, impaired immunologic status, diabetes mellitus, or extreme age, as well as patients who have undergone an extensive invasive procedure.

Treatment consists of control of the infectious process, early administration of antibiotics, fluid-volume replacement, and oxygen. Diuretics, sodium bicarbonate, vasoconstrictors, vasodilators, inotropic agents, or heparin may also be indicated. Corticosteroids may be used, but their use is controversial. A monoclonal antibody may be administered to reduce endotoxins.

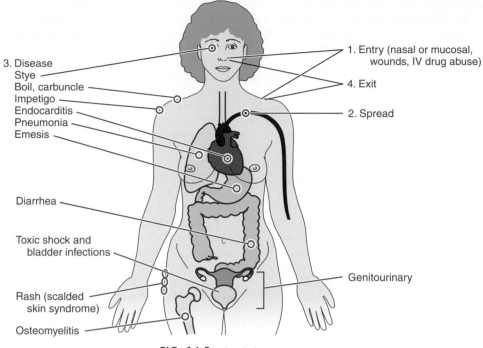

3. Disease
Stye
Boil, carbuncle
Impetigo
Endocarditis
Pneumonia
Emesis

Diarrhea

Toxic shock and
bladder infections

Rash (scalded
skin syndrome)

Osteomyelitis

1. Entry (nasal or mucosal,
wounds, IV drug abuse)

4. Exit

2. Spread

Genitourinary

FIG. 14-5   *Staphylococcus aureus.*

Bacterial Disease Examples

Tuberculosis. Tuberculosis (TB) is caused by the acid-fast gram-positive bacterium *M. tuberculosis.* Tubercle bacilli usually infect the lungs (pulmonary TB), but they may be present in joints, kidneys, ovaries, or other organs. Acute miliary tuberculosis may be seen in an abdominal procedure as generalized peritonitis. *M. tuberculosis* is an opportunistic organism. Individuals at high risk for TB include persons immunosuppressed from human immunodeficiency virus (HIV) infection, corticosteroid therapy, chemotherapy, or malnutrition.

Persons with diabetes mellitus, cirrhosis, alcoholism, silicosis or other lung disease, or prolonged contact with an actively infected person are also at risk. The tubercle bacillus can remain dormant, encased in a hard shell, for years after exposure. Because the bacillus may become airborne by droplets from the respiratory tract, the disease must be monitored and controlled to prevent cross-infection. Unsuspected active cases and inactive carriers represent a particular hazard. Patients with acute disease are isolated and placed on respiratory secretion precautions for approximately 2 weeks after initiation of treatment.

Therapy is long-term (usually 6 to 12 months of drug therapy). Isoniazid (INH) and rifampin most effectively kill reactive bacilli and prevent reactivation. Pyrazinamide, ethambutol, and streptomycin also may be used for multidrug therapy; some other drugs that are less effective and have more side effects may be indicated. *M. tuberculosis* mutates and may become resistant to a single-drug or multidrug therapy regimen. Multidrug-resistant tuberculosis (MDR-TB) can be fatal, especially in human immunodeficiency virus (HIV)-infected persons.

The following is recommended in the care of surgical patients who have active TB:

- Postpone elective surgical procedures, if possible, until the patient shows a response to drug therapy (i.e., is no longer infectious as confirmed by a negative sputum smear).
- Use disposable anesthesia equipment to the extent possible. Reusable equipment must be sterilized or undergo high-level disinfection immediately after use. A bacterial filter on the endotracheal tube or at the expiratory side of the breathing circuit may be useful in reducing the risk of contamination of anesthesia equipment or the discharge of tubercle bacilli into ambient air.
- Use respiratory isolation precautions for patients with TB-positive sputum culture. This includes putting a mask on the patient during transport to the operating room (OR). The transporter also wears a TB-filtering mask. OR team members should wear face-fitting masks that filter particles of 1 mm at a 95% efficiency level (i.e., a disposable high-efficiency particulate air [HEPA] filtered mask, valveless dust-mist respirator, or dust-fume-mist filtered respirator). Powered respirator masks equipped with HEPA filters may be worn during high-risk procedures such as bronchoscopy, endotracheal intubation, and tracheal suctioning.
- Perform the surgical procedure at a time when other patients and a minimum number of staff members are present in the OR suite (i.e., at the end of the day's schedule, if possible). Keep OR doors closed and traffic to a minimum.
- Sterilize critical items (i.e., those entering the bloodstream or body cavity); semicritical items (i.e., those in contact with mucous membranes only) may be sterilized or undergo high-level disinfection with a tuberculocide.

- Move the patient into an isolation room that has negative pressure ventilation with a local exhaust and HEPA air filtration and/or ultraviolet radiation lamps.
- Screen high-risk patients, and test personnel at least annually. Testing includes a chest x-ray film and skin test. Exposed personnel should be retested every 6 months.

TB is the leading fatal infectious disease in the world. In many facilities, yearly TB testing of all OR personnel is mandatory. The most accurate test is the Mantoux test, which is administered by injecting 0.1 mL of purified protein derivative (PPD) of tubercle bacillus subcutaneously in the forearm to form a small wheal under the skin. The site is examined in 24 to 72 hours. Redness, itching, and induration of 8 to 10 mm at the site of injection are considered a positive or a significant reaction.

Further testing and chest x-ray films may be performed before treatment can begin. Reaction of less than 8 mm at the site of injection is considered an insignificant or negative reading, and no further action is needed.

Sexually Transmitted Diseases. Any sexually active person who has multiple partners is at risk for acquiring a sexually transmitted disease. In addition to those previously discussed (hepatitis B virus [HBV], HIV, and herpes simplex virus [HSV] infections), gonorrhea, syphilis, and chlamydia are transmitted by sexual contact. Transmission can occur also from contact with secretions containing the causative organism, such as those a health care provider might encounter through a cut or broken skin.

Gonorrhea. *Neisseria gonorrhoeae* most often infects the genitourinary tract, but it may infect the rectum, pharynx, or conjunctiva. Burning, itching, and pain around the vaginal or urethral orifice with purulent discharge are characteristic symptoms. If untreated, the infection can spread to cause inflammation within the peritoneal cavity and septicemia. Disseminated infection is more common in women than in men. Gonorrhea is treated with penicillinase-inhibiting antibiotics. Generally, patients should be treated simultaneously for presumptive chlamydial infections.

As a prophylactic measure, a one-time instillation of silver nitrate, erythromycin 0.5% ophthalmic ointment, or tetracycline 1% ophthalmic ointment may be administered within 1 hour after birth to protect the neonate against potential contamination by vaginal secretions of an infected mother. Single-use tubes or ampules are preferable to multiple-use tubes to prevent cross-contamination between newborns. A newborn with a known gonorrheal infection will need further antibiotic treatment.

According to the National Institutes of Health (NIH), 30% of gonorrhea isolates are resistant to penicillin or tetracycline, or both.

Syphilis. Routine screening for syphilis in hospitalized patients and couples applying for marriage licenses is a thing of the past. However, the incidence of syphilis is on the increase again. *Treponema pallidum* is a blood-borne spirochete that may infect any organ system. Syphilis is characterized by distinct stages of effects over a period of years if it is untreated by antibiotics. Congenital syphilis

results from prenatal infection unless the infected mother is treated within the first 4 months of pregnancy.

In the first stage (primary syphilis), a lesion on the skin or mucous membrane, most commonly around the anogenital region, quickly forms a chancre. This is a painless ulceration that exudes fluid laden with spirochetes. The chancre heals spontaneously within 40 days. During the second stage (secondary syphilis), spirochetes migrate from the chancre throughout the bloodstream. The disease can remain contagious for as long as 2 years during this stage. The third stage (tertiary syphilis) may not develop for many years. When it does, secondary lesions may damage or destroy tissues and body structures, including the heart and CNS, with ensuing mental disability or death.

Chlamydia. Chlamydial infection is caused by *Chlamydia trachomatis* (bacteria). It is the most prevalent sexually transmitted disease—more common than gonorrhea and syphilis. It is transmitted only by person-to-person contact. It occurs more often in men than in women but women are more frequently asymptomatic than are men.

Chlamydia can cause epithelial tissue inflammation, ulceration and scarring of the urethra and rectum, and damage to reproductive organs. Pelvic inflammatory disease (PID) is a serious complication in women. Asymptomatic salpingitis is a major cause of tubal infertility or ectopic pregnancy. Exposure of infants to *C. trachomatis* in the birth canal can cause neonatal conjunctivitis and pneumonia.

Viruses

A virus is not an independent cell unit and is not capable of autonomous metabolism. It is an obligate intracellular parasite that is confined to living in a host cell, such as a somatic cell, or a bacterium. As a bacteriophage, a virus can attach itself to a bacterium and create an opening. While still attached, the nucleic acid of the viral capsule enters the bacteria. The empty capsule remains attached to the bacteria.

Once the virus is inside the host cell, regardless of the cell type, it uses the cell's genetic contents and metabolic machinery for replication. New viruses are passed out the cell membrane, and they in turn attach to other cells to repeat the replication process. Some viruses engorge the cell, causing it to rupture and thus dispersing the virus into the host's body.

During viral infection, the host cell reacts to invasion by producing an inflammatory response, antibodies, and interferon to slow the progression of viral replication. Some cellular immunity is developed (e.g., in mumps, chickenpox). Some viruses can attach to nerve cells and undergo activation, deactivation, and reactivation cycles, such as in herpes simplex types I and II (herpes simplex virus). Some of the nerve cells destroyed by viral invasion include motor neurons, which when damaged cannot be repaired or replaced, such as in polio.

Until the discovery of viruses as a separate entity by Dmitri Iwanowski (1864-1920) in 1892, viruses were identified only by the diseases they caused. Martinus Beijerinck (1851-1931) made significant contributions to scientific knowledge by expanding the knowledge of viruses. The virus species can usually be identified by the specific alterations in structure and function effected in the host cell as seen under electron microscopy. Other diagnostics include detection of viral antigen, nucleic acid, or antiviral antibody in the serum.

Characteristics

- *Structure.* Viruses are composed of a protein capsule but have no true cellular components other than nucleic acid. They are categorized by the morphologic core structure of their nucleic material—either DNA or ribonucleic acid (RNA) (not both)—and the presence or absence of an envelope. They can mutate. Viruses are extremely small and are visible only by electron microscope.
- *Life cycle.* A virus must have a living biologic host cell. The virus enters a host cell and uses the host's genetic and other cellular protein material for replication.
- *Transmission.* Infection can be transmitted through blood and body fluids of animals and humans. Some viruses can be transmitted by insect bites, such as ticks or mosquitoes; other viruses are transmitted by the fecal-oral route. Direct contact of virus with nonintact skin or mucous membranes can allow entry.

Viral Disease Examples

Hepatitis Infection. Viruses can produce several types of acute and chronic inflammation of the liver. The pathogens causing viral hepatitis create an occupational hazard to health care providers. A patient may be in an acute stage of the infection but more commonly is an unknown carrier of one and occasionally two of the viruses that can cause hepatitis.

Hepatitis A. Hepatitis A virus (HAV) infection is an acute illness that is usually brief but can last for several months. It is spread by oral ingestion of contaminated water and food, especially shellfish, and by fecal contaminants. It is most infectious during the 2 weeks before the onset of symptoms and until after the first week of jaundice. The incubation period is 14 to 90 days, with an average of 28 days. Immune globulin may be effective if given within 2 weeks of exposure.

HAV infection is the most common type of viral hepatitis and causes critical disease if it occurs in combination with other types of hepatitis. HAV infection as a single entity is not a health care–associated problem because it does not have a chronic carrier state. It is usually self-limiting and does not typically cause chronic liver damage. A vaccine is available for areas where HAV is endemic.

Hepatitis B. Hepatitis B virus (HBV) infection is a major health care–associated problem. Carriers are a main source of cross-infection. Hepatitis B surface antigen is the carrier state of HBV. This can be harbored for prolonged periods of up to 15 years and has been found in practically all body fluids of infected persons. It is transmitted percutaneously or permucosally by blood, saliva, semen, and other body fluids. It is not found in feces or urine, according to the U.S. Department of Health and Human Services.

The incubation period is 60 to 90 days before mild to severe symptoms become apparent. Chronic hepatitis, cirrhosis, or liver carcinoma may develop. A liver transplant may be necessary.

Serologic tests are used to diagnose infection, detect carriers, and monitor high-risk persons. Patients who have undiagnosed hepatitis, who fail to reveal they have chronic hepatitis, or who are asymptomatic carriers can transmit the virus to health care providers. Perioperative, emergency department, blood bank, laboratory, and hemodialysis unit personnel are especially at risk. HBV surface antigen is easily transmitted by direct contact with blood and body fluids via a needle-stick or break in the skin, such as a minor cut or hangnail, or via a splash into the mucosa of the eye, nose, or mouth.

HBV can be transmitted by fomites, through sexual intercourse, and from an infected mother to a neonate during birth.

Preexposure immunization over a period of 6 months through a series of three injections of 10 mg (1 mL) of recombinant vaccine against HBV is recommended for all persons at risk. The injections are given in the deltoid muscle because injection in the gluteal muscle has been shown to not produce immunity. After exposure, such as after an accidental needle-stick, both the vaccine and hepatitis B immune globulin are given. Since 1991 the Occupational Safety and Health Administration (OSHA) has mandated that health care facilities make these immunizations available to personnel. The series may need to be repeated in 7 years if the titer falls below a detectable level in the serum.

Hepatitis C. Hepatitis C virus (HCV) is a bloodborne RNA virus. Recipients of multiple transfusions or chronic hemodialysis, intravenous drug users, and health care workers are at risk. Persons with acute HCV infection are asymptomatic but have a higher mortality if they are simultaneously exposed to HAV. A screening test detects the presence of antibodies in the blood. Incubation varies from 2 weeks to 6 months. The infection may progress insidiously in a carrier for as long as 25 years. Immediate HCV postexposure treatment consists of immune globulin injections.

Persons who become infected with HCV have a 40% to 60% chance of becoming chronic carriers and may be treated with interferon and ribavirin. Newer treatments approved by the U.S. Food and Drug Administration (FDA) in 1998 include Rebetron (combined interferon A and ribavirin) injections for 6 months. Women should avoid pregnancy while taking this drug.

HCV infection can precipitate chronic hepatitis, cirrhosis, and liver cancer. A liver transplant may be needed. Mortality rates associated with HCV infection exceed 10,000 deaths per year. This form of hepatitis may surpass HIV infection in the number of new cases reported each year. An estimated 4 million persons in the United States have HCV infection. There is no cure, although 15% recover without lasting effects.

Hepatitis D. Hepatitis D virus (HDV) infection coexists with HBV infection or superinfects an HBV carrier. A defective RNA virus, HDV requires HBV for its survival and replication in both acute and chronic forms. HDV infection is communicable during all phases of active infection. It can lead to necrotizing liver disease and death. The majority of patients developing this complication of HBV infection are intravenous drug abusers who used contaminated needles. Immunization against HBV will also prevent hepatitis D.

Hepatitis E. Hepatitis E virus (HEV) infection is common in Asia, Africa, and Mexico. The incubation period is 15 to 64 days, with an average of 25 to 42 days in different epidemics. The characteristics of HEV are similar to those of HAV, and there are no specific serologic tests for HEV at this time. HEV infection is spread via the fecal-oral route through contaminated water or food or from poor sanitation conditions. Current immunoglobulins do not provide protection. HEV infection has no known chronic carrier state, and full recovery in infected persons can usually be expected. The best protection is proper handwashing.

Hepatitis G. Hepatitis G virus (HGV) infection is rare (2000 cases diagnosed per year). Most infected persons have no clear symptoms. It is transmitted by infected blood, and exposure to HCV increases mortality associated with the disease.

Herpes Infection. Related DNA viruses that form eosinophilic intranuclear inclusion bodies are collectively called herpesviruses. The viral infections they cause may be acute and highly contagious, or they may remain latent for many years even if antibodies are in circulation.

Herpes Simplex Infection. Herpes simplex virus (HSV) is the pathogen of herpes simplex infections. These cutaneous infections may cause localized eruptions, similar to blisters, on the border of the lips or external nares, in the mouth, or in the genital or anal region. Transmission is by direct contact with vesicle fluid from lesions or with saliva. The infection may be transmitted to the neonate during passage through an infected birth canal. HSV also can cause cutaneous eczema, acute stomatitis, keratoconjunctivitis, acute retinal necrosis, and meningoencephalitis. Herpes simplex infections are common in HIV-infected and other immunocompromised patients.

Patients who have a history of HSV infection may be treated with oral acyclovir preoperatively to prevent an outbreak in the surgical wound. This prophylaxis is particularly important for patients who are having facial procedures, such as a chemical peel or face-lift.

Herpetic Whitlow. Herpetic whitlow, a herpesvirus infection of the fingers, is transmitted by direct contact with oral secretions from a person with active herpesvirus or from an asymptomatic carrier. Entry of the virus into the host is via a cut or break in the skin or in nail folds. Herpetic whitlow is an occupational hazard to nurses, physicians, dentists, and anesthesia providers.

Cytomegalovirus Infection. Cytomegalovirus (CMV) may infect salivary glands or viscera, causing enlargement of cells. Transmission can be by direct contact with body fluids, secretions, and excretions. CMV infection usually is asymptomatic in a healthy person, but it is an opportunistic pathogen in immunosuppressed patients with HIV infection or acquired immunodeficiency syndrome (AIDS). Lymphadenopathy, enteritis, and pneumonitis may persist. Chorioretinitis and blindness may result in the end-stage of infection. CMV infection may also be associated with hepatitis. CMV may infect arterial smooth muscle cells, stimulating them to pro-liferate, which can contribute to the formation of atherosclerotic plaque.

CMV is the most common cause of congenital viral infection; it may be transmitted from an asymptomatic mother during pregnancy. A CMV-infected infant may develop neurologic problems. Latent CMV may become reactivated after organ transplantation. The incidence of primary and reactivated CMV infection is fairly high after renal, cardiac, and bone marrow transplantation.

Human Papillomavirus Infection. Condylomas (venereal warts) are caused by the human papillomavirus (HPV) and are transmitted through vaginal, anal, or oral-genital sexual contact. The infectious process appears as accumulations of warts over the perineal and/or anogenital surface. HPV infection in women can lead to cervical carcinoma. More than 200 varieties have been identified. Some subtypes have been associated with an increased incidence of cervical cancer. Not all of them are visible or pigmented. Some patients are infected simultaneously with multiple varieties. HPV vaccine is recommended by the CDC as routine prophylaxis for girls as young as nine years of age and all sexually active females up to age 25 years.

Treatment for venereal warts includes cryotherapy with liquid nitrogen, electrosurgical removal, CO_2 laser ablation, chemical peel with trichloroacetic acid (TCA), and/or topical application of medication (podophyllum 10% to 25% in a benzoin tincture, podofilox 0.5% solution or gel, or imiquimod 5.0% cream). Patients with wart accumulations of 0.5 to 1 cm² respond to topical applications. Patients with larger areas greater than 10 cm² may require staged surgical intervention.

Some infections are extensive, and the treatment may leave the patient with chronic reflexive neurologic pain, such as vulvodynia. Patients should be advised that their sexual partners also need to be evaluated for venereal warts. Most of the topical medications have not been approved for safe use during pregnancy.

Human Immunodeficiency Virus Infection. Human immunodeficiency virus (HIV) clearly represents a worldwide threat to public health that is unprecedented in modern times. Since this virus was introduced into the United States in the late 1970s, the resultant infection has spread at an alarming rate via contaminated blood and infected persons. Clinical problems in seropositive patients began appearing in 1978. Because of its effect on the immune system and its unknown origin when first reported in 1981, this infection became known as acquired immunodeficiency syndrome (AIDS). In 1983 researchers at the Institut Pasteur in Paris isolated the lymphadenopathy-associated virus (LAV). In 1984 a similar retrovirus called human T-cell lymphotropic virus type III (HTLV-III) was reported by the National Institutes of Health in Bethesda, Maryland. Since 1986, LAV and HTLV retroviruses causing AIDS or related illnesses have been known collectively as HIV.

Retroviruses synthesize DNA from RNA, a reversal of the usual process. As a result of this reversal process, there is a rapid rate of mutation, making resistance to antiviral drugs a major problem. Normally when a virus enters the body, helper T lymphocytes (T cells) release proteins that activate the immune system to produce antibodies against the virus and macrophages to attack the virus. HIV is different from other viruses in that it attacks the cell membrane of these white blood cells. When the virus penetrates the T cell membrane, the viral RNA and enzyme are released into the T cell cytoplasm and converted into DNA. This newly formed DNA penetrates the T cell nucleus, causing replication of the HIV virus. The cell dies, and the virus is released into the bloodstream to attack other helper T lymphocytes and macrophages, thus compromising the immune system.

HIV can live and reproduce in macrophages without stimulating the production of antibodies, because the viral composition resembles the host cell. HIV will survive in blood and any body fluid that contains white blood cells. The primary routes of transmission are through sexual intercourse and by direct contact with blood and blood products. HIV may be transmitted to the fetus by the blood of an infected mother or to the neonate via breast milk. HIV is not transmitted by casual contact with an infected person. The virus is relatively fragile and easily destroyed outside the body.

After exposure, antibodies may not be identified through serologic testing for 6 to 12 weeks, and detection can be delayed for up to 18 months or longer. Enzyme immunoassays (EIAs) and the Western blot analysis are used to test for the presence of antibodies. Blood banks test donor blood for HIV antibodies. Transplant donors also are tested. Blood screening for HIV has been routine in the United States since 1985, thus decreasing the potential for transmission by blood transfusion. Seropositive blood is destroyed, and the donor is notified.

The incubation period before symptoms of infection develop ranges from 6 months to 5 years or longer. Persons in whom the antibody is identified are considered infected and infective. They are classified by physical findings.

Acute Infection. The acute stage of HIV infection lasts 2 to 3 weeks. Signs and symptoms may be specific to an opportunistic infection or disease, but marked fatigue, prolonged diarrhea, weight loss, dry cough, enlarged lymph nodes, fever, and night sweats are striking features. Infections are primarily viral, mycobacterial, and fungal in origin. Oral candidiasis lesions (thrush) may be the first observable symptom. *Pneumocystis jiroveci* (formerly known as *Pneumocystis carinii* pneumonia), an unusual lung infection caused by a fungal parasite, is quite common.

Other common infections are CMV, HSV, cryptococcosis, and *Mycobacterium avium-intracellulare* complex disease. The patient may survive one infection only to succumb to another. Prophylactic drug therapy aims to prevent or delay the onset of infections. Malignancies and lymphomas also may develop.

Acquired Immunodeficiency Syndrome. As the HIV infection progresses, the cell-mediated immune system is irreversibly compromised. As concentration of the virus gradually increases, the patient becomes symptomatic for clinical manifestations of AIDS. Clinical diagnosis of AIDS requires a positive test for HIV antibodies, any one of the specified opportunistic infections, and a lowered T cell count. AIDS is not a well-defined disease but rather a state of immune dysfunction.

AIDS causes persistent destruction of the helper T lymphocytes (white blood cells that stimulate production of antibodies), resulting in profound immunosuppression (diminished resistance to infection and disease). The acronym AIDS helps to define the disease process:

Acquired. HIV has passed from one person to another by blood or body fluid in direct cell-to-cell contact; infection is not hereditary except through transplacental transfer from an infected mother to a fetus.

Immune. The normal defense system protects the body against certain diseases and opportunistic infections; immunity depends on the production of antibodies.

Deficiency. The immune system becomes compromised (i.e., immunosuppressed against opportunists); the host is unable to protect the person with no previous history of immunodeficiency against opportunists.

Syndrome. A group of symptoms or laboratory evidence indicates the presence of a particular disease, abnormality, or infection; seroconversion is positive for HIV antibodies. *P. jiroveci* pneumonia is the most common opportunistic respiratory infection. *M. avium-intracellulare* complex, the most common AIDS-related bacterial infection, is a leading cause of the wasting syndrome (i.e., loss of body fat and weight). Kaposi's sarcoma, a vascular tumor, is the most common malignancy. HPV and HSV infection may be present. Neurologic disease may cause dementia. Lymphomas and opportunistic infections of the brain, spinal cord, and peripheral nerves are not uncommon.

Asymptomatic Infection. The patient may be completely asymptomatic of infection but tests seropositive for HIV antibodies, which confirms the presence of virus in the body.

Persistent Generalized Lymphadenopathy. Swelling or enlargement of lymph nodes suggests cellular immune dysfunction. Prolonged infection with HIV may occur without the formation of HIV antibodies.

HIV-Related Clinical Manifestations. Originally referred to as AIDS-related complexes, a variety of health conditions suggest an impaired immune system. The patient who does not have one of the specific opportunistic infections but is seropositive for HIV antibodies does not technically have AIDS. An infectious disease, such as tuberculosis, and some cancers may be a result of a deteriorating immune system. AIDS may develop within a year of seroconversion.

A patient may be infected with HIV but may not yet test positive. Health care providers who have a valid reason to be concerned that they may have been infected may request to be tested. Few health care providers seroconvert from a single needle-stick or splash of blood on mucous membranes. Handling all needles and sharp instruments carefully and using barriers to avoid direct contact with blood and body fluids are the best measures to prevent work-related transmission of HIV. An HIV inhibitor such as zidovudine may be given immediately after exposure. A vaccine has not been developed for immunization. Antiviral agents interfere with the life cycle of the virus. Immune-modulating agents stimulate function of the suppressed immune system.

Prions. Transmissible spongiform encephalopathy (TSE) is a family of protein diseases that cause fatal neurologic disorders. Infection is through an unconventional route. A neurologic cellular protein referred to as a prion causes the disease. Exposure to a prion through direct contact with neurologic tissue, incidental inoculation with neurologic biologic matter, implantation through contaminated instrumentation, and possibly a genetic autosomal dominant predisposition are theorized sources. Ingestion of food contaminated with neurologic material, such as cerebrospinal fluid, is also considered a possible route of transmission. Known forms of TSE that affect humans and animals include the following:

Human forms:
- Creutzfeldt-Jakob disease (CJD) (human)
  - New variant Creutzfeldt-Jakob disease (vCJD): not known to science before 1994 suspected to be transmitted by eating infected cattle. The gut absorbs the iron storage protein ferritin of the consumed meat that binds with the prions.
  - Sporadic CJD: most common type. No known cause and is suspected to arise spontaneously.
  - Genetic CJD: very rare. Caused by aberrant gene.
  - Iatrogenic CJD: caused by cross infection during medical or surgical intervention. Can be passed by contaminated surgical instruments. Transmission has been documented by blood transfusion and human growth hormone treatments.

Animal forms:
- Bovine spongiform encephalopathy (BSE) (cattle)
- Scrapie (sheep)

Creutzfeldt-Jakob Disease. Although rare, CJD is a progressive, fatal neurodegenerative disease characterized by dementia, myoclonus (muscle spasms), and multifocal neurologic signs and symptoms.

It was first described in 1920 by German psychiatrists Hans Gerhard Creutzfeldt and Alphonse Maria Jakob. Thought to be associated with genetic factors that influence susceptibility to the formation of abnormal neurologic protein, the condition may be dormant for more than 30 years before the onset of symptoms around the age of 65 years. The disease then progresses rapidly, leading to coma and death, usually within 2 years of onset of symptoms.

CJD is not the same as vCJD or BSE. Diagnosis is made on the basis of a characteristic electroencephalogram (EEG) and brain biopsy positive for protein prion accumulation with neuron destruction. The disease is not seen on computed tomography (CT), magnetic resonance imaging (MRI), or positron emission studies (PET) scans. Autopsies of the brains of patients with suspected Alzheimer's disease revealed that 13% had undiagnosed CJD, and the tissue sampled resembled that of other TSE-infected mammals.

CJD is not living tissue but is still a particularly virulent protein substance. The prions are resistant to deactivation or destruction by heat, chemicals, radiation, freezing, drying, and conventional detergents.

In 2005, STERIS Corporation released a product (Hamo™ 100) that quickly removes prion contamination from surgical instruments with the exception of aluminum and endoscopes (both rigid and flexible). The product is available in the U.K. but has not yet been cleared for use in the USA. Hamo™ 100 is nonflammable, but is irritating to skin, eyes, and the respiratory system. The product can be used in automated washer systems or for manual instrument washing. PPE must be worn. The product is water soluble and can be disposed of in the sanitary sewer system.[2]

Studies have shown that items contaminated with prion material can cause infection many years after initial contamination. One study demonstrated that brain probes caused CJD in an animal subject two years after being used in a contaminated patient. Current literature recommends the following for deactivating prions before handling contaminated items for processing:
1. Soak contaminated items in sodium hydroxide for 2 hours.
2. Immediately follow soak with steam sterilization in an autoclave, using one of the following steam methods:
   a. 60 minutes in a gravity displacement sterilizer at 270° F (132° C)
   b. 18 minutes in a prevacuum sterilizer (longer than normal cycles) at 274° F (134° C) before routine cleaning

Sterilization of tissue that has been fixed with formalin is impossible. Serious attention should be given to the cleaning processes for contaminated items before they are safe for handling or safe for use on other patients. Several manufacturers have developed disposable instruments specific to handling suspected CJD tissue. The process of soaking in sodium hydroxide followed by steam autoclaving is deleterious to surgical instruments and the autoclave, according to the CDC. Autoclaving an instrument immersed in the chemical can release a gaseous form of sodium hydroxide that may be harmful to humans.

Standard Precautions for prevention of bloodborne exposure must be strictly observed. A bloodborne source has been confirmed in the U.K. At least two confirmed cases of transmission through blood transfusion have been identified. Human illness has been demonstrated after ingestion of beef from BSE-contaminated cattle. As a precaution the FDA recommends that individuals who have spent 6 months or more in the United Kingdom since 1980 defer from donating blood and body tissues for transplantation.

Leukoreduction with the Pall Leukotrap[3,4] of blood products has been implemented in the U.K. to remove the white cells and prions from the blood supply and has decreased the risk of contamination by 45%.

Contaminated neurologic tissue sources include dural grafts, corneal transplants, and human growth hormone. Prion contamination has been found in tonsil tissue, lymphatics, Peyer's patches in the bowel, and the spleen. Suction canister contents and used cleaning solutions should not be disposed of in the sanitary sewer system. All biologic material should be disposed of according to facility policy and procedure.

[2]www.steris.com.
[3]www.pall.com.
[4]Saunders C: In vitro evaluation of the Pall Leukotrap affinity prion reduction filter as a secondary device following primary leukoreduction, *Int J Transfus Med* 89(4):220-228, 2005.

Postexposure Prophylaxis for Transmissible Spongiform Encephalopathy. Any percutaneous exposure to known or suspected TSE-infected CNS tissue should be irrigated with 0.5% sodium hypochlorite. Skin exposure requires a thorough hand scrub with sodium hydroxide. Mucous membrane exposure should be followed by cleansing with soap and water. To date, no known direct transmission from person to person has been reported in surgery. (More information about CJD and current treatments can be found at www.cjd.ed.ac.uk.)

Fungi

More than 100,000 species of fungi have been identified. Not all fungi are pathogenic (causing mycosis). A *Penicillium* variety is used to make the antibiotic penicillin and to give flavor to Roquefort cheese. The blue color of the cheese is caused by collections of spores.

The body responds with an inflammatory response to tissue invasion by a fungus. Respiratory responses include hypersensitivity reaction to fungal antigens. According to statistics compiled by the CDC, the number of health care–associated fungal (mycotic) infections doubled between 1980 and 1990.

Fungal infections are classified according to the degree of tissue involvement and mode of transmission.

Characteristics

* *Structure.* Fungi are plantlike structures that lack chlorophyll and therefore are unable to photosynthesize. True fungi are nonmotile. Fungi are eukaryotic and range in size from microscopic to large mushroom forms. Yeast species are single cell but cling together with like cells. Fungi are aerobic. Molds are multicellular and reproduce by airborne spores that can be inhaled.
* *Life cycle.* A fungus grows as a mold (filamentous, spore forming) or a yeast (round, budlike cells). Molds can reproduce sexually and asexually by forming spore sacs. Yeasts produce buds. A parasitic saprophyte that thrives in a dark, damp, aerobic, warm environment, a fungus lives on decaying material. It can produce toxins referred to as aflatoxins and mycotoxins, found in moldy foodstuffs.
* *Transmission.* Infection can be transmitted by spores in direct contact with the respiratory system, nonintact skin, or mucous membranes.

Fungal Disease Examples

* *Superficial.* Dermatophytes such as tinea (ringworm). Localized to skin, hair, and nails, *Candida albicans* (thrush and vaginitis), athlete's foot.
* *Subcutaneous.* Confined to the dermis and subcutaneous tissue.
* *Systemic.* Infections of internal organs can gain entry via intestinal tract, intravenous line, or lungs. Respiratory fungal diseases include aspergillosis *(Aspergillus fumigatus),* histoplasmosis (*Histoplasma capsulatum,* commonly found in bat and bird excreta), cryptococcosis (*Cryptococcus neoformans,* found in pigeon excreta).
* *Opportunistic. Pneumocystis* pneumonia (*P. jiroveci,* which was originally thought to be a protozoan; DNA and RNA studies showed it was a red yeast fungus possibly carried on dogs).

Protozoa

Although microscopic, protozoa are relatively large. They grasp and ingest food particles and are motile. Protozoa have many diverse pathogenic mechanisms, although most types are not harmful to healthy humans. Protozoa become pathogenic as a result of opportunistic infection. Each species has a distinct reproductive cycle. Some parasitic protozoa reproduce only in a living host, such as in a female mosquito of the genus *Anopheles* (e.g., *Plasmodium malariae*).

Other species of protozoa living free in watery environments split by binary fission to form two daughter cells. Cryptosporidiosis (*Cryptosporidium parvum* from calves) and toxoplasmosis (*Toxoplasma gondii* from domestic cats) are examples of parasitic diseases that currently cause diseases in humans living in contemporary cities.

Characteristics

* *Structure.* Protozoa are animal-like parasites that are single-cell microorganisms without a morphologically distinct cell wall. They are eukaryotic with chromosomes and aerobic.
* *Life cycle.* Protozoa reproduce sexually (in a sanguineous host) or by binary fission (free in nature). They are capable of walling off and resist drying out by becoming cystic. They can be reactivated by moisture and prefer to live in a watery environment. Larger and more complex than bacteria, they ingest decaying organic matter. They have some diffusion through the cell membrane.
* *Transmission.* Contact is through ingestion of a cyst in soil or water, the fecal-oral route, or more commonly a bug bite. Dissemination is commonly bloodborne directly to major organs. There may be direct contact with the organism through mucous secretions from the genitourinary tract.

Protozoan Disease Examples

Intracellular

* Bloodborne protozoa passed by insect vectors include *P. malariae* that is found in red blood cells (RBCs) and liver cells.
* A localized parasitic infestation passed by the sandfly is leishmaniasis (nonhealing skin lesions; the leishmania organism lives in macrophages).
* A parasite from cats is *T. gondii.*

Extracellular

* Intestinal protozoa acquired free in nature include *Giardia lamblia* (enteritis), which is commonly misdiagnosed because symptoms mimic colitis.
* Genitourinary protozoa include *Trichomonas vaginalis.* Vulvovaginitis or urethritis can be transmitted through sexual contact or fomites.
* Amebic dysentery protozoa include *Sarcodina* and *Entamoeba* species.
* *Trypanosoma cruzi* (South American: Chagas disease can be extracellular and intracellular; lives in macrophages and muscle cells) and *T. rhodesiense* (African sleeping sickness) (parasite lives freely in blood)

Helminths

Adult helminths (worms) are not true microorganisms but are considered parasites in humans and animals. Most adult worms are visible to the naked eye, but the eggs and larvae are microscopic. Symptoms are increased as the number of worms increases. The host responds by increasing immunoglobulin E (IgE) and macrophage levels in the blood to fight the invasion. The eggs and larvae are very irritating to tissues, causing intense granulomatous inflammation.

Large volumes of invading worms can cause mechanical obstruction of lumens, such as in the gastrointestinal tract, or tunnel-through organs, such as the heart or lungs. Many intestinal varieties cause nutritional and/or hematologic depletion of the host. If a worm dies while in the host's tissue, it becomes encased in inflammatory exudate. Helminths may be found in immigrant communities or in populations living in rural farmlands with feces in the soil. Young children may acquire pinworms through fecal-oral ingestion in daycare or school settings.

Characteristics

- *Structure.* Morphologically more complex than protozoa, helminths can be round and tubular (nematodes), flat (cestodes), or flat and large (trematodes).
- *Life cycle.* Helminths are hermaphrodites. Eggs are laid in a host and are passed through excreta. Eggs hatch, becoming larvae and reentering a host by penetration or introduction through a vector. Larvae mature in the host, becoming adults capable of self-reproduction. They can become bloodborne and lymph-borne.
- *Transmission.* Introduced by insect bites, some can self-penetrate host tissues and skin and some are acquired by ingesting undercooked flesh from an infected animal or shellfish. Fecal-oral route transmission of eggs and/or larvae is common. Wading in contaminated water permits penetration of skin by active larvae.

Helminth Disease Examples

- Nematode diseases include intestinal pinworms and hookworms, and trichinosis in skeletal muscle of pigs. Filarial worms cause filariasis (elephantiasis), which is transmitted by fly or mosquito bites and becomes bloodborne.
- Cestode diseases include intestinal tapeworms.
- Trematode diseases include bloodborne flukes.

ANTIMICROBIAL THERAPY

Antimicrobial drugs or agents are adjuvants to, not substitutes for, strict adherence to aseptic and sterile techniques. Perioperative patients receive antibiotics or antimicrobials in several ways in the operating room. Routes for administration include:

- PO administration preoperatively or postoperatively
- IV administration
- Irrigation and lavage
- Implantable disks or timed-release base (i.e., bone cement with timed-release beads)
- Topical solutions or ointments
- Surgical skin prep

Antibiotics

Antibiotics act by killing bacteria (bactericidal) or inhibiting the growth of bacteria (bacteriostatic). The following actions are examples of how select antibiotic groups work against microorganisms:

1. Inhibition of cell wall synthesis
   a. Penicillins
   b. Cephalosporins
   c. Carbopenems
   d. Vancomycin
   e. Monobactams
2. Inhibition of protein synthesis
   a. Macrolides
   b. Tetracyclines
   c. Aminoglycosides
   d. Chloramphenicol
   e. Sodium fusidate
3. Inhibition of nucleic acid synthesis
   a. Sulphonamides
   b. Quinolones
   c. Nitroimidaxoles

To be effective, the bacteria must be sensitive to the activity of the antibiotic. Some antibiotic classes are broad spectrum and attack many aerobic and anaerobic bacteria; others selectively destroy specific species. Antibiotics do not affect viruses and many fungi and yeasts. Antibiotic categories are listed in Table 14-3.

The incidence of allergic reactions to antibiotics is relatively high. Patients should be questioned about allergies and known reactions before any drug is administered and should be closely watched for signs of toxicity as evidenced by skin rash, gastrointestinal disturbance, renal disorder, fever, or blood dyscrasias.

The efficacy of antibiotics is greatly reduced when multiple organisms are involved in an infection and if a biofilm has formed. Antibiotics are usually given as follows:

1. Therapeutically to eliminate sensitive viable organisms during a clinical course of infection and in grossly contaminated and traumatic wounds. The choice of antibiotic and the duration of therapy should be determined by clinical factors (i.e., pathogen, severity and site of infection, and clinical response). A broad-spectrum drug may be given while awaiting results of culture and sensitivity tests.
2. Prophylactically to prevent the development of infection. Prophylaxis implies that the microorganism is attacked by the antimicrobial agent when it harbors in tissue before colonization takes place. A prophylactic antibiotic is given before surgical intervention, bacterial invasion, or clinically evident infection. These agents are effective as supplements to host defense mechanisms in selected patients. Antibiotic prophylaxis is recommended as follows:
   a. For procedures associated with brief exposure to possible infection; evidence indicates that antibiotics can reduce infection (e.g., cystoscopy after cystitis).
   b. For procedures not frequently associated with infection but when occurrence would have disastrous or life-threatening consequences (e.g., clean wounds; insertion of a prosthetic implant such as a heart valve, vascular graft, or total joint replacement).
   c. For procedures associated with a high risk of infection. Organisms are predictable and susceptible to

TABLE 14-3	Antibiotic Categories and Related Toxicity	
Antibiotic Categories	**Caution and Considerations**	**Drug Examples**
Aminoglycoside	Nephrotoxic, ototoxic, aggravates myasthenia gravis	Gentamycin, Tobramycin, and Streptomycin
Carbapenem	Renal excretion	Imipenem, Meropenem
Cephalosporin	Renal excretion 10% cross-reaction to penicillins	1st generation: Cephalexin 2nd generation: Cefuroxime 3rd generation: Ceftazidime 4th generation: Cefepime
Sulphonamide and trimethoprim	Blood dyscrasias	Co-trimoxazole, erythromycin, Gantrisin, Septra, and Bactrim
Fluoroquinolone	Renal excretion; decreased effectiveness of antiseizure medication; interferes with theophylline, glyburide, and warfarin	1st generation: cinoxacin 2nd generation: ciprofloxacin 3rd generation: levofloxacin 4th generation: trovafloxacin
Chloramphenicol	Marrow suppression, aplastic anemia, hazardous in breast milk	Chloromycetin
Tricyclic glycopeptide	Ototoxic, nephrotoxic	Vancomycin
Tetracycline	Discoloration of bones or teeth in children under age 8, nephrotoxicity, rare hepatotoxicity	Demeclocycline, Doxycyline, and Minocyline
Macrolide	Jaundice and hepatitis, can prolong cardiac Q-T interval, hazardous in breast milk	Clindamycin, Azithromycin
Penicillin		Ampicillin, Amoxicillin, Augmentin, Piperacillin, Azlocillin, Ticarcillin, Carbenicillin, and Timentin
Nitroimidazole	Peripheral neuropathy, intolerance to alcohol, hazardous in breast milk	Metronidazole
Nitrofurantoin	Hazardous in breast milk	Macrobid
Monobactams	Hepatotoxic, marrow toxic	Aztreonam

antibiotics (e.g., clean-contaminated wounds such as a biliary tract with obstruction; transection of the colon).

The probability of infection is determined in the first few hours after bacterial invasion, when capillary permeability and host inflammatory response are at a peak immediately after bacterial contamination. Therefore, timing and duration of drug administration are crucial. To be effective, the prophylactic antibiotic must be present in adequate concentration in tissues at the time of wound creation or contamination.

Studies are under way in the prevention of biofilm formation on implants and the potential for disrupting biofilm in situ. Antibiotic hydrogel coatings are being tested on the surfaces of several types of implantable medical and surgical devices. The mechanism is not merely a timed release, but a stimulated release in response to ultrasonic waves. Unnecessary antibiotic exposure is avoided, but is there if needed. This provides a more controlled distribution in the site of implantation. Ciprofloxuin is one antibiotic hydrogel undergoing testing against *Pseudomonas aeruginosa* at this time.[5]

Selection of the appropriate drug and early use are pertinent factors (Table 14-4). The antibiotic regimen is governed by the site of the surgical procedure, potential pathogens to be found, and the patient's history of drug sensitivities. The metabolism and excretion of the drug should be considered as well as any inherent toxicities. The CDC recommends the following:

- Except for cesarean section, parenteral antibiotic prophylaxis should be started within 1 to 2 hours before a surgical procedure to produce a therapeutic level during the surgical procedure and should not be continued for more than 48 hours. A 12-hour limit is

TABLE 14-4	Selection of Antibiotics According to Gram Stain Reaction

AEROBIC BACTERIA
Amikacin
Ciprofloxacin
Aztreonam
Gentamycin
Ceftriaxone
Tobramycin

ANAEROBIC BACTERIA
Chloramphenicol
Metronidazole
Clindamycin

ANAEROBIC-AEROBIC COVERAGE
Ampicillin-Sulbactam
Imipenem-Cilastin
Cefotan
Piperacillin-Tazobactam
Ticarcillin-Clavulanate
Cefoxitin
Ceftizoxime

[5]Norris et al: Ultrasonic-activated antibiotic hydrolgels retards device-related biofilms. *Antimicrobial Agents Chemo* 49:4272-4279, 2005.

desirable for most types of wounds. Parenteral use for more than 24 hours increases the risk of antibiotic toxicity and development of resistant strains of bacteria or superinfection and does not further reduce the risk of infection.

- For cesarean section, prophylaxis usually is given intraoperatively after the umbilical cord is clamped.
- Oral, absorbable prophylactic antibiotics should not be used to supplement or extend parenteral prophylaxis. They should be limited to 24 hours before the surgical procedure when used prophylactically in colorectal operations.
- Topical antimicrobial products used in the wound should be limited to agents that will not cause serious local or systemic side effects.

Resistance to Antibiotic Therapy

Antibiotic resistance is a serious problem costing more than $30 billion in the United States. A drastic change in the pattern of life-threatening infections has occurred since the advent of broad-spectrum antibiotics and penicillinase-resistant penicillins. Many of the products used in health care end up in the water supply, causing conditions supportive of an increased antibiotic resistance in environmental microorganisms.

Gram-negative bacilli, both aerobic and anaerobic, deeply concern clinicians, because the incidence of infections by bacteria of supposedly low virulence (e.g., *Serratia* and *E. coli* organisms) is increasing. These microorganisms are capable of causing deep, latent infections, rapidly colonize, and are transferred among individuals by hands or equipment. Many of these organisms develop plasmid-mediated resistance to antibiotics. This means that a bacterium carrying genetic particles (plasmids) that allow it to replicate will be resistant to it. Resistance can be inherent or acquired. Mechanisms by which bacteria resist antibiotic action include but are not limited to the following:

1. Inherent resistance
   a. Bacterium does not absorb the antibiotic by forming an impermeable biofilm membrane.
   b. Bacterium is able to physically expel, or pump out, the antibiotic.
   c. Bacterium can render the antibiotic ineffective by chemical or enzymatic means.
   d. Bacterium can alter the molecular or ribosomal target of the antibiotic.
2. Acquired resistance
   a. Vertical evolution: a bacterium spontaneously mutates and imparts a chromosome to a member of its own bacterial population.
   b. Horizontal evolution: a bacterium with a resistant gene releases that resistant gene to a different bacterial type.

Methicillin-Resistant Staphylococcus aureus.
Methicillin-resistant *S. aureus* (MRSA) is not plasmid-mediated. However, it is resistant not just to methicillin, a penicillin, but to other categories of antibiotics as well. This resistance has probably developed as a result of overuse of these broad-spectrum agents. Clinically, MRSA poses an important health care–associated problem, whether by infection of patients or colonization in health care workers. Vancomycin, a highly toxic antimicrobial drug, seems to be effective against MRSA.

Vancomycin-Resistant Enterococci.
Vancomycin-resistant enterococci (VRE) have flourished since 1989. Studies have shown that VRE genes can be passed on to other gram-positive cocci, such as vancomycin-resistant *Streptococcus pneumoniae* and *S. aureus* (VRSA). Cases of VRSA have been reported in Japan. The CDC is currently compiling statistics on gram-positive vancomycin resistance. Previous treatment with vancomycin or multiantimicrobial therapies increases the risk for VRE. The greatest routes for spread of VRE are the hands of caregivers and contaminated equipment. According to the CDC, prevention of VRE includes but is not limited to the following:

- Education of the staff
- Prevention of transmission by isolating known colonized or infected patients
- Early detection of colonization or infection with VRE
- Screening of all enterococci isolated from blood and body substances (except urine) for vancomycin resistance
- Prudent use of vancomycin

Approved antimicrobial agents have been shown to be effective for the cleaning and disinfection of medical devices and environmental surfaces used in the care of antibiotic-resistant patients. The CDC has not issued time lines for periods of isolation, or contact precautions for VRE-infected patients, but three successive negative cultures, 1 or more weeks apart, is one possible guideline that has been used by some institutions.

Antifungal and Antiviral Drugs

Fungal and viral infections can be problematic. Topical antifungal drugs usually control fungus. *C. albicans,* for example, can lead to a fatal opportunistic systemic infection. Candicidin is a specific fungicide for this organism.

Viruses are not usually a risk to a healthy patient undergoing an elective procedure. Hepatitis and HIV present a unique challenge because they are potential threats to the caregiver. Knowledge of the medication and the disease it treats may be required for perioperative patient education. Dosages will vary. Examples of available antiviral agents include but are not limited to the following:

- Ribavirin for respiratory syncytial virus infection
- Zidovudine/dideoxyinosine for HIV infection
- Ganciclovir for CMV infection
- Acyclovir/famciclovir/valacyclovir for HSV infection
- Rimantadine/amantadine for influenza
- Didanosine for retrovirus infection
- Lamivudine for retrovirus infection
- Stavudine for retrovirus infection

Microorganisms in Mass Casualty and Bioterrorism

Health care workers should have a basic familiarity with microorganisms associated with bioterrorism. Many terrorist acts against populated areas have resulted in mass casualties that enter the hospital systems. In many circumstances, the hospital system will be the first agency to recognize clusters of infections that signal a biologic terrorist attack. Each facility should have a response and reporting plan in place as a first responder to bioterrorism.[6] Agents used in bioterrorism are listed in Box 14-3. (This list is current as of first quarter 2006.)

Perioperative personnel should be aware that in the event of a mass casualty patients may arrive at the facility in a biologically contaminated state. The facility should have a plan for decontamination of these patients before permitting them to enter the general patient population. (Additional information is available at www.ahrq.gov under the search terms for mass casualty.)

---

[6]www.cdc.gov large section of PDF documents pertaining to bioterrorism and hospital responses. Additional resources can be found at www.pbs.org/nova/bioterror.

BOX 14-3	Microbiologic Agents used in Bioterrorism

Anthrax	Plague
Botulism	Q Fever
Cholera	Smallpox
Glanders	Tularemia

Bibliography

Ellis K: The effort to protect instrumentation from tough infectious agents such as biofilm and CJD prions, *Infect Control Today* 9(2):24-27, 2005.

Llewelyn CA et al: Possible transmission of variant CJD by blood transfusion, *Lancet* 363:417-421, 2004.

McDonald M: Mandatory reporting of HAIs: What is your role? *Infect Control Today* 9(5):8-10, 2005.

McKibben L, et al: Guidance on public reporting of healthcare-associated infections: Recommendation of the healthcare infection control practices advisory committee, *AJIC* 33(4):217-226, 2005.

Meyers F: A quandary over contact precautions, *Infect Control Today* 9(6):84-88, 2005.

Oteo J et al: Antimicrobial resistant invasive *Escherichia coli,* Spain, *Emerg Infect Dis* 11(4):546-553, 2005.

Paulson DS: Persistent and residual antimicrobial effects: Are they important in the clinical setting? *Infect Control Today* 9(4):30-36, 2005.

Paulson DS: Efficacy of preoperative antimicrobial skin preparation solutions on biofilm bacteria, *AORN Journal* 81(3):491-506, 2005.

Pyrek KM: HICPAC issues guidance document on mandatory reporting of HAIs, *Infect Control Today* 9(5):18-23, 2005.

Roark J: HICPAC revises isolation and TB guidelines, *Infect Control Today* 9(3):12-16, 2005.

Roark J: Microbiology 101 for the ICP, *Infect Control Today* 9(2):38-40, 2005.

Saunders P, et al: In-vitro evaluation of the PALL Leukotrap Affinity Prion Reduction Filter as a secondary device following primary leukoreduction, *Vox Sanguinis* 89:220-228, 2005.

Trautner BW, Darouiche RO: Role of biofilm in catheter-associated urinary tract infection, *AJIC* 32(3):177-183, 2004.

Chapter 15

Principles of Asepsis and Sterile Techniques

CHAPTER OBJECTIVES

After studying this chapter, the learner will be able to:
- Define aseptic technique.
- Define sterile technique.
- Describe the transmission of microorganisms.
- List several principles of standard precautions.
- Discuss the obligation of the team to practice aseptic and sterile techniques.

CHAPTER OUTLINE

KEY TERMS AND DEFINITIONS

Aerosol   Dispersion of fine mist, droplets, or particulate matter into air (*vt:* aerosolize, to become airborne).

Antisepsis   Prevention of sepsis by the exclusion, destruction, or inhibition of growth or multiplication of microorganisms from body tissues and fluids.

Antiseptics   Inorganic chemical compounds that combat sepsis by inhibiting the growth of microorganisms without necessarily killing them. They are used on skin and tissue to arrest the growth of endogenous microorganisms (resident flora), and they must not destroy tissue.

Asepsis   Absence of microorganisms that cause disease; freedom from infection; exclusion of microorganisms. Not the same as sterile.

Aseptic technique   Methods by which contamination with microorganisms is prevented (alternate term *aseptic practice,* to maintain asepsis).

Barrier   Material used to reduce or inhibit the migration or transmission of microorganisms in the environment. Barriers include attire of personnel, drapes over furniture and patients, packaging of supplies, and filters in ventilating system.

Carrier   Person who has potentially pathogenic microorganisms on or in his or her body and disperses them into the environment without becoming ill from the pathogen.

Contaminated   Soiled or infected by microorganisms.

Cross-contamination   Transmission of microorganisms from patient to patient and from inanimate objects to patients and vice versa.

Decontamination   Cleaning and disinfecting or sterilizing processes carried out to make contaminated items safe to handle.

Disinfection   Chemical or mechanical destruction of most pathogens rendering an object safe to handle.

Fomite   Inanimate object that may be contaminated with infectious organisms and serves to transmit disease.

Irreducible minimum   Microbial burden cannot get any lower. Item is sterile to its highest degree.

Isolation   Special precautions taken to prevent the transmission of microorganisms from specific body substances.

Pathogenic   Producing or capable of producing disease.

Pathogenic microorganisms   Microorganisms that cause infectious disease. They can invade healthy tissue through some power of their own or can injure tissue by a toxin they produce.

Sepsis   Severe toxic febrile state resulting from infection with pyogenic microorganisms, with or without associated septicemia.

Spatial relationships   An awareness of sterile, unsterile, clean, and contaminated areas and their proximity to each. This includes the height of scrubbed team members in relation to each other and the sterile field. The circulating nurse must be aware of his or her closeness to the sterile field and of the appropriate means to control environmental contaminants.

Spore   A protective casing formed by a bacterium. These must be destroyed to produce sterility of that item.

Standard precautions   Procedures followed to protect personnel from contact with the blood and body fluids of all patients (formerly referred to as universal precautions).

Sterile   Free of living microorganisms, including all spores.

Sterile field   Area around the site of incision into tissue or site of introduction of an instrument into a body orifice that has been prepared for the use of sterile supplies and equipment. This area includes all furniture covered with sterile drapes and all personnel who are properly attired in sterile garb.

Sterile technique   Methods by which contamination with microorganisms is prevented to maintain sterility throughout the surgical procedure.

Terminal sterilization and disinfection   Procedures carried out for the destruction of pathogens at the end of the surgical procedure in the OR or in other areas of patient contact (e.g., postanesthesia care unit [PACU], intensive care unit [ICU], nursing unit).

Unsterile   Inanimate object that has not been subjected to a sterilization process; the outside wrapping of a package containing a sterile item; a person who has not prepared to enter the sterile field (*syn:* nonsterile).

HISTORICAL BACKGROUND

In ancient times, demons and evil spirits were thought to be the cause of pestilence and infection. The strange methods used to drive them away were replaced with purification by fire. Heat is still used today as one means of destroying microorganisms.

Not until Ignaz Semmelweis (1818-1865) advocated the value of handwashing and Louis Pasteur (1822-1895) taught his germ theory did physicians begin to study the cause of infections and the means of controlling them. Robert Koch (1843-1910), who isolated the tubercle bacillus, advocated the use of bichloride of mercury as an antiseptic. These events triggered interest in antisepsis.

Pasteur's work was pursued by Joseph Lister (1827-1912), the English surgeon who became known as the "Father of Modern Surgery." Because the relationship between bacteria and infection was now known, he searched for a chemical that could combat bacteria and surgical infections. He was the first to use a carbolic solution on dressings, which reduced the mortality of his patients to some degree. Lister believed infections were airborne.

In 1865 he started to use carbolic spray in the operating room (OR). He then used it in the wound, on articles in contact with the wound, and on the hands of the surgical team. The result was a notable decrease in mortality, but the carbolic solution caused wound necrosis and skin irritation in patients and team members. The solution also had an anticoagulant effect, which made hemostasis difficult. Not all surgeons were convinced of the value of surgical antiseptics. It was not until 1879, at a medical meeting in Amsterdam, that Lister's antiseptic principles of surgery were truly accepted by the medical profession.

German surgeons played a role in the transition from antisepsis to asepsis. Gustav Neuber (1850-1932) introduced mercuric chloride in 1886 to clean his apron, and he advocated scrubbing the furniture with disinfectant and wearing gowns, boots, and caps. He eventually sterilized everything that came into contact with wounds. The first steam sterilizer was introduced in Germany in 1886. Surgeons began to accept that all things coming into contact with a wound should be sterile. Aseptic technique evolved into sterile technique through the refinement of surgical technique, the use of a controlled environment, precise housekeeping methods, and aseptic precautions to protect patients and personnel from infection.

WHAT IS THE DIFFERENCE BETWEEN ASEPSIS AND STERILE TECHNIQUE?

Aseptic and sterile techniques are based on sound scientific principles and are carried out primarily to prevent the transmission of microorganisms that can cause infection. Microorganisms are invisible but are present in the air and on animate and inanimate objects.

To prevent infection, all possible measures are taken to create and maintain an aseptic environment for the patient. Infection that is acquired during the course of health care may occur in the surgical site or as a complication unrelated to a surgical procedure. A postoperative infection is a very serious, potentially fatal complication that may result from a single break in sterile technique. Therefore, the basis of prevention is the knowledge of causative agents and their control, as well as the principles of aseptic and sterile techniques. To effectively apply the principles of asepsis, environmental control, and sterile techniques discussed in this chapter, the meaning of terms related to aseptic technique must first be understood. The terms *aseptic* and *sterile* are not synonymous, although aspects of both are closely related. An object can be aseptic without being sterile.

Asepsis literally means "without infection," and it implies the absence of pathogenic microorganisms that cause infection. It is impossible to exclude all microorganisms from the environment, but for the safety of both patients and personnel, every effort is made to minimize and control these microorganisms. The methods by which microbial contamination is prevented in the environment are referred to as aseptic techniques.

Aseptic technique is used to protect both the patient and the caregiver. These practices are the key to the containment of microorganisms. Practices involving aseptic technique include the following:

- Items in use may be sterile or unsterile. Unsterile gloves may be used to pick up bloody sponges from the sponge bucket. Sterile gloves are used within a sterile field.
- Items are used for an individual patient only. A disposable sigmoidoscope is disposed of after use in patient care. A disposable item should not be washed and reused for another patient.
- Items are not always used within a sterile field. The brush used in surgical scrub is not considered sterile at any time during its use, yet aseptic practice in surgery requires the hands to be cleaned before donning a sterile gown and gloves.
- Contamination is contained. If the oral suction tip falls to the floor, it is discarded and a new one is obtained even though the mouth is not considered part of the sterile field. The soiled tip would not be picked up and placed back into the patient's mouth.
- Reusable items must be terminally sterilized or high-level disinfected before reuse. A stainless steel reusable sigmoidoscope will be decontaminated and terminally sterilized after use. Although it is not used under sterile conditions, it would be negligent to use an item for another patient that may have a bioburden.
- Items are not necessarily stored in a sterile condition. When a reusable item is processed after use, it may be

stored in an unwrapped state if it is not to be used within a sterile field.

- Aseptic technique is sometimes referred to as clean technique.

Sterile technique refers to creating and working within the sterile field. To protect the patient during invasive procedures, microorganisms in the sterile field are kept to an irreducible minimum. The patient is at risk for infection any time tissues are interrupted or instrumentation is introduced into the vascular system. Sterile items should be used to prevent the introduction of pathogens into the patient's body.

- Items used are sterile without exception.
- Items used have been stored in sterile conditions.
- Contamination is avoided or remedied immediately.
- Reusable items are rendered sterile before reuse.

TRANSMISSION OF MICROORGANISMS

People remain the major source of microorganisms in the environment. In the OR, the surgical team is the most common source of transmission, followed by contaminated instrumentation. Everything on or around a human being is contaminated by the body in some way. The action and interaction of personnel and patients also contribute to the prevalence and dispersion of microorganisms.

There are many sources of contamination in the OR environment. Transmission-based precautions should be implemented in the perioperative environment and in any area with the potential to transmit potentially pathogenic microorganisms. Transmission-based precautions are described in Box 15-1. Perioperative personnel are concerned primarily with protecting the environment of the OR suite because surgical procedures should be performed under optimal aseptic conditions. Two areas in the OR suite are most critical for the introduction and spread of microorganisms:

- Semirestricted areas
- Restricted areas

Most microorganisms grow in a warm, moist host, but some aerobic bacteria, yeasts, and fungi can remain viable in the air and on inanimate objects. Advances in aseptic technique and infection control include the following:

- Operating room ventilation, humidity, and temperature controls
- Sterilization, decontamination, and disinfection methods
- Improved barriers between sterile, clean, and contaminated surfaces
- Surgical technique
- Antimicrobial prophylaxis

Despite advances, surgical-site infections (SSIs) continue to cause significant morbidity and mortality in surgical patients. Emergence of resistant microorganisms is complicated by patients with comorbid disease and the increasing numbers of implants and transplants. Microbiologic considerations and specific microorganisms that concern the perioperative team are described in Chapter 14.

Factors to consider when evaluating the reasons for the emergence of resistant microorganisms include the following:

- Inadequate doses of antibiotic

| BOX 15-1 | Transmission-Based Precautions |

AIRBORNE
The use of special air handlers and ventilation and respiratory protection is recommended for susceptible people. Contaminated air currents can settle on or be inhaled by those who are susceptible.

Particles smaller than 5 mm may carry airborne droplet nuclei. Examples of airborne diseases include varicella, tuberculosis, and rubeola.

DROPLET
A distance of more than 3 feet from the source patient is recommended. Masks should be worn by those closer than 3 feet and should be worn by the source patient during transport. Droplet particles are larger than 5 mm and are disseminated during coughs, sneezes, and talking. Droplets do not travel more than 3 feet and are not suspended in the air. Examples of droplet diseases include diphtheria, mumps, pertussis, and influenza.

CONTACT
The use of gloves when coming into contact with items contaminated with blood or body substances is recommended. Gowns are recommended if there is a potential for contamination of clothing.

Cleaning and disinfecting patient care equipment after use protects other patients.

Data from U.S. Department of Health and Human Services (www.hhs.gov) and Centers for Disease Control and Prevention (www.cdc.gov).

- Improper selection of antibiotic
- Previous use of ineffective antibiotic
- Sequestered infectious site in biofilm or retained foreign body

Inadequate infection control practices

HUMAN-BORNE SOURCES OF CONTAMINATION

Skin

The skin of patients, OR team members, and visitors constitutes a microbiologic hazard. Sebaceous (oil) and sudoriferous (sweat) glands contain abundant resident microbial flora, many of which have the potential to become pathogenic if colonized in greater-than-average numbers or if colonized on a weakened host. In an average individual, an estimated 4000 to 10,000 viable contaminated particles are shed by the skin each minute. Some disperse up to 30,000 particles per minute; these individuals are referred to as shedders. Shedders are densely populated with virulent organisms, such as *Staphylococcus aureus,* and shed contaminated skin cells into the environment.

Patients who are shedders have a much higher incidence of infection at the surgical site. On all individuals, the major areas of microbial shedding include the head, neck, axillae, hands, groin, perineum, legs, and feet. Cosmetic detritus and body powders are also laden with potential pathogens. Microbial shedding is contained effectively by appropriate antiseptic cleansing and maximum skin coverage.

The following are key points for all personnel entering the OR:

- Bathe daily with soap that contains an antibacterial agent.
- Wash hands before entering the OR suite and after every patient contact to prevent infection and cross-infection. This handwashing technique involves vigorously rubbing together all surfaces of well-lathered, soapy hands, followed by rinsing under a stream of water.
- Don clean OR attire for each entry into the OR suite. Unsterile team members should wear long sleeves.
- Cover any cuts and abrasions. Open wounds on the skin are portals for infection, and infected wounds can disseminate microorganisms.
- Wear gloves when handling blood, body fluids, or tissue specimens, and wash hands after removing sterile and unsterile gloves.

Hair

Hair is a gross contaminant and a major source of staphylococci. The extent to which the microbial population is attracted to and shed from hair is directly related to the length and cleanliness of the hair. Hair follicles and filaments harbor resident and transient flora. Hair can become a mechanical irritant in wound healing and cause a foreign body tissue reaction. Hair should be shampooed frequently. Clean caps or hoods are worn to cover hair completely, including facial hair. Hair should be contained at all times in semirestricted and restricted environments.

Nasopharynx

Microorganisms forcibly expelled by talking, coughing, or sneezing give rise to bacteria-laden dust and lint as droplets settle on surfaces and skin. Carriers harbor many organisms, most notably group A streptococci and *S. aureus,* without experiencing the harmful physical effects of infection. Surgeons and anesthesia providers may be carriers more so than other caregivers because of their intimate contact with patients' respiratory tracts.

Shedders and carriers may be identified through nasopharyngeal culturing. Some departments, such as obstetrics and the newborn nursery, may require routine periodic cultures as a condition of employment. When multiple patients develop the same or similar postoperative infections, infection control teams at the facility actively seek the source of the infection.

Masks are worn in all restricted areas to cover the nose and mouth and should be changed after caring for each patient. Masks protect the wearer and the patient. Coughing and sneezing explode droplets into the environment, and therefore people with a respiratory infection should not be permitted in the OR suite. Talking should be kept to a minimum.

Human Error

Direct person-to-person contact is the most common route of transmission. Human error is an exogenous source of contamination, and it is not to be underestimated. Failure to follow the principles and applications of sterile and aseptic techniques places the patient and personnel at risk—a risk that could be prevented. Errors should be readily admitted and corrected.

Cross-Infection

Every patient in the OR should be considered to be a potential source of infection. Standard precautions and routine aseptic techniques are observed whether or not a patient is known to have an infectious condition. All patients should be treated as though they have a known infection. Care, caution, and conscientiousness on the part of all team members are essential at all times. Thorough handwashing after every patient contact is important.

NONHUMAN FACTORS IN CONTAMINATION

Fomites

Contaminated particles are present in the dust that rests on inanimate objects such as furniture, OR surfaces (e.g., walls, floors, cabinet shelves), equipment, computer keyboards, cabinet handles, supplies, and fabrics. Covert contamination may result from improper handling of equipment such as anesthesia apparatus or intravenous (IV) lines and fluids. Contamination also may result from the administration of unsterile medications or the use of unsterile water to rinse sterile items. Any unsterile item placed within the sterile field causes contamination and increases the risk of infection.

In maintaining an aseptic environment, the following key points should be considered:

- Prompt disinfection and decontamination of used equipment and reusable supplies.
- Prompt disinfection of OR surfaces (e.g., disinfecting furniture and floors, disposing of waste and laundry).
- Separation of clean and soiled items. Sterile storage areas are physically separated from decontamination areas.
- Proper packaging and storing of supplies. External shipping cartons should be removed before bringing supplies beyond the unrestricted area in the OR suite. Insects and rodents can gain entrance to the suite in corrugated cartons.
- Placement of dust covers over sterile items during transport and while in prolonged storage.

Air

The perioperative environment contains thousands of particles per cubic foot of air. During a long surgical procedure, the particle count can rise to more than 1 million particles per cubic foot. Air and dust are vehicles for transporting particles laden with microorganisms. Heat rises, and therefore the lights and other heat-generating equipment of the OR produce convective up-currents. Personnel walking about the room can generate airborne contamination; every movement increases the potential for infection of the surgical site. Traffic should be kept to an absolute minimum. Particulates bearing microorganisms become airborne and settle in an open wound.

Between 80% and 90% of the microbial contaminations found in an open surgical site come from ambient (room) air. Beta-hemolytic streptococci have been directly traced from contaminated personnel and contamination of a patient. The actual microorganism was recovered from the room air.[1]

Microorganisms have an affinity for horizontal surfaces, of which the floor is the largest. From the floor, micro-organisms are projected into the air. Endogenous flora from the patient's skin, oropharynx, tracheobronchial tree, and gastrointestinal tract, as well as exogenous flora, also are significant. Microorganisms from patients or carriers settle on equipment and flat surfaces and then become airborne. Airborne particles increase significantly during the activity before incision and after wound closure. Relief personnel create significant air currents. The potential for contamination increases each time the door to the OR opens and closes.

An effective ventilation system is essential to prevent patients and personnel from breathing potentially contaminated air, which can predispose them to infection.

SOURCES OF INFECTION

The incidence and types of infections that occur in surgical patients may be the result of a preexisting localized infectious process, a systemic communicable disease, or an acquired perioperative complication.

Community-Acquired Infection

Community-acquired infections are natural disease processes that developed or were incubating before a patient's admission to the hospital or ambulatory care facility.

Communicable Infection

Systemic bacterial, viral, or fungal infections may be transmitted from one person to another. These infections are discussed in detail in Chapter 14.

Spontaneous Infection

Examples of localized infections that require surgical diagnosis and treatment for management or that occur as adjuvant to medical therapy include acute appendicitis, cholecystitis, and bowel perforation with peritonitis. Therapy consists of identification of the infection site and causative microorganism, excision or drainage, prevention of further contamination, and augmentation of host resistance.[1]

Health Care–Acquired Infection (HAI)

An infection is considered hospital associated or acquired (i.e., nosocomial) during the course of health care if it was neither present nor incubating when the patient was admitted.

Approximately 35% of all nosocomial *S. aureus* infections develop in surgical patients. They may occur as complications of surgical or other procedures performed on uninfected patients. They may occur also as complicating infections in organs unrelated to the surgical procedure that occur with or as a result of postoperative care. The majority of nosocomial infections are related to instrumentation of the urinary and respiratory tracts. Microbial colonization is the

[1]CDC *Guideline for prevention of surgical site infection*, 1999, www.cdc.gov.

primary component of nosocomial infection. The potential for SSIs can be conceptualized in the following equation[1]:

$$\frac{\text{Dose of contamination} \times \text{virulence}}{\text{Resistance of the host}} = \text{Risk of SSI}$$

The following are examples of HAI:
- Urinary tract and respiratory tract infections and infected pressure and stasis ulcers
- Cellulitis and abscess formations in pressure sores
- Thrombophlebitis, which is a regional extension of postoperative intravenous infection
- Bacteremia and septicemia, the postoperative systemic infections that result from dissemination of microorganisms into the bloodstream from a distributing focus
- Septicemia caused by intravascular catheters
- Persistent infections at the site of surgical implants

Exogenous. An exogenous nosocomial infection is acquired from sources outside the body, such as personnel or the environment. Cross-contamination occurs when organisms are transferred to the patient from another individual or inanimate object.

Endogenous. An endogenous infection develops from sources within the body. Most postoperative wound infections result from seeding by endogenous microorganisms. Disruption of the balance between potentially pathogenic organisms and host defenses permits the invasion of microorganisms for which the patient is the primary reservoir. For example, abdominal sepsis may result from enteric flora if the intestine is perforated or transected.

Criteria for Defining a Surgical-Site Infection. According to the Centers for Disease Control and Prevention (CDC) an SSI is the most common type of infection reported. Mortality associated with surgical patients with infection is commonly linked to death from sepsis 77% of the time. Hospital stay was significantly increased, thereby exposing the weakened patient to increased risk of additional infections. A synopsis of the criteria for defining an SSI as described by the CDC is presented in Table 15-1.

ASEPTIC TECHNIQUE AND ENVIRONMENTAL CONTROLS

Control of the environment is a necessary part of overall infection prevention. The inanimate and animate environment of the OR suite presents a risk for the transmission of microorganisms. The aim of a microbiologically controlled environment is to keep contamination to a minimum. The key to controlling microorganisms lies in the knowledge of their favorable living conditions. Best practices in asepsis should be rooted in prevention of proliferation and spread of microorganisms

AORN (Association of periOperative Registered Nurses) has developed standards and recommended practices for achieving the optimal aseptic practices in the care of perioperative patients. These guidelines are intended to give direction and information for the formulation of institutional policies. Individual hospital policies and procedures

TABLE 15-1	Criteria for Defining a Surgical-Site Infection (SSI) According to the CDC (1999)	
Superficial Incisional SSI	**Deep Incisional SSI**	**Organ/Space SSI**

Infection occurs within 30 days of the surgical procedure. Infection involves only skin or subcutaneous tissue of the incision and at least one of the following from the superficial incision unless the wound is culture negative:
1. Purulent drainage with or without laboratory confirmation, from the incision
2. Organisms isolated from an aseptically obtained culture of fluid or tissue
3. At least one of the following signs or symptoms of infection:
  a. Pain or tenderness
  b. Localized swelling
  c. Redness or heat
  d. Surgeon deliberately opens the incision
4. Diagnosis of superficial incisional SSI by the surgeon or physician
Do not report the following conditions as superficial SSI:
1. Stitch abscess (minimal inflammation and discharge) confined to the points of suture penetration
2. Infection of episiotomy or newborn circumcision site (these have separate criteria)
3. Infected burn wound
4. Incisional SSI that extends into the fascial and muscle layers
	Infection occurs within 30 days after the procedure if no implant is left in place or within 1 year if an implant is left in place and the infection appears to be related to the procedure. Infection involves deep soft tissues (e.g., fascial and muscle layers) of the incision and at least one of the following unless the site is culture negative:
	1. Purulent drainage from the deep aspects of the incision, but not theorgans or compartments
	2. A deep incision spontaneously dehisces or deliberately opened by the surgeon because of:
	  a. Fever >100.4° F (38° C)
	  b. Localized pain
	3. Diagnosis of deep SSI by physician or surgeon
	Additional factors:
	1. Report combined superficial and deep infections as deep SSI
	2. Report organ space or deep infection that drains through the incision as deep SSI
		Infection occurs within 30 days after the procedure if no implant is left in place or within 1 year if an implant is left in place and the infection appears to be related to the procedure. Infection involves any part of the anatomy (e.g., organs or spaces) other than the incision that was opened or manipulated during an operation and at least one of the following:
		1. Purulent drainage from a drain that is placed through a stab wound into the organ or space
		2. Organisms are isolated from an aseptically obtained culture of fluid or tissue in the organ or space
		3. An abscess or other evidence of infection involving the organ or space that is found by direct examination or by radiograph

reflect variations in the physical environment and in clinical situations that determine the degree to which these recommended practices can be implemented. All health care facilities should incorporate into their policies and procedures the recommendations for infection control from the CDC, as well as the regulations for the prevention of exposure to bloodborne pathogens from the Occupational Safety and Health Administration (OSHA).

The perioperative environment is designed both to optimize function and safety and protect patients from sources of contamination. The surgical suite includes specific areas for traffic, support systems, administration, communication, and storage as described in Chapter 10. Traffic patterns are designed to flow smoothly and to prevent backtrack and crossover traffic. Clean and soiled activities, areas, and personnel and sterile and unsterile supplies should be distinctly separated.

Impervious barriers such as sterile drapes, gowns, and gloves protect sterile areas, isolate surgical sites, and keep the number of microorganisms to an irreducible minimum. These barriers must remain impervious to the passage of microorganisms under ordinary operating conditions.

Procedures are established to use barriers effectively against microorganisms from any potential source of contamination.

Environmental Services/Housekeeping

Housekeeping practices that use the most effective supplies, techniques, and equipment available are a most important aspect of infection control. Good housekeeping techniques should reduce microbial flora by approximately 90%. Housekeeping procedures include cleaning and disinfecting the perioperative environment, handling soiled laundry, and disposing of solid waste. Disinfectants are used in combination with thorough mechanical cleaning. These procedures are performed by environmental service personnel under supervision and are carried out according to established practices, policies, and schedules as described in Chapter 12. Of primary concern are locations that by design or construction are difficult to clean (e.g., lavatories, workrooms) and areas that may be touched by patients or personnel.

Any equipment requiring water in its operation can support microbial growth, especially if the water is not changed frequently. Unsterile water, the universal solvent and transporter, can support, maintain, and protect almost every contaminant produced by human beings. Water especially supports the growth of gram-negative bacilli, including *Serratia* and *Pseudomonas*. Airborne aerosolized particles produced during hand scrubs can contaminate the area around the scrub sink. Disinfectants reduce the contamination potential of unsterile cleaning water.

The following housekeeping points are especially relevant to infection control and the prevention of cross-infection and are listed to emphasize the importance of aseptic environmental control:

- The faucet head should be of a type that does not hold water and should be removed for terminal sterilization. Containers for antimicrobial handwashing agents should be disassembled, cleaned, and terminally sterilized before refilling.
- No surface should remain wet, which would support microbial growth and the formation of biofilm.
- Organic debris should be promptly removed from walls and other surfaces with a disinfectant to prevent drying and airborne contamination.
- Lights should be cleaned after every procedure. Overhead tracks should be cleaned upon completion of the day's schedule.
- The entrance to the OR suite and the floors in corridors and rooms should be cleaned at the end of the day's schedule.
- Housekeeping equipment should be cleaned and dried for storage. Moisture and darkness are conducive to microbial growth.
- Disposable trash should be separated into infectious and noninfectious waste and put in impervious receptacles.
- Service elevators rather than chutes should be used to remove soiled laundry and waste/trash from the OR suite. Chutes become grossly contaminated with airborne particles and are a fire hazard.
- Waste should be contained at the source of origin to prevent aerosol generation during handling. Contaminated waste is decontaminated and/or sterilized before compaction or disposal in the general environment. Incineration is the most effective means of waste disposal, especially of infectious wastes. However, health care facilities must comply with local, state, and federal regulations for contamination control and waste disposal.
- Adequate time must be allowed between patients for proper terminal disinfection of the OR. A patient must not be assigned to an inadequately cleaned OR, which could be a source of an SSI.
- All areas and equipment throughout the perioperative environment should be cleaned on a scheduled basis as defined by institutional policy. These areas include the grills, vents, and filters of the air-conditioning system; storage shelves and cabinets; lighting fixtures; walls; and other areas in offices, lounges, dressing rooms, storage areas, workrooms, and corridors. Handles of cabinets and push plates of doors should be cleaned several times daily.

Control of Airborne Contamination

Air currents and movement in the OR should be kept to a minimum to prevent airborne contamination. Viable microorganisms from the air settle on horizontal surfaces. Proper cleaning of these surfaces helps to control this contamination. The ventilating system and efforts to minimize air turbulence and contaminants also are important factors. Doors to the OR should remain closed during the procedure to maintain a positive pressure atmosphere.

Air-Conditioning System. When properly designed, installed, and maintained, a conventional air-conditioning system effectively reduces the number of airborne organisms by removing dust and aerosol particles. Air contaminated by dust and lint is removed as fresh, clean outside air is supplied. Recirculation of filtered air at a minimum rate of 15 volume exchanges per hour, at least three of which are fresh air, is considered safe and economical as recommended by the American Institute of Architects in collaboration with the U.S. Department of Health and Human Services (HHS), 1996. However, fire codes in some states require 100% outside fresh air. All air, whether recirculated or fresh, is filtered before entering the OR. The system uses high-efficiency particulate air (HEPA) filters to remove particles larger than 0.3 μm.

Air enters from a ceiling vent, is diluted, and passes out through vents at floor level. Filters are located downstream from the air-processing equipment so microorganisms will not be drawn into the room. The system maintains a positive pressure if the doors to the room remain closed.

Laminar Air System. Often referred to as ultraclean airflow, a special air-handling system for the filtration, dilution, and distribution of air may be installed in one or more ORs. High-risk procedures such as total joint replacement, cardiac surgery, and organ transplantation are performed in this environment. Laminar airflow is a controlled, unidirectional, positive pressure stream of air.

From a ceiling diffuser, clean air flows downward at a high velocity, progressively decreasing as it flows radially outward. The controlled airstream entraps particulate matter and microorganisms. The flow returns to the system and passes through a prefilter to remove gross particles. It then passes through a HEPA filter that traps and eliminates more than 99% of all particles larger than 0.3 μm, including virtually all bacteria and most viruses. A rate of 100 to 400 air changes per hour is possible; most systems deliver approximately 240. The flow can be directed vertically or horizontally. Studies have shown that ultraclean air and antimicrobial prophylaxis used together can decrease SSI. The same studies, however, indicated that antimicrobial prophylaxis alone decreased SSI more than the use of ultraclean air.

To augment the laminar airflow system, sterile team members wear a total body exhaust gown, which resembles a spacesuit and covers the entire body. Air is piped into the headpiece and removed through filtered tubes. The hood or helmet is equipped for hearing and speaking. A mask is not used. Negative pressure is maintained under the gown by a vacuum hose. The system provides body cooling for the wearer.

Laminar airflow with a total body exhaust system reliably reduces bacterial contamination at the wound site. Although an ultraclean air system provides microbe-free air (no more than one organism per cubic foot) with minimal air turbulence, it is not a substitute for meticulous surgical technique. The decrease in particle count does not significantly reduce the rate of infection at the surgical site. It is an adjunct to controlling airborne contamination.

Doors. The doors to the OR should be kept closed except as necessary for passage of the patient and personnel and supplies and equipment. If the door is left open, the positive air pressure in the room equalizes with the negative air pressure in the hallway. Disrupted pressurization mixes the clean air of the OR with the corridor air, which has a higher microbial count. Cabinet doors should remain closed.

Traffic and Movement. Traffic in and out of the OR is kept to a minimum. Only essential personnel should be allowed inside the OR. The amount of activity in the room increases as the number of people present increases. This in turn increases the potential for contamination as a result of the shedding and air turbulence that carries microbes to the wound. Movement in the OR should be reduced to a minimum.

Lint. Agents are added to the final rinse during laundering to minimize the lint that results from the friction of woven fibers against each other. Disintegrated paper from disposable nonwoven products is another source of lint on fabrics. Therefore paper products should not be discarded in the same receptacle as soiled reusable woven fabrics.

Isolation Precautions

The isolation of patients by diagnosis or body substance is related to the mode of transmission of pathogenic microorganisms (i.e., air, droplet, contact). A patient with a communicable disease could need emergency surgery and perioperative personnel should know about appropriate patient handling and exposure precautions. A communicable disease such as tuberculosis (TB) could be diagnosed via bronchoscopy.

Isolation precautions and guidelines are discussed in detail in hospital procedure books and in the CDC "Guideline for Isolation Precautions in Hospitals." There are different methods of isolation technique:

* Category-specific isolation precautions for patients with suspected or confirmed communicable disease transmitted either by droplets via the airborne route (e.g., pulmonary tuberculosis) or by enteric excretions, drainage, or secretions
* Disease-specific isolation precautions for contact with patients known to be infected with specific pathogens
* Body-substance isolation precautions incorporating standard precautions for contact with all body substances of all patients, regardless of the diagnosis (all patients are considered contaminated)
* Protective isolation for immunosuppressed patients

The purpose of these precautions is to prevent the transmission of pathogenic microorganisms. Isolation and barrier techniques protect both personnel and other patients. Each hospital may incorporate into its procedures whichever methods are most appropriate for its particular needs and patient population.

The perioperative staff should be informed that a patient requires isolation precautions before that patient comes to the OR. Some situations, such as TB requires the use of HEPA masks for the staff. A sticker on the patient's chart and bed indicates the type of hospital isolation. For most patients the same precautions apply in the OR as on the patient care unit, and a commonsense approach is used. In all types of isolation, the most important control measure is thorough handwashing before and after close patient contact; after handling contaminated objects, body fluids, and excretions; and between patients. Isolation techniques must not be implemented in a way that causes the patient to feel victimized. Patients should be educated to understand that the isolation protects them as well as the caregiver and they must comply with the regimen.

STANDARD PRECAUTIONS

As established by the CDC and enforced by OSHA, standard precautions (formerly referred to as universal precautions) protect health care workers from contact with blood and body fluids of all patients. Standard precautions include considerations for the following:

* All body fluids
* Handwashing
* Barrier clothing
* Handling of used patient care equipment and linen
* Occupational exposure to bloodborne pathogens
* Patient placement

Recommendations for standard precautions have been modified to reflect routes of transmission. The format for the CDC's identification of routes of transmission includes airborne, droplet, and contact precautions. The potential for becoming infected through skin exposure depends on colonization, duration of contact, the presence of skin lesions on the hands, and immune status. Standard precautions supplement other recommended practices for environmental controls and are the minimum precautions for all invasive procedures. An invasive procedure involves any entry into body tissues or cavities in any procedural environment. Standard precautions are in effect for any procedure during which bleeding occurs or for which the potential for bleeding or exposure to body substances exists. Standard precautions involve the following:

1. *Protective barriers and personal protective equipment (PPE).* Appropriate barriers, such as PPE, prevent contact of the skin and mucous membranes with blood and body substances. PPE and other barrier materials must prevent blood and other fluids from passing through or reaching the wearer's clothing or body. The type of PPE used depends on the task and the degree of anticipated exposure. Examples include gloves, eyewear, gowns, hair covers, and masks.
   a. Gloves reduce contamination of hands. Intact gloves, both sterile and unsterile, are used. Latex,

vinyl, and other materials are used in the manufacturing of these gloves. Care is taken to avoid natural rubber latex (NRL) when either the patient or the caregiver has a latex sensitivity. Vinyl may be more permeable to some viruses than is latex.

(1) Sterile gloves are worn for procedures that involve the invasion of body tissues when a sterile field is created.

    (a) Double-gloving does not prevent puncture wounds but may be appropriate for procedures in which the risk of glove tears is high. Comfort is improved with double-gloving if the wearer dons larger gloves under the regular size worn. The larger glove creates a narrow air cushion that prevents constriction caused by wearing two sets of gloves of the same size. With double-gloving, the exterior glove has a mechanical squeegee effect on a sharp object as it punctures its surface. The innermost glove further squeegees material from the sharp object, which reduces the potential numbers of microorganisms that come into contact with the wearer.

    (b) Sterile glove liners may provide protection from glove tears and skin cuts, particularly when working with heavy orthopedic equipment. Double-gloving also may substantially reduce the risk of exposure from the seepage of blood and fluid through gloves onto hands during long procedures or in the presence of voluminous blood loss. No glove is 100% impervious.

(2) Unsterile latex or vinyl examination gloves are worn for procedures that do not require a sterile field, such as handling specimens, placentas, newborns, and contaminated items (e.g., sponges). Powdered gloves leave a residue that may carry latex particles.

(3) General-purpose utility gloves are worn for cleaning instruments and for decontaminating and housekeeping procedures involving potential blood contact. These heavy-duty gloves may be decontaminated and reused.

(4) Gloves are changed after every contact with patients or contaminated items. Latex and vinyl gloves are discarded. Washing gloves between patient contacts is not an acceptable practice.

(5) Hands are washed immediately after glove removal. All gloves have microscopic holes and may be permeable to certain substances or microorganisms. The mechanical and chemical actions of handwashing significantly decrease the risk associated with the permeability of glove materials.

b. Masks protect personnel from aerosols and patients from droplets. They are worn for all invasive procedures. Specialty masks to filter laser plume are commercially available. The mask should be changed immediately if grossly contaminated by a splash of blood or body fluid. Patients with a known infectious process such as varicella, tuberculosis, or rubeola should wear a HEPA mask during transport to and from the OR.

c. Eyewear with side shields protects the mucous membranes of the eyes, and full face shields protect the mucous membranes of the eyes, nose, and mouth. They are worn for procedures in which blood, bone chips, amniotic fluid, and the aerosol of other body fluids may splash or be projected into the eyes. Goggles with enclosed sides and chin-length face shields offer better protection than do simple eyeglasses.

d. Gowns or aprons made of fluid-resistant material protect the wearer from a splash with blood and body fluids. A plastic apron may be worn under a woven fabric gown. Impervious gowns offer better protection. Disposable impervious gowns are preferred.

e. Shoe covers or boots protect the wearer when gross contamination on the floor can be anticipated. Grossly soiled shoe covers or knee-high disposable boots are removed before the wearer leaves the room.

2. *Prevention of puncture injuries.* Needles, knife blades, and sharp instruments present a potential hazard for the handler and user. Skin may be punctured or cut if caution is not taken. Specific recommendations for handling disposable surgical needles, syringes and needles, and knife blades (collectively referred to as sharps) include the following:

a. Do not manipulate sharps by hand. Use an instrument, such as a heavy hemostat, to attach and remove the scalpel blade. Arm the needle directly from the suture packet when possible. Do not bend or break an injection needle. Pass needles in a needle holder or use a "neutral zone" to transfer sharps on field. Sharp instruments and needles may be passed on a tray or magnetic mat for a hands-free technique rather than from hand to hand. Remove instruments from the surgical field after use, and return them to the Mayo stand or instrument table promptly.

b. Do not recap used injection needles except with a recapping safety device.

c. Do not remove the needle from a disposable syringe by hand after use. If a needle must be changed, use a hemostat or other instrument to exchange a hypodermic needle.

d. Place all used sharps in a puncture-resistant container for disposal.

3. *Management of puncture injuries.* If a glove is torn or punctured, remove the puncturing sharp or instrument from the sterile field immediately and change the glove promptly, using the open-glove method. If the skin is punctured or cut, remove both gloves immediately. If both gloves are not removed, the risk of introducing microorganisms from the remaining contaminated glove is increased. Squeeze the

skin to release blood. Wash out contaminants under running water with an antiseptic; then irrigate the wound with a virucidal disinfectant such as an iodophor, bleach, or peroxide. Report the incident immediately, and document all actions on the appropriate forms. Baseline testing may be necessary for the punctured individual and the patient. These actions are necessary to protect the employee and the patient should either party seroconvert to a positive status at a later date.

4. *Oral procedures.* Although transmission by saliva is unlikely, contact with blood-contaminated saliva and gingival fluid is expected during dental and surgical procedures in the oropharyngeal cavity. Mouth protection, Ambu bags, and/or other ventilation devices should be available for emergency airway resuscitation. Respiratory secretions coughed up during endotracheal procedures are often infectious.

5. *Care of specimens.* All specimens of blood, body fluids, and tissues should be contained to prevent leaking during transport to the laboratory. The outside of the container should be clean. The circulating nurse, while wearing gloves, needs to disinfect the outside of a culture tube handed from the sterile field or a container if it has been contaminated. Care is taken not to get blood and body fluids on the pathology requisition slip.

6. *Decontamination.* All instruments are thoroughly cleaned before sterilization or high-level disinfection. The surfaces of furniture and floors are cleaned and decontaminated with a detergent-disinfectant. Blood or body fluids that have spilled on the floor during a procedure should be wiped up immediately and the area decontaminated. Gloves, masks, and eyewear are worn for cleaning procedures.

7. *Laundry.* Soiled woven fabrics should be handled as little as possible and are transported to the laundry in leak-proof bags. All laundry is considered contaminated and should be handled only by gloved hands. Laundry should be washed in water at 160° F (71.1° C) or higher with 50 to 150 parts per million (ppm) of chlorine bleach. Temperatures lower than 160° F (71.1° C) can be used for washing laundry if the appropriate antimicrobial detergent is used. Commercial dry cleaning uses chemicals that reduce the transmission of pathogens. Home laundering of surgical scrub suits may not consistently meet parameters for adequate disinfection.

8. *Waste.* Blood and suctioned fluids may be safely poured down a drain that is connected to a sanitary sewer. A solidifying agent can be added to disposable suction containers to disinfect the produce and convert it into solid waste. Trash is disposed of by incineration or sent to a sanitary landfill in sealed containers as required by local ordinances or state regulations. Trash bags must be leak-proof and of sufficient thickness and strength to ensure integrity during transport. For disposal purposes, waste may be differentiated as either infectious or noninfectious. Bags are either color-coded (e.g., red for infectious waste) or labeled as biohazard.

9. *Handwashing.* Thorough handwashing with an approved antimicrobial agent after every contact with a patient, contaminated items, or suspected contamination protects both the patient and personnel, and it cannot be overemphasized.

10. *No touching of mucous membranes.* Eating and drinking are prohibited in any area where there is a risk for exposure. Applying lip balm or cosmetics or adjusting contact lenses in the perioperative environment significantly increases the risk of exposure. Hand-to-mouth and hand-to-eye contact can contribute to microbial transmission.

11. *Prophylaxis.* Perioperative personnel are encouraged to know their human immunodeficiency virus (HIV), hepatitis B virus (HBV), and hepatitis C virus (HCV) antibody status. The disclosure of a positive status to the appropriate facility is recommended. Personnel who participate in invasive procedures are at risk for bloodborne exposure and should have the HBV immunization series. Personnel who choose not to have the immunization series should sign a release stating the declination. Experts disagree about the need for booster injections after 7 years to maintain the antibody titer.

For personal protection and for the safety of patients, all health care providers should be familiar with policies and procedures and must understand the need for standard precautions. A health care provider should report a blood or body fluid exposure as defined by policy. The surgeon and first assistant usually are at greatest risk. Similarly, a patient should be informed of any incident in which he or she is exposed to the blood of a health care provider.

APPLICATION OF STERILE TECHNIQUE

Sterile technique prevents the transfer of microorganisms into body tissues during invasive procedures. Freshly incised or traumatized tissue can become infected easily, regardless of the area of the body. Intact skin and mucous membranes are the body's first line of defense against infection, but a portal for microorganisms is created if the integrity of the skin is interrupted.

Levels of Sterility and Disinfection

Depending on their intended purpose and body contact, the items and equipment for patient care are classified into the following categories described by Spaulding according to the level of sterility necessary for safe patient care use:

- *Critical.* Any item entering the body tissues underlying the skin and mucous membranes must be sterile (i.e., free of microorganisms, including spores). These items are handled using sterile technique to maintain sterility.
- *Semicritical.* Sterility is less critical for items that come into contact with intact skin or mucous membranes. These items are clean and safe to handle (i.e., mechanically cleaned and disinfected to reduce microorganisms, but unsterile). Some items are disinfected immediately before use and are handled using aseptic technique to prevent contamination before use. Other items are terminally sterilized, but sterility is not maintained during use.

- *Noncritical.* Items that will come into contact with only intact skin or mucous membranes in an area remote from the surgical site may be cleaned, terminally disinfected, and stored unsterile between patient uses. No special technique in handling is observed.

Surgical procedures are performed under sterile conditions; contamination with microorganisms is prevented to maintain sterility throughout the procedure. A sterile field is created around the site of incision into tissues or the site of introduction of sterile instruments into a body orifice. Conversely, all materials and equipment used during a surgical procedure are terminally decontaminated and sterilized after use with the assumption that every patient is a potential source of infection for other persons.

It is essential that all members of the perioperative team know the common sources and mechanisms of contamination by microorganisms in the perioperative environment. The practices of sterile and aseptic techniques are the particular responsibility of everyone caring for the patient in the OR. All members of the OR team must be vigilant in safeguarding the sterility of the sterile field. Any contamination must be remedied immediately.

PRINCIPLES OF STERILE TECHNIQUE

Sterile technique is the foundation of modern surgery. The patient is the center of the sterile field, which includes the personnel wearing sterile attire and the areas of the patient, operating bed, and furniture that are covered with sterile drapes. Strict adherence to the recommended practices of sterile technique reflects the surgical conscience of the perioperative team and is mandatory for the safety of the patient and personnel in the environment. The principles of sterile technique are applied under the following conditions:

- In preparation for an invasive procedure by sterilization of necessary materials and supplies
- In preparation of the sterile team to handle sterile supplies and intimately contact the surgical site by scrubbing, gowning, and gloving
- In the creation and maintenance of the sterile field, including skin preparation and draping of the patient
- In the maintenance of sterility throughout the entire surgical procedure. Breaches in sterility are remedied immediately.
- In terminal sterilization and disinfection at the conclusion of the surgical procedure

Only Sterile Items Are Used Within the Sterile Field

Items such as sterile instrument sets, drapes, sponges, and basins are obtained from the sterile core. If absolutely necessary, items such as unwrapped instruments may be steam-sterilized immediately before the surgical procedure and taken directly from the sterilizer to the sterile field. This rapid steam sterilization method is referred to as flashing and should be used only if no other alternative is available.

Every person who dispenses a sterile item to the field must be sure of its sterility and of its remaining sterile until used. Proper packaging, sterilizing, delivery to the field, and handling should provide such assurance. If there is any doubt about the sterility of any item, it should be considered not sterile and therefore should not be used. The phrase "when in doubt, throw it out" applies to this situation. Examples of questionably sterile items include, but are not limited to, the following:

- If a sterilized package is found in a contaminated area (e.g., the general unsterile workroom, the locker room).
- If uncertain about the actual timing or operation of the sterilizer. Items processed in a suspect load are considered unsterile. Other items processed in that load may need to be recalled to the processing department for reprocessing (e.g., the external process monitor has irregular color changes).
- If an unsterile person or object comes into close contact with a sterile table and vice versa.
- If a sterile table or unwrapped sterile items are not under constant observation (e.g., a sterile field under a table cover is not directly visible).
- If the integrity of the packaging material is not intact.
- If a sterile package wrapped in a material other than plastic or another moisture-resistant barrier becomes damp or wet. Humidity in the storage area or moisture on hands may seep into the package.
- If a sterile package wrapped in a pervious woven material drops to the floor or other area of questionable cleanliness. These materials allow the implosion of air into the package. A dropped package is considered contaminated on the outside. If the wrapper is impervious and the area of contact is dry and intact, the item may be transferred to the sterile field. Packages that have been dropped on the floor should not be put back into sterile storage.

Sterile Personnel Are Gowned and Gloved

Gowns are considered sterile only from the chest to the level of the sterile field in the front, and from 2 inches above the elbows to the cuffs on the sleeves (Fig. 15-1). When wearing a gown, only the area that can be seen in front down to the level of the sterile field should be considered sterile. Keep in mind that the level of the patient's surgical site actually establishes the level of the sterile field (Fig. 15-2). Usually this does not extend below waist level. The following practices are observed:

- Self-gowning and gloving should be done from a separate sterile surface to avoid dripping water onto sterile supplies or a sterile table. Closed gloving technique is preferred for the person who is establishing the sterile field and gowning and gloving others.
- The stockinette cuffs of the gown are enclosed beneath sterile gloves. The stockinette is absorbent and retains moisture, and therefore this part of the gown does not provide a microbial barrier. The cuff permits the transfer of microorganisms. Once the cuff has been contained within the closed glove, it should not be pulled back over the hand for any re-gloving procedure because it is contaminated. Re-gloving should be performed using the open-assisted gloving technique. Another sterile team member can assist with this process as necessary.
- Sterile people must keep their hands in sight at all times and at or above waist level or the level of the sterile field (Fig. 15-3).

• Hands are kept away from the face, and the elbows are kept close to the sides. The hands are never folded under the arms because of perspiration in the axillary region. The neckline, shoulders, and back also may become contaminated with perspiration. The back of the gown is not under constant observation and therefore is considered contaminated.

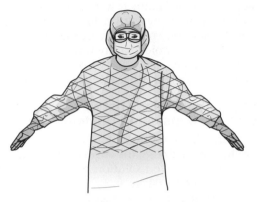

FIG. 15-1   Zones of sterility on front of gown. The zones of sterility can change based on position of draped patient and sterile team.

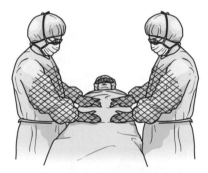

FIG. 15-2   Zones of sterility when standing at sterile field with patient as the baseline for the level of the sterile field.

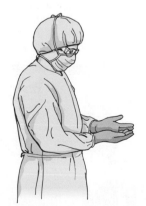

FIG. 15-3   Sterile personnel keep hands in sight at or above waist or level of sterile field. Gowns are considered sterile only in front from chest to level of sterile field, and the sleeves from above elbows to cuffs.

• Sterile people are aware of the height of team members in relation to each other and the sterile field. Changing levels at the sterile field is avoided. The gown is considered sterile only down to the highest level of the sterile working field. If a sterile person must stand on a platform to reach the surgical site, the standing platform should be positioned before this person steps up to the draped area. Sterile personnel should sit only when the entire procedure will be performed at this level. If one person on the team sits, the entire team should be seated (Fig. 15-4).

Tables Are Sterile Only at Table Level

Because tables are sterile only at table level, OR personnel must adhere to the following:

• Only the top of a sterile, draped table is considered sterile. The edges and sides of the drape extending below table level are considered contaminated. The Mayo stand, when covered by a sterile drape may be placed over the sterile field. Minimal contact is had with the underside of the Mayo drape.

• Anything falling or extending over the table or operating bed edge, such as a piece of suture or suction tip, is contaminated. The scrub person does not touch the part hanging below the level of the established sterile field.

• When unfolding or applying a sterile drape, it is unfolded away from the sterile person and the part that drops below the table surface is not brought back up to table level. Once placed, the drape is not moved or shifted.

• Cords, tubing, and other materials are secured on the sterile field with a nonperforating clip to prevent them from sliding over the edge of the operating bed.

Sterile Personnel Touch Only Sterile Items or Areas; Unsterile Personnel Touch Only Unsterile Items or Areas

• Sterile team members maintain contact with the sterile field by means of sterile gowns and gloves.

• The unsterile circulating nurse does not directly contact the sterile field.

• Supplies are brought to sterile team members and opened by the circulating nurse using aseptic technique. The circulating nurse ensures a sterile transfer to the sterile field. Only sterile items touch sterile surfaces.

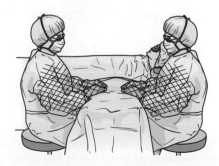

FIG. 15-4   Seated team for upper extremity procedure. The zones of sterility change based on the placement of the team in relation to the type of surgical procedure.

Unsterile Personnel Avoid Reaching over the Sterile Field; Sterile Personnel Avoid Leaning over an Unsterile Area

- The unsterile circulating nurse never reaches over a sterile field to transfer sterile items.
- The circulating nurse holds only the lip of the bottle over the basin when pouring solution into a sterile basin to avoid reaching over a sterile area (Fig. 15-5). He or she should avoid making contact with the bottle and the basin and avoid splashing solutions. The entire contents of the bottle should be dispensed in one pouring motion. If some of the solution is not poured, it is considered contaminated and may not be recapped for later use or dispensed to another sterile basin. Once the cap is off, it is considered contaminated. The solution may be saved for cleaning the patient's skin after the surgical site is undraped.
- The scrub person sets basins or medicine cups to be filled at the edge of the sterile table; the circulating nurse stands a safe distance away from the edge of the table to fill them. Medications are drawn up in a syringe, the needle removed and the drug dispensed to the cup without aerosolization. It is unsafe to dispense the drug via syringe and needle because the needle could accidentally injure a team member or cause an aerosolization of a drug that a team member might be sensitive to.
- The team uses sterile light handles for manipulation and adjustment of the surgical lights.

- The surgeon or team member steps away from the sterile field to have perspiration removed from the brow.
- The scrub person drapes an unsterile table by:
  - Unfolded drape. Placing the drape over the unsterile surface nearest self first and carefully completing the coverage of the far side. This protects the front of the gown from coming into contact with the unsterile surface being covered. Gloved hands are protected by cuffing a drape over them (Fig. 15-6).
  - Folded drape. Unfolding toward self first to protect the gown when working with a folded drape (Figs. 15-7 through 15-9). When completing the coverage, the rest of the drape is unfolded away from self.
- The scrub person stands back from the unsterile table when draping it to avoid leaning over an unsterile area.

The Edges of Anything That Encloses Sterile Contents Are Considered Unsterile

The boundaries between sterile and unsterile areas are not always rigidly defined (e.g., the edges of wrappers on sterile packages and the caps on solution bottles). The following precautions should be taken:

- When opening sterile packages, a margin of safety is always maintained. The inside of a wrapper is considered sterile to within 1 inch of the edges. The circulating nurse opens the top flap away from self, then

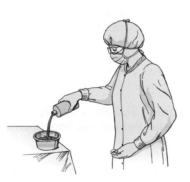

FIG. 15-5   Circulating nurse pouring sterile solution into sterile basin. Note that only lip of bottle is over the basin. Unsterile person avoids reaching over sterile field.

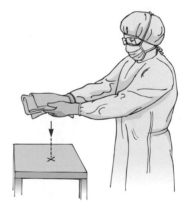

FIG. 15-7   Draping large unsterile table. Scrub person holds sterile fan-folded table drape high and drops it on the center of table, standing back from table to protect gown.

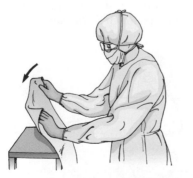

FIG. 15-6   Sterile scrub person draping a small table. Sterile personnel avoid reaching over unsterile field. The scrub person therefore drapes unsterile table first toward self, then away. Gown is protected by distance, and hands are protected by cuffing drape over them.

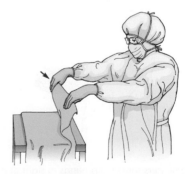

FIG. 15-8   Scrub person unfolding sterile table drape. Scrub person stands back from unsterile table and unfolds drape first toward self. Note that hands are inside sterile cover to protect them.

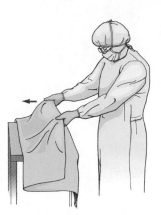

FIG. 15-9   Scrub person continuing to unfold sterile table drape. Hands are inside sterile cover for protection. Scrub person may now move closer to table because the first part of unfolded drape now protects gown.

turns the sides under. The ends of the flaps are secured in the hand so they do not dangle loosely. The last flap is pulled toward the person opening the package, thereby exposing the package contents away from the unsterile hand.

- Sterile personnel lift contents from packages by reaching down and lifting them straight up, holding their elbows high.
- The flaps on peel-open packages should be pulled back, not torn, to expose the sterile contents. The contents should not be permitted to slide over the edges. The inner edge of the heat seal is considered the line of demarcation between sterile and unsterile. The sterile item should be presented to the scrub person. Flipping can cause air turbulence, and the item may miss its mark and fall to an unsterile area. Staplers and similar devices should not be flipped, because they may be damaged by impact with the table and may misfire when used.
- If a sterile wrapper is used as a table cover, it should amply cover the entire table surface. Only the interior and surface levels of the cover are considered sterile.
- After a bottle of sterile solution is opened, the contents are either used or discarded. The cap cannot be replaced without contaminating the pouring edges.
- Steam reaches only the area within the gasket of a sterilizer. Instrument trays should not touch the edge of the sterilizer outside the gasket when being removed after flash sterilization.
- When using a rigid closed container system with an inner sterile basket, the edges of the rigid outer container are not sterile. The inner basket is carefully lifted out by the scrub person and set on the sterile field. Sterile items should never be dispensed into the rigid container, because the risk of contamination by the edges is high.

The Sterile Field Is Created as Close as Possible to the Time of Use

The degree of contamination is proportionate to the length of time that sterile items are exposed to the environment. Precautions must be taken as follows:

- Sterile tables are set up just before the surgical procedure. There is not an established time period or duration wherein the table is considered sterile or unsterile. Setting up as close to the time of use is in the best interest of the patient.
- It is virtually impossible to uncover a table of sterile contents without a potential for contamination. Covering sterile tables for later use is not recommended. The sterile field is not in direct vision and is not considered sterile.
- A covered table is not under observation at all times.
- It is not appropriate to set up a room and leave it unattended. Taping the door shut is not a guarantee of continued sterility.

Sterile Areas Are Continuously Kept in View

Inadvertent contamination of sterile areas must be readily visible. To ensure this principle, the following steps must be taken:

- Sterile personnel face sterile areas.
- Someone must remain in the room to maintain vigilance when sterile packs are opened in a room or a sterile field is set up. Sterility cannot be ensured without direct observation. An unguarded sterile field should be considered contaminated.
- Covered tables are not in view and may pose questionable sterility issues.

Sterile Personnel Keep Well Within the Sterile Area

Sterile persons allow a wide margin of safety when passing unsterile areas and observe the following rules:

- Sterile personnel stand back at a safe distance from the operating bed when draping the patient.
- Sterile personnel pass each other back to back at a 360-degree turn (Fig. 15-10).
- Sterile personnel turn their backs to an unsterile person or area when passing.
- Sterile personnel face a sterile area to pass it.
- Sterile personnel ask an unsterile individual to step aside rather than risk contamination.
- Sterile personnel stay within the sterile field. They do not walk around or go outside the room.
- Movement within and around a sterile area is kept to a minimum to avoid contamination of sterile items or personnel.

Sterile Personnel Keep Contact with Sterile Areas to a Minimum

To keep contact with the sterile areas to a minimum, sterile personnel observe the following rules:

- Sterile personnel do not lean on sterile tables or on the draped patient. Leaning on the patient can cause injury to tissues and structures.
- Sitting or leaning against an unsterile surface is a break in technique. If the sterile team sits to operate, they do so without proximity to unsterile areas.

Unsterile Personnel Avoid Sterile Areas

Unsterile personnel maintain an awareness of sterile, unsterile, clean, and contaminated areas and their proxi-

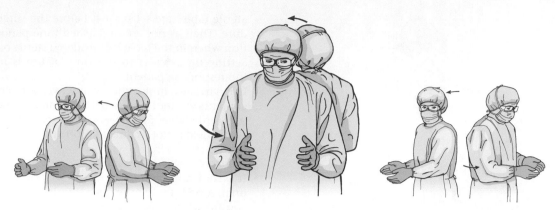

FIG. 15-10   Sequence of one sterile person going around another. They pass each other back to back, keeping well within the sterile area and allowing a margin of safety between them.

mity to each. They must be aware of their closeness to the sterile field. A wide margin of safety must be maintained when passing sterile areas by observing the following rules:

- Unsterile personnel maintain a distance of at least 1 foot (30 cm) from any area of the sterile field.
- Unsterile personnel face and observe a sterile area when passing it to be sure they do not touch it.
- Unsterile personnel never walk between two sterile areas (e.g., between sterile instrument tables).
- The circulating nurse restricts to a minimum all activity near the sterile field.

Destruction of the Integrity of Microbial Barriers Results in Contamination

The integrity of a sterile package or sterile drape is destroyed by perforation, puncture, or strike-through. Strike-through is the soaking of moisture through unsterile layers to sterile layers or vice versa. Ideal barrier materials are resistant to abrasion and impervious to permeation by the fluids or dust that transports microorganisms. The integrity of a sterile package and the appearance of the process monitor must be checked for sterility just before opening.

To ensure sterility, the following precautions should be taken:

- Sterile packages are laid only on dry surfaces.
- If a sterile package wrapped in absorbent material becomes damp or wet, it is discarded or wrapped in fresh wrappers and resterilized. The package is considered unsterile if any part of it comes into contact with moisture.
- Drapes are placed on a dry field.
- If solution soaks through a sterile drape to an unsterile area, the wet area is covered with impervious sterile drapes or towels.
- Packages wrapped in woven fabric or paper should cool after being removed from the sterilizer and before being placed on a cold surface; this prevents steam condensation and the resultant contamination.
- Sterile items are stored in clean, dry areas.
- Sterile packages are handled with clean, dry hands.
- Undue pressure on sterile packs is avoided to prevent forcing sterile air out and pulling unsterile air into the pack. Peel packs should be stored on their sides to

prevent pressure that could rupture the integrity of the package.

Microorganisms Must Be Kept to an Irreducible Minimum

Sterile technique in the surgical site is an ideal to be approached; it is not absolute. All microorganisms in the environment cannot be eliminated, but this does not obviate the necessity for strict sterile technique. There is general agreement about the following:

- Skin cannot be sterilized. Skin is a potential source of contamination in every invasive procedure. Inherent body defenses usually can overcome the relatively few organisms remaining after preparation of the patient's skin. Microorganisms on the face, neck, hair, hands, and arms of the OR team and patient are a hazard. All possible means are used to prevent the entrance of microorganisms into the wound. Preventive measures include the following:
  - Mechanical washing and chemical antisepsis is used to remove or inactivate transient and resident flora from the skin around the surgical site of the patient and from the hands and arms of sterile team members.
  - Gowning and gloving of the OR team is accomplished without contamination of the sterile exterior of gowns and gloves.
  - Sterile gloved hands do not directly touch the skin and then touch deeper tissues. Instruments used in contact with skin are discarded and not reused.
  - If a glove is torn or punctured by a needle or instrument, it is changed immediately. The puncturing needle or instrument is removed from the sterile field.
  - A sterile dressing should be applied to the surgical site before the drapes are removed to reduce the risk of the incision being touched by contaminated hands or objects.
- Some areas cannot be scrubbed. When the surgical site includes the mouth, nose, throat, or anus, the number of microorganisms present is great. Various parts of the body, such as the gastrointestinal tract and vagina, usually are resistant to infection by the flora that normally inhabit these parts. However, the following

steps may be taken to reduce the number of microorganisms in these areas and prevent them from scattering:

- The surgeon makes an effort to use a sponge only once and then discards it.
- The gastrointestinal tract (especially the colon) is contaminated, and measures are used to prevent spreading this contamination.
- Irrigation and suction may be employed to remove gross debris.
- Aseptic technique is generally used, but if the vascular system of the patient is entered, the items in use should be sterile.
- Infected areas are grossly contaminated. The team avoids disseminating the contamination.
- Air is contaminated by dust, droplets, and shedding. The following environmental control measures are used:
  - Drapes placed over the anesthesia screen or attached to IV poles at the head of the bed separate the anesthesia area from the sterile field.
  - Movement around the sterile field is kept to a minimum to avoid air turbulence.
  - To avoid the dispersion of lint and dust, drapes are not flipped, fanned, or shaken.
  - Talking is kept to a minimum in the OR. Moisture droplets are expelled with force into the mask during the process of articulating words.
  - OR attire is worn properly: the mask covers the nose and mouth, the hair is completely covered, and body covers are close fitting. Unsterile personnel should wear long-sleeved warm-up jackets with knitted cuffs. Fronts of jackets should be completely buttoned.

NO COMPROMISE OF STERILITY

There is no compromise with sterility. In clinical practice, an item is considered either sterile or unsterile. Team members should always be as certain of sterility as possible. That certainty rests on the fact that the necessary conditions have been met and that all factors in the sterilization process have been observed. Obviously it is impossible to prove that every package is free from bacteria, but a single break in technique can compromise the life of a patient.

OR personnel must maintain the high standards of sterile technique they know are essential. Every individual is accountable for his or her own role in infection control. The patient should be considered an extension of the caregiver's own body. The patient is completely trusting the team to provide safe care and protection from infection. This is a solemn obligation, with moral implications.

Bibliography

AORN (Association of periOperative Registered Nurses): *AORN standards, recommended practices, and guidelines,* Denver, 2006, The Association.

Department of Health and Human Services Centers for Disease Control and Prevention: *Guideline for isolation precautions in hospitals,* www.cdc.org

Department of Health and Human Services Centers for Disease Control and Prevention: *Guideline for prevention of SSI,* 1999, www.cdc.org

Finney J: When a needle stick occurs, *SSM* 6(3):41-43, 2000.

Pournoor J: New scientific tools to expand the understanding of aseptic practices, *SSM* 6(4):28-31, 2000.

Preston RM: Infection control nursing. Aseptic technique: Evidence-based approach for patient safety, *Brit J Nurs* 14(10):540-546, 2005.

Roark J: Maintaining the sterile field: A roundtable of expert advice, *Infect Control Today* 9(1):16-20, 2005.

Ward S: Infection prevention and the surgical conscience, *SSM* 6(3):6, 2000.

Chapter 16

Appropriate Attire, Surgical Hand Cleansing, Gowning and Gloving

CHAPTER OBJECTIVES

After studying this chapter, the learner will be able to:
- Identify the components of appropriate operating room attire worn in specific areas of the surgical suite.
- Identify the components of personal protective equipment (PPE) donned before performing surgical hand cleansing.
- Identify the sterile parameters of a surgical gown.
- Demonstrate the correct method of gowning and gloving before establishing the sterile field.
- Demonstrate the appropriate method of changing a contaminated glove during a surgical procedure.
- Demonstrate the proper method for removing a contaminated gown and gloves.

CHAPTER OUTLINE

KEY TERMS AND DEFINITIONS

Antimicrobial agent   Antiseptic soap or cleanser used for cleaning the skin of patients and caregivers that has a fast-acting, broad-spectrum action to reduce the count of microorganisms before a surgical procedure.

Attire   Appropriate operating room attire consists of body covers such as a two-piece pantsuit, head cover, mask, and shoe covers (shoe covers are used as appropriate).

Barrier   Physical or mechanical obstacle between a person and a hazardous substance or microorganism.

Gowning   Applying a sterile gown to self or other member of the sterile team.

Gloving   Applying or donning gloves using one of the following methods:

Open gloving.   A method of self-applying gloves while the hands are exposed. This is how gloves are reapplied after a contaminated glove is removed by the circulating nurse.

Closed gloving.   A method of self-applying gloves while the hands are concealed within the cuffs of a sterile gown.

Open-assisted gloving.   A method for applying sterile gloves to another person who has his or her hands exposed through the cuffs of a sterile gown.

Double-gloving.   The wearer applies two pair of sterile gloves. The inner gloves should be one half size larger than the outer glove to create a comfortable air cushion. Wearing two gloves of the same size can cause compression of the median nerve and aggravate carpal tunnel syndrome in some susceptible people.

Hand hygiene   Method of cleansing hands using an alcohol-based rub.

Indicator gloves   Specialized gloves that change color, commonly green when punctured.

Personal protective equipment (PPE)   Eyewear, mask, hair cover, shoe covers, gown, apron, and/or gloves worn to prevent airborne, droplet, or contact-based transmission of potentially hazardous substances or microorganisms between caregiver and patient.

Scrub suit   Attire intended for wear in the operating room.

Sterile attire   Consists of basic appropriate attire for the operating room with the addition of sterile gown and sterile gloves.

Subungual   Under the fingernails.

Surgical hand cleansing (surgical scrub)   Process by which the hands and arms of the team are rendered clean by mechanical and chemical action before a surgical procedure.

HISTORICAL BACKGROUND

The evolution of special operating room (OR) attire as an adjunct to asepsis paralleled the development of aseptic and sterile techniques in the latter half of the nineteenth century. Many surgeons of that time continued to perform surgical procedures while wearing street clothes under pus- and blood-encrusted aprons despite the expansion of germ theory knowledge.

One of the earliest mentions of specific OR attire appeared in a nurse's training handbook that advised the nurse to bathe before a surgical procedure, to take a carbolic bath before laparotomy, and to wear long sleeves and a clean apron for the surgical procedure. Although the apron has long since given way to the present scrub attire, long sleeves are again recommended for anesthesia providers and circulating nurses to reduce the shedding of microorganisms and to protect them from contact with body substances.

The first use of caps and sterile gowns occurred in Germany while English surgeon Joseph Lister's (1827-1912) principles of antiseptic surgery were still being debated. In some ORs, bacteria-laden, infection-causing woolen suits and Prince Albert coats were replaced by OR garb made of sterilizable material that lessened the introduction of pathogenic microorganisms into the wound. The use of sterile gowns antedated the routine use of caps, gloves, and masks, although in 1883 Gustav Neuber (1850-1932) insisted that team members wear caps also.

Emphasis on personal cleanliness expedited acceptance of special OR attire, but these standards were not rigidly practiced in all hospitals. Various styles of turbans and shower cap–style head coverings were worn from about 1908 to the 1930s, when hair was generally acknowledged to be an attraction for and shedder of bacteria.

In Fig. 16-1, a short-sleeved surgical gown is depicted from a 1917 catalog. The team sometimes wore gowns and rubber gloves but often operated without caps or masks. Charles Mayo and his team were photographed in 1913 operating in surgical gowns, caps, and masks. Early caps and masks are shown in Fig. 16-2. The onlookers, however, wore only white coats over street attire. Early photographs show the surgeon in a gown, cap, gloves, and a mask below his nose; the instrument nurse in a gown and head cover but no mask;

and the anesthetist and other nurses in gowns but regular nurses' caps. Standards of attire did not exist at that time.

In 1897 American surgeon William Halsted (1852-1922), chief of surgery at Johns Hopkins, designed a semicircular instrument table to separate himself, in sterile gown and gloves, from observers in street clothes who watched him operate (Fig. 16-3).

Rubber surgical gloves were introduced, not to protect the patient but to protect the wearer's hands from the harsh, irritating antiseptic solutions and hand soaks of the 1870s and 1880s. The use of gloves was not popularized until the 1890s, when Halsted's scrub nurse, Caroline Hampton (whom he later married), complained of dermatitis. Dr. Halsted had rubber gloves with gauntlets molded for her use. One of his assistants began to wear gloves routinely for surgical procedures in 1896, although Halsted himself is known for popularizing the use of gloves to protect patients from the bacteria of ungloved hands. In 1896 Johann von Mikulicz (1850-1905), a pioneering Romanian surgeon, advocated the wearing of cotton gloves also, but these were soon found to lack the qualities of impermeable rubber gloves for infection control. Disposable latex gloves, introduced about 1958, were a welcome innovation that saved countless hours of daily glove reprocessing, repairing, and sterilizing.

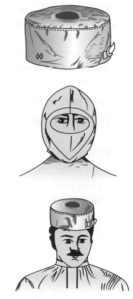

FIG. 16-2 Old-style surgeon's cap and mask. Note hole on top of the cap for heat escape.

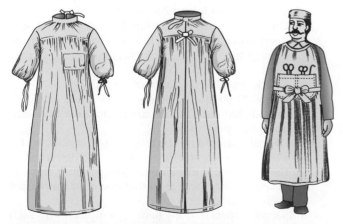

FIG. 16-1 Surgeon's gown from 1917 Powers and Anderson catalog.

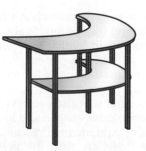

FIG. 16-3 Semicircular instrument table.

Gauze masks were advocated by Mikulicz in 1897, when the droplet theory of infection was demonstrated. However, it was not until 1926, when wound infections yielded the same organisms as found in the noses and throats of surgeons and nurses, that masks became obligatory. Although gauze masks were routinely worn, their efficiency decreased rapidly during wearing from saturation with respiratory secretions and saliva. Often the nose was not properly covered.

In 1924 one of the surgical nursing texts described the attire of the OR nurses: the circulating nurse wore an OR cap, but no mask, and a gown with a pocket for a pad and pencil; the scrub nurse wore both a mask and a gown, but had extra pockets in front for the surgeon's instruments. By the 1930s and 1940s, scrub dresses began to replace nurses' regular uniforms, heretofore worn under the sterile gown. Observers in the OR were gowned, capped, and masked. In the 1960s, full skirts were replaced by close-fitting scrub dresses and pantsuits that reduced the hazard of brushing against a sterile table when near or passing by it.

In 1950, as safety restrictions became more rigid, OR personnel were required to change shoes when entering the OR suite and to wear those shoes only when within the suite. Those shoes had conductive contacts that grounded the wearer, preventing the potential for igniting explosive anesthetics. Shoe covers became popular both as a method of keeping the shoes clean and for preventing dissemination of soil from the shoes. Personnel not wearing conductive shoes could wear conductive shoe covers with long strips of conductive material that made contact with the wearer's bare foot inside the sock. These conductive strips left black marks on the skin that were difficult to remove.

APPROPRIATE OPERATING ROOM ATTIRE

Purpose of Appropriate Attire

Sebaceous and sweat glands in and around hair follicles over the entire surface of the body contain microorganisms that are continually shed into the environment. The purpose of OR attire is to provide effective barriers that prevent the dissemination of microorganisms to patients and protect personnel from blood and body substances of patients. OR attire has been shown to reduce microbial shedding from more than 10,000 particles per minute to 3000, or from 50,000 microorganisms per cubic foot to 500 and to prevent contamination of the surgical site and sterile field by direct contact.

Definition

OR attire consists of body covers such as a two-piece pantsuit, head cover, mask, and shoe covers, as appropriate. Each has an appropriate purpose to combat sources of contamination exogenous (external) to the patient. A sterile gown and gloves are added to this basic attire for sterile team members at the sterile field. Appropriate attire is a part of aseptic environmental control that also protects personnel against exposure to communicable diseases and hazardous materials. Personal protective equipment (PPE) such as eyewear and other protective items are worn by personnel as appropriate for anticipated exposure to blood and body fluids.

Considerations for Appropriate Attire

The OR should have specific written policies and procedures for proper attire to be worn within the semi-restricted and restricted areas of the OR suite. The dress code should include aspects of personal hygiene important to environmental control. Protocol is strictly monitored so that everyone conforms to established policy, such as the following:

1. Dressing rooms located in the unrestricted area adjacent to the semirestricted area of the OR suite are reached through the outer unrestricted corridor. Street clothes are not worn beyond the unrestricted area.

2. Only approved, freshly laundered attire intended for use in the OR is worn within the semirestricted and restricted areas. This policy applies to everyone entering the OR suite, both professional and nonprofessional personnel and visitors.

   a. Clean, fresh attire is donned each time on arrival in the OR suite and as necessary at other times if the attire becomes wet or grossly soiled. Blood-stained or soiled attire, including shoe covers, is not only unattractive but can also be a source of cross-contamination. Soiled attire is not worn outside the OR suite.

   b. An adequate supply of clean scrub suits should always be available and laundered daily, preferably in the hospital's laundry facilities. It should not be taken home for laundering because standardized sanitation processes may not be followed. The risk for contamination of family members might be increased if clothing were contaminated with resistant microorganisms (e.g., prions causing Creutzfeldt-Jakob disease, or *Mycobacterium tuberculosis* causing tuberculosis [TB]).

   c. Masks should be changed between patients and whenever wet or soiled.

3. OR attire should not be worn outside the OR suite or outdoors. This protects the OR environment from microorganisms inherent in the outside environment and protects the outside from contamination normally associated with the OR. Before leaving the OR suite, everyone should change to street clothes. Surgeons who wear scrubs back and forth to the office place their patients at risk for exposure, and their appearance is unprofessional.

   a. On occasion, such as for lunch breaks, a single-use cover gown or other jacket may be worn over OR attire outside the suite. The practice of wearing cover gowns is not encouraged. After a gown is worn, it should be placed in a laundry hamper or if it is disposable it should be discarded. Some hospitals provide lab coats. These are completely buttoned and worn only once.

   b. OR attire should not be hung or put in a locker for wearing a second time. It should be discarded in the trash or put in a laundry hamper after one use, as appropriate. Shoes should be stored on the bottom shelf or under the locker.

4. Impeccable personal hygiene is emphasized. Each person should bathe daily with an antimicrobial and apply deodorant as appropriate. Body odor is the result

of microorganisms in the hair-bearing areas of the body. This becomes unpleasant when confined to an OR while wearing a gown and gloves under hot lights. This is augmented when working with pediatric or geriatric patients where the room temperature has been intentionally elevated for patient care.

a. A person with an acute infection, such as a cold or sore throat, should not be permitted within the OR suite. Personnel with cuts, burns, or skin lesions should not scrub or handle sterile supplies because serum, a bacterial medium, may seep from the eroded area. An open skin lesion may be a portal of entry for cutaneous contact with bloodborne pathogens.

b. Some sterile team members who are known carriers of pathogenic microorganisms should be treated with appropriate antibiotics until nasopharyngeal culture findings are negative.

c. Fingernails should be kept short (i.e., should not extend past the fingertips). Routine manicures prevent cracked cuticles and hangnails. Subungual areas harbor the majority of microorganisms on hands. Fresh nail polish on short, healthy nails may not alter the microbial count on fingernails. Polish may seal crevices. However, damaged nails and chipped or peeling polish may provide a harbor for microorganisms. Studies have shown that artificial nails and other enhancers harbor organisms, especially fungi and gram-negative bacilli. These are prohibited from wear in the OR.

d. Jewelry, including rings and watches, should be removed before entering semirestricted and restricted areas. Organisms may be harbored under rings, thus preventing effective handwashing. Necklaces or chains can grate on the skin, increasing desquamation. They might break and fall into a wound or contaminate a sterile field. Pierced-ear studs should be confined within the head cover. Dangling earrings are inappropriate in the OR.

e. Facial makeup should be minimal.

f. Eyewear or spectacles should be wiped with a cleaning solution before each surgical procedure and secured to the face with a head-strap to prevent slippage.

g. External apparel that does not serve a functional purpose should not be worn. Identification badges should be secured to prevent their contact with the sterile field or equipment used for patient care.

h. Hands are washed frequently and thoroughly to remove bioburden. Washing before and after using the restroom can reduce the risk of self-contamination. Using hand cream regularly helps prevent chapped, dry skin. Bacteriostatic varieties may help reduce microbial counts on the skin. Hand sanitizer can be of benefit in reducing flora.

5. Comfortable, supportive shoes should be worn to minimize fatigue and for personal safety. Shoes should have enclosed toes and heels. Clogs may not provide a safe surface for fast walking or running during an emergency, especially while pushing a crash cart. Cloth shoes do not offer protection against spilled fluids or sharp items that may be dropped or kicked. Shoes are cleaned frequently, whether or not shoe covers are worn.

Components of Appropriate Attire

Each item of OR attire is a specific means for containment of or protection against the potential sources of environmental contamination, including skin, hair, and nasopharyngeal flora and microorganisms in air, blood, and body substances. Scrub suits and head covers are worn by all personnel in the semirestricted areas of the OR suite. Masks also are worn in the restricted areas. Additional items, such as protective eyewear, gloves, and shoe covers, are worn during a surgical procedure and for protection during hazardous exposure.

Body Cover. Everyone dons attire intended for use within a semirestricted or restricted area (e.g., scrub suit). A variety of scrub suits, either two-piece pantsuits or one-piece coveralls, are available in either a solid color or an attractive print. All should fit the body snugly. Pantsuits confine organisms shed from the perineal region and legs more effectively than do dresses; 90% of bacterial dissemination originates from the perineum. Pantyhose do not contain this shedding and may in fact increase it by constant friction.

Shirt and waistline drawstrings are tucked inside pants to avoid their touching sterile areas. Microorganisms multiply more rapidly beneath a covered area. A tunic top that fits snugly may be worn on the outside of pants. The scrub suit should be changed as soon as possible whenever it becomes wet or visibly soiled.

Those who will not be sterile team members should wear long-sleeved jackets with front closures over a scrub suit. The sleeves help contain shedding from axillae and arms and help protect from biologic contamination caused by splashes. The jacket should be closed to prevent a bellows effect and the possibility of brushing against the sterile field during movement.

A one-piece coverall, head cover, mask, and shoe covers are convenient garb for a visitor whose presence in the OR will be brief (e.g., pathologist, laboratory personnel). These coveralls are usually made of white disposable tear-resistant material and resemble jumpsuits with a zipper down the front.

Some facilities provide body cooling units for the team that consist of a reusable vest that is connected to a portable cooling device. These are useful during procedures where the room is warmed for patients at risk for hypothermia.[1]

Head Cover. Because hair is a gross contaminant, a cap or hood is put on before the scrub suit to protect the garment from contamination by hair. All facial and head hair is completely covered in the semirestricted and restricted areas. Various types of lightweight caps and hoods are available. Most of them are made of disposable, lint-free, nonporous, nonwoven fabrics. If hair is long, a bouffant-style hat or

---

[1]Information about personal cooling vests for intraoperative use can be obtained from Shafer Enterprises, LLC-Cool Vest, Suite 200, 10 Andrew Drive, Stockbridge, GA 30281.

hood is worn to cover the neck area. Headgear should fit well so that it confines and prevents escape of any hair.

Some facilities permit the wearing of reusable cloth bouffant-style caps. These should be freshly laundered daily. Skullcaps do not cover the entire head, and hair can shed from the inferior edges. Hair should not be combed while one is wearing a scrub suit. Anyone with a scalp infection should be excluded from the OR and treated.

Shoe Covers. Shoe covers may be worn in the semi-restricted and restricted areas as needed to protect from blood and fluid. Knee-high impervious styles will protect the wearer from spills into or onto shoes during procedures wherein extensive fluid irrigation and/or blood loss can be anticipated. Some surgeons wear plastic or rubber boots. The legs of scrub pants are tucked into boots.

Studies have not shown a significant correlation between footwear and wound infection. However, the flow of traffic is one critical factor in airborne dispersal of microbes from the floor. Unprotected street shoes can increase floor contamination and conversely carry biologic material from the OR. Shoes restricted to wear in the OR are preferable in reducing microbial transfer from the outside into the OR suite. Protective gloves should be worn to change shoe covers whenever they become wet, soiled, or torn. Shoe covers can inadvertently become soiled and harbor microorganisms. They should be removed before entering the dressing room area and must be removed before leaving the OR suite.

Mask. A single mask is worn in the restricted area to contain and filter droplets containing microorganisms expelled from the mouth and nasopharynx during breathing, talking, sneezing, and coughing. Some tight-fitting masks also effectively reduce exposure to submicron particles by filtration of inhaled air. Many masks filter about 99% of particulate matter larger than 5 mm in diameter but only about 45% to 60% of particles 0.3 mm in diameter. Aerosolized particles and viruses dispersed in laser and electrosurgical plume or by power instruments may be this small. Masks provide some protection to the sterile team members from bloodborne pathogens that may splash or spray toward the nose or mouth. Wearing double masks forms a barrier instead of a filter and may actually cause expulsion of airborne particles to escape from the cheek folds.

Reusable cotton masks are obsolete; they filter ineffectively as soon as they become moist. Contemporary disposable masks of soft, clothlike material in very fine synthetic fiber materials fulfill the following essential criteria:

- They are at least 95% efficient in filtering microbes from droplet particles in exhalations and also filter inhalations. A fluid-resistant mask is advantageous.
- They are cool, comfortable, and nonobstructive to respiration.
- They are nonirritating to the skin. Disposable masks are made of polypropylene, polyester, or rayon fibers. Some have fiberglass filters. If a person is sensitive to one type, he or she should try another brand.
- Mask styles include rectangle shapes with four strings or cup-shaped, formed masks with an elastic band that fits around the head.

- High efficiency particulate air (HEPA) filtration masks are cup shaped and are worn when working with patients who have tuberculosis (TB). The patient should wear a mask during transport as well.
- Laser masks are high-filtration masks worn when plume from laser or electrosurgical unit is in the environment. These masks filter airborne viruses.

Some experts believe that masks should be worn to protect team members rather than to protect patients from moisture droplets. However, current practice recommendations of AORN (Association of periOperative Registered Nurses) are that masks be worn at all times in the restricted area of the OR suite—where sterile supplies will be opened and scrubbed personnel may be present—including areas where scrub sinks are located. Masks should always be worn in the OR itself, whether or not a surgical procedure is in progress. Masks are worn on entering the room before, during, and after the surgical procedure (i.e., from setup through cleanup). This includes terminal cleaning at the end of the day and restocking of supplies. The policy in some OR suites may be less restrictive. All team members, departmental staff, and visitors should follow the institution's written policy.

To be effective, a mask filters inhalations and exhalations. Therefore it is worn over both the nose and the mouth. To be effective, air must pass only through the filtering system; thus the mask needs to conform to facial contours to prevent leakage of expired air. Venting, the drawing of air back and forth, can occur along the sides, top, and bottom of the mask. The inside of the mask is covered with droplets from the mouth and nose and should not be touched with the hands.

Masks are designed with pleats or are conical, like a cup, for a close fit, but improper application can negate their efficiency. The strings should be tied tightly, if this is the method of securing the mask, to prevent the strings from coming loose during the surgical procedure. The upper strings are tied at the back of the head; the lower strings are tied behind the neck (Fig. 16-4). The strings are never crossed over the head, because this distorts the contours of the mask along the cheeks. Masks have an exterior pliable metallic strip that can be bent to contour the mask over the bridge of the nose. A close-fitting mask or a small strip of nonallergenic tape over the nosepiece also helps avoid fogging of eyewear. To prevent cross-infection, personnel should do the following:

1. Handle the mask only by the strings, thereby keeping the facial area of a fresh mask clean and the hands uncontaminated by a soiled mask. Do not handle the mask excessively.
2. Never lower the mask to hang loosely around the neck, never place the mask on top of the head, and never place the mask in a pocket. Avoid disseminating microorganisms.
3. Promptly discard the mask into the proper receptacle on removal. Remask with a fresh mask between patients.
4. Change the mask frequently. Do not permit the mask to become wet. Limit talking to a minimum.

If a sneeze is eminent, one should step back away from the field and sneeze directly into the mask without turning the head sideways. Expelled air will be forced out the sides

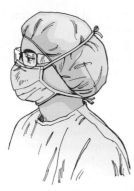

FIG. 16-4   Mask covers nose and mouth and conforms to facial contours. Upper strings are tied at back of head; lower strings are tied behind neck.

of the mask and directly into the sterile field through the vent if the head is sideways. The purpose of the mask is to filter air through the filtration material. Ideally, stepping away from the field and turning the head 180 degrees with the back of the head to the field may minimize exposure of the field. It may be necessary to remove the gown, gloves, and mask.

The hands should be washed with antimicrobial soap before and after cleaning the nose and applying a new mask. The hands should be rescrubbed before donning a sterile gown and gloves.

Personal Protective Equipment. Personnel should be protected from hazardous conditions in the semirestricted and restricted areas. Depending on the exposure that will be encountered, protective attire should be worn. The type and characteristics of this attire depend on the task and degree of exposure anticipated. Protective attire does not allow blood or other potentially injurious materials to reach the inner clothing, skin, or eyes. Other considerations concerning protective attire are as follows:

1. Aprons
   a. A decontamination apron worn over the scrub suit protects against liquids and cleaning agents during cleaning procedures. It should be a full-front barrier.
   b. Fluid-proof aprons are worn by sterile team members under permeable reusable sterile gowns when extensive blood loss or irrigation is anticipated. They should be lightweight and full front.
   c. Lead aprons worn under sterile gowns protect against radiation exposure during procedures performed under fluoroscopy or image intensification or when personnel are exposed to radioactive implants.
2. Eyewear
   a. Eyewear or a face shield is worn whenever a risk exists of blood or body substances from the patient splashing into the eyes of sterile team members. Bone chips and splatter can be projected from bone-cutting instruments. Several styles of goggles and eyeglasses with top and side shields fit securely against the face. Antifog goggles fit over prescription eyeglasses. A combination surgical mask with a visor eye shield or a chin-length face shield is another option. Care is taken that the lower edge of the face shield does not touch the front of the gown. Side shields applied to spectacles may not be adequate protection for random splashes.
   b. Laser eyewear is worn for eye protection from laser beams. Lenses of the proper optical density for each type of laser should be available and worn. An extra pair should be placed on the outer door for personnel who may need to enter the room during the procedure.
   c. Protective eyewear, preferably a face shield, should be worn by personnel handling or washing instruments when this activity could result in a splash, spray, or splatter to the eyes or face. Eyewear should be worn when cleaning the room to avoid splashing chemical germicides into eyes during mopping or cleaning.
   d. Eyewear or a face shield that becomes contaminated should be decontaminated or discarded promptly.
3. Gloves
   a. Nonsterile latex or vinyl gloves are worn to handle any material or items contaminated by blood and body substances. Gloves should be worn only during the period of contact, not continuously. Gloves are never washed between patient contacts; they are discarded. Clean objects and sterile packages should not be handled with contaminated gloves. Avoid opening cupboard doors while wearing soiled gloves.
   b. Sterile gloves are worn by sterile team members and for all invasive procedures. Sterile glove liners may be worn over or under gloves to protect the hands from cuts caused by heavy instrumentation. Liners can be worn between two layers of gloves and should be one half size larger to prevent constriction.
   c. Lead and radiation protective gloves may be needed for protection from scatter during ionizing radiation exposure for diagnostic and therapeutic procedures that use real-time imaging. The surgeon may wear natural rubber gloves impregnated with lead for procedures performed under fluoroscopy. The lead is not in direct contact with skin. Lead gloves are available in powdered and nonpowdered styles.

   When evaluating radiation protective gloves, be sure to note whether they are protective when used in direct radiation beams or if they are intended for use as protection from scatter. Not all radiation protective gloves are intended for use in direct beams. Radiation protective gloves without lead are commercially available.[2]

---

[2]www.hospitalmanagement.net describes specialty gloves and their composition. Additional information is available at www.medline.com/Products/Gloves/surgeonsgloves.htm in .pdf (Adobe Acrobat) format. Acrobat Reader can be downloaded free from www.nvo.com/delphipro.

d. Utility gloves are worn for cleaning and house-keeping duties. Sterile and nonsterile single-use disposable latex and vinyl gloves are discarded after use. They should not be washed and reused. Soaps and surfactants decrease the surface tension of the gloves and increase the risk of wicking through microscopic holes in the gloves. Hands are washed after gloves are removed.

Surgical Gown. A sterile gown is worn over the scrub suit to permit the wearer to enter the sterile field. It prevents intercontamination between the wearer and the field and differentiates sterile (scrubbed) from nonsterile (unscrubbed) team members. The gown should provide a protective barrier from strike-through (i.e., migration of microorganisms from the skin and scrub suit of the wearer to the sterile field and the patient, and penetration of blood and body substances from the patient to the scrub suit and skin of the wearer).

Both reusable and disposable gowns, in a variety of styles, are in use. Although the entire gown is sterilized, the back is not considered sterile nor is any area below the level of the sterile field, once the gown is donned. Wraparound sterile gowns that provide coverage to the back by a generous overlap are recommended. These gowns are secured at the neck and waist before the sterile flap is brought over the back and secured by ties at the side or front. A sterile vest put on over the gown covers any exposed back area of scrub attire but does not render the back sterile.

The cuffs of gowns are knitted stockinette to snugly fit wrists. The cuffs are not fluid impervious and cause wicking from the wearer's body sweat. Sterile gloves cover the cuffs of the gown to prevent moisture from the wearer from contaminating the sterile field. Changing a contaminated glove by pulling the cuff back down over the hand and employing the closed gloving method renders the gloves contaminated because the sterile surface is now exposed to the wearer's body moisture.

Gowns should be resistant to penetration by fluids and blood and should be comfortable without producing excessive heat buildup. Most single-use disposable gowns are made of spun-laced fiber or nonwoven, moisture-repellent materials. Some of these are reinforced with plastic on the forearms and front. Reusable gowns should be made of a densely woven, moisture-repellent material. Some reusable gowns are a cotton-polyester blend. Tightly woven 100% polyester gowns are impervious to moisture. Seams of the gowns should be constructed to prevent penetration of fluids. Loosely woven, 140-thread-count, all-carded cotton muslin or similar-quality permeable material is not a barrier to microbial migration.

Sterile team members may not need a reinforced barrier gown for every procedure; the scrub person usually can safely wear a single-layer impervious gown. The surgeon and first assistant are at greatest risks during procedures when blood loss will be more than 20 mL or when the time will exceed 2 hours. The amount of blood and fluid on the outside of the gown is a critical factor in strike-through by wicking. Bloodborne pathogens can penetrate fabric without visible strike-through. The forearms are the most frequently contaminated areas. Therefore, the surgeon and first assistant should wear a gown with at least reinforced or plastic-coated sleeves for these procedures.

Woven textile gowns withstand about 75 launderings and sterilizing cycles before appreciable deterioration of the finish occurs. Monitoring the number of uses is necessary to remove the gown from use at the sterile field when it is no longer an effective barrier. Also, an additional rinse cycle may be required in the laundering process to remove residual detergent that could adversely affect the fabric. Mechanical damage from sharp instruments or snags will destroy the integrity of the gown, jeopardizing its purpose. The gown should be changed if it is punctured or torn during the surgical procedure. Textile gowns can be patched only with heat-applied vulcanized mending fabrics.

All woven and some nonwoven gowns are not flame-retardant. Fire-resistant gowns should be worn for laser surgery and preferably when electrosurgery is used.

Special attire often is worn with ultraclean laminar airflow systems. A body exhaust gown envelops the wearer from the top of the head to within about 16 inches (40 cm) of the floor. If a gown that fits closely at the neck is used, a rigid facemask or helmet is worn. With both types of gowns, an exhaust system is attached for body cooling and airflow. Powered coolant vests for wear under scrub attire are commercially available.

Surgical Gloves. Sterile gloves complete the attire for sterile team members. They are worn to permit the wearer to handle sterile supplies and tissues of the surgical site. Surgical gloves are made of natural rubber latex, synthetic rubber, thermoplastic elastomers, neoprene, vinyl, or polyethylene. Disposable latex gloves are worn most frequently. Latex is a polymeric membrane of natural rubber with an infinite number of holes between lattices. However, it is a better barrier than vinyl, which may allow permeation of blood and fluids over prolonged exposure. Selection of surgical gloves worn during specific procedures depends on the following:

- Length of the surgical procedure
- Type of surgical procedure
- The need to double-glove
- Stresses to which the glove is exposed
- Chemical exposure to the gloves during the surgical procedure
- Caregiver and patient sensitivity
- Individual preference

Latex gloves of varying thickness, with a minimum of 0.1 mm, can be chosen to meet the needs of the surgeon for tactile sensation. Latex contains protein antigen and is cured with agents that may cause an allergic dermatitis or systemic anaphylaxis. Hypoallergenic milled gloves that do not contain these sensitizers are available. Latex gloves labeled "hypoallergenic" do not always prevent reaction in a highly sensitive person. Several varieties of synthetic nonlatex sterile gloves (e.g., those made of neoprene) are available commercially. Sterile team members should not wear latex gloves if the patient has a known latex sensitivity or allergy.

Gloves are packaged in pairs with an everted cuff on each to protect the sterile outer surface of the glove during donning. The inner sterile paper wrap of the disposable glove package protects the sterility of the gloves when they are removed from the peel-pack outer wrap. Before opening, the package should be inspected for damage or wetness, which indicates contamination. When the inner paper is unfolded, the wearer finds the right glove to the right and the left glove to the left, both with palm sides up (Fig.16-5).

Both inner and outer glove surfaces may be prelubricated with an absorbable dry cornstarch powder before the sterilization process to facilitate donning and to prevent adhesion of the glove surfaces. During donning, this powder is aerosolized into the room air and affects people other than the wearer, including the patient. Although considered absorbable and inert in tissue, the powder may cause serious complications, such as starch granulomas, adhesions, or peritonitis if it is introduced into wounds. Consequently, it is important to remove the powder from the outside of the gloves after donning them. They may be thoroughly wiped with a sterile, damp towel or rinsed with sterile saline. Immersion in a splash basin should be avoided because the powder clumps and accumulates on the surface of the water and redeposits on the surface of the glove. Latex protein allergens can adhere to powder, thus providing another potential route of exposure or sensitization if the powder is aerosolized during a rinsing process. Latex coated on the inside with a hydrogel lubricant allows smooth donning of gloves without the hazard of glove powder.

Surgeons frequently puncture their gloves, most often on the index finger of the nondominant hand. Glove puncture and minute holes in gloves are hazardous to both patients and team members. Seepage under the glove poses a threat to a team member if his or her skin is not intact. The risk of blood contamination of the fingers increases the longer the glove is worn. If a sterile glove is punctured or torn, it should be changed immediately to prevent escape of microorganisms from the wearer's skin and seepage of blood and body substances from the patient into the glove.

The scrub person should not be intimidated by politely informing the surgeon or any sterile team member of having a potentially contaminated glove. This is an important part of surgical conscience. The circulating nurse will obtain new gloves and dispense them to the sterile field. The circulator should don nonsterile gloves to remove contaminated gloves from a sterile team member.

Microbial colonization may be minimized if latex gloves are impregnated with an antiseptic, and gloves with colored puncture indicators are commercially available. High-molecular-weight polyethylene orthopedic gloves resist punctures and tears.

Some sterile team members prefer to double-glove (wear two pairs of sterile gloves). Double-gloving is recommended for long procedures.[3] The gloves do not need to be of the same variety or composition, but they both need to be sterile. The inner pair of sterile gloves should be applied using the closed gloving method and should be a half size larger than the outside glove to create a cushion of air. The outer sterile glove should be the wearer's normal size and can be applied using any sterile method. Wearing two pairs of gloves in the same size can cause compression on the median nerve, resulting in carpal tunnel syndrome in susceptible people.

Some sterile team members wear sterile glove liners for protection from scalpel cuts or instrument tears. These do not protect the hands from needlesticks. Liners are usually worn between two pairs of sterile surgical gloves, usually a half size larger than usual so that they will not cause constriction. The liners may be made of polymer fibers or a Kevlar metal mesh. Some are disposable; others may be reprocessed and sterilized with steam or ethylene oxide.

Petrolatum-based lotions or lubricants should not be used on the hands before donning latex gloves. Hydrocarbons will penetrate latex, causing a change in its physical characteristics, including tear resistance. Gloves with aloe vera inner coating are commercially available from Medline.

Criteria for Surgical Attire

Surgical attire should be as follows:

- An effective barrier to microorganisms. Both reusable woven and disposable nonwoven materials are used. The design and composition should minimize microbial shedding.
- Made of closely woven material void of dangerous electrostatic properties. The garment should meet National Fire Protection Association standards (NFPA-56A), including resistance to flame.
- Resistant to blood, fluids, and abrasion to prevent penetration by microorganisms.
- Designed for maximal skin coverage.
- Hypoallergenic, cool, and comfortable.
- Nongenerative of lint. Lint can increase the particle count of contaminants in the OR.
- Made of a pliable material to permit freedom of movement for the practice of sterile technique.
- Able to transmit heat and water vapor to protect the wearer.
- Colored to reduce glare under lights. Various types of clothes in colorful prints that fulfill the necessary criteria are both attractive and functional.
- Easy to don and remove.

SURGICAL HAND AND SKIN CLEANSING

Surgical hand cleansing (also called the surgical scrub) is the process of removing as many microorganisms as possible from the skin of the hands and arms by mechanical washing and chemical antisepsis before participating in a surgical procedure. The surgical hand and arm cleansing is done

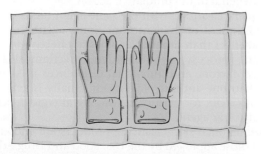

FIG. 16-5 Gloves on unfolded open wrapper: right glove to right, and left glove to left, palm sides up.

[3]Tanner P: Double gloving to reduce surgical cross-infection, *Cochrane Review* 4, 2005.

just before gowning and gloving for each surgical procedure. Despite the antimicrobial component of the hand- and arm-cleansing process, skin is never rendered sterile. Consider that the tap water used in the rinse is from the public water system. This water is not sterile and can in itself grow microbial cultures. The process of scrubbing is not a sterile procedure.

Microbiology of the Skin

The skin is inhabited by the following organisms:

- Transient organisms acquired by direct contact. Usually loosely attached to the skin surface, they are almost completely *mechanically* removed by thorough washing with soap and water.
- Resident organisms below the skin surface in hair follicles and in sebaceous and sweat glands. They are more adherent and therefore more resistant to removal. Their growth is inhibited by the *chemical* phase of the surgical hand-cleansing process. Resident skin flora represent the microorganisms present in the hospital environment. They are predominantly gram-negative microorganisms, but some are coagulase-positive staphylococci. Prolonged exposure of skin to contaminants yields a more pathogenic resident population (i.e., capable of causing infection).

In scrubbing, the skin is cleansed of as many microorganisms as possible. Two properties are employed for surgical hand or skin cleansing:

1. Mechanical. The mechanical properties remove soil and transient organisms with friction.
2. Chemical. The chemical properties reduce resident flora and inactivate microorganisms with an antimicrobial or antiseptic agent.

In a brushless/waterless surgical skin-cleansing method, the antimicrobial chemical properties of the hand gel kill microorganisms. Many gel-type surgical skin cleansers have a lasting antimicrobial effect for several hours after application. Users of this product should wash hands with soap and water to remove gross soil followed by thorough drying with a paper towel before applying the surgical hand cleansing gel. The gel is alcohol based and should be completely dry before donning the sterile gown and gloves.

Purpose

The purpose of surgical hand and arm cleansing is to remove or deactivate soil, debris, natural skin oils, hand lotions, and transient microorganisms from the hands and forearms of sterile team members. More specifically, the purposes are as follows:

- To decrease the number of resident microorganisms on skin to an irreducible minimum
- To keep the population of microorganisms minimal during the surgical procedure by suppression of growth
- To reduce the hazard of microbial contamination of the surgical wound by skin flora

Scrub Sink

Adequate scrubbing and handwashing facilities should be provided for all operating team members. The scrub room is adjacent to the OR for safety and convenience. Scrub sinks with automatic sensor controls or foot- or knee-operated faucets are preferred to eliminate the hazard of contaminating the hands after hand- and arm washing. Protective eyewear should be worn when performing a surgical scrub. Aerosolization from the scrub brush can cause chemicals to be dispersed into the user's eyes.

The sink should be deep, wide, and low enough to prevent splashes. Aerated faucets prevent splatter. A sterile gown cannot be donned over damp scrub attire without resultant contamination.

Scrub sinks should be used only for scrubbing or handwashing. They should not be used to clean or rinse contaminated instruments or equipment. Bioburden could inadvertently be transferred to personnel who scrub in the vicinity.

Equipment

Debris should be removed from the subungual area of each finger. Plastic, single-use, disposable nail-cleaning products are available and are usually supplied with disposable scrub brushes. Reusable nail cleaners are not recommended. Orangewood sticks are not used to clean under the fingernails because the wood may splinter and harbor *Pseudomonas* organisms.

Sterilized reusable scrub brushes or disposable sponges may be used. Biologic material may be difficult to remove from reusable brushes. If reusable brushes are taken from the dispenser in which they were sterilized, each brush should be removed without contaminating the others.

Single-use disposable products may be a brush-sponge combination. Some are impregnated with antiseptic-detergent agents. Disposable products are individually packaged. The brush should not cause skin abrasion. The scrubbing solution is dispensed onto the brush or sponge by a foot pedal from a container attached or adjacent to the sink. Six drops (about 2 to 3 mL) of solution is sufficient to generate a lather for the scrub procedure. Waste of antiseptic solution should be avoided.

Antimicrobial Skin-Cleansing Agents

Various antimicrobial soaps are used for surgical hand cleansing. The following are desirable characteristics of antimicrobial agents:

- Broad spectrum
- Fast acting and effective
- Nonirritating and nonsensitizing
- Prolonged action (i.e., leaves an antimicrobial residue on the skin to temporarily prevent growth of microorganisms)
- Independent of cumulative action

Frequent cleansing with the same agent tends to inhibit reestablishment of resident flora. Some agents have more residual effect than others. Variables in effectiveness of the cleansing process are bioburden, mechanical factors, chemical factors, and individual differences in skin flora. More than one antimicrobial agent usually is available in the scrub room for personnel who are allergic or sensitive to a particular agent.

Antimicrobial skin-cleansing products are chosen from among those approved by the U.S. Food and Drug Administration (FDA) for surgical hand scrubs. Each product has a specific antimicrobial agent. Antiseptics alter the physical or chemical properties of the cell membrane of microorganisms, thus destroying or inhibiting cellular function.

When an individual scrubs with a brush and antimicrobial agent, the soap decreases the surface tension of the skin, thus permitting the shed cells to be rinsed away with the tap water. The mechanical property physically removes debris and the antimicrobial agent chemically acts on the microorganisms to inhibit or kill them.

Brushless/waterless hand cleansers do not use mechanical action or friction. There is no water rinse to physically remove microorganisms; the main action is chemical. That is why a simple hand washing and drying is recommended to remove gross soil before using a surgical hand cleansing gel.

The Centers for Disease Control and Prevention (CDC) indicates that most of the studies performed to date have focused on measuring hand bacterial counts and not on the impact of any scrub agent choice on surgical-site infection.[4]

Chlorhexidine Gluconate.
A 4% aqueous concentration of chlorhexidine gluconate (CHG) in a soap base or 0.5% in alcohol exerts an antimicrobial effect against gram-positive and gram-negative, fungal, and viral microorganisms. It reacts poorly against TB microorganisms. Antimicrobial residues tend to accumulate on the skin with repeated use and produce a prolonged effect. This agent produces effective, intermediate action and cumulative reductions of resident and transient flora. The residual effect is maintained for more than 6 hours. CHG is rarely irritating to the skin, but it is highly ototoxic and is irritating if splashed in the eye. It can cause permanent corneal damage. Caution should be observed when scrubbing with this agent. It is used in several of the brushless/waterless hand cleansers.

The alcohol-based chlorhexidine preparation is effective if the hands are coated in the solution for 20 to 30 seconds after mechanical cleansing. Brushless/waterless surgical hand cleansers contain this product. The alcohol evaporates rapidly and has minimal odor. Personnel with reactive airway conditions should be aware of minor volatile qualities when using this product. Allow the product to dry thoroughly before donning gowns and gloves.

Iodophors.
A povidone-iodine complex in detergent fulfills the criteria for an effective surgical scrub. It is available in concentrations of 10%, 7.5%, 2%, and 0.5%. Iodophors are intermediate-acting antimicrobial agents against gram-positive and gram-negative, TB, fungal, and viral microorganisms. Iodophors have minimal residual effect, but this is not sustained for a prolonged period (over 6 hours). Iodophors can be irritating to the skin. Anyone allergic to iodine should not scrub with these agents.

Triclosan.
A solution of 1% triclosan is a nontoxic, nonirritating, intermediate antimicrobial agent that inhibits growth of a wide range of gram-positive and gram-negative and TB microorganisms. Triclosan does not work as well against fungi. Antiviral action is unknown. It develops a prolonged cumulative suppressive action when used routinely. The agent is blended with lanolin cholesterols and petrolatum into a creamy, mild detergent. It

may be used by personnel sensitive to other antiseptics, although it can be absorbed through intact skin. Triclosan is less effective than are chlorhexidine gluconate and iodophors.

Alcohol.
Ethyl or isopropyl alcohol (60% to 90%) is rapidly antimicrobial against all microorganisms. It is volatile and does not have residual activity. It is nontoxic but has a drying effect on skin. Alcohol preparations, usually in a foam, contain emollients to minimize drying. If other agents cannot be used because of skin sensitivity, mechanical cleansing with soap to remove transient organisms may be followed by cleansing with an alcohol-based skin cleanser.

Hexachlorophene.
In concentrations up to 3%, hexachlorophene is most effective after buildup of cumulative suppressive action. The action is slow but effective against most gram-positive bacteria; it has poor action against all other microorganisms. Its high potential for neurotoxicity makes it unsuitable for routine use. Hexachlorophene is available by prescription only.

Parachlorometaxylenol.
Used in a concentration of 1% to 3.75%, parachlorometaxylenol does not substantially reduce microorganisms immediately. It does not produce sustained residual activity. Its antimicrobial activity can be altered significantly by the composition of the antiseptic product. Efficacy data should be reviewed before these products are used for surgical scrubs.

Preparation for Surgical Hand Cleansing
General Preparations
1. The skin and nails should be kept clean and in good condition, and the cuticles should be uncut. If hand lotion is used to protect the skin, a non–oil-based product is recommended. Oil can weaken the integrity of gloves.
2. Fingernails should not reach beyond the fingertips to avoid glove puncture.
3. Fingernail polish should not be chipped or cracked. Freshly applied polish may be worn if permitted by facility policy.
4. Artificial nails harbor microorganisms such as bacteria and fungi and are inappropriate for scrub personnel.
5. All jewelry is removed from the fingers, wrists, and neck. Jewelry harbors microorganisms.

Opening the Gown and Gloves
The double-wrapped gown package contains one sterile folded gown and towel. The outer wrap is a peel-pouch and the inner wrap is envelope style. The gown is folded inside out to facilitate donning. The folded gown resembles a thick book with the main fold as its binding. A folded woven fabric or disposable paper towel for drying the hands is packed on top of the gown. The towel is folded into a square or rectangle with one corner turned down for ease of grasping without disturbing the entire gown-towel assembly.

The gown package is opened before the glove package. It is opened on a separate surface from the main sterile field. The gown inner wrapper is removed from the peel pouch and is opened to create a temporary sterile field of its own.

The gloves will be double-wrapped in a peel pouch and folded paper. The peel pouch is opened and the paper-wrapped gloves can be dispensed to the side of the gown on the inner aspect of the sterile gown wrapper. Ideally, if another surface is available, the glove wrapper can be opened in its entirety to fashion a temporary sterile area for the purpose of donning the gloves.

Preparations Immediately Before Surgical Hand Cleansing

1. Be sure all hair is covered by headwear. Pierced-ear studs should be contained by the head cover. They are a potential foreign body in the surgical site.
2. Adjust the disposable mask snugly and comfortably over the nose and mouth.
3. Clean spectacles if worn. Adjust and secure protective eyewear or the face shield comfortably in relation to the mask and spectacles.
4. Adjust water to a comfortable temperature.

Surgical Hand and Arm Scrub with a Brush

A vigorous 2- to 5-minute scrub with a reliable agent is effective. A counted brushstroke method is equally effective in decreasing the microbial count on the skin. Prolonged scrubbing raises resident microbes from deep dermal layers and is therefore counterproductive. Care should be taken not to abrade the skin during the scrub process. Denuded areas allow the entry of microorganisms. Too short a scrub may be equally ineffectual.

Every member of the surgical team should scrub according to a standardized written procedure. The time required may be based on the manufacturer's recommendations for the agent used and documentation of the product's efficacy in the scientific literature. A copy of the procedure should be posted in every scrub room.

Subsequent scrubs should follow the same procedure as the initial scrub of the day. When gloves are removed at the end of the surgical procedure, the hands are considered contaminated and should be immediately washed with soap and water. Resident microorganisms multiply rapidly in the warm, moist environment under the gloves. Hands should be washed as soon as the gloves are removed, but they will become contaminated as soon as contact is made with any inanimate items.

Personnel who scrub should think of their fingers, hands, and arms as having four sides or surfaces. Both methods follow an anatomic pattern of scrubbing: the four surfaces of each finger, beginning with the thumb and moving from one finger to the next, down the outer edge of the fifth finger, over the dorsal (back) surface of the hand, then the palmar (palm) surface of the hand, or vice versa, from the small finger to the thumb, over the wrists and up the arm, in thirds, ending 2 inches (5 cm) above the elbow. Because the hands are in most direct contact with the sterile field, all steps of the scrub procedure begin with cleaning the fingernails and hands and end with the elbows.

During and after scrubbing, keep the hands higher than the elbows to allow water and suds to flow from the cleanest area—the hands—to the marginal area of the upper arms.

Take care not to slip in water that may have dripped to the floor during the process. A waterproof mat is suggested in front of the sink. Protective eyewear should be worn to protect from antiseptic solution splashes.

Brushless/Waterless Surgical Hand Cleansing

AORN recommends that personnel who use a brushless/waterless surgical hand and arm cleansing should wash hands before applying the antiseptic solution. The antiseptic does not remove debris from under the nails and hands.

Most brushless cleansing agents have an alcohol base with an antimicrobial ingredient such as CHG or triclosan. Care is taken to allow the agent to completely dry before donning the sterile gown and gloves. All products of this nature should be used as directed by the manufacturer. Each product has a specific application process and drying protocol.

GOWNING AND GLOVING

The sterile gown is put on after drying the hands and arms with a sterile towel, immediately after the surgical hand and arm cleansing. If using the gel antiseptic surgical hand cleanser, the arms and hands must air dry before donning the sterile gown. The sterile gloves are put on immediately after gowning.

Purpose

A sterile gown and gloves are worn to exclude skin as a possible contaminant and to create a barrier between the sterile and nonsterile areas.

General Considerations

1. The scrub person gowns and gloves from a surface separate from the main sterile field using the closed gloving method and then gowns and gloves the surgeon and the rest of the sterile team using the open assisted gloving method.
2. Gown packages preferably are opened on a separate table from other packages to avoid any chance of contamination from dripping water.
3. Splashing water on scrub attire during the surgical scrub should be avoided because moisture may contaminate the sterile gown.

Drying the Hands and Arms

The hands and arms are dried as follows:

1. Reach down to the opened sterile gown package and pick up the towel with one hand by one corner. Be careful not to drip water onto the pack. Contamination can occur.[4] Be sure no one is within arm's reach (Fig. 16-6). Be aware of the environment to prevent contamination.
2. Grasp the opposing corner of the towel with the other hand and open the towel full-length. Use one end

---

[4]Heal JS et al: Bacterial contamination of surgical gloves by water droplets spilt [sic] after scrubbing, *J Hosp Infect* 53(2):136-139, 2003. This article describes that droplets contained *Micrococcus*, a coliform and coagulase-negative staphylococcus. The paper wrapper of the gloves was found to be permeable to gram-negative bacteria.

of the towel to dry one hand and arm. Use a circumferential motion to rub in one direction from hand to upper arm. Don't rub back and forth (Fig. 16-7). Bend slightly forward to avoid letting the towel touch the attire.

3. To dry the second arm, hold the dry end of the towel in the opposite hand and use a circumferential motion to dry the hand and all areas of the arm to the elbow.

4. Discard the towel with the hand that is currently holding it without letting it touch the scrub suit. Do not wad it and toss it across the room to the laundry hamper or trash.

Gowning and Gloving Techniques

The scrub person will don the gown before the gloves. The scrub person may don gloves in one of two ways: by the *closed gloving* technique or by the *open gloving* technique. The closed gloving method is preferred for establishing the initial sterile field by the scrub person. Properly executed, the closed gloving method affords assurance against contamination when donning gloves, because no bare skin is exposed in the process because the bare hands do not extend through the cuffs of the gown.

The open gloving method is used when changing a glove during a surgical procedure or when donning gloves for procedures not requiring gowns. Assisted open gloving technique is used by the scrub person to help other sterile team members don gowns and gloves before entering the sterile field.

Gowning

1. Reach down to the sterile pack and lift the folded gown directly upward (Fig. 16-8). This is like picking up a book by its binding. Take care not to touch the sterile gown wrapper because the gloves will be opened up completely on this surface after the gown is on.

2. Step back away from the table into an unobstructed area to provide a wide margin of safety while gowning.

3. Holding the folded gown like a book by its binding, carefully locate the neckline and the armholes.

4. Holding the inside front of the gown just at the armholes with both hands, let the gown unfold, keeping the inside of the gown toward the body and the hands in the armholes. Do not touch the outside of the gown with bare hands. If the top of the gown drops downward inadvertently, discard the gown as contaminated. Never reverse a sterile gown if the wrong end is dropped toward the floor.

5. Extend both arms into the armholes simultaneously as the gown and its sleeves unfold (Fig. 16-9).

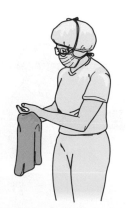

FIG. 16-6   Scrub person preparing to gown removes hand towel on top of gown from opened package.

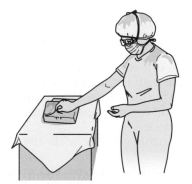

FIG. 16-7   Scrub person, holding towel away from body, dries only scrubbed areas, starting with hands. He or she avoids contaminating hands on areas proximal to elbows, and then discards towel.

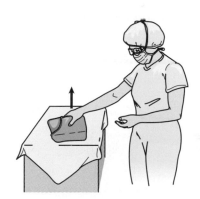

FIG. 16-8   Scrub person, picking up gown below neck edge, lifts it directly upward and steps away to avoid touching edge of wrapper. Note that sterile inside of wrapper covers table. Gown is folded inside out.

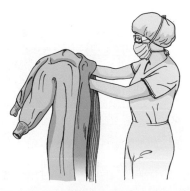

FIG. 16-9   Scrub person, putting on gown, gently allows the gown to unfold away from body and then slips arms into sleeves without touching sterile outside of gown with bare hands.

6. The circulating nurse, standing behind the scrub, brings the gown over the shoulders by reaching inside to the shoulder and arm seams. The gown is pulled on, leaving the cuffs of the sleeves extended over the hands. Do not push the hands through the cuffs. The back of the gown is securely tied at the waist first, followed by the neckline. The circulating nurse takes care not to pull the gown so snug that the cuffs are pulled back exposing the hands (Figs. 16-10 and 16-11).

If the gown is wraparound style, the sterile flap to cover the back is not touched until the scrub person has donned the gloves. A sterile gown may be wrapped around for a "tie in" in various ways:

1. Reusable gown. The wraparound ties are secured to the front of the gown by a single hitch knot. With sterile gloved hands, pull the knot open. Take the longer right tie in the right hand and the shorter left tie in the left hand. Hold on to the left tie. Hand the long right tie to a sterile team member who remains stationary.

    Allowing a margin of safety, turn around toward the left, thereby completely covering the back with the extended flap of the gown. Take the long right tie from the sterile person and tie it to the short left tie on the left side of the gown. Do not place the long right tie under an object on the sterile field to tie yourself

in. This causes the back to be turned to the field. It is best to have a sterile person tie you in.

2. Disposable gown. The ends of the ties are covered by a disposable paper tag. Disengage the left short tie from the tag with the left hand. Hold on to the left tie. The tag will remain attached to the long right tie. Hand the tag with the right tie still attached to the circulating nurse, taking care to protect the hands and not disconnect the tag. Turn toward the left, closing the gown flap in the back. Grasp the long right tie about 4 to 6 inches from the tag that the circulating nurse is holding, and pull the tie out of the paper tag. The circulating nurse discards the tag. Tie the long right tie to the short left tie at the side of the gown.

3. If either of the ties drops at any time, the circulating nurse retrieves both ties and secures them behind the scrubbed person's back because the dropped tie is contaminated.

Closed Gloving Technique

Gloving by the Closed Gloving Technique

During the closed gloving process the scrub person keeps the hands inside the cuffs of the sterile gown. At first this seems tricky, but with practice the technique will become more refined and quick. Remember to keep the hands inside the cuffs at all times.

1. If the gloves are still in the folded inner paper wrapper, they need to be opened. Using the cuff-covered hands, place the wrapper in front of you like a book. Open the two sides. There is an inner fold to the glove wrapper. With the two cuff-covered hands grasp the lower inner corners of the bottom fold. Lift both corners open and fold under at the same time. When this method is used the wrapper will remain open and not fall closed during the gloving process.

2. Extend the right forearm with the palm upward (supinated).

3. With the cuff-covered left hand, pick up the right glove from the inner wrap of the glove package by grasping the fingers, lifting straight up, and placing on the right palm thumb side down. The glove fingers will be pointing toward the body (Fig. 16-12).

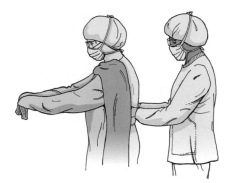

FIG. 16-10 Circulating nurse, pulling gown on for closed gloving technique, reaches inside gown to sleeve seams and pulls gown on, leaving cuffs of sleeves extended over hands.

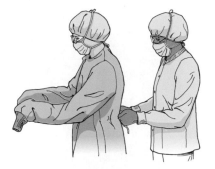

FIG. 16-11 Circulating nurse completes pulling on scrub person's gown, secures ties on inside of back at waist first, and then closes fastener at neck, taking care not to cause the scrub person's hand to protrude through the knitted cuffs.

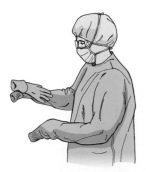

FIG. 16-12 For closed gloving technique, using left hand and keeping it within cuff of sleeve, gowned scrub person picks up right glove. Palm of glove is placed against palm of right hand, grasping top edge of glove cuff above palm.

4. Grasp the edges of the glove cuff with the cuffed left hand and the opposite edge with the cuffed right hand. Peel the glove over the right cuffed hand, over the end of the right sleeve and wiggle the fingers to extend them into the glove covered hand. The cuff of the glove is now over the stockinette cuff of the gown, with the hand still inside the sleeve (Figs. 16-13 and 16-14).

5. Grasp the cuff of the right glove and underlying gown sleeve with the covered left hand (Fig. 16-15). Pull the glove on over the extended right fingers until it completely covers the stockinette cuff.

6. Glove the left hand in the same manner, reversing hands. Use the gloved right hand to pull on the left glove (Figs. 16-16, 16-17, and 16-18). Be sure that the entire cuff of each sleeve is contained within the sterile glove.

Open Gloving Technique

Gowning for the Open Gloving Technique. Gowning for the open gloving method is the same as for the closed gloving method. The only difference is that the scrubbed person extends the hands all the way through the cuffs and sleeves. The hands are totally exposed outside the cuffs (Fig. 16-19). This method is not preferred for the person establishing the sterile field.

Gloving by the Open Gloving Technique. The open gloving method uses a skin-to-skin, glove-to-glove technique. The hand, although scrubbed, is not sterile and must

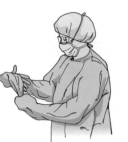

FIG. 16-13 Back of cuff is grasped in left hand and turned over right sleeve and hand.

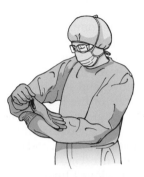

FIG. 16-16 Using gloved right hand, left glove is picked up and placed with palm of glove against palm of left hand. Back of cuff is grasped above palm in right hand and turned over left sleeve and hand.

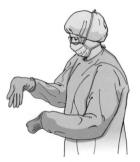

FIG. 16-14 Cuff of glove is now over stockinette cuff of sleeve, with hand still inside sleeve.

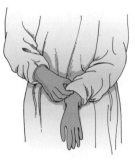

FIG. 16-17 Cuff of left glove is now over stockinette cuff of sleeve, with hand still inside sleeve.

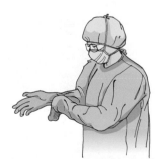

FIG. 16-15 Top of right glove and underlying sleeve of gown are grasped with left hand. By pulling sleeve up, glove is pulled onto hand.

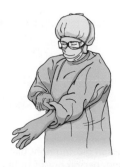

FIG. 16-18 Top of left glove and underlying gown sleeve are grasped with right hand, and sleeve is pulled up, pulling glove onto hand.

not contact the exterior of the sterile gloves. The everted cuff on the gloves exposes the inner surfaces. The first glove is put on with the skin-to-skin technique, bare hand to inside cuff. The sterile fingers of that gloved hand then may touch the sterile exterior of the second glove (i.e., glove-to-glove technique).

The procedure is as follows:

1. With the left hand, grasp the inner edge of the cuff of the right glove and lift from the wrapper. Take care not to touch the inner aspect of the wrapper or the sterile exterior portions of the glove.
2. Align the fingers of the right hand, and insert the right hand into the glove, pulling it on, leaving the cuff turned well down over the hand. Be sure to keep the thumb adducted into the palm of the hand until it is well inside the confines of the glove. Do not adjust the cuff. This will be done as a last step (Fig. 16-20).
3. Slip the fingers of the sterile gloved right hand under the everted cuff, on the sterile side of the left glove. Pick up the glove, and step back (Fig. 16-21).
4. Align the fingers of the left hand and insert the left hand into the left glove, keeping the thumb adducted until well inside the glove. Pull the left glove on all the way, unfolding the cuff, and enclosing the knitted left cuff at the wrist (Fig. 16-22).
5. With the sterile gloved fingers of the left hand, pull the cuff of the right glove up and over the cuff of the right sleeve. Avoid touching the bare wrist. Sterile surfaces may touch only sterile surfaces (Fig. 16-23).

Assisted Gowning and Gloving of a Team Member

A team member in sterile gown and gloves, usually the scrub person, may assist the surgeon or another team member in gowning and gloving by taking the following steps:

1. Open the hand towel, and lay one end on the freshly scrubbed team member's right hand, being careful not to touch the hand.

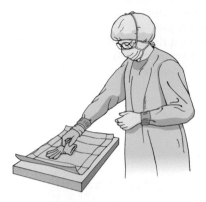

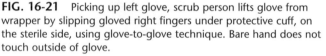

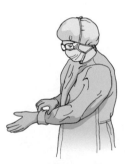

FIG. 16-21   Picking up left glove, scrub person lifts glove from wrapper by slipping gloved right fingers under protective cuff, on the sterile side, using glove-to-glove technique. Bare hand does not touch outside of glove.

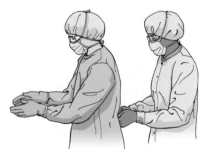

FIG. 16-19   For open gloving technique, circulating nurse fastens back of scrub person's gown. Note that hands extend through stockinette cuffs intentionally.

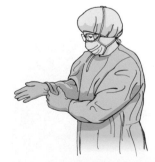

FIG. 16-22   The gloved fingers of right hand touch only the sterile side of left glove cuff near wrist to pull the cuff up and over the knitted cuff of the gown. Contact with exposed skin would contaminate right glove. The left cuff must be completely covered in this maneuver.

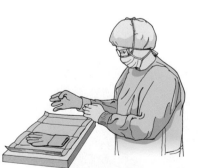

FIG. 16-20   Scrub person gloving right hand with open gloving technique. With left hand, person grasps right glove on folded-back cuff and lifts it directly up and away from wrapper. Right hand is inserted directly into glove opening. Note that left hand touches only cuff or inside of glove, which is skin-to-skin technique.

FIG. 16-23   The fingers of the completely gloved left hand are inserted under the sterile side of the cuff of the right glove. The cuff of the right glove is pulled up and over the knitted cuff of the gown. The cuff must be completely covered in this maneuver.

Do not hand a towel from a bloody back table or hand a towel with contaminated gloves or any instrument from the active sterile field. The biologic contamination is a hazard. The circulating nurse can open a separate gown and towel package for additional persons who need to enter the sterile field. Each person can pick up his or her own towel from the opened package. The scrub person can help with the remaining gowning and gloving procedure without touching any surface of the gown or gloves that would come in contact with the wearer's skin or clothing.

2. Lift the gown, and unfold it carefully with the sterile outside toward you and the unsterile inside toward the person being gowned, holding it open at the shoulders and neckline by cuffing over the hands.

   Do not hand a gown from a back table when the case is in progress. The drapes and gowns on the field in progress are considered biologically contaminated and could contaminate the wearer.

3. Keeping your hands on the sterile side of the gown under a protective cuff of the neck and shoulder area, offer the inside of the gown for the team member to don. He or she slips the arms into the sleeves. Take care not to let the sleeves make contact with unsterile areas.

4. Release the gown when it is secured by the person being gowned. The team member holds arms outstretched while the circulating nurse pulls the gown onto the shoulders and adjusts the sleeves so that the cuffs are properly slid back to expose the hands. In doing so, the circulating nurse touches only the inside of the gown at the seams.

Gloving a Team Member

1. Offer the right glove first. Pick up the right glove, and grasp it firmly with the fingers of both hands under the everted cuff on the sterile side. Hold the palm of the glove toward the person being gloved.

2. Stretch the cuff sufficiently open to allow for passage of the right hand. Avoid touching the hand by holding your thumbs out (abducted) (Fig. 16-24).

3. Exert upward pressure as the person slides the hand into the glove. Don't allow the hand to drop below the level of the sterile field.

4. Pull the glove cuff up and over the cuff of the right sleeve. Enclose the entire cuff.

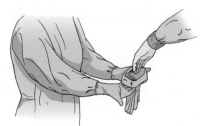

FIG. 16-24 Open assisted gloving of another team member is performed by holding the right glove open with the palm facing toward the person being gloved. Scrub person keeps thumbs extended (abducted) to avoid being touched by bare hands of person donning gloves.

5. Repeat for the left hand. The person being gloved can facilitate the process by supinating the gloved right hand and flexing the fingers like a hook to hold open the cuff of the glove being donned.

6. If a sterile vest is needed, hold it for the surgeon to slip the hands into the armholes. Be careful not to contaminate the gloves at the neck level. If the gown is a wraparound, assist the person to tie in. Remember that the back of the gown is not considered sterile even if a sterile vest is worn. The back is not considered sterile because it is not in the field of vision of the sterile team.

Removing or Changing Contaminated Gown and Gloves

Occasionally a contaminated gown must be changed during a surgical procedure. This means that both gown and gloves must be removed and changed. The circulating nurse obtains sterile gowns and gloves for personnel needing to change. The gown is always removed first, followed by the gloves. The contaminated team member steps away from the field, and the circulating nurse unfastens the neck and waist ties of the soiled gown. The contaminated person grasps the front of the gown at the shoulders below the neckline (Fig. 16-25, *A*). The gown is pulled off inside out by the wearer and rolled off away from the body (Fig. 16-25, *B* and *C*).

The gloves are removed using a glove-to-glove and then skin-to-skin technique. The cuffs of the gloves usually turn down as the gown is pulled off the arms. A *glove-to-glove*, then *skin-to-skin* technique is used to protect the clean hands from the contaminated outside of the gloves, which bear blood and body fluid of the patient (Fig. 16-26). The gloves are removed as follows:

1. Grasp the cuff of the left glove with the gloved fingers of the right hand, and pull it off inside out.

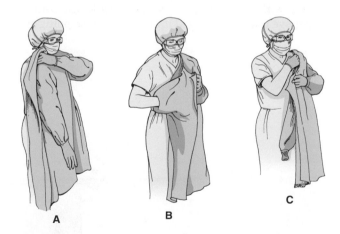

FIG. 16-25 Sequence of scrub person removing soiled gown at end of surgical procedure. The gown is removed before the gloves. Clean arms and scrub suit are protected from contaminated outside of gown. Do not reach behind the gown to untie the back strings. Have someone untie the back. **A,** With gloves on, grasp the front shoulder of gown and pull forward. **B,** In pulling gown off arms, be sure that gown sleeve is turned inside out to prevent contamination of scrub attire. **C,** The other shoulder is grasped with the other hand, and gown is removed entirely by pulling it off inside out and rolling it away from body.

2. Slip the ungloved fingers of the left hand under the cuff of the right glove, and slip it off inside out.
3. Discard the gloves in a trash receptacle.
4. Wash hands.

This is the same manner in which a gown and gloves are removed at the completion of the surgical procedure. Contaminated gowns and gloves are disposed of immediately in the appropriate biohazard receptacle.

When a sterile team member becomes contaminated during a case, rescrubbing is not necessary to re-gown and re-glove to reenter the sterile field. If only a sleeve is contaminated, a sterile sleeve may be put on over the contaminated one. If the person is not planning to reenter the sterile field, he or she should wash the hands immediately after removing the gloves.

Managing Contaminated Gloves or Objects During the Surgical Procedure

Contamination of the gown and gloves depends on the nature of contamination and whether or not the scrub person is double-gloved. Any puncture of a glove requires a complete glove change, even if double-gloved.

Contamination When Wearing Two Sets of Gloves

The contaminated outer glove can be removed leaving the sterile under glove intact. A new second pair of gloves can be applied over the remaining gloves. If the nature of the contamination is a puncture, both sets of gloves are considered contaminated and must be removed. Re-gloving is accomplished by employing the open gloving method.

Contamination When Wearing a Single Set of Gloves

A second glove can be applied over top of a superficially contaminated glove by using the open glove method. If covering with a second glove is not possible, the contaminated glove must be changed immediately. If stepping away

immediately is not feasible, the contaminated hand and any object involved in the contamination should be held away from the sterile field for the circulating nurse to remove.

The glove is changed as follows:

1. Turn away from the sterile field and request a new pair of sterile gloves from the circulating nurse. Re-gloving should take place from a surface separate from the main sterile field.
2. Extend the contaminated hand to the circulating nurse who, wearing protective gloves, grasps the contaminated objects and sets them aside. The circulating nurse then grasps the outside of the contaminated glove cuff about 2 inches (5 cm) below the top of the glove, closer toward the palm, and pulls the glove off inside out. Care is taken not to snap the glove, creating an aerosol.
3. Preferably, a sterile team member gloves another. If this is not possible, step aside and glove the hand using the open gloving technique.

The closed gloving technique is inappropriate for a glove change during a surgical procedure because contamination of the new glove by the porous cuff of a gown in use is inevitable. The hand will be contaminated by the knitted cuff of the gown, which has absorbed body sweat. The contaminated cuff may not be pulled down over the hand because the cuff is contaminated by shed skin cells.

The only way closed gloving is acceptable is for the scrub person to remove both the contaminated gown and gloves and another sterile gown is donned before re-gloving using the closed gloving method. The scrub person should change his or her own gloves before gowning and gloving another team member to avoid exposing the team member to contamination.

Bibliography

American Health Consultants: To brush or not to brush? CDC issues new hand-washing guideline, *Same Day Surg* 26(1):4-6, 2002.

AORN (Association of periOperative Registered Nurse): *AORN standards, recommended practices, and guidelines,* Denver, 2006, The Association.

Cohen ML: Proper hand washing protocols, *SSM* 6(3):21-28, 2000.

Dix K: Apparel in the hospital: What to wear where? *Infect Control Today* 9(3):28-30, 2005.

Dwividi AJ et al: Effects of surgical gloves on postoperative peritoneal adhesions and cytokine expression in a rat model, *Am J Surg* 188(5):491-494, 2004.

Gruendemann BJ, Bjerke NB: Is it time for brushless scrubbing with alcohol-based agent? *AORN J* 74(6):859-860, 862-873, 2001.

Hoffman RS et al: Surgical glove-associated diffuse lamellar keratitis, *Cornea* 24(6):699-704, 2005.

Kovach TL: Managing infection during handwashing with a newly patented activated triclosan technology, *Infect Control Today* 6(4):38-39, 2002.

Larson E: Hygiene of the skin: when is clean too clean? *Emerg Infect Dis* 2(7):1-6, 2001.

Newman JL, Hanuman BJ: Waterless antimicrobial hand disinfection, *SSM* 6(3):36-39, 2000.

Paulson DS: Hand scrub products: Performance versus clinical relevance, *AORN J* 80(2):225-234, 2004.

Petty L et al: Surgical gloves in the perioperative setting, *Dissector* 33(1):13-18, 2005.

Stein B: Coated gloves may be good for infection control as well as damaged ands, *Infect Control Today* 9(6):28-30, 2005.

Twomey C: Double gloving: A risk reduction strategy, *Joint Commission J Qual Patient Safety* 29(7):369-378, 2003.

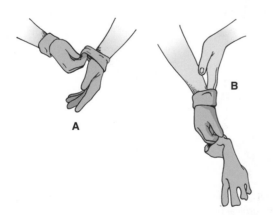

FIG. 16-26 Sequence of scrub person removing soiled gloves at end of surgical procedure. First, glove-to-glove technique **(A)** and then skin-to-skin technique **(B)** is used to protect "clean" hands from contaminated outside of gloves. Gloves are turned inside out for removal. The first glove is contained within the second glove. Avoid snapping gloves, which can cause aerosolization of contamination and latex particles.

Chapter 17

Decontamination and Disinfection

CHAPTER OBJECTIVES

After studying this chapter, the learner will be able to:
- Describe the steps in decontamination.
- List Spaulding's classifications of patient care items.
- Compare and contrast the three levels of disinfection.
- Discuss how an instrument is rendered safe for handling.
- Identify three safety issues associated with the use of chemical disinfectants.

CHAPTER OUTLINE

KEY TERMS AND DEFINITIONS

Bactericide Kills gram-negative and gram-positive bacteria unless specifically stated to the contrary (*adj:* bactericidal). Action may be specific to a species of bacteria.

Bacteriostatic Inhibits growth of bacteria.

Bioburden Degree of microbial load on an item before sterilization.

Biofilm Microbial load attached to a surface in a fluid environment. Microbes in a slime adhere to surfaces of all kinds of moist material, such as implantable metals, plastics, and tissue, causing antibiotic resistance.

Decontamination Process by which chemical or physical agents are used to clean inanimate, noncritical surfaces. A specific contact time is not specified. A low-level disinfectant is commonly used for this purpose. If a known organism, such as HBV, *Mycobacterium tuberculosis*, or HIV, is present on the surface, an intermediate-level disinfectant should be used.

Deionized water Water that has been processed through synthetic cation-anion resins to remove the positive or negatively charged ions.

Disinfection Chemical or physical process of destroying most forms of pathogenic microorganisms except bacterial spores; used for inanimate objects but not on tissue. The degree of disinfection depends primarily on the strength of the agent, the nature of the contamination, and the purpose for the process.
- **High-level disinfection** Process that destroys all microorganisms except high numbers of bacterial spores.
- **Intermediate-level disinfection** Process that inactivates vegetative bacteria, including *M. tuberculosis,* and most fungi and viruses but does not kill bacterial spores.
- **Low-level disinfection** Process that kills most bacteria, some viruses, and some fungi but does not destroy resistant microorganisms, such as *M. tuberculosis* or bacterial spores.

Distilled water The process of evaporating water and creating condensation from the steam that is collected for future use.

Fungicide Kills fungi.

Passivation Rendering the metallic surface of a surgical instrument resistant to corrosion or accumulation of mineral deposits.

Pasteurization Not a method of sterilization. This heating process kills many pathogenic microorganisms that are found in biosubstances such as milk or wine.

Sanitizer Chemical used on inanimate surfaces to reduce the number of bacteria to a safe level.

Sporicide Kills spores.

Virucide Kills viruses.

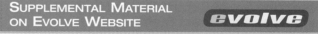

SUPPLEMENTAL MATERIAL ON EVOLVE WEBSITE

http://evolve.elsevier.com/BerryKohn
- Content Updates
- Glossary
- Full Set of Perioperative Flash Cards
- Interactive Key Term Flash Cards
- Student Activities
- WebLinks

CENTRAL SERVICE PERSONNEL

Central service (CS) personnel entrusted with the care, cleaning, assembly, and processing of patient care equipment to the appropriate degree of safety require specific training and credentialing. Training entails learning thousands of surgical instruments and their care. CS personnel need to know and understand all methods of instrument processing such as decontamination, disinfection, and sterilization. The role of the CS technician requires attention to detail.

Credentialing of Central Service Personnel

New Jersey is the first state to pass legislature requiring certification for CS personnel. Personnel currently holding positions in CS have until 2009 to become certified. New hires will have 3 years from the date of hire to attain the credential. Certification signifies that an individual professional has attained specific knowledge and skill in a specific professional practice. It sets a standard for performance and raises the bar for expectations in the profession. (Information about certification of CS personnel can be found at www.sterileprocessing.org.)

The Certification Board of Sterile Processing and Distribution (CBSPD) is the only sterile processing certification program that is accredited by the National Commission for Certifying Agencies. Five levels of certification are offered: technician, supervisor, manager, surgical instrument processor, and ambulatory surgery. The Ambulatory Surgery Sterile Processing Technician exam was implemented in 2005 because a job analysis survey indicated significant differences in practice between ambulatory surgery processing areas and hospital sterile processing departments.

Certified CS individuals are recertified through examination or by continuing education credits. Becoming certified encourages individuals to seek additional training that exemplifies certification level knowledge. Periodic competency testing should be incorporated into performance assessment. (An example of central service personnel competency testing can be found at www.apic.org.)

Coordination of Central Service Staff and Operating Room Staff

The relationship between CS staff and operating room (OR) staff is complex and synergistic. The OR staff relies on the CS staff to provide complete instrumentation processed to the appropriate degree of safety for patient use. The CS staff relies on the OR staff to return used sets in a safe-to-process condition without the risk of concealed blades or other sharps that pose a risk for injury during preparation for processing. Each person has a stake in the intricate coordination of preparing for a surgical procedure. Mutual respect and cooperation between the two specialty areas is in the best interest of safe and efficient patient care.

INSTRUMENT CLEANING AND DECONTAMINATION

Decontamination of instrumentation is performed in a designated area by specially trained personnel immediately after completion of the surgical procedure. The scrub person can facilitate the instrument decontamination process by wiping instruments as they are used on the sterile field and then opening the instruments completely before placing in a tray for return to the processing area. Enzymatic foam or solution can applied to the instruments to prevent debris from drying during transport to the central service area. All instruments on the table during a surgical procedure require decontamination and disinfection before processing to the required level of safety for patient use. The processing of endoscopes is discussed in Chapter 32.

Decontamination combines mechanical or manual cleaning and a physical or chemical microbicidal process. Prerinsing, washing, rinsing, and disinfecting/sterilizing is done in the processing department to render the instrumentation safe for handling by CS personnel. After the formal decontamination process the instrumentation can be assembled into sets by the CS technician and processed for use by the OR staff. Methods and procedures for decontamination and disinfection vary according to the item to be processed and the recommended agent used in processing. Personal protective equipment (PPE) should be worn at all times while using chemical disinfecting agents.

Prerinsing/Presoaking

The purpose of prerinsing or presoaking is to prevent blood and debris from drying on instruments or to soften and remove dried blood and debris. The circulating nurse can prepare a basin or plastic bin (with a cover) of enzymatic solution for the scrub person. For a short immersion period, instruments may be presoaked in the following:

- A triple proteolytic enzymatic detergent. Proteolytic enzymes dissolve blood and debris, and the detergent removes dissolved particulate from the surfaces of instruments, including otherwise inaccessible areas such as lumens. Enzyme-impregnated tubular sponges are commercially available from companies such as Ruhof for cleaning endoscopes and tubular instruments used in adipose and greasy tissues. (More information is available at www.ruhof.com.)
- An enzymatic agent diluted per manufacturer's instructions.
- Water with a low-sudsing, near-neutral detergent. The detergent should be compatible with the local water supply.
- Plain, clean, demineralized distilled water.
- Sodium hypochlorite (chlorine bleach) is corrosive; however, it is used as a presoak in suspected or potential prion disease such as transmissible spongiform encephalopathy (TSE). Instruments should not be soaked in any chlorine compound for more than 1 hour and should not be autoclaved with chlorine solution because of the formation of toxic chlorine gas.
  - Soaking in a phenolic, guanidine thiocyanate, or sodium hydroxide is an alternative, but chlorine bleach is the most reliable in reducing the prion titer within 1 hour. These chemicals are extremely corrosive and are not appropriate for use on endoscopes.
  - STERIS corporation has developed Hamo 100. This is an alkaline prion inactivating and removal detergent that is a corrosive potassium hydroxide solution. It cannot be used with soft metal or anodized aluminum. Hamo 100 is not recommended for use with rigid or

flexible endoscopes. This product has been released for use in Europe, but not currently approved for use in the United States.

Prerinsing or presoaking instruments with enzymatic solution in the OR can make further processing more efficient. Instruments should not be cleaned in scrub sinks or utility sinks in the substerile room. Instruments in an enzymatic soak solution should be transported to the processing department in a covered container.

Manual Cleaning

If a washer-sterilizer or washer-decontaminator is not available, instruments are washed by hand in the processing area. The purpose of manual cleaning is to remove residual blood and debris before terminal sterilization or high-level disinfection.

Delicate and sharp instruments should be handled separately. Microsurgical and ophthalmic instruments should be cleaned and dried by hand; they are not put in a washer-sterilizer. Because moisture is conducive to corrosion, these instruments should not remain wet for long periods. Complex instruments require complete disassembly before cleaning. Other instruments require special care. For example, the outside surfaces of powered instruments must be cleaned, but these instruments cannot be immersed in liquid. Some powered equipment requires lubrication as part of the cleaning process.

Personnel in the processing area wear personal protective equipment (PPE) such as caps, gloves, waterproof aprons, and face shields to prevent accidental spray from contaminated body fluids and chemical cleaning solutions.

The following steps should be observed when cleaning instruments manually:

1. Fill the washing sink with clean, warm water to which a noncorrosive, neutral pH, low-sudsing, free-rinsing detergent has been added.
    a. Detergent should be compatible with the local water supply. The mineral content of water varies from one area to another; a water softener may be used in the system routinely to minimize mineral deposits. Regardless of the water content, the detergent should be anionic or nonionic and have a pH as close to neutral as possible. An alkaline detergent (pH more than 8.5) can stain instruments; an acidic detergent (pH less than 6) can corrode or pit them.
    b. Proteolytic enzymatic detergents dissolve blood and protein and remove dissolved debris from crevices. These detergents are effective in a wide range of water qualities.
    c. Liquid detergents are preferable because they disperse more completely than do solids. Dilute the concentration before contact with instruments to avoid corrosion and staining. Do not pour liquid or put solid detergents directly on instruments.
2. Wash instruments carefully to guard against splashing and creating aerosols.
    a. Use a soft brush to clean serrations and box locks. A soft-bristle toothbrush may be used to clean ophthalmic, microsurgical, and other delicate instruments. Keep instruments totally submerged while brushing to minimize aerosolizing microorganisms.
    b. Use a soft cloth to wipe surfaces. A nonfibrous cellulose sponge will prevent damage to delicate tips.
    c. Remove bone, tissue, and other debris from cutting instruments.
    d. Never scrub surfaces with abrasive agents such as steel wool, wire brushes, scouring pads, or powders. These agents will scratch and may remove the protective finish on metal, thus increasing the likelihood of corrosion. The finish on stainless steel instruments protects the base metal from oxidation.
3. Rinse instruments thoroughly in distilled or deionized water at the temperature recommended by the manufacturer. Some enzymes can be inactivated by extreme temperatures. The water should not exceed 140° F (60° C) to prevent burns of the skin. Inadequate rinsing can leave a surface residue that can stain instruments.
4. Load instruments into the appropriate trays for terminal sterilization or into containers for high-level disinfection.
    a. Put instruments back into sterilization racks or replace the protective guards as appropriate.
    b. Arrange instruments that can be steam-sterilized in sterilizer trays for the washer-sterilizer or washer-decontaminator. The unwrapped tray is terminally steam-sterilized to make it safe for handling.
    c. Unless an automatic cleaning, disinfecting, and sterilizing machine is available, immerse lensed instruments that are heat sensitive in a high-level disinfectant after manual cleaning.
    d. Follow the manufacturer's instructions for the proper decontamination, cleaning, lubrication, and terminal sterilization of powered instruments.

Washer-Sterilizer/Washer-Decontaminator

Mechanical cleaning and terminal sterilization/decontamination can be accomplished in an automated washer-sterilizer or washer-decontaminator. Precleaning takes place before instruments are placed in any automated machine.

A washer-sterilizer requires instruments to be prewashed by hand in germicidal solution at 110° F (43.3° C) before being placed in the machine. All bioburden must be removed for the washer-sterilizer cycle to be effective. The temperature of the washer-sterilizer ranges from 250° to 280° F (121° to 138° C) and would cause coagulation and crusting of protein. The instruments should be thoroughly rinsed. At the end of the cycle, the instruments may be safely handled without gloves. The sets can be assembled and prepared for routine sterilization. A cycle in a washer-sterilizer makes the instruments safe to handle with the bare hands, but does not render instruments safe for immediate patient use or sterile storage.

A washer-decontaminator cleans with a spray-force action. It is similar to the washer-sterilizer in that the cycle includes a cold-water prerinse to loosen blood and protein, an alkaline low sudsing detergent wash, a neutral rinse, and finally, steam and heat. A washer-decontaminator does not reach the same temperature as a washer-sterilizer. It cleans at a maximum temperature of 140° to 180° F (60° to 82° C), rendering the instrument safe to handle without gloves at the end of the cycle. Some models incorporate ultrasonic capabilities and lubrication for select loads. The sets can be assembled and prepared for routine sterilization when the process is complete.

An indexed washer-decontaminator has several chambers. The instrument tray automatically passes from chamber to chamber like a car wash. It is indexed for the prerinse, ultrasonic cleaning, wash, rinse and lubrication, and drying cycles. The multiple chambers of the indexed washer-decontaminator can process several trays simultaneously.

Instruments should be arranged in perforated trays for processing in the washer-sterilizer or washer-decontaminator. The following steps should be observed when arranging the instruments:

1. Place heavy instruments in a separate tray or in the bottom of a tray, with smaller, lightweight instruments on top.
2. Turn instruments with concave surfaces, such as curettes and rongeurs, with the bowl side down; this facilitates drainage of the concave surface. Be certain that bone and tissue are removed from these surfaces during precleaning.
3. Open the box locks and pivots of hinged instruments to expose maximum surface area.
4. Disassemble complex instruments that can be disassembled without tools (e.g., stapling devices).
5. Position sharp or pointed instruments carefully on top of other instruments to prevent contacts that could damage the cutting edges or surfaces of other instruments. An alternative is to either place sharp instruments in a separate tray or terminally sterilize them after manual cleaning. Fine, delicate instruments should never be put in a washer-sterilizer or washer-decontaminator because the mechanical agitation will damage them.
6. Always arrange instruments neatly. They should not be randomly piled on top of one another.

Ultrasonic Cleaning

Surgical instruments vary in configuration from smooth surfaces, which respond to most types of cleaning, to complicated devices that contain box locks, serrations, grooves, blind holes, and interstices that are difficult to clean. Using high-frequency sound waves, ultrasonic energy thoroughly cleans by a process of cavitation. These sound waves generate tiny bubbles in the solution of the ultrasonic cleaner. The bubbles are small enough to get into the serrations, box locks, and crevices of instruments that are impossible to clean by other methods. The bubbles expand until they become unstable and collapse in on themselves. This implosion generates minute vacuum areas that dislodge, dissolve, or disperse soil.

For ultrasonic cleaning, precleaned and decontaminated instruments are completely immersed in the cleaning solution. The tank should be filled to a level of 1 inch (2.5 cm) above the top of the instrument tray. Suitable detergent, as specified by the manufacturer, is added. The temperature of the water should be between 100° and 140° F (37.7° and 60° C) to enhance the effectiveness of the detergent, but it should not be extremely hot, which would coagulate protein material on instruments. Instrument trays should be designed for maximum transmission of sonic energy. An important

relationship exists between wire gauge, opening size, and sonic frequency. A large mesh of small wire size transmits more energy than heavy wire with narrow spacing.

The solution is degassed by the ultrasonic energy. Gas, which is present in most tap water, impedes the transmission of sonic energy. An electrical generator supplies electrical energy to a transducer. The transducer converts the electrical energy into mechanical energy in the form of vibrating sound waves that are not audible to the human ear because they are of such high frequency. The presence of excess gas prevents the cleaning process from being fully effective, because the cavitation bubbles fill with gas and the energy released during implosion is reduced. Tap water should be degassed for 5 minutes or longer each time it is changed. The solution should be changed at least once per shift and whenever the detergent solution is visibly soiled. The inside of the tank should be cleaned between fillings.

An ultrasonic cleaner is not a sterilizer like the washer-sterilizer. The ultrasonic process uses mechanical and chemical action to process the instrumentation, but the instrument does not go through a sterilization process that renders the item safe for handling. The terminal sterilization function is performed separately in a different machine.

Most surgical instruments, including ophthalmic instruments, microinstruments, glassware, rubber goods, and thermoplastics, can be definitively cleaned by this method to remove the tiniest particles of debris from crevices. The manufacturer's instructions must be carefully followed. In general, these instructions include the following:

1. Arrange instruments with heavy instruments at the bottom of the tray and lightweight instruments on top.
2. Open the box locks and pivots of hinged instruments. Disassemble instruments as appropriate.
3. Protect cutting edges from other instruments. Fine, delicate microsurgical and ophthalmic instruments may be damaged by vibrations or contact with each other. Some small units may be suitable for delicate instruments.
4. Separate dissimilar metals. Do not mix stainless steel instruments with other metals because electrolysis with resultant etching may occur.
5. Do not clean plated instruments in an ultrasonic cleaner. Cavitation will accelerate the rupture and flaking of plating. Plated instruments are not suitable for use in surgery. The surface coating of the instrument could potentially flake or peel during use and leave particles in the patient's tissues.
6. Rinse instruments thoroughly in hot deionized water after the cleaning cycle to remove any surface debris and detergent residue.
7. Dry instruments promptly and completely before reassembling or storing. Instruments will corrode, spot, or stain if they are stored with trapped moisture.

Lubrication

All instruments with moving parts should be lubricated after cleaning. This is particularly important after ultrasonic cleaning, because the sonic energy removes all lubricant. Instruments are immersed in an antimicrobial water-soluble lubricant that is steam penetrable. The antimicrobial properties help prevent microbial growth in the lubricant bath, which can be reused for up to 7 days. A water-soluble lubricant deposits a thin film deep in box locks, hinges, and crevices but does not interfere with sterilization. Some lubricants also contain a rust inhibitor to prevent electrolytic mineral deposits.

Mineral oil, silicones, and machine oils are not used to lubricate instruments because they leave a residue that interferes with steam or ethylene oxide sterilization. Oiling any surgical instrument constitutes a break in technique by introducing a nonsterile item into a sterile field during its use in patient care. Oil deposits can be left in patient's tissues.

The lubricant should be used according to manufacturer's instructions for dilution, effectiveness, and exposure. To use most lubricants, instruments are completely immersed for 30 to 45 seconds; they are dipped and then allowed to drain dry. The solution is not rinsed or wiped off; excess solution can be shaken off. The thin film will evaporate during steam sterilization. This process is sometimes referred to as "milking" the instrument, because the solution is white and opaque like milk.

Inspecting and Testing

Each instrument must be critically inspected after each cleaning. Instruments with movable parts should be inspected and tested after lubrication. Each instrument should be completely clean to ensure effective sterilization, and each should be inspected for proper function. The following key points should be observed when inspecting an instrument after cleaning:

- Check hinged instruments for stiffness. Box locks and joints should work smoothly. Stiff joints are usually caused by inadequate cleaning. Lubrication eases stiffness temporarily. If box locks are frozen, leave the instruments in a water-soluble lubricant bath overnight, and then gently work the jaws back and forth. Reinspect the instrument for cleanliness and function.
- Test forceps for alignment. A forceps that is out of alignment can break during use. Close the jaws of the forceps slightly; if they overlap, they are out of alignment. The teeth of forceps with serrated jaws should mesh perfectly. Hold the shanks in each hand with the forceps open, and try to wiggle them. If the box lock has considerable play or is very loose, the forceps will not hold tissue securely. If a surgeon continues to use it, jaw misalignment will occur and impair the effectiveness of the forceps.
- Check the ratchet teeth. Ratchet teeth are subject to friction and metal-to-metal wear by the constant strain of closing and opening. Ratchets should close easily and hold firmly. To check this, clamp the forceps on the first tooth only. Hold the instrument at the box lock and tap the ratchet teeth lightly against a solid object. If the forceps springs open, it is faulty and should be repaired. A forceps that springs open when clamped on a blood vessel or duct is hazardous to the patient and is an annoyance to the surgeon. The ratchets must hold.
- Check the tension between the shanks. When the jaws touch, a clearance of $\frac{1}{16}$ to $\frac{1}{8}$ inch (1.5 to 3 mm) should be visible between the ratchet teeth of each shank.

This clearance provides adequate tension at the jaws when closed. The misalignment of hinged instruments is a common problem that occurs primarily as a result of misuse. The instrument needs to be repaired or replaced if the teeth or serrations do not mesh perfectly or if the jaws overlap.

- Test needle holders for needle security and precision. Clamp an appropriate-size needle in the jaws of the needle holder, and lock it on the second ratchet tooth. If the needle can be turned easily by hand, the needle holder needs repair. Using a needle holder for placement of a blade on a scalpel handle can cause the jaws of a needle holder to loosen.
- Test scissors for correctly ground and properly set blades. The blades should cut on the tips and glide over each other smoothly. Use tissue/operating scissors to cut through four layers of gauze at the tip of the blades (or through two layers if the scissors are less than 4 inches [10 cm] long). The scissors should cut with a fine, smooth feel and a minimum of pressure. Tissue scissors should not be used to cut dressings or tape.
- Electrical insulation should be intact on all reusable electrosurgical equipment. Split insulation can cause inadvertent tissue damage during use.
- Inspect the edges of sharp and semisharp instruments such as trocars, needles, chisels, osteotomes, rongeurs, and adenotomes for sharpness, chips or dents, and alignment. Remove any questionable items from service, and send for repair or replacement. Shards of metal could be deposited in patient's tissue during use.
- Inspect microsurgical instruments under a magnifying glass or microscope to check alignment and to detect burrs on tips and nicks on cutting edges. The exact alignment of teeth on fine-tooth forceps is an absolute necessity. Microscopic teeth are very easily bent. Be certain that these instruments are thoroughly dry. A chamois is useful for drying to prevent snagging delicate tips.
- Check pins and screws of reusable staplers to be sure they are secure and intact. They can become loose or fall out during ultrasonic cleaning as a result of vibration.
- Flatten or straighten malleable instruments such as retractors and probes. Weakened or cracked items should be immediately replaced.
- Self-retaining retractors should provide free motion and sliding of the retracting blades. They should attach, slide, and detach easily. The tilts and ratchets should slide and hold as appropriate. All screws, wing nuts, and removable parts should be inspected for stripped threads.
- Demagnetize instruments by passing them back through a magnetic field. Although this is not a common occurrence, instruments can become magnetized.
- Unclean or questionable instruments should be returned to the cleaning area for ultrasonic cleaning. Instruments in poor working condition should be removed from the processing area. A place is usually designated in the OR suite or in the CS department for the collection of instruments for repair. A defective instrument should be tagged as unsafe for use and not be allowed to remain in circulation.

Instrument Marking for Identification

New instruments may be marked for identification before they are put in service. Some manufacturers will imprint identification numbers or bar codes with a laser when their instruments are purchased. The surface of the instrument should not be etched or engraved by personnel in the department. Etching and engraving causes destruction of the instrument surface that permits trapped microorganisms and spores.

Some facilities affix specialized heat-stable tape to instruments to color-code them by sets or specialty. These tapes must withstand cleaning and sterilizing without peeling. They must be replaced if they loosen. The tape is wrapped around the circumference of the handle but should not overlap. The edges should just meet. The presence of marking tape allows debris to accumulate in the folds. Worn or peeling tape leaves an adhesive residue on the instrument that is hard to remove and attracts debris. The tape manufacturers have commercial tape-removal systems available for purchase. The kits include a tape cutter and solvent that is safe for use on instruments.

Instrument processing departments may find that a loose-leaf binder containing pictures and descriptions of each instrument is useful for the identification of specialty set contents. This process can be cumbersome and time consuming because manufacturers use different numbers and names for similar devices.

Repairing or Restoring versus Replacing Instruments

Instruments in poor working condition inhibit the surgeon and create a serious hazard for the patient. Instruments should be repaired at the first sign of damage or malfunction. If an instrument breaks during a procedure, all pieces should be accounted for in their entirety. A lighted magnifying lens is a useful central service tool for examining instrumentation.

Repair

Even with normal usage, the blades of scissors and the edges of other cutting instruments become dull over time, just as kitchen knives do at home. Steam sterilization causes the softening of the metal that in turn dulls the edge. Cutting instruments must be sharp. For this reason, scalpel blades are disposed of after a single patient use. Osteotomes, chisels, gouges, and meniscotomes can be sharpened by specialty companies that use handheld hones or a honing machine designed for this purpose. Some specialty instrument repair companies will come to the facility in a mobile van fully equipped with all the machines and tools needed to recondition and repair surgical instruments. Scissors, curettes, rongeurs, and reamers should be frequently rotated for sharpening. OR personnel are not qualified to sharpen or repair surgical instruments.

Drill bits and saw blades should be single use items. Reuse and processing causes the cutting edges to rip tissue instead of cutting. Stiff joints or frozen box locks are the result of inadequate cleaning or corrosion caused by trapped moisture or a corrosive substance. The instrument should be repaired before the box lock cracks and the instrument must be replaced.

After repeated use, instruments eventually wear, misalign, and stiffen. Parts such as inserts, screws, or springs may need to be replaced. The life of many instruments can be extended by preventive maintenance or prompt repair.

Restoration and Resurfacing

Instruments may become spotted, stained, corroded, pitted, or rusted. Some surface discoloration will appear with normal use, but the unusual or severe buildup of deposits may impair function or sterilization. The color of a stain may help identify a problem that needs to be corrected:

- Light or dark water spots (from mineral content in tap water or condensate in sterilizer caused by inadequate drying)
- Rust-colored film (from iron content or softening agents in steam pipes)
- Bluish gray stain (from some chemical sterilizing or disinfecting solutions)
- Brownish stain (from polyphosphate cleaning compounds that are incompatible with local water supply, leaving a chromic oxide film on instruments)
- Purplish black stain (from detergents that contain ammonia or from amines in steam lines)
- Rust deposits (from inadequate cleaning or drying, agents not thoroughly rinsed, electrolytic deposits from exposed metal under chipped chrome plating onto stainless steel, or residues in textile wrappers; avoid the use of plated instruments in surgery; these are not surgical grade instruments)

Blood, saline solution, and detergents that contain chloride can cause pitting if they are not rinsed promptly and thoroughly. Detergents with high or low pH can destroy the protective chromium oxide layer on stainless steel.

If an instrument has been damaged, the surface can be repolished and passivated by the manufacturer to restore the integrity of the finish.

Replacement

Broken instruments must be replaced if they are beyond repair or restoration. With normal use, good-quality surgical instruments have an expected life of at least 10 years. Using these precise tools for only their intended purpose cannot be overemphasized. Misuse and abuse are the most common causes of instrument breakage. Use of a lightweight instrument on heavy tissue causes the jaws to bend or "spring." Using a needle holder to load and disarm knife blades can damage the jaws.

Instrument counts and accountability activities in the OR help prevent instruments from being discarded into trash or sent to the laundry. Replacing instruments that have been needlessly damaged is an unnecessary expense for the OR. Repairing the laundry equipment can be an additional expense. Personnel could be injured by instruments that protrude through trash bags and puncture the skin. Some facilities have had extreme instrument losses and have installed metal detectors in the trash room. These are valid reinforcements for accountability for instrumentation in the OR.

DISINFECTION OF ITEMS USED IN PATIENT CARE

Disinfection differs from sterilization by its lack of sporicidal power. Theoretically, all items used in the sterile field should be sterilized. Surfaces of items that will penetrate or separate tissue or invade the intravascular system must be sterile to prevent the introduction of potentially harmful microorganisms into the patient's body. Items that cannot be sterilized by conventional sterilization methods discussed in Chapter 18 are disinfected to eliminate as many microorganisms as possible.

Some specialized instruments and equipment cannot be sterilized between each patient use or will not withstand a sterilization process. Disinfection may be the only alternative. Disinfection can be accomplished with chemical and physical agents. The application and selection of disinfecting agents depend on the level of importance of the item as used in patient care, risk of exposure to biologic material, or environmental contamination.

Chemical agents used for disinfection of the environment or instrumentation are prepared and maintained for use according to the manufacturer's recommendations. Care is taken not to over-dilute the solution by immersing wet items. Anything placed into the solution must be absolutely dry to prevent inactivity of the chemical properties. Dip sticks are commercially available to test the concentration and efficacy of the solution before use. Care is taken to note the correct use and shelf life of mixed solutions. A reconstituted chemical container should be labeled with the date of mixing and date of expiration. It should remain covered at all times and PPE should be worn any time the solution is used. Disposal of used or expired solution may be subject to special handling to meet federal environmental guidelines.

Spaulding's Classification of Patient Care Items

Earle H. Spaulding, a well-known microbiologist, developed a classification system in 1968 to determine the appropriate processing method to attain the desired level of disinfection required for patient care items. This system was adopted and later modified by the Centers for Disease Control and Prevention (CDC). Spaulding's classifications are still true in the twenty-first century.

- Critical items must be sterile because they enter sterile tissue, break the mucosal barrier, or come into contact with the vascular system. Examples include surgical instruments, endoscopic accessories that cut tissue, catheters, implants, and needles. Sterilization is required for critical items. High-level chemical disinfection should not be confused with chemical sterilization. Some of the same chemicals used for disinfection are used for longer times in higher concentrations to cause sterilization.
- Semicritical items come into contact with nonintact skin and mucous membranes and require high-level disinfection, although they also may be sterilized. Examples include respiratory therapy equipment, anesthesia equipment, bronchoscopes, colonoscopes, gastroscopes, sigmoidoscopes, and cystoscopes.
- Noncritical items are used in contact only with intact skin. Intermediate or low-level disinfection is adequate. Examples include blood pressure cuffs, furniture, linens, bedpans, and eating utensils.

Levels of Disinfection

Disinfection is the process of destroying or inhibiting growth of pathogenic microorganisms on inanimate objects. It reduces the risk of microbial contamination but does not provide the same level of assurance as sterilization because all spores are not killed. Disinfection levels are classified by the effectiveness of the process (i.e., the ability of the agent to kill microorganisms) as follows:

- High-level disinfection. Kills all bacteria, viruses, and fungi. The process may kill spores if contact time is sufficient and other conditions are met. A high-level disinfectant should be used if a semicritical item is disinfected rather than sterilized for use in contact with nonintact skin or mucous membranes. Some chemicals used in high-level disinfection can produce sterilization if they are allowed to remain in contact with the surface of the item for the time specified by the manufacturer. For example, exposure of a clean item to 2% glutaraldehyde for 20 minutes at 68° F (20° C) produces high-level disinfection. The item is then rinsed with sterile distilled water.

  NOTE: High-level disinfection *is not effective* against Creutzfeldt-Jakob disease (CJD; also including new variant CJD), which is a transmissible spongiform encephalopathy (TSE). The agent that causes CJD is not a living microorganism like a bacteria or virus. It is a protein, referred to as a prion, that is extremely difficult to remove and inactivate. Prions and other specific microorganisms are discussed in detail in Chapter 14.
- Intermediate-level disinfection. Kills most bacteria, viruses, and fungi on noncritical items. The process does not attack spores. It does inactivate *Mycobacterium tuberculosis.*
- Low-level disinfection. Kills most vegetative bacteria, fungi, and the least resistant viruses on noncritical items, including human immunodeficiency virus (HIV).

A record of the agent, concentration, and time of exposure should be maintained for semicritical items that have undergone high-level disinfection (see sample in Fig. 17-1).

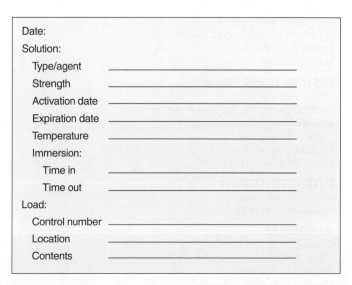

Date:
Solution:
  Type/agent _____
  Strength _____
  Activation date _____
  Expiration date _____
  Temperature _____
  Immersion:
    Time in _____
    Time out _____
Load:
  Control number _____
  Location _____
  Contents _____

FIG. 17-1 Record for sterilization or high-level disinfection with chemical solutions.

The level of disinfection that can be achieved depends on the type and concentration of the agent, contact time, and bioburden. Items that are disinfected are patient safe for their intended uses to minimize risks of infection for the patient. An all-purpose disinfectant does not exist. The best housekeeping agents are not the best disinfectants and vice versa.

METHODS OF DISINFECTION

Methods of disinfection include manual wiping with a chemical-impregnated cloth or sponge, soaking by total immersion, and processing by flush-through machinery. The method employed depends on the desired resultant level of disinfection.

Chemical Disinfectants

Chemical agents for disinfection are registered with the Pesticide Regulation Division of the Environmental Protection Agency (EPA) to be sold in interstate commerce. An EPA registration number is granted only when requirements of laboratory test data, toxicity data, product formula, and label copy are approved. Any chemical agent accepted for use by a facility should have a copy of the material safety data sheet (MSDS) readily available in the event of a spill or exposure as required by the Occupational Safety and Health Administration (OSHA).

Disinfectants are labeled with the chemical properties and appropriate warnings of precautions. The labels must be read, and directions for dilution and/or use must be followed. The product label should indicate several salient points important to the selection of the appropriate agent for the desired task. The user should read the label before use. Sample labeling information is listed in Box 17-1. Isopropyl alcohol, sodium hypochlorite, formaldehyde, glutaraldehyde, and phenol are considered hazardous chemicals. Some other chemicals can cause contact dermatitis. Gloves should be worn when handling all chemical agents.

To be labeled for hospital use, a chemical disinfectant should be proven effective against *Staphylococcus aureus* (gram positive), *Salmonella choleraesuis* (gram negative), and *Pseudomonas aeruginosa* (gram negative); these are the most resistant gram-positive and gram-negative organisms. The agent can be classified as a hospital disinfectant without being pseudomonacidal, but the label is required to say whether it is effective against *Pseudomonas* organisms. Influences on efficacy of the solution can be found in Box 17-2.

The EPA defines a disinfectant as an agent that kills growing or vegetative forms of bacteria. The terms *germicide* and *bactericide* may be used synonymously with the term *disinfectant* according to this definition. However, *M. tuberculosis* has a waxy envelope that makes it comparatively resistant to aqueous germicides. Effective agents against *M. tuberculosis* should be labeled tuberculocidal. Agents also are labeled regarding whether they kill fungi (fungicide), viruses (virucide), and/or spores (sporicide). Agents effective enough to be labeled tuberculocidal will kill HIV. Those that meet the EPA testing requirements may be labeled specifically as HIV virucides. Hepatitis B virus (HBV) cannot be adapted to laboratory testing, but it is known to survive exposure to many disinfectants.

The most common liquid chemical disinfectants used in the perioperative environment are listed in Table 17-1. With few exceptions, most liquid chemical disinfectants are not sporicides. Analysis of the label statements helps determine whether a product is appropriate for a specific purpose in the OR. Items disinfected by chemical agents for patient care require removal of the agent before the item is safe for use on a patient. Items need to be rinsed with clear water until the chemical is removed. The sterility of the rinse water depends on the intended use of the item. Sterile and high-level disinfected items will require the use of sterile water as a rinse. Semicritical and noncritical items can be rinsed with tap water.

BOX 17-1	**Information to Look for on a Disinfectant Label**

INFORMATION ABOUT ACTIVE INGREDIENT
Trade and generic name
Concentration or strength
Environmental Protection Agency (EPA) registration number

WARNINGS
Toxicity alert
Cautionary statement
Treatment for untoward exposure
Poison control listing
Hotline number

INSTRUCTIONS FOR USE
Dilution information
Personal protective equipment requirements
Intended use
Surfaces safe for use
Method of application
Duration of necessary contact

INTENDED ACTION
Antimicrobial activity
Residual action (if any)

AFTERCARE
Of equipment
Of treated surface
Of cleaning supplies
Disposal or storage of unused product
Biodegradability and effects in the natural environment

BOX 17-2	**Influences on the Efficacy of Disinfectants on Patient Care Items**

Concentration of the solution
Temperature of the solution
Shelf life and storage of solution
Compounded agents in the solution
Precleaning and drying of item before immersion
Degree of bioburden and biofilm on the surface of the item
Composition and surface texture of item
Duration of contact with the agent
Humidity of the environment
Temperature of the environment
Diluent's pH and mineral content

TABLE 17-1	Common Liquid Chemical Disinfectants							
Disinfectant Agent	Level of Disinfection	Timing	Virucidal	Fungicidal	Sporicidal	Mycobacterium (Tuberculocidal)	Hazards	Notes
ALCOHOL, 70%-95% Ethyl	Intermediate level	10-30 minutes for both	Yes, but not all lipid viruses, HAV	Yes	No	Yes	All forms are flammable	Bactericidal but not bacteriostatic. Ineffective against spores.
Isopropyl	Intermediate level		Yes, but not enteroviruses	Yes	No	Yes		Denatures proteins. Harms rubber and plastic. Combined with other disinfectants to form a tincture that can extend the bactericidal action. Rapid evaporation. Used in skin antisepsis.
ALDEHYDE							Toxic: skin, eye, and respiratory irritant	
Aqueous acidic 2%	High level	20-90 minutes at 20°-25° C	Yes	Yes	No	Yes; very slow	OSHA exposure limit is 0.05 ppm. Can cause respiratory irritation	Excellent materials compatibility. Local regulations may restrict disposal of used product. Inexpensive to use. Manual soaking costs an average of $0.25 per load.
Glutaraldehyde								
Banicide 3.5%	Sterile	10 hours at 25° C	Yes	Yes	Yes	Yes		30-day reuse period
	High level	45 minutes at 25° C						
Cidex activated alkaline 2.4% dialdehyde	Sterile	10 hours at 25° C	Yes	Yes	Yes	Yes		Coagulates blood and tissue. Activated alkaline form has shelf life of 14 to 30 days. Concentration level must be monitored.
	High level	45 minutes at 25° C	Yes	Yes	Some	Yes		
Cidex OPA- (0.55%) ortho-phthalaldehyde	High level	12 minutes at 20° C	Yes	Yes	Some, but improves when the pH is increased to 8. Scopes pass sporicidal test at 32 hours at 20° C	Yes; superior action	No known irritations	Requires no activation and remains more stable over a wide range of pH (3-9). Stains protein gray; 14-day reuse period. Concentration level must be monitored.

Continued.

TABLE 17-1   Common Liquid Chemical Disinfectants—cont'd

Disinfectant Agent	Level of Disinfection	Timing	Virucidal	Fungicidal	Sporicidal	Mycobacterium (Tuberculocidal)	Hazards	Notes
Cidex OPA- (5.75%) ortho-phthalaldehyde concentrate	High level	5 minutes at 50° C			Scopes pass sporicidal test at 32 hours at 50° C			Used in an automated endoscope high-level disinfector by EvoTech Integrated Endoscope Disinfection System.
PHENOL COMPOUND								
1.64% with 0.95% glutaraldehyde (Sporicidin)	Sterile	12 hours at 25° C	Yes	Yes	Yes	Yes		Effective in presence of organic matter. Leaves an active residue. Maximum reuse period 7 days.
	High level	20 minutes at 25° C	Yes, but limited	Yes	No	Yes		
QUATERNARY AMMONIUM COMPOUNDS (QUATS)								
C0.1%-2% concentration	Low	10 minutes	Limited; lipophilic only	Yes	No	No	No odor and low toxicity	Easily inactivated by organic debris. Effective in temperatures up to 212° F. Most effective in alkaline solution. Neutralized by detergents and hard water. Nonirritating and noncorrosive. Inexpensive. Inactivated by use with gauze pads. Surface disinfection.
HALOGENS							Toxic and corrosive	
Chlorine and chlorine compounds such as sodium hypochlorite	Low to high based on concentration and pH	10-30 minutes	Yes	Yes	Limited	Yes	Do not autoclave chlorine solutions; will vaporize and cause free chlorine gas inhalation hazard	Ethyl alcohol 60% can be added to increase kill potential. Oxidizes metallic objects. 1:10 dilution of 6% chlorine bleach (household bleach) contains 6000 ppm available chlorine. Combines with protein and decreases in effectiveness. Premixed solution can be stored in cool place in a light-proof container.

TABLE 17-1	Common Liquid Chemical Disinfectants—cont'd							
Disinfectant Agent	Level of Disinfection	Timing	Virucidal	Fungicidal	Sporicidal	Mycobacterium (Tuberculocidal)	Hazards	Notes
Iodophors (Wescodyne)	Low at a wide range of pH	10-30 minutes	Yes	Yes	No	Yes		Alcohol can be added to extend effectiveness in a solution of 1:10 in 50% ethyl alcohol. Vaporizes in hot water (120°-125° F). Reduced action in presence of protein. Inactivated iodophor loses brown-yellow color. Becomes clear when deactivated.
PERACETIC ACID								
STERIS 0.2%	Sterile	12-30 minutes at 50°-56° C	Yes	Yes	Yes	Yes, even at low temperatures. Can be a fire hazard at high temperatures when dry	Wear PPE if risk of contact to skin, eyes, or mucous membranes	Used in STERIS processing as a single-use liquid chemical sterilant. No residue. Uses filtered tap water for rinse. Can corrode metallics. Approximately $6 per cycle. No special disposal requirements. Protect from light and heat.
SPOROX HYDROGEN PEROXIDE								
7.5%	Sterile	6 hours at 20° C	Yes	Yes	Yes	Yes	Wear PPE to protect eyes	Requires no activation. Has no special disposal instructions.
	High level	30 minutes at 20° C	Yes	Yes	Some	Yes		Must monitor minimal effective concentration. Maximum reuse period 21 days. May enhance removal of organic debris. Not effective as a disinfectant in presence of organic matter.

HAV, Hepatitis A virus; *OSHA,* Occupational Safety and Health Administration; *ppm,* parts per million; *PPE,* personal protective equipment.

Factors to be considered in the selection of an agent include the following:

1. Microorganisms, particularly bacteria and viruses, differ markedly in their resistance to liquid chemical disinfectants. Factors influencing the microbial response include the structure and design of the item to be disinfected, the active ingredient of the chemical, pH, hardness of the water, exposure time, and extent of precleaning before processing. Resistance levels of select microorganisms are described in Table 17-2.

2. Disinfectants differ widely in the level of microbicidal action they produce and mechanisms involved. All are protoplasmic poisons that can coagulate or denature cell protein, oxidize or bind enzymes, or alter cell membranes. In-use culture testing must determine the number of viable microorganisms after an agent is used for the intended purpose.

3. The nature of the microbial contamination influences the results of chemical disinfection. Bacteria, spores, fungi, and viruses are present in air and on surfaces throughout the environment. However, organic soil, such as blood, plasma, pus, feces, and tissue, absorbs germicidal molecules and inactivates some chemicals. Therefore good physical precleaning before disinfetion helps reduce the number of microorganisms and maintain the effectiveness of the disinfectant.

4. Requirements of the chemical agent vary.
   a. Housekeeping products should be detergent-disinfectants that meet the following requirements for both cleaning and disinfection:
      (1) They must be effective against a broad spectrum of microorganisms, including *P. aeruginosa* and *M. tuberculosis,* preferably in the presence of organic soil.
      (2) They must be compatible with tap water for dilution.
      (3) They must be low-foaming and prevent waterborne deposits.
      (4) They must rinse easily and not leave a residual film that could affect electrical conductivity.
      (5) They should be nontoxic and nonirritating to patients and personnel.
      (6) They should be virtually odorless.
   b. Instrument and equipment disinfectants should be registered by the EPA and should kill as many species of microorganisms as possible to decontaminate items effectively for handling by personnel or for preparing semicritical items for patient use, such as stethoscopes and monitors.

5. The kill time is correlated with the concentration of the agent and the number of microorganisms present. Most disinfectant chemicals are used in aqueous solution. Water brings the chemical and microorganisms together. Without this water reaction, the process stops. Increasing the concentration of the chemical may shorten exposure time but not necessarily.
   a. All tap water has *Pseudomonas* bacteria in it. The pH, calcium, and magnesium in hard tap water can inactivate disinfectants. Therefore deionized water may be recommended for use in dilution.

TABLE 17-2   Resistance Levels of Select Microorganisms

Minimal Resistance	Intermediate Resistance	High Resistance
LIPID VIRUSES	**NONLIPID VIRUSES (HYDROPHILIC)**	**BACTERIAL ENDOSPORES**
Influenza	Echovirus	Gram positive
Rubeola	Parvovirus	*Bacillus subtilis*
Cytomegalovirus (CMV)	Hepatitis A virus	*Bacillus stearothermophilus*
Human immunodeficiency virus (HIV)	Rhinovirus	*Clostridium tetani*
Herpes simplex virus types 1 and 2 (HSV)	Poliovirus	*Bacillus anthracis*
Hepatitis B virus (HBV)	Coxsackievirus	*Clostridium botulinum*
Hepatitis C virus (HCV)		*Clostridium perfringens*
Respiratory syncytial virus (RSV)		*Clostridium difficile*
Epstein-Barr virus (EBV)		Gram negative
		Coxiella burnetii
VEGETATIVE LIPID-COATED BACTERIA	**FUNGI**	**MYCOBACTERIA**
NON-ENDOSPORE FORMING		
Gram positive	*Trichophyton* species	*Mycobacterium bovis*
Staphylococcus aureus	*Cryptococcus* species	*Mycobacterium tuberculosis*
Staphylococcus epidermidis	*Candida* species	*Mycobacterium leprae*
Streptococcus groups A and B		
Pseudomonas aeruginosa		
Salmonella choleraesuis		
Corynebacterium diphtheriae		
Gram negative		
Haemophilus influenzae		
Helicobacter pylori		

Knowledge of microbial resistance to decontamination, disinfection, and sterilization is important in selecting method to use during reprocessing.

b. The temperature of hot water may make chemical agents unstable.

c. Disinfectants should be premixed in required concentrations and stored in properly labeled containers to ensure that personnel use the product in the correct concentration.

d. Instruments are completely submerged for the maximum time recommended by the manufacturer of the product used.

e. All instruments should be clean and dry when put into solution. Drippy, wet items will dilute the solution and change the concentration of a chemical agent.

6. The composition of items to be disinfected varies. Nonporous items, such as metal instruments, are more easily disinfected than are porous materials.

7. The method of application influences the effectiveness of the chemical agent.

a. Direct application of a liquid disinfectant, either by mechanical action for housekeeping purposes or by immersion for instrument disinfection, is the most effective method of applying chemicals to the surface of inanimate objects.

b. Aerosol spray from a pressurized container is an effective method of spot disinfection on smooth surfaces and into crevices not otherwise accessible.

c. Fogging is the process of filling the air in a room with an aerosolized disinfectant solution in an attempt to control microbial contamination. Action on airborne contaminants is temporary because the agent dispersed through the air settles on surfaces or is exhausted through the ventilating system. This method is potentially toxic to personnel and patients. Unless all surfaces are completely covered by a layer of the disinfectant solution for the minimum exposure period, disinfection is incomplete. Fogging is impractical and too ineffective to be an acceptable method of disinfection in OR suites.

8. Disinfection should be done immediately before and after use or contamination. All patients are considered to be potential carriers of microbial contamination. Therefore adequate bactericidal and virucidal disinfection is needed before and after every invasive procedure.

9. The shelf life and safe storage after reconstitution are other factors to be considered. Room temperature and exposure to lighting may be factors in efficacy.

Alcohol. Ethyl or isopropyl alcohol, 70% to 95%, kills microorganisms by coagulation of cell proteins.

Effectiveness

- It may be used as a housekeeping disinfectant for damp-dusting furniture and lights or wiping electrical cords without leaving a residue on treated surfaces. It is nonstaining.

- It can disinfect semicritical instruments. To prevent corrosion of metal, 0.2% sodium nitrite is added.

- It is bactericidal, pseudomonacidal, and fungicidal in a minimum of 10 minutes' exposure by total immersion. It is not sporicidal.

- It is tuberculocidal and virucidal for most viruses (except hydrophilic viruses), including HIV, in a minimum of 15 minutes' exposure. Isopropyl 70% to 95% ethyl alcohol is effective against HBV.

Precautions

- The pattern of effectiveness of 95% isopropyl alcohol on HBV is irregular because it evaporates rapidly and does not have prolonged moist contact with the microorganism. It should not be used for cleaning up blood or body fluid spills because it is inactivated in the presence of biologic matter.

- It is volatile; it will act only as long as it is in solution. Alcohol becomes ineffective as soon as it evaporates, and it loses its microbicidal activity below a concentration of 50%; it should be discarded at frequent intervals.

- It is inactive in the presence of organic soil. It does not penetrate skin oil that lodges on instruments through handling.

- It will blanch asphalt floor tiles.

- It cannot be used on lensed instruments with cement mountings because it dissolves cement.

- With long exposure, it will harden and swell plastic tubing and items, including polyethylene.

- It is flammable, so it is stored in a cool, well-ventilated area.

- It is a skin irritant.

Chlorine Compounds. Inorganic chlorine is valuable for the disinfection of water. Chlorine compounds kill microorganisms by the oxidation of enzymes. Sodium hypochlorite (household bleach), 1:10 dilution of 5.25%, is a low-level disinfectant. Concentration may range up to 1:100, or 500 parts per million (ppm). Sodium dichloroisocyanurate (Presept disinfectant tablet) has a lowered pH, which enhances its microbicidal action. Chlorine compounds are limited to housekeeping disinfection.

Effectiveness

- Chlorine compounds are housekeeping disinfectants for spot cleaning of blood and body fluid spills and for cleaning of floors and furniture.

- They are bactericidal, fungicidal, and tuberculocidal and have a virucidal effect on HIV, HBV, and other viruses.

Precautions

- Sodium hypochlorite is unstable and dissipates rapidly in the presence of organic soil. A dilution is prepared daily.

- The odor may be objectionable. It can be a respiratory irritant.

- Chlorine is corrosive to metal; it cannot be used for instrument disinfection and decontamination.

- Chlorine compounds are potentially carcinogenic if combined with formaldehyde.

Formaldehyde. Formaldehyde kills microorganisms by coagulation of protein in cells. The solution may be 37% formaldehyde in water (Formalin) or 8% formaldehyde in 70% isopropyl alcohol. Formaldehyde is not used for housekeeping purposes as a surface disinfectant.

Effectiveness

- It is a high-level instrument disinfectant. To prevent corrosion of metal, 0.2% sodium nitrite is added.

- It is bactericidal, pseudomonacidal, and fungicidal in a minimum of 5 minutes' exposure.

- It is tuberculocidal and virucidal in a minimum of 10 minutes in alcohol solution and in a minimum of 15 minutes in aqueous solution.
- It is sporicidal in a minimum of 12 hours.

Precautions

- Fumes are irritating to the eyes and mucous membranes.
- Fumes are potentially carcinogenic.
- It is toxic to tissues, so instruments are thoroughly rinsed with sterile distilled water before use.
- Because rubber and porous materials may absorb formaldehyde, they should not be disinfected in this agent.

Glutaraldehyde. An aqueous solution of glutaraldehyde kills microorganisms by denaturation of protein. It is most commonly used in an activated 2.0% to 2.4% solution that can be reused for the specified period of activation. Both alkaline and acid solutions are available for high-level disinfection of critical and semicritical items. A 1:16 dilution is not considered a high-level disinfectant; a 2% solution is. Glutaraldehyde is not used for housekeeping purposes.

Effectiveness

- It is a noncorrosive high-level disinfectant for endoscopes and lensed instruments.
- It is a safe high-level disinfectant for most plastic and rubber items, such as those used for administering anesthetic agents or respiratory therapy.
- It is bactericidal, pseudomonacidal, fungicidal, and virucidal, including against HIV and HBV, in a minimum of 10 minutes' exposure at a temperature between 68° and 86° F (20° and 30° C).
- It is tuberculocidal. Variations in formulations of products available affect the exposure time and temperature of the solution, especially after reuse. A 2% solution at 77° or 86° F (25° or 30° C) may be 100% tuberculocidal in 45 to 90 minutes, depending on the formulation. Label instructions of the manufacturer should be followed.
- Most of the products labeled as cold sterilants are sporicidal in a minimum of 10 hours' exposure at room temperature.
- Some products can be reused in closed containers or in an automatic machine for a period of activation specified by the manufacturer.
- It remains active in the presence of organic matter; it does not coagulate protein material.

Precautions

- Thorough and careful cleaning in a mild detergent is essential to remove organic debris and reduce microbial contamination. Detergent is rinsed off, and the item is dried before immersion.
- Items are completely immersed and lumens are filled with solution for no longer than 24 hours.
- Items are thoroughly rinsed before use.
- Glutaraldehyde may be retained by woven polyester catheters and be an irritant to mucous membranes.
- Odor and fumes may be irritating to the eyes, throat, and nasal passages. The solution should be kept covered and used in a well-ventilated area.
- Its shelf life is limited after activation.

Iodophors. A complex of free iodine with detergent kills microorganisms through a process of oxidation of essential enzymes. An iodophor is an effective low- to intermediate-level disinfectant. The iodine-detergent complex enhances the microbicidal activity of free iodine and renders it nontoxic, nonirritating, and nonstaining when used as directed. The concentration varies among the products available. The manufacturer's instructions for use should be followed.

Effectiveness

- Iodophors are used as housekeeping disinfectants for surfaces such as floors, furniture, and walls. Iodine is effective as long as it is wet. An aqueous solution is more effective for cleaning than is an alcohol solution because it dries more slowly.
- An iodophor may be used as a semicritical instrument disinfectant. To prevent corrosion of metal, 0.2% sodium nitrite is added.
- Iodophors are bactericidal, pseudomonacidal, and fungicidal in a minimum of 10 minutes' exposure in a concentration of 450 ppm of iodine or a minimum of 20 minutes' exposure in a concentration of 100 ppm of iodine.
- They are tuberculocidal and virucidal, including against HIV and HBV, in a minimum of 20 minutes' exposure with a minimum concentration of 450 ppm of iodine. They are not sporicidal.

Precautions

- Some iodophors are unstable in the presence of hard water or heat and are inactivated by organic soil.
- Iodine stains fabrics and tissue; however, this is reduced or is temporary when iodine is used as an iodophor.

Phenolic Compounds. Derivatives of pure phenol kill microorganisms mainly by coagulation of protein. Depending on the phenol coefficient and species of organisms, phenolic compounds may cause rapid lysis of cells, leakage of cell constituents without lysis, or death by denaturing enzymes. Pure phenol, obtained from coal tar, is an extremely caustic agent and dangerous to tissue. Derivatives are used as low-level disinfectants, usually with a minimum of a 2% phenolic compound in an aqueous or detergent solution. Phenolic compounds are used primarily for housekeeping purposes.

Effectiveness

- Phenolic compounds may be used as housekeeping disinfectants for cleaning surfaces such as floors, furniture, and walls. Phenolics retain a safe level of activity in the presence of heavy organic soil.
- They are the disinfectants of choice when dealing with fecal contamination. They have good stability and remain active after mild heating and prolonged drying. Subsequent application of moisture to dry surfaces can redissolve the chemical so that it becomes bactericidal again.
- They are tuberculocidal.

Precautions

- Tissue irritation precludes use for semicritical instruments that will come into contact with skin and mucous membranes (e.g., anesthesia equipment).
- Personnel should wear gloves when cleaning with these products to avoid skin irritation.
- Rubber and plastics may absorb phenol derivatives.
- The product may have an unpleasant odor.

- Pure phenol is inactivated by the application of alcohol.

Quaternary Ammonium Compounds.
"Quats," as these compounds are often called, cause gradual alteration of cell membranes to produce leakage of protoplasm of some microorganisms, primarily vegetative bacteria. These compounds possess detergent properties and are used to sanitize noncritical surfaces. Benzalkonium chloride, one of the most widely used of these compounds, should be used in a concentration of 1:750.

Effectiveness
- They are rarely used as housekeeping disinfectants for surfaces such as floors, furniture, and walls.
- For low-level, noncritical instrument disinfection, 0.2% sodium nitrite is added to the solution to prevent corrosion of metal.
- They are bactericidal, pseudomonacidal, fungicidal, and lipid virucidal in a minimum of 10 minutes' exposure. They are nonirritating to skin.
- There is no buildup on surfaces. They are not inactivated by hard water.

Precautions
- The microbicidal effect can be reversed by adding a neutralizer, such as soap.
- They are not effective against tuberculosis or hydrophilic viruses, such as poliovirus.
- The active agent can be selectively absorbed by fabrics, thus reducing the strength perhaps to an ineffectively low level. Gauze or a towel must not be put in the basin used for immersing instruments.
- Compounds are inactivated in the presence of organic soil.

Hydrogen Peroxide
Effectiveness
- It is rapidly bactericidal, virucidal, fungicidal, and tuberculocidal.
- It is useful for disinfection of noncritical items.

Precautions
- It is inactivated by blood.

Physical Disinfectants

Boiling Water.
Boiling water cannot be depended on to kill spores. Heat-resistant bacterial spores will withstand water boiling at 212° F (100° C) for many hours of continuous exposure. Inactivation of some viruses, such as those associated with hepatitis, is uncertain.

If no other method of sterilization or disinfection is available, boiling water can be rendered more effective by adding sodium carbonate to make a 2% solution, which reduces the hydrogen-ion concentration. At sea level the recommended boiling time for disinfection is 15 minutes. Rubber goods and glassware must not be boiled in sodium carbonate because it is destructive to both. If sodium carbonate is not used, the minimum boiling period is 30 minutes. At high altitudes the boiling time is increased to compensate for the lower temperature of boiling water.

Pasteurization.
High-level disinfection process, sometimes referred to as pasteurization, can be used for items such as reusable respiratory devices and anesthesia breathing circuits to render them safe for patient use.

Pasteurization is a method of hot water decontamination/disinfection performed with chlorine detergents and low temperatures. Although not a sterilization process, exposure to hot water (140° to 180° F [60° to 82° C]) for 30 minutes kills microorganisms without killing spores.

Anesthesia hoses, masks, and fluted breathing bags are positioned in the pasteurization unit on special pegs and hooks that permit total immersion and full surface contact of the sprayer arms. Time and temperature are closely monitored to provide high-level disinfection. The pasteurization process takes approximately 1 hour to complete, followed by air-drying in a specially filtered cabinet. The items must be completely dry before being placed in storage. The average pasteurization unit can process up to 10 complete anesthesia circuits in one cycle.

Ultraviolet Irradiation.
Ultraviolet (UV) rays at wavelengths of 240 to 480 nm photochemically transform nucleic acid bases to denature deoxyribonucleic acid (DNA) and proteins. Generated by low-pressure mercury vapor bulbs, UV lights produce nonionizing radiant energy in sufficient wavelengths and intensity for low-level disinfection. The rays can kill select vegetative bacteria, fungi, and lipoprotein viruses on contact in air or water.

The practical usefulness of UV irradiation is very limited, however, because the rays must make direct contact with the organisms and may actually support life for some varieties. Microorganisms are in a constant state of motion in the air currents of the ventilating system and in water. Moving across the ray of UV light, pathogens may be exposed for too short a time for effective contact with the radiant energy. The average UV lamp produces 45 microwatts per cubic centimeter. Many microorganisms require application of UV lights at 2000 to 100,000 microwatts per cubic centimeter to be effective.

UV lights have been installed in a few ORs to decrease airborne microorganisms to low levels. UV rays can cause skin burns, similar to sunburn, and conjunctivitis. Therefore, when working under exposure to UV rays, protective skin coverings and goggles or a visor over the eyes are worn. These lights may be turned on only when the room is unoccupied to reduce airborne and surface contamination.

UV irradiation is used in conjunction with activated carbon 5-micron filters for water purification. UV irradiation kills bacteria but does not remove impurities. The filtration process is followed by exposing water flowing at a constant rate and temperature to a 5-watt UV lamp. This produces purified, not sterile, water. UV irradiation is not sporicidal, and HBV can survive exposure to it.

DISPOSABLE PRODUCTS

Disposable products can be useful in the OR. It is sometimes easier to discard a contaminated item after use than to clean and process it. The use of disposable products has become popular, but consideration of the logistics of using them includes determination of the benefits and/or consequences of their use and their reuse.

The production of disposable products often involves the use of natural resources and potential industrial damage to the earth's environment. Disposal of the contaminated item by incineration or in landfills can pose similar problems. Many issues concerning economy, including labor costs, storage, and delivery need to be evaluated on an individual basis. Economy may be shown with the use of disposable products.

Considerations for the Use of Disposable Products

A disposable product is used once with reasonable assurance of safety and effectiveness. Most disposables are patient-charge items (i.e., the cost of these items is added to the patient's bill). Use of patient-charge items requires specific and accurate recordkeeping.

Most surgical computer systems send all the estimated items into a case cart system with an estimated charge sheet. The case cart usually contains only the items needed for a routine procedure. If the total complement of items is used during the procedure, the disposables are already charged in the system. This saves personnel time and money by having much of the paperwork done in advance. This process facilitates flat-rate costing by procedure.

If a disposable item remains completely intact (is not opened or used in any way), it can be returned to stock. The cost of the item is then removed from the patient's charge sheet in the computer, using a process referred to as charging by exception. The cost is removed by personnel in the stock room, and the patient is not charged. The item is then electronically credited to stock for future use in the departmental inventory. Bar code technology is very useful for inventory tracking. Many manufacturers have included a bar code on their packaging.

Conversely, taking an item from the stock room without accounting for it in the computer system will leave an inaccurate number of items available for actual use. Planning for other cases depends on having correct numbers of disposables available for use. The system will know when an item is really available only if the records are complete and up-to-date.

Advantages

- When a sterile item is required, proper packaging and sterility must be ensured. Sterility is guaranteed by reliable manufacturers as long as the integrity of their packages is maintained. Industry conforms to far more rigid standards of quality control than onsite conditions permit. All sterilized products are tested for sterility before they are distributed to purchasers.
- Single-use items, such as urinary and suction catheters, are aesthetically more acceptable to patients. More important, disposable products eliminate a potential source of cross-contamination.
- Items such as needles and safety razors ensure more comfort for the patient because they are always new and sharp. Proper function is thus ensured.
- Standardized service at reduced cost per unit may be provided. Sponges are precounted and sterilized, for example. Packs and trays become standardized and can be customized.
- Loss and breakage in reprocessing reusable items are eliminated.

- Labor costs of processing supplies are reduced, particularly in the tedious, meticulous cleaning and packaging.
- The need for expensive mechanical cleaning equipment is eliminated.
- Contaminated used items can be contained for safe disposal. Handling is minimal, and processing is eliminated.

Disadvantages

- Costly waste occurs if sterile items are contaminated by carelessness or are unnecessarily opened. Extreme care is needed in opening packages to maintain sterility. Handling should not compromise the integrity of wrappings and pose a threat to the maintenance of sterility.
- Flexibility in complying with requests of individual physicians for special setups can be complicated. No allowance is made for deviation from custom packs. Procedures need to be standardized to conform to available items and sets.
- If a defect is found in one package, it may extend throughout the total lot, requiring replacement of the total supply on hand. Each lot is numbered for identification and recall if a problem arises.
- The circulating nurse may have to open an increased number of individually packaged items if the custom pack is not adequate.
- In the event of a sudden increase in use, adequate inventory may not be readily available.
- Potentially unstable products, such as some disposable trays containing medications, may carry an expiration date. Unless oldest products are used first, unnecessary costs are incurred if a product must be discarded because its time of reliability has expired. All dated products should be routinely checked for expiration.
- Environmental ecology may be affected by incineration or disposal in landfills. Some medical waste is regulated by local and federal laws.

Other Considerations

Some other considerations regarding the use of disposable products include the following:

- Some hospitals have saved money by reducing their labor force through conversion to as many totally disposable systems as possible, such as intravenous therapy, drapes, and special procedure trays. In some geographic areas where efficient labor may be readily available at minimum wage, disposable products are more costly than labor. However, if professional personnel are being used for reprocessing supplies, use of disposable products will enable them to spend more time giving more care to patients and less time on processing supplies.
- Proper and safe storage facilities should be provided. More storage space or more frequent deliveries may be required to maintain adequate inventories of disposable products.
- Disposal may be an ecologic problem. Used items are taken to an incinerator, compactor, or other safe waste-disposal area. Waste should not be allowed to accumulate in the OR suite or in other hospital areas.
- Disposables opened but unused or exposed to patients in any way can be set aside for orientation or practice sessions or donated to nursing schools. Care is taken not to use

anything from a sterile field that has been used in a surgical procedure. Cases that are set up and immediately canceled are ideal for salvaging items for learning situations.

Reusing/Reprocessing Disposable Single-Use Products/Devices

Manufacturers use extensive controls and testing procedures to ensure cleanliness, nontoxicity, nonpyrogenicity, biocompatibility, sterility, and function of disposable products. All items must be safe and effective for their intended patient uses. The manufacturer guarantees product stability and sterility for a single use only.[1]

In this era of cost containment, salvage of undamaged disposable items may be attempted. The risks of salvaging items should be evaluated seriously. The health care facility assumes legal responsibility for items it chooses to reuse, reprocess, and resterilize. The manufacturer cannot be held liable for the efficacy of a disposable product or one intended for single use if the user chooses to reprocess it. The burden of liability rests with the processor.

Reuse. Reuse of a used, disposable, single-use item requires cleaning, packaging, and sterilizing if it will be reused as a sterile item. Some products degrade with use. Many manufacturers have not tested their products for more than one use. To reuse a product, the product should be tested to validate patient safety. Patients have the right to know that they are using a reused single-use product. They should not be charged the cost of a new item.

Reprocessing. Repackaging and resterilizing unused sterile disposable items may be hazardous. These are items that were opened and not needed, or they are clean but have been contaminated in some way (i.e., the original packaging is not intact). Many of these items are very expensive, and salvage seems to be an acceptable alternative. The manufacturer must provide written instructions for resterilization of unused but contaminated items by onsite personnel. Many of these items are heat sensitive. Services that reprocess and resterilize some types of clean, unused, and undamaged products are available. Such services must guarantee product stability and sterility.

Resterilization. The sterilization process must not alter the characteristics of any part of the product, regardless of whether it is intended to be disposable or reusable. Some products are labeled "do not resterilize." This instruction means that the product will be damaged in the process of resterilization. The manufacturer's recommendations should be followed if any reprocessing is performed.

---

[1]www.fda.gov is a good source for documentation concerning the regulation of reprocessing single-use devices. Manufacturers guarantee safe use of a single-use device for one patient; however, questions of safety and liability associated with reprocessing continue to be raised in select circumstances.

Safety Considerations. Patient safety should be the prime concern in the decision to reuse, reprocess, or resterilize a disposable item. Several questions should be answered:

- Is the item a noncritical/noninvasive device? Critical items, particularly those that will enter or be in contact with the bloodstream or mucous membranes, present the greatest risks of adverse effects. Disposables of this type should not be reprocessed.
- Is the item really clean? Many porous materials cannot be thoroughly cleaned after use. If these are not adequately cleaned, microbial growth can predispose patients to infection. Lumens of catheters and tubing are especially difficult to clean. Biologic debris interferes with the sterilization process.
- Is the item nontoxic or nonpyrogenic after cleaning and reprocessing? Residues from some cleaning compounds and sterilizing processes are toxic. Chemicals can be retained by the item during reprocessing.
- Is the item truly sterile? The sterilization method should be appropriate for materials in the item and in the packaging. The packaging material should allow penetration of the sterilant to all surfaces of the item and should prevent contamination during storage. Sterility should be verified by biologic testing for each type of product that is resterilized.
- Is the integrity of the product maintained? Physical and/or chemical characteristics may be altered by cleaning agents, the cleaning process, or resterilization. Some materials deteriorate or become brittle, which can affect function.
- Is the number of times an item has been reprocessed tracked and controlled? The manufacturer's written instructions should include the number of times the product may safely be reused or sterilized if the item can be reprocessed. The user should ensure that this number is not exceeded. The manufacturer has no control after a product leaves the factory. If the item is not in its original package, pertinent product information may not be immediately available.
- Is the item traceable? Reprocessing of any implantable item, such as synthetic mesh or graft material, should be controlled by lot numbers. The lot number on the product when first obtained from the manufacturer corresponds only with the processes at the point of controlled production. If the product is reprocessed onsite, the lot number is no longer valid because the same controls are not in place for subsequent sterilization. Many variables can alter the safety of the product for reuse. Any patient receiving this implantable material after reprocessing is not getting the same level of care as the first patient for whom it was opened.
- Is the item being charged for twice? How are charges determined? Charging full price for a used item is not ethical.

If in doubt about the appropriateness of a reprocessed item, it should not be reused. With or without written instructions from the manufacturer, the health care facility is liable for product safety, stability, and sterility of any item it processes and sterilizes.

Bibliography

AORN (Association of periOperative Registered Nurse): *AORN standards, recommended practices, and guidelines,* Denver, 2006, The Association.

Cozad A, Jones RD: Disinfection and the prevention of infectious disease, *Am J of Infect Control* 31(4):243-254, 2003.

Camardella E: Cleaning patient care equipment and surfaces, *Infect Control Today* 9(6):50-52, 2005.

Davoren M, Fogarty AM: Ecotoxicological evaluation of the biocidal agents sodium o-phenylphenol, sodium o-benzyl-p-chlorophenol, and sodium p-tertiary amylphenol, *Ecotoxicol Environment Safety* 60(2):203-212, 2005.

Dix K: Chemical selection for cleaning and disinfection, *Infect Control Today* 9(6):26-28, 2005.

Dix K: The ABCs of reprocessing: Educating sterile processing staff, *Infect Control Today* 9(6):42-44, 2005.

Ellis K: Mandatory certification: Raising the CS bar, *Infect Control Today* 9(6):46-48, 2005.

LeTexier RA: Optimum cleaning and disinfecting of surgical instruments, *Infect Control Today* 6(4):14, 2002.

Kimsey J, Barton J: The sterile processing factory goal: 100 percent, *Infect Control Today* 9(4):70-78, 2005.

Meyer B: Approaches to prevention, removal, and killing of biofilms, *Intl Biodeterioration and Biodegradation* 51(4):249-253, 2003.

Muscarella LF: FDA labeling of liquid chemical sterilants: Are modifications needed? *Infect Control Today* (2):50, 2002.

Rudin D: Efficacy against infectious prions in instrument reprocessing, *Infect Control Today* 10(3):16-18, 2006.

Rutala WA, Weber DJ: New disinfection and sterilization methods, *Emerging Infect Dis* 7(2):1-14, 2001.

Rutala WA, Weber DJ: Uses of inorganic hypochlorite (bleach) in healthcare facilities, *Clin Microbiol Rev* 10(4):597-610, 1997.

Chapter 18

Sterilization

CHAPTER OBJECTIVES

After studying this chapter, the learner will be able to:
- Define the term *sterilization*.
- List three methods of sterilization.
- Describe the process for preparing an item for sterilization.
- Identify the primary hazards associated with each type of sterilization.
- Discuss sterilization process monitors.
- Discuss the use of a case cart system.

CHAPTER OUTLINE

KEY TERMS AND DEFINITIONS

Aeration   Warm circulating air is used to remove ethylene oxide sterilant gas from packages in a special chamber.

Bowie-Dick test   Used in a prevacuum sterilizer to test the efficacy of the air removal cycle.

Case cart   System of gathering and delivering instruments and supplies to the perioperative environment. Some models include provision for the return of instruments and contaminated items to the appropriate decontamination area after the surgical or interventional procedure.

Custom packs   Prepackaged collections of disposable supplies, drapes, sponges, and containers prepared by the manufacturer or the distributor according to specific instructions and requests by a particular service at a facility.

Flash sterilization   A rapid method of steam sterilizing properly prepared instruments for immediate use. These instruments are not wrapped. Flash sterilization is not the preferred method of sterilization.

Gravity displacement sterilizer   A steam sterilizer that uses steam in a downward motion to remove air from the sterilizing chamber. Air exits near front l-ower drain. Can be high speed or pulsing.

Indicator   A device used by health care personnel to monitor sterilization exposure conditions. Biologic indicators are the best indicators that parameters are adequate to kill microorganisms. Chemical indicators are not proof of sterility, but they signify that the item was exposed to the parameters necessary for sterilization.

Prevacuum sterilizer   A faster steam sterilizer that removes air by a vacuum before filling the chamber with steam. Also known as dynamic air removal steam sterilization.

Process challenge pack   A prepackaged unit consisting of dense materials and sterilization indicators used to test the effectiveness of the steam sterilizer.

Rigid container   An instrument case that seals and locks. Instruments are placed in a rigid container for sterilization.

Sterile   Microorganisms are at an irreducible minimum.

Sterilization   Processes by which all pathogenic and nonpathogenic microorganisms, including spores, are killed. This term refers only to a process capable of destroying all forms of microbial life, including spores. The sterilizer is a piece of equipment used to attain either physical or chemical sterilization. The agent used must be capable of killing all forms of microorganisms.

Terminal cleaning   Thorough cleaning and disinfection of the perioperative environment at the end of use.

Terminal sterilization   Procedures carried out for the destruction of pathogens at the end of the surgical procedure in the OR or in other areas of patient contact (e.g., postanesthesia care unit [PACU], intensive care unit [ICU], patient care unit).

Turnover   Activity geared toward cleaning and preparation of the operating room between cases for the next patient's arrival.

Wet pack   Internal aspect of the sterile package remains moist or damp after passing through all sterilization parameters. Indicates a nonsterile item.

Wicking   Passage of fluids through a material by passive action. Also referred to as capillary action or strike-through.

SUPPLEMENTAL MATERIAL ON EVOLVE WEBSITE   *evolve*

http://evolve.elsevier.com/BerryKohn
- Content Updates
- Glossary
- Full Set of Perioperative Flash Cards
- Interactive Key Term Flash Cards
- Student Activities
- WebLinks

HISTORICAL BACKGROUND

By the end of the nineteenth century, the concepts of Semmelweis, Pasteur, Lister, Nightingale, Neuber, and others were established to control the operating room (OR) environment. Surgeons had moved out of the front parlors and into hospitals. Disinfectants were used to clean furniture, floors, and walls. Antiseptic solution or green soap was used to clean the skin of patients and members of the perioperative team. The team wore gowns and gloves.

Heat-resistant bacteria were demonstrated in 1876. In the 1880s, sterilization by boiling was introduced. Everything used during a surgical procedure was boiled, including linens, dressings, and gowns. Around 1886, the German surgeon Ernst von Bergmann (1863-1907) and his associates introduced the steam sterilizer, which was a great improvement over his previous method of soaking surgical supplies in bichloride of mercury. Surgeons soon learned that steam under pressure was necessary to raise the temperature sufficiently to kill heat-resistant microorganisms and spores. Vacuum-type pressure sterilizers and dry heat sterilizers followed.

Used as a fumigant for insects in the early twentieth century, ethylene oxide (EO or EtO) was recognized as an antibacterial agent around 1929, when it was used to sterilize imported spices. It has been used as a sterilizing agent in industry and in hospitals since the 1950s, when Dr. Charles Phillips published a series of articles about its effectiveness. Sterilization by irradiation has since been developed and is used for the sterilization of commercially prepared surgical supplies.

Chemical sterilants began with carbolic sprays and mercurial compounds. Although not the method of choice, these products underwent many changes to improve their safety and efficacy. Instruments that could not be heat sterilized posed a problem for the surgeon. Glutaraldehyde, introduced in 1963, was the first chemical solution approved by the Environmental Protection Agency (EPA) as a sterilant for heat-sensitive instruments.

STERILIZATION VERSUS DISINFECTION

Pathogenic microorganisms, as well as those that do not normally invade healthy tissue, are capable of causing infection if introduced mechanically into the body. Standardized procedures that are based on accepted principles and practices are necessary for the sterilization or disinfection of all supplies and equipment used for patient care in the perioperative environment. Following established protocols for instrument processing helps minimize the patient's risk for infection of the surgical site.

A sterile item has been exposed to a sterilization process to render it free of all living microorganisms, including spores. As long as sterility is maintained, this process renders items safe for contact with nonintact tissue and for exposure to the vascular system without transmitting infection. The sterilization process should provide assurance that an item can be expected to be free of known viable pathogenic and nonpathogenic microorganisms, including spores. For items and materials that cannot be sterilized, disinfectants are used to kill as many microorganisms in the environment as possible. (Decontamination and disinfection are described in Chapter 17.)

STERILIZATION

Bacterial spores are the most resistant of all living organisms because of their capacity to withstand external destructive agents. Although the physical or chemical process by which all pathogenic and nonpathogenic microorganisms (including spores) are destroyed is not absolute, supplies and equipment are considered sterile when all parameters have been met during a sterilization process.

Reliability Parameters for Sterilization

Two types of parameters are considered for the reliability of sterilizing methods: product-associated parameters and process-associated parameters.

Product-Associated Parameters

- *Bioburden.* The degree of contamination with microorganisms and organic debris
- *Bioresistance.* Factors such as heat and/or moisture sensitivities and product stability
- *Biostate.* The nutritional, physical, and/or reproductive phase of microorganisms
- *Bioshielding.* Characteristics of the packaging materials
- *Density.* Factors affecting penetration and evacuation of the agent

Process-Associated Parameters

- Temperature
- Humidity/moisture/hydration
- Time
- Purity of the agent and air, and the residual effects or residues
- Saturation/penetration
- Capacity of the sterilizer and the position of items within the chamber

Methods of Sterilization

Reliable sterilization depends on the contact of the sterilizing agent with all surfaces of the item to be sterilized. Selection of the agent used to achieve sterility depends primarily on the nature of the item to be sterilized. The time required to kill spores in the available equipment then becomes critical. Sterilization processes are either physical or chemical, and each method has its advantages and disadvantages. The following are available sterilizing agents (sterilants):

1. Thermal (physical)
   a. Steam under pressure/moist heat
   b. Hot air/dry heat
2. Chemical
   a. Ethylene oxide gas
   b. Formaldehyde gas and solution
   c. Hydrogen peroxide plasma/vapor
   d. Ozone gas
   e. Acetic acid solution
   f. Glutaraldehyde solution
   g. Peracetic acid 0.2% solution
   h. Hypochlorous acid (electrochemical conversion process)
3. Radiation (physical)
   a. Microwave (nonionizing)
   b. X-ray (ionizing)

Sterilization Cycle

The time required to achieve sterilization is referred to as the process cycle, which includes the following:

- Heat up and/or penetration of the agent
- Kill time (i.e., exposure to the agent)
- Safety factor for bioburden
- Evacuation or dissipation of the agent

Monitoring the Sterilization Cycle

To ensure that instruments and supplies are sterile when used, it is essential that the sterilization process be monitored. The general considerations are mentioned in the following sections. Specific tests are discussed later in this chapter with each method of sterilization.

Administrative Monitoring. Work practices are supervised. Written policies and procedures are strictly followed by all personnel responsible for sterilizing and handling sterile supplies. If sterility cannot be achieved or maintained, the system has failed. Policies and procedures pertain to the following:

- Decontaminating, terminally sterilizing, and cleaning all reusable items; disposing of disposable items in the appropriate manner
- Packaging and labeling items
- Loading and unloading the sterilizer
- Operating the sterilizer
- Monitoring and maintaining the records of each cycle
- Adhering to safety precautions and preventive maintenance protocol
- Transporting sterile packages to the sterile storage room. Cart should be enclosed and have a solid bottom
- Storing sterile items
- Handling sterile items ready for use
- Making a sterile transfer to a sterile field at the point of use
- Tracking and recalling items if an item in a particular load is not safe for use

Mechanical Indicators. Sterilizers have gauges, thermometers, timers, recorders, and/or other devices that monitor their functions. Most sterilizers have automatic controls and locking devices, and some have alarm systems that are activated if the sterilizer fails to operate correctly. Records are reviewed and maintained for each cycle. Test packs or special diagnostics are run at least daily, as appropriate for the type of sterilizer, to monitor the functions of each sterilizer. Such tests can identify processing errors.

The manufacturer of the sterilizer provides a manual for the comprehensive care and maintenance of the sterilizing device. Reliable operation depends on the following:

- Routine maintenance that consists of daily inspections and scheduled cleanings per the manufacturer's recommendation. All gaskets, gauges, graph pens, drain screens, paper rolls, ink cartridges, and charting devices should be repaired or replaced by qualified personnel as needed.
- Preventive maintenance (PM) that includes periodic calibration, lubrication, and function checks by qualified personnel on a scheduled basis. Each PM should be documented.

Chemical Indicators. External indicator tape, labels, or paper strips should be clearly visible on the outside of every package to differentiate between sterilized and unsterilized items. The indicator helps monitor the physical conditions within the sterilizer to alert personnel to malfunctions, human errors in packaging, or improper loading of the sterilizer.[1]

An internal indicator/integrator may be placed inside a package in a position most likely to be difficult for the sterilant to penetrate. If a chemical reaction of the indicator does not show the expected results, the item should not be used. Indicators do not establish the sterility of an item; they indicate only that process parameters have been met.

Biologic Indicators. Positive assurance that sterilization conditions have been achieved can be obtained only through a biologic control test. A biologic indicator is a preparation of living spores that are resistant to the sterilizing agent. The preparation may be supplied in a self-contained system (e.g., dry spore strips) or in sealed vials or ampules of spores in suspension.

To perform the test, a biologic unit that has been exposed to the sterilant and an unprocessed biologic unit (control) from the same lot number are incubated for the same period of time. If sterilization has occurred, the processed biologic unit will not grow any microorganisms. The unprocessed biologic control unit will grow microorganisms and display a change in color. If the unprocessed biologic unit fails to grow microorganisms, its spores have been inactivated. In such a case, the processed unit also may have been inactive before processing; thus the biologic test is rendered invalid. The entire load is considered unsterile when either the test indicator or the control is in question. Test indicators and controls should be interpreted by qualified personnel.

Each sterilization process requires biologic testing at regular intervals.[2] Consecutive biologic monitors should be run each time the sterilizer is calibrated, repaired, or relocated. Biologic testing involves incubation according to the manufacturer's recommendations. The bacterial spores used for biologic monitoring and testing intervals include:

- *Bacillus stearothermophilus* at 131° to 140° F (55° to 60° C) tests steam under pressure daily and with each load of implants (also known as *Geobacillus stearothermophilus*).
- *Bacillus subtilis* at 95° to 98.6° F (35° to 37° C) tests dry heat and ethylene oxide with every load.
- *B. subtilis* testing is performed daily for low-temperature hydrogen peroxide plasma.
- Peracetic acid sterilizers are tested according to the manufacturer's recommendations. The user can employ commercial spore strips for use during the cycle but may want to test rinse water as a secondary measure.

A rapid-readout biologic indicator specifically for monitoring a high-speed pressure steam sterilizer with a gravity displacement cycle is based on the fluorometric detection of a *B. stearothermophilus*–bound enzyme rather than on spore

[1]The FDA defines a chemical sterilization indicator as a device used by health care personnel to measure one or more parameters of the sterilization process, 21 CFR §880.2800(b).
[2]The FDA defines a biologic indicator as a device used by health care personnel to measure sterilization effectiveness, 21 CFR §880.2800(a).

growth. The enzyme becomes fluorescent yellow within 60 minutes as the spores are killed.

Biologic indicators need to conform to the testing standards of the United States Pharmacopeia (USP). A control test is performed at least weekly in each sterilizer (Table 18-1). Many hospitals monitor on a daily basis; others test each cycle. Every load of implantable devices is monitored, and the implant should not be used until negative test results are known. All test results are filed in a permanent record for each sterilizer.

ASSEMBLY OF INSTRUMENT SETS

The weight of instruments and density of metal mass is distributed in the tray to allow steam penetration for sterilizing and revaporization for drying. A large tray distributes instruments so they make minimum contact with one another. The size, design, and density of instruments are more important than their weight. The conditions necessary for steam sterilization are difficult to achieve in exceedingly heavy sets. Trays should not be overloaded. To assemble instrument sets for sterilization, the following steps should be performed:

1. Make sure the instruments are thoroughly dry.
2. Unless contraindicated, place an absorbent towel or foam in the bottom of the tray to absorb condensate, as for a rigid container with vacuum valves.
3. Count instruments as they are placed in the tray, and record the number of each type. A preprinted form is often used for this purpose. This form is placed in the tray before wrapping and sterilization so the circulating nurse and scrub person can verify the baseline count. The form can be folded in half and placed in a peel pouch or in a folded towel to prevent ink from transferring to the instruments during processing.
4. Arrange the instruments in a definite pattern to protect them from damage and to facilitate their removal for counting and use. Follow the instrument book or other listing of instruments to be included.

TABLE 18-1 Guidelines for the Use of Chemical and Biologic Indicators*

AAMI	AHA	AORN	CDC	JCAHO
CHEMICAL				
Purpose: To indicate items exposed to the sterilization process; to monitor one or more sterilization parameters; to detect failures in packaging, loading, or sterilizer function. Indicators do not verify sterility.				
Placement				
External: On all packages except if internal indicator is visible. Internal: In center or area least accessible to sterilant within each package	With each package; can be used inside or on outside	External: Visible on every package. Internal: Inside each package	External: Attached to each package. Internal: Inside large pack	With each package, no designation to inside or outside
BIOLOGIC				
Purpose: To document efficacy of sterilization process by killing resistant spores; to ensure that all process parameters are met; to detect nonsterilizing conditions in sterilizer.				
Steam				
Frequency: At least weekly, preferably daily. Placement: Positioned in cold point in test pack, normally bottom front of sterilizer	Frequency: Once a day	Frequency: At least once a week, preferable daily, and with each load of implants	Frequency: At least once a week, and with each load of implants	Frequency: At least weekly (daily is recommended), or with each load if sterilization activities are performed less frequently or if load contains implantable or intravascular material
Ethylene oxide				
Frequency: Every load. Placement: Inside pack in geometric center of load	Frequency: Every load	Frequency: Every load	Frequency: At least once a week, and with each load of implants	Frequency: At least weekly (daily is recommended), or with each load if sterilization activities are performed less frequently or if load contains implantable or intravascular material

*All organizations require that indicators and integrators be used routinely.

5. Place heavy instruments, such as retractors, in the bottom of the tray.
6. Open the hinges and box locks on all hinged instruments.
7. Place ring-handled instruments on stringers or holders designed for this purpose. The curved jaws of hemostatic forceps and clamps should point in the same direction from smallest to largest. Instruments should be grouped by style and classification (e.g., six straight hemostats, six curved hemostats). Do not band instruments together with rubber bands. Steam cannot penetrate through or under the bands to make contact with instrument surfaces.
8. Place sharp and delicate instruments on top of other instruments. They can be separated with an absorbent material or left in a sterilizing rack with the blades and tips suspended. The blades of scissors, other cutting edges, and delicate tips should not touch other instruments. If the instrument has a protective guard, leave it on. Tip-protecting covers or instrument-protecting plastic sleeves should be made of material that is steam-permeable and does not melt or deform with heat.
9. Place concave or cupped instruments with the cupped surfaces down so that water condensate does not collect in them during sterilization and drying.
10. Disassemble all detachable parts. Some parts, such as screws and springs, can be put in a peel pouch that is left open. Sealed pouches may not process correctly during the sterilization process.
11. Separate dissimilar metals. For example, brass knife handles and malleable retractors should be separated from stainless steel instruments. Preferably, put each metal in a separate tray, or separate metals with absorbent material.
12. Place instruments with a lumen, such as a suction tip, in as near a horizontal position as possible. These instruments should be tilted as little as possible to prevent the pooling of water condensate.
13. Distribute weight as evenly as possible in the tray. Some trays have dividers, clips, and pins that attach to the bottom, which help prevent instruments from shifting and keep them in alignment.
14. Wrap the tray, or place it in a rigid container. Check woven textile wrappers for holes or abrasion. Sequentially double-wrap in a woven or nonwoven material, or use a double-thickness wrap in a single-fold configuration.
15. Place a chemical sterilization indicator on the outside wrapper or container. A combined chemical/biologic integrator may also be placed inside the tray.
16. Label the sets appropriately with their intended use (e.g., basic set), the date sterilized, and the control number.

PACKAGING INSTRUMENTS AND OTHER ITEMS FOR STERILIZATION

To be effective, the sterilizing agent must come into direct contact with all surfaces of every instrument. Therefore, instruments must be packaged (individually or in sets) in such a way to allow adequate exposure to the sterilant, to prevent air from being trapped and moisture from being retained during the sterilization process, and to ensure sterile transfer to the sterile field.

The majority of surgical instruments are made of stainless steel and can be sterilized by steam under pressure. Effective steam sterilization involves the direct contact of all surfaces with steam and the revaporization of water condensate to produce a dry, sterile instrument.

Instrument Packaging

For sterilizing and transporting, instruments are put in a closed container or wrapped individually. Instruments placed in open trays are wrapped as sets. Instruments may be sterilized unwrapped in a high-speed pressure sterilizer immediately before use, may be prepared in advance as for a case cart, or may be retained in sterile core storage until needed.

Packaging Considerations. The packaging materials for all methods of sterilization should do the following:
- Permit penetration of the sterilizing agent to achieve sterilization of all items in the package.
- Allow the release of the sterilizing agent at the end of the exposure period and allow adequate drying or aerating.
- Withstand the physical conditions of the sterilizing process.
- Maintain integrity of the package at varying atmospheric and humidity levels. In dry climates or at high altitudes, some packaging materials are susceptible to rupture during sterilization or dry out and crack in storage.
- Provide an impermeable barrier to microorganisms, dust particles, and moisture after sterilization. Items must remain sterile from the time they are removed from the sterilizer until they are used.
- Cover items completely and easily and fasten securely with tape or a heat seal that cannot be resealed after opening. Seal integrity should be tamperproof. A margin of at least 1 inch (2.5 cm) is considered a standard for safety on all sealed packages. Pins, staples, paper clips, or other penetrating objects must never be used to seal packages, because these cannot be removed without destroying the integrity of the package and contaminating the contents. Scissors should not be used to cut off the end of a package. Contents cannot be drawn out over this cut end because the contents would be contaminated by the edge of the packaging material. For the same reason, packages are never torn open below a seal.
- Resist tears and punctures in handling. If accidental tears and holes do occur, they must be visible.
- Permit identification of the contents and evidence of exposure to a sterilizing agent. Chemical indicator tapes or strips on the outside of packages change color during exposure to a sterilization process. They do not indicate sterility, only that the package has been sufficiently exposed to a given parameter to change the color of the indicator. Indicators show that all parameters have been met.
- Be free of toxic ingredients and nonfast dyes.
- Be lint-free or low-linting.
- Protect the contents from physical damage.

- Permit easy removal of the contents with transfer to the sterile field without contamination or delamination (separation into layers).
- Be economical.

Packages should be wrapped far enough away from sterile storage areas so that mixing sterile and nonsterile packages is not possible. Cabinets that contain nonsterile items should be labeled conspicuously. A procedure for sending items to and receiving items from the sterilizer should be set up so that sterile and nonsterile packages can never be confused en route. This procedure must be understood by everyone. External indicator tape or plastic tabs that have darkened stripes or dots demonstrate that the package has passed through the parameters for sterilization.

Packages may be wrapped with nonwoven or woven materials sequentially in two layers. Double-thickness wrapping in one layer without using the sequential method is also acceptable. The wrappers can be stitched around the edges or bonded/fused together. Aseptic presentation to the sterile field is the prime consideration. Each facility should determine which method and material is best suited to the clinical environment.

Items are enclosed with all corners of the wrapper folded in. Either a square or an envelope fold may be used (Figs. 18-1 and 18-2).

- *Sequential wrapping with two wrappers.* An item is wrapped in one wrapper, the package is wrapped in a second wrapper. A cuff turned back on the first fold of each wrapper provides a margin of safety to prevent contamination when opening after sterilization. Packages can be fastened securely with chemical indicator tape.
- *Single wrap.* An item is wrapped in a single wrap that is of double thickness. The package is sealed with chemical indicator tape.

Packaging Materials and Methods. Packaging materials must be compatible with the sterilization process. The following materials may be safely used to wrap items for steam sterilization because they permit steam penetration, adequate air removal, and adequate drying.

Woven Fabrics. Reusable woven fabrics are commonly referred to as muslin or linen. When no other alternative is available, a 140-thread-count, carded, 100% cotton muslin is used. Steam sterilizer cycles are based on a time-temperature profile of 140-thread-count muslin. This type of fabric is not moisture resistant and is used in a double thickness. Two pieces are sewn together on the edges only, with a blind hem and without cross-stitching, so the wrapper is free of holes. This wrapper should withstand between 50 and 75 launderings before becoming too worn to be a microbial barrier. A laundering mark-off system is helpful to monitor the number of times a wrapper has been used. The manufacturer should provide information about the number of launderings and sterilization cycles the wrapper can withstand.

Before resterilization, woven fabrics are laundered to rehydrate them. The moisture content of the woven material affects steam penetration and prevents superheating during the sterilization process. The fabric should be stored at a room temperature of 64° to 72° F (18° to 22° C) and in a relative humidity of 35% to 70%. Before use, the woven fabric is inspected for holes and patched with vulcanized patches if necessary. Fabric may create free-floating lint in the OR.

Nonwoven Fabrics. Nonwoven fabrics are a combination of cellulose and rayon with strands of nylon randomly oriented through it or they are a combination of other natural and synthetic fibers bonded by a method other than weaving. These fabrics have the flexibility and handling qualities of woven materials and are available in several weights. Lightweight is used in four thicknesses; medium weight is the most economical for wrapping items in two thicknesses; and heavy-duty weight is used when a single wrap is used for wrapping supplies for sterilization. Packages are wrapped in the same manner as woven fabrics. Nonwoven fabrics provide an excellent barrier against microorganisms and moisture during storage after sterilization. They are disposable and virtually lint-free. Some manufacturers provide a recycling service for nonwoven wrappers.

Peel Packs or Pouches. Peel pouches and tubes made of a combination of paper on one side and clear plastic film on the other are satisfactory for wrapping single instruments, odd-shaped items, and small items. For sterile presentation, a peel-open seal may be preformed on one end. The open end is either heat sealed or closed with indicator tape after the item is inserted. All air is expressed from the package before sealing. Self-sealing pouches with adhesive flaps that do not require heat sealing also are available.

The sequential packaging of supplies in a smaller pouch into a larger pouch is not routinely necessary. However, this method may be useful for keeping multiple small items together, such as a set of bone screws. The aseptic presentation of tiny parts to the sterile field without dropping items on the floor can be accomplished with sequential packaging. The manufacturer's instructions should be consulted if sequential peel pouches will be used.

Sealants and Labeling. Chemical indicator tape is used to seal packages such as peel pouches and wrapped items. Steam-sensitive tape resembles tan masking tape and reveals dark stripes when exposed to steam sterilizing conditions. Gas-sensitive tape is light green and reveals dark stripes after exposure to gas sterilizing conditions. Peel pouches are usually heat-sealed and have an indicator area or dot that changes color in response to steam or gas exposure. They may be sealed with steam- or gas-sensitive tape. These sealants are not indicators of sterility but are a visual means by which to validate exposure to sterilant conditions.

The sealing tape on the outside of the package should be labeled with a dark marker that is resistant to moisture, bleeding-through, or smearing. Preprinted labels may be used instead. The date of processing and a load number should be attached to each package. These forms of identification are helpful in tracking and locating items that have been processed in batches. A recall of items may be necessary if the sterility of a particular load is in doubt.

Wrapped Trays. To allow steam penetration around instruments and to prevent air from being trapped in the tray, trays cannot be solid. Therefore, instruments are placed in

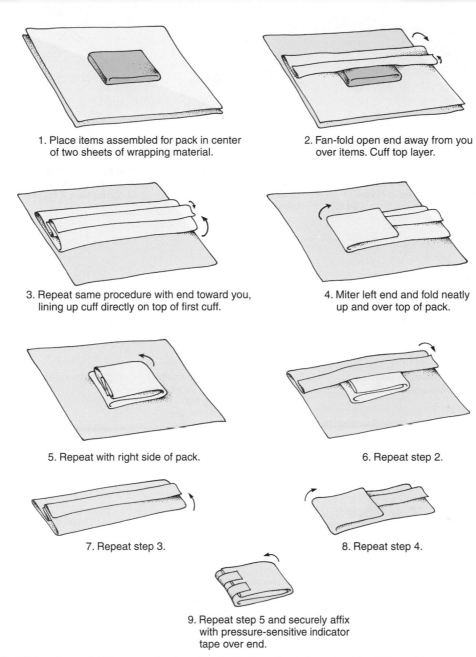

1. Place items assembled for pack in center of two sheets of wrapping material.

2. Fan-fold open end away from you over items. Cuff top layer.

3. Repeat same procedure with end toward you, lining up cuff directly on top of first cuff.

4. Miter left end and fold neatly up and over top of pack.

5. Repeat with right side of pack.

6. Repeat step 2.

7. Repeat step 3.

8. Repeat step 4.

9. Repeat step 5 and securely affix with pressure-sensitive indicator tape over end.

FIG. 18-1   Square fold for wrapping item for sterilization. Single-layer (double-thickness) heavy wrap may be applied in a nonsequential manner.
(Modified from the Association for the Advancement of Medical Instrumentation: *Good hospital practice: Steam sterilization and sterility assurance*, ANSI/AAMI ST46-1993, Arlington, Va, 1993, American National Standards Institute.)

open trays with mesh or perforated bottoms. Absorbent towels or foam may be placed in the bottom of the tray and over instruments to absorb condensate and protect instruments from snagging in the perforations. Trays are sequentially double-wrapped in woven or nonwoven wrappers. They must be allowed to cool and dry at the end of the sterilizing cycle before they are handled.

Rigid Closed Containers. A metal or plastic rigid closed container system may be used for sterilizing instruments singly or in sets. A stainless steel mesh or perforated basket lined with foam porous padding nests in the rigid container. The lid is affixed to the container base by metal snap locks. Plastic break-away shrink bands secure the flip locks and act as chemical external indicators by changing color. The body of the container is labeled with the contents. A load-identifying label is affixed to the container before processing.

Most styles of closed containers have single-use unidirectional air filters in the lid and bottom. These filters are changed each time the container is processed. The closed container is placed into the steam sterilizer so the steam can penetrate through the bottom and lid. Some containers do

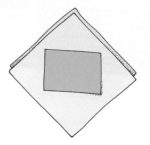

1. Place two wrappers on flat surface with one point toward you. Place item to be wrapped in center of wrapper with its length parallel to you.

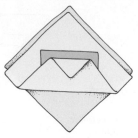

2. Fold corner nearest you over item until it is completely covered. Fold corner back toward you 2 to 3 inches.

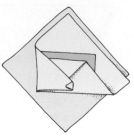

3. Fold left side of wrapper over and parallel to item. Fold end of corner back 2 to 3 inches.

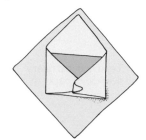

4. Repeat with right side. Lap center folds at least ¹/₂ inch.

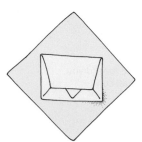

5. Tuck in side edges of remaining corner to eliminate any direct opening to item. Bring top corner down to bottom edges and tuck in, leaving point for opening.

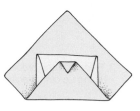

6. Repeat step 2.

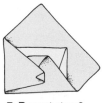

7. Repeat step 3.

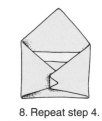

8. Repeat step 4.

9. Bring point of wrapper completely around package and seal with appropriate tape.

FIG. 18-2 Envelope fold for wrapping item for sterilization. Single-layer (double-thickness) heavy wrap may be applied in a nonsequential manner.
(Modified from the Association for the Advancement of Medical Instrumentation: *Good hospital practice: Steam sterilization and sterility assurance*, ANSI/AAMI ST46-1993, Arlington, Va, 1993, American National Standards Institute.)

not have vents in the bottom. The manufacturer of the closed container system should establish the processing temperature and time.

After the sterilization process is complete, the container is placed on a firm, dry surface adjacent to the sterile table. The circulating nurse breaks the shrink band seal by flipping open the locks and then lifts the lid toward himself or herself. The outer rigid container is not considered sterile. The scrub person carefully reaches into the container without touching it and grasps the handles of the sterile inner basket, lifting it straight up and out. The sterile basket containing the instruments can be placed on the sterile back table. Sterile supplies are not to be opened into the rigid container, because the edges are not considered sterile. Condensate in the bottom of the nonvented closed container is considered sterile because it is not permeable to the capillary action associated with other packaging methods.

Specialized Tray Sets. A manufacturer may supply a fitted case or rack for a set of instruments or implants, such as orthopedic devices. These cases or racks help protect the instruments and keep them separated for sterilization and use. These cases or racks are double-wrapped before sterilization; they are not the same as rigid closed containers.

THERMAL STERILIZATION

Heat is a dependable physical agent for the destruction of all forms of microbial life, including spores. It may be used moist or dry. The most reliable and commonly used method of sterilization is steam under pressure.

Steam Under Pressure (Moist Heat Sterilization)

Heat destroys microorganisms, and this process is hastened by the addition of moisture. Steam in itself is inadequate for sterilization. Pressure that is greater than atmospheric pressure is necessary to increase the temperature of steam for the thermal destruction of microbial life. Moist heat in the form of steam under pressure causes the denaturation and coagulation of protein or the enzyme-protein system within cells.

Direct saturated steam contact is the basis of the steam sterilization process. For a specified time and at a required temperature, the steam must penetrate every fiber and reach every surface of the items to be sterilized. When steam enters the sterilizer chamber under pressure, it condenses on contact with cold items. This condensation liberates heat, simultaneously heating and wetting all items in the load and thereby providing the two requisites: moisture and heat. This sterilization process is spoken of in terms of degrees of temperature and time of exposure—not in terms of pounds of pressure. Pressure increases the boiling temperature of water but in itself has no significant effect on microorganisms or steam penetration.

Exposure time depends on the size and contents of the load and the temperature within the sterilizer. At the end of the cycle, revaporation of water condensate must effectively dry contents of the load to maintain sterility; the water is dried from the sterilized pack or item.

The vegetative forms of most microorganisms are killed in a few minutes at temperatures ranging from 130° to 150° F (54° to 65° C); however, certain bacterial spores will withstand a temperature of 240° F (115° C) for more than 3 hours. No living thing can survive direct exposure to saturated steam at 250° F (121° C) for longer than 15 minutes. As the temperature of the steam is increased, the time of exposure may be decreased. A minimum temperature-time relationship is maintained throughout all portions of the load to accomplish effective sterilization. Prions (pronounced *pree-ons*) such as those that cause Creutzfeldt-Jakob disease (CJD) are not a living plant, animal, or virus. They are infectious protein material and must be steam sterilized for a minimum of 1 hour at 270° F (132° C) after soaking in sodium hydroxide at room temperature for 1 hour. If a prevacuum sterilizer is used, the item can be processed for 18 minutes at 274° F (134° C) after the 1-hour exposure to sodium hydroxide.

Advantages of Steam Sterilization

- Steam sterilization is the easiest, safest, and surest method of onsite sterilization. Heat- and moisture-stable items that can be steam sterilized without damage should be processed with this method.
- Steam is the fastest method; its total time cycle is the shortest.
- Steam is the least expensive and most easily supplied agent. It is piped in from the facility's boiler room. An automatic, electrically powered steam generator can be mounted beneath the sterilizer for emergency standby when steam pressure is low.
- Most sterilizers have automatic controls and recording devices that eliminate the human factor from the sterilization process as much as possible when operated and cared for according to the recommendations of the manufacturer.

- Steam leaves no harmful residue. Many items such as stainless steel instruments withstand repeated processing without damage.

Disadvantages of Steam Sterilization

- Precautions must be used in preparing and packaging items, loading and operating the sterilizer, and drying the load.
- Items need to be clean, free of grease and oil, and not sensitive to heat.
- Steam must have direct contact with all areas of an item. It must be able to penetrate packaging material, but the material must be able to maintain sterility.
- The timing of the cycle is adjusted for differences in materials and sizes of loads; these variables are subject to human error.
- Steam may not be pure. Steam purity refers to the amount of solid, liquid, or vapor contamination in steam. Impurities can cause wet or stained packs and stained instruments.

Types of Steam Sterilizers. Sterilizers that are designed to use steam under pressure are often referred to as autoclaves to distinguish them from sterilizers that use other agents. Personnel charged with the responsibility of operating steam sterilizers must fully understand the principles and operation of each type. They must be aware of the problems that cause malfunction, which include attaining the sterilization temperature and maintaining it for the required period of time, trapped air, and dirty traps.

Gravity Displacement Sterilizer. The metal construction of the gravity displacement sterilizer contains two shells (either round or rectangular) that form a jacket and a chamber. Steam fills the jacket that surrounds the chamber. After the door is tightly closed, steam enters the chamber at the back, near the top, and is deflected upward. Air is more than twice as heavy as steam. Thus by gravity, air goes to the bottom and steam floats on top. Steam, entering under pressure and remaining above the air, displaces air downward (both in the chamber and in the wrapped items) and forces it out through a discharge outlet at the bottom front. The air passes through a filtering screen to a waste line. A thermometer located at this outlet below the screen measures the temperature in the chamber. When steam has filled the chamber, it begins to flow past the thermometer (Fig. 18-3). The timing of the sterilizing period starts only when the thermometer reaches the desired temperature.

When air is trapped in the chamber or in wrapped items, the killing power of steam is decreased in direct proportion to the amount of air present. Because the vital discharge of air from the load always occurs in a downward direction, never sideways, all supplies are prepared and arranged to present the least possible resistance to the passage of steam downward through the load from the top of the chamber. Air and steam discharge lines are kept free of dirt, sediment, and lint.

Many gravity displacement steam sterilizers operate on a standard cycle of 250° to 254° F (121° to 123° C) at a pressure of 15 to 18 pounds per square inch (psi). The size and contents of the chamber determine the exposure period; the minimum exposure time is 15 minutes. Exposure time

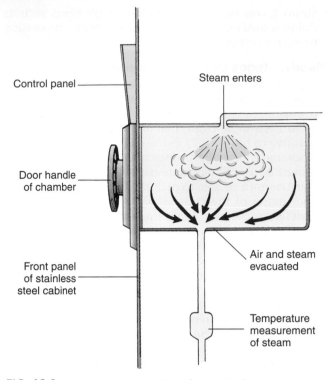

Control panel

Steam enters

Door handle
of chamber

Front panel
of stainless
steel cabinet

Air and steam
evacuated

Temperature
measurement
of steam

FIG. 18-3 Schematic cross section of steam-under-pressure sterilizer. Steam enters at top of chamber to displace air or enters after air is withdrawn by vacuum. Air and steam are evacuated at bottom of chamber. Temperature of steam is measured in air-steam drain line near vent.

the sterilizing steam is admitted. The desired degree of vacuum is achieved by means of a pump and a steam-injector system.

A prevacuum period of 8 to 10 minutes effectively removes the air to minimize the steam penetration time. The steam injector preconditions the load and helps eliminate air from the packages. As a result, the sterilizing steam almost instantly penetrates to the center of the packages when admitted to the chamber, because the air has been vacuum-pumped out. If the items in the load are easily penetrable and the sterilizer is functioning properly, there is no demonstrable time difference between complete steam penetration of large or small and tight or loose packages. Therefore, the maximum capacity of the sterilizer can be used.

A postvacuum cycle draws moisture from the load to shorten the drying time. The Bowie-Dick test is performed daily to ensure that the air vacuum pump is functioning properly.

Temperatures in the prevacuum sterilizer are controlled at 270° to 276° F (132° to 135.5° C) at a pressure of 27 psi. Some prevacuum sterilizers with computer-controlled pulsing air evacuation systems reach temperatures between 275° and 286° F (135° and 141° C). All items are exposed to a temperature of at least 270° F (132° C) for a minimum of 4 minutes. A complete cycle takes approximately 15 to 30 minutes, depending on sterilizer capacity.

Flash/High-Speed Pressure Sterilizer. A flash/high-speed pressure sterilizer may have either a gravity displacement or a prevacuum cycle; the gravity displacement cycle is the most common (Table 18-2). The flash/high-speed pressure sterilizer operates at a pressure of 27 psi at sea level (or a maximum of 22 psi at 5000 feet above sea level) to increase the temperature in the chamber to between 270° and 275° F (132° and 135° C).

The minimum exposure time at this temperature is 3 minutes for unwrapped, nonporous, uncomplicated stainless steel items without lumens. When porous items or instruments with instrument marking tape or lumens are included in the load, timing is increased to 4 minutes or longer in a prevacuum sterilizer and to 10 minutes or longer in a gravity displacement sterilizer.

may vary if a closed sterilization container system is used. Some air-powered instruments may require longer exposure periods at different temperatures. The manufacturer's instructions included with the instrumentation should be consulted for the recommended times and settings for steam sterilization.

Prevacuum Sterilizer. In this high-vacuum sterilizer, air is almost completely evacuated from the chamber before

TABLE 18-2	Flashing Unwrapped Instruments for Immediate Use After Cleaning With Approved Instrument Cleanser		
Item	Gravity Displacement	Prevacuum	Notes
Stainless steel Nonporous No lumens	3 minutes at 270° F (132° C)	3 minutes at 270° F (132° C)	Items must be clean, disassembled, open box locks; 30 pounds per square inch Use chemical indicator
Porous lumens Mixed loads	10 minutes at 270° F (132° C)	4 minutes at 270° F (132° C)	Items must be clean, disassembled, open box locks; 30 lb/psi Lumen should be flushed with water and sterilized wet Use chemical indicator
Complex device Saws or drills	Follow steam and dry times Most require longer times at temperatures between 120° and 32° F (48.9° and 55.6° C)	Follow steam and dry times Most require shorter steam exposure and longer dry times at temperatures between 120° and 132° F (48.9° and 55.6° C)	Refer to manufacturer's recommendations Use chemical indicator

BOX 18-1	Content of Flash Sterilization Record

- Date
- Time
- Patient name or number
- Load contents
- Sterilizer identification number
- Cycle parameters (time, temperature, pressure)
- Indicator verification (chemical and/or biologic)

With these cycles, the entire time for starting, sterilizing, and opening the sterilizer is a minimum of 6 to 7 minutes. The process should be documented for the record (Box 18-1). Steam should be maintained in the jacket at all times.

Flash sterilizers should not be used for routine sterilization of complete instrument sets. Flash sterilization in a high-speed pressure sterilizer should be used only in urgent, unplanned, or emergency situations (e.g., individual items inadvertently dropped or forgotten) for which no alternative method exists. The Association of periOperative Registered Nurses (AORN) indicates that one or more step in the decontamination and sterilization processes may be skipped leading to surgical infection and that all instruments should be thoroughly washed and dried before processing. Closed container flash pans/trays should be used if flashing is unavoidable.[3]

Specially designed surgical suites with in-room sterilizers may provide an acceptable form of flash sterilization. Items to be permanently implanted in the body are not flash sterilized for immediate use unless the results of biologic monitoring are immediately available. Sterility is not ensured without the results of biologic test indicators.

Container systems are available for flash sterilization to protect items during transfer from the sterilizer to the sterile field. The manufacturer of the container should provide scientific evidence of its suitability for the sterilizer in use.

A high-speed pressure sterilizer used for the flash sterilization of unwrapped instruments is physically located in or immediately adjacent to the OR (e.g., the substerile room). A sterile transfer is made from the sterilizer to the sterile field. Transferring the sterilized item to the sterile field without contaminating it is difficult. The following methods may be used for transporting the sterilized instrument to the sterile field:

1. If the OR is connected to the substerile room containing the sterilizer, the sterile scrub person may enter the substerile room, retrieve the sterilized item, and return to the sterile field. The sterile scrub person takes great care not to contaminate his or her gown or gloves in the process. The scrub person uses folded sterile towels for protection from contact burns from the hot tray.

2. The circulating nurse may use a special open flash sterilization tray with a detachable handle. With this method, the tray is sterilized with the instrument inside. The inside of the tray is considered sterile. The outside surface is considered contaminated and is not placed in direct contact with the sterile field. When the cycle is complete, the circulating nurse attaches the nonsterile handle to the outside front of the tray and carries it to the scrub person, who in turn retrieves the sterile item without touching the edges of the tray.

Closed varieties are commercially available that allow an item to be flash sterilized in a covered container. The outside is considered contaminated, but the inside is considered sterile. The circulating nurse removes the lid toward self, touching only the edges. The scrub person reaches inside to remove the sterile item.

Precautions. With all types of steam sterilizers, the following precautions are taken to ensure safe operation:

NOTE: Most steam sterilizers are automatically ready for immediate use. Older models are described for facilities that need additional instruction.

1. Turn on the valve for steam in the jacket before use. Steam may be kept in the jacket throughout the day. (It may be turned off at the end of the surgical schedule if departmental policy indicates this practice.) The jacket maintains heat, so do not touch the inside of the chamber when loading. Check the sterilizer; not all of them have a steam jacket.
2. Never put heat-sensitive items into a steam sterilizer of any type; they will be destroyed.
3. Close the door tightly before activating either the automatic or the manual controls.
4. Unless it is an automatically controlled device, do not set a manually operated timer until the desired temperature registers on the thermometer and recording graphic chart. Thermometers, not pressure gauges, are the guides for sterilization.
5. Open the door only when the exhaust valve registers zero. Stand behind the door and open it slowly to avoid the steam that may escape around the door.
6. Wash the inside of the chamber according to the manufacturer's directions and with manufacturer-approved solution, rinse it with tap water, and dry it with a lint-free cloth every day. Remove and clean the filtering screen daily. Flush the discharge lines weekly with a hot solution of trisodium phosphate: 1 ounce (30 mL) to 1 quart (1000 mL) of hot water. Follow the flush with a rinse of 1 quart (1000 mL) of tap water. Ruhof makes a very efficient descaling cleanser.
7. Wipe the gasket daily with a lint-free cloth, and check for signs of wear and defects.
8. Provide routine preventive maintenance, including the evaluation of steam and air purity. The amount of solid, liquid, or vapor contamination in the steam is minimal. An ineffective air filter may contaminate a load when air is drawn into the chamber at the end of the cycle. A defective steam trap or clogged exhaust line can cause malfunction. Make sure the thermometer is correctly calibrated.

[3]AAMI/CDV-3 ST79 document: Comprehensive guide to steam sterilization and sterility assurance in health care facilities, 2006. This document combines the four previous flash sterilization standards (ST37, ST42, ST46, and ST33).

Preparing Items for Steam Sterilization. For effective steam sterilization, organic material and debris are first removed. Items are thoroughly rinsed and dried after cleaning and before sterilization.

Surgical Instruments. Special attention is given to cleaning surgical instruments before sterilization. Most instruments are made of metal, but many are difficult to clean. Instruments with removable parts should be disassembled, box locks should be opened, and heavy instruments should be placed on the bottom levels of the tray, with lighter instruments on top. The tray contents should be evenly distributed and not exceed the weight set forth by the manufacturer.

Powered Equipment. Powered equipment should be placed in the cases provided by the manufacturer after appropriate decontamination and lubrication.

Basin Sets. If they are nested (placed one inside another), basins and solid utensils are separated ½ inch by porous material, such as toweling. This permits the permeation of steam via wicking around all surfaces and the condensation of steam from the inside during sterilization. Sponges and drapes are not packaged in basins because steam could be deflected from penetrating fabrics. Basin sets should not exceed 7 pounds.

Drape Packs. Freshly laundered woven fabric drapes and gowns are fan-folded or rolled loosely to provide the least possible resistance to the penetration of steam through each layer of material. Packs must not exceed a maximum size of 12 × 12 × 20 inches (30 × 30 × 50 cm) and must not weigh more than 12 pounds (5.5 kg). Drapes are loosely criss-crossed so they do not form a dense, impermeable mass. Pack density should not exceed 7.2 lb/ft (see Box 18-2 for the calculation of density). The inner aspect of the outside wrapper becomes the temporary sterile field when the pack is opened. An impervious sterile barrier drape should be placed on the instrument table before the sterile field is established for the procedure. The drapes are transferred to the table with the impervious barrier drape.

Rubber Goods and Thermoplastics. A rubber or Silastic sheet or any other impervious material should not be folded for sterilization because steam can neither penetrate it nor displace air from the folds. It should be covered with a piece of gauze fabric or toweling of the same size, loosely rolled, and then wrapped. For example, a layer of roller gauze is rolled between layers of an Esmarch bandage.

The mechanical cleaning of tubing, including catheters and drains, is a factor in reducing the microbial count inside the lumen. A residual of distilled water should be left in the lumen of any tubing that is to be steam sterilized by gravity displacement. The residual becomes steam as the temperature rises, which helps displace air in the lumen and increase the temperature within it. (This is not necessary in a prevacuum sterilizer.) The tubing should be coiled without kinks. Keep in mind that disposable tubing is generally preferred because of the complexities associated with cleaning tubing.

Detachable rubber or plastic parts should be removed from instruments and syringes for cleaning and sterilizing. Rubber surfaces should not touch metal, glassware, or each other during sterilization; this prevents melting or sticking and permits steam to reach all surfaces. Rubber bands should not be used around solid items because steam cannot penetrate through or under rubber.

Wood Products. During sterilization, lignocellulose resin (lignin) is driven out of wood by heat. This resin may condense onto other items in the sterilizer and cause reactions if it gets into the tissues of a patient. Therefore, wooden items are individually wrapped and separated from other items in the sterilizer.

Repeated sterilization dries wood so that during sterilization it adsorbs moisture from the saturated steam. As the water content of the saturated steam decreases, the steam becomes superheated and loses some of its sterilizing power. Because of this problem, the use of wood products that require steam sterilization should be minimized, and their repeated sterilization is avoided.

All Items. Whether washed by hand, in a washer-sterilizer or washer-decontaminator, or in an ultrasonic cleaner, all items with detachable or separable parts are disassembled for cleaning, packaging, and sterilizing. Except for perhaps the lumen of tubing, all items are cleaned and dried before steam sterilization. Manuals (which often contain photographs) or index file cards are available in the room in which supplies are packaged; these materials provide ready reference during preparation and for wrapping single items, packs, or trays. Instructions are strictly followed to ensure safety in sterilizing items.

Loading the Sterilizer. All packages are positioned in the chamber to allow free circulation and steam penetration and to prevent the entrapment of air or water. A gravity displacement sterilizer is loaded so that steam can displace air downward and out through the discharge line. Wire mesh or perforated metal shelves separate layers of packages. Shelves may be contained within the chamber on sliding racks or on a transfer carriage. The shelves are loaded and rolled into the sterilizer. Floor loaders are easier to manage than off-floor carriage racks. Steam sterilizers should be loaded as follows:

BOX 18-2	Calculation of Density of Drape Pack

$$\frac{\text{Size of pack (inches)}}{1728 \ (\text{in/ft}^2)} = \text{Cubic feet of pack}$$

$$\frac{\text{Weight of pack (lb)}}{\text{Cubic feet of pack}} = \text{Density factor (lb/ft}^3)$$

Example:

$$\frac{12'' \times 12'' \times 20''}{1728 \ (\text{in/ft}^2)} = 1.666 \ \text{ft}^3$$

$$\frac{12 \ \text{lb}}{1.666 \ \text{ft}^3} = 7.2 \ \text{lb/ft}^3 \ (\text{maximum density})$$

1. Flat packages of textiles are placed on the shelf on edge so flat surfaces are vertical as shown in Figure 8-4. Instrument trays and closed container systems with perforated bottoms may be laid flat.
2. Large packs are placed 2 to 4 inches apart in one layer only on a shelf. Small packages may be placed on the shelf above with 1 or 2 inches between them. If small packages are placed one on top of another, they should be crisscrossed.
3. Packages must not touch the chamber walls, floor, or ceiling.
4. Rubber goods are placed on edge, loosely arranged and in one layer to a shelf; this allows free steam circulation and penetration. No other articles should be with the rubber goods.
5. Basins and solid containers are placed on their sides to allow air to flow out of them. They should be placed so that if they contained water all of it would flow out. If being sterilized in a combined load with fabrics, basins and containers should be placed on the lowest shelf.
6. Solutions are sterilized alone. At the completion of the sterilization cycle, the steam should be turned off and the temperature allowed to decrease to 212° F (100° C) before the exhaust is opened; the selector should be set to slow exhaust. This prevents the solutions from boiling over. Allow the pressure gauge to reach zero before opening the door so caps will not pop off.

Timing the Load. The timing of a sterilization cycle begins when the desired temperature is reached throughout the chamber. If the sterilizer does not have an automatic timing device with a buzzer that sounds at the end of the cycle, a manual timer can be set after the proper temperature has been reached to time the load and to alert personnel when the cycle is completed.

Materials that need different lengths of exposure to ensure sterilization in a gravity displacement sterilizer should not be combined in the same load if the maximum time needed will be destructive to some items. Items may be sterilized either wrapped or unwrapped and either alone or in combination with other items. The time of exposure varies according to these factors and the temperature of the steam. The minimum time standards, which are calculated after effective steam penetration of porous materials and the rate of heat transfer through wrapping materials, are listed in Table 18-3.

Most sterilizers are equipped with a graphic recorder and automatic electromechanical or microcomputer time-temperature controls. Some sterilizers print out a computer record to document each load. The time and temperature for each load are recorded for a 24-hour period. The record of each load should be checked before unloading to be certain that the desired temperature was achieved. Also, the temperature being recorded should be checked daily against the thermometer to see that the recording arm is working properly.

Drying the Load. After the sterilizer door is opened, the load of wrapped packages is left untouched to dry for 15 to 60 minutes. The time required for drying depends on the type of sterilizer and the type of supplies in a load. Large packages require a longer time than small ones. The packages are then unloaded onto a table or cart containing wire mesh shelves padded with absorbent material. Warm packages laid on a solid, cold surface become damp from steam condensation and thus contaminated by strike-through (capillary action).

Packages are observed for water droplets on the exterior or interior and for absorbed moisture in the package. Packs wrapped in moisture-permeable materials that have water droplets on the outside or inside are unsafe for use because the moisture can be a pathway for microbial migration into the package via capillary action. A package should be considered contaminated if it is wet when opened for use. Packages should be completely dry after cooling at a room temperature of 68° to 75° F (20° to 24° C) for a minimum of 1 hour.

Biologic Testing of the Steam Sterilizer. Biologic test packs for steam sterilizers vary according to the type of sterilizer being tested. Each steam sterilizer is tested at least weekly for routine monitoring and as needed for a challenge test. Many hospitals test sterilizers daily. Because of the variations in sterilizers, the appropriate test is used for each type of sterilizer.

Gravity Displacement Sterilizer. With a gravity displacement sterilizer, the test pack is placed on edge in the lower front of the load. This is the coldest area and therefore represents the greatest challenge in sterilization. The chamber is fully loaded. The contents of the test pack may be any of the following:

- The equivalent of three woven fabric gowns, 12 towels, 30 gauze sponges (4 × 4 inches), 5 laparotomy tapes/sponges (12 × 12 inches), and 1 woven fabric drape sheet. Two biologic indicators are placed in the center of the pack, with a chemical indicator placed one towel above or below them. The pack is double-wrapped. It should be approximately 12 × 12 × 20 inches (30 × 30 × 50 cm) and should weigh 10 to 12 pounds.
- The equivalent of 16 freshly laundered reusable huck towels or absorbent towels in good condition, each

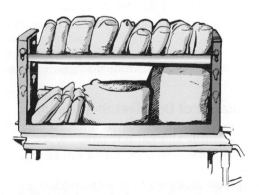

FIG. 18-4 Proper loading of gravity displacement steam sterilizer; packs should be placed on edge, and the rack should not be overloaded. Steam must completely surround and penetrate every package in all sterilizers.

TABLE 18-3	Minimum Exposure Time Standards for Steam Sterilization After Effective Steam Penetration and Heat Transfer		
	Gravity Displacement		**Prevacuum**
Materials	250° F (121° C)	270° F (132° C)	270° F (132° C)
Basin sets, wrapped	20 minutes	Not applicable	4 minutes
Basins, glassware, and utensils, unwrapped	15 minutes	Not recommended	3 minutes
Instruments, with or without other items, wrapped as set in double-thickness wrappers	30 minutes	Not applicable	4 minutes
Instruments, unwrapped but with other items, including towel in bottom of tray or cover over them	20 minutes	10 minutes	4 minutes
Instruments, completely unwrapped	15 minutes	3 minutes	3 minutes
Drape packs, 12 × 12 × 20 inches (30 × 30 × 5 cm) maximum size, 12 lb (5.5 kg) maximum weight	30 minutes*	Not applicable	4 minutes
Fabrics, single items wrapped	30 minutes*	Not applicable	4 minutes
Rubber and thermoplastics, including small items and gloves but excluding tubing, wrapped	20 minutes*	Not applicable	4 minutes
Tubing, wrapped	30 minutes	Not applicable	4 minutes
Tubing, unwrapped	20 minutes	Not applicable	4 minutes
Sponges and dressings, wrapped	30 minutes	Not applicable	4 minutes
Solutions, flask	(Slow exhaust)	Not applicable	Automatic selector determines correct temperature and exposure period for solutions
75-mL flask	20 minutes		
250-mL flask	25 minutes		
500-mL flask	30 minutes		
1000-mL flask	35 minutes		
1500-mL flask	45 minutes		
2000-mL flask	45 minutes		

*Fabrics and rubber more rapidly with repeated sterilization for prolonged periods in gravity displacement sterilizer.

approximately 16 × 26 inches (40 × 66 cm), folded 9 × 9 inches (23 × 23 cm), and stacked with a biologic indicator in the center. The pack is taped to provide a density of 12 lb/ft³, and it should weigh 3 pounds.
• An equivalent commercial test pack.

Prevacuum Sterilizer. With a prevacuum sterilizer, the contents of the test pack with biologic indicators can be the same as for a gravity displacement sterilizer. In addition, a Bowie-Dick test is conducted daily, usually on the first run of the day, to check for air entrapment in the prevacuum sterilizer. A biologic indicator may be put into this test pack. The test pack is placed horizontally on the bottom shelf at the front, near the door, and over the drain of an empty prevacuum chamber. The test pack consists of the following:
• Between 24 and 44 absorbent towels folded in a stack no smaller than 9 × 12 × 11 inches (23 × 30 × 28 cm)
• One Bowie-Dick test sheet placed in the center of the stack
• One double-thickness wrapper

Flash/High-Speed Pressure Sterilizer. For this type of sterilizer, the biologic indicator can be put in the bottom of a tray of unwrapped instruments. It should be positioned in the lower front of the chamber.

Dry Heat Sterilization

Dry heat in the form of hot air is used primarily to sterilize anhydrous oils, petroleum products, and talc, which steam and ethylene oxide gas cannot penetrate. The destruction of microbial life by dry heat is a physical oxidation or slow burning process that involves coagulating the protein in cells. Higher temperatures are required in the absence of moisture because the microorganisms are destroyed through a very slow process of heat absorption by conduction.

Advantages of Dry Heat Sterilization
• Hot air penetrates certain substances that cannot be sterilized by steam sterilization or another method.
• Dry heat is a protective method of sterilizing some delicate, sharp, or cutting-edge instruments. Steam may erode or corrode cutting edges.

Disadvantages of Dry Heat Sterilization
• A long exposure period is required, because hot air penetrates slowly and possibly unevenly.
• The time and temperature required will vary for different substances.
• Overexposure may ruin some substances.

Types of Dry Heat Sterilizers
Mechanical Convection Oven. The most efficient and reliable dry heat sterilizer is an electrically heated, mechanical

convection hot air oven. A blower forces hot air in motion around items in the load to hasten the heating of substances and to ensure a uniform temperature in all areas of the oven.

Early models operated at 320° to 340° F (160° to 171° C) for 1 to 2 hours. Faster portable tabletop models are available; these run at 375° to 400° F (190.5° to 204° C), with total cycle times of 6 minutes for unwrapped items and 12 minutes for wrapped ones. Optional cooling chambers are also available.

Gravity Convection Oven. A conventional gravity displacement steam sterilizer chamber can be used for dry heat sterilization. Heat is provided by steam in the jacket only; this heat may not be evenly distributed throughout the chamber. The hot air rises initially and by gravity displaces cooler air at the bottom of the chamber. The maximum temperature that can be obtained is 250° F (121° C) or 270° F (132° C) in a high-pressure gravity displacement sterilizer. To ensure adequate heat conduction through all items, the exposure period is a minimum of 6 hours and preferably overnight.

Preparing Items for Dry Heat Sterilization

Oils. The amount of oil—including mineral oil and lubricating oil for electrically powered or air-powered instruments—put into a container should not exceed 1 ounce (30 mL). The depth of the oil is preferably not more than 1/4 inch (6.35 mm). The greater the depth, the longer the exposure period.

Talc. A maximum of 5 g to 1 ounce of talc may be spread out in a glass container so the depth of the layer does not exceed 1/4 inch (6.25 mm). The lid is secured, with the cap screwed tightly on the bottle or jar, and a dry heat process chemical indicator is affixed to the bottle. The sterilizing cycle for a gravity convection oven (steam sterilizer with steam in the jacket only) should be a minimum of 9 hours at 250° F (121° C) or 6 hours at 270° F (132° C).

An average quantity of 2 to 3 g of talc is usually needed as an intrapleural sclerosing agent. This smaller quantity may be evenly distributed inside a sealed glassine envelope or peel pouch, which is then inserted into a second envelope or pouch. The talc should not accumulate into a mass exceeding 1/4 inch (6.25 mm); the package should lie flat in the sterilizer. Prepackaged sterile talc is commercially available.

Packaging Materials for Dry Heat Sterilization

Glass. Petri dishes, ointment jars, flasks, small bottles, or test tubes can be used for dry heat sterilization. Caps or lids are affixed or screwed tightly onto containers.

Stainless Steel Boats or Trays. Covers must fit tightly. They can be held in place with indicator tape.

Aluminum Foil. Foil conducts heat rapidly.

Woven Fabric and Peel Pouches. These materials can be used for wrapping instruments if the temperature in the chamber will not exceed 400° F (204° C). Powders and talc can be put in double glassine envelopes.

Loading the Sterilizer. When loading a dry heat sterilizer, it is necessary to allow space between the items and along the chamber walls so the hot air can circulate freely. The chamber is never loaded to full capacity.

Timing the Load. The time of exposure in a dry heat sterilizer varies depending on the characteristics of individual items, the layer depth in containers, and the temperature in the sterilizer. The timing of exposure begins when the thermometer registers the desired temperature. Items are exposed for the following minimum periods, assuming the amount in each container is kept to a minimum and the sterilizer is loaded according to the manufacturer's recommendations:

- 6 minutes at 400° F (204° C), unwrapped
- 12 minutes at 375° F (190.5° C), wrapped
- 1 hour at 340° F (171° C), wrapped or unwrapped
- 2 hours at 320° F (160° C), wrapped or unwrapped
- 3 hours at 285° F (140° C), wrapped or unwrapped
- 6 hours at 250° F (121° C), wrapped or unwrapped

Biologic Testing of the Dry Heat Sterilizer. Biologic indicators with spores of *B. subtilis* are used to monitor the dry heat process. Commercially prepared spore strips in glassine envelopes should be used. Each load should be tested and the items quarantined until negative results are confirmed.

CHEMICAL STERILIZATION

The only chemicals used for sterilization are those that are registered as a sterilant by the EPA. They may be approved for use in either a gaseous, plasma, or liquid state.

Ethylene Oxide Gas Sterilization

Ethylene oxide gas is used to sterilize items that are sensitive to heat or moisture. EO or EtO is a chemical alkylating agent that kills microorganisms (including spores) by interfering with the normal metabolism of protein and reproductive processes, resulting in cell death. Used in the gaseous state, EO must have direct contact with microorganisms on or in the items to be sterilized. The cost is about $7.35 per load.

EO is highly flammable and explosive in air and therefore must be used in an explosion-proof sterilizing chamber in a controlled environment. When handled properly, EO is reliable and safe for sterilization, but the toxic emissions and residues of EO present health hazards to personnel and patients. Therefore, the environment in which EO is used is constantly monitored for unsafe exposure levels. Employee exposure records are required by law to be retained for 30 years.

EO gas sterilization depends on four parameters, each of which may be varied. Consequently, EO sterilization is a complex, multiparameter process. Each variable affects the other dependent parameters:

1. Concentration of EO gas. Liquefied EO is supplied in high-pressure metal cylinders or disposable cartridges. In the sterilization process, air is withdrawn from the chamber and the EO enters as gas under pressure. The only means for controlling EO concentration is to operate the sterilizer according to the manufacturer's instructions. The operating pressure of the cycle influences the rate of gas diffusion through the items to

be sterilized. The absorbency of the items and packaging materials influences the concentration of the gas. EO gas may be diluted or used in pure form:

a. CFC-12, also referred to as 12/88. This is a mixture of 12% ethylene oxide in 88% chlorofluorocarbon (CFC) by weight. Because CFCs cause destruction of the stratospheric ozone shield that protects the earth, 24 nations (including the United States) have signed the Montreal Protocol, agreeing to reduce the production of CFCs. Since 2000, CFCs are no longer produced in the United States.

b. HCFC-124 (trade name: Oxyfume 2000 Sterilant Gas). HCFC-124 can be used in sterilizers that formerly used CFC. Conversion to this replacement gas requires minor changes in the sterilizing pressure and time, and more gas is used than with CFC. Manufacturers of EO gas sterilizers are researching alternative ozone shield–compatible flame retardants that can be used with no or only a minimal change in procedures and equipment. This product will start a phase-out process in 2004, with complete halt to production by 2030 in the United States. European countries have called for its ban by 2003—12 years sooner than originally planned.

c. 100% EO. Unit-dose cartridges of 67 g or 134 g pure EO are used in small self-contained sterilizers. Because pure EO is highly flammable, only a small number of cartridges are kept in inventory.

d. EO/CO_2, referred to as 10/90. This is a mixture of 10% ethylene oxide in 90% carbon dioxide. Because of the great pressure differential between EO and carbon dioxide, maintaining a uniform mix is difficult. A high-pressure cycle must be used, and therefore not all devices can be sterilized safely in this mixture.

2. Temperature. Temperature influences the destruction of microorganisms and affects the permeability of EO through cell walls and packaging materials. Higher density items and loads require a longer heat-up time. As temperature is increased, exposure time can be decreased. Gas sterilizers operate at temperatures ranging from 85° to 145° F (29° to 63° C). The uppermost limit for many heat-sensitive plastic materials is 140° F (60° C). The temperature in the chamber is raised by the injection of saturated steam.

3. Humidity. Moisture is essential in achieving sterility with EO gas. Desiccated or highly dried bacterial spores are resistant to EO gas; they must be hydrated. The moisture content of the immediately surrounding atmosphere and the water content within organisms are important to the action of EO gas. Therefore, to hydrate the items during preparation, the relative humidity of the room in which the items are packaged and held for sterilization should be at least 50% and must not be less than 30%. The ability of the item and packaging material to absorb moisture affects the humidification and diffusion of gas during the sterilization process. A humidity level of 30% to 80% is maintained throughout the cycle; excessive moisture will inhibit sterilization. Saturated steam provides the necessary humidity.

4. Time. The time required for the complete destruction of microorganisms is related primarily to the concentration and temperature of the gas. The cleanliness of items, type of materials, arrangement of load, and rate of penetration also influence exposure time. Drawing an initial vacuum at the start of the cycle aids in penetration of the gas.

Advantages of EO Gas Sterilization

1. EO gas is an effective substitute agent to use with most items that cannot be sterilized by heat, such as plastics with low melting points.

2. EO gas provides an effective method of sterilization for items that steam and moisture may erode; it is non-corrosive and does not damage items.

3. EO gas completely permeates all porous materials; it does not penetrate metal, glass, and petroleum-based lubricants. Whether or not it penetrates oils, liquids, or powder depends on the amount in the containers. If the material is spread thin, the gas will penetrate; it will not go through bulk. EO gas sterilization is not recommended for oils, liquids, and powder (including talc).

   Solutions in glass ampules can be sterilized in EO because the gas does not penetrate glass. But a glass vial with a rubber stopper must not be put in the sterilizer because the gas will penetrate the rubber and may react with the drugs in solution, causing a potentially harmful chemical reaction.

4. Automatic controls preclude human error by establishing proper levels of pressure, temperature, humidity, and gas concentration. The sterilizer is operated according to the manufacturer's instructions.

5. EO gas leaves no film on items.

6. EO gas sterilization is used extensively in the preparation of commercially available, packaged, presterilized items because packaging materials that prolong storage life can be used.

Disadvantages of EO Gas Sterilization

1. EO gas sterilization is a complicated process that is carefully monitored.
   a. An item that can be safely steam sterilized should never be gas sterilized.
   b. Biologic tests, chemical indicators, sterilizer operation, and maintenance records should be reviewed to verify the adequacy of every cycle.
   c. Implants should not be used until the results of biologic testing are known (a minimum of 48 hours).
   d. Items are completely aerated before use to eliminate harmful residues.

2. EO sterilization takes longer than steam sterilization; it is a long, slow process.

3. EO gas requires special, expensive equipment. Gas is somewhat expensive per cycle.

4. Items that absorb EO gas during sterilization, such as rubber, polyethylene, or silicone, require an aeration period (Table 18-4). Air admitted to the sterilizer at the end of the cycle only partially aerates the load.

5. Toxic by-products can be formed in the presence of moisture droplets during the exposure of some plastics, particularly polyvinyl chloride.

TABLE 18-4	Minimum Aeration Times After Ethylene Oxide Sterilization at Different Temperatures		
	Ambient Room Air	Mechanical Aerator	
Materials	**65°-72° F (18°-22° C)**	**122° F (50° C)**	**140° F (60° C)**
Metal and glass			
Unwrapped	May be used immediately		
Wrapped	2 hours	2 hours	2 hours
Rubber for external use—not sealed in plastic	24 hours	8 hours	5 hours
Polyethylene and polypropylene for external use—not sealed in plastic	48 hours	12 hours	8 hours
Plastics except polyvinyl chloride items—not sealed in plastic	96 hours (4 days)	12 hours	8 hours
Polyvinyl chloride	168 hours (7 days)	12 hours	8 hours
Plastic and rubber items—those sealed in plastic and/or those that will come in contact with body tissues	168 hours (7 days)	12 hours	8 hours
Internal pacemaker	504 hours (21 days)	32 hours	24 hours

6. Repeated sterilization can increase the concentration of the total EO residues in porous items. These increased levels can be hazardous unless the gas can be dissipated.

7. EO is a vesicant when in contact with skin and mucous membranes.
   a. Liquid EO may cause serious burns if not removed immediately by thorough washing.
   b. Gloves made of neoprene, polyvinyl fluoride, nitryl or butyl rubber, or other material known to be impermeable to EO penetration should be worn for handling sterilized packages before aeration. If thick cotton gloves are worn, they should be placed in the aerator between uses.
   c. Personnel who wear contact lenses, especially soft lenses, should wear protective goggles when working around EO sterilizers to avoid eye irritation.

8. Inhaled EO gas can be irritating to mucous membranes. It is a colorless gas, but its presence is easily detectable by odor. Overexposure causes nasal and throat irritation. Prolonged exposure may result in nausea, vomiting, dizziness, difficulty breathing, and peripheral paralysis.
   a. Immediately after the completion of each cycle, the sterilizer door should be opened approximately 2 inches and the area cleared of all personnel for 15 minutes before unloading.
   b. Loading carts should be pulled, not pushed, from the sterilizer to the aerator. Air currents flowing over the load may accumulate a residual gas that could be inhaled.

9. Long-term exposure to EO is known to be a potential occupational carcinogen, causing leukemia. It is also a mutagen, causing spontaneous abortion, genetic defects, chromosomal damage, and neurologic dysfunction.
   a. The standards of the Occupational Safety and Health Administration (OSHA) limit an employee's exposure to ethylene oxide to 1 part per million (ppm) of air averaged over an 8-hour period to an active level of 0.5 ppm, and to a short-term limit of 5 ppm averaged over a 15-minute period. These exposure limits are referred to as permissible exposure limits (PELs). The short-term limit addresses exposure to bursts of gas, such as when opening a sterilizer. Breathing zone sampling is performed daily throughout an 8-hour shift on at least one employee for each job classification of exposed personnel. Passive dosimeter badges are the most popular monitoring devices for personnel. Chromographs and other types of detectors are used for continuous gas analysis of the environment.
   b. EO gas is vented from the sterilizer to the outside atmosphere to avoid personnel exposure. Audible and visual alarm systems should be installed to indicate a failure in the ventilation system. Most sterilizers have an exhaust hood over the sterilizer door.
   c. The sterilizer door has locking and sealing mechanisms. The integrity of the seals is checked regularly. Automatic controls must function properly so the door cannot be opened until the gas is evacuated from the chamber.

Types of EO Gas Sterilizers. The capacity of EO chambers varies from approximately 2 ft (57.5 L) in a tabletop size of 12 × 12 × 24 inches (30 × 30 × 60 cm) to very large floor-loading units that are 28 × 67 × 78 inches (72 × 180 × 198 cm). These chambers automatically control gas concentration, temperature, humidity, and time. Most models have vacuum pumps to evacuate air from the chamber and steam ejectors to humidify and increase temperature. Microcomputer controls and digital printouts of cycle parameters provide evidence of proper operation. A purge cycle follows the timed gas-exposure cycle to vent the chamber of airborne residual gas. Some chambers are a combination sterilizer/aerator, which eliminates the need for personnel to handle the load immediately after sterilization; the load is removed only after aeration.

Preparing Items for EO Gas Sterilization

All Items. All items to be sterilized with EO gas are thoroughly cleaned and dried. Detachable parts are disassembled, and syringes are separated. Impermeable items such as caps, plugs, and stylets are removed. All items must be completely dry.

Lumens. Any tubing or other item with a lumen should be blown out with air to force it dry before packaging, because water combines with EO gas to form ethylene glycol, a harmful acid that causes hemolysis of red blood cells in the patient.

Lensed Instruments. Endoscopes with cemented optical lenses require special cement for EO gas sterilization.

Lubricated Instruments. All traces of lubricant, especially petroleum-based lubricants, should be removed before sterilization. EO cannot permeate the film of the lubricant.

Cameras. As a permanent record or teaching aid, photographs are sometimes taken at the surgical site with a sterile, specially constructed camera. Some cameras and film can be sterilized with EO gas. The film is loaded before packaging for sterilization.

Packaging Materials for EO Gas Sterilization.

The type and thickness of the wrapper, the size and shape of the package, and the porosity of the contents used influence the time it takes for the EO gas to penetrate. Items wrapped for EO gas sterilization should be tagged for gas to prevent them from being inadvertently steam sterilized and damaged. Materials used for wrapping items are permeable to EO gas and water vapor and allow effective aeration. The materials discussed in the following sections are acceptable.

Woven Fabric. Reusable double-thickness woven fabrics are used as they are for steam, with the same advantages and disadvantages.

Nonwoven Fabric. Tyvek spunbonded olefin and other high-density polyethylene fabrics are highly permeable to EO and moisture. These single-use disposable wrappers offer the same advantages as the nonwoven fabrics described for use in steam, but not all of them can be used interchangeably; the cellulose/nylon/rayon combination should be used only for steam sterilization. Packages should be sequentially single-wrapped or double-wrapped or the material used according to the manufacturer's recommendations.

Peel Packs and Pouches.

Double-wrapping may not allow adequate penetration of the gas and moisture. Peel pouches with either coated or uncoated paper on one side and coated Mylar on the other are generally acceptable for most gas sterilizers, and they allow visualization of contents. The manufacturer's instructions should be checked.

Materials not to be used for EO sterilization because of inadequate permeability include nylon, polyvinyl chloride film, saran, polyester, polyvinyl alcohol, cellophane, and aluminum foil. Combinations of materials that make a package insufficiently permeable for adequate humidification, gas penetration, and aeration are avoided.

Loading the Sterilizer.

All packages are positioned in the chamber to allow free circulation and penetration of gas. Overloading creates conditions that can slow the penetration of EO gas, moisture, and heat. Air space should be provided between the chamber ceiling and the uppermost packages in the load, and packages should not touch the chamber walls and floor. Packages should not be stacked tightly; space is allowed between them. If paper or plastic pouches are used, the packages are placed on edge, with the plastic side of one facing the paper side of another.

Timing the Load.

The timing of the EO cycle varies depending on the size of the chamber, the contents of the load, gas concentration, temperature, and humidity. For example, a cool cycle at 99° F (37° C) may require more than 5 hours, whereas the same load at 131° F (55° C) may take less than 3 hours. The instructions provided by the manufacturer of the sterilizer should be followed closely.

Aerating Items After EO Gas Sterilization.

EO gas exerts toxic effects on living tissue. Therefore after EO gas sterilization, adequate aeration is absolutely essential for all absorbent materials that will come into contact with skin or tissues, either directly or indirectly. Residual products after sterilization can include the following:

1. *Ethylene oxide.* Porous materials, such as plastic, silicone, rubber, wood, and leather, absorb a certain amount of gas that must be removed. The thicker the walls of items, the longer the aeration time required. Residual EO gas in plastic tubing or in parts of a heart-lung pump oxygenator causes hemolysis of blood. Rubber gloves or shoes worn immediately after exposure can cause irritation or burns on skin. The following are acceptable limits for residual EO:
   a. 25 ppm for blood dialysis units, blood oxygenators, heart-lung machines, and all implants
   b. 250 ppm for all topical medical devices
2. *Ethylene glycol.* Ethylene glycol is formed by a reaction of EO gas with water or moisture; this reaction leaves a clear or brownish oily film on exposed surfaces. This substance causes hemolysis of the red blood cells. It also can cause irritation to the mucous membranes if left on plastic or rubber endotracheal tubes or airways. The following are acceptable limits of ethylene glycol:
   a. 250 ppm for blood dialysis units, blood oxygenators, heart-lung machines, and all implants
   b. 1000 ppm for all topical medical devices
3. *Ethylene chlorohydrin.* This by-product is formed when a chloride ion is present to combine with EO, such as in polyvinyl chloride plastic. Rubber, soft nylon, and polyethylene items that have been in contact with saline solution or blood can retain enough chloride ions to cause this reaction in the presence of moisture. To avoid this hazard, disposable products should be discarded after use. The following are acceptable limits of ethylene chlorohydrin:
   a. 25 ppm for blood dialysis units, blood oxygenators, heart-lung machines, and all implants
   b. 250 ppm for all topical medical devices

Residuals are expressed as the weight of EO gas remaining in the item divided by the weight of the item. For example, 25 ppm in a device weighing 2500 g (approximately 5.5 pounds) equals 0.01 mg of EO. Residues cannot be removed by rinsing items in water or liquids.

To purge residual gas, air is admitted into the chamber at the end of the sterilization cycle. In sterilizers with a pulse-purge cycle, the air is admitted and immediately removed as many as six times in 30 minutes. Additional aeration is required for all wrapped and porous items. Aeration to diffuse any residual products may be accomplished with ambient (room) air or preferably with an aerator chamber designed for this purpose.

Manufacturers of products suitable for EO sterilization should provide written instructions for the sterilizing cycle and for aerating. The available recommendations are followed. Polyvinyl chloride is one of the most difficult materials to aerate. If the composition of an item is not known, the minimum time for polyvinyl chloride should be followed (see Table 18-4). Aeration time depends on the following:

- Composition, density, porosity, weight, and configuration of the item
- Packaging material
- Sterilizing conditions, such as the size of the load, the nature of the items in it, and variable required factors
- Aeration conditions, such as ambient versus mechanical airflow and temperature
- Acceptable limits of residual products for the intended use of the item, such as external application or internal implantation

Aeration at an elevated temperature enhances the dissipation rate of absorbed gas, which results in faster removal. The entire load on the sterilizer carriage can be transferred into an aerator. A blower system draws air in from the outside to the heater in the upper part of the chamber to maintain a minimum rate of four air exchanges per minute. The aerator is vented to the outside atmosphere. Items cannot be safely used until they have been completely aerated.

All materials remain in the aerator for 8 hours at 140° F (60° C) to 12 hours at 120° F (50° C) or longer, depending on temperature and the instructions of the manufacturer of the aerator or item. In a combination sterilizer/aerator, aeration time varies according to temperature and airflow (e.g., 12 hours at 130° F [55° C] or 32 hours at 100° F [38° C]).

If an aerator is not available, packages may be moved on a cart or in a basket from the sterilizer into a well-ventilated clean storage area that has at least 10 air exchanges per hour. The cart should be pulled, not pushed, to this area to avoid being downwind of the EO gas adhering to the wrappers. Aeration time is prominently noted on the cart or basket. At a room temperature controlled between 65° and 72° F (18° and 22° C), a minimum aeration time of 168 hours (7 days) is required for polyvinyl chloride and plastic and rubber items sealed in plastic packages and for porous items that:

1. Come into direct contact with blood
2. Are implanted, inserted, or applied to body tissues
3. Are used for assisted respiration

Unwrapped, nonporous metal and glass may be handled immediately. Wrapped metal should be aerated for at least 2 hours. Intravenous or irrigation fluids in plastic containers must not be stored in a room where gas-sterilized items are aerating, because the residual diffusing gas could be absorbed through the plastic.

Biologic Testing of the EO Gas Sterilizer. Biologic indicators carrying spores of *B. subtilis* are used to monitor EO gas sterilizers. Each sterilizer is tested in each load. Every load containing implantable devices should be tested. An implant should not be used until the test results are negative. The manufacturer's recommendations should be followed for the use of biologic test packs for EO gas sterilizers.

Hydrogen Peroxide Plasma Sterilization

Hydrogen peroxide can be activated to create a reactive plasma. Plasma has been described as the fourth state of matter, being not a liquid, gas, or solid. It can be produced through the action of either a strong electrical or magnetic field, somewhat like a neon light. The cloud of plasma created consists of ions, electrons, and neutral atomic particles that produce a visible pink glow. Free radicals of the hydrogen peroxide in the cloud interact with cell membranes, enzymes, or nucleic acids to disrupt the life functions of microorganisms. The plasma and vapor phases of hydrogen peroxide are highly sporicidal, even at a low concentration and temperature. The sterilizer chambers are simple in design, but the process of the sterilization cycle differs with the method used to convert hydrogen peroxide into plasma or vapor. Plasma technology uses an oxidation process that can be corrosive to some polymers and adhesives. This can cause problems with some lensed instruments.

This method is used for sterilization of metal and nonmetal surgical devices at low temperatures in a dry environment. This method works well for instruments that have diffusion-restricted spaces, such as box locks on clamps. Instruments with lumens have specific requirements:

- Metallic or nonmetallic instruments with lumens of 6 mm or larger and lengths of 310 mm or shorter can be processed.
- Stainless lumens larger than 3 mm and shorter than 400 mm are safely processed.

Advantages of Hydrogen Peroxide Sterilization

- The process is dry and nontoxic.
- The by-products of oxygen and water vapor are safely evacuated into the room atmosphere.
- Aeration is not necessary.
- A low temperature allows the safe sterilization of some heat-sensitive items.
- Plasma has significantly less effect on metal than does steam sterilization; corrosion does not occur on moisture-sensitive microsurgical and powered instruments.
- The sterilizer is simple in design and connects to standard electrical outlets.

Disadvantages of Hydrogen Peroxide Sterilization

- Metal trays block radiofrequency waves and cannot be used.
- Hydrogen peroxide is not compatible with cellulose (i.e., woven textiles with cotton fibers and paper products). This causes a decrease in the sterilant concentration by absorbing the vapors.
- Nylon becomes brittle after repeated exposure to hydrogen peroxide sterilization.
- This method is not approved in the United States for use with flexible endoscopes with lumens.

Low-Temperature Gas Plasma Sterilizers

STERRAD by Advanced Sterilization Products. This sterilizer connects to a standard electrical outlet. The supplies are placed in the chamber, and a strong vacuum is created. A solution of water and 58% hydrogen peroxide is vaporized by radiofrequency energy to create a pink, glowing reactive plasma. The reactive particles in the plasma are maintained at 104° F (40° C) and sterilize the heat- and moisture-sensitive load in approximately 1 hour. No aeration is necessary because the by-product is primarily oxygen and water. The cycle will automatically abort if the sterilant concentration is not adequate.

Vapor Phase Sterilizer. A vacuum is created in the chamber for delivery of a cold vapor of hydrogen peroxide at 39° to 46° F (4° to 8° C). A vacuum exhausts vapor at the end of the cycle. The cost to run is about $8 per load.[4]

Considerations for Hydrogen Peroxide Sterilization

- All items are thoroughly clean, free of organic debris, and dry.
- Items are wrapped in nonwoven polypropylene. Tyvek peel pouches may be used.
- Trays are placed flat on the shelf for penetration. Peel pouches are stood on the side. Nothing should rest on the walls of the chamber.
- The timing of the cycle varies with the process, capacity of the chamber, and contents of the load. The manufacturer's instructions are followed. May take more than 75 minutes to run a load.
- Biologic indicators with spores of *B. subtilis var. niger* are used to monitor the hydrogen peroxide process.

Ozone Gas Sterilization

Ozone sterilizes by oxidation, a process that destroys organic and inorganic matter. It penetrates the membrane of cells, causing them to explode. Ozone has been used to purify water since the early twentieth century. Ozone is a metastable gas that can be generated easily from oxygen and water at the point of use. No special outlet or water supply is required. No special cartridges or canisters of a chemical are needed. This is a low-temperature method of sterilization that has been in use in industry for more than 100 years.

Safety of ozone gas exposure is measured in permissible exposure limits (PELs). OSHA has set limits as 0.1 ppm per 8-hour period. The PEL is not to exceed 0.3 ppm/15 minutes. Severe pulmonary edema will result at levels of 0.3 ppm exposure for 30 minutes. Personnel using ozone sterilization do not encounter the gas in its intact state. The gas is converted back to water and oxygen at the end of the cycle before the unit can be opened. There is only one setting for all cycles, so the risk for error in operating the machine is minimized.

The FDA has cleared ozone sterilizers for use on plastic, metal and some rigid lumens.[5] Cellulose packaging cannot be used. Nonwoven pouches or vented closed container systems are used for instrumentation in ozone sterilizers.

The 125L ozone sterilizing machine was developed in Canada and approved for sale in 2005. Skytron will be marketing the unit in the United States. (More information can be found at www.tso3.com.)

The ozone sterilizer works in four phases over a period of 4.5 hours:

- Cold water vapor is humidified. About 75 mL per load O_2 is electrically charged to create O_3, which is ozone. Ozone has a bluish color.
- The water vapor and O_3 combine in the chamber. One oxygen atom is released from the O_3 molecule to combine with and deactivate microorganisms.
- The water vapor, ozone, and free oxygen molecule are vented into a catalytic converter that separates out the water and oxygen (H_2O and O_2) for discharge into the drain and room air.

Advantages of Ozone Gas Sterilization

- The sterilizer generates its own agent using hospital-grade oxygen, water, and the electrical supply. It is simple and inexpensive to operate. The cost is less than $1 per load.
- Ozone gas sterilization provides an alternative to EO gas sterilization of many heat- and moisture-sensitive items.
- Ozone gas sterilization does not affect anodized aluminum, titanium, chromium, silicone, neoprene, and Teflon.
- Aeration is not necessary; ozone leaves no residue and converts to oxygen in a short time.
- Low temperature is safer for heat sensitive instrumentation.

Disadvantages of Ozone Gas Sterilization

- Ozone can be corrosive. It will oxidize steel, iron, brass, bronze, zinc, nickel, and copper.
- It destroys natural rubber, such as latex, natural fibers, and some plastics.
- Not used to sterilize implants or flexible endoscopes at this time.
- Not used to sterilize sealed glass ampules.
- Each cycle takes 4.5 hours.
- Pure ozone damages proteins and fatty acids and is harmful if inhaled in its intact state.

Considerations for Ozone Sterilization. Preparing items, packaging, loading the sterilizer, and timing the cycle are done according to the instructions provided by the manufacturer of the sterilizer. *B. stearothermophilus* biologic indicator challenge packs (also known as *Geobacillus stearothermophilus*) are used to monitor the process and are recommended for each cycle. Prion destruction studies in process are promising because the protein oxidation properties of ozone have been successful in the presence of brain tissue testing.[6] (A comprehensive self-study module on ozone technology can be found online at www.continuinged.purdue.edu/iahcsmm/pdf/Lesson83.pdf.)

Chemical Sterilants in Solution

Liquid chemical agents registered as sterilants by the EPA provide an alternative method for sterilizing minimally invasive heat-sensitive items if a gas or plasma sterilizer is not available or if the aeration period makes EO gas sterilization impractical. Items are categorized as critical, semicritical, and noncritical according to the risk of infection to the

---

[4]www.devicelink.com/mddi/archive/04/01/027.html.
[5]Lumens tested included lengths of 25 to 60 cm. Diameters tested were 2 to 4 mm.

[6]Refer to ozone sterilization white paper at www.tso3.com for study results.

patient. Items that enter tissue or the vascular system are considered critical and should be sterile. Items are sterilized with a liquid sterilant by immersing them in solution for the required time specified by the manufacturer to be sporicidal (i.e., to kill spores). All chemical solutions have advantages and disadvantages, and each sterilant has specific assets and limitations. (Additional information is available at www.fda.gov.)

Advantages of Chemical Sterilants

* The solution has a low surface tension; it penetrates into crevices and is readily rinsed from items.
* It is noncorrosive, nonstaining, and safe for instruments that can be immersed in a chemical solution.
* It does not damage lenses or cement on lensed endoscopes.
* It is not absorbed by rubber or plastic.
* It has low volatility and is stable for the time specified by the manufacturer.

Disadvantages of Chemical Sterilants

* Prolonged exposure to a chemical sterilant may be necessary for sterilization.
* Some chemical sterilants have hazardous effects associated with exposure.
* Even if a chemical has low toxicity and irritation, items must be thoroughly rinsed in sterile distilled water before use.
* Failure to adequately rinse an endoscope can cause a chemically induced colitis.
* Sterile transfer is difficult, because items are wet.
* Chemically sterilized items cannot be held in long-term sterile storage.
* The solution can become diluted during use if an item is wet when placed in it.

Types of Chemical Sterilants. In addition to EPA registration, chemical sterilants are approved by the U.S. Food and Drug Administration (FDA) as a method of sterilization for critical items that are heat sensitive and can be immersed. The manufacturer is responsible for providing processing instructions on the container label, and the user is obligated to follow the instructions.

Acetic Acid. Acetic acid mixed with a solution of salts (Bionox) kills microorganisms by a process of oxidation to denature proteins. The process takes 20 minutes at a room temperature of 77° F (25° C). The solution is supplied in unit doses for each cycle.

Formaldehyde. A 37% aqueous solution (formalin) or 8% formaldehyde in 70% isopropyl alcohol kills microorganisms by coagulating protein in the cells. The solution is effective at room temperature. Formaldehyde has a pungent odor and is irritating to the eyes and nasal passages. Its vapors can be toxic.

Glutaraldehyde. According to the FDA, a 2.4%, 2.5%, or 3.4% aqueous solution of activated buffered alkaline glutaraldehyde kills microorganisms by the denaturation of protein in cells. The solution is activated by adding a powdered buffer to the liquid. Alkaline glutaraldehyde solu-

tion changes pH and gradually loses its effectiveness after the date of activation. The expiration date specified by the manufacturer is marked on the container when activated (e.g., 14 or 28 days for aqueous Cidex–activated dialdehyde solution). The solution is reusable until this date, after which it is discarded according to EPA requirements. In most locales it may be discarded into the sanitary sewer, where it is bioxidized by sewer microorganisms into glutaric acid and then into carbon dioxide and water.

Most manufacturers claim that glutaraldehyde is a sterilant at 10 hours and a high-level disinfectant at 25 to 30 minutes, although the long-life varieties require 90 minutes to attain the same level of disinfection. These solutions are effective at a room temperature of 77° F (25° C).

Glutaraldehyde vaporizes rapidly and must remain covered to retain its concentration parameters. The fumes may have a mild odor and can be irritating to the eyes, nose, and throat. OSHA has established an exposure limit of 0.2 ppm in room air averaged over 8 hours. A glutaraldehyde exposure monitor should be worn by personnel who are at risk. Nitrile or butyl rubber or polyethylene gloves are worn to prevent skin sensitivity and contact dermatitis. Double-gloving with latex provides protection. Neoprene and polyvinyl chloride gloves are not protective.

The concentration of glutaraldehyde in solution should be monitored. A test strip or kit of reagents is used for testing the concentration before and after each use. If the solution has become diluted below 1.5%, it is ineffective and should be discarded.

Peracetic Acid. A proprietary (STERIS) chemical formulation of 35% peracetic acid, hydrogen peroxide, and water inactivates critical microbial cell systems. Peracetic acid is an acetic acid plus an extra oxygen atom that reacts with most cellular components to cause cell death. The mechanism may vary with each type of cell (e.g., vegetative bacterial spores, mycobacterium). The sterilant is supplied in unit doses for each cycle and is diluted during the sterilization process to 0.2% peracetic acid solution. During the 20- to 30-minute sterilization process, the solution is heated to 122° to 131° F (50° to 55° C) as it passes through the self-contained processing chamber. All items and internal components of the STERIS unit are submerged in the heated sterilant.

On completion of the sterilizing cycle, the sterilant is discharged into the sanitary drain. The used chemical is not considered a hazardous material by the EPA. The instruments are automatically rinsed in tap water that is filtered through two external prefilters and a 0.22-mm internal microfiltration system. The smallest known bacterium, *Pseudomonas diminuta,* is unable to pass through the pores in this filter system. (This is the same method used by pharmaceutical manufacturers to make sterile injectable medications.)

The STERIS unit uses a standard tap water supply, a sanitary drain, and a 110-volt electrical connection. This tabletop unit has a printout to document each cycle. Periodic maintenance includes filter changes based on the chemical components of the external water supply. Biologic monitoring according to the manufacturer's recommendation is performed daily with a commercially prepared spore strip containing *B. subtilis* or *B. stearothermophilus.*

Hypochlorous Acid. Hypochlorous acid is derived from electrochemical activation of a brine solution. Although technically a high-level disinfectant (HLD), it kills many spores on well-cleaned endoscopes and other heat-sensitive items. This technique was approved in late 2002 by the FDA. Sterilox liquid chemical HLD system is nontoxic and environmentally safe. The 10-minute process is a single-use design that requires a base unit with inflows of water and electricity that connects to an endoscope processor. Salt tablets (400 grain) and a water conditioner are added at the beginning of the cycle. No special handling or precautions are required.

Containers for Chemical Sterilant in Solution. A large bin with a perforated inner tray (nested) and lid is used with chemical sterilant solutions at room temperature. With chemical sterilization, items are completely immersed and the lumens filled with sterilant solution. The outside of the bin is labeled with the product name, date of activation, date of expiration, and initials of the person who mixed the solution. The inside of the bin, inner tray, and its lid should be kept sterile throughout the duration of use of that batch of solution. The lid should remain on the bin to prevent evaporation of the solution and to minimize vaporization of the solution. Evaporation changes the concentration of the mix and will alter the sterilant properties. Formaldehyde and glutaraldehyde solutions are used in a well-ventilated room.

Preparing Items for Sterilization by Chemical Immersion. Items should be clean and free of organic debris and blood. Items should be washed thoroughly in a nonfilming soapy solution, rinsed, and thoroughly dried before placing them in the chemical sterilant. Lumens should be dried with jets of forced air. The solution will become diluted and lose effectiveness if other solutions such as water are added. No biologic material should be permitted to contaminate the solution.

Timing the Immersion Cycle. The time required for sterilization varies with the sporicidal activity of the chemical agent. The FDA has published a chart with brand names and timetables on the Internet. Below is an example of chemical sterilants and time ranges:

- Acetic acid (20 minutes at 77° F [25° C] in a processing unit)
- Glutaraldehyde (10 to 12 hours at 77° F [25° C]; concentrations of 1.12% to 3.4%; specialized processors using glutaraldehyde 2.5% take 7 hours and 40 minutes at 95° F [35° C])
- Hydrogen peroxide 1% to 7.5% (3 to 8 hours at 68° F [20° C])
- Peracetic acid (12 minutes at 122° to 132° F [50° to 56° C])

A load control record of the items sterilized in solution is kept as for other methods of sterilization (see the sample record in Box 18-1).

Rinsing After Immersion. At the completion of the exposure period, all items are thoroughly rinsed in sterile distilled water before use. This step is automatic with the STERIS

unit and other automatic endoscope processors. Sterile gloves are worn to transfer items from the chemical sterilant solution bin to a second sterile bin for rinsing. Items should then be dried with a sterile towel before being transferred to or placed on a sterile field. Items being terminally sterilized should be completely dry before placing in storage. Flexible endoscopes should be hung from a rack so the lumens are in a straight configuration—not coiled.

RADIATION STERILIZATION
Microwave Sterilization
The nonionizing radiation of microwaves produces hyperthermic conditions that disrupt life processes. This heating action affects water molecules and interferes with cell membranes. Microwave sterilization uses low-pressure steam with the nonionizing radiation to produce the localized heat that kills microorganisms. The temperature is lower than conventional steam, and the cycle is faster—as short as 30 seconds. Metal instruments can be sterilized if placed under a partial vacuum in a glass container. Small tabletop units may be useful for rapid sterilization of a single instrument or a small number of instruments. Current models have a small chamber size—1 to 3 ft^3.

Gamma Ray and Beta Particle Sterilization
Some commercially available products are sterilized by irradiation. Ionizing radiation produces ions by knocking electrons out of atoms. These electrons are knocked out so violently that they strike an adjacent atom and either attach themselves to it or dislodge an electron from the second atom. The ionic energy that results becomes converted to thermal and chemical energy. This energy kills microorganisms by disrupting the deoxyribonucleic acid (DNA) molecule, thus preventing cellular division and the propagation of biologic life.

The principal sources of ionizing radiation are beta particles and gamma rays. Beta particles are free electrons and are transmitted through a high-voltage electron beam from a linear accelerator. These high-energy free electrons penetrate matter before being stopped by collisions with other atoms. Thus their usefulness in sterilizing an object is limited by the density and thickness of the object and by the energy of the electrons. They produce their effect by ionizing the atoms they hit, producing secondary electrons that in turn produce lethal effects on microorganisms.

Cobalt-60 is a radioactive isotope capable of disintegrating to produce gamma rays and is the most commonly used source for irradiation sterilization. Gamma rays are electromagnetic waves and have the capability of penetrating to a much greater distance than do beta particles before losing their energy from collisions. Because they travel at the speed of light, they must pass through a thickness of several feet before making sufficient collisions to lose all of their energy.

Irradiation sterilization with beta particles or gamma rays is limited to industrial use. Depending on the strength of the source, the product is exposed to radiation for 10 to 20 hours. Ionizing radiation penetrates most materials to sterilize reliably. However, the physical properties of some materials are altered by exposure to ionizing radiation, thus limiting its use. Irradiation can be used to sterilize heat- and moisture-sensitive items because the rays have a very low temperature effect on materials and because the process is dry. Because gamma rays can penetrate large bulky objects, cartons ready for shipment can be sterilized in the cobalt-60 irradiator; this is cost-effective for the manufacturer.

Ionizing radiation is the most effective sterilization method. No residual radiation is generated. The process may be monitored with biologic indicators using *Bacillus pumilus*. However, products can be released for use on the basis of dosimetry (measurements of radiation dose) without the quarantine periods required for biologic testing. It is commonly used for commercially prepared single-use disposable items such as catheters, syringes, IV sets, and gloves.

CONTROL MEASURES

With the exception of items sterilized in a high-speed pressure flash steam sterilizer for immediate use or by immersion in a chemical solution, all items are wrapped before sterilization. The integrity of the packaging material is maintained before use and during storage. Packages are labeled so the contents are known (unless they are visible through the packaging material). The label also includes the conditions of sterilization. A chemical indicator on the exterior of each package verifies exposure to a sterilization process.

Load Control Number

Whether sterilized on- or off-site, a load control number should be imprinted on or be part of the label on every package of sterile items. This number designates the sterilization equipment used, the cycle, and the sterilization date. For sterilizers with microcomputer processor printouts, a label gun correlates the same control number for every package put in the load. Load control numbers are used to facilitate the identification and retrieval of supplies, if necessary, in the event of a sterilization failure. A load control number should also be assigned to items immersed in a chemical sterilant.

The sterilization date can be recorded as a Julian date (day 1 through 365) or as a Georgian date (month, day, year). The package may be stamped with the date of sterilization as it is removed from the sterilizer. The date also may be written or affixed on the package when it is wrapped. Monthly, color-coded machine-labeling systems may be used. Peel-off bar code labels also help to control inventory and patient charges for items.

Wet Packs

All sterilizing methods in which humidity, usually steam, is a parameter of the process potentially present the hazard of producing wet packages. Microorganisms migrate easily through moisture when a pathway is provided from outside to inside a package. Water droplets may be visible on the outside or inside, or absorbed moisture may be seen or felt. Unless the wrapper is completely impermeable to water, a pack should be considered unsterile and unacceptable for use if it is wet. A stain on a wrapper may indicate that moisture was present and has dried. The cause of the wet pack is investigated and promptly corrected. Reprocessing is necessary for a wet package or a load with one or more wet or suspect packages.

Closed container systems with nonvented bottoms may have some retained condensate after processing. This retained moisture within the closed tray is not considered contamination because the container is sealed and impermeable to capillary action. The condensate is considered sterile.

Causes/Conditions of Wet Packs. Excessive moisture may be related to the steam itself, to the load, or to the sterilizer.

Wet Steam. If the steam is abnormally wet, water droplets may form on the outside or inside of packages, and absorbent materials will become soaked with moisture. At the boiling point, water becomes steam. Saturated steam contains as much water in the vapor state as physically possible (98%) and minimal liquid water (2% water droplets). In a steam sterilizer, pressure increases the temperature to raise the boiling point to 250° F (121° C) or above at a pressure of 15 pounds or more above atmospheric pressure at sea level. The temperature of steam does not increase above the boiling point at normal atmospheric pressure in other types of sterilizers. If steam loses water vapor, it can achieve a higher temperature at the same pressure, thus becoming superheated. In steam sterilization, superheating decreases the effectiveness of steam to kill microorganisms.

The dryness (purity) of steam depends on the amount of water in the vapor state in proportion to the amount of solid, liquid, or vapor contamination. This contamination can come from particles in the boiler, steam lines, or sterilizer; from chemical additives in the water; or from moisture in the load. When steam contacts cold surfaces, a lowering of its temperature reverts steam to water, producing condensation on surfaces and raising the temperature of the remaining vapor, which causes superheating of the steam. Dry, dehydrated textiles and other porous materials will absorb water from steam, which changes the proportion of the water content of steam and causes superheating. The water content of steam should not fall below 97% during the sterilization cycle. Below this level, items in the load can become supersaturated with water and subsequent drying will be inadequate.

Characteristics of the Load. Many factors affect the penetration of the sterilant through the load. The following characteristics are reiterated for emphasis:

1. Items are cleaned before they are packaged. Nonporous items must be dry. Porous materials, such as woven fabrics, are hydrated (i.e., humidified) but not wet.
2. Basins are separated by absorbent material and positioned on the side rim so the water condensate will drain out.
3. Heat penetrates different materials at different rates. For even heating of the load, it is preferable not to mix materials. For example, a load may contain only instrument sets and metals or only packs of fabrics.
4. The density of a pack must allow the circulation of air, moisture, and sterilant within the pack. Porous items should not be wrapped tightly.
5. The permeability of packaging materials varies. A water droplet on an impermeable wrapper may not be a problem, but it can be absorbed by an adjacent package with a permeable wrapper.

6. Because condensation diffuses at different rates, the drying and cooling cycle depends on the materials in the load. Packages should not be handled until this cycle is complete.

Sterilizer Malfunctions. Clogged drains, steam traps and air filters, inoperable control valves, worn gaskets, and a dirty chamber can cause the sterilizer to malfunction. Routine cleaning and preventive maintenance techniques are imperative.

Reprocessing Wet Packs. Wet packs are disassembled and the items properly dried and repackaged before resterilization. Reusable woven fabrics should be sent to the laundry and are relaundered before use. Damp or wet fabrics will cause superheating during steam sterilization.

Shelf Life

Sterility is event related; it is not time elated unless the package contains unstable components such as drugs or chemicals. Storage conditions are established to maintain the integrity of the package. An item is considered sterile on the basis of the following events:

- Handling of the package during transport and storage (i.e., the prevention of contamination and physical damage)
- Integrity, type, and configuration of packaging material
- Conditions of storage

Specific written policies should address the handling and storage of all stored sterile supplies. Expiration dates should be placed on a tray that contains medications or other unstable supplies. Most commercially sterilized products are considered sterile indefinitely or as long as the integrity of the package is maintained. An expiration date put on the label by the manufacturer indicates the maximum time the manufacturer can guarantee product stability and sterility on the basis of test data approved by the FDA.

Integrity of Packaging Material and Handling. The method of sterilization establishes the type of packaging material that may be used. Shelf life is affected by the permeability and density of the material, the type of closure used, and the method by which the package is handled. The following are considerations regarding the integrity of packaging materials:

1. An item is no longer considered sterile after an accidental puncture, tear, or rupture of the package. Paper may become brittle and crack.
2. Squeezing or crushing a package may force air out and draw unsterile air in, thus contaminating the contents. Packages wrapped in woven fabrics should be handled carefully and not packed tightly together for storage.
3. The accidental wetting of a package contaminates the contents. It is necessary to avoid the following:
   a. Handling the package with moist or wet hands
   b. Handling the package with soiled gloves
   c. Placing the package on a wet surface
4. The density of nonwoven fabrics and plastic materials protects the integrity of the package.

5. Heat- or self-sealed pouches protect the contents from dust.
6. Commercially packaged sterilized items are usually considered sterile until the package is opened or damaged or the stability of the product becomes outdated.

Dust Cover. A sealed, airtight plastic bag protects a sterile package from dust, dirt, lint, moisture, and vermin during storage. After sterilization and immediately after aerating or cooling to room temperature, infrequently used items may be sealed in plastic 2 to 3 mil thick. A dust cover will protect the integrity of the package.

Storage Conditions. The maintenance of sterility is related to the event and is not based on time. How sterile packages are handled and stored is as important as how long they can remain sterile. The following guidelines are helpful in maintaining the sterility of a package during storage:

1. Storage areas are clean and free of dust, lint, dirt, and vermin. Routine cleaning procedures are followed for all areas in the perioperative environment.
2. All sterile items should be stored under conditions that protect them from the extremes of temperature and humidity. Prolonged storage in a warm environment at high humidity can cause moisture to condense inside packages and thus destroy the microbial barrier of some packaging materials. Ventilating and air-conditioning systems with filtered air should maintain a temperature below 80° F (26° C) and a relative humidity between 30% and 60%. Ten air exchanges per hour are recommended.
3. Packages should be allowed to cool to room temperature before being put into storage to avoid condensation inside the package.
4. Peel pouches should be stored on their sides to minimize the pressure from items stacked on top of them.
5. For open shelving, the highest shelf should be at least 18 inches (46 cm) below the ceiling and 8 to 10 inches (20 to 25 cm) above the floor. Closed cupboards are preferred.
6. Sterile storage areas should have controlled traffic patterns.

Rotation of Supplies. When the standard number of packages kept sterile is adjusted according to daily needs, packages seldom need to be held for prolonged storage periods. In the interest of economy and good management, a stock supply of day-to-day items should be regulated to have enough for the busiest day, with used items replenished daily. Many items are seldom used, yet several are kept sterile at all times. These supplies should be sterilized, or commercially sterilized items ordered, only in quantities sufficient to ensure prompt use and rapid turnover.

Sterile supplies should be checked daily for the integrity of the packages. Some items deteriorate with repeated sterilization or prolonged storage (e.g., latex items). Any sterile packages that become contaminated are reprocessed and resterilized. Older supplies should always be used first to minimize storage. The acronym FIFO (first in/first out) is helpful to remember for the rotation of supplies—particularly sterile supplies.

CUSTOM PACKS

A custom pack is a preassembled collection of disposable supplies sterilized as a single unit. The components are specified by the user (i.e., the OR's specifications) for a particular procedure or specialty or a surgeon's preferences. These components are assembled and sterilized by a custom pack supplier or the manufacturer. A pack assembled by a manufacturer will have an assortment of products in a specific category, such as a kit of sutures, ligating clips, and skin staplers or a custom pack of disposable drapes. Many custom packs have approximately 100 diversified items needed for a specific type of surgical procedure, such as a pack for an open-heart procedure. Care should be taken in handling packs because damage to or contamination of a custom pack may waste many sterile items.

The assembler sterilizes packs with either ethylene oxide gas or gamma radiation. All components of the pack must be compatible with the sterilization method. The assembler must adhere to government manufacturing regulations for testing to guarantee product stability and sterility and package integrity. Using custom packs may be cost-effective for the health care facility, and the following indirect savings are shared by the materials management department and the OR:

1. Personnel time (labor costs) for handling supplies is reduced.
   a. It reduces turnover time between procedures by saving time spent gathering and opening supplies. The circulating nurse has more time for direct patient care activities.
   b. It reduces setup time for the scrub person. Items can be prearranged in order of use and with components in proximity, such as suction tubing with a tip.
   c. It facilitates transport of supplies into storage or into a case cart system.
2. Storage space requirements are consolidated by storing supplies in bulk rather than individually.
3. Inventory control is facilitated.
   a. It simplifies listing of items in inventory. The supplier may maintain a computerized information system of usage and inventory levels.
   b. It reduces inventory. A minimal backup of supplies can be maintained.
   c. It reduces lost patient charges. The circulating nurse can process one charge for the custom pack rather than itemizing items.
4. Standardization is encouraged by incorporating the basic items routinely used by surgeon(s) into custom packs. This helps standardize preparations.
5. The infection rate may be decreased. The physical activity of opening supplies can disperse lint and dust into the air. Opening fewer packages decreases this potential environmental hazard.
6. Less environmental waste is generated by packaging material. Fewer disposable wrappers are used.

Many custom pack processors have addressed the problem of changes in surgeons' preferences by offering to supply the packs in small quantities. Changes are incorporated into new stock, thus decreasing the number of pack contents that may not be used. Some manufacturers will replace older or damaged packs for new stock. Evaluation of pack usefulness is ongoing and may change as the types and complexity of surgical procedures change.

Case Cart System

Most facilities use a surgery case cart system to gather and deliver supplies for each surgical procedure. These sterile and nonsterile supplies are selected according to standard routines and the individual surgeon's preferences. For the system to be efficient, good communication must exist among the staff in the OR and the central processing department (CPD). The surgeon's preference data should be current in the computer. Personnel in CPD prepare the case carts with the required supplies and instrument sets according to computerized schedules, preference cards, and case cart pull sheets (Fig. 18-5). Designated clean elevators connect these respective areas in the two departments if they are not located on the same floor.

The majority of the drapes and disposables will be contained within the custom pack that is on the cart as designated by the facility. This saves time in opening supplies for the case. The items on the cart are patient charge items. Inventory lists that are supplied with the carts may be used for patient charges and inventory control. A bar code or other computer label system may be used to facilitate these functions. Any items not used or opened during the procedure are returned to stock and credited to the patient's account. Some carts are designed to serve as the instrument table during the surgical procedure.

After use, the cart is loaded with the contaminated instrument sets and taken back to the decontamination area. Unopened sterile supplies are not placed on the contaminated cart. They are returned separately. The cart and its contaminated supplies are enclosed during transport to the decontamination area. Usually the decontamination and reprocessing of OR instruments and equipment are done in areas separated from supplies used in other hospital depart-

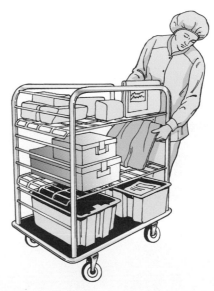

FIG. 18-5 Surgery case cart being loaded for transport to the operating room.

ments. This prevents mixing expensive surgical instruments with those of hospital grade supplied to other units. The personnel assigned to the surgery case cart areas should be familiar with the supplies needed for each surgical procedure, how surgical instruments are used, and the proper method of cleaning and sterilizing each. Surgical technologists frequently are assigned to sterile processing because of their technical background.

Bibliography

Ames H: Sterility assurance through quality control, *Infect Control Today* 9(3):18-20, 2005.

Amsco technique manual, Erie, Pa, 1993, American Sterilizer.

AORN (Association of periOperative Registered Nurses): *AORN standards, recommended practices, and guidelines,* Denver, 2006, The Association.

Association for the Advancement of Medical Instrumentation: *AAMI standards and recommended practices for sterilization,* vol 1, Sterilization, Arlington, Va, 1992, American National Standards Institute.

Association for the Advancement of Medical Instrumentation: *Chemical sterilants and sterilization methods: A guide to selection and use (TIR7-008-HM),* Arlington, Va, 1990, American National Standards Institute.

Association for the Advancement of Medical Instrumentation: *Good hospital practice: Flash sterilization–steam sterilization of patient care items for immediate use,* Arlington, Va, 1992, American National Standards Institute.

Dix K: Sterile instrument packs: handle with care, *Infect Control Today* 6(8):24, 2002.

Gardner M: Flash sterilization: A questionable practice requires proper usage, *Infect Control Today* 6(4):20-22, 2002.

Jenkins B: Standard guidelines for sterile processing vs. common practice, *Infect Control Today* 9(4):83-86, 2005.

Lind N: Problems and pitfalls in the sterilization process, *SSM* 6(4):33-35, 2000.

Mayworm D: What you need to know about EtO, *Outpatient Surg* 11(3):67-73, 2001.

Mosley G: Overcoming the complexities of instrument sterilization, *Mat Manage Health Care* 14(11):26-28, 2005.

Pyrek KM: Time vs. event: Preserving sterile package integrity, *Infect Control Today* 6(4):16, 2002.

Reichert M, Young J: *Sterilization technology for the health care facility,* Gaithersburg, Md, 1993, Aspen.

Scmidt-Bies M: Good sterilization practices in outpatient and office-based practices, *SSM* 6(4):42-47, 2000.

Tager IB, et al: Chronic exposure to ambient ozone and lung function in young adults, *Epidemiology* 16(6):751-759, 2005.

Chapter **19**

Surgical Instrumentation

CHAPTER OBJECTIVES

After studying this chapter, the learner will be able to:
- Identify the use and function of each type of surgical instrument.
- Demonstrate the appropriate methods for passing each type of instrument.
- Understand the rationale and methods of decontamination of instrumentation.
- Demonstrate the assembly and passing of sharps.

CHAPTER OUTLINE

KEY TERMS AND DEFINITIONS

Anodized Dull blackened surface. The instrument is exposed to conditions that cause an oxide coating that is relatively impenetrable to atmospheric oxygen. Instruments can be anodized to reduce reflections. Tints and dyes can be added during the process.
Atraumatic Without injury.
Crushing Destructive effects of specific instruments. Some procedures require the use of crushing clamps.
Dilation Enlarging an opening in a progressive manner.

Dissection Process of separating tissues through anatomic planes by using sharp or blunt instrumentation.
Grasping Holding in a traumatic or atraumatic manner.
Occlusion Closing a lumen for the purpose of the procedure. The closure can be permanent or temporary.
Retraction Stabilizing a tissue layer in a safe position for exposure of a part. A retractor can be manual or self-retaining.
Sharp Instrument with a cutting edge or pointed tip(s) that is used to cut or dissect tissue. These items include blades, scissors, needles, and other dissection devices.
Traumatic Causing injury by penetration or crushing.
Trocar A device used for penetration of tissue layers. It is commonly used for percutaneous endoscopy. It is used as a temporary pathway for gases, fluids, other instrumentation, or the removal of an organ or substance.

HISTORICAL BACKGROUND

Perhaps as early as 10,000 BC, prehistoric man fashioned tools to cut human flesh for the purpose of either inflicting wounds or repairing them. Early writings describe cutting tools. The Incas of Peru used razor-sharp flint and sharpened animal teeth. The Code of Hammurabi (circa 1900 BC) describes a bronze lancet. The Egyptian Ebers papyrus mentions blades made of flint, reed, and bronze used around 1900 to 1200 BC. Hippocrates (460-377 BC) advocated heating the tips of rounded and pointed blades.

During the pre-Christian era in India, Shusruta made grasping tools designed for extracting objects such as arrowheads. Many of these tools were in the form of animal or bird heads, such as a toothed forceps that resembled a crocodile or a smooth forceps that was shaped like the bill of a heron. He described more than 100 instruments, including scalpels, lancets, saws, bone cutters, trocars, and needles.

In the first century AD, Celsus described the use in Rome of scalpel handles with blunt dissecting ends, knives, saws, forceps, and clamps with locking handles, probes, and hooks for retraction. These crude and often heavy instruments were the armamentarium of medicine through the Dark and Middle Ages. Ambroise Paré (1510-1590) was the first to grasp blood vessels with a pinching instrument (the predecessor of the hemostat used today).

In the United States, amputations were the surgical trademark of the Civil War (1861-1865). In some instances these amputations were performed on kitchen tables with crude heavy knives and instruments, and table forks were even used as retractors.

Through the eighteenth and nineteenth centuries, surgical tools were made by skilled silversmiths, coppersmiths, and woodworkers. Some instruments had beautifully carved ivory, bone, or wood handles, and the surgeon kept them in velvet-lined cases. When sterilization became accepted around the turn of the twentieth century, instruments made entirely of metals such as carbon steel, silver, and brass replaced those with ornate handles. The velvet cases gave way to sterilizer trays. The development of stainless steel in the 1900s enhanced the art and craft of precision surgical instruments. Craftsmen—primarily in Germany, Sweden, France, England, Pakistan, and the United States—continue to provide the surgical instruments needed to extend the capabilities of the surgeons' hands.

Hippocrates wrote that the size, weight, and delicacy of an instrument ought to be well suited for its purpose. Consequently, instrument modifications vary from the strength needed for bone work, to the length needed to reach the depths of body cavities, to the delicacy needed to handle structures even under the microscope. All instruments are designed to provide a necessary tool to perform a basic surgical maneuver. The variations are numerous.

Surgical instrumentation is critical to the surgical procedure. The performance of the operating room (OR) team is enhanced when team members know each instrument by name, know how each is safely handled, and know how each is used. Preparing the instrument for appropriate processing will prolong its use in patient care and decrease the costs for repair and replacement.

FABRICATION OF METAL INSTRUMENTS

Although some surgical instruments are made of titanium, cobalt-based alloy (Vitallium), or other metals, the vast majority are made of stainless steel. The alloys used must have specific properties to make them resistant to corrosion when exposed to blood and body fluids, cleaning solutions, sterilization, and the atmosphere. The manufacturer chooses the alloy for its durability, functional capacity, and ease of fabrication for the intended purpose.

Stainless Steel

Stainless steel is an alloy of iron, chromium, and carbon. It may also contain nickel, manganese, silicon, molybdenum, sulfur, and other elements to prevent corrosion or to add tensile strength. The formulation of the steel plus the heat treatment and finishing processes determine the qualities of the instrument. Chromium in the steel makes it resistant to corrosion. Carbon is necessary to give steel its hardness, but it also reduces the corrosion-resistant effects of chromium. Iron alloys in the 400 series (low in chromium and high in carbon) are most commonly used for the fabrication of surgical instruments.

Steel is milled into blanks that are forged, spun, drawn, die cast, molded, or machined into component shapes and sizes. These components are assembled by hand, then heat-hardened (tempered) and buffed radiograph and/or fluoroscopy techniques are used to detect any defects that may occur as a result of the forging or machining operations. The stress and tension must be in balance; that is, the instrument must have the flexibility to withstand the stresses of normal use. The temper of the steel determines this balance.

The instrument is then subjected to processes that protect its surfaces and minimize corrosion. Oxidation of the surface chromium by a process called passivation forms a hard chromium oxide layer. Nitric acid removes carbon particles and promotes the formation of this surface coating. Polishing creates a smooth surface for the continuous layer of chromium oxide. Passivation continues to form this layer when the instrument is exposed to the atmosphere and oxidizing agents in cleaning solutions. The term *stainless* is a misnomer. Steel does not tarnish, rust, or corrode easily; but some staining and spotting will occur with normal use.

Stainless steel instruments are fabricated with one of three types of finishes before passivation:

1. A mirror finish is shiny and reflects light. This highly polished finish tends to resist surface corrosion, but the glare can be a distraction for the surgeon or an obstruction to visibility.
2. An anodized finish, sometimes referred to as a satin finish, is dull and nonreflective. Protective coatings of chromium and nickel are deposited electrolytically and reduce glare. This type of finish is somewhat more susceptible to surface corrosion than is a highly polished surface, but the corrosion is usually easily removed.
3. An ebony finish is black, which eliminates glare. The surface is darkened by a process of chemical oxidation. Instruments with an ebony finish are used in laser surgery to prevent beam reflection. In other surgical

procedures, instruments with an ebony finish may offer the surgeon better color contrast because they do not reflect the color of tissues.

Titanium

In comparison to stainless steel, the metallurgic properties of titanium are excellent for the manufacture of micro-surgical instruments. Titanium is nonmagnetic and inert. Titanium alloy is harder, stronger, lighter in weight, and more resistant to corrosion than is stainless steel. A blue anodized finish of titanium oxide reduces glare.

Vitallium

Vitallium is the trade name for an alloy of cobalt, chromium, and molybdenum. This inert alloy has the strength and corrosion-resistant properties suitable for some orthopedic devices and maxillofacial implants. Instruments made of Vitallium must be used when these devices are implanted. In an electrolytic environment such as body tissues, metals of different potentials can cause corrosion if they come into contact with each other. Therefore, an implant of a cobalt-based alloy is not compatible with instruments that are iron-based alloys (stainless steel) and vice versa.

Other Metals

Although most instruments are made of steel alloys, other metals are used. Some instruments are fabricated from brass, silver, or aluminum. Tungsten carbide is an exceptionally hard metal used for laminating some cutting blades or as inserts on the functional tips or jaws of some instruments.

Plated Instruments

A shiny finish can be put on a basic forging or tooling of an iron alloy. Chromium, nickel, cadmium, silver, and copper are used for coating or flash-plating. When deposited directly on the steel, any of these metals is prone to rupturing, chipping, and spontaneous peeling. It is difficult to keep plated instruments from corroding, and rust can form beneath the plating. Plated instruments are used infrequently today.

CLASSIFICATION OF INSTRUMENTS

Various basic maneuvers are common to all surgical procedures. The surgeon dissects, resects, or alters tissues and/or organs to restore or repair bodily functions or body parts. Bleeding must be controlled during the process. Surgical instruments are designed to provide the tools the surgeon needs for each maneuver. Whether they are small or large, short or long, straight or curved, sharp or blunt, all instruments can be classified by their function. Because the nomenclature is not standardized, the names of specific instruments must be learned in the clinical practice setting. All instruments should be used only for their intended purpose, and they should not be abused.

Cutting and Dissecting

Cutting instruments have sharp edges. They are used to dissect, incise, separate, or excise tissues. These instruments should be kept separate from other instruments, and the sharp edges should be protected during cleaning, sterilizing, and storing. To prevent injury to the handler and damage to the sharp edges, proper precautions are necessary to take during the handling or disposing of all sharps, blades, or scalpels.

Scalpels. The type of scalpel most commonly used has a reusable handle with a disposable blade. Most handles are made of brass; the blades may be made of carbon steel. Blades vary by size and shape (Fig. 19-1); handles vary by width and length (Fig. 19-2). Blades with a numeric prefix of "1" as in a "10" series (e.g., 10, 11, 12, and 15) fit handle size number 3 or 7. Blades with a numeric prefix of "2" as in "20" series (e.g., 20, 22, or 25) fit handle size number 4. Disposable scalpels also are available.

The blade is attached to the handle by slipping the slit in the blade into the grooves on the handle. An instrument, never the fingers, is used to attach and detach the blade; this instrument, usually a heavy hemostat or Kelly clamp, should not touch the cutting edge. Needle holders are not designed to load scalpel blades and can become misaligned. The following are descriptions of blade and scalpel combinations:

- Number 10 blades are rounded toward the tip and are often used to open the skin.
- Number 11 blades have a linear edge with a sharp tip. Can be used to make the initial skin puncture for tiny deep incisions.
- Number 12 blades have a curved cutting surface like a hook. Commonly used for tonsillectomy.
- Number 15 blades have a short rounded edge for shallow short controlled incisions.
- Number 20 blades are shaped similar to number 10 blades but larger.
- An assortment of blades with angulations and configurations for specific uses, such as a Beaver blade, also are used (Fig. 19-3). These blades insert into a special universal handle that secures by turning a screw-in collar (Fig. 19-4).

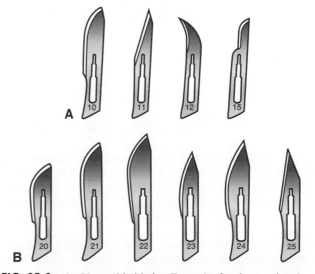

FIG. 19-1 **A,** Disposable blades: Ten series for the number 3 scalpel. Blade sizes 10, 11, 12, and 15. **B,** Twenty series for the number 4 scalpel. Blade sizes 20, 21, 22, 23, 24, and 25.

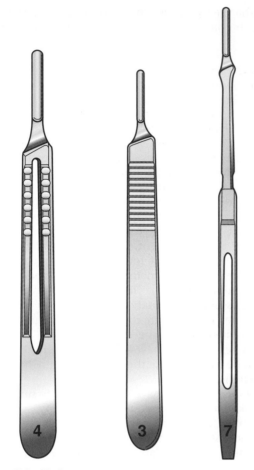

FIG. 19-2   Most common scalpels. 4, 3, and 7.

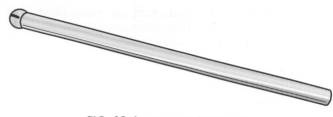

FIG. 19-4   Beaver scalpel handle.

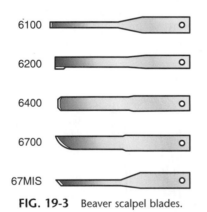

FIG. 19-3   Beaver scalpel blades.

Knives. Knives come in various sizes and configurations. Like a kitchen paring knife, they usually have a blade at one end that may have one or two cutting edges. The knives are designed for very specific purposes (e.g., cataract knife). Other types of knives have detachable and replaceable blades (e.g., adenotome, dermatome). A knife blade may be incorporated into a multifunctional instrument, such as a gastro-intestinal anastomosis (GIA) stapler that cuts and staples tissue.

Scissors. The blades of scissors may be straight, angled, or curved, as well as either pointed or blunt at the tips (Fig.

19-5). The handles may be long or short. Some scissors are used only to cut or dissect tissues; others are used to cut other materials. To maintain sharpness of the cutting edges and proper alignment of the blades, scissors should be used only for their intended purpose:

- Tissue/dissecting scissors must have sharp blades. The type and location of tissue to be cut determines which scissors the surgeon will use. Blades needed to cut tough tissues are heavier than those needed to cut fine, delicate structures. Curved or angled blades are needed to reach under or around structures. Handles to reach deep into body cavities are longer than those needed for superficial tissues (Fig 19-5, *A*).
- Suture scissors have blunt points to prevent structures close to the suture from being cut. The scrub person may use scissors to cut sutures during preparation if needed (Fig. 19-5, *B*).
- Wire scissors have short, heavy blades. Wire scissors are used instead of suture scissors to cut stainless steel sutures. Heavy wire cutters are used to cut bone fixation wires (Fig 19-5, *C*).
- Short jaw sharp tipped scissors for deep areas such the nasal cavity (Fig. 19-5, *D*)
- Sharp-tipped angled scissors with short jaws for vascular surgery (Fig. 19-5, *E*)
- Dressing/bandage scissors are used to cut drains and dressings and to open items such as plastic packets (Fig. 19-5, *F*).
- Small scissors with specially shaped tips such as tenotomy scissors (Fig. 19-5, *G*)

Bone Cutters and Debulking Tools. Many types of instruments have cutting edges suitable for cutting into or through bone and cartilage. These instruments include chisels, osteotomes, gouges, rasps, and files (Fig. 19-6). Some have moving parts, such as rongeurs and rib cutters. Others, such as drills, saws, and reamers, are powered by air or electricity. The purpose of these instruments is to decrease the bulk of firm tissue.

Other Sharp Dissectors. Sharp dissection to cut tissue apart or to separate tissue layers may be accomplished with other types of sharp instruments:

- *Biopsy forceps and punches.* A small piece of tissue for pathologic examination may be removed with a biopsy forceps or punch. These instruments may be used through an endoscope (Fig. 19-7).

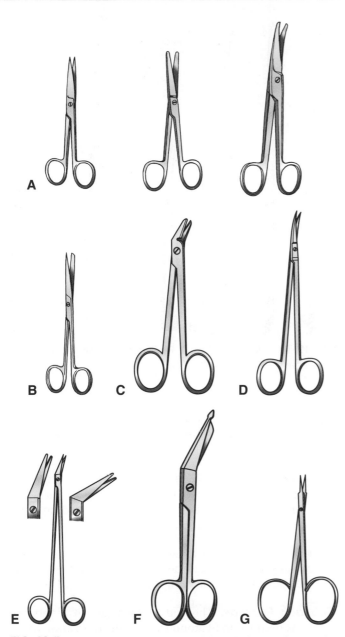

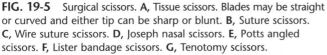

FIG. 19-5 Surgical scissors. **A,** Tissue scissors. Blades may be straight or curved and either tip can be sharp or blunt. **B,** Suture scissors. **C,** Wire suture scissors. **D,** Joseph nasal scissors. **E,** Potts angled scissors. **F,** Lister bandage scissors. **G,** Tenotomy scissors.

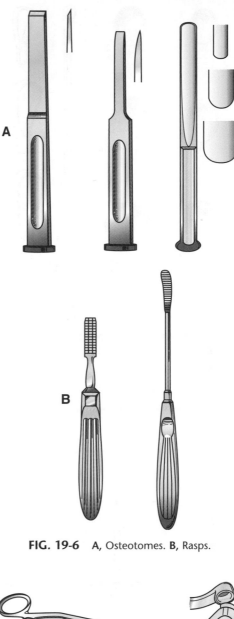

FIG. 19-6 **A,** Osteotomes. **B,** Rasps.

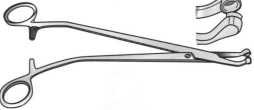

FIG. 19-7 Punch biopsy instrument.

- *Curettes.* Tissue or bone is removed by scraping with the sharp edge of the loop, ring, or scoop on the end of a curette (Fig. 19-8).
- *Snares.* A loop of wire may be put around a pedicle to dissect tissue such as a tonsil. The wire cuts the pedicle as it retracts into the instrument. The wire is replaced after use (Fig 19-9).

Blunt Dissectors. Friable tissues or tissue planes can be separated by blunt dissection. The scalpel handle, the blunt sides of tissue scissors blades, and dissecting sponges may be used for this purpose (Fig. 19-10).

Grasping and Holding

Tissues should be grasped and held in position so the surgeon can perform the desired maneuver, such as dissecting or suturing, without injuring the surrounding tissues (Fig. 19-11).

Delicate Forceps. Fine tissues such eye tissue are held with delicate forceps (Fig. 19-11, *A*).

Adson Forceps. Forceps are used to pick up or hold soft tissues during closure (Fig. 19-11, *B*).

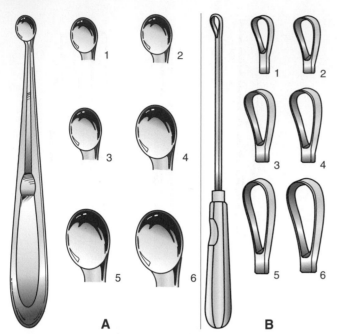

FIG. 19-8   Tissue curettes. **A,** Soft and compact tissue curettes. **B,** Uterine curettes.

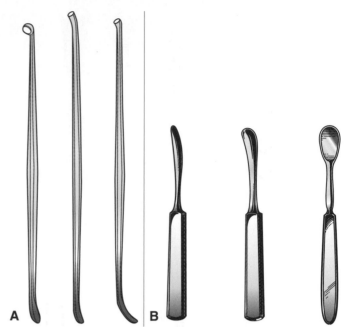

FIG. 19-10   Blunt dissectors. **A,** Penfield blunt dissectors and tamps. **B,** Periosteal elevators.

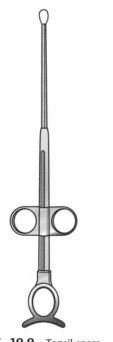

FIG. 19-9   Tonsil snare.

Bayonet Forceps. Forceps are angled like a bayonet to prevent the user's hand from occluding vision in a small space (Fig. 19-11, *C*).

Smooth Forceps. Also referred to as thumb forceps or pick-ups, smooth forceps resemble tweezers. They are tapered and have serrations (grooves) at the tip. They may be straight or bayonet (angled), short or long, and delicate or heavy. Smooth forceps will not injure delicate structures (Fig. 19-11, *D*).

Toothed Forceps. Toothed forceps differ from smooth forceps at the tip. Rather than being serrated, they have a single tooth on one side that fits between two teeth on the opposing side or they have a row of multiple teeth at the tip. Heavy types are sometimes referred to as rat-toothed forceps. Toothed forceps provide a firm hold on tough tissues, including skin. Finer versions have delicate teeth for holding more delicate tissue (Fig. 19-11, *E*).

Allis Forceps. An Allis forceps has a scissors action. Each jaw curves slightly inward, and there is a row of teeth at the end. The teeth hold tissue gently but securely (Fig. 19-12, *A*).

Babcock Forceps. The end of each jaw of a Babcock forceps is rounded to fit around a structure or to grasp tissue without injury. This rounded section is circumferentially fenestrated (Fig. 19-12, *B*).

Lahey Forceps. The tips of the Lahey forceps are sharp points for grasping tough organs or tumors during excision (Fig. 19-12, *C*).

Stone Forceps. Either curved or straight forceps are used to grasp calculi such as kidney stones or gallstones. These forceps have blunt loops or cups at the end of the jaws.

Tenaculums. The curved or angled points on the ends of the jaws of tenaculums penetrate tissue to grasp firmly, such as when a uterine tenaculum is used to manipulate the uterus. Tenaculums may have a single tooth or multiple teeth, such as a Jacob tenaculum (Fig. 19-13). Some uterine tenaculums have a built-in uterine cannula or probe elevator tip, such as a Hulka tenaculum (Fig. 19-14). A uterine cannula, or probe, can be used during laparoscopy to raise the uterus

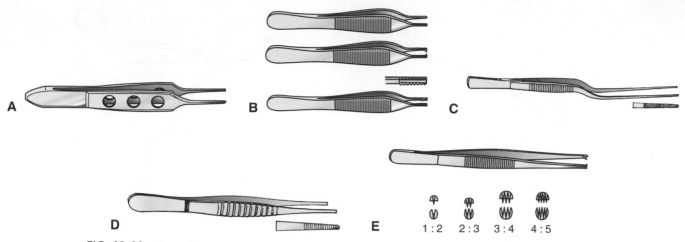

FIG. 19-11   Tissue forceps. **A,** Bishop eye or forceps. **B,** Adson forceps. **C,** Bayonet forceps. **D,** Smooth forceps. **E,** Forceps with teeth.

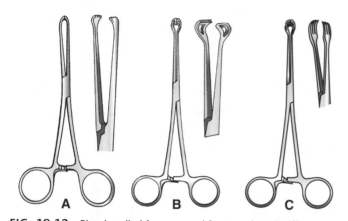

FIG. 19-12   Ring-handled forceps used for grasping. **A,** Allis forceps. **B,** Babcock forceps. **C,** Lahey forceps.

into the visual field (Fig. 19-15). The cannula tip is inserted into the cervical os as the tenaculum is clamped on the anterior aspect of the cervix. Dye or contrast media can be instilled through the cannula into the uterine cavity to visualize tubal patency or the inner configuration of the uterine cavity.

Bone Holders. Grasping forceps, Vise-Grip pliers, and other types of heavy holding forceps stabilize bone (Fig. 19-16).

Clamping and Occluding

Instruments that clamp and occlude are used to apply pressure. Some clamps are designed to crush the structure as the instrument is applied. Other clamps are noncrushing and are used to occlude or secure tissue.

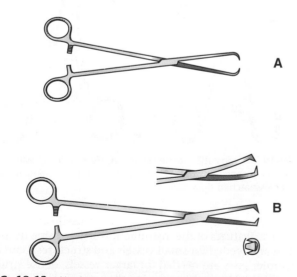

FIG. 19-13   Uterine cervix graspers. **A,** Single-tooth uterine tenaculum. **B,** Jacob multitooth uterine tenaculum.

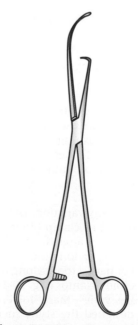

FIG. 19-14   Hulka uterine elevator and tenaculum.

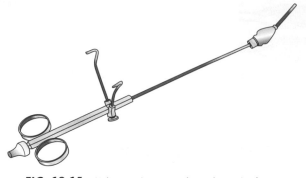

FIG. 19-15   Kahn uterine cannula and manipulator.

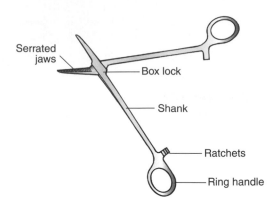

FIG. 19-17   Anatomy of a ring-handled clamp.

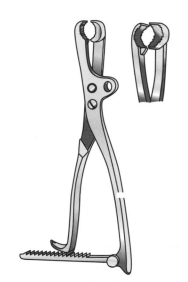

FIG. 19-16   Lambotte bone holding forceps.

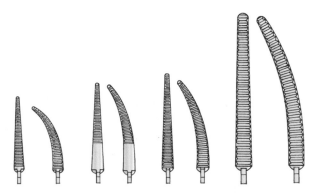

FIG. 19-18   Crushing clamps. Jaws may be straight or curved. Tips may be pointed or rounded. Serrations may be horizontal or longitudinal. Jaws and handles may be long or short.

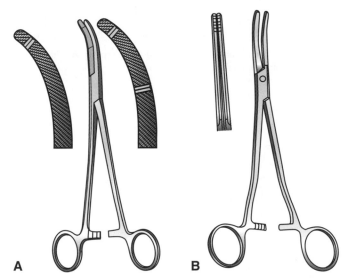

FIG. 19-19   Hemostatic uterine clamps. **A,** Heaney clamp with teeth along crosshatched jaw. **B,** Hysterectomy clamp with longitudinal jaw and crosshatched tips.

Hemostatic Forceps. Most clamps used for occluding blood vessels have two opposing serrated jaws that are stabilized by a box lock and controlled by ringed handles. When the box locks are closed, the handles remain locked on ratchets. Most ring handled instruments have a common design (Fig. 19-17). The length of the shanks or jaws may vary according to the intended function of the instrument.

Hemostats. Hemostats are the most commonly used surgical instruments and are used primarily to clamp blood vessels. They have a crushing action. Hemostats have either straight or curved slender jaws that taper to a fine point. The serrations are longitudinal or horizontal inside the jaws (Fig. 19-18).

Crushing Clamps. Many variations of hemostatic forceps are used to crush tissues or clamp blood vessels. The jaws may be straight, curved, or angled, and the serrations may be horizontal, diagonal, or longitudinal. The tip may be pointed or rounded or have a tooth along the jaw such as on a Heany or hysterectomy clamps (Fig. 19-19). The length of the jaws and handles varies. Many forceps are named for the surgeon who designed the style, such as the Kocher and the Ochsner clamps (Fig. 19-20).

Some instruments are designed to be used on specific organs. The features of the instrument will determine its use. Fine tips are needed for small vessels and structures. Longer and sturdier jaws are needed for larger vessels, dense structures, and thick tissue. Longer handles are needed to reach structures deep in body cavities.

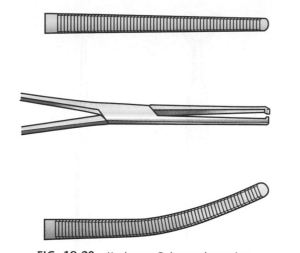

FIG. 19-20   Kocher or Ochsner clamp tips.

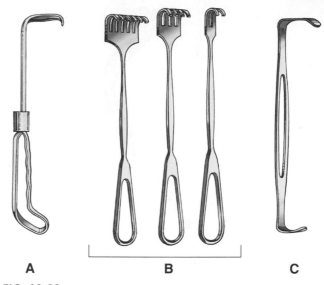

FIG. 19-22   Manual retractors. **A,** Solid blade appendiceal retractor. **B,** Volkmann rake retractors (tips can be sharp or blunt). **C,** Double-ended Army-Navy retractor.

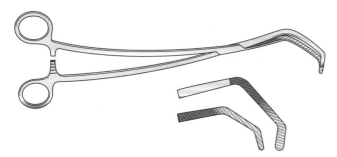

FIG. 19-21   Noncrushing vascular clamp.

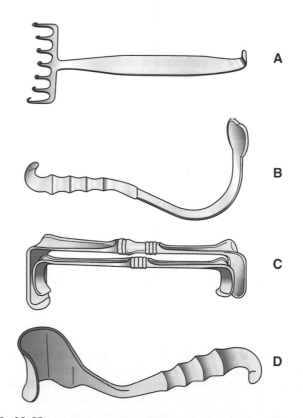

FIG. 19-23   Manual specialty retractors. **A,** Freeman face-lift retractor. **B,** Harrington Sweetheart liver retractor. **C,** Double-ended Eastman retractor. **D,** Mayo retractor.

Noncrushing Vascular Clamps. Noncrushing clamps are used to occlude peripheral or major blood vessels temporarily, which minimizes tissue trauma. The jaws of these types of clamps have opposing rows of finely serrated teeth. The jaws may be straight, curved, angled, or S-shaped (Fig. 19-21).

Exposing and Retracting

Soft tissues, muscles, and other structures should be pulled aside for exposure of the surgical site.

Handheld Retractors. Most retractors have a blade on a handle (Fig. 19-22). The term *blade* should not be confused with scalpel. Retractors are not intended for cutting or dissecting. The blades vary in width and length to correspond to the size and depth of the incision. The curved or angled blade may be solid or pronged like a rake. These blades are usually dull, but some are sharp. Some retractors have blades at both ends rather than a handle on one end (Fig. 19-23). Other retractors have traction groves for slippery surfaces such as the tongue (Fig. 19-24). Handheld retractors are usually used in pairs, and they are held by the first or second assistant.

Malleable Retractors. A malleable retractor is a flat length of low-carbon stainless steel, silver, or silver-plated copper that may be bent to the desired angle and depth for retraction (Fig. 19-25).

Hooks. Single, double, or multiple very fine hooks with sharp points are used to retract delicate structures. Hooks are commonly used to retract skin edges during a wide-flap dissection such as a face-lift or mastectomy (see Figure 19-23, *A;* Freeman face-lift retractor). Some styles of hooks have ball tips, which cause less trauma to tissues (Fig. 19-26).

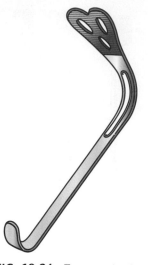

FIG. 19-24   Tongue retractor.

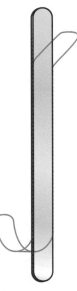

FIG. 19-25   Malleable "ribbon" retractor bends to the shape of the body part to be retracted. Widths vary.

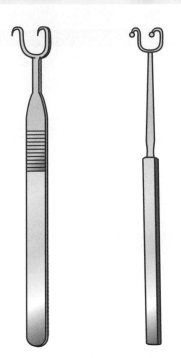

FIG. 19-26   Double skin hooks depicted as sharp and ball-tipped.

Self-Retaining Retractors. Holding devices with two or more blades can be inserted to spread the edges of an incision and hold them apart (Fig. 19-27). For example, a rib spreader holds the chest open during a thoracic or cardiac procedure. A self-retaining retractor may have shallow or deep blades. Some retractors have ratchets or spring locks to keep the device open; others have wing nuts to secure the blades. Some retractors have interchangeable blades of different sizes. Some self-retaining retractors can be attached to the operating bed for stability (Fig. 19-28).

Suturing or Stapling

Suture materials, surgical needles, and surgical staples are discussed in detail in Chapter 28. Only the instruments required for suture placement are mentioned here.

Needle Holders. A needle holder is used to grasp and hold curved surgical needles. Most needle holders resemble hemostatic forceps; the basic difference is the shortness of the jaws (Fig. 19-29). A needle holder has short, sturdy jaws for grasping a needle without damaging it or the suture material. The jaws are usually straight, but they may be curved or angled; the inside surfaces of the jaws also may differ. In addition, the handles may be long to facilitate needle placement in surgical sites such as the pelvis or chest. For example, the fine jaws of the needle holders used for ophthalmic surgery and microsurgery may be either diamond-cut or crosshatched, and the configuration of the handles is different; the jaws are squeezed together by a spring action. The size of the needle holder should match the size of the needle (i.e., heavy jaws for large needles and slim jaws for small needles) (Fig. 19-30). A needle holder should not be placed on a magnetic pad because it may become magnetized.

Tungsten Carbide Jaws. Tungsten carbide is a hard metal. Jaws with an insert of solid tungsten carbide with diamond-cut precision teeth are designed specifically to eliminate the twisting and turning of the needle in the needle holder (Fig. 19-31). These diamond-jaw needle holders can be identified by the gold plating on the handles.

Crosshatched Serrations. The serrations on the inside surface of the jaws are crosshatched rather than grooved, as in a hemostat. Crosshatching provides a smoother surface and prevents damage to the needle.

Smooth Jaws. Some surgeons prefer needle holders that have jaws without serrations. These needle holders are used with small needles, such as those used for plastic surgery.

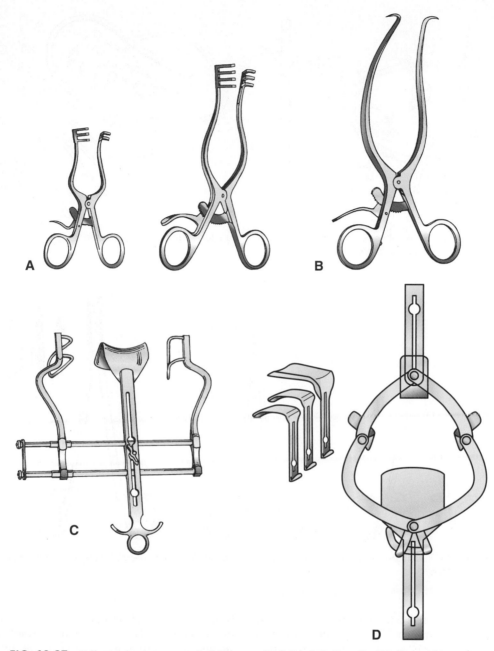

FIG. 19-27 Self-retaining retractors. **A,** Weitlaners. **B,** Gelpi. **C,** Balfour. **D,** O'Sullivan-O'Connor.

Staplers. Whether reusable or disposable, all surgical staplers are bulky, heavy instruments. Reusable staplers have many moving parts and are disassembled for cleaning and assembled at the sterile field before use. Sterile, single-use disposable staplers that are completely assembled eliminate the many problems associated with reusable instruments. The staples are usually made from titanium, stainless steel, or absorbable material.

Clip Appliers. Individual staples can be placed with a preloaded or single clip applier. These clips are used to mark tissue and to occlude vessels or small lumens of tubes (Fig. 19-32). Powered or manual styles are available. Endoscopic clip appliers have been used for many years with laparoscopic tubal occlusion for reproductive sterilization.

Terminal End Staplers. Terminal end staplers are designed for closing the end of a hollow organ (e.g., bowel, stomach) with a double staggered line of staples. The stapler is L-shaped and is positioned across the end of the hollow organ to be closed or the tissue to be amputated. A pin is positioned in the stapler head to contain the tissue neatly, and the instrument is closed and fired. A scalpel is used to trim the tissue extruding from the end of the closed instrument. The stapler is opened, and the staple line is inspected for integrity. Some types of terminal end staplers have articulating ends for placement across hard-to-reach areas, such as the vaginal cuff during a hysterectomy (Fig. 19-33, *A*).

Internal Anastomosis Staplers. Internal anastomosis staplers are designed to connect hollow organ segments to

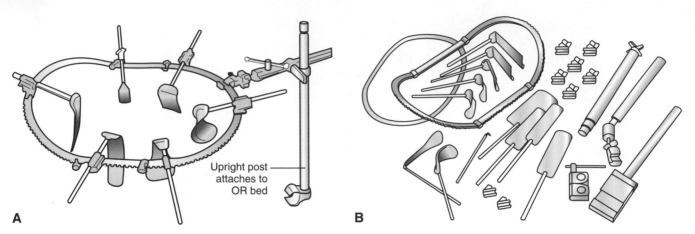

FIG. 19-28 Bookwalter bed-mounted self-retaining retractor. **A,** Bookwalter retractor assembled. **B,** Bookwalter retractor disassembled.

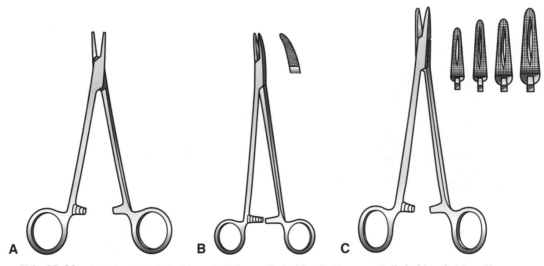

FIG. 19-29 Standard needle holders. **A,** Crile needle holder. **B,** Heaney needle holder. **C,** Mayo Hegar needle holder.

fashion a larger pouch or reservoir. Two tube-shaped organs are aligned side by side, and one fork of the two-forked stapler is positioned in each opening. The instrument is fired, and the tubes are stapled along the adjoining lengths. A trigger is pulled, and a knife blade traverses between the two sets of double staple lines, creating a longitudinal opening on the inside of the anastomosed organ segments. Intestinal pouches can be fashioned in this manner. Some styles of side-to-side staplers do not have a self-contained knife. Endoscopic styles are available (Fig. 19-33, *B*).

End-to-End Circular Staplers. End-to-end circular staplers are designed to staple two hollow, tubular organs end to end to create a continuous circuit. These staplers are commonly used for bowel anastomosis after resection. The instrument can be inserted via the rectum or inserted through a small incision in the wall of one limb of the tubes to be anastomosed. The ends of the tubes are positioned over the distal and proximal tips of the stapler and are secured with circumferential pursestring sutures. The end of the stapler is closed, with the tissue of the tied ends completely enveloped in the closure. The instrument is fired, a double row of staples is placed, and a circular knife automatically trims the excess rim from the joined tubes. The instrument is opened, and the trimmed rims (donuts) are examined for circular integrity. These trimmed rims should be carefully separated and identified as proximal and distal tissue for the pathologist; the margins may be examined for the presence or absence of cancer cells. End-to-end staplers may be curved or straight (Fig. 19-33, *C*).

Viewing

Surgeons can examine the interior of body cavities, hollow organs, or structures with viewing instruments and can perform many procedures through them.

Speculums. The hinged, blunt blades of a speculum enlarge and hold open a canal (e.g., vagina, rectum [Fig. 19-34] or a cavity (e.g., nose [Fig. 19-35]). An ear speculum is like a funnel (Fig. 19-36).

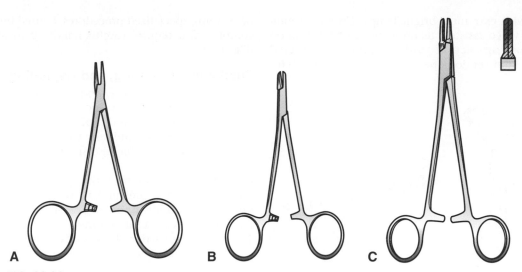

FIG. 19-30   Standard small needle holders. **A,** Webster smooth jaw needle holder. **B,** Derf snub-jaw needle holder. **C,** Ryder narrow tip needle holder.

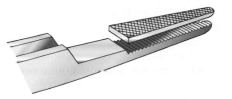

FIG. 19-31   Tungsten carbide insert in jaws of needle holder, with diamond-cut teeth, is designed to eliminate needle twisting and turning.

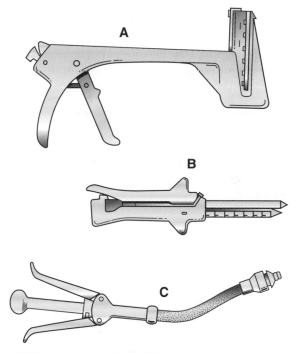

FIG. 19-33   Internal staplers. **A,** Terminal end stapler. **B,** Internal anastomosis stapler. **C,** End-to-end stapler.

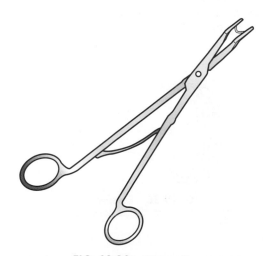

FIG. 19-32   Clip applier.

Endoscopes. The round or oval sheath of an endoscope is inserted into a body orifice or through a small skin incision. Each type of endoscope is designed for viewing in a specific anatomic location. Many accessory instruments are used through endoscopes. Endoscopic procedures are discussed in each surgical specialty chapter of this text.

Hollow Endoscopes. In a hollow endoscope, the rigid hollow sheath permits viewing in a forward direction through the endoscope. The sheath is made of brass, stainless steel, or plastic. A light carrier supplied by a fiberoptic cable provides illumination.

Lensed Endoscopes. Lensed endoscopes have either rigid or flexible sheaths, and they have an eyepiece with a telescopic lens system for viewing in several directions. Lighting is provided through fiberoptic cable and an electric light source with extremely bright lamps. Used in combination with video-assisted technology, computerization permits recording action videos and still digital photography. Many endoscopes have working channels for performing specialized procedures. Lensed instruments are complex and require careful handling to avoid damage (Fig. 19-37).

Suctioning, Irrigating, and Aspirating

Blood, body fluids, tissue, and irrigating solution may be removed by mechanical suction or manual aspiration. Reusable suction tips and aspiration devices have lumens that are difficult to terminally clean and sterilize. Many of these items are available in disposable models.

Suction. Suction involves the application of pressure (less than atmospheric pressure) to withdraw blood or fluids, usually for visibility at the surgical site. An appropriate style tip is attached to sterile tubing; many tips are disposable. The style of the suction tip depends on where it is to be used and the surgeon's preference (Fig. 19-38).

Poole Abdominal Tip. The Poole abdominal tip is a straight hollow tube with a perforated outer filter shield. It is used during abdominal laparotomy or within any cavity in which copious amounts of fluid or pus are encountered. The outer filter shield prevents the adjacent tissues from being pulled into the suction apparatus. This outer shield is completely removable.

Frazier Tip. The Frazier tip is a right-angle tube with a small diameter. It is used when encountering little or no fluid except capillary bleeding and irrigating fluid, such as in brain, spinal, plastic, or orthopedic procedures. The Frazier tip keeps the field dry without the need for sponging. One model has a connection for an electrosurgical unit, and the tip can be used for fulguration. A fiberoptic cable can be attached to another model. The vacuum exerted by the suction is controlled by a small hole that is covered by the thumb in the handgrip of the Frazier.

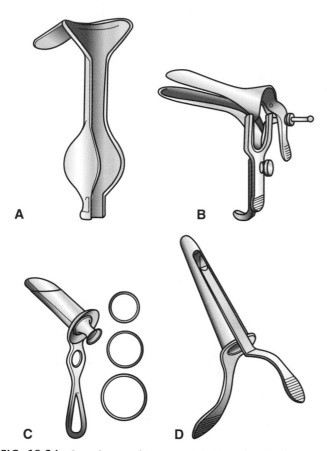

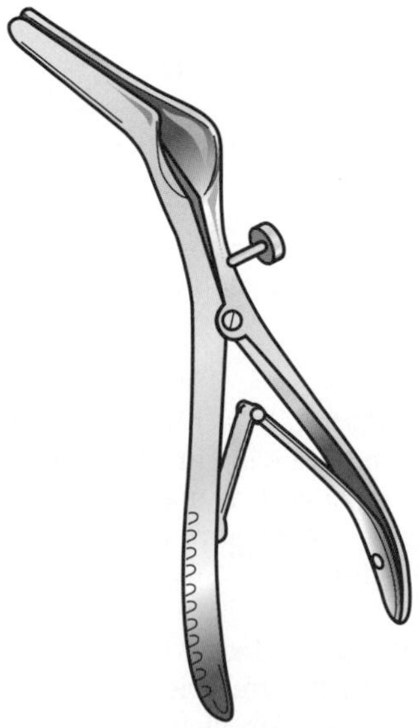

FIG. 19-34 Speculums and anoscopes. **A,** Auvard vaginal speculum. **B,** Graves vaginal speculum. **C,** Hirschman anoscope. **D,** Brinckerhoff anoscope.

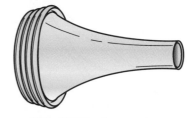

FIG. 19-36 Ear speculum.

FIG. 19-35 Nasal speculum.

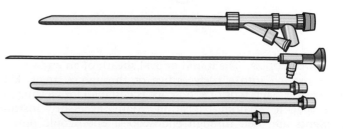

FIG. 19-37 Rigid and lensed endoscopes.

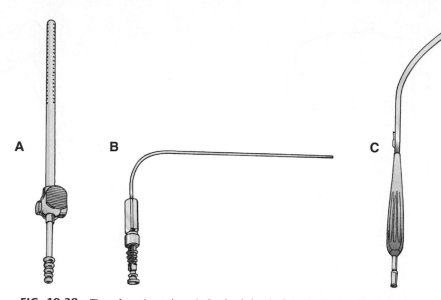

FIG. 19-38   Tips of suction tubes. **A,** Poole abdominal tip. **B,** Frazier tip. **C,** Yankauer tip.

Yankauer Tip. The Yankauer tip is a hollow tube that has an angle for use in the mouth or throat. Large quantities of blood and fluid can be suctioned quickly with a Yankauer tip, which is useful for visualization during ruptured aneurysms. Reusable Yankauer suction tips have a removable end cap that screws on. This must be accounted for at the end of the procedure. It is easily lost in a patient.

Autotransfusion. A double-lumen suction tip is used to remove blood for autotransfusion.

Aspiration. Blood, body fluid, or tissue may be aspirated manually to obtain a specimen for laboratory examination or to obtain bone marrow for transplantation. Suction is often performed with a needle and syringe.

Trocar. A trocar may be needed to cut through tissues for access to fluid or a body cavity. A trocar has two parts—a sharp obturator and a sheath. The sharp obturator with the sheath is used to perforate the tissues. When the trocar is in place the obturator is removed, leaving the sheath in place and creating a stented tunnel for drainage of fluids, introduction of instrumentation, or instillation of medication. Some trocars have suction ports, such as is used for draining the gallbladder (Fig. 19-39).

Endoscopic instruments may be manipulated through special trocars that have valves for insufflation, irrigation, and aspiration. Endoscopy and the eight essentials associated with endoscopic procedures are described in detail in Chapter 32.

Cannula. A cannula with a blunt end and perforations around the tip may be used to aspirate fluid without cutting into tissue. Cannulas also are used to open blocked vessels or ducts for drainage or to shunt blood flow from the surgical site.

Dilating and Probing

A dilator is used to enlarge orifices and ducts, such as dilation of the uterine cervix (Fig. 19-40). A probe is used to explore a structure or to locate an obstruction. Probes are used to explore the depth of a wound or to trace the path of a fistula. Tunneling devices can be used to make a passage for a vascular graft or shunt.

Measuring

Rulers, depth gauges, and trial sizers are used to measure parts of the patient's body (Fig. 19-41). Some of these devices are used to determine the precise size needed for an implant, such as a joint or breast prosthesis.

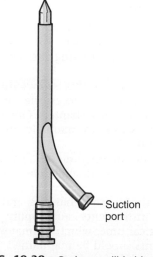

Suction port

FIG. 19-39   Oschner gallbladder trocar.

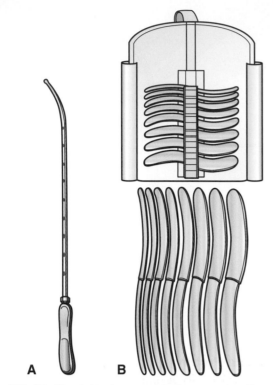

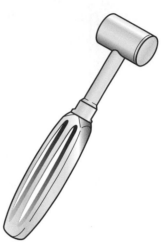

FIG. 19-42　Mallet.

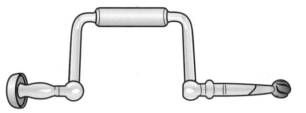

A　　**B**

FIG. 19-40　**A**, Uterine sound. **B**, Hegar uterine dilators.

FIG. 19-43　Hudson brace for manual drilling into skull.

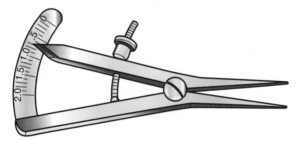

FIG. 19-41　Calipers.

Accessory Instruments

Many accessories are used in addition to the basic instruments previously discussed. For example, a mallet may be needed to drive a cutting instrument into bone (Fig. 19-42).

Screwdrivers are used to affix screws into bone. Each surgical specialty has its own accessories, many of which are described in the specialty chapters. One example is the Hudson brace that is used to manually drill through the cranium (Fig. 19-43).

Of the thousands of instruments available, surgeons choose those that are most suitable to meet their particular needs. Differences in the size, curvature, or angulation of jaws or blades; in the length of handles; and in the weight and shape of the instruments can simplify, improve, and even shorten surgical time, which ultimately benefits the patient. Instruments should be maintained to provide the specific function each has been designed to do.

Microinstrumentation

Improved outcomes of surgical intervention using microsurgical techniques are to a great extent the result of the miniaturized precision instrumentation developed in association with the performance of these delicate procedures. The instruments are extremely fine, delicate, and miniature enough to handle in the very small working area. Manipulation becomes more difficult with increased size or bulk and weight. As with techniques, instruments are constantly being improved. Surgeons work with manufacturers to develop appropriate instruments, suture materials, and needles. Many surgeons purchase the instruments of their choice. Whether owned by the surgeon or the facility, microinstruments require exacting care to maintain desired function.

Instruments are designed to conform to hand movements under the microscope. They must permit secure grasp, ease of holding and manipulation, and fulfillment of their intended purpose. They are shaped to not obscure the limited field of view. Although these factors are important criteria for any instrument, they are especially vital for microinstruments. Everyone assisting in or setting up for microsurgical procedures must know the identification and functions of these unique instruments. Design is coincident to function.

Material and Surface. Microinstruments are made of stainless steel or titanium. Titanium alloy is considerably stronger yet lighter weight than stainless steel. Some microinstruments are malleable for desired angling. Some are disposable. All are extremely vulnerable to abuse.

Finishes of at least the portions of instruments exposed to light in the surgical field are deliberately dulled during manufacture to reduce glare, which is both annoying and tiring to the surgeon. Titanium microinstruments have a dull blue finish.

Shape and Tips. Microinstruments are shorter than standard instruments and often are angulated for convenience of approach and avoidance of obstruction of the surgical field.

Instrument tips have minimal separation, which is compatible with their function. Finger pressure and movement necessary to close wide tips are undesirable, because they may induce tremor.

Handles. Handles are designed for a secure and comfortable grasp, with a diameter comparable to that of a pen or pencil. Minimal diameter between fingers facilitates feel and accuracy of manipulation. Double-handled instruments (scissors, needle holders) have a slightly larger diameter than single-handled ones (razor knife). The shape of the handle is also important for manipulation. For example, instruments that are rotated between fingers when in use, such as forceps, must be turned easily. Their handles therefore are rounded or have six sides like a pencil (Fig. 19-44). Those that are not rotated have finger grips or are flattened. Ring-handled instruments are not practical in microsurgery.

Many instruments, particularly scissors and some needle holders, have spring handles that return tips to the open position between cutting or grasping functions (Fig. 19-45). The distance from hinge to tip will vary according to function. Proper spring tension can be easily ruined by mishandling.

Handles should be long enough for comfort in the working position but must not extend beyond the working distance to contact the unsterile objective of the microscope. The maximum length of most microinstruments is about 4 inches (100 mm). Gripping surfaces should be functionally located to prevent fingers from slipping during manipulation. These surfaces serve as a guide to accurate finger positioning. The gripping area may have a six-sided, round, knurled, or flat and serrated surface.

Primary Uses. Appropriate instrumentation is used for specific types of procedures. Although all surgical instruments are structured for a definitive use, the function of microinstruments is even more restricted. Tissue can be severely injured by use of an improper or imperfect instrument. Instruments, too, can be damaged by use on inappropriate tissue. Primary use includes cutting (knives, scissors, saws), exposure (spatulas, retractors), gross and fine fixation (forceps, clamps), and suture and needle manipulation (needle holders). Instruments must not be used for manipulations other than the intended purpose.

Knives. Edges of razor, diamond, and dissecting knives have different degrees of sharpness and thickness of blades that are appropriate to the cutting function of each (i.e., to make penetrating or slicing incisions). A clean cut is desired to minimize trauma and tissue destruction.

Scissors. Like knives, scissors are designed to make a specific type of incision related both to the plane and to thickness. Incisions are vertical, horizontal, or of a special configuration, such as curved or two-planed. Use is governed by hinging and blade relationship. Scissors are hinged to cut vertically or obliquely. Cutting is usually done by the distal part of blades for better control. Some scissors come

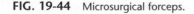

1mm
straight

1mm
ring tips

FIG. 19-44 Microsurgical forceps.

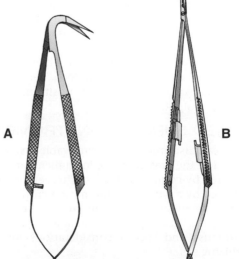

A

B

FIG. 19-45 Microsurgical instruments with spring handles.
A, Scissors. **B,** Needle holder.

in pairs with right and left curves. Often a part number inscribed by the manufacturer on the handle will be an even number for a right-handed instrument and an odd number for a left-handed one. Blades may be sharp or blunt, long or short, and straight or angulated. Available with straight or curved blades, microsurgical scissors have a spring-type handle (see Fig. 19-45, *A*).

Powered Instruments. Microsurgical air-powered drills and saws vary in sizes and shapes. They have a fingertip control; some have an optional foot control.

Spatulas and Retractors. Spatulas and retractors are used to draw tissue back for better exposure or protection. Nerve hooks and elevators also are used for these purposes.

Forceps. Straight and curved forceps may be toothed or smooth. They have light spring action and minimal tip separation. Teeth of some tissue forceps may be as small as $\frac{1}{250}$ inch (0.03 mm) in diameter. Therefore, many tips are barely visible to the unaided eye. Toothed forceps are used for grasping tissue but never for grasping needles or sutures. Smooth forceps are used for tying delicate ligatures and sutures. For stability of grasp and avoidance of injury to the suture strand, the tips of the forceps should be absolutely parallel and have perfect apposition of grasping surfaces. Suture should be grasped firmly but without trauma, often from a slippery surface. Other smooth forceps are used on friable tissues. Bipolar forceps are used for electrocoagulation.

Clamps. Mosquito hemostats and various clamps are used for vascular occlusion and for approximation of edges of tissues such as nerves and vessels. Crushing of vessels should be avoided.

Needle Holders. Microsurgical needle holders are used only for suturing, not ligating, because the very fine suture materials would break if they were tied with a needle holder. They should be used to hold only minute microsurgical needles so as not to alter alignment. Handles are round to permit easy rotation between fingers. Some have spring handles. Although a lock on a needle holder may cause tips to jerk when engaged or released, some have a holding catch for use in deep wounds to prevent loss of small needles (see Fig. 19-45, *B*). Needle holders held closed by finger pressure, rather than by a catch, firmly hold a needle shaft yet permit easy adjustment of the needle position. The tips can be curved or straight.

POWERED SURGICAL INSTRUMENTS

Most surgical instruments have movable parts that are manipulated by the surgeon. Some instruments are pneumatically powered by compressed air or nitrogen or are electrically powered by a battery or alternating current. Powered surgical instruments are complex assemblies of gears, rotating shafts, and seals. They require special handling during preparation and use and special considerations for cleaning and sterilizing.

Powered instruments are used primarily for precision drilling, cutting, shaping, and beveling bone. They also may be used for skin grafts and to abrade skin. Powered instru-

ments increase speed and decrease the fatigue caused by manually driven drills, saws, and reamers. The instrument may have rotary, reciprocating, or oscillating action. Rotary movement is used to drill holes or to insert screws, wires, or pins. Reciprocating movement (a cutting action from front to back), and oscillating movement (a cutting action from side to side) are used to cut or remove bone or skin. Some instruments have a combination of movements and can be changed from one to another by adjusting controls.

Depending on the function desired, the surgeon chooses a drill, burr, blade, reamer, or abrader of appropriate size. These accessories attach securely into the handpiece. Small drill bits, burrs, cutting blades, and abraders may be disposable.

The heat generated by powered instruments can damage bone cells. Blood loss from bone is reduced by the tiny particles that these high-speed instruments pack into the cut surfaces. The speed of these instruments may disperse a fine mist of blood and bone cells. For this reason, the Occupational Safety and Health Administration (OSHA), the Centers for Disease Control and Prevention (CDC), and the American Academy of Orthopaedic Surgeons recommend wearing at least protective eyewear; a face shield or spacesuit-type headgear should be considered if splatter is anticipated.

Unless the instrument is carefully controlled, tissue can be unintentionally caught in a rapidly spinning drill or oscillating saw or the instrument may cut more than desired. When a powered instrument is being used, particularly one with a rotating movement, all team members must be very careful to keep their hands away from the blade. Most powered instruments have a safety mechanism on the handpiece. Some are operated by foot pedals.

Power Sources

The type of power used by an instrument determines the accessories that are needed to operate the instrument.

Air-Powered Instruments. Air-powered instruments are small, lightweight, free of vibration, and easy to handle for pinpoint accuracy at high speeds. Compared with electrical instruments, they cause minimal heating of bone because they operate at a faster and higher speed.

In operating air-powered instruments, medical-grade compressed air or pure (99.97%) dry nitrogen is either piped into the OR or supplied from a cylinder tank on a stable carrier. The pressure must be set and monitored by the operating pressure gauges of the regulator. The correct pounds per square inch (psi), as determined by the manufacturer, is set after the instrument is assembled and turned on. The operating pressure is usually within a range of 70 to 160 psi, and storage pressure in the cylinder is at least 500 psi. Excessive pressure can damage the instrument and the hose that connects it to the regulator. A broken air hose under pressure can whip out of control and injure personnel or the patient.

Electrically Powered Instruments. Electrically powered instruments such as saws, drills, dermatomes, and nerve stimulators are potential explosion hazards in the OR. Most of the motors are designed to be explosion-proof. All must have spark-proof connections.

Because of the heat generated when using electrical instruments, the surgeon usually has the assistant use a bulb syringe to drip saline solution on the area to cool the bone and wash away particles. Care must be taken so the syringe does not touch the blade, especially if it is glass. Plastic syringes are less hazardous.

Battery Power. Some battery-operated instruments are cordless and have rechargeable batteries in the handpiece. Others have cords that attach to a battery charger, which is plugged into an electrical outlet. The batteries are charged and sterilized for use on the sterile table.

Alternating Current. Power switches should be off before cords are plugged into electrical outlets. The power supply cord should be connected to the outlet before anesthetic gases are administered and should not be disconnected during anesthesia administration. The anesthesia provider should be alerted that electrical equipment will be used. The scrub person may be able to disconnect the instrument from its power source when it is not in use so a team member cannot inadvertently activate it. Many of these instruments are activated by foot pedals. The circulator can move the foot pedal away from the surgeon until it is needed.

Sonic Energy. Some instruments are activated by sonic energy to move cutting edges in a linear direction. This is a power assist without the rotary motion and high speed of other electrically powered instruments.

Handling Powered Instruments

Before any new or repaired powered instrument is put into use, the biomedical technician should verify that the instrument is functioning according to the manufacturer's specifications. Powered instruments are not without some inherent dangers. Key points in handling powered instruments include the following:

1. Set the instrument and attachments alone on a small sterile table when they are not in use. This provides added protection from inadvertent activation.
2. Handle and store the air hose or electrical power cord with care. A broken air hose can whip out of control. A broken electrical cord can short-circuit the instrument. Always inspect the hose and cord for cracks and breaks.
3. To prevent inadvertent activation, assemble the appropriate handpiece, attachments (e.g., blades, drills, reamers), and power source with the safety mechanism in position. Always be certain that attachments are completely seated and locked in the handpiece.
4. Test whether the instrument is in working condition before the surgeon is ready to use it and before it is applied to the patient. To prevent inadvertent activation, the safety mechanism must be set in position until ready to use and when changing attachments.

Cleaning and Sterilizing Powered Instruments

Powered instruments should always be operated, cleaned, and sterilized according to the manufacturer's directions for use and care. Each instrument has different cleaning, lubricating, packaging, and sterilizing requirements because

of its various component parts. The bioburden is determined by the size, design, complexity, and condition of the instrument; the degree of contamination during use; and subsequent decontaminating and cleaning procedures. Microorganisms can become entrapped around the seals on rotating shafts. For instruments with a specific biologic challenge, manufacturers test in the area most difficult to sterilize and recommend sterilization cycles accordingly. The following general guidelines apply to the care of all powered instruments:

1. Clean and decontaminate the instrument immediately after use to maintain optimal function.
   a. During the surgical procedure, the scrub person should wipe off any organic debris between uses.
   b. The accessories are disassembled for cleaning.
   c. The air hose should remain attached to the handpiece during cleaning. The air hose and electrical cord should be wiped with detergent, damp cloth, and dry towel.
   d. The motor is not immersed in liquid. The power mechanism cannot be cleaned in a basin of solution or put in a washer-sterilizer, a washer-decontaminator, or an ultrasonic cleaner. The surface of the instrument is wiped with a mild detergent, and caution is used to prevent solution from entering the internal mechanism. The detergent is wiped off with a damp cloth, and the mechanism is dried with a lint-free towel.
2. Lubricate the instrument as recommended by the manufacturer.

HANDLING INSTRUMENTS

Surgical instruments are expensive and represent a major investment. Surgical procedures have become more complicated and intricate, and as a result, instruments have become more complex, more precise in design, and more delicate in structure. Abuse, misuse, inadequate cleaning or processing, or rough handling can damage and reduce the life expectancy of even the most durable instrument, and the cost of repair or replacement becomes unnecessarily high. Instruments do deteriorate from normal use, but with proper care an instrument should have a life of 10 years or more.

Setting Up the Instrument Table

Standardized basic sets of sterile instruments are selected for each specific surgical procedure. A set is a group of instruments that may include all appropriate classifications of instruments or the instruments needed for a specific part of the procedure (e.g., a gallbladder set). The surgeon may prefer some specific instruments that are wrapped separately or added to the instrument set.

Instruments are usually prepared, wrapped, and sterilized several hours before the surgical procedure so they are dry and cool for safe handling. Instruments are sometimes steam sterilized immediately before use, but this method is not recommended as a routine practice. The instruments may be kept in an enclosed rigid container, or they may be sterilized in an unwrapped tray.

Exposed sterile instruments are never transported through corridors. The sterilizer may be located in the substerile room or in the OR. The scrub person or circulator may lift the tray from the sterilizer, depending on the physical location of the sterilizer in relation to the OR. The scrub person should not go beyond the confines of the OR, but this is the practice in some suites in which the sterilizer is immediately adjacent to the door of the substerile room. In lifting a tray from the sterilizer, the scrub person takes care not to brush the sleeves or the front of his or her sterile gown against the sterilizer. The circulator must not reach over the sterile instruments when lifting the tray or over the sterile table when placing it. The exterior of the sterilizing container is not considered sterile if handled by the nonsterile circulator.

When removed from the sterilizer, the instruments are hot. Condensate must not contaminate the sterile table cover. The tray can be set on the large basin in the ring stand if handled by the sterile scrub person.

The scrub person counts all instruments, sponges, and sharps with the circulator before setting up the Mayo stand and instrument table. Key points in handling instruments before the surgical procedure include:

1. Handle loose instruments separately to prevent interlocking or crushing.
   a. Instruments are never piled one on top of another on an instrument table; they are laid side by side. Close the box locks on the instrument to avoid entanglement.
   b. Microsurgical, ophthalmic, and other delicate instruments are vulnerable to damage through rough handling. Tip protectors are removed during setup.
   c. Metal-to-metal contact should be avoided or minimized. Scalpel blades should not be set in a metal basin. The edges can become dull, and small chips of metal can become dislodged and inadvertently transferred to the patient during irrigation.
2. Inspect instruments such as scissors and forceps for alignment, imperfections, cleanliness, and working condition. Remove any malfunctioning instrument from the set. It should be labeled and sent for repair. Replace it in the set with a correctly functioning instrument before processing. If the procedure is in process, the circulator can obtain a sterile replacement and remove the broken instrument from the room. Be sure to reconcile the count sheet.
   a. Scalpel blades should be properly set in handles using a heavy instrument, not fingers.
   b. Teeth and serrations should align exactly.
   c. Tips should be straight and in alignment.
   d. Scissors should be snug and sharp in action.
   e. Cannulas should be clear and without obstruction. Stylets should be removed.
3. Sort instruments neatly by classifications.
4. Keep ring-handled instruments together with the curvatures and angles pointed in the same direction.
   a. Hang ring handles over a rolled towel or over the edge of the instrument tray or container.
   b. Remove instrument stringers or holders if used to keep box locks open during processing.
   c. Close box locks on the first ratchet.
5. Leave retractors and other heavy instruments in a tray or container, or lay them out on a flat surface of the table.

6. Protect sharp blades, edges, and tips. They should not touch anything. Take care not to perforate the sterile table cover.
   a. Sets of instruments, such as osteotomes or microsurgical instruments, may be in sterilization racks so that the blades and tips are suspended. These instruments can remain in racks during the initial table setup and until they are needed during the surgical procedure.
   b. Tip-protecting covers or instrument-protecting plastic sleeves should be removed and discarded before the instruments are used on the patient. Most covers and sleeves are not radiopaque and could become a retained foreign body.
   c. If they are not in a rack, handles should be supported on a rolled towel or gauze sponge. This keeps the blades and tips of microinstruments suspended in midair for easy visualization.

Handling Instruments During the Surgical Procedure

Efficient instrument handling throughout the surgical procedure is the hallmark of an efficient scrub person. Key points in handling instruments during the surgical procedure include the following:

1. Know the name and appropriate use of each instrument. Using fine instruments for heavy tissue damages the instrument.
2. Handle instruments individually. Tangled instruments are hard to separate in an emergency.
   a. If several instruments of the same type will be needed in rapid succession (e.g., hemostats to clamp subcutaneous vessels), three or four may be picked up at one time, but they are passed individually to the surgeon and/or assistant.
   b. Instruments with sharp edges and fine tips are more susceptible to damage than are standard instruments. The edges are easily dulled, and the tips are easily bent or broken. Extreme caution is necessary to prevent catching the tips of microinstruments on any object that could bend them.
3. Hand the surgeon or assistant the correct instrument for each particular task. Remember the following principle: Use for the intended purpose only.
   a. Avoid placing fingers in the instrument rings as the instrument is passed. The instrument may inadvertently drop or snag on drapes, causing an untoward injury to the patient or a team member. The instrument may fall to the floor, thus becoming damaged and contaminated.
   b. Many surgeons use hand signals to indicate the type of instrument needed. An understanding of what is taking place at the surgical site makes these signals meaningful.
   c. Select instruments appropriate to the location of the surgical site; short instruments are used for superficial work, and long ones are used for work deep in a body cavity. Experience will facilitate instrument selection according to the surgeon's preference and need.

d. Many instruments are used in pairs or in sequence. When the surgeon clamps and/or cuts tissue, he or she will usually request suture. After using suture, the surgeon or assistant will need scissors to cut or a hemostat to hold the end of the strand as a tag.

e. Hand instruments around the incisional area, not directly over it, to prevent possible injury.

f. A knowledge of anatomy is useful for determining which instrument is needed.

4. Pass instruments decisively and firmly. When the surgeon extends his or her hand, the instrument should be slapped or placed firmly into his or her palm in the proper position for use. In general, when passing a curved instrument, the curve of the instrument aligns with the direction of the curve of the surgeon's hand. The following points should be remembered when passing an instrument to the surgeon:

a. If the surgeon is on the opposite side of the operating bed, pass across right hand to right hand (or with the left hand to a left-handed surgeon).

b. If the surgeon or assistant is on the same side of the operating bed and to the right, pass with your left hand; if the surgeon or assistant is to your left, pass with your right hand.

c. Hemostatic forceps are held near the box lock by the scrub person and passed by rotating the wrist clockwise to place the handle directly into the surgeon's waiting hand (Fig. 19-46).

d. Clip appliers are held between the fingers by the hinged joint during loading and passing. Placing fingers in the rings may cause the clip to be discharged unintentionally. The loaded applier is passed so the rings automatically pass over the surgeon's finger in a position of function for rapid use.

e. Sharp and delicate instruments may be placed on a flat surface for the surgeon to pick up. This technique avoids potential contact with items such as cutting blades, sharp points, and needles in hand-to-hand transfer. Always protect the hands when manipulating sharp instruments. Some surgeons prefer to have all instruments placed on a magnetic pad or other flat surface to avoid hand-to-hand transfers (i.e., a free-hand technique).

5. Watch the sterile field for loose instruments. After use, remove them promptly to the Mayo stand or instru-

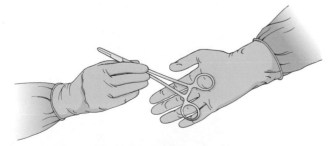

FIG. 19-46 Passing an instrument. Tip is visible; hand is free. Handle is placed directly into waiting hand. Avoid placing fingers in the rings as the instrument is passed.

ment table. The weight of instruments can injure the patient or cause postoperative discomfort. Keeping instruments off the field also decreases the possibility of their falling to the floor.

6. With a moist sponge, wipe blood and organic debris from instruments promptly after each use.

a. Demineralized, sterile distilled water should be used to wipe instruments. Saline, blood, and other solutions can damage surfaces, causing corrosion and, ultimately, pitting.

b. Blood and debris that are allowed to dry on surfaces, in box locks, and in crevices increase the bioburden that could be carried into the surgical site.

c. A nonfibrous sponge should be used to wipe off microsurgical, ophthalmic, and other delicate tips. This type of sponge prevents the snagging and breaking of delicate tips, and the potential for lint is decreased. Commercial microsurgical instrument wipes are available.

7. Flush the suction tip and tubing with sterile distilled water periodically to keep the lumens patent. Use only a few milliliters of solution if using irrigating fluids from the surgical field. Keep a tally of the amount used to clear the suction line, and deduct this amount from the total used to irrigate the surgical site. Accurate accounting of the solutions used for patient irrigation is necessary when determining the amount of blood lost during the surgical procedure.

8. Remove debris from electrosurgical tips to ensure electrical contact. Disposable abrasive tip cleaners are helpful for maintaining the conductivity and effectiveness of the surface of the tip. Avoid using a scalpel blade to clean electrosurgical tips, because the debris may become airborne and contaminate the surgical field.

9. Place used instruments that will not be needed again (except sharp, cutting, delicate, or powered instruments) into a tray or basin during or at the end of the surgical procedure.

a. Blood and gross debris are removed before actual cleaning.

b. Carelessly dropping, tossing, or throwing instruments into a basin causes damage.

c. Instruments that have been wiped can be immersed in a basin of sterile demineralized distilled water, not saline solution. The sodium chloride in saline solution and in blood is corrosive and can damage instrument surfaces. Bloody instruments should not soak in a basin of solution for a prolonged period.

d. Heavy instruments such as retractors should not be placed on top of tissue and hemostatic forceps and other clamps. Place them in a separate tray.

e. Reusable sharps should be kept separate from other instruments of the same or similar size to prevent injury to instrument processing personnel.

f. Keep instruments accessible for final counts.

Dismantling the Instrument Table

Whether used or unused, all instruments on the instrument table are considered contaminated and must be promptly and properly decontaminated/cleaned, inspected, terminally sterilized, and prepared for subsequent use. Wearing gloves, a gown, a mask, and protective eyewear, the scrub person prepares instruments for the cleaning process. Instruments are cleaned in a designated instrument processing area, not in the OR. Key points in handling instruments when dismantling the instrument table include the following:

1. Check drapes, towels, and table covers to be sure that instruments do not go to the laundry or into the trash. A final quick count is a safeguard.
2. Collect instruments from the Mayo stand and any other small tables, and collect those that may have been dropped or passed off the sterile field.
3. Separate delicate, small instruments and those with sharp or semisharp edges for special handling.
4. Disassemble all instruments with removable parts to expose all surfaces for cleaning.
5. Open all hinged instruments to expose box locks and serrations.
6. Separate instruments of dissimilar metals. Instruments of each type of metal should be cleaned separately to prevent electrolytic deposition of other metals.
7. Flush cold, distilled water through hollow instruments or channels, such as suction tips or endoscopes, to prevent organic debris from drying.
8. Rinse off blood and debris with demineralized distilled water or an enzymatic detergent solution.
9. Follow the procedures for preparing each instrument for decontamination or terminal sterilization. Procedures vary depending on the type of instrument and its components and on the equipment available and its location.
   a. Some air-powered instruments can be lubricated with a sterile lubricant after sterilization and just before use.
   b. Some manufacturers supply lubricant (usually a silicone oil).
   c. Some instruments must be run after lubrication to disperse the lubricant through the mechanism.
10. Wrap the instrument for sterilization.
    a. Some manufacturers supply sterilizing cases. These cases can be wrapped in woven or nonwoven material.
    b. The instrument must be disassembled.
    c. The sharp edges of accessories must be protected.
    d. Hoses or cords should be loosely coiled.
11. Sterilize the instrument in steam unless contraindicated by the manufacturer.
    a. A prevacuum sterilizer removes entrapped air and allows steam to access the internal mechanism; this type of sterilizer is therefore preferred to a gravity displacement sterilizer.
    b. Exposure time depends on the type of sterilizer, the design and complexity of the instrument, and packaging. In a gravity displacement sterilizer at 250° F (121° C), exposure time may be as long as 1 hour.
    c. Sterilization of an unwrapped instrument in a gravity displacement sterilizer at 270° F (132° C) must provide exposure that is long enough to sterilize the internal mechanism (usually at least 15 minutes).
    d. Ethylene oxide gas sterilization should be used only if the instrument cannot withstand the heat or moisture of steam sterilization. The instrument must be free of all traces of lubricant. The manufacturer should specify the aeration time.

Bibliography

AORN (Association of periOperative Registered Nurses): *AORN standards, recommended practices, and guidelines,* Denver, 2006, The Association.

Association for the Advancement of Medical Instrumentation: *AAMI standards for the sterilization of patient care items for immediate use,* Arlington, Va, 1996, The Association.

Gardner M: Instrument knowledge: Testing instruments and making the grade, *Infect Control Today* 6(9):20, 2002.

Junge T: Heavy metals: Metallurgy primer, *Surg Tech* 34(4):22-29, 2002.

Maresca TA, Wikander N: Beyond testing and repairing instruments, *Infect Control Today* 7(4):18-20, 2003.

Prephan L: Surgical instrument availability, *AORN J* 81(5):1017-1022, 2005.

Pyrek KM: Preventative maintenance extends life of surgical instruments, *Infect Control Today* 6(12):20-22, 2002.

Rohrlach G: Answers supplied: handing scalpels and other sharps to the surgeon, *Br J Periop Nurs* 11(1):9, 2001.

Vrancich A: Instrumental care, *Materials Manage* 12(3):22-25, 2003.

Chapter 20

Specialized Surgical Equipment

CHAPTER OBJECTIVES

After studying this chapter, the learner will be able to:
- Distinguish between monopolar and bipolar electrosurgical units and applications.
- List the basic elements of electrosurgical safety.
- Identify three basic types of lasers.
- Describe the tissue effects of the different types of laser light in vivo.
- Identify potential safety hazards associated with high technology in patient care.

CHAPTER OUTLINE

KEY TERMS AND DEFINITIONS

Terms Associated With Electrosurgery

Active electrode   Apparatus used to deliver electric current to the surgical site.

Bipolar unit   Current is delivered to the surgical site and returned to the generator by forceps. One side of the forceps is active; the other side is inactive. The current passes only between the tips of the forceps.

Blended current   Current that divides tissue and controls some bleeding.

Coagulating current   Current that passes intense heat through the active electrode used to sear vessels and control bleeding.

Current   Flow of electrical energy.

Cutting current   Current that arcs between tissue and the active electrode to divide tissue without coagulation.

Electrosurgical unit (ESU)   Generator, foot pedal, cords, active electrode, and inactive dispersive electrode designed to safely deliver electric current through tissue.

Generator   Machine that produces electric current by generating high-frequency radio waves.

Ground   Conducting connection between the generator, the patient, and the earth.

Inactive dispersive electrode   Apparatus used to return current from the patient back to the generator; also referred to as inactive electrode, return electrode, or patient plate.

Monopolar unit   Current flows from the generator to the active electrode, through the patient to the inactive dispersive electrode, and returns to the generator.

Terms Associated With Laser Surgery

Emissions   Surgical lasers emit nonionizing radiation, heat, and debris.

Laser   Acronym for light amplification by stimulated emission of radiation. Light, concentrated and focused, stimulates atoms to emit radiant energy when activated.

Laser beam   Light beams, either pulsed or continuous, go through a medium to produce lasing effect. The beam has three distinct characteristics:
- **Coherent** Light beams are sustained over space and time because electromagnetic waves are in same frequency and energy phase with each other.
- **Collimated** Light beams are parallel.
- **Monochromatic** Light beam is one color because waves are all the same length in the electromagnetic spectrum.

Laser plume   Carbonized cell fragments, toxic hydrocarbons, viruses, and noxious fumes can be dispersed from tissues exposed to the laser beam. Vaporization converts solid tissue to smoke and gas. This plume (smoke) is evacuated to maintain visibility and also to minimize the hazard of inhalation by personnel.

Medium   Gases, synthetic crystals, glass rods, liquid dyes, free electrons, and semiconductors are used to produce the lasing effect.

Power   All lasers have a combination of duration, intensity, and output of radiation when wavelengths are activated.

Source   Power to energize the light beam may be electrical, radiofrequency, or optical.

Wavelength   Electromagnetic waves transfer energy progressively from point to point through a medium. The wavelength is the distance traveled along the electromagnetic spectrum. Radiation penetration differs at different wavelengths. Each laser has a different wavelength and color, depending on the medium the light beam passes through.

Terms Associated With Microsurgery

Beam splitter   Attachment to the microscope that splits light; one part is reflected laterally, and the other part is relayed upward to the binocular tube; percentage can be 50/50 or 30/70. The greater portion may be directed to a camera or video system.

Binocular   Using two eyes to see in stereoscopic vision.

Coaxial illumination   The light path follows the same direction as the visual image.

Contraves stand   Series of weights used to balance some microscopes.

Depth of field   Distance of focus.

Diopter   Power of the lens to assist vision by refractive correction of reflected light.

Focal length   Distance between the lens and the object in focus.
Microscope   Equipment that uses a series of lenses to magnify very small objects.
Monocular   Using one eye for vision. Depth of field is absent; the image is two-dimensional.
Objective   Power of the lens that determines the focal distance of vision.
Ocular   Eyepiece lens that multiplies the basic magnification of the microscope.
Pupillary distance   Measurement between the pupils of the eyes; used to position the binocular eyepieces.
Stereopsis   Vision with two eyes that enables objects to appear three-dimensional.
Working distance   Physical space between the objective lens of the microscope and the surgical field.
Zoom   To change the range of focus in continuous magnification; the change can be closer or more distant.

SUPPLEMENTAL MATERIAL ON EVOLVE WEBSITE   *evolve*

http://evolve.elsevier.com/BerryKohn
- Content Updates
- Glossary
- Full Set of Perioperative Flash Cards
- Interactive Key Term Flash Cards
- Student Activities
- WebLinks

USING SPECIALIZED EQUIPMENT IN SURGERY

Advances in technology have made possible the complex surgical techniques of the present. Technology may be defined as the branch of knowledge that deals with the creation and use of technical means for scientific purposes. In the context of surgery, technology refers to a system that uses devices as well as people to perform specific tasks. Continuing research will further enhance technology. New devices are usually adjuncts to or extensions of devices or techniques already in use. To enhance their use in patient care, perioperative team members constantly need to learn about new equipment and its applications.

The focus of technology used in patient care is improvement of care beyond human capability. Users of multiple technologic devices in the OR need to be acutely aware of safety. One aspect of safety in this environment is paying attention to the patient as a physical being as well as to the devices used in care. Equipment used in concert with patient care includes but is not limited to the following:
- Anesthesia machine
- Defibrillators
- Monitors
- Sterilizing machinery
- Warming and cooling devices
- Surgical headlights
- Pressurized fluid delivery systems

Before handling new equipment, patient care personnel on the perioperative team should be knowledgeable about its care and use. Some surgical procedures use more than one of these technologies (e.g., laser surgery through an attachment to the operating microscope).

Preparing and handling these expensive pieces of equipment are major responsibilities of perioperative nurses and surgical technologists. In addition, all OR personnel should be aware of and safeguard against hazards associated with equipment. The perioperative environment should be safe for patients and personnel.

Safety points to consider when using equipment in the OR:
- Has the equipment been serviced on a routine schedule?
- Has the equipment had calibration testing?
- Has the equipment been cleaned or processed to the degree of safety for patient use?
- Are the cords and attachments connected properly?
- Are foot pedals in a secure position for safe use?
- Are reusable components in serviceable condition?
- Are disposable components in stock in the appropriate sizes?
- Are adjunct devices and machines in proper working order?
- Are alarms in working order?
- Are power sources available?
- Is the team knowledgeable about the correct sequence for powering up and using the equipment?
- Have policies and procedures for equipment use been developed and provided to the OR team?

All equipment in the OR has an individual asset tag number. The asset number is a combination of alphanumeric figures used to identify the particular unit. When documenting the use of equipment in the OR the identifying number is placed in the patient's record. Some departments log all asset tags in a master log and assign a simple unit-identifying number or letter that corresponds to the equipment in use. This simplifies documentation.

If any equipment is not in good working order, it must be taken out of service immediately and tagged for repair. It should not put back into service until the biomedical department clears it for use. Some manufacturers will provide loaners when equipment is out for repair. Information on the service tag of malfunctioning equipment should include:
- Name of person reporting
- The date of report
- Description of the problem
- Any other information that may be pertinent

ELECTROSURGERY

HISTORICAL BACKGROUND

The ancient practice of pouring boiling oil into a wound or searing it with hot irons to stop bleeding and infection was extreme. Patients usually were crippled if they survived. Surgeons continued to use these techniques, however, long after Ambroise Paré discredited their use in the sixteenth century. They recognized that application of heat accelerates the natural chemical reaction of blood to hasten clotting. This eventually led to the development of electrocautery (direct contact of an electrically heated wire with tissue). Still in use, pencil-size battery-operated cautery units provide hemostasis by using a self-contained battery to heat a cauterizing wire. These are used primarily in plastic surgery.

Electrosurgery, by contrast, delivers high-frequency oscillating electric currents through tissue between two electrodes to coagulate or cut tissue.

In 1906 Lee DeForest, the physicist commonly known as the "Father of Radio," discovered by accident that a high-frequency electric current could sever tissue with only slight traces of generated heat. In conjunction with his vacuum tube generator, he patented an electrode that cut tissue with an electric arc created at the point of a dull blade. Referred to as cold cautery, the device was used successfully by pioneers like Boston neurosurgeon Harvey Cushing (1869-1939).

Working with Cushing, W.T. Bovie, also a physicist, developed the first spark-gap tube generator in the 1920s. This became the universal basis of electrosurgical units (ESUs), often referred to as "Bovies" until the 1970s, when solid-state units became available. These solid-state units use transistors, diodes, and rectifiers to generate current. The spark-gap generator continues to be used in urology.

Principles of Electrosurgery

Electric current can be used to cut or coagulate most tissues. The initial incision is made by a scalpel to prevent charring and scarring of skin. Electrosurgery can then be used on fat, fascia, muscle, internal organs, and vessels. High-frequency alternating or oscillating electric currents move at more than 20,000 cycles per second (10,000 for radiofrequency). ESUs operate at frequencies between 100,000 and 10,000,000 Hz. This current can be passed through tissue without causing stimulation of muscles or nerves. The heat produced is a direct result of resistance to its passage through tissue.

The density of electric current flowing through a point of contact in tissue elevates temperature sufficiently to cause destruction of cells by dissolution of their molecular structure. The amount of heat produced by any amount of resistance is proportional to the current squared. For example, doubling the current increases the heat produced fourfold. Conversely, the amount of heat produced by any amount of current is directly proportional to resistance; doubling the resistance doubles the heat produced. Therefore, current should be concentrated in a small area of high resistance to produce the high temperature required for electrosurgery, which is approximately 2000° F (1093° C).

Electrosurgical Unit

To complete the electric circuit to coagulate or cut tissue, current flows from a generator (electrosurgical power unit) to an active electrode, through tissue, and back to the generator via an inactive dispersive electrode (also known as return electrode). Electrosurgery is used to a greater or lesser extent in all surgical specialties. Several different units are available. Some have selective uses; others are adaptable to many types of surgical procedures. Personnel should be familiar with the manufacturer's detailed manual of operating instructions for each type used.

Generator. The machine that produces high-frequency or radio waves is the generator or power component of the ESU. Some generators are grounded. This means that the machine acts as a ground to earth. Current returns to the machine, but if the circuit is broken, the current will find an alternate route back to earth, such as through metal in contact with a body. A balanced-output generator is referenced to earth. An isolated generator offers the advantage of a non–ground-seeking circuit. The flow of current is isolated and restricted to active and dispersive electrodes, and the current returns directly back to the generator. With an isolated generator, if the circuit is broken, current will not flow.

Solid-state generators are transistorized and use diodes (semiconductors) and rectifiers (devices that change alternating current [AC] to direct current [DC]) to produce current. They usually operate at a lower output than spark-gap generators and have safety features such as return monitors to prevent burns and electrocution. Both solid-state and spark-gap generators provide two separate circuits within the housing of the machine. Controls on the outside of the housing allow selection of desired characteristic of current. The current may be identical in frequency, power (voltage), and amount (amperage) but vary in quality. Quality depends on the difference in damping (the pattern of waveforms by which oscillations diminish after surges of power). This difference determines tissue reaction to the current.

Coagulating Current. A damped waveform has a continuous pattern of surges of current that rapidly diminishes to short periods, or gaps, in which no current is delivered. This is produced by the spark-gap circuit. Damped current coagulates tissue. As it approaches the active electrode, the density of current increases to produce an intense heat, which sears the ends of small or moderate-size vessels to control bleeding on contact. Attempts to coagulate large vessels can result in an extensive burn and necrosis. Excess charring interferes with wound healing and may provide a medium for infection.

Cutting Current. An undamped waveform, which is produced by a vacuum tube oscillator, does not diminish but retains a constant output of high-frequency current. Undamped current cuts tissue. This continuous current forms an arc between tissues and an active electrode that is intense enough to divide fibrous tissue as it moves along lines of deep incision before sufficient heat builds up to coagulate adjacent tissues.

Blended Current. Undamped current can be blended with damped current to add a coagulating effect to the cutting current. At the same time that it cuts through or across tissue, cutting current accomplishes some coagulation of cells on the surface of the incision and prevents capillary bleeding. Some solid-state generators have a setting for blend or hemostasis for this function. This blend can also be achieved by a slightly damped waveform from a spark-gap generator.

Argon Enhanced. Argon gas can be incorporated into a monopolar ESU to create a path between the tissue and the electrode. The gas is inert and noncombustible and is easily ionized by the electrical current. Argon is heavier than air and creates less plume. The argon-enhanced ESU tip is held at a 60-degree angle and does not contact the tissue during coagulation, thereby causing less tissue damage. The ESU and gas stream are passed over tissue. Care is taken not to cause the gas to enter large open vessels because of the risk of gas embolism.

Controls. The type and amount of current are regulated by controls on the generator. Most units provide up to 400 watts of power. It is seldom necessary to use full-power settings. A safe general rule for the circulating nurse is to start with the lowest setting of current that accomplishes the desired degree of coagulation or cutting and then increase the current at the surgeon's request. The surgeon selects the type of current to be used with either a foot pedal or hand control switch. The circulating nurse verbally confirms and documents the power settings before the generator is activated. The generator should be designed to minimize unintentional activation.

In solid-state units the power output is isolated to prevent overheating and is equipped with a warning buzzer and/or light to warn of too high a setting or a break in the circuit. Flow of current to and from the generator should be balanced. A return electrode monitoring system measures and compares current flowing from the active electrode with current returning from the inactive dispersive electrode. The generator deactivates if continuity in the electrical circuit is disrupted or inadequate in some units. Safety features should be tested before each patient use, and the generator should be periodically inspected by biomedical engineering department personnel.

The generator may be mounted on a portable stand. It should be moved carefully to avoid tipping. The machine should be cleaned before and after use. Unintentional activation or failure may occur if liquid or debris enters the generator. The facility may be held responsible for a defect causing patient injury. The generator should have an identification number. This should be recorded in the patient's record to verify the equipment used. This identification number also provides a means of maintaining records of routine inspections and maintenance. Operational instructions should be on or attached to every unit. Personnel using this equipment should be trained and knowledgeable in its use.

Active Electrode. The sterile active electrode directs flow of current to the surgical site. The style of the electrode tip (i.e., blade, loop, ball, or needle) will be determined by the type of surgical procedure and current to be used. The electrode tip may be fixed into or detachable from a pencil-shaped handle, or it may be incorporated into a tissue forceps or suction tube. It is attached to a conductor cord, which is connected to the generator. The scrub person hands the end of the conductor cord off of the sterile field to the circulating nurse, who attaches it to the generator. The cord should be long and flexible enough to reach between the sterile field and the generator without stress. It should be free of kinks and bends that could deviate current flow.

When the unit is not in actual use, although connected, the electrode tip should be kept clean, dry, and visible. It may be kept in an insulated holster/container attached to the drape over the patient to avoid the possibility of a fire being started by someone on the team inadvertently stepping on the foot switch or activating the hand control.

The surgeon places the active electrode tip on the tissue and then activates the foot switch or hand control to transfer electric current from the generator to the tissue. Some hand switches are color-coded to identify coagulating and cutting functions. Some generators produce a buzzing sound that varies in pitch, depending on which current is being used.

Charred or coagulated tissue should be removed from the tip, because charred tissue absorbs heat and decreases the effectiveness of current. This can be done by scraping the tip on a disposable tip cleaner. Some specialized bipolar tips are wiped with hydrogen peroxide. Using a scalpel blade should be avoided because the debris may become airborne, creating a biologic hazard. Coated Bovie tips have a Teflon surface and need only a wipe with a damp Raytec for cleaning.

Rather than placing the tip directly on tissue, bleeding vessels may be clamped with hemostats or smooth-tipped tissue forceps. As little extraneous tissue as possible should be clamped to minimize damage to adjacent tissue. Vessels are coagulated when any part of the metal instrument is touched with the active electrode; this is frequently referred to as "buzzing."

To avoid arcing, the active electrode should be in contact with the instrument before electric current is applied. The person holding it should have a firm grip on as large an area of instrument as possible and avoid touching the patient. The active current should not be applied for more than 3 seconds. Inadvertent patient injury can occur if the metal instrument is in contact with retractors or other instrumentation placed in the surgical field. Low-voltage cutting current should be used. Current can burn through surgical gloves if these precautions are not taken.

The active electrode and cord may be disposable. Reusable active electrodes should be inspected for damage before reprocessing and before use at the sterile field.

Inactive Dispersive Electrode (Return Electrode). Electric current will flow to ground or a neutral potential. Therefore, a proper channel should be provided to disperse current and heat generated in tissue. The inactive electrode disperses high-frequency current released through the active electrode and provides low current density return from tissues back to the generator. Resistance from the patient to the generator and from the generator to the wall electrical outlet should be less than 1 ohm. ESUs have either monopolar or bipolar mechanisms or both to direct the flow of electric current.

Bipolar Units. With bipolar units the dispersive electrode is incorporated into forceps used by the surgeon. One side of the forceps is the active electrode through which current passes to tissues. The other side is inactive. Output voltage is relatively low. Current flows only between the tips of the forceps, returning directly to the generator. Current does not disperse itself throughout the patient, as it does in monopolar units. This provides extremely precise control of the coagulated area. A dispersive pad or return electrode is not needed because current does not flow through the patient.

Monopolar Units. With monopolar units the electric current flows from the generator to the active electrode, through the patient to an inactive dispersive electrode, and returns back to the generator (Fig. 20-1). Power is greater than through bipolar forceps. Because current supplied by the generator is dispersed from the active electrode, it seeks completion of the electrical circuit to ground or a neutral potential through the patient's body. An inactive dispersive electrode is used. One form of a patient return electrode adhesive pad is placed in direct contact with skin (Fig. 20-2). The contact area must exceed 100 mm^2 or have a diameter greater than 1.2 cm. Disposable styles are flexible to mold to the appropriate body surface. They need to maintain uniform body contact to be effective. Pads should be checked for dry spots before placement.

MEGADYNE manufactures a reusable return electrode, MEGA 2000, that measures 720 square inches and is not adherent to the patient's body. This large pad is placed in a plastic sheath underneath the bed sheet on the OR bed. The patient makes contact with the pad over most of the contact surface through the bed sheets. This style of return electrode is useful when there is not a suitable site for an adherent pad, such as in a burn patient. Positioning in lithotomy can be difficult with this type of electrode. Imaging can be distorted if used under the patient during fluoroscopy. The cord attaches to the generator in the patient return electrode socket.

In both models of dispersive electrodes, the current returns to the generator via a conductor cord. This cord should be long and flexible enough to reach without stress on attachments to the electrode or generator. Attachments to both the pad and the generator should be secure. Unless it is disposable, the cord should be checked before use for wire breakage or fraying. Reusable cords should be inspected by biomedical engineering department personnel periodically for electrical integrity.

The dispersive electrode is properly placed and connected to the generator to avoid an electrical burn to the patient. The following safeguards are taken:

1. The dispersive electrode should be as close as possible to the site where the active electrode will be used to minimize current through the body.

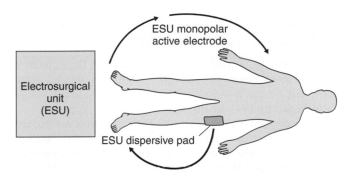

FIG. 20-1 Path of electric current from electrosurgical unit (ESU).

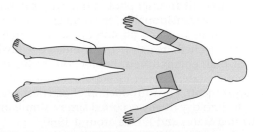

FIG. 20-2 Placement of electrosurgical unit (ESU) dispersive electrode.

2. The patient should be in the desired position before the dispersive electrode is applied to prevent its becoming dislodged or buckled during patient positioning. Do not remove or reposition the disposable dispersive electrode because the integrity of the adhesive will be altered. A new electrode is used each time.
3. The dispersive electrode should never be cut to fit.
4. The dispersive electrode should cover as large an area of the patient's skin as possible in an area free of hair or scar tissue, both of which tend to act as insulation. An area may need to be shaved. The surface area affects heat buildup and dissipation. Avoid areas where bony prominences might result in pressure points, which in turn can cause current concentration. Place the pad on a clean, dry skin surface over or under as large a muscle mass area as possible. The gel conduction material on the pad is cold and sticky to the touch; a patient who is awake should be forewarned of its application.
5. The dispersive electrode should not be placed on skin over a metal implant, such as a hip prosthesis, because current could be diverted to the implant and generate excessive heat. Any area that overlies an implant is a former surgical site and is not suitable for placement of a dispersive electrode.
6. The integrity of the package of a disposable dispersive electrode should be inspected before use. Do not use the electrode if the package is damaged or has been previously opened.
7. Special care should be taken to ensure that the cord does not become dislodged. Do not put a safety belt over the electrode or cord. The connector should not create a pressure point on the patient's skin.
8. The connection between the dispersive electrode and generator should be secure and made with compatible attachments. If the return circuit is faulty, the ground circuit may be completed through inadvertent contact with the metal operating bed or its attachments. This is referred to as an alternative pathway for the current. If the dispersive pad surface area is too small, current passing through an exposed area of skin in contact with metal will create intense heat. For example, one such contact point could be the thigh touching a leg stirrup while the patient is in the lithotomy position. A serious full-thickness burn can occur.
9. A dispersive electrode is not used with bipolar generators.

The circulating nurse should record on the patient's chart the type and/or location of the dispersive electrode, the condition of the patient's skin before and after electrosurgery, the generator identification number, and the settings used. Some institutions also require documentation of the dispersive electrode lot number.

Safety Factors

Electrical burn through the patient's skin is the greatest hazard of electrosurgery. These burns are usually deeper than flame burns, causing widespread tissue necrosis and deep thrombosis to the extent that débridement and grafting may be required. Not all deep thermal injury is immediately apparent.

Isolated circuits for ESUs and return electrode monitoring systems, if used, virtually eliminate these burns. Perioperative personnel should be aware of hazards and safeguard against injury to the patient. In addition to the precautions noted for preparing the ESU and for positioning the dispersive electrode used with monopolar units, other precautions should be taken as follows:

1. Electrosurgery should not be used in the mouth, trachea, around the head, or in the pleural cavity when high concentrations of oxygen or nitrous oxide are used. During some procedures such as eye surgery, oxygen is administered via nasal cannula or mask. Oxygen builds up under the drapes and sets the stage for a combustible situation. Flame-retardant drapes can conceal a fire in a confined space. Safety regulations for use with all inhalation anesthetic agents are followed.

2. Electrocardiogram electrodes should be placed as far away from the surgical site as possible. Burns can occur at the site of electrocardiogram electrodes and other low-impedance points from invasive monitor probes if current diverts to alternate paths of least resistance.

3. Rings and other jewelry should be removed. Metallic jewelry, including that used in body piercing, presents a potential risk of burn for the patient from diverted currents from the monopolar unit with either an isolated or ground-referenced output.

4. Flammable agents such as alcohol should be used with great care in skin preparation. If they are used, the skin surface should be completely dry before draping. Volatile fumes and vapors may collect in drapes and ignite when the electrosurgical or cautery unit is used.

5. If another piece of electrical equipment is used in direct contact with the patient at the same time as the ESU, connect it to a different source of current if possible. The cutting current of the ESU may not work if another piece of electrical equipment is on the same circuit. The ESU may interfere with the operation of some equipment, such as older models of cardiac monitors. The isolated power system of solid-state generators may prevent these problems.

6. Monopolar electrosurgery may disrupt operation of an implanted cardiac pacemaker. New models of cardiac pacemakers are unaffected by monopolar ESU generators. Check with the pacemaker manufacturer regarding compatibility. The bipolar ESU may be used, because the current does not pass through the patient's body and return to the generator. The patient is continuously monitored. A defibrillator should be on standby in the OR.

7. Connection of a bipolar active electrode to a monopolar receptacle may activate current, causing a short circuit. Plugs on cords should be differentiated to prevent misconnections of active and inactive electrodes.

8. Secure the active electrode handle in an insulated holster/container when not in use. Do not immerse an active electrode in liquid.

9. To prevent fire, only moist sponges should be permitted on the sterile field while the ESU is in use. This includes using moist sponges during the use of battery-operated pencil cautery. Dry sponges can ignite.

10. Investigate a repeated request for more current. The dispersive electrode or connecting cord may be at fault and should be checked first, followed by the handpiece connection. Shock to those touching the patient may result. The patient may be burned at the dispersive pad site.

11. For safety of the patient and personnel, follow instructions for use and care; these appear on the machine or in the manual provided by the manufacturer that accompanies each ESU. Grasp and pull only the plugs, not cords, when disconnecting attachments from the generator or the power source. Position the power cord away from the team to avoid tripping team members. Avoid rolling equipment over the power cord. Disposable cords should not be cut with scissors.

12. Any malfunctioning ESU should be labeled with the problem and taken out of service until cleared for use by biomedical engineering department personnel.

13. The patient and personnel should be protected from inhaling plume (smoke) generated during electrosurgery. A suction evacuator device should be placed as close to the source of plume as possible to maximize evacuation of smoke and enhance visibility at the surgical site.

Electrosurgery causes more patient injuries than any other electrical device used in the OR. Most incidents are caused by personnel error.

LASER SURGERY

The term *laser* is an acronym for light amplification by stimulated emission of radiation.

HISTORICAL BACKGROUND

Einstein's theory, purported in 1917, explaining the difference between spontaneous and stimulated emission of light, eventually led to the development of the laser. This development began in 1940 in the Soviet Union.

Lasers depend on the capacity of atoms to become excited when struck by a quantum of electromagnetic energy known as a photon. Photons are the basic units of radiation that constitute light. When struck by a photon, the electrons of the atom move to a high energy level. On spontaneous return to a lower energy level toward normal ground state, these electrons emit another photon that will strike another atom also in the transitional pumped-up energy state. This reaction produces a second photon of the same frequency. This sets up a chain reaction of stimulated emission of photons at high energy levels. Production of this reaction in a sustained state, known as population inversion, was technically difficult. The introduction of practical lasers into scientific technology finally occurred almost simultaneously in the United States and Russia around 1960.

The laser as a surgical instrument was developed in the United States. The first surgical laser, the ruby laser, was used in ophthalmology for retinal hemorrhages. As scientists discovered that other materials could be electrically stimulated to produce lasers in a variety of wavelengths, the CO_2 and argon gas surgical lasers were developed in the mid-1960s. The argon laser replaced the ruby laser for use in ophthalmology. Not until after Jako adapted the CO_2 laser to the operating microscope in 1972 did lasers truly become viable adjuncts to the surgical arena.

Physical Properties of Lasers

The laser focuses light on atoms to stimulate them to a high point of excitation. The resulting radiation is then amplified and metamorphosed into the wavelengths of laser light. This light beam is monochromatic (one color), because all of the electromagnetic waves are the same length and collimated, or parallel to each other. The light is totally concentrated and easily focused. Unlike conventional light waves, which spread and dissipate electromagnetic radiation by many different wavelengths, the coherence of the laser beam is sustained over space and time with wavelengths in the same frequency and energy phase.

Lasers may emit their energy in brief, repeating emissions that have a duration of only an extremely small fraction of a second. These are pulsed laser systems. Or they are capable of producing continuous light beams; these are continuous-wave lasers. All lasers have a combination of duration, level, and output wavelengths of radiation emitted when activated. Power density, the irradiance, is the amount of power per unit surface area during a single pulse or exposure. This is expressed as watts per centimeter squared. Regardless of beam characteristics, components of a laser system are the same (Fig. 20-3). These components include the following:

- A medium to produce a lasing effect of the stimulated emission. Gases, solid rods or crystals, liquid dyes, and free electrons are used. Each produces a different wavelength, color, and effect.
- A power source to create population inversion by pumping energy into the lasing medium. This may be electrical or radiofrequency power or an optical power source such as a xenon flash lamp or another laser.
- An amplification mechanism to change random directional movement of stimulated emissions to a parallel direction. This occurs within an optical resonator or laser cavity, which is a tube with mirrors at each end. As photons traveling the length of the resonator reflect back through the medium, they stimulate more atoms to release photons, thus amplifying the lasing effect. The power density of the beam determines the laser's capacity to cut, coagulate, or vaporize tissue.

- Wave guides to aim and control the direction of the laser beam. The optical resonator has a small opening in one end that permits transmission of a small beam of laser light. The smaller the beam, the higher its power density will be. Fiberoptic wave guides or a series of rhodium reflecting mirrors then direct the beam to tissue. The wave mode may be continuous, pulsed, or a Q-switched single pulse of high energy.
- Backstops to stop the laser beam from penetrating beyond the expected impact site and affecting nontargeted tissue. Quartz or titanium rods will stop the beam.

Types of Lasers

Lasers use argon, carbon dioxide, holmium, krypton, neodymium, phosphate, ruby, or xenon as their active medium. When delivered to tissues, laser light can be absorbed, reflected, transmitted, or scattered, depending on the characteristics of the laser and the type of tissue. Only absorbed light produces thermal effects in tissue. Thermal penetration varies according to the ratio of absorption versus scattering. Energy absorbed at the surface will destroy superficial cells; further penetration extends cell destruction in surrounding tissues. The wavelength of the laser light, power density, rate of delivery of energy, and exposure time will vary the effects on tissue. Energy density is based on the laser's wattage, beam or spot size, and time of exposure. The spot size depends on the laser fiber size and distance of the tip from tissue; it increases and becomes defocused as fiber is moved farther from tissue. Variables in tissue reaction are listed in Box 20-1.

Laser beams cut, vaporize, or coagulate tissue. Coagulative effect causes collagen bonding and welding of tissue surfaces. Each laser has selective uses. Laser light colors vary from the visible, near-ultraviolet range to the invisible, far-infrared range of the electromagnetic spectrum (Fig. 20-4). Wavelengths also vary, providing different radiation penetration depths. Lasers are commonly used in conjunction with the operating microscope and/or an endoscope. The surgeon selects the appropriate laser for the tissue to be incised, excised, or coagulated.

Argon Laser. Argon ion gas emits a blue-green light beam in the visible electromagnetic spectrum at wavelengths of 450 and 530 nm. This wavelength passes through water and clear fluid, such as cerebrospinal fluid, with minimal absorption. It is intensely absorbed by the brown-red pigment of hemoglobin in blood or melanin in pigmented tissue and converted into heat. Thermal radiation penetrates to a depth of 1 or 2 mm in most tissue.

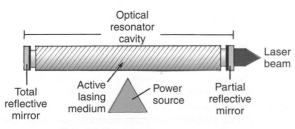

FIG. 20-3 Basic laser components.

BOX 20-1	Factors Associated With Tissue Reaction to Laser Light

- Type of laser (wavelength)
- Intensity of laser focus
- Duration of application
- Depth of penetration
- Type of tissue (color and composition)

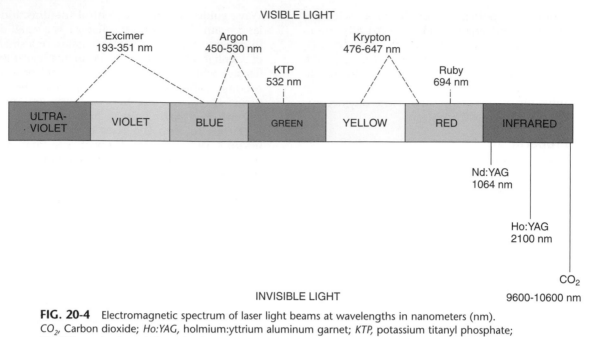

VISIBLE LIGHT

FIG. 20-4   Electromagnetic spectrum of laser light beams at wavelengths in nanometers (nm). *CO₂,* Carbon dioxide; *Ho:YAG,* holmium:yttrium aluminum garnet; *KTP,* potassium titanyl phosphate; *Nd:YAG,* neodymium:yttrium aluminum garnet.

The argon laser operates from electrical power. A water-cooling system is often required to dissipate heat generated in the argon medium.

The argon laser beam usually is transmitted through a flexible quartz fiberoptic wave guide that is 200 to 600 mm in diameter. This can be directed to a handpiece or through an endoscope or operating microscope. Most argon laser machines deliver a nonfocused beam that vaporizes tissue poorly and scatters more radiation than other types of lasers. Irradiance may vary from less than 1 watt to 20 watts, depending on the model.

Argon lasers coagulate bleeding points or lesions involving many small superficial vessels, such as a port-wine stain. They are used primarily to destroy specific cutaneous lesions while sparing adjacent tissue and minimizing scarring. Argon lasers may be used to treat vascular lesions and remove plaque and to coagulate superficial vessels in mucosa, such as in the gastrointestinal tract. They are also used in ophthalmology, otolaryngology, gynecology, urology, neurosurgery, and dermatology.

Carbon Dioxide Laser. Using a mixture of carbon dioxide (CO_2), nitrogen, and helium molecular gases, the CO_2 laser emits an invisible beam from the mid- to far-infrared range of the electromagnetic spectrum at wavelengths of 9600 and 10,600 nm. This wavelength is intensely absorbed by water. It raises water temperature in cells to the flash boiling point, thus vaporizing tissue. Vaporization is the conversion of solid tissue to smoke and gas. This plume should be evacuated or suctioned through a filter device from the site of lasing. The intense heat of the CO_2 laser also coagulates vessels as it cuts through them. It penetrates the surface to a depth of 0.1 to 0.2 mm per application to tissue, with minimal thermal effect to surrounding tissue.

The CO_2 laser operates from electrical power. The machine has a self-contained cooling system. The CO_2 laser beam should be delivered in a direct line of vision. It can be directed through a rigid endoscope, but it cannot be transmitted through a fiberoptic wave guide because its longer wavelength prevents conduction through crystal fibers. It is transmitted through an operating microscope or an articulating arm with a series of mirrors. The articulating arm allows precise focus and direction of the beam to a pencil-like handpiece. CO_2 lasers have a helium-neon (HeNe) laser coaxial target beam that superimposes the invisible carbon dioxide beam to provide a visible red aiming light. The wave generated may be continuous or pulsed. Irradiance can vary from less than 1 watt to up to 300 watts. A portable handheld laser tube with a hollow needle to deliver the carbon dioxide beam is available for use in vascular surgery and microsurgery.

The vaporization and hemostatic actions of the CO_2 laser are of value to the surgeon in treating soft tissue and vascular lesions. Large or small masses of tissue can be removed rapidly and efficiently. The CO_2 laser cannot be used in a fluid environment. The peritoneal cavity is insufflated with gas before the beam is directed through an endoscope. This laser is used primarily in otolaryngology, gynecology, plastic surgery, dermatology, neurosurgery, orthopedics, and cardiovascular and general surgery.

Excimer Laser. When organic molecular bonds are broken up by a photochemical reaction, cool laser energy is emitted. Short wavelengths in the ultraviolet to visible blue-green spectrum are produced by gas used in the excimer laser combining with a halide medium. Argon fluoride produces a wavelength of 193 nm; krypton fluoride, 248 nm; xenon chloride, 308 nm; and xenon fluoride, 351 nm. These gases are extremely toxic. The beams they produce offer precision in cutting and coagulating without thermal damage to adjacent tissue. Excimer lasers have been developed for use in ophthalmology, peripheral and coronary angioplasty, orthopedics (to cut bone), and neurosurgery.

Free Electron Laser. Free electrons, which are not bound to a specific atom, pass from a particle accelerator through a series of magnets to create a light beam. The beam can be tuned anywhere within the electromagnetic spectrum from ultraviolet to infrared. The free electron laser (FEL) produces light waves as a series of rapid superpulses of high energy and short duration, with minimal thermal damage. These light waves can fragment calculi. The FEL can be used also for precise cutting of tissues.

Holmium:Yttrium Aluminum Garnet (Ho:YAG) Laser. A crystal that contains holmium, thulium, and chromium elements increases the wavelength of YAG laser energy to 2100 nm. This invisible beam in the mid-infrared range of the electromagnetic spectrum is absorbed by tissues containing water. Combined with high-energy pulsed delivery, it penetrates less deeply into tissue than does the neodymium (Nd):YAG laser for more precise cutting and less generalized heating of tissue. It may be used percutaneously through a laser fiber threaded through a hollow needle or be delivered through a fine fiberoptic fiber. It may be used in a fluid medium. It acts on water in cells without char or extensive tissue damage. Approved for use in all joints except the spine, the Ho:YAG laser is useful in orthopedics to cut, shape, and sculpt cartilage and bone and to ablate soft tissues.

Krypton Laser. The krypton ion gas laser emits a red-yellow light beam in the visible electromagnetic spectrum at wavelengths of 476.2 to 647.1 nm. It is intensely absorbed by pigment in blood and retinal epithelium. The krypton laser resembles the argon laser in construction and use. It operates from electrical power and is water cooled. Used in ophthalmology, it is more versatile than the argon laser in selective photocoagulation of the retina.

Nd:YAG Laser. Neodymium, yttrium, aluminum, and garnet (Nd:YAG) constitute the solid-state crystal medium from which the light beam of this laser emanates. This invisible beam in the near-infrared range of the electromagnetic spectrum has a wavelength of 1064 nm. It is poorly absorbed by hemoglobin and water but is intensely absorbed by tissue protein. The wavelength penetrates to a depth of 3 to 7 mm to denature protein by thermal coagulation and shrinkage of tissue beneath the surface.

The Nd:YAG laser operates from electric current through the optical power source of xenon flash lamps. It must have an air, carbon dioxide, or water cooling system.

The Nd:YAG laser beam can be transmitted through a flexible quartz fiber, 200 to 600 mm in diameter, which passes through a rigid endoscope. It can also be transmitted through a fiberoptic wave guide to a handpiece or a flexible endoscope or be focused through an operating microscope. An aiming light of blue xenon or red neon-helium may be used in conjunction with the Nd:YAG beam. Sapphire or ceramic tips allow direct contact with tissue for

cutting and vaporizing without diffuse coagulation, using less than 25 watts of power. These tips are available on handheld scalpels or to fit on the ends of fibers for endoscopic use. Many of these tips are reusable; some are for single use only.

The Nd:YAG laser has the most powerful coagulating action of all the surgical lasers. Its continuous or pulsed wave penetrates deeper into tissues than do other lasers (i.e., up to 2 cm) and will coagulate large vessels (up to 4 mm). It is used to coagulate and vaporize large volumes of tissue. This versatile laser has applications in rhinolaryngology, urology, gynecology, neurosurgery, orthopedics, and thoracic and general surgery.

For ophthalmology, the Nd:YAG laser uses a Q-switching mode to store energy in a resonator during pumping action, followed by release of a single short pulse of high energy. This does not burn tissue but disrupts it with minute shock waves.

Potassium Titanyl Phosphate Laser. The solid-state potassium titanyl phosphate (KTP) crystal emits a visible green light at a wavelength of 532mm. This laser produces less power than CO_2 or Nd:YAG lasers but can be focused to a smaller diameter for precision work, such as in the middle ear. KTP absorbs most effectively into red or black tissue for coagulation. The beam can be directed by a handpiece at or in contact with tissue or through a rigid or flexible fiberoptic fiber or micromanipulator. The beam cuts, vaporizes, or coagulates tissue with minimal lateral thermal damage and plume. Cooling gases are not necessary, but the system should be water cooled. Instruments are available that provide both KTP and Nd:YAG wavelengths selected by a button on the control panel or that pass the Nd:YAG beam through the KTP crystal. Many accessories are available for specific applications in all surgical specialties. The KTP laser has good cutting properties.

Ruby Laser. The ruby solid-state crystal laser emits a visible red light at a wavelength of 694 nm. A synthetically machined crystal rod is placed in a resonator cavity with a xenon flash lamp that when activated creates the optical pumping to produce the ruby laser beam. Blood vessels and transparent substances do not absorb this beam. A pulsed system, the ruby laser is capable of generating large fields of energy on impact. This shock wave effect can injure internal tissues and bone. Irradiance is 1 watt. Originally used in ophthalmology, the ruby laser currently is used primarily to eradicate port-wine stain lesions of the skin.

Tunable Dye Laser. Fluorescent liquid dyes or vapors can produce lasing energy. When exposed to intense laser light, usually an argon beam, dye absorbs light and fluoresces over a broad spectrum from ultraviolet to the far-infrared range. The laser may be delivered interstitially, endoscopically, externally, or retrobulbarly. A tunable prism can adjust the laser wavelength from 400 to 1000 nm, in either continuous or pulsed mode, for the specific dye in use.

The argon tunable dye laser system emits a blue-green beam at a wavelength of 430 to 530 nm from an argon laser that pumps a rhodamine B dye laser to produce a red laser beam at a wavelength of approximately 630 nm for selective destruction of malignant tumor cells. A dye laser tuned to 577 nm can be used on vascular lesions. Other wavelengths, such as through copper vapor, may be used to treat skin lesions or superficial tumors, such as of the bladder wall. The site can be repeatedly treated as long as cells remain photosensitive. This tunable dye laser is used most commonly for photodynamic therapy.

Photodynamic Therapy. For photodynamic therapy, the patient is injected 24 to 48 hours before laser therapy with a photosensitive drug that is absorbed by normal and malignant tissue. Normal tissue gradually releases the drug, but abnormal tissue retains it. The abnormal photosensitive tissue is destroyed when exposed to the laser beam. Normal adjacent tissue appears sunburned but is not permanently damaged. All dyes used with tunable dye lasers are potentially toxic and are handled with caution.

Safety Factors

All surgical lasers present hazards to patients and to the OR team. This equipment should be used in accordance with established regulations, standards and recommended practices, manufacturer's recommendations, and institutional policies. Laser safety is based on knowledge of the specific laser to be used, its instrumentation, its mode of operation, its power densities, its action in tissues, and its risks.

Regulatory Agencies. Lasers are classified as medical devices and are subject to regulation. The Code of Federal Regulations' Performance Standards for Light Emitting Products provides specifications for manufacturers of medical laser systems.

National Center for Devices and Radiological Health. The National Center for Devices and Radiological Health (NCDRH) is the regulatory section of the U.S. Food and Drug Administration (FDA) in the Department of Health and Human Services (HHS). More than 250 types of lasers are regulated by the FDA. Those intended for medical and surgical use come under the jurisdiction of medical device regulations. They are categorized as class III, subdivision class 4, because lasers are potentially hazardous (Box 20-2).

Manufacturers must verify that their products meet all safety requirements of the federal standard. They must receive approval from the NCDRH to market or test a laser for a particular clinical application or use, and they must comply with labeling requirements.

American National Standards Institute. The American National Standards Institute (ANSI) is a voluntary organization of experts who determine industry consensus standards in technical fields. The standard developed specifically for laser safety in health care facilities is intended for all users. Existing federal legislation and state laser safety regulations are based on the ANSI standard. Simply stated, this standard implies that every health care facility that uses surgical lasers must establish and maintain an adequate program for control of laser hazards. This program shall include provisions for the following:
- *Laser safety officer.* This person should have authority to suspend, restrict, or terminate operation of a laser

---

BOX 20-2 | **Medical Device Regulations**

FDA CLASSIFICATION OF MEDICAL DEVICES
Medical devices were classified in 1976 by the FDA according to their safety factors.

Class I
Subject to general controls

Class II
Devices for which general controls are not enough

Class III
Implants and life support devices

CLASSIFICATION OF LASERS
Lasers are classified according to potential hazard of exposure.

Class 1
Enclosed system, considered safe based on current medical knowledge; no light emission escapes the enclosure

Class 2
Limited to visible light (400-780 nm). Output power is 1 mW or less. Momentary viewing (0.25-second maximum permissible exposure) is not considered hazardous. Staring into the beam is not recommended. Protective eyewear of the correct optical density should be worn.

Class 3A
Emitted laser viewed directly through collecting optics would cause permanent eye damage. Output power is 0.5 mW or less. Protective eyewear of the correct optical density should be worn.

Class 3B
Continuous laser light with 0.5-watt or less output can cause permanent eye damage. Exposure to the beam should be avoided. Protective eyewear of the correct optical density should be worn.

Class 4
Laser light produced is hazardous to skin and eyes. Strict control measures are enforced. Protective eyewear of the correct optical density should be worn.

FDA, U.S. Food and Drug Administration.

---

system if hazard controls are inadequate. A laser safety committee, often a subcommittee of the OR committee, may appoint this surveillance officer.
- *Education of users.* A safety training program must ensure that all users, including surgeons, perioperative nurses, surgical technologists, and biomedical engineers and technicians, are knowledgeable of correct operation, potential hazards, and control measures.
- *Protective measures.* Protective measures are for patients, personnel, and the environment.
- *Management of accidents.* Management includes reporting accidents and developing plans of action to prevent a future occurrence.

Occupational Safety and Health Administration. The Occupational Safety and Health Administration (OSHA) is concerned primarily with the safety of health care workers. The agency can enforce ANSI standards.

State and Local Agencies. State regulations and local ordinances vary. Knowledge of and compliance with any requirements should be established.

Policies and Procedures. Specific policies and procedures related to use of lasers should be written by the laser safety committee before a laser program is instituted. These policies and procedures will need to be revised or updated when new equipment is installed. Applicable policies include, but are not limited to, the following:

1. Credentialing and clinical practice privileges of medical staff. Physicians authorized to use a laser should be required to complete a postgraduate laser course in their specialties. Hands-on experience and a preceptorship with a qualified user also should be required. The physician must have training for each type and wavelength of laser. A list of approved physicians should be available to the perioperative staff. Scheduling privileges should be denied to those surgeons who are not appropriately credentialed.

2. Initial and ongoing educational laser use and safety programs for perioperative personnel. Perioperative personnel should have thorough knowledge and understanding of laser equipment, laser physics, tissue reactions, applications, and safety precautions.

3. Continuous quality improvement. A program of continuous quality improvement includes appropriate care, use, and maintenance of equipment and prevention of laser-related accidents.

4. Documentation. The surgeon, procedure, type of laser used, length of use, and wattage should be recorded in the patient's medical record. This information, plus the patient's name, should also be recorded in the OR log.

Patient Safety. The surgeon must explain laser surgery and its potential complications to the patient before obtaining written consent. Some lasers are considered investigational devices by the FDA. The patient must sign a specific consent form permitting experimental use and data collection. With all lasers, appropriate precautions (including protection of the patient's eyes, skin, and tissue surrounding the target area from thermal burns) are taken to ensure patient safety as follows:

1. The eyes and eyelids should be adequately protected from the specific laser beam in use.
   a. Patients who are awake must wear the same type of safety glasses or goggles as those worn by the laser team.
   b. The eyelids can be taped shut on patients who are under general anesthesia.
   c. Eye pads moistened with saline solution should be taped securely in place for procedures around the head and neck, except for ophthalmic procedures and those using the Nd:YAG laser. Nonflammable material, such as aluminum foil with the reflective side down, can be taped over the eyes for Nd:YAG laser procedures. Moistened eye pads will not stop this laser beam.
   d. Protective shields should be used on the eyes during ophthalmic procedures. Corneal eye shields can

be applied directly onto anesthetized eyes to protect corneal tissue.

2. Antiseptics used for skin preparation should be nonflammable.
   a. Aqueous solutions are safest, but they can retain laser heat if they are allowed to pool on or around skin. The skin should be thoroughly dry before the laser is activated.
   b. Alcohol and tinctures are flammable and volatile when wet. Vapors must not accumulate under drapes because they can ignite.

3. The immediate area around the incision and/or tissue surrounding the target site should be protected from thermal injury. Flammable materials are avoided or safeguarded to prevent fire.
   a. Flame- or fire-resistant drapes should be used. Metallic foil and polypropylene laser-retardant and ignition-resistant drapes are available. Polypropylene and plastic incise drapes can melt if a laser beam strikes them. Woven and nonwoven fabrics can ignite.
   b. Woven textile or cellulose-based absorbent nonwoven towels saturated with sterile normal saline solution or water should be placed over fabric drapes around the incision before the laser is used.
   c. The laser handpiece should be laid on a moistened surface. The laser tip is extremely hot and may shatter if placed in contact with a cold surface.
   d. Moistened sponges, towels, or compressed patties should be placed around target tissue except when the Nd:YAG laser is used. Sponges and other material should be removed from tissue near the target site of the Nd:YAG laser because wetting will not stop this beam and they could be ignited.
   e. The rectum should be packed with a moistened sponge to prevent methane gas, which is potentially explosive, from escaping from the intestinal tract during use of a laser in the perineal area. Placement of the sponge in the anal orifice and removal of the rectal packing should be recorded as part of the sponge count.

4. Anesthetic agents should be noncombustible. Nonflammable anesthetics and oxygen mixed with nonflammable agents are administered in a closed system.
   a. Oxygen and nitrous oxide concentrations around the head should be as low as possible during use of a laser in the aerodigestive tract (i.e., oral, laryngeal, bronchial, or esophageal procedures).
   b. Flexible metallic or insulated silicone endotracheal tubes are preferred for aerodigestive tract procedures. Laser-approved varieties are commercially available. If used, red rubber tubes are wrapped with reflective aluminum or copper tape to prevent ignition. Polyvinyl chloride (PVC) endotracheal tubes should not be used because they ignite easily. The endotracheal tube cuff should be inflated with saline solution, which may be tinted with methylene blue to facilitate detection of a leak.

5. The teeth should be covered during oropharyngeal procedures to protect against reflective radiation.

6. Patients who are awake may wear a protective high-filtration mask during CO_2 laser ablation, such as of condylomata (venereal warts), to prevent inhaling airborne material into the lungs. An intubated patient is not considered at risk for respiratory contamination.

7. Postoperative instructions should include care of a healing thermal skin wound.

Personnel Safety. Exposure to nonionizing laser radiation can be hazardous for personnel. Precautions are taken to avoid eye and skin exposure to direct or scattered radiation and inhalation of plume. Some facilities require laser personnel to have baseline retinal screening performed before working in the laser unit.

Eye Protection. The eye is the organ most susceptible to laser injury. Different laser wavelengths affect eyes differently: argon and Nd:YAG lasers will be absorbed by retina, and the CO_2 laser will be absorbed by the cornea. Therefore, safety glasses or goggles of the correct optical density are worn at all times while the laser is in use. Optical density is the ability of the lens to absorb a specific wavelength (Table 20-1). The color of the lens is not the protective feature of the eyewear. Each type of wavelength requires protective eyewear of a specific optical density as recommended by the manufacturer of the laser. The following considerations apply to eye protection:

1. Protective eyewear is available outside the room near posted signs designating the specific type of laser in use. Only people with appropriate eye protection are admitted in the room while the laser is in use.
   a. All protective eyewear (i.e., safety glasses, goggles) must shield the wearer's eyes from the top, bottom, and sides of the visual field.
   b. Goggles will fit over eyeglasses, or prescription lenses of the correct optical density can be obtained. Contact lenses do not provide eye protection.
   c. Scratches on the lens or breaks in the frame can negate eye protection.
2. Lens covers with filter caps are available for optical eyepieces of endoscopes and operating microscopes. Their use does not eliminate the need for the entire team to wear eye protection.

TABLE 20-1	Optical Density Necessary for Protective Eyewear

Optical Density	Transmission of Light (% of Wavelength)*
0	1
1	0.1
2	0.01
3	0.001
4	0.0001
5	0.00001
6	0.000001

*Light transmission is measured with a spectrophotometer to calculate the optical density needed for protective eyewear.

Skin Protection. Skin sensitivities can develop from overexposure to ultraviolet radiation. Skin also can be burned from exposure to direct or reflected laser energy. These hazards are minimized if personnel are alert to precautions for environmental safety. Other personnel safety precautions reduce risks and include the following:
- Metallic jewelry should not be worn. It could absorb heat or reflect the beam.
- Fire-resistant gowns may be worn.

Laser Plume. Toxic substances, including carcinogens and viruses, may become airborne from vaporization of tissues, especially from CO_2 and Nd:YAG lasers. The smoke produced, referred to as laser plume, contains water, carbonized particles, mutated deoxyribonucleic acid (DNA), and intact cells. It may have a distinct odor.

Laser plume should not be inhaled. One gram of plume is equivalent to smoking six cigarettes. Smoke evacuation from the site of lasing and high-filtration masks prevent personnel from inhaling plume. Removal of plume also enhances visibility at the target site for the surgeon. Plume can bend or refract the beam, thus inadvertently causing injury to adjacent tissues. The following precautions should be taken:

1. A mechanical smoke evacuator or suction with a high-efficiency filter should be turned on before or at the same time as the laser and should be run during activation and for 20 to 30 seconds after the laser is deactivated. The tip should be placed as close as possible, at least within 2 inches (5 cm), to the lasing site of tissue vaporization.
   a. Several types of mechanical smoke evacuators are available. Many systems have charcoal filters.
   b. Charcoal filters in most evacuators are changed regularly. Gloves and a mask are worn when handling contaminated filters.
2. Masks should be tight-fitting and should filter particles as small as 0.1 mm.

Environmental Safety. Only properly trained personnel are authorized to participate in laser surgery. Others should be made aware of its hazards. The following considerations apply to environmental safety:

1. Warning signs (e.g., Laser Surgery in Progress) should be posted on the outside of all OR doors when the laser is in use. The design, symbols, and wording on the warning sign should be specific for the type of laser in use.
2. Walls and ceilings should have nonreflective surfaces. Glass, as in windows, cabinet doors, and/or the x-ray viewing box, should be covered with nonreflective material to stop beams when lasers other than CO_2 lasers are used. CO_2 laser beams are absorbed by glass.
3. Warning labels on the machine, affixed by the manufacturer, must indicate points of danger to avoid personnel exposure to laser radiation.
4. The machine should be prepared, checked, and tested before the patient is brought into the room. A preoperative checklist is helpful. Any malfunction should be reported immediately, and the equipment should not be used until it is in proper working order.

5. When not in use, the machine should be kept on the "standby" setting with the beam terminated in a beam stop of highly absorbent, nonreflecting, fire-resistant material to avoid accidental activation. It should be turned off and locked with a key when left unattended. Only authorized personnel should have access to the key.

6. The foot switch should be operated by the surgeon who delivers the laser energy to the tissue. The foot pedal can be covered when not in use so that the surgeon will not inadvertently activate the laser. Foot pedals for other equipment should be moved away while the laser is in use. The laser pedal can then be removed after use.

7. Nonreflective instruments should be used in or near the beam. These instruments may be of a dull blue titanium alloy or an ebonized or anodized stainless steel. These finishes defocus and disperse the laser beam. Reflective instruments can cause burns or start fires.

8. Fire is a potential hazard that must not be underestimated. Personnel should be aware of fire safeguards and adhere to precautions for their own and the patient's safety.
   a. A basin of sterile water or normal saline solution should be readily available at the sterile field.
   b. A halon fire extinguisher should be available.
   c. Oxygen concentration in the room should be as low as possible. Oxygen leaking from the side of a patient's facemask can be ignited by the laser beam. The anesthesia provider should be knowledgeable about flash points and fire retardation when the laser is in use.
   d. Liquids should not be placed on the machine. A spill could act as a conductor and short-circuit the mechanism.

9. Electrical codes and standards should be enforced to avoid electrical hazards. An isolation transformer is recommended for a high-power laser power source to avoid dangerous overload of the existing OR power system. Electrical circuitry must provide adequate amperage for power requirements. Preferably, the laser has its own dedicated circuit.

10. The manufacturer's instructions for operation, care, handling, and sterilization of the laser system should be followed. Proper care of lasers and accessory equipment is essential to patient, personnel, and environmental safety.

Laser Team

A laser team should be designated to carry out the duties that are different from those of the traditional OR team. This team may include the following personnel:

1. Clinical laser nurse. The responsibilities of the clinical laser nurse are different from those of the circulating nurse. Duties include the following:
   a. Preparing and teaching the patient preoperatively, intraoperatively, and postoperatively.
   b. Bringing laser equipment to the OR and checking it. The chassis and the floor around it should be inspected for water leak. Using sterile technique, the clinical laser nurse and scrub person calibrate the laser as appropriate.
   c. Covering windows, posting signs, and distributing appropriate protective eyewear.
   d. Covering the patient's eyes.
   e. Positioning the laser foot pedal for the surgeon's convenience and removing it after use.
   f. Operating the key switch and monitoring activation of the laser. The wattage and exposure time are set according to the surgeon's orders. These should be repeated before and after adjusting controls.
   g. Cleaning and checking laser fibers after use and preparing them for sterilization.
   h. Completing the laser log.
   i. Collaborating with the laser safety officer and biomedical engineer and/or technician to ensure safe use of laser equipment.

2. Biomedical technician. The biomedical technician provides preventive maintenance and handles minor problems with the laser system. A log of laser use and maintenance is maintained.

3. Camera operator. Endoscopic procedures performed under video control may require an additional sterile team member to operate the camera attached to the endoscope while the surgeon controls the laser fiber.

Advantages of Laser Surgery

Surgical lasers emit nonionizing radiation. This radiation is selectively absorbed by different tissues with resultant penetration and destruction at the focal point but with differential thermal protection of surrounding tissues. Lasers offer the surgeon and the patient many advantages over other surgical techniques, including the following:

- Precise control for accurate incision, excision, or ablation of tissue. The laser beam is precisely focused for localized tissue destruction. The depth of radiation penetration is precisely regulated by the duration of focus, power density, and type of tissue.
- Access to areas inaccessible to other surgical instruments through minimally invasive techniques. The beam can be directed through endoscopes or deflected off of rhodium reflector mirrors.
- An unobstructed view of the surgical site. The laser beam comes in contact with tissue to be cut, coagulated, or vaporized. It can be directed through the operating microscope.
- Minimal handling of and trauma to tissues. Traction on target tissue is unnecessary.
- A dry, bloodless surgical field. The laser beam simultaneously cuts and coagulates blood vessels, thus providing hemostasis in vascular areas.
- Minimal thermal effect on surrounding tissue. Essentially no permanent thermal necrosis of tissue occurs beyond 100 mm from the edge of the area incised. This minimizes postoperative pain.
- Reduced risk of contamination or infection. The laser beam vaporizes microorganisms, thus essentially sterilizing the contact area.
- Prompt healing with minimal postoperative edema, sloughing of tissue, pain, and scarring.

• Reduced operating time. Because procedures can be done more quickly, both anesthesia time and operating time are shorter. Many procedures can be done without general anesthesia. Many are done in ambulatory care facilities.

Disadvantages of Laser Surgery

• The costs to start and maintain a program are high. Equipment, instrumentation, supplies, and staff education are expensive initial investments. Most aspects need frequent updates and maintenance.
• Decisions should be made about the use of disposable versus reusable supplies and the effect on patient care. Most reusable supplies are fragile and should be replaced on a regular basis.
• Liability may increase as the number of users increases. Specific credentialing and continuing education require planning and are time consuming.

MICROSURGERY

The simplest magnifying instrument consists of a single lens with relatively high magnification (e.g., a magnifying glass or a jeweler's lens). Surgeons requiring lesser magnification than that provided by the microscope use an operating loupe. This simple lens magnifies approximately two times. It attaches to a headband or to the surgeon's spectacles. Loupe surgery terminates where microsurgery begins. From loupe surgery and refinements of the binocular microscope, microsurgery has evolved.

HISTORICAL BACKGROUND

Use of the microscope has been an essential modality in scientific investigation for centuries. Pioneers such as Dutch microscopist Anton van Leeuwenhoek (1632-1723), who in 1680 developed the compound microscope, which magnified objects 270 times, contributed to the adoption of the germ theory. Objects as small as protozoa and bacteria could be seen only through a light microscope, just as viruses can be seen only through the more recently developed electron microscope.

Optician Joseph Jackson Lister (1786-1869), father of the English surgeon who introduced antiseptic surgery, perfected the achromatic lens to eliminate color aberrations in the compound microscope. Ernest Abbe (1840-1905) did further work in the nineteenth century to improve refraction through immersion of the lens in oil and concentration of illumination (1886). A basic system for binocular eyepieces was devised in 1902.

A microscope was first used for clinical surgery in 1921 when Nylen operated on patients with chronic otitis in Sweden. He used a monocular microscope. Subsequently, as binocular magnification, adequate illumination, and stable support were added, otolaryngology became the first surgical specialty to routinely use a microscope.

Ophthalmologists were the first to use the stereoscopic biomicroscope, commonly referred to as a slit lamp, in clinical examination to magnify objects in three dimensions. The principles applied to the biomicroscope led to the development of an operating microscope in 1953. Ophthalmologists quickly expanded applications and indications for ocular microsurgery. Most other specialties were slow to implement its use.

The first of the current operating microscopes was developed in 1960 by the Zeiss Instrument Company in collaboration with Julius Jacobson, a vascular surgeon in New York. Jacobson developed microsurgical instruments, introduced microvascular techniques, and began using the term *microsurgery.* Thus began the development of clinical applications of microsurgery in every surgical specialty.

Technique of Microsurgery

Performance of surgical procedures while directly viewing the surgical field under magnification affords surgeons greater visual acuity of small structures. The microscope provides a more limited, although more readily visible, surgical field. All things look considerably different under magnification. Tissues not otherwise visible can be manipulated.

Use of microsurgical instrumentation and techniques is not simply a matter of adapting formerly learned conventional methods for use under the microscope. The techniques themselves for handling instruments, sutures, and tissues are different and infinitely more complex, precise, and time consuming because of the meticulous skill involved. Coordination must be adapted to working with minute materials in a field of altered perception and position. Proficiency and facility in using the operating microscope entail laboratory practice in movements and manipulation of instruments and suture materials under various magnifications.

Divergence from tactile-manual to vision-oriented techniques requires that the surgeon and assistants pay maximum attention to detail. The most common maneuvers for placing and manipulating instruments, making an incision with scissors, and tying sutures involve a combination of several basic movements:

• *Compression-decompression.* To close scissors and forceps
• *Rotation.* To insert a needle, to cut, to extract, to engage or disengage
• *Push-pull, direct, or linear.* To incise with a razor knife

The surgeon also must be able to maintain a steady, stationary position during remote activation of equipment such as a laser beam. It is advisable that surgeons and assistants do no manual labor for at least a day before operating. Drinking coffee the morning of surgery may decrease steadiness in some individuals. Very little tremor is tolerable in microsurgery.

Advantages of Microsurgery

Microsurgery provides unique advantages in the restoration of wholeness and function of the body, such as restitution of hearing, vision, tactile sensation, circulation, and/or motion. It is used in many surgical specialties to improve precision of already-established surgical procedures and to permit successful performance of procedures previously not possible. For example, blood vessels less than 3 mm in exterior diameter can be sutured. Nerves can be anastomosed. Replantation of amputated parts and some reconstructive surgery are possible only under magnification. In general, microsurgery allows the following:

• Dissection and repair of fine structures through better visualization

- Adaptation of surgical procedures to individual patient requirements (variation in anatomic landmarks is more distinct with magnification)
- Diminution of surgical trauma and complications because of safer dissection
- Superior focal lighting of the surgical field, particularly in deep areas

Operating Microscope

Compound microscopes use two or more lens systems or several lenses grouped in one unit. The operating microscope is a compound binocular instrument. Interchangeable objective lenses combined with interchangeable eyepieces allow a wide range of magnification and working distances adjustable to the surgeon's needs.

The operating microscope uses light waves for illumination. These waves are bent as they pass through the microscope, causing the image seen by the viewer's eye to be magnified.

The users must understand the parts and their functions. Basically, all operating microscopes incorporate the same essential components: an optical lens system and controls for magnification and focus, an illumination system, a mounting system for stability, an electrical system, and accessories.

Optical Lens System. The ability to enlarge an image is known as magnifying power. This is the ratio of the size of the image produced on the viewer's retina by magnification to the size of the retinal image when the object is viewed without optical aid. To create a distinct image, adjacent images must be separated. An indistinct image remains unclear no matter how many times it is magnified. The ability to discern detail is known as resolving power.

Components. The heart of the optical system is the body, which contains the objective lens (lens closest to the object). The head or binocular oculars (eyepieces) through which the surgeon looks are physically and optically attached to the body. The optical combination of the objective lens and the oculars determines the magnification of the microscope (Fig. 20-5).

Objective lenses are available in various focal lengths ranging from 100 to 400 mm, with intervening increases by 25-mm increments. The 400-mm lens provides the greatest magnification. The designation of the objective lens enumerates the working distance (the distance from the lens to the surgical field). Distances vary from 6 to 10 inches (15 to 25 cm). For example, a 200-mm lens will be in focus at a working distance of 200 mm, or approximately 8 inches (20 cm).

The oculars serve as magnifying glasses used to examine the real image formed by the objective. Most objectives are achromatic so that the true color of tissues can be viewed in sharp detail. The binocular arrangement provides stereoscopic viewing. Stereopsis is basically achieved through binocular viewing, wherein each eye has a slightly different positional view of the object under examination. The observer's brain then combines the two dissimilar images taken from points of view a little distance apart, thus producing a perception of a single three-dimensional image. If

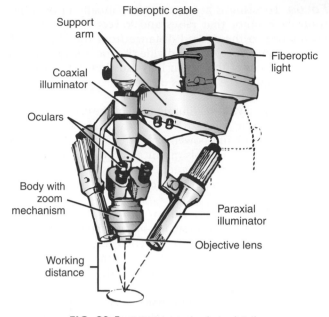

FIG. 20-5   Microscope body in detail.

the user is wearing corrective lenses, the eyepieces are set to zero. If the user needs corrective lenses but is not wearing them, he or she should preset the eyepieces to a position of visual comfort and acuity before draping the microscope. Detachable rubber eyecups for the eyepieces are commercially available for the user's comfort.

Magnification. The ability of the microscope to magnify depends on the design and quality of the parts in addition to the resolving power. The total magnification is computed by multiplying the enlarging power of the objective lens by that of the lenses of the oculars. The depth of the field, which is the vertical dimension within which objects are seen in clear focus, decreases with increases in magnification of power. Likewise, the width of the field of view narrows as the power of magnification increases. For example, at 20× magnification, the field of view narrows to $\frac{1}{2}$ inch (10 mm, or less than 1.25 cm). Vertical viewing of the surgical field is extremely important, particularly in higher magnification ranges. It allows the surgeon more effective use of the increasingly limited depth of field.

In more complex microscopes, a third set of lenses is interposed between the oculars and the objective lens to provide additional magnification in variable degrees as desired by the surgeon. A continuously variable system of magnification for increasing or decreasing images is possible with a zoom lens. Most surgeons prefer a faster, easier-to-handle zoom lens to a simpler turret magnifier that manually changes magnification by fixed increments. The zoom lens is usually operated by a foot control that permits the surgeon to change magnification without removing the hands from the surgical field. The popular range of magnification in the zoom microscope is from 3.5× to 20× magnification. At 3.5× magnification, the depth of the field is about 0.01 inch (2.5 mm); at 20× magnification, the depth is about $\frac{1}{25}$ inch (1 mm). Some microscopes magnify to 40 times.

Focus. Focusing is accomplished manually or by a foot-controlled motor that raises and lowers the body of the microscope to the desired distance from the object to be viewed. Some microscopes divide the focus into gross and fine. The focus of the ocular lens usually is set at zero; the surgeon adjusts the focus as desired.

Illumination System. Illumination of the operating microscope uses light waves. The shorter the wavelength, the greater the resolving power. The intensity of illumination can be varied by controls mounted on the support arm of the body. The operating microscope has two basic sources of illumination: paraxial and coaxial.

Paraxial Illuminators. One or more light tubes (paraxial illuminators) contain tungsten or halogen bulbs and focusing lenses. The illuminators are attached to the mounting of the body of the microscope in a position to illuminate the field of view. Light is focused to coincide with the working distance of the microscope.

One of the paraxial illuminators may be equipped with a diaphragm containing a variable-width slit aperture. This device permits a narrow beam of light to be brought into focus on the objective field. This slit image assists the surgeon in defining depth perception (i.e., in ascertaining the relative distance of objects within the field—which are closer, which are farther).

Coaxial Illuminators. With fiberoptic coaxial illuminators, light is transmitted through the optical system of the microscope body. This type of illumination is called coaxial because it illuminates the same area in the same focus as the viewing, or objective, field of the microscope. The fiberoptic system provides intense, though cool, light that protects the patient's tissues and the optics of the microscope from excessive heat. The light intensity ranges from 600 to 2250 foot-candles without creating shadows. Reflected glare may be a problem. Frequent wound irrigation with a cool solution is necessary to avoid tissue damage from radiant energy during long procedures.

If a fiberoptic system is not used for coaxial illumination, a heat-absorbing filter must be interposed in the illumination system. Direct heat from a high-intensity source can damage and even burn tissues. Tungsten and halogen bulbs are used in some housings.

Another type of optical prism assembly provides a larger area of coaxial illumination with a brighter light than that obtained with fiberoptic light bundles. Known as liquid light, it uses ionic, inorganic saline solution with quartz glass inserts inside a flexible aluminum spiral tube insulated with a polyvinyl chloride coating. Light is conducted throughout the cross section of the liquid, unlike the light provided by a fiberoptic bundle.

Mounting Systems. The stability of the microscope is of paramount importance. The body, the optical portion, is mounted on a vertical column that may be supported by the floor, ceiling, or wall, or by attachment to the operating bed. The body of the microscope is attached to the column by a hinged arm and a central pivot. The mounting permits positioning as desired. It may be adjusted horizontally or vertically, rotated on its axis, and tilted at different angles. The microscope can be aimed in any direction. The objective is aimed at the principal surgical site.

Floor and ceiling mounting systems are the most popular and versatile. All microscopes must have a locking mechanism to immobilize the microscope body over the surgical field.

Floor Mount. The base of the vertical support, which rests on the floor, has retractable casters for ease in moving the entire instrument. When the base is lowered to working position, it is locked into position (Fig. 20-6).

The base should be properly positioned in relation to the operating bed before the anesthetic is administered or the patient is prepped. To maintain balance and control, one should gently push (not pull) the microscope when moving it. Jarring or banging the scope should be avoided, since the lenses may dislocate and obscure vision. The brake should be released or casters activated before the microscope is moved. The arms should be folded close to the column with all of the attachments locked into place. Cords should be out of the way. Observation tubes should not be used as handles. Force should never be used in moving the microscope or in applying attachments; one should look for the problem instead. A floor-based microscope with column support is placed to the left of a right-handed surgeon. The base should not interfere with foot controls or power cables. It should be clear of any table attachments.

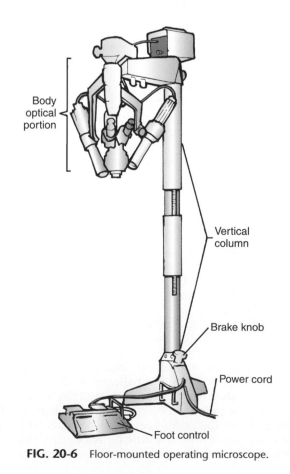

Body optical portion

Vertical column

Brake knob

Power cord

Foot control

FIG. 20-6 Floor-mounted operating microscope.

Some microscopes use a Contraves stand. This is a counterbalanced weight system used to position the operating microscope in a suspended position over the surgical field. The weights are set and locked according to the type of attachments on the body of the microscope. The balance is set before activating the power switch.

As a safety factor, the base must not be moved when the microscope is positioned over the patient, because it is top-heavy. Gross adjustments, such as height in relation to the surgical field and focus, are made with the microscope swung away from the patient. The operating bed height, chair, and armrest heights are adjusted at the same time that gross adjustments are made. Fine focusing and adjustments are done after the microscope is in position for the surgical procedure. The assistant's microscope is adjusted to the same focus as that of the surgeon. During prepping and draping, the microscope is rotated out of position and then brought over the surgical field for the procedure.

Ceiling Mount.

A ceiling mount, either a fixed or track-mounted model, provides freer floor space. The fixed unit is suspended from a telescoping column attached directly to the ceiling. Vertical support of a track-mounted unit is suspended from a ceiling rail. It can be moved out of the way when not in use (Fig. 20-7). The microscope is positioned and focused after the patient is anesthetized. A ceiling-mounted instrument is operated by a control panel on a wall (on-off switch) and by foot controls for focusing, magnifying, raising, and lowering.

A ceiling mount is generally very stable, but it is only as stable as the supporting ceiling. Mechanical devices adjacent to the OR, such as air-conditioning units, may cause vibration. The microscope should be vibration-free. A ceiling mount permits the same flexibility of positioning as a floor mount.

The vertical support has a memory stop mechanism that can be preset for a preselected operating bed height. This setting should be checked and adjusted for each operating bed position change. The mechanism is a safety factor to prevent accidental lowering of the microscope at high speed too close to the patient. High-speed lowering should be done away from the patient until the memory stop is reached. As with the floor-mounted instrument, gross adjustments are never made over the patient. Fine adjustment and focusing are done after the microscope is over the surgical field.

Wall Mount.

The microscope is bracketed by a flexible arm to a stable wall. The swing-arm extension permits proper positioning.

Operating Bed Mount.

Smaller microscopes may be mounted on the framework of the operating bed. This system has many disadvantages and thus is not popular.

Electrical System.

The same precautions are observed with the operating microscope as with any electrical equipment in the OR. Switches and wall interlocks should be explosion-proof. Circuits are protected from overload by breaker relays and fuses. All light controls should be in the off position when the power plug is inserted or removed from the wall outlet to avoid short-circuiting or sparking. A red pilot light illuminates on the control panel when the electrical power is on.

Accessories.

A number of accessories are available to enhance the versatility of microsurgery. The value of a good microscope is negated without proper ancillary equipment.

Assistant's Binoculars.

A separate optical body with a nonmotorized, hand-controlled zoom lens can be attached to the main microscope body for use by the assistant (Fig. 20-8). This mechanism can be focused in the same plane as the surgeon's oculars. Its field of view may not coincide exactly with that of the surgeon. This can be rectified by using a beam splitter, which takes the image from one of the surgeon's oculars and transmits it through an observer tube, thereby providing the assistant with an identical image of the surgeon's view (see Fig. 20-8). This is particularly important in critical areas where a difference of 1 or 2 mm is crucial.

Assistant's binocular co-observer tubes can be placed on the body of the microscope so that the assistant can work and observe from the same side of the operating bed as, at a right angle to, or directly opposite the surgeon. Binocular tubes (tiltable, straight, or inclined) can be attached on the right or left side of the body of the microscope. A dual viewing bridge, the quadroscope, is attached when the surgeon and assistant sit opposite each other. They have exactly the

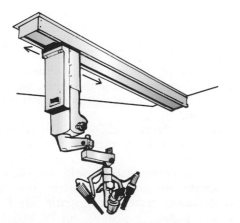

FIG. 20-7   Ceiling track-mounted microscope.

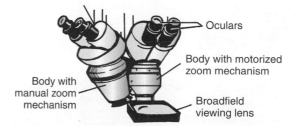

Oculars

Body with motorized zoom mechanism

Body with manual zoom mechanism

Broadfield viewing lens

FIG. 20-8   Surgeon's microscope on right with assistant's binoculars attached on left.

same view of the field with this accessory. Binoculars should be appropriately placed on the microscope body before the surgical procedure begins.

Broadfield Viewing Lens. A low-power magnifying glass is used for grasping needles or for getting an overall view of the field adjacent to the objective. This lens attaches to the front of the body of the surgeon's ocular (see Fig. 20-8).

Couplings. Couplings allow versatility in positioning the microscope for specific applications. An automated mechanism, the X-Y attachment, provides precision in controlling small movements of the microscope in the field of view. A coupling piece lets surgeons change the angle for side-to-side or front-to-back viewing. A universal tilt coupling can be integrated into the X-Y coupling.

Cameras. Still photographic, motion picture, videotape, and television cameras may be attached to the beam splitter, permitting filming of the surgical procedure (Fig. 20-9). The camera unit should be in the upright position when connected to the operating microscope. It may require the use of a stronger illumination source. One should check to ensure film is in the camera by trying to rewind the film cartridge holder. The patient's and surgeon's names, the date, and the time are documented on the film or video cartridge to prevent mixing recorded images among patients. The use of recording equipment may require special patient consent in some institutions. The recorded procedure is useful in assisting, teaching, and research.

Laser Microadapter. Laser beams can be directed through the operating microscope. The microscope and laser head couplings should be perfectly aligned in the grooves and protrusions on the metal adapters. A screw and locking pin secure the coupling. In the operating position, the laser head is at approximately a 60-degree angle to the microscope. It will not fire in a horizontal or upside-down position. The microadapter must have a compatible lens with a focal length of 200, 300, or 400 mm so that the surgeon can properly adjust the focal point of the laser beam. A CO_2 laser with electronic components that delivers milliwatt energy may be used to vaporize tissues or weld tissues together. Other types of lasers are directed through fiberoptics. To protect the

surgeon's eyes, filter caps over optics should be the appropriate optical density for the wavelength of the laser being used. The entire team and patient must wear eye protection of the appropriate optical density when the laser is in use.

Remote Foot Controls. Simple microscopes are manually operated. It is more convenient for the surgeon to use motorized foot controls for functions such as focus, zoom, and tilt. Foot controls may be activated by switches of the push-button type, heel-to-toe, or side-to-side motion. The number of switches corresponds to the number of motor-controlled functions. There may be additional foot switches for the camera or for other nonmicroscope-associated equipment, such as cryosurgical, bipolar electrosurgical, or laser units.

Switches may be separated by a vertical bar to prevent inadvertent contact. The bar also serves as a footrest for the surgeon. Because the surgeon and assistant usually are seated during microsurgical procedures, the height of the operating bed must permit them adequate knee room to operate foot controls.

Microscope Drape. The entire working mechanism and support arm of the microscope are encased in a sterile drape. Draping the entire microscope permits it to be brought into the sterile field so that the surgeon can position the body and adjust the optics. Disposable drapes that are heat resistant, lint-free, nonreflective, transparent, and quiet are available to fit the configuration of all microscopes and attachments. The scrub person slides the drape over the body of the microscope, with hands protected as for draping a Mayo stand. The circulating nurse helps guide the drape toward the vertical column and secures it. The scrub person secures the drape to the oculars. Sterile lens covers or rubber bands may be supplied with the drape for this purpose.

If it is not heat resistant, a plastic drape may cause heat buildup beneath it that can damage the microscope. A heat guard may be applied over the light source, or heat may be evacuated through an opening in the top of the drape.

Care of the Microscope

Persons responsible for the microscope should consult the manufacturer's manual. Any malfunction should be reported to the OR manager or appropriate person who can arrange for repair service. A checklist to verify care and functioning of various parts before the surgical procedure is helpful. Everyone who assists with microsurgery must know how to set up, position, and otherwise care for the microscope as follows:

1. The microscope should be damp-dusted before use.
    a. External surfaces, except the lenses, are wiped with a clean cloth saturated with detergent-disinfectant solution.
    b. Casters or wheels should be clean to reduce contamination and prevent interference with mobility.
2. Lenses should be cleaned according to the manufacturer's recommendations only, to avoid scratching or damage to antireflective lens coating. Most manufacturers recommend sterile distilled water and lens paper. They must not be soaked in any solution.

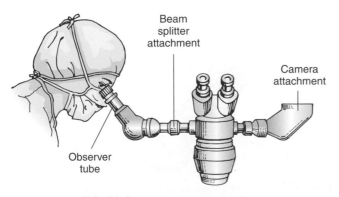

Beam splitter attachment

Camera attachment

Observer tube

FIG. 20-9   *Microscope accessories.*

3. The circulating nurse should prepare the microscope.
   a. When changing oculars, do not drop or fingerprint lenses. Avoid stripping the threads of screw mounts by seating the optics and turning in a counterclockwise direction until the threads align. Proceed by turning in a clockwise motion until secure. Take care not to overtighten. Right turns tighten; left turns loosen.
   b. Both hands should be used for attaching observation tubes, which are heavy.
   c. Extra lamp bulbs and fuses should be on hand. The circulating nurse must know where they are stored and how to change them. It is advisable to check bulbs periodically to avoid the necessity of replacing them during a procedure. New bulbs should be inserted if a long procedure is anticipated. Bulbs should be changed with the power off.
   d. Check electrical connections for proper fit or wire fraying. Take special care of power cables to prevent accidental breakage from heavy equipment rolling over them.
   e. Check that all knobs are secured after the microscope is in operating position.
   f. Place foot controls in a convenient position so that the surgeon does not have to search for them.
4. The microscope and accessories should be properly stored. Store away from traffic but close to areas where used.
   a. Openings into the microscope body for attachment of accessory devices, such as the observer tube, should be closed with covers provided by the manufacturer when not in use to prevent accumulation of dust.
   b. Lenses and viewing tubes should be protected.
   c. The microscope and attachments should be enclosed in an antistatic plastic cover when not in use to keep them free from dust.
   d. Power cords should be neatly coiled for storage.

General Considerations in Microsurgery

Patient. The patient is prepared as for a standard surgical procedure. He or she should be positioned comfortably and safely with the operating bed locked in position. The surgical site is immobilized if possible.

Anesthesia. If a general anesthetic is to be administered, the anesthesia provider should be informed in advance of the surgeon's intention to use the microscope. This is especially pertinent in procedures in which patient movements under light anesthesia could result in disaster. In addition, the anesthesia provider's position in relation to the patient should be considered to allow room for the microscope. The anesthesia provider should be aware that microsurgical procedures will take somewhat longer.

With local anesthesia, the patient should be instructed to lie quietly and to tell the anesthesia provider or circulating nurse of a desire to move. Many patients sleep during the procedure. A startle reflex on awakening or unexpected movement is especially hazardous in microsurgery, wherein the surgeon's mobility and field of view are limited. If the patient jerks or turns, he or she literally may move out of the surgeon's hands and often out of view of the microsurgical field. Therefore, the patient should be closely monitored.

Stability of the Surgical Field. A vital factor for successful microsurgery is stability of the surgical field, microscope, and surgeon's hands. The complete microsurgical unit consists of the operating bed with the patient, the microscope, and the surgeon's chair. These should be functionally positioned in relation to each other so that major adjustments need not be made during the surgical procedure. The surgeon and circulating nurse should check that all components are properly placed before the incision is made.

Armrests and Chair. It is important that the surgeon's hands be adequately supported, because a shift of even $\frac{1}{25}$ inch (1 mm) can alter the precision of motion, particularly at high magnifications. Support of the surgeon's arm should be continuous from shoulder to hand to give stability and to minimize tremor, especially in fine finger movements. A detachable, sterile, padded wrist support such as the Chan wrist rest may be affixed to the operating bed for eye procedures.

A chair with hydraulic foot controls for raising or lowering provides the necessary forearm support by means of attached armrests. These armrests are individually draped. Mayo stand covers are convenient. Armrests can be moved independently to a variety of levels and positions. They are secured in the desired position. The surgeon should be in a comfortable position to work.

Duties of the Scrub Person

Although a stabilized situation is crucial, a second fundamental necessity is for the surgeon to keep his or her eyes on the field of view through the microscope at all times. Looking away from the field requires readjustment of vision to the field. Cooperation and coordination by the scrub person in carrying out the following duties will prevent the surgeon's distraction from the surgical site:

1. Set up the Mayo stand and instrument table without touching the tips of instruments. Leave protective covers on them until they are needed for use. Holders are available to keep instrument tips in the air and to keep them separated. Microinstruments are handled individually. They are more susceptible to damage than are standard instruments. Edges are easily dulled, and fine tips are easily bent or broken. Extreme caution is necessary not to catch tips on any object that could bend them.
2. Place instruments on the Mayo stand in anticipated order of use. Place the Mayo stand and instrument table conveniently to the surgeon's hand so that he or she does not have to look around the microscope.
3. Pass instruments by placing them in the surgeon's hand in position for use, and guide the hand toward the surgical field so that the surgeon may keep his or her eyes on the field.
4. Keep debris (e.g., blood, mucus, suture ends) from the tips of instruments by wiping them gently on a nonfibrous sponge or lint-free gauze. Replace them in their original position on the Mayo stand, not touching each other.

5. Assist efficiently but never put hands in the surgical field unless requested to do so.
6. Understand the need for slow dissection at times. Do not let attention stray; observe the video monitor if one is available.

The increased time needed for use of the operating microscope can be minimized by adequate preparation and efficient assistance. Each team member should thoroughly understand the microscope and every aspect of microsurgical techniques.

Team members can be kept up-to-date by inservice explanation of new instruments and demonstration of the microscope. It is extremely helpful and contributory to understanding for the surgeon to show perioperative team members anatomic structures and instruments through the microscope. A comparison of microinstruments with standard instruments under the microscope is always a revelation.

A television monitor is advantageous in providing the scrub person and anesthesia provider continuous observation of the surgical procedure. All members should be completely familiar with instrumentation. Not only are instruments then properly cared for, but even more important, surgical time is reduced.

ULTRASONOSURGERY

Ultrasonosurgery, also referred to as cytoreductive debulking surgery, is useful in removing or reducing tumors in highly vascular, delicate tissue such as the brain, liver, kidney, and spleen. The original prototypes of ultrasonic equipment were developed in 1967 to fragment and aspirate cataracts. An ultrasonic aspirator, such as the Cavitron, simultaneously fragments, irrigates, and aspirates tissue. During the fragmentation process, sterile fluid passes through the handpiece to emulsify target tissue. The emulsified tissue is aspirated and collected in a closed-container system.

A transducer in the handpiece converts electrical energy into mechanical motion. Ultrahigh-frequency sound waves produce vibrations at the tip. These vibrations are of the same physical nature as sound but with frequencies above the range of human hearing. Ultrasound has a frequency greater than 30,000 Hz. The vibrating tip of the ultrasonic aspirator fragments tissues at the cellular level. When the tip contacts tissue, vapor pockets within high-water-content cells cause cell walls to separate and collapse. The ultrasonic aspirator is used to disrupt tissues, or tracts, particularly in the central nervous system. It is also used to emulsify tumors with minimal mechanical trauma to surrounding nerves and blood vessels. A device that combines electrosurgery with ultrasonic dissection also allows coagulation during resection and aspiration of a tumor mass.

An ultrasonic probe can be inserted through an endoscope to fragment renal or ureteral calculi (i.e., kidney stones). A suction channel is incorporated into the probe to aspirate fragments as stone is pulverized by ultrasonic energy.

INTEGRATED TECHNOLOGIES

As mentioned, several technologies may be used for minimally invasive surgical procedures. Video-assisted laser endoscopy allows the surgeon to remove organs and tumors and to ablate or repair tissues without making a major incision. An endoscope is introduced into a body cavity through a small incision. The viewing area from the telescopic lens of the scope is magnified from a video camera to a video screen. While viewing the screen, the surgeon can direct a laser beam through the endoscope to the target tissue. (Endoscopy is described in detail in Chapter 32.)

Other instrumentation may be introduced through adjacent small incisions for dissection, ligation, and suturing. These instruments can be manipulated while the surgeon looks through the endoscope or at a monitor. Manipulations may be observed with use of fluoroscopy or a video camera. Ultrasonic and thermal probes, electrosurgical electrodes, and laser beams can be directed through endoscopes. Laser beams can also be directed through the operating microscope.

Lasers and microscopes may be controlled by computerized systems. Computers can automatically scan tissues to select target tissue for the laser beam. Operating microscopes may contain voice-activated minicomputers that manipulate controls for fine adjustments, thus eliminating foot and hand switches.

Bibliography

Anderson K: Safe use of lasers in the operating room: What perioperative nurses should know, *AORN J* 79(1):171-182, 2004.

AORN (Association of periOperative Registered Nurses): *AORN standards, recommended practices, and guidelines,* Denver, 2006, The Association.

Ball KA: *Lasers: The perioperative challenge,* Denver, AORN Inc, 2004.

Lee JL: How to buy an OR microscope, *Outpatient Surg* 11(3):41-44, 2002.

Moses K: *How do you know if your equipment is safe to use?* Healthcare Technology Horizons, supplement to AAMI publications, 2005.

Morino M et al: Ultrasonic versus standard electric dissection in laparoscopic colorectal surgery: A prospective randomized trial, *Ann Surg* 242(6):897-901, 2005.

Pyrek KM: Education in electrosurgery technology is key for patient safety, *Infect Control Today* 6(7):18-22, 2002.

Sheridan RL et al: Noncontact electrosurgical grounding is useful in burn surgery, *J Burn Care Rehab* 24(6):400-401, 2003.

Ulmer B: Use of electrosurgery in the perioperative setting, *Plastic Surg Nurs* 22(4):173-178, 2003.

Chapter 21

Preoperative Preparation of the Patient

CHAPTER OBJECTIVES

After studying this chapter, the learner will be able to:
- Discuss the importance of preoperative preparation.
- Describe the content of preoperative patient teaching.
- List several preoperative assessment factors relevant to all presurgical patients.
- Identify the key elements in a successful presurgical interview.

CHAPTER OUTLINE

KEY TERMS AND DEFINITIONS

Anxiety   Emotional state characterized by subjective feelings of tension, apprehension, and/or worry. The autonomic nervous system is activated.

PAT   Preadmission testing area where preoperative patients are assessed.

Presurgical holding area   An area within the perioperative environment where the patient waits immediately before entering the operating room.

SUPPLEMENTAL MATERIAL ON EVOLVE WEBSITE   *evolve*

http://evolve.elsevier.com/BerryKohn
- Content Updates
- Glossary
- Full Set of Perioperative Flash Cards
- Interactive Key Term Flash Cards
- Student Activities
- WebLinks

HISTORICAL BACKGROUND

For centuries before the proliferation of operating rooms (ORs) in hospitals, surgical procedures were performed on battlefields, in barber chairs, and on kitchen tables. Hospitals focused on the care of the poor, crippled, chronically ill, and insane until the eighteenth and nineteenth centuries. Even then, and on into the early twentieth century, many surgeons operated in their offices and in the homes of their patients. Nurses were dispatched to the homes to prepare a suitable room and to prepare the patient for the surgeon.

From the late nineteenth century, the achievements in surgery as a medical discipline can be attributed to an increase in the understanding of physiology, the introduction of safe anesthetics and methods of blood transfusion, the development of antimicrobials, and the management of the patient before, during, and after invasive procedures. As surgeons moved into the OR arenas of hospitals, nurses became responsible for physically preparing patients for surgical procedures. In the early 1900s, patients were admitted 4 or 5 days before the procedure; by the late 1930s, this time was reduced to 24 hours or less.

From around 1920, nursing leaders advocated the importance of both the physiologic and the psychological preparation of surgical patients. The individual needs of patients were recognized but were not emphasized in nursing education until the 1940s. During the 1950s, patient teaching became a limited part of preoperative preparation as surgeons recognized the value of early ambulation. It was not until the 1960s and 1970s that nursing research studies validated a link between preoperative preparation and postoperative recovery. The risk of postoperative physiologic complications can be reduced by teaching deep breathing, coughing, and leg exercises and by preparing the patient for early ambulation. Attention to the patient's preoperative psychosocial and spiritual needs also has important consequences for the management of postoperative pain and the promotion of desired outcomes.

Studies showed that patients who received structured preoperative teaching had a smoother postoperative recovery. During those decades, OR nurses were encouraged to visit patients preoperatively and prepare them psychologically for the surgical experience by helping alleviate their fears and anxieties and by teaching appropriate postoperative behaviors. This visit could take place at the bedside the day before the scheduled procedure.

In 1983, amendments to the Social Security Act established a prospective hospital reimbursement system for

Medicare patients. This system is based on diagnosis-related groups (DRGs), which have changed the time and place of the preoperative preparation of most surgical patients who require postoperative hospital support services. It has also stimulated the development of ambulatory surgery (i.e., minimally invasive procedures). The number of surgical procedures performed in ambulatory care facilities and on patients admitted to the hospital the same day of surgery increases annually.

HOSPITALIZED PATIENT

Regardless of the physical setting in which an invasive or surgical procedure will be performed, each patient should be adequately assessed and prepared so that the effect and potential risks of the surgical intervention are minimized. This involves both physical and emotional preparation. Perioperative caregivers should establish a baseline for the patient's preoperative condition so that changes that occur during the perioperative/perianesthesia care period can be easily recognized.

Although most patients undergoing a surgical procedure are admitted the same day of surgery, some are admitted to the hospital 1 or more days before the scheduled procedure. The acuity of illness or the patient's general health status, as well as the surgical procedure to be performed, will influence whether the patient should be admitted to the hospital preoperatively or can arrive on the day of the procedure. Radiologic, endoscopic, or other diagnostic studies may be performed to confirm the medical diagnosis. Systemic disease or chronic illness, such as diabetes or heart disease, should be under control to the extent possible preoperatively.

Most patients who will remain in the hospital postoperatively are admitted the day of the surgical procedure. Often referred to as AM or morning admission, TCI (to come in), or TBA (to be admitted), these patients may be prepared for the procedure in a same-day admission unit before transferring to the OR suite. (Some facilities have a preoperative check-in area within the OR suite.) From the OR, some patients may go to the postanesthesia care unit (PACU) to recover from anesthesia before being transferred to a patient care unit; others are transferred directly from the OR to the intensive care unit (ICU). The magnitude of the surgical procedure and the patient's postoperative needs for complex care will determine when the patient can be discharged safely to home.

PREOPERATIVE PREPARATION OF ALL PATIENTS

Specific activities such as the preoperative history and physical examination are completed and documented before the patient arrives in the OR. This process can be performed before admission to the hospital or ambulatory care facility; other activities are performed when the patient arrives. The preoperative physical preparation is designed to help all patients overcome the stresses of anesthesia, pain, fluid and blood loss, immobilization, and tissue trauma. Preparation often begins before the patient's hospital admission with the institution of nutritional or drug therapy. An attempt is made to bring all patients to their best possible physical status before surgery. Appropriate consultations, such as a cardiac workup, are sought when necessary.

Preadmission Procedures

Some of the preoperative preparations can be performed in the surgeon's office. Patients are then referred to the preoperative testing center of the hospital or ambulatory care facility. Tests and records should be completed and available before the patient is admitted the day of the surgical procedure. Preadmission tests (PATs) are scheduled according to the guidelines of each facility. Some tests are acceptable only for a 30-day period or are repeated before admission. The preoperative preparations include the following:

1. Medical history and physical examination. These are performed and documented by a physician, nurse practitioner, physician assistant (PA), or the registered nurse first assistant (RNFA). The preoperative nurse establishes the baseline for the patient's vital signs (Fig. 21-1).
2. Laboratory tests. Testing should be based on specific clinical indicators or risk factors that could affect surgical management or anesthesia. Tests include age, gender, preexisting disease, magnitude of surgical procedure, and type of anesthesia. Ideally these tests should be completed 24 hours before admission so the results are available for review. Some facilities perform laboratory studies the morning of the procedure.
   a. Hemoglobin, hematocrit, blood urea nitrogen (BUN), and blood glucose may be routinely tested for patients ages 60 years or older.
   b. Hematocrit is usually ordered for women of all ages before the administration of a general anesthetic.
   c. Complete blood count and blood chemistry profile may be indicated. Differential, platelet count, activated partial thromboplastin time, and prothrombin time also may be ordered.
   d. Urinalysis may be indicated by the type of surgical procedure, medical history, and/or physical examination.
3. Blood type and crossmatch. If a transfusion is anticipated, the patient's blood is typed and crossmatched. Many patients prefer to have their own blood drawn and stored for autotransfusion. Patients should be advised that blood banks charge an additional fee to store and preserve blood for personal use. Even if the patient is to have an autotransfusion, his or her blood should still be typed and crossmatched in the event that additional transfusions are needed. If the patient refuses to accept blood transfusions, the appropriate documentation of refusal should be completed according to the policies and procedures of the facility.
4. Chest radiographic study. A preoperative chest x-ray study is not routinely required for all patients. It may be required by facility policy or medically indicated as an adjunct to the clinical evaluation of patients with cardiac or pulmonary disease and for smokers, patients age 60 years or older, and cancer patients.
5. Electrocardiogram (ECG). If the patient has known or suspected cardiac disease, an ECG is mandatory. Depending on the policy of the facility, an ECG may be routine for patients ages 40 years or older.

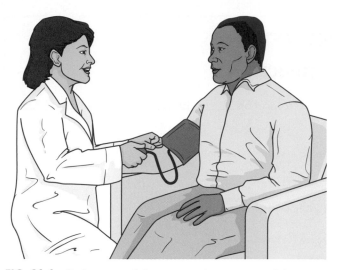

FIG. 21-1 Performance of the preoperative assessment is important to establish a health baseline. Vital signs, height in centimeters, weight in kilograms, and review of systems should be done.

6. Diagnostic procedures. Special diagnostic procedures are performed when specifically indicated (e.g., Doppler studies for vascular surgery).

7. Written instructions. The patient should receive written preoperative instructions to follow before admission for the surgical procedure. These instructions should be reviewed with the patient in the surgeon's office or in the preoperative testing center (Fig. 21-2).

   a. To prevent regurgitation or emesis and aspiration of gastric contents, the patient should not ingest solid foods before the surgical procedure. These instructions are usually stated as "NPO after midnight." (NPO is the Latin abbreviation for nil per os, or nothing by mouth.) Solid foods empty from the stomach after changing to a liquid state, which may take up to 12 hours. Clear fluids may be unrestricted until 2 to 3 hours before the surgical procedure but only at the discretion of the surgeon or anesthesia provider in selected patients. NPO time usually is reduced for infants, small children, patients with diabetes, and older adults prone to dehydration.

   b. The physician may want the patient to take any essential oral medications that he or she normally takes. These can be taken as prescribed with a minimal fluid intake (a few sips of water) up to 1 hour before the surgical procedure.

   c. The skin should be cleansed to prepare the surgical site. Many surgeons want patients to clean the surgical area with an antimicrobial soap preoperatively. Patients who will undergo a surgical procedure on the face, ear, or neck are advised to shampoo their hair before admission, because this may not be permitted for a few days or weeks after the procedure.

   d. Nail polish and acrylic nails should be removed to permit observation of and access to the nailbed

during the surgical procedure. The patient should be advised to uncover at least one fingernail if the anesthesia provider will use these monitoring devices during the procedure. Either the finger or toe can be used when a digit is desired, but the finger is usually more accessible.

   Some sensors are adhesive and can be placed on an earlobe or across the bridge of the nose. The nailbed is a vascular area, and the color of the nailbed is one indicator of peripheral oxygenation and circulation. The oxisensor (optode) of a pulse oximeter may be attached to the nailbed to monitor oxygen saturation and pulse rate. A finger cuff may be used for continuous blood pressure monitoring. Nail polish or acrylic nails inhibit contact between these devices and the vascular bed.

   e. Jewelry and valuables should be left at home to ensure safekeeping. If electrosurgery will be used, patients should be informed that all metal jewelry, including wedding bands and religious artifacts, should be removed to prevent possible burns. Loss prevention is a consideration as well.

   f. Patients should be given other special instructions about what is expected, such as when to arrive at the surgical facility. A responsible adult should be available to take the patient home if the procedure, medication, or anesthetic agent renders the patient incapable of driving. Family members or significant others should know where to wait and where the patient will be taken after the surgical procedure.

8. Informed consent. The physician should obtain informed consent from the patient or legal designee. After explaining the surgical procedure and its risks, benefits, and alternatives, the surgeon should document the process and have the patient sign the consent form. This documentation becomes part of the permanent record and accompanies the patient to the OR. Policy and state laws dictate the parameters for ascertaining an informed consent.

9. Nurse interview. A perioperative/perianesthesia nurse should meet with the patient to make a preoperative assessment. Ideally, an appointment with the perioperative nurse is arranged when the patient comes to the facility for preoperative tests. Through physiologic and psychosocial assessments, the nurse collects data for the nursing diagnoses, expected outcomes, and plan of care.

   From the assessment data and nursing diagnoses, the nurse establishes expected outcomes with the patient. The nurse develops the plan of care, which becomes a part of the patient's record. The nurse reviews the written preoperative instructions and consent form with the patient to assess the patient's knowledge and understanding. The nurse also provides emotional support and teaches the patient in preparation for postoperative recovery. Before or after the interview, the patient may view a videotape to reinforce information.

GETBETTER HOSPITAL
PREOPERATIVE INSTRUCTIONS

Your doctor has scheduled your surgery to be performed at Getbetter Hospital on _____ (day)_____ (date) at _____ AM/PM. Please arrive at _____ AM/PM.

If you develop a cold, flu, or illness before surgery or cannot keep your surgery appointment, please call your surgeon.

DIETARY RESTRICTIONS

- Avoid alcoholic beverages and cigarette smoking for at least 24 hours before surgery.
- Finish dinner the evening before surgery no later than 8 PM.
- Nothing to eat or drink after midnight the night before surgery.
  (This includes candy, gum, mints, Lifesavers, ice chips, and water.)
- Eating or drinking may result in the delay or cancellation of surgery.
- Medications to be taken the day of surgery _____ with sip (1 ounce) of water.
- Medications *not* to be taken the day of surgery _____ .

FOR YOUR SAFETY AND COMFORT

- No makeup—it may cause eye irritation or corneal abrasions while under anesthesia.
- Remove nail polish and artificial nails from at least one finger on each hand—oxygen is measured by placing a sensor on your finger tip.
- Do not bring valuables or jewelry—jewelry must be removed before surgery.
- Dress simply in loose-fitting clothes (sweatsuits are ideal).

UPON YOUR ARRIVAL

- Report to Main Lobby Admissions Desk.

AFTER YOUR SURGERY

- No driving, operating of heavy machinery, heavy physical activity, or decision making for 24 hours after receiving an anesthetic.
- If you are returning home on the same day as your surgery, make arrangements for a responsible adult to accompany you. Your operation cannot be performed if a responsible adult is not with you.
- Call your surgeon for postoperative appointments.

If you have any questions, do not hesitate to call the <u>Preadmission Testing Unit</u> at xxx-xxx-xxxx or <u>The Department of Anesthesia</u> at xxx-xxx-xxxx.

Patient signature: _____

RN signature: _____

FIG. 21-2   Sample written preoperative instructions for the patient.

10. Anesthesia assessment. An anesthesia history and physical assessment are performed before a general or regional anesthetic is administered. The history may be obtained by the surgeon, and/or the patient may be asked to complete a questionnaire for the anesthesia provider in the surgeon's office or in the preoperative testing center. An interview by an anesthesia provider or nurse anesthetist may be conducted before admission if the patient has a complex medical history, is high risk, or has a high degree of anxiety. All patients should understand the risks of and alternatives to the type of anesthetic to be administered. After discussion with the anesthesia provider, the patient should sign an anesthesia consent form.

A preoperative phone call by a perioperative nurse to the patient several days in advance of the scheduled surgical procedure may prevent cancellation because of inadequate preoperative testing. Testing requirements are reviewed with the patient, and arrangements for additional tests can be made as needed. The importance of preoperative preparations is reiterated, especially NPO status and the availability of a responsible adult for transportation home after the surgical procedure (if having ambulatory surgery).

Evening Before an Elective Surgical Procedure

In addition to the preadmission procedures described, the surgeon may write specific orders for other appropriate preoperative preparations. All preadmission assessment and testing procedures may be performed after the patient is admitted to a surgical unit before the surgical procedure. Some patients may require the following:

1. Bowel preparation. "Enemas till clear" may be ordered when it is advantageous to have the bowel and rectum empty (e.g., gastrointestinal procedures such as bowel resection or endoscopy, and surgical procedures in the pelvic, perineal, or perianal areas). An intestinal lavage with an oral solution that induces diarrhea may be ordered to clear the intestine of feces. Solutions such as GoLYTELY or CoLyte normally will clear the bowel in 4 to 6 hours. Because potassium is lost during diarrhea, serum potassium levels should be checked before the surgical procedure. Geriatric, underweight, and malnourished patients are prone to other electrolyte disturbances from intestinal lavage.
2. Bedtime sedation for sleep in select circumstances.

Preoperative Visit by the Perioperative/Perianesthesia Nurse

The patient should be assessed preoperatively. Every effort should be made through supportive measures to minimize the potential hazards of adverse psychosocial distress. Ideally this assessment takes place before the day of the surgical procedure; its purpose is to alleviate anxiety and fears. Factual information and clarification of misunderstandings will be helpful in this regard, as will the opportunity for the patient to express his or her feelings.

The broadened scope of perioperative nursing encompasses the phases of preoperative and postoperative care that contribute to the continuity of patient care. Preoperative visits to patients are made by RNFAs or perioperative/perianesthesia nurses skilled in interviewing and assessment. These interviews afford nurses an opportunity to learn about the patients, establish rapport, and develop a plan of care before the patients are brought to the *perioperative environment*.

Pros of Preoperative Visits. The advantages of preoperative visits with patients include the following:

1. An experienced perioperative/perianesthesia nurse is well qualified to discuss a patient's OR experience. The nurse can orient and prepare the patient and family for the procedure and for the postoperative period.
2. The perioperative/perianesthesia nurse can review critical data before the procedure and assess the patient before planning care. The surgical site is marked by the surgeon or surgeon's designee.

3. Visits improve and individualize intraoperative care and efficiency and prevent needless delays in the OR.
4. Visits foster a meaningful nurse-patient relationship. Some patients are reluctant to reveal their feelings and needs to someone in a short-term relationship.
5. Visits make intraoperative observations more meaningful by establishing a baseline for the measurement of patient outcomes.
6. Visits contribute to patient cooperation and involvement by facilitating communication. Mutual goals and expected outcomes are more easily developed.
7. Visits enhance the positive self-image of the perioperative nurse and contribute to job satisfaction, which in turn reduces job turnover and is thus a benefit to the hospital. Because of increased patient contact, visits make perioperative and perianesthesia nursing more attractive to those who enjoy patient proximity and teaching.

Cons of Preoperative Visits. The disadvantages associated with preoperative visits include:

1. Cost-containment measures may not provide adequate staffing or allow time to visit patients.
2. The admission of patients on the day of the surgical procedure or late the day before the procedure makes the timing of visits difficult.
3. Visits may produce friction among different team factions if the program is not well planned and executed.
4. Repetitious use of interviewing terminology may lead to a lack of enthusiasm and spontaneity on the part of nurse interviewers.
5. If the nurse's interviewing skills are not practiced, patients may feel their privacy is being invaded.
6. Barriers to visits may arise from the nurse's inability to do the following:
   a. Verbalize and communicate effectively.
   b. Handle or accept a patient's illness.
   c. Handle emotionally stressed persons.
   d. Understand cultural, ethnic, and value system differences.
   e. Function efficiently outside of his or her customary environment.
   f. Recognize how personal beliefs and biases can influence objectivity.

Interviewing Skills. Interviewing is a form of verbal interaction and is a valuable tool for obtaining information. The interview can be directive and structured with predetermined questions in a specific, predetermined order that limits responses. An example of a directive question is, "Have you had a surgical procedure before?" A nondirective interview gives the patient more of an opportunity to respond openly. An example of a nondirective question is, "Tell me about your previous surgical experience." The choice of technique depends on the information desired.

Determine the level of patient understanding about the surgical procedure. One method is to ask, "Can you tell me what we will be doing for you during your surgical procedure?" Some patients will not be able to articulate the terms or adequately describe the procedure. Direct inquiry about specific procedures may be necessary, but give the patient plenty of opportunities to describe in his or her own words what the anticipated procedure is.

A structured interview is valuable in learning about an individual's health history. The unstructured interview gives a portrait of the patient's emotional reactions, concerns, and personality. An effective preoperative interview usually includes questions about both facts and feelings. The informal observation of nonverbal behavior is an essential component of the interview. The setting should be conducive to communication, and all questions should be relevant. The interviewer should be able to handle the situation with spontaneity, judgment, and tact. The interview should be meaningful to both the patient and the nurse.

Structured Preoperative Visits

1. Review the patient's chart and records. Focus on medical and nursing diagnoses and the surgical procedure to be performed. Collect any information relevant to planning care in the OR. If the patient is admitted to the hospital, discuss the assessment data and the plan of care with the unit nurses before visiting the patient. Nursing data include the following pertinent information; these baseline parameters are essential for accurate intraoperative and postoperative assessment.
   a. Biographic information (name, age, gender, family status, ethnic background, educational level, patterns of living, previous hospitalization and surgical procedures, religion).
   b. Physical findings (vital signs; height; weight; skin integrity; allergies; the presence of pain, drainage, or bleeding; state of consciousness and orientation; sensory or physical deficits; assistive aids or prosthetics).
   c. Special therapy (tracheostomy, inhalation therapy, hyperalimentation).
   d. Emotional status (understanding, expectations, specific problems concerning comfort, safety, language barrier, and other concerns).
2. Choose an optimal time and place without interruptions.
   a. Patients who will be admitted on the day of the surgical procedure may be interviewed in the preoperative testing center several days before the surgical procedure. If this is not feasible, a telephone call to the patient may provide an alternative means of contact.
   b. Patients who have been admitted to the hospital may be visited on a patient care unit the day before the surgical procedure. The best time to visit a patient is early evening—after dinner and before visiting hours.
   c. Allow adequate time for the interview, usually 10 to 20 minutes unless the patient has complex problems or special needs that require more time. Give the patient time to think and respond and to ask questions.
   d. If the patient is in acute physical or psychological distress, offer support and consider rescheduling the visit. The visit may need to be canceled or conducted through a family member or significant other. An emergency surgical patient may be assessed in the preoperative holding area.
   e. Do not conduct the interview on the morning of the procedure unless there is no other choice. Patients are not psychologically receptive to preoperative teaching at this time. Premedicated patients may be susceptible to suggestions such as "You will have minimal discomfort after the surgical procedure."
3. Greet the patient by introducing yourself and explaining the purpose of the visit. Tell the patient that the visit is a routine part of care so the patient does not feel singled out because of his or her medical diagnosis. Unless specifically requested to use a first name, demonstrate respect at all times by addressing the patient by his or her last name, preceded by Mr., Mrs., or Ms. Terms such as honey, dear, or sweetheart are unacceptable. Children are usually addressed by their given first name unless the family uses a nickname.
   a. Put the patient at ease. Sit close so the patient can easily see and hear you.
   b. Secure the patient's attention and cooperation. Establish eye contact.
   c. Speak first with the patient alone (unless the patient is a small child, an individual who needs an interpreter, or an individual who is mentally impaired). This affords the patient privacy so he or she may feel free to talk. Then, if the patient is willing, the family may be invited to participate and ask questions. The family should be present during the preoperative teaching to learn how to assist the patient postoperatively.
   d. Allow the patient to maintain self-respect and dignity.
   e. Instill confidence in the patient by having a neat appearance and a positive attitude. Establish rapport by demonstrating warmth and genuine interest. Avoid displaying an authoritative manner.
   f. Use language at the patient's level of development, understanding, and education.
4. Obtain information by asking about the patient's understanding of the surgical procedure.
   a. Assess the patient's level of information and understanding and check its accuracy to determine whether further instruction or clarification is needed. Ask questions such as, "What has your surgeon told you about the surgical procedure?" Correct any misconceptions about the surgical procedure as appropriate within the scope of nursing.
   b. Permit the patient to talk openly. The objective is to gather data that will generate the plan of care to be implemented by the perioperative team.
   c. Direct questions should be used with caution and are not suitable for collecting all objective data. Construct open-ended questions to elicit information more detailed than one-word answers.
   d. Listen attentively. To preserve self-esteem, the patient may tell you what he or she thinks you want to hear. A patient's statement that ends in a question may be either a request for more information or an expression of a feeling or attitude.
5. Orient the patient to the environment of the OR suite, and interpret policies and routines.
   a. Tell the patient the scheduled time of the surgical procedure, the approximate length of the procedure,

and the probable length of stay in the PACU. Explain the procedures that will be performed in the preoperative holding area before the surgery, if this is the routine.

b. Ask the patient if family members or friends will be at the facility during the surgical procedure. They should be informed how early to be there to see the patient before sedation is given. Tell the patient and family where the waiting room is located.

c. Tell the patient that the family will be updated on the progress of the surgical procedure and informed when he or she arrives in the PACU, if this is hospital policy. Communicating the progress of the procedure, especially if it is prolonged, provides emotional support and decreases the family's anxiety.

6. Review the preoperative preparations that the patient will experience.

a. Familiarize the patient with whom and what will be seen in the perioperative environment. Many perioperative nurses wear OR attire and laboratory coats with name tags when they visit patients, which familiarizes patients with the way they will see personnel the next day. Attire should be changed if the nurse reenters the OR suite after the visit.

b. Use discretion regarding how much the patient should know and wants to know. Use words that do not evoke an anxiety-inducing state of mind. Do not use words with unpleasant associations, such as knife, needle, or nausea.

c. Postoperative recovery begins with preoperative teaching, but keep the explanations short and simple. Excessive detail can increase patient anxiety, which reduces the attention span.

d. Give practical information about what the patient should expect, such as withholding fluids, drowsiness, and/or dry mouth caused by preoperative medications; transportation to the OR and the holding area; and where he or she will be taken after the surgical procedure. Instruct the patient not to hesitate to ask for assistance at any time. Explain any other relevant special precautions.

e. Give the basic reasons for procedures and regulations; this reduces patient anxiety. With children and older adults, the nurse may have to repeat information as a reinforcement.

f. Explain only the procedures of which the patient will be aware.

g. If patient will be going to the ICU after the procedure, tell the family what they will see there, such as monitors and machines.

7. Tell the patient that an anesthesia provider will visit to discuss specific questions relative to anesthesia, if this is routine.

8. Answer the patient's questions about the surgical procedure in general terms. Refer specific questions to the surgeon.

a. Be honest and responsible in communications about a proposed diagnostic or surgical procedure. Complement, but do not overlap, the surgeon's area of responsibility. Do not be unrealistic, falsify the truth, or give false reassurances to the patient or family.

b. Be extremely cautious about spelling out specific details of the treatment, procedure, and postoperative care unless you have been thoroughly briefed by the surgeon in charge. Surgeons individualize and tailor their plan of care to their own techniques and to the patient's needs, and certain forms of therapy may be controversial. Continual interdisciplinary communication is essential.

c. If unable or unprepared to answer a legitimate question, tell the patient that the concern will be answered by the appropriate personnel. For example, say, "I don't know, but I'll get that information for you." Then be certain to follow up with an answer.

9. Encourage the patient and family to discuss their feelings or anxieties regarding the surgical procedure and anticipated results.

a. Motivate and assist the patient and family to gain perspective, objectivity, awareness, and insight. A skilled professional nurse will know how to discourage wishful thinking for miraculous cures while communicating an understanding of their fears and wishes for an uncomplicated, fast recovery.

b. Observe emotional reactions.

c. As an interviewer, be objective about personal feelings. Listen to what the patient is asking without feeling threatened. Do not superimpose personal feelings onto what the patient is actually expressing. Empathy is appropriate in this environment.

d. Acknowledge the effect of the procedure on the patient's sexuality, if appropriate. Allow the patient to express personal feelings without evoking shame or guilt. Include the family or significant others as the patient desires.

e. Try to help the patient solve his or her own problems when possible. Ask open-ended questions that help explore a subject or feelings, but do not probe to elicit specific responses. Do not destroy the patient's coping mechanism; encourage an appropriate one. The visit is not a structured psychiatric counseling session.

f. Listen to the anxieties of the patient, family, or significant others in a realistic time frame, and get others to follow through as necessary. Do not attempt too full an agenda, but sort out what is legitimate. You cannot solve all problems in 20 minutes. For example, say, "I'll share this information with someone who can help you with this problem." Use a colleague's expertise to assist you or to make a proper referral.

g. Comfort the patient, and convey a sense of security and trust. Use touch as appropriate. Touch has a positive effect on physiologic parameters, such as respiration and circulation, and it can lower heart rate and blood pressure. Its calming effect can improve perceptual and cognitive abilities. It establishes rapport, provides reassurance, and conveys warmth, empathy, encouragement, and support. Touch should be comfortable. A perceptive nurse can tell when a patient resents being touched; respect the patient's feelings. Patients with decreased visual acuity appreciate the assurance that touch can give, but always speak first to avoid startling the patient.

h. Reassure the patient that he or she will not be alone but will be constantly attended by competent perioperative team members. Try to increase the patient's trust and confidence in the team as a whole.

i. Allow time to deal with the patient's questions or concerns. Ask the patient, "Do you have any other concerns?" Never bring a patient's feelings into the open and then cut off the conversation. Do not interrupt, interrogate, or belittle an expressed fear or seemingly irrelevant topic. All questions are significant to the patient. Answer the questions honestly, and try to resolve concerns.

10. Identify any special needs of the patient that will alter the plan for intraoperative care. The preoperative visit is the time for a total assessment to guard against a traumatic experience for the patient.

   a. Observe any physical characteristics of the patient that might affect positioning or require special setups. The plan of care will include considerations for extra tall, obese, or left-handed patients. For example, an intravenous (IV) infusion should be started in the right arm of a left-handed person to minimize the limitation of manual dexterity.

   b. Observe the patient for physical limitations such as pain on moving, an amputated extremity, paralysis, or sensory loss. This information enables the circulating nurse to anticipate how much cooperation to expect from the patient and how much additional help may be needed. A pad of paper and pencil may be needed to communicate with a patient who is unable to speak or hear. In certain instances, an interpreter may be needed.

   c. Ask the patient whether he or she wears any type of prosthetic device. Explain, per accepted hospital policy, that the device should be removed before the surgical procedure either at the bedside or in the OR. Explain that jewelry should be removed.

   d. Determine how a preexisting medical condition should be managed in the OR. For example, it is important that the circulating nurse know about the presence of an implanted pacemaker. Monopolar electrosurgery could cause certain models of pacemakers to malfunction and monopolar electrosurgery would therefore be contraindicated.

   e. Know the patient's special requests. Placing a note on the front of the chart is one method of relaying temporary information about a patient's special requests. These notes are not part of the permanent record.

11. Offer the patient reassurance when possible, and maintain an attitude of hope. Avoid using phrases such as "Everything will be all right" or "You are okay." Reinforce the concept that the team will provide good care.

   a. Help both yourself and the patient turn negative feelings into positive, useful responses.

   b. Offer realistic hope, but do not minimize the seriousness of the surgical procedure.

12. Use audiovisual materials to supplement the interview, if available and appropriate.

   a. Written instructions with photographs or drawings are useful for explaining procedures and equipment. These can be presented in a booklet or pamphlet that the patient can keep and share with family members or significant others.

   b. Videotapes, slide/tape programs, DVDs, or films help to reinforce the preoperative teaching.

Preoperative Teaching. Teaching is a function of nursing practice and embraces perception, thought, feeling, and performance. During the preoperative visit, the perioperative nurse supplements the instructions of the other perioperative team members and gives information unique to the patient's specific surgical procedure. The perioperative nurse teaches patients how to participate in their own postoperative recovery. Patients must have a readiness to learn. Preoperative teaching should take place at three levels:

1. Information. Explanations of procedures, patient care activities, and physical feelings that the patient may encounter during the perioperative experience help the patient identify what is happening and what to expect. Such explanations also enhance patient satisfaction with care.

2. Psychosocial support. Interactions enhance coping mechanisms to deal with anxiety and fears and provide emotional comfort.

3. Skill training. Guided practice of specific tasks to be performed by the patient in the postoperative period can decrease anxiety, hasten recovery, and help prevent complications.

Effective Teaching. Patient teaching involves emotional energy on the part of the nurse. It can produce behavioral changes in patients as they become better prepared, both physically and emotionally, for the surgical procedure. They also learn how to use the health care system. Learning self-help has a positive effect. Discharge planning begins during preoperative teaching. The patient knows what to expect and where to go for help after discharge if needed, such as a support group.

Patient teaching may be conducted in an informal, individual manner or in a formal, group instructional setting. In conjunction with other team members, the nurse-instructor should first formulate attainable learning objectives with the patient's input. The development of learning objectives is based on the assessed level of the patient's emotional receptivity and mental capacity.

The nurse also assesses, by observation and elicited response, factors such as the patient's developmental level, sight, hearing, and acceptance of his or her problem. Before beginning an explanation, the nurse should verify what the patient already knows, needs to know, and wants to know. An understanding relationship with the patient facilitates the teaching-learning experience.

The nurse assists family members to cope with the situation to the extent of their ability. The success or failure of treatment often depends on what happens after the patient leaves the hospital. The family's knowledge and understanding of the patient's needs, their coping skills, and their willingness to help are important factors in recovery. Teaching should be presented at the family members' level of particular resources and knowledge base. Other points to consider include the following:

1. Arrange the environment so that a teaching-learning exchange can take place; a quiet, undisturbed environment and proper timing are important.
2. Language is the fundamental tool for education. Use understandable terms. Do not equate intelligence level with educational level. The nurse is accountable for what is taught.
3. Set priorities, and teach what is significant and appropriate to the patient's particular needs.
   a. Break down instructions into manageable steps; for example, instruct the patient to deep breathe and then cough while he or she splints the site of the surgical incision with a pillow.
   b. Put content into a logical sequence of activities to facilitate learning. For example, to avoid the possibility of an inappropriate dosage, instruct the patient to write down the time he or she takes the medication when at home.
   c. Give the reasons for and the benefits of specific activities. For example, the movement of legs and toes and ambulation postoperatively, unless contraindicated, aid circulation and prevent venous stasis.
   d. Adapt the teaching method and timing to the specific situation. The patient may reject teaching not relevant to the immediate present. For example, a patient about to have a heart valve replacement procedure may listen to instructions but may actually be concentrating on the fact that his or her heart is going to be cut open.
   e. Do not overburden the patient with a multitude of facts.
4. Recognize the patient's need to know. This recognition, not pressure, should be the motivating factor in learning.
5. To evaluate understanding, ask the patient to repeat in his or her own words what has been explained during the instructional session and to demonstrate deep breathing and leg exercises.
6. Written information is helpful in reviewing verbal instruction. Go over the material with the patient, and test his or her comprehension by asking questions. A patient who is experiencing pain or anxiety or who is under the influence of medication may not fully understand verbal communication.
7. As the resource person, be consistent, concise, and organized. Repeat instructions to help the patient retain them.

Patients who receive preoperative instructions from and interact with the perioperative nurse may experience less apprehension, better tolerate the surgical procedure, and seem more secure and comfortable postoperatively. Patients usually remember what has been taught. They react more positively to their perioperative experience than do patients who have not been given the benefit of this interaction.

At the end of the preoperative assessment and teaching session, the perioperative nurse should not depart from the patient abruptly but should briefly summarize the events that have taken place. The patient should be left with the understanding that a postoperative visit may be made after the procedure, if this is the policy.

Preoperative Visit by the Anesthesia Provider

The anesthesia provider is knowledgeable in the pathophysiology of disease as it pertains to anesthetic agents. Participation in the patient's preoperative preparation can reduce intraoperative complications. If the patient has been admitted the evening before the surgical procedure, the anesthesia provider usually assesses the patient if he or she is scheduled for anesthesia. Otherwise the patient may be seen before admission in the preoperative testing center, in the same-day procedures unit, or in the preoperative holding area. All patients should be evaluated before the anesthetic is administered.

Judgment and skill are important in the selection of agents and in the administration of anesthesia, but firsthand knowledge of the patient is extremely valuable. The anesthesia provider visits the patient to seek information and to establish rapport, inspire confidence and trust, and alleviate fear. Preparation for anesthesia begins with this visit.

Before meeting the patient, the anesthesia provider reviews the patient's past and present medical records. If recent laboratory or other test reports are not in the chart, all decisions and the surgical procedure are delayed until all essential information is available. Special attention is given to past surgical procedures and any disease or complicating processes, especially those involving vital organs.

After introducing himself or herself to the patient, the anesthesia provider does the following:

1. Obtains a history pertinent to the administration of anesthetic agents by questioning the patient about past anesthetic experiences, allergies, adverse reactions to drugs, and habitual drug usage (Fig. 21-3). Tranquilizers, cortisone, reserpine, alcohol, herbal preparations, and recreational drugs, for example, influence the course of anesthesia. Smoking habits, genetic and metabolic problems, and reactions to previous blood transfusions also influence the choice of anesthetic.

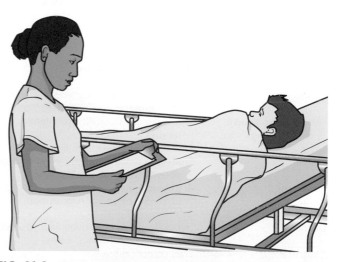

FIG. 21-3   The anesthesia provider assesses the patient and plans the anesthetic for the surgical procedure.

Patients are advised to report all herbal supplements, because they can cause serious complications such as bleeding. (Table 21-1 describes common herbs and dietary supplements.) The American Society of Anesthesiologists (ASA) cautions about herbal remedies and the serious complications that can ensue.

2. Evaluates the patient's physical, mental, and emotional status to determine the most appropriate type and amount of anesthetic agent(s).
   a. Examines the patient as necessary to obtain the information desired, with particular interest in the heart and lungs.
   b. Palpates the needle insertion site and observes for skin infection if a regional block anesthesia is contemplated.
   c. Assesses the patient's mental state and cognitive ability subjectively, and observes for signs of anxiety.
3. Investigates the patient's cardiac reserve and observes for signs of dyspnea or claudication during a short exercise tolerance test, if indicated.
4. Asks about teeth. If indicated, explains that dental work may be damaged inadvertently during airway insertion.

5. Evaluates the patient's physique for possible technical difficulties in the administration of the anesthetic. The patient will be asked to move the head and neck in a natural range of motion. The oropharynx will be assessed.
   a. A short, stout neck may cause respiratory problems or difficult intubation. A stiff neck or unstable cervical spine such as from rheumatoid arthritis can make intubation difficult or dangerous, especially in a geriatric patient. Fiberoptic laryngoscope and/or awake intubation may be necessary.
   b. Active athletic and obese patients require more anesthetic than do inactive patients.
   c. The patient's accurate weight should be known in both kilograms and pounds because the dosage of many medications is calculated from body weight. Most dosages are calculated in milligrams per kilogram.
6. Explains his or her preference of anesthetic, pending the surgeon's approval, and informs the patient what to expect concerning anesthesia. The patient's wishes are considered, if expressed.
7. Tells the patient or asks about restricted or prohibited oral intake before anesthesia, and gives the reasons for these restrictions. IV therapy is explained.

TABLE 21-1	Examples of Common Herbal and Dietary Supplements and Potential Complications	
Herbal or Dietary Supplement	**Action and Potential Complications**	**Notes on Patient Usage**
St. John's wort	Prolonged sedative effect, photosensitivity, peripheral neuropathy, interferes with metabolism of some antibiotics, calcium channel blockers, and warfarin	Antidepressant, antiinflammatory, possibly antiviral
Ginkgo biloba	Bleeding, anticoagulant	Improves circulation and memory
Ginseng	Hypertension and tachycardia, hypoglycemia, bleeding	Boosts vitality, stimulant, enhances sexuality
Vitamin E	Bleeding, slows wound healing and collagen repair	Prevents heart disease
Vitamin A (beta carotene converts to vitamin A in the body)	Can cause complications in pregnancy	Reverses the adverse effects on wound healing caused by steroid use, enhances healing, boosts immune system, fights infection, fights inflammation
Vitamin C	Potential for kidney stones and anemia in toxic state; can interfere with vitamin B_{12}; water-soluble: excreted readily via kidneys	Enhances wound healing
Garlic	Bleeding, hypotension, hypoglycemia, antithrombotic, antiplatelet	Lowers cholesterol, prevents heart disease, fights infection
Fish oil	Bleeding, hypotension	Prevents heart disease
Bromelain (found in pineapple stems)	No known complications	Antiinflammatory, digestive aid
Echinacea	Liver complications, interferes with immunosuppression, can cause transplant rejection	Antiinfective, fights common cold, enhances wound healing
Ephedra (also known as Ma Huang)	Cardiovascular instability, palpitations, hypertension, seizures	Appetite suppressant, respiratory treatment, boosts energy
Kava	Prolonged sedative effect, liver toxicity	Sedative, antiepileptic
Valerian	Prolonged sedative effect, can go through withdrawal, potentiated by alcohol, nausea	Sedative, sleep aid, muscle relaxant
Black cohosh	Bradycardia, peripheral dilation, hypotension	Alternative to estrogen replacement
Ginger	Bradycardia, bleeding, hypotension	Antiemetic, digestive aid, cough suppressant, relieves menstrual cramps
Licorice	Hypokalemia and dysrhythmia, hypertension, bleeding, can affect electrolytes, edema	Digestive aid
Chaparral	Liver complications	Alternative anticancer therapy
Chamomile	Potential allergy, bleeding, can affect electrolytes	Digestive aid, antiinflammatory, antiinfective

8. Discusses preoperative sedation in relation to the time the surgical procedure is scheduled to begin.
9. Reassures the patient that constant observation will be maintained during the surgical procedure and in the immediate postoperative period. Also explains the methods of monitoring vital functions.
10. Explains the risks of anesthesia without causing the patient undue stress.
11. Answers the patient's questions and allays his or her fears related to anesthesia.

After this visit with the patient, the anesthesia provider does the following:

1. Estimates the effect of the necessary positioning during the surgical procedure on the patient's physiologic processes.
2. Records preliminary data on the anesthesia chart.
3. Writes preanesthesia orders, including times for medication administration.
4. Writes a summary of the visit and the proposed anesthetic management of the patient on the physicians' progress note. This summary has medicolegal value if a problem subsequently develops, and it is also necessary for regulatory accreditation, such as for the state or the Joint Commission on Accreditation of Healthcare Organizations (JCAHO).
5. Assigns the patient a physical status classification for the purpose of anesthesia, as per the taxonomy adopted by the ASA.
   a. Class I theoretically includes relatively healthy patients with localized pathologic processes. An emergency surgical procedure, designated E, signifies additional risk. For example, a hernia that becomes incarcerated changes the patient's status to Class I-E.
   b. Class II includes patients with mild systemic disease (e.g., diabetes mellitus controlled by oral hypoglycemic agents or diet).
   c. Class III includes patients with severe systemic disease that limits activity but is not totally incapacitating (e.g., chronic obstructive pulmonary disease or severe hypertension).
   d. Class IV includes patients with an incapacitating disease that is a constant threat to life (e.g., cardiovascular or renal disease).
   e. Class V includes moribund patients who are not expected to survive 24 hours with or without the surgical procedure. They are operated on in an attempt to save their life; the surgical procedure is a resuscitative measure, as in a massive pulmonary embolus. The patient may or may not survive the surgical procedure.
   f. Class VI includes patients who have been declared brain dead but whose organs will be removed for donor purposes. Mechanical ventilation and life support systems are maintained until the organs are procured.
6. Consults with the surgeon and other physicians (e.g., a cardiologist) about a patient who has been assigned a Class III, IV, or V status. Considers the critical nature of the surgical procedure in relation to the risks of anesthesia.

   a. In elective situations, the surgical procedure is postponed until anesthesia will be less hazardous (e.g., after acute respiratory infection or cardiac decompensation).
   b. In emergency situations, ideal practices may be altered or disregarded to meet the exigencies of the situation. For example, if a patient is hemorrhaging, there is no time to wait to replace a low red blood count. A multiple trauma victim with a full stomach may need a nasogastric tube inserted and suction applied, an endotracheal intubation while awake, or spinal anesthesia as applicable, and he or she may undergo a surgical procedure despite food ingestion.

In addition to the preoperative assessment of the patient and the administration and maintenance of the intraoperative anesthetic, the anesthesia provider may see the patient postoperatively. He or she has a responsibility to inform the patient of any unfavorable reaction to a medication or agent so that the patient is forewarned and can report these reactions to other physicians and anesthesia providers in future experiences.

Before Leaving for the Operating Room

Before the patient goes to the OR suite, his or her physical and emotional status and vital signs should be assessed and recorded by the nurse on the surgical unit or in the same-day admission unit. Any untoward signs and symptoms and extreme apprehension are reported to the surgeon, because they could affect the patient's intraoperative course. The following preparations are made:

1. The patient puts on a clean hospital gown. The surgeon permits some patients to wear underpants or pajama pants if the lower body segment is not part of the surgical site. This is helpful in adolescents and patients who are very embarrassed and uncomfortable. Any clothing removed in OR should be placed in a clear plastic bag and labeled with the patient's name, date, and surgeon's name.

   Menstruating patients should use a sanitary napkin if they will be under general anesthesia for more than 2 hours. Tampons can be used if they will not remain in place for more than a few hours total. The presence of a tampon should be clearly noted in the chart so it is not forgotten if the surgery becomes more extensive and longer in duration. The circulating nurse should be informed verbally about the patient's menses so confusion does not arise if vaginal bleeding is noted.

2. Jewelry is removed for safekeeping. If a wedding ring cannot be removed, it is taped loosely or tied securely to prevent loss. The patient may be permitted to keep a religious symbol, but the patient should understand this may be removed during the surgical procedure. Document the personal items and their disposition in the chart before, during, and after the procedure.

3. Unless otherwise ordered, dentures and removable bridges are removed before the administration of the general anesthetic to safeguard them and to prevent them from obstructing respiration. Dentures are per-

mitted during local anesthesia, especially if the patient can breathe more easily with them in place. Some anesthesia providers prefer that securely fitting dentures be left in place to facilitate the airway maintenance. Dentures are necessary to retain facial contours for some plastic surgery procedures. Dentures removed in the OR should be labeled and taken to PACU for placement in the patient's mouth during the postprocedure period.

4. All removable prostheses (e.g., eye, extremity, contact lenses, hearing aids, eyeglasses) are removed for safekeeping. In some instances the patient may be permitted to wear eyeglasses or a hearing aid to the OR. The circulating nurse safeguards them and sends them to the PACU with the patient. Contact lenses are removed before the administration of a general anesthetic because they may become dry and cause corneal abrasions.

    The patient's personal property is safeguarded to prevent loss or damage. Jewelry and valuables can be given to the family or sent to the hospital safe. The clothing of ambulatory surgery patients can be stored in a locker. The clothing of TCI patients can be sent to the room or unit where the patient will be admitted postoperatively. Be sure that all items are bagged and clearly marked with the patient's name and date. Document the disposition of all patient belongings.

5. Long hair may be braided. Wigs should be removed, or in special cases, covered with a surgical cap. Hairpins are removed to prevent scalp injury.

6. Antiembolic stockings or elastic bandages may be ordered for the lower extremities to prevent embolic phenomena. The stockings are applied before abdominal or pelvic procedures; for patients who have varicosities, are prone to thrombus formation, or have a history of emboli; and for some geriatric patients. They also are often applied for long procedures.

7. The patient voids to prevent overdistention of the bladder or incontinence during unconsciousness. This is especially important for abdominal or pelvic procedures in which a large bladder may be traumatized or may interfere with adequate exposure of the abdominal contents. The time of voiding is recorded. Double-check that a urine specimen is not needed before discarding the urine. When indicated, an indwelling Foley catheter is usually inserted in the OR after the patient has been anesthetized. Some urologic procedures require a full bladder, such as urodynamics (UD) with cystometrography (CMG) or electromyography (EMG); therefore, the patient should not void preoperatively.

8. If ordered, an antibiotic is given 1 hour preoperatively to establish and reach a therapeutic blood level of antibiotic prophylaxis intraoperatively. This may be a one-time dose or may be continued into the postoperative period. If cultures or specimens are obtained during the surgical procedure, a notation should be made on the pathology specimen sheet to indicate antibiotic use.

9. Preanesthesia medications are given as ordered. Their purpose is to eliminate apprehension by making the patient calm, drowsy, and comfortable. Patients who receive a preanesthesia medication should be cautioned to remain in bed and not to smoke. Many of the drugs cause drowsiness, vertigo, or postural hypotension. Therefore the side rails on the bed should be raised and the call bell placed within the patient's reach.

10. The patient, bed, and chart are accurately identified, and identifications are fastened securely in place. Allergies should be prominently noted on the chart and patient's wristband.

A preoperative checklist helps ensure that the patient has been properly prepared. If preparation is inadequate, the surgical procedure may be canceled. All essential records, including the plan of care or the clinical care map, must accompany the patient.

Emotional Preparation. By fulfilling spiritual and psychosocial needs, the caregiver helps to provide the preoperative patient with as much peace of mind as possible. Understandably, the patient's tension level rises as the time for the surgical procedure approaches. The better prepared the patient is emotionally, the smoother his or her postoperative course will be. If the patient has not seen his or her cleric or the hospital chaplain and makes such a request, the nurse should make every effort to contact that person for the patient.

Family members or significant others should be permitted to stay with the patient until he or she goes to the OR suite. Some hospitals permit parents to accompany infants and children into the OR suite. After leaving the patient, the family should be directed to the waiting area.

TRANSPORTATION TO THE OPERATING ROOM SUITE

Patients may be taken to the OR suite approximately 30 to 45 minutes before the scheduled time of the procedure. For safety, they are commonly transported via a transport stretcher or wheelchair. If a stretcher is used, it should be pushed from the head end so the patient's feet go first. Rapid movements through corridors and around corners may cause dizziness and nausea, especially if the patient has been medicated. The attendant at the head end can observe for vomiting or respiratory distress. The patient may be more comfortable if the head end of the stretcher is raised.

If transporting by wheelchair, the patient should be instructed not to help with door opening and to keep hands on the lap. A blanket or sheet should be placed on the seat of the chair and a cover over the lap for modesty. It is inappropriate for bare buttocks to be seated on the uncovered surface of the wheelchair. Take care with tubing such as IVs or catheters so they do not get tangled in the wheels. Drainage bags should be maintained below the level of the bladder to prevent reflux infection.

Some ambulatory patients may be permitted to walk to the OR. They are given foot protection such as slippers to prevent injury. The slippers should be skid-proof on the bottom. Paper slippers may be unsafe. They do not protect from injury or slippage. The slippers may need to be removed for the procedure but should be retained until the end of the procedure and returned to the patient for use within the facility.

Ideally, certain elevators are designated "For OR Use Only," which ensures privacy and minimizes microbial contamination. The patient should be comfortable, warm, and safe during transport. Side rails are raised, and restraint straps are applied. The patient should be instructed to keep his or her arms, hands, and fingers inside the side rails during transport to avoid injury when going through doorways.

IV solution bags hung on poles during transportation are attached securely and placed at the foot of the bed away from the patient's head; this minimizes the danger of injury to the patient if the container should fall. Gentle handling is indicated to prevent dislodging IV needles or indwelling catheters. Parent(s) sometimes are permitted to accompany a child. If the patient has a language barrier or is profoundly deaf, an interpreter may accompany him or her to the OR and stay until the induction of anesthesia.

ADMISSION TO THE OPERATING ROOM SUITE

Presurgical Holding Area

The patient is brought through the outer corridor to the holding area by transport personnel where he or she remains until taken to the OR. In some facilities, this holding area is in the PACU in a designated space on one end of the unit that is not occupied by patients who are recovering from anesthesia. This can be an advantage because many of the nurses in the holding area also perform patient care in the PACU area. This can promote familiarity between the patient and the nurse.

Some conditions justify bringing patients to the OR suite in their beds. Such conditions include patients in traction, patients on Stryker frames, or cardiac patients who cannot be moved until transferred to the operating bed. A patient on a Stryker or similar frame may undergo surgery while on the frame. The surgeon chooses the course that best benefits the individual patient.

Beds, stretchers, and frames are stabilized by personnel and by locking the wheels when a patient is moved or is permitted to move from one surface to another. Mattresses also should be stabilized. An adequate number of personnel and a transfer device should be available to ensure patient safety during transfer between surfaces. The patient's head, arms, and legs are protected. When using a transfer roller or other device, a minimum of four people is required to control the head, foot, and both sides of the patient.

Some hospitals have individual rooms for anesthesia induction. The patient waits in this room and is administered an anesthetic before being taken into the OR.

Admission to the Presurgical Holding Area. The holding area nurse greets the patient by name and introduces himself or herself. The nurse stands next to the midsection of the stretcher so the patient can comfortably see him or her. The holding area nurse does the following:

1. Places a warm blanket on the patient, verifies patient identification, and notifies the individual at the surgery control desk that the patient is in the holding area.

2. Verifies the surgical procedure, site, and surgeon verbally with the patient and/or family as appropriate. Some facilities require that the surgical site be physically marked with indelible ink or the surgeon's initials. Some facilities use a sticker applied to the spot. Take care that the sticker does not get rubbed off or moved.
3. Reviews the patient's chart for completeness (Fig. 21-4).
   a. Medical history and physical examination
   b. Laboratory reports
   c. Consent forms and documentation of consents
      (1) Informed consent data
      (2) General consent to treat
      (3) Anesthesia consent
4. Measures the vital signs and blood pressure.
5. Verifies allergies and medication history.
6. Checks skin tone and integrity.
7. Verifies physical limitations.
8. Notes the patient's mental state.
9. Puts a cap on the patient to protect his or her hair (in case vomiting occurs), for purposes of asepsis, and to help prevent hypothermia. Patients who are bald are required to wear a head covering to prevent heat loss and dander shed.
10. Notifies the individual at the surgery control desk when the patient is ready for transport to the OR. The patient is under constant observation by the patient care staff until transported from the surgical department to another patient care unit or discharged.

The holding area nurse records pertinent findings in the perioperative patient care record. If a perioperative patient assessment has not been performed, the holding area nurse will assess the patient, formulate the nursing diagnoses and expected outcomes, and prepare an individualized plan of care or initialize the care map.

Preanesthesia Preparations. The anesthesia provider or surgeon may wish to talk with the patient before sedation

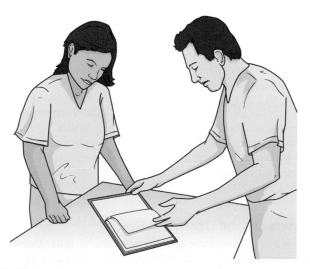

FIG. 21-4   The holding room nurse reviews the patient's chart for completeness.

is given. The surgeon should mark the actual surgical site with his or her initials with an indelible marker. The patient should be informed about all procedures before they are initiated. The following procedures may need to be completed before the induction of anesthesia; some or all of these procedures can be performed in the preoperative holding area if there are adequate facilities for patient privacy:

- Removal of body hair, if ordered.
- Marking of surgical incision sites such as for plastic surgery of the face and torso.
- Insertion of IV access. Be sure the placement does not interfere with the surgical site. Avoid the operative side of the body if possible.
- Insertion of invasive hemodynamic monitoring lines, as appropriate.
- Administration of the preanesthesia medication and other drugs such as preoperative antibiotics, as ordered. The preanesthesia medication can precipitate respiratory depression and hypotension, and the perioperative nurse should be alert and take prompt action for airway maintenance if necessary. The holding area should be equipped for cardiopulmonary resuscitation. An emergency or code blue button should be accessible to summon help at all times.

The anesthesia provider may perform regional blocks in the holding area. All procedures performed in the holding area are documented on the patient's chart.

Despite the activities around them, patients may feel more alone in a holding area than in any other location. Time passes slowly, and anxiety can increase. An anxious patient looks to the nurse for comfort, reassurance, and attention. A compassionate expression in the eyes and voice and a reassuring touch of the hand can convey concern and understanding to the patient.

If the patient is drowsy, unnecessary conversation should be avoided. The nurse should answer questions and see to the patient's comfort. The patient should be kept warm, or the blanket should be turned down if he or she is too warm. An extra pillow should be placed under the patient's head or under an arthritic knee. Dry lips should be moistened, if appropriate. Any delay or unusual circumstances should be explained to the patient and family.

A quiet, restful atmosphere enables the patient to gain full advantage of the premedication. Some holding areas and ORs have piped-in recorded music, which diverts attention from the many other sounds in the environment. Music with a slow, easy rhythm and a low volume is most conducive to relaxation. Familiar music is more pleasing and relaxing, because the patient can associate it with pleasant experiences. Some facilities provide earphones or headsets so patients can listen to the music of their choice. Earphones also muffle extraneous noises and conversations. Ideally, the patient should have a choice in selecting the music or in having no music at all; this is the advantage of individual headsets over piped-in systems.

Transfer to the Operating Room

When everything is ready, the circulating nurse comes to the holding area for the patient. It is advantageous if this person is the perioperative nurse who made the preoperative visit, because the patient will appreciate seeing a familiar face. Before transporting the patient into the OR, the circulating nurse has several important duties to fulfill:

1. Greet the patient, and validate his or her identity (Fig. 21-5).
   a. The circulating nurse should introduce himself or herself if he or she has not previously met the patient. The patient should be addressed as Mr., Mrs., or Ms.—not by the first name. It is appropriate to ask the patient to state and/or spell his or her name. The patient should be asked his or her full name and date of birth.
   b. When the patient arrives at the facility, an identifying wristband is put on in the admitting office. The perianesthesia nurse checks the band before the patient leaves for the OR. The circulating nurse compares the information on the wristband, including the identification number, with the information on the chart and with the information on the surgical schedule: name, anticipated surgical procedure, time, and surgeon. An allergy band and other notification band (e.g., Do Not Resuscitate [DNR]) should be checked at the same time.
   c. Identification on the stretcher or bed ensures the patient's return to the same stretcher or bed after surgery, if this is the procedure. If the patient is an infant or child, the identification tag on the crib should be out of his or her reach. Always validate the identity of a child with a parent. Ask what procedure is being performed.
   d. Verification of the surgical procedure, site, and surgeon with the patient provides reassurance that this is the correct patient. The patient's own words should be documented on the chart. The circulating nurse should note the presence of the surgeon's identifying mark on the surgical site. If the patient is heavily sedated, the surgeon may be asked to help identify the patient.
2. Check the side rails, restraining straps, IV infusions, and indwelling catheters.
3. Observe the patient for any reaction to the medication.

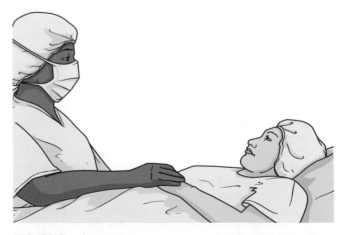

FIG. 21-5   The circulating nurse greets and identifies the patient.

4. Observe the patient's anxiety level.
5. Check the history and physical examination data, laboratory tests, radiograph reports, and consent form(s) or documentation in the patient's chart.
6. Review the plan of care or care map.
   a. Pay particular attention to allergies and any previous unfavorable reactions to anesthesia or blood transfusions.
   b. Become familiar with this patient's unique and individual needs.

The patient is taken into the OR after the surgeon sees him or her and the anesthesia provider is ready to receive the patient. The main preparations for the procedure should be complete so the circulating nurse can devote undivided attention to the patient.

Before the Induction of Anesthesia. The anesthesia provider also has immediate preanesthesia duties, such as the following:

1. Checking and assembling equipment before the patient enters the room. Airways, endotracheal tubes, laryngoscopes, suction catheters, labeled prefilled medication syringes, and other items are arranged on a cart or table.
2. Reviewing the preoperative physical examination, history, and laboratory reports in the chart.
3. Making certain that the patient is comfortable and secure on the operating bed.
4. Checking for denture removal or any loose teeth. The latter may be secured with a 2-0 silk tie and taped to the patient's cheek to prevent possible aspiration.
5. Checking to be certain that contact lenses have been removed.
6. Asking the patient when he or she last took anything by mouth, including medications.
7. Checking the patient's pulse, respiration, and blood pressure to obtain a baseline for the subsequent assessment of vital signs while the patient is anesthetized.
8. Listening to the heart and lungs, and then connecting ECG monitor leads and attaching the pulse oximeter and other monitoring devices (Fig. 21-6).
9. Starting the IV access. This may be done in the holding area or in an induction room. Some patients arrive with an IV line in place.
10. Preparing for and explaining the induction procedure to the patient. If properly premedicated, the patient should be able to respond to simple instructions.

Circulating Nurse's Role During Induction. The patient's welfare and individual needs take priority over all other activities before and during the induction of anesthesia. The patient is the most important person in the OR. If the circulating nurse gives more attention to the equipment than to the patient, the patient may feel abandoned. In addition, the monitoring equipment is not the best indicator of patient condition. At this time of stress, the patient wants the physical presence of a trusted, competent, and compassionate person.

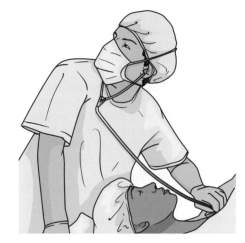

FIG. 21-6   The anesthesia provider preparing for induction of anesthesia.

The patient expects the circulating nurse to be cognizant of his or her problems and conditions and willing to help relieve them. The patient will perceive the circulating nurse's attitude as one of either acceptance or rejection. Consequently, the behavior of the circulating nurse affects the patient in either a positive or a negative way. Positive actions include spending time with and staying close to the patient (distance may be interpreted as disapproval), paying attention to the patient's needs and discomfort, looking directly at the patient when he or she speaks, touching the patient with kindness, and appearing poised, confident, and professional. Negative actions include frowning, ignoring the patient, and failing to respond to the patient's feelings or needs. The way in which something is said and done is as important as what is said and done.

Human beings react through their senses. The positive effect of touch is a helpful nonverbal communication in establishing nurse-patient rapport within a short time. Touch communicates caring. A gentle touch can bridge a language barrier by establishing human contact. Holding a patient's hand warmly or laying a hand on an arm during the induction of anesthesia or a painful procedure can do much to alleviate anxiety and elicit trust.

A smile has been called the universal language. Even though the circulating nurse is wearing a mask, his or her eyes can convey a smile or hope. Likewise, they can reveal anger or hostility. Physiognomy, the ancient Chinese art of discovering qualities of the mind and temperament from the expression of facial features, still has relevance. Facial expressions, eye contact, and body movements have either a positive or a negative effect on the patient. Warmth and caring can be conveyed by a pleasant manner and by the expression of the eyes.

Although routine procedures for care and teaching have been established, each patient deserves personalized care in the face of a disruptive life experience. The circulating nurse should not become insensitive to patients because of depersonalized procedures and routines or his or her own prejudices. The patient must not be treated as inanimate or anonymous or categorized by the disease or surgical procedure. The patient is a living, feeling person, not "Dr. Brown's hysterectomy," "the cardiac in Room 4," or "the arthritic I need help to move." Jargon such as this is depersonalizing, demoralizing, offensive, and totally unacceptable. The goal of perioperative patient care is to combine efficiency with caring.

The protection of modesty, dignity, and privacy is essential regardless of whether the patient is conscious or unconscious. Unnecessary exposure should be avoided. The gown and cotton blanket protect modesty and keep the patient warm. The OR door should be kept closed for privacy; this is also important in terms of aseptic technique. Surgical procedures may be viewed only by authorized personnel who have a definite function. All privileged information is kept confidential.

Patients are unnerved by stimuli such as strange odors and disturbing sights. A used, unclean operating room, with its soiled linen, instruments, equipment, unconscious patients, and bright lights, can be frightening. Patients feel isolation amid the hustle and bustle of activity, and a lack of team preparedness increases the patient's stress level. The patient may feel embarrassment from body exposure, and loud noises such as voices, inappropriate conversation, staff disagreements, clattering instruments, crumpling paper, and sterilizer noises contribute to the atmosphere of fear perceived by the patient.

Anxiety and preoperative sedation tend to alter the patient's ability to interpret events objectively. The patient may relate everything heard to himself or herself, even though he or she may not actually be the subject of the conversation, and he or she may misinterpret or react unfavorably. Hearing is the last sense lost when becoming unconscious. It is not known at precisely what moment a person can no longer hear and interpret what is said, but it is known that patients remain aware of their environment much longer than their seemingly unconscious state would indicate.

A lack of consideration can destroy the patient's confidence in the team. An overheard thoughtless comment can create a lasting traumatic memory and fear. Negative recall can induce anxiety in similar future experiences. Therefore, team members should think before speaking and should not converse near the patient while excluding him or her from the conversation. Sedation does not imply exclusion. The patient may be aware of conversation, even if he or she appears to be asleep! Out of the patient's hearing, conversation should pertain only to the work at hand. The OR is not the place for social discourse.

Time is of the essence to keep anesthesia and procedure time to a minimum, and it is a protective factor to provide as little disturbance to physiologic homeostasis as possible. However, efficiency and safety must not be sacrificed for speed. Safety is the prime concern. The OR suite imposes a high degree of vulnerability on patients and on the entire staff. Patients lack the power to defend and protect themselves during a surgical intervention; therefore, the circulating nurses are their advocates and protectors. They provide supportive care and safeguard patients from emotional and physical harm by maintaining constant vigilance. Circulating nurses can minimize the potential hazards in the following manner:

- Never leave a sedated patient unguarded. In addition to causing mental anguish from a feeling of abandonment, an unattended patient may fall or be injured by equipment.
- Correctly identify patients, surgical sites, and medications. An incorrect surgical procedure on a patient or an error in medication is usually the result of inadequate identification.
- Create, maintain, and control an optimally therapeutic environment in the OR. This involves control of the physical environment, such as temperature, humidity, and personnel. Traffic flow in and out of the room should be kept to a minimum. The more movement and talking, the greater the microbial count in the room. Once the patient is in the OR, it should be kept quiet so the effects of sedation are not counteracted. A tranquil, relaxed atmosphere is conducive to team concentration and orderly functioning so all can go well. The standards of ethical conduct should be strictly enforced.

The effect inherent in any type of surgical intervention can be reconciled when the patient has hope and confidence in the caregivers. Nurses are the central figures in patient care and can do much to relieve fear and provide security. Preoperative preparations can influence the outcome of the surgical procedure.

Bibliography

American Society of PeriAnesthesia Nurses: *Standards of perianesthesia nursing practice,* Thorofare, N.J., 1998, The Society.

AORN (Association of periOperative Registered Nurses): *AORN standards, recommended practices, and guidelines,* Denver, 2006, The Association.

AORN (Association of periOperative Registered Nurses): *Perioperative nursing data set: Tthe perioperative nursing vocabulary,* Denver, 2000, The Association.

Barnes S: Patient preparation: the physical assessment, *J Perianesth Nurs* 17(1):46-47, 2001.

Barnes S: Preparing for surgery: providing the details, *J Perianesth Nurs* 16(1):31-32, 2001.

Flanagan K: Preoperative assessment: safety considerations for patients taking herbal products, *J Perianesth Nurs* 16(1):16-26, 2001.

Iacono M: Informed consent, *J Perianesth Nurs* 15(3):180-181, 2000.

Kiernan M: Minor surgery in general practice: avoiding the pitfalls, *J Commun Nurs* 3(10):50-51, 1997.

Kopanski JE: A solution for wrong site surgery, *SSM* 7(2):12-14, 2001.

Kumar NB et al: Perioperative herbal supplement use in cancer patients: Potential implications and recommendations for presurgical screening, *Cancer Control* 12(3):149-157, 2005.

Munro H, D'Errico C: Parental involvement in perioperative anesthetic management, *J Perianesth Nurs* 15(6):397-400, 2000.

Murphy JM: Preoperative considerations with herbal medicines, *AORN J* 69(1):173-183, 1999.

Quinn DD, Schick L: *Perianesthesia nursing core curriculum,* ed 4, St Louis, 2004, Saunders.

Wren KR et al: Use of complementary and alternative medications by surgical patients, *J Perianesth Nurs* 17(3):170-177, 2002.

Chapter 22

Diagnostic Procedures and Oncologic Considerations

CHAPTER OBJECTIVES

After studying this chapter, the learner will be able to:
- List several invasive diagnostic tests.
- List several noninvasive diagnostic tests.
- List several interventional procedures that incorporate diagnostics.
- Describe several aspects of patient care associated with diagnostic testing.
- Discuss the role of diagnostics in oncology

CHAPTER OUTLINE

KEY TERMS AND DEFINITIONS

Anaplasia   Change in cellular differentiation and orientation that causes a more primitive structural appearance and function. Anaplastic cell changes are characteristic of malignancy.

Biopsy   Procedure for obtaining a representative tissue sample for gross and/or microscopic examination. The specimen can be obtained surgically or by other means.

Brachytherapy   Placement of radioactive material inside of or close to a tumor. Radioactive elements are introduced through catheters inserted into the tumor.

Cancer   Broad term that describes any malignant tumor within a large class of diseases. More than 100 different forms of cancer are known, each with histologic variations. Cancerous tumors are divided into two broad groups:
- **Carcinoma**   Malignant tumor of epithelial origin that affects glandular organs, viscera, and skin.
- **Sarcoma**   Malignant tumor of mesenchymal origin that affects bones, muscles, and soft tissue.

Chemotherapy   Use of chemical or pharmacologic agents to treat diseases, such as cancer.

Contrast medium   Use of a substance in the creation of density on a radiographic imaging device; radiopaque contrast injected or instilled to outline an organ or a structure. A radiolucent substance, such as air, can help define a hollow space, such as a ventricle of the brain.

Cytoreductive surgery   Mechanical reduction in cell volume at the tumor site by sharp or blunt tissue dissection. Vessel- and nerve-sparing procedures include the use of an ultrasonic aspirator and hydrostatic pulsed lavage.

Immunotherapy   Use of agents that stimulate or activate the body's own host defense immune system to combat disease.

Interventional radiology   Invasive procedures performed under radiologic control. Examples include balloon angioplasty, coronary artery stent placement, and inferior vena cava filter placement.

Neoplasm   Atypical new growth of abnormal cells or tissues, which may be malignant or benign.

Nuclear medicine study   Diagnostic test performed using radioactive substances to image a body part or system.

-oma   Suffix denoting a tumor or neoplasm.

Palliation   Measures taken to decrease the negative effects of a terminal or moribund condition. This is not considered a cure, but a temporary solution to a problematic situation. Examples include removing an obstruction or attempts to preserve fertility in the face of cancer.

Pathologic examination   A series of tests and examinations conducted by a pathologist to determine the cause of changes in the structure or function of a body part or tissue.

Percutaneous   Directed through the skin and tissues of the external body surface. Diagnostics, treatments, or tissue removal can be performed by direct percutaneous routes.

Plethysmography   Procedure to determine variations in blood flow between parts.

Scintigraphy   Recording of the emissions of radiologic substances as they are collected or secreted by tissues and/or organs in body.

Smear   A sample of tissue cells or fluid aspirated or scraped from a mucous membrane or a potentially pathologic site. The material is stained and studied for cellular components to make a diagnosis.

Stereotaxis   Computerized localization of a lesion.

Tomography   Computerized method of imaging a structure in layers.

Tumor   Any neoplasm in which cells are permanently altered but have the capability of growth and reproduction. A tumor consists of two elements: the tumor cells themselves and a supporting framework of connective tissue and vascular supply.

- **Benign tumor** Aggregation of cells that closely resemble those of the parent tissue of origin. The tumor usually grows slowly by expansion, is localized, and is surrounded by a capsule of fibrous tissue.
- **Malignant tumor** Progressively growing tumor that originates from a specialized organ such as the lung, breast, or brain, or a tumor localized to a specific body system such as bone, skin, lymph nodes, or blood vessels.

SUPPLEMENTAL MATERIAL ON EVOLVE WEBSITE   *evolve*

http://evolve.elsevier.com/BerryKohn
- Content Updates
- Glossary
- Full Set of Perioperative Flash Cards
- Interactive Key Term Flash Cards
- Student Activities
- WebLinks

HISTORICAL BACKGROUND

Early diagnostic testing was surrounded by myths and legends. Most diseases were not detected until they became symptomatic or caused death. Primitive practitioners diagnosed illness as punishment from evil spirits and effected treatment by determining which taboo had been breached. One method of diagnosis was to rub a small animal over the surface of the body and then dissect it to observe the configuration of its internal organs.

Hippocrates used a format of history taking and physical examination that consisted of placing an ear on the patient's chest to hear heart and breath sounds. Other tests included smelling and tasting body fluids. Palpation was used for ascertaining body temperature and sampling the pulse. His philosophy was to study the patient, not the disease.

The discovery of the microscope and other tools of diagnosis improved patient outcomes by revealing previously unknown causes of disease and illness. In the sixteenth century Ambroise Paré performed routine autopsies after death to determine the cause of illness. He learned much about anatomy and physiology from studying the dead.

In 1895 German physics professor Wilhelm Conrad Roentgen discovered x-rays. An electromagnetic wave with a short wavelength was emitted from a small screen that was placed near a cathode ray tube. He was able to see the bones in his hand. He termed the mysterious ray *x-ray,* because x always represented an unknown quotient in science. He published his results and did not seek to patent his discovery. Boston was the first city in the United States to boast an x-ray machine for the diagnosis of physical disease. The use of the x-ray was extended to multiple body systems, including active physiology (e.g., the study of blood and urine flow during angiography and voiding cystometrics).

In 1927 Egas Moniz, a Portuguese physician, was the first to perform cerebral angiography. In 1929 in Germany, Werner Forssman catheterized the right atrium by passing a ureteral catheter into it through a vein in the right arm. He was not successful in his attempt to inject a radiopaque substance through the catheter to visualize the pulmonary vessels. In 1931 Moniz was able to visualize the right chambers of the heart and pulmonary vessels using Forssman's technique. Poor visualization and unfavorable reactions of patients to the contrast media discouraged pioneers in this procedure. By 1937 Robb and Steinberg had worked out the precursors to the cardiopulmonary visualization techniques as they are used today.

DIAGNOSING PATHOLOGY

Diagnosis of a pathologic disease, anomaly, or traumatic injury is established before a surgical procedure is undertaken. Many modalities and techniques help surgeons assess each individual patient problem, guide them through the surgical procedure, and help them verify the results of surgical intervention. The term *diagnosis* refers to the art or the act of determining the nature of a patient's disease. Diagnostic procedures can be classified as follows:

- *Noninvasive.* Noninvasive techniques use equipment placed on or near the patient's skin but outside body tissues.
- *Invasive.* Invasive techniques use equipment placed into a body cavity or vessel and/or use substances injected into body structures.
- *Interventional.* Interventional techniques involve invasive diagnostics and procedures performed in a specialty department, such as in radiology.

Perioperative nurses and surgical technologists should be familiar with the modalities and equipment necessary to assist with diagnostic procedures in the operating room (OR) and interventional departments.

PATIENT CARE CONSIDERATIONS FOR DIAGNOSTIC PROCEDURES

1. Patients should be assessed for their physical condition and any metal implants, pacemakers, infusion pumps, sensitivities, and allergies.
2. Clear instructions should be given verbally and in writing before the test is performed.
3. Preprocedure preparations should be confirmed before the patient begins testing.
4. Explanations of procedures should be given to patients to allay fears and to ensure their understanding of the value of the procedure in making a diagnosis. Before the procedure begins, an explanation should be given of the equipment being used and of the necessity to remain quiet while films are being taken.
5. Sterile and aseptic techniques of invasive procedures are strictly observed.
6. Some surgical procedures are performed with the patient positioned on a fluoroscopic table equipped with an image intensifier for radiographic visualization of anatomic structures as the surgical procedure progresses. Positioning aids should be used as compatible with the machinery.
7. The x-ray tube or C-arm that will extend over the surgical site should be free from dust. It should be damp-dusted with a disinfectant solution before the patient arrives and the surgical procedure begins. It may be covered with a sterile drape or sleeve before it is moved over the sterile field.

8. Time, distance, and shielding are the key factors in minimizing radiation exposure. Personnel should stand at least 6 feet (2 m) away from the x-ray beam and/or wear lead aprons or sternal and gonadal shields. Patients should be protected with gonadal shields if possible.

9. A stock of routine supplies should be kept on a portable cart if procedures are done in the radiology department or other interventional area. In general, the following items should be readily available:
   a. Sterile tray for the specific procedure
   b. Skin preparation tray and solutions
   c. Intravenous (IV) administration sets and solutions
   d. Local anesthetic agents, needles, and syringes
   e. Radiopaque contrast material
   f. Sterile gowns, gloves, drapes, and dressings

10. The following emergency equipment should be readily available:
   a. Cardiac resuscitation equipment, including a defibrillator and emergency medications
   b. Oxygen supply, Ambu bag, and tubing

11. Patients should be carefully observed and monitored during all procedures for any change in condition. If a procedure is done with the patient under local anesthesia, a qualified registered nurse should monitor the patient's vital signs. A stand-by anesthesia provider should be available to check the patient's physiologic status as needed.

PATHOLOGIC EXAMINATION

Clinical pathology is the use of laboratory methods to establish a clinical diagnosis of a disease by examining tissue and organs. Surgical pathology is the study of alterations in body tissues removed by surgical intervention.

Biopsy

The removal of tissue or fluid for diagnosis is referred to as a biopsy. Biopsy specimens can be obtained by many invasive methods. The pathologist determines and/or confirms the diagnosis by histologic examination (the study of tissue) and cytologic analysis (the study of cells).

Smear. Cells and small pieces of tissue are suspended in liquid and smeared on glass microscope slides. The specimen is "fixed" by being sprayed with fixative or immersed in liquid. The fixed slide is then stained and examined under a microscope by the pathologist or specially trained technician. This technique is useful for the examination of fine needle aspirate or scrapings. Smears can be examined within minutes after they have been obtained from the patient. Instant diagnosis is possible in many cases.

Aspiration Biopsy. Fluid is aspirated through a 22- to 25-gauge needle placed in a lesion, such as a cyst or abscess, or in a joint or body cavity. Fine needle aspiration biopsies are done most commonly to obtain cells from solid lesions in the breast, thyroid, neck, lymph nodes, or soft tissues. The needle is manipulated in the mass while suction is placed on the syringe. Several hundred cells are drawn into the syringe. The cells can be chemically fixed and then examined under the microscope. Aspiration biopsies can be performed under computed tomography (CT) or ultrasonic guidance with minimal local anesthesia.

Bone Marrow Biopsy. A trocar puncture needle or aspiration needle is placed into bone, through a small skin incision or percutaneous puncture. The sternum and iliac crest are common sites for bone marrow aspiration. Patients with abnormal blood counts or unusual blood morphology can benefit from cytologic studies of bone marrow.

Local anesthesia to the level of the periosteum is necessary. In obese patients a spinal needle may be needed to reach this depth. After satisfactory anesthesia, a larger-bore needle is introduced into the marrow space and the specimen is aspirated. The aspiration may feel painful to the patient, because the bone is not numb. A core sample of bone may be obtained at this time for pathologic examination.

Percutaneous Needle Biopsy. Tissue is obtained from an internal organ or solid mass by means of a hollow needle inserted through the body wall. Percutaneous puncture into a lesion may be guided by fluoroscopy under image intensification, by ultrasound, or by CT scanning. Special needles are used; some types are disposable.

Punch Biopsy. An instrument with a 3- to 4-mm circular, sharp, hollow tip is used to sample skin lesions in a cookie-cutter manner. The plug of tissue is sent for pathologic study. The circular wound is usually closed with 4-0 suture and heals without incident. Dermatologists or plastic surgeons use this method for skin biopsy.

Brush Biopsy. Stiff brushes of nylon or steel are passed through an endoscope to the interior of the respiratory tree or urinary tract. Tissue samples are collected as the brush rubs against the target organ. Smears are made on glass slides; the tip of the brush is then cut off and placed in formalin for a minimum of 1 hour for fixation. The slides and fixed tissue are subjected to histologic studies for *diagnosis.*

Excisional Biopsy. A mass or entire structure is cut from the body. The advent of fine needle aspiration has decreased the need for full excisional biopsy with the exception of a friable organ or a breast mass. In diagnosing lymphoma, an entire lymph node is necessary for adequate diagnosis. Some excisional biopsies can be performed endoscopically (Fig. 22-1).

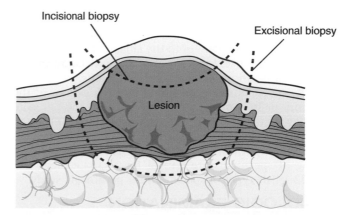

FIG. 22-1 Comparison between incisional and excisional tissue biopsies.

Incisional Biopsy. A portion of a mass is removed. Soft tissue masses incised for diagnosis include muscle, fat, or other connective tissue (see Fig. 22-1).

Frozen Section. Special preparation and examination of tissue can determine whether it is malignant and whether regional nodes are involved. When the surgeon removes a piece of tissue and wants an immediate diagnosis, it is placed in a basin or specimen container without any added preservative, such as formalin or normal saline solution. Formalin or normal saline solution will alter the freezing process used in the specialized pathologic study. The circulating nurse should alert the pathologist that his or her services will be needed. In some facilities the pathologist comes to the OR suite to do a frozen section, which takes only a few minutes. When the tissue examination is complete, the pathologist will report the results directly to the surgeon in the OR.

The patient's level of consciousness should be considered during report of pathologic results, especially if the patient is awake. The use of speakerphones should be avoided for patient confidentiality. If a malignant lesion is present and the individual situation calls for it, the surgeon proceeds with a radical resection of the affected organ or body area. In some situations, additional tissue is needed for diagnosis.

Permanent Section. The specimen is placed in fixative, commonly formalin, for several hours to cause the cells to become firm. The fixed specimen is placed in a machine that removes all of the water from the tissues, replacing it with paraffin. When this process is complete, the specimen is embedded into a block of wax. It is placed in a microtome and is sliced tissue-paper thin and floated in a bath of water. The slices are placed on glass slides, where the paraffin is dissolved with solvent and the water is restored to the tissue on the slide. The slices readily accept dyes and stains used for diagnosis. Permanent section is the best diagnostic biopsy tool. Box 22-1 lists several tissue dyes and stains used in diagnostic procedures.

Surgical Specimens

All tissue removed during the surgical procedure is sent to the pathology laboratory for verification of the diagnosis. Any unidentifiable or unusual item removed from a patient should be sent for identification by the pathology department. Some examples include removal of retained surgical items, such as instruments, sponges and towels. Any questionable item should be sent to the lab and documented by the circulating nurse. Facility policy and procedure should delineate disposition of all surgical specimens.

Tissue specimens may be stored in a refrigerator in the laboratory or in some other location within the OR suite until they are taken to the pathology department at the end of each day's schedule of surgical procedures or at intervals during the day. Correct solutions for storage and correct labeling of specimens are critical for accurate diagnosis. Table 22-1 lists types of specimens for pathologic study.

RADIOLOGIC EXAMINATION

An x-ray is a high-energy electromagnetic wave capable of penetrating various thicknesses of solid substances and

| BOX 22-1 | Surgical Dyes and Tissue Stains |

DYES
Blue
   Trypan blue
   Isosulfan blue
   Methylene blue
   Indigo carmine
   Cyanosine
Green
   Brilliant green
   Indocyanine green
Red
   Congo red
   Carmine
Yellow
   Fluorescein sodium
Purple
   Crystal violet
   Gentian violet
Black
   India ink

STAINS
Brown-yellow
   Lugol's (iodine)
   Monsel's (ferric)

affecting photographic plates. X-rays are generated on a vacuum tube when high-velocity electrons from a heated filament strike a metal target (anode), causing it to emit x-rays. The image obtained by the use of x-rays may be referred to as an x-ray film, roentgenogram, radiograph, or other -gram name associated either with the specific technique used to obtain the photograph or with the anatomic structures identified (e.g., mammogram). Most facilities have eliminated the use of x-ray film and have changed to a digital format.

X-rays are also used for diagnostic imaging with fluoroscopy, computed tomography (CT), and digital radiography. Computerized radiologic images may be stored on diskettes.

Types of Radiologic Equipment and Accessories

Many hospitals have one or more rooms within the OR suite that are equipped for diagnostic as well as intraoperative radiologic procedures. In some facilities, OR personnel are cross-trained to assist with diagnostic and interventional procedures in the radiology department.

Contrast Media. Agents composed of nonmetallic compounds or heavy metallic salts that do not permit passage of radiant energy are radiopaque. When exposed to x-rays, the lumina of body structures filled with these agents appear as dense areas. Radiopaque contrast media frequently used for the procedures to be described are listed in Box 22-2. Some of these agents are fluorescent dyes. Most contain iodine. A history of sensitivity to substances that contain iodine, such as shellfish, or other allergies must be obtained before these agents are injected. A test dose of 1 or 2 mL may be given before the dose required for x-ray study. The

TABLE 22-1	Specimen Types and Considerations for Handling		
Specimen Type	**Test**	**Preparation**	**Example**
Fluid	Bacteriology	Anaerobic or aerobic on culture swab in sterile tube	Exudate
	Virology	Fresh, in sterile container	Cerebrospinal fluid
	Cytology	Fresh or added solution of pathologist's choice in sterile container	Cell washings, urine
	Genetic studies	Fresh, in sterile container	Amniotic fluid
	Cell count	Fresh, in sterile container	Semen for infertility study
Tissue	Permanent section	Fresh or added solution of pathologist's choice in sterile container	Diseased organ
	Frozen section	Fresh, in sterile container. No saline.	Margin of malignant lesion
	Biopsy	Fresh or solution of pathologist's choice in sterile container	Suspicious lesion
	Hormonal assay	Fresh, in sterile container	Breast tissue
	Donor tissue	Fresh or added solution of pathologist's choice	Cadaver skin
	Calculi	Dry, in sterile container	Gallstone
	Ova	Fresh or added solution of surgeon's choice	Human egg for preservation
	Muscle	Fresh, extended in special clamp in sterile container	Test for malignant hyperthermia
Nonbiologic specimen	Foreign body	Fresh, in sterile container	Glass fragments
	Projectile from crime scene	Dry, in nonmetallic container	Bullet
	Clothing of crime or accident victim	Dry, in porous paper	Underclothes of rape victim
	Explanted prosthesis	Dry, in sterile container	Orthopedic screws or plates

patient should be observed for allergic reaction throughout the procedure. Signs of reaction may include the following:
- Red rash over face and chest
- Extreme agitation
- Sudden elevation of body temperature
- Complaints of muscle, joint, and back pain
- Respiratory distress
- Tachycardia
- Hypotension
- Blood-tinged urine
- Convulsions
- Loss of consciousness
- Cardiac arrest

Radiolucent Gases. Filtered room air, oxygen, nitrogen, carbon dioxide, or a combination of gases may be injected into body spaces or structures that normally contain fluid other than blood. Gases are radiolucent (i.e., transparent to x-rays). Thus gas-filled spaces appear less dense on x-ray film than do surrounding tissues.

Radiologic Table. The tabletop the patient lies on is made of acrylic or some other radiolucent material (Fig. 22-2). Some operating beds have a Bakelite top that fits over the length of the table and permits insertion of the x-ray cassette at any area. For fluoroscopy with image intensification, the entire top must be radiolucent because the image intensifier is positioned underneath the table. If the entire operating bed is not radiolucent, the foot section can be lowered and a radiolucent extension attached that will accommodate specialized x-ray machinery.

Cassette. The lightproof holder for x-ray film is referred to as a cassette. The patient is positioned between the x-ray tube and the cassette. Holders for cassettes may be built into or attached to the operating bed. Intraoperative x-rays may require the use of a sterile disposable cassette cover. If a sterile cover is unavailable, a sterile Mayo stand cover may be substituted. In some circumstances, a cassette may be slid under a patient on the OR table. Care is taken not to contaminate the sterile drapes. Many facilities have discontinued the use of x-ray film and have converted to digital format.

Processing Equipment. Conventional x-ray equipment projects a black-and-white image on x-ray film that is developed by a chemical process. Some OR suites have a darkroom where x-ray film is developed after exposure so that the surgeon can see results of the study without excessive delay. An automatic processor in which film can be developed within 90 seconds to 3 minutes may be available.

Fixed X-Ray Equipment. A fixed overhead x-ray tube with housing may be mounted on a ceiling track for unrestricted movement of the x-ray beam into the desired position over the patient. When not in use, it can be moved against a wall and retracted toward the ceiling. Some units are fixed to specially designed tables, such as the urologic table for cystoscopic examinations. The controls are in an adjacent room or behind a lead shield and are activated by the radiologist or radiology technician.

BOX 22-2 | Radiopaque Contrast Media

Barium sulfate for gastrointestinal studies

Diatrizoate meglumine, injectable:
- Cardiografin for angiography and aortography
- Hypaque Meglumine, 30%, for urography and computed tomography (CT)
- Hypaque Meglumine, 60%, for urography, cerebral and peripheral angiography, aortography, venography, cholangiography, hysterosalpingography, and splenoportography

Diatrizoate sodium, injectable:
- Hypaque sodium, 25%, for urography and CT
- Hypaque sodium, 50%, same uses as for Hypaque Meglumine, 60%

Diatrizoic acid, injectable, used as meglumine and sodium salts:
- Hypaque-M, 75%, for angiocardiography, angiography, aortography, and urography
- Renografin for cerebral angiography, peripheral arteriography and venography, cholangiography, splenoportography, arthrography, discography, urography, and CT
- Renovist for aortography, angiocardiography, peripheral arteriography and venography, venacavography, and urography

Ethiodized oil (Ethiodol) for splenoportography and CT

Iodipamide meglumine, injectable:
- Cholografin Meglumine for cholangiography and cholecystography
- Renovue for IV excretory urography
- Sinografin for hysterosalpingography

Iohexol (Omnipaque) for myelography

Iophendylate (Pantopaque) for myelography

Ioversol (Optiray) for arteriography and CT

Metrizamide (Amipaque) for myelography and CT

Propyliodone (Dionosil) for bronchography

Sodium iothalamate (Angio-Conray) for arteriography

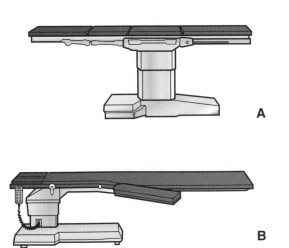

FIG. 22-2   Pedestal bases. **A,** Central. **B,** Eccentric for C-arm image intensifier placement.

Portable X-Ray Machine. An x-ray tube mounted on a portable electric- or battery-powered generator of a non-explosive design may be moved from one room to another in the OR suite and postanesthesia care unit (PACU). A portable x-ray machine offers the advantages of flexibility in scheduling procedures and availability for when and where it is needed.

Portable x-ray machines can be a source for cross-contamination. All portable equipment should be thoroughly disinfected before being brought into the OR/PACU and again after use. It should be stored within the perioperative environment between uses. Portable x-ray machines are used for intraoperative angiography, cholangiography, orthopedic localization, and urologic contrast procedures.

Intraoperative images require the x-ray machine to be in proximity to the sterile field and could cause contamination. A few options to prevent contamination include draping the machine with a specialized drape or temporarily placing a sterile towel over the site to be imaged. Extreme care is taken to prevent contamination when the towel is removed. Reasons for intraoperative x-ray imaging include performing diagnostic examinations with contrast media or looking for a lost surgical object.

In the PACU the portable x-ray machine is used for immediate (stat) chest and kidney-ureter-bladder (KUB) films. X-ray films can be used to check the location of implants and delayed passage of contrast medium through an organ system.

Fluoroscope. Similar to an x-ray generator, a fluoroscope has an additional screen, composed of fluorescent crystals, which lies in contact with a photocathode. When an x-ray beam passes through this screen, it fluoresces. Fluorescent light sets electrons free from an adjacent photocathode to produce an electron image. Rather than this image of body structures being photographed on x-ray film, it is reproduced as a digital image on a luminescent screen. Known as fluoroscopy, examination under a fluoroscope allows visualization of both form and movement of internal body structures. Fluoroscopy is used frequently for both pre-operative and intraoperative procedures.

It is an invasive technique, because a fluorescent substance must be injected or a radiopaque device inserted. When exposure time is prolonged to perform a procedure with visual fluoroscopic control (e.g., cardiac catheterization), fluoroscopy exposes the patient and personnel to radiation at higher levels than do conventional x-rays. Personnel must wear lead aprons during fluoroscopy even though a lead shield is part of the installation. Patients in the vicinity should be protected with gonadal and thyroid shields.

Image Intensifier. The image intensifier is used with the fluoroscope. It amplifies the image onto a monitor screen. The surgeon activates the image intensifier with a foot pedal. Clarity of the image is an aid in diagnosis, particularly of vascular, urologic, neurologic, and bone disorders. The surgeon can observe the progression of an injected fluorescent substance as it moves through internal structures or the placement of a device, such as a catheter, into the body. When connected to other closed-circuit television facilities, the image can be transmitted to other rooms for teaching purposes. In addition, the image can be filmed for a permanent record and for teaching. The monitoring screen may be mounted on the ceiling above the operating bed to save space in the OR, or it may be portable.

Mobile C-Arm Image Intensifier. Designed primarily for orthopedic procedures, foreign body and calculi localization, and catheter placement, mobile image intensifiers offer the same advantages and disadvantages as do portable x-ray machines. The C-arm, so named because of its shape (see Fig. 13-2), keeps the image intensifier and x-ray tube in alignment; the intensifier is directly under the tube. It can be moved from an anterior to a lateral position. Utility of the mobile C-arm image intensifier is enhanced when the system is capable of making electronic radiographs for permanent records. An additional formatting device is required for this function.

Computerized Digital Subtraction Processor. After IV injection of a radiopaque contrast medium, the computerized digital subtraction x-ray imaging system visually records perfusion within the cardiovascular system (e.g., extracranial and intracranial vessels).

Initially, before contrast medium is injected, fluoroscopic body images are converted to digital data for storage in a memory unit in the processor. Termed the *mask image,* these digitized data are integrated into single or multiple video frames. The video signal is logarithmically amplified and digitized. The mask image is electronically subtracted from subsequent images with the contrast medium. This process removes unwanted background, thus providing optimal visualization of vessels with contrast density that cannot be achieved by other image intensifiers. The resultant images (digital radiographs) are displayed on a video screen and can be recorded on diskette or videotape.

Radiologic Diagnostic Procedures

Chest X-Ray. Most surgeons consider a chest x-ray film as an extension of the patient's history and physical examination if it is clinically necessary. An x-ray study of the chest may be part of the admission procedure for elective surgical patients to rule out unsuspected pulmonary disease that could be communicable or would contraindicate the use of inhalation anesthetics.

This procedure may be routine for patients older than 40 years. It is always a part of the diagnostic workup in patients with suspected or symptomatic pulmonary abnormalities if they will be undergoing general anesthesia.

X-Ray Studies for Trauma. In addition to being an aid in determining the extent of traumatic injury, x-ray films and scans may be entered as legal evidence in a court of law to establish injuries sustained by the patient or to justify medical care given. Conventional noninvasive x-ray images will show the following:

- Fractures of bones
- Presence and location of some types of foreign bodies (e.g., bullets)
- Air or blood in the pleural cavity
- Gas or fluid in the abdominal cavity
- Outline of abdominal and chest organs and any deviation from normal size or location

Mammography. A technique for projecting an x-ray image of soft tissue of the breast, mammography is the most effective screening method for early diagnosis of small, nonpalpable breast tumors. Mammography may be performed in conjunction with ultrasonography if the woman has fibrocystic breasts and difficult-to-palpate masses less than ¼ inch (0.5 cm) in diameter.

Three views of each breast are exposed to conventional x-rays. The procedure may be somewhat painful for the woman, because compression is needed for radiologic imaging. Tumors appear on the mammogram as opaque spiculated areas or, occasionally, as areas of calcification. The radiologist places a small, BB-like radiolucent bead with crosshairs over a suspicious area. Another x-ray film of this area is obtained. Fine needle aspiration may be performed under ultrasonic guidance to gather cells for cytologic study.

Patient Teaching. Women 35 to 40 years of age should have a baseline screening mammogram. Between the ages of 40 and 50 years, they should have additional screening films yearly or every other year as recommended by their physician. After the age of 50 years, every woman should have a yearly mammogram.

Mammography is not contraindicated in women with breast implants. The technician obtaining the radiograph should be informed of previous breast surgeries, hormone replacement therapy, and augmentation mammoplasty. Special breast-imaging techniques are employed to displace an implant or to obtain an x-ray film of extremely dense breast tissue.

Men with suspicious breast lesions or pronounced gynecomastia should have mammographic screening to rule out cancerous tissue.

Every patient should be taught breast self-examination and practice it every month as a baseline diagnostic test. Early diagnosis is the best chance for a cure. Figure 22-3

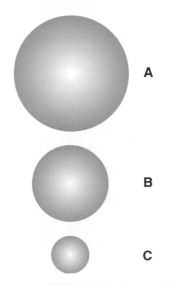

FIG. 22-3   Average-size lumps found by breast self-examination (BSE). **A,** Woman not practicing BSE. **B,** Woman practicing occasional BSE. **C,** Woman practicing monthly BSE. *(From Fortunato NM, McCullough SM: Plastic and reconstructive surgery, St Louis, 1998, Mosby.)*

depicts the average sizes of masses discovered in patients who do and do not practice breast self-examination.

Stereotactic Core Breast Tissue Biopsy. A needle biopsy device may be used in conjunction with mammography to obtain a tissue specimen from a lesion seen on the mammogram. The patient is positioned prone on a special table with her breasts placed through a biopsy porthole. Imaging equipment is used to stereotactically isolate breast lesions that may not be palpable. Percutaneous needle biopsies are performed with the patient under local anesthesia.

Computed Tomography. In CT, special complex and expensive equipment uses an x-ray beam in conjunction with a computer. Because the x-ray beam moves back and forth across the body to project cross-sectional images, the technique is referred to as computed tomography (CT), computed axial tomography (CAT), or simply scanning. It produces a highly contrasted, detailed study of normal and pathologic anatomy. The x-ray tube and photomultiplier detectors rotate slowly around the patient's head, chest, or body for 180 degrees in a linear fashion along the vertical axis. The computer processes the data and constructs a three-dimensional or two-dimensional picture on a black-and-white monitor or in colors that correspond to the density of tissue. Structures are identified by differences in density. This picture is photographed for a permanent record. The computer also prints out on a magnetic disk the numerical density values related to the radiation-absorption coefficients of substances in the area scanned. The radiologist uses this printout to determine whether a substance is fluid, blood, normal tissue, bone, air, or a pathologic lesion. The exact size and location of lesions in the brain, mediastinum, and abdominal organs are identified.

CT becomes an invasive procedure when a radiopaque contrast medium is injected IV to enhance visualization of the vascular and renal systems. Oral diluted barium contrast can be used to examine the gastrointestinal tract. Tissue biopsy can be performed under CT guidance. Needle aspiration can be performed under direct CT visualization.

CT exposes the patient to ionizing radiation and a potential allergic reaction to contrast medium, if used. To ensure proper use of this complex equipment, as well as to protect the patient from excessive or unnecessary radiation, the procedure is done under the supervision of a qualified radiologist.

Ventriculography. Ventriculography is the radiographic study of the ventricles after injection of gas directly into the lateral ventricles of the brain. It may be used to evaluate a patient with signs of increased intracranial pressure as a result of blockage of cerebrospinal fluid circulation. Ventricular needles or catheters are inserted into one or both lateral ventricles through holes made in the skull. The ventricular needle has a blunt, tapered point that prevents injury to the brain as it is inserted into the ventricle. Openings on the side near the point permit removal of spinal fluid and injection of gas. If the patient is an infant whose suture lines in the skull are not yet closed, needles are inserted through these.

The entire ventriculographic procedure may be done in the OR. Otherwise, the holes are drilled and the ventricular needles or an intraventricular catheter is inserted and the patient is then transferred to the radiology department or special procedures room within the OR suite. If a lesion is identified, the diagnostic procedure may be followed immediately by a surgical procedure because of the possibility of a further increase in intracranial pressure. If the patient is returned to the unit after the procedure, sterile ventricular needles should accompany the patient. If intracranial pressure becomes too great after gas injection, a needle can be inserted to remove the gas.

Arthrography. Arthrography is the study of a joint after the injection of gas or contrast medium into it. Conventional x-ray films show only the bony structure of a joint. Through injection of a dye or gas, injury to cartilage and ligaments may be visualized. A double-contrast study uses both gas and contrast, which is particularly useful in knee arthrograms.

Angiography and Arteriography. Angiography is a comprehensive term for studies of the circulatory system after injection of a radiopaque substance to permit visualization of the venous blood vessel system. These procedures are useful in the differential diagnosis of arteriovenous malformations, aneurysms, tumors, vascular accidents, or other circulatory abnormalities caused either by traumatic injury or by an acquired structural disease.

Intraoperative studies often are essential to assess the results of vascular reconstruction. Angiography is one method of assessment to confirm the position and patency of an arterial or venous graft or the quality of a restored vessel lumen. Intraoperative angiography frequently is indicated for these assessments in the peripheral vessels of extremities. After insertion of a bypass graft or endarterectomy, patency of the graft or vessel is checked by pulsations and also by arteriography to examine the arterial blood vessels of the circulatory system.

Angiography is also used at the time of the surgical procedure to identify vascularity or the exact location of some types of lesions in the extremities, brain, and thoracic and abdominal cavities. After venous injection of radiopaque contrast medium, radiologic studies are done. Techniques and equipment to be used will vary according to the specific procedure, but all types of angiography have the following features in common:

1. Access to the vessel (either an artery or vein) to be injected with a radiopaque contrast medium may be made by a percutaneous puncture or a cutdown. An IV drip is maintained when the latter approach is used.
   a. Cannulated needles with or without a radiopaque plastic catheter, similar to those used for IV infusions, may be used for a percutaneous puncture to penetrate an artery or vein. To prevent backflow of blood, cannulated needles have an obturator that remains in place until the contrast medium is injected. Long catheters have a guidewire to assist threading through the vessel.
   b. A Seldinger (18-gauge) needle has a sharply beveled inner cannula and a blunt outer cannula. The

blunt end of the outer cannula prevents trauma to the vessel. After insertion, the inner cannula is replaced with a guidewire and the outer cannula is removed. A 20-cm vessel dilator sheath (which is approximately 8 inches long) is threaded over the guidewire to create a track for a radiopaque catheter.

After the dilator sheath is removed, the catheter is positioned and the guidewire is withdrawn. This method is generally preferred for angiography because blood vessels other than the one punctured can be injected with contrast medium.

   c. A Cournand needle has a curved, flanged guard that contours to the body. It is particularly useful in carotid arteriography to hold the needle in position in the neck during injection.

   d. A Robb cannula is blunt, with a large lumen and a stopcock at the hub. It is inserted via a cutdown and is used with a Robb syringe that has a large opening in the tip for fast injection.

   e. A Sheldon needle has an occluded point with an opening at 90 degrees to the lumen. When the vertebral artery is entered, a right-angle injection is made into the lumen of the artery.

2. The amounts of radiopaque contrast substances injected into blood vessels are computed for infants and children according to weight. In adults the amount is measured so that it can be repeated safely for more exposures if necessary. Radiopaque agents dissipate very rapidly in the bloodstream.

3. Radiopaque contrast material should be warmed to body temperature to prevent precipitation and to reduce viscosity.

4. If awake, the patient should be told to expect a warm feeling and possibly a burning sensation when the contrast medium is injected. Procedures may be done with the patient under local anesthesia.

5. Sterile plastic tubing, 30 inches (76 cm) long with a syringe on one end and an adapter on the other, is connected to the needle or catheter in the vessel to prevent jarring from the pressure of injection and to keep the hands of the operator out of the x-ray beam.

6. An automatic injector may be used instead of injecting contrast medium by hand. This device correlates injection and x-ray exposure. When an automatic injector is used, special high-pressure nylon tubing is used that does not pull apart with pressure. When this tubing is used, a stopcock is placed on the end for closing it off at the syringe connection, because nylon tubing cannot be clamped.

7. Automatic radiologic seriogram equipment takes rapid multiple exposures while the contrast medium is in sufficient concentration to visualize the vessels. It can be set at 0.5- to 2-second intervals to take multiple pictures in succession.

8. Digital subtraction angiography converts the x-ray beam into a video screen image. A small amount of contrast medium is injected IV. Vessel catheterization is unnecessary, and less contrast medium is used. This procedure may be done on an ambulatory basis.

Bronchography. Study of the tracheobronchial tree is performed by instillation of a contrast medium to aid in the diagnosis of bronchiectasis, cancer, tuberculosis, and lung abscess or to detect a foreign body. The location of a lesion can be determined and the surgical procedure planned accordingly. The procedure should be explained in detail to the patient, because cooperation is necessary to accomplish the desired result. This radiologic study may be done in conjunction with bronchoscopy. In most patients, bronchoscopy is performed alone without the use of a bronchographic contrast medium.

Cholangiography. In addition to preoperative diagnostic x-ray studies, some surgeons routinely request radiologic studies in conjunction with cholecystectomy or cholelithotomy to identify gallstones in the biliary tract. Other surgeons selectively include cholangiography at the time of the surgical procedure in patients in whom they suspect stones might be present or retained in the bile ducts. Conventional x-ray equipment or an image intensifier may be used for these intraoperative studies.

The basic difference between preoperative and intraoperative cholangiography is the site of administration of the radiopaque contrast medium. For preoperative invasive cholangiography, the contrast medium injected IV through percutaneous venipuncture is excreted by the liver into the bile ducts. During open surgical procedures, the medium is injected directly into bile ducts.

Gastrointestinal X-Ray Studies. Studies are performed to identify lesions in the mucosa of the gastrointestinal tract, such as an ulcer, stricture, or tumor. Inflammatory lesions and partial or complete obstructions also may be identified. Barium sulfate is either swallowed by the patient or instilled by enema to outline the lumina of segments of the tract to be studied. These studies are done in the radiology department, but surgeons often refer to films during the surgical procedure. Care is taken not to use natural latex rubber enema tubing for this procedure if the patient is sensitive to latex.

Myelography. Lesions in the spinal canal are studied by myelography. It is helpful to localize a filling defect, spinal cord tumor, or herniated nucleus pulposus. Most surgeons do not rely entirely on this method of diagnosis; the patient's symptoms and signs are important in making a final diagnosis. Arachnoiditis is a potential complication of intrathecal injection of iophendylate (Pantopaque). Therefore a water-based contrast medium such as metrizamide (Amipaque) may be preferred.

Urography. Urography is a comprehensive term for radiologic studies of the urinary tract. Most procedures are performed in the radiology department, but some are done in conjunction with cystoscopic examinations. Urographic studies are described as follows:

• *Cystography.* The study of the bladder after instillation of a contrast medium. It is valuable in detecting ureterovesical reflux, a malfunction of the sphincter valves.

• *Cystourethrography.* The study of the bladder and urethra to determine whether there is an obstruction or abnormality in contour or position. X-ray films may be taken as contrast medium is injected into the bladder or when the patient voids the material.

- *Intravenous pyelography (IVP).* The study of structures of the urinary tract and kidney function. Contrast medium is introduced into the circulatory system by rapid IV injection or slow IV infusion drip. It is excreted through the kidneys. X-ray films are taken at carefully timed intervals. If the medium is poorly excreted through the kidneys, the last film may be taken as late as 24 hours after injection. Tomograms also may be taken while the contrast material is still in the urinary tract. These procedures are done in the radiology department rather than in the cystoscopy room.
- *Retrograde pyelography.* The study of the shape and position of the kidneys and ureters. Contrast medium is injected through catheters placed in each ureter. This procedure is used to visualize the renal pelves and calyces.
- *Voiding cystourethrography.* The study of contour and patency of the urethra. Contrast medium may be instilled into the bladder. X-ray films are taken as the patient voids. The medium must flow well but be viscous enough to distend the urethra and provide good detail on the x-ray film. If the patient is anesthetized, a very viscous contrast medium is injected into the urethra and films are taken. Because the female urethra is quite short, the latter technique is of little value in female patients.

Incidental X-Ray Films. An unanticipated need for an x-ray film occurs when a sponge, needle, or instrument is unaccounted for at the time the final count is taken during wound closure. An x-ray film will confirm whether the item is still in the patient. Unless the patient's condition demands immediate wound closure, a film may be taken before closure is completed.

Interventional Radiology

The radiologist may work in collaboration with the surgeon to insert catheters for infusion of cytotoxic and pharmacologic drugs, dilation, or embolization of vessels or organs. Cardiac catheterization, angioplasty, and stent placement are performed in an interventional radiology department. Biopsies may be performed percutaneously under radiologic C-arm control. Foreign bodies and thrombi may be extracted.

MAGNETIC RESONANCE IMAGING

Magnetic resonance imaging (MRI) was introduced in hospitals in the United States in 1981. Unlike CT scanning, MRI does not use radiation. The patient lies flat inside a large electromagnet. In this static magnetic field the patient is exposed to bursts of alternating radiofrequency energy waves. The magnetic nuclei of hydrogen atoms in the water of body cells are stimulated from their state of equilibrium. As nuclei return to their original state, they emit radiofrequency signals. These signals are converted by a digital computer into two-dimensional color images displayed on a monitor and recorded on film. Cross-sectional views of the head and all body soft tissue planes can be obtained. A computer software system has been developed that produces three-dimensional images.

MRI is based on the magnetic properties of hydrogen in the body rather than on the radiodensity of calcium, which is the basis of radiology. MRI looks at both the body's structure and function. It defines soft tissues in relationship to bony and neurovascular structures. It distinguishes between fat, muscle, compact bone and bone marrow, brain and spinal cord, fluid-filled cavities, ligaments and tendons, and blood vessels. The major applications of MRI are detection of tumors, inflammatory diseases, infections, and abscesses and evaluation of functions of the cardiovascular and central nervous systems and other organs.

MRI paramagnetic IV contrast media, such as gadopentetate, are sometimes used to localize tumors in the central nervous system. These media do not contain iodine, and allergic reactions are rare. All metals can cause artifacts that distort MRI scans—some more so than others. Titanium ligating clips, for example, create less distortion than do ferromagnetic (iron) or stainless steel clips. Iron-containing pigments used in tattoos and permanent eyeliner can alter the image produced. The magnetic field can cause ferromagnetic components of implants, such as pacemakers and cochlear implants, to malfunction. The magnetic field will also disable metallic devices in the area, such as cardiac monitors, infusion pumps, and wristwatches.

Some patients feel a sense of claustrophobia in a conventional MRI machine (Fig. 22-4). The procedure lasts from 30 to 90 minutes, and the patient must remain still. As the magnets switch on and off, a banging noise echoes through the chamber. Ear plugs and cassette players help reduce the sound. Newer open MRI technology has decreased the feeling of being closed in and has decreased the noise level caused by the scanning (Fig. 22-5).

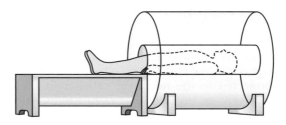

FIG. 22-4   Conventional closed magnetic resonance imaging (MRI).

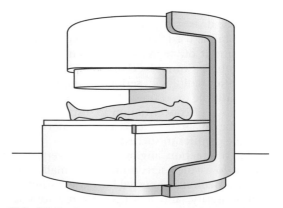
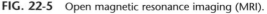

FIG. 22-5   Open magnetic resonance imaging (MRI).

MRI is used during select neurosurgical procedures since the advent of open units. Dedicated MRI interventional rooms permit the use of MRI during the actual surgical procedure. It is critical to prevent any magnetic metallic equipment or instrumentation from being used in the vicinity of the MRI. The literature reports instances of severe patient injury caused by objects such as a metal oxygen tank being pulled into the field by the powerful magnets.

NUCLEAR MEDICINE STUDIES
Radionuclides

Radioactive isotopes used in medicine are referred to as radionuclides. A nuclide is a stable nucleus of a chemical element, such as iodine, plus its orbiting electrons. A nuclide bombarded with radioactive particles becomes unstable and emits radiant energy; it becomes a radionuclide.

Radionuclides that emit electromagnetic energy are used for diagnostic studies to trace the function and structure of most organs of the body. They may be given by the oral, intracavitary, or IV route, including slow IV infusion. These agents may be used to visualize specific areas rather than radiopaque contrast media in some of the procedures previously described. They are particularly useful in studies of the bone marrow, liver, spleen, biliary tract, thyroid, brain, urinary tract, and peripheral vascular system. Because they provide better quantification of arrival times for vascular perfusion above and below lesions, radionuclides may be a more accurate index of the functional significance of a lesion than are other radiopaque contrast media.

Total-Body Scanning

Total-body scanning does not refer to CT but to a radiologic scanning procedure after IV injection of a radionuclide material. Uptake of the radionuclide within the tissues depends on blood flow. Therefore the imaging procedure may be delayed for several hours after the dose is given—not because it takes long for the material to localize in a tumor or inflammatory lesion, where the uptake is high, but because differentiation is achieved after washout from normal structures.

Scanning may include the whole body or only areas of specific interest. Total-body scanning includes identification of structures in the skeletal and vascular systems for diagnosis of a pathologic process such as metastatic bone tumors or thrombotic vascular disease. The scanner can be angled for many views of the same structure.

Scintigraphy and Lymph Node Mapping

Distribution of gamma radioactivity, such as from gallium-67 citrate, may be determined by an external scintillation detector. This is referred to as scintigraphy; the record produced is a scintigram or scintiscan. A sterile probe may be used intraoperatively to count gamma emissions from cancer cells. A radionuclide, such as iodine-125, and specific antibodies for antigen-producing tumors are injected approximately 3 weeks before the surgical procedure. The computerized display unit emits an auditory signal when the probe detects radioactivity in tissue.

Lymphoscintigraphy (Sentinel Node Sampling). Spread of cancer from the primary tumor starts with cells entering an adjacent lymph node. This node is referred to as the sentinel lymph node. Some patients have multiple sentinel nodes in some areas of the body. The degree of tumor progression is measured, and the prognostics of the disease can be predicted by evaluating the findings in the sentinel node(s). It is possible to detect spread to other nodes in the area. If the sentinel node is disease-free, it can be assumed that the cancer has not spread to other nodes in the area.

Lymphoscintigraphy uses technetium-99m sulfur colloid, which is an isotope that emits gamma rays as it spontaneously degrades. The isotope is injected around the primary tumor and taken up by the lymphatics. A high-resolution gamma camera follows the isotope's path. Images are captured on digital media until the sentinel node is visualized. An excisional biopsy is performed in the OR.

Some surgeons prefer to use isosulfan blue dye, which is selectively picked up by lymphatic vessels, to visually observe the location of the sentinel node. The dye is injected 1 hour before the excisional biopsy. Care is taken not to transect the lymphatic vessels that carry the dye—other tissue could be stained, and the location of the node in question would be obscured. The excised specimen is sent to the laboratory for fixation or frozen section. Before permanent slides are made, the specimen is stored in the nuclear medicine department for 2 or 3 days until the isotope has degraded to normal. At this point, the permanent slide is sent to the pathology department for further diagnosis.

Positron Emission Tomography

Positron emission tomography (PET) is a form of nuclear imaging that combines elements of CT scanning and nuclear scanning to create a picture representing the brain or other organ structure. The radioisotopes used emit positrons that cause pairs of gamma rays to be discharged. The rays are detected by the scanner and are relayed to a computer that converts them into cross-sectional, three-dimensional color images. PET studies provide detailed measurements of biochemistry and physiologic activity. They are used to study blood flow and metabolic functions, primarily in the brain and heart. Higher metabolic activity appears red, lesser activity appears yellow, still lesser activity appears green, and the least activity appears blue.

A PET scan can be used with fludeoxyglucose-F18 to identify and localize lymph node activity. Metastasis can be detected, and/or the patient's response to therapy can be assessed. This method is costly because the radioisotopes have a short half-life. The patient is placed on a table that slides into a tubelike opening. A similar form of scan is the single photon emission computed tomography (SPECT) scan, which is done with a rotating gamma camera and is commonly used in brain, liver, and cardiac imaging.

ULTRASONOGRAPHY

Ultrasonography uses vibrating high-frequency sound waves in the frequency of 20,000 to 10 billion cycles per second, beyond the hearing capability of human ears, to detect alterations in anatomic structures or hemodynamic properties within the body. The basic component of any diagnostic ultrasound system is its specialized transducer, which is a piezoelectric crystal. The transducer converts electrical impulses to ultrasonic waves at a frequency greater than

1 million cycles per second. These ultrasonic frequencies are transmitted into tissues through a transducer placed on the skin.

A water-soluble gel is applied to the skin to maintain airtight contact between the skin and the transducer, because ultrasonic waves do not travel well through air. A portion of the transmitted ultrasonic waves is reflected back as real-time images to a receiving crystal. The transducer, connected to a microprocessing computer, is held on the skin long enough to obtain a graphic recording of the reflected high-frequency sound waves. Uniform imaging of a wide range of body tissues is possible. Ultrasound is not effective in the presence of bone or gases in the gastrointestinal tract.

Whether used as a preoperative or intraoperative diagnostic technique, ultrasonography is a rapid, painless, noninvasive procedure that distinguishes between fluid-filled and solid masses.

Ultrasonic frequencies are reflected when the beam reaches target anatomic structures of different densities and acoustic impedance. The reflected signal is picked up by the transducer/receiver as an echo. The intensity of the returning echo is determined not only by the angle formed between the ultrasound beam and the reflecting surface of the anatomic structure but also by the acoustic properties of that surface. The resulting echo is described in terms of time and intensity and displayed on a computerized monitor for immediate interpretation of movements and dimensions of structures.

The image can be recorded on videotape or printed to provide a permanent record known as an echogram or sonogram. Sonograms can be obtained on multiple planes. Ultrasonography is a useful adjunct in the diagnosis of the following:

* *Space-occupying lesions in the neonatal brain.* The echoencephalogram will show a shift of the brain caused by tumor.
* *Lesions in the breast, thyroid, and parathyroid glands and in abdominal and pelvic organs.* Ultrasound can distinguish between a cystic and a solid tumor mass in the kidney, pancreas, liver, ovary, and testis. It is the best imaging method in patients with gallbladder disease.
* *Emboli (air, blood, or fat).* Ultrasonography is particularly useful in the early diagnosis of pulmonary embolism. Fat embolus syndrome can develop after long bone fractures.
* *Fetal maturation.* Fetal head size is an aid in the determination of fetal maturation. This can be measured by ultrasound before an elective cesarean section (C-section) or to determine the need for a C-section if the head is too large for vaginal delivery. Ultrasonography is also used to determine the position of the fetus and placenta, to identify gender, and to detect fetal abnormalities.
* *Cardiac defects.* Structural defects, insufficient valvular movement, and blood flow volumes within the heart chambers and myocardium can be detected. This diagnostic technique is known as echocardiography. The echo probe is inserted into the esophagus to obtain a transesophageal echocardiogram (TEE) or placed over the chest for a two-dimensional effect. The esophageal method is useful during open heart surgery.

Doppler Studies

Blood flow velocity and pressure measurements are possible with ultrasound, because moving blood cells produce a sufficient interface with surrounding vessels to independently reflect high-frequency sound waves. The Doppler ultrasonic velocity detector emits a beam of 5 to 10 megahertz (MHz) that is directed through the skin into the bloodstream. A portion of the transmitted ultrasound is reflected from moving particles in the blood. Known as the Doppler effect, the reflected sound wave changes in frequency because the source of the sound is in motion. This shift in frequency is proportional to the velocity of the blood flow.

Originally introduced for use in detecting obstruction in arterial blood flow, the Doppler instrument is used extensively to locate and evaluate blood flow patterns in peripheral arterial and venous diseases or defects:

* *Arterial disease.* Detection of altered hemodynamics in arterial flow is significant in diagnosis of obstructive or occlusive arterial lesions. For example, the Doppler instrument will indicate regions in the neck where carotid artery blood flow to the brain is obstructed by atherosclerosis. A surgical procedure can be performed to remove or bypass the obstruction to prevent the patient from suffering a cerebrovascular accident (stroke). It also may help the surgeon determine the appropriate level of lower extremity amputation for ischemia caused by peripheral arterial occlusive disease. It is useful in diagnosis of aortoiliac aneurysms.
* *Venous disease.* Occlusion of superficial or deep veins and the presence of incompetent valves can be located and identified by sounds made by the flow of blood through the peripheral venous system. This qualitative information of abnormal venous hemodynamics in patients with varicose veins and thrombotic disease helps the surgeon plan surgical intervention.

Intraoperative Ultrasonography

A sterile ultrasound transducer probe or scan head may be placed on tissue to evaluate vascularity or density. A pathologic condition can be diagnosed or localized. The handheld transducer must make an acoustic coupling with tissue. Tissues are moistened with sterile normal saline solution, acoustic gel, or peritoneal fluid (if the transducer is placed in the abdomen). The flexible transducer cable is attached to the ultrasound machine, which has a visible display screen.

Permanent recordings of images may be made on a videocassette incorporated into the machine. The sound waves may be either continuous or pulsed. A 7.5-MHz focused transducer generally is used. Ultrasonography is less time-consuming and requires less tissue manipulation than do other intraoperative diagnostic procedures and does not expose the patient to radiation and contrast medium.

Hemodynamics

Ultrasound imaging is used to evaluate the adequacy or restoration of blood flow during vascular reconstruction procedures, such as of peripheral vessels in the lower extremities, hepatic and portal shunts, and carotid arteries. A TEE may be obtained during coronary revascularization by placing the transducer in the esophagus. Doppler instruments are frequently used to assess blood flow through reconstructive tissue flaps and grafts and microvascular anastomoses.

Air Embolus

The Doppler instrument can be used to monitor patients during, neurosurgery, open heart surgery or during procedures on the great vessels in the chest to detect the escape of air into the circulation. Air entering an artery to the brain (cerebral air embolism) or venous system may cause brain damage or death. An air embolus of 50 mL causes severe dysrhythmias; however, 300 mL can be fatal. If an air embolus is detected at the time it occurs, therapy can be initiated immediately.

Right atrial air embolus is corrected by placing the patient's head lower than the heart (Trendelenburg's position) and introducing a multilumen right atrial catheter through a central venous line into the superior vena cava and into the right atrium.[1] The air can be manually removed by the anesthesia provider with a large syringe.[2]

Localization of Lesions

Ultrasound imaging is used for intraoperative localization of subcortical brain lesions, spinal cord lesions, pancreatic and hepatic tumors, pelvic masses, and lesions in other soft tissues to determine whether the lesion is resectable. The exact location of gallbladder and kidney stones can also be identified.

Percutaneous Puncture

The direction and depth of needle punctures to locate lesions in various abdominal organs, such as a pancreatic cyst, can be determined by following the ultrasound that is continuously visualized on the monitor. The echo from the tip of the needle is easily visible on the scope when the lesion is entered. These procedures are performed to aspirate cytologic specimens for diagnosis.

SENSORY EVOKED POTENTIAL

Sensory evoked potential (SEP), used to measure neural pathways, involves placement of multiple recording electrodes over peripheral nerves or the scalp and ears. The evoked potentials generated in response to stimulation are recorded. Components of the computerized system provide sensory stimulation; acquisition, amplification, and filtering of electrophysiologic signals; signal processing; and display, measurement, and storage of SEP waveforms. These noninvasive measurements may be taken preoperatively to assist in the diagnosis of a pathologic condition, such as acoustic neuroma. The techniques may be used also for intraoperative monitoring to assess the status of the central nervous system. Multimodality evoked potentials aid in assessment of patients with trauma. Three modalities are used:

1. *Somatosensory evoked potential.* An objective evaluation of peripheral and central neural pathways. Pairs of surface or needle skin or scalp electrodes are placed in desired patterns over the appropriate peripheral nerves

and areas of the spinal cord and cerebral cortex. These electrodes record somatosensory responses elicited on application of electrical stimuli, such as to the peroneal peripheral nerve at the knee or from over the spinal column or scalp. These impulses along neural pathways are charted to determine if the nerve is functioning properly or if a lesion is impeding impulses to the brain. Testing time can range from 45 minutes to 4 hours, depending on the number of peripheral nerves stimulated and sites necessary to assess neural pathways.

2. *Auditory brainstem evoked potential.* A test of the eighth cranial nerve and the auditory pathway to the cerebral cortex. The patient, wearing headphones or earphones, responds to auditory clicks or tones. Multiple electrodes on the scalp and ears record responses. This study is used to assess the physiologic condition of the brainstem and the patient's hearing threshold.

3. *Visual evoked potential.* A test of responses to visual pattern-reversal stimulation of the optic nerve and its associated pathways to the cerebral cortex. The patient receives stimuli via a television monitor or special eye goggles. Multiple electrodes on the scalp and ears record the evoked potentials.

PLETHYSMOGRAPHY

In plethysmography, pressure-sensitive instruments placed on an organ or around an extremity record variations in volume and pressure of blood passing through tissues. Pen-recorded tracings reflect pulse wave impulses transmitted from moving currents within arteries and veins. These impulses may be measured, computed by electronic circuits, and displayed as digitized data. Plethysmography does not identify the exact anatomic location, extent, or characteristics of vascular disease. It will quantitatively measure the rate of blood flow or degree of vascular obstruction. Four techniques are used:

1. *Oculoplethysmography.* A technique for determining hemodynamically significant carotid artery stenosis or cerebrovascular obstruction. The instrument is placed on each eyeball to record pulse waves emanating from the cerebrovascular system.

2. *Strain-gauge plethysmography.* A technique to evaluate altered venous hemodynamics in deep venous thrombosis and varicose veins. Two pneumatic cuffs are placed on the leg snugly around the thigh and calf, or ankle and great toe. A mercury strain gauge attached to the plethysmograph is secured around the leg or foot between the two cuffs. Cuffs are inflated sequentially for distal arterial occlusion and proximal venous occlusion. Changes in blood flow volume are measured as the gauge detects changes in the circumference of the calf or foot caused by sequential inflation and deflation of the pneumatic cuffs.

3. *Venous impedance plethysmography.* A technique to measure venous reflux in the lower extremity. Impedance electrodes are attached to the calf under a pneumatic boot. As the boot is inflated, blood is forced proximally out of the veins. Tissues are compressed, causing a concomitant increase in impedance and decrease in calf volume.

---

[1] www.cardioconsult.com/anatomy.
[2] www.gasnet.org. This website requires registration and is free to all users.

4. *Cutaneous pressure photoplethysmography.* A technique to identify peripheral arterial occlusive disease. An infrared light source in a handheld photoplethysmograph probe is applied to the skin with increasing pressure until the pulse is occluded. Infrared light is absorbed by blood. The intensity of the reflected light changes as the volume of blood increases as pressure is released. The probe measures the ability of the vascular system to force arterial blood into skin tissue.

ENDOSCOPY

Direct visualization within body cavities and structures aids in determination of the appropriate course of therapy for many conditions.

Diagnostic endoscopy frequently is performed in conjunction with radiologic studies or to obtain specimens for pathologic examination. A tissue staining dye and/or radiopaque contrast material may be injected through the endoscope or an accessory before radiologic studies. Fluid and secretions may be withdrawn for culture or chemical analysis. Biopsy specimens are frequently obtained.

Direct visualization alone may confirm the presence or absence of a suspected lesion or abnormal condition. This may be enhanced by an ultrasonic transducer at the end of a flexible fiberoptic scope. Endoscopic diagnosis often provides the information necessary to proceed with an open procedure or to cancel an anticipated surgical procedure. Small video capsules can be swallowed to allow visualization of the small intestine.

Endoscopy is described in detail in Chapter 32, and specific endoscopic procedures are discussed in subsequent chapters when they are pertinent to diagnostic and surgical procedures in the appropriate surgical specialties.

DIAGNOSING AND TREATING THE PATIENT WITH CANCER

Oncology is the study of scientific control over neoplastic growth. It concerns the etiology, diagnosis, treatment, and rehabilitation of patients with known or potential neoplasms. A neoplasm is an atypical growth of abnormal cells or tissues that may be a benign or malignant tumor.

Cancer is a broad term that encompasses any malignant tissue change. The exact cause of cancer is unknown. Cancerous tumors can be caused by exposure to chemical toxins, ionizing radiation, chronic tissue irritation, tobacco smoke, ultraviolet rays, viral invasion, and genetic predisposition. Studies have shown that immunosuppression may contribute to the incidence of cancer by altering biochemical metabolism and cellular enzyme production. Other research has shown that dietary influences, such as nitrates, salt-cured or smoked foods, and high-fat diets, may contribute to cancer in certain individuals.

Both malignant and benign neoplasms consist of cells that divide and grow uncontrollably at varied rates. The stimulus for growth can be intrinsic (e.g., hormonal) or extrinsic (e.g., exposure to external elements). Neoplastic overgrowth or the invasion of surrounding tissue causes dysfunction and may eventually cause the death of the patient.

TABLE 22-2	Comparison of Benign and Malignant Tumors
Benign	**Malignant**
CHARACTERISTICS	
Expansive	Invasive
Localized	Spreads to distant sites
Encapsulated	No capsule
Slow growth	Rapid growth
Resembles parent tissue	Varied differentiation
Normal cell reproduction	Disorganized cell reproduction
Organized mitoses	Abnormal mitoses
EFFECT ON PATIENT	
Pain uncommon	Severe pain common
Little nutritional effect unless mechanical obstruction is involved	Cachexia, nausea, and vomiting

Table 22-2 compares the characteristics and effects of benign and malignant tumors. Four characteristics distinguish malignant from benign tumors, with a malignant tumor having the following characteristics:

- It is anaplastic. Cancer cells resemble normal cell forms but are morphologically and functionally differentiated from the normal tissue of origin. They vary in size, shape, and texture.
- It infiltrates and destroys adjacent normal tissue.
- It grows in a disorganized, uncontrolled, and irregular manner, usually increasing in size both rapidly and perceptibly within weeks or months.
- It has the power to metastasize. Cancer cells migrate from the primary focus to another single focus or to multiple foci in distant tissues or organs via lymphatic or vascular channels.

Clinical Signs and Symptoms of Cancer

According to the American Cancer Society, the following are the clinical signs and symptoms of cancer:
- Palpable mass or abnormal thickening of tissue
- Abnormal bleeding or discharge
- Obvious change in a wart or mole
- Lesion that does not heal
- Steady decrease in weight, appetite, and energy
- Chronic cough
- Change in bowel or bladder habits

Potential Causes of Cancer

The early detection of cancer decreases the incidence of morbidity and mortality. A screening examination may identify a neoplasm before clinical symptoms develop. Recommended cancer screening examinations are listed in Table 22-3. (More screening information can be found on the American Public Health Website at www.apha.org.)

Risk-Related Factors

Risk factors for cancer include the following:
- Age, gender, or racial, genetic, or hereditary predisposition. Table 22-4 identifies neoplasms associated with familial cancer syndromes.

TABLE 22-3	Cancer Screening Examinations	
Sex	**Age**	**Frequency of Examination**
PELVIC EXAMINATION BY PALPATION AND INSPECTION		
Female	18-40 years More than age 40	Every 1-3 years Every year
PELVIC EXAMINATION BY PALPATION AND INSPECTION, INCLUDING PAP SMEAR AND HPV TESTING		
Female	Start at age 18 or at age of onset of sexual activity if younger	Yearly; may be performed less frequently on advice of physician if patient has had three negative Pap smears in 3 consecutive years
ENDOMETRIAL TISSUE SAMPLE		
Female	At menopause or sooner at recommendation of physician	Sample for baseline in high-risk patient
BREAST SELF-EXAMINATION		
Female and male	Start at age 18 and throughout life span	Female: monthly after menses or at same time each month after menopause Male: monthly
CLINICAL BREAST EXAMINATION		
Female	Start at age 18 and throughout life span	Corresponds with pelvic examination sequence unless patient has a previous history of breast disease or is at high risk for breast disease
MAMMOGRAPHY		
Female	Baseline at age 35, yearly after age 40	Frequency after baseline is individualized according to age, health, and risk factor analysis by physician; mammography, when performed, should precede clinical breast examination so that data analysis will be complete
TESTICULAR SELF-EXAMINATION BY PALPATION AND INSPECTION		
Male	Start at age 16 and throughout life span	Monthly
PROSTATE		
Male	More than age 50; start at age 40 for men at high risk	Yearly, prostate-specific antigen (PSA) blood test
DIGITAL RECTAL EXAMINATION		
Male and female	More than age 40	Yearly; frequency may vary according to individual risk factors or the recommendation of physician
STOOL GUAIAC EXAMINATION		
Male and female	More than age 50	Yearly; age and frequency may vary according to symptoms and the recommendation of physician
SIGMOIDOSCOPY OR COLONOSCOPY		
Male and female	More than age 50	Every 3-5 years or according to the advice of physician; age and frequency may vary in the presence of risk factors or individual symptoms; colonoscopy may be advised according to risk factors
GENERALIZED PHYSICAL WITH HEALTH COUNSELING Includes palpation of thyroid, gonads, and lymphatics, as well as inspection of oral mucosa		
Male and female	More than age 20	Every 3 years
Male and female	More than age 40	Every year

- Exposure to carcinogens (cancer-producing agents) such as tobacco smoke, coal tar, ionizing radiation, ultraviolet rays, and chemicals. Table 22-5 lists examples of chemical carcinogens.
- Predisposition from specific environmental conditions or acquired conditions or diseases. Table 22-6 gives examples of viral-mediated carcinogens.

Extent of Disease

Carcinoma In Situ. In carcinoma in situ, normal cells are replaced by anaplastic cells but the growth disturbance of epithelial surfaces shows no behavioral evidence of invasion and metastasis. This cellular change is noted most often in stratified squamous and glandular epithelium. Carcinoma in situ is also referred to as intraepithelial or preinvasive

TABLE 22-4	Familial Cancer Syndromes
Syndrome	**Associated Neoplasm**
AUTOSOMAL DOMINANT GENE	
Familial polyposis coli	Adenocarcinoma of colon, adenomatous polyps
Gardner syndrome	Adenocarcinoma of colon, musculoaponeurotic tumors
Peutz-Jeghers syndrome	Adenocarcinoma of small intestine, colon, ovary
Neurofibromatosis	Neurofibroma, neurogenic sarcoma, pheochromocytoma
Multiple endocrine neoplasia (MEN type I), or Wermer syndrome	Pituitary, pancreatic islet cells, parathyroid glands
Multiple endocrine neoplasia (MEN type IIA), or Sipple syndrome	Thyroid, parathyroid glands, pheochromocytoma
Multiple endocrine neoplasia (MEN type IIB)	Thyroid, parathyroid, pheochromocytoma, mucosa ganglioneuromas
AUTOSOMAL RECESSIVE GENE	
Xeroderma pigmentosum	Basal and squamous cell carcinoma of skin, malignant melanoma
Ataxia-telangiectasia	Acute leukemia, lymphoma, some gastric cancers

TABLE 22-5	Examples of Chemical Carcinogenesis
Chemical	**Site of Neoplasm**
ALKYLATING AGENTS	
Nitrogen mustard, cyclophosphamide, chlorambucil	Leukemia, urinary bladder
Vinyl chloride	Angiosarcoma of liver
POLYCYCLIC HYDROCARBONS	
Tar, soot, oils	Skin, lung
AROMATIC AMINES AND AZO DYES	
α-Naphthylamine, benzidine	Urinary bladder
FOOD PRODUCTS	
Saccharin	Urinary bladder
Aflatoxin (mold on peanuts)	Liver
Betel nuts	Oral mucosa
MEDICATION	
Androgenic metabolic steroids	Liver
Diethylstilbestrol	Vagina
Phenacetin	Renal pelvis
INORGANIC COMPOUNDS	
Chromium	Lung
Nickel	Lung, nasal sinuses
Asbestos	Serosal membranes, lung
Arsenic	Skin

TABLE 22-6	Viral-Mediated Carcinogenesis
Viral Family	**Type of Neoplasm**
DNA-ASSOCIATED	
Papilloma (condyloma)	Squamous papilloma and squamous cell carcinoma
Hepatitis B	Hepatocellular carcinoma
HERPESVIRUS	
Epstein-Barr	Burkitt's lymphoma, nasopharyngeal carcinoma
Cytomegalovirus	Kaposi sarcoma
Herpes simplex type II	Uterine cervical carcinoma
RNA-DEPENDENT	
Human T cell lymphotrophic type I (retrovirus C)	T cell leukemia, lymphoma

DNA, Deoxyribonucleic acid; *RNA,* ribonucleic acid.

cancer. Common sites for in situ carcinoma include the following:

- Uterine cervix
- Uterine endometrium
- Vagina
- Anus
- Penis
- Lip
- Buccal mucosa
- Bronchi
- Esophagus
- Eye
- Breast

Localized Cancer. Localized cancer is contained within the organ of its origin.

Regional Cancer. In regional cancer, the invaded area extends from the periphery of the organ or tissue of origin to include tumor cells in adjacent organs or tissues (e.g., the regional lymph nodes).

Metastatic Cancer. In metastatic cancer, the tumor extends by way of lymphatic or vascular channels to tissues or organs beyond the regional area.

Disseminated Cancer. In disseminated cancer, multiple foci of tumor cells are dispersed throughout the body.

Tumor Identification System

A standardized tumor identification system, which includes classification and staging, is essential for establishing treatment protocols and evaluating the end result of therapy. Hospitals maintain a tumor registry of patients to evaluate therapeutic approaches to specific types of tumors. Classification includes the anatomic and histologic description of a tumor, whereas staging refers to the extent of the tumor. There are three basic categories of the tumor identification system:

- Primary Tumor
- Regional Nodes
- Distant Metastases

The TNM categories are identified by pretreatment clinical diagnosis, tissue biopsy, and/or histopathologic examination after surgical resection of the tumor. Numeric subscripts are used to describe the findings; for example, bronchogenic carcinoma $T_1 N_0 M_0$ means a primary tumor in the lung without positive regional nodes or distant metastases. If a positive lymph node is identified in the area, it is indicated in a subscript (e.g., $T_1 N_1 M_0$). If a metastatic site also is diagnosed, it too is indicated in the subscript (e.g., $T_1 N_1 M_1$). The subscripts correspond to the number of separate tumors at the identified primary site, positive lymph nodes, or metastatic sites (Box 22-3). Other staging systems are referred to in the literature as stages I, II, III, and IV. After treatment, the estimation of residual tumor volume is indicated by the letter R.

Monitoring Tumor Markers

Tumor markers are serum studies used to measure specific enzymes emitted by tumor cells. Elevated tumor markers in the patient's blood and tissues can help determine the patient's treatment and prognosis. Table 22-7 describes common blood tests for serum tumor markers and their implication in cancer prognostication.

CANCER TREATMENT

Cancer is a systemic disease and is treated based on location and cell type. Therapy is curative if the disease process can be totally eradicated, but the success of therapy depends largely on early diagnosis. Tumors are classified to determine the most effective therapy. When a cure is not possible, palliative therapy relieves symptoms and improves quality of life but does not cure the disease.

TABLE 22-7	Common Serum Tumor Markers	
Test	**Value**	**Indication**
Carcinoembryonic antigen (CEA)	0-2.5 ng/mL	Colorectal
Alpha-fetoprotein (AFP)	10 ng/mL	Testicular Liver
Human chorionic gonadotropin (HCG)	0-1 ng/mL	Choriocarcinoma Testicular
Prostate-specific antigen (PSA)	0-4 mcg/L (>40 yr)	Prostate

Before beginning therapy, a patient with cancer undergoes an extensive pretreatment workup. Each form of cancer therapy has certain advantages and limitations. Several factors affect a patient's response to treatment: host factors, clinical stage of malignancy, and type of therapy. The patient is followed carefully to determine the effectiveness of treatment at routine intervals.

Adjuvant Therapy

Surgical resection, endocrine therapy, radiation therapy, chemotherapy, immunotherapy, hyperthermia, or combinations of these procedures are used in the treatment of cancer. The surgeon or oncologist determines the most appropriate therapy for each patient. When determining the most appropriate therapy, the following are considered:

- Type, site, and extent of tumor and whether lymph nodes are involved
- Type of surrounding normal tissue
- Age and general condition of the patient, including nutritional status and whether other diseases are present
- Whether curative or palliative therapy is possible

Surgical Resection and Palliation

Surgical resection is the modality of choice to remove solid tumors. The resection of a malignant tumor is, however, localized therapy for what may be a systemic disease. Each patient is evaluated and treated individually, and the surgical procedure is planned appropriately for the identified stage of disease. Depending on localization, regionalization, and dissemination of the tumor, the surgeon selects either a radical curative surgical procedure or a salvage palliative surgical procedure.

Surgical debulking, in which the tumor is partially removed, may be the procedure of choice for some types of surgically incurable malignant neoplasms. With surgical debulking, the intent is not to cure but to make subsequent therapy with irradiation, drugs, or other palliative measures more effective and thereby extend survival. In planning the surgical procedure, the surgeon considers the length of expected survival, the prognosis of surgical intervention, and the effect of concurrent diseases on the postoperative result.

Accessible primary tumors are often treated by excision. An extremely wide resection may be necessary to avoid recurrence of the tumor. The pathologist is able to make judgments about questionable margins by evaluating frozen

---

BOX 22-3	Tumor Identification Scale

PRIMARY TUMOR

TX	Primary tumor discovered by the detection of malignant cells in secretions or cell washings but not directly visualized
T_0	No evidence of primary tumor
Tis	Tumor (carcinoma) in situ
T_1	Tumor is 2 cm or less at largest dimension
T_2	Tumor is larger than 2 cm at largest dimension
T_3	Tumor directly invades surrounding tissue
T_4	Tumor invades surrounding tissue and adjacent structures, such as blood vessels or bone

REGIONAL LYMPH NODES

NX	Unable to assess nodes
N_0	No regional lymph node metastasis
N_1	Metastasis to ipsilateral nodes or direct extension to nodes
N_2	Metastasis to contralateral nodes

DISTANT METASTASIS

MX	Distant metastasis cannot be assessed
M_0	No distant metastasis
M_1	Distant metastasis confirmed

POSTTREATMENT RESIDUAL TUMOR

RX	Unable to assess residual tumor
R_0	No residual tumor
R_1	Microscopic residual tumor
R_2	Macroscopic residual tumor

sections while the surgical procedure is in progress. The pathologist's findings guide the surgeon during resection so that residual tumor is not left in the patient. The specimen is also tested after permanent section fixation in the pathology laboratory. Final results are available in 2 to 3 days.

Many surgical procedures are performed for ablation of tumors by primary resection. In addition, a lymphadenectomy (removal of local lymph nodes) may be performed as a prophylactic measure to inhibit the metastatic spread of tumor cells via lymphatic channels. These nodes are tested to determine the extent of tumor cell spread. Other modalities of therapy may be administered preoperatively, intraoperatively, and/or postoperatively to reduce or prevent a recurrence or metastasis.

Preservation of Reproductive System

Females and males of reproductive age with cancer who are facing radiation therapy are at risk for becoming sterile as a result of treatment. Gonadal shields are used whenever possible. Males can donate sperm for cryopreservation and later use it for in vitro fertilization or artificial insemination. In some circumstances females can have a laparoscopic procedure to relocate their ovaries to a deeper or medial location in the pelvis where they will experience little or no exposure to radiation. Other palliative surgical interventions are described in Box 22-4.

Endocrine Therapy

Tumors arising in organs that are usually under hormonal influence (e.g., breast, ovary, and uterus in female patients; prostate and testes in male patients) may be stimulated by hormones produced in the endocrine glands. Cellular metabolism is affected by the presence of specific hormone receptors in tumor cells: estrogen and/or progesterone in a female, and androgens in a male.

Certain breast, endometrial, and prostatic cancers depend on sex hormones for growth and maintenance. Therefore the recurrence or spread of disease may be slowed by therapeutic hormonal manipulation. Endocrine manipulation does not cure, but it can control dissemination of the disease if the tumor progresses beyond the limits of effective surgical resection or radiation therapy.

BOX 22-4   Palliative Oncologic Surgical Procedures

- Reduction of tumor to prevent obstruction (debulking)
- Reduction of tumor cells to aid effectiveness of chemotherapy
- Treatment of oncologic emergencies such as hemorrhage or compression
- Removal of enlarged organs such as the spleen
- Repair of perforations in irradiated parts such as the rectum
- Removal of a hormone-producing part such as a gonad or other gland
- Removal of a diseased organ such as the uterus, prostate, or breast
- Insertion of a nutritional support device such as a feeding gastrostomy or total parenteral alimentation line
- Pain control such as nerve blocks or the severing of a neural pathway or receptor site

---

Hormonal Receptor Site Studies. Identifying the hormonal dependence of the primary tumor through studies of the receptor site is a fairly reliable way of selecting patients who will benefit from preoperative or postoperative endocrine manipulation. After a positive diagnosis of cancer, either by a frozen section biopsy or by pathologic permanent sections, the surgeon will probably request a receptor site evaluation of a primary breast, uterine, or prostatic tumor.

The tissue specimen removed by surgical resection should be sent fresh or in saline. It should not be placed in formalin preservative solution because doing so will alter the receptor cells enough to negate the hormonal study.

Endocrine Ablation. Since 1896, surgeons have described positive clinical responses in patients with metastatic breast cancer after treatment by endocrine ablation—the surgical removal of endocrine glands. If the surgeon plans to eliminate endocrine stimulation surgically in a patient with a known hormone-dependent tumor, all sources of the hormone should be ablated chemically, hormonally, or surgically.

- *Bilateral adrenalectomy and oophorectomy.* Both adrenal glands and/or ovaries may be resected to prevent the recurrence of endocrine-derived cancer. These may be removed as a one-stage surgical procedure (i.e., bilateral adrenalectomy/oophorectomy). If two separate surgical procedures are preferred, the bilateral oophorectomy precedes the bilateral adrenalectomy, except in menopausal women in whom only the latter surgical procedure may be indicated.
- *Bilateral adrenalectomy and orchiectomy.* After prostatectomy for advanced carcinoma of the prostate, both testes may be removed (i.e., bilateral orchiectomy) to eliminate androgens of testicular origin. Bilateral adrenalectomy also may be indicated.

Hormonal Therapy. Hormones administered orally or via injection can alter cell metabolism by changing the systemic hormonal environment of the body. For hormones to be effective, tumor cells must contain receptors. Hormones must bind to these receptors before they can exert an effect on cells.

- *Antiestrogen therapy.* Patients with medical contraindications to endocrine ablation may receive antiestrogen therapy. An estrogen antagonist deprives an estrogen-dependent tumor of the estrogen necessary for its growth. Nafoxidine and tamoxifen (Nolvadex) are synthetic nonsteroidal drugs that inhibit the normal intake of estrogen at estrogen receptor sites; they are taken orally.
- *Corticosteroids.* Prednisone, cortisone, hydrocortisone, or some other preparation of corticosteroids may be administered as an antiinflammatory agent along with the chemotherapeutic agents given to control disseminated disease.

Photodynamic (Laser) Therapy

For photodynamic therapy (also referred to as photoradiation), an argon tunable dye laser is used to destroy malignant cells by photochemical reaction. A photosensitive drug, either hematoporphyrin derivative (HPD) from bovine blood (Photofrin) or purified dihematoporphyrin ether, is absorbed by malignant and reticular endothelial cells.

The photosensitive drug is injected intravenously via venipuncture or Hickman catheter 24 to 48 hours before the photodynamic therapy and is taken up by cells to make them fluorescent and photosensitive. It remains longer in malignant cells than in normal cells before being excreted from the body. When exposed to light from an argon laser, the tunable rhodamine B dye laser produces a red beam of approximately 630 nm. Other dyes, such as dicyanomethylene, may produce different wavelengths. HPD in cells absorbs the laser light, which leads to a photochemical reaction that causes tissue-oxygen molecules to release cytotoxic singlet oxygen and destroy tumor cells. Depending on tumor site, the laser can be delivered interstitially, endoscopically, externally, or retrobulbarly.

Photodynamic therapy may be used to debulk tumors of the eye, head and neck, breast, esophagus, gastrointestinal tract, bronchus, and bladder. The tunable dye laser also may be used to diagnose tumor cells. The OR should be darkened or have shades to block outside daylight during the laser treatment. The patient is cautioned to avoid exposure to sunlight or other sources of ultraviolet light both after injection of the dye and postoperatively. Photosensitivity is the primary side effect of the dye and may last 4 to 6 weeks.

Radiation Therapy

Radiation is the emission of electromagnetic waves or atomic particles that result from the disintegration of nuclei of unstable or radioactive elements. The treatment of malignant disease with radiation may be referred to as radiation therapy, brachytherapy, or radiotherapy. Ionizing radiation is used for this type of therapy, which involves the use of high-voltage radiation and other radioactive elements to injure or destroy cells. Like surgical resection and photodynamic therapy, radiation therapy is localized therapy that is applicable for a limited number of specific tumors.

Ionizing Radiation. Ionization is the physical production of positive and negative ions capable of conducting electricity. Ionizing radiation is radiation with sufficient energy to disrupt the electronic balance of an atom. When disruption occurs in tissue cells or extracellular fluids, the effect can range from minor changes to profound disturbances. Radiation may come either from particles of the nuclei of disintegrating atoms or from electromagnetic waves that have no mass. Types of ionizing radiation include:

- *Alpha particles.* Alpha particles are relatively large particles that have a very slight penetrating power. They are stopped by a thin sheet of paper. They have dense ionization but can produce tremendous tissue destruction within a short distance.
- *Beta particles.* Beta particles are relatively small, are electrical, and travel with the speed of light. They have greater penetrating properties than do alpha particles. Their emissions cause tissue necrosis, and they produce ionization, which has destructive properties.
- *Gamma rays and x-rays.* Gamma rays and x-rays are electromagnetic radiations of short wavelength but high energy, and they are capable of completely penetrating the body. They affect tumor tissue more rapidly than normal tissue. These types of rays are stopped by a thick lead shield. Protons ranging in energy from 30 kilovolts

(kV) to 35 million electron volts (eV) are available for the treatment of various cancers. Gamma rays are emitted spontaneously from the nucleus of an atom of a radioactive element.

Implantation of Radiation Sources

All radiation sources for implantation are prepared in the desired therapeutic dosages by personnel in the nuclear medicine department. Many types of sources are used to deliver maximum radiation to the primary tumor. No single type is ideal for every tumor or anatomic site.

Interstitial Needles. Interstitial needles are hollow sheaths and are usually made of platinum or Monel metal. Radium salts or radionuclides are encased in platinum or platinum-iridium short units or cells, which in turn are sealed in the metal sheath of the needle for implantation into tumor tissue. A needle may contain one or several short units or cells of the radiation source, depending on the length of needle to be used. Needles vary in length from 10 to 60 mm, with a diameter of 1 to 2 mm. The choice of length depends on dosage and on the area involved. Dosage is measured in milligram-hours, which can be converted to rads.

The interstitial needles, which usually contain cesium-137, are implanted in tumors near the body surface or in tissue accessible enough to permit their use (e.g., vagina, cervix, tongue, mouth, neck). In certain patients, stereotactic techniques are used to implant needles for the irradiation of brain tumors.

In the OR, these needles are inserted at the periphery of and within the tumor. One end of the needle is pointed, and the other end has an eye for a heavy (size 2) suture. Needles are threaded to prevent loss while in use and to aid in removal. After the surgeon inserts the needles, the ends of the sutures are tied or taped together and are taped to the skin in an adjoining area or secured to buttons.

Depending on the anatomic site, a template may be used to position and secure the needles. A template consists of two acrylic plates that are separated by rubber O-rings and held together with screws. The plates have holes for insertion of the interstitial needles. The template remains in place until the needles are removed. Depending on the planned dosage to the tumor bed, needles are usually left in place for 4 to 7 days.

Interstitial Seeds. Sealed radionuclide seeds may be implanted permanently or temporarily. Because they have a short half-life, gold seeds are permanently implanted, most commonly into the prostate, lungs, or pancreas. Seeds containing cesium-137, iridium-192, or iodine-125 implanted directly into tumor tissue are removed after the desired exposure.

Seeds are useful in body cavities, in localized areas, and in tumors that are not resectable because of their location near major vessels or the spinal cord. Because they are small, the seeds can be placed to fit a curved area without requiring immobilization. However, they may move about if there is much motion.

Radionuclide seeds are 7 mm or less in length, are 0.75 mm in diameter, and have a wall 0.3 mm thick. The length of the seed depends on the desired dosage. Seeds can be inserted with or without an invasive surgical procedure. They may be strung on a strand of suture material or placed in a hollow plastic tube with sealed ends. With a needle attached, the strand or tube is woven or pulled through the tumor. Seeds in a plastic tube may be inserted through a hollow needle, such as a catheter through a trocar. Empty tubes may be inserted in the OR and afterloaded (i.e., the seeds are put into the tube at a later time and place). A microprocessor-controlled machine that pulls wire attached to radioactive material through the tube may be used for remote afterloading.

Brachytherapy. The term *brachytherapy* comes from a Greek term meaning "short-range treatment." Tiny titanium cylinders that contain a radioactive isotope are implanted to deliver a dose of radiation from the inside out that kills cancer cells while sparing healthy tissue. Brachytherapy is performed for many types of cancers including breast and prostate (see Fig. 7.5).

Brachytherapy is useful for delivering higher cell-killing doses in shorter periods than conventional radiation treatments. The capsules are placed under ultrasound guidance. A rapid delivery system that uses a catheter with a balloon on the tip has been developed to treat breast cancer smaller than 3 cm. The catheter is placed into the breast tissue during tumor excision, and the balloon is expanded with water. Twice per day for 4 to 5 days a high-dose radiation pellet is placed inside the catheter to treat the tissue. When the treatment period is complete, the catheter and pellet are removed. Patient selection includes those with clear margins of the tumor and with less than three affected lymph nodes.

Intracavitary Capsules. A sealed capsule of radium, cesium-137, iodine-125, yttrium-192, or cobalt-60 may be placed into a body cavity or orifice. The capsule may be a single tube of radioactive pins fixed in a tandem loader or a group of individual capsules, each of which contains one radioactive pin. Commonly used to treat tumors in the cervix or endometrium of the uterus, a capsule is inserted via the vagina for treatment of the uterine body.

In a patient with cervical cancer, an instrument such as an Ernst applicator is used. A metal or plastic tube with radioactive pins is inserted in the uterus. Metal pins are used in conjunction with heat. The tube is attached to two vaginal ovoids, each of which contains a radioactive pin, that are placed in the cul-de-sac around the cervix. This type of application delivers the desired dosage in a pear-shaped volume of tissue, which includes the cervix, corpus, and tissue around the cervix but spares the bladder and rectum from high doses of radiation.

A blunt intracavitary applicator is used to position the parts. The applicator is held securely and remains fixed to ensure proper dosage to the tumor without injuring the normal surrounding structures. For stabilization, the surgeon may suture the applicator to the cervix, and vaginal packing also is used. Two different methods of application are used for inserting the radiation source: afterloading techniques and preloading techniques.

Afterloading Techniques. Afterloading techniques afford the greatest safety for OR personnel. In the OR, a cold, unloaded, hollow plastic or metal applicator, such as the Fletcher afterloader, is inserted into or adjacent to the tissues that will receive radiation. After x-ray verification of correct placement, the radiation source is loaded into the applicator at the patient's bedside.

Preloading Techniques. Preloading techniques require insertion of the "hot" radiation capsule in the OR by the surgeon. OR personnel should not be permitted in the OR during this procedure. To deliver a uniform dose to the desired area, the surgeon inserts an adjustable device designed to hold the radiation source in proper position in the tissues (e.g., the Ernst applicator). The bladder and rectum are held away from the area with packs to avoid undesired irradiation. To calculate the necessary dosage, the surgeon uses x-ray films of the pelvis to check the position of the radiation source and to measure its distance from critical sites.

All preparations for insertion are made by nursing team members before they leave the room. (They wait in the substerile room during insertion.) Preparations include setting the sterile table with vaginal packing, antibiotic cream for packing, radiopaque solutions for x-ray studies, and a basin of sterile water; placing the x-ray cassette on the operating bed and notifying the radiology technician; obtaining the radiation source; positioning the patient; and putting a radiation sheet on the patient's chart and a card on the stretcher.

Intracavitary Colloidal Suspensions. Sterile radioactive colloidal suspensions of gold or phosphorus are used as palliative therapy to limit the growth of metastatic tumors in the pleural or peritoneal cavities. Radioactive colloidal gold-198 is most commonly used; it has a half-life of 2.7 days. It also may be instilled within the bladder. The effect of these suspensions is caused by the emission of beta particles that penetrate tissue so slightly that radioactivity is limited to the immediate area in which the colloidal suspension is placed. A trocar and cannula are introduced into the pleural or peritoneal cavity, and the colloidal suspension is injected through the cannula from a lead-shielded syringe. After use, these instruments are stored in a remote area until the decay of radioactivity is complete.

Intraoperative Radiation Therapy. During a surgical procedure, a single high dose of radiation may be delivered directly to an intraabdominal or intrapelvic tumor or tumor bed to provide an additional palliative or localized means of control. Normal organs or tissues can be shielded from exposure. Radiation may also be used after resection of the bulk of the tumor.

An orthovoltage unit may be installed in a lead-lined OR for performing intraoperative radiation therapy. The sterile Lucite cone is placed directly over the tumor site. All team members leave the room during treatment. In some hospitals the patient is transported from the OR to the radiation therapy department. After exposure to a megavoltage electron beam, the wound may be closed in the treatment area or the patient may be returned to the OR for further surgery and/or wound closure. The open wound is covered with a sterile drape during transport, and sterile technique is used for closure.

Stereotactic Radiosurgery. Gamma Knife technology was developed in Sweden in the early 1950s by surgeon Lars Leksell and Borje Larsson, PhD. They experimented with guiding devices and proton beams. Cobalt-60 was found to be most effective in the treatment of brain tumors and was selected as the energy source for the Gamma Knife. In 1975 the device was used to treat brain tumors in humans.

With stereotactic radiosurgery, fiberglass fixation pins are used to apply a base ring (the Leksell head frame) to the patient's head preoperatively. Two small rods are placed in the ear canals to stabilize the head frame during fixation. Care is taken not to injure the ear canal or tympanic membrane during this process. A calibrated ring is affixed to the frame to form X, Y, and Z coordinates to localize the brain lesion. The frame and ring sit within a larger helmet that aims the radiation at the tumor.

The Gamma Knife delivers highly concentrated doses of gamma rays to inoperable or deep-seated vascular malformations or brain tumors 1 to 10 cm^3 in size. The localized area is determined by precision stereotaxis. The neurosurgeon places the patient's head, with the Leksell head frame and localizing ring, into the collimator helmet so that the focusing channels direct 201 pinpointed cobalt-60 beams to the tumor. (The radiation sources are housed in a large spherical chamber that is housed within a special room.) The patient is placed on a sliding bed that accommodates and aligns with the helmet as it enters the spherical chamber. The Gamma Knife process lasts 3 to 4 hours. During the procedure, the patient is in video and voice communication with the perioperative team. All personnel leave the room during treatment because of the intensity of the radiation and its cumulative effects.

Effects of Radiation Therapy on the Perioperative Patient

The patient may be undergoing several treatment modalities and may experience the specific tissue and systemic effects of each. The perioperative nurse should understand how radiation affects the patient and how it affects the attainment of desired outcomes. The plan of care should include consideration for the potential side effects of radiation therapy. Box 22-5 describes the patient's responses to the physiologic effects of radiation.

Chemotherapy

Either alone or in combination, a variety of chemotherapeutic agents is capable of providing measurable palliative remission or regression of primary and metastatic disease, with a decrease in the size of the tumor and no new metastases. In some instances a complete response, with the disappearance of all clinical evidence of the tumor, is achieved.

The trend is toward earlier and greater use of adjuvant chemotherapy. More than one agent may be administered to enhance the action of another cytotoxic or antigenic substance. Adjuvant therapy is designed to maximize the benefits of each agent in the combination while avoiding overlapping toxicities. The following factors are important in determining the ability of tumor cells to respond to chemotherapy:

- *Size and location of the tumor.* The smaller the tumor, the easier it will be to reach cells. The mechanism for the passage of drugs into the brain differs from that for other body organs.
- *Type of tumor.* For example, cells of solid tumors in the lung, stomach, colon, and breast may be more resistant than cells in the lymphatic system.
- *Combinations of adjuvant therapy.* In select patients, chemotherapy may be used as an adjunct to all other types of therapy. Precise scheduling of dosages is necessary to attain effective results.
- *Specific biochemical requirements of the tumor.* Agents are selected according to the appropriateness of their structure and function. More than one agent is usually given.
- *State of life cycle of the cancer cells.* Cancer cells and normal cells go through the same life-cycle phases. An understanding of this phenomenon is necessary for understanding chemotherapy.

Indications for Chemotherapy

Patients who are at risk for or who have systemic signs of advanced or disseminated disease (generally indicated by extranodal involvement) may be candidates for preoperative or postoperative chemotherapy.

Preoperative Chemotherapy. The objective of preoperative chemotherapy may be to shrink the tumor sufficiently to permit surgical resection. Adjuvant radiation therapy may be used in combination with chemotherapy to increase tumor regression and necrosis. Agents may also eliminate subclinical microscopic metastatic disease.

BOX 22-5   Physiologic Effects of Radiation Therapy

EXTERNAL BEAM
Gastroenteritis
Nausea and vomiting
Diarrhea
Menstrual irregularities
Miscarriage
Sexual dysfunction
Fatigue
Cystitis
Erythema
Skin desquamation
Decreased circulation

INTERNAL IMPLANTS
Bleeding tendency
Increased infections
Sexual dysfunction

INTRACAVITARY IMPLANTS
Bleeding
Infection
Sexual dysfunction

INTRAOPERATIVE RADIATION
Anorexia
Nausea and vomiting

Postoperative Chemotherapy. Surgical resection followed by regional chemotherapy often can control local disease to keep a tumor in remission. Residual metastatic disease may be treated with systemic chemotherapy to cure the patient or to prolong life. Multiple doses may be given over a long period (several months to a year or more) to delay or eliminate recurrence of the tumor.

Delivery Devices for Chemotherapeutic Agents

The method of chemotherapy administration depends on the extent of dissemination or localization of the tumor cells and on the agent or combination of agents selected. Agents can be instilled locally into a target site by continuous infusion, injected intramuscularly or intrathecally, infused by intravenous push or drip, or ingested orally.

A patient with widely disseminated metastatic disease usually receives systemic chemotherapy via the intravenous, intramuscular, or oral route. Agents may be infused regionally for patients whose tumor cannot be removed because of its location (e.g., a primary or metastatic tumor in the liver). The patient may come to the OR for insertion of an indwelling catheter or implantable infusion pump of the brain.

Infusion Catheters. An indwelling infusion catheter may be placed percutaneously or directly into a vein, artery, or body cavity. Continuous or intermittent infusion of the chemotherapeutic agent can be maintained by means of a portable infusion pump attached to the catheter, or the catheter may be used on an intermittent basis.

Central Venous Catheter. Under local anesthesia, a long-term Hickman, Quinton, Groshong, or other central venous catheter is inserted percutaneously through a particular blood vessel and into the right atrium of the heart. The catheter also may be used for hyperalimentation. Varieties include single-, double-, and triple-lumen styles and require heparinized saline flushes between uses (Fig. 22-6). Groshong catheters have a self-closing distal tip, do not require heparinization, and are available in single-, double-, and triple-lumen styles. Therefore the Groshong catheter

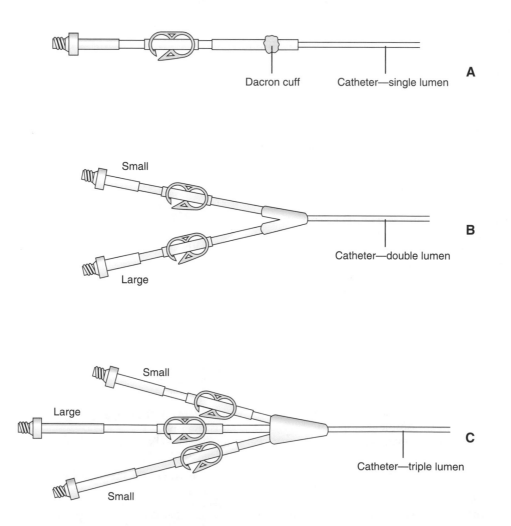

FIG. 22-6 Intravenous catheters for long-term intravascular access. **A,** Hickman and Broviac single-lumen catheter for intravenous (IV) fluids or total parenteral nutrition (TPN). **B,** Hickman and Leonard multipurpose dual-lumen catheter for IV fluids or blood sampling. **C,** Hickman triple-lumen catheter for IV fluids, TPN, and blood administration.

can be used for patients with bleeding tendencies without the same risk associated with added heparinization. Sterile normal saline for injection is used to flush the line between uses.

Short-term subclavian catheters in double- and triple-lumen styles can be used for the administration of chemotherapeutic agents and total parenteral nutrition (TPN). These types of catheters require heparin flushes between uses.

Hepatic Artery Catheter.
Hepatic Artery Catheter. Hepatic artery catheterization may be performed to establish regional chemotherapy to treat primary or metastatic disease of the liver. With the use of a local anesthetic, the catheter may be inserted percutaneously into the left axillary artery and threaded into the common hepatic artery. This technique eliminates the need for a laparotomy to cannulate the hepatic arteries. However, some patients have variant anatomy that requires a dual-catheter delivery system. Vascular reconstruction, ligation, and/or occlusion of an artery may be necessary for local/regional perfusion. Regardless of the method of catheterization, an infusion pump is attached to the catheter(s) to deliver the cytotoxic agent to the tumor.

Intraperitoneal Catheter. Intraperitoneal chemotherapy permits the delivery of high concentrations of an agent to an ovarian or colorectal tumor without exposing normal tissues systemically. With the use of a local anesthetic, a Tenckhoff catheter is inserted into the peritoneal cavity. An incision in the anterior abdominal wall is usually located just lateral to the right or left of the rectus abdominis muscle at the level of the umbilicus. The anterior rectus sheath is incised to allow a Verres needle to penetrate the peritoneum. To prevent the catheter from kinking, air is injected before the catheter is placed in the peritoneal cavity. A subcutaneous tunnel is made between the initial incision and stab wound to secure the catheter. A Dacron cuff is embedded in the subcutaneous tissue to anchor the catheter in place. The agent exits the peritoneal cavity via the portal circulation.

Infusion Devices. Devices with reservoirs for the chemotherapeutic agent are implanted into body tissues.

Subcutaneous Infusion Port. With the use of a local anesthetic, a venous access device is implanted subcutaneously for continuous or intermittent injections of cytotoxic agent(s), TPN, or blood products. Depending on the manufacturer, the device consists of a plastic or silicone rubber self-sealing port on a plastic or stainless steel reservoir (Fig. 22-7). The catheter attached to the reservoir is inserted into a central vein, hepatic artery, peritoneal cavity, or epidural space. A tunnel is created from the point at which the catheter enters the vessel, cavity, or space to a subcutaneous pocket (Fig. 22-8). The pocket is made wherever necessary to stabilize the port. The reservoir is sutured to the underlying fascia. A Huber needle with a 90-degree-angle tip is used to enter the port for heparinizing and infusing agents (Fig. 22-9). Extension tubing may connect the needle to an infusion pump for continuous infusion. After use, the port is flushed with 10 mL of sterile normal saline followed by

3 to 10 mL of heparinized saline (100 units/mL). Thrombosis and infection are potential complications of long-term venous access devices and catheters.

Implantable Infusion Pump. With the patient under local, regional, or general anesthesia, an infusion catheter is placed into an artery, vein, body space, spine, or ventricle for localized chemotherapy to a tumor in the liver, head, neck, or brain. The infusion pump device is implanted in a subcutaneous pocket created in the abdominal wall, beneath the clavicle, or under the scalp. The titanium, stainless steel, and silicone rubber device resembles a hockey puck and delivers the agent by means of a bellows device (Infusaid) or by radio signals (Medtronic). The inner reservoir is filled with the cytotoxic agent. When the reservoir is collapsed by pressure, the agent is infused into the catheter. The pump is warmed initially to activate the fluorocarbon propellant in the chamber around the reservoir. It is placed over a bony prominence for support when refilling.

The drug is replenished periodically by percutaneous injection. A bolus can be administered through a side port on the pump. These implanted infusion devices also are used to control severe systemic conditions such as diabetes, thromboembolic disease, or pain from a malignancy. Insulin, heparin, or morphine is infused, respectively.

Perioperative Care of the Patient With Cancer

Malignant tumor cells can be disseminated by manipulation of tissue. Because of their altered nutritional and physiologic status, patients with cancer also may be highly susceptible to the complications of postoperative infection. To minimize these risks, the following specific precautions are taken in the surgical management of patients with cancer:

1. The skin over the site of a soft tissue tumor should be handled gently during hair removal and antisepsis. Vigorous scrubbing could dislodge underlying tumor cells; this is avoided by the use of "no-touch" techniques. With vascular tumors, manipulation during positioning or skin preparation could cause vascular complications such as emboli or hemorrhage. The no-touch technique means that the tumor is handled as little as possible during its removal. Radiated skin is very fragile.
2. Gowns, gloves, drapes, and instruments may be changed after a biopsy (e.g., a breast biopsy) before incision for a radical resection (e.g., a mastectomy). The tumor is deliberately incised to obtain a biopsy for diagnosis.

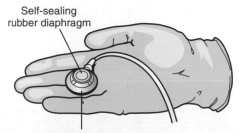

FIG. 22-7 Implantable subcutaneous infusion port.

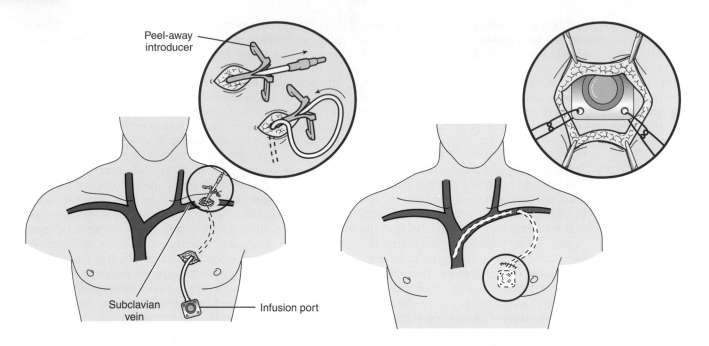

Peel-away introducer

Subclavian vein

Infusion port

FIG. 22-8 Placement of an implantable subcutaneous infusion port.

3. Instruments placed in direct contact with tumor cells may be discarded immediately after use. Even when the tumor appears to be localized, most cancers have disseminated to some degree. Therefore some surgeons prefer to use each instrument once and then discard it.
4. Some surgeons prefer to irrigate the surgical site with sterile water instead of sterile normal saline solution to cause the destruction of cancerous cells by crenation. This practice is common during mastectomy.
5. As a prophylactic measure, antibiotics are administered preoperatively, intraoperatively, and postoperatively to provide an adequate antibacterial level to prevent wound infection.
6. Time-honored precautions such as handling tissue gently, keeping blood loss to a minimum, and avoiding an unduly prolonged surgical procedure influence the outcome for the patient.

During a long surgical procedure, messages should be conveyed periodically to the patient's anxiously waiting family members or significant others to reassure them that

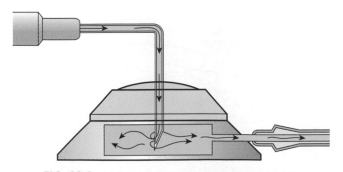

FIG. 22-9 Huber needle with a 90-degree-angle tip.

their loved one is receiving care from a concerned perioperative team.

Teaching Patients Risk Avoidance Behaviors

Patient education should include information about avoiding cancer-causing behaviors and how to minimize the risk for cancer. Behaviors to discuss include the following:

- Avoiding smoking and exposure to smoke. The Department of Health and Human Services reports that exposure to cigarette smoke is responsible for 83% of all cases of lung cancer. Each year more than 100,000 children 12 years of age and younger begin smoking, which leads to habitual use. Secondhand smoke, referred to as environmental tobacco smoke (ETS), has been implicated in the development of cancer in nonsmoking people who are exposed to smoke on a regular basis.
- Increasing dietary intake of fiber and low-fat foods. Antioxidants such as vitamins C and A may reduce an individual's risk for developing cancer. High-fat diets have been implicated in the development of breast, colon, and prostate cancers. According to reports of the American Cancer Society, 35% of cancer deaths are related to dietary causes and are possibly preventable. A desirable weight should be maintained, and obesity should be avoided. Excessive alcohol intake should also be avoided.
- Minimizing sun exposure, especially between the hours of 10:00 AM and 3:30 PM. Sun exposure has been shown to be the major cause of skin cancer, especially melanoma. Severe sunburn in childhood may be linked to the development of skin cancer later in life. Certain medications, such as tranquilizers, antidiabetic agents, diuretics, antiinflammatory agents, and antibiotics, can predispose an individual to sunburn. Certain cosmetic products, such as tretinoin (Retin-A) and alpha-hydroxy

acid are extremely reactive to sunlight and can increase the risk of sunburn within 30 minutes of exposure. Tanning booths also can be hazardous to the skin.

- A waterproof sunscreen lotion with a sun-protection factor (SPF) of at least 15 should be applied whenever sun exposure is likely. Sun-blocking products of SPF 30 to 45 are preferred. The sun-blocking product should provide protection from both ultraviolet A and ultraviolet B (UVA, UVB) rays. (UVA rays can increase the damage caused by UVB rays.) Sunscreen should be applied at least 30 minutes before going outdoors and reapplied every hour thereafter.

- Having regular checkups, especially yearly checkups after 40 years of age. Knowing the warning signs of cancer may promote prompt diagnosis and treatment. Signs to consider in young children include frequent swelling (lymphadenopathy) or bruising, unexplained headaches or fevers, dramatic weight loss or gain, and localized pain.

Self-examination of the skin, breast, and testes may reveal an early sign of cancer and should be performed on a routine monthly basis.

Bibliography

Butler SA et al: Computer-aided detection in diagnostic mammography, *Am J Roentgenol* 183(5):1511-1515, 2004.

Jacobs DS et al: Capsule staining as an adjunct to cataract surgery: *A report from the American Academy of Ophthalmology* 113(4):707-713, 2006.

Carroll CM: Eye on diagnostics: Sorting out breast biopsy options, *Nursing* 36(3)70-71, 2006.

Del Ojo L et al: Is magnetic resonance imaging safe in cardiac pacemaker recipients? *Pacing Clin Electophysiol* 25(2):274-278, 2005.

Fletcher JG et al: CT colonography: Unraveling the twists and turns, *Curr Opin Gastroenterol* 21(1):90-98, 2005.

Kidwell C: MRI replaces CT for stroke evaluation, *Medscape Gen Med* 7(4):22, 2005.

Marshall A: As patients seek whole-body CT imaging, who's is charge? *Clin News* 7(9):1, 22, 2003.

Russell L: Intraoperative magnetic resonance imaging safety considerations, *AORN* 77(3):590-592, 2003.

Scott S, Schlaff W: Laparoscopic oophoropexy prior to radiation therapy in an adolescent with Hodgkin's disease, *J Adolesc Gynecol* 18(5):355-357, 2005.

Shaw N et al: Magnetic resonance spectroscopy as an imaging tool for cancer: A review of the literature, *JAOA* 106(1):23-26, 2006.

Youssef IM, Abdel-Dayem HM: Breast cancer and the role of sentinel lymph node localization, *J Womans Imag* 6(3):114-124, 141-144, 2004.

Chapter **23**

Surgical Pharmacology

CHAPTER OBJECTIVES

After studying this chapter, the learner will be able to:
- Calculate drug dosages in the perioperative environment.
- List common drugs used in surgery.
- Identify drug sources and the effect on patient use.
- Demonstrate drug handling in a sterile environment.

CHAPTER OUTLINE

KEY TERMS AND DEFINITIONS

Ampule   Sealed glass tube containing a drug. Tip is scored for removal by snapping off. Drug is removed by a sterile syringe and filter needle to prevent aspiration of glass shards.

Antagonist   One drug is used to alter or stop the effect of another drug.

Conversion   Standard scale of equivalents used to measure between metric, English, and apothecary.

Diagnostic drug   Used to perform a medical test or confirm a pathogenic condition.
- **Dye**   Colored solution used to identify structures with gross vision.
- **Stain**   Chemical used in solution to tint cellular structures for microscopic study.
- **Contrast medium**   Radiopaque solution used during radiography or fluoroscopy to define structures on film or digital media.

Diluent   Liquid used to decrease the concentration of a substance.

Gas   A non-solid, non-liquid form of a chemical.

Generic   Chemically equivalent drugs formulated as substitutes for brand-name products.

Hypodermic   Below the skin.

Infusion   Flow of a drug directly into the circulatory system.

Inhalant   Drug that is taken in like a breath then absorbed through the respiratory tract.

Injection   Insertion of a drug directly into the tissues using a syringe and needle.

Loading dose   The first dose of a series given in a larger quantity than the subsequent doses.

Localized drug effect   The physiologic response to a drug is in a select area of the body and not carried to other regions in an effective form.

Pharmacokinetics   The actions and disposition of a chemical in the body.
- **Absorption**   The drug is taken in by the cells of the body.
- **Distribution**   The drug is evenly absorbed by the entire body.
- **Metabolism**   The drug is used throughout the body and broken down by major organs.
- **Excretion**   The drug is released from the body in naturally excreted substances.

Placebo   An inert substance given to a patient to stimulate the power of suggestion of effectiveness. Commonly used as a control in experimental medicine.

Potentiation   A synergistic action of one drug against another to cause an increased response by the body.

Preventive drug   Chemical or biologic preparation given with the intent of avoiding a disease state.

Reaction to a drug   The physiologic response of the body when exposed to a drug. The response can be positive or negative.
- **Sensitivity**   Physiologic mechanisms are triggered by exposure to small doses of a given drug.
- **Allergy**   Physiologic defense mechanisms are triggered by exposure to a drug or chemical causing a potentially life-threatening response.
- **Anaphylaxis**   Severe physiologic response to exposure to a drug or chemical causing a definite threat to the patient's life.

Receptor site   Location in the body that acts in response to a chemical stimulus. Some drugs act by blocking a receptor site and prevent naturally produced chemicals from bonding.

Side-effect   A secondary reaction that occurs in response to administration of a drug.

Systemic drug effect   The physiologic response to a drug is manifest in the entire body.

Tolerance   The physiologic response caused by prolonged use of large quantities of a drug that makes average doses ineffective.

Toxic   A level of any given drug that causes a negative or possibly fatal physiologic response.

Vial   A vacuum-sealed glass or plastic container of medication that is sealed by a rubber stopper. The drug is removed by a sterile syringe and needle.

HISTORICAL BACKGROUND

Pharmaceutical history extends to the beginning of time. Fossils found near Neanderthal digs point to the use of plants as medicinals. The ancient Egyptians recorded the use of medications in 3000 BC. Babylonian clay tablets from 2600 BC describe diseases and the use of formulated treatments.

In Greek mythology, the immortal centaur (half man, half horse) Chiron was the first to use medicines to heal battle-scarred warriors. Chiron trained Asklepios, who was the first physician, in the healing arts. Several words were derived from the name Chiron, which means chiral: the polarization of light from one hand to the other. Later forms of the term became chiropracty, which refers to the manipulation by hand of the body's joints and muscles for health. The term *chirurgery,* evolved into the word *surgery,* which means to heal by the hands.

PHARMACOLOGY BASELINES

The main purpose of this chapter is to highlight the drugs specifically used in perioperative patient care. This chapter is not intended to be an all-inclusive pharmacologic resource. (Drugs used in patient care areas other than the perioperative environment can be reviewed at www.globalrph.com/druglist.htm. This site has most of the common drugs and dosages listed in chart form.)

Many drugs and pharmaceutical substances require special preparation and handling in the surgical environment. Some of these preparations are found only in the operating room (OR), and their proper use is based on sterile technique, precise actions, and extreme caution.

Safe drug and pharmaceutical administration in the OR is practiced according to the seven rights of medication administration in any setting:
  • Right patient
  • Right drug
  • Right time
  • Right dose
  • Right route
  • Right reason
  • Right documentation

Patient assessment will provide information about the patient's health and general condition. The patient's history may require a change in the plan of care or clinical path for the intraoperative care period. Allergies are assessed and documented, and reactions are prevented.

Prescription items in the OR are more than drugs and medications. Surgical pharmacology encompasses many chemicals ranging from dyes to adhesives, most of which are not used in any other patient care area. All of the specialized items require special handling within the confines of the sterile field. Other items used in the OR include gaseous materials and surgical-site closure materials.

Pregnancy Classifications

The safe administration of any drug to a pregnant woman requires knowledge of how the drug might affect a developing fetus. All drugs, chemicals, and solutions in surgery have a pregnancy classification, including solutions such as bacteriostatic water that has a pregnancy classification of "C." The risks should be identified before any drug is administered to a pregnant or possibly pregnant woman. Pregnancy classifications are as follows:
  • A No known risk
  • B No risk shown in humans
  • C Possible risk
  • D Positive risk
  • E Contraindicated

Drug Development

New drugs take many years to become available for patient use. According to the Office of Research and Development of the Pharmaceutical Manufacturers Association, it takes almost 12 years for a drug to be discovered and placed into use. Safety and efficacy testing on animals and laboratory simulation takes an average of $3\frac{1}{2}$ years to complete. It is estimated that only 1 of every 1000 compounds is actually tested in human trials. Each potential drug is filed with the U.S. Food and Drug Administration (FDA) in an Investigational New Drug (IND) application. A series of clinical trials are performed on humans, who have given informed consent as follows:
  • *Phase I clinical trial:* 20 to 80 healthy individuals for a period of 1 year. The drug is studied for safety in dosage, duration of action, absorption, distribution, metabolism, and excretion.
  • *Phase II clinical trial:* 100 to 300 people with actual disease process for which the drug is proposed treatment for a period of 2 years. The drug is studied for effectiveness and tolerability. Adverse reactions are monitored.
  • *Phase III clinical trial:* 1000 to 3000 patients in multiple health care settings participate. The drug is monitored to validate effectiveness and safety.
  • *Phase VI postmarket surveillance:* After the drug is on the market, the manufacturer monitors the users for therapeutic and nontherapeutic effects and reports to the FDA.

Clinical trial results are reported yearly to the FDA. Only one in five drugs ever completes the three-clinical-trial process. The long period needed for the clinical trials permits the researchers to observe for long-term effects of the compound. Upon completion of the clinical trial phases, the drug manufacturer submits a New Drug Application (NDA). Once approved by the FDA, the new drug is made available for physicians to prescribe. The approval process takes between 6 and 29 months to complete.

Drug Names

Drugs have three names. The first name, which is the chemical name, describes the chemical components such as molecular and atomic structure of the drug. It is not commonly used when referencing the drug.

The second name is the official name, referred to as generic and given to the compound by the initial manufacturer. The generic name is derived from the chemical name and is not capitalized. The drugs are listed in the United States Pharmacopeia (USP) and the National Formulary (NF) according to the generic names.

For the third name, the drug company who is selling the drug will assign a copyrighted trade name, or a brand name, which is proprietary. The trade name is capitalized and designated by a registration mark (®).

Mathematics Baselines

Decimals. Numbers to the left of the decimal are whole numbers. Numbers to the right of the decimal are decimal fractions and are read according to their place value:

0.1	one-tenth
0.01	one-hundredth
0.001	one-thousandth
0.0001	one–ten thousandth

Addition of Decimals

1. Write numbers in column with the decimals vertically aligned.
2. Place the decimal in the answer beneath the decimal in the problem.

Example: Add 1.33, 4.0, 2.146, and 0.03

```
   1.33
   4.0
   2.146
 + 0.03
   7.506
```

Subtraction of Decimals

1. Write numbers in column with the decimals vertically aligned.
2. Subtract and place the decimal in the answer beneath the decimal in the problem.

Example: Subtract 0.025 from 15.838

```
  15.838
 −0.025
  15.813
```

Multiplication of Decimals

1. Find the product of the numbers.
2. Total the number of decimal places in the multiplicand and in the multiplier.
3. Mark off the total decimal places in the product, and insert a decimal.

Example: Multiply 2.05 by 0.2

```
    2.05 (multiplicand)
 ×  0.2 (multiplier)
   0.410 (product with three decimal places marked off
         [answer])
```

When the number of decimal places to be marked off goes beyond the numbers in the product, add a zero in each place.

To multiply a decimal by 100, 1000, 10,000, move the decimal to the right as many places as there are zeros in the multiplier.

Example: Multiply 0.25 by 100. There are two zeros, so move the decimal two places to the right: 025., or 25

To multiply a decimal by 0.1, 0.01, 0.001, move the decimal to the left as many places as there are decimal places in the multiplier.

Example: Multiply 0.25 by 0.1. There is one decimal place, so move the decimal one place to the left: 0.025

If the decimal must be moved farther than there are numbers, add a zero for each decimal place.

Division of Decimals To divide a decimal by a whole number:

1. Write the problem.
2. Place a decimal in the quotient directly above the decimal in the dividend.
3. Solve the quotient.

Example: Divide 0.1 by 50

```
        0.002
(divisor) 50)0.100 (dividend)
```

To divide a whole number or decimal by a decimal:

1. Move the decimal in the divisor to the right until the divisor is a whole number.
2. Move the decimal in the dividend to the right as many places as you moved the decimal in the divisor.
3. Place the decimal in the quotient directly above the (moved) decimal in the dividend.
4. Solve the quotient.

Example: Divide 0.225 by 0.5

```
       0.450
 0.5)0.225
```

To divide a decimal by 10, 100, 1000, and so on, move the decimal to the left as many places as there are zeros in the divisor.

Example: Divide 0.25 by 1000. There are three zeros, so move the decimal three places to the left: 0.00025

To divide a decimal by 0.1, 0.01, 0.001, and so on, move the decimal to the right as many places as there are decimal places in the divisor.

Example: Divide 0.25 by 0.1. There is one decimal place, so move the decimal one place to the right: 02.5, or 2.5

Percent. The word *percent* means part of 100. Twenty-five percent (25%) means 25 parts of 100, or 25/100; also written as the decimal 0.25. Percent indicates a fraction in which the denominator is 100.

Fractions. A fraction represents a part of a whole number. If a circle is divided into four equal parts, each part is ¼ of the circle, as seen in Figure 23-1. The numerator is 1 and the denominator is 4. The line between 1 and 4 means divide.

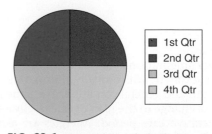

FIG. 23-1 Parts of the whole (fractions).

Common Denominator. Unlike denominators cannot be added or subtracted. Common denominator means the fractions have the same denominator.

Reduce a Fraction to Lowest Terms. Determine the largest number that divides evenly into both numbers; when the fraction cannot be reduced any further, it is in its lowest terms.

Example: Reduce to lowest terms: 20/80

Both numbers are divisible evenly by 20: 20 × 20 × 1, and 80 × 20 × 4

Therefore the lowest terms of 20/80 × 1/4.

Improper Fraction. ⁵⁄₄ is an improper fraction; when reduced to its lowest terms, it becomes 1¼, a mixed number.

Ratio and Proportion

Ratio. We use ratios to compare two things. If we have 6 hemostats and 4 scissors, the ratio is termed 6:4 (stated *six to four*). Any two sets of quantified items (numbers of things) can be put into ratio format for comparison. The ratio concept can be expressed as "to," colon, or as a fraction. *Example:*

6:4

6 to 4

6/4

In pharmacology the use of a ratio is expressed in relatively equal terms. For example if there is 1 ounce of medicine, it is the same as 30 mL of medicine. It is expressed as (1 oz is to 30 mL) and written as 1 oz : 30 mL. A ratio is one way of saying that 1 oz is equal to 30 mL.

Proportion. When we compare two ratios or need to solve for an unknown quantity to make the ratios balance the process uses the following format:

1 oz : 30 mL = 2 oz : X mL (stated: 1 ounce is to 30 milliliters as 2 ounces is to X milliliters.)

The outer numbers are referred to as the extremes and the inner numbers are referred to as the means. The problem is solved by equalizing the formula. That is why an equal sign connects the two ratios.

Notice that the order of the formula follows ___oz : ___mL = ___oz : ___mL.

The quantities need to be expressed in the same order on both sides of the equation.

Here is one method of using ratios and proportions. (1) Multiply the extremes. (2) Multiply the means. (3) Divide the left side by the right side with X. (NOTE: Think of the phrase *"X goes into"* because the number next to the X goes into the number on the other side of the equal sign to get the answer.

1 oz : 30 mL = 2 oz : X mL	Multiply the extremes.
1 × X = 2 × 30	Multiply the means.
1X = 60	Divide the number on the
X = 60	right side by the number
Therefore:	on the left side with the X.
1 oz : 30 mL = 2 oz : 60 mL	The product is 60.

Using ratio and proportion is a good way to solve most medication problems for mixing solutions in the OR;

however, several measurements from the conversion chart must be known to complete the formula. For example: knowing that 1 ounce is the same as 30 milliliters is important to finding out that 2 ounces is 60 milliliters.

If the ratio is X mL : 2 pints (stated as X milliliters is to one pint) the problem is to solve for X or how many milliliters is in one pint. This is how to use ratio and proportion to solve this problem. Knowing the baseline conversion of 500 mL: 1 pint is the key to solving for X. Here is how to set up the formula:

500 mL : 1 pint = X mL : 2 pints
1000 = 1X
(remember the phrase "X goes into") (1000 is divided by 1)
1000 = X

Answer 500 mL : 1 pint = 1000 mL : 2 pints

Pharmacologic Conversions

Medications are measured in metric, English/household, or apothecary equivalents. Each unit of measure has a designated accepted abbreviation. Standardization of abbreviations is important for prevention of error in dosage caused by misinterpretation.

Accepted Abbreviations. Documentation of medication in the OR is done by using a series of abbreviations and symbols. Standardization of the abbreviations used is important for accuracy. Most of these are expressed in Latin terminology. Common uses include the abbreviations in Box 23-1.

Weights and Measures. Converting dosages between metric, English/household, or apothecary systems is done by calculating with a standard set of measures (Table 23-1). Tables are commonly used for conversions of units between systems. Table 23-2 is representative of the most common conversions used in the OR.

CONSIDERATIONS IN SURGICAL PHARMACOLOGY

Pharmaceuticals used in the OR are not limited to medicines in the ordinary concept of medication. Sources for surgical pharmaceuticals can be living matter from a biologic source or compounded from some other natural or synthetic mixture. Some surgical pharmacologic materials remain inside the body permanently (e.g., an implant), and some are systemically absorbed.

Items procured from the pharmacy require special handling within the sterile field. Care is taken not to expose the patient to an allergen or any substance that can cause a sensitivity reaction.

Handling Drugs and Pharmacologic Materials in Surgery

Drugs and pharmaceuticals are given to the scrub person for use in the field by a physician or circulating nurse who is a registered nurse (RN). The surgeon requests a drug or pharmaceutical either verbally or in writing for use during surgery, and the circulating nurse obtains it from the pharmacy or stock. The circulating nurse validates the integrity

BOX 23-1	Abbreviations for the Administration of Medications

Meaning	Abbreviation
After meals	pc
Before meals	ac
Hour of sleep	hs
Right eye	OD
Left eye	OS
Both eyes	OU
Right ear	AD
Left ear	AS
Both ears	AU
By mouth	per os (PO)
Nothing by mouth	NPO
Quantity sufficient	qs
As needed	prn
As desired	ad lib
Drop	gt
Twice per day	bid
Three times per day	tid
Four times per day	qid
Every day	qd
Liter	L
Milliliter	mL
Cubic centimeter	cc
Grains	gr
Gram	g
Kilogram	kg
Milligram	mg
Ounce	oz
Pint	pt
Quart	qt
Pound	lb
Micron	μm
Microgram	mcg (or μg)

of the package or container, checks the expiration date, checks for patient allergy or contraindication, and shows the complete label to the scrub person for verification. As the drug is dispensed to the field, the circulating nurse should say the drug name and concentration out loud. The drug or material is dispensed to the sterile field in one of the following ways:

- Solutions for irrigation are poured in their entirety into a sterile basin. If the contents are not completely dispensed, the bottle is not recapped and saved for later use. Once the bottle is opened, the lip of the bottle has rendered the contents unsterile once pouring has started. Do not splash or create an aerosol.
- Products in peel packs may be dispensed directly to the field, or the scrub person can take the item with a forceps from the opened package as it is held open by the circulating nurse.
- Drugs in vials (Fig. 23-2) for injection should be removed from the vial by the circulating nurse with a syringe (Fig. 23-3) and an 18- or 19-gauge hypodermic needle (Fig. 23-4). The scrub person should place a sterile glass or plastic medicine cup near the edge of the table.

Metal medicine cups are not advised for some drugs, because they may bind with the metallic substance. Popping off the cap of the vial usually contaminates the lip, and pouring over that lip renders the drug contaminated.

- After the circulating nurse withdraws the drug from the vial, he or she removes the injection needle and carefully delivers the drug through the syringe into the medicine cup. The needle is removed because dispensing via the needle creates an aerosol that can cause exposure to an allergen.
- The circulating nurse should use a filter when withdrawing drugs from a glass ampule (Fig. 23-5). Shards of glass can get into the solution and inadvertently be injected into a patient.
- Ointments and creams should be purchased in unit-dose tubes. Multidose tubes are easily contaminated. If such a tube is used, $\frac{1}{2}$ inch of the ointment or cream should be squeezed out into the trash before any is used for the current patient. The sterility is questionable.

The scrub person should not use a needle and syringe to pierce the rubber stopper on the bottle as the circulating nurse holds it over the field. This places the nurse at risk for needlestick injury. The circulating nurse should not deliver the drug through the needle, because it creates an aerosol in the room.

The drug should be labeled as soon as it is received into the sterile field. The container and the syringe (Fig. 23-6) should be clearly marked with the name and concentration of the drug. According to the Joint Commission on Accreditation of Healthcare Organizations (JCAHO) the content of the sterile field drug label should include the first three of the following list and all five on the following list if prepared for used and not yet dispensed to the sterile field:

1. Drug name
2. Strength
3. Amount if not apparent by markings on the container
4. Expiration date if not used within 24 hours
5. Expiration date if expiration occurs within 24 hours

Only approved abbreviations should be used. (These can be found in Box 23-1.) Sterile labels and sterile marking pens are commercially available and come packed in many custom packs. If these types of labels are not used in the facility, wound closure strips, such as Steri-Strips, and a sterile marking pen can be used. The scrub person should say the name of the drug as he or she hands the syringe to the surgeon. Some facilities have practices such as placing the syringe cap in the medicine cup to denote a certain drug. This practice is strongly discouraged because it is not a universal practice and can lead to patient harm.

The circulating nurse documents the delivery of the drug to the sterile field and its usage. The actual dose given to the patient should be recorded on the operating room record and relayed to the anesthesia provider to avoid any incompatibility with medicines given during anesthesia.

The circulating nurse takes great care in the access of double or triple lumen central venous lines. Some of the connectors can be misconnected to a harmful infusion if universal adapters are used. Intravascular catheters should not be compatible with other infusion devices.

TABLE 23-1	Drug Measurement Abbreviations with JCAHO "Do Not Use List"	
Unit of Measure	**Approved Abbreviation**	**JCAHO's "Do Not Use List" with Rationale**
millimeter	mm	
meter	m	
inch	in	
gram	g	
microgram	mcg	μg too easily confused with mg.
kilogram	kg	
pound	lb	
degrees Fahrenheit	° F	
pint	pt	
gallon	gal	
grain	gr	
centimeter	cm	
foot/feet	ft	
milligram	mg	
milliliter	mL	Do not use cc. Too easily mistaken for "u" as in units.
liter	L	
ounce	oz	
degrees Celsius (Centigrade)	° C	
quart	qt	
tablespoon	tbsp	
teaspoon	tsp	
unit	unit	Do not abbreviate as "U."
drop or drops	gt or gtt	Do not use abbreviations for right, left, or both eyes or ears. Write out in full terms "right," "left," or "both eyes" or "both ears."

TABLE 23-2	Basic Weights and Measures in Pharmacology	
Metric	**Household/English**	**Apothecary**
FLUID MEASURE		
4 L/4000 mL	1 gal	1 gal
1 L/1000 mL	1 qt/32 oz/2 pt	32 oz (no pleural for pints)
500 mL	1 pt/16 oz/2 cups	16 oz
250 mL	1 cup/8 oz	8 oz
30 mL	1 oz	1 oz/8 dr
15 mL	1 tbsp/3 tsp	225 gtt/m
5 mL	1 tsp	75 gtt/m
1 mL		15 gtt/m
0.0667 mL		1 gt/m
MASS WEIGHT		
1 mg/1000 mcg		1/60 gr
60 mg		1 gr
1 g		15 gr
4 g		60 gr
1000 g/1 kg	2.2 lb	
	16 oz/1 lb	12 oz
MEASURE OF SIZE		
1 m/1000 mm	3.281 ft	
10 mm/1 cm		
2.54 cm	1 in	
	12 in/1 ft	
	3 ft/1 yd	

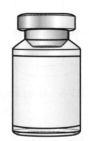

FIG. 23-2   Drug vial with rubber stopper and plastic cap in place.

L, Liter; *mL,* milliliter; *cc,* cubic centimeter; *gal,* gallon; *qt,* quart; *oz,* ounce; *pt,* pint; *dr,* dram; *tbsp,* tablespoon; *tsp,* teaspoon; *gt,* drop; *gtt,* drops; *m,* minim; *mg,* milligram; *mcg,* microgram; *g,* gram; *kg,* kilogram; *lb,* pound; *gr,* grain; *oz,* ounce; *m,* meter; *mm,* millimeter; *cm,* centimeter; *ft,* foot; *in,* inch; *yd,* yard.

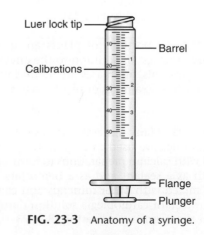

FIG. 23-3   Anatomy of a syringe.

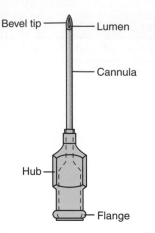

FIG. 23-4   Anatomy of a hypodermic needle.

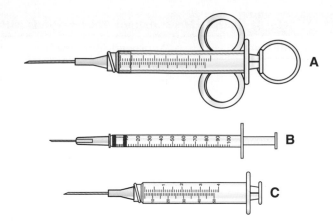

FIG. 23-6   **A,** Control syringe. **B,** One-milliliter syringe used for insulin or tuberculosis (TB) testing. **C,** Standard syringe.

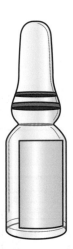

FIG. 23-5   Drug ampule.

SURGICAL DRUG AND PHARMACEUTICAL SOURCES

Biologic Sources

Biologic sources for drugs can be found in glands, body fluids, organs, fats, and cells of living entities.

Animal Sources. Animals are used for the manufacturing of drugs. Examples of animals used in the production of pharmaceuticals are found in Box 23-2.

Plant Sources. All portions of plants are used for the manufacturing of drugs. In addition to the anatomic parts of the plant, gums, oils, and bases are used as vehicles for drug administration. Examples of plant usage are found in Box 23-3.

Mineral Sources. Many minerals such as calcium, potassium, and chlorides are used intraoperatively. Fibrinogen can be mixed with calcium preparations to form an adhesive that acts both as a sealant and as a hemostatic material. Potassium is mixed with other minerals and chemicals to form a cell protectant cardioplegia solution during cardiac surgery when the heart is not beating (Box 23-4).

BOX 23-2	Animal Sources of Drugs

BOVINE
  Hemostatic agent
  Blood substitute (Hemopure)
  Insulin
PORCINE
  Hemostatic agent
  Biologic dressing
  Insulin
EQUINE
  Serum vaccine
  Hormones (estrogen)
  Pericardial implant
OVINE
  Suture
  Lanolin
  Hyaluronidase ophthalmic
FISH
  Protamine
REPTILIAN
  Antivenom (antivenin)
  Ancrod
  Exenatide (Byetta)
HUMAN
  Blood
  Blood fraction
  Tissue:
  • Reconstruction
  • Biologic dressing
  Semen
  Hormones (growth hormone)
  Human source extraction:
  • Human skin equivalent
  Hemoglobin-based oxygen carrier (PolyHeme)

Synthetic and Semisynthetic Sources

Chemical Sources. Replication of natural drugs from synthetic sources is common. Narcotic pain medications resembling the action of opioids are used for postoperative patients.

BOX 23-3	Plant Sources of Drugs

Leaves (atropine from belladonna leaves, indigo carmine)
Blossom (opium poppy, colchicine from crocus)
Seed (arabic)
Fruit (cranberry)
Tubers/roots (ginseng) and rhizomes (valerian, gentian)
Sap (aloe, gum arabic preservative)
Bark (aspirin, quinine, cascara)
Wood-extract
Resin (benzoin)
Fungi (some antibiotics)
Herbs (tranquilizers)
Cellulose fibers (hemostatic)

BOX 23-4	Minerals Used as Drugs

Multivitamins contain: calcium, iron, copper, magnesium, selenium, zinc
Potassium is replaced after diuretic administration
Iodine is used in contrast media and radioactive markers
Sodium and chloride balance body fluids

Engineered Protein from Plant, Animal, and Chemical Combinations. Skin substitute, pharmaceuticals, and blood products have been manufactured using biologic material as their base. Skin has been cultured for use in wound repair. Blood cells from bovine and human sources have been engineered for use in humans as an oxygen-carrying medium.

PHARMACOLOGIC FORMS USED IN SURGERY

Box 23-5 gives examples of select surgical medications. Drugs used in surgery are found in many forms, ranging from liquids to solids. Routes of drug administration can be found in Box 23-6.

Liquids

A variety of solutions and liquids are used within the sterile field and nonsterile fields before, during, and after the surgical procedure. These can be used topically or as an injection. Uses of solutions include the following:

- Irrigations: Ringer's lactate, saline, water
- Tumescence: Fluid mixed with epinephrine, placed under the skin with a special cannula and pressurized delivery system to make the skin firm for liposuction
- Expansion media: Sterile water, glycine, or saline to create a working space for endoscopy
- Biologic adhesives: To adhere delicate tissues together
- Perfusion: For cardioplegia (cardiac cell nutrient and preservation during heart stoppage for heart surgery)
- Preservatives and fixatives: For tissues and specimens
- Medications: For injection in a sterile field
- Caustics: Phenols to remove cell layers
- Skin cleansers and degreasers: For skin prep

BOX 23-5	Examples of Drugs Used in Surgery
Classification	**Drugs**
ANTIINFECTIVE	
Antibiotics	*Aminoglycosides*
	Gentamicin
	Kanamycin
	Neomycin
	Streptomycin
	Tobramycin
	Cephalosporins
	Cefazolin
	Cefonicid
	Cefotaxime
	Quinolones
	Ciprofloxacin
	Macrolides
	Erythromycin
	Penicillins
	Ampicillin
	Penicillin G potassium
	Amoxicillin
	Mezlocillin
	Carbenicillin
	Ticarcillin
	Tetracyclines
	Doxycycline
	Tetracycline
	Sulfonamides (antimicrobial)
	Sulfamethoxazole
	Glycylcycline
	Tygacil
	Lipopeptides
	Daptomycin
	Oxazolidinones
	Linezolid
	Ketolide
	Telithromycin
AUTONOMIC NERVOUS SYSTEM AGENTS	
Adrenergic Agonists	*Alpha- and beta-adrenergic agonists*
	Epinephrine
	Isoproterenol
Adrenergic Antagonists	*Antidysrhythmics*
	Propranolol
Anticholinergics	*Muscarinics*
	Atropine sulfate
	Glycopyrrolate
	Scopolamine
Anticoagulants	*Anticoagulants*
	Heparin
	Warfarin
	Enoxaparin
	Protamine
ANTICOAGULANTS AND COAGULANTS	
Antiplatelet Agents	Aspirin
	Ticlopidine
Coagulant Hemostatics	Thrombin

Continued

BOX 23-5	Examples of Drugs Used in Surgery—cont'd

Classification	Drugs
CENTRAL NERVOUS SYSTEM AGENTS	
Analgesics	*Narcotics*
	Morphine
	Meperidine
	Fentanyl
BENZODIAZEPINES	
Antianxiety Medications	*Sedatives*
	Diazepam
	Lorazepam
	Midazolam
THROMBOLYTICS	
Thrombolytics	Streptokinase
	Urokinase
	Alteplase
SURGICAL DYES AND CONTRAST	
Dyes	Methylene blue
	Indigo carmine
	Brilliant green
	Gentian violet
Contrast Media	Iohexol
	Vasovist MRI contrast
	Diatrizoate meglumine
Tissue Stains	Lugol's iodine solution (aka Schiller's solution)
	Monsel's ferric solution

BOX 23-6	Routes for Administration of Drugs

Oral
Sublingual
Nasogastric
Gastric tube
Rectal
Vaginal
Topical
Transdermal
Inhalation
Parenteral
Subcutaneous
Intramuscular
Intravenous
Intraarticular
Endotracheal
Intraarterial
Intracardiac
Intradermal
Intraperitoneal
Intraosseous
Intrathecal
Umbilical artery or vein

Solids

Many preoperative and postoperative oral medications are in pill or tablet form. Patients are instructed in their use and about how much water they are permitted to have to swallow them. Small children can be given a medicated pacifier or lollipop that contains preoperative medication, such as a sedative.

Hemostasis can be obtained using woven sheets of hemostatic material. Other sheets of specialized material can be used for adhesion prevention when placed around internal organs.

Suppositories are sometimes used as an adjunct to rectal surgery. Some surgeons place a belladonna suppository in the rectum to slow peristalsis and allow healing after hemorrhoidectomy. Timed-release medications such as antibiotics can be implanted in bead form in orthopedic cement during prosthetic joint procedures. Gynecologic procedures can include placement of timed-release rings of contraception medication in the uterine cervix.

Orthopedic surgeons commonly use bone cement impregnated with antibiotic pellets or beads when placing implants into bone. Some of these antibiotic beads are time release.

Powder. Pharmacologic materials in powder form are commonly used in the OR in both dry and diluted forms. Dry powders and fibers used for hemostasis, such as bovine collagen, are applied dry and resorbed by the body in that form. Antibiotic powders are diluted in saline before being used as irrigants in the surgical site or before administration intravenously (IV). Sterile talc and tetracycline powder can be placed in solution for a sclerosant action in poudrage of the pleural cavity for the treatment of pleural effusion.

Semisolid

Creams and lotions are commonly used during surgical procedures. Ideally, the product should be double-wrapped and the inner sterile packaging should be placed directly on the sterile field. Many semisolids are supplied in multidose packages and are dispensed to the field carefully without contaminating the rest of the material in the package or tube. Drugs supplied in multidose tubes should have the first half inch of the product squeezed out into the trash before dispensing a portion to the field for use.

Lubricants are used for many procedures intraoperatively. Most are water-soluble, but those with a petroleum, lanolin, or oil base are not. Postoperatively, petroleum- or oil-based nonadherent dressings are placed on some surgical sites.

Gases

Few substances are used in the OR as gaseous forms. Nitrous oxide, nitrogen, carbon dioxide, medical air, and oxygen are the main gases found in the OR. Of these five gases, nitrous oxide, medical air, and oxygen are administered to the patient in drug-related form through the respiratory tree. Nitrogen is used to power drills and saws and carbon dioxide is used to create a working space during an endoscopic procedure, but they are not used as drug forms. Compressed gas cylinders have a valve opening that turns to the left to open (turn on) and to the right to close (turn off).

A simple mnemonic to use to remember which direction to turn for which function is: Be sure to turn it RIGHT OFF after use and check to see it's not LEFT ON.

Volatile substances are passed through special vaporizers and warmers to become gaseous drugs used during general anesthetic delivery.

Medical Gas Terminology

- *Cylinder:* Metal container designed to hold compressed medical gases at a high pressure
- *Cryogenic vessel:* Metal container designed to hold liquefied compressed medical gases at extremely low temperatures
- *Compressed medical gas:* Any liquefied or vaporized gas alone or in combination with other gases
- *Concentrator:* Stand-alone unit that extracts oxygen from room air and delivers concentrated oxygen at a continuous flow rate
- *Regulator:* Mechanism that controls the flow of a medical gas

Bibliography

Alexander JW: Nutritional pharmacology in surgical patients, *Am J Surg* 183(4):349-352, 2002.

AORN: *Drug information handbook for perioperative nurses,* Denver, AORN and Lexi-Comp, 2006.

Ang-Lee MK, Moss J, Yuan CS: Herbal medicines and perioperative care, *JAMA* 286(2):208-216, 2001.

Goldman P: Herbal medicines today and the roots of modern pharmacology, *Ann Intern Med* 135(8):594-600, 2001.

Rosenthal MH: Intraoperative fluid management—When and how much? *Chest* 115(Suppl 5):106-112, 1999.

Turkoski BB: Fighting infection: An ongoing challenge, Part I, *Orthop Nurs* 24(1):40-46, 2005.

Wilson BA, Shannon MT, Stang CL: *Prentice Hall nurse's drug guide 2005,* Upper Saddle River, NJ, 2005, Prentice Hall.

Chapter 24

Anesthesia: Techniques and Agents

CHAPTER OBJECTIVES

After studying this chapter, the learner will be able to:
- Identify three methods of general anesthesia.
- Describe the physiologic effects of general anesthesia.
- Discuss the purpose for cricoid pressure.
- Differentiate between general and regional anesthesia.
- List key points in providing safety for the anesthetized patient.

CHAPTER OUTLINE

KEY TERMS AND DEFINITIONS

Amnesia   Loss of memory.
Analgesia   Relief of pain by altering perception of painful stimuli; acts on specific receptors in the nervous system. Does not alter consciousness.
Anesthesia   Loss of feeling or sensation, especially loss of the sensation of pain with loss of protective reflexes.
Anoxia   Absence of oxygen.
Anticholinergic   Antagonist to action of parasympathetic and other cholinergic nerve fibers.
Apnea   Suspension or cessation of breathing.
Conduction anesthesia   Loss of sensation in a region of the body produced by injecting an anesthetic drug along the course of a nerve or a group of nerves to inhibit conduction of impulses to and from the area supplied by that nerve or nerves (block anesthesia, nerve block anesthesia).

Depolarization   Neutralization of polarity; reduction of differentials of ion distribution across polarized semipermeable membranes, as in nerve or muscle cells in the conduction of impulses; to make electrically negative.
Dysrhythmia   Ineffective rhythm, as of heart rate or brain waves; term used interchangeably with arrhythmia.
Emergence   Return of consciousness, sensation, and reflexes after general anesthesia.
Endotracheal   Within the trachea. An endotracheal tube may be placed in the trachea to maintain a patent airway during loss of consciousness.
Epidural anesthesia   Loss of sensation below the level of peridural injection of an anesthetic drug into the epidural space in the spinal canal for relief of pain in the lower extremities, abdomen, and pelvis without loss of consciousness.
Extubation   Removal of an endotracheal tube.
Fasciculation   Abnormal skeletal muscle contraction in which groups of muscle fibers innervated by the same neuron contract together.
Hypercapnia   Excessive amount of carbon dioxide in the blood; may also be termed hypercarbia.
Hypnotic   Drug or verbal suggestion that induces sleep.
Hypothermia   State in which body temperature is lower than the physiologic normal (i.e., below 95° F [35° C]).
Hypoxia, hypoxemia   Oxygen deficiency; state in which an inadequate amount of oxygen is available to or utilized by tissue; inadequate tissue oxygenation.
Induction   Period from the beginning of administration of an anesthetic until the patient loses consciousness and is stabilized in the desired plane of anesthesia.
Intrathecal injection   Instillation of solution, such as an anesthetic drug, into the subarachnoid space for diffusion in spinal fluid, as for spinal anesthesia.
Intubation   Insertion of an endotracheal tube.
Laryngospasm   Involuntary spasmodic reflex action that partially or completely closes the vocal cords of the larynx.
Local anesthesia   Loss of sensation along specific nerve pathways produced by blocking transmissions of impulses to receptor fibers. The anesthetic drug injected depresses sensory nerves and blocks conduction of pain impulses from their site of origin. The patient remains conscious, with or without IV sedation.
Moderate sedation   (formerly known as intravenous conscious sedation [IVCS]). Depressed level of consciousness produced by IV administration of pharmacologic agents. The patient retains the ability to continuously maintain a patent airway independently and to respond to physical or verbal stimulation. Sedation may relieve anxiety and produce amnesia. Also referred to as moderate sedation.
Narcosis   State of arrested consciousness, sensation, motor activity, and reflex action produced by drugs.

Narcotic Drug derived from opium or opium-like compounds, with potent analgesic effects associated with significant alteration of mood and behavior.

Nerve block Loss of sensation produced by injecting an anesthetic drug around a specific nerve or nerve plexus to interrupt sensory, motor, or sympathetic transmission of impulses.

Paco$_2$ Arterial carbon dioxide tension (partial pressure of carbon dioxide in arterial blood). Normal: 35 to 45 torr.

Pao$_2$ Arterial oxygen tension (partial pressure of oxygen in the arterial blood); degree of oxygen transported in the circulating blood. Normal: 80 to 100 torr.

pH Expression for hydrogen ion concentration or acidity. In blood, alkalemia: values above 7.45; acidemia: values below 7.35; normal: 7.4.

Tachycardia Excessive rapidity of heart action, heartbeat. Pulse rate is higher than 100 beats per minute.

Tachypnea Abnormally rapid rate of breathing.

Regional anesthesia Loss of sensation in a specific body part or region produced by blocking conductivity of sensory nerves supplying that area. The anesthetic drug is injected around a specific nerve or group of nerves to interrupt pain impulses. The patient remains conscious, with or without IV sedation. Regional anesthetic techniques include nerve, intrathecal, peridural, and epidural blocks.

Sedative Pharmacologic agent (drug) that suppresses nervous excitement, allays anxiety, and produces a calming effect. Benzodiazepines, barbiturates, and opioids (narcotics) are the most commonly used drugs for conscious sedation.

Spinal anesthesia Loss of sensation below the level of the diaphragm produced by intrathecal injection of an anesthetic drug into the subarachnoid space without loss of consciousness.

Topical anesthesia Depression of sensation in superficial peripheral nerves by application of an anesthetic agent directly to the mucous membrane, skin, or cornea.

SUPPLEMENTAL MATERIAL ON Evolve WEBSITE — *evolve*

http://evolve.elsevier.com/BerryKohn
- Content Updates
- Glossary
- Full Set of Perioperative Flash Cards
- Interactive Key Term Flash Cards
- Student Activities
- WebLinks

THE ART AND SCIENCE OF ANESTHESIA

Anesthesiology is the branch of medicine and nursing that is concerned with the administration of medication or anesthetic agents to relieve pain and support physiologic functions during a surgical procedure. It is a specialty that requires knowledge of biochemistry, clinical pharmacology, cardiology, and respiratory physiology. The American Society of Anesthesiologists (ASA), founded in 1905 and incorporated in 1936 has defined anesthesiology as the practice of medicine dealing with the management of procedures for rendering a patient insensible to pain during surgical procedures and with the support of life functions under the stress of anesthetic and surgical manipulations.

The purpose of this chapter is to acquaint the surgical team with several processes associated with the delivery and maintenance of anesthesia and how the team works together to provide a safe surgical procedure for the patient.

All perioperative team members should be readily available to assist the anesthesia provider as needed. Continuing education is advised for the entire team. (Internet websites included with links to educational information, such as Gas Net, http://gasnet.med.yale.edu and The Virtual Anesthesia Machine http://vam.anest.ufl.edu, are excellent free resources.) Links on the Virtual Anesthesia Machine website offer other forms of simulated learning such as difficult airway management for a signup fee.

HISTORICAL BACKGROUND

During the time of Nero (AD 37-68), Greek and Roman surgeons gave their patients a mixture of wine and vinegar. Called a "potion of the condemned," the mixture was used to relieve anguish such as that suffered during crucifixion. These surgeons also experimented with a form of local anesthesia by placing a carbonate stone directly over the surgical site and pouring vinegar over it; they noted a numbing sensation, resulting from the formation of carbon dioxide.

Sleep-producing inhalants were first used by the Egyptians and Arabs, who concocted many potions from plants such as poppy and hemlock. Sponges saturated in these solutions were held to the patient's nostrils. Death often resulted from them and from root juices used as reviving agents, because dosage was unregulated and drug action unknown. The Egyptians and Assyrians produced unconsciousness by pressing on the carotid vessels in the neck, causing cerebral anoxia.

Army surgeons have always contributed to medical advancement. Ambroise Paré (1510-1590) dulled the pain of his soldiers in the sixteenth century by compressing blood vessels and nerves near the surgical area. At this time also, half-frozen soldiers were found to have a higher pain threshold. Refrigeration anesthesia was revived in 1941 for use in amputations during World War II.

Joseph Priestley (1733-1804), an English chemist, experimented with oxygen and nitrous oxide, setting the stage for modern anesthesia. This combination and ether were first used at parties for entertainment. Traveling chemists administered these agents to induce incoherence and giddy laughter, hence the term laughing gas. The anesthetic properties were realized when injuries sustained during inhalation of these agents were not felt.

Crawford Williamson Long (1815-1878), a physician in Georgia, administered the first ether anesthetic in 1842 for the painless removal of a tumor of the neck, but he did not publish the results of this and subsequent cases until 1849. In 1846, however, two Boston dentists, William T.G. Morton and Horace Wells, used nitrous oxide for tooth extraction. In October of that year, Morton first demonstrated ether for surgical anesthesia before an astounded group of clinicians; a new era in surgery was born. Oliver Wendell Holmes (1804-1894), an American physician as well as professor of anatomy and literature, devised the term *anesthesia* from the Greek words meaning "negative sensation."

The first nurse anesthetist of record was Catherine S. Lawrence, who with other nurses gave anesthesia during the Civil War (1861-1865). According to the Anesthesia

Nursing website the first "Official Nurse Anesthetist" was Sister Mary Bernard at St. Vincent Hospital in Erie, Pennsylvania, in 1878.[1] The first school for nurse anesthesia was started in 1909 in Portland, Oregon, by Agnes McGee. The coursework was 6 months in duration and sparked the opening of 19 additional schools between 1912 and 1920. Many physicians attended these schools because few physician-oriented schools were available.

Sir James Simpson (1811-1870), a Scottish obstetrician, instituted the use of chloroform anesthesia in 1847. In the late nineteenth and twentieth centuries, surgical procedures within the abdomen, thorax, and cranium evolved with administration of ether and chloroform for anesthesia as demonstrated by John Snow (1813-1858), an English physician and epidemiologist. He administered chloroform to Queen Victoria during childbirth. Development of the surgical specialties was concurrent with the refinement of anesthesia methods and instrumentation.

Purification of drugs such as morphine, the invention of the hollow needle in the 1850s, and the development of gas machines hastened the finding of new anesthetic techniques and agents. Endotracheal anesthesia, first used by open tracheotomy, was developed by German physician Friedrich Trendelenburg (1844-1924). The development of the laryngoscope by American laryngologist Chevalier Jackson (1865-1949) greatly aided intubation.

American surgeons George Crile (1864-1943) and Harvey Cushing (1869-1939) developed methods for monitoring and supporting the patient's physiology during anesthesia. Agatha Hodgkins, RN, was Dr. Crile's nurse anesthetist. Hodgkins opened Lakeside Hospital School of Anesthesia in Cleveland, Ohio, under the direction or Dr. Crile for the administration of newer, and perhaps, safer inhalants, such as nitrous oxide. Hodgkins was later responsible for the first meeting of the American Association of Nurse Anesthetists (AANA) in 1931. The purpose of the meeting was to establish a national qualifying examination and creating a stand for accreditation of nurse anesthesia schools. The first examination took place in 1945, and standardized accreditation began in 1952.

Crile's studies on surgical shock and blood pressure emphasized the importance of keeping accurate records of the patient's condition during the surgical procedure. He found that ether and chloroform could lead to surgical shock and preferred nitrous oxide.

In 1896 Cushing brought to the United States from Italy one of the first sphygmomanometers invented and founded the basis for opioid administration during (unconscious/unaware) anesthesia.

The use of muscle-paralyzing agents, such as curare in 1942 in Montreal, required the use of endotracheal intubation for safe administration. Education and qualifications of anesthesia providers included the complexities of respiratory physiology. Postanesthesia care units (PACUs) were developed to monitor the patient who had received general anesthesia. Special techniques such as hypothermia and extracorporeal circulation opened new vistas. Complex

---

[1]www.anesthesia-nursing.com. A good site for anesthesia nursing history and photographs.

BOX 24-1	ASA Classifications

- Class I theoretically includes relatively healthy patients with localized pathologic processes. An emergency surgical procedure, designated E, signifies additional risk. For example, a hernia that becomes incarcerated changes the patient's status to class I-E.
- Class II includes patients with mild systemic disease (e.g., diabetes mellitus controlled by oral hypoglycemic agents or diet).
- Class III includes patients with severe systemic disease that limits activity but is not totally incapacitating (e.g., chronic obstructive pulmonary disease or severe hypertension).
- Class IV includes patients with an incapacitating disease that is a constant threat to life (e.g., cardiovascular or renal disease).
- Class V includes moribund patients who are not expected to survive 24 hours with or without the surgical procedure. They are operated on in an attempt to save their life; the surgical procedure is a resuscitative measure, as in a massive pulmonary embolus. The patient may or may not survive the surgical procedure.
- Class VI includes patients who have been declared brain dead but whose organs will be removed for donor purposes. Mechanical ventilation and life support systems are maintained until the organs are procured.

procedures lasting 6 to 24 hours are not uncommon using these techniques.

Salient features of modern anesthesia include assessment of patients preoperatively; selection of appropriate agents and techniques; management of induction, maintenance, and emergence processes; and continuous monitoring of vital functions during anesthesia. ASA and AANA have established guidelines and standards for safely administering and monitoring anesthesia care. ASA also developed the taxonomy for classifying patients by physical status from class I, the lowest risk, to class VI, the highest risk (Box 24-1). Historically, specialists in anesthesia have been advocates of patient safety and risk management.

With the proliferation of pain clinics, anesthesia providers are essential members of multidisciplinary teams concerned with management of acute and chronic pain. Because of their familiarity with anesthetic drugs, nerve pathways, and nerve block techniques, anesthesia providers are well qualified to assess and treat pain. Pain management is discussed in greater detail in Chapter 30.

TYPES OF ANESTHESIA

Anesthesia may be produced in a number of ways:

- General anesthesia: Pain is controlled by general insensibility. Basic elements include loss of consciousness, analgesia, interference with undesirable reflexes, and muscle relaxation.
- Balanced anesthesia: The properties of general anesthesia (i.e., hypnosis, analgesia, and muscle relaxation) are produced, in varying degrees, by a combination of agents. Each agent has a specific purpose. This often is referred to as neuroleptanesthesia.
- Local or regional block anesthesia: Pain is controlled without loss of consciousness. The sensory nerves in one area or region of the body are anesthetized. This is

- sometimes called conduction anesthesia. Acupuncture is sometimes used.
- Spinal or epidural anesthesia: Sensation of pain is blocked at a level below the diaphragm without loss of consciousness. The agent is injected in the spinal canal.

CHOICE OF ANESTHESIA

Selection of anesthesia is made by the anesthesia provider in consultation with the surgeon and the patient. The primary consideration with any anesthetic is that it should be associated with low morbidity and mortality. Choosing the safest agent and technique is a decision predicated on thorough knowledge, sound judgment, and evaluation of each individual situation. The anesthesia provider uses the lowest concentration of anesthetic agents compatible with patient analgesia, relaxation, and facilitation of the surgical procedure. An ideal anesthetic agent or technique suitable for all patients does not exist, but the one selected should include the following characteristics:

- Provide maximum safety for the patient
- Provide optimal operating conditions for the surgeon
- Provide patient comfort
- Have a low index of toxicity
- Provide potent, predictable analgesia extending into the postoperative period
- Produce adequate muscle relaxation
- Provide amnesia
- Have a rapid onset and easy reversibility
- Produce minimum side effects

The patient's ability to tolerate stress and adverse effects of anesthesia and the surgical procedure depends on respiration; circulation; and function of the liver, kidneys, endocrine system, and central nervous system (CNS). The following factors are important:

- Age, size, and weight of the patient
- Physical, mental, and emotional status of the patient
- Presence of complicating systemic disease or concurrent drug therapy
- Presence of infection at the site of the surgical procedure
- Previous anesthesia experience
- Anticipated procedure
- Position required for the procedure
- Type and expected length of the procedure
- Local or systemic toxicity of the agent
- Expertise of the anesthesia provider
- Preference of the surgeon and patient

ANESTHESIA STATE

Both the central and the autonomic nervous systems play essential roles in clinical anesthesia. The CNS exerts powerful control throughout the body. The effect of anesthetic drugs is one of progressive depression of the CNS, beginning with the higher centers of the cerebral cortex and ending with the vital centers in the medulla. The cerebral cortex is not inactive during deep anesthesia. Afferent impulses continue to flow into the cortex along primary pathways and to excite cells in appropriate sensory areas. Also, the cerebral cortex is integrated with the reticular system. The brain represents approximately 2% of body weight but receives about 15% of cardiac output. Various factors cause alterations in cerebral blood flow and are of considerable importance in anesthesia. These factors are oxygen, carbon dioxide, temperature, arterial blood pressure, drugs, the age of the patient, anesthetic techniques, and neurogenic factors.

The autonomic nervous system is equally important because of its role in the physiology of the cardiovascular system, the anesthesia provider's ability to block certain autonomic pathways with local analgesic agents, specific blocking effects of certain drugs, and the sympathomimetic and parasympathomimetic effects of many anesthetic agents.

The anesthesia state involves control of motor, sensory, mental, and reflex functions. The anesthesia provider constantly assesses the patient's response to stimuli to evaluate specific anesthetic requirements. Specific drugs are used to achieve the desired results: amnesia, analgesia, and muscle relaxation.

KNOWLEDGE OF ANESTHETICS

Anesthesia involves the administration of potentially lethal drugs and gases. Interactions of these with human physiology can be profound. Using discerning observation, astute deduction, and meticulous attention to the minutiae, the anesthesia provider provides skilled induction, careful maintenance of anesthesia, and prophylaxis to avoid postoperative complications. Being responsible for vital functions of the patient, the anesthesia provider must know physical and chemical properties of all gases and liquids used in anesthesia. These properties determine how agents are supplied, their stability, systems used for their administration, and their uptake and distribution in the body. Important factors are diffusion, solubility in body fluids, and relationships of pressure, volume, and temperature. The synthesized general anesthetic agents are nonflammable, in contrast with the older agents.

Perioperative and PACU nurses need to be cognizant of the pharmacologic characteristics of the most commonly used anesthetics and techniques. Anesthesia and surgical trauma produce multiple systemic effects, which are continually monitored throughout the perioperative care period. The type and level of anesthesia will vary according to the type of surgery being performed. These types are described as follows:

1. *Minimal or light sedation (anxiolysis):* A drug-induced state during which patients respond normally to verbal command. Although cognitive function and coordination may be impaired, ventilatory and cardiovascular functions are unaffected.
2. *Moderate sedation/analgesia (formerly known as conscious sedation):* A drug-induced depression of consciousness during which patients can respond purposefully to verbal commands, either alone or accompanied by light tactile stimulation. No interventions are required to maintain a patent airway, and spontaneous ventilation is adequate.
3. *Deep sedation/analgesia:* A drug-induced depression of consciousness during which patients cannot be easily aroused but respond purposefully after repeated or painful stimulation. The ability to independently maintain ventilatory function may be impaired. Patients may require assistance to maintain a patent airway, and spontaneous ventilation may be inadequate.

4. *Full anesthesia:* General anesthesia and regional anesthesia. General anesthesia is a drug-induced loss of consciousness during which patients cannot be roused, even by painful stimulation. The ability to independently maintain ventilatory function is often impaired. Patients often require assistance to maintain a patent airway, and positive pressure ventilation may be required because of depressed spontaneous ventilation or drug-induced depression of neuromuscular function. Cardiovascular function may be impaired.

GENERAL ANESTHESIA

Anesthesia is produced as the CNS is affected. Association pathways are broken in the cerebral cortex to produce more or less complete lack of sensory perception and motor discharge. Unconsciousness is produced when blood circulating to the brain contains an adequate amount of the anesthetic agent. General anesthesia results in an unconscious, immobile, quiet patient who does not recall the surgical procedure.

Most anesthetic agents are potentially lethal. The anesthesia provider must constantly observe the body's reflex responses to stimuli and other guides to determine the degree of CNS, respiratory, and circulatory depression during induction and the surgical procedure. No one clinical sign can be used as a reliable indication of anesthesia depth. Continuous watching and appraisal of all clinical signs, in addition to other available objective measurements, are necessary. In this way the anesthesia provider judges the level of anesthesia, referred to as light, moderate, or deep, and provides the patient with optimal care (Table 24-1).

The three methods of administering general anesthetic are inhalation, IV injection, and rectal instillation. The latter method is not commonly used, except occasionally in pediatrics, because retention and absorption in the colon is unpredictable. Control of each method varies.

Induction of General Anesthesia

Induction involves putting the patient safely into a state of unconsciousness. Figure 24-1 depicts the levels of unconsciousness associated with general anesthesia. A patent airway and adequate ventilation must be ensured. If one is not already running, an intravenous (IV) infusion is started. The anesthesia provider should wear gloves for venipuncture. A nasogastric tube may be inserted to decompress the gastrointestinal tract and evacuate stomach contents.

Preoxygenation. The anesthesia provider may have the patient breathe pure (100%) oxygen by facemask for a few minutes. This provides a margin of safety in the event of airway obstruction or apnea during induction, with resultant hypoxia.

Loss of Consciousness. Unconsciousness is induced by IV administration of a drug or by inhalation of an agent mixed with oxygen. Because the technique is rapid and simple, an IV drug usually is preferred by anesthesia providers and often is requested by patients.

Intubation. A patent airway must be established to provide adequate oxygenation and to control breathing of the unconscious patient. The patient's tongue and secretions can obstruct respiration in the absence of protective reflexes. The anesthesia provider evaluates the airway for the risk of difficult intubation using the Mallampati classification chart (Fig. 24-2). Other measurements include thryomental distance, neck flexion/extension range, and the ability to prognath (protrude the mandible). An oropharygeal airway, nasopharyngeal airway, laryngeal mask, endotracheal tube, or endobronchial tube (for lung procedures) may be inserted.

TABLE 24-1	Depth of General Anesthesia		
From	To	Patient's Responses	Patient Care Considerations
Induction of general anesthesia and beginning and/or IV drug of inhalant	Begins to lose consciousness; will have recall. Bispectral state 100	Drowsy, dizzy, amnesic	Close OR doors. Keep room quiet. Stand by to assist. Initiate cricoid pressure if requested.
Loss of consciousness: excitement phase	Relaxation, light hypnosis; low probability of recall. Bispectral state 70 to 50	May be excited, with irregular breathing and movements of extremities; susceptible to external stimuli (e.g., noise, touch)	Restrain patient. Remain at patient's side, quietly, but ready to assist anesthesia provider as needed.
Surgical anesthesia stage of relaxation	Loss of reflexes: depression of vital functions. Bispectral state 40: maintenance range	Regular respiration; contracted pupils; reflexes disappear; muscles relax; auditory sensation lost	Position patient and prepare skin only when anesthesia provider indicates this stage is reached and under control.
Danger stage: vital functions too depressed	Respiratory failure; possible cardiac arrest. Bispectral state 0	Not breathing; little or no pulse or heartbeat	Prepare for cardiopulmonary resuscitation.

IV, Intravenous; *OR,* operating room.

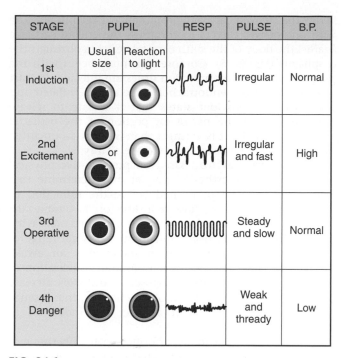

STAGE	PUPIL		RESP	PULSE	B.P.
	Usual size	Reaction to light			
1st Induction				Irregular	Normal
2nd Excitement	or			Irregular and fast	High
3rd Operative				Steady and slow	Normal
4th Danger				Weak and thready	Low

FIG. 24-1   Levels of unconsciousness associated with general anesthesia.

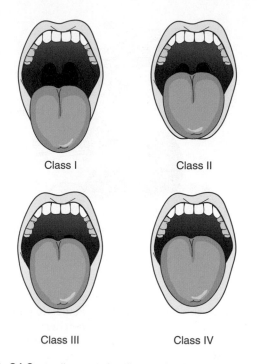

Class I   Class II

Class III   Class IV

FIG. 24-2   Mallampati classification for difficult intubation.

Physiologic indicators of a difficult airway include the following:

- Inability to open the mouth. Patients with previous jaw surgery may have jaw wires in place. Wire cutters should be immediately available in the event of a return to surgery.
- Immobility of the cervical spine. Patients with vertebral disease or injury may not have full range of motion necessary for intubation.
- Chin or jaw deformities. Patients with small jaws or chin may have a difficult airway. Edentulous patients commonly have some bone loss that alters facial contours.
- Dentition can be an issue if the patient has loose teeth or periodontal disease. A tooth can be aspirated during the airway maintenance process.
- Short neck or morbid obesity (Fig. 24-3).
- Pathology of the head and neck such as tumors or deformity. An enlarged tongue can be an obstruction to a full view of the glottis.

- Previous tracheostomy scar, which can cause a stricture.
- Trauma.

Intubation is insertion of an endotracheal tube between vocal cords, usually with an oral tube by direct laryngoscopy. A nasotracheal tube may be inserted by blind intubation or with a direct approach using Magill forceps to guide the tube through the pharynx (Fig. 24-4). Epistaxis can be a complication of nasal airway use. This method is contraindicated in anticoagulated patients. Tubes may be made of metal, plastic, silicone, or rubber. Most styles for adult sizes have a built-in cuff that is inflated with a measured amount of air, water, or saline after insertion, to completely occlude the trachea.

The anesthesia provider is informed if a laser will be used in the mouth or throat so that a laser-resistant endotracheal tube can be inserted. The endotracheal tube must be securely fixed in place to prevent irritation of the trachea and to maintain ventilation. The anesthesia provider should wear a mask and protective eyewear to prevent secretions from splashing in the eyes during intubation. An oropharyngeal suction tip and tubing should be kept close at hand.

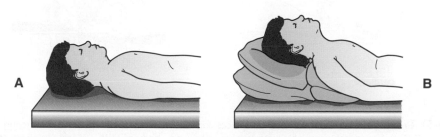

FIG. 24-3   Short neck or morbid obesity. **A,** Supine position. **B,** Sniffing position.

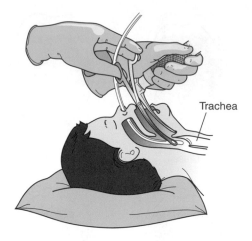

FIG. 24-4 Nasotracheal intubation with a Magill forceps.

Neuromuscular blocking agents are given before intubation to relax the jaw and larynx. Pediatric patients and patients susceptible to malignant hyperthermia may experience jaw tightness, which is referred to as masseter muscle rigidity (MMR) or trismus. Intubation during induction and extubation during emergence from anesthesia are precarious times for the patient. The patient may cough, jerk, or experience laryngospasm from tracheal stimulation. Cardiac dysrhythmias may occur. Hypoxia is a potential complication. Hypoxia commonly precedes dysrhythmia.

Aspiration is also a hazard, particularly in a patient with a full stomach or with increased intraabdominal or intracranial pressure. Any patient who arrives in operating room (OR) unconscious or who is a victim of trauma should be treated as though he or she has a full stomach. Pregnant patients and obese patients should also be considered in this category because of increased intraabdominal pressure in the supine position and possible decreased gastric motility.

Cricoid Pressure. The circulating nurse may be asked to apply pressure to the cricoid cartilage to occlude the esophagus and immobilize the trachea. Referred to as the Sellick's maneuver, this action prevents regurgitation and aspiration of stomach contents. The cricoid cartilage forms a complete ring around the inferior wall of the larynx below the thyroid cartilage prominence. Exerting pressure with one or two fingers to compress the cricoid cartilage against the body of the sixth cervical vertebra obstructs the esophagus (Fig. 24-5). Compression must begin with the patient awake before induction drugs are injected. It must continue until the endotracheal tube cuff is inflated and the anesthesia provider states that it is safe to release pressure. This is the narrowest portion of the pediatric airway. If the patient is younger than 8 years, an uncuffed tube is used to prevent damage to the airway.

Awake Intubation. Based on preoperative physical assessment, the anesthesia provider may determine that intubation must be performed before the induction of general anesthesia (i.e., "awake intubation"). Acromegaly, an anterior larynx, an enlarged tongue, a limited oral cavity, jaw fixation, a short neck, and limited cervical range of motion are the most common indications for awake intubation. These conditions may inhibit visualization of the vocal cords by direct laryngoscopy and thus increase the potential risk of airway obstruction in the absence of protective reflexes, such as after the induction of anesthesia.

Awake intubation can be performed with a fiberoptic or rigid laryngoscope for direct visualization of vocal cords after the administration of IV sedation and application of a topical spray anesthetic to the posterior pharynx. The anesthesia provider may inject a local anesthetic around the laryngeal nerve to suppress the patient's gag and cough reflex. Usually two anesthesia providers work together during awake intubation. After the patient is sedated and the topical anesthetic agent is applied, one anesthesia provider inserts the endotracheal or nasotracheal tube as the second anesthesia provider gives a rapid-acting barbiturate to induce general anesthesia.

Key Points During Induction. Induction of general anesthesia is a crucial period requiring maximum attention from the OR team. The following key points are critical to the patient's welfare:

1. The circulating nurse should remain at the patient's side during induction to provide physical protection and emotional support, assist the anesthesia provider as needed, and closely observe the monitors.

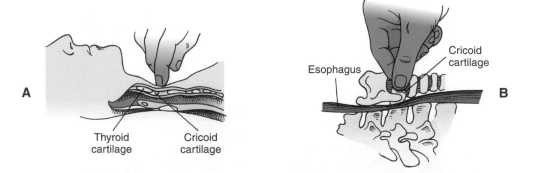

FIG. 24-5 Cricoid pressure. **A,** Index finger displaces cricoid cartilage posteriorly, thus obstructing esophagus. **B,** Two-finger technique obstructs esophagus between body of sixth cervical vertebra and cricoid cartilage.

2. Although induction is quiet and uneventful for most patients, untoward occurrences are possible. Excitement, coughing, breath holding, retching, vomiting, irregular respiratory patterns, or laryngospasm can lead to hypoxia. Secretions in air passages from irritation by the anesthetic can cause obstruction and dysrhythmias. Induction is gentle and not so rapid as to cause physiologic insult. To prevent these events, the patient must not be stimulated. (Avoid venting steam from the sterilizer in the adjacent substerile room, clattering instruments, or opening paper wrappers. Do not move or begin prepping the patient until the anesthesia provider says it is safe to do so.)

3. Precautions to be taken during induction include continuous electrocardiogram (ECG) monitoring, use of a precordial chest stethoscope, and having resuscitative equipment, including a defibrillator, readily available.

4. Induction is individualized. For example, an obese or pregnant patient may be induced with the head raised slightly to avoid pressure of the abdominal viscera against the diaphragm. The patient is placed flat, however, if the blood pressure begins to drop.

5. Small children need gentle handling. The circulating nurse can help the anesthesia provider make the induction period less frightening by staying close to the child. Sometimes a drop of artificial flavoring (e.g., orange, peppermint) put inside the facemask facilitates the child's acceptance of it. Parents are often allowed in for induction according to the institution's policy. After induction, the parent is escorted back to the waiting area.

6. The speed of induction depends on the potency of the agent, administration technique, partial pressure administered, and the rate at which the anesthetic is taken up by blood and tissues.

Maintenance of General Anesthesia

The anesthesia provider attempts to maintain the lightest level of anesthesia in the brain compatible with operating conditions. The following are five objectives of general anesthesia:

1. *Oxygenation:* Tissues, especially the brain, must be continuously perfused with oxygenated blood. The color of the blood, amount and kind of bleeding, and pulse oximetry are indicators of the adequacy of oxygenation. Controls on the anesthesia machine and monitors of vital functions keep the anesthesia provider aware of the patient's condition.

2. *Unconsciousness:* The patient remains asleep and unaware of the environment during the surgical procedure.

3. *Analgesia:* The patient must be free of pain during the surgical procedure.

4. *Muscle relaxation:* Muscle relaxation must be constantly assessed to provide necessary amounts of drugs that cause skeletal muscles to relax. Less tissue manipulation is required when muscles are relaxed.

5. *Control of autonomic reflexes:* Anesthetic agents affect cardiovascular and respiratory systems. Tissue manipulations and systemic reactions to them may be altered by drugs that control the autonomic nervous system.

Anesthesia Machine. General anesthesia is maintained by inhalation of gases and IV injection of drugs. An anesthesia machine is always used to deliver oxygen-anesthetic mixtures to the patient through a breathing system.

The anesthesia machine includes sources of oxygen and gases with flowmeters for measuring and controlling their delivery; devices to volatilize and deliver liquid anesthetics; a gas-driven mechanical ventilator; devices for monitoring the electrocardiogram (ECG), blood pressure, inspired oxygen, and end-tidal carbon dioxide; and alarm systems to signal apnea or disconnection of the breathing circuit. Breathing tubes of corrugated rubber or plastic carry gases from the machine to the facemask and breathing system. The reservoir (breathing) bag compensates for variations in respiratory demand and permits assisted or controlled ventilation by manual or mechanical compression of the bag. Sterile disposable sets containing tubing, a mask, a Y-connector, and a reservoir bag are commercially available in conductive and nonconductive materials.

Machine design includes fail-safe alarm systems to prevent delivery of a hypoxic gas mixture and to reduce the possibility of human error or mechanical failure. Reference to a daily machine performance checklist by the anesthesia provider before induction should be routine as recommended by the U.S. Food and Drug Administration (FDA) in 1986. Studies have shown that many complications associated with the administration of anesthetic could have been avoided if the equipment had been checked before use.

All anesthesia machines have the following features (Fig. 24-6):

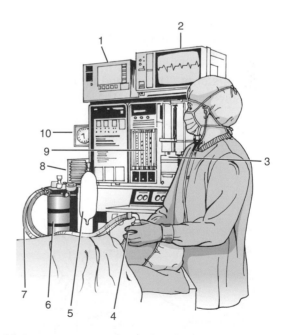

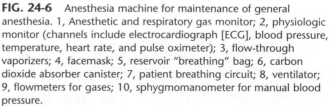

FIG. 24-6 Anesthesia machine for maintenance of general anesthesia. 1, Anesthetic and respiratory gas monitor; 2, physiologic monitor (channels include electrocardiograph [ECG], blood pressure, temperature, heart rate, and pulse oximeter); 3, flow-through vaporizers; 4, facemask; 5, reservoir "breathing" bag; 6, carbon dioxide absorber canister; 7, patient breathing circuit; 8, ventilator; 9, flowmeters for gases; 10, sphygmomanometer for manual blood pressure.

1. Sources of oxygen and compressed gases (Fig. 24-7). These may come from piped-in systems, but mounted oxygen tanks are necessary in the event of failure of systems.
2. Means for measuring (flowmeters) and controlling (reservoir bag) delivery of gases.
3. Means to volatilize liquid (vaporizer) and deliver (breathing tubes) anesthetic vapor or gas.
4. Device for disposal of carbon dioxide (carbon dioxide absorption canister).
5. Safety devices:
   a. Oxygen analyzers
   b. Oxygen pressure interlock system or equivalent to automatically shut off the flow of gases in the absence of oxygen pressure
   c. End-tidal carbon dioxide monitors
   d. Pressure and disconnect alarms to notify the anesthesia provider if the flow of oxygen and gases becomes disproportional
   e. Pin-index safety system to release excess gases
   f. Gas scavenger system to collect exhaled gases

Waste Gases. The elimination of waste gas, vented through an exhaust valve into a waste gas scavenger system, controls pollution of the room air. Nitrous oxide and halogenated agents can escape into room air if they are not directed through the scavenger system. Substantial amounts may be an occupational health hazard to OR team members. Valves on the machine and tubing connections should be checked daily and must be secure for the system to work properly. Room air should be monitored. This may be done by an infrared spectrophotometer, for example, to monitor the escape of gases from the patient's exhalations and from the anesthetic delivery system. Passive dosimeters may be used to monitor air in team members' personal breathing spaces.

Inhalation Systems. The method for administration of inhalation anesthetics through the anesthesia machine

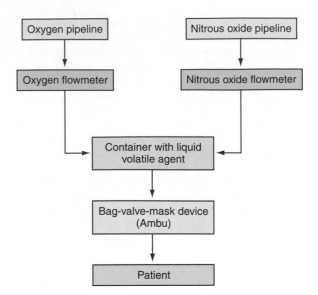

FIG. 24-7   Minimum number of components needed for an anesthesia gas machine.

can be classified as semiclosed, closed, semiopen, or open (Fig. 24-8):

- *Semiclosed system:* The most widely used system, a semiclosed system permits exhaled gases to pass into the atmosphere so that they will not mix with fresh gases and be rebreathed. A chemical absorber for carbon dioxide is placed in the breathing circuit. This reduces carbon dioxide accumulation in blood. Induction is slower but with less loss of heat and water vapor than with open methods.
- *Closed system:* A closed system allows complete rebreathing of expired gases. Exhaled carbon dioxide is absorbed by soda lime or a mixture of barium and calcium hydroxide (Baralyme) in the absorber on the machine. The body's metabolic demand for oxygen is

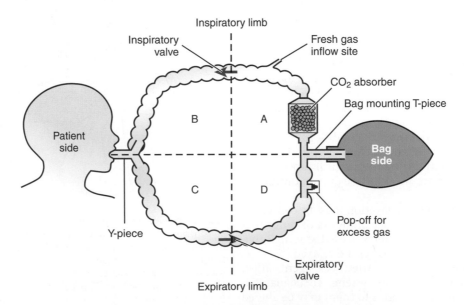

FIG. 24-8   Complete anesthesia breathing circuit.

met by adding oxygen to the inspired mixture of gases or vapors. This system provides maximal conservation of heat and moisture. It reduces the amount and therefore the cost of agents and reduces environmental contamination.

- *Semiopen system:* With the semiopen system some exhaled gas can pass into surrounding air but some returns to the inspiratory part of the circuit for rebreathing. The degree of rebreathing is determined by the volume of flow of fresh gas. Expired carbon dioxide is not chemically absorbed.
- *Open system:* In an open system, valves direct expired gases into the lower portion of the canister, where they are removed by vacuum. The patient inhales only the anesthetic mixture delivered by the anesthesia machine. The composition of the inspired mixture can be accurately determined. However, anesthetic gases are not confined to the breathing system. High flows of gases are necessary, because resistance to breathing varies. Water vapor and heat are lost. Inspired gases should be humidified for respiratory mucosa to function properly, especially for children and during long surgical procedures.

Administration Techniques. Inhalation gases and vapors can be delivered from an anesthesia machine via a facemask, laryngeal mask, or endotracheal tube. Respirations must be assisted or controlled.

Mask Inhalation. Anesthetic gas or vapor of a volatile liquid is inhaled through a facemask attached to the anesthesia machine by breathing tubes. The mask must fit the face tightly to minimize escape of gases into room air. Significant leakage occurs around an ill-fitting mask, particularly in the area above the nose. Several sizes should be available.

Laryngeal Mask. An airway can be maintained by inserting a laryngeal mask into the larynx. This flexible tube has an inflatable silicone ring and cuff. When the cuff is inflated, the mask fills the space around and behind the larynx to form a seal between the tube and the trachea. The method does not protect against regurgitation and aspiration. Reusable and disposable styles are commercially available (Fig. 24-9). The mask is selected for use by size of the patient as follows:

- Size 1: 0 to 6.5 kg
- Size 2: 6.5 to 20 kg

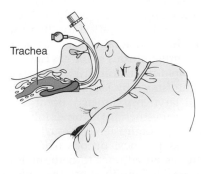

FIG. 24-9 Laryngeal mask airway.

- Size 2.5: 20 to 30 kg
- Size 3: 30 to 70 kg
- Size 4: 70 to 80 kg
- Size 5: 80 kg or greater

Endotracheal Administration. Anesthetic vapor or gas is inhaled directly into the trachea through a nasal or oral tube inserted between the vocal cords by direct laryngoscopy. The tube is securely fixed in place to minimize tissue trauma. The patient is given oxygen before and after suctioning of a tracheal tube. Advantages of endotracheal administration are the following:

- It ensures a patent airway and control of respiration. Secretions are easily removed from the trachea by suctioning. Positive pressure can be given immediately by pressing the reservoir bag on the machine without danger of dilating the stomach.
- It protects the lungs from aspiration of blood, vomitus of gastric contents, or foreign material.
- It preserves the airway regardless of the patient's position during the surgical procedure.
- It interferes minimally with the surgical field during head and neck procedures.
- It helps minimize the escape of vapors or gases into the room atmosphere.

Intubation and extubation can cause tracheal stimulation. The patient may cough, jerk, or develop spasms of the larynx (laryngospasm). Other potential complications of endotracheal administration include the following:

- *Trauma to the teeth, pharynx, vocal cords, or trachea:* Postoperatively the patient may experience sore throat, hoarseness, laryngitis, and/or tracheitis. Laryngeal edema is more common in children than in adults. Ulceration of the tracheal mucosa or vocal cords may cause granuloma.
- *Cardiac dysrhythmias:* Cardiac dysrhythmias may occur in light anesthesia or be caused by suctioning through the endotracheal tube.
- *Hypoxia and hypoxemia:* Hypoxia is a common complication during intubation and extubation. Endotracheal tube suctioning can cause hypoxemia.
- *Accidental esophageal or endobronchial intubation:* The latter results in ventilation of only one lung.
- *Aspiration of gastrointestinal contents:* This is a hazard in a patient with a full stomach or a patient who has increased intraabdominal or intracranial pressure. It can also occur in a patient with intestinal obstruction who is extubated before protective reflexes return.

Controlled Respiration. Respirations may be assisted or controlled. Assistance, to improve ventilation, may easily be given by manual pressure on the reservoir (breathing) bag of the anesthesia machine. Assisted respiration implies that the patient's own respiratory effort initiates the cycle. Controlled respiration may be defined as the completely controlled rate and volume of respirations. The latter is best accomplished by means of a mechanical device that automatically and rhythmically inflates the lungs with intermittent positive pressure, requiring no effort by the patient. Gas moves in and out of the lungs. The combination of a volume preset ventilator with an assist mechanism maintains the integrity of the respiratory center. Controlled respiration is initiated after the anesthesia provider has produced apnea by hyperventilation or administration of respiratory depressant drugs or a neuromuscular blocker.

Controlled ventilation is used in all types of surgical procedures, especially in lengthy ones. The anesthesia provider's artificial control of respiration or the patient's respiratory efforts influence the minute-to-minute level of anesthesia. Advantages of controlled respiration are the following:

- It provides for optimal ventilation.
- It allows for selective lung deflation for thoracic procedures.
- It provides access to deep regions of the thorax and upper abdomen.
- It permits deliberate production of apnea to facilitate surgical manipulation below the diaphragm, ligation of deep vessels, or obtaining radiographic films.

The patient is taken off the respirator gradually near the end of the surgical procedure, and spontaneous respiration resumes. Assisted ventilation may be continued postoperatively after lengthy procedures until reflexes and spontaneous respirations return.

Inhalation Anesthetic Agents. Inhalation is a controllable method of administration because uptake and elimination of anesthetic agents are accomplished mainly by pulmonary ventilation and selective organ metabolism. The anesthetic vapor of a volatile liquid or an anesthetic gas is inhaled and carried into the bloodstream by passing across the alveolar membrane into the general circulation and on to the tissues.

Ventilation and pulmonary circulation are two critical factors involved in the process. Each can be affected by components of the anesthetic experience, such as a change in body position, preanesthetic medication, alteration in body temperature, or respiratory gas tensions.

In inhalation anesthesia, the aim is to establish balance between the content of the anesthetic vapor or gas inhaled and that of body tissues. The blood and lungs function as the transport system. Anesthesia is produced by the development of an anesthetizing concentration of anesthetic in the brain. The depth of anesthesia is related to concentration and biotransformation (see Table 24-1).

Pulmonary blood-gas exchange is important to tissue perfusion. Defective gas exchange can cause hypoxemia and respiratory failure. It also interferes with delivery of the anesthetic. Potent inhalation agents, such as myocardial depressants, affect oxygenation. Most of them induce a dose-related hypoventilation. The deeper the anesthesia, the more depressed ventilation becomes. Surgical stimulation partially corrects depression, but respiration must be controlled to keep oxygen and carbon dioxide exchange constant to prevent hypoventilation and cardiac depression.

Although the respiratory system is employed for distribution of the anesthetic, it also must carry on its normal function of ventilation (i.e., meeting tissue demands for adequate oxygenation and elimination of carbon dioxide and helping maintain normal acid-base balance). The amount of anesthetic vapor inspired is influenced by the volume and rate of respirations. Gas or vapor concentration and the rate of delivery are also significant. Pulmonary

circulation is the vehicle for oxygen and anesthetic transport to the general circulation. The large absorptive surface of the lungs and their extensive microcirculation provide a large gas-exchanging surface. In optimal gas exchange, all alveoli share inspired gas and cardiac output equally (ventilation-perfusion match). Because respiratory and anesthetic gases interact with pulmonary circulation, alveolar anesthetic concentrations are rapidly reflected in circulating blood.

Alveolar concentration results from a balance between two forces: ventilation that delivers the anesthetic to the alveoli and uptake that removes the anesthetic from the alveoli. Certain factors influence uptake of the anesthetic and thus induction and recovery. Uptake has two phases:

1. *Transfer of anesthetic from alveoli to blood:* The rate of transfer is determined by the solubility of the agent in the blood, the rate of pulmonary blood flow (related to cardiac output), and the partial pressure of the anesthetic in arterial and mixed venous blood.
2. *Transfer of anesthetic from blood to tissues:* Factors influencing uptake by individual tissues are similar to those for uptake by blood. They are the solubility of the gas in tissues, the tissue volume relative to the blood flow (flow rate), and the partial pressure of the anesthetic in arterial blood and tissues. Tissues differ, thus uptake of the anesthetic differs. Highly perfused tissues (heart) equilibrate more rapidly with arterial tension than does poorly perfused tissue (fat), which has a slow rise to equilibrium and retains anesthetic longer.

Elimination of the anesthetic is affected by the same factors that affected uptake. As an anesthetic is eliminated, its partial pressure in arterial blood drops first, followed by that in tissues.

The most important factors influencing safe administration of any anesthetic are the knowledge and skill of the anesthesia provider. A perfect agent has not been found, and no agent is entirely safe. Commonly used agents are listed in Table 24-2. Advantages and disadvantages are relative.

Synthesis of potent, nonflammable, halogenated, volatile liquids has replaced cyclopropane and ether, which are highly flammable agents. All inhalation agents are administered with oxygen. Volatile liquids are vaporized for inhalation by oxygen, which acts as a carrier, flowing over or bubbling through liquid in the vaporizer on the anesthesia machine. The oxygen picks up 0.25% to 5% concentration of the halogenated agent. Known sensitivity to halogenated agents or a history significant for the risk of malignant hyperthermia is a contraindication for their use.

Nitrous Oxide. Generally used as a nonvolatile adjunct to an IV drug, nitrous oxide gas can be inhaled for a comfortable, rapid induction. It has a pleasant, fruitlike odor and is administered by facemask. Relaxation is poor. Excitement and laryngospasm may occur. It is the only true gas in use for anesthesia. The other inhalants used are liquid volatile drugs administered through a vaporizer.

Because it lacks potency, nitrous oxide is rarely used alone but rather as an adjunct to barbiturates, narcotics, and other IV drugs. In combination, the concentration of potent drug is reduced, thereby lessening circulatory and

TABLE 24-2	Most Commonly Used General Anesthetic Agents

Generic Name	Trade Name	Administration	Characteristics	Uses
INHALATION AGENTS				
Nitrous oxide	None	Inhalation	Inorganic nonvolatile gas; slight potency; pleasant, fruitlike odor; nonirritating; nonflammable but supports combustion; poor muscle relaxation	Rapid induction and recovery; short procedures when muscle relaxation unimportant; adjunct to potent agents. Should be mixed with 30% oxygen to prevent hypoxia.
Halothane	Fluothane	Inhalation	Halogenated volatile liquid; potent; pleasant odor; nonirritating; cardiovascular and respiratory depressant; incomplete muscle relaxation; potentially toxic to liver	Rapid induction; wide spectrum for maintenance; depth of anesthesia easily altered; rapid reversal. Rarely used.
Enflurane	Ethrane	Inhalation	Halogenated ether; potent; some muscle relaxation; respiratory depressant	Rapid induction and recovery; wide spectrum for maintenance. Rarely used.
Desflurane	Suprane	Inhalation	Halogenated liquid with low solubility, desflurane has faster uptake by inhalation and elimination	Not used for induction with children. Can be used for maintenance in adults and children.
Sevoflurane	Ultane	Inhalation	Volatile liquid form, nonflammable and nonexplosive; noted for its rapid induction and rapid emergence qualities	Used for adults and children. Rapid elimination.
Isoflurane	Forane	Inhalation	Halogenated methyl ether; potent; muscle relaxant; profound respiratory depressant; metabolized in liver	Rapid induction and recovery with minimal aftereffects; wide spectrum for maintenance.
INTRAVENOUS AGENTS				
Thiopental sodium	Pentothal sodium	Intravenous	Barbiturate; potent; short acting with cumulative effect; rapid uptake by circulatory system; no muscle relaxation; respiratory depressant	Rapid induction and recovery; short procedures when muscle relaxation not needed; basal anesthetic.
Methohexital	Brevital	Intravenous	Barbiturate; potent; circulatory and respiratory depressant	Rapid induction; brief anesthesia.
Propofol	Diprivan	Intravenous	Alkylphenol; potent short-acting sedative-hypnotic; cardiovascular depressant	Rapid induction and recovery; short procedures alone; prolonged anesthesia in combination with inhalation agents or opioids.
Ketamine	Ketaject, Ketalar	Intravenous, intramuscular	Dissociative drug; profound amnesia and analgesia; may cause psychologic problems during emergence	Rapid induction; short procedures when muscle relaxation not needed; children and young adults.
Fentanyl	Sublimaze	Intravenous	Opioid; potent narcotic; metabolizes slowly; respiratory depressant	High-dose narcotic anesthesia in combination with oxygen
Sufentanil	Sufenta	Intravenous	Opioid; potent narcotic, respiratory depressant	Premedication; high-dose narcotic anesthesia in combination with oxygen.
Fentanyl and droperidol	Innovar	Intravenous	Combination narcotic and tranquilizer; potent; long acting	Neuroleptanalgesia
Diazepam	Valium	Intravenous, intramuscular	Benzodiazepine; tranquilizer; produces amnesia, sedation, and muscle relaxation	Premedication; awake intubation; induction.
Midazolam	Versed	Intravenous, intramuscular	Benzodiazepine; sedative; short-acting amnesic; central nervous system and respiratory depressant	Premedication; conscious sedation; induction in children

respiratory depression. Because exposure can be an occupational hazard for personnel, measures are taken to minimize levels of nitrous oxide in room air.

Advantages. When nitrous oxide is used in combination with other forms of inhalants and IV drugs, excessive depth of anesthesia is avoided. Nitrous oxide is rapidly cleared from the circulation. The incidence of nausea and vomiting is minimal. The gas has a rapid uptake and elimination and few aftereffects except headache, vertigo, and drowsiness. It causes minimal physiologic change; adverse effects can be quickly reversed. It is an excellent analgesic for procedures not producing severe pain.

Disadvantages. Nitrous oxide can cause bowel distention and increased volume in other air pockets. The use of nitrous oxide can cause displacement of tympanoplasty grafts or increased intracranial pressure. It should not be used during laparoscopy. There is no muscle relaxation. There is possible excitement or laryngospasm. Hypoxia is a hazard. There is a depressant effect on myocardial contractility.

Halothane (Fluothane). An infrequently used halogenated hydrocarbon, halothane reduces myocardial oxygen consumption more than it depresses cardiac function. Halothane was used in a wide spectrum of all types of surgical procedures for adults and children except routine obstetrics, when uterine relaxation is not desired. It is a profound uterine relaxant.

Because its metabolites have a possible effect as a hepatotoxin, some anesthesia providers avoid repeated administration within an arbitrary time (e.g., 3 months) in adults. Recent jaundice and known or suspected liver disease (past or present) are usually contraindications to its use. It is contraindicated in patients who are susceptible to malignant hyperthermia. Malignant hyperthermia is covered in depth in Chapter 31.

Advantages. Halothane is nonflammable, potent, versatile, chemically stable, and rapid, and it has a smooth induction.

Disadvantages. Halothane is potentially toxic to the liver and has a profound effect on body temperature control; it may cause hypothermia. Complete elimination of halothane takes some time.

Enflurane (Ethrane). A nonflammable, stable, halogenated ether, enflurane is similar in potency and versatility to halothane. Enflurane is used in a wide spectrum of procedures.

Advantages. Enflurane has a rapid induction and recovery with minimal aftereffects. Pharyngeal and laryngeal reflexes are obtunded easily, salivation is not stimulated, and bronchomotor tone is not affected. The cardiac rate and rhythm remain relatively stable, although caution is advised when it is used with epinephrine. Muscle relaxation is produced, but small supplementary doses of muscle relaxants may be required; nondepolarizing relaxants are potentiated by enflurane.

Disadvantages. Enflurane has a pungent odor. Respiration and blood pressure are progressively depressed with deepening anesthesia. Although biotransformation (metabolism) of enflurane is less than what occurs with other halogenated agents, small amounts of fluoride ion are released. Severe renal disease is a contraindication to use. At deeper levels, an electroencephalographic (EEG) pattern resembling seizures may occur. The agent is absorbed by rubber.

Isoflurane (Forane). Isoflurane comes closer to ideal than other inhalation agents and is most commonly used. Isoflurane is a nonflammable, fluorinated, halogenated methyl ether similar to halothane and enflurane, yet different. It is a more potent muscle relaxant, but unlike the others, it protects the heart against catecholamine-induced dysrhythmias. Heart rhythm is remarkably stable with a slightly elevated rate. The blood pressure drops with induction but returns to normal with intraoperative stimulation. A dose-related lowering of the blood pressure occurs, but cardiac output is unaltered, mainly as a result of increased heart rate. Isoflurane potentiates all commonly used muscle relaxants, the most profound effect occurring with the nondepolarizing type.

Isoflurane is used for induction and maintenance in a wide spectrum of procedures except routine obstetrics. Isoflurane produces uterine relaxation. Safety to the mother and fetus has not been established. Because the drug is metabolized in the liver, it may be given to patients with minimal renal disease.

Advantages. There is less cardiac depression; there is increased cardiac output with a wide margin of cardiovascular safety. Isoflurane does not sensitize the myocardium to the effects of epinephrine. There are no central nervous system (CNS) excitatory effects. There is rapid induction and, especially, rapid emergence with minimal aftereffects (less postoperative nausea and confusion). Isoflurane is innocuous to organs; it has low organ toxicity because of its low blood solubility and minimal susceptibility to biodegradation and metabolism. It provides superb muscle relaxation. Pharyngeal and laryngeal reflexes are easily obtunded. Isoflurane depresses bronchoconstriction; it may be used in patients with asthma and patients with chronic obstructive pulmonary disease.

Disadvantages. Isoflurane is expensive. It is a profound respiratory depressant and reduces respiratory minute volume. Respirations must be closely monitored and supported. Assisted or controlled ventilation is used to prevent respiratory acidosis. In the absence of intraoperative stimulation, the blood pressure may drop as a result of peripheral vasodilation. Cerebral vascular resistance decreases, cerebral blood flow increases, and intracranial pressure rises but is reversible with hyperventilation. Secretions are weakly stimulated.

Desflurane (Suprane). A nonflammable, volatile liquid with low solubility, desflurane has faster uptake by inhalation and elimination than do halothane and isoflurane. Desflurane is used in induction and maintenance of anesthesia in adults. It may be used for maintenance in infants and children, but it is not used for induction because of its potential for causing coughing and laryngospasm. Because it has a high vapor pressure, desflurane is delivered only through a vaporizer specifically designed for this agent. Desflurane vaporizers require electrical power to heat the liquid. It works well for ambulatory surgery patients because of the rapid emergence at the end of the case.

Advantages. There is rapid emergence and recovery from anesthesia. Desflurane resists biotransformation (metabolism) and degradation; it produces few urinary metabolites. The dosage of nondepolarizing muscle relaxants to maintain neuromuscular blockade may be reduced.

Disadvantages. Desflurane has a pungent odor that may be irritating during induction. Increasing alveolar concentration may lower the blood pressure, which may be corrected by reducing the inspired concentration. Hemodynamic effects, including an elevated heart rate, preclude use of desflurane by itself in a patient with cardiovascular disease; it may be combined with IV opioids or benzodiazepines.

Sevoflurane (Ultane). Sevoflurane is a volatile liquid used for inhalation anesthesia. It is nonflammable and nonexplosive. Noted for its rapid induction and rapid emergence qualities, it is commonly used for induction and maintenance of general anesthesia.

Advantages. Sevoflurane is used as an inhalant anesthetic for adults and pediatric patients. It is rapidly eliminated by the lungs.

Disadvantages. Sevoflurane may cause glycosuria and proteinuria when used for long procedures at low flow rates.

Intravenous Anesthetic Agents.
IV anesthesia became popular with the introduction in the 1930s of ultrashort-acting barbiturates. A drug that produces hypnosis, sedation, amnesia, and/or analgesia is injected directly into the circulation, usually via a peripheral vein in the arm. Diluted by blood in the heart and the lungs, the drug passes in high concentration to the brain, heart, liver, and kidneys—the organs of highest blood flow. Concentration in the brain is rapid. With recirculation, redistribution occurs in the body, decreasing cerebral concentration. Dissipation of effects depends on redistribution and biotransformation. Because removal of drug from the circulation is impossible, safety in use is related to metabolism. It is advisable for the anesthesia provider to give a small test dose at induction.

Oxygen is always given during IV and inhalation anesthesia. A barbiturate, dissociative agent, or narcotic may be given (see Table 24-2). Each has advantages, disadvantages, and contraindications. They may be supplemented with other drugs.

Thiopental (Pentothal). Thiopental sodium is a sedative-hypnotic used as an IV induction agent and a supplement to regional anesthesia. This drug can be used as a safe adjunct for intubation in head injuries. Cerebral perfusion pressure is maintained while decreasing elevated intracranial pressure. Thiopental is also used as a cerebral protectant in barbiturate narcosis.

Repeated doses are cumulative because of high lipid solubility. Systemic vascular resistance is decreased, causing lowered arterial pressure and lower cardiac output. Decreases uterine blood flow in pregnant patients.

Advantages. Onset of action is within 30 seconds. Short acting duration 5 to 30 minutes depending on body mass. Can be used as an anticonvulsant.

Disadvantages. Contraindicated in status asthmaticus. Lower doses are required in the elderly and high-risk surgical patients.

Contraindications. Should not be used in patients who are sensitive to the drug.

Propofol (Diprivan). An ultrashort-acting alkylphenol, propofol is a sedative-hypnotic that produces anesthesia. It is used for rapid induction and maintenance of anesthesia for short procedures. It can be used also in combination with inhalation agents or opioids for prolonged anesthesia. Propofol is supplied in a sterile, milky soybean, oil-in-water emulsion. In low doses it produces sedation (i.e., drowsiness, decreased responsiveness). Continued IV administration leads to hypnosis and unconsciousness. Propofol is twice as potent as thiopental sodium.

Propofol is used for general anesthesia for ambulatory surgery patients and for maintenance of moderate sedation during local and regional anesthesia. It is acceptable for patients who are allergic to barbiturates or who have porphyria.

Advantages. Propofol is rapidly distributed, metabolized, and eliminated. Emergence is very rapid, with few postoperative side effects. Can be used for postoperative nausea and vomiting (PONV).

Disadvantages. Propofol produces dose-related cardiorespiratory depression. Cardiovascular depressant action will decrease the blood pressure. Its hypotensive effect is potentiated by narcotics. The solution supports rapid growth of microorganisms if the infusion pump or syringes become contaminated. Moderate to severe pain may be felt at the injection site in the small vein of the hand or forearm; the larger antecubital vein should be used, or the site should be injected with lidocaine.

Contraindications. Propofol is used with caution in geriatric, debilitated, and hypovolemic patients. It is not recommended for pediatrics, obstetrics, and some neurosurgical procedures. Patients with egg lecithin or soybean sensitivities may experience an allergic reaction.

Ketamine (Ketalar, Ketaject). General anesthesia may be produced by a phencyclidine derivative to produce a state referred to as dissociative anesthesia. The drug acts by selectively interrupting associative pathways of the brain before producing sensory blockage. This permits a surgical procedure on a patient who appears to be awake (i.e., eyes are open, may move) but who is anesthetized (i.e., unaware, amnesic).

Ketamine may be given IV or intramuscularly (IM) to yield profound analgesia. It is swiftly metabolized. Individual response varies, depending on the dose, route of administration, and age. Because of a dose-response relationship, careful patient selection and dose selection are important. Ketamine is used alone or with nitrous oxide. Anticholinergics may be given to decrease hypersalivation.

Ketamine is used mainly in children between the ages of 2 and 10 years and in adults younger than 30 years for short procedures not requiring skeletal muscle relaxation, for plastic and eye procedures when combined with local agents, for diagnostic procedures, as an induction agent before other general agents are used, and to supplement nitrous oxide when adequate respiratory exchange is maintained. For longer procedures, repeated doses are given that may prolong recovery time. If relaxation is needed, muscle relaxants and controlled ventilation are indicated.

Advantages. Ketamine has a rapid induction. Respirations are not depressed unless the drug is administered too rapidly or in too large a dose. A mild stimulant action on the cardiovascular system may elevate the blood pressure. The effects of ketamine are potentiated by narcotics and barbiturates.

Disadvantages. Psychological manifestations (e.g., delirium, vivid imagery, hallucinations, unpleasant dreams) may occur during emergence. These can be reduced by giving preanesthetic diazepam and by allowing the patient to lie quietly and undisturbed during recovery except for essential procedures. Reactions are more common in adults than in children. IV thiopental sodium or diazepam may be given to treat emergence delirium.

Low-dose ketamine (1 mg/kg) has been used as an induction agent for obstetric procedures because of rapid onset, intense analgesia and amnesia, and minimal fetal effects. With its cardiovascular-stimulating properties, it is useful in hypovolemic and hypotensive patients, allowing the use of high oxygen concentration, both in obstetric and trauma procedures.

Contraindications. Ketamine is contraindicated in procedures involving tracheobronchial stimulation, because pharyngeal and laryngeal reflexes are usually active. If the drug is used alone, mechanical stimulation of the pharynx should be avoided. Other contraindications include pregnancy, hypertension, increased intracranial pressure, intraocular procedures, and previous cerebrovascular accident, because this agent increases cerebrospinal fluid and intraocular pressure.

Adjunctive Drugs Used in Anesthesia

Many drugs are used to supplement nitrous oxide, halogenated inhalation agents, and IV drugs to maintain amnesia and analgesia, control hypertension, attenuate the extent of postoperative respiratory depression, or maintain or control other effects of general anesthesia. These drugs must be carefully controlled to avoid adverse drug interactions. For example, morphine sulfate and nitrous oxide have a synergistic action with thiopental sodium (i.e., when they are given together, each potentiates the action of the other). Therefore they are given concomitantly with caution because of their combined respiratory depressant effect.

Some drugs are given preoperatively, during induction, and/or intraoperatively. Adjunctive drugs are used primarily for analgesia and amnesia or to counteract side effects of anesthesia. Some are particularly useful for ambulatory surgery patients, because they are short acting.

Narcotics. Historically, natural opiates and synthetic opioids have been given to produce analgesia and sedation preoperatively and postoperatively. In addition, they are used intraoperatively as supplemental agents and/or in combination with oxygen for complete anesthesia for short procedures and in patients with little cardiovascular reserve. Cardiovascular depression must be avoided in these patients. Halogenated agents are contraindicated in patients with liver and renal disease and malignant hyperthermia risk.

The most popular narcotics for general anesthesia are the opioids fentanyl (Sublimaze), sufentanil (Sufenta), alfentanil (Alfenta), and meperidine (Demerol), and the opiate morphine sulfate. Although they are analgesics, to reliably achieve anesthesia, markedly larger doses of narcotics are needed (e.g., 10 to 30 times as much morphine [3 to 8 or more mg/kg body weight]). High doses of fentanyl range from 50 to 100 mg/kg body weight. The drugs may be given in bolus doses or continuously via IV infusion in combination with inhalant anesthesia. Surprisingly, side effects seem to occur less frequently as the potency of narcotics increases.

Some drugs work as agonists to each other. An agonist is a drug or a combination of drugs given to augment each other. In some circumstances, lower doses of each can be given to achieve the desired effect. They reduce adverse physiologic responses to the stress of the surgical procedure, such as increased work of the heart, potential dysrhythmias, sodium and water retention, and increased blood glucose levels. Narcotics produce a dose-related respiratory depression. The respiratory effects of narcotics are as follows:

- Reduction of responsiveness of the CNS respiratory centers to carbon dioxide (less stimulation)
- Impairment of respiratory reflexes and alteration of rhythmicity (prolonged inspiration, delayed expiration)
- Reduction in the respiratory rate before reduction in the tidal volume
- Production of bronchoconstriction (morphine, meperidine) or rigidity of the chest wall (fentanyl)
- Impairment of ciliary motion

Factors that influence narcotic respiratory actions include age, pain, sleep, urinary output, other drugs, intestinal resorption, and disease.

The neurophysical state obtained by use of large doses of narcotics is not the same as "the general anesthesia state" resulting from use of volatile inhalation agents such as halothane. Narcotics are more selective in action. Narcotics do not produce muscle relaxation. Conversely, they cause an increase in muscle tone. Neuromuscular blocking agents can block or treat this action or rigidity.

After high-dose narcotic anesthesia, patients are awake and pain-free, with adequate though not good ventilation. These patients need careful monitoring by a well-trained PACU staff because narcotization after large doses of narcotics can occur rapidly in an apparently awake and responsive patient. The patient can hypoventilate, become hypoxic, and stop breathing when intraoperative stimuli cease. The vital signs, pupils, and skin color must be monitored.

Clinical signs of narcotic toxicity are pinpoint pupils, depressed respiration, and reduced consciousness. A narcotic antagonist is given to reverse narcotic-induced hypoventilation. Antagonists are used to block cellular receptor sites that bind to a drug. The potential for delayed toxicity after IM injection of narcotics, as opposed to IV administration, exists because absorption from muscle mass may be irregular.

Narcotic Reversal (Narcotic Antagonist). A narcotic antagonist neutralizes or impedes the action of another drug (i.e., reverses its effects). For example, narcotics produce a dose-related respiratory depression that can be reversed by opiate antagonists. These drugs are given IV, IM, or subcutaneously (subQ).

Naloxone (Narcan). A specific narcotic antagonist, naloxone reverses respiratory depression caused by narcotics. It has no respiratory or circulatory action of its own in the presence or absence of a narcotic or other agonist-antagonist. Complications can include hypertension and tachycardia if naloxone is combined with opioids. Naloxone has a shorter duration of action than the narcotic being reversed. Respiratory depression can occur. Initial dose is 0.4 to 2 mg diluted in 10 mL normal saline titrated IV in 1-mL increments every 2 to 3 minutes as needed until adequate reversal is attained. Narcan can be administered subQ or IM.[2]

Flumazenil (Romazicon). Flumazenil is a benzodiazepine antagonist used for complete or partial reversal after general anesthesia or conscious sedation. The duration of action is shorter than the action of the drugs being reversed, and resedation can occur. Initial dose is 0.2 mg IV over 15 seconds. May repeat in 1-minute intervals up to a total dose of 1 mg. If resedation occurs, dose may be repeated but not to exceed 3 mg in 1 hour.

Muscle Relaxants. Skeletal muscle relaxant drugs, referred to as neuromuscular blockers, facilitate muscle relaxation for smoother endotracheal intubation and working conditions during the surgical procedure. Their use has eliminated the need for deep inhalation anesthesia to produce relaxation. Administered IV in small amounts at intervals, they interfere with the passage of impulses from motor nerves to skeletal muscles. They act primarily at autonomic receptor sites, the neuromuscular junction, and at prejunctional and postjunctional acetylcholine-binding sites, causing paralysis of variable duration. They also can affect transmission of impulses at preganglionic and postganglionic endings in the autonomic nervous system.

Neuromuscular blockers paralyze all skeletal muscles, including the diaphragm and accessory muscles of respiration. Therefore, the chief danger in their use is that they decrease pulmonary ventilation, causing respiratory depression. They also may cause circulatory disturbance. Special attention to anesthesia depth, ventilation, and electrolyte balance is required.

The anesthesia provider must constantly verify the degree of paralysis present by noting the amount of relaxation of the abdominal wall or the limpness of extremities or by using a nerve stimulator connected to the patient through needle electrodes. The use of neuromuscular blockers requires surgeon–anesthesia provider teamwork and communication. Use of these drugs always presents the hazard of overdosage, a danger alleviated by the anesthesia provider's familiarity with the surgeon's technique and the requirements of the particular surgical procedure; thus the anesthesia provider can regulate the dosage of anesthetic and relaxant necessary to produce the conditions required at the appropriate time. For example, a major use of neuromuscular blockers is in intraabdominal procedures.

At different times during the surgical procedure, blockade may be more or less essential. Although tightness of tissues and inadequate exposure may be a result of factors other than relaxation, it is helpful to the anesthesia provider to be told before pertinent action, such as closure of the peritoneum, is taken. Inadequate muscle relaxation makes closure difficult. Controlled respiration during upper abdominal manipulation can prevent descent of the diaphragm into the surgical field.

Neuromuscular blockers are classified as nondepolarizing or depolarizing. Although theoretically they are antagonistic, combinations are used. They may widen the scope of less potent anesthetics, such as nitrous oxide, or lessen the overall amount of anesthetic needed. Depolarizing and nondepolarizing drugs behave differently; depolarizers stimulate, whereas nondepolarizers inhibit autonomic receptors. Duration of action should be balanced against duration of effect on ventilation.

Nondepolarizing Neuromuscular Blockers. Nondepolarizing neuromuscular blockers act on enzymes to prevent muscle contraction. They produce tetanic electrical impulses that gradually fade, but they do not cause muscular fasciculation on IV injection. Their effects are decreased by anticholinesterase drugs, acetylcholine, epinephrine, and depolarizing neuromuscular blockers. Action is potentiated by halogenated inhalation agents and some aminoglycoside antibiotics. Interactions with other drugs can result in delayed recovery. For example, antibiotics may act synergistically to produce prolonged paralysis, such as occurs when the peritoneal cavity is irrigated with an antibiotic solution or antibiotic is injected IV. Box 24-2 lists some antibiotics that can potentiate neuromuscular blockers.

Synergism also occurs with local and inhalation anesthetic agents. They are useful for patients on mechanical ventilators. Nondepolarizing blockers may be referred to as competitive antagonists. A peripheral nerve stimulator is useful for assessing neuromuscular transmission as a guide to the dosage, degree and nature of the blockade, and evidence of muscle-response recovery during and after the use of nondepolarizing agents. The anesthesia provider can choose from several drugs.

BOX 24-2	**Antibiotics that Can Potentiate Neuromuscular Blocking Agents**

AMINOGLYCOSIDES	**MISCELLANEOUS ANTIBIOTICS**
Streptomycin	Polymyxin A
Gentamicin	Polymyxin B
Tobramycin	Colistin
Kanamycin	Lincomycin
Amikacin	Clindamycin
Netilmicin	Tetracycline

BETA-LACTAMS
Penicillin G
Penicillin V
Piperacillin

---

[2]AORN: *Drug information handbook for perioperative nursing*, AORN and Lexi-Comp, Denver, 2006.

Short-Acting Neuromuscular Blocking Agents
Mivacurium (Mivacron): Blockade lasts 15 to 20 minutes. It has minimal cardiovascular effect but can cause skin flushing.

Intermediate-Acting Neuromuscular Blocking Agents
- *Atracurium (Tracrium):* With a duration of action of about 30 minutes, atracurium metabolizes more quickly than the other blockers, which may be an advantage in patients with liver or renal disease. Repeated doses are not cumulative. Atracurium causes histamine release, vasodilation, and hypotension.
- *Cisatracurium (Nimbex):* Cisatracurium can cause bradycardia, hypotension, and skin flushing.
- *Vecuronium (Norcuron):* Similar to pancuronium, vecuronium has a shorter duration of action and is more potent. It does not noticeably increase the heart rate or blood pressure unless it is combined with opioids.
- *Rocuronium (Zemuron):* With a rapid onset of action, rocuronium facilitates intubation. The duration of action is about 30 minutes, with minimal overall effect on cardiovascular stability. Can be reversed with neostigmine. Tachycardia is possible. Rocuronium interacts with some antibiotics including gentamicin, neomycin, and polymyxin B. Must be refrigerated.

Long-Acting Neuromuscular Blocking Agents
- *Tubocurarine (Curare):* Obtained from plants, tubocurarine was used centuries ago by South American Indians for poison arrows. The poison caused death by suffocation from respiratory paralysis. The effects of tubocurarine on the neuromuscular junction were first described in 1856. Blocking transmission of nerve impulses to muscle fibers results in paralysis, predominantly of voluntary muscles. d-Tubocurarine releases histamine. Autonomic blockade can cause vasodilation, hypotension, and histamine release. Tubocurarine is used as pretreatment if succinylcholine is used, to decrease the possibility of fasciculation.
- *Gallamine (Flaxedil):* Similar in action and duration to d-tubocurarine, gallamine does not cause hypotension or bronchospasm. It may increase arterial pressure and cause tachycardia. It is contraindicated in patients with iodide and sulfide allergies.
- *Metocurine (Metubine):* Metocurine iodide produces less hypotension and releases less histamine than does d-tubocurarine. It is contraindicated in patients with iodide allergy.
- *Pancuronium (Pavulon):* Pancuronium is similar in action to d-tubocurarine but about five times more potent. It has a vagolytic action that may raise the blood pressure, pulse rate, and heart rate. It can cause dysrhythmia if used with digoxin.
- *Pipecuronium (Arduan):* Pipecuronium can cause decreased arterial pressure with moderate histamine release.

Depolarizing Neuromuscular Blockers. Depolarizing neuromuscular blockers have the opposite effect of the nondepolarizing drugs. They stimulate autonomic receptors. For example, they cause muscular fasciculation (i.e., involuntary muscle contractions). These contractions, the result of depolarization of nerve-muscle end plate, are seen after injection. They are followed by fatigue. Drugs may be given IM, but IV use is more common.
- *Succinylcholine (Anectine, Quelicin, Sucostrin):* An ultrashort-acting synthetic drug with an onset of action in seconds, succinylcholine produces paralysis for up to 20 minutes. It is used primarily for endotracheal intubation. A dilute solution may be used to provide continuing muscle relaxation. Repeated IV administration may effect changes in the heart rate and rhythm (i.e., bradycardia and ventricular dysrhythmias) until the drug is metabolized by enzymes. Muscle pain may occur after use unless fasciculation is prevented by a small preliminary dose of a nondepolarizing agent. Succinylcholine is contraindicated in patients with a known or suspected history of malignant hyperthermia. It can cause increased intracranial and intraocular pressures.
- *Decamethonium (Syncurine):* A very potent synthetic with a rapid onset and short duration of action, decamethonium is not cumulative and has little effect on vital systems. It is used for deep relaxation of a short duration, such as for endoscopy, treatment of laryngeal spasm, abdominal closure, and endotracheal intubation. It is excreted through the kidneys. Prolonged blockade may result if decamethonium is given to a patient in renal failure.

Muscle Relaxant Reversal Agents (Cholinergics)
- *Neostigmine (Prostigmin):* Neostigmine inhibits the destruction of acetylcholine released from parasympathetic nerves. It is used to reverse nondepolarizing neuromuscular blocking agents. Use with care in patients with bronchial asthma, bradycardia, seizure disorders, coronary artery disease, and hyperthyroidism. Monitor vital signs, particularly respirations, carefully, and have atropine close at hand. Neostigmine is not for use in patients with peritonitis or bowel or urinary obstruction.
- *Edrophonium (Tensilon):* Edrophonium works as a curare antagonist to reverse the nondepolarizing neuromuscular blocking action. It has a rapid onset, but short duration. It is contraindicated in bowel or urinary tract obstruction. Monitor vital signs, and have atropine immediately available.

Monitoring the Depth of Anesthesia
The anesthesia provider monitors the level of anesthesia, balancing doses of medications, throughout the surgical procedure. Bispectral Index (BIS) is a compact system for monitoring the effects of anesthesia on the brain. The BIS monitor allows the anesthesia provider to accurately track the patient's level of consciousness by using an electrode applied to the patient's forehead that sends electroencephalogram (EEG)-like signals to a small monitor. The readout is a single number ranging from 100 (wide awake) to zero (absence of brain activity).

The device can be used as a stand-alone unit or be integrated into other monitoring devices. The result of its use is decreased amounts of anesthetic administration and a faster postoperative return to alertness. The BIS monitor is not a substitute for clinical judgment and does not detect cerebral ischemia or blood pressure. (More information is available on the Internet at www.aspectms.com.)

Emergence from General Anesthesia

The anesthesia provider attempts to have the patient as nearly awake as possible at the end of a surgical procedure. Pharyngeal and laryngeal reflexes must be recovered to prevent aspiration and respiratory obstruction. The degree of residual neuromuscular blockade must be determined and treated if necessary for respiratory adequacy. The action of nondepolarizing muscle relaxants may be reversed with antagonists, such as long-acting neostigmine (Prostigmin) or pyridostigmine (Regonol), or short-acting edrophonium (Tensilon, Enlon). These anticholinesterase drugs are accompanied or preceded by atropine to minimize side effects, such as excessive secretions and bradycardia.

Extubation is delayed until spontaneous respiration is ensured. The endotracheal tube is carefully removed when this maneuver is deemed safe. A patent airway and adequate manual or mechanical ventilation are maintained until full recovery. In the absence of a means of respiratory control, such as when a maxillofacial procedure endangers the airway, the endotracheal tube may be left in place.

Vomiting and restlessness may accompany emergence. Slight cyanosis, stertorous respiration, rigidity, and shivering are not uncommon as a result of a temporary disturbance of body temperature–regulating mechanisms, thus altering circulation to the skin and muscles. Administering oxygen and pain medication and applying warm blankets help relieve these after-effects. The anesthesia provider should flush the patient's lungs with oxygen to minimize exhalation of gases in the PACU.

BALANCED ANESTHESIA

Balanced anesthesia has become a widely used technique to achieve physiologic homeostasis, analgesia, amnesia, and muscle relaxation. A combination of agents is used with many possible variations, depending on the condition of the patient and requirements of the procedure. The technique is especially useful for preventing CNS depression in older and poor-risk patients.

Induction

Induction can be accomplished with a thiobarbiturate derivative (thiopental [Pentothal], methohexital [Brevital]), diazepam (Valium), midazolam (Versed), or other induction agent. Oxygen is administered in physiologic quantities. Neuromuscular blockers permit control of ventilation while providing muscle relaxation during intubation.

Maintenance

Different combinations of narcotics and neuroleptic drugs (tranquilizers) are administered IV, whether they are used alone or in combination with inhalation agents. Neuroleptics reduce motor activity and anxiety; produce a detached, apathetic state; and potentiate hypnotic and analgesic narcotic effects. The dosage can be regulated to produce the desired state.

Emergence

Residual effects of narcotics or muscle relaxants may require reversal by antagonists during and/or at the conclusion of the surgical procedure. Other precautions are taken as for any patient emerging from general anesthesia.

CONTROLLED HOMEOSTASIS

Functions controlled by homeostatic mechanisms include body temperature, heartbeat, blood pressure, electrolyte balance, and respiration. These parameters may be altered by anesthetic and other pharmacologic agents and by physiologic stresses during surgical manipulations. In the hands of a skilled anesthesia provider, adjunctive methods of control may be used concurrently with the administration of general anesthesia, but only when the expected outcomes will outweigh the inherent risks.

Induced Hypothermia

Hypothermia is an artificial, deliberate lowering of body temperature below the normal limits (Box 24-3). It reduces the metabolic rate and oxygen needs of the tissues in conditions causing hypoxia or during a decrease or interruption of circulation. Bleeding is also decreased, and less anesthetic is needed. The patient can therefore better tolerate the surgical procedure.

Hypothermia may be used as follows:

- For direct-vision intracardiac repair of complex congenital defects in infants and in other cardiac procedures (most common usage)
- After cardiac resuscitation, to decrease oxygen requirements of vital tissues and limit further damage to the brain after anoxia
- In treatment of hyperpyrexia and some other nonsurgical conditions, such as hypertensive crisis
- To increase tolerance in septic shock
- In neurosurgery, to decrease cerebral blood flow, cerebrospinal fluid volume, and venous and intracranial pressures
- To aid in transplantation of organs

Attaining Hypothermia. To achieve hypothermia, heat must be lost more rapidly than it is produced. The following methods may be used:

- *Surface-induced hypothermia:* External cooling of infants and small children weighing less than 20 pounds (10 kg) may be attained by immersion in ice water, packing the body in ice, or alcohol sponging. A hypothermia/hyperthermia machine with a cooling blanket or mattress is used for adults and larger children.

BOX 24-3	Hypothermia

Normal core temperature: 98.2° to 99.9° F (36.8°-37.7° C)
Systemic hypothermia may be:
  Light: 98.6° to 89.6° F (37°-32° C)
  Moderate: 89.6° to 78.8° F (32°-26° C)
  Deep: 78.8° to 68° F (26°-20° C)
  Profound: 68° F (20° C) or below
Sensorium fades at: 91° to 93° F (33°-34° C)

- *Internal cooling:* A decreased or interruption of blood flow can be achieved by placing sterile iced saline slush packs around a specific internal organ or by irrigation of cold fluids within a body cavity, such as intraperitoneal lavage. The cold cardioplegia technique combines cold from saline slush with drugs injected into coronary arteries for myocardial protection during heart surgery. Drugs may also be used to lower metabolism and to increase resistance to shivering during cooling.
- *Systemic hypothermia:* The bloodstream is cooled by diverting blood through heat-exchanging devices of extracorporeal circulation and returning it to the body by a continuous flowing circuit (e.g., core cooling by cardiopulmonary bypass or IV administration of cold fluids). Systemic hypothermia is used in adults and larger children to 78.8° F (26° C). Oxygen consumption and metabolism of different organs vary, making uniform hypothermia impossible. The temperature is not deliberately lowered below about 84.5° F (29° C) unless arrest of the heart is desired by means of deep hypothermia (below 78.8° F [26° C]). This is accompanied by perfusion of the rest of the body with the extracorporeal circulation method, permitting an open, motionless dry field while the blood flow is interrupted. A noncontracting heart requires very little oxygen.

The patient is progressively rewarmed at the close of the surgical procedure until the temperature is 95° F (35° C) or until consciousness returns. Sometimes a degree of hypothermia is maintained for a day or two postoperatively to allow the patient to adapt more readily. Oxygen therapy and intubation, if advised, are part of postoperative care.

Complications in the Use of Hypothermia. Hypothermia carries many inherent risks. Primarily it affects the myocardium, decreasing its resistance to ventricular fibrillation and predisposing the patient to cardiac arrest. This is more likely to happen with deep hypothermia or during manipulation of the heart itself. Other dangers are heart block, effects on the vascular system, atrial fibrillation, embolism, microcirculation stasis, undesired downward drift of temperature, tissue damage, metabolic acidosis, and numerous effects on other organs and systems.

Time is required for cooling and rewarming. Shivering and vasoconstriction, normal defenses of the body against cooling, can be problems during the use of hypothermia. This muscle activity greatly increases oxygen needs. Shivering can be overcome by the administration of a muscle relaxant drug or IV injection of chlorpromazine or an analgesic such as meperidine.

Rewarming can be accomplished by circulating warmed blood by means of extracorporeal circulation or by using a heating mattress with circulating fluid and warm blankets. If external heat is applied, care should be taken not to burn the patient. Rewarming carries potential problems such as reactive bleeding or circulatory collapse. If the patient is rewarmed too rapidly, vasodilation causes the blood pressure to drop. Organ ischemia can occur from severe shivering. These superficial and systemic events impair perfusion (oxygenation) of tissues. "Rewarming shock" may be prevented by slow warming, adequate oxygenation, and prevention of massive sudden vasodilation or vasoconstriction associated with shivering.

Induced Hypotension

Induced, deliberate hypotension is the controlled lowering of arterial blood pressure during anesthesia as an adjunct to the surgical procedure. Hypotensive anesthesia is used to shorten the operating time, reduce blood loss and the need for transfusion, and facilitate dissection and visibility, especially of tumor margins in radical procedures. Visible vessels are ligated, even in the absence of active bleeding.

Adequate oxygenation of blood and tissue perfusion in vital organs (heart, liver, kidneys, lungs) and in the cerebrum must be maintained to prevent damage. The degree and duration of hypotension must be carefully controlled so that the state can be rapidly terminated at any time.

Naturally, controlled hypotension is not indicated as a routine procedure. It is used only when the expected gain for a particular patient requiring a specific surgical procedure outweighs the risks. Hypotension may be specifically induced for the following:

- Surgical procedures in which excessive blood loss is anticipated, such as spinal surgery, to decrease gross hemorrhage or venous oozing.
- Surgical procedures on the head, face, neck, and upper thorax, especially radical dissection, in which the position of the patient allows blood to pool in dependent areas and reduces venous return to the heart and cardiac output.
- Neurosurgical procedures when control of intracranial vessel hemorrhage may be difficult. It reduces leakage, makes an aneurysm less turgid and prone to rupture, decreases blood loss in the case of rupture, and facilitates placement of ligating clips.
- Surgical procedures in which blood transfusions should be avoided, such as when compatible blood is unavailable or transfusion is against the patient's religious belief.
- Surgical procedures on the spine or posterior torso. Blood loss is decreased in the prone position.
- Total hip replacement.

Attaining Hypotension. Several techniques will produce hypotension. The blood pressure may be lowered chemically by direct arterial or venous dilators or by ganglionic blocking drugs. Perfusion pressure drops in proportion to a decrease in vascular flow resistance, but adequate tissue blood flow exists. Fine adjustment of the desired level of hypotension can be achieved by mechanical maneuvers—namely, alterations in body position or changes in airway pressure, control of the heart rate or blood volume, or addition of other vasoactive drugs in conjunction with hypotensive drugs. Properly used, these maneuvers can reduce the total dose of potentially toxic drugs needed for maintenance of hypotension.

Methods to produce hypotension include:

1. Deep general anesthesia with halothane or isoflurane, followed by a vasodilator, produces the desired minute-to-minute effect. With increased concentration, halogenated agents produce hypotension as a result of myocardial and peripheral vascular depression.

2. Sodium nitroprusside is a potent, fast-acting vasodilator that reduces virtually all resistance in vascular smooth muscle (resistance vessels). It also reduces preload and afterload of the heart and pulmonary vascular resistance. To achieve safe arterial pressure control, administration is via a calibrated drug pump. The acid-base status and blood cyanide level are determined frequently to guard against metabolic acidosis and nitroprusside-induced cyanide and thiocyanate toxicity.

3. Nitroglycerin, primarily a vasodilator, directly dilates capacitance vessels. It reduces preload and improves myocardial perfusion during diastole—a protection against potential ischemia. Nitroglycerin for IV infusion (Nitrostat), after dilution in 5% dextrose or physiologic saline, dilates both venous and arterial beds. Arterial pressures are reduced. Nitroglycerin migrates into plastic. To avoid its absorption into plastic parenteral solution containers, dilution and storage are done in glass parenteral solution bottles. A special nonabsorbing infusion set prevents loss of nitroglycerin.

4. Trimethaphan (Arfonad) blocks sympathetic ganglia, which results in relaxation of resistance and capacitance vessels and reduces arterial pressure.

5. Fentanyl may be used as a basal anesthetic for hypotension. The blood pressure can be maintained at the desired level by the addition of a small amount of a volatile agent. Fentanyl lowers arterial pressure; volatile agents reduce cardiac output.

6. Other drugs such as verapamil, nifedipine, phentolamine, tetrodotoxin, or adenosine triphosphate may be used.

Safe lower limits of arterial pressure may vary. Average values are 50 mm Hg mean and 65 to 70 mm Hg systolic, with lower values for short periods only.

Precautions in the Use of Hypotension. Potential complications of hypotensive anesthesia include cerebral or coronary ischemia or thrombosis, reactionary hemorrhage, anuria in acute renal failure, delayed awakening, and dermal ischemic lesions. Primary contraindications are vascular compromise to any vital organ system or the brain. Precautions include the following:

- Careful selection of the patient
- Preoperative cardiac, renal, and hepatic evaluation of the patient to avoid circulatory insufficiency in vital organs
- Selection of an appropriate but not arbitrary level of blood pressure
- Administration and evaluation by expert anesthesia providers
- Use for only a short time and lowering of blood pressure only enough to obtain the desired result
- Maintenance of blood volume at an optimal level by continuous infusion
- Controlled ventilation with adequate oxygenation via an endotracheal tube, because hypotension increases susceptibility to hypoxia
- Extensive monitoring: ECG, core temperature, esophageal stethoscopy, urinary output, central venous pressure and arterial catheters, and electrophysiologic brain monitoring or EEG via BIS monitoring

Normovolemic Hemodilution Technique

Intraoperative normovolemic hemodilution has been used in cardiac surgery for several decades but more recently as an adjunct technique in major surgery when large blood loss is anticipated. It is especially useful in infants and children and in patients who, for religious or personal reasons, do not accept administration of blood products.

At the beginning of the surgical procedure, whole blood is withdrawn from the patient to a hematocrit of 14% to 15% and replaced with three times the volume of a balanced electrolyte solution to maintain intravascular volume. This diluted blood is transparent, giving the surgeon a clearer, almost bloodless field. This may decrease operating time. The patient is maintained under controlled hypotension with halothane anesthetic and a supplemental narcotic. The body temperature may be lowered to 89.6° F (32° C) or below for moderate hypothermia to help protect vital organs against hypoxia and hypotension.

After significant blood loss has ceased, the patient's own blood is reinfused. Diuresis is stimulated to remove electrolyte solution. Normovolemic hemodilution can make a difficult surgical procedure easier and in some patients makes an otherwise impossible resection possible.

CARE OF THE ANESTHETIZED PATIENT

Anesthetic agents and drugs vary in potency. Therefore they differ in the amount of analgesia, amnesia, or muscle relaxation produced. Each patient's ability to detoxify anesthetic agents and to tolerate physiologic stress differs. Impairment of pulmonary function accompanies general anesthesia to some degree. General anesthesia is usually more complicated than local or regional anesthesia.

Considerations

The anesthesia provider keeps the surgeon informed of significant physiologic changes detected by monitoring vital functions. The following should be considered:

1. A deficit in pulmonary and/or cardiac functions is detrimental to the patient's physiologic status. Abnormalities of pulmonary ventilation and diffusion influence the course of anesthesia and diminish tolerance to stress or the insults from the anesthetic and the procedure.
   a. Respiratory patterns vary from breath holding and apnea to deep breathing and tachypnea.
   b. Drug action affecting respiratory stimulation or depression is related to changes in oxygen tension (Pao_2) or arterial carbon dioxide tension ($Paco_2$).
   c. Hypoxia, anemia, and decreased cardiac output may produce inadequate tissue oxygenation. Subnormal cardiac reserve or oxygen-transporting ability, combined with anemia or hypoxia in an arteriosclerotic patient, for example, can be lethal.
2. Circulation is affected both centrally and peripherally. Individual agents are associated with characteristic hemodynamic patterns. Generally, the agents are circulatory depressants that reduce arterial pressure, myocardial contractility, and cardiac output.

3. The liver is affected by general agents (e.g., the rate of visceral blood flow). Alterations in liver function tests may follow anesthesia. Halogenated hydrocarbons have been associated with hepatotoxicity. The liver metabolizes many anesthetic agents and other medications.

4. Kidney function is affected by disturbances in systemic circulation, since kidneys normally receive 20% to 25% of the cardiac output. A reduced renal plasma flow and glomerular filtration rate depress renal functions related to hemodynamics and to water and electrolyte excretion. Oliguria, with reduced sodium and potassium excretion, accompanies induction. Postoperative fluid retention may result from a reduction in urine volume from anesthesia, intraoperative trauma, and the use of narcotics. In the absence of renal disease, changes in renal function are usually transitory and reversible. Endocrine effects on renal function during anesthesia are important. Many drugs and agents are excreted by the kidneys.

5. Biotransformation of agents varies with metabolites excreted by the kidneys. Urinary excretion of IV agents may be slow and unpredictable. Studies indicate that nitrous oxide may be exhaled as long as 56 hours after anesthesia, and metabolites of halothane have been recovered from patients' urine as long as 20 days after anesthesia.

6. Agents may cause nausea, emesis, or systemic complications.

General anesthesia may be contraindicated for the following:

- Elective procedures on patients who are medically at high risk or severely debilitated.
- Elective procedures during the first 5 months of pregnancy. Some anesthesia providers avoid general anesthesia because of unknown teratogenic effects of inhalation anesthetics.
- Emergency surgical procedures on patients who have recently ingested food or fluids. Gastric suction and awake intubation are indicated if the surgical procedure cannot be delayed.

Intraoperative Awareness

Although seemingly anesthetized, the patient may be aware of conversations, noises, and even pain. Is it possible to imagine anything more terrifying than to feel intraoperative maneuvers but be unable to communicate this discomfort? Intraoperative awareness varies, depending on the type of procedure and depth of anesthesia. Monitoring techniques, such as BIS monitoring, may decrease the incidence of intraoperative awareness.

The common use of narcotics and muscle relaxants as adjuncts has consequently decreased the amount of anesthetic used to induce and maintain unconsciousness. This is particularly true in balanced anesthesia. As a result, studies have shown evidence of intraoperative awareness (i.e., recall), consciously or unconsciously, of events and sounds during a state of anesthesia. Even though the patient may not consciously recall or remember the experience, unconsciously it may affect behavior and attitudes postoperatively. Subconscious memory may cause anger, generalized irritability, anxiety, repetitive nightmares, preoccupation with death, or physiologic complications.

Patient awareness of pain is rare in the hands of skilled anesthesia providers. However, hearing is the last sensation to surrender to anesthesia. Therefore perioperative caregivers should be constantly aware of the patient's vulnerability to auditory stimuli, including conversations and room noise. Even potent amnesic drugs may not totally block recall of stimuli, especially disturbing stimuli.

Safety Factors

Team members, especially the anesthesia provider and the circulating nurse, must be constantly aware of potential trauma to the patient, since he or she is unable to produce a normal response to painful or injurious stimuli. The circulating nurse assists the anesthesia provider during the extubation of the patient at the conclusion of the surgical procedure. Although safety factors are stressed throughout the text, important factors in the care of the anesthetized patient are reiterated here for emphasis:

1. The patient's position is changed slowly and gently to allow circulation to readjust (i.e., to compensate for physiologic changes caused by motion or position).

2. Proper positioning and padding are important to avoid pressure points, stretching of nerves, or interference with circulation to an extremity.

3. The patient's chest must be free for adequate respiratory excursion during the surgical procedure. The airway must be patent. Leaning on the patient during the procedure can cause permanent injury. Remember that the patient under the drapes is unable to complain!

4. The lungs must be adequately ventilated intraoperatively and postoperatively by either voluntary or mechanical means. Anesthetic agents are basically depressants that affect the vasomotor and respiratory centers, predisposing the patient to postoperative respiratory complications.

5. The anesthesia provider assesses the patient assists in transferring the patient to a stretcher or bed, safeguarding the head and neck, when it is safe to move the patient. The anesthesia provider calls the count and initiates the move from operating bed to transport cart. The transfer is made carefully and gently to avoid strain on ligaments or muscles of the patient and the caregivers. The relaxed, unconscious patient is adequately supported.

6. The anesthesia provider gives the PACU nurse a verbal report, including specific problems in regard to this patient, and completes records before the transfer of responsibility. The circulating nurse gives a report of preoperative baselines and intraoperative care to the PACU nurse. The PACU hand off exchange report is described in detail in Chapter 30.

CARE OF GENERAL ANESTHESIA EQUIPMENT

The anesthesia equipment is a potential vector in the spread of infection. The anesthesia provider may become the victim of an acquired infection from contact with a patient's body fluids or blood. Studies have found that nearly 20% of anesthesia providers have had hepatitis B infections.

Standard Precautions

The need for anesthesia staff to strictly adhere to standard precautions (formerly known as universal precautions) while caring for patients and equipment should be emphasized. Gloves should be worn to prevent skin contact with patient's blood and body fluids, such as when starting the IV infusion, when intubating and/or extubating, or when suctioning the patient. Protective eyewear should be worn to prevent a splash in the eye. Hands should be washed and the mask should be changed between patient contacts. Needles must be handled carefully without recapping to avoid accidental needle sticks. All anesthesia equipment that has come in contact with mucous membranes, blood, or body fluids is cleaned, disinfected, or sterilized after use to render it safe for handling and for subsequent patient use. Disposable items are discarded in the appropriate receptacles.

Hazards of Equipment

Anesthesia techniques encompass the use of drugs for parenteral administration and gases and volatile liquids for inhalation administration by means of anesthesia machines. These machines and their component parts (reservoir bags, canisters, connecting pieces, ventilators) accumulate large numbers of microorganisms during use. Consequently, the parts that come in contact with the patient's skin or respiratory tract are sources of cross-contamination. Inhalation, exhalation, and the forcible expulsion of secretions create moist conditions favorable to the survival and growth of a multitude of organisms (streptococci, staphylococci, coliform bacteria, fungi, yeasts). Therefore the anesthesia circuit can become a veritable reservoir for microorganisms and a pathway for transmission of disease. When the apparatus is used on a patient with a known respiratory disease, such as tuberculosis, the risk increases.

All used accessories must be terminally cleaned and either undergo high-level disinfection or sterilization before reuse, because clinical respiratory cross-infection has been traced to contaminated apparatus. Valves of the breathing circuit become contaminated from essentially healthy patients at an average rate of 35 organisms per minute. *Pseudomonas aeruginosa* has been cultured from carbon dioxide absorption devices. Many microorganisms accumulate in valves and air passages and in soda lime canisters. Although the alkalinity of soda lime inhibits many organisms, it is neither a dependable germicide nor an effective mechanical filter nor is it meant to be one. Respiratory therapy equipment, mechanical ventilators, resuscitators, and suction machines and bottles present the same problems. Resistant strains of organisms, as well as opportunists, have caused health care–associated infections. Patient-to-patient infection must be eliminated. The following are points to remember:

- The patient's respiratory tract is a portal of entry for pathogenic organisms and a source of delivering pathogens into the environment.
- The respiratory tract loses some of its inherent defense mechanisms during anesthesia.

- Aseptic precautions are necessary to prevent needless exposure of air passages to foreign, potentially pathogenic organisms from equipment and hands of anesthesia personnel.
- Anesthesia machines and equipment, unless properly treated, increase the danger of airborne contamination and contact transmission of pathogenic microorganisms capable of causing postoperative wound infections and systemic infections.

In the presence of tuberculosis or a virulent respiratory infection, the anesthesia provider should wear a gown and strictly adhere to standard precautions. Some contacts require donning a mask with high-efficiency particulate air (HEPA) filters. The patient should wear a mask during transportation and until induction of anesthesia.

Disposable Equipment

Disposable equipment warrants use for reasons of safety, efficiency, and convenience. Presterilized, disposable airways, endotracheal tubes, tracheotomy tubes, breathing circuits, masks and canisters (with soda lime sealed in the plastic), and spinal trays reduce the hazard of cross-infection. They are especially recommended for the compromised host and the bacteriologically contaminated patient. Single-use components of the anesthesia system are discarded after use. Needles are disposed of in puncture-resistant containers.

Care of Reusable Equipment

All parts of patient-exposed, reusable equipment must be thoroughly cleaned after every use to prevent pulmonary complications. Thorough cleaning to remove organic debris and drying must precede any high-level disinfection or sterilization process. All items that can be sterilized should be sterilized. Manufacturers strive to make the machines that cannot be sterilized more amenable to adequate terminal cleaning and freedom from microorganisms. The following points should also be considered:

1. The anesthesia machine should be disinfected immediately whenever it is soiled by blood and secretions.
2. The surfaces of anesthesia machines, carts, or cabinets should be disinfected after each patient use. The specific work area used for airways, endotracheal tubes, and other items should also be cleaned. The top of a cart or tray should be draped with a disposable impervious material that is changed between patients. All equipment for maintenance of the airway should be set up on and returned to this drape.

    Disposable items should be discarded in suitable containers after use. Reusable equipment must be set aside after use for terminal cleaning and testing, thereby diminishing the risk of contaminating clean equipment needed for subsequent patients. A biohazard disposal container should be placed by the anesthesia machine.
3. Monitoring equipment, including ECG and other electrodes and blood pressure cuffs, should be cleaned with a detergent-disinfectant when contaminated and preferably after each use.
4. All equipment that comes in contact with mucous membranes of the patient and the inside of the breath-

ing circuit must be terminally cleaned and sterilized, preferably, or undergo high-level disinfection:

a. Endotracheal tubes, stylets, airways, laryngoscope blades, facemasks, and suction equipment should be sterile for each patient. Suction catheters and tubing should be sterile, single-use disposable items.

b. Disposable breathing circuits are preferred to reusable equipment because of the complexities of cleaning and maintaining cleanliness. The interior of reusable breathing circuits remains sterile if they stand unused in their normal position on the machine, but contamination rapidly occurs when the circuits are used on patients. The parts of the circuit nearest the patient are the most heavily contaminated. Therefore reusable corrugated hoses, breathing tubes, and reservoir bags are sterilized or undergo high-level disinfection between each patient use.

c. Items located farther away, such as circle systems and ventilators, are cleaned and sterilized according to a regular schedule—at least once or twice a month.

5. For cleaning, an automated process is available for decontamination. Machines wash equipment in mild detergent and hot water, and rinse and dry it. Some machines incorporate a chemical disinfection cycle. If automatic equipment is not used, anesthesia and respiratory therapy equipment must be disconnected and manually cleaned before sterilization. Prompt immersion in a detergent-disinfectant solution prevents crusting of secretions. Tubing takes a long time to dry. Commercial dryers are available.

6. Sterilization methods:

a. Steam is the preferred method for all heat-stable materials.

b. Ethylene oxide is used for materials that are deteriorated by heat, such as rubber, plastics, mechanical ventilators, and electronic equipment. Thorough aeration, according to the manufacturer's recommendations, is necessary before use to remove all residual gas from the material sterilized. Otherwise, facial burns, laryngotracheal inflammation, and obstruction or bilateral vocal cord paralysis may be caused by use of the equipment.

c. Buffered glutaraldehyde solution does not impair conductivity of antistatic rubber. Although its use is the least convenient method, it is preferred if ethylene oxide is not available for heat-sensitive items. The manufacturer's recommendations should be followed for a 100% kill of *Mycobacterium tuberculosis* by immersion methods. When glutaraldehyde is used, the items must be thoroughly rinsed with sterile water because tap water contains microorganisms and pyrogens.

7. Sterile packaged equipment should be stored in a closed, clean, and dry area. Anesthesia and respiratory therapy equipment should be kept sterile until used.

8. Policies and procedures regarding processing of equipment should be written, available, and reviewed annually.

Checking Anesthesia Equipment

Inhalation systems are tested biologically at regular intervals and checked daily for proper functioning. Preventive maintenance is essential to avoid mechanical failures, which could be fatal. Goals for quality control are to ensure that equipment is available and that it performs reliably when needed. The anesthesia machine and its components should be checked and serviced only by qualified personnel.

LOCAL AND REGIONAL ANESTHESIA

Local and regional anesthetic techniques are used to decrease intraoperative stimuli, thereby diminishing stress response to surgical trauma. Injected at or near the nerves of the surgical site, the anesthetic drug temporarily interrupts sensory nerve impulses during manipulation of sensitive tissues.

When a local anesthetic drug is used, the patient usually remains conscious. Local infiltration anesthesia is particularly advantageous for procedures performed in ambulatory surgery settings from which the patient is discharged to home soon after completion of the procedure. Oral, IM, or IV sedation may be given to relieve anxiety and to produce amnesia. IV sedation is commonly used and is referred to as moderate sedation.

Anesthetic may be administered locally during general anesthesia for postoperative pain control. When injected before the incision is made, the patient's nervous system is preempted from sensory stimulation associated with the initial trauma of incision. Some surgeons elect to inject local anesthesia drugs before the skin is closed for additional delay of sensory stimulation associated with postoperative pain.

Regional blocks are useful for more extensive procedures. Regional anesthesia may be used, with or without moderate sedation, when general anesthesia is contraindicated or undesired. Nerve blocks, intrathecal blocks, peridural blocks, and epidural blocks are examples of regional anesthesia techniques. These techniques block conduction of pain impulses from a specific area or region. The anesthetic drug is injected around a specific nerve or group of nerves to prevent pain of the surgical procedure.

Local anesthetics and regional blocks, with or without supplementary sedation, are administered as the anesthetic of choice for many diagnostic and therapeutic surgical procedures.

HISTORICAL BACKGROUND OF REGIONAL ANESTHESIA

Historically, the Incas used the coca leaf for local pain relief. Anthropologists have found evidence that liquid derivatives were used for trephination (creating holes in the skull). More formalized experimentation with cocaine began in 1860. European physicians found it had a numbing effect on the tongue and caused the pupils to dilate. Theories of the day held that cocaine had potential as a replacement for morphine. Sigmund Freud (1856-1939), an Austrian psychiatrist, and an ophthalmology student performed experiments in the use of cocaine as a local anesthetic for the eye. Freud also experimented with cocaine as a substitute for chemically dependent patients. Unfortunately, the patients ultimately became addicted to cocaine.

Leonard Corning (1855-1923), an American neurologist, experimented with cocaine as a local infiltrate in the spinal column. In 1885 he successfully induced spinal anesthesia and published a textbook on the subject of local anesthesia the following year. Epidural techniques were developed by two French physicians in 1901. August Bier (1861-1949), a German surgeon, continued the experimentation and the use of regional anesthesia in Europe. His technique of regional anesthesia using double tourniquets was introduced in 1908.

Refinement of other drugs followed and was strongly enhanced by the isolation of epinephrine by John Abel (1857-1938), an American pharmacologist. Heinrich Braun (1847-1911), a German surgeon, used epinephrine mixed with cocaine for local anesthesia during nasal and urologic surgery. He found that the tissues bled less and a lower concentration of the drug could be safely used. Local agents procaine (1904) and lidocaine (1948) advanced the use of local anesthesia by many practitioners.

Modern refinements and the development of additional drugs for injection have increased the use of local and regional anesthesia for surgical procedures.

PREPARATION OF THE PATIENT

Preparation of the patient who will receive a local or regional anesthetic depends on the extent of the procedure to be performed and on the anticipated technique of administration. Although it is anticipated that the patient will remain conscious, it is sometimes desirable or necessary to supplement the local or regional anesthesia with moderate sedation. Careful preoperative assessment, history taking, and a clear explanation of what to expect are part of the preparatory process. (More information can be found at www.nursingnet.org.)

Preoperative assessment of the patient who is scheduled for a procedure provides baseline data and identifies risk factors. Data that should be documented include the following:
- Baseline vital signs, blood pressure, laboratory values, and results of ECG monitoring and any other tests that were performed.
- Weight, height, and age; dosage of some drugs is calculated on the basis of body weight in kilograms (mg/kg of body weight). Some drugs are contraindicated for age extremes (i.e., pediatric or geriatric patients).
- Current medical problem(s) and history of medical events, including a history of substance abuse.
- Current medications or drug therapy, such as insulin for diabetes or hypertensive drugs.
- Allergy or hypersensitivity reactions to previous anesthetics or other drugs.
- Mental status, including emotional state and level of consciousness.
- Communication ability; a patient with hearing impairment or language barrier may be unable to understand verbal instructions during the procedure or to respond appropriately.

Preoperative orders regarding the time when the patient should cease taking anything by mouth vary with the circumstances; 6 to 8 hours before the surgical procedure is the usual minimum for adults. If possible, the adult patient is instructed to remain on nothing-by-mouth (NPO) status after midnight. Some patients are permitted a few sips of water to take oral medications, such as hypoglycemics or antihypertensives.

Many ambulatory surgical patients scheduled for same-day procedures have no premedication and are permitted to walk to the OR. Some facilities require the use of a stretcher or wheelchair for transport. The patient should be transported via a stretcher if sedated.

INTRAOPERATIVE PATIENT CARE

The patient must be able to respond cooperatively and to maintain respiration unassisted. The patient needs careful observation throughout the surgical procedure and for a period afterward for signs and symptoms of delayed reaction or complications. The care the patient will need depends on the type and length of the procedure, the amount of sedation given, and the type and amount of local anesthetic used. Psychologic support and reassurance are given before and during the surgical procedure. The patient should be told what to expect and what is expected of him or her. The patient should be monitored by qualified personnel and observed for adverse effects of the medication or the procedure.

LOCAL ANESTHESIA

The surgeon injects the anesthetic drug or applies it topically. The anesthesia provider is not in attendance for this method. Supplemental agents should be available for analgesia or anesthesia, if necessary, or for adverse reactions (Table 24-3). Resuscitative equipment, suction, and oxygen must be at hand before administration of any anesthetic. Qualified personnel should be immediately available to assist in the event of an emergency.

Administration of Local Anesthesia

In the absence of an anesthesia provider, a qualified registered nurse is responsible for monitoring the patient's physiologic status and safety during local anesthesia. This should be the only activity assigned to this nurse for the duration of the procedure. He or she should not perform circulating duties simultaneously. The circulating nurse who assumes the responsibility for patient monitoring should have the knowledge, skill, and ability to use and interpret data from monitoring equipment. The circulating nurse also should be able to recognize signs and symptoms of abnormal reactions to local anesthetic drugs and to provide interventions to prevent further complications.

The patient who is under local anesthesia requires observation of physiologic changes in pulse, blood pressure, oxygenation, and respiration. Baseline data obtained during preoperative assessment are compared with intraoperative and postoperative findings. The vital signs, including blood pressure, pulse, and respirations, are continuously monitored. Monitoring devices may include an electrocardiograph and pulse oximeter. Monitoring equipment is used

TABLE 24-3	Comparison of Toxicity and Allergy Caused by Local Anesthetic Drugs
Toxic Reaction	**Allergic Reaction***
Symptoms vary depending on the drug	Immediate localized reaction followed by generalized body reaction
SUBJECTIVE	
Dizziness, somnolence, paresthesia, nausea, visual/speech problems	Sense of uneasiness, pruritus, agitation, paresthesia
OBJECTIVE	
Decreased breathing rate and depth, muscle twitches, tremors, slurred speech, seizures, vomiting unconsciousness, coma	Erythema, urticaria, wheals
VASOVAGAL	
Dysrhythmias, bradycardia, vasodilation, hypotension, myocardial depression, cardiac arrest	Coughing, sneezing, wheezing, bronchospasm, hypotension, hypovolemia, vasodilation, cardiovascular collapse, cardiac arrest
TREATMENT	
Supportive, airway management; need intravenous (IV) line; Trendelenburg position; muscular contractions are treated with diazepam (Valium)	Especially with amino ester type: airway management, IV fluids, epinephrine, diphenhydramine, and steroids as needed

*Not common with amino amide.

to assess the patient's physiologic status in combination with direct observation.

Data from monitoring and direct observation are documented at frequent intervals and with any significant event, such as the injection of medication or the removal of a specimen. The patient is monitored for reaction to drugs and for behavioral and physiologic changes. It is important for the circulating nurse to be aware of the maximum dosages of local anesthetics in milligrams per kilogram of body weight. The total amount of anesthetic and supplementary drugs administered is also recorded in the patient's record. AORN has established recommended practices for the care of patients receiving local anesthesia. Policies and procedures should be in place to delineate patient care, monitoring activities, and documentation during the use of local anesthetics.

Moderate Sedation (Formerly Known as Intravenous Conscious Sedation)

During procedures performed with the patient under local anesthesia, mild sedation may be given by IV infusion. Moderate sedation refers to a mild to moderate depressed level of consciousness that allows the patient to maintain a patent airway independently and to respond appropriately to verbal instructions or physical stimulation. A benzodiazepine, such as midazolam (Versed) or diazepam (Valium), is most commonly given either alone or in combination with a narcotic and atropine or scopolamine. Benzodiazepines provide amnesia with sedation, but they also may cause respiratory depression and fluctuations in blood pressure and heart rate and rhythm.

All team members need to understand the objectives and desired effects of moderate sedation. If the primary objective is to allay the patient's anxiety and fear, the therapeutic effects of the drugs given should produce relaxation and some degree of amnesia. Because consciousness is maintained, the patient has intact protective reflexes to respond to physical stimuli. The patient also can easily be aroused with verbal commands as necessary. In this state, vital signs may fluctuate to a minimal extent. Documen-

tation in the patient's record should reflect evidence of continuous assessment and identification of any untoward or significant reactions during administration of local anesthesia with moderate sedation.

The Perioperative Nurse's Role During Local Anesthesia and Moderate Sedation

The patient under moderate sedation should be monitored continuously for cardiac status, blood pressure, pulse, respiration, and oxygen saturation. Monitoring devices may include but are not limited to an electrocardiograph and pulse oximeter. In the absence of an anesthesia provider, a qualified registered nurse should be assigned to monitor the patient's physiologic state. This registered nurse should not be assigned to simultaneously circulate and should be competent in the use and interpretation of monitoring devices.

An anesthesia provider should be in attendance to monitor those patients whose physiologic status is unstable. Policies and procedures should be in place that address the registered nurse's competency in patient monitoring and the nurse's role during the use of moderate sedation.

Monitored Anesthesia Care (MAC)

When an anesthesia provider's presence is necessary, the surgical procedure is scheduled as monitored anesthesia care (MAC), attended local, or anesthesia standby. Terminology may vary at different institutions. Patients with particular medical problems or age-extreme patients (pediatric or geriatric) may require supervision by anesthesia personnel.

Patients receiving a local anesthetic because they are too ill to undergo general anesthesia should have an anesthesia provider in attendance. The type and length of procedure also may be factors that influence the surgeon's request for an anesthesia provider to be available to give and monitor moderate sedation. The anesthesia provider may initiate and maintain a regional nerve block, such as an axillary brachial plexus block for hand surgery. Moderate sedation and regional blocks with MAC have gained popularity for ambulatory surgery.

Monitoring the Patient Receiving a Local Anesthetic

The extent of monitoring, determined in consultation with physicians in the department of surgery and anesthesiology where applicable, depends on the seriousness of the procedure, sedation required, and/or patient's condition. The circulating nurse assigned to monitor the patient receiving a local anesthetic, with or without moderate sedation, continuously attends the patient. This nurse does not have other responsibilities during the surgical procedure. *AORN Standards, Recommended Practices, and Guidelines* provides guidance for the circulating nurse in monitoring the patient receiving a local anesthetic and the patient receiving moderate sedation. The guidelines may be summarized briefly as follows:

1. The patient is monitored for reaction to drugs and for behavioral and physiologic changes. The circulating nurse should recognize and report to the physician significant changes in the patient's status and be prepared to initiate appropriate interventions.
2. The nurse attending the patient should have basic knowledge of the function and use of monitoring equipment, ability to interpret information, and working knowledge of resuscitation equipment. The nurse should have appropriate training and knowledge in pharmacology and the application of the drugs used in the patient's care.
3. Accurate reflection of perioperative care should be documented on the patient's record.
4. Institutional policies and procedures in regard to patient care, including monitoring, should be written, reviewed annually, and readily available. This information should be included in orientation and inservice programs. It should include policies regarding permissible drug administration and emergency interventions by the nurse.

In addition to preoperative assessment and postoperative evaluation for a continuum of care, intraoperative activities include determining and documenting the patient's baseline physiologic status before administration of sedatives, analgesics, and anesthetic drugs and monitoring the patient throughout the procedure. Parameters include but are not limited to the following:

- Blood pressure
- Heart rate and rhythm
- Respiratory rate
- Oxygen saturation by pulse oximetry
- Body temperature
- Skin condition and color
- Mental status and level of consciousness

Baseline vital signs are taken when the patient arrives in the OR. These are compared with admission vital signs. Vital signs are taken continually before injection of a drug and at 5- to 15-minute intervals after injection. Changes in the patient's condition are reported to the surgeon immediately. If an adverse reaction occurs, emergency measures should be instituted on request as per policy. These may include maintaining a patent airway, starting oxygen therapy when clinically indicated, and administering IV therapy per the physician's order.

Considerations in the Selection of Local Anesthetics

A local anesthetic depresses superficial peripheral nerves and blocks conduction of pain impulses from their site of origin. Regional nerve blocks interrupt conduction of pain impulses from a specific area or region. These techniques may be employed, with or without moderate sedation, when general anesthesia is contraindicated. As with any anesthetic agent, local anesthetics offer advantages in some circumstances but have disadvantages and are contraindicated in others.

Advantages

- Use of local anesthetic agents can minimize the recovery period. The patient can ambulate, eat, void, and resume normal activity.
- Use of local anesthetic requires minimal equipment and is economical.
- Loss of consciousness does not occur unless anesthesia is supplemented with additional drugs.
- Local anesthesia avoids the undesirable effects of general anesthesia.
- Local anesthesia is suitable for patients who recently ingested food or fluids (e.g., before an emergency procedure).
- Local anesthesia is useful for ambulatory patients having minor procedures.
- Local anesthesia is ideal for procedures in which it is desirable to have the patient awake and cooperative.

Disadvantages

- Local anesthesia is not practical for all types of procedures. For example, too much drug would be needed for some major surgical procedures; the duration of anesthesia is insufficient for others.
- There are individual variations in response to local anesthetic drugs.
- Rapid absorption of the drug into the bloodstream can cause severe, potentially fatal reactions.
- Apprehension may be increased by the patient's ability to see and hear. Some patients prefer to be unconscious and unaware.

Contraindications. Local anesthesia is generally contraindicated in patients with the following:

- Allergic sensitivity to the local anesthetic drug.
- Local infection or malignancy at the site of injection, which may be carried to and spread in adjacent tissues by injection. A bacteriologically safe injection site should be selected.
- Septicemia. In a proximal nerve block, a needle may open new lymph channels that drain through a region, thereby causing new foci and local abscess formation from the perforation of small vessels and escape of bacteria.
- Extreme nervousness, apprehension, excitability or inability to cooperate because of mental state or age.

SPINAL AND EPIDURAL ANESTHESIA

Intraspinal injection of an anesthetic drug is a technique of regional anesthesia performed by a person who has been properly trained and has acquired the necessary

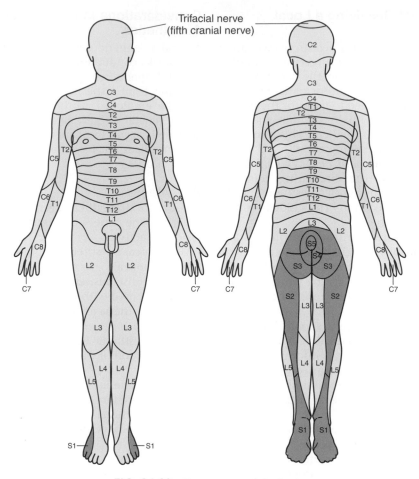

FIG. 24-10   Dermatomes of the body.

skill. Regional anesthesia is delivered to select areas, referred to as dermatomes, to affect motor and sensory nerves as desired (Fig. 24-10). The patient's dermatome levels can be tested by touch and by asking the patient to move his or her extremities. Dermatome level T12 is near the iliac crest, T10 is near the umbilicus, and T6 is near the xiphoid.

Assessment of the patient's level of consciousness, pulse, respirations, and blood pressure is essential for early detection of hypotension associated with high spinal anesthesia. If regional anesthesia extends above the level of T4, a full sympathetic block may follow, causing cardiorespiratory arrest. Ventilatory support equipment and naloxone should be immediately available.

Choices in Regional Drugs

The choice of drug depends on factors such as the duration, intensity, and level of anesthesia desired; the anticipated surgical position of the patient; and the surgical procedure (Fig. 24-11). Patient factors include the anesthetic history, physical condition, and preference of the patient and surgeon. The duration of action depends on physiologic and metabolic factors. The addition of a vasoconstrictor, usually epinephrine 1:200,000, prolongs the duration. Diffusion of the drug into the cerebrospinal fluid (CSF) is affected by solubility, molecular weight, and

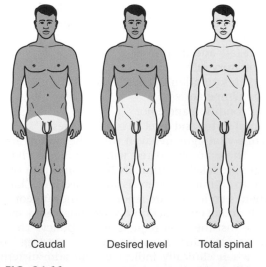

Caudal   Desired level   Total spinal

FIG. 24-11   Levels of spinal and epidural anesthesia.

TABLE 24-4	Local and Regional Anesthetic Agents				
Generic Name	Trade Name(s)	Uses	Concentration	Duration of Effect (Hours)	Maximum Dosage
AMINO AMIDES					
Bupivacaine	Marcaine Sensorcaine	Local infiltration* Regional block* Surgical epidural	0.25%-0.50%	2 to 3	400 mg
Dibucaine	Nupercaine Percaine Cinchocaine	Local infiltration Peripheral nerves	0.05%-0.1%	3 to 3½	30 mg
Etidocaine	Duranest	Peripheral nerves Epidural	0.5%-1%	2 to 3	500 mg
Lidocaine	Xylocaine Lignocaine	Topical Infiltration* Peripheral nerves* Nerve block* Spinal Epidural	2%-4% 0.5% 1%-2%	½ to 2	200 mg or 4 mg/kg 500 mg or 7 mg/kg when mixed with vasocontrictor
Mepivacaine	Carbocaine	Infiltration Peripheral nerves Epidural	0.5%-1% 1%-2%	½ to 2	500 mg
Prilocaine	Citanest	Infiltration Peripheral nerves Regional block Epidural	1%-2% 2%-3%	½ to 2½	600 mg
Ropivacaine	Naropin	Infiltration Field block Nerve block Epidural Postoperative pain management Not used for Bier block	0.2% 0.5% 0.75% 1%	2½ for surgical analgesia; 6 to 10 for surgical nerve block	200 mg for analgesia; 300 mg for nerve block
AMINO ESTERS					
Chloroprocaine	Nesacaine	Infiltration* Peripheral nerves* Nerve block* Epidural Topical	0.5% 2% 2% 2%-3% 4%-10%	¼ to ½ ½	1000 mg 200 mg or 4 mg/kg body weight
Cocaine					
Procaine	Novocain	Infiltration Peripheral nerves Spinal	0.5% 1%-2%	¼ to ½	1000 mg or 14 mg/kg body weight
Tetracaine	Cetacaine Pontocaine	Topical Spinal	2% 1%	2 to 4	20 mg

*Epinephrine may be used.

volume. Glucose may be added to make the drug heavier than CSF (hyperbaric). Anesthesia diminishes as the drug is absorbed into the systemic circulation. The most commonly used anesthetic drugs for spinal and epidural anesthesia are listed in Table 24-4.

The anesthesia provider determines the placement site of the injection needle according to the bony landmarks of the spine (Fig. 24-12). The spinal and epidural drugs are injected using specially designed needles with angles and lumens that are specific to the type of anesthesia being delivered (Fig. 24-13).

Spinal Anesthesia

Spinal anesthesia, also referred to as an intrathecal block, causes desensitization of spinal ganglia and motor roots. The agent is injected into the CSF in the subarachnoid space of the meninges (the three-layered covering of the spinal cord) using a lumbar interspace in the vertebral

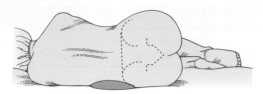

FIG. 24-12 Landmarks used for epidural or spinal anesthesia.

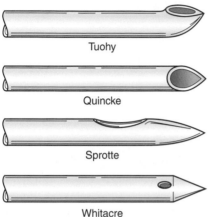

Tuohy

Quincke

Sprotte

Whitacre

FIG. 24-13 Physical characteristics of four different spinal and epidural needles (not to scale).

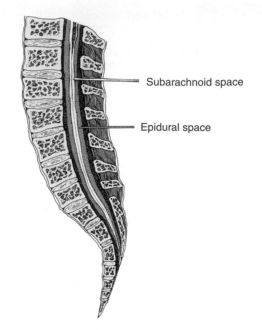

Subarachnoid space

Epidural space

FIG. 24-14 Agent is injected into subarachnoid space for spinal anesthesia or into epidural space for epidural anesthesia.

column (Fig. 24-14). The subarachnoid space is located between the pia mater (the innermost membranous layer covering the spinal cord) and the arachnoid (the thin, vascular, weblike layer immediately beneath the dura mater, which is the outermost sheath covering the spinal cord). Spinal ganglia, motor nerve roots, and blood vessels pass through the meninges. The drug diffuses into the CSF around ganglia and nerves before it is absorbed into the bloodstream. Absorption into nerve fibers is rapid.

Spinal anesthesia is often used for abdominal (mainly lower) or pelvic procedures requiring relaxation, inguinal or lower extremity procedures, surgical obstetrics (cesarean section without effect on the fetus), and urologic procedures. It is preferred for patients with alcoholism, substance abusers, or obese or muscular patients (who would need large doses of general anesthetic and muscle relaxant), and for emergency surgical procedures on patients who have eaten recently. It is also used in the presence of hepatic, renal, or metabolic disease, because it causes minimal upset of body chemistry.

The level of anesthesia attained depends on various factors, such as the patient's position during and immediately after injection; CSF pressure; site and rate of injection; volume, dosage, and specific gravity (baricity) of the solution; inclusion of a vasoconstrictor, such as epinephrine; spinal curvature; interspace chosen; uterine contractions with labor; and coughing or straining, which can inadvertently raise the level. Spread of the anesthetic is controlled mainly by solution baricity and patient position. The period immediately after injection is decisive; the anesthetic is

becoming "fixed" (i.e., absorbed by the tissues and unable to travel). Further control of the anesthetic level is attained by tilting the operating bed at that time. The direction of tilting depends on whether the drug is hyperbaric (specific gravity greater than that of spinal fluid) or hypobaric (lighter than spinal fluid). Isobaric anesthetics (same weight as spinal fluid) are made hyperbaric by the addition of 5% or 10% dextrose to the anesthetic before injection.

Immediately after the anesthetic is injected, the anesthesia provider carefully tests the level of anesthesia by pinprick, touch, or nerve stimulation, tilting the bed as necessary to achieve the desired level for the surgical procedure. After anesthetic fixation and with the anesthesia provider's permission, the patient is placed in surgical position. The patient is asked to relax and let the team turn him or her. Straining or holding the breath can alter the position of the dural sac and precipitate hypotension or an inadvertent rise in the level of anesthesia. The incision is not made until it is certain that anesthesia is adequate. Supplementation of spinal anesthesia is necessary if anesthesia or muscular relaxation is insufficient or the patient is unduly apprehensive. Sometimes the patient is given moderate sedation but can still be roused.

Choice of Agent. The drug used depends on various factors such as the duration, intensity, and level of anesthesia desired, the anticipated surgical position of the patient, and the surgical procedure.

Duration of Agent. The variable duration of anesthesia depends on physiologic and metabolic factors. It is prolonged by the addition of a vasoconstrictor. Anesthesia diminishes as the agent is absorbed into the systemic circulation.

Spinal Anesthesia Procedure. For injection, the patient is placed in the position desired by the anesthesia provider, depending on patient condition, solution baricity, and level of anesthesia to be produced:

- *Lateral position:* The patient lies on the side with the back at the edge of the operating bed. The knees are flexed onto the abdomen, and the head is flexed to the chest. The hips and shoulders are vertical to the operating bed to prevent rotation of the spine (Fig. 24-15).
- *Sitting position:* The patient sits on the side of the operating bed with the feet resting on a stool. The spine is flexed, with the chin lowered to the sternum; the arms are crossed and supported on a pillow on an adjustable table or Mayo stand (Fig. 24-16).

The circulating nurse or an anesthesia technician supports and reassures the patient in an aligned position and assists the anesthesia provider as possible. Attention to asepsis is extremely important. The anesthesia provider dons sterile gloves before handling sterile items. Sterile disposable spinal trays eliminate the need for cleaning and sterilizing of reusable equipment. They also avoid the hazards of sterilizing ampules. The dates on the drugs supplied by the manufacturer should be checked.

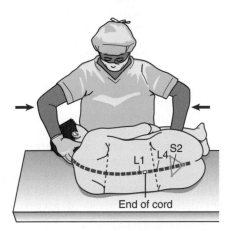

FIG. 24-15   Spinal block—lateral position.

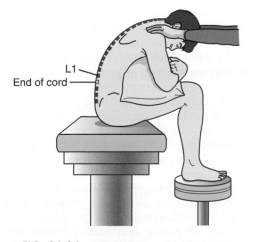

FIG. 24-16   Spinal block—sitting position.

A spinal tray usually contains the following:
- Fenestrated drape.
- Ampules of local anesthetic, spinal anesthetic, vasoconstrictor drug, 10% dextrose.
- Gauze squares, forceps, and antiseptic solution. Some kits include disposable skin prep sponges on plastic applicator sticks.
- Needles: 25-gauge hypodermic needle for infiltration of local anesthetic into the skin; 22-gauge × 2-inch (5-cm) needle for IM injection, blunt 18-gauge needles for mixing drugs, 22- or 26-gauge × 3½-inch (9-cm) spinal needle with stylets for intrathecal injection.
- Syringes: 5-mL syringes for spinal anesthetic, 10-mL syringes for hypobaric solutions, 2-mL syringes for superficial anesthesia.

The puncture site is cleansed with an antiseptic solution and draped with a fenestrated drape. Advise the patient that the prep solution will feel cold and wet. Before the skin is penetrated, the patient should be told that the skin will be numbed with local anesthetic and the spinal needle will be inserted. This prevents the startle effect of the needlestick in the patient. The blood pressure is checked before, during, and after spinal anesthesia because hypotension is common.

Advantages. The patient is conscious if desired. The procedure can be performed with moderate sedation as necessary. Throat reflexes are maintained; breathing is quiet, without airway problems because the respiratory system is not irritated. The bowel is contracted. Muscle relaxation and anesthesia are excellent if the procedure is properly executed.

Disadvantages. Spinal anesthesia produces a circulatory depressant effect: hypotension, and stasis of blood as a result of interference with venous return from motor paralysis and arteriolar dilation in the lower extremities. A change in body position may be followed by a sudden drop in blood pressure; after fixation of the anesthetic, a slight elevation of the feet and legs may increase venous return to the heart. The agent cannot be removed after injection. Nausea and emesis may accompany cerebral ischemia, traction on viscera and peritoneum, or premedication. There is possible sensitivity to the agent and danger of trauma or infection. The patient has all senses present, such as hearing, sight, and smell, and is able to speak.

Complications. Transient or permanent neurologic sequelae from cord trauma, irritation by the agent, lack of asepsis, and loss of spinal fluid with decreased intracranial pressure syndrome are potential complications. Examples include spinal headache; auditory and ocular disturbances, such as tinnitus and diplopia; arachnoiditis; meningitis; transverse myelitis; cauda equina syndrome (failure to regain use of the legs or control of urinary and bowel functions); temporary paresthesias, such as numbness and tingling; cranial nerve palsies; and urinary retention. Late complications include nerve root lesions, spinal cord lesions, and ruptured nucleus pulposus.

True spinal headache caused by a persistent CSF leak through the needle hole in the dura usually responds to supine bed rest, copious oral or IV fluids, and systemic analgesia. Refractory postspinal headache may be treated by an epidural blood patch: 5 to 10 mL of the patient's own blood is administered at the puncture site. This usually affords prompt relief.

If a high level of anesthesia is reached, extreme caution is essential to prevent respiratory paralysis ("total spinal"), an emergency situation requiring mechanical ventilation until the level of anesthesia has receded. Respiratory arrest, although rare, is thought to be a result of medullary hypoperfusion caused by a sympathetic block. Apnea also can be produced by respiratory center ischemia resulting from precipitous hypotension.

The anesthesia machine, oxygen, and IV line must bein readiness before injection. Constant vigilance of respiration and circulation is critical. The blood pressure and heart rate are monitored and maintained at normal levels.

Epidural Anesthesia

The terms *epidural, peridural,* and *extradural* are used synonymously. The epidural space lies between the dura mater, the outermost sheath covering the spinal cord, and the walls of the vertebral column. It contains a network of blood vessels, lymphatics, fat, loose connective tissue, and spinal nerve roots. Injection is made into this space surrounding the dura mater (see Fig. 24-14). The drug diffuses slowly through the dura mater into CSF. Anesthesia is prolonged while the drug is absorbed from CSF into the bloodstream. The spread of anesthetic and duration of action are influenced by the concentration and volume of solution injected (total drug mass) and the rate of injection. The anesthetic diffuses toward the head (cephalad) and toward the coccyx (caudad). In contrast to spinal anesthesia, patient position, baricity, and gravity have little influence on anesthetic distribution. The high incidence of systemic reactions is attributed to absorption of the agent from the highly vascular peridural area and the relatively large mass of anesthetic injected. Epinephrine 1:200,000 is usually added to retard absorption. Approaches used for epidural anesthesia and analgesia include thoracic, lumbar, and caudal approaches. Skin and ligaments are infiltrated with a local anesthetic agent before the epidural catheter is placed.

The management and sequelae of epidural anesthesia are similar to those of spinal anesthesia. An epidural approach may be used for lower extremity, abdominal, urologic, anorectal, vaginal, or perineal procedures. It is used commonly for postoperative pain management and in obstetrics during labor and delivery or during and after cesarean section. The patient is attended constantly by a qualified registered nurse once the block is initiated for analgesia. Vital signs should be monitored at regular intervals, and any deviation of level of consciousness, pulse, respirations, or blood pressure should be reported immediately to the anesthesiologist. Use of an apnea monitor may be indicated. In an obstetric patient, the fetal heart rate should be electronically monitored continuously because the patient is insensitive to uterine contractions.

Epidural narcotic analgesia may provide sustained postoperative relief or control of pain in patients with intractable or prolonged pain. This may be administered by a percutaneous indwelling epidural catheter, an implanted epidural catheter with infusion port or reservoir and pump, or an implantable infusion device. A patient may come to the OR for placement of an epidural catheter or pump device for ongoing pain management.

An epidural catheter for administration of a narcotic for prolonged postoperative pain relief, usually for 2 or 3 days, may be inserted before induction of general anesthesia, for postoperative use. Morphine, fentanyl, sufentanil, and buprenorphine are the drugs most commonly used for prolonged pain relief. Although probability of respiratory depression is less when the epidural route is used as compared with spinal narcotics, use of an apnea monitor is advisable. Side effects include nausea and vomiting, urinary retention, and pruritus. Epidural narcotics block pain at the level of opiate receptors in the dorsal horn of the spinal cord, not in the brain, so the patient is mentally alert and able to ambulate.

Thoracic and Lumbar Approaches. The thoracic and lumbar approaches are peridural blocks. Equipment is similar to that for a spinal block with the addition of a 19-gauge × 3½-inch (9-cm), thin-walled needle with a stylet with a rigid shaft and a short, beveled tip to minimize the danger of inadvertent dural puncture. Insertion of a catheter allows repeated injections for continuous intraoperative and postoperative epidural anesthesia, requiring additional needles, stopcocks, and a plastic catheter in the setup.

Caudal Approach. The caudal approach is an epidural sacral block. Epidural injection is through the caudal canal, desensitizing nerves emerging from the dural sac. The patient position for injection is prone with the hips flexed, sacrum horizontal, and heels turned outward to expose the injection site. The sacral area is prepared and draped, with care taken to protect the genitalia from irritating solution. The left lateral position is used in the pregnant patient. The spread of agents in epidural anesthesia is enhanced in pregnancy, atherosclerosis, and advanced age.

The tray includes the addition of a 20- to 24-gauge × 1½ inch (4-cm) spinal needle with a stylet. Commercial sets are available.

Advantages. Compared with spinal anesthesia, epidural anesthesia has a decreased incidence of hypotension, headache, and potential for neurologic complications, although a higher failure rate is reported.

Disadvantages. There is less controllable height of anesthesia; it is a more difficult technique; there is a greater area of potential infection from anaerobic organisms with the caudal approach; it is unpredictable; it is time consuming (i.e., a longer time is required for complete anesthesia); a larger amount of agent is injected; continuous technique may slow the first stage of labor.

Complications. Intravascular injection, accidental dural puncture and total spinal anesthesia, blood vessel puncture and hematoma, profound hypotension, backache, and transient or permanent paralysis (paraplegia) are possible complications. The patient may suffer hypoxia, respiratory arrest, and/or cardiac arrest.

TECHNIQUES OF ADMINISTRATION OF LOCAL OR REGIONAL ANESTHESIA

Topical Application

The anesthetic is applied directly to a mucous membrane, to a serous surface, or into an open wound. A topical agent is often applied to the respiratory passages to eliminate laryngeal reflexes and cough, for insertion of airways before induction or during light general anesthesia, or for therapeutic and diagnostic procedures such as laryngoscopy or bronchoscopy. It is also used in the urethral meatus for cystoscopy. Mucous membranes readily absorb topical agents because of their vascularity. The onset of anesthesia occurs within minutes. The blood level of a topical agent may equal the same level obtained by IV injection. The duration of anesthesia is 20 to 30 minutes. If a spray or atomizer is used, it should contain a visible reservoir so that the quantity of drug administered is clearly observed, because droplets vary in size, causing variations in dosages.

Preanesthetic anticholinergics are important before topical application within the respiratory tract. Saliva can dilute the topical anesthetic and prevent adequate duration of contact with mucous membranes. Also, a dry throat is necessary to prevent aspiration until the anesthetic effect has disappeared and throat reflexes have returned. Adverse reactions to topical anesthetic agents are uncommon when dosage is carefully controlled. Sudden cardiovascular collapse can occur, more commonly after topical anesthesia of the respiratory tract.

Topical local anesthetic ointment may be used on the skin surface before establishing IV access. The ointment should be applied and allowed to remain in contact with the skin for several minutes to an hour for optimal effect. A transparent cover dressing may be placed over the application point to prevent accidental smearing of the medication. Care is taken to prevent contact with the eyes and other mucous membranes.

Cryoanesthesia

Cryoanesthesia involves blocking local nerve conduction of painful impulses by means of marked surface cooling (i.e., freezing) of a localized area. It is used in such brief procedures as the removal of warts or noninvasive papular surface lesions. Cryotherapy units are commercially available.

Simple Local Infiltration

The agent is injected intracutaneously and subcutaneously into tissues at and around the incisional site to block peripheral sensory nerve stimuli at their origin. It is used before suturing superficial lacerations or excising minor lesions.

Regional Injection

The agent is injected into or around a specific nerve or group of nerves to depress the entire sensory nervous system of a limited, localized area of the body. The injection is at a distance from the surgical site. A wider, deeper area is anesthetized than with simple infiltration. There are several types of regional blocks.

Nerve Block. A selected nerve is anesthetized at a given point. Nerve blocks are performed to interrupt sensory,

motor, and/or sympathetic transmission. Blocks may be used preoperatively, intraoperatively, and postoperatively to prevent pain of the procedure; diagnostically to ascertain the cause of pain; or therapeutically to relieve chronic pain. Blocks are useful in various circulatory and neurosurgical syndromes, such as reflex sympathetic dystrophy (RSD). For prolonged pain relief (e.g., during a long procedure or to treat chronic pain associated with disease or trauma), a continuous infusion or incremental injections through a catheter may sustain regional anesthesia. Some examples of blocks are as follows:

1. Surgical blocks
   a. Paravertebral block of the cervical plexus for procedures in the area between the jaw and the clavicle
   b. Intercostal block for relatively superficial intra-abdominal procedures, such as drain placement
   c. Brachial plexus or axillary block for arm procedures
   d. Median, radial, or ulnar nerve block for the elbow or wrist
   e. Hand and digital block for fingers (an additive vasoconstrictor, such as epinephrine, is not added to the local agent because necrosis can result from inadequate circulation to the digit)
   f. Blocks in other specific areas, such as a penile block for circumcision in adults
2. Diagnostic or therapeutic blocks
   a. Sympathetic nerve ganglion block to produce desired vasodilation by paralysis of the sympathetic nerve supply to the constricting smooth muscle in the artery wall
   b. Stellate ganglion block to increase circulation in peripheral vascular disease in the head, neck, arm, or hand
   c. Paravertebral lumbar block to increase circulation in the lower extremities
   d. Celiac block for relief of abdominal pain of pancreatic origin

Bier Block. A Bier block is a regional IV injection of a local anesthetic to an extremity below the level of a double-cuffed tourniquet (Fig. 24-17). The extremity is elevated. Blood is drained from the extremity by wrapping it from distal to proximal with a rubber compression Esmarch bandage as the limb is held up. The upper (proximal) cuff is inflated to stop blood flow after the extremity has been exsanguinated (Fig. 24-18). The arm is lowered and the Esmarch bandage is removed. Local anesthetic is injected into the IV catheter (Fig. 24-19). When the anesthetic takes effect over the limb, the lower (distal) cuff of the tourniquet is inflated. When the lower cuff is fully inflated, the upper (proximal) cuff is released. The patient feels less discomfort related to the tourniquet, because the lower cuff is over an anesthetized region.

On release of the tourniquet at the conclusion of the surgical procedure, entry of a bolus of the remaining drug and metabolic waste into systemic circulation may cause cardiovascular or CNS symptoms of toxicity, such as blindness. A Bier block is used for upper extremity procedures and for those that last an hour or less.

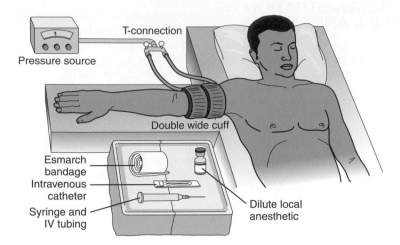

FIG. 24-17   Intravenous regional block—equipment for Bier block using double tourniquet.

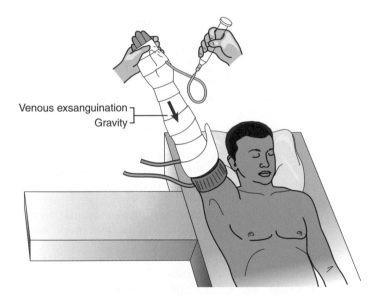

FIG. 24-18   Intravenous regional block—venous exsanguination with Esmarch bandage before inflation of upper tourniquet.

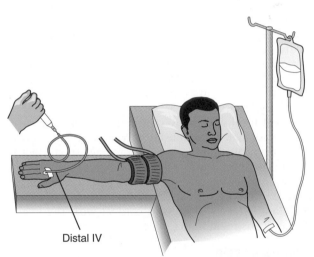

FIG. 24-19   Intravenous regional block—Esmarch is removed. Drug is injected intravenously and lower cuff inflated. Upper cuff is deflated.

Field Block. The surgical site is blocked off with a wall of anesthetic drug. A series of injections into proximal and surrounding tissues will provide a wide area of anesthesia, as in an abdominal wall block for herniorrhaphy.

Complications of Blocks. Each type of block carries unique complication potential. Examples of complications include the following:

- *Intercostal blocks:* Pneumothorax, atelectasis, total spinal anesthesia, air embolism, transverse myelitis
- *Brachial plexus blocks:* Pneumothorax, hemothorax, recurrent laryngeal nerve paralysis, phrenic paralysis, subarachnoid injection, Horner syndrome (axillary approach may be preferred to interscalene approach)
- *Stellate ganglion blocks:* pneumothorax
- *Celiac blocks:* Large vessel perforation, pancreatic injury, total spinal anesthesia

ACTIONS OF LOCAL AND REGIONAL ANESTHETICS

Local and regional anesthetics interfere with the initiation and transmission of nerve impulses by interacting with the membranous sheath that covers nerve fibers. By physical and biochemical mechanisms, drugs retard and stop the propagation of nerve impulses, eventually blocking conduction.

Drug Pharmacodynamics

The duration of action depends not only on pharmacologic properties of drugs but also on the volume and concentration of the solution and its systemic interactions. Drugs vary in potency, penetration, rapidity of hydrolysis or destruction, and toxicity.

Conduction Velocity. Nerve fibers vary in their susceptibility to drugs. The larger the fiber, the greater the concentration required. The least amount and lowest concentration to achieve the desired effect should be administered. Conduction of a peripheral stimulus is blocked at its origin by topical application or local infiltration of the drug. Transmission of stimuli along afferent nerves from the surgical site is blocked in regional anesthesia. Conductive pathways in and around the spinal cord are blocked for spinal and epidural anesthesia.

Blocking Quality. Drugs of high potency, minimal systemic activity, and prompt metabolism and those that lack local irritation are most effective. Blocking qualities include the following:

- Latency time between administration and maximum effect
- Duration of action
- Regression time between beginning and end of pain perception

Sensory nerves are blocked initially. Motor nerves also are affected, with resultant paralysis of both voluntary and involuntary muscles. Some degree of vasodilation occurs with all local and regional use of anesthetic drugs except cocaine.

Absorption Rate and Additives. Local blood flow, vasodilation, and vascularity of tissues can markedly influence local anesthetic action and systemic absorption of drugs. Fibrous tissue and fat in some injection sites act as diffusion barriers and nonspecific binding sites. Additives to slow uptake include:

- *Epinephrine (Adrenalin):* A catecholamine, epinephrine is a potent stimulant. When combined with an anesthetic drug, it causes vasoconstriction to slow circulatory uptake and absorption, thus prolonging anesthesia. It is used to counteract cardiovascular depressant effects of large doses of local anesthetic. It also decreases bleeding, which is a desired effect in many surgical procedures. A concentration of epinephrine that is 1:1000 (1000 mg/1000 mL × 1 mg/mL) to 1:200,000 (0.005 mg/mL) may be optimal for absorptive and hemostatic purposes. Epinephrine is premixed in commercially prepared solutions. If it is added to an anesthetic drug, it is best to do so with a calibrated syringe to avoid overdosage. Epinephrine can produce an acute adrenergic response: nervousness, pallor, diaphoresis, tremor, palpitation, tachycardia, and hypertension. The patient receiving epinephrine should be well oxygenated.
- *Sodium bicarbonate:* A small amount of carbonation can be added to local anesthetic agents. The carbonation lowers the pH of the solution, causing it to cross the cell membrane more readily. Alkalization results in decreased pain on injection. One potential problem with the addition of bicarbonate is that it may precipitate in the local anesthetic solution.
- *Dextran:* Anesthetic solutions with a pH higher than 8 can be mixed with dextran for prolongation of the localized anesthetic effect.

Toxicity. Allergic reactions to anesthetic drugs can occur but are rare. Toxic reactions occur when the concentration of drug in the blood affects the CNS. Slurred speech, numbness of the tongue, blurred vision, and tinnitus are symptoms of toxicity that can progress to drowsiness and confusion. The maximum recommended dosage for each drug should not be exceeded. Severe toxic reaction can quickly lead to cardiovascular collapse. In topical anesthesia, extremely rapid systemic absorption from the mucous membranes explains the relatively high frequency of toxic reactions. In local or regional anesthesia, inadvertent intravascular injection and use of fairly large quantities in highly vascular areas will contribute to local anesthetic toxicity.

Pharmacologic Agent Overview

Many different local or regional anesthetic drugs are in use. All are direct myocardial depressants, but the CNS effects precede this depression. Detoxification occurs in the liver. They differ in structure and therefore in action. These drugs are hydrochloride salts of weak bases in solution. They are categorized by chemical structure as amino amides and amino esters (see Table 24-4).

Amino Amides. Amino amides are metabolized in the liver by enzymes and are excreted by the kidneys. Patients with hepatic disease may become toxic with normal dosages because of ineffective metabolism. The amides include the following:

- *Ropivacaine (Naropin):* One of the newest local anesthetics on the market, ropivacaine is used for field blocks, nerve blocks, epidurals, and postoperative pain control epidural applications. Four strengths are available: 0.2% (2 mg/mL), 0.5% (5 mg/mL), 0.75% (7.5 mg/mL), and 1% (10 mg/mL). Epidural administration may result in hypotension and bradycardia.
- *Lidocaine (Xylocaine):* Probably the most widely used agent, this potent anesthetic slowly hydrolyzes in circulating plasma. It undergoes hepatic degradation and is pregnancy category C. Dosage should be reduced if hepatic function or blood flow is impaired. Its major advantages are a rapid onset of anesthesia and lack of local irritant effect. Allergic reactions are rare. Used extensively for surgical procedures and dentistry, it has moderate potency and a moderate duration of action. For infiltration: 0.5%; for peripheral nerves: 1% to 2% with vasoconstrictor additive; maximum dose: 500 mg or 7 mg/kg body weight. It is a good topical anesthetic, although it is not as effective as cocaine. For topical use in the respiratory tract: 2% to 4%; maximum dose: 200 mg without vasoconstrictor additive. It is commonly used topically before intubation. Clinical indications of lidocaine toxicity usually are related to the CNS such as complaints of circumoral and tongue numbness. Excessive doses can produce myocardial and circulatory depression. Toxic IV dose is 250 mg.
- *Mepivacaine (Carbocaine):* Similar to lidocaine, mepivacaine takes effect rapidly but produces a 20% longer duration of anesthesia. It has moderate potency and a moderate duration of action. It is commonly employed for infiltration and nerve block. It produces minimal tissue irritation and few adverse reactions. Epinephrine may not be added to it because of its duration of action.

For infiltration: 0.5% to 1%; for peripheral nerves: 1% to 2%; maximum dose: 500 mg.

- *Bupivacaine (Marcaine, Sensorcaine):* Four times more potent than lidocaine, bupivacaine has high potency of long duration. The onset of anesthesia is slow, but the duration is two to three times longer than that of lidocaine or mepivacaine, with toxicity approximate to that of tetracaine. Cumulation occurs with repeated injection. The drug affords prolonged pain relief after caudal block for rectal procedures. It is contraindicated for obstetric paracervical block and epidural anesthesia and for a Bier block. For local infiltration or a regional block, with or without epinephrine: 0.25% to 0.50%; maximum dose: 175 mg per dose without epinephrine or 225 mg with epinephrine 1:200,000 to a total dose of 400 mg.
- *Prilocaine (Citanest):* With prilocaine the onset of anesthesia is slower than with lidocaine, but the duration of action is longer. It is particularly useful for patients with diabetes or cardiovascular disease. It is used without epinephrine. For infiltration: 1% or 2%; for regional blocks and peripheral nerves: 2% or 3%; maximum dose: 600 mg.
- *Etidocaine (Duranest):* The onset of anesthesia is slower than that of lidocaine, but the block is of greater potency and toxicity, with a longer duration of action. For peripheral nerves: 0.5% to 1%; maximum dose: 500 mg.
- *Dibucaine (Nupercaine, Percaine, Cinchocaine):* Dibucaine is a very potent drug with a high rate of systemic toxicity. The onset is slow, and the duration of action is long. For infiltration and peripheral nerves: 0.05% to 0.1%; maximum dose: 30 mg.

Amino Esters. Amino esters are hydrolyzed in plasma by pseudocholinesterase enzymes produced by the liver. Para-aminobenzoic acid (PABA), a factor in the vitamin B complex, is a product of this metabolism. Some patients are allergic to PABA. The esters include the following:

- *Cocaine:* The first known local anesthetic, introduced in 1884, cocaine is a crystalline powder with a bitter taste in solution. It is the most toxic of the local drugs and, in contrast to all but lidocaine, is a vasoconstrictor and a CNS stimulant. Cocaine reduces bleeding and shrinks congested mucous membranes. It causes temporary paralysis of sensory nerve fibers, produces exhilaration, lessens hunger and fatigue, and stimulates pulse and respiratory rates. Administration is by topical application only, because of its high toxicity; the solution rapidly penetrates mucous membrane and spreads into highly vascular tissue. Absorption is self-limiting because of vasoconstrictive properties associated with the drug. Epinephrine should not be added. When applied to the throat, cocaine abolishes throat reflexes. The patient is awake and can cooperate, but its limited use and possible addiction are disadvantages.

    Cocaine is used topically in 4% concentration for anesthesia of the upper respiratory tract (nose, pharynx, tracheobronchial tree) in 1- to 2-mL amounts on a cotton pattie. Untoward reactions may occur rapidly in response to even a very small amount of the drug. Maximum dose: 200 mg or 1.5 mg/kg body weight. Cocaine is metabolized by the liver and excreted by the kidneys. It should be used with caution in patients with impaired liver or kidney function. It is contraindicated in pregnancy because it decreases uterine blood flow.

- *Procaine (Novocain):* Procaine is similar to cocaine but less toxic. Concentrations used: 0.5% for infiltration; 1% to 2% for peripheral nerves. It is injected subcutaneously, intramuscularly, or intrathecally. It has low potency, is of short duration, and is ineffective topically. Its advantages include minimal toxicity, easy sterilization, low cost, and lack of local irritation. Newer agents are used more frequently. Maximum dose: 1000 mg (1 g) or 14 mg/kg body weight.
- *Chloroprocaine (Nesacaine):* Chloroprocaine is possibly the safest local anesthetic from the standpoint of systemic toxicity because of its fast metabolism. It has moderate potency of short duration. It is rapidly hydrolyzed in the plasma. Its action is fast, but it is not active topically. When used in obstetrics, it does not alter neurobehavioral responses of newborn infants in any detectable way. For infiltration: 0.5%; for peripheral nerves: 2%; maximum dose: 1000 mg (1 g).
- *Tetracaine (Cetacaine):* With tetracaine, the onset of analgesia is slow but the duration of its effect is longer than that of many other drugs. It has high potency of long duration. It is also more toxic systemically because of the slow rate of destruction in the body, but low total dosage tends to reduce the chances of reaction. It is not used for local tissue infiltration or nerve block. Tetracaine in 2% solution is used only for topical anesthesia on accessible mucous membranes such as the oropharynx. Maximum dose: 20 mg. Tetracaine is used primarily for spinal anesthesia.

COMPLICATIONS OF LOCAL AND REGIONAL ANESTHESIA

Minor or transient complications of local and regional anesthesia are common. Serious complications, although rare, are usually permanent. Complications may be caused by the mechanical effect of needles or pharmacologic effect of the drug administered. As with general anesthesia, the prevention of complications requires patient assessment and preparation, knowledge of anatomy and physiology, and attention to detail. Proper choice of drug, equipment, and constant monitoring are as necessary in local and regional anesthesia as in general anesthesia. Complications of local and regional anesthesia may be summarized briefly as local effects, systemic effects, and effects unrelated to the anesthetic drug.

Local Effects

Tissue trauma, hematoma, ischemia, drug sensitivity, and infection can be minimized by the use of proper drugs and equipment, sterile technique, avoidance of local anesthetics with vasoconstrictors in sites with smaller vascular structures (digits, penis), and avoidance of repetitive injection that promotes trauma, edema, tissue necrosis, and infection.

Systemic Effects

Systemic effects are primarily cardiovascular, neurologic, or respiratory (e.g., hypotension, seizure, respiratory depression). Drug interactions also are systemic. After high blood levels, toxicity that affects more than one system may occur. Blood levels depend on the amount of drug used, its physical characteristics, the presence or absence of vasoconstrictors, and the injection site. For example, because of vascularity of surrounding tissue, intercostal blocks produce higher anesthetic blood levels in a shorter time than do axillary or epidural blocks. Absorption and the blood level of drugs are related to their uptake and rate of removal from the circulation. A linear relationship exists between the amount of drug administered via a given route and the resultant peak anesthetic blood level.

Predisposing Factors for Hypersensitivity

True hypersensitivity that produces an allergic response can occur, but it is less frequent than reactions from overdosage of pharmacologic agents. The following may predispose a patient to hypersensitivity:

- *Immunologic sensitization:* Allergies are thought to be more common with the amino esters than with the amide group of compounds. An allergic reaction to the preservative in some solutions, such as methylparaben, also is possible. Some local anesthetics release histamine, which is the basis of an allergic response. True allergy, mediated by antigen-antibody reaction, can cause anaphylaxis, urticaria (skin wheals), dermatitis, itching, laryngeal edema, and possibly cardiovascular collapse.
- *Overdosage:* An excessive amount of drug may enter the bloodstream if the injection exceeds maximum dose or is absorbed too rapidly. The IV route is the most dangerous route of injection, because histamine is released into the systemic circulation. The injection site is also pertinent. Hazardous sites involve vascular areas of tracheobronchial mucosa, and tissues of the head, neck, and paravertebral region. The least hazardous areas are subcutaneous tissue of the extremities and trunk (abdominal wall and buttocks).

Precautions

Extraordinary precautions must be taken for a patient with a history of any allergies, hypersensitivities, or reactions to previous anesthetics or other drugs. Atopic individuals, those with a hereditary tendency or with multiple allergies, may be more prone to adverse reactions to anesthetics or other drugs. Prediction of allergic reactions is unreliable. If testing for sensitivity to specific drugs is done, it is executed cautiously under well-controlled conditions.

Precautions for preventing adverse drug reactions in all patients include the following:

1. Assessing the patient's preoperative physiologic and psychological condition to determine potential problems and abnormal stress responses:
   a. Identify all medications the patient has recently received or is currently taking, including any history of substance abuse. If local anesthesia is planned, ask the patient if he or she has ever had local anesthesia at the dentist's office and if there were any adverse effects.
   b. Question the patient about known or suspected previous drug reactions. Any chemically related drug is not given.
   c. Help the patient cope with anxiety and fears by giving preoperative instructions and answering questions.
2. Handling drugs with care. Before administering or placing drugs on the sterile table:
   a. Read the label carefully. Check the expiration date.
   b. Discard the ampule or vial if the label is not completely legible or has been disturbed.
   c. Open, unlabeled, undated, multiple-use vials should be discarded and not used.
   d. Observe the solution for clarity, and discard any suspicious ampule or vial.
3. Administering drugs selected by a physician in appropriate concentrations and dosages for anesthesia and moderate sedation:
   a. Give the minimum effective concentration and smallest volume needed. Adjust the precise amount to the weight of the patient in kilograms as appropriate.
   b. Limit the total amount of drug injected or applied to prescribed safe limits. Sterile single-dose ampules and prefilled syringes are recommended.
   c. Inject slowly to retard absorption and avoid overdosage. Use incremental titration of drug.
   d. Pull back on the syringe plunger frequently while injecting tissues to be sure the solution is not entering a blood vessel inadvertently. Intravascular injection of an anesthetic drug can release histamine into the systemic circulation, causing an anaphylactoid (nonimmunologic) reaction.
   e. Exercise caution with drugs that depress respiratory or cardiovascular functions, such as sedatives, when the upper dose limit of the anesthetic drug is used.
   f. Provide continuous IV access for administering drugs for moderate sedation or adverse reactions. An IV line should be established in case of adverse reaction or inadvertent intravascular injection or bolus of anesthetic. A heparin lock device or infusion of IV fluids may be used to maintain continuous access.
   g. Cease administration of the drug immediately at the sign of any sensitivity.
   h. Record the drug name, dosage, route, time, and effects of all drugs or pharmacologic agents used.
4. Monitoring patient continuously:
   a. Observe the patient, including facial expressions, and note responses to conversation and the patient's state of alertness.
   b. Assess the patient's physical signs and symptoms, such as skin color and temperature. Use assessment knowledge and skill, and avoid total reliance on monitoring equipment.
   c. Monitor the patient's vital signs as appropriate (ECG, blood pressure, pulse, oxygen saturation, and respiration).

d. Know resuscitation measures and be able to assist or initiate them as necessary, as per institutional policies and procedures. Basic cardiac life support certification (BCLS) is required of all registered nurses who monitor patients. Advanced cardiac life support certification (ACLS) is preferred.

Signs and Symptoms of Systemic Reactions

Signs and symptoms of systemic reaction may be CNS stimulation or depression. Conversely, stimulation may be followed by depression and cardiovascular collapse (see Table 24-3). The cardiovascular system seems more resistant than the CNS to toxic effects of local anesthetics. The seizure threshold may differ enormously in individual patients, as may the relationship of the dose to signs and symptoms of CNS effect. For example, lidocaine usually produces drowsiness before a convulsion, whereas bupivacaine may cause sudden seizure, disorientation, decreased hearing ability, paresthesias, muscle twitching, or agitation in a wide-awake patient without premonitory signs. Hypercapnia or hypoxemia from hypoventilation lowers the seizure threshold.

Toxicity of local anesthetics is manifested primarily by CNS effects resulting from high blood levels. Signs and symptoms of systemic reaction include but are not limited to the following:

- *Stimulation:* Talkativeness, restlessness, incoherence, excitation, tachycardia, bounding pulse, flushed face, hyperpyrexia, tremors, hyperactive reflexes, muscular twitching, focal or grand mal convulsions
- *Depression:* Drowsiness; disorientation; decreased hearing ability; stupor; syncope; rapid, thready pulse or bradycardia; apprehension; hypotension; pale or cyanotic, moist skin; coma
- *Other signs and symptoms:* Nausea, vomiting, dizziness, blurred vision, sudden severe headache, precordial pain, extreme pulse rate or blood pressure change, angioneurotic edema (wheeze, laryngeal edema, bronchospasm), rashes, urticaria, severe local tissue reaction

Systemic reactions or undesired effects of moderate sedation used in combination with local anesthetics may include slurred speech, agitation, combativeness, unarousable sleep, hypotension, hypoventilation, airway obstruction, and apnea. Other signs and symptoms may be related to specific drugs.

Benzodiazepines and sedatives used in moderate sedation may cause somnolence, confusion, diminished reflexes, depressed respiratory and cardiovascular function, and coma. Nystagmus (involuntary eye movements), which may be normal with large doses of diazepam (Valium), may be an abnormal reaction with other drugs. Opioids (narcotics) may cause nausea and vomiting, hypotension, and respiratory depression.

Treatment of Adverse Reactions. Treatment of an adverse reaction is aimed at preventing respiratory and cardiac arrest. Treatment must be prompt. ACLS protocol may be needed.

Administration of the agent thought to produce the reaction is stopped immediately at the first indication of reaction. Therapy is generally supportive, the specifics dictated by clinical manifestations. Treatment consists of the following:

1. Maintaining oxygenation of vital organs and tissues with ventilation by manual or mechanical assistance to give 100% oxygen with positive pressure. Tracheal intubation may be indicated.
2. Reversing myocardial depression and peripheral vasodilation before cardiac arrest occurs. The patient is supine with the legs elevated. IV fluid therapy is begun, and a vasoconstrictor drug may be given IV or IM for hypotension or a weak pulse, which are signs of progressive circulatory depression. The choice of vasopressor is suggested by the signs and symptoms, and the drug is used with caution. Drugs that may be used include the following:
   a. Epinephrine (IV) counteracts hypotension, bronchoconstriction, and laryngeal edema. It also stimulates beta- and alpha-adrenergic receptors and inhibits further release of mediators. It increases arteriolar constriction and force of the heartbeat. When appropriate, application of a tourniquet or subcutaneous injection of epinephrine in an area of drug injection may delay absorption of toxic drug.
   b. Ephedrine and other vasoconstrictors such as phenylephrine (Neo-Synephrine) or mephentermine (Wyamine) cause peripheral vasoconstriction, increased myocardial contraction, and bronchodilation.
   c. Antihistamines block histamine release but generally are not advocated.
   d. Steroids enhance the effect of epinephrine and inhibit further release of histamine. The effect is not immediate, and use is directed toward late manifestations of allergic response.
   e. Isoproterenol (Isuprel) is used predominantly in asthma and heart attacks; it is a bronchodilator.
   f. Antagonist drug may be given in situations in which the causative agent is identified.
3. Stopping muscle tremors or convulsions if they are present, since they constitute a hazard for further hypoxia, aspiration, or bodily injury. Diazepam in 5-mg doses or a short-acting barbiturate is given IV to inhibit cortical irritation.

For patients in whom the adverse response is caused by hypersensitivity, the previous measures are applicable. However, aminophylline may be administered to help alleviate bronchospasm, hydrocortisone (IV) to combat shock, and sodium or potassium iodide (IV) to reduce mucosal edema.

The perioperative nurse who is monitoring the patient must know resuscitation measures and be able to assist in or initiate them when necessary. An emergency cart with emergency resuscitative drugs and a defibrillator should be immediately available to the room where local or regional anesthetic with or without moderate sedation is administered. The following equipment should be in the room and ready for use:

- Oxygen and positive pressure breathing device (e.g., Ambu bag and mask)
- Oral and nasopharyngeal airways and endotracheal tubes in an assortment of sizes

- Cardiac and oxygen saturation monitoring equipment
- Suction

Unrelated Effects. A nerve deficit, such as pain or neuritis that occurs in the postoperative period may be related to a preexisting condition such as multiple sclerosis. Alternatively, it may be from a cause unrelated to the anesthetic drug, such as faulty positioning; trauma from retractors; a tourniquet inflated for an inordinately long period, resulting in ischemia or pressure on peripheral nerves; or an improperly applied cast. Less common causes involve bleeding around the nerve or reaction to epinephrine.

ALTERNATIVES TO CONVENTIONAL ANESTHESIA

When local or regional anesthesia may be contraindicated but consciousness is desirable, acupuncture or hypnoanesthesia may offer alternative methods to control pain. An altered state of awareness of painful stimuli may be advantageous in selected patients.

Hypnosis

Hypnoanesthesia refers to hypnosis used as a method of anesthesia. Hypnosis produces a state of altered consciousness characterized by heightened suggestibility, selective wakefulness, reduced awareness, and restricted attentiveness. Although hypnosis has a long history of misuse, modern application by highly trained medical specialists is appropriate. Hypnoanesthesia, although seldom used, has been successfully employed in adult and pediatric patients. Motivation and concentration on the part of the patient are important factors. The method may be combined with the use of a small dose of a chemical anesthetic or muscle relaxing drug. Hypnosis should not be used indiscriminately in place of standard treatment.

Hypnosis may be used as a therapeutic aid in very selected patients in the following situations:
- When chemical agents are contraindicated (patient may be kept pain-free, asleep or awake, without toxic side effects)
- As an adjunct to chemical anesthesia to decrease the amount of anesthesia needed
- When it is desirable to free the patient from certain neurophysical effects of an anesthetic
- When anxiety and fear of anesthesia are so great as to contribute to serious anesthetic risk
- When posthypnotic suggestion may be valuable in the postoperative period
- When it is desirable to raise the pain threshold
- When it is desirable to have the patient respond to questions or commands

Hypnoanesthesia is advantageous for changing burn dressings and debridement of wounds and for patients with severe respiratory or cardiovascular disease or multiple drug allergies. The anesthesia provider must establish rapport with the patient preoperatively so that the patient will listen to and obey hypnotic commands. Hypnosis is a time-consuming method and is unreliable as compared with chemical anesthesia.

Acupuncture

The ancient Chinese art of acupuncture has been practiced for more than 5000 years. Its acceptance by Western medical practitioners is fairly recent. Acupuncture is a

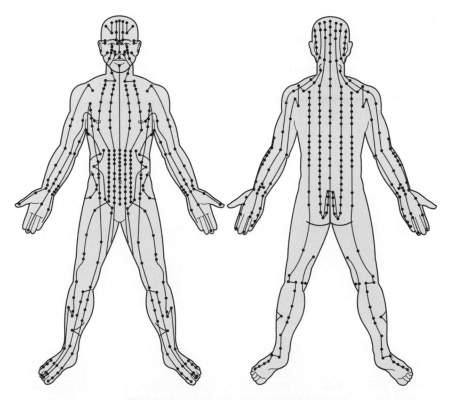

FIG. 24-20 Meridians for acupuncture.

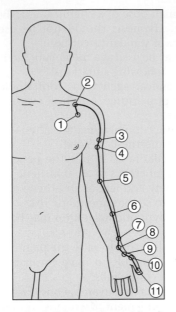

FIG. 24-21   Example of *Chi* points in meridian line used in acupuncture for treatment of the left lung.

technique of providing intense stimulation at meridian points, or planes of energy referred to as *Chi* (Fig. 24-20). This stimulation prompts the brain to release endorphins and other chemicals that can relieve or block pain. Some meridians are associated with prevention of nausea and vomiting postoperatively. An example of *Chi* points in a meridian line for the lung is depicted in Figure 24-21.

Stimulation is effected by manually rotating or applying electric current to very-fine-gauge needles inserted into meridian points. When acupuncture is used for anesthesia, a minute electric current is used to speed and enhance analgesia or anesthesia in the desired body region. The meridian points generally correspond to the area where the somatic nerve supply is located. It is a time-consuming technique. It may be used immediately after premedication is given to reduce postoperative nausea and vomiting after short procedures with the patient under general anesthesia.

Acupuncture is gaining popularity in surgical and dental procedures and for postoperative or intractable pain. The patient remains conscious. Procedures are limited to use by physicians or appropriate personnel under their direct supervision in keeping with acceptable standards of medical practice.

Bibliography

AORN (Association of periOperative Registered Nurses): *AORN standards, recommended practices, and guidelines,* Denver, 2006, The Association.

Arbous MS et al: Impact of anesthesia management characteristics on severe morbidity and mortality, *Anesthesiology* 102(2):257-268, 2005.

Chernyak G et al: Perioperative acupuncture and related techniques, *Anesthesiology* 102(5):1031-1049, 2005.

Dawson JS: Bispectral index monitoring, *Anesth Intens Care* 32(1): 28-30, 2004.

Forestier F et al: Propofol and sufentanil titration with the bispectral index to provide anesthesia for coronary artery surgery, *Anesthesiology* 99(2):334-346, 2003.

Halaszynski TM et al: Optimizing perioperative outcomes with efficient preoperative assessment and management, *Crit Care Med* 32(4):S76-86, 2004.

Ianchulev SA, Comunate ME: To do or not to do a preinduction check-up of the anesthesia machine, *Anesth Analg* 102(4): 1290-1291, 2005.

Nguyen MT et al: Pediatric imaging: Sedation with an injection formulation modified for rectal administration, *Radiology* 221(3):760-762, 2001.

Odom-Forren J, Watson DS: *Practical guide to moderate sedation/ analgesia,* St Louis, 2005, Elsevier.

Russo H, Bressolle F: Pharmacodynamics and pharmacokinetics of thiopental, *Clinical Pharm* 5(2):95-134, 1998.

Sawyer RJ, von Schroeder H: Temporary blindness after acute lidocaine toxicity, *Anesth Analg* 95(1):224-226, 2002.

Schulz-Stubner SB, Boezaart AH: Regional analgesia in the critically ill, *Crit Care Med* 33(6):1400-1407, 2005.

Schwartz AJ: Learning the essentials of epidural anesthesia, *Nursing 2006* 36(1):44-50, 2006.

Sherman KJ et al: The practice of acupuncture: Who are the providers and what do they do? *Ann Fam Med* 3(2):151-158, 2005.

Slowikowski RD, Flaherty SA: Epidural analgesia for postoperative orthopaedic pain, *Orthop Nurs* 19(1):23-31, 2000.

White SM: Consent for anesthesia, *J Med Ethics* 30(3):286-290, 2004.

Coordinated Roles of the Scrub Person and the Circulating Nurse

CHAPTER OBJECTIVES

After studying this chapter, the learner will be able to:
- Describe the activities of the scrub person.
- Describe the activities of the circulating nurse.
- Discuss the preliminary care of the patient by the circulating nurse.
- Differentiate between counting and being accountable for items used in patient care.

CHAPTER OUTLINE

SUPPLEMENTAL MATERIAL ON EVOLVE WEBSITE *evolve*

http://evolve.elsevier.com/BerryKohn
- Content Updates
- Glossary
- Full Set of Perioperative Flash Cards
- Interactive Key Term Flash Cards
- Student Activities
- WebLinks

DIVISION OF DUTIES

The circulating nurse and the scrub person should plan their duties so that through coordination of their efforts, the sterile and unsterile parts of the surgical procedure move along simultaneously. From the time the scrub person starts the surgical scrub until the surgical procedure is completed and dressings are applied, an invisible line separates the duties of the scrub person (Box 25-1) and the circulating nurse (Box 25-2), which neither person may cross. In this chapter, the duties of the two positions are listed sepa-

rately, but a spirit of mutual cooperation is essential to move the schedule of surgical procedures efficiently and to serve the best interests of the patient.

As a coordinated, systematic effort, the scrub person and the circulating nurse should complete the preparation of the environment as described in Chapter 12, whether it is for the first case of the day or for a subsequent case performed during the course of the day. Establishing a system for performance of roles helps to minimize the risk for human error.[1] Both caregivers should double-check the needs for the procedure before the patient arrives at the room. Table 25-1 contains a systematic checklist of the case flow and case-related activities for the scrub person. Table 25-2 contains a systematic checklist of the case-flow and patient care activities for the circulating nurse.

SETTING UP THE ROOM

Both the circulating nurse and the scrub person set up the room and position equipment. One suggested room arrangement is illustrated in Figure 25-1. The case cart and the room furniture are checked by both people as a team. The duties and activities change when the patient arrives at the room. The circulating nurse begins working with the patient, and the scrub person continues readying the room. The following activities are performed together before the patient arrives:

1. Place a clean sheet, lift sheet, armboard covers, and safety straps on the operating bed. Put a pressure-reducing mattress or gel pads on the bed if needed to relieve pressure during a long procedure. A warming or cooling blanket may be needed to heat or cool the patient during a long procedure. Obtain special equipment, such as table appliances, pillows, or padding, needed to position and protect the patient.
2. Obtain appropriate patient monitoring equipment. Sequential compression devices may be indicated.

---

[1]The Agency for Healthcare Research and Quality (AHRQ) supports the premise that systems and standardization help minimize human factors that result in medical error and patient or staff injury (www.ahrq.gov).

BOX 25-1   Role of the Scrub Person as Part of the Sterile Team

PREPARES
Sterile instruments and supplies
Works in concert with the circulating nurse to set up the OR
Surgeon's specific procedural needs
Procedure specific needs
Hemostatic techniques
Suture and closure materials

STERILE TECHNIQUE
Scrubs, gowns, and gloves using the closed gloving method
Establishes the sterile field
Facilitates the surgical procedure
Anticipates the needs of the sterile team
Gowns other team members using the open-assisted gowning and gloving technique

ADAPATABILITY
Remedies any breach of sterile technique
Requests and prepares material needed by surgeon
Keeps the sterile field neat and functional

ACCOUNTABILITY
Establishes baseline counts with circulating nurse
Informs the circulating nurse of items placed inside patient
Double-checks items dispensed to the sterile field
Labels all medication containers and delivery devices
Reports volume of drug administered to patient for documentation by circulating nurse

SAFETY
Manages sharps
Prevents retained foreign objects in the patient
Reconciles counts and is accountable for items used in the surgical procedure

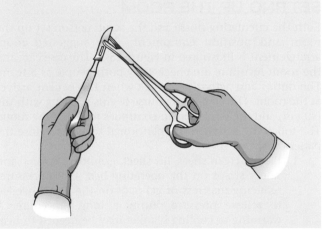

BOX 25-2   Role of the Circulating Nurse as Part of the Nonsterile Team

INDIRECT PATIENT CARE
Assists with OR preparation
Opens sterile supplies
Prepares medication for use in OR
Maintains patient confidentiality
Communication with surgical services personnel
Pretests equipment
Plans postoperative care
Initiates discharge planning

DIRECT PATIENT CARE
Patient identification
Patient assessment
Identification of correct surgical site
Transfers patient between cart and bed
Assists the anesthesia provider
Provides skin antisepsis
Provides thermoregulation
Prevents electrosurgical injury
Collaborates with patient fluid intake and output
Monitors vital signs as needed
Provides dressings and drains

COORDINATES
Plans for each member of the sterile team to enter the sterile field
Positioning, prepping, and draping
Connection of surgical machinery
Laboratory tests
Multidisciplinary teams
Diagnostic activities
Emergency response to patient crisis
Communication with patient's significant others

ANTICIPATES
Sequence of the procedure
Needs of the sterile team
Breaches of sterile technique
Hemostatic needs
Radiation (ionizing and nonionizing) protection for sterile team
Potential for patient's physiologic changes
Wound class at conclusion of the procedure
Patient responses to care
Significant other's response to patient's condition

ACCOUNTABILITY
Validates implants
Documents patient care
Hands off report to postoperative care giver
Specimen care and reporting
Promotes a culture of safety
Accountability for instruments, sponges, and sharps
Patient's advocate
Evaluates patient outcomes

3. Obtain any specialized equipment that will be needed, such as an electrosurgical unit (ESU), smoke evacuator, pneumatic tourniquet, laser, or operating microscope, and check/test for proper function. Have the appropriate attachments and adjunctive supplies in the room.

4. Gather protective devices such as x-ray–protective gowns and/or lead screens and laser eyewear of the correct optical density as needed.

TABLE 25-1	Systematic Activities for the Scrub Person

Baseline Systematic Activity	Systematic Critical Thinking Activity

Room Setup
- Plan for patient to enter the room without contaminating the setup
- Plan for position of patient, surgeon, and anesthesia provider

Determine the position of the surgeon and preference for positioning of the scrub person before setting up table.

Case Cart Contents
- Instrument set(s)
- Custom pack
- Gowns
- Sterile towels
- Prep supplies
- Additional soft goods

Check cart contents. Inspect package integrity.
Check for each item listed on case cart sheet.
Record preference changes on case cart sheet for computer update.

Items to Have Available
- Suture
- Sponges
- Pack of towels
- Gloves
- Staplers
- Dressing

Have extra preferred suture in the room.
Extra sponges may be needed.

Table Setup
- Open the main custom drape pack. The outer wrapper is the sterile table drape.
- Determine which part of the table will be closest to the draped patient and establish this area as the working end of the table. Sharps and suture should be opened on to this location.
- Open remaining items into a position of function. Inspect package integrity.
- Do not open items into closed container system. Edges are unsterile.
- Don eyewear.
- Open gown and gloves for self before performing hand and arm cleansing.
- Don gown and gloves using closed glove procedure. Remember to tie in.
- Set up the working end of the table according to position of patient.
- Plan to pass off cords in one direction.
- terile marker and labels are placed on the sterile instrument table near the working end.
- Place items once. Do not leave trash on the field.

The surgical site on the patient is the "ground zero" for the establishment of the level of the sterile field.
Stack drapes in order of use and place away from main instrument setup area of sterile table.
Create towel roll(s) for instrument stringers. Align stringer on the roll with shortest instruments closest to the working end of the table.
Instrument ratchets are open on the table and closed on the Mayo stand.
Establish baseline: Count instruments, sharps, and sponges with circulating nurse.
Plan for exchange of scalpel by no touch technique.

Mayo Stand Setup
- Drape the Mayo stand. Cover surface with one unfolded towel to protect from perforation by sharps.

Mayo setup: 2 scalpels, 3 scissors (1 curved and 1 straight Mayo and 1 Metzenbaum), 4 curved Crile hemostats, 2 medium pick ups, 4 Allis forceps, and 2 small skin retractors (Army Navy)
2 Light handles, suction tubing and suction tip (Yankauer), electrosurgical unit (ESU) pencil and holder, tip cleaner, and sponges.

Medication and/or Chemicals on the Sterile Instrument Table
- Place labeled medication cups near edge of field.
- Validate all medications and solutions with circulating nurse.

Label syringes and administration devices.

Irrigation and Fluids on the Sterile Instrument Table
- Place labeled basins near edge of sterile field.
- Label all delivery devices.

Normal saline or other isotonic solution for irrigation.
Sterile water for instrumentation.

Patient Positioning
Stand clear and remain sterile because positioning is a nonsterile activity.

Note the presence of safety restraints as the second set of eyes.
Drapes and blankets can obscure safety straps.

Team Gowning
- Assist team to gown and glove using the open assisted method.
- Contaminated gloves are changed using the open method. Circulating nurse will remove contaminated gloves. Scrub person will re-glove the individual.

Do not pass any towels or gowns from the sterile field during the procedure. Biologic contamination is present.

Continued

TABLE 25-1	Systematic Activities for the Scrub Person—cont'd

Baseline Systematic Activity	Systematic Critical Thinking Activity
Patient Draping • Prep solution must be completely dry • Patient is draped to establish the level of the sterile surgical field before instrument tables are positioned for use.	Some surgeons use towel clips to secure drapes. Nonperforating styles are preferred. Some surgeons suture or staple specialty drapes in place.
Procedure Start and Flow • Position Mayo stand. • Position sterile instrument table. • Hand off ESU cords, tubing, and cables to circulating nurse. • Apply light handles. • Two sponges on field adjacent to incision. • Provide scalpel for skin (place skin knife aside on working end immediately after use; disarm and reload as time permits). • Provide ESU for hemostasis (keep in holder when not in use). • Clean the ESU pencil tip. • Keep instrumentation free of debris with moist sponge. • Trade one-for-one sponges and needles. • Open soiled sponges completely before discarding into sponge bucket.	Initiate timeout before skin scalpel is provided. • Correct patient • Correct site • Correct procedure Inform circulating nurse if any uncounted item has been brought into the surgical field. Reconcile all counts by starting at the patient and working toward Mayo stand and then to instrument table. Count sponges and sharps at each cavity within cavity closure. Do closing counts of sponges sharps and instruments during surgical site closure. Contain pathology specimen in closed container as possible before passing to gloved circulating nurse.
Dressings and Drains • Double-check type of dressing material before circulating nurse dispenses to field. • Dressing is placed over surgical site after incision is cleaned. • Disconnect tubing and cords from field. • Drapes are removed by rolling them off and away from the patient after placement of the surgical site dressing.	Wet sponge followed by dry sponge to clean closed incision. Wound closure strips may be placed over subcuticular closure. Dressing is positioned over cleaned incision before removal of drapes. Skin surrounding the dressing area is cleaned with wet and dry sponges before tape is applied.
Procedure Completion All reusable instruments are opened or disassembled and placed in bins for decontamination in the processing area. Enzyme solution or foam may be applied before transit.	Remove the Bovie tip and place in sharps container. Disarm scalpels. Open all instrument ratchets and box locks and place in mesh tray.
Room Break-down • When patient leaves the room the table can be broken down completely. • Dispose of sharps in sharps container. • Remove light handles. • Case cart is reloaded with used instrument trays and reusable equipment. • Don exam gloves after removing gown and gloves and washing hands. • Transport the case cart to the processing area.	**Trash Disposal** Biologic trash into biohazard containers Clean trash into regular garbage receptacle Linen into hampers Remove contaminated gown first followed by gloves using peel off glove to glove–skin to skin method. Wash hands with soap and water after removing gloves. All case-specific equipment should be cleaned with antiseptic and returned to storage.

5. Position the operating bed under the overhead operating spotlight fixture. Orient the head of the bed according to the type of procedure to be performed. Patient positioning for some procedures requires the anesthesia provider to be located at the patient's side instead of at the head of the bed. Anesthesia personnel should be responsible for moving the anesthesia equipment to the proper position. The hoses and connections should be checked each time the anesthesia machine is moved. The circulating nurse and scrub person are not trained in this checking procedure.

6. Test the overhead operating light to check focus and intensity, and pre-position it as much as possible.

Do not leave the light turned on. The light should be positioned in relationship to the location of the surgeon at the operating bed and to that part of the patient's anatomy that will be encountered during the surgical procedure. The circulating nurse should know how to change the lightbulb in case a bulb burns out during a procedure. Newer lights have replacement bulbs in place that activate if one bulb burns out.

7. Connect and check the suction between the receptacle canisters and the wall outlet to be certain suction functions at maximum vacuum. Some facilities use inline filters for specialized equipment. The filters are changed between cases. Gloves and

TABLE 25-2	Systematic Activities for the Circulating Nurse

Baseline Systematic Activity for all Cases	Systematic Patient Care

Patient Assessment and Safety

Assess for patient identity and correct site information concerning the planned procedure. Note the presence of correct site markings.
Assess physiologic and psychologic status.
- Labwork
- Current medications and herbals
- Allergies and sensitivities
- Last intake by mouth
- Location of family or significant other

Talk to the patient and determine understanding of the procedure.
Check the paperwork/chart/computer for consents, tests, and family contact information.
Check for films, digital information, or scans for use during the procedure.
Consult with anesthesia provider and surgeon for information exchange.

Room Setup
- Ensure a clear path for emergency equipment.
- Plan for adequate positioning of the anesthesia provider.
- Check the operating bed for correct position.
- Make sure lights are in working order.

All necessary positioning aids are available.
Plan for entrance of patient without impeding the process of setup or contamination.
Plan setup for position of instrument table in relation to surgical field.

Standard Room Equipment
- Appropriate operating bed with armboards
- Patient transfer device
- Sequential compression device
- Two IV poles
- Patient-warming device
- Mayo stand
- Instrument table
- Prep stand
- Monopolar ESU and dispersive electrode
- Suction collection apparatus
- Platform steps for team

Check equipment (suction and ESU) for proper function.
Place equipment in a position of function. Plan for cords and tubing to be passed off in one direction.
Avoid having cords and cables as "trip hazards" if lights are lowered for endoscopy.

Case Cart Contents
- Instrument set(s)
- Custom pack
- Gowns
- Sterile towels
- Prep supplies
- Additional soft goods

Check cart contents. Inspect package integrity.
Check for each items listed on case cart sheet.
Record preference changes on case cart sheet for computer update.

Items to Have Available
- Suture
- Sponges
- Sterile towels
- Gloves
- Staplers
- Dressings

Have a few sizes available. Only open if necessary.
Charge only for items used.

Table Setup
- Place packs to be opened on clean dry table surface.
- Do not open items into closed container system. Edges are unsterile.
- Open adequate gowns and gloves for surgeon and first assistant.
- Tie gowns of team.
- If blades are opened separately, inform scrub person of location on the field.

Open sterile packs in a position of function.
Establish and document baseline: Count instruments, sharps, and sponges with scrub person.
Provide additional sterile supplies as needed by scrub person.

Medication and/or Chemicals on the Sterile Field
- Obtain medications and/or chemicals for sterile field using patient identification number.
- Dispense medications without aerosolization.
- Draw up with needle and syringe. Remove needle before delivering drug to field.

Validate medication type and dose with the scrub person.
Validate total amount given and administered.
Charge only for drugs used on sterile field.

Irrigation on the Sterile Field
- Obtain solutions of appropriate temperature for sterile field.
- Dispense solutions without aerosolization.

Dispense normal saline or other isotonic solution to the field after verifying the date, name, and seal integrity.

Continued

TABLE 25-2	Systematic Activities for the Circulating Nurse—cont'd

Baseline Systematic Activity for all Cases	Systematic Patient Care
Assisting the Anesthesia Provider • Assist with positioning during regional anesthesia. • Stand at patient's side during induction of general anesthesia.	Help anesthesia personnel with IV or intubation if needed. Prepare to apply cricoid pressure as needed during intubation.
Patient Positioning • Don nonsterile gloves. • Provide positioning devices as appropriate. • Adequate exposure of surgical site • Appropriate safety restraints • Apply dispersive electrode after patient is positioned. Do not cut or reapply.	The anesthesia provider will indicate when it is safe to start positioning and prepping. The anesthesia provider and surgeon will determine the appropriate safe position for the surgical procedure.
Skin Prep: Determine Patient Potential for Skin Sensitivity • One-step • Two-step	Open and set up appropriate skin prep materials. Expose the surgical site without undue exposure. Protect nontarget areas from pooling.
Procedural Positioning of Equipment and Team • Assist scrub person to move sterile table adjacent to surgical field. • Attach cords, cables, and tubing to appropriate devices. • Place suction canister in direct view of anesthesia provider. • Provide standing platforms/steps as needed	Scrub person will hand off cords and cables in one direction. Determine machine settings per surgeon. Scrub person will place sterile Mayo stand over sterile field.
Procedure Start and Flow • Initiate the timeout, verifying the patient name, procedure, and correct site. • Prepare specimens for pathology. • Communicate with family or significant other within acceptable parameters for patient privacy.	**Documentation** • Procedural times and timeout • Additional items not in the baseline count added to field or placed in patient • Handle specimen containers wearing exam gloves. • Family updates as appropriate
Dressings and Drains • Dispense dressing materials to sterile field at end of procedure. • Don nonsterile gloves to clean skin edges after patient is undraped. • Tape dressings. Avoid affixing to hairy surface.	One-step prep should not be removed.
Procedure Completion • Reconcile closing count with scrub person. Begin count from surgical field on patient to Mayo stand to instrument table. Sponges in sponge bucket are counted in increments of size and initial packaging amounts. • Prepare hand-off report for postprocedural area nursing staff. • Transport patient to postprocedural area with anesthesia provider.	Give hand-off report to RN in postprocedural area. • Patient name and age • Allergies or sensitivities • Current procedure and type of anesthesia • Location of incisions, dressings, and drains • Pertinent comorbidity • Special needs (language, vision, hearing) • Location of family or significant other • Any procedure-specific information

personal protective equipment are worn to prevent contact with harmful microorganisms when changing these filters.

8. Place a waterproof laundry bag or antistatic plastic bag in the laundry hamper frame for disposal of reusable woven fabric items.

9. Place appropriately marked receptacles in the room for safe disposal of biohazardous items, such as sharps, disposable drapes, or other biologically contaminated materials. Clean trash containers should be available for noncontaminated trash. Many hospitals do not have in-house incinerators and pay per the pound to have biohazard trash hauled away. Mixed clean and biohazard trash disposal is an unnecessary expense.

10. Line each kick bucket and wastebasket with an impervious plastic liner with a cuff turned over the edge.

11. Arrange furniture with those pieces that will be draped to become part of the sterile field at least 18 inches (45 cm) away from walls or cabinets. They should be kept side by side, away from the laundry hamper, trash container, anesthesia equipment, doors, and paths of traffic.

12. If a case cart system is used, all or most of the needed supplies should be on the cart. Check to ascertain that everything is there and that the wrappings are intact. Position the case cart near the instrument table. Collect additional instruments and supplies, according to the preference card or case cart sheet and from cabinets in the room or from another supply area within the operating room (OR) suite.

13. Obtain an appropriate set of sterile, wrapped instruments from one of the cart shelves and place on top of the case cart.

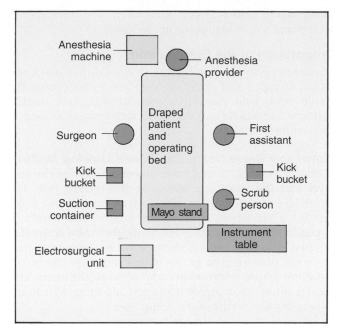

FIG. 25-1 Arrangement of the operating room showing sterile field, team members, and unsterile equipment.

14. Place the sterile, wrapped drape pack (or custom pack) on the instrument table so that when opened, the wrapper will adequately drape the table and the drapes will be in their proper place. Open the drape pack first to establish a sterile place to open other sterile items. A splash basin can be opened onto the field as a catch basin for opening small packages.

15. Select the correct-size gloves and gowns for each member of the sterile team. A prep table can be opened as a sterile gown table. The extra gloves can be opened into the basin on the sterile table.

16. Select the initial sutures to have ready for the surgeon. Open only those needed to begin the case, such as free ties. These can be opened into the sterile basin on the main field near the working end of the table. Place unopened but probably needed sutures on top of the case cart for opening as the case progresses.

17. Open the instrument set. If it is a wrapped set, open the wrapper on top of the case cart. If the instrument set is in a closed container, open the container by lifting the lid straight up and tilted back toward your body. Place the opened lid on the bottom shelf of the case cart. Do not open any supplies into a rigid instrument container, because the edges are not considered sterile.

Opening Sterile Supplies

The doors to the room should be shut to maintain positive pressure, and each team member present should be wearing appropriate OR attire. Before any sterile supplies are opened, the integrity of each package must be checked for tears and watermarks. If either is present, the package is unsafe to use. The process monitor should also be checked. Open packages as follows:

1. Remove tape from packages wrapped in woven fabric wrappers. Laundry machinery can be damaged by wads of tape becoming lodged in the mechanisms. Few facilities use woven wrappers. The tape should be opened by breaking the seal on paper or nonwoven material. Removing tape strips from paper-wrapped items increases the risk of tearing the wrapper and exposing the contents to contamination. Check the external chemical indicator tape to be certain the item has been exposed to a sterilization process.

2. Open the drape pack, instrument set, and gown pack on their own individual surfaces so that the inside of each inner wrapper becomes a sterile table cover.

   For an envelope-folded wrapper, open the first flap of the wrapper away from yourself. The area touched falls below table level, and the inside of the wrapper remains sterile. Each flap will look triangular. Do not reach over the inside of the sterile table cover or contents of the pack. Pull open each side by pulling the side flaps open, one at a time. Lift the final edge of the wrapper toward you to complete the opening of the sterile field.

   For a square side-folded wrapper, open one side, followed by the other side, in a sideways motion so both sides are over the edge of the table. The front and back flaps can be difficult. Both team members should do this step together—one person stands on one side of the table, and the second person stands on the opposite side. Each (simultaneously) grasps a lower edge of both the front and back flaps and opens both flaps together to complete the opening of the pack.

   For a square front-back-folded wrapper, the steps for the envelope fold are followed in the same sequences. Each flap will look square. The final square flap will be brought toward your body to create the field (Fig. 25-2).

   a. If packs or sets have sequential double wrappers, both layers are opened by the person opening supplies by following the same sequences twice. The outer wrapper is considered the dust cover, and the inner wrapper the sterile barrier. The person opening the inner wrapper need not be sterile.

   b. Open other packages, such as sponges, gloves, and sutures, maintaining a sterile transfer to the appropriate sterile table. Touch only the outside of the outer wrapper. Avoid reaching over sterile contents and the sterile table. Enclose your hand in the wrapper to the extent possible. Do not slide the inner package over the edge of the peel-pack pouch. Sutures and blades should be opened on to the working edge of the table.

   c. If small peel packages are sequentially double-wrapped (i.e., a peel package inside a peel package), only the outer wrapper is removed. Usually the inner wrapper contains several smaller parts that may accidentally fall off the table when dispensed.

   d. Instruments processed in rigid, closed container systems are opened by breaking the seal on the lid and raising it up and away from the tray. The inner basket of instruments is considered sterile,

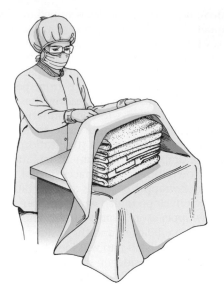

FIG. 25-2 Opening square-fold sterile pack. Wrapper is lifted back while keeping hands on the outside. Hands are in folded cuff to avoid contaminating contents of pack. Area touched falls below unsterile table level; sterile inside of wrapper (now table cover) remains sterile.

but the container itself is not. Sterile soft goods, sutures, and other individually wrapped items should not be opened into this pan, because the edges are not considered sterile.

e. If a sterile package is dropped, the item may be considered safe for immediate use only if it is enclosed in an impervious material and the integrity of the package is maintained.

f. Mechanical items such as staplers should not be flipped onto the field. The mechanisms can be damaged and may malfunction when used in patient care. Do not open these items until a sterile team member can take them directly from the inner aspect of the package.

g. Blades should be opened on the working end of the sterile field. The scrub person should be aware of exactly where these are opened. Do not open other items near the blades. Do not open blades into the basins. This dulls the cutting surface. This location should be standardized for systematic safety for the scrub person.

3. The gown and gloves for the scrub person are opened on the Mayo stand or small table separate from the main sterile field. The person establishing the sterile field should not gown and glove from the main field because the risk of contamination is higher than gowning and gloving from a separate surface.

4. The circulating nurse assists the anesthesia provider with patient care preparations as the scrub person sets up the sterile field after scrubbing, gowning, and gloving.

SCRUB PERSON DUTIES

When all supplies have been obtained and opened and the room is ready for the patient's arrival, the scrub person prepares for the surgeon's arrival. At all times, the integrity

of the sterile field is closely monitored. The principles of asepsis and sterile technique are followed.

Preparation of the Sterile Field

The scrub person should be sure that his or her gown and gloves are open and ready on a surface separate from the sterile field. Don protective eyewear with side shields. Perform a complete surgical hand cleansing according to the facility procedure.

Gown and Glove Using the Closed Gloving Method.
If double-gloving, wear gloves one size larger as the first layer and the usual size gloves as the second pair. The larger size underneath provides an air pocket and helps prevent a sensation of tightness around the hands. If hypoallergenic gloves are worn, these should be donned as the first pair, with generic gloves worn as the outside pair. Wipe the powder from gloves with a moist sponge before handling drapes, instruments, and other sterile items. This sponge should be completely opened and dropped into the sponge bucket as part of the count.

When establishing the main sterile field, drape unsterile tables according to the standard departmental setup procedure with drapes from the drape pack. Most facilities will consider the outer wrap of the custom pack as the main sterile table cover. The scrub person may need to drape and set a small table for the patient's skin prep, but more commonly the circulating nurse opens and prepares a disposable or prepackaged prep tray. A second instrument table may be needed for extensive surgical procedures or special types of instrumentation (e.g., tables for preparation of an implant or organ for transplant).

When draping an unsterile table with a separate sterile table drape, unfold it toward yourself to cover the front edge of the unsterile table first; this minimizes the possibility of self-contamination from the edge of the table. Unfold the remainder of the sterile table drape over the surface of the table and away from yourself. The edges are allowed to fall over the ends of the table and are considered contaminated below the tabletop. Avoid leaning over the table.

Place the remaining contents of the drape pack on a corner of the instrument table if they are not prepositioned in a convenient place on the table drape. Place them once—do not keep moving things from one side to another. Custom packs usually contain disposable supplies that are nested within each other and require minimal handling when setting up the field. Reusable woven fabric drapes may be arranged within the drape pack according to the size or direction of the folds. A standard number of each item is contained within a drape pack. The basic drape pack usually contains, at a minimum, the following items:
- One Mayo stand cover
- Four to eight towels
- Two to four medium drape sheets (optional)
- One fenestrated sheet

Draping the Mayo Stand

When draping the Mayo stand, drape both the frame and the tray. The Mayo stand cover is like a long plastic pillowcase with a single sheet of nonwoven fabric that will lie on the flat surface that will hold instruments. It is fan-folded with a wide cuff to protect gloved hands. With hands in the cuff, support the folds of the drape on the arms, in the bend of the elbows, to prevent it from falling below waist level (Fig. 25-3). While sliding the cover on the Mayo stand, place a foot on the base of the stand to stabilize it (Fig. 25-4). Some sterile custom packs contain an impervious plastic disposable Mayo tray as the bottom layer of the pack. At some facilities, a stainless steel Mayo tray is wrapped snugly and sterilized separately. The tray can be set into the draped Mayo stand.

Setting Up the Basin Sets. If reusable basin sets are used, leave the large solution basin in the ring stand and take the remainder of the basins to the instrument table. The wrapper on the basin set serves as the cover for the ring stand with the large basin. Fabric or paper towels separate the basins. The fabric towels can be folded and placed on the stack of towels on the sterile field. They can be used for wiping instruments or cleaning the patient at the end of the procedure.

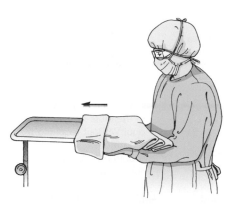

FIG. 25-3 Starting to drape Mayo stand. Scrub person's hands are protected in cuff of drape. Folds of drape are supported on arms, in bend of elbows, to prevent their falling below waist level. Foot is placed on base of stand to stabilize it.

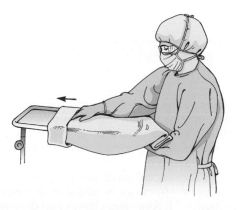

FIG. 25-4 Completing draping of Mayo stand. Hands are protected in cuffs.

Many facilities have discontinued the use of ring stands because they are usually lower than the established sterile field (i.e., the instrument table and the draped patient bed). The use of basins as "splash basins" is discouraged, but a few surgeons still prefer to use them to wash their gloved hands at the start of the case or during the case as blood and debris accumulate on glove surfaces.

If basins are used for this purpose, the circulating nurse should fill them with sterile normal saline and remove them from use when the water is grossly dirty. Each time someone rinses their gloves in the basin, the powder and debris resettle on the gloved surfaces and can be transferred back to the patient, causing foreign body granulomas.

The preferred methods for removing powder or blood from gloves is either to use a sterile towel or sponge moistened with sterile saline or to pour sterile saline directly over the gloved hands. The basin should not be permitted to sit after being used to remove glove powder; it should be emptied into the dirty sink in the utility room by the circulating nurse. Any counted sponge should be unfolded and dropped into the sponge bucket for counting.

Some facilities use the large solution basin directly on the sterile field to collect and rinse used instruments. Only distilled sterile water should be used for this purpose because saline is corrosive. Disposable custom packs usually contain plastic basins that can remain on the sterile instrument table.

Separate 1- or 2-L–sized basins are arranged close to the working edge of the instrument table for holding sterile warm irrigation solution (usually Ringer's lactate or normal saline), for securing the specimen after it is procured, and for moistening sponges. All basins and containers should be clearly labeled to identify their contents. The practice of dipping sponges into the irrigation solution should be discouraged because this releases lint into the solution, which in turn can be introduced into the patient during irrigation. Lint can contribute to foreign body reactions and granulomas in the tissues of the patient. An Asepto syringe can be used to moisten sponges with warm saline in their own basin.

The basin set also may contain solution cups for the skin preparation table and/or a basin specifically intended for trash (waste suture packaging) disposal. Attaching a trash bag to the side of the table compromises the sterility of the field because the bag hangs lower than the sterile table surface. If these bags are used, the inside is not considered sterile because it is below the level of the sterile field. These bags can be hazardous if a needle becomes ensnared in the suture debris and perforates the thin exterior surface of the bag. It could puncture the scrub person during handling.

Arranging the Instrument Table

Arrange other instruments and items on the instrument table (Fig. 25-5). Table 25-3 describes the "Eight P's" of table and room organization, which can help the scrub person and circulating nurse improve the efficiency of the setup procedure and the case flow.

The instruments for each surgical procedure are selected and placed according to standard basic sets and the preferences of the surgeon. Instruments of suitable size, shape,

TABLE 25-3	The "Eight P's" of Operating Room and Sterile Field Setup and Management	
The Eight "P's" to Consider When Preparing for a Surgical Procedure*	Environment Considerations for the Circulating nurse	Sterile Field Considerations for the Scrub Person
PROPER PLACEMENT Items should be placed so they will not need to be moved during the procedure.	Suction canisters, tourniquet, and the electrosurgical unit (ESU) need to be stationary. The operating lights should be directed toward the field.	The Mayo stand and instrument table should not be moved during the procedure. Drapes may not be moved on the patient's skin.
PROPER FUNCTION Items should be tested for safety and usefulness before they are needed, to prevent delay in the case.	Test the ESU, tourniquet, laser, and other equipment before the patient enters the room.	Test the efficiency of instruments (e.g., scissors, needle holders, clamps) as they are needed.
PLACE IT ONCE Items should not be manipulated during the procedure. Energy and attention should not be diverted to resetting the field.	The operating bed should be in the right place for the procedure. The dispersive electrode should not be moved or displaced.	When setting up the field, each item (e.g., a basin) should be placed where it will be used during the procedure with minimal handling.
POINT OF CONTACT Items used within the field could cause harm or be rendered useless if they do not reach the intended point of contact.	The circulating nurse should evaluate the delivery of items to the sterile field. Some items (e.g., staplers) should be handed; others can be transferred in other ways.	The scrub person should be aware of the passing of instruments and how they are securely placed in the waiting hand of the surgeon or first assistant.
POSITION OF FUNCTION Items should be positioned so they will be usable during the procedure.	The use of a C-arm, laser with articulating arm, or microscope should be preplanned so they may be positioned while the procedure is in progress.	When passing instruments, they should be placed in the surgeon's hand in a usable way. For example, the curve of the instrument should match the curve of the hand.
POINT OF USE Items should be as close to the area of use as possible.	Pour solutions directly into the basins, open and hand sponges or sutures directly to the scrub person as they are needed.	Basins should be placed close to the edge of the table so the circulating nurse can pour without requiring the basin to be repositioned. The ESU pencil holder should be close to the field for safe containment of the tip.
PROTECTED PARTS Items and surfaces should be rendered safe for the patient and the team.	Cords, cables, and tubing should be secured and appropriately directed away from the field. Pad the operating bed and patient as appropriate. Use safety belts.	Apply jaw liners to instruments during setup. Hand instruments with care to avoid causing injury with the tip or sharp surface. Do not lay items on or against the patient's body.
PERFECT PICTURE Items within and around the field should not be at risk for causing harm or becoming damaged. The environment should not be cluttered.	The entire room should appear neat and tidy. The door should be closed, and the temperature and humidity should be appropriate. Forethought to having a clear path for the crash cart or emergency equipment is essential.	The sterile field should remain neat and orderly, with instruments and supplies within easy sight and reach. Consistent setup fosters a sense of comfort and confidence in the scrub role.

*The examples used for each "P" will vary according to the type of procedure and equipment, the position of the patient, and the surgeon's preference. The Eight P's apply to both the scrub person and the circulating nurse.

strength, and function are needed for each step of the surgical procedure. The styles and numbers of instruments are dictated by the type of surgical procedure. Standardization of instrument sets is cost effective and supports the use of a system for counting and accounting for instruments during the procedure.

Arranging the Mayo Stand

Arrange on the Mayo stand the instruments and accessory items needed to create the primary incision and control initial bleeders. A few of each classification of instruments and sponges, may be put on the Mayo stand initially. If a local anesthetic will be used, one or two labeled syringes with appropriate sized hypodermic needles also are needed.

One possible setup of the Mayo stand is illustrated in Figure 25-6. As the surgical procedure progresses, additional instruments and supplies can be added or deleted as necessary. Long-handled forceps and clamps and deep retractors can be substituted for those used on superficial structures. The Mayo stand should be kept neat throughout the surgical

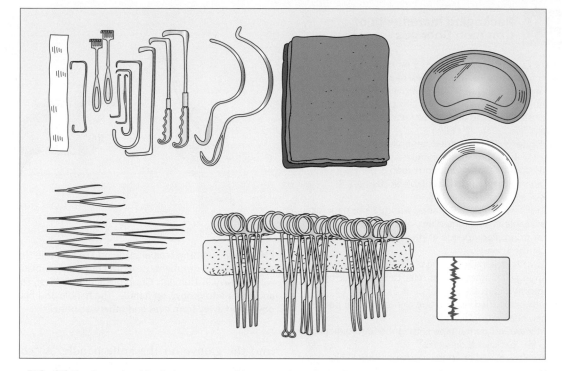

FIG. 25-5   Example of basic instrument table setup. Contents will vary according to the type of surgical procedure.

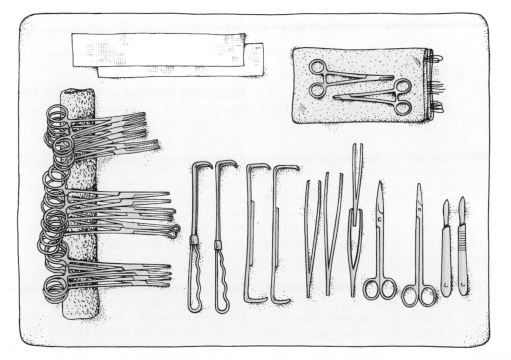

FIG. 25-6   Example of setup for Mayo stand.

procedure. Do not overload it with sponges and sharps. The needle counting magnet or box should not be kept on the Mayo because it is easily bumped during the procedure and could discharge needles into the surgical field.

Establishing Baselines

The scrub person should count sponges, surgical needles, other sharps, and instruments with the circulating nurse according to established facility policy and procedure. After

BOX 25-3   Packaging Increments of Common Sponges

Sponges are packaged in increments of 5 or 10 and are imbedded with a radiopaque strip. The incremental complement is bound with a paper band or wound onto a cardboard holder or Styrofoam holder. Towels can be specially packed in counted increments for use within the body as retractor padding or as a visceral retainer.

1. Raytec or Raytex with embedded radiopaque string 10 per pack (aka: 4 × 4s, 4 × 8s, pusher, gauze sponge).
2. Laparotomy sponge with radiopaque loop 5 per pack (aka: lap tape, lap sponge, lap pad) available in sizes 4 × 8, 12 × 12, 8 × 36, 18 × 18, 8 × 108.
3. Tonsil sponges with long radiopaque string: 5 per pack (aka: tampon) available in small, medium, and large. Available without the string. Radiopaque element is embedded within the fabric of the sponge.
4. Cottonoids with radiopaque strings: 10 per pack (aka: patties or neuro sponges). Some facilities refer to cottonoids by their size in length in inches (i.e., ½, 1, 2, or 3).
5. Peanuts with embedded radiopaque element: 5 per pack (aka: pusher, cherry, or dissector).
6. Kitner tightly wound dental tape with embedded radiopaque element: 5 per pack (aka: dissector).
7. Surgical towels with radiopaque element in blue, white, or blue. Commercially packaged in counted increments of 3 or 5. Not used as drapes.

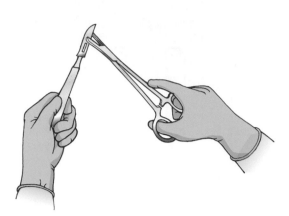

FIG. 25-7   Putting scalpel blade on knife handle. To avoid injury, always use an instrument; never use fingers. The blade is attached with a heavy instrument. Grasp blade at its widest, strongest part, and slip it into groove on handle. The handle and blade are pointed down and away from eyes and other personnel.

completing the initial baseline count with the circulating nurse, a few appropriate-size sponges for the initial incision are placed on the Mayo stand. Many different types of precounted sponges and special towels are available (Box 25-3). The gauze sponges may be opened to their full length or left folded. Fix two or three sponges on sponge forceps (if these will be used), but leave the forceps on the instrument table. Sponges and counting procedures are discussed later in this chapter.

Managing Sharps

After completing the baseline counts with the circulating nurse, the scrub person should secure surgical needles and all other sharps, including knife blades. Blades should be opened onto a consistent spot on the field that is agreed upon by everyone who scrubs and circulates. This will help avoid inadvertent cuts to the fingers of the scrub person, who may be unaware of where blades have been opened onto the field.

Surgical needles and sharps should never be loose on the Mayo stand. If eyed reusable needles are used, each needle must be inspected for cleanliness, burrs, and integrity of the eye before threading. Disposable needles are preferred.

Loading Scalpels

Put blades on knife handles. To avoid injury, always use an instrument, such as a heavy Kelly clamp, to attach the blade; never use the fingers. Avoid using a needle holder because this can weaken the jaws. Holding the cutting edge down and away from the eyes and other personnel in the room, grasp the widest and strongest part of the blade above the notch with the heavy clamp, and slip the blade

into the groove on the knife handle. A "click" indicates the blade is in place. To prevent damage to the blade, the instrument should not touch the cutting edge of the blade (Fig. 25-7).

Scalpels should be loaded early in the setup procedure. This is a good habit to acquire because in emergency surgery the surgeon could be opening the patient while the setup ensues. Time can mean a patient's life. The counting process is handled differently during emergency life and death procedures and is sometimes aborted in favor of a radiographic examination.

Preparing Sutures and Ties for Use

Prepare sutures in the sequence in which the surgeon will use them. The surgeon may ligate (tie off) large blood vessels with a suture ligature shortly after the incision is made, unless electrosurgery is preferred to seal vessels. Prepare ligatures (freehand ties) first if they will be used. Remove suture material from the packet, unless the packet is designed for single-strand dispensing. When trimming the ties to size, work over the instrument table and hold on to the ends of the suture material to prevent strands from dropping over the edge of the table and thus becoming contaminated.

Dispensing reels, relay packets, or strands of ligating material can be placed in a suture book (an old pet name for a fan-folded towel), with the ends extended far enough for rapid extraction. Place the largest size in the bottom layer along the fold that is farthest away when placed on the Mayo stand. The next smaller size is placed in the next layer so that the ends are not overriding those below; if three sizes are prepared, the medium size can be placed midway between the other two. The smallest size will be along the closest fold. The suture book may be placed on the Mayo stand with the ends of the strands on the stand, not over the edges, and toward the sterile field. To prevent possible contamination, strands are pulled out toward the surgical field, never away from it.

A few packets of suture may be opened and prepared for suturing (sewing or stitching). Seldom is it necessary to prepare large amounts of suture material in advance. Suture materials, preparation, and handling are discussed in detail in Chapter 28.

Handling Medications and Solutions on the Sterile Field

Make labels for the sterile container and the syringe. Sterile labels and marking pens are commercially available for labeling containers for medications, radiopaque dyes, and other solutions used in the sterile field. Labeling should include the name and strength of the solution. An appropriate label should be placed on syringes, basins, and medicine cups to prevent inadvertent use of the wrong solution in the wrong manner.

Medications and solutions are dispensed to the sterile field by the circulating nurse after confirming drug identification with the scrub person. The solution basins and medicine cups should be placed near the edge of the sterile field. If a local anesthetic is to be used, the circulating nurse will dispense the drug to the field after drawing it into a syringe. The drug is not dispensed to the field through the needle because it becomes aerosolized and could exposed susceptible people. It is not wise to point a needle for any reason in the interest of safety.

Syringes and Their Handling

Fill the labeled syringe and attach an appropriate-size needle, and put it on the Mayo stand. This will be the first thing the surgeon will use after the patient is draped. State the type and percentage of the solution when handing the syringe to the surgeon. Some facilities use a "no touch" technique. This means that the filled syringe is placed in a basin or tray for the surgeon to retrieve. Do not recap any needle by hand. Place near the working end of the table with the needle pointing away from yourself.

Syringes with needles are used for injection and aspiration, and syringes without needles (e.g., Asepto) are used for irrigation. Most hospitals use sterile disposable syringes and needles. Glass syringes and reusable needles in the same models and sizes are occasionally used.

When using a sterile syringe, be very careful not to touch the plunger, even while wearing gloves. Contamination of the plunger contaminates the inner wall of the barrel and thus the solution that is drawn into it. Glove powder and other debris can act as a contaminant and cause a foreign body reaction. Care is taken to determine if the patient is at risk for latex sensitivity. Nonlatex injection and irrigation syringes are commercially available, and reusable sterile glass syringes are available at many facilities.

The following types of syringes are commonly used for injection or aspiration:

- *Luer-Lok tip:* This type of syringe has a tip that locks over the needle hub. It is used whenever pressure is exerted to inject or aspirate fluid. Sizes range from 2 to 100 mL.
- *Ring control:* This type of syringe has a Luer-Lok tip. The barrel has a thumbhold and two fingerholds, which give the surgeon a secure grip when injecting with only one hand. Sizes range from 3 to 10 mL.

- *Luer slip tip:* This type of syringe has a plain, tapered tip that may not give a secure connection on a needle hub. It is necessary when using some catheter adapters or a rubber connection for aspiration. Sizes range from 1 to 100 mL.

The size of injection needles is designated by length and gauge. Gauge is the outside diameter of a needle, which gets smaller as the number gets larger (e.g., a 30-gauge needle is smaller than a 20-gauge needle). Although numerous sizes of needles are available, only a few representative sizes and their uses are mentioned here:

- $\frac{1}{2}$ inch (12.7 mm) × 30 gauge, for intradermal local anesthetic
- $\frac{3}{4}$ inch (19 mm) × 24 or 25 gauge, the usual needle for any subcutaneous injection
- $1\frac{1}{2}$ inches (3.8 cm) × 22 gauge, for subcutaneous or intramuscular injection
- 2 inches (5 cm) × 18 or 20 gauge, for aspiration
- 4 inches (10 cm) × 20 or 22 gauge, for deep injections into joints or for intracardiac injections

The following types of syringes are used for irrigation:

- Bulb with tapered barrel: With this type of syringe (commonly referred to by the trade name Asepto syringe), a plastic or rubber bulb is attached to the neck of the barrel. The barrel has a tapered or blunt end (like a turkey baster) and can be made of plastic or glass. It is used for one-hand control of irrigation during many types of surgical procedures. This type of syringe has a solution capacity of $\frac{1}{4}$ to 4 ounces (7.6 to 118 mL).
- Tapered bulb without barrel: This type of syringe is a one-piece bulb that tapers to a blunt end. It is used to irrigate small structures, and it may be used for suctioning nasal and oral fluids from neonates during deliveries by cesarean section or used for neurosurgery. This variety is usually disposable because it is not possible to clean the interior of the bulb after use.

To fill an irrigation Asepto syringe, depress the bulb, submerge the end in solution, and release the bulb. The bulb will reinflate, thus drawing solution into the syringe. Take care not to let the bulb express its contents into the air while withdrawing it from the solution. Warm, not hot, solution generally is used for irrigation; check the temperature before giving the syringe to the surgeon. Irrigating solution may be stored in a warmer maintained at a temperature that ranges from 98.6° to 122° F (37° to 50° C). For use, solution usually should not exceed body temperature.

After the Surgeon and Assistant(s) Scrub

Gown and glove the surgeon and assistant(s) as soon after they enter the room as possible, if this is routine procedure. This procedure should take precedence over other setup activities, but do not interrupt a sharps, instrument, or sponge count to do so; such interruptions lead to incorrect counts. The surgeon and assistant(s) may take their gowns from a separate table that has been set up for this purpose. The scrub person should always glove the remainder of the team by the assisted open-glove method. The team should never take towels, gowns, or gloves from the primary sterile field.

Draping the Patient

After the patient is positioned and prepped, assist in draping according to the type of procedure and the surgeon's preference. Many surgeons use towels secured with towel clips to square off the incision. To prevent reaching over the unsterile operating bed, go to the same side of the table as the surgeon to hand towels and towel clips. For hard-to-drape areas, skin towels may be held in place with sutures or staples rather than clips.

Some surgeons use self-adhering plastic incise sheeting directly over the squared-off incision site; the adherent sheeting may be plain or impregnated with iodophor. To apply this adherent drape, stand on the opposite side of the operating bed to assist as the surgeon positions the adherent surface over the patient's prepped skin. A large sheet of paper will be pulled from the sticky surface as the sheet adheres to the patient. The circulating nurse should take the paper from the sterile team member and discard it.

The fenestrated drape sheet is placed over this. During the draping process, care is taken not to allow sterile gloves to touch unsterile surfaces. Drapes are cuffed over the hands as they are positioned. Drapes are not to be moved or repositioned once they are placed.

Once a perforating towel clip has been fastened through a drape, do not remove it, because the points are contaminated and the drape now has holes. If it is necessary to remove a perforating towel clip, discard it from the field and cover the punctured area with another sterile drape or towel. A transparent wound dressing can be stuck over a pinhole from a towel clip in an urgent situation. Nonperforating ball-tip towel clips are preferred for securing drapes.

After draping is completed, bring the Mayo stand into position over the patient, making sure it does not rest on the patient. Position the instrument table at a right angle to the operating bed. Assist the surgeon in securing sterile light handles for adjustment of the operating light. The beam of light should pass the surgeon's right ear and center at the tip of the index finger of his or her right hand (or left hand for a left-handed surgeon).

Lay a towel or magnetic pad for instruments below the fenestration (opening) in the drape, and lay two dry sponges on the pad. Use a nonperforating clamp to attach suction tubing and ESU cords to drapes. Some drapes have loopholes for threading suction tubing and ESU wire through. Allow ample length to reach both the incision area and the equipment. Drop the ends off the side of the operating bed nearest the unit to which the circulating nurse will attach them. It is helpful to have the cables and tubing directed over the same side of the field.

Starting the Surgical Procedure

Initiate a timeout to validate correct site and correct patient. Pass the skin knife to the surgeon (Fig. 25-8), and pass a hemostat and suction to the assistant. When passing the knife, take care to direct the blade away from yourself and all other personnel. Hold the hand pronated, with thumb apposed against the tip of the index finger, and flex the wrist. Eye contact is recommended when passing the scalpel. Some surgeons do not want the knife handed to them but prefer to use a no-passing technique for sharps. When using

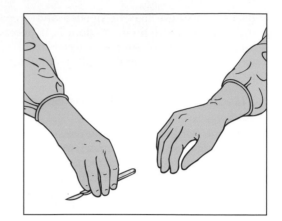

FIG. 25-8 Passing the knife with the blade down and protected. The scrub person's hand is pronated.

the no-passing technique, lay the knife on an instrument towel, magnetic pad, or tray for the surgeon to pick up. The surgeon will replace the knife onto this surface or tray after the incision is made. The scrub person should not allow the scalpel to remain on the field after its use.

Because skin cannot be sterilized, the initial skin scalpel is considered contaminated, whether or not the surgeon has cut through an adhering plastic skin drape. It is removed from the handle and a fresh blade applied in readiness. The skin incision exposes deep skin flora of the hair follicles and sebaceous gland ducts. If an existing scar is excised, it may be sent to the pathology department as a specimen for gross identification. Some surgeons discard this tissue. Determine the surgeon's preferences and the facility policies.

Hand up sterile towels or lap sponges if requested for covering skin at the edges of the incision. Open and drop soiled sponges into the appropriate sponge receptacle for counting, and add clean sponges to the field. If sponges or tapes are added by the circulating nurse during the surgical procedure, break the paper bands and count all of them aloud before use. Do not mix types of sponges and tapes on the table. Keep them separated for ease of identification and tracking.

The tip of the ESU pencil becomes hot and could burn the patient or a team member. Accidental activation can occur if pressure is exerted on the handpiece; this can cause ignition of the draping material or dry sponges. Therefore attach a container (holder/holster) to the drape with a nonperforating clip for containment of the ESU pencil. When not in use, the tip of the ESU pencil is cleaned on a tip polisher/scraper and placed into the holder. The ESU tip should not be cleaned with a scalpel blade. The char should not be permitted to fall into the patient.

If the instrument towel on the sterile field becomes bloody, do not remove it but cover it with a fresh, sterile towel. Stick with the "place it once" principle. Remember that drapes should not be repositioned once they have been placed. Take care not to lay the clean towel over a sponge or instrument.

If the surgeon uses a sterile towel as packing within the wound as a retractor pad or visceral retainer, this is relayed to the circulating nurse and the number of towels is tracked with all other counted items. The circulating nurse is informed when the packing towel is removed, and it is accounted for at the conclusion of the procedure. The practice of using towels for packing is discouraged unless a mechanism is in place for accounting for their removal from the patient at the end of the procedure. Commercially precounted and packed disposable towels with radiopaque

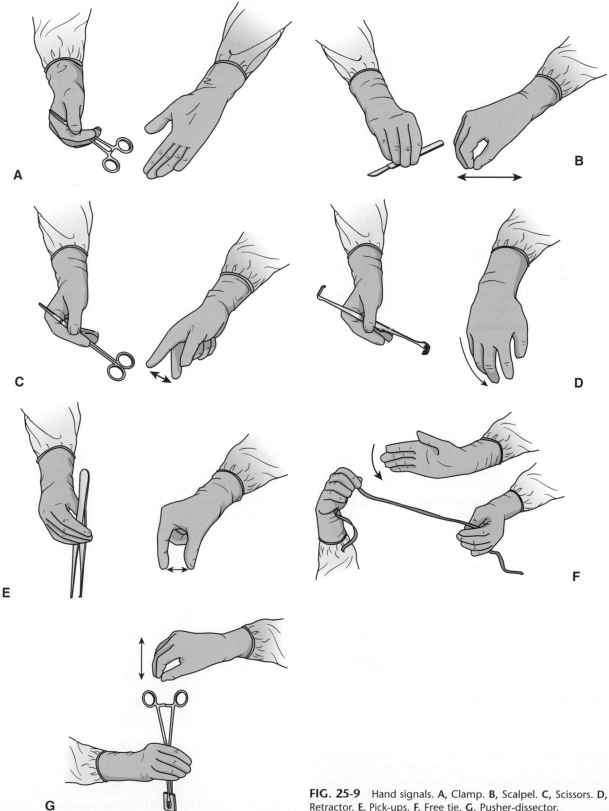

FIG. 25-9 Hand signals. **A,** Clamp. **B,** Scalpel. **C,** Scissors. **D,** Retractor. **E,** Pick-ups. **F,** Free tie. **G,** Pusher-dissector.

markers are available from several manufacturers. Most reusable towels are processed in-house and do not have radiograph-detectable markers.

Watch the field, and try to anticipate the needs of the surgeon and assistant. Keep one step ahead of them in passing instruments, sutures, and sponges and in handing up the specimen basin. Notify the circulating nurse if additional supplies are needed or if the surgeon asks for something not on the table. Ask quietly or signal to the circulating nurse for supplies to avoid distracting the surgeon. Consideration is given to the patient who has received a local or regional anesthetic and may be awake.

When bleeding is obvious, the surgeon needs a hemostatic forceps and/or the ESU pencil. If the bleeding is in a deep wound, the extended ESU pencil tip may need to be attached quickly. After making a deep stitch, the surgeon may want to tag the ends of the suture with a hemostat. Scissors are needed for cutting the suture. Some surgeons use hand signals to indicate the type of instrument needed (Fig. 25-9). These universal signals eliminate the need for talking, but such signs should be clearly understood. An understanding of what is taking place at the surgical site makes these signals meaningful.

Pass instruments in a decisive and positive manner. When instruments are passed properly, surgeons know they have them; their eyes do not need to leave the surgical site. When the surgeon extends his or her hand, the instrument should be placed firmly into his or her palm in the proper position for use (Fig. 25-10). Return instruments to the Mayo stand or instrument table promptly after use. Their weight or a sharp tip could injure the patient.

Keep instruments as clean as possible. Wipe blood and organic debris from them with a moist sponge. Remove debris from electrosurgical tips with the tip polisher/scraper. To keep the suction tip and tubing patent, periodically flush the suction tip with a few milliliters of saline or sterile water. Keep track of the amount of solution used to clear the line, and inform the circulating nurse. The volume of fluid in the suction canister may be confused with blood loss.

Place a ligature in the surgeon's hand. The surgeon keeps both eyes on the field and does not reach for a ligature except to hold out a hand to receive it. Draw a strand out of the suture book and toward the sterile field, grasp both ends, and place the strand securely with an upward sweep in the surgeon's outstretched hand. The end of a ligature may be placed in a long curved forceps, such as Adson tonsil forceps or a right-angled clamp, in a maneuver referred to as a "tie on a passer" (Fig. 25-11). This method is used when the structure will be circumferentially tied off instead of being sutured, such as a vessel in the mesentery. When handing a tie on a passer, place the forceps in the surgeon's hand in the same manner used to pass any hemostatic forceps. Trail the end of the ligature until it is taken by the surgeon or the assistant during the tying procedure. Be ready with the suture scissors as appropriate.

At all times during the surgical procedure, have ready a fine and a heavy suture on needles placed in needle holders. Load the needle into the needle holder in a left- or right-hand manner according to the hand dominance of the surgeon or the direction of the suturing motion (Fig. 25-12). After handing a suture to the surgeon, hand the suture scissors to the assistant and immediately prepare another suture just like it. The surgeon will probably need a forceps for manipulation of tissue during the suturing process. Account for each needle in its entirety as the surgeon finishes with it, because a suture or needle can break. Check the integrity of the needle as it is returned in the needle holder. Tell the surgeon immediately if a needle is broken so that all pieces can be retrieved.

Repeat the size of a suture or ligature when handing it to the surgeon as appropriate. Obviously, this repetition is not necessary if the surgeon is using a long series of interrupted sutures or many ligatures in rapid succession. Use good judgment. Be logical in selecting the instruments used for suturing. Give the surgeon long needle holders to work deep in a cavity; short ones may be used for surface work. Give the assistant a needle holder to pull the needle through tissue for the surgeon. Have scissors ready when the knot is tied. Hemostatic forceps are sometimes used to secure the ends of multiple interrupted sutures placed in rapid succession. Often the knot tying and cutting take place after all sutures are in position, especially during closure.

Remove the waste ends of suture material from the field, Mayo stand, and instrument table, and place them in the

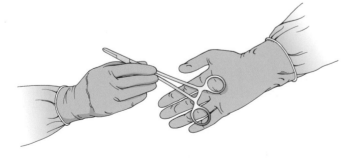

FIG. 25-10 Passing a ringed instrument. The scrub person holds the instrument by the hinge and avoids entangling fingers in the rings. Tip is visible, and handle is free. Handle is placed firmly and directly into waiting hand. A soft snap may be heard as the instrument contacts the waiting gloved hand.

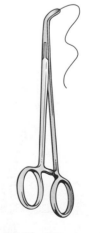

FIG. 25-11 Tie on a passer.

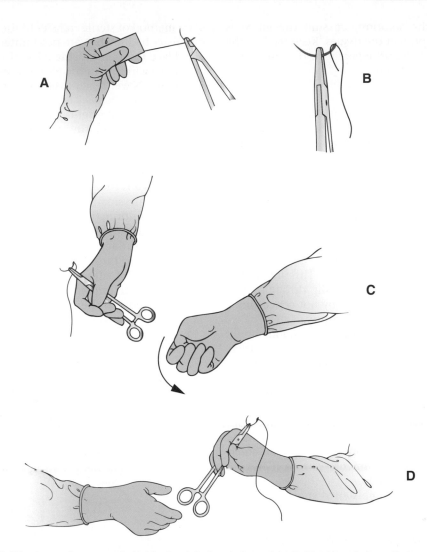

FIG. 25-12 A, Loading a needle holder for right-handed suturing. **B,** Right-handed needle in needle holder. **C,** Hand signal for suture on a needle. **D,** Passing right-handed needle.

trash disposal container. Put used needles on a magnet, numbered needle foam box, or in a needle rack (or other container for this purpose) until the needle count is complete. Follow established institutional policy and procedure for securing sharps during the surgical procedure.

Save and care for all tissue specimens according to policy and procedure. Some facilities require that all tissue removed from a patient, including exudates, be sent for pathologic examination. Therefore it is advisable to send all tissue to the laboratory even though it may appear to be of no value for examination or diagnostic purposes. Any other unusual item such as a retained foreign object should be sent to pathology for accession.

Specimens are put in a specimen basin or another container. Never put a large clamp on a small specimen; this may crush cells and make tissue identification difficult. Some specimens have borders or margins that the surgeon will mark with specific sutures as tags for the pathologist's identification of and attention to certain areas. Keep the specimen basin on the field until all tissue has been removed or all contaminated items have been placed in it. Specimens

designated as right or left should be kept separate in clearly marked containers (e.g., tonsils). Keeping bilateral specimens separated helps prevent confusion if part of the tissue sample is found to be positive for cancer.

When handing a specimen from the field to the circulating nurse, hand it in a basin or appropriate container; never place it on a surgical sponge. Tell the circulating nurse exactly what the specimen is, if there are any identifying notations for the pathologist, or if the specimen is to have special testing (e.g., frozen section). If there are any doubts about the specimen's identification, markers, or processing, ask the surgeon for clarification.

Before closure, the surgeon may request several liters of fresh, warm irrigation solution[2] to rinse the abdomen (or smaller amounts to irrigate other surgical wounds). Some surgeons may pour the irrigation directly from the basin, and others may request an Asepto syringe. If a Poole suction

---

[2]Temperature of the solution should not exceed 110° F (44° C), which is the average temperature used for bathing.

is used to evacuate the solution, be sure the guard is slipped over the tip to protect the tissues. Keep track of the amount of irrigation used, and report it to the circulating nurse for the permanent record.

During Closure

Alert the circulating nurse that closure is about to begin, and hand up the wound closure suture materials. In accordance with established procedures, count sponges, sharps, and instruments with the circulating nurse as the surgeon begins closure of the wound. Verify with the surgeon and circulating nurse that intraabdominal or other cavity-packing materials and towels have been removed.

As time permits, clear unnecessary instrumentation from the Mayo stand, leaving a pair of tissue forceps (pick-ups), suture scissors, and four hemostats or Allis clamps. Place unneeded instruments and supplies on the instrument table in the original set position. This makes the instrument count easier than trying to dig through a pile of jumbled instruments. It is also safer by not concealing a sharp tip that could cause a puncture injury.

The instrumentation setup and the Mayo stand should remain sterile until the patient has left the room. Cardiac arrest, laryngospasm, hemorrhage, premature drain extraction, or other emergencies can occur in the immediate postoperative-postanesthesia period. Even though sterile instrument sets are nearby, valuable time can be lost in reopening sterile supplies, and every second counts in an emergency situation. Regardless of their previous use, instruments on the Mayo stand can be used for an emergency intervention. These instruments can be lifesaving until other ones become available.

Have a clean, warm, saline-moistened sponge ready to wash blood from the area surrounding the incision as soon as skin closure is completed. Have the sterile dressings ready. Radiopaque sponges are never to be used as dressings. After the dressing is in place, the team will undrape the patient. Place the soiled drapes in the appropriate receptacle—not on the instrument table or Mayo stand. The surrounding skin needs to be cleaned before the dressing can be secured with tape.

CIRCULATING NURSE DUTIES

Before entering the OR at the beginning of the day, circulating nurses should wash their hands and arms as required by institutional policy and procedure, but they do not don sterile gowns and gloves. The circulating nurse is an unsterile team member. Personnel who wear sterile attire touch only sterile items; those who are not sterile touch only unsterile items. The circulating nurse should assist the sterile scrub person by providing and opening sterile supplies needed to prepare for arrival of the patient and the surgeon. The circulating nurse should test all equipment before bringing the patient into the room.

After the Scrub Person Scrubs

Fasten the back of the scrub person's gown and assist with the wrap-around tie. Check with the scrub person to see if additional supplies or instruments are needed. Open the remaining packages of sterile supplies (e.g., syringes, suction tubing, sutures, sponges, gloves) as needed. Use an appro-

priate method of sterile transfer to the sterile field. Methods of transfer include but are not limited to the following:

1. Place the item on the edge of the sterile instrument table with the inside of the wrapper everted over your hand. Never reach over the sterile field and shake an item from its package.
2. Expose the contents so the scrub person can remove the item from the wrapper or package by using a forceps or by grasping the item (Fig. 25-13). The scrub person avoids touching the unsterile outside. Remember that the sterile boundary of a peel-open package is the inner edge.
3. Flip only small, rigid items (e.g., suture), and do so with caution (Fig. 25-14). Flipping an item from a package may result in the item missing the intended sterile surface and landing on the floor. Flipping creates air turbulence and thus is the least preferred method of sterile transfer. Larger items, such as staplers or implants, can become contaminated or damaged and therefore are never flipped.

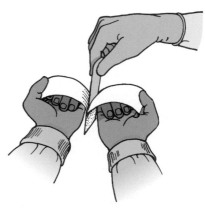

FIG. 25-13 Scrub person taking contents from suture packet opened and held by circulating nurse. Scrub person avoids touching unsterile outer wrapper.

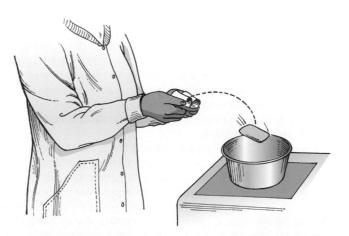

FIG. 25-14 Flipping a packet of suture to the sterile field.

BOX 25-4	Brief Physical Assessment That Can Be Performed by the Circulating Nurse During the Check-in Period Before Entering the Operating Room*

Review of Body Systems (Brief History)	Head-to-Toe Assessment (Brief Physical)
Is the patient a reliable historian, or is a family member translating or communicating on his or her behalf?	Is the patient here for a scheduled procedure, urgent or emergent care, or possibly a redo from an earlier surgery? This may alter the needed supplies for the case.
Is the patient taking any medication on a regular basis (e.g., heart or blood pressure medications)? This should include vitamins, hormones, or herbal preparations.	Is the patient a child or adult? Is a parent present?
Does the patient have any allergies? What are the patient's reactions when exposed to the offending substance? Is the reaction localized or systemic?	Observe the color of the patient's skin and body tissues.
When was the patient's last meal and oral intake? If this is an emergency, what were the foods in this meal. Red foods may falsely imply gastrointestinal bleeding if the patient vomits.	Listen to the sound of the patient's voice as he or she speaks. Is it raspy or breathless? Is the patient coughing? Note any odors on breath or body.
Has the patient ever had any surgery before? This may reveal a condition that requires special positioning or other modification to the standard plan of care.	Touch the patient's skin as the dialog progresses. Is it cool, hot, damp, dry, or in any other condition? This assessment can be performed as part of shaking hands. Does the patient have a weak or strong handshake or grasp? Is the patient shaky?
Has the patient experienced any complications during previous surgeries?	Is there eye contact, and do the eyes move appropriately? Is one or the other eyelid drooping? Is the patient crying?
Does the patient wear contact lenses or prosthetic parts?	Does the patient have enough physical coordination to point to the surgical site? Has the correct site been marked per facility policy and procedure?
Does the patient have any trouble moving limbs?	Does the patient appear to understand what is being said? Can the patient speak and respond appropriately?
Is the patient extremely large or small? This may indicate the need for additional instruments or a weight-appropriate operating bed.	Does the patient have a Foley catheter or an ostomy? Is the patient continent?
Is the patient aware of the procedure being performed?	Are intravenous fluids running? Is the line infusing? Are additives in the container?
Are laboratory studies and blood work reports included with the chart? Are they current?	Is the correct surgical site marked with the surgeon's initials?

*Most of these assessment activities can be performed simultaneously in just a few minutes and may lead to additional nursing diagnoses that require a modification of the plan of care.

Check the list of suture materials and sizes on the surgeon's preference card, but verify with the surgeon before opening packets. Avoid opening suture packets in advance that may not be used. The surgical procedure might be canceled at the last minute or the patient's condition may warrant something different, and then the sutures would be wasted. If the surgeon's need for sutures cannot be anticipated and further instructions have not been given, dispense one or two packets ahead of actual need during the surgical procedure. Once the surgical procedure is started, additional suture can be dispensed to the field, preventing waste.

Pour warmed solution[3] (usually normal saline or Ringer's lactate) into the round solution basin on the instrument table for irrigation and moistening sponges. Pour sterile water into the instrument basin if one is used. For the skin preparation using a two-step prep, pour a small amount of antiseptic agent into the solution cups or prep set on the

prep table and obtain sterile gloves for the person doing the prep.

To establish a baseline of table contents for the record, count sponges, sharps, and instruments with the scrub person in the manner as described in facility policy and procedure. Record this number immediately on the tally sheet or wipe-off board to begin the ongoing tally. Leave a sufficient space for the listing of items that may be added during the procedure. The baseline instrument counts will be recorded on the instrument tray sheet packed with the set.

After the Patient Arrives

The circulating nurse attends to the patient while the scrub person continues to prepare the instrument table for the arrival of the surgeon. Although time is limited during the check-in process, the circulating nurse should perform a brief assessment of the patient. Assessment data about the patient's health status that can be gathered without using equipment or taking an extraordinary amount of time are listed in Box 25-4.

[3]Not to exceed 110° F (44° C).

Greet and identify the patient, introduce yourself, and identify your title and role. Offer the patient a blanket from the warming cabinet. Check the wristband for identification by name and number. Ask the patient to verbally identify himself or herself and (in his or her own words) describe an understanding of the surgical procedure. Many patients have similar-sounding names, and a spelling by the patient may be indicated. If the surgical site is designated left or right, validate the area by having the patient point to the spot. Double-check this spot against the permanent record and the scheduled procedure. The correct surgical site should be marked by the surgeon's initials with an ink marker. If the patient is a minor or is unable to respond, this process is performed in the presence of a parent or legal guardian. Check the plan of care and the patient's chart for pertinent information, including consent and lab work. Immediately report any discrepancies or questions to the surgeon and anesthesia provider.

Verify any allergies or environmental and/or chemical sensitivities the patient may have. These may be identified by an additional wristband and by a special notation on the patient's chart. Ask the patient to describe his or her reaction to the drug or substance.

Be sure the patient's hair is covered with a cap; this prevents dissemination of microorganisms and protects the hair from being soiled. Loosen the neck and back ties on the patient's gown, and untuck the blanket from the foot of the transport stretcher. Align the transport cart with the locked operating bed, and lock the wheels. Ask the anesthesia provider or other personnel to stand on the opposite side of the bed as the patient moves over. Assist the patient as needed, taking care that the patient's gown, blanket, intravenous (IV) infusion tubing, and catheter drainage tubing are not caught between the stretcher and the operating bed. Protect the patient's modesty, and use good body mechanics. Additional personnel should be summoned to help if the patient is unable to move himself or herself. If the patient requires the use of a patient roller device, ensure that adequate personnel are available to assist with the move from one surface to the other (see Fig. 13-1).

After the patient has transferred to the operating bed, apply the safety belt over the thighs 2 to 3 inches above the patient's knees, and place his or her arms on armboards. The safety belt should be placed over the blanket so it is visible, and it should not impair circulation to the extremities. Avoid placing additional blankets over the belt because there is no way to be sure the belt is secure if it is not visible. Other considerations include the following:

1. The patient's legs should not be crossed. A small pillow may be placed under the patient's knees to decrease strain on the lower back. Patients at risk for pressure injury should have gel sacral and heel protectors applied.
2. Remove the patient's arm from the sleeve of the gown before securing it to the armboard. The angle of abduction of the arm on the armboard should not exceed 90 degrees—a right angle with the body. The brachial nerve plexus can be damaged by lengthy, severe abduction of the arm.

Help the anesthesia provider as needed. Apply and connect monitoring devices, and assist with IV infusion,

induction, and intubation as necessary. Some facilities have anesthesia technicians to assist the anesthesia provider. Before the patient arrives, the anesthesia technician will obtain the following equipment:

- Unsterile gloves for the person who will do a percutaneous venipuncture. Sterile gloves are required for a venous cutdown or insertion of arterial monitoring lines.
- A tourniquet to help expose the vein for percutaneous insertion. An unsterile Penrose drain is sometimes used for this purpose.
- Sponges saturated with antiseptic solution for skin preparation. Thorough skin antisepsis is imperative.
- A sterile IV administration tubing set and Angiocaths. A cutdown tray may be needed.
- 1½-inch (3.8-cm) × 20- or 21-gauge Angiocaths, which generally are used for IV fluids when blood transfusion is not anticipated; 1½-inch (3.8-cm) × 18-gauge or 2-inch (5-cm) × 20-gauge needles are used when blood transfusion is anticipated.
- Adhesive tape strips to firmly secure the needle or catheter and tubing to the patient's skin, which prevents motion that may traumatize the vein or cause microorganisms to enter into the skin wound. If the patient is sensitive to adhesives, paper tape may be used.
- A stopcock to regulate or stop the flow of solution through the tubing into the vein. Ports should remain covered until needed to prevent microbial migration into the system.
- IV crystalloid solutions, which include normal saline, dextrose, 5% or 10%, in water (D5W), dextrose in 0.25% saline, Ringer's lactate solution, dextrose in Ringer's lactate solution.

When prolonged postoperative fluid therapy or hyperalimentation is anticipated, an inert, nontoxic, radiopaque, plastic, single-, double-, or triple-lumen catheter is inserted through either a venipuncture through the skin (percutaneous insertion) of the neck or subclavian area or a cutdown through a skin incision to expose the vein. A venous cutdown is performed in other selected situations: for central venous pressure monitoring or if superficial veins are thrombosed or if they are superficially collapsed as a result of shock or prolonged preoperative IV therapy.

A venous cutdown is a sterile procedure that creates an open wound. Sterile gloves, drapes, and a tray of sterile instruments and sutures are needed. Assorted sizes of IV catheters should be available so the anesthesia provider can choose the size best suited to the vein. A soft, pliant catheter takes the contour of the anatomy and is not easily dislodged by movement of the patient. The long-term IV access port will be sutured to the skin.

Check the expiration date, and gently squeeze the plastic IV bag to detect leaks. Check the solution for clarity or discoloration; a cloudy solution is contaminated. A registered nurse or physician must check the label on the container before the solution is administered. All solutions given are charted and monitored to see that they are infusing at the proper speed. Usually this is the responsibility of the anesthesia provider.

Some vascular or radiologic imaging procedures require the use of IV solutions on the sterile field for use in intravascular injection. A plastic bag decanter is used to pour the solution into a basin on the field. The solution should be labeled as IV saline or IV Ringer's. Sometimes heparin or contrast medium is added. The dosage should be indicated on the labeled container.

During the Induction of General Anesthesia

Remain at the patient's side during the induction of anesthesia. Assist the anesthesia provider during induction and intubation.

Maintain a quiet environment. Tactile or auditory stimulation may produce excitement in the patient during induction. Hearing is the last sense lost. A strong startle reaction to sound can provoke life-threatening cardiac dysrhythmias or laryngospasms in any patient. Undue stimulation while the patient is under light anesthesia should be avoided. A quiet, undisturbed induction makes for a much safer and easier maintenance of and recovery from anesthesia. The patient should not be positioned or prepped until the anesthesia provider indicates that it is okay to do so.

After the Patient Is Anesthetized

Attach the anesthesia screen and other table attachments as needed. Reposition the patient only after the anesthesia provider says the patient is anesthetized to the extent that he or she will not be disturbed by being moved or touched. If the patient is to be placed in the prone position, be sure a transport cart remains outside the door for the duration of the case in the event of an emergency. In the event of cardiac arrest or other emergency, the patient will need to be rapidly turned to a supine position for treatment.

If an ESU is to be used, place the dispersive electrode pad in contact with the patient's skin (Fig. 25-15). Avoid scar tissue and hairy or bony areas. If an excessively hairy area is to be used for the electrode, a small area is dry-shaved. A wet shave may prevent the electrode from adhering to the skin surface. Expose the appropriate area for skin preparation and/or Foley catheter insertion. Turn the blanket downward and the gown upward neatly to make a smooth area around the surgical site. Other areas are exposed only as necessary. Before prepping and draping begins, note the patient's position to be certain all measures for his or her safety have been observed. Double-check the safety belt for security. The circulating nurse or first assistant then prepares the patient's skin with antiseptic solution

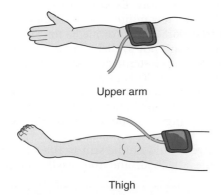

Upper arm

Thigh

FIG. 25-15 Dispersive electrode placement.

using the one-step or two-step method. All prep solutions should be completely dry before the patient is draped.

Turn on the overhead spotlight over the site of the incision. Preoperative medication affects the protective pupillary reflex, and therefore bright light should not be focused on the patient before he or she is asleep or the eyes are covered.

Bag and discard the sponges from a reusable prep tray immediately after use. Prep sponges are not detectable on radiograph examination. Because they are not included in the sponge count, they are not discarded in the kick bucket. A totally disposable prep tray may be bagged for disposal with trash at the completion of the surgical procedure. This is not considered a biohazard, but eyewear should be worn to prevent splashes or aerosolization.

After the Surgeon and Assistant(s) Scrub

Assist with gowning the team. Reach inside the gown to the shoulder seam. If a closed gloving technique is used, pull the gown sleeves only so far that the hands remain covered by the knitted cuffs. If an open technique is used, pull each sleeve over the hands so the gown cuffs are at the wrists. Fasten the waist tie first, followed by the neck closure. Securing the back of the gown in this order allows the upper body more freedom of motion for gloving. The scrub person will assist with open-assisted gloving of the team.

The circulating nurse, as a nonsterile person, should stand by to help with the wrap back tie-in of the gown. The gowned person holds the short tie in the left hand and the long tie attached to a cardboard tab in the right hand. The cardboard tab with the long tie is handed to the nonsterile person. The nonsterile person does not actually touch the long tie—only the cardboard tab. The sterile person still holding the short tie slowly turns away from the nonsterile person, causing the long tie to cross over the back of the gown at the waist. The sterile person carefully takes the long tie from the cardboard tab the nonsterile person is holding and ties the two ends together at the waist front. The nonsterile person discards the cardboard tab.

After gloving, the surgeon and assistant(s) should wipe their gloves with a sterile damp towel to remove glove powder. If the surgeon rinses his or her gloves in a splash basin, the basin should be removed from the sterile field immediately after use; this prevents powder from being carried into the surgical wound if the gloves are rinsed of blood and debris during the surgical procedure.

Observe for any breaks in sterile technique during draping. Stand near the head end of the operating bed to assist the anesthesia provider in fastening the drape over the anesthesia screen or around an IV pole next to the armboard. The drainage bag of the Foley catheter should be placed in view of the anesthesia provider and the circulating nurse.

The scrub person will move the sterile Mayo stand into position over the table. The circulating nurse will move the instrument table into position, being careful not to touch the sterile surface of the drapes. Place steps or platforms for team members who need them, or place sitting stools in position for the team that needs to operate while seated. If one person sits, the entire team should be seated to protect the level of the sterile field.

Position kick buckets (sponge buckets) on each side of the operating bed. Connect suction, the ESU cord, the dispersive electrode cable, or any other powered equipment to be used. If possible, these cords should be directed off the same side of the operating bed to avoid creating a stumbling hazard. Place foot pedals within easy reach of the surgeon's right foot. Tell the surgeon which foot pedal is placed by which foot (if more than one is used), and confirm and document the desired settings on all machines.

During the Surgical Procedure

Some surgeons want the circulating nurse to communicate updates with family or significant others throughout the procedure. Document the time and the calls in the perioperative nurses' notes.

Be alert to anticipate the needs of the sterile team, such as adjusting the operating light, removing perspiration from brows, and keeping the scrub person supplied with sponges, sutures, warm saline, and other necessary items. Ideally, the circulating nurse watches the surgical procedure closely enough to see when routine supplies are needed and gives them to the scrub person without being asked. The circulating nurse should know how to use and care for all supplies, instruments, and equipment and be able to get them quickly. This is particularly important in emergency situations, such as cardiac arrest or hemorrhage.

Stay in the room. Send a runner for supplies if at all possible. Inform the scrub person if you must leave to get something. Be available to answer questions, obtain supplies, and assist team members.

Keep discarded sponges carefully collected, separated by sizes, and counted according to the number they are packaged in. Sponge forceps or gloves are used to handle and count sponges. Soiled sponges should be placed in untied clear plastic bags away from traffic, cabinets, and doors but in full view of the scrub person and anesthesia provider. The bags are not tied, in the event a recount must be done.

Assist the surgeon and the anesthesia provider to monitor blood loss. Weigh sponges if requested to do so. Scales can be brought into the OR for this purpose. Estimate the blood volume in the suction container by subtracting irrigation and body fluids from the total volume in the container. Determinations of total blood volume may be used for estimation of the surgical blood loss. Obtain blood products for transfusion from the refrigerator as necessary, or send a patient care assistant to the blood bank. If the patient's own blood will be recovered for intraoperative autotransfusion, obtain the necessary equipment.

Know the condition of the patient at all times. Inform the OR manager of any marked changes, unanticipated additional procedure, or delays. In a busy department it may be necessary to rearrange the schedule.

Prepare and label specimens for transport to the laboratory. An error in labeling a tissue specimen or culture could cause an inaccurate diagnosis or improper therapy or necessitate another operation. Each container is labeled with the patient's name, identification number, and type and site of specimen. Accompanying the specimen is a requisition that specifies the laboratory test requested by the surgeon. The requisition includes the date, name of the surgeon, preoperative and postoperative diagnoses, surgical procedure, desired test, and tissue to be examined, including its source. Specimens taken from bilateral aspects of the body, such as tonsils should be separated and labeled as left and right. This is important if there is a potential for the diagnosis of cancer.

Specimen containers may be plastic containers, waxed cardboard cartons, or glass jars with preservative solution. AORN recommended practices suggest that the specimen container be part of the sterile setup so the container can be closed on the field minimizing the handling of biohazardous material.[4] The closed, labeled container is placed into a plastic bag or additional container for transport to the laboratory.

The handling of specimens should be kept to a minimum and only while wearing gloves and appropriate personal protective gear, such as eyewear. Use care to avoid contaminating the outside of a specimen container. If it is contaminated, wipe it with an antiseptic solution. Always wash hands thoroughly after removing gloves that have been worn to handle specimens. If instruments are used for handling, be careful not to tear, crush, or damage tissue. The routine care for each type of tissue specimen may vary as follows:

* Pathology tissue specimens should not be allowed to dry out. Saline or a solution of aqueous formaldehyde (10% formalin) is commonly used as the fixative until the specimen is processed further in the laboratory. Some pathology laboratories prefer moistening the specimen with sterile normal saline. Check for the preference of the laboratory that will be examining the specimen. Fresh tissue and frozen sections are not placed in preservative solution.
* Cultures should be refrigerated or sent to the laboratory immediately. Cultures that are immediately placed into media can be stored in an incubator. Cultures are obtained under sterile conditions. The tips of swabs must not be contaminated by any other source. The circulating nurse may hold the tube with gloved hands, but swabs are handled only by sterile team members. OR and laboratory personnel must be protected from contamination. If the tube is handed off the sterile field, the circulating nurse (wearing gloves) can hold open a small plastic bag into which the scrub person drops the tube.
* Cultures for suspected anaerobic pathogens require immediate attention. Exposure to room air may kill anaerobes in a few minutes. Most laboratories provide special transport devices or media for their survival. If such devices are not available, purulent material can be aspirated into a sterile disposable syringe through a disposable needle. This needle is removed and placed with counted sharps on the instrument table. Air is expelled away from the field, and the syringe is capped with the syringe tip supplied with the syringe; the syringe is then sent immediately to the laboratory. The syringe should not be sent to the laboratory with the needle attached, and the needle should not be

[4]*AORN standards, recommended practices, and guidelines 2006.*

recapped by hand because of the potential for a needlestick injury.

- Smears and fluids should be taken to the laboratory as soon as possible. These may be placed on glass slides or drawn into evacuation tubes.
- Stones are placed in a dry container so they will not dissolve.
- Foreign bodies should be sent for accession according to policy, and a record is kept for legal purposes. The description and the disposition of the object are recorded. A foreign body may be given to the police, surgeon, or patient, depending on legal implications, policy, or the surgeon's wishes.
- Amputated extremities are wrapped in plastic before sending them to a refrigerator in the laboratory or morgue. Avoid placing the amputated limb in the patient's field of vision. Most patients needing amputation have spinal or epidural anesthesia for the procedure. The sight of the body part may cause emotional distress in the patient. The patient may request that an amputated extremity be sent to a mortuary for preservation for burial with his or her body after death. This request must be noted on the requisition sent to the laboratory. Refer to institutional policy and procedure for the care of amputated limbs.

As required, complete the documentation in the patient's chart, permanent OR records, and requisitions for laboratory tests or chargeable items. Information to be included in the documentation of direct intraoperative care is shown in Box 25-5.

During Closure

Count sponges, sharps, and instruments with the scrub person. Report counts as correct or incorrect to the surgeon. Complete the count records. Collect used sponges for disposal in the appropriately marked receptacles.

If another patient is scheduled to follow (TF), the following procedures should be observed:

1. Phone or ask the clerk-receptionist to call the unit where the next patient is waiting and request that preoperative medication be given if ordered; this should be done at least 1 hour to 45 minutes before the scheduled time of the surgical procedure. This procedure usually is not necessary for the first scheduled patient of the day but is important for subsequent patients when the exact time of the surgical procedure is uncertain. For these patients the anesthesia provider usually orders medication or antibiotics "on call."
2. Send a nursing assistant or transporter for the patient, or notify the unit to transport the patient. The patient should be in the OR suite 30 minutes before the anticipated time of incision. If a holding area is included in the OR suite, the patient may arrive earlier to receive the preoperative medication there.

Check the surgeon's preference card or case cart sheet for the next procedure. Collect supplies that will be needed, and get them organized to the extent possible. These supplies can be assembled in the substerile room or left in a cabinet. They cannot be put on furniture in the room until it is cleaned after completion of the current

---

BOX 25-5	Documentation by the Circulating Nurse of Direct Intraoperative Patient Care

- Initial assessment of the patient on arrival to the OR. The identity of the patient and verification of the procedure should be validated. Correct surgical site should be marked by surgeon's initials.
- The significant times, such as arrival, start, completion, and room exit times.
- Disposition of sensory aids or prosthetic devices accompanying the patient on arrival in the operating room (OR).
- Position, surgical safety devices, and/or restraints used during the surgical procedure.
- Placement of monitoring and electrosurgical unit (ESU) electrodes, tourniquets and other special equipment and identification of units or machines used, as applicable. The settings and duration of use should be recorded.
- The names and times of all personnel in the room for the procedure.
- The type of anesthetic administered, and by whom.
- The surgical site preparation, the antiseptic agent administered, and by whom.
- Medications, solutions, and doses administered, and by whom.
- Timeout validation of site, patient, and procedure.
- A description of the actual surgical procedure performed.
- Contact with the patient's family or significant others.
- Type, size, and manufacturer's identifying information (lot numbers) of prosthetic implants, or the type, source, and location of tissue transplants or inserted radioactive materials.
- Use of radiograph or imaging.
- Disposition of tissue specimens and cultures.
- Correctness or incorrectness of surgical counts (if incorrect, the remedial measures to locate the lost item).
- Placement of drains, catheters, dressings, and packing. Output is recorded if receptacle is emptied in the OR.
- Wound classification is designated at the end of the procedure.
- Charges to patient for supplies, according to hospital routine.
- Piece of equipment sent from OR with patient to unit (e.g., tracheotomy set that accompanies patient after thyroidectomy, wire scissors if patient has had teeth wired together). These items are to be returned.
- Disposition of the patient after leaving the OR.
- Any unusual event or complication.

---

surgical procedure. Advance preparation for the following case may vary if a case cart system is used. Prepare for room cleanup so that minimal time is expended between surgical procedures:

1. Remove radiographs from the view box, place them in an envelope, and take them to the designated area to be returned to the radiology department. Digital displays should be cleared.
2. Obtain the washer-sterilizer tray, instrument tray, and other items necessary for the cleanup procedure. Place them on top of case cart for the scrub person to break down table when the current patient leaves the room.

Send for a postanesthesia care unit (PACU) stretcher or an intensive care unit (ICU) bed as appropriate, or prepare the patient's stretcher or bed with a clean sheet; follow whatever is the institutional procedure. Obtain a transfer monitor and oxygen tank with tubing if needed. Also alert patient care assistants and housekeeping personnel that the surgical procedure is nearing completion so they can be ready to assist in room turnover as needed. This helps shorten the downtime between surgical procedures. Be as systematic as possible so steps are not omitted.

After the Surgical Procedure Is Complete

Assist with securing the dressing(s) over the surgical wound and managing the surgical drainage systems. The scrub person should roll the drapes off the patient and clean the surrounding skin before the outer layer of dressing is secured with the appropriate type of tape. Open the neck and back closures of the surgeon's and assistants' gowns so they can remove them without contaminating themselves.

See that the patient is clean. Wash off body substances or plaster. Put on a clean, warm gown and blanket. Have a patient care assistant bring in the clean transport cart or bed. Check the patient's name on the stretcher or bed if it is the procedure to return the patient to the same one used for transport to the OR suite. Align the cart with the operating bed, and lock the wheels. Remove the arm and leg safety belts and table appliances.

A lifting frame or patient roller is a great help in moving unconscious and obese patients. The Davis patient roller consists of a series of rollers that are mounted in a frame long enough to accommodate the trunk of an adult patient. The edge of the roller is placed under the lift sheet and the patient's side. With the patient's head and feet supported by separate team members, the lift sheet is pulled and the patient is rolled onto the stretcher or bed (see Fig. 13-1). A *minimum of four people* is required to move the patient with this device: one to lift the head, one to lift the feet, one beside the stretcher or bed to pull, and one beside the patient to lift him or her from the operating bed. The action of all four people should be synchronized, and the count of three is called by the anesthesia provider. The following precautions should be taken in lifting or rolling an unconscious patient:

1. Protect the IV, drains, and urinary drainage bag. Secure IV solution bags on an IV pole. It is preferable to attach the IV pole near the foot end of the stretcher or bed, where there is less danger of injury to the patient if the bag or IV pole should fall or break.
2. Use the lift sheet to support the arms at the sides so the arms do not dangle.
3. The anesthesia provider guards the head and neck from injury and calls the count for the move.
4. Lift or roll the patient gently and slowly to avoid circulatory depression.

After the patient is safely on the transport cart, remove the lift sheet by logrolling the patient gently from side to side. Brush burns result if the fabric is pulled from under the patient. Place the patient in a comfortable position that is most conducive to the maintenance of respiration and circulation. The appropriate position may vary with the type of surgical procedure; usually the patient should:

- Be supine after a laparotomy, with the head of the stretcher elevated 15 degrees, especially if he or she is still intubated
- Be semiprone after a tonsillectomy, for drainage, if extubated

- Be lateral, on the affected side, after transthoracic surgical procedures, thus splinting the side, usually extubated
- Have the affected extremity supported on a pillow

Raise the side rails before the patient is transported out of the OR. Be sure the completed chart and proper records accompany the patient, and send other supplies as indicated (e.g., tracheostomy obturator). Help transport the patient to the PACU or patient care unit.

Patient Transfer from the Operating Room

During transport, the patient should be constantly observed by someone familiar with his or her condition. If the patient has had local anesthesia, the circulating nurse and transporter may accompany the patient during the return to an ambulatory unit. If the patient has had general anesthesia, the anesthesia provider and circulating nurse should accompany him or her during transport to the PACU, where they give a verbal hand-off report to the PACU nurse. This postoperative report is important for the continuity of care. A concise verbal report from the anesthesia provider and/or circulating nurse includes the following:

- Name and age of the patient
- Type of surgical procedure and name of the surgeon
- Type of anesthesia and name of the anesthesia provider
- Vital signs (baseline, preoperative, and intraoperative), including current body temperature
- Types and locations of drains, packing, and dressings
- Preoperative level of consciousness and current status
- Medications given preoperatively and intraoperatively, as well as those regularly taken by prescription or self-medication
- Medical history, including previous surgical procedures
- Allergies and responses to allergens, substance sensitivity
- Positioning on the operating bed and devices attached to the skin
- Complications during the surgical procedure
- Intake and output, including IV fluids and blood
- Location of the waiting family or significant others
- Special considerations:
- Sensory and/or physical impairments; eyewear, hearing aids, dentures, or other personal property brought to the OR is returned to the patient when the level of consciousness is appropriate
- Language barrier and level of understanding
- Use of tobacco, alcohol, and/or addictive drugs
- Orders such as "no code," "do not resuscitate (DNR)," or "do not attempt resuscitation"

SPONGE, SHARPS, AND INSTRUMENT COUNTS

The counting of sponges, needles and other sharps, and instruments has been mentioned throughout this chapter. These supplies are crucial to the surgical procedure and must be accounted for throughout every procedure, regardless of size or function. Items are counted before and after use. The types and numbers of sponges, needles and other sharps, and instruments vary for each surgical procedure.

Accountability is a professional responsibility that rests primarily on the scrub person and the circulating nurse. The surgeon and patient rely on the accuracy of this accountability by the team. There are several reasons why it is important for the scrub person and circulating nurse to count and be accountable for all items used during the procedure (Box 25-6). Counts are performed for patient and personnel safety, infection control, and inventory purposes. A needle, instrument, sponge, tape, or towel left in the wound after closure is a possible cause for a lawsuit after a surgical procedure. Containment and control are also important for infection control.

A retained foreign object made of woven textile is referred to as a gossypiboma or a textiloma. A foreign body unintentionally left in a patient can be the source of wound infection or disruption. The longer the object remains in the body, the more it incorporates ingrowth of tissue. An abscess can form, and fistulas may develop between organs. The foreign body reaction may be immediate or may be delayed for years. Diagnosis is sometimes difficult and costly, and removal of the object usually requires major surgery. The literature reports the removal of some retained sponges through laparoscopic surgery if they are discovered before adhesions develop.

A contaminated sponge or needle that is unaccounted for at the close of procedure could also inadvertently come into contact with the personnel who clean the room, process instruments, launder the linens, or transport the trash. Blood or body fluids are sources of pathogens such as human immunodeficiency virus (HIV) or hepatitis B virus (HBV). A surgical pattie that has become saturated with cerebrospinal fluid during a neurologic case may also be contaminated with Creutzfeldt-Jakob disease (CJD).

Inventory control is monitored by accounting for the instrument set in its entirety. Counting ensures that expensive instruments such as towel clips and scissors are not accidentally thrown away or discarded with the drapes. Injury to laundry and housekeeping/environmental services personnel by the contaminated sharp edges of surgical instruments, blades, and needles is a risk. Surgical instruments also can cause major damage to equipment in the laundry services. Unfortunately, some facilities have felt a need to install metal detectors in the trash and soiled linen areas to monitor for missing instruments.

Counting Procedures

A counting procedure is a method of accounting for items put on the sterile table for use during the surgical procedure. Sponges, sharps, and instruments should be counted and/or accounted for on all surgical procedures. This includes any materials introduced into the patient during the procedure, such as rectal or vaginal packs or sterile towels used to pack off or retain viscera.

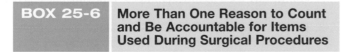

BOX 25-6	More Than One Reason to Count and Be Accountable for Items Used During Surgical Procedures

- Item can be lost in patient's body, causing the need for additional surgery.
- Item can be lost in trash or linen, causing harm to other personnel.
- Item can be lost from inventory, resulting in high replacement costs.

Items used during organ procurement procedures should be accounted for in their entirety in the same manner as for any surgical procedure. Respect for the donor should be as important to the surgical team as respect for any patient.

Initial Count When the Tray Is Assembled

The person who assembles and wraps items for sterilization will count them in standardized multiple units. Some facilities enclose a copy of this tray inventory count sheet in the instrument set. In commercially prepackaged sterile items (e.g., sponges, disposable towels), this count is performed by the manufacturer.

Baseline Count During Setup for the Surgical Procedure

The scrub person and the circulating nurse together count all items before the surgical procedure begins and during the surgical procedure as each additional package is opened and added to the sterile field. These initial counts provide the baseline for subsequent counts. Any item intentionally placed in the wound, such as towels, is recorded. A useful method for counting is as follows:

1. As the scrub person touches each item, he or she and the circulating nurse number each item aloud until all items are counted. There is no need to be disruptive when performing this task. Each pack of sponges will be bound with a paper band that is broken only as each bundle is counted. The presence of an intact paper band indicates that bundle has not been counted yet. Count them one bundle at a time.
2. The circulating nurse immediately records the count for each type of item on the count record or wipe-off board. Preprinted forms are helpful for this purpose.
3. Additional packages should be counted away from counted items already on the table in case it is necessary to repeat the count or to discard an item.
4. Counting should not be interrupted. The count should be repeated if there is uncertainty because of interruption, fumbling, or any other reason.
5. If either the scrub person or the circulating nurse is permanently relieved by another person during the surgical procedure, the incoming person should verify all counts before the person being relieved leaves the room. Personnel who perform the final counts are held accountable for the entire count.

Closing Counts (First Closing Count)

Counts are taken in three areas before the surgeon starts the closure of a body cavity or a deep or large incision:

1. Field count: Either the surgeon or the assistant assists the scrub person with the surgical field count. Additional items (e.g., vaginal or rectal packing, sterile towels used as intraabdominal packing) are accounted for at this time. This area should be counted first. Counting this area last could delay closure of the patient's wound and prolong anesthesia.
2. Table count: The scrub person and the circulating nurse together count all items on the Mayo stand and instrument table. The surgeon and assistant may be suturing the wound while this count is in process.

3. Floor count: The circulating nurse counts sponges and any other items that have been recovered from the floor or passed off the sterile field to the kick buckets. These counts should be verified by the scrub person.

Final Count (Second Closing Count)

The final count is performed to verify any counts and/or if institutional policy and procedure stipulates additional counts before any part of a cavity or a cavity within a cavity is closed. A final count may be taken during subcuticular or skin closure. The circulating nurse totals the field, table, and floor counts. If the final counts match the totals on the tally sheet, the circulating nurse tells the surgeon the counts are correct. A count should be reported to the surgeon as correct only after a physical count by number actually has been completed. Intentionally exposing the patient to x-rays is not a replacement for the physical count.

The circulating nurse documents on the patient's record what was counted, how many counts were performed and by whom, and if the counts were correct or incorrect. There is no need to write all the tallies on the permanent record. A registered nurse should participate to verify that all counts are correct, but the personnel actually performing the counts are responsible for the accuracy of the counts. The counting procedure, the outcome, and participating personnel should be documented according to institutional policy and procedure.

Omitted counts because of an extreme patient emergency should be recorded on the patient's record, and the event should be documented according to institutional policy and procedure. If a sponge or sponges are intentionally retained for packing or if an instrument intentionally remains with the patient, the number and type should be documented on the patient's record. Any time a count is omitted, refused by a surgeon, or aborted, the reason should be fully documented.

Records can be subpoenaed and admitted as evidence in court. The accountability for all items used during the surgical procedure is placed on the scrub person and the circulating nurse, who jointly perform the counting procedures as defined by institutional policy and procedure. The surgeon and the first assistant facilitate the counting process. It is not the job of the surgeon or the first assistant to actively perform the counts or sign the count reconciliation sheet.

Incorrect Count

A specific policy and procedure for any count that is incorrect should be defined by each institution and should include but not be limited to the following:

1. The surgeon is informed immediately.
2. The entire count is repeated.
3. The circulating nurse searches the trash receptacles, under the furniture, on the floor, in the laundry hamper, and throughout the room.
4. The scrub person searches the drapes and under items on the table and Mayo stand.
5. The surgeon searches the surgical field and wound.
6. The circulating nurse should call the immediate supervisor to check the count and assist with the search.

7. After all search options have been exhausted, policy should stipulate that a radiograph film be taken before the patient leaves the OR. The surgeon may wish a radiograph be taken at once, with a portable machine, to determine whether the item is in the wound. Alternatively, the surgeon may prefer to complete the closure first because of the patient's condition or because there is reasonable assurance, based on wound exploration that the item is not in the patient. Unfortunately, patients' incisions have been reopened after complete closure to retrieve retained objects, such as sponges.
8. The circulating nurse should write an incident report and document on the OR record all efforts and actions to locate the missing item, even if the item is located on the radiograph. This report has legal significance for verification that an appropriate attempt was made to find the missing item. If the item is not found on the radiograph, the report brings to the attention of personnel the need for more careful counting and the control of sponges, sharps, and instruments.

SPONGES

Sponges are used for absorbing blood and fluids, protecting tissues, applying pressure or traction, and for blunt dissection. Many different types of sponges are available. All sponges on the sterile table and field should be radiopaque. A radiopaque thread or marker made of a barium substance is incorporated into commercially manufactured sponges.

Types of Sponges

The following list is representative of the types of sponges used:

1. Gauze sponges (which are called "swabs" in some countries) are supplied sterile, precounted, and folded. When opened out to a single ply during blunt dissection, fibers along the raw edges could become foreign bodies in the wound. These are also called Raytec or Raytex sponges. All are packed in groups of 10 and bound with a paper band.
2. Laparotomy tapes, also called lap pads, tapes, or packs, are used for retaining the viscera and keeping them moist and warm. Tapes are either square or oblong and have a loop of blue twill tape sewn on one corner. A small radiopaque marker is sewn into one corner of the tape. A metal or plastic radiopaque ring, approximately 1½ inches (3.8 cm) in diameter, may be attached on this twill tape. If rings are used, they remain outside the edges of the incision while the tape is inside. Normal saline or Ringer's lactate is commonly used to moisten tapes. Tapes are packaged in groups of five.
3. Dissecting sponges have a self-contained, radiograph-detectable element incorporated into the weave.
   a. Peanut sponges are very small, ovoid gauze sponges used for blunt dissection or absorption of fluid in delicate procedures. They are clamped into the tip of an Adson or right-angle clamp during use. They are packaged in groups of five.
   b. Kitner dissectors are small cylindrical rolls of heavy cotton dental tape that are held in a Kelly or Kocher

(Oschner) clamp for use during blunt dissection. They are packaged in groups of five.

c. Tonsil sponges are soft, ball-shaped, cotton-filled gauze sponges with an attached cotton thread. They are held in a forceps for use. These come in several sizes and are held in the tip of a forceps to use. They are packaged in groups of five.

4. Compressed absorbent cottonoids (also known as patties) are small squares or rectangles made of compressed rayon or cotton; they are very absorbent and resemble a strip of felt. They are moistened with Ringer's lactate or a topical hemostatic agent, such as thrombin, for use on delicate structures such as the nerves, brain, and spinal cord.

They are pressed out flat after moistening and before handing them to the surgeon. The surgeon will pick up the cottonoid with a forceps (commonly bayonet forceps) and apply it to the area of intended use. Some surgeons will use cottonoids to apply intranasal anesthetic such as cocaine. Cottonoids have a radiopaque element and a thread attached so they can be located in the wound. These range in size from $\frac{1}{4} \times \frac{1}{4}$ inch to 1×3 inches.

5. Towels are occasionally but not universally used for protecting the viscera. The scrub person and circulating nurse are responsible for accounting for the tracking and retrieval of towels or anything placed in the patient. The scrub person informs the circulating nurse that a towel has been used for packing or protecting viscera, and the circulating nurse documents the event. This does not mean that all towels used in draping are part of the count—only those towels placed *inside the patient.*

During the first closing count at the conclusion of the case, the circulating nurse checks with the scrub person to verify that the towel has been removed before closure. Disposable varieties of sterile, precounted, packaged towels with radiograph-detectable elements are commercially available. Towels can be white, blue, or green. Some have twill-tape tags with rings like those on lap tapes.

Retained surgical towels have been the subject of several liability suits. Case law demonstrates that the hospital, on behalf of the scrub person and the circulating nurse, has been successfully sued in these cases, while the surgeon has been exonerated (*Good Samaritan Hospital v. Dr. Ramondelli;* Court of Common Pleas, Montgomery, Ohio, 1997). The premise for these findings is based on the fact that the scrub person and circulating nurse are responsible for the counts and the fact that the surgeon relies on their accurate performance in this role. Everything temporarily placed inside the patient must be accounted for at the conclusion of the case.

Counting Sponges

Radiopaque, radiograph-detectable gauze sponges, tapes, towels, dissecting sponges, and cottonoid patties are counted in multiples of 5 or 10 per package. The types of sponges and number of different sizes should be kept to a minimum. To count them, the scrub person will do the following:

1. Hold the entire pack of sponges of whatever type, including tapes, in one hand. The thumb should be over the edges of the folded sponges.
2. Break the paper band. Breaking the band is a good way to designate which stacks have been counted and which ones have not.
3. Shake the pack gently to separate the sponges and loosen the twill-tape tails on tapes.
4. Pick each sponge separately from the pack with the other hand, and number it aloud while placing it in a pile on the sterile instrument table.

If a pack contains an incorrect number of sponges, the scrub person should hand the entire pack to the circulating nurse for removal from the room. There should be no attempt to correct errors or to compensate for discrepancies. The pack should be removed from the room and not used.

Methods of Accounting for Sponges

Regardless of the types and numbers of sponges counted, various methods may be used to help ensure that one is not misplaced or left in the patient.

By the Scrub Person

1. Keep sponges, tapes, peanuts, and other such materials separated on the instrument table and far away from each other and from any draping material, especially towels.
2. Keep sponges far away from small items (e.g., needles, hemostatic clips) that might be dragged into the wound by a sponge or tape.
3. Do not give the surgeon or assistant a sponge to wipe the powder off his or her gloves. It may end up in the laundry hamper or trash. Use a sterile towel instead if at all possible.
4. Do not cut sponges or tapes. It may be hard to account for the item in its entirety.
5. Do not remove the radiopaque thread or marker. Either the marker or the sponge could be lost.
6. Never mix sponges and tapes in a solution basin at the same time; this prevents the danger of dragging a small sponge unknowingly into the wound along with a tape.
7. Do not give the pathologist a specimen on a sponge to take from the room; instead, put the specimen in a basin or on a towel.
8. Discard all soiled sponges into the kick bucket after completely opening them and leave no more than two clean sponges on the sterile field at a time. Put up clean ones before removing soiled ones on an exchange basis as part of a systems approach to error prevention.
9. Do not be wasteful of sponges. Besides the economy factor, the more sponges that are used, the more there are to count and the greater the chance for error.
10. Once the peritoneum is opened or the incision is made and extends deep into a body cavity (where a sponge could be lost), four alternative precautions can be taken:
    a. Remove all Raytec sponges from the field, and use only tapes. Rings, if used, hang outside, over the edges of the wound.
    b. Use folded Raytec sponges on sponge forceps only. Completely unfold and open each one before dropping into the sponge bucket.

c. Give laparotomy sponges to the surgeon one at a time on an exchange basis.

d. Dissectors are given one at a time clamped inside the tip of an instrument on an exchange basis. Bloody dissector sponges are replaced into the Styrofoam holder after use. When the complement of five is soiled, the entire holder with the bloody dissectors is dropped into the sponge bucket for the circulating nurse to package.

11. With the circulating nurse, count sponges and tapes added during the surgical procedure before moistening or using them. Break the paper band to signify they have been counted.

13. Do not add or remove sponges from the surgical field during a sponge count until the count is verified as complete and correct. Before beginning the final count, place one or two tapes or sponges on the field for use while the count is being taken.

By the Circulating Nurse

1. To prevent the possibility of confusion in the count, nonradiopaque gauze sponges used on different trays (e.g., spinal, shave, or prep trays) should be bagged and moved away from the field before the incision is made.

2. Each discarded sponge should be examined briefly to be sure no saturated sponges are tangled with them. To avoid the transmission of bloodborne pathogenic organisms, wear gloves and protective eyewear to separate sponges for counting, stacking, and bagging.

3. Count and bag sponges in the same increment in which they are supplied, such as groups of 5 or 10 of like sponges. These numbers should be recorded on the sponge count record and counted. The bagged units are not tied shut or discarded into the trash. The bags are placed aside in full view of the scrub person and the anesthesia provider until the end of the case and all the numbers are reconciled. The anesthesia provider will be observing for blood loss on the sponges.

4. Give additional sponges or tapes to the scrub person when it is convenient for him or her to count them. The scrub person breaks the paper band as the bundle is counted. Broken paper bands are a signal that that particular pack has been counted. The scrub person separates each sponge and counts them, and the circulating nurse records the numbers immediately.

5. Give dressings to the scrub person after the final sponge count. Radiopaque sponges are not used for dressings because they could distort a postoperative radiograph of the site.

6. Do not discard or remove counted sponges from the room for any reason until the patient is out of the room.

SHARPS

Sharps include surgical needles, hypodermic needles, knife blades, electrosurgical needles and blades, and safety pins. Each item must be accounted for. Surgical needles are the most difficult to track and are used in the largest quantity. All surgical needles and other sharps are counted as they are added to the sterile table and/or separated from other instruments in the instrument tray.

Surgical Needle Counts

Surgical needles are used for suturing. The type will determine the method of transfer to the sterile table:

1. Reusable eyed needles put in a needle rack or a suture book are uniformly counted into sets in multiples of two or three of each type and size the surgeon will need. These needles are usually packaged and sterilized separately from the instrument sets. Most facilities have converted to disposable free needles and no longer reuse needles.

2. Disposable suturing needles are precounted, packaged, and sterilized by the manufacturer. The label will specify whether the sterile pack contains single or multiple needles. Closure materials are discussed in detail in Chapter 28.

Counting Needles and Other Sharps

Each needle or packet containing needles is separated for individual counting. Suture packets containing swaged needles can remain unopened. The count is taken according to the label on each packet. Some packets contain multiple needles. The scrub person verifies the count when the packet is opened.

Methods of Accounting for Sharps

If a needle or blade has broken, both the scrub person and the circulating nurse must make sure all pieces are recovered or accounted for. Sometimes the risk of retrieving a piece of a sharp or needle is more hazardous than letting it encapsulate in tissue. The surgeon makes this determination.

Many smaller-gauge needles do not appear easily on radiograph unless the technician uses special density calculations. Needles, knife blades, safety pins, and other small sharps should never be left loose on the Mayo stand, because they could be dragged into the incision or knocked onto the floor. Smallness of the needle is not a valid reason to fail to account for each one.

By the Scrub Person

1. Leave needles swaged to suture material in their inner folder or dispenser packet until the surgeon is ready to use them. These folders or packets can be placed in a fold of the suture book or secured on the Mayo stand or the working end of the table. Suture packets can remain sealed until the scrub person anticipates their use, thus minimizing the number of loose, unused needles on the sterile table.

2. Give needles to the surgeon on an exchange basis; that is, one is returned before another is passed. Account for each needle as the surgeon finishes with it.

3. Use needles and needle holders as a unit. The following is a good rule: No needle on the Mayo stand without a needle holder, and no needle holder without a needle.

4. Secure used needles and sharps in a needle counting box until after the final count. Many methods for efficient handling are available:

a. Sterile adhesive pads with or without magnets facilitate counting and safe disposal. When a large number of swaged needles will be used, the scrub person and circulating nurse may determine the number of needles a pad will hold and work out a unit system.

When this maximum number is reached and counted by both, the pad or box is closed and handed off to the gloved circulating nurse, who will place the container with the other countable items off the field. This method eliminates the hazard of handling extreme amounts of loose needles on the instrument table. Disposable plastic boxes of various sizes for the containment of sharps are commercially available.

   b. Used eyed needles can be returned to the needle rack. The use of reusable suture needles is not encouraged because they become dulled with use and could harbor microorganisms if not properly cleaned.

By the Circulating Nurse

1. Open only the necessary number of packets of sutures with swaged needles. Overstocking the instrument table not only is wasteful but also complicates the needle count.
2. Counted sharps should not be taken from the OR during the surgical procedure. If a scalpel with a counted knife blade is given to a pathologist to open a specimen, the scalpel must remain in the room after gross examination of the specimen; it is not to be taken to the laboratory with the specimen.
3. A sharp is passed off the sterile field if it punctures, cuts, or tears the glove of a sterile team member. These sharps are retained and added to the table and field counts to reconcile the final sharp count. An empty specimen cup is a good container for a loose sharp.
4. A magnetic roller may be used to locate a surgical needle or blade that has dropped on the floor.

INSTRUMENTS

Surgical tools and devices are designed to perform specific functions that include cutting or dissecting, grasping and holding, clamping and occluding, exposing, or suturing. For each basic maneuver, an instrument of suitable size, shape, strength, and function is needed. Variation in the style and number of instruments will be dictated by the type of surgical procedure and, to some extent, by the personal preferences of the surgeon.

Counting Instruments

Instrument counts are recommended for all surgical procedures. Specific written policies and procedures are followed without deviation. To count instruments, the scrub person should do the following:

1. Remove the top rack of instruments from the instrument tray or container and place it on a rolled towel or over the lip of a tray or container. Instruments are counted as they are assembled in standardized sets. Groups of even numbers of each of the basic clamps facilitate handling and counting.

   Some facilities permit "cluster counting," which is a method of counting all scissors, pick-ups, needle holders, retractors, and other like groups together without having to name each item with its formal name. For example, the tray may contain two pairs each of three different types of scissors. This cluster would be counted as "six scissors" instead of two Mayo, two Metzenbaum, and two suture scissors. This can speed up the count. If an item is not accounted for in the cluster, an itemized individual count ensues.

2. Expose all instruments left in the tray for counting. Remove knife handles, towel clips, tissue forceps, and other small instruments from the tray, and place them on the instrument table. Do not put instruments on the Mayo stand until they are counted; they can be put on the stand as they are being counted.
3. Account for all detachable and disassembled parts. These must be counted or accounted for during assembly and once again during disassembly at the end of the case.
4. Recover and retain all pieces of an instrument that breaks during use. A replacement instrument is added to the count sheet.
5. After the initial count is taken, count any instruments added to the table, with one exception. If the circulating nurse decontaminates and sterilizes an instrument that has dropped to the floor or has been passed off the table, an adjustment in the count is unnecessary. Instruments that are recovered from the floor or passed off the table and not sterilized are retained by the circulating nurse and reconciled at the closing count.

Simplifying Instrument Counts

Counting is easier if the number and types of instruments are reduced and if standardized sets are streamlined. Inform the OR manager if unused, unnecessary instruments are routinely included in basic sets. Keep the surgeons' preference cards up-to-date. Instruments peculiar to specific surgical procedures or surgeons can be wrapped separately and added to the basic set only when needed.

Standard count sheets for each basic instrument set will facilitate the counting process. The sheet accompanies the set. The person who prepares the set verifies the initial count as listed. The circulating nurse can check the items as they are counted with the scrub person.

EFFICIENCY OF THE OPERATING ROOM TEAM

A discussion of the duties of the scrub person and the circulating nurse would not be complete without consideration of efficiency, productivity, and work habits. Therefore, efficiency depends primarily on individual effort and the working relationship among team members.

Productivity

Productivity and efficiency go hand in hand. Productivity is directly related to what a person does and how he or she does it. Productivity is also the quantity and quality of work (output) in relation to the costs in terms of labor and time (input). Labor costs can amount to as much as 60% of the OR budget. To be productive, perioperative nurses and surgical technologists should develop their psychomotor skills, competencies, and mental capacities. This requires an accurate perception of the factors and conditions that affect the patient, surgeon, and other team members. The concept of situational awareness means staying in touch with the environment and thinking ahead in preparing for and participating in the surgical procedure. Productivity is enhanced by a person's ability to do the following:

1. Organize work efficiently and effectively. Efficiency is important to minimize the length of time during which a patient is anesthetized and the anxious family is waiting.
2. Work rapidly with precision and dexterity. Learn to follow directions quickly and accurately, and give attention to the smallest detail. Carelessness creates waste and unnecessary hazards for the patient and team.
3. Adapt to changes or unexpected situations quickly, calmly, and efficiently. A change in diagnosis during the surgical procedure may require an altogether different setup and a different surgical approach from the one anticipated. Emergencies will arise. Knowing what to do and why to do it in a particular way decreases the anxiety of rapid performance. Exercise good judgment, and learn to prioritize actions and function competently under pressure.
4. Anticipate the needs of the surgeon and the team, and keep one step ahead. The surgeon becomes distracted if handed the wrong instrument or is made to wait for supplies. Be alert and try to anticipate procedural needs logically.
5. Maintain physical and emotional stamina. Situational awareness can be compromised by fatigue, poor physical health, and emotional distress. Be sensitive to the health and well-being of other team members.

Time and Motion Economy

Time is money; do not waste it. Know the policies and procedures, and follow them efficiently. Learn to do things right the first time, and continue to do them that way; time is wasted in correcting errors. Motions should be productive.

Time Is Costly. Time is an important element in the OR. If time is wasted between surgical procedures, the day's schedule is slowed down and later procedures are delayed. The surgeons' time is wasted, and they then tend to come late because they anticipate delays. The patients and families become anxious during these delays.

Workers with poor time-management skills tend to become less efficient and drift into poor work habits. Common sense is a great ally. Take time to stop and think. Is there a quicker, easier, or more efficient way of doing the job without compromising technique? Most work habits can be improved. Analyze them in a methodic manner.

Recognizing that a problem exists is the first step toward solving that problem. Gather the facts needed to support the desirability of adopting alternatives. Seek to develop more efficient and more economical work methods.

Associations. Each patient, surgeon, and surgical procedure is unique, but all have commonalities. A logical thought process will simplify the necessary OR preparations for the patient and the surgeon. Supplies and equipment must be ready before the procedure can begin.

Association is a great aid to memory and organization of work. With association, the mention of one article brings to mind the others used with it. For instance, the scrub person knows a suture calls for a tissue forceps to the surgeon, a needle holder to the assistant, and then scissors. Watch for and try to establish associations to increase efficiency. Think of the order in which instruments and supplies are going to be needed, and do first things first (e.g., prepare sutures for closing deep tissue layers before preparing sutures for the skin).

To be proficient, know the organization of work and the relative importance of the factors in accomplishing it. If, as the patient is being prepped, the surgeon requests stainless steel retention sutures for closure instead of the usual sutures, the circulating nurse should realize there is plenty of time to get these sutures after the other duties have been completed. Before getting these closing sutures, the circulating nurse must perform the duties necessary to start the surgical procedure; for example, tie the gowns, supervise the draping, adjust the Mayo stand and instrument table, and connect the ESU and suction. When getting these steel sutures, association tells the circulating nurse to also get wire scissors and bumpers or bridges.

Motion Economy. Wasted motion not only is time consuming but also adds to physical fatigue. Fatigue is the result of body movement. Ten principles of motion economy can reduce fatigue from physical activity and improve personal levels of efficiency:

1. Motion should be productive. Once the steps in a procedure are learned, work to increase speed and the psychomotor skill needed to perform them. Make each movement purposeful; avoid rushed or disorganized motions. Work quietly and quickly. Work as fast as possible without sacrificing accuracy and technique for speed.

   The corollary to this principle is a place for everything and everything in its place. Keep an orderly work area to avoid fumbling and rehandling items. If everything has a place and is in its place, supplies are easily obtained by instinct when needed. A neat and orderly work area is one of the first requirements for productive motions. Consider the workflow so that minimal motions can be made to accomplish productive work.
2. Motions should be simple. Body movements should be confined to the lowest classification with which it is possible to perform work properly. Movements of the upper extremity are classified into five levels:
   a. Class 1 involves the fingers. The knuckle provides the pivot for motion for such tasks as fingering through a card file, turning a setscrew on an instrument, and using a pair of scissors.
   b. Class 2 involves both the hand and the fingers. The wrist is the pivot for motion for tasks such as passing instruments, counting sponges, and picking up or writing on an intraoperative record.
   c. Class 3 includes the forearm. The elbow is used as a pivot to open a peel-open package, unfold drapes, and unwrap small supplies. More effort and time are expended in the third and succeeding classifications, because the movements of any one class involve the movements of all classes

preceding it. It takes longer and requires more effort to turn the pages of a procedure book or a patient's chart than to thumb through a file of surgeons' preference cards.

d. Class 4 includes the upper arm. The shoulder pivot is used when opening a door, setting up the Mayo stand, and prepping a patient.

e. Class 5 adds the torso. The trunk bends or stretches to lift a patient, take supplies from a low shelf or drawer, hang an IV bag, or count the sponges in a kick bucket.

Upper extremity work should be arranged to reduce work to the lowest possible classification. Finger motion is the least fatiguing, and shoulder motion is the most fatiguing. The scrub person should be positioned at the operating bed so that elbow, wrist, and finger motions can be used. To prevent prolonged shoulder motion for both of them, he or she should be positioned opposite the surgeon so that both can work with their elbows at their sides.

It is quicker for the circulating nurse to stretch to hang an IV bag than to take time to use finger action to loosen the set screw on an IV pole, lower it with shoulder movement, hang the bag with elbow action, and repeat the sequence in reverse. However, stretching is more fatiguing. Increasing fatigue causes slower motion as the day progresses. Maybe 30 seconds was saved with the first patient of the day, but what happens to the last patient of the day? Time is lost because energy wanes.

3. Motions should be curved. Motions should follow curved rather than straight paths whenever possible. A circular motion to clean the flat surfaces of furniture is less fatiguing than straight push-and-pull strokes.

4. Motions should be symmetric. Motions should be rhythmic and flow smoothly; when possible, both hands should be used symmetrically. Damp cloths in both hands, going in opposing circles, will get flat surfaces cleaned faster and easier.

5. Work should be within grasp range. To avoid changes in body position, all work materials should be arranged so they are within grasp range. Grasp range is within the radius from the pivot point of the elbow or shoulder, either horizontally or vertically. The minimum grasp range is within the radius of the arcs formed with only the forearms extended, using the elbows as pivot points on the horizontal plane (Fig. 25-16). The optimum grasp range is within the area where the left-hand and right-hand arcs overlap. This is the area in which two-handed work, such as putting a needle in a needle holder, can be performed most conveniently. The maximum grasp range is within the arcs formed from the shoulder pivots. The overlapping of these arcs is the maximum extent at which two-handed work can be performed within reach without changing body position.

The Mayo stand should be placed over the operating bed at a height and in a position within

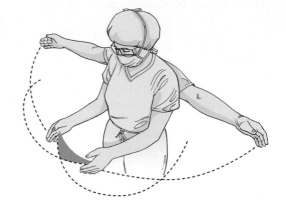

FIG. 25-16 Grasp ranges. Minimum range is within radius of arcs formed with only forearms extended, using elbows as pivotal points. Optimum range is within area where arcs of hands overlap. Maximum range is within the arcs formed from shoulder pivots.

the minimum and optimum grasp range of the scrub person. It must not rest on the patient, but it can be lowered to an inch or two above the patient.

The instrument table should be positioned as close as possible to the horizontal plane within maximum grasp range. Instruments or supplies that require two-handed work should be placed on the Mayo stand and instrument table as close to the optimum grasp range as possible.

6. Hands should be relieved of work. Hands should be relieved of any work that can be performed more advantageously by other parts of the body. Many electrical instruments have foot pedals to facilitate operation.

7. Work materials should be prepositioned. Supplies can be arranged for convenient use and minimal handling. Drapes are packaged in order of use so they do not need to be handled by the scrub person, except to move the stack to a corner of the instrument table, until ready to use. Instruments can be arranged in containers so that all of them do not need to be removed until needed.

Economize time and effort by placing items on the instrument table and Mayo stand in the order in which they will be used, and put them in their proper places without rearranging them. Arrange instruments on the Mayo stand in position to hand to the surgeon or assistant.

In passing an instrument, place it in the surgeon's hand in the position in which it will be used so that readjustments will not be necessary. Grasp the instrument with the thumb and the first two fingers, far enough away from the handle so the surgeon can grasp it. Hand a needle in a needle holder in the same way, supporting the suture so it does not drag; hand it with the needle pointing in the direction in which the surgeon will start to use it. Hand thumb forceps so the surgeon can grasp the handle; do the same with retractors.

8. Gravity should be used. Dispensers for scrub sponges and brushes operate on the principle that

gravity should be used whenever possible. Cabinets for smaller packages in the sterile supply room can be vertical and divided into appropriate-size slots. These cabinets can be filled from the top and dispensed from the bottom of each slot. This method is convenient, saves space, and ensures that older items are used first. Shelves for large, heavy packs can be slanted slightly to facilitate handling. Gravity-feed and drop-delivery installations eliminate or reduce motions. The quickest way to dispose of an object is to drop it. Because this also may be the quickest way to break or contaminate the object, the application of this principle requires good judgment.

9. Supplies should be combined. Items should serve two or more purposes whenever possible. For example, sterilizer chemical indicator tape serves a dual purpose: to hold the package closed and to show if it has been exposed to a sterilization process. And only inches, not a yard, of tape accomplish the job. Disposable kits and trays are purchased, or sets are made up of reusable items so that all the supplies and materials needed for a procedure are combined into a single unit. This eliminates opening many separate packages.

10. The worker should be at ease. Tiring body motions or awkward or strained body postures should be avoided. A pleasant, quiet environment is less fatiguing, has fewer psychologic and physiologic adverse effects on team members, and enhances greater efficiency.

Economical Use of Supplies and Equipment

As the cost of supplies increases, circulating nurses and scrub persons should be conscious of ways in which to eliminate wasteful practices. For example, throw away disposable items only. Avoid throwing away reusable items.

The OR suite is one of the most expensive departments of a hospital. Adequate instruments and supplies are necessary for patient care, and cost is not always the primary consideration. Economy becomes a hazard when exercised beyond the point of safety. Nevertheless, supplies do not need to be used lavishly just because they are available. Remember the principles mentioned in the following sections.

"Just Enough Is Enough." The varieties and numbers of instruments and supplies needed for each surgical procedure can be kept to a minimum. If the procedure book and surgeons' preference cards are kept up-to-date, articles no longer used can be eliminated. Items to "have available" are not opened unnecessarily. The following procedures should be observed:

1. Pour just enough antiseptic solution for the two-step skin preparation according to the manufacturer's recommendation; it takes only a small amount. Do not open a bottle unnecessarily for a small amount if you know the remainder will not be used.
2. Follow the procedures for draping to provide an adequate sterile field without wasting disposable draping material.

3. Do not open another packet of sutures for the last stitch unless absolutely necessary. A few leftover pieces are usually long enough to complete the closure.
4. Suction tubing, syringes, hypodermic needles, drains, catheters, extra drapes, and other such materials are kept sterile and available. Supplies should be opened only as needed—not routinely "just in case" they may be needed.
5. Do not soak too much plaster or fiberglass casting material when helping with cast applications. Keep just ahead of the surgeon. Ask if more is needed before soaking an extra roll.
6. Turn off lights when they are not needed.
7. Separate trash into contaminated and noncontaminated waste. Contaminated waste is processed at a cost per pound.

Use Supplies and Equipment for Intended Use

1. Use operating bed appliances according to the manufacturer's instructions for positioning and stabilizing patients.
2. Use unsterile gloves for unsterile procedures in which the use of gloves is for hand protection. Open sterile gloves for sterile procedures only.
3. Do not use hemostats to clamp drapes or tubing; doing so ruins both the hemostat and the tubing. Use a stopcock or a special tubing clamp for tubes, and use a nonpiercing towel clip to secure drapes.
4. Give the assistant a needle holder for pulling needles through tissue for the surgeon. A hemostat can be ruined by using it for this purpose, and the needle can be damaged.
5. Use wire scissors for cutting wire, tissue scissors for cutting tissue, dressing scissors for cutting drains and dressings, and suture scissors for cutting sutures.

Avoid Damage. Handle all supplies and equipment carefully to avoid damage and breakage:

1. Slip off the patient's gown sleeve before the preoperative IV infusion is started. This prevents having to cut off a wet, soiled gown at the completion of the surgical procedure.
2. Rotate sterile and older supplies to prevent items from deteriorating or the integrity of packaging from being compromised.
3. Take special care to preserve the edges of sharp instruments.
4. Follow established procedures for the proper sterilization and care of instruments, electrical equipment, and other materials. If uncertain how to sterilize or care for any equipment, find out; do not ruin items by guessing. Items for gas sterilization should be tagged "for gas" or "heat sensitive" to help prevent the possibility of inadvertent steam sterilization. Moisture-sensitive items like surgical cameras should be labeled as such.
5. Check drapes to be certain that instruments are not discarded in disposable drapes or sent to the laundry. At the end of the surgical procedure, the scrub person should look for instruments, needles, and equipment before discarding drapes. This is part of the inventory control reason for counting instruments.

6. If an instrument or piece of equipment is defective, immediately remove it from use. Tag the device with a description of the problem, and report the malfunction promptly for corrective action. In addition, report a surgeon's complaints about the function or quality of an instrument or equipment.
8. Adhere to the routine preventive maintenance schedule for equipment.

Bibliography

AORN (Association of periOperative Registered Nurses): *AORN standards, recommended practices, and guidelines,* Denver, 2006, The Association.

Barrow CJ: Use of x-ray in the presence of an incorrect needle count, *AORN J* 74(1):80-81, 2001.

Beyea SC: The ideal state for perioperative nursing, *AORN J* 73(5):897-901, 2001.

Clark SG, Slavik NS: Surgical instrument loss control, *SSM* 7(5):12-14, 2001.

Heffernan JP et al: Gossypiboma and recurrent bladder neck contracture after retropubic prostatectomy and bilateral pelvic lymph node dissection, *J Urol* 157(4):1356-1357, 1997.

Matson K: The critical "nurse" in the circulating nurse role, *AORN J* 73(5):971-975, 2001.

Patterson P: How ORs decide when to count instruments, *OR Manager* 16(4):11-14, 2000.

Pezzella AT: Hand signals in surgery, *AORN J* 63(4):769-771, 1996.

Reeder JM: Being there: Supporting health professionals involved in medical errors, *SSM* 7(5):40-41, 43-44, 2001.

Voss SJ: Creating a safety culture, *SSM* 7(5):6, 8-9, 2001.

Wanzer LJ, Dunlap KD: Medical errors, *SSM* 7(5):17-22, 24-27, 2001.

Chapter 26

Positioning, Prepping, and Draping the Patient

CHAPTER OBJECTIVES

After studying this chapter, the learner will be able to:
- Identify the safety hazards associated with moving a patient from one surface to another.
- List the anatomic considerations for positioning.
- Describe the effects of positioning on the patient's body systems.
- Identify key elements of preoperative skin preparation of patients.
- Discuss the implications of chemical and mechanical actions of prepping the patient.
- Describe how a patient is draped using sterile technique.

CHAPTER OUTLINE

KEY TERMS AND DEFINITIONS

Abduct   Move away from the body.
Adduct   Move toward the body.
Anterior   In front of.
Antiseptic solution   Topical cleansing chemical used to decrease the microbial count on the skin surface.

Body habitus   Generalized physiologic configuration of the patient's size, weight, and shape.
Caudad   Toward the foot of the patient.
Cephalad   Toward the head of the patient.
Circumduct   Rotate a joint in a circumferential axis (usually a ball joint).
Circumferential   The surface area of the patient's skin that encompasses a limb or other rounded tissue area.
Deep   Below the surface layers.
Distal   Away from the core.
Dorsal   Back of a part.
Extend   Flatten a joint (zero-degree flexion).
Flexion   Bend at a normal joint, close the angle of the joint.
Hyperabduction   Move away from the body in a line more than a safe 90-degree angle.
Hyperadduction   Move toward the body and crossing over the neutral plane of the body.
Hyperextend   Move beyond the normal flattening of a joint axis.
Inferior   Below or beneath.
Lateral   Toward the side of the patient.
Medial   Toward the midline.
Posterior   Behind.
Prone   Face down.
Proximal   Closer to the core.
Reverse Trendelenburg's position   Head-elevated position.
Superficial   On the surface.
Superior   Above.
Supine   Face up.
Trendelenburg's position   Head-down position.
Ventral   Front surface.

SUPPLEMENTAL MATERIAL ON EVOLVE WEBSITE   *evolve*

http://evolve.elsevier.com/BerryKohn
- Content Updates
- Glossary
- Full Set of Perioperative Flash Cards
- Interactive Key Term Flash Cards
- Student Activities
- WebLinks

HISTORICAL BACKGROUND

The surgical team of the early 1900s was very resourceful. Planning patient care did not always involve the use of hospital equipment in an established facility. The surgical nurse had to know how to convert a living room, dining room, or kitchen into an operating room (OR) at a moment's notice. This included providing for patient positioning and preparing draping materials. Many of these materials were personally sewn by the nurse and brought into the patient's home.

The historical methods of patient positioning were not standardized for safety or comfort. Surgical procedures were commonly performed with the patient in a seated position and with people in the room holding him or her down. This method of restraint was common because anesthetics were not always available. Lithographs depict patients lying on unpadded tables, such as those used for meals. Chairs turned upside down were used as backrest for the patient, and the foot of the table was placed up on blocks to facilitate the Trendelenburg's position. Some drawings illustrate dogs at the surgeons' feet.

Skin preparation was important as a means of preventing infection. Potash soap was used to soften the keratin layers and hair on the surface of the skin, and a razor was used to scrape away the softened material. In hard-to-cleanse areas, a poultice was placed 3 hours preoperatively to macerate the skin and make removal of the top layers easier. In the operating room, the area was wiped down with 1:5000 solution of bichloride of mercury to complete the antiseptic skin-cleansing process. Areas of mucous membrane, such as the vagina or rectum, were cleansed with potash soap and hot water followed by alcohol or hydrogen peroxide rinse. All perineal hair was removed by shaving. The urinary meatus was cleansed with alcohol or bichloride of mercury 1:1000 before placing a urinary catheter. Bichloride of mercury was found to be absorbed through the skin and was replaced in 1914 by iodine preparations.

PRELIMINARY CONSIDERATIONS

Positioning for a surgical procedure is important to the patient's outcome. Proper positioning facilitates preoperative skin preparation and appropriate draping with sterile drapes. Positioning requires a detailed knowledge of anatomy and physiologic principles, as well as familiarity with the necessary equipment. Safety is a prime consideration.

Patient position and prep are determined by the procedure to be performed, with consideration given to the surgeon's choice of surgical approach and the technique of anesthetic administration. Factors such as age, height, weight, cardiopulmonary status, and preexisting disease condition (e.g., arthritis, allergies) also should be incorporated into the plan of care. Preoperatively, the patient should be assessed for alterations in skin integrity, for joint mobility, and for the presence of joint or vascular prostheses. The expected outcome is that the patient will not be harmed by positioning, prepping, or draping for the surgical procedure.

Efficiency of the patient preparation process can be attained by organizing activities in a logical sequence. Table 26-1 illustrates how to coordinate and organize patient preparation activities.

The main objectives for any surgical or procedural positioning are as follows:
- Optimize surgical-site exposure for the surgeon.
- Minimize the risk for adverse physiologic effects.
- Facilitate physiologic monitoring by the anesthesia provider.
- Promote safety and security for the patient.

Responsibility for Patient Positioning

The selection of the surgical position is made by the surgeon in consultation with the anesthesia provider. Adjustments are made as necessary for the administration and monitoring of anesthetic and for maintenance of the patient's physiologic status. The circulating nurse or first assistant may be responsible for placing the patient in a surgical position, with guidance from the anesthesia provider and the surgeon. In essence, patient positioning is a shared responsibility among all team members. The anesthesia provider has the final word on positioning when the patient's physiologic status and monitoring are in question.

In cases of complex positioning or positioning patients who are obese, the plan of care includes the need for additional help in lifting and/or positioning. Special devices or positioning aids may be necessary. The weight tolerance of the mechanism and balance of the operating bed should be considered. The manufacturer's recommendations should be consulted for guidance in selecting the appropriate bed. To avoid questions or confusion, the weight tolerance should be clearly labeled on every operating bed.

Timing of Patient Positioning and Anesthetic Administration

Moving the patient from the transport stretcher to the operating bed or vice versa requires that both surfaces are securely locked and stable. Someone should be stationed on the far side of the receiving surface to prevent the patient from tumbling off the edge. For any patient under the influence of an anesthetic agent or narcotic medication, personnel should be at the head, foot, and both sides of the patient to prevent dependent parts from sliding off the table. The neck of the patient's gown should be untied to prevent entanglement and choking as the patient moves or is moved from one surface to another.

After transfer from the transport stretcher to the operating bed, the patient is usually supine (face up on his or her back; a few exceptions apply and will be explained later in this chapter). Privacy is maintained by a warm cotton blanket, and the thigh strap is positioned in clear sight of the entire team. The patient may be anesthetized in a supine position and then repositioned for the surgical procedure. Some patients are positioned and then anesthetized if their physiologic status requires special care. If the patient is having a procedure performed while in a prone position and under general anesthesia, he or she is anesthetized and intubated on the transport stretcher. A minimum of four people is required to place the patient safely in the prone position on the operating bed. Commonly, more personnel are required for a safe transfer between surfaces when the patient is fully under anesthesia.

Text continued on p. 497

TABLE 26-1   Planning the Organization of Patient Positioning, Prepping, and Draping

Type of Procedure	Positioning	Catheterization	Prep Sequence	Drape Tips
ABDOMINAL Anterior chest, epigastrium, umbilicus, pelvis Laparoscopy	Supine with arms tucked at sides or secured on armboards. Thigh strap is secured. Legs remain flat. Small pillow under knees to take pressure off lower back. Trendelenburg's position can increase intraocular and intracranial pressure. Blood pressure and cardiac output decrease. Reverse Trendelenburg's position decreases intracranial pressure. Place padded footboard on lower bed segment to support feet. Lateral tilt can be used to elevate the surgical site.	Catheter is placed before the abdomen is cleansed. The urinary drainage bag is placed in view of the anesthesia provider. Female is frog-legged for the catheterization procedure. Support legs to prevent extreme external rotation. Complex patients may require ureteral catheters placed preoperatively. This utilizes a cystoscopy setup, two ureteral catheters, and a ureteral catheter drainage bag.	Hair is removed during the prep process as desired by the surgeon. Umbilicus is cleansed in sequence as preferred by the surgeon. Urinary meatus is prepped as part of the catheterization process. Abdominal cleansing begins at surgical site and proceeds to the periphery in a circular motion. Avoid pooling of prep solutions under the patient. Thigh strap is secured after the prep. Before draping, be sure that leg strap is placed over a blanket so it is visible to entire team.	The dispersive electrode for electrosurgical unit is placed when patient is in the final resting position for the procedure. Do not cut or reposition the electrode. Some surgeons like the surgical site squared off with towels. Some surgeons prefer medium sheets placed above and below the abdominal incision before placing a fenestrated sheet. Some surgeons prefer a clear or impregnated incise sheet. Fenestrated laparotomy sheet is positioned over the surgical site. Additional drapes may be needed to cover the armboards if the laparotomy sheet does not have arm flaps.
Combined abdominal and perineal Abdominal, epigastrium, pelvis Laparoscopy Genitourinary	Patient is anesthetized in the supine position unless epidural or spinal is used. Thigh strap is secured during induction. Lithotomy with arms tucked at sides or secured on armboards. Take care not to crush digits in table break. No strap on abdomen. Stirrups should be padded, and the legs should be elevated and lowered simultaneously. Legs are secured in stirrups with straps. Pulses should be checked after placement in the stirrups (e.g., popliteal, posterior tibial, dorsalis pedis). Sequential compression devices should remain functional and tubing unobstructed. Lithotomy position increases autotransfusion from legs. Lowering the legs decreases blood pressure.	Foley catheter is placed before the abdomen is cleansed. The drain bag is placed in view of the anesthesia provider. Rectal irrigation for colon procedures (if necessary) is performed after the catheterization and before the perineal cleansing prep. An impervious, nonsterile, under buttocks drape should be used to deflect runoff prep solution into a kick bucket. Complex patients may require ureteral catheters placed preoperatively. This utilizes a cystoscopy setup, two ureteral catheters, and a ureteral catheter drainage bag.	Urinary meatus is prepped as part of the catheterization process. Hair is removed during the prep process as desired by the surgeon. Perineum is prepped first, including the vagina, followed by the rectum. Abdominal cleansing begins at surgical site and proceeds to the periphery in a circular motion. Thigh strap is secured after the prep. Before draping, be sure that leg strap is placed over a blanket so it is visible to entire team.	The dispersive electrode for electrosurgical unit is placed when patient is in the final resting position for the procedure. Do not cut or reposition the electrode. Under buttocks, sterile drape is placed first, followed by leggings. Some surgeons like the surgical site squared off with towels. Some surgeons prefer a clear or impregnated incise sheet. Fenestrated laparotomy sheet is positioned over the surgical site. Additional drapes may be needed to cover the armboards if the laparotomy sheet does not have arm flaps. Some surgeons request a sterile drape over the exposed perineum until that portion of the procedure is started. Laparoscopic procedures may require perineal access during the abdominal phase of surgery.

Position/Procedure	Positioning	Catheterization	Prep	Draping
LATERAL Thorax, kidney, hip	Patient is anesthetized in the supine position unless epidural or spinal is used. Thigh strap is secured during induction. Patient is positioned on the side after the catheter is placed. Padded beanbag vacuum positioning devices may be used. Legs are slightly flexed with pillow between knees. Lower leg is flexed more for stability. Axillary roll is placed under lower axilla. Arms are supported on armboards perpendicular to body. Use wide body strap over the hip and narrow belt loosely over lower leg. Some surgeons prefer to use wide adhesive tape secured to the bed. Table may be flexed to elevate the surgical site.	Catheterization is performed in the supine position. Catheter is placed before the patient is positioned and before the surgical site is cleansed. The drain bag is placed in view of the anesthesia provider. Female is frog-legged for the catheterization procedure. Complex patients may require ureteral catheters placed preoperatively. This utilizes a cystoscopy setup, two ureteral catheters, and a ureteral catheter drainage bag.	Hair is removed during the prep process as desired by the surgeon. Cleansing begins at surgical site and proceeds to the periphery in a circular motion.	The dispersive electrode for electrosurgical unit is placed when patient is in the final resting position for the procedure. Do not cut or reposition the electrode. Some surgeons like the surgical site squared off with towels. Some surgeons prefer a clear or impregnated incise sheet. Fenestrated laparotomy sheet is positioned over the surgical site.
EXTREMITY Shoulder, arm, wrist, leg, foot	*Upper:* Elbow and distal to elbow may require a hand table attachment as a work surface. Sterile or nonsterile tourniquet may be placed. Shoulder procedures may require the patient to be in a supine posture. *Lower:* *Supine:* Special orthopedic table may be used with support for unaffected limb and traction for affected limb. *Lateral:* Standard operating bed can be used.	Some patients with lower extremity fractures or joint replacements may require a Foley catheter. Placement of the Foley catheter may require additional help in holding the female's legs in position. Frog-legging is not advised with lower extremity fractures. Procedures lasting longer than 2 hours may require a urinary catheter to monitor intake and output.	Extremity is suspended above the surface of the operating bed. Hair is removed as desired by physician. Prep will be circumferential. Prevent backflow of prep solution from clean to dirty. Prep from incision to periphery.	The dispersive electrode for electrosurgical unit is placed when patient is in the final resting position for the procedure. Do not cut or reposition the electrode. Do not place electrode on affected leg. Some surgeons like a sterile stockinette placed over the freshly prepped extremity. When a nonsterile tourniquet is used, a plastic impervious drape is placed around the distal aspect of the cuff to protect from prep solution. U-drapes and split sheets are commonly used to isolate the surgical site from the nonaffected areas.
SITTING Cranial, neck, ear, anterior face, throat, posterior cervical area Abdominoplasty	Patient is anesthetized in the supine position unless epidural or spinal is used. Thigh strap is secured during induction. *Many seated variations:*	Foley catheter is placed with the patient supine before placement into a seated position. Take care not to allow the catheter to kink when repositioning the patient.	Hair is removed during the prep process as desired by the surgeon. Patient may want long head hair saved in a plastic bag for personal reasons. Always do this for pediatric patients and their parents.	The dispersive electrode for electrosurgical unit is placed when patient is in the final resting position for the procedure. Do not cut or reposition the electrode. Cranial procedures employ a fenestrated sheet with round aperture. Disposable sheets commonly have an incise sheet built in.

Continued

TABLE 26-1	Planning the Organization of Patient Positioning, Prepping, and Draping—cont'd			
Type of Procedure	Positioning	Catheterization	Prep Sequence	Drape Tips
	Operating bed is in semi- or high Fowler's position, with the back of the bed elevated between 10 and 45 degrees. Leg break is slightly 5 to 10 degrees flexed to prevent the patient from sliding down. *Sequential* compression devices should remain functional and tubing unobstructed to decrease venous pooling in legs. A bed pillow is placed over the patient's midsection (or over bed table); the arms are placed over the tap. Safety strap is placed lightly but securely over the thighs. Footboard may be used to maintain position of feet at right angles to legs. Intracranial pressure is decreased in the seated position. Abdominal closure for abdominoplasty is facilitated by the flexed body position.	Drainage bag should be placed in clear view of anesthesia provider.	Cleansing begins at surgical site and proceeds to the periphery in a circular motion. Take extreme care not to get prep solution into eyes, nose, mouth, or ears. Clear plastic dressing materials can be placed over the facial orifices of the patient under general anesthesia to prevent exposure. Some surgeons prefer cotton balls placed in the patient's ears.	Most have an inferior drainage pouch to catch runoff irrigation. Facial and anterior neck procedures require wrapping the head in a towel drape to isolate scalp hair from the field. Full sheets or split sheets can be used to cover the body.
PRONE Rectal spinal, posterior thorax, cervical	Patient is anesthetized in the supine position on the transport cart unless epidural or spinal is used. Thigh strap is secured on posterior aspect of calves to prevent leg flexion. Chest rolls or frame prevent constriction of chest and abdomen.	Foley catheter is placed with the patient supine before placement into the prone position. Drainage bag is placed in the view of the anesthesia provider.	Hair is removed during the prep process as desired by the surgeon. Cleansing begins at surgical site and proceeds to the periphery in a circular motion.	Some surgeons like the surgical site squared off with towels. Some surgeons prefer a clear or impregnated incise sheet. Fenestrated laparotomy sheet is positioned over the surgical site. Additional drapes may be needed to cover the armboards if the laparotomy sheet does not have arm flaps.
Modified spinal procedure prone/kneeling	Protect genitalia and breasts from compression and shearing force. Gel pads under knees and dorsum of foot to protect the toes. Some special kneeling spinal tables have fabric boots that are fastened around the patient's feet. Kneeling tables have padded positioner boards that rest against the patient's buttocks for stabilization.			

Several factors influence the time at which the patient is positioned: the site of the surgical procedure; the age and size of the patient; the technique of anesthetic administration; and if the patient is conscious, pain on moving. The patient is not moved, positioned, or prepped until the anesthesia provider indicates it is safe to do so.

Preparations for Positioning

Before the patient is brought into the OR, the circulating nurse should do the following:

1. Review the proposed position by referring to the procedure book and the surgeon's preference card in comparison with the scheduled procedure.
2. Ask the surgeon for assistance if unsure how to position the patient.
3. The circulating nurse will assess for any patient-specific positioning needs.
4. Check the working parts of the operating bed before bringing the patient into the room.
5. Assemble and test all table attachments and protective pads anticipated for the surgical procedure and have them immediately available for use at the bedside. Box 26-1 lists areas that may need specific attention during padding.
6. Review the plan of care for unique needs of the patient.

Safety Measures

Safety measures, including the following, are observed while transferring, moving, and positioning patients:

1. The patient is properly identified before being transferred to the operating bed, and the surgical site is affirmed according to facility policy. This may require some form of initialing the site or marking with a specific symbol. Some facilities require the surgeon to label the correct site.
2. The patient is assessed for mobility status. This includes determination of the patient's ability to transfer between the transport stretcher and the operating bed. Do not plan to have the patient move his or her self toward an affected limb or toward the blinded eye.
3. The operating bed and transport vehicle are securely locked in position, with the mattress stabilized during transfer to and from the operating bed. Velcro strips or other means should be employed to maintain the stability of the mattresses of the two surfaces.
4. Two people should assist an awake patient with the transfer by positioning themselves on each side of the patient's transfer path. The person on the side of the transport stretcher assists the patient in moving toward the operating bed. The person on the opposite side prevents the patient from falling over the edge of the operating bed. Untie the ties of the patient's gown, and take care not to allow the patient's gown or blanket to become lodged between the two surfaces or under the bottom of a moving patient. Maintain the patient's dignity at all times.
5. Adequate assistance in lifting unconscious, anesthetized, obese, or weak patients is necessary to prevent injury. A minimum of four people is recommended, and transfer devices and lifters may be used. The patient is moved on the count of three, with the anesthesia provider giving the signal. Sliding or pulling the patient may cause dermal abrasion or injury to soft tissues. Dependent limbs can cause a counterbalance and cause the patient to fall to the floor. Examination gloves should be worn if the patient is incontinent or offers other risk of exposure to blood and body substances.
6. The anesthesia provider guards the head of the anesthetized patient at all times and supports it during movement. The head should be kept in a neutral axis and turned as little as possible to maintain the airway and cerebral circulation.
7. The physician assumes responsibility for protecting an unsplinted fracture during movement.
8. The anesthetized patient is not moved without permission of the anesthesia provider.
9. The anesthetized patient is moved slowly and gently to allow the circulatory system to adjust and to control the body during movement.
10. No body part should extend beyond the edges of the operating bed or contact metal parts or unpadded surfaces.
11. Body exposure should be minimal to prevent hypothermia and preserve dignity.
12. Movement and positioning should not obstruct or dislodge catheters, intravenous (IV) infusion tubing, oxygen cannulas, and monitors.
13. The armboard is protected to avoid hyperextending the arm or dislodging the IV cannula. The surface of the armboard pad and the mattress of the operating bed should be of equal height. Hyperabduction is avoided to prevent brachial plexus stretch.
14. When the patient is supine (on the back), the ankles and legs must not be crossed. Crossing the ankles and legs creates occlusive pressure on blood vessels and nerves, and pressure necrosis may occur. The patient would be at risk for deep vein thrombosis (DVT).

BOX 26-1	**Body Areas That Need Padding During Positioning**

SUPINE POSITION
Occiput
Heels
Elbows
Sacrum

PRONE OR OTHER "FACE DOWN" POSITION
Anterior knees of kneeling patient
Face (particularly the forehead) and ears
Dorsum of foot to protect toes
Genitalia and breasts

LATERAL POSITION
Face and ears
Medial knees
Axilla
Ankles and feet
Arms

15. When the patient is prone (on the abdomen), the thorax is relieved of pressure by using chest rolls (subclavicle to iliac crest) to facilitate chest expansion with respiration. The chest rolls should be adequately secured to the table to prevent shifting. The abdomen should remain dependent to decrease abdominal venous pressure. Padding should be placed at the dorsum of the feet to prevent pressure on the toes. In the event of cardiac arrest, a transport cart should be available for immediate emergency repositioning into the supine position and subsequent resuscitation.

16. When the patient is positioned lateral (on the side), a pillow is placed lengthwise between the legs to prevent pressure on bony prominences, blood vessels, and nerves. This also relieves pressure on the superior hip.

17. During articulation of the operating bed, the patient is protected from crush injury at the flex points of the operating bed.

18. When the operating bed is elevated, the patient's feet and protuberant parts are protected from compression by overbed tables, Mayo stands, and frames. An adequate clearance of 2 to 3 inches is maintained.

19. Surfaces should not create pressure on any body part. Alternating or pressure-relieving surfaces should be used. Rolled blankets and towels can create pressure because they do not allow for relief of compression at the contact surface. A gel pad or other alternating pressure pad should be used. Figure 26-1 depicts the tissue layers as they are compressed against a bony prominence.

ANATOMIC AND PHYSIOLOGIC CONSIDERATIONS

A patient's tolerance of the stresses of the surgical procedure depends greatly on normal functioning of the vital systems. The patient's physical condition is considered, and proper body alignment is important. Criteria are met for physiologic positioning to prevent injury from pressure, crushing, pinching, obstruction, or stretching. Each body system is considered when planning the patient's position for the surgical procedure. Complications of positioning are listed in Box 26-2.

Respiratory Considerations

Unhindered diaphragmatic movement and a patent airway are essential for maintaining respiratory function, preventing hypoxia, and facilitating induction by inhalation. Chest excursion is a concern because inspiration expands the chest anteriorly. Some positions limit the amount of mechanical excursion of the chest. Some hypoxia is always present in a horizontal position because the anteroposterior diameter of the ribcage and abdomen decreases. The tidal volume, the functional residual capacity of air moved by a single breath, is reduced by as much as one third when a patient lies down, because the diaphragm shifts cephalad. Therefore, there should be no constriction around the neck or chest.

The patient's arms should be at his or her side, on armboards, or otherwise supported—not crossed on the chest unless this is absolutely necessary for the procedure. Patients have additional respiratory compromise if they are obese, smoke, or have pulmonary disease.

Circulatory Considerations

Adequate arterial circulation is necessary for maintaining blood pressure, perfusing tissues with oxygen, facilitating venous return, and preventing thrombus formation. Occlusion and pressure on the peripheral blood vessels are avoided. Body support and restraining straps must not be fastened too tightly. Anesthetic agents alter normal body circulatory mechanisms, such as blood pressure. Some drugs cause constriction or dilation of the blood vessels, which is further complicated by positioning.

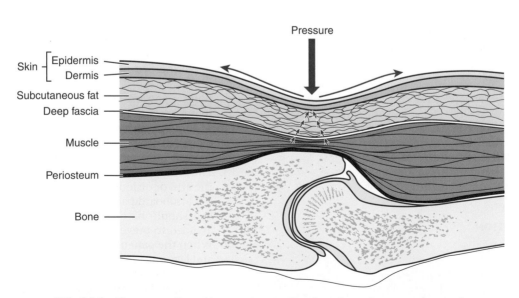

FIG. 26-1   Tissues are affected by pressure, causing deep tissue damage and necrosis.

BOX 26-2	Complications Caused by Positioning

Hemodynamic instability by orthostatic position
Poor ventilation by thoracic compression
Peripheral nerve injury caused by compression or stretch
Tissue damage from crush or shearing force
Ischemia of hair-bearing scalp, causing bald spots
Compartment syndrome
Pressure necrosis
Digit amputation in table bends
Blindness from optic nerve ischemia
Corneal abrasion
Ischemic limbs from arterial occlusion
Venous emboli
Vertebral injury
Panic attacks and feelings of claustrophobia in awake patient

Peripheral Nerve Considerations

Prolonged pressure on or stretching of the peripheral nerves can result in injuries that range from sensory and motor loss to paralysis and wasting. The extremities, as well as the body, should be well supported at all times. The most common sites of injury are the divisions of the brachial plexus and the ulnar, radial, peroneal, and facial nerves; the axons may be stretched or disrupted. Extremes of position of the head and arm greater than 90 degrees can easily injure the brachial plexus. If the patient is improperly positioned, the ulnar, radial, and peroneal nerves may be compressed against bone, stirrups, or the operating bed.

Arthroscopy leg holders and tourniquets can cause crushed or transected nerve injury. Femoral nerve injury can be caused by retractors during pelvic procedures. Sciatic nerve injury may be caused by tissue retraction or manipulation during hip surgery or extremes of lithotomy position. Facial nerve injury may result from a head strap that is too tight or from manually elevating the mandible too vigorously to maintain the airway.

Musculoskeletal Considerations

A strain on muscle groups results in injury and/or needless postoperative discomfort. An anesthetized patient lacks protective muscle tone. If the head is extended for a prolonged time, the patient may suffer more pain from the resulting stiff neck than from the surgical wound. Care is taken not to hyperextend a joint, which not only causes postoperative pain but also may contribute to permanent injury to an extremity. Elderly or debilitated patients with osteoporosis or other bone disease may suffer fractures.

When turning a patient, always keep the spine in alignment by grasping the shoulder girdle and hip in a logrolling fashion. Do not turn or elevate a patient by grasping only a hip and twisting the spine. Proper body alignment is maintained.

Soft Tissue Considerations

Body weight is distributed unevenly when the patient lies on the operating bed. Weight that is concentrated over bony prominences can cause skin pressure ulcers and deep tissue injury. These areas should be protected from constant external pressure against hard surfaces, particularly in patients who are thin or underweight. In addition, tissue that is subjected to prolonged mechanical pressure (e.g., a fold in the skin under an obese or malnourished patient) will not be adequately perfused. Wrinkled sheets and the edges of a positioning or other device under the patient can cause pressure on the skin. Foam pads are not adequate to relieve pressure, because they compress and do not alternate pressure. Towels and sheet rolls do not relieve pressure because they are unyielding to the patient's body weight. Gel pads are preferred. According to the *AORN Standards, Recommended Practices, and Guidelines* (2006), positioning devices should maintain normal capillary interface pressure of 23 to 32 mm Hg or less to prevent pressure injuries. Blood flow and tissue perfusion are restricted at higher pressures.

Pressure injuries are more common after surgical procedures that last 1 hour or longer. During lengthy procedures, the head and other body parts should be repositioned if possible. Patients who are debilitated, poorly nourished, and diabetic are at particularly high risk for pressure ulcers and alopecia (permanent bald spots from pressure).

Accessibility of the Surgical Site

The surgical procedure and patient condition determine the position in which the patient is placed. To minimize trauma and operating time, the surgeon must have adequate exposure of the surgical site.

Accessibility for Anesthetic Administration

The anesthesia provider should be able to attach monitoring electrodes, administer the anesthetic and observe its effects, and maintain IV access. The patient's airway is of prime concern and must be patent and accessible at all times. The anesthesia provider needs to assess urinary output, blood loss, and irrigation use at all times. Consideration for visibility of measuring devices and drainage bags should be incorporated in the plan for positioning.

Individual Positioning Considerations

If a patient is extremely obese (e.g., the torso occupies the width of the operating bed), his or her arms may be placed on armboards. Heavy-duty operating beds are available with side extenders to accommodate wide patients. Patients with arthritis or previous joint surgery may need special individualized care because of limited range of motion in their joints. A patient who has cardiac problems or is obese may experience orthopnea or dyspnea when lying flat.

Pediatric patients, especially infants, require less operating bed length. Some surgeons like the foot portion of the bed lowered to decrease the length of the working surface for accessibility.

EQUIPMENT FOR POSITIONING
Operating Bed

Many different operating beds with suitable attachments are available, and practice is necessary to master the adjustments. Operating beds are versatile and adaptable to a number of diversified positions for many surgical specialties; orthopedic, urologic, and fluoroscopic tables are often used for specialized procedures. Figure 26-2 depicts a typical

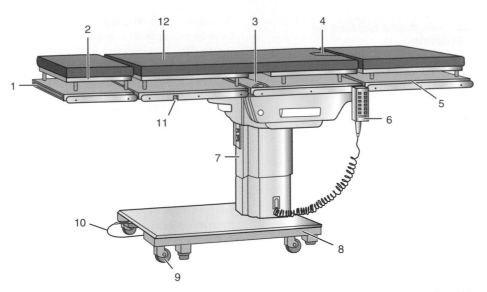

FIG. 26-2 General-purpose operating bed. *1,* Movable head section; *2,* x-ray cassette tunnel; *3,* kidney elevation bar; *4,* perineal cutout; *5,* lower extremity section; *6,* control box; *7,* pedestal; *8,* base; *9,* casters; *10,* power cord; *11,* side rails; *12,* pads.

general-purpose operating bed. The patient's body habitus may require the use of a specialty operating bed with an increased weight limit. The manufacturer's recommendations should be consulted for the operation of each model of operating bed.

Most operating beds consist of a rectangular metal top measuring 79 to 89 inches long by 20 to 24 inches wide (201 to 225 cm × 51 to 61 cm) that rests on an electric or hydraulic lift base. Some models have interchangeable radiopaque tops for various specialties. The surface of the operating bed is divided into three or more hinged sections: the head, the body, and the leg sections. The joints of the operating bed are referred to as breaks. Each hinged section can be manipulated, flexed, or extended to the desired position in a procedure called "breaking the operating bed." Figure 26-3 shows the range of flexibility of an average general-purpose operating bed.

Some operating beds have a metal body elevator plate between the two upper sections that may be raised up to 5½ inches (14 cm) to elevate an area for a gallbladder or kidney procedure. Care is taken when using this elevator because this can decrease the ability of the chest to expand during ventilation. The head section is removable, which permits the insertion of special headrests for cranial procedures. An extension may be inserted at the foot of the operating bed to accommodate an exceptionally tall patient. A radiopaque cassette loading top extends the length of the bed and permits the insertion of a radiograph cassette holder at any area. A self-adhering, sectional, conductive rubber mattress (at least 3 inches [8 cm] thick) covers the surface of the operating bed. Gel-filled alternating surface mattress and pads are commercially available to cover the surface of the operating bed.

Standard operating beds have controls for manipulation into desired positions. Some beds are electrically controlled by either remote hand- or foot-control switches or a lever-operated electrohydraulic system; older operating beds are controlled with manual hand cranks. Most electric styles have a rechargeable battery that can be used for several weeks without recharging. The desired section(s) of the operating bed surface can be articulated by setting the selector control on "back," "side," "foot," or "flex." By activating other selector controls, the surface of the operating bed may be tilted laterally up to 28 degrees from side to side and raised or lowered in its entirety. A tiltometer indicates the degree of tilt between horizontal and vertical for variations in Trendelenburg's position. Most styles offer between 30 and 40 degrees of Trendelenburg's position full-table tilt down or up. All operating beds have a brake or floor lock for stabilization in all positions.

Special Equipment and Bed Attachments

The equipment used in positioning is designed to stabilize the patient in the desired position and thus permit optimal exposure of the surgical site. All devices are clean, free of sharp edges, and padded to prevent trauma or abrasion. Each operating bed has attachments for specific purposes. Many positioning devices to protect pressure points and joints are commercially available. If they are reusable, they are washable; some may be terminally sterilized for asepsis between uses.

Safety Belt (Thigh Strap). To restrain leg movement during surgical procedures, a sturdy, wide strap of durable material (e.g., nylon webbing, conductive rubber) is placed and fastened over the thighs, above the knees, and around the surface of the operating bed. Placement in this location prevents the large muscle groups of the legs from flexing and causing the patient to fall from the operating bed. Some straps are attached at each side of the bed and fastened together at the center. This belt should be secure but not so tight that it impairs circulation; the circulating nurse should be able to pass two fingers between the strap and the patient. Placement of the belt depends on body position. To prevent

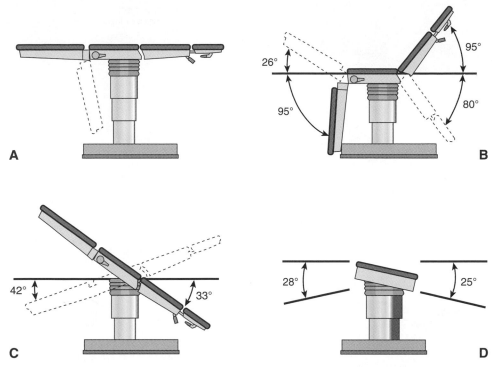

FIG. 26-3   Flexibility range of general-purpose operating bed. **A,** Lower extremity section lowered. **B,** Range of positions for raised and lowered body and lower extremity sections. **C,** Trendelenburg's position and reverse Trendelenburg's position. **D,** Lateral tilt.

injury to underlying tissue, padding (e.g., a blanket) should be placed between the skin and the belt. The strap should be placed over, not under, this blanket for easy visualization before prepping and draping.

The safety belt is used during surgical procedures except for certain positions (e.g., lithotomy and seated). Belting across the patient's abdomen during the lithotomy position can cause compression of the abdominal structures. The safety belt is used before and after the procedure, when the patient's legs are in the down position.

Anesthesia Screen. A metal bar attaches to the head of the operating bed and holds the drapes from the patient's face. It is placed after the induction of anesthesia and the positioning of the patient and is used to separate the nonsterile from the sterile area at the head of the bed. The bar is adjustable and allows rotation or angling. Some facilities use two IV poles to secure the drapes at the head of the bed. Special procedures may require the use of an overbed table that mounts in the same fashion as an anesthesia screen. The socket attachments are secured to the side rail of the bed and are locked onto the frame of this table (Fig. 26-4).

Lift Sheet (Drawsheet). A double-layer sheet is placed horizontally across the top of a clean sheet on the operating bed. After the patient is transferred to the operating bed, his or her arms are enclosed in the lower flaps of this sheet, with the palms against the sides in a natural position and the fingers extended along the length of the body. The upper flaps are brought down over the arms and tucked under the patient's sides. The sheet should not be tucked under the

sides of the mattress, because the combined weight of the mattress and the patient's torso may impair circulation or cause nerve torsion. The full length of each arm is supported at the patient's side, protected from injury, and secured. In addition, a plastic, curved shield, referred to as a sled, can be used to protect and secure the arms from injury (Fig. 26-5). Tucking the patient's arms helps to prevent inadvertent pressure from upright bars of anesthesia screens, table attachments, or stationary retractor poles (Fig. 26-6).

The patient should be told that these methods are used to support the arms when he or she is anesthetized and relaxed. The word *restraint* is avoided. At the end of the surgical procedure, this sheet—if not soiled or wet—may be used to lift the patient from the operating bed.

Armboard. Armboard(s) are used to support the arm(s) if IV fluids are being infused, if the arm or hand is the site of the surgical procedure, if the arm at the side would interfere

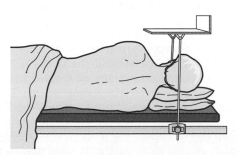

FIG. 26-4   Overbed table attachment.

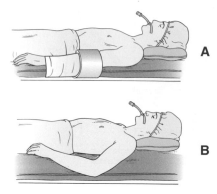

FIG. 26-5 The patient's arms can be placed at the sides with the lift sheet pulled over the length of the arm and tucked under the patient's body. **A,** Correct way to secure arm at patient's side. **B,** Incorrect placement of patient's arm results in ulnar nerve injury.

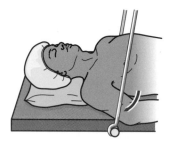

FIG. 26-6 Tucking the arms can prevent accidental compression against an upright post attached to the bed frame.

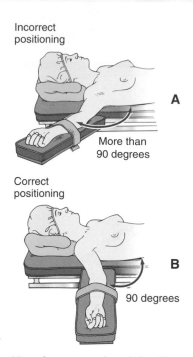

FIG. 26-7 Position of arm on armboard should not exceed 90 degrees or injury to the brachial plexus may result. **A,** Incorrect positioning. **B,** Correct positioning.

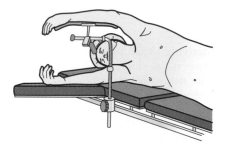

FIG. 26-8 Double armboard with elevated arm positioner.

with access to the surgical area, if space is inadequate on the operating bed for the arm to rest beside the body (as with an obese patient), or if the arm requires support (as in the lateral position). The armboard is padded to a height that is level with the operating bed. To prevent ulnar nerve pressure and abnormal shoulder rotation, the patient's arm is placed palm up (supinated), except when the patient is in the prone position. The armboard has adjustable angles, but the arm is never abducted beyond an angle of 90 degrees from the shoulder, or brachial nerve plexus injury may occur from hyperabduction (Fig. 26-7). A self-locking type of armboard is safest to prevent displacement.

Double Armboard. With a double armboard, both arms are supported, with one directly above the other in lateral position. This type of armboard resembles the wings of a biplane and is sometimes called an airplane support or overbed arm support. Both levels of the armboard are padded (Fig. 26-8).

Wrist or Arm Strap. Narrow straps at least 1½ inches (3.8 cm) wide are placed around the wrists to secure the arms to the armboards. The straps are secured without pressure or a tourniquet effect to the hands or arms. Tubing and monitoring lead wires should not be kinked or dislodged.

Upper Extremity Table. For a surgical procedure on an arm or hand, an adjustable extremity table may be attached to the side of the operating bed and used in lieu of an arm-

board. This attachment is sometimes referred to as a hand table. Some types of extremity tables slip under the mattress proximal to the surgical site and extend perpendicular to the patient's arm, with the distal end supported by a metal leg. Some models attach directly to the operating bed and require no additional floor support.

A solution drain pan may fit into some extremity tables. After skin preparation or irrigation, the pan is removed and the top panel is reinserted to cover the opening. A firm foam-rubber pad is placed on the table and draped to receive the arm, which is then draped. The upper extremity table provides a large, firm surface for the surgical procedure. The surgeon and sterile team usually sit for these types of procedures. If one team member sits, the entire team should sit to maintain the level of the sterile field.

Shoulder Bridge (Thyroid Elevator). When a shoulder bridge is used, the head section is temporarily removed and a metal bar is slipped under the mattress between the head and body sections of the operating bed. The bridge can be raised to hyperextend the shoulder or thyroid area for surgical accessibility. This position can be achieved also by placing a towel or blanket roll transversely under the shoulders, which causes the neck to hyperextend. A perpendicular towel roll can be placed between the shoulders to cause the shoulders to fall back bilaterally, which elevates the sternum.

Shoulder Braces or Supports. Adjustable, well-padded concave metal supports are occasionally used to prevent the patient from slipping when the head of the operating bed is tilted down, such as in the Trendelenburg's position. Braces should be placed equidistant from the head of the operating bed, with a ½-inch (13-mm) space between the shoulders and the braces to eliminate pressure against the shoulders. The braces are placed over the acromion processes, not over the muscles and soft tissues near the neck. To avoid nerve compression, a shoulder brace is not used when the arm is extended on an armboard; in such cases, ankle straps may be used to stabilize the patient. Many surgeons have modified positioning routines to avoid the use of shoulder braces because of inadvertent nerve injury.

Body Rests and Braces. Body rests and braces are made of metal and have a foam-rubber or gel pad covered with conductive, waterproof fabric. These devices are placed in metal clamps on the side of the operating bed and are slipped in from the edge of the operating bed against the body at various points to stabilize it in a lateral position.

Lateral Positioner (Kidney Rests). Kidney rests are concave metal pieces with grooved notches at the base, and are placed under the mattress on the body elevator flexion of the operating bed. They are slipped in from the edge of the operating bed and placed snugly against the body for lateral stability in the side-lying kidney position. Even though the kidney rest is padded, care should be taken so that the upper edge of the rest does not press too tightly against the body. Some operating beds have built-in kidney rests that are raised and lowered electrically or by a hand crank.

Anteroposterior positioner frames attach to the bed in the socket attachments for use during spinal endoscopy. All other aspects of positioning should be considered, such as arms, legs, neck, and head (Fig. 26-9).

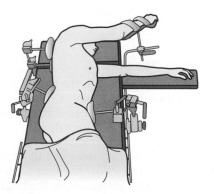

FIG. 26-9 Anteroposterior positioning frames for lateral positioning.

Body (Hip) Restraint Strap. With a body restraint strap, a wide belt with a padded center portion (to protect the skin) is placed over the patient's hips and secured by hooks to the sides of the operating bed. This strap helps to hold the patient securely in the lateral position. Some surgeons prefer to use 2- to 3-inch wide bands of adhesive tape to secure the shoulders and hips of patients in the lateral position. A towel can be placed over the patient's skin before the tape is applied. The ends of the long strips of tape are secured to the underside of the operating bed. Care is taken not to cause compression, stretching, or folding of the skin under the tape.

Positioning for Anal Procedures with Adhesive Tape. For anal procedures, the patient is placed in a prone position (Kraske position). To separate and retract the buttocks, a piece of 3-inch (7.5-cm) adhesive tape is placed on each buttock, 4 inches (10 cm) lateral to the surgical site. For greater security of tape adhesion, benzoin or adhesive liquid is applied to each buttock before the tape strips are applied. Each end of the tape is fastened to the frame of the operating bed.

Adjustable Arched Spinal Frame. An adjustable arched spinal frame consists of two padded arches mounted on a frame that is attached to the operating bed. The patient is placed in the prone position with his or her abdomen over this device (referred to as a Wilson frame). The pads extend from the shoulders to the thighs, with the abdomen hanging dependently between the arches. The desired degree of flexion for spinal procedures is achieved by adjusting the height of the arch by means of a crank. Other types of frames are available (Fig. 26-10).

Stirrups. Metal stirrup posts are placed in holders, one on each side rail of the operating bed, to support the legs and feet in the lithotomy position. The feet are supported by canvas or fabric loops that suspend the legs at a right angle to the feet. These are sometimes called candy cane or sling stirrups (Fig. 26-11).

During extensive surgery, special leg holders may be used to support the lower legs and feet. Also available are metal or high-impact-plastic knee-crutch stirrups that can be adjusted for knee flexion and extension. Even if well padded, these stirrups may create some pressure on the back of the knees and lower extremities and may jeopardize the popliteal vessels and nerves. Gel and foam pads are available for patient protection when stirrups are used (Fig. 26-12).

Metal Footboard. The footboard can be left flat as a horizontal extension of the operating bed or raised perpendicular to the operating bed to support the feet, with the soles resting securely against it. It is padded when the patient is placed in reverse Trendelenburg's position.

Headrests. Padded headrests are used with supine, prone, sitting, or lateral positions. They attach to the operating bed to support and expose the occiput and cervical vertebrae. The head is held securely but without the pressure that could cause pressure injury to the ears or optic nerve ischemic blindness. Headrests can be shaped like a donut or horse-

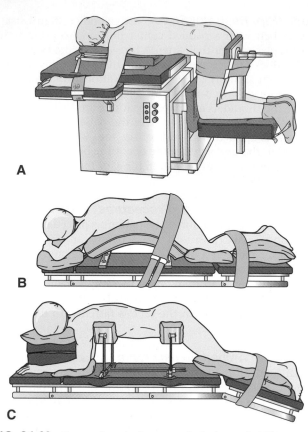

FIG. 26-10   Frames for spinal surgery. **A,** Andrews. **B,** Wilson. **C,** Four-poster.

shoe for head and neck procedures; other styles are flat or concave to stabilize the head and neck in alignment. Nonpadded metal headrests have sterile skull pins that are inserted into the patient's head for neurologic procedures (Fig. 26-13).

Accessories. Various sizes and shapes of pads, pillows, and bead bags (beanbags) that fit various anatomic structures are used to protect, support, or immobilize body parts. Foam rubber, polymer pads, silicone gel pads, vacuum-shaped bags, and other accessories are covered with washable materials unless designed for single-patient use.

A donut (a ring-shaped foam-rubber or silicone gel pad) may be used during procedures on the head or face to keep the surgical area in a horizontal plane. Donuts are used also to protect pressure points such as the ear, knee, heel, or elbow. Protectors made of foam rubber, polymers, silicone gel, or other material also may be used to protect the joints from pressure. Many other types of protectors are available.

Bolsters are used to elevate a specific part of the body (e.g., Kraske pillow to elevate the buttocks for anal procedures). Solid rolls of blankets or firm foam under each side of a patient's chest, referred to as chest rolls, raise the chest off the operating bed to facilitate respiration. Large 2- or 3-L water bags also can be used for this purpose as well as for axillary elevation during lateral positioning. Commercially available bolsters and elevating pads are commonly used. Because patients may have a latex sensitivity, the manu-

facturer's literature should be checked for latex content (Fig. 26-14).

Pressure-Minimizing Mattress. To minimize pressure on bony prominences, peripheral blood vessels, and nerves during prolonged surgical procedures (more than 2 hours for the average patient, less for a debilitated patient), an alternating pressure mattress is put over the mattress on the operating bed before the patient arrives. This may be a positive-pressure air mattress, a circulating-water thermal mattress, a foam-rubber mattress (with indentations similar to an egg crate), a gel pad, or a dry polymer pad. Unless designed to be placed next to a patient's skin, pressure mattresses and thermal blankets used to induce hypothermia or hyperthermia should be covered with an absorbent sheet or thin pad. Folds and creases in the covering should be avoided to prevent pressure indentations in the skin. The manufacturer's instructions should be followed in using these devices.

Surgical Vacuum Positioning System. With the surgical vacuum positioning system, soft pads filled with tiny plastic beads are placed under or around the body part to be supported. Suction is attached to the vacuum port on the pad; as air is withdrawn, the pad becomes firm and molds to the patient's body. The suction is then disconnected. A vacuum is created inside the pad, causing the beads to press together. Friction between the beads prevents them from moving; this creates a solid mass that keeps its molded shape. Various sizes and shapes of pads provide firm support while relieving pressure points. To change the patient's position during the surgical procedure, the valve on the pad is squeezed until the pad is slightly soft. The patient is repositioned, and suction is applied to remold the pad. A pressure-reduction gel pad or other protection should be placed between the patient and the vacuum positioning device.

SURGICAL POSITIONS

Many positions are used for surgical procedures; the most commonly used positions are discussed in the following sections. If IV fluids will be infused in the arm during the surgical procedure, the arm is placed on an armboard. This fact is assumed in the following discussion, because IV fluids are usually given. If electrosurgery is used, the dispersive return electrode should be placed after the patient is in position for the surgical procedure and the electrode should not be moved, shifted, or cut to size. Take care not to kink catheter tubing or dislodge monitoring devices during positioning.

Supine (Dorsal) Position

Figure 26-15 shows the patient in the supine position—the most natural position for the body at rest. The patient lies flat on the back with the arms secured at the sides with the lift sheet, and the palms extend along the side of the body in their natural resting position. The elbows may be protected with plastic sleds. The legs are straight and parallel and are in line with the head and spine; the hips are parallel with the spine. A safety belt is placed across the thighs 2 inches above the knees. Small positioning pads may be placed under the head and popliteal area to relieve pressure on the

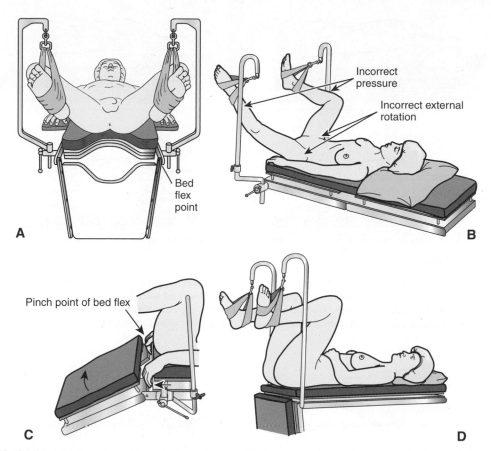

FIG. 26-11 **A,** Correct use of candy cane stirrups with feet suspended in cloth slings. **B,** Legs should not rest on stirrup posts or lower leg nerve injury could result. **C,** Hands should be positioned away from bed flex points. **D,** Correct flexion of legs in stirrups.

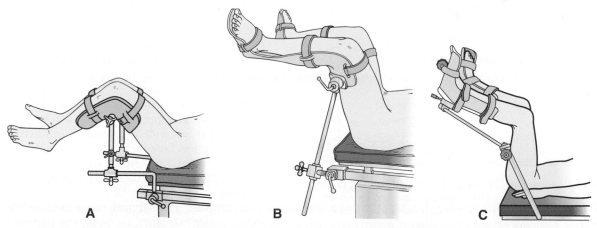

FIG. 26-12   Additional types of stirrups. **A,** Urologic stirrups. **B,** Stirrups used for abdominoperineal and obstetric procedures. **C,** Allen-style stirrups.

spine as needed. The heels are protected from pressure by a pillow, gel pad, or donut. The feet must not be in prolonged plantar flexion, or nerve stretch injury could result. To prevent footdrop, the soles may be supported by a pillow or padded footboard.

The supine position is used for procedures on the anterior surface of the body, such as abdominal, abdominothoracic,

and some lower extremity procedures. Modifications of the supine position are used for specific body areas:
- *Procedures on the face or neck:* The neck may be slightly hyperextended by lowering the head section of the operating bed or by placing a shoulder roll. With the patient in the supine position, the head may be supported in a headrest or donut and/or turned toward the unaf-

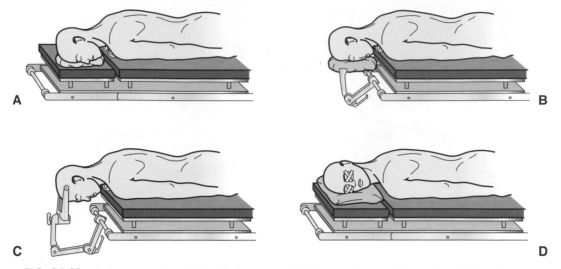

FIG. 26-13   **A,** Prone position with face in foam or gel-filled donut head positioner ring. **B,** Horseshoe head holder used for prone or supine procedures. **C,** Mayfield headrest with sterile metal pins inserted into patient's scalp for stability. **D,** Prone position with head placed on pillow. Patient can experience ear compression using this method. Donut should be used in place of pillow to allow for zero pressure on ear.

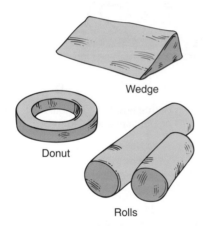

Wedge

Donut

Rolls

FIG. 26-14   Common positioning pads.

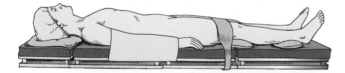

FIG. 26-15   Supine position. Patient lies straight on back, face upward, with arms at sides, legs extended parallel and uncrossed, and feet slightly separated. Strap is placed above knees. Head is in line with spine. Note small pillow under ankles to protect heels from pressure. Arms are secured with lift sheet or placed on armboards.

fected side. The eyes are protected from injury, laser light, or irritating solutions by shields, goggles, or nonallergenic tape. During skin preparation and the surgical procedure, contact lenses should be removed, and the eyes should be lubricated with ophthalmic gel and secured with eye pads taped in place. The eyes should be inspected periodically by the anesthesia provider during the case and at the end of the surgical procedure.

- *Shoulder or anterolateral procedures:* With the patient in the supine position, a small sandbag, water bag, roll, or pad is placed under the affected side to elevate the shoulder off the operating bed for exposure. The length of the body is stabilized to prevent the spine from rolling or twisting. Hips and shoulders should be kept in a straight plane. The operating bed also can be tilted laterally to elevate the affected part.
- *Dorsal recumbent position:* For some vaginal or perineal procedures the patient is in the supine position except that the knees are flexed upward and the thighs are slightly externally rotated. The soles of the feet rest on the operating bed. Pillows may be placed under the knees if needed for support.
- *Modified dorsal recumbent (frog-leg) position:* For some surgical procedures in the region of the groin or lower extremity, the patient is in the supine position except that the knees are slightly flexed with a pillow or wedge support beneath each leg (Fig. 26-16). The thighs are widely externally rotated, and the soles of the feet face each other. The blanket is placed over the lower legs, and the safety strap is placed anterior to the shins to secure the legs from sliding forward.
- *Arm extension:* For surgical procedures of the breast, axilla, upper extremity, or hand, the patient is placed in the supine position; the arm on the affected side is placed on an armboard or upper extremity table extension that locks into position at a right angle to the body. The affected side of the body is close to the edge of the operating bed for access to the surgical area. If the axilla is involved, the arm is placed even with the lower edge of the armboard for accessibility. Hyperextension of the arm is avoided to prevent neural or vascular injury, such as brachial plexus injury or occlusion of the axillary artery. The armboard is well padded.

A modification of this position may be used for patients in hypovolemic shock. Many anesthesia providers prefer to keep the trunk level and to elevate the legs by raising the lower part of the operating bed at the break under the hips. Others prefer to tilt the entire operating bed downward toward the head. Either position reduces venous stasis in the lower extremities and promotes venous return.

Reverse Trendelenburg's Position

With reverse Trendelenburg's position, the patient lies on his or her back in the supine position (Fig. 26-18). The entire operating bed is tilted 30 to 40 degrees so the head is higher than the feet; a padded footboard is used to prevent the patient from sliding toward the tilt. The thigh safety belt is positioned 2 inches above the knees. Small pillows may be placed under the knees. A small pillow or donut may stabilize the head.

This position is used for thyroidectomy to facilitate breathing and to decrease blood supply to the surgical site (blood will pool caudally). It is also used for laparoscopic gallbladder, biliary tract, or stomach procedures to allow the abdominal viscera to fall away from the epigastrium, giving access to the upper abdomen.

Venous stasis can cause complications, and prevention of deep vein thrombosis is an important consideration. The use of sequential compression devices, antiembolic stockings, or foot pumps is suggested to improve venous return.

Fowler's Position

With the Fowler's position, the patient lies on his or her back with the buttocks at the flex in the operating bed and the knees over the lower break. The foot of the operating bed is lowered slightly, flexing the knees. The body section is raised 45 degrees, thereby becoming the backrest. Arms may rest on armboards parallel to the operating bed or on a large, soft pillow on the lap. Care is taken that the arms do not fall dependent from the body during the procedure. The safety belt is secured 2 inches above the knees. The entire operating bed is tilted slightly with the head end downward to prevent the patient from slipping toward the foot of the operating bed. Feet should rest on the padded footboard to prevent footdrop. For cranial procedures, the head is supported in a headrest.

In this position, the operating bed looks like a modified armchair. This position may be used for shoulder, nasopharyngeal, facial, and breast reconstruction procedures (Fig. 26-19). Complications of this position include air embolus

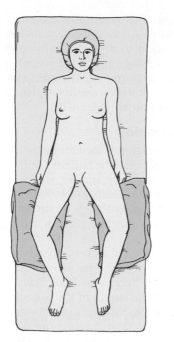

FIG. 26-16   Modified dorsal recumbent position. Patient lies on back with arms at sides. Knees are slightly flexed, with a pillow under each. Thighs are externally rotated. Referred to as frog-legged.

Trendelenburg's Position

With the Trendelenburg's position, the patient lies on his or her back in the supine position with the knees over the lower break of the operating bed (Fig. 26-17). The knees must bend with the break of the operating bed to prevent pressure on the peroneal nerves and veins in the legs. The entire operating bed is tilted approximately 40 degrees downward at the head, depending on the surgeon's preference. The foot of the operating bed is lowered to the desired angle.

Trendelenburg's position is used for procedures in the lower abdomen or pelvis when it is desirable to tilt the abdominal viscera away from the pelvic area for better exposure. Although surgical accessibility is increased, lung volume is decreased and the heart is mechanically compressed by the pressure of the organs against the diaphragm. Intracranial pressure is increased. Therefore the patient remains in this position for as short a time as possible. In returning to a horizontal position, the leg section should be raised first and slowly while venous stasis in the legs is reversed. The entire operating bed is then leveled.

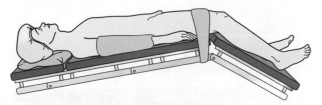

FIG. 26-17   Trendelenburg's position. Note knees are over lower break in operating bed, with knee strap above knees. Arms are secured. Shoulder braces are not usually needed with this method of Trendelenburg's position.

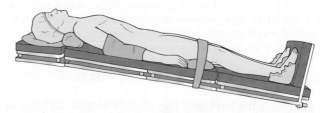

FIG. 26-18   Reverse Trendelenburg's position, with soft roll under shoulders for thyroid, neck, or shoulder procedures. *(From Meeker MH, Rothrock JC: Alexander's care of the patient in surgery, ed 11, St Louis, 1999, Mosby.)*

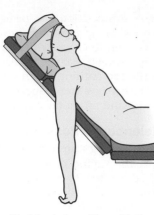

FIG. 26-19 Modified Fowler's position with the shoulder dependent over the edge of the bed for shoulder procedure. Sometimes referred to as the captain's chair.

into the venous system, pelvic pooling or venous stasis, hypotension, positional orthopedic injury, and tissue pressure injury and necrosis.

If an air embolus should enter the patient's right atrium, he or she is immediately repositioned in the left lateral position and the bed is lowered into steep Trendelenburg's position. This emergent posture is referred to the Durant position or Durant maneuver. This immediate action causes the air embolus to move from the right ventricular outflow tract. A central venous catheter is placed into the right atrium by the anesthesiologist to withdraw the air bubble and restore cardiac function.

Sitting Position. With the sitting position, the patient is placed in the Fowler position except that the torso is completely in an upright position. The shoulders and torso should be supported with body straps but not so tightly that respiration and circulation are impeded. Pressure points (especially ischial tuberosities) are padded to reduce the risk of sciatic nerve damage. The flexed arms rest on a large pillow on the lap or on a pillow on an adjustable table in front of the patient (see Fig. 26-4; this table attachment can be secured in the bed sockets in front of the patient as a padded armrest). The head is seated forward in a cranial headrest for neurosurgical procedures. A padded footboard may be placed to maintain the patient's feet in an upright position and deter sliding down on the bed.

This position is used on occasion for some otorhinologic and neurosurgical procedures. Air embolism is a potential complication and is treated in the same manner as described in the Fowler position. Antiembolic stockings or sequential compression devices are used to counteract postural hypotension and decrease venous pooling in the extremities and pelvis.

Beach Chair or Modified Sitting Position. With the beach chair or modified sitting position, the patient is supine with the back and legs slightly elevated. The entire spine is somewhat contoured with the angle of flexion at the hip decreased. Both the head and the feet are elevated 10 to 20 degrees above the level of the heart. The arms are placed across the abdomen, and the safety belt is secured

over the thighs. This position is used for several nose and throat procedures. Abdominoplasty closure is performed by using this position to bring the skin edges closer together after resection of large redundant skin flaps. The xiphoid-pubic distance is shortened. The arms can be secured with the lift sheet if the hands are not at risk for crush injury at the bed flexion points (Fig. 26-20).

Lithotomy Position

The lithotomy position is used for perineal, vaginal, urologic, and rectal procedures. The patient's buttocks rest along the break between the body and leg sections of the operating bed. A padded metal footboard is used as an operating bed extension so the patient's legs do not extend over the foot of the operating bed before placing the legs in the upright position.

Stirrups are secured in sockets on each side of the operating bed rail at the level of the patient's upper thighs. They are adjusted at equal height on both sides and at an appropriate height for the length of the patient's legs to maintain symmetry when the patient is positioned. After the patient is anesthetized, the safety belt is removed and the patient's legs are raised simultaneously by two people (Fig. 26-21). Each person grasps the sole of a foot in one hand and supports the calf at the knee area with the other. The knees are flexed, and the legs and feet are placed inside the stirrups. For sling, or candy cane stirrups, the feet are placed in the fabric slings of the stirrups at a 90-degree angle to the abdomen. One padded loop encircles the sole; the other padded loop goes around the ankle.

Simultaneous movement as the knees are flexed is essential to avoid straining the lower back. If the patient's legs are properly placed, undue abduction and external rotation are avoided. The leg or ankle must not touch the metal stirrup. Padding is placed as necessary. If the legs are put in stirrups before the induction of anesthesia, the patient can identify discomfort and pressure on the back and/or legs. The positioning procedure is similar for other types of stirrups. The level of the lithotomy position needed for the surgical procedure is determined by the surgeon (Fig. 26-22).

After the patient's legs are placed in the stirrups, the lower section of mattress is removed and the lower section of the operating bed is lowered. The buttocks must not extend beyond the edge of the operating bed, which would strain the lumbosacral muscles and ligaments as the weight of the body rests on the sacrum.

The hands should not extend along the operating bed, where they could be injured in the table flex point, referred

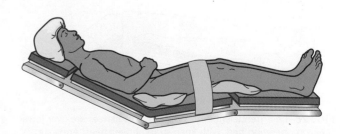

FIG. 26-20 Beach chair position. The arms are typically placed across the abdomen, and a safety strap is across the thighs.

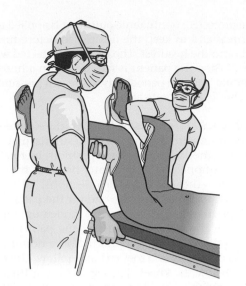

FIG. 26-21 Lithotomy position. Patient is on back with foot section of operating bed lowered to right angle with body on operating bed. Knees are flexed and legs are elevated to the degree necessary for the type of surgical procedure. Note that buttocks are even with edge of the operating bed and that sometimes a roll is needed under the buttocks to elevate the hips above the level of the bed.

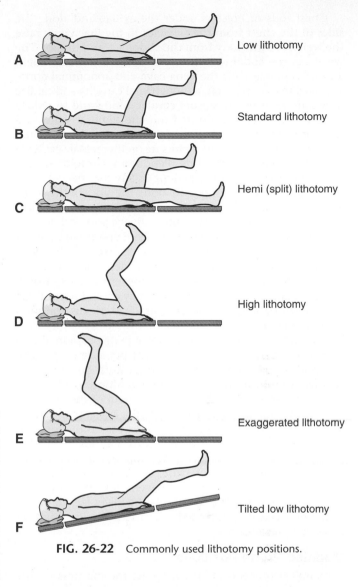

A Low lithotomy
B Standard lithotomy
C Hemi (split) lithotomy
D High lithotomy
E Exaggerated lithotomy
F Tilted low lithotomy

FIG. 26-22 Commonly used lithotomy positions.

to as the break, during manipulation of the operating bed or movement of the patient. Hands have been crushed in the break as the leg section of the operating bed was raised at the conclusion of the surgical procedure. Arms may be placed on armboards or loosely cradled over the lower abdomen and secured by the lower end of the blanket. Arms must not rest directly on the chest, which could impede respiration. Lung compliance is decreased by pressure of the thighs on the abdomen, which hinders the descent of the diaphragm.

Blood pools in the lumbar region of the torso, especially during prolonged surgical procedures in lithotomy. Antiembolic stockings may be worn, or legs may be wrapped in sequential compression devices or foot pumps during the surgical procedure to prevent the formation of thrombi or emboli. The legs should be checked periodically for distal pulses, skin color, and evidence of edema. In the lithotomy position, nerve damage or compartment syndrome can occur from direct pressure and/or ischemia of the muscles, which compromises the viability of tissues.

At the conclusion of the surgical procedure, the leg section of the operating bed is raised and the lower section of the mattress is replaced. The patient's legs are removed simultaneously from the stirrups and lowered slowly to prevent hypotension as blood reenters the legs and leaves the torso. To prevent wide abduction of the thighs, the legs are fully extended and brought together as they are lifted from the stirrups. The safety belt should be reapplied over the thighs during the patient's emergence from anesthesia.

Prone Position

Prone position is used for all procedures with a dorsal or posterior approach (Fig. 26-23). When the prone position is used, the patient is anesthetized and intubated in the supine position on the locked transport stretcher. The patient's

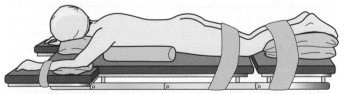

FIG. 26-23 Prone position. Patient is placed on abdomen. Chest rolls are placed under axillae and sides of chest to the level of the iliac crest to facilitate respiration. Knees should be padded and a pillow is placed under dorsum of feet.

arms are along his or her sides. When the anesthesia provider gives permission, the patient is slowly and cautiously shifted toward the operating bed in the supine position and then turned onto the abdomen onto the operating bed. The patient's body is rotated as if rolling a log; a team of at least four to six people is needed to maintain body alignment during this transfer. The anesthesia provider controls the patient's head and airway while the rest of the patient's body is moved by the team.

Chest rolls or bolsters under the axillae and along the sides of the chest from the clavicles to the iliac crests raise the weight of the body from the abdomen and thorax. The weight of the abdomen will fall away from the diaphragm and keep pressure off the vena cava and abdominal aorta. This facilitates respiration, although vital capacity and cardiac index are reduced. To ensure cardiac filling and to reduce hypotension, venous return from the femoral veins and inferior vena cava is uninterrupted. Female breasts should be moved laterally to reduce pressure on them. Male genitalia should be free from pressure. Pendulous skinfolds should not be crimped under the patient in any manner.

The arms may lie supported along the sides of the body, with the palms up or inward toward the body. An alternate position is to place the arms into a diver's pose by lowering them toward the floor and rotating them upward in a natural range of motion. The armboards are reversed on the table, pointing toward the anesthesia provider. The elbows are padded and are slightly flexed to prevent overextension, and the palms are down. The arms may extend beyond the head, but not so far as to cause brachial plexus compression or stretch.

The head can be turned to one side or positioned face down on a padded donut to prevent pressure on the ear, eye, and face. Clearance of the airway must be ensured. A serious complication of the prone position is blindness caused by ischemia of the vascular system of the eye.[1]

A pillow or padding under the anterior aspect of the ankles and the dorsa of the feet prevents pressure on the toes and elevates the feet to aid venous return. Do not permit the patient's toes to extend beyond the foot of the bed. Donuts under the knees prevent pressure on the patellae. The safety belt is placed over the calves to prevent flexion of the lower legs. Care is taken not to compress the lower legs. An additional belt can be positioned over the posterior thighs as an added precaution.

Modified Prone Positions

For surgical procedures on the spine, the mattress on the operating bed is adjusted so the hips are over the break between the body and leg sections. A large, soft pillow is placed under the abdomen. The upper break of the operating bed is flexed, and the operating bed is tilted so the surgical area is horizontal. Some surgeons prefer a special assembly for the orthopedic operating bed, such as an adjustable arch (Wilson frame), a Hastings frame, or an Andrews frame for spinal surgery. The patient is carefully lifted and properly positioned on a special table or frame. The patient may be placed in a prone, extreme forward sitting, or kneeling position with the torso at a right angle to the thighs. The lower legs, at right angles at the knees, rest on the foot extension, which is at a 90-degree angle. The midsection of the abdomen is allowed to hang free. This allows the anesthesia provider to use the hypotensive anesthetic technique for hemostasis.

For neurosurgical procedures, the head rests in a cranial headrest to expose the occiput and cervical vertebrae. The eyes are protected; ophthalmic ointment is applied to protect the corneas and to keep the lids closed before turning the patient onto the headrest. The ears are protected with foam support. When the patient is face down on a headrest, the head should be raised periodically to prevent pressure necrosis of the cheeks and forehead.

Kraske (Jackknife) Position. With the Kraske position, the patient remains supine until anesthetized and is then turned onto the abdomen (prone position) by rotation. The hips are positioned over the center break of the operating bed between the body and leg sections. Chest rolls or bolsters are placed to raise the chest if the patient is under general anesthesia. The arms are extended on angled armboards with the elbows flexed and the palms down. The head is to the side and is supported on a donut or pillow. The dorsa of the feet and toes rest on a pillow. The safety belt is placed below the knees. The leg section of the operating bed is lowered the desired amount (usually about 90 degrees), and the entire operating bed is tilted head downward to elevate the hips above the rest of the body.

The patient is well balanced on the operating bed (Fig. 26-24). For procedures in the rectal area (e.g., pilonidal sinus, hemorrhoidectomy), the buttocks are retracted with wide tape strips. Because of the dependent position, venous pooling occurs cephalad (toward the head) and caudad (toward the feet). It is very important to return the patient slowly to horizontal from this unnatural position.

Knee-Chest Position. The knee-chest position is used for sigmoidoscopy or culdoscopy. For this position, an extension is attached to the foot section. The operating bed is flexed at the center break, and the lower section is broken until it is at a right angle to the operating bed. The patient kneels on the lower section; the knees are thus flexed at a right angle to the body.

The upper portion of the operating bed may be raised slightly to support the head, which is turned to the side. The arms are placed around the head with the elbows flexed, and a large soft pillow is placed beneath them. The chest rests on the operating bed, and the safety belt is placed above the knees. The entire operating bed is tilted head downward so the hips and pelvis are at the highest point—a modified jackknife position.

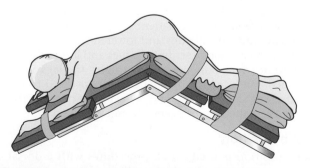

FIG. 26-24 Kraske (jackknife) position. *(From Meeker MH, Rothrock JC: Alexander's care of the patient in surgery, ed 11, St Louis, 1999, Mosby.)*

---

[1] *AHRQ Mortality and Morbidity Report,* June 2005, describes permanent vision loss caused by retinal ischemia during surgical positioning. www.webmd.ahrq.gov.

Lateral Positions

For lateral positioning, the operating bed remains flat. The patient is anesthetized and intubated in the supine position and then turned to the unaffected side. In the right lateral position, the patient lies on the right side with the left side up (for a left-sided procedure); the left lateral position exposes the right side (Fig. 26-25).

The patient is turned by no fewer than four people to maintain body alignment and achieve stability. The patient's back is drawn to the edge of the operating bed. The knee of the lower leg is flexed slightly to provide stabilization, and the upper leg is flexed to provide counterbalance. The flexed knees may require padding to prevent pressure and shearing force. In addition, a large, soft pillow is placed lengthwise between the legs to take pressure off the upper hip and lower leg and therefore prevent circulatory complications and pressure on the peroneal nerve. The ankle and foot of the upper leg should be supported to prevent footdrop. Bony prominences are padded. For added stability, a safety belt and/or a 3-inch (7.5-cm)-wide tape is placed over the hip.

The patient's arms may be placed on a padded double armboard, with the lower arm palm up and the upper arm slightly flexed with the palm down. Blood pressure should be measured from the lower arm. As an alternative, the upper arm can be positioned on a padded Mayo stand. A water bag or pressure reduction pad under the axilla protects neurovascular structures. The shoulders should be in alignment.

The patient's head is in cervical alignment with the spine. The head should be supported on a small pillow between the shoulder and neck to prevent stretching the neck and brachial plexus and to maintain a patent airway (Fig. 26-26).

Referred to synonymously as the lateral, lateral decubitus, or lateral recumbent, this position is used for access to the hemithorax, kidney, or retroperitoneal space. This position contributes to physiologic alterations. Respiration is affected by differing gas exchange ratios in the lungs. Because of gravity, the lower lung receives more blood from the right side of the heart; the lower lung therefore has increased perfusion but less residual air because of mediastinal compression and the weight of the abdominal contents on the diaphragm. Positive pressure to both lungs helps

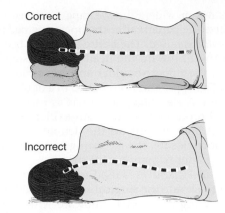

FIG. 26-26 Proper alignment of spinal column in lateral position.

control respiratory changes. Circulation is also compromised by pressure on the abdominal vessels. In the right lateral position, compression of the vena cava impairs venous return.

Sims Recumbent Position. With the Sims recumbent position (a modified left lateral recumbent position), the patient lies on his or her left side with the upper leg flexed at the hip and knee; the lower leg is straight. The lower arm is extended along the patient's back, with the weight of the chest on the operating bed. The upper arm rests in a flexed position on the operating bed. This position may be preferred for an endoscopic examination performed via the anus in obese or geriatric patients.

Kidney Position. With the kidney position, the flank region is positioned over the kidney elevator on the operating bed when the patient is turned onto the unaffected side (Fig. 26-27). The short kidney rest is attached to the body elevator at the patient's back. The longer rest is placed in front at a level beneath the iliac crest to minimize pressure on the abdominal organs. Both rests are well padded. In an obese patient, folds of abdominal tissue may extend over the end of the anterior rest and be bruised if caution is not taken. The operating bed is flexed slightly at the level of the iliac crest so the body elevator can be raised as desired to increase space between the lower ribs and iliac crest.

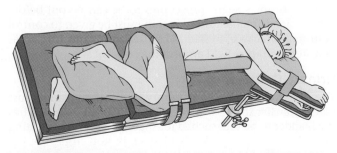

FIG. 26-25 Left lateral position is when the patient is lying on the left side. Note strap across hip to stabilize body. Pillow between legs relieves pressure on lower legs. Both legs are flexed slightly to alleviate any pressure or stretch. Note that bed is flat, not flexed. Right lateral is directly the opposite position.

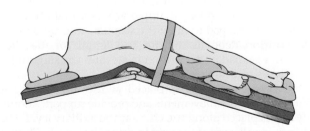

FIG. 26-27 Right kidney position for a procedure on the right kidney. Patient is in lateral position with kidney region over operating bed break, or body elevation bar. The table is flexed. Note strap across hip to stabilize body, raised kidney elevator for hyperextending surgical site, and pillow between legs. The lower leg is flexed more than the upper leg. Patient's side is horizontal from shoulder to hip. The arm is supported by a double airplane armboard (not shown).

A body strap or wide adhesive tape is placed over the hip to stabilize the patient after the operating bed is flexed and the elevator is raised. The entire operating bed is tilted slightly downward toward the head until the surgical area is horizontal; the upper shoulder and hip should be in a straight line. The upper arm is supported in a double airplane-style armboard. A water bag or gel pad is used to support the chest and protect the breasts. An axillary roll may be placed to take body weight off the deltoid muscle in the shoulder. Before closure, the operating bed is straightened to allow better approximation of tissues.

The term *kidney position* is used to designate the lateral flexion used to elevate the surgical site. It should be clearly documented as right or left to indicate which kidney is elevated for the procedure. The kidney position is used for procedures on the kidney and ureter; this position is not well tolerated. Skin and underlying tissue can be damaged by excessive pressure during flexion of the operating bed. Operating bed flexion combined with use of the kidney elevator may cause cardiovascular responses. Blood tends to pool in the lower arm and leg. Circulation is further compromised by increased pressure on the abdominal vessels when the kidney elevator is raised. The spine is stressed in a lateral flexed position and can cause strain on the vertebral structures.

Lateral Jackknife Position. For positioning in the lateral jackknife position, the patient is first placed in the lateral position, and then the operating bed is flexed at the level of the patient's flank or lower ribs. The operating bed is tilted so the torso is level; this drops the legs into a dependent position.

Similar to the kidney position already described, the lateral jackknife position is not well tolerated. Blood tends to pool in the legs. Extreme operating bed flexion into a lateral jackknife position may occlude the inferior vena cava, causing venous obstruction. Pulmonary compliance is reduced, making ventilation difficult.

Lateral Chest (Thoracotomy) Position. Modifications of the lateral position are used for unilateral transthoracic procedures with a lateral approach. After the patient is turned onto the unaffected side and positioned as described for the lateral position, a second strap may be placed over the shoulder for stability unless doing so would interfere with skin preparation. The arms may be extended on a double armboard, or the lower arm is extended on an armboard with the palm up while the upper arm is brought forward and down over a pad to draw the scapula from the surgical area. Position depends on site and length of the chest incision. A gel pad under the axilla elevates the surgical site and relieves pressure on the lower arm.

One lateral body rest is placed at the lumbar area to facilitate respiratory movements and provide support. Another body rest is placed along the chest at the axillary level. This body rest is well padded to avoid bruising the breasts. Vacuum positioning devices or bolsters may be used instead of body rests. The shoulders and hips should be level. Slightly lowering the head of the operating bed assists postural drainage during the surgical procedure. This position is restrictive to the cardiopulmonary system, especially if used for a prolonged period.

Anterior Chest Position. For thoracoabdominal procedures with an anterior approach, the positioning is more supine than for the lateral chest position. After the patient is anesthetized, a water bag or gel pad is placed under the lower axilla; another pillow or wedge is placed behind the buttocks and spine to support the torso. The upper knee is flexed slightly, and a large, soft pillow is placed beneath it to relieve strain on the abdominal muscles and upper hip.

The operating bed can be tilted laterally to raise the incisional site. A safety belt is placed across the hip and another above the knees. The lower arm on the unaffected side is supported at the side by an armboard. The upper arm on the affected side is padded well and bandaged loosely to the anesthesia screen above the patient's head. To avoid injury to the brachial plexus, the arm must not be hyperextended or hyperabducted. The head of the operating bed is lowered slightly for postural drainage.

MODIFICATIONS FOR INDIVIDUAL PATIENT NEEDS

Anomalies and physical defects are accommodated according to each patient's needs. Whether the patient is unconscious or conscious, the avoidance of unnecessary exposure is an essential consideration for all patients. The patient's position should be observed objectively before skin preparation and draping to see that it adheres to physiologic principles. Protective devices, positioning aids, and padded areas should be reassessed before draping, because they could have shifted during the skin preparation procedure or during insertion of an indwelling urinary catheter. Careful observation of patient protection and positioning facilitates the expected outcome.

Documentation

The circulating nurse should document any preoperative limitations in the patient's range of motion, the condition of the skin before and after the surgical procedure, and the position in which the patient was positioned during the surgical procedure—including the use of special equipment. Personnel performing the positioning should be listed by name, role, and title.

PHYSICAL PREPARATION AND DRAPING OF THE SURGICAL SITE

The type of surgical procedure to be performed, the age and condition of the patient, and the preferences of the surgeon will determine specific procedures to be carried out before the incision is made. Consideration must be given to control of urinary drainage, to skin antisepsis, and to establishment of a sterile draped field around the surgical site.

Urinary Catheterization

The patient should void to empty the urinary bladder just before transfer to the OR suite unless the procedure requires the bladder to be full, such as for special bladder tone testing procedures. If the patient's bladder is not empty or the surgeon wishes to prevent bladder distention during a long procedure or after the surgical procedure, urinary catheterization may be necessary after the patient is anesthetized. An indwelling Foley catheter may be inserted by a member of the team. This maintains bladder decompression to avoid trauma during a lower abdominal or pelvic procedure, to permit accurate measurement of output during or after the surgical procedure, or to facilitate output and healing after a surgical procedure on genitourinary tract structures. Catheterization is performed before the patient is positioned for the surgical procedure, except for a patient who will remain in the lithotomy position. The Foley catheter should be inserted before the vaginal and/or abdominal skin preparation to prevent perineal splash to the surgical site. The vagina can be prepped immediately after the Foley catheter is placed. Gloves should be changed and a new prep set used for the abdominal skin prep.

Urinary tract infection can be caused by contamination or trauma to structures during urinary catheterization. Sterile technique must be maintained. A sterile, disposable catheterization tray is used unless the patient is being prepared for a surgical procedure in the perineal or genital area. For these latter procedures, a sterile catheter and lubricant may be added to the perineal skin preparation setup. For other surgical procedures, the perineal and meatal areas should be cleansed with an antiseptic agent to reduce microbial flora and remove gross contaminants before the catheterization procedure. Sterile gloves are donned using open glove technique (Fig. 26-28).

The catheter should be small enough to minimize trauma to the urethra and prevent necrosis of the meatus; usually a size 16 or 14 French (Fr) catheter is inserted in a woman, and a 16 or 18 Fr catheter is inserted in a man. Care is taken to note whether the patient is sensitive to latex. Many Foley catheters are composed of latex and could cause a reaction in susceptible patients. Silicone catheters are commercially available.

The balloon size may be 5 or 30 mL (5 mL is used most frequently in adults); 10 mL of sterile water is needed to properly expand a 5-mL balloon, to compensate for volume required by the expansion channel. Foley catheters have a Luer-Lok valve over the lumen to the expansion channel that is filled using a Luer-Lok syringe. Foley catheter manufacturers do not recommend testing the balloon before insertion. They maintain that doing so causes the balloon to weaken. The balloon is tested in the factory at the time of manufacture.

The hand used to spread the labia or stabilize the penis is considered contaminated and should not be used to handle the catheter or prep sponges (Fig. 26-29). To facilitate insertion and minimize trauma, the tip of the catheter is lubricated with a sterile water-soluble lubricant. Urine will start to flow when the catheter has passed into the bladder. The balloon of a Foley catheter is expanded with sterile water only after urine is seen in the tubing, and the bladder is allowed to drain. If difficulty is encountered during catheter insertion, especially in a geriatric male patient with an enlarged prostate, the catheter should not be forced into the urethra. One should stop the catheterization procedure and request help from the surgeon. A firm catheter stylet may be needed to pass the catheter through the prostatic segment of the urethra to minimize trauma to the structures.

The catheter is attached to a sterile drainage system and drainage bag is positioned in the direct view of the anesthesia provider. The tubing is later attached to the patient's

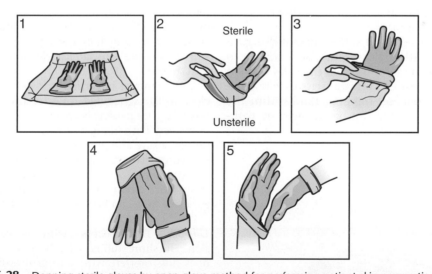

FIG. 26-28   Donning sterile gloves by open glove method for performing patient skin preparation or catheterization. (1) Open sterile glove wrapper. Gloves will be in a face-up position with a short pre-rolled cuff. (2) To glove the right hand: Grasp the inner aspect of the right cuff with the bare left forefinger and thumb. Take care to touch only the inner cuff surface with bare skin. The outer surface of the glove is sterile. (3) Slide right hand into the opening of the glove, taking care not to touch the outer sterile surface. Do not adjust cuff once the glove is on. This will be done later. (4) To glove the left hand: Using gloved right hand, slide gloved fingers under the inner sterile aspect of the left cuff. Steady the fingers of the right hand as the bare left hand is slid into the glove. The left cuff is straightened by the right fingers as the final act of donning the glove. (5) Use the sterile fingers of the left hand on the sterile aspect of the right glove to slide the remaining right glove cuff into position. Do not touch the inner aspect (the skin side) of either glove with the outer sterile gloved surface.

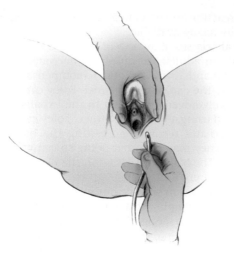

FIG. 26-29   Female urinary catheterization.
(From Davis JH et al: Essentials of clinical surgery, St Louis, 1991, Mosby.)

leg with enough slack in it to prevent tension or pull on the penis or urethra at the conclusion of the case (Fig. 26-30).

Attention is paid to the catheter and tubing during positioning of the patient for the surgical procedure to prevent compression or kinking. Dependent loops of tubing should not be permitted to hang on the floor. This could cause a trip hazard. If the container must be raised above the level of the bladder during positioning, the tubing is clamped or kinked until the container can be lowered and secured under the operating bed to avoid contamination by retrograde or backward flow of urine.

If the catheter is to be removed at the end of the surgical procedure, don examination gloves and use a syringe to withdraw and measure the solution from the Foley balloon expansion port. Cutting the end off with scissors may cause the inflation port to collapse, trapping fluid within the expanded balloon. The urethra can be damaged by withdrawing the expanded balloon.

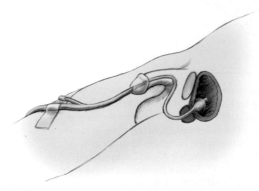

FIG. 26-30   Secure the urinary catheter.
(From Davis JH et al: Essentials of clinical surgery, St Louis, 1991, Mosby.)

PRINCIPLES OF PATIENT SKIN PREPARATION

The purpose of skin preparation is to render the surgical site as free as possible from transient and resident microorganisms, dirt, and skin oil so that the incision can be made through the skin with minimal danger of infection from this source.

Many surgeons prefer to have their patients bathe with antimicrobial soap the morning of the surgical procedure. The patient should be advised to avoid the use of body emollients, oils, creams, and lotions after washing. Some products decrease the efficacy of antimicrobial soap, and other products prevent adherence of electrodes to the skin.

The perioperative nurse should assess the patient's skin before, during, and after the prepping process. It is important to document the condition of the patient's tissues, noting lesions and other markings as appropriate. Abnormal skin irritation, infection, or abrasion on or near the surgical site might be a contraindication to the surgical procedure and is reported to the surgeon. Patients who have been involved in accidents or injured during the commission of a crime may be bearing physical marks or materials important to the investigation. Objective description of injuries that may include sketches on the record is part of the chain of evidence. Any material on the patient's person could be evidence and should be handled according to facility policy.

PRELIMINARY PREPARATION OF THE PATIENT'S SKIN
Hair Removal

Hair removal can injure skin and many surgeons no longer request hair removal. Hair surrounding the surgical site may be so thick that removal is necessary. Hair may be removed with clippers, by applying a depilatory cream, or by shaving with a razor. Hair may interfere with exposure, closure, or dressing. It may also prevent adequate skin contact with dispersive electrosurgical electrodes or electrocardiograph (ECG) leads.

Hair removal is carried out per the surgeon's order as close to the scheduled time for the surgical procedure as possible. The patient is covered to expose only the area to be shaved. Bath blankets are useful for preventing unnecessary exposure and prevent excess body heat loss during the procedure. The patient may be shaved in the OR after the anesthetic has been administered. Care is taken to not let stray hair remain in the surgical field. A wide piece of adhesive tape can be used to collect stray hair.

Clippers. Electric clippers with fine teeth cut hair close to the skin. The short stubble, usually about a millimeter in length, does not interfere with skin antisepsis or exposure of the surgical site. Clipping can be done using short strokes against the direction of hair growth. The blade lies flat against the skin surface. After use, a reusable blade assembly is disassembled, cleaned, and terminally sterilized. The clipper handle is cleaned and disinfected. Cordless handles with rechargeable batteries are available. Disposable clipper heads are preferred over reusable styles for sharpness and optimal function.

Depilatory Cream. Hair can be removed by chemical depilation before the patient comes to the OR suite. A preliminary skin patch is tested on a forearm before general application. If the patient is not sensitive, a thick layer of cream is applied over the hair to be removed. Depilatories should not be used around the eyes or genitalia. After the cream has remained on the skin for the required time, usually about 20 minutes, it is washed off. The hair comes off in the cream. The skin is intact and free from cuts, but any evidence of irritation should be documented.

Razor. Shaving should be performed as near the time of incision as possible if this method is used. Avoid making nicks and cuts in the skin. Gloves should be worn to prevent blood exposure if a nick should occur. Nicks made immediately before the surgical procedure (i.e., up to 30 minutes) are considered clean wounds. However, nicks and abrasions made several hours before the procedure may present as inflamed wounds at the time of surgical incision. The surgeon should be notified if the skin is not intact at the surgical site. This could be cause for cancellation of the surgical procedure. The time lapse between the preoperative shave and the surgical procedure may increase the risk of postoperative infection.

Wet shaving is preferable to dry shaves, which can leave the skin abraded. Soaking hair in lather allows keratin to absorb water, making hair softer and easier to remove. A sharp, clean razor blade should be used. The skin is held taut and is shaved by stroking in the direction of hair growth. Blades are discarded in the appropriate sharps container. If disposable razors are not used, the razor, minus the blade, is decontaminated and terminally sterilized between uses.

Skin Degreasing

The skin surface is composed of cornified epithelium with a coating of secretions that include perspiration, oils, and desquamated epithelium. These surface sebaceous lubricants are insoluble in water. Therefore, a skin degreaser or fat solvent may be used to enhance adhesion of ECG or other electrodes. It also may be used before skin preparation to improve adhesion of self-adhering drapes or to prevent smudging of skin markings. Isopropyl alcohol and acetone are effective fat solvents. A fat-solvent emollient is incorporated into some antiseptic agents. Some solvents, such as alcohol, are flammable and must be allowed to completely dry before draping. Vapors can become a fire hazard if trapped beneath surgical drapes.

SURGICAL SKIN CLEANSING FUNDAMENTALS

Before beginning the positioning and prepping sequence, ask the patient to verbally state the location and to point to and touch the site if possible. The correct site should have been marked with indelible ink before the patient is brought to the OR, as part of the identification process. Before amputation of an extremity, expose the opposite limb also for comparison. Check with the surgeon, the permit, and the notes in the chart. Confirm that the correct area is identified by the surgery schedule as well. Double-check the radiographs to be sure they have not been hung in the view box backward.

After the patient is anesthetized and positioned on the operating bed, the skin at the surgical site and an extensive area surrounding it is exposed and cleansed with an anti-septic agent immediately before draping. Towels should be tucked in at the patient's sides to catch any runoff. The two-step skin preparation employing scrub soap and paint is performed wearing sterile gloves. The one-step prep is essentially a layer of alcohol-based solution performed while wearing nonsterile examination gloves. The end result of antisepsis of the skin is essentially the same. Keep in mind that skin is never sterile regardless of surgical cleansing method employed.

Care is taken when prepping areas of the body that may be delicate or potentially harmful to the patient, such as carotid arteries, occluded vessels, tumor masses, distended abdomens, traumatic wounds, eyes, ears, trachea, and questionably stable tissues. Areas marked by the surgeon preoperatively should be gently cleansed, so as not to wash off the markings. Some surgeons use surgical marking pens or surgical dyes, such as methylene blue, brilliant green, or alcohol-based gentian violet. Others may use heavy-duty black markers to delineate the surgical site.

Setup and Procedure for a Two-Step Prep

Some disposable skin preparation trays include gloves, disposable towels, prep sponges, and cotton-tipped applicators. Some disposable trays have containers of premeasured antiseptic cleansing solution (Fig. 26-31). Disposable trays without antiseptic agents can be packaged sterile or unsterile. These are referred to as dry trays and require the addition of the antiseptic cleansing solution of choice. If prepackaged disposable trays are not used, a sterile table is prepared by the scrub person with the following sterile items:

- Small table drape to create the sterile field.
- Sterile gloves.
- Two absorbent towels are used to prevent pooling under body parts along the sides of the area and to define the upper and lower limits of the area to be prepped.
- Two or three small basins for solutions (antiseptic scrub detergent, antiseptic paint solution, and sterile water or alcohol if requested by the surgeon). About 1 or 2 ounces of solution in each basin usually is sufficient.
- Gauze sponges (nonradiopaque), which may be 4 × 8 inches (10 × 20 cm) for large areas and 4 × 4 inches (10 × 10 cm) or 3 × 3 inches (7.5 × 7.5 cm) for small areas. These are not counted sponges from the instrument

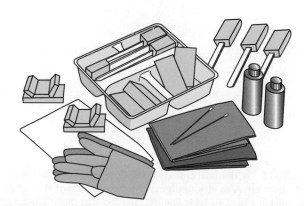

FIG. 26-31 Contents of a two-step prep tray depicted with textured sponges.

table and should be discarded in a trash container separate from the sponge bucket. Textured foam sponges may be preferred.

• Cotton-tipped applicators as necessary.

The antiseptic solutions are poured into each of the basins. One-half ounce of warm sterile water is added to the scrub soap basin to allow sudsing action of the agent.

Sterile gloves are donned by the person doing the prep using the open glove method for the two-step prep. A sterile setup is commonly used. Studies have shown that a clean but unsterile setup may be used for intact skin without compromising antimicrobial activity. Skin is mechanically cleansed and chemically decontaminated to reduce skin flora.

The surgical site is bordered by sterile towels after donning the sterile gloves. The sides of the patient are protected by towels to prevent runoff of excess solution. The cotton-tipped applicators are dipped into the soapy solution and used to cleanse the umbilicus if the umbilicus is part of the surgical site. The soiled applicators are discarded into the trash. Several sponges are placed into the soapy solution, and several are placed into the paint solution. A few sponges are reserved for use at the end of the prep if the surgeon incorporates an alcohol rinse. Each sponge is squeezed into the corresponding basin as to not soak the patient and the surrounding bed linens.

The soapy antiseptic sponges are used to mechanically and chemically cleanse the skin in a circular or linear motion from the incisional site to the periphery (Fig. 26-32). The soap decreases the surface tension of the skin and permits the sponge to pick up and remove dirt and microbes from the skin. The sponge should not backtrack over the already prepped area. Each sponge is discarded in the trash after use and not placed in the sponge bucket. A towel is used to blot the soap from the site. It is fully opened and placed over the site and carefully lifted off without rubbing or dragging the fabric over the cleansed area.

The paint-style antiseptic solution is applied in the same manner, using a circular motion from the incisional site to the periphery. This solution is not blotted or wiped off. It should be allowed to dry. If the surgeon prefers, an alcohol sponge is sometimes used to complete the prep procedure. If alcohol is used, it is allowed to dry completely before drapes are applied, to minimize the risk of fire from trapped vapors.

Setup and Procedure for a One-Step Prep

A one-step prep is a self-contained unit that is constructed of a sponge applicator tip (like a shoe polish dauber) and a chamber containing antiseptic solution (Fig. 26-33). The unit is packed in a blister pack with two cotton-tipped applicators. A pack of sterile towels is opened and used to tuck in at the patient's sides and periphery of the surgical site. When taken from the package, the applicator is not handled under sterile conditions. The user wears nonsterile examination gloves to prevent the solution from getting on his or her hands. The product should not be permitted to come into contact with reusable equipment such as basins because it will not readily wash off.

To apply the prep solution, the unit is compressed at the working end to break the seal of the inner chamber and allow the solution to saturate the applicator tip. The cotton-tipped applicators are dipped into the saturated sponge and used to clean the umbilicus; these cotton-tipped applicators are then discarded. The sponge end is inverted and allowed to become the applicator end. The area to be prepped is painted in the same stroke direction as for a two-step prep. These one-step prep antiseptics have a thicker texture and dry like shellac and are not blotted off in any manner after application. The risk of pooling is minimized with these products because of their consistency. They mechanically hold cells in place over the skin surface and chemically kill microorganisms.

The manufacturer recommends not removing the product after the procedure but, instead, allowing it to wear off over time to provide a lasting antisepsis for up to 3 days. Alcohol can be used to remove the product if necessary, or remover solution is commercially available. A package insert includes patient take-home instructions about the product and the purpose for its presence on the skin.

The chemical action is the actual antiseptic agent (iodophor or chlorhexidine) in combination with an alcohol base.

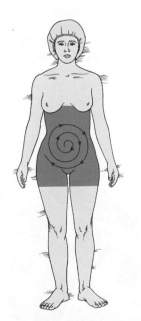

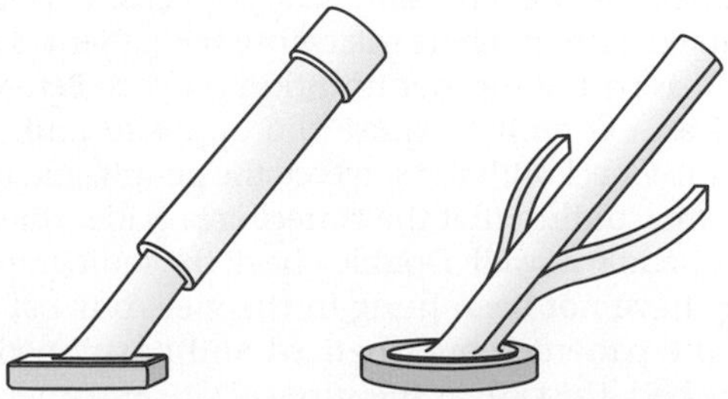

FIG. 26-32 Abdominal antiseptic skin preparation. Patient is in supine position. Area includes breast line to upper third of thighs, from table line right to table line left. Shaded area shows anatomic area to be cleansed with antiseptic. Arrows within area show direction of motion for skin preparation.

FIG. 26-33 One-step prep applicator.

The alcohol base can pose a fire hazard if not permitted to dry completely before draping. These items should not be heated in any way. They contain an ampule that can pressurize and explode in the presence of heat.

Prepping Areas Considered Contaminated

Umbilicus. Although the umbilicus is considered a contaminated area, prepping this central area of the abdomen after the surgical site can cause contamination. Some surgeons prefer the umbilicus to be cleaned with cotton-tipped swabs before the main incision. This prevents debris from the contaminated site splashing on the freshly prepped incision. This is a logical conclusion.

Stoma. Intestinal stomas are contaminated with fecal material and intestinal flora. The stoma should be isolated with a sterile clear plastic adhesive dressing and prepped last. If the stoma is to be incorporated with the surgical incision, it is prepped and dried last and covered by a sterile clear plastic adhesive dressing to prevent fecal material from entering the wound. Some surgeons pack the open end of the stoma with a Betadine-soaked radiopaque sponge. This sponge should be accounted for in the count tally at the end of the procedure. A nonradiopaque gauze sponge should not be used in the sterile field because it could become misplaced and be unaccounted for in the procedure.

Other Contaminated Areas. Other areas such as draining sinuses, skin ulcers, the vagina, and the anus are considered contaminated areas also. In all of these, the general rule of scrubbing the most contaminated area last with separate sponges applies. Use logic when determining the sequence for surgical prepping.

Foreign Substances. Adhesive, grease, tar, and similar foreign materials are removed from skin before the area is mechanically cleansed with an antiseptic agent. A nonirritating solvent should be used to cleanse the skin. The solvent should be nonflammable and nontoxic. Do not allow the solution to collect underneath the patient. Take care that the foreign substance in itself is not hazardous or flammable. Some chemicals can ignite when exposed to water or moisture.

Traumatic Wounds. In the preparation of an area in which the skin is not intact because of a traumatic injury, wound irrigation may be part of the skin preparation procedure. The wound may be packed or covered with sterile gauze while the area around it is thoroughly scrubbed and shaved if necessary. The extent and type of injury will determine the appropriate procedure. Protective gloves, eyewear, and a mask should be worn during the irrigation.

Solutions irritating to a denuded area must not be used. Small areas may be irrigated with warm sterile normal saline, with a bulb syringe. When a bulb syringe is used, care must be taken not to force debris and microorganisms deeper into the wound. The wound is irrigated gently to dislodge debris and flush it out. Soft nylon brushes are sometimes used.

Copious amounts of warm sterile solutions may be needed to flush out a large wound. A container of warm sterile normal saline or Ringer's lactate solution attached to IV tubing can be hung on an IV pole near the area to be copiously irrigated. If the area is on an extremity, a sterile irrigating pan with a wire screen fitted over the top is placed under the extremity. During irrigation, solution runs from the wound into the pan. A piece of tubing connected to an outlet on the pan carries the irrigating solution into a kick bucket on the floor near the table.

It may be necessary to place dry towels or sheets under the patient if the area has not been protected during irrigation. A moisture-proof pad placed under the wound before irrigation will help channel solutions into a drainage pan.

Debridement of the wound (excision of all devitalized tissue) usually follows irrigation. The surgeon may request to have sterile tissue forceps and scissors on the prep table for removal of nonviable tissue.

Areas Prepared for Grafts. Separate setups are necessary for skin preparation of recipient and donor sites before skin, bone, or vascular grafting procedures. The donor site is usually scrubbed first.

The donor site for a skin graft should be scrubbed with a colorless antiseptic agent so that the surgeon can properly evaluate the vascularity of the graft postoperatively. The recipient site for skin grafts is usually more or less contaminated (e.g., after a burn or other traumatic injury). Items used in preparation of the recipient site must not be permitted to contaminate the donor site. Also, microorganisms on the skin of the donor site must not be transferred to a denuded recipient site.

ANTISEPTIC SOLUTIONS

The infection control committee usually determines the chemical antiseptic or antimicrobial agent(s) to be used in the OR for skin preparation. Products selected by the committee are commonly the same ones selected for use as hand and skin antisepsis of the sterile team. The maximum concentration of a germicidal agent that can be used on skin and mucous membranes is limited by the agent's toxicity for these tissues. The ideal antiseptic skin cleansing agent should have the following qualities:

- It has broad-spectrum antimicrobial action and rapidly decreases the microbial count. It should be virucidal and be active against protozoa and yeasts.
- It can be quickly applied and remains effective against microorganisms.
- It can be safely used without skin irritation or sensitization. It should be nontoxic.
- It effectively remains active in the presence of alcohol, organic matter, soap, or detergent.
- It should be nonflammable when dried for use with laser, electrosurgical, or other high-energy devices.

Chlorhexidine Gluconate

Chlorhexidine gluconate was discovered in 1950 in England. A solution of 2% to 4% chlorhexidine gluconate is used as an antiseptic skin cleansing soap preoperatively. A tincture of 0.5% chlorhexidine gluconate in 70% isopropyl alcohol (Hibitane) is sometimes used. A broad-spectrum, rapid-acting antimicrobial agent, it binds to negative charges on microbial cell walls to produce irreversible damage and death. It has minimal activity against yeasts, spores, and tuberculosis. It is effective against most viruses.

Activity is adversely affected by traces of soap and is reduced in the presence of organic matter. If chlorhexidine is used in combination with personal soaps and shampoos for preoperative bathing, it is inactivated. The patient should be instructed to shampoo his or her hair with personal shampoo and thoroughly rinse before applying chlorhexidine as a body wash. Body lotion should not be applied after bathing, since this will nullify the residual bacteriostatic properties of the compound. The patient should be instructed to keep chlorhexidine out of the eyes and ears.

This agent is not absorbed through intact skin but binds with mucous membranes. It significantly reduces and maintains a reduction of microbial flora, such as bacteria and yeasts, for at least 4 hours. The prolonged effect is inhibited if chlorhexidine is combined with iodine preparations. Its activity increases at elevated temperature because it binds with the stratum corneum. It is available either tinted for color demarcation of the skin area being prepped or non-tinted if the surgeon needs to observe the skin color. Because it is an irritant to the eyes and ototoxic, it is contraindicated for facial antisepsis. If chlorhexidine gets on clothing, chlorine bleach is avoided because it will permanently stain the fabric. Clothing should be rinsed with cold water until all traces of the product have been removed.

Iodine and Iodophors

Discovered in 1812, iodine was first used in wound care in 1839. A solution of 1% or 2% iodine in water or in 70% alcohol is an excellent antiseptic. However, potential hazards of skin irritations and burns led to a decline in its use. If used, iodine should dry and then be rinsed off with 70% alcohol to neutralize the damaging effect.

Iodophors are iodine compounds that may be combined with detergents. Povidone-iodine has a surfactant, a wetting and dispersive agent, in an aqueous solution such as Betadine surgical scrub—a commonly used detergent form of iodophor. The detergent form should be rinsed off. Iodophor solution without detergent can be used for rinsing. Iodophor in 70% alcohol also is available. Iodophors are excellent cleansing agents that remove debris from skin surfaces while slowly releasing iodine. They are broad-spectrum antimicrobial agents that have some virucidal and sporicidal activity. Iodophors are relatively nontoxic and virtually nonirritating to skin or mucous membranes.

The brown film left on the skin after application of the solution clearly defines the area of application. This should not be wiped off because microbial activity is sustained by the release of free iodine as the agent dries and color fades from the skin. It should remain on the skin for at least 2 minutes. To hasten drying of the skin, alcohol may be painted on the area without friction before a self-adhering drape is applied. The alcohol must not be permitted to pool and must be completely dry before draping.

Iodophors are not to be used to prep the skin of patients who are sensitive or allergic to iodine or seafood. Shellfish, for example, contains iodine. The association with an actual allergy is more an issue with systemic problems as opposed to topical sensitivity.

The type of preparation, concentration of iodine, and presence of surfactants affect the microbial activity of products. Povidone-iodine complexes are available in solution, spray, or gel forms. Tinctures are in solution. The manufacturer's instructions are strictly followed for the product in use. The concentration of povidone-iodine may be altered by evaporation if the solution is warmed. Skin irritation may be caused by an increase in iodine concentration. The manufacturer's recommendations should be followed.

Alcohol

Isopropyl and ethyl alcohols are broad-spectrum agents that denature proteins in cells. A 70% concentration with continuous contact for several minutes is satisfactory for skin antisepsis if the surgeon prefers a colorless solution that permits observation of true skin color. Because alcohol coagulates protein, it is not applied to mucous membranes or used on an open wound. Isopropyl alcohol is a more effective fat solvent than is ethyl alcohol. Both are volatile and flammable. They must not pool around or under the patient, especially if an electrosurgical unit (ESU) or laser will be used. Vapors can accumulate under the drapes and become an explosion hazard.

Triclosan

A solution of 0.25% to 3% triclosan is a broad-spectrum antimicrobial agent that can be used for surgical antisepsis.[2] Triclosan is chemically related to hexachlorophene and is pregnancy category C. It interferes with the enzymes needed for fatty-acid synthesis in bacterial cells.

It is incorporated into many over-the-counter products used by consumers, such as deodorants and bath soaps. It is blended with oils and lanolin in a mild detergent. Cumulative suppressive action develops slowly only with prolonged routine use. It is considered nontoxic and safe for use on the face, but do not allow the solution to enter the eyes or other denuded tissues. Studies are under way to determine the efficacy of triclosan in dentifrice preparations as a plaque-control agent. Triclosan containing agents include Septisol 0.25% triclosan manufactured by STERIS, and Dial Liquid Gold 3% triclosan from the Dial Corporation, a subsidiary of the Henkel Group.

Parachlorometaxylenol

Originally developed in 1948 in Europe as a hair conditioner, parachlorometaxylenol (PCMX) has bactericidal properties useful for skin antisepsis. It is effective against some fungi, tuberculosis, and viruses. PCMX has residual properties with repeated use. It is nontoxic to the skin, eyes, and ears.

SKIN PREPARATION FOR SPECIFIC ANATOMIC AREAS
Head and Neck
Eye
1. The eyebrows are never shaved or removed unless the surgeon deems this essential. Eyebrows do not grow back completely or evenly.

---

[2]www.cdc.gov, Guideline for Prevention of SSI, *Federal Register* 20(4):257, 1999.

2. The eyelashes may be trimmed, if ordered by the surgeon, with fine iris scissors coated with sterile water-soluble lubricant to catch the lashes.
3. The eyelids and periorbital areas are cleansed with a nonirritating antiseptic agent, commonly triclosan detergent, and then rinsed with warm sterile water. The prep starts centrally and extends to the periphery (i.e., from the center of the lid to the brow and cheek).
4. The conjunctival sac is flushed with a nontoxic agent, such as sterile normal saline, with a bulb syringe. Some surgeons use a dilute iodophor solution (not the detergent). The patient's head is turned slightly to the affected side. The solution is contained with sponges or an absorbent towel. Care must be taken to prevent prep solution from entering the patient's eyes or ears.

   Chlorhexidine is contraindicated for facial preps. Iodophors are used with caution around the eyes. Chlorhexidine gluconate and iodophors can cause corneal damage if accidentally introduced into the eyes or can cause sensorineural deafness if the agent enters the inner ear (e.g., through a perforated tympanic membrane).

Ears, Face, or Nose
1. Usually it is not easy to define the area with towels. As much of the surrounding area is included as is feasible and consistent with aseptic technique. Skin surfaces should be cleansed at least to the hairline.
2. Cotton applicators are used for cleansing the nostrils and external ear canals.
3. Protect the eyes with a piece of sterile plastic sheeting. If the patient is awake, ask that the eyes be kept closed during the prep. Cotton balls should be placed in the ears to prevent runoff.

Neck
1. One sterile towel is folded under the edge of the blanket and gown, which are turned down almost to the nipple line.
2. The area includes the neck laterally to the table line and up to the mandible, tops of the shoulders, and chest almost to the nipple line.
3. For combined head and neck surgical procedures, include the face to the eyes; the shaved areas of the head, ears, and posterior neck; and the area over the shoulders.

Chest and Trunk
Lateral Thoracoabdominal Area
1. The gown is removed. The blanket is turned down well below the lower limit of the area to be prepared. A towel is folded under the edge of the blanket.
2. The arm is held up during the prep.
3. Beginning at the site of incision, the area may include the axilla, chest, and abdomen from the neck to the iliac crest. For a surgical procedure in the region of the kidney, it extends up to the axilla and down to the pubis. The area also extends beyond midlines, anteriorly and posteriorly, and may include the arm to the elbow (Fig. 26-34).

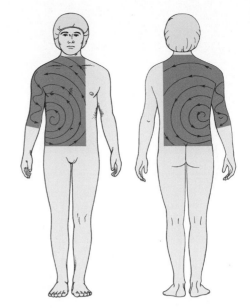

FIG. 26-34 Lateral thoracoabdominal antiseptic skin preparation. Patient is in lateral position. Area includes axilla, chest, and abdomen from neck to iliac crest. Area extends beyond midline, anteriorly and posteriorly.

Chest and Breast
1. The anesthesia provider turns the patient's face toward the unaffected side.
2. One towel is folded under the blanket edge, just above the pubis. Another is placed on the operating bed under the shoulder and side.
3. The arm on the affected side is held up by grasping the hand and raising the shoulder and axilla slightly from the operating bed.
4. The area includes the shoulder, upper arm down to the elbow, axilla, and chest wall to the table line and beyond the sternum to the opposite shoulder (Fig. 26-35).

Shoulder
1. The anesthesia provider turns the patient's face toward the opposite side.
2. A towel is placed under the shoulder and axilla.
3. The arm is held up by grasping the hand and elevating the shoulder slightly from the operating bed.
4. The area includes the circumference of the upper arm to below the elbow, from the base of the neck over the shoulder, scapula, and chest to the midline.

Rectoperineal Area
1. With the patient in lithotomy position, a moisture-proof pad is placed under the buttocks and extends to the kick bucket that receives solutions and discarded sponges.
2. The area includes the pubis, external genitalia, perineum and anus, and inner aspects of the thighs (Fig. 26-36).
3. Begin the scrub over the pubic area, scrubbing downward over the genitalia and perineum. Discard the sponge.

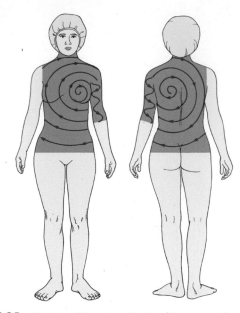

FIG. 26-35 Chest and breast antiseptic skin preparation. Area includes shoulder, upper arm down to elbow, axilla, and chest wall to table line and beyond sternum to opposite shoulder. If patient is in lateral position, back is prepped also.

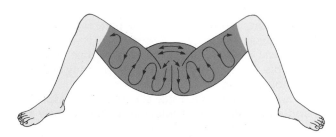

FIG. 26-36 Rectoperineal and vaginal antiseptic skin preparation. Area includes pubis, vulva, labia, perineum, anus, and adjacent area, including inner aspects of upper third of thighs. The inner aspect of the vagina is prepped after the external vulva is prepped. The anus is prepped last.

4. The inner aspects of the upper third of both thighs are scrubbed with separate sponges working from groin to distal aspect of thigh.
5. The anus is prepped last.
6. The rectoperineal area is prepped before the abdomen, using a separate prep set and gloves if an abdominal approach is planned.

Vagina

1. Sponge forceps should be included on the preparation table for a vaginal prep, because a portion of the prep is done internally. A disposable vaginal prep tray, with sponge sticks included, is available.
2. With the patient in lithotomy position, a moisture-proof pad is placed under the buttocks and extends to the kick bucket that receives solutions and discarded sponges.
3. A towel is folded under the edge of the blanket above the pubis.

4. Urinary catheterization is performed if indicated. Vaginal and anal flora should not be permitted to enter the sterile environment of the urinary bladder.
5. The external area includes the pubis, vulva, labia, perineum, anus, and adjacent area, including inner aspects of the upper third of the thighs (see Fig. 26-36).
6. Begin over the pubic area, scrubbing downward over the vulva and perineum. The inner aspects of the thighs are scrubbed with separate sponges from the labia majora outward.
7. The vagina and cervix are cleansed with sponges on sponge forceps or disposable sponge sticks. The cleansing agent should be applied generously in the vagina, because vaginal mucosa has many folds and crevices that are not easily cleansed.
8. After thoroughly cleansing the vagina, wipe it out with a dry sponge to prevent the possibility of the fluid entering the peritoneal cavity during the surgical procedure on pelvic organs.
9. The anus is prepped last to prevent intestinal florae from entering the vaginal vault.

Extremities

1. A moisture-proof pad should be placed on the operating bed under an extremity to retain runoff solution. This is removed after the prep so that the bed will be dry under the surgical site. The extremity is supported by personnel wearing sterile gloves and remains elevated until sterile drapes are applied under and around the prepped area.
2. A full extremity prep may be done in two stages to provide adequate support to joints and to ensure that all areas are scrubbed. It may include the foot for hip, thigh, knee, and lower leg procedures.
3. Caution must be taken to prevent solution from pooling under a tourniquet. The padding will absorb the solution and could cause tissue maceration. If a nonsterile pneumatic tourniquet is used, it is positioned before the prep and protected by a sterile clear plastic drape. A towel tucked under the tourniquet cuff absorbs excess solution. This is removed before the tourniquet is inflated.

Upper Arm

1. A towel is placed under the shoulder and axilla.
2. The arm is held up by grasping the hand and elevating the shoulder slightly from the operating bed.
3. The area includes the entire circumference of the arm to the wrist, the axilla, and over the shoulder and scapula.

Elbow and Forearm

1. A towel is placed under the shoulder and axilla.
2. The arm is held up by grasping the hand.
3. The area includes the entire arm from the shoulder and axilla to and including the hand.

Hand

1. Towels may be omitted. The anatomy of the hand furnishes sufficient landmarks to define the area, and towels are apt to slip over the scrubbed area.

2. The arm must be held up by a gloved person supporting it above the elbow so that the entire circumference can be scrubbed.
3. The area includes the hand and arm to 3 inches (7.5 cm) above the elbow.

Hip

1. One towel is placed under the thigh on the operating bed. Another towel is placed on the abdomen and folded under the edge of the gown, just above the umbilicus.
2. The leg on the affected side is held up by supporting it just below the knee.
3. The area includes the abdomen on the affected side, the thigh to the knee, the buttocks to the table line, the groin, and the pubis (Fig. 26-37).

Thigh

1. One towel is placed under the thigh on the operating bed. Another towel is placed on the abdomen and folded under the edge of the gown, just below the umbilicus.
2. The leg is held up by supporting the foot and ankle.
3. The area includes the entire circumference of the thigh and leg to the ankle, over the hip and buttocks to the table line, the groin, and the pubis. Take care not to allow the solution to pool under the patient's buttocks.

Knee and Lower Leg

1. A towel is placed over the groin.
2. The leg is held up by supporting it at the foot.
3. The area includes the entire circumference of the leg and extends from the foot to the upper part of the thigh (Fig. 26-38).

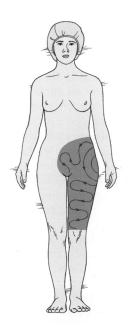

FIG. 26-37 Hip antiseptic skin preparation. Area includes abdomen on affected side, thigh to knee, buttock to table line, groin, and pubis.

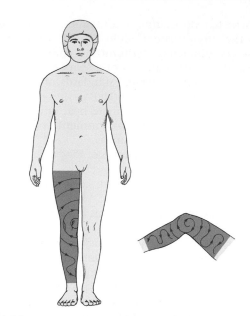

FIG. 26-38 Knee and lower leg antiseptic skin preparation. Area includes entire circumference of affected leg and extends from foot to upper part of thigh. Upper extremity is prepped in the same manner.

Ankle and Foot

1. Towels are omitted.
2. The foot is held up by supporting the leg at the knee. A leg-holder device is useful.
3. The area includes the foot and entire circumference of the lower leg to the knee.

DOCUMENTATION

Details of the preoperative skin condition and preparation should be documented in the patient's intraoperative record. These should include but are not limited to the following:

- The condition of the skin around the surgical site and placement sites of any electrodes
- Hair removal, if done, including the method and location, and areas for attachment of monitors or electrodes
- Antiseptic solutions, fat solvents, irrigating solutions, and any other agents used
- The skin area prepped and skin reaction, if any
- The name of the person who did the prep

DRAPING

Draping is the procedure of covering the patient and surrounding areas with a sterile barrier to create and maintain an adequate sterile field. An effective barrier eliminates or minimizes passage of microorganisms between nonsterile and sterile areas. Criteria to be met in establishing an effective barrier are that the material must be:

- Blood and fluid resistant to keep drapes dry and prevent migration of microorganisms. Material should be impermeable to moist microbial penetration (i.e., resistant to strike-through). Resistant to tearing, puncture, or abrasion that causes fiber breakdown and thus permits microbial penetration.

- Lint-free to reduce airborne contaminants and shedding into the surgical site. Cellulose and cotton fibers can cause granulomatous peritonitis or embolize arteries.
- Antistatic to eliminate risk of a spark from static electricity. Material must meet standards of the National Fire Protection Association (NFPA).
- Sufficiently porous to eliminate heat buildup so as to maintain an isothermic environment appropriate for the patient's body temperature.
- Drapable to fit around contours of the patient, furniture, and equipment.
- Dull, nonglaring to minimize color distortion from reflected light.
- Free of toxic ingredients, such as laundry residues, and nonfast dyes.
- Flame resistant to self-extinguish rapidly on removal of an ignition source. This is a concern with use of lasers, electrosurgical units (ESUs), and other high-energy devices that provide an ignition source at the sterile field. Drapes become fuel for a fire. Some materials are more flammable than others; some are fire-retardant.

DRAPING MATERIALS
Self-Adhering Sheeting

Sterile, waterproof, antistatic, and transparent or translucent plastic sheeting may be applied to dry skin.

Incise Drape. The entire clear plastic drape has an adhesive backing that is applied to skin. This may be applied separately, or the sheeting may be incorporated into the drape sheet. The skin incision is made through the plastic.

Antimicrobial incise drapes have an antimicrobial agent impregnated in the adhesive or the polymeric film. A film coated with an iodophor-containing adhesive, for example, slowly releases active iodine during the surgical procedure to effectively inhibit proliferation of organisms from the patient's skin. The antimicrobial may be triclosan or another agent that does not contain iodine. The skin may be prepped with alcohol and allowed to dry before the drape is applied. Time is a factor in microbial accumulation from resident bacteria. Antimicrobial incise drapes are used, particularly for procedures lasting more than 3 hours, to sustain suppression.

Towel Drape. The plastic sheeting has a band of adhesive along one edge. Used as a draping towel, it will remain fixed on skin without towel clips. This is advantageous when clips might obscure the view of a part exposed to x-rays during the surgical procedure. It also is used to wall off a contaminated area, such as a stoma, from the clean skin area to prevent spilling contents and causing infection or chemical irritation.

Aperture Drape. Adhesive surrounds a fenestration (opening) in the plastic sheeting. This secures the drape to the skin around the surgical site, such as an eye or ear. Caution is used in applying this type of drape around the face of a patient who is awake. The patient must have breathing space. Some patients experience claustrophobia. Fabric towels may not feel as confining.

Advantages of Self-Adhering Drape Material

- Resident microbial flora from skin pores, sebaceous glands, and hair follicles cannot migrate laterally to the incision.
- Microorganisms do not penetrate the impermeable material.
- Landmarks and skin tones are visible through the transparent plastic.
- Inert adhesive holds drapes securely, eliminating the need for towel clips and possible puncture of the patient's skin.
- Plastic sheeting conforms to body contours and has elasticity to stretch without breaking its adhesion to skin.

Some self-adhering drapes have sufficient moisture-vapor permeability to reduce excessive moisture buildup that could macerate the skin and/or loosen adhesive. A nonporous material should not cover more than 10% of the body surface because it may interfere with the patient's thermal regulatory mechanism of perspiration evaporation. The heat-retaining property of plastic causes the patient to perspire excessively, but its nonporous nature prevents evaporation.

This material is used in the following manner:
1. The usual skin preparation is done.
2. The scrubbed area must be dry. It may dry by evaporation, or excess solution may be blotted or wiped off with a sterile sponge or towel. Alcohol may be applied after an iodophor scrub to hasten drying by evaporation.
3. Transparent plastic material is applied firmly to the skin, with the initial contact along the proposed line of incision. The drape is smoothed away from the incision area.
4. Regular fabric drapes are applied over the plastic sheeting unless plastic is incorporated into the fenestrated area of the drape.

Nonwoven Fabric Disposable Drapes

Most nonwoven disposable materials are compressed layers of synthetic fibers (i.e., rayon, nylon, or polyester) combined with cellulose (wood pulp) and bonded together chemically or mechanically without knitting, tufting, or weaving. This material may be either nonabsorbent or absorbent. Polypropylene and foil also are used. Those fabrics that comply with criteria for establishing an effective barrier have the following advantages as disposable drapes:

- They are moisture-repellant; they retard blood and aqueous fluid moisture strike-through to prevent contamination. Not all nonwoven fabrics have this characteristic; only nonabsorbent materials or those laminated with plastic are impermeable to moisture.
- They are lightweight, yet strong enough to resist tears.
- They are lint-free unless cellulose fibers are torn or cut.
- Contaminants are disposed of along with drapes.
- They are antistatic and flame-retardant for OR use.
- They are prepackaged and sterilized by the manufacturer, which eliminates washing, mending, folding, and sterilizing processes.

Some drapes have a reinforced area of multiple layers surrounding the fenestration. The outer layer absorbs fluids, but the underneath layer is impermeable to strike-through. An antimicrobial may be incorporated into this reinforced area. Other drapes have an impermeable layer around the fenestration. Drapes that are completely laminated with a plastic layer may be used for an extremity or for instrument table covers. They are not used over the entire body of the patient because of their heat retention property.

Many nonwoven drapes have pouches or troughs incorporated close to the fenestration or along the sides of the drape to collect fluids, such as amniotic fluid. The pouch may have drainage ports, or fluid may be suctioned out. Some drapes also have pockets, skid-resistant instrument pads, and/or devices for holding cords incorporated in them (Fig. 26-39).

Laser-Resistant Drapes. Nonwoven drapes that contain cellulose ignite and burn easily. Polypropylene drapes will not ignite, but they can melt. An aluminum-coated drape may be safest for use with lasers, especially around the oxygen-enriched environment of the head and neck area.

Thermal Drape. An aluminum-coated plastic body cover reflects radiant body heat back to the patient to reduce intraoperative heat loss. A sterile, nonconductive, radiolucent thermal drape may be used as the final drape. The patient may be wrapped in nonsterile reflective covers (Thermadrape) in the preoperative holding area. These may remain in place through the surgical procedure under standard sterile drapes and during postoperative recovery in the postanesthesia care unit (PACU). A reflective blanket or thermal drape is recommended when more than 60% of the body surface can be covered and when the surgical procedure will last more than 2 hours.

Nonwoven, disposable drapes are supplied prepackaged and presterilized by the manufacturer. A sterile package may contain a single drape, or it may have all of the drapes needed for a procedure, including towels, a Mayo stand and instrument table covers, and gowns. Unused disposable drapes and gowns should not be resterilized unless the manufacturer provides written instructions for reprocessing.

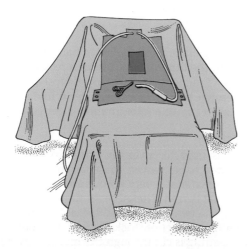

FIG. 26-39 Fenestrated laparotomy drape sheet with reinforcement around fenestration.

Woven Textile Fabrics

The thread count and finish of woven natural fibers determine the integrity and porosity of reusable fabrics. Tightly woven textile fabrics may inhibit migration of microorganisms. Cotton fibers swell when they become wet. This swelling action closes pores or interstices so that liquid cannot diffuse through tightly woven fibers. The fabric can be treated to further repel fluids (i.e., be impermeable to moisture strike-through). Reusable drapes may be made of 270- or 280-thread-count pima cotton with a Quarpel finish. This fluorochemical finish combined with phenazopyridine or a melanin hydrophobe produces a durable water-resistant fabric. However, this fabric has essentially the same heat-retaining qualities as plastic lamination, so it cannot be used for complete patient draping. This treated material can be used as reinforcement around fenestrations in otherwise untreated drapes.

Tightly woven 100% polyester reusable fabrics are hydrophobic (repel water droplets) but allow vapor permeation. Other reusable fabrics with different construction but similar barrier properties may be used.

The following points about reusable woven textile drapes should be considered:

- Material must be steam-penetrable and must withstand multiple sterilization cycles.
- When packaged for sterilization, drapes must be properly folded and arranged in sequence of use. Drapes may be fan-folded or rolled.
- Material must be free from holes and tears. The person who folds the drape is responsible for inspecting it for holes. Those detected may be covered with heat-seal patches. Tears or punctures (e.g., from towel clips or sharp instruments) compromise barrier qualities of drapes.
- Drapes should be sufficiently impermeable to prevent moisture from soaking through them. Moisture has a wicking action that can cause migration of microorganisms.
- Reusable fabrics must maintain barrier qualities through multiple launderings. Densely woven, treated cotton will become moisture permeable after about 75 washings; untreated cotton will become moisture permeable after as few as 30 washings. Repeated drying, ironing, and steam sterilizing also alter fabric structure. The number of uses, washings, and sterilizing cycles should be recorded, and drapes that are no longer effective as barriers should be taken out of use.

STYLE/TYPE OF DRAPES
Towels

Disposable or reusable sterile towels may be used to outline, or square off the surgical site after prepping the skin. The folded edge of each towel is placed toward the line of incision to square it off. Towels are usually packaged in groups of four by the inhouse laundry and can be secured with nonperforating towel clips or may be sutured or stapled to skin. Radiopaque towels in counted packages are commercially available. Some disposable types have adhesive strips to hold them in place.

Surgical towels are traditionally used as draping material and therefore are not routinely considered counted items.

However, if a surgical towel is placed in the surgical incision, it becomes an item that must be accounted for and is listed by the same mechanism that is in place to track any other counted items.

The scrub person reports to the circulating nurse that a towel has been placed in the incision. The circulating nurse writes down the number of towels placed inside the patient on the count tally sheet or wipe-off board. At the conclusion of the surgical procedure the scrub reports how many towels have been removed and the number is validated by the circulating nurse during the final count. Counts are documented as correct or incorrect per facility policy.

The literature is replete with horror stories about surgical towels that carelessly become retained foreign objects when the team fails to account for them. Anything that becomes part of the incisional packing is considered a counted item.

Fenestrated Sheets

The drape sheet has an opening (fenestration) that is placed to expose the anatomic area where the incision will be made. Many styles of disposable nonwoven or reusable woven fabrics are available for specific uses. The size, direction, and shape of the fenestration vary to give adequate exposure of the surgical site. The sheet is long enough to cover the anesthesia screen at the head and extend down over the foot of the operating bed. Fenestrated sheets are usually marked to indicate the direction in which they should be unfolded. This may be an arrow or label designating the top or head, bottom or foot. It is wide enough to cover one or two armboards.

Reinforcement around the fenestration (see Fig. 26-39) for both nonwoven and woven fabrics provides an extra thickness to minimize the passage of microorganisms by capillary action to the sterile field. The reinforced area is usually 24 inches (60 cm) wide.

The drapes described are basic styles of fenestrated sheets.

Laparotomy Sheet. The laparotomy sheet is often referred to as a lap sheet; the longitudinal fenestration is placed over the surgical site on the abdomen, back, or a comparable area (see Fig. 26-37). The opening is large enough to give adequate exposure in the usual laparotomy. The sheet is at least 108 × 72 inches (274 × 183 cm).

Thyroid Sheet. The thyroid sheet is the same size as a laparotomy sheet. The fenestration is transverse or diamond shape and is positioned closer to the top of the sheet over the neck area.

Chest Sheet. The chest sheet is similar to a laparotomy sheet except that the fenestration provides for a larger exposure. It is used for chest and breast procedures.

Hip Sheet. The hip sheet is similar to the laparotomy sheet but somewhat longer to completely cover the orthopedic fracture table.

Perineal Sheet. The perineal sheet is of adequate size to create a sterile field with the patient in the lithotomy position. Some styles have large leggings incorporated into it to cover the legs in stirrups. It may have one or two openings to accommodate the perineum and/or rectum.

Laparoscopy Sheet. A laparoscopy sheet is a combination laparotomy and perineal sheet. It is used for gynecologic laparoscopy in lithotomy or combined abdominoperineal resection with the patient in the lithotomy position.

Separate Sheets

Although fenestrated sheets are used for most surgical procedures, they are not always practical. The openings may be much too large for small incisions, such as taking specimens for biopsies or procedures on the hands or feet. Smaller, separate sheets may be used for these purposes, leaving exposed only the small surgical area, or for providing additional drapes on the surgical field. Many of these are disposable.

Split Sheet. The split sheet is the same size as a laparotomy sheet. Rather than being fenestrated, one end is cut longitudinally up the middle at least one third the length of the sheet to form two free ends (tails). The upper end of this split may be in the shape of a U. Adhesive strips on each tail approximately 8 inches (20 cm) from the end of the split adhere together to snug the drape around an extremity or head. Shorter styles have adhesive strips the full length of the inner aspect of the tails for circumferential wrapping.

Minor Sheet. The minor sheet is 36 × 45 inches (91 × 114 cm). It has many uses. Wrapped around an extremity, it permits the extremity to remain on the sterile field for manipulation during the surgical procedure. It is used under an arm to cover an armboard for shoulder, axillary, arm, or hand procedures.

Medium Sheet. The medium sheet is about 36 × 72 inches (91 × 183 cm). It is used to drape under legs, as an added protection above or below the surgical area, or for draping areas in which a fenestrated sheet cannot be used.

Single Sheet. The single sheet is 108 × 72 inches (274 × 183 cm). Folded lengthwise, it is placed above the sterile field to shield off the anesthesia provider and anesthesia machine or other equipment near the patient's head or operating bed. A single sheet also is used to cover the patient and operating bed below the surgical area around the face.

Leggings. Leg drapes are supplied in pairs to cover the legs of a patient in the lithotomy position. A rectangle, approximately 36 × 72 inches (91 × 183 cm), is closed on two sides to form a tentlike pocket. One open edge is folded into a cuff to protect gloves from contamination during application.

Stockinette

Stockinette is used to cover an extremity. This seamless tubing of stretchable woven material contours snugly to the skin. The material is very porous and absorbent, so it is not a microbial barrier. Therefore, it may be covered with a layer of plastic. A two-ply tubular disposable drape is available that has an inner layer of stockinette and an outer layer of vinyl. An opening is cut through the material over the line of incision. Edges may be secured with a plastic incise drape before the incision is made, or it may be clipped to the wound edges after the incision. Rolled elastic ACE or Coban bandage is sometimes used for this purpose. Care is taken to use nonlatex materials for patients sensitive to latex.

PRINCIPLES OF DRAPING

The entire team should be familiar with the draping procedure because draping is a very important step in the preparation of the patient for a surgical procedure. The scrub person should be knowledgeable and ready to assist with draping. The scrub person is responsible for seeing that necessary articles are arranged in proper sequence on the instrument table.

The person responsible for draping the patient may vary, as do materials and styles of drapes used to create a sterile field. The surgeon or assistant usually places the self-adhering incise drape and/or towels and towel clips to outline the surgical site. The scrub person assists with placing the remainder of the drapes.

During any draping procedure, the circulating nurse should stand by to direct the scrub person as necessary and to watch carefully for breaks in technique. A contaminated drape or exposure of a nonsterile area is a potential source of infection for the patient.

Basic principles regarding draping are as follows:

1. Place drapes on a dry area. The area around or under the patient may become damp from solutions used for skin preparation. The circulating nurse removes damp items or covers the area to provide a dry field on which to lay sterile drapes.
2. Allow sufficient time to permit careful application.
3. Allow sufficient space to observe sterile technique. Do not reach across a nonsterile surface.
4. Handle drapes as little as possible.
5. Never reach across the operating bed to drape the opposite side; go around it.
6. Take towels and towel clips, if used, to the side of the operating bed from which the surgeon is going to apply them before handing them to him or her.
7. Carry folded drapes to the operating bed. Watch the front of the sterile gown; it may bulge and touch the nonsterile operating bed or blanket on the patient. Stand well back from the nonsterile operating bed.
   a. Hold drapes high enough to avoid touching nonsterile areas, but avoid touching the overhead operating light.
   b. Hold a drape high until it is directly over the proper area, and then lay it down where it is to remain. Once a sheet is placed, do not adjust it. Be careful not to slide the sheet out of place when opening the folds.
   c. Protect gloved hands by cuffing the end of the sheet over them. Do not let gloved hands touch the skin of the patient.
8. In unfolding a sheet from the prepped area toward the foot or head of the operating bed, protect the gloved hand by enclosing it in a turned-back cuff of sheet provided for this purpose. Keep hands at table level.

9. If a drape becomes contaminated, do not handle it further. Discard it without contaminating gloves or other items.
   a. If the end of a sheet falls below waist level, do not handle it further. Drop it, and use another.
   b. If in doubt as to its sterility, consider a drape contaminated.
   c. If a drape is incorrectly placed, discard it. The circulating nurse peels it from the operating bed without contaminating other drapes or the prepped area.
10. A towel clip that has been fastened through a drape has its points contaminated. Remove it only if absolutely necessary, and then discard it from the sterile setup without touching the points. Cover the area from which it was removed with another piece of sterile draping material.
11. If a hole is found in a drape after it is laid down, the hole must be covered with another piece of draping material or the entire drape discarded.
12. A hair found on a drape must be removed, and the area must be covered immediately. Although hair can be sterilized, the source of a hair is usually unknown when it is found on a sterile drape. It would cause a foreign body tissue reaction in a patient if it got into the wound. Remove the hair with a hemostat, and hand the instrument off the sterile field; cover the area with a towel or another piece of draping material.

PROCEDURES FOR DRAPING THE PATIENT

Draping procedures establish the sterile field. Standardized methods of application should be practiced using adequate draping materials. The most common procedures are discussed here merely to elaborate the principles. The following details procedures using only absorbent woven draping materials, because it is more complex to establish a microbial barrier with them. The draping procedure is simplified when single-thickness impermeable materials are used. A procedure book should be consulted for specific draping procedures.

Laparotomy

The term *laparotomy* refers to an incision through the abdominal wall into the abdominal cavity. All flat, smooth areas are draped in the same manner as the abdomen. These areas include the neck, chest, flank, and back. The draping procedure is as follows:

1. Hand up four towels and towel clips. With practice, these can be held in the hands at the same time and separated one by one as the surgeon takes them. Go to the side of the operating bed on which the surgeon is draping to avoid reaching over the nonsterile table. The surgeon places these towels within the prepped area, leaving only the surgical area exposed.
2. Hand one end of a fan-folded medium sheet across the operating bed to the assistant, supporting the folds, keeping the sheet high, and holding it taut until it is opened; then lay it down. Place this medium sheet below the surgical site with the edge of it at the skin

edge, covering the draping towel. This sheet provides an extra thickness of material under the area from the Mayo stand to the incision, where instruments and sponges are placed, and closes some of the opening in the laparotomy sheet if necessary. This sheet may be eliminated if a self-adhering incise drape or impermeable drapes are used.

3. Place a laparotomy sheet with the opening directly over the prepped area outlined by the towels, in the direction indicated for the foot or head of the operating bed (Fig. 26-40). Drop the folds over the sides of the table. However, if an armboard is in place, hold the folds at table level until the sheet is opened all the way. Open it downward over the patient's feet first and then upward over the anesthesia screen (Fig. 26-41). Sheets with appropriate fenestrations are used to expose the surgical site.
   a. For the neck, use a thyroid sheet.
   b. For the chest, with the patient in either the supine or lateral position, use a breast sheet.
   c. For the flank, with the patient in the kidney position for transverse incision, use a kidney sheet.
   d. For the back, use a laparotomy sheet, the same as for the abdomen.
4. Place a large, single sheet crosswise on the operating bed above the fenestrated site. This sheet provides an extra thickness above the area and closes some of the opening in the laparotomy sheet if necessary. It also covers the armboard if one is in use. A single sheet may be needed for this latter purpose even if an impermeable laparotomy sheet is used.

Head

An overhead instrument table may be positioned over the patient for neurologic procedures. The table drape is extended down over the patient's shoulders to create a continuous sterile field between the instrument table and the surgical site. The draping procedure is as follows:

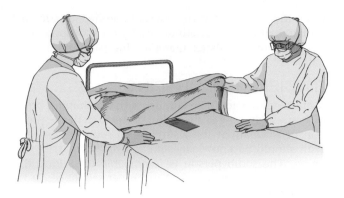

FIG. 26-41 Unfolding upper end of laparotomy sheet over anesthesia screen. Note that hands approaching unsterile area are protected in cuff of drape and that sheet is stabilized with other hand.

1. The surgeon places four towels around the head and secures them with towel clips or affixes them in place with sutures or skin staples. Towel clips and staples are not used if radiographs will be taken during the surgical procedure.
2. Hand one end of a fan-folded medium sheet to the assistant. Holding it taut, unfold and secure it over the head end of the operating bed below the surgical site at the skin edge of the draping towel.
3. Place a fenestrated sheet with the opening over the exposed skin area of the head. Unfold the sheet across the front edge of the overhead table, and secure it before allowing the remainder of the drape to drop over the head of the operating bed toward the floor. Some disposable fenestrated head sheets have transparent plastic adhesive incise sheeting to cover the incisional site. The incise sheet may be impregnated with iodophor for additional wound protection during the procedure.

Face

Even if the surgical site is unilateral, the surgeon may want the entire face exposed for comparison of skin lines. The draping procedure is as follows:

1. The surgeon places a drape under the head while the circulating nurse or assistant elevates the head. This drape consists of an open towel placed on a medium sheet. The center of the towel edge is 2 inches (5 cm) in from the center of the sheet edge. The towel is drawn up on each side of the face, over the forehead or at the hairline, and fastened with a small, nonperforating towel clip. This leaves the desired amount of the face exposed.
2. Hand up three additional towels and four towel clips. These towels frame the surgical site.
3. Place a medium sheet just below the site. This sheet must overlap the one under the head.
4. A fenestrated drape may be placed to complete draping.
5. Cover the remainder of the foot of the operating bed, as necessary, with a single sheet.

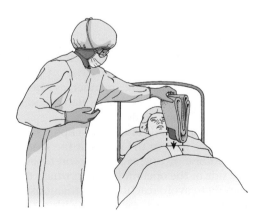

FIG. 26-40 Draping with sterile laparotomy sheet. Scrub person carries folded sheet to table. Standing far back from operating bed, with one hand, scrub person places the fenestration of the sheet on patient so that opening in sheet is directly over prepped skin area. A second sterile team member helps complete the opening of the drape over the body from the opposite side of the table.

If the patient is receiving inhalation anesthesia, use a minor sheet instead of a towel on a medium sheet for the first drape under the head. A minor sheet is large enough to draw up on each side of the face and to enclose the endotracheal tube and oropharyngeal monitoring probes from the anesthesia machine for a considerable distance, thus keeping them from contaminating the sterile field.

If the surgical procedure on the face is unilateral, the anesthesia provider may sit along the unaffected side, near the patient's head, with the anesthesia screen placed on the same side of the operating bed.

Skin staples or sutures may be used to affix towels around the contours of the face and neck of the patient under general anesthesia. Each staple or stitch overlaps the skin and edge of the drape.

Eye

After skin preparation, the unaffected eye is protected by covering it with a sterile eye pad before draping the patient. The draping procedure is as follows:

1. The surgeon places two towels and a medium sheet under the head while the circulating nurse holds the head up, as described for a face drape. One towel is drawn up around the head, exposing only the eyebrow and affected eye, and fastened with a clip without pressure on the eyes.
2. Hand up four towels and towel clips to isolate the affected eye. Some surgeons prefer a self-adhering aperture drape.
3. Cover the patient and remainder of the operating bed below the surgical area with a single sheet.

If local anesthetic will be administered, the drapes are raised off of the patient's nose and mouth to permit free breathing. A Mayo stand or anesthesia screen positioned over the lower face before the draping is one method used to elevate the drapes. Oxygen, 6 to 8 L/min, can be supplied under the drapes by tube or nasal cannula. Take extreme caution that oxygen does not build up under the drapes. An ignition source such as a cautery or laser could spark a fire beneath the drapes.

For a microsurgical procedure, a sterile, padded, U-shaped steel wrist rest for the surgeon and assistant is fastened to the head of the operating bed. Towels are put around the patient's head before the rest of the facial and body draping is completed.

If irrigation will be used, a plastic fenestrated drape is placed over the four towels to keep them dry if an aperture drape is not preferred.

Ear

The basic draping procedure is the same as for draping a face or eye, except that only the affected ear is exposed. The head will be turned toward the unaffected side. Oxygen can be supplied under the drapes, as previously described. The anesthesia provider is usually positioned at the side of the operating bed near the patient's face.

Chest and Breast

While the arm is still being held up by the assistant after skin preparation:

1. Place a minor sheet on an armboard, under the patient's arm, extending the sheet under the side of the chest and shoulder. The prepped arm is lowered to the sterile draped armboard. The distal portion of the arm may be encased in sterile stockinette so that the arm can be manipulated during the surgical procedure.
2. The patient's body is draped with a sterile medium sheet.
3. Hand up towels and towel clips; five or six are required.
4. Apply a breast sheet so that the axilla is exposed for anticipated axillary dissection.

Shoulder

While the arm is still being held up by the assistant after skin preparation:

1. Place medium sheets over the chest and under the arm.
2. Place a minor sheet under the shoulder and side of the chest.
3. The surgeon outlines the surgical site with towels and secures them with clips.
4. Place a minor sheet over the patient's chest, covering the neck. Keep this sheet even with the edge of the towel that borders the surgical site laterally.
5. Wrap the arm in a minor sheet or encase it in sterile stockinette, and secure it with a sterile gauze or elastic bandage. At this point, a sterile team member relieves the unsterile person who has been holding the arm.
6. Place a medium sheet above the area, and secure these sheets together with towel clips.
7. A laparotomy or breast sheet may be used. Pull the arm through the opening. Or a single sheet may be placed above the area, and the foot of the operating bed is covered with a medium sheet.

Elbow

While the arm is still being held up by the unsterile assistant after skin preparation:

1. Place a sterile medium sheet across the chest and under the arm, up to the axilla.
2. The surgeon defines the surgical area on the upper (proximal) arm by placing a towel around the upper arm and securing it with a towel clip.
3. Wrap the hand in a sterile towel. At this point, a sterile team member relieves the unsterile person who has been holding the arm by grasping the wrapped hand, maintaining the arm in an elevated position.
4. The hand is grasped with a sterile stockinette, which is pulled down over the entire arm toward the axilla, over the surgical site. An elastic bandage is wrapped around the arm starting at the distal end (hand) to the proximal area (axilla).
5. Place a medium sheet across the chest, on top of the arm, even with the towel on the upper arm and covering it. Secure this sheet around the arm with a towel clip.
6. An extremity sheet is drawn over the hand and the arm. The extremity sheet is opened in its entirety across the patient's body.

Hand

While the arm and hand are still being held up after skin preparation:

1. Place an impervious minor sheet, folded in half, on the extremity table.
2. The surgeon places a towel around the lower arm, limiting the exposed area to the affected hand, and secures it with a towel clip.
3. Pull stockinette over the hand and up over the length of the arm. At this stage in draping, the unsterile person is relieved of holding the arm. The draped arm is laid on the draped extremity table.
4. Place a minor sheet across the extremity table just above the surgical site.
5. Place an extremity sheet over the hand. Do not drop folds below the level of the armboard. Open the sheet across the patient's body toward the feet first. Attach the top end to the IV poles at the head of the bed.

Perineum

With the patient in the lithotomy position for a genital, vaginal, or rectal procedure:

1. Place a medium sheet under the buttocks. The circulating nurse can grasp the underside and assist in placement. With the patient's legs elevated in stirrups, this drape hangs below the level of the operating bed and covers the lowered section of the operating bed.
2. Slide legging over each leg, protecting the gloved hands in the folded cuffs.
3. The anus is covered if it is not part of the surgical site. An adhesive towel drape may be used for this purpose.
4. Place a medium sheet across the abdomen, from the level of the pubis, extending over the anesthesia screen or attached to IV poles at the head of the bed.
5. A fenestrated perineal sheet may be used rather than a medium sheet over the abdomen. To use a perineal sheet with built-in leggings, hand one end of the sheet to the assistant, opening out folds, and draw the leggings over the feet and legs simultaneously. The hands are kept on the outside of the sheet to avoid contaminating the gloves and gown.

Hip

The patient is in a lateral position. If the leg will be manipulated during the surgical procedure, while the leg is still being held up after skin preparation:

1. Place a medium sheet on the operating bed under the leg, up to the buttock.
2. Place another medium sheet on the operating bed, overlapping the first one, to cover the unaffected leg. Some surgeons prefer to use an incise sheet or a lower extremity stockinette.
3. The surgeon wraps the foot and leg with an elastic bandage, covering the stockinette. The leg, held up to this point, is laid on the operating bed.
4. Place a minor sheet lengthwise of the operating bed on each side of the exposed area, even with the skin. The sheets under the leg and above the site do not overlap. Some surgeons prefer to draw the leg through

the opening of a hip sheet or place a split sheet under the leg with the tails crossed over it toward the patient's head.
5. Place a medium sheet above the exposed area. Secure these last three sheets with towel clips.
6. Place a single sheet above the surgical area and over the anesthesia screen.

If manipulation of the leg is not necessary during the surgical procedure, drape the same as for a laparotomy, using a hip sheet instead of a laparotomy sheet.

Knee

While the leg is still being held up after skin preparation:

1. Place a medium sheet lengthwise on the operating bed, under the leg, up to the buttock. Take care not to contaminate sterile gloves on the unsterile tourniquet if used.
2. Place another medium sheet on the operating bed, overlapping the first sheet, to cover the unaffected leg.
3. The surgeon limits the sterile field above the knee by placing a towel around the leg and securing it with a towel clip.
4. Lay a minor sheet on the sterile sheets under the leg. The person who has been holding the leg lays it on this minor sheet. The surgeon wraps the leg in the minor sheet and secures it with a sterile bandage. Stockinette may be preferred for this step.
5. Place a medium sheet above the exposed area, at the skin edge, over the draping towel and fasten it with a towel clip.
6. Place a laparotomy or extremity sheet, with the opening on the foot and the longer part of the sheet toward the head of the operating bed. Open it, and draw the leg through the opening. A split sheet may be used.

Lower Leg and Ankle

While the leg is still being held up after skin preparation:

1. Place a medium sheet under the leg and over the unaffected leg to above the knees.
2. The surgeon limits the sterile field by placing a towel around the leg above the area of the intended surgical site and securing it with a towel clip.
3. Put stockinette over the foot and draw it up over the leg to above the skin edge of the towel. The person who has been holding the leg is relieved, and the leg is held by a sterile team member.
4. Place a medium sheet above the surgical area, and secure it around the leg with a towel clip.
5. Place a laparotomy, extremity, or split sheet with the leg drawn through the opening.
6. Cover the remainder of the operating bed over the anesthesia screen with a single sheet as necessary.

Foot

The general method of draping a foot is the same as that for the hand. While the foot is still being held up after skin preparation:

1. Place a medium sheet on the operating bed under the foot.

2. The surgeon limits the exposed area to the foot by placing a towel around the ankle and securing it with a towel clip.
3. Enclose the foot in stockinette. A sterile team member relieves the unsterile person who has been holding the leg.
4. Place a medium sheet above the foot, and secure it around the ankle with a towel clip.
5. Place a laparotomy or extremity sheet with the opening over the foot and longer part of the sheet toward the head of the operating bed.

DRAPING OF EQUIPMENT

A pneumatic tourniquet frequently is used to control bleeding during surgical procedures on the upper and lower extremities. A nonsterile tourniquet cuff is placed around the extremity before skin preparation and is covered by the draping material. An impervious towel that delineates the upper limit of the surgical area is placed around the extremity below the tourniquet cuff.

Equipment that is brought into the sterile field but cannot be sterilized must be draped before it is handled by sterile team members. The following applies to draping of equipment:

1. Tailored, disposable, clear plastic drapes are available to cover equipment, such as the operating microscope and the C-arm, so that they can be manipulated in the sterile field by the sterile team.
2. If radiographs are to be taken during the surgical procedure, a cassette holder may be placed on the operating bed, under the mattress, before the patient is positioned, prepped, and draped. The circulating nurse raises the edge of the sterile drape for the radiology technician to place and remove the x-ray cassette. The cassette may be covered with a sterile Mayo stand cover or specially designed disposable cover and placed on sterile drapes when a lateral view is needed.
3. Cords, cables, attachments, and tubing that are not sterile are inserted into sterile plastic sleeves before they are placed on the sterile field.

Nonsterile equipment that must stand near the sterile field is isolated from the sterile area by a barrier drape. IV poles frequently are used to attach drapes to shield off power-generating sources of mechanical and electrical equipment, such as electrosurgical and cryosurgical units, fiberoptic lighting units, and air-powered or electrical instruments. The drape over the patient or a separate single sheet is extended from the operating bed upward in front of or over the nonsterile equipment. The circulating nurse fastens the drape to IV poles on each side of the equipment that stands above the level of the sterile field or near it.

Heat-generating equipment must have adequate ventilation to dissipate heat. Impermeable, heat-retaining materials cannot completely encase these units. Ends of fiberoptic light cables should not make prolonged contact with drapes, or a fire may result.

Some nonsterile equipment, of necessity, will be moved over the sterile field. The sterile field is protected by additional draping material as follows:

1. Sterile disposable drapes are available to cover radiograph equipment and image intensifiers.
2. When ready to move an x-ray tube or image intensifier over the sterile field, cover the field with a sterile minor sheet. The circulating nurse will discard this sheet after use, because it is considered contaminated.
3. Photographic equipment and video cameras should be draped as much as feasible when used over the sterile field. Some video cameras fit directly into the headlamp of the surgeon and require no special draping.

PLASTIC ISOLATOR

A plastic isolator (a clear plastic shield on one side of or completely over the operating bed) may be used to exclude microorganisms from the environment immediately surrounding the patient. It may isolate a patient who is highly susceptible to infection, such as a burned or immunosuppressed patient, or it may isolate a patient with a gross infection and provide protection for others. In the OR, plastic isolators are used to isolate the sterile field from both room air and the OR team and thus exclude microorganisms normally in the OR environment.

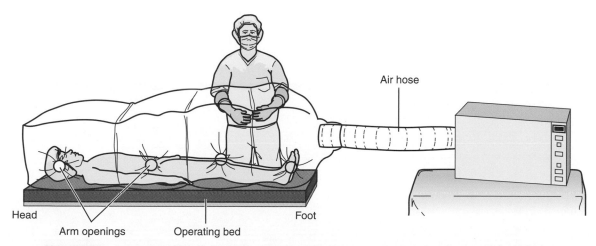

FIG. 26-42 Surgical isolation bubble. Base of bubble attaches to operating bed over the prepped and draped patient. Creates a sterile environment.

The portable, lightweight, optically transparent surgical isolator forms a bubble over the patient when inflated. This surgical isolation bubble system (SIBS) has two elements: a filter/blower unit and a prepackaged sterile disposable bubble. Its floor provides a sterile drape that adheres to prepped skin around the incision site. Built into the sides are ports (armholes) through which the team works and a port for passing sterile supplies from the circulating nurse (Fig. 26-42).

A patient isolation drape may be used that is a modification of the total isolator. It isolates the sterile field from equipment, such as the C-arm image intensifier used for hip procedures. The drape is suspended from a steel frame on one side of the special orthopedic table but does not enclose the patient. The drape may have an incise portion that may be impregnated with a time-released iodophor. Storage holsters and irrigation pouches are commonly incorporated into the side. Care is taken not to perforate through the plastic surface when placing items in the pouches.

Bibliography

AORN (Association of periOperative Registered Nurses): *AORN standards, recommended practices, and guidelines,* Denver, 2006, The Association.

Belkin NL: Barrier drapes and their impact on surgical site infections, *Infect Control Today* 6(5):56-58, 2002.

Iqbal J, Wilson B: What's new in surgical drapes? *Outpatient Surg* March, 41-43, 2000.

Knight KA: Understanding the needs of morbidly obese patients, *Nurs Spect* 16(10):26-27, 2004.

Martin JT, Warner MA: *Positioning in anesthesia and surgery,* ed 3, Philadelphia, 1996, Saunders.

McEwen D: Intraoperative positioning of surgical patients, *AORN J* 63(6):1059-1063, 1066-1075, 1077-1079, 1996.

Richardson C: Use of leg positioning holders, *Brit J Periop Nurs* 14(3):127-130, 2004.

Senn N: *A nurse's guide for the operating room,* ed 2, Chicago, 1905, Chicago Medical Book Company.

Schultz A: Predicting and preventing pressure ulcers in surgical patients, *AORN J* 81(5):985-994, 2005.

Shields JA, Nelson CM: Acute Hypoxemia after repositioning of patient: A case report, *AANA Journal* 72(3):207-210, 2004.

Smith AA: *The operating room: primer for pupil nurses,* ed 1, Philadelphia, 1918, Saunders.

Susanti R: Air embolism after intravenous injection of contrast material, *South Med J* 92(9):930-933, 1999.

Warnshuis FC: *Principals of surgical nursing: A guide to modern surgical technic,* Philadelphia, 1918, Saunders.

Williams H, Reeves F: Anesthetic techniques and positioning: implications for perioperative nurses, *Semin Perioper Nurs* 7(1):14-20, 1998.

Chapter 27

Physiologic Maintenance and Monitoring of the Perioperative Patient

CHAPTER OBJECTIVES

After studying this chapter, the learner will be able to:
- Identify pertinent body systems that should be monitored during a surgical procedure.
- Discuss the differences between invasive and noninvasive means of patient monitoring.
- Discuss why personnel monitoring a patient should be knowledgeable about the monitoring devices used.
- Describe how monitoring parameters provide information about interrelated body systems.

CHAPTER OUTLINE

KEY TERMS AND DEFINITIONS

Core temperature   Temperature inside the body.
Expiration   Exit of waste gases from the body through the mouth and nose.
External respiration   Exchange of gases between the lungs and blood at the alveolar level.
Hemodynamics   Study of blood circulation, blood pressure, peripheral vascular physiology, and cardiac function.
Internal respiration   Exchange of gases between the blood and cells at the capillary/tissue level.
Monitoring   Observing, evaluating, and reporting physiologic function.
Pulse   Palpable sensation of blood passing through an artery.
Respiration   Exchange of oxygen and carbon dioxide at the molecular level.
Sinus rhythm   Electrical impulse in the heart that originates at the sinoatrial node of the right atrium of the heart, passes through the atrioventricular node at the atrial-septal junction, and continues down the length of the Purkinje fibers in the ventricular septum, causing contraction of the ventricles.
Ventilation/inspiration   Bringing air into the lungs through the mouth and nose.

SUPPLEMENTAL MATERIAL ON EVOLVE WEBSITE   *evolve*

http://evolve.elsevier.com/BerryKohn
- Content Updates
- Glossary
- Full Set of Perioperative Flash Cards
- Interactive Key Term Flash Cards
- Student Activities
- WebLinks

HISTORICAL BACKGROUND

Iatrophysics is the study of the application of the principles of mechanics to human physiology. As early scientists and physicians learned more about anatomy and physiology, assessment of precise physiologic measurements improved patient care. The most significant discovery of the seventeenth century was cardiopulmonary circulation. In 1628 English physiologist William Harvey (1578-1657) described the circulation of blood through the body. Spanish physician Michael Servetus (1511-1553) had paved the way by describing theories of pulmonary circulation through the lungs. Conceptually, these discoveries disproved theories developed by the Roman "Father of Physiology" Claudius Galen (130-200) that blood flowed between the heart chambers via pores. Earlier myths included the belief that blood actually originated in the heart and was pumped one drop at a time.

Expanding knowledge of circulation and its effects on the body led to the ability to monitor physiologic function. Italian physicist Galileo Galilei (1564-1642) experimented with temperature measurement in 1592. His theories were followed by those of Santorio Santorio (1561-1637), who developed a prototype of a thermometer. Dutch physician Herman Boerhaave (1668-1738) was the first to use a thermometer in clinical practice and taught that clinical discussions of patient condition improved the outcome of treatment. The glass thermometer as used in current practice was developed by Clifford Allbutt in 1870.

Monitoring techniques began to improve with the development of the sphygmomanometer for the measurement of blood pressure in 1896 by Italian physician Scipione Riva-Rocci (1863-1943). The development of watches with second hands allowed physicians to count a patient's pulse and respirations.

Techniques for monitoring patients have improved significantly over the past decade. Automated monitoring devices have become more sensitive and accurate. Electrocardiographic (ECG) monitors, blood pressure machines, and pulse oximeters display the patient's hemodynamics electronically. Specialized probes measure core temperature, and skin patches measure surface temperature without the use of a glass thermometer. Appropriate monitoring techniques can assist the perioperative team in patient care.

IMPORTANCE OF PATIENT MONITORING

The development of successful, controllable anesthesia has made modern surgery possible. Because anesthesia is an adjunct to most surgical procedures, familiarity with various anesthetic agents, their interaction with certain drugs, and their potential hazards is a necessity. The perioperative nurse responsible for patient monitoring may detect the onset of complications and help avert an undesired outcome.

Working with anesthesia providers in the perioperative environment gives the learner an unparalleled opportunity to master immediate resuscitative measures and their effectiveness, as well as an understanding of the care of unconscious and critically ill patients. For example, the learner daily observes endotracheal intubation, ventilatory control, insertion of arterial and venous cannulas, fluid replacement, and sophisticated hemodynamic monitoring.

No surgical procedure is minor. Surgery and anesthesia impose on the patient certain inescapable risks, even under supposedly ideal circumstances. Overall, however, the anesthetic-related surgical mortality rate is relatively low. Preexisting patient factors, such as age and/or medical condition, and those related to the circumstances of the surgical procedure, such as type, duration, and elective versus emergency procedure, are more significant in determining surgical mortality. The American Society of Anesthesiologists (ASA) has established standards for basic perioperative monitoring. Specialization in monitoring equipment and the use of computers to record monitoring data are facets of contemporary anesthesia practice.

MONITORING PHYSIOLOGIC FUNCTIONS

Preoperative patient assessment establishes a baseline and provides valuable information by which intraoperative and postoperative patient care is planned and evaluated. Establishing a preoperative baseline enables the caregiver to be alerted to changes in the patient's physiologic condition that may require prompt attention.

Surgical and anesthesia techniques have become increasingly complex, allowing many critically ill patients of all ages to undergo surgical procedures. The anesthesia provider carefully monitors the patient's condition through the entire perioperative process and keeps the surgeon informed of important changes.

Monitoring implies keeping track of vital functions. During extensive surgery with the patient under anesthesia, the body is subjected to physiologic stress. Bleeding, tissue trauma, potent drugs, large extravascular fluid shifts, multiple transfusions, and a surgical position that may inhibit breathing and circulation all contribute to altered physiology. These factors can induce significant cardiopulmonary dysfunction.

Evaluation of the patient's responses to these stressors includes observation, auscultation, and palpation. The assessment is enhanced by the use of electronic or mechanical devices that reveal physiologic trends and subtle changes and indicate responses to therapy. Most of this equipment is expensive and is incorporated into the anesthesia machine. Compact, precise devices with miniaturized circuitry, better visibility, and easier maintenance are incorporated

into portable models that allow for continued monitoring after the patient leaves the operating room (OR).

Computers improve and expedite analysis of data. They are sophisticated data collection and management tools to assist in physiologic assessment, diagnosis, and therapy. Clinical computers vary from single-function devices to complex, multifunction, real-time systems that acquire, store, and display data; organize information; display trends; and perform calculations.

Personnel using electronic and computerized monitoring equipment must understand its use and function, be experienced in its interpretation, and be able to determine equipment malfunction easily. Instrumentation should augment, not replace, careful observation of the patient. Monitoring equipment can be inaccurate. Information from monitors should be compared with physical assessment data. Perioperative nurses involved with patient monitoring should remain current in the knowledge of physical assessment and the use of the equipment in use. Periodic competency testing should be performed. Written policies, procedures, and guidelines should be available for reference.

The spectrum of monitoring devices is broad. It ranges from noninvasive to invasive. Noninvasive monitors do not penetrate the body or a body orifice. Conversely, invasive monitors penetrate skin or mucosa, or they enter a body cavity. Some parameters can be measured by both noninvasive and invasive methods. Perioperative nursing responsibilities may include assisting with sophisticated hemodynamic monitoring to evaluate the interrelationship of blood pressure, blood flow, vascular volumes, physical properties of blood, heart rate, and ventricular function. Detection of early changes in hemodynamics allows prompt action to maintain cardiac function and adequate cardiac output. Monitoring facilitates rapid, accurate determination of decreased perfusion. It reflects immediate response to therapeutic measures and stress.

Invasive Hemodynamic Monitoring

Hemodynamics is the study of the movement of blood. Measurements of cardiac output and intracardiac pressures provide information related to functions of the heart and other major organ systems.

Invasive hemodynamic monitoring uses basic physiologic principles to detect and treat a wide variety of abnormalities. Its purpose is to avoid problems in high-risk patients and to accurately diagnose and treat patients with established life-threatening disorders. It involves direct intravascular measurements and assessments by means of indwelling catheters connected to transducers and monitors. Pressures and forces within arteries and veins are converted to electrical signals by the transducer, a device that transfers energy from one system to another. These electrical signals are then processed and amplified by the monitor into a continuous waveform displayed on an oscilloscope or monitoring screen that reproduces images received via the transducer; or the monitor may digitally display the values. These measurements yield specific information that is otherwise not usually attainable or as accurate. Although these measurements may be pertinent in guiding patient care, they present additional risks because obtaining them requires invasion of the great vessels or heart. The benefits of invasive monitoring must be balanced against the risks.

Various types of equipment, monitors, and catheters are in use. Everyone caring for patients with invasive monitors must have knowledge of anatomy and physiology and understanding of the entire monitoring circuit. Every precaution must be taken to ensure patient safety. Strict adherence to policies and procedures, manufacturers' instructions for use, and sterile technique is absolutely essential to minimize complications and misinterpretation of data that could lead to errors in therapy.

Indwelling arterial, venous, and intracardiac catheters permit rapid, accurate assessment of physiologic alterations in high-risk patients. Intravascular access is justified because of the high yield of information with minimal discomfort to patients. But hemodynamic monitoring techniques must not be abused. Cardiac dysrhythmias, thrombosis, embolism, and infection are serious, sometimes fatal, complications of intravascular cannulation. Some facilities require the patient to sign an informed consent form before insertion of an invasive catheter.

Intravascular Cannulation. Intravascular catheters usually are inserted before induction of anesthesia by a physician or a certified registered nurse anesthetist (CRNA). They may be inserted percutaneously or by cutdown, depending on the type of catheter, intended purpose(s), and location of the vessel to be cannulated. Intracardiac catheters may be placed under fluoroscopic control, or their position may be verified on a chest radiograph after insertion. In addition to their use in hemodynamic monitoring, intravenous (IV) catheters can be used to administer blood, drugs, and nutrients. Catheters may be inserted into the right atrium or pulmonary artery via the vena cava through a subclavian, jugular, brachial, or femoral vein.

Intraarterial catheters are inserted for direct pressure measurements and to obtain blood for arterial blood gas (ABG) analyses. Potential sites for cannulation include the radial, ulnar, axillary, brachial, femoral, and dorsalis pedis arteries. The radial artery is most commonly used if ulnar circulation to the hand is adequate. A Doppler ultrasonic device may be used to determine a dominant artery and to locate a weakly palpable one. When radial artery dominance exists, the ulnar, brachial, or other artery is used. As a precaution, adequacy of perfusion to the extremity below the catheter should be established before insertion, in case thrombosis or occlusion occurs. A radial artery distal to a brachial artery previously used for cardiac catheterization is avoided because of the possibility of distorted pressures or occlusion. Some physicians cannulate the femoral artery if the catheter is to remain in place for more than 24 hours. The incidence of thrombosis is lower when a large vessel is used. Thrombosis may result from irritation of the vessel wall or hypercoagulation or inadequate flushing of the catheter and line. The larger the catheter in relation to the arterial lumen, the greater the incidence of thrombosis. Other complications of arterial cannulation include embolic phenomena, blood loss from a dislodged catheter or disconnected line, bruise or hematoma formation, arteriovenous fistula or aneurysm formation, systemic infection, and ischemic fingers from arterial spasm.

Intravascular Catheters. Most catheters are radiopaque and have centimeter calibrations. They are flexible. They may be made of silicone, polyethylene, polyvinyl chloride, polytetrafluoroethylene (Teflon), or polyurethane. Those with soft, pliable tips are safer than are stiff catheters. Shearing of a vessel with extravascular migration of the catheter has occurred from stiffness and sharpness of the catheter and movement of the patient. Soft catheters must be introduced over a guidewire or by flow-directed balloons. The catheter and related introducer, guidewire, and caps may be supplied as a prepackaged sterile kit.

Many catheters have a heparin coating to prevent clot formation. Polyurethane or other uncoated catheters are available for the patient who is allergic to heparin. The catheter is kept open with a slow, continuous infusion. Routine flushing of the catheter is necessary. Normal saline may be used if heparin is unnecessary or contraindicated. Continuous-flush devices with fast-flush valves release small amounts of solution. Limited pressure diminishes the possibility of ejecting a large clot. The catheter usually is fast-flushed both hourly and after blood samples are withdrawn. Air bubbles in the line must be avoided. After flushing, the drip rate in the drip chamber is checked.

A catheter may have a single lumen or two or three lumens. The catheters discussed are used for hemodynamic monitoring of the following:

- ABGs and pressure via a single-lumen intraarterial catheter
- Central venous pressure via a central venous, Hickman, or Broviac catheter
- Pulmonary artery pressures via a pulmonary artery or Swan-Ganz catheter

Catheter Insertion. Catheter insertion is a sterile procedure. The necessary sterile supplies should be collected before the patient arrives. Although catheters are different, the technique for insertion is basically the same for all types. Insertion is a team effort. The circulating nurse's responsibilities may vary but usually include the following:

1. Explain the procedure and reassure the patient. If the patient will be awake, sedation may be ordered.
2. Document the patient's vital signs and pulse distal to the selected insertion site. If the pulse weakens after cannulation, circulation may be inadequate in an extremity and the catheter may need to be removed.
3. Position the patient as appropriate.
   a. For radial artery cannulation, affix the forearm to an armboard with the hand supinated and wrist dorsiflexed to an angle of 50 to 60 degrees over a towel. Avoid extreme dorsiflexion; this can obliterate the pulse. Tape the thumb to the armboard to stabilize the artery at the wrist.
   b. For subclavian or jugular vein insertion, place the patient in a 25- to 30-degree Trendelenburg's position to reduce the potential for air embolism. Elevate the scapular area with padding or a rolled towel underneath the shoulders to allow the physician to identify anatomic landmarks and locate the vein more easily. Turn the patient's head away from the insertion site.
4. Prepare the skin per routine procedure. Wearing sterile gloves, the physician then drapes the area. Warn the patient if his or her face will be covered.
5. Inform the patient, if awake, that he or she may have a burning sensation for a few seconds when the

local anesthetic is injected before the area becomes numb. Explain that pressure, but not pain, may be felt during insertion. The skin and subcutaneous tissues are infiltrated with a local anesthetic because the skin is incised to facilitate entrance of the catheter. A cutdown, or opening of the skin and tissues to access a vein, may be necessary.

6. Assist the physician as appropriate. Be familiar with and follow the manufacturer's directions for the brand of catheter and monitoring equipment used.

7. Make sure the connections between the catheter and infusion line are secure after the catheter has been inserted and properly placed. The catheter is sutured in place to prevent inadvertent advancement or removal and is taped to the skin. Lumens on the three-way stopcock and catheter may be capped to prevent fibrin deposits and retrograde contamination.

8. Connect the catheter line to the transducer or monitor, and take baseline pressure readings.

9. Dress the puncture site. An antibacterial ointment may be put around the site. Tape must not apply pressure directly over the insertion site or catheter. A transparent dressing is preferable. The catheter beneath it must not be bent or curled.

10. Take the patient's vital signs. Using a sphygmomanometer with the blood pressure cuff on the opposite arm from the insertion site, check the blood pressure to compare with the monitor's pressure reading to verify the monitor's accuracy. The monitor will probably read higher systolic and lower diastolic pressures than the blood pressure cuff readings.

11. Document the procedure and initial readings. Include the insertion site; type and gauge of catheter; type of infusion solution and amount of heparin, if added; flow rate and pressure; pulse before and after insertion; tolerance of the procedure; color, sensation, and warmth of the area distal to the insertion site; time of insertion; and names of insertion team members.

Frequent checks of circuitry and calibrations are necessary to validate the recorded data. Conscientious attention to every detail is mandatory during catheter insertion and monitoring.

Drawing Blood Samples. When the arterial or venous catheters are in place, the perioperative nurse may be asked to collect blood samples for analysis or to take measurements, although this is not universal practice. These procedures require special training, skill, and knowledge of equipment and hazards involved.

Samples for ABG measurements are sometimes drawn from an indwelling catheter line kept open by a continuously running infusion. The tubing incorporates a plastic three-way stopcock, usually close to the catheter insertion site. One lumen of the stopcock goes to the infusion solution, one to the cannulated vessel, and one to outside air. The last-mentioned one is normally closed or covered with a sterile cap, or a sterile syringe is kept inserted in the lumen to prevent bacteria and air from entering. With a three-way stopcock, two of the three lumens are always open.

In drawing blood samples from an indwelling catheter, always use strict sterile technique. Blood may be drawn

through a stopcock on a single-lumen catheter or from one lumen of a multilumen catheter. A sterile ABG monitoring kit with administration tubing and pressure transducers may be used for intraarterial pressure monitoring. The manufacturer's instructions should be followed for turning the stopcock to draw blood samples and to flush lines. Drawing blood from a multilumen catheter is simplified when an injection port can be used. The basic procedure is similar to the following, using a stopcock (always wipe the stopcock or end of the catheter with alcohol before entering the system):

1. Wear sterile gloves. A sterile heparinized syringe is used to prevent the blood samples from clotting. To heparinize, draw 1 mL of aqueous heparin 1:1000 into a 10-mL syringe. While rotating the barrel, pull the plunger back beyond the 7-mL calibration. With the syringe in an upright position, slowly eject the heparin and air bubbles while rotating the barrel.

2. Attach a sterile 5-mL syringe to the stopcock lumen going to outside air. Turn off (close) the infusion lumen. This automatically opens the line between the patient and the syringe. Aspirate to clear the line of fluid, and close the lumen to the patient. Discard this diluted sample.

3. Quickly attach the sterile heparinized syringe to a lumen to outside air, and open the lumen to the patient. This closes the lumen to the infusion, permitting aspiration of undiluted blood for analysis. Arterial pressure forces blood into the syringe. Withdraw 3 to 5 mL of blood. Hold the barrel, as well as the plunger, of the syringe to avoid their separation. Cap the syringe for placement in a properly labeled specimen bag.

4. Close the lumen to the patient, and flush the line and stopcock by letting the infusion solution run through them to prevent clot formation inside the catheter wall or stopcock, which could result in arterial embolization.

5. Close and recap the lumen to outside air (being careful not to contaminate the cap), thereby restarting the infusion to the patient. Regulate the infusion rate with the clamp on the infusion tubing.

6. If air bubbles are in the syringe, remove them. Send the samples immediately to the laboratory. If more than 10 minutes elapses between blood drawing and analysis, the analysis cannot be considered accurate. In the event of delay, the syringe with blood should be immersed in ice immediately and refrigerated at near-freezing temperature. Iced specimen bags may be used.

7. Attach the appropriate laboratory slips that include information such as the patient's name and location, the time and date, and whether the patient is receiving oxygen supplement or breathing room air.

Physiologic Parameters Monitored

Noninvasive methods can be used to monitor some cardiopulmonary and neural functions and to determine body temperature and urinary output (Box 27-1). Both noninvasive and invasive techniques are used for monitoring hemodynamic parameters to show minute-to-minute changes in physiologic variables. Normal ranges of hemodynamic parameters are given in Table 27-1.

BOX 27-1	Noninvasive Methods of Monitoring Vital Functions

CARDIOPULMONARY FUNCTIONS

Blood pressure (BP)—Measurement of pressure exerted against arterial vessel walls to force blood through circulation.

Capnometry—Measurement of end-tidal concentration of carbon dioxide, by exposing expired air to infrared light.

Cardiac index (CI)—Measurement of cardiac output in relation to body surface, by using ultrasound.

Chest radiograph study—Determination by radiology of the position of intravascular catheters and endotracheal or chest tubes.

Echocardiogram—Assessment of intraventricular blood volume by observing two-dimensional color images of the beating heart produced by an ultrasonic probe placed in the esophagus.

Electrocardiogram (ECG)—Recording of electrical forces produced by the heart to evaluate changes in rhythm, rate, or conduction.

Near-infrared reflectance—Determination of the amount of oxygen in hemoglobin being delivered to the brain, by using a niroscope (NIRS).

Pulse oximetry—Determination of arterial hemoglobin oxygen saturation by measuring the optical density of light passing through tissues.

Respiratory tidal volume (V_T)—By using a respirometer, measurement of the volume of air moved with each respiration.

Stethoscopy—Detection of cardiac rate and rhythm and pulmonary sounds, by auscultation.

Total blood volume (TBV)—Measurement of plasma and red blood cell volumes, by using an electronic device.

NEURAL FUNCTIONS

Electroencephalogram (EEG)—Recording of electrical activity in the brain.

Evoked potentials—Recording of electrical responses from the cerebral cortex after stimulation of a peripheral sensory organ.

OTHER FUNCTIONS

Temperature—Measurement of core body temperature, by using a thermometer probe.

Urinary output—Measurement of urine to assess renal perfusion, by using an indwelling catheter attached to a calibrated collection device.

TABLE 27-1	Hemodynamic Monitoring Parameters

Parameter	Abbreviation	Normal Range for Adults
Arterial oxygen content	Cao_2	17-20 mL/dL blood
Blood pressure	BP	Systolic 90-130 mm Hg
		Diastolic 60-85 mm Hg
Cardiac index	CI	2.8-4.2 L/min/m²
Cardiac output	CO	4-8 L/min
Central venous pressure	CVP	2-8 mm Hg, 3-10 cm H_2O
Cerebral perfusion pressure	CPP	80-100 mm Hg
Coronary perfusion pressure	CPP	60-80 mm Hg
Ejection fraction	EF	60%-70%
Glomerular filtration rate	GFR	80-120 mL/min
Heart rate	HR	60-100 beats/min
Intracranial pressure	ICP	0-15 mm Hg
Left ventricular end-diastolic pressure	LVEDP	8-12 mm Hg
Mean arterial pressure	MAP	70-105 mm Hg
Mean pulmonary artery pressure	MPAP	9-19 mm Hg
Oxygen saturation in arterial blood	Sao_2	95%-97.5%
Oxygen saturation in mixed venous blood	Svo_2	75%
Partial pressure of carbon dioxide in arterial blood	$Paco_2$	34-45 mm Hg (torr)
Partial pressure of oxygen in arterial blood	Pao_2	80-100 mm Hg (torr)
Partial pressure of oxygen in venous blood	Pvo_2	40 mm Hg (torr)
Pulmonary artery pressure	PAP	Systolic 15-25 mm Hg
		Diastolic 8-15 mm Hg
Pulmonary capillary wedge pressure	PCWP	6-12 mm Hg
Right atrial pressure	RAP	3-6 mm Hg
Right ventricular pressure	RVP	Systolic 15-25 mm Hg
		Diastolic 0-5 mm Hg
Stroke volume	SV	60-130 mL/beat
Systemic vascular resistance	SVR	800-1600 dyne/sec/cm
Total blood volume	TBV	8.5%-9% of body weight in kg
Venous oxygen content	Cvo_2	15 mL/dL blood

Electrocardiogram. Every heartbeat depends on the electrical process of polarization. Muscles in the heart wall are alternately stimulated and relaxed. An ECG is a recording of electrical forces produced by the heart and translated as waveforms (Fig. 27-1). It shows changes in rhythm, rate, or conduction, such as dysrhythmias; appearance of premature beats; and block of impulses. An ECG does not provide an index of cardiac output (CO). Cardiac monitoring has become standard procedure in the OR and postanesthesia care unit (PACU).

Cardiac monitoring systems generally consist of a monitor screen; a cathode ray oscilloscope, on which the ECG is continuously visualized; and a printout system, which transcribes the rhythm strip to paper to permit comparison of tracings and provide a permanent record. The printout may be controlled or automatic. A heart rate meter may be set to print out a rhythm strip and sound an alarm if the rate goes above or below a preset figure. Lights and beepers may provide appropriate visual and audible signals of the heart rate. Monitor leads or electrodes are attached to the chest and/or extremities. These electrodes detect electrical impulses that the heart generates. Connecting lead wires and cables transmit them to the cardiac monitor. A complete cardiogram includes 12 different leads, but usually only two or three electrodes are used. Careful placement of leads is important to show waves and complexes on the ECG rhythm strip. Leads to the anterior, lateral, or inferior cardiac surfaces, where ischemia most often occurs, provide myocardial ischemia monitoring. Use of multiple leads allows better definition of dysrhythmia and ischemia—the main reason for cardiac monitoring in the OR. The choice of leads is made by the anesthesia provider or by the surgeon in unattended local anesthesia.

In placing disc electrodes, the underlying skin must be clean and dry for adequate adherence. The sites are shaved, if necessary, because hair can interfere with adherence. The skin is abraded slightly with a gauze pad or rough material to facilitate conduction. The paper backing is peeled off the disc. As much as possible, avoid touching the adhesive. The conductive gel within the gauze pad at the center of the disc is checked. If it is not moist, another is used. The electrode is placed on the desired site, adhesive side down, and secured tightly by applying pressure. One begins at the center and moves outward to avoid expressing gel from beneath the electrode. Placing gel over a bony area is avoided because bone will interfere with conduction.

One ECG tracing is taken as a baseline before induction of anesthesia. An ECG is especially valuable during induction and intubation, when dysrhythmias are prone to occur. Early detection and rapid identification of abnormal rhythms and irregularities of the heart's actions permit treatment to be more specific. Tracings may show changes related to the anesthetic itself or to oxygenation, coronary blood flow, hypercapnia (increased $Paco_2$), or alterations in electrolyte balance or body temperature. The ECG tracing becomes a flat line when heart action ceases, but preceding tracings may define the type of cardiac arrest, which is of value in treatment. It is beyond the scope of this text to

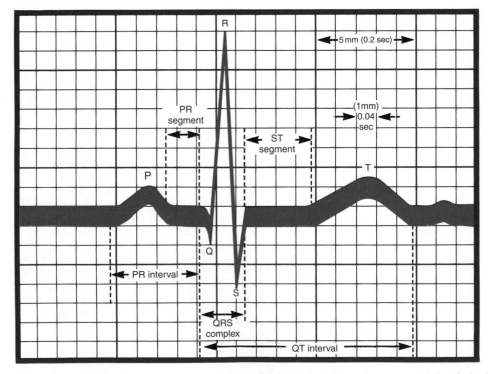

FIG. 27-1 Electrocardiogram complex. P wave before each QRS complex represents atrial depolarization. PR interval of sinus rhythm occurs between each P wave and R wave. PR segment represents conduction of impulse through atrioventricular (AV) node, bundle of His, bundle branches, and Purkinje fibers. QRS complex following each P wave represents ventricular depolarization and occurs at regular intervals, but rate can vary. T wave represents ventricular repolarization.

describe normal and abnormal cardiac rhythms interpreted by the ECG. However, perioperative nurses who monitor patients under local anesthesia should become familiar with them. Box 27-2 shows the characteristics of sinus rhythm, and Fig. 27-2 shows an example of sinus rhythm in each of 12 leads.

ECG monitors should be insensitive to electrical interference. Occasionally, recording may be affected by a high-frequency electrosurgical unit. If a tracing problem occurs, lead contacts, the integrity of the leads, and the choice of monitoring axis are checked.

The ECG monitor may be connected to a computer for analysis and storage of data. From the ECG readings, a device within the computer may be able to measure the amount of blood being pumped by the heart. This gives a continuous assessment of pumping capacity and CO. Impedance cardiography also provides data based on the mechanical activity of the heart. This is also a noninvasive computer-assisted measurement of CO—an alternative to the thermodilution technique.

Echocardiogram. Sound waves from a sonar-like device provide two-dimensional color images of the beating heart. An ultrasonic probe on the end of a small gastroscope is

BOX 27-2	Characteristics of Sinus Rhythm

- P wave is present before each QRS complex.
- There is equal space between P wave and R wave (PR interval) in each complex.
- QRS complex follows each P wave (ratio 1:1).
- P wave and QRS complex occur at regular intervals (rate can vary).

placed in the esophagus during the surgical procedure. Also referred to as transesophageal echocardiography, this form of echocardiogram can help the anesthesia provider immediately assess intraventricular blood volumes. This can be useful information for the surgeon during cardiac surgery.

Stethoscopy. Auscultation of the chest (listening to the chest) detects both cardiac rate and rhythm and pulmonary sounds. A stethoscope is taped over the precordium (the region over the heart and stomach at the level of the diaphragm), or a pressure-sensitive detector may be placed within the patient's esophagus. With the trachea protected by a cuffed endotracheal tube to prevent aspiration, the

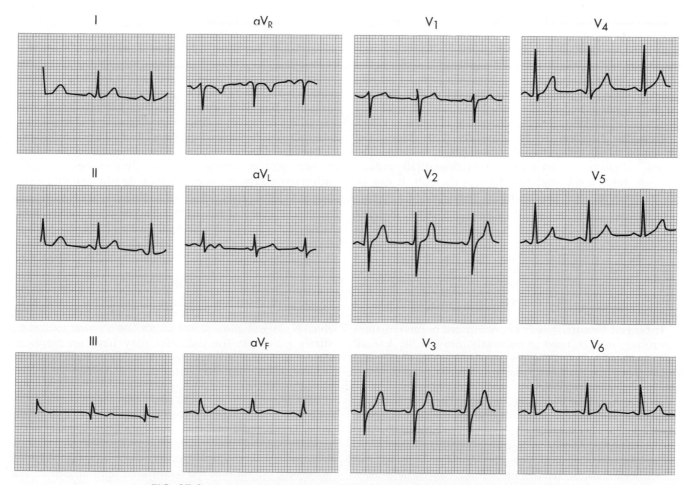

FIG. 27-2   Example of normal sinus rhythms as they appear in each of 12 leads.
(From Kinney MR et al: Andreoli's comprehensive cardiac care, ed 8, St Louis, 1996, Mosby.)

stethoscope is inserted into the esophagus to the level of the heart. Esophageal stethoscopy is especially valuable during thoracic and abdominal procedures, when auscultatory monitoring is ineffective because of tissue manipulation or movements of the members of the operating team.

Arterial Blood Pressure. Blood pressure (BP) signifies the pressure exerted against vessel walls to force blood through the circulation. Evaluation of BP during anesthesia requires consideration of blood volume, CO, and the state of the sympathetic tone of the vessels. Tissue perfusion is dependent on these factors. Arterial BP is used to assess hemodynamic and respiratory status during every surgical procedure, with very few exceptions. BP measures contraction of the heart (systolic pressure) and relaxation of the heart between contractions (diastolic pressure). Blood is forced through the arteries between contractions. Pressure is higher during systole and lower during diastole. Many factors can cause BP to vary. It is measured in millimeters of mercury (mm Hg). Normal range is 90 to 130 mm Hg systolic and 60 to 85 mm Hg diastolic.

The arm used for measurements should be opposite the one cannulated for IV fluid therapy or invasive monitoring and should be protected from contact with team members standing beside the operating bed. BP readings can be obtained by indirect or direct methods, either intermittently or continuously.

Sphygmomanometer. A pneumatic cuff is wrapped around the circumference of the upper arm. When the cuff is inflated, measurements are obtained on the sphygmomanometer as the cuff deflates. Through a stethoscope placed over an artery distal to the cuff, the systolic pressure is heard when blood begins to flow through the artery. The diastolic pressure is noted by a change in sound. This is an indirect, noninvasive method for intermittent monitoring of BP.

Doppler Ultrasonic Flowmeter. With ultrasound, BP can be monitored automatically at preset intervals. The Doppler ultrasonic flowmeter monitor automatically inflates the cuff, takes a reading, and deflates the cuff. It can be programmed to sound an alarm if systolic pressure reaches a preset high or low level. The readings are more accurate than with sphygmomanometer pressure cuff monitoring, because the ultrasonic transducer amplifies blood flow sounds. Automated, noninvasive BP monitors function well in a noisy environment. However, they do not provide continuous BP measurement or detect extremely low pressures. Frequent inflations of the cuff can bruise the skin, especially of geriatric patients.

Infrared Beams. Noninvasive infrared beams (Finapres technique) may be used to indirectly monitor BP. A small cuff fits on a finger. The beams from the cuff shine through tissue. They continuously measure arterial pressure from one heartbeat to the next.

Direct Arterial Pressure. From an invasive modality, beat-to-beat direct pressures are obtained through an artery, usually the radial or femoral, via an indwelling catheter inserted percutaneously. A very slow drip of slightly heparinized saline keeps the catheter open. The fluid-filled tubing from the catheter is connected to a mechanical electric transducer. The transducer is attached to an amplifier. A waveform of the amplified pulse, which represents force imposed on the transducer, is displayed. The monitor also converts waveforms into numerical measurements of systolic and diastolic rates. An alarm sounds if deviations are significant.

Mean Arterial Pressure. Mean arterial pressure (MAP), calculated by most monitors and shown on digital display, portrays perfusion pressure of the body. This is significant in evaluating myocardial perfusion. Normal MAP is between 70 and 105 mm Hg. Direct intraarterial pressure monitoring is valuable in patients with major multiple trauma or burns, inaccessibility of an extremity, unstable vital signs, or inaudible BP. Other indications are complex, extensive procedures, such as a cardiopulmonary bypass with an open chest; major vascular surgery with large potential fluid shifts or blood loss; total hip replacement; and major neurosurgery with the patient in the sitting position. Also included are patients in shock or with preexisting cardiac or pulmonary disease who must undergo major surgery. Direct pressure monitoring is necessary in deliberate hypotensive anesthesia, as well as in treatment of hypotensive or hypertensive crisis with continuous infusion of vasopressor or hypertensive drugs.

Blood Gases and pH. Monitoring of tissue perfusion is indispensable in evaluating pulmonary gas exchange and acid-base balance. Measurements are considered in relation to other parameters, such as vital signs, venous pressure, and left atrial pressure. Oxygen and carbon dioxide in blood exert their own partial pressures (P). Measurements are expressed in millimeters of mercury or torr. They may be differentiated as arterial (Pa) or venous (Pv). The gas being measured is identified. The partial pressure of oxygen is expressed as Po_2, or specifically in arterial blood as Pao_2 and in venous blood as Pvo_2. Oxygen saturation (So_2) in arterial blood (Sao_2) is expressed in percentages. The partial pressure of carbon dioxide is specified as $Paco_2$ or $Pvco_2$. (See Table 27-1 for normal ranges.) Monitoring techniques can be either noninvasive or invasive.

Pulse Oximetry. A pulse oximeter measures arterial oxyhemoglobin saturation (Sao_2). It provides a reading within seconds by measuring optical density of light passing through tissues. A sensor probe is clipped on each side of a pulsating vascular bed. Fingers, toes, earlobes, and the bridge of the nose are suitable sites. The patient's skin should be clean and dry. An area with fingernail polish should be avoided or the polish removed. Skin integrity under the sensor must be intact.

The sensor must be maintained flush with the skin surface and positioned so that the light source and photodetector are in direct alignment. The sensor is attached to an oximeter, which is plugged into a power source. Some power sources are battery powered. The oximeter may have an earphone adapter and an alarm system. The alarm is usually set for audible alert within 10 seconds if the oxygen saturation falls below the preset range.

Wavelengths of red (660 nm) and infrared (940 nm) light pass through tissues from the light source side of the probe. Light is picked up by a receptor in the sensor on the opposite side of the tissue. The oximeter continuously calculates the amount of oxygen present in the blood by processing the ratio of red to infrared light absorbed. The presence of oxygen in hemoglobin influences this absorption (oxyhemoglobin).

The oximeter reading should remain above 95%. A reading less than 90% probably signifies developing hypoxia. Some patients have significant respiratory disease and have prolonged trends of low readings. Oximeters give no information about the retention of carbon dioxide and are not indicators of respiratory failure caused by carbon dioxide retention. In some circumstances the readings that indicate gas exchange can be altered by the administration of supplemental oxygen.[1]

Falsely high readings may occur in cigarette smokers, because carbon monoxide (carboxyhemoglobin) can prevent red blood cells from picking up oxygen. Carboxyhemoglobin closely resembles oxyhemoglobin and is perceived by the sensor to be oxygenated. These cells may absorb light from the oximeter, however, so the reading may be higher than the actual Sao_2. Other factors may influence reliability, such as shielding of the sensor, excessive ambient light, patient movement, or intravascular dyes. Patients undergoing a surgical procedure with local anesthesia may exhibit an average consistent with 2% of baseline oxygenation.[2]

Oximeter readings should always be compared with patient assessment. (Information about competency testing for the use of pulse oximetry can be found at the National Institutes of Health [NIH] website: www.cc.nih.gov/nursing.)

Niroscope. Oxygen reserves in the brain can be assessed with a near-infrared reflectance scope (NIRS), which is a noninvasive technique. A specific form of infrared light passes through the skull. The portion of light reflected back to sensors outside the skull is measured to determine the amount of oxygen in the hemoglobin being delivered to the brain. The niroscope provides a continuous reading of the brain's oxygen reserves.

Capnometry. Changes in exhaled carbon dioxide reflect changes in respiration, circulation, or metabolism. Capnometry measures end-tidal concentration of carbon dioxide. Normal concentration is 38 torr (5%). Carbon dioxide production is in direct relationship to cellular metabolism. Monitoring carbon dioxide can detect the onset of inadvertent hypothermia or malignant hyperthermia. Capnometry, a noninvasive technique, also can detect anesthesia equipment problems, inadvertent esophageal intubation, inadequate neuromuscular blockage, air embolus, or a ventilation-perfusion problem.

A mainstream or sidestream adapter is placed in the breathing circuit as close to the facemask as possible so that expired carbon dioxide will approximate alveolar concentration. The analyzer, attached to the adapter, exposes expired air to infrared light. The amount of light absorbed by carbon dioxide determines the end-tidal concentration. A sidestream analyzer can be used to monitor patients receiving local or regional anesthesia by placing the sampling end of the tubing in the patient's nostril or mouth.

A capnographic waveform printout provides data to evaluate respiratory rate and rhythm. Some gas monitors continuously measure carbon dioxide, oxygen, and nitrous oxide parameters of the patient's airway. Digital values are displayed on the monitor.

Optode. An optode is an optical fiber inserted through an 18- or 20-gauge radial artery cannula. The tip contains chemicals that react to oxygen, carbon dioxide, and acidity of the blood. The optode is connected to a monitor that generates light through the fiber. The chemicals produce luminosities that vary in intensity for oxygen and carbon dioxide. These are measured. Readings are instantaneously and continuously shown on a digital display. Precautions must be taken to maintain sterile technique with this equipment as with other methods of percutaneous radial artery cannulation.

Direct Arterial Blood Analysis. Blood samples may be drawn intermittently from arterial or venous indwelling catheters. ABG determinations of Pao_2, Pco_2, and So_2 monitor adequacy of oxygenation and carbon dioxide elimination. This is especially important in patients requiring mechanical ventilation. The tidal volume, respiratory rate, and concentration of oxygen can be appropriately adjusted. ABG monitoring also permits laboratory analyses of pH, base excess, bicarbonate, and electrolytes to evaluate metabolic processes and acid-base status. Differentiation of respiratory or metabolic acidosis or alkalosis is a guide to appropriate treatment. Samples may be taken also for other analyses (e.g., glucose or coagulation factors).

Hypoventilation, uneven ventilation in relation to blood flow, impairment of diffusion, and venous-to-arterial shunting lead to anoxemia unless oxygen in inspired air is increased. Hypoventilation of the whole lung or a major portion leads to retention of carbon dioxide and predisposes the patient to cardiac dysrhythmias. Disturbances of acid-base balance have many serious consequences in many organs. They must be corrected to achieve normal physiologic functioning.[3]

Central Venous Pressure. Because it accurately measures right atrial BP, which in turn images right ventricular BP, central venous pressure (CVP) assesses function of the heart's right side. It measures the pressure under which blood returns to the right atrium. It reflects pressure in the major veins as blood returns to the heart. In other words, CVP represents the amount of venous return and filling pressure of the right ventricle. This information helps determine the patient's circulatory status.

CVP monitoring also aids in evaluating blood volume and the relationship between circulating blood volume and the pumping action of the heart (i.e., adequacy of volume presented to the heart for pumping). Therefore, CVP monitoring is a useful guide in blood or fluid administration to avoid circulatory overload in patients having limited cardiopulmonary reserve. Too great or too rapid replacement can cause pulmonary edema. Generally, a low CVP indicates that additional fluid can be given safely. CVP monitoring may be used during shock or hypotension to judge the adequacy of blood replacement. However, CVP is not a measure of blood volume per se or of CO.

[1]Fu ES, et al: Supplemental oxygen impairs detection of hypoventilation by pulse oximetry, *Chest* 126(5):1552-1558, 2004.
[2]Larson MJ, Taylor RS: Monitoring vital signs during outpatient Moh's and post Moh's reconstructive surgery performed under local anesthesia, *Dermatol Surg* 30(5):777-783, 2004.

[3]Fu, et al: 2004.

Indications for CVP monitoring include major surgical procedures in patients with preexisting cardiovascular disease, in surgical procedures in which large-volume shifts are anticipated (e.g., open heart surgery), in critically ill patients (e.g., massive trauma), in surgical procedures in which venous air emboli are a risk (e.g., craniotomy in sitting position), and in rapid administration of blood or fluid.

Although CVP monitoring provides valuable data for assessing the adequacy of vascular volume, it only indirectly reflects the function of the left side of the heart. There is no direct relationship between right and left ventricular filling pressures. Because of the distensibility (compliancy) of the pulmonary blood vessels, the lungs can accept a marked increase in blood flow before significant congestion appears. Backup of blood caused by impaired function of the left ventricle and a subsequent increase in pulmonary vascular resistance (PVR) may occur before this increased pressure affects the right side of the heart, as exhibited by CVP values. Thus CVP does not correlate with left-sided heart performance in patients with left ventricular dysfunction or pulmonary congestion.

Central Venous Cannulation. CVP may be monitored with a single-lumen or multilumen radiopaque catheter. A double- or triple-lumen Hickman or Broviac catheter is used most commonly. The right atrial lumen of a Swan-Ganz pulmonary artery catheter also can be used to obtain CVP readings. The lumens are labeled and color-coded on multilumen catheters.

The catheter is inserted, preferably percutaneously through a subclavian vein. A brachial, external or internal jugular, or femoral vein may be used or, by cutdown, the antecubital vein. If the patient is awake, he or she is asked to bear down (Valsalva maneuver) as the vein is punctured. This increases intrathoracic pressure and counteracts negative pressure from the vein, thus reducing the possibility of air embolism.

The catheter is threaded through the vein and advanced into the superior vena cava or right atrium. This may be done under fluoroscopy, or a chest radiograph may be taken to verify accurate placement of the catheter tip.

The catheter may be attached to a transducer and monitor. Pressure readings are expressed in millimeters of mercury (mm Hg). The catheter can be attached to a fluid-filled manometer that measures pressure in centimeters of water (cm H$_2$O). To set up this line, the IV solution bag is connected to the tubing; the manometer is inserted into the line by attaching it to the stopcock between the IV tubing and the extension tubing; air is expelled from the line, and the line is clamped; and the manometer is secured upright to an IV pole. The hub of the catheter lumen is connected to the stopcock. Connections to the three-way stopcock should be taped to prevent inadvertent disconnection and air leaks. Cyclic variations in intracaval venous pressure occur; pressure becomes negative during atrial filling and respiratory inspiration. Sucking of air into the system during negative venous pressure can result in an air embolus.

Baseline measurement is taken as soon as the catheter is in place and attached to the monitor. This is also a presumptive check for proper placement of the cannula tip. Because expansion of the lungs increases intrathoracic pressure and deflation decreases it, fluid in the manometer should fluctuate with each breath. To obtain a CVP reading on the manometer, adjust the scale to zero level with the patient's right atrium. The lumen of the stopcock to the catheter is shut off, allowing the IV fluid to run into the manometer to the desired level. The infusion is shut off, and the catheter is opened. After obtaining the reading, the infusion lumen to the catheter is opened to keep the line open.

Electronic transducer systems provide continuous monitoring of venous pressure. Continuous monitoring supplies good measurement of the right side of the heart and portrays the trend of heart function that is more valuable than are isolated readings obtained with a manometer. CVP values may vary somewhat, but normal readings range from 2 to 8 mm Hg, or 3 to 10 cm H$_2$O.

Multilumen central venous catheters provide access for administration of drugs, blood, fluids, and hyperalimentation. Blood can be removed for blood gas analyses or autotransfusion. These catheters also provide access for removal of air embolus.

Pulmonary Artery Pressure Monitoring. Because a pulmonary artery catheter measures function of both the right and the left sides of the heart, it provides faster, more accurate indication of impending left ventricular failure than does CVP alone. Pressures of the left side of the heart are reflected in pulmonary artery and pulmonary capillary wedge pressures, measured by the pulmonary artery catheter. This is more sensitive to rapid changes in the cardiovascular system than is CVP and is more sensitive to the ability of the heart to accommodate fluid loads. Measurement of pulmonary pressures enables precise, rapid assessment of the left ventricle's ability to eject adequate CO. Continuous evaluation of left ventricular function is extremely important in patients whose left-sided heart dysfunction has a greater direct effect on CO, circulating volume, and respiratory function than does impaired right-sided heart function. Data procured include PAP, pulmonary capillary wedge pressure (PCWP), right atrial pressure (RAP), and CO computation. These pressures reveal the hemodynamic status of cardiovascular and pulmonary functions. They also serve as guidelines for administration of fluids, diuretics, or cardiotonic drugs to obtain optimal CO.

Indications for pulmonary artery monitoring include preexisting cardiac or pulmonary disease in a patient undergoing a major vascular, intraabdominal, or neurosurgical procedure, and a potential risk of development of cardiopulmonary instability from the stress of the surgical procedure. Other conditions may include shock, burns with large fluid shifts, renal failure with low CO, or pulmonary emboli. Pulmonary artery catheters may be used in patients who require long-term monitoring. Some multipurpose catheters may be used with ventricular and atrial pacing wires in patients with heart block or severe bradycardia. These catheters may be used to measure CO in patients with intracardiac shunts or during titrated drug administration.

Contraindications to invasive pulmonary catheter monitoring are abnormal cardiac anatomy in the patient, inadequate monitors, or lack of personnel trained in the use of the monitors.

Pulmonary Artery Cannulation. Various pulmonary artery catheters are available. The number of lumens varies from two to five, depending on the range of functions desired. These catheters are used with transducers for monitoring. The type of transducer varies according to the balloon flotation device in the catheter.

In setting up the monitoring system, the manufacturer's instructions must be followed explicitly. All equipment, including the oscilloscope, should be checked. The stopcocks and flush devices in the lines to the transducer head(s) need to be attached. Preassembled tubing systems and disposable transducer domes are commercially available. If the patient also will have a peripheral arterial line, two transducers and a triple stopcock manifold are needed. Simultaneous monitoring of PAP and RAP is thus possible. The transducer dome is back-flushed. The monitor should be balanced and calibrated according to the manufacturer's directions. There must be no air bubbles remaining in the lines or system.

Before the catheter is inserted, the physician inspects it for defects and tests the balloon for leakage by inflating it, submerging it in sterile saline solution, and watching for air bubbles. The balloon must then be deflated. Moistening the catheter tip with saline solution or lidocaine reduces the possibility of venospasm at insertion.

Vital signs are taken before insertion of the catheter. An ECG should be monitored for dysrhythmias during insertion. With the introducer set, the catheter is inserted and advanced rapidly to prevent kinking or knotting. It is advanced through the vein into the inferior or superior vena cava and on into the right atrium. Continued manipulation irritates or damages vessel walls. Watching the increment markings on the side helps determine how far the catheter has advanced. It is possible to keep pushing the catheter while it is not going into the right place. It can coil up and knot in the ventricle.

When the catheter tip reaches the right atrium and a right atrial waveform appears on the oscilloscope screen or readout strip, the balloon is inflated slowly with air with a tuberculin syringe to enable it to float with the flow of blood. The balloon is never inflated without a visible oscilloscope trace. If the patient is awake, a voluntary cough confirms the position of the catheter in the thoracic cavity if the right atrial wave fluctuates. The amount of air is specified by the manufacturer (usually about 1.3 to 1.5 mL). Overinflation could rupture the balloon. Carbon dioxide is used for balloon inflation in patients with intracardiac shunts. If the balloon ruptures in arterial circulation, carbon dioxide is more soluble than ambient (room) air in blood. A feeling of resistance should accompany inflation. Absence of resistance is a sign of a ruptured balloon; inflation should be stopped immediately. Fluid is never used for inflation, because it would prevent proper catheter flotation and complete deflation.

Passing through the tricuspid valve, the catheter enters the right ventricle. A typical right ventricular waveform should appear. If dysrhythmia develops or is persistent, a bolus of lidocaine may be injected. Then after the catheter floats through the pulmonary semilunar valve into the pulmonary artery, a pulmonary artery tracing should appear on the monitor. This waveform has a steep upstroke at the beginning from right ventricular ejection and opening of the pulmonic valve, followed by a dicrotic notch on the downstroke at the closing of the pulmonic valve. Pulmonary artery blood flow carries the balloon into one of the artery's smaller branches. When the vessel diameter becomes too narrow for it to pass, the balloon wedges in the vessel and occludes it. A PCWP waveform should appear. After recording of this wedge pressure, the physician permits the balloon to deflate passively; air is not aspirated with the syringe.

The catheter will then slip back into the main branch of the pulmonary artery. A PAP waveform should reappear on the monitor. Thus the physician depends on these sequential characteristic pressure waveforms to reveal the catheter tip's location at all times. The circulating nurse records pressure at each location. The catheter remains in the pulmonary artery with the balloon deflated, continuously recording the PAP, except when a PCWP reading is desired. The balloon may be ruptured if a PAP waveform persists and a PCWP reading is unobtainable or if resistance is not felt with an attempt to inflate the balloon. A radiograph is taken to confirm the catheter position. In the case of rupture, the catheter may be left in place to record the PAP, provided that it has not slipped back to the right ventricle. The physician may also elect to remove it. The balloon is always inflated during catheter advancement and deflated during catheter withdrawal.

To prevent an air embolus after catheter insertion, the catheter must not be attached to the monitoring system until all air has been expelled. All lines and transducers should be checked for secure connections and patency. Each transducer's balancing port must be leveled with the patient's right atrium. RAP, PAP, and PCWP waveforms, as well as the patient's response to the procedure, must be documented.

Swan-Ganz Thermodilution Catheter. The No. 7 Swan-Ganz thermodilution catheter has four separate lumens or passages within its outside wall. It is versatile and widely used. It is $43\frac{1}{4}$ inches (110 cm) long, with 10-cm increments marked on the side to permit observation of how far the catheter has advanced during insertion. Like all pulmonary artery catheters, it is a balloon-tipped flotation catheter that is inserted into a major vein and advanced to the inferior or superior vena cava. When inflated, the thin latex balloon at the tip permits the catheter to float with the flow of blood through the right atrium, tricuspid valve, right ventricle, pulmonary semilunar valve, and pulmonary artery and to wedge in a small pulmonary artery branch (arteriole) for recording the PCWP during occlusion of the vessel. When the balloon is not inflated, the catheter lies in the pulmonary artery to record the PAP. It is essential to achieve proper catheter placement to minimize the risk of vessel damage and complications, as well as to validate pressure readings.

The end of the catheter inserted in the patient is referred to as the distal end; the opposite one is the proximal end. The proximal end has several external ports that provide access to the lumens used in patient monitoring. The pulmonary artery port is used for monitoring PAP and PCWP. A syringe is connected to the balloon port for the desired balloon inflation. The thermistor port is used for CO calculation. The right atrial port is used for measuring RAP. This port also can be used to administer fluids or can be connected to a flush system for maintenance of catheter patency. For CO measurement, normal saline or dextrose solution is injected into the cardiovascular system via the proximal lumen. The pulmonary artery and right atrial ports should be labeled.

The catheter has four separate lumens or passages. The pulmonary artery lumen, the largest and most distal, terminates in the opening at the catheter's tip. With proper catheter positioning, this opening lies in the pulmonary artery. In this position with the balloon deflated, pulmonary artery systolic, diastolic, and mean pressures are recorded on the monitor. These are indicative of pulmonary function. When the balloon is inflated and the catheter migrates to a pulmonary artery branch to wedge, the PCWP is recorded. PCWP is sometimes referred to as pulmonary artery wedge pressure (PAWP) or pulmonary artery occlusion pressure (PAOP). Occlusion of a pulmonary artery branch creates a no-flow system, thereby blocking blood flow from the right side of the heart to the lungs and permitting pressure equilibration in the pulmonary vascular bed distal to the catheter. Occlusion of an arteriole and low resistance of the pulmonary systems give a pressure measurement equal to the left atrial pressure (LAP), which in turn is equal to the left ventricular end-diastolic pressure (LVEDP). To prevent pulmonary infarction, ischemia, or hemorrhage from prolonged wedging, the balloon is always deflated immediately after a reading is taken. The catheter will float back into the main pulmonary artery. The pulmonary artery lumen can provide blood samples for blood gas measurements and mixed venous blood, which is also of value in judging cardiac function.

The balloon lumen opening, permitting inflation and deflation, is about 1 cm from the catheter tip. When inflated, the balloon surrounds, but does not cover, the opening in this tip.

The thermistor lumen opening is about 4 cm from the catheter tip. This lumen contains temperature-sensitive wires that run its length and transmit the temperature of blood flowing over them from the thermistor to the computer used to determine CO by the thermodilution technique.

The proximal right atrial lumen opening is about 30 cm from the catheter's tip. This opening lies in the right atrium to monitor RAP when the catheter is in place.

Interpretation of Pressures. The range of normal pressure values may vary slightly from one authority to another. Characteristic waveforms appear on the oscilloscope or screen, depending on the location of the catheter tip during insertion and continuous monitoring. These waveforms must be watched carefully to ascertain that the catheter is in the desired position. The catheter enters the right atrium via the vena cava.

Right Atrial Pressure. Normal RAP is 3 to 6 mm Hg. RAP reflects right atrial filling diastolic pressure, equivalent to CVP and right ventricular end-diastolic pressure (RVEDP)—pressure at the end of filling just before contraction. A rise in RAP may indicate right or left ventricular failure, volume overload (hypovolemia), or air embolism. A fall in RAP may indicate vasodilation, hypovolemia, or peripheral blood pooling.

Right Ventricular Pressure. Normal right ventricular pressure (RVP) is 15 to 25 mm Hg systolic and 0 to 5 mm Hg diastolic. A rise in RVP may indicate mitral insufficiency,

congestive heart failure, hypoxemia, or left ventricular failure.

Pulmonary Artery Pressure. Normal PAP is 15 to 25 mm Hg systolic and 8 to 15 mm Hg diastolic; the mean is 9 to 19 mm Hg. These pressures estimate venous pressure in the lungs, as well as mean filling pressure of the left atrium and left ventricle. They reflect right ventricular function unless the patient has pulmonary stenosis, because commonly the pulmonary artery systolic pressure approximates the right ventricular systolic pressure. Changes in pulmonary artery systolic and mean pressures indicate changes in PVR. Alterations in PVR occur in hypoxemia, respiratory insufficiency, pulmonary edema, pulmonary emboli, shock, or sepsis. Thus these pressures are indices of pulmonary function. A rise in PAP may indicate left ventricular failure; increased pulmonary arteriolar resistance, as in pulmonary hypertension and hypoxia; or fluid overload.

Pulmonary Capillary Wedge Pressure. Normal pressure is 6 to 12 mm Hg. Pulmonary artery diastolic pressure and PCWP are prime determinants of function of the left side of the heart, because they reflect LVEDP just before the left ventricle contracts, except in patients with mitral valve impairment.

Normally, when the mitral valve between the right atrium and right ventricle is open (ventricular diastole), flow of blood from the pulmonary artery to the pulmonary veins and left side of the heart is unimpeded. Then pressures throughout the pulmonary circulation and left side of the heart are comparable. Because PCWP usually approximates LAP, an indicator of left heart function, it is an important determinant of left ventricular preload. Intraoperative monitoring of PCWP usually can give early disclosure of left ventricular dysfunction. A rise in PCWP may indicate left ventricular failure, mitral insufficiency, pulmonary hypertension, fluid overload, or pulmonary congestion. A rise also may occur during anesthesia induction. A fall in PCWP may indicate a reduction in LVEDP and CO, or hypovolemia.

Complications of Pulmonary Artery Catheter Monitoring. Invasion of the great vessels and heart carries many inherent perils. Probably the most common during insertion is cardiac dysrhythmia, especially premature contractions. Other problems include local or systemic infection (septicemia, endocarditis), thrombus formation, pulmonary emboli, pulmonary infarction, pneumothorax, hemothorax, major vessel or heart chamber perforation, kinking or knotting of the catheter, balloon rupture, postoperative bleeding, or erroneous diagnosis from misinterpretation of data.

Although rare, pulmonary artery perforation is very serious. Predisposing factors are pulmonary hypertension, anticoagulation, hyperthermia, or an overinflated balloon or catheter. Hemoptysis and sudden hypotension are signs and symptoms of pulmonary artery rupture. Equipment for endobronchial intubation, chest tube insertion, and surgical intervention must be available.

Complications that are potentially life-threatening increase markedly after 48 to 72 hours of indwelling catheterization. The physician must be notified of any change in patient status. Catheter withdrawal is performed by and at the discretion of a physician. To prevent injury to the heart valves, the balloon is slightly inflated until the catheter is withdrawn to the right atrium. Then the balloon is completely deflated for withdrawal. Dysrhythmias may occur. Pressure is applied to the insertion site to prevent bleeding. The pulse and BP are checked before and after withdrawal. A postwithdrawal dressing is applied. The patient is monitored for at least 24 hours.

In addition to patient problems, monitoring problems may arise. Each requires a specific intervention. A major problem is a damped pressure or PAP waveform. This means decreased amplitude in pressure tracings or loss of sharpness in the image that suggests a defect in the circuit. Common causes are air in the system or blood in the transducer; loose connections; a kinked, overwedged, or malpositioned catheter; falling systolic pressure in the patient; or a clot in the monitor system. If the last-mentioned cause is suspected, one should gently try to aspirate blood. If no blood can be aspirated, the catheter should not be flushed. Flushing could dislodge a clot. The physician should be notified; he or she may withdraw the catheter.

Another problem involves a sudden change in configuration of a pressure tracing. Potential causes include the following:

- The transducer is not at the right atrial level.
- The transducer is in need of calibration.
- The transducer connection to the catheter is not secure.
- The catheter is no longer in proper position.
- There is a loss of pressure in the pressure bag.

If a PCWP waveform persists after a reading, the balloon may not be completely deflated or the distal catheter tip may be caught in the wedge position, requiring immediate attention. Circulating nurses should be familiar with the appropriate interventions in both patient problems and monitoring problems, in addition to being knowledgeable about the causes and preventive measures. Only in this way can patient safety be maximized in invasive monitoring.

Cardiac Output. CO is measured by the thermodilution technique to determine liters of blood pumped per minute by the left ventricle into the aorta. Normal resting value is 4 to 8 liters per minute (L/min). A known amount of fluid at a known temperature is injected into a lumen of an arterial catheter, and a temperature gradient at a point downstream is measured via a second lumen. Iced-cold or room-temperature physiologic saline solution or 5% dextrose in water (10 mL) generally is used. Blood flow supplies the thermal dilution; for example, saline mixes with blood in the superior vena cava or right atrium, depending on the catheter location, reducing the temperature of blood in the heart. The cooled blood flows past a transistorized intravascular thermistor in the thermodilution catheter that detects changes in blood temperatures that are then used to compute CO. When the solution is injected via the proximal right atrial lumen of a pulmonary artery Swan-Ganz catheter, a digital display of CO is seen within 4 to 5 seconds.

CO reflects the mechanical activity of the heart and represents total blood flow to all tissues and vascular shunts. It depends on the heartbeat rate, the contractile strength of the heart muscle (myocardial contractility), the peripheral resistance of vessels, and venous return. Inotropic agents such as digitalis or epinephrine increase contractility and CO

except in patients with loss of functioning ventricular muscle (e.g., after myocardial infarction or an aneurysm of the left ventricle). Agents such as beta-blockers decrease the work of the heart by reducing contractility and CO. Calculation of the left ventricular stroke work index reflects pumping ability. During systole, the ventricle does not totally eject the blood received during diastole. The amount of blood ejected with each contraction is referred to as the stroke volume (SV). Normal resting SV is 60 to 130 mL per beat. Determinants of the SV are the LAP, afterload, contractile state of the myocardium, and LVEDP. The ejection fraction (EF), a commonly used indicator of ventricular function, is the percentage value of the SV. Normal EF is 60% to 70%. Major SV determinants of CO are preload, contractility, and afterload. Only in limited circumstances does adjustment of the heart rate therapeutically enhance CO.

Preload, the amount of blood in the ventricle at the end of diastole, may be referred to as left ventricular end-diastolic volume (LVEDV) or filling pressure (LVEDP). Assessment of changes in volume by measurement of changes in filling pressure helps to describe cardiac function. The Starling principle concerns the relationship between volume, stretch, and contractility. It relates myocardial fiber length to the force of the contraction. The greater the preload and stretch of myocardial fibers, the greater the subsequent contraction, thereby increasing the SV until at some point ventricular failure commences. Fiber overstretch weakens contractions. As the pumping ability decreases, the left ventricle is unable to empty completely. Residual blood, combined during diastole with incoming oxygenated blood from the pulmonary veins and left atrium, increases workload and elevates the left ventricular volume and pressure. As ventricular efficiency declines, CO falls. Unpumped blood in the left ventricle backs up into the left atrium and pulmonary circulation, increasing these pressures. Pulmonary edema and respiratory insufficiency result as fluid is impelled into the alveoli. The CVP catheter measures the right-sided heart preload; the pulmonary artery catheter measures left atrial and left ventricular end-diastolic pressures.

Cardiac function may be classified as normal, compromised, or failing. In normal hearts, maximum ventricular performance seems to be achieved at 8 to 12 mm Hg filling pressure. In compromised hearts, this pressure is higher.

A reduced CO results in decreased perfusion of the capillary circulation. During hemorrhage, when circulating blood volume is reduced, the resulting diminished venous return and preload lead to a lowered CO. Atrial fibrillation also can modify the filling of the ventricles. Venous dilation contributes to pooling of blood, with subsequent decreased venous return to the heart. Low CO states result from reduced preload, as in hypovolemia, venous dilation, or cardiac tamponade; reduced contractility, as from anesthetic drugs, ischemia, infarction, or cardiac decompensation; dysrhythmias; or increased afterload, as in hypertension, pulmonary emboli, or an elevated or diminished heart rate. Body position can influence circulation, as can age, body surface area, oxygen consumption, body temperature, basal metabolic rate, and activity. Thus many factors can affect CO.

Afterload indicates the resistance the heart must overcome to eject blood into the systemic circulation. This impedance to flow is called systemic vascular resistance (SVR).

Left ventricular pressure must exceed pressure in the aorta to open the aortic valve and force blood from the heart into the circulation. Afterload, not a direct measure, is deduced by calculating the SVR. An elevated afterload can produce increased left ventricular wall tension in an attempt to generate adequate intracavitary ventricular pressure to overcome resistance and permit systolic ejection. The subsequent increase in myocardial oxygen demand must be met, or ventricular function deteriorates. Diminution of afterload reduces wall tension, thereby improving ventricular contraction. Improving cardiac function involves cost in myocardial oxygen consumption. Augmenting CO by increasing the heart rate and contractility increases myocardial oxygen consumption. Improving CO by augmenting preload or by reducing afterload results in relatively little oxygen cost to the myocardium.

A comprehensive view of cardiac function can be obtained by measurements of filling pressure, CO, and calculation of peripheral resistance. Repeated measurements offer evaluation of treatment.

Cardiac Index. The cardiac index (CI) assesses the heart's ability to meet the body's need for oxygen and other nutrients. With noninvasive ultrasound, the CI measures CO in relation to body surface. A CI less than 2 L of blood per minute per square meter of body surface identifies high risk for untoward cardiovascular events during or after anesthesia. The BP may drop; irregular heartbeats may develop. If these adverse events are anticipated, they can be prevented or treated.

Total Blood Volume. Blood volume is useful in determining the total amount of blood replacement required. An accurate method of total blood volume (TBV) measurement involves measuring plasma and red blood cell volumes separately and then adding the results together. To measure red blood cell volume, cells are tagged with detectable, nontoxic, radioactive chromium, subsequently injected intravenously, and counted after an appropriate mixing time. Or radioactive iodinated human serum albumin, in standard-dose packages, can be injected, mixed, and counted. Counting may be done rapidly by an electronic device. This technique may be used in place of estimation of blood loss.

Respiratory Tidal Volume. The respiratory tidal volume (V_T), the volume of air moved with each respiration, may be measured with a respirometer placed on the expiratory limb of the anesthesia machine or mechanical ventilator. Alarms may be incorporated to signal disconnection, failure to cycle, or excessive pressure.

Body Temperature. The body continuously produces heat through metabolic activities and loses heat through convection, evaporation, conduction, and radiation. The production of heat causes increased oxygen consumption by the body's cells. When the rate of heat production is equal to the rate of loss, a heat balance of constant core body temperature is maintained. Core temperature is that of the interior of the body as opposed to the body surface temperature. Normal core temperature ranges from 98° to 100° F (36.8° to 37.7° C).

Under anesthesia, the average adult loses 0.9° to 2.7° F (0.5° to 1.5° C); the greatest loss occurs during the first hour, through convection from exposure to the environment, through evaporation via respiration, through conduction from contact with cool surfaces, and through radiation from tissues. Intraoperative hypothermia, or core temperature less than 96° F (36° C), is a common complication of surgery under general anesthesia, especially in pediatric and geriatric patients. Some anesthetic agents inhibit heat production; halogenated agents cause vasodilation that contributes to surface cooling; muscle relaxants prevent shivering, which is a thermoregulatory protective reflex. Other factors can change core temperature. Hyperthermia (retention of heat) may be caused by premedication, drapes, a closed anesthesia breathing circuit, or fever from sepsis. Physical reactions are not seen in the anesthetized patient. Therefore, the body temperature should be continuously monitored for metabolic changes.

Electronic telethermometers with dial or digital readouts measure body and surface temperatures with thermistor or thermocouple probes. A core temperature probe can be inserted into a body orifice (i.e., nasopharynx, esophagus, bladder, rectum). An esophageal probe measures body temperature at the level of the right side of the heart and is responsive to changes in body heat. A rectal probe responds slowly to changes in body temperature and can be inaccurate because of the presence of stool. These probes are available in various sizes and have flexible tips; some are disposable. The sensor of a bladder probe is in the tip of a sterile Foley catheter. A sterile catheter probe may also be inserted into the pulmonary artery. A probe can be placed on the tympanic membrane via the external auditory canal of the ear. This measures temperature closest to the hypothalamus, which is the thermoregulatory center in the brain.

Skin surface probes have either small tips or discs that are attached to the skin, often on an extremity, with an adhesive-backed foam pad. Cutaneous liquid crystal thermography, with temperature-sensitive chemicals laminated within an adhesive plastic strip, may be used for surface monitoring. The strip is usually applied to the forehead; its chemicals visibly change color with a temperature variation. Proximity to major arteries, insulation from the external environment, and the location of an inflammatory process and the surgical site are considerations in the choice of the temperature monitoring site.

Urinary Output. Urinary output can be measured by an indwelling Foley catheter attached to a calibrated collection bag. The sterile disposable collection system must be below the level of the bladder to prevent distention and allow flow without reflux. Output is valuable in assessing effective blood volume and fluid administration, except when a diuretic is given. Volume, electrolytes, osmolarity, and pH are important.

A reduction in urinary volume may indicate reduced renal perfusion. Oliguria can result from stress of the surgical procedure, antidiuresis from the anesthetic agent, impending renal failure, or reduced volume of circulating blood. Urinary output greater than 30 to 60 mL/hr usually shows adequate intravascular volume and BP.

The collecting system should be able to accurately measure a half-hour output between 1 and 200 mL and provide observation of the urine. Hemoglobinuria can be a manifestation of transfusion of incompatible blood. An electronic monitoring system is available with digital display of data that can be fed into a computer. The system records output in milliliters for both the present and the immediately past hours. It also shows the number of minutes elapsed in the current hour. Early warning of possible cardiovascular or renal problems is facilitated by visual alert signals if urine flow falls below 15 mL/hr or ceases.

Chest Radiograph. A chest radiograph essential for checking the position of the pulmonary artery (Swan-Ganz) catheter, CVP line, endotracheal tube, and chest tube and for observing changes in the lungs and heart during the perioperative care period.

Electroencephalogram. Electrical activity of the nervous system reflects neurologic function. Therefore, electrophysiologic monitoring provides information about the functional integrity of the central nervous system during anesthesia and is especially valuable in patients undergoing high-risk neurosurgical, cardiac, vascular, or orthopedic procedures. Electrodes placed on the scalp transmit the electrical signals, alpha rhythms, from brain activity. Alpha rhythms normally occur at a rate of 8 to 13 waves per second. On the electroencephalogram (EEG) these wave patterns vary among individuals in response to anesthetics, drugs, and pathologic and physiologic changes. They reveal the presence of organic brain damage, abnormal physiologic alterations, and actions of drugs.

Regional cerebral blood flow correlates well with EEG activity. Computer analysis offers visual recognition of cerebral hypoperfusion or ischemia. The EEG is used particularly in surgical procedures involving expected localized brain ischemia caused by intentional surgical occlusion. An EEG also is a means of determining cessation of circulation, an index of expected prognosis, and brain vitality.

Scalp electrodes (cups or discs of silver/silver chloride, gold, or tin) are fixed in place with conductive gel. Or subdermal platinum electrodes can be used. Electrodes are placed over areas of cerebral cortex according to a system that uses measurements of head circumference, distance between the ears, and distance from the nasion (point where the sagittal plane intersects the frontonasal suture) to the inion (external protuberance of the occipital bone). The small neurophysiologic signals recorded are amplified for analysis and display. Multiple channels are necessary to detect regional versus global alterations in function. As many as 8 to 32 channels may be recorded simultaneously.

Paper records or strip-charting provides comparisons of EEG activity during crucial periods with the activity seen before anesthesia induction or surgical manipulation. Methods of EEG analysis that permit automated pattern recognition and alarm generation enhance monitoring in the OR or intensive care unit (ICU). Devices are available that process EEG signals to simplify and facilitate the complex EEG analysis.

Cerebral Function Monitor. The cerebral function monitor provides trend recording of amplitude and amplitude variability for a single channel of the EEG and is useful mainly for detecting marked global alterations in EEG activity during cardiopulmonary bypass, induced hypotension, or metabolic coma. During carotid endarterectomy, paired monitors can detect EEG asymmetries. Although they simplify monitoring, they may be less sensitive to ischemia than the 16-channel-strip–chart recording.

Compressed Spectral Array. Compressed spectral array (CSA) programs may give a time-compressed mountain-and-valley representation of brain activity. The mountains move to the left with slower brain activity and to the right with faster activity. CSA helps determine if the brain is ischemic because of a lack of contralateral circulation during vascular surgery, such as carotid endarterectomy. This type of computerized EEG can be run on general-purpose minicomputers or microcomputers.

Neurometrics Monitor. A neurometrics monitor is also a single-channel device for displaying processed EEG signals. From 4 to 32 minutes of EEG can be seen at one time, but trends are less easily seen.

Bispectral Index Monitoring. Bispectral index (BIS) monitoring is a noninvasive method of monitoring the anesthesia level through processed EEG parameters. An electrode patch is placed on the patient's forehead, and the brain signals are relayed to a monitor. Readings are displayed as a single number (100 [wide awake] to 0 [absence of brain electrical activity]) and indicate the level of anesthesia. The results are reduced drug use, faster wake-up time, and decreased risk of patient awareness during the surgical procedure. This potentially translates into faster discharge for ambulatory surgery patients.

Evoked Potentials. Sensory information (sight, sound, smell, taste, touch) evokes an electrical response when it reaches the brain. Evoked potentials are those electrical responses recorded from the cerebral cortex after stimulation of a peripheral sensory organ. A computer is programmed to average the brain's repetitive responses to the stimuli. The computer displays these as waves on a video screen or prints them on a plotter.

Auditory Evoked Potentials. A clicking sound is delivered in the ear to stimulate the auditory nerve. Brain waves are recorded by the evoked potential computer. The evoked potentials can be used to assess function of the auditory nerve (e.g., during removal of acoustic neuroma). Because the auditory nerve enters the brainstem, evoked responses provide an indirect assessment of brainstem activity.

Somatosensory Evoked Potentials. Intraoperative monitoring of somatosensory evoked potentials is used to continuously assess spinal cord function and to protect the cord from injury during orthopedic or neurosurgical procedures on the spine or spinal cord. Because hypotension increases the insult of direct pressure on the cord and heightens damage to cord function, the spinal cord is monitored when induced hypotension is employed for spinal surgery. Impulses generated below the site of the surgical procedure travel over lateral afferent neural pathways and through the operative spinal area and are recorded by electrodes at brain level. Abnormal brain responses are marked by changes in the arrival time of electrical impulses or amplitude of the waves on a graph. Change in latency and amplitude of the recorded signal, which normally averages 30 to 50 evoked responses, alerts the team to the danger of spinal cord compression or ischemia. Corrective measures taken immediately can prevent serious sequelae. Evoked responses then return to normal.

Bibliography

Davis JW et al: Are automated blood pressure measurements accurate in trauma patients? *J Trauma Injury Infect Crit Care* 55(5):860-863, 2003.

Eisenbacher S, Heard L: Capnography in the gastroenterology lab, *Gastroenterol Nurs* 28(2):99-105, 2005.

Fu ES et al: Supplemental oxygen impairs detection of hypoventilation by pulse oximetry, *Chest* 126(5):1552-1558, 2004.

Kwagyan J et al: The impact of body mass index on pulse pressure in obesity, *J Hypertens* 23(3):619-624, 2005.

Larson MJ, Taylor RS: Monitoring vital signs during outpatient Mohs and post-Mohs reconstructive surgery performed under local anesthesia, *Dermatol Surg* 30(5):777-783, 2004.

Oparil S, Miller AP: Gender and blood pressure, *J Clin Hypertens* 7(5):300-309, 2004.

Pruitt WC, Jacobs M: Interpreting arterial blood gases: Easy as ABC, *Nursing 2004* 34(8):50-53, 2004.

Schneider G et al: Detection of consciousness by electroencephalogram and auditory evoked potentials, *Anesthesiology* 103(5):934-943, 2005.

Sugino S et al: Forehead is as sensitive as finger pulse oximetry during general anesthesia, *Can J Anesth* 51(5):432-436, 2004.

Chapter 28

Hemostasis, Implants, and Wound Closure

CHAPTER OBJECTIVES

After studying this chapter, the learner will be able to:
- Describe mechanical methods of hemostasis.
- Describe chemical methods of hemostasis.
- Describe thermal methods of hemostasis.
- Identify several absorbable sutures.
- Identify several nonabsorbable sutures.
- List several different types of needles.

CHAPTER OUTLINE

Historical Background, p. 547
Hemostasis, p. 548
Wound Closure, p. 557

KEY TERMS AND DEFINITIONS

Allogeneic graft   Tissue taken from the same species for implantation into a different individual of the same species.
Approximation   Bringing the edges of an incision together
Autologous graft   Tissue taken from one area of a person's body for implantation into another area of the same person's body.
Hematoma   Accumulation of blood and fluid in the wound that can promote infection and delay wound healing.
Hemostasis   Control of arterial and/or venous bleeding in the surgical site.
Implant   Process of placing material or tissue into a surgical site.
Ligature   A strand of suture material used to tie or bind. Suture ligature is a free tie. Tie on a passer is a tie held in the tip of a clamp
Prosthesis   Artificial part worn on the outside or implanted inside the body.
Suture   A strand of material used for sewing tissue together or ligating a structure.
Xenograft   Tissue taken from one species for implantation into another species.

HISTORICAL BACKGROUND

The story of hemostasis and sutures, in some measure, is the story of surgery itself. Many kinds of materials were used in the past, and many of the same materials are used today, to close or cover wounds.

The first written description of sutures, which were probably made of linen, to approximate wound edges is in the Edwin Smith papyrus from the sixteenth century BC. The *Shusruta Samhita*, an ancient Indian classic written between 600 and 1000 BC, refers to plaited horsehair, cotton, strips of leather, and fibers from tree bark for use as sutures. These and other writings dating back to 2000 BC refer to strings and animal tendons for ligating and suturing. In AD 30, Celsus referred to the use of twisted sutures.

Galen (AD 130-220) mentioned the use of animal gut sutures for the primary closure of wounds in Roman gladiators, although he recommended silk when it could be obtained. Previous knowledge of ligatures seems to have been lost until Galen wrote of using them to stop bleeding after trying all other methods known at the time.

Mohammedan religious laws required caravan leaders to carry sutures and needles to care for injuries. Sometimes camel hair was used for sutures. Arabian surgeons used harp strings. Rhazes (circa AD 854-930) of Persia is credited with first employing kit strings to suture abdominal wounds. In Arabic, a kit is a fiddle. The fiddle strings, referred to as kitgut, were made from sheep intestines (ovine source), which were twisted and dried in the sun. The term *catgut* is believed to have evolved from its origin as kitgut. Suture material is still made from sheep or beef intestine but is more accurately called surgical gut today.

Sutures fell into disuse during the Middle Ages, accompanying a general regression in surgical technique. Their use was revived by Ambroise Paré (1510-1590), a French army surgeon. He ligated arteries to stop the bleeding after amputations.

Early in the nineteenth century Dr. Philip Syng Physick (1768-1837) found that the body absorbs sutures made from animal tissue. Probably the first surgeon to realize this, Physick was the first American to use catgut extensively. He also fashioned a curved needle for circumventing an artery.

Catgut sutures were used in the early nineteenth century by English surgeons. However, Joseph Lister (1827-1912) is credited with sterilizing and chromicizing them. Only since Lister's time have wound closure techniques been brought to an advanced state of development.

Many materials have been used as ligatures and sutures through the centuries, including gold, silver, and tantalum wire; silk; silkworm gut; horsehair; kangaroo tendon; cotton; and linen. The synthetic polymers developed in the twentieth century resulted in the demise of many of these materials for use as surgical sutures. Polymer chemistry has revolutionized the manufacture of sutures, although older styles of sutures continue to be widely used.

Needles were first swaged (i.e., permanently attached to the suture material) in 1928. Today more than a hundred shapes, sizes, and types of surgical needles are swaged to the suture materials that are in common use.

Although surgical stapling is considered to be an innovation of the twentieth century, the concept of mechanically holding tissues together dates back to antiquity. The *Shusruta Samhita* describes the use of termites to hold wound edges in apposition. The termite would bite through the skin at the wound site and, with subsequent beheading, would hold the wound edges together with its pincers. Ancient Egyptians and some modern South American tribes used ant jaws. East Africans closed wounds with acacia thorns. These insects and plants were the forerunners of the skin staplers used today.

The first internal stapler was introduced in Budapest by Professor Hamer Hültl in 1908 for closing the stomach. This was followed in 1924, also in Hungary, by a mechanical device for gastrointestinal anastomosis developed by Aladar von Petz. Although cumbersome and heavy, weighing over 7 pounds (3.2 kg), the von Petz clamp received worldwide acceptance. The Russians subsequently became the leaders in the field of stapling tissue with their refinements in instrumentation during the 1950s. Most of the reusable staplers currently in use are available through patents licensed from the former Soviet Union. A disposable skin stapler was introduced in 1978, and disposable internal staplers have been available since 1980.

HEMOSTASIS

Hemostasis, the arrest of a flow of blood or hemorrhage, is essential to successful wound management. The mechanism is coagulation, or the formation of a blood clot. The clotting of blood takes place in several stages by enzyme reaction.

Hemostatic Process

When severed by incision or traumatic injury, a blood vessel constricts and the ends contract somewhat. Platelets rapidly clump and adhere to connective tissue at the cut end of a constricted vessel. Interaction with collagen fibers causes platelets to liberate adenosine diphosphate (ADP), epinephrine, and serotonin from their secretory granules. In turn, ADP causes other platelets to clump to the initial layer and to each other, forming a platelet plug. This may be sufficient in small vessels to provide primary hemostasis.

The reaction of plasma from vessels with connective tissue cells at the site of injury activates clotting factors and causes a series of other reactions. Prothrombin, normally present in blood, reacts with thromboplastin, which is released

when tissues are injured. Prothrombin and thromboplastin, along with calcium ions in the blood, form thrombin. This requires several minutes. Thrombin unites with fibrinogen, a blood protein, to form fibrin, which is the basic structural material of blood clots. This last reaction is very rapid.

The fibrin strands reinforce the platelet plug to form a resilient hemostatic plug capable of withstanding arterial pressure when the constricted vessel relaxes. Massive thrombosis within the vessels would occur once coagulation was initiated, if it continued. However, fibrin is digested during the process. The products of this digestion, as well as antithrombins normally present in blood, act as anticoagulants. The coagulation mechanism rapidly and efficiently inhibits excessive blood loss so that excessive coagulation does not occur (Fig. 28-1).

Bleeding During a Surgical Procedure

Two types of bleeding occur during surgical procedures: pulsating arterial bleeding and venous oozing from denuded or cut surfaces. Although the need to control gross bleeding is obvious, insidious but continuous loss of blood from small veins and capillaries can become significant if oozing is uncontrolled. Complete hemostasis, gentle tissue

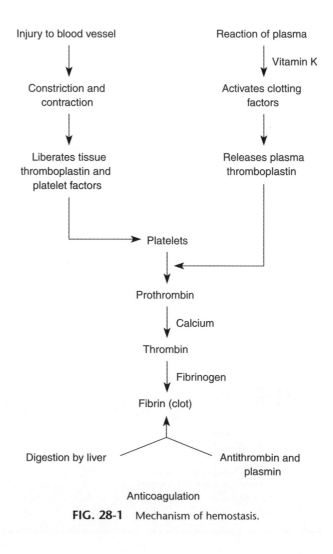

FIG. 28-1 Mechanism of hemostasis.

handling, elimination of dead space, precise wound closure, and a protective wound dressing are essential to minimize trauma to tissue and to enhance healing.

Incomplete hemostasis may cause the formation of a hematoma. A hematoma is a collection of extravasated blood in a body cavity, space, or tissue caused by uncontrolled bleeding or oozing. It may be painful and firm to the touch. Some hematomas require evacuation to prevent infection; others reabsorb with time.

Methods of Hemostasis

Numerous agents, devices, and sophisticated pieces of equipment are used to achieve hemostasis and wound closure. These various methods can be classified as chemical, mechanical, or thermal.

Chemical Methods of Hemostasis

Absorbable Gelatin. Available in either powder or compressed pad form, gelatin (Gelfoam) is an absorbable hemostatic agent made from purified porcine gelatin solution that has been beaten to a foamy consistency, dried, and sterilized by dry heat. As a pad, it is available in an assortment of sizes that can be cut as desired without crumbling. When it is placed on an area of capillary bleeding, fibrin is deposited in the interstices and the sponge swells, forming a substantial clot.

The gelatin sponge is not soluble; it absorbs 45 times its own weight in blood. It is denatured to retard absorption, which takes place in 20 to 40 days. It is frequently soaked in thrombin or epinephrine solution, although it may be used dry after compression.

Before a gelatin sponge is handed to the surgeon, it is dipped into warm saline, if used without thrombin or epinephrine, and pressed between the fingers or against the sides of the basin to remove air from it. The same procedure is used with thrombin or epinephrine solution, but then the sponge is dropped back into the solution and allowed to absorb solution back to its original size.

In powder form, gelatin is mixed with sterile saline to make a paste for application to cancellous bone to control bleeding or to denuded areas of skin or muscles to stimulate growth of granulation tissue.

Absorbable Collagen. Hemostatic sponges (Collastat, Superstat, Helistat) or felt (Lyostypt) of bovine collagen origin are applied dry to oozing or bleeding sites. The collagen activates the coagulation mechanism, especially the aggregation of platelets, to accelerate clot formation. The material dissolves as hemostasis occurs. Any residual will absorb in the wound. Because of an affinity for wet surfaces, it must be kept dry and should be applied with dry gloves or instruments. Absorbable collagen is contraindicated in the presence of infection or in areas where blood or other fluids have pooled. It is applied directly to the bleeding surface as supplied from the sterile package. Do not let this material accumulate in the skin incision because it will create a mechanical barrier to healing causing scars.

Microfibrillar Collagen. Available in compacted nonwoven web form or in loose fibrous form, microfibrillar collagen (Avitene, Instat) is an absorbable topical hemostatic agent. It is produced from a hydrochloric acid salt of purified bovine corium collagen. It is applied dry. When it

is placed in contact with a bleeding surface, hemostasis is achieved by adhesion of platelets and prompt fibrin deposition within the interstices of the collagen.

Tissue cohesion is an inherent property of the collagen itself. It functions as a hemostatic agent only when it is applied directly to the source of bleeding from raw, oozing surfaces, including bone and friable tissues, or directly to active bleeding from irregular contours, from crevices, and around suture lines. Firm pressure is applied quickly with a dry gauze sponge, which is held either by the fingers in accessible areas or by a sponge forceps in less accessible areas. It is important that the material be compressed firmly against the bleeding surface before excessive wetting with blood can occur. Effective application is evidenced by a firm, adherent coagulum with no break-through bleeding from either the surface or edges. Excess material should be removed from around the site without re-creating bleeding. The remaining coagulum absorbs during wound healing.

Oxidized Cellulose. Absorbable oxidation products of cellulose are available in the form of a pad of oxidized regenerated cellulose in a knitted fabric strip that is of low density (Surgicel) or high density (Surgicel Nu-Knit). These products are applied dry and may be sutured to, wrapped around, or held firmly against a bleeding site or laid dry on an oozing surface until hemostasis is obtained. When oxidized cellulose comes into contact with whole blood, a clot forms rapidly. As it reacts with blood, it increases in size to form a gel and stops bleeding in areas in which bleeding is difficult to control by other means of hemostasis.

Except in situations in which packing is required as a lifesaving measure, only the minimal amount required to control capillary or venous bleeding is used. If left on oozing surfaces, it will absorb ten times its own weight with minimal tissue reaction.[1] It is not recommended for use on bone unless it is removed after hemostasis, because it may interfere with bone regeneration. Oxidized regenerated cellulose has some bactericidal properties, but it is not a substitute for antimicrobial agents. Oxidized cellulose is inactivated in the presence of thrombin.

Zeolite Beads (QuikClot). Trauma patients may arrive in the OR packed with zeolite beads used for emergency hemostasis by emergency squads in the field. The intact bag can be placed into the wound. Pressure is applied. It is packaged in 3.5-ounce mesh bags wrapped in foil. The large volume is necessary to have enough to fill a traumatic wound.[2]

The beads are derived from a form of volcanic pumice that has an exothermic reaction in the presence of moisture. The beads absorb the water from blood and reach temperatures around 140° F to 155° F. The OR team removes the bead-pack as part of the trauma surgery because the beads are not biodegradable and could cause a foreign body

---

[1]The FDA advises that absorbable hemostatic agents should not be left in areas where pressure is exerted over neural or bony areas. The force of the pressure causes damage to nerves, particularly in the area of the spinal cord causing intractable pain and disability; www.fda.gov.
[2]Studies were done with prepacked QuikClot in 3.5-ounce quantities. This volume was shown effective in bisected femoral artery and vein. Time is lost in opening multiple packs.

reaction. Copious room temperature irrigation is required to prevent or minimize exothermic reaction at the surface of the wound near the skin edges during removal.

QuikClot is approved by the U.S. Food and Drug Administration (FDA) for uncontrolled emergency bleeding and is used for eviscerating wounds. The foil-wrapped packet can be stored in warm or cool temperatures and has a shelf life of 3 years. Prolonged exposure to the air diminishes the effectiveness of the product once opened. American troops have been deployed for combat with this product since 2005.[3]

Oxytocin. Oxytocin is a hormone produced by the pituitary gland. It can be prepared synthetically for therapeutic injection. During cesarean section, oxytocin (10 units) may be directly injected into the uterine muscle to cause contraction after delivery of the baby and placenta. It is a systemic agent used to control hemorrhage from the uterus, rather than a local hemostatic agent per se. Oxytocin is sometimes used to induce labor. It also causes contraction of the uterus after delivery of the placenta.

Ergonovine, another oxytoxic drug commonly referred to as ergotrate maleate, can be used to treat uterine bleeding after childbirth or abortion after the delivery of the placenta. It causes sustained uterine contractions over a period of 3 hours. The drug is derived from ergot, a form of rye. Ergotrate should be stored in cool, dry area and protected from light.

Phenol and Alcohol. Some surgeons use a cotton-tipped swab dipped in 95% phenol to cauterize tissue when cutting across the lumen of the appendix. Phenol is caustic and coagulates proteins, and in high concentration it is so caustic that it can cause severe burns. It is neutralized with 95% alcohol.

Styptics. A styptic is an agent that checks hemorrhage by causing vasoconstriction. Styptics have the disadvantage of being rapidly carried away by the bloodstream.

Epinephrine. A hormone of the adrenal gland, epinephrine (Adrenalin) is prepared synthetically for use as a vasoconstrictor to prolong the action of local anesthetic agents or to decrease bleeding. Used in some local anesthetic agents to constrict the vessels locally, epinephrine keeps the anesthetic concentrated within the area injected and reduces the amount of bleeding when the incision is made. It is rapidly dispersed, leaving little local effect. Within the incision, gelatin sponges soaked in 1:1000 epinephrine may be applied to bleeding surfaces. These are especially useful in ear and microsurgical procedures in which localized hemostasis is critical.

Silver Nitrate. Crystals of silver nitrate in 20% to 50% solution or mixed with silver chloride and molded into applicator sticks are applied topically. Both an astringent and an antimicrobial, silver nitrate is commonly used in the treatment of burns or other moist wounds. Silver nitrate can be used to seal areas of previous surgical incisions that are left open to heal by secondary intention. Silver nitrate should not be used on the face because it may cause discoloration of the skin. The staining darkens to black in the presence of light.

Silver nitrate 1% solution is sometimes used in the eyes of newborns as gonorrhea prophylaxis. Two drops are placed in the lower conjunctival sac. Eye prophylaxis is required by all states in the United States.

Ferric Subsulfate 20% (Monsel's Solution). Can be used to create hemostasis over denuded areas caused by shave biopsies of the skin or anorectal or uterine cervix punch biopsies. Ferric subsulfate is applied by a cotton swab and causes the vessels to occlude by denaturing protein.

Aluminum Chloride 30%. Applied with a cotton swab to cause the formation of coagulum over a denuded area. Not as effective as Monsel's solution and does not cause skin discoloration. Area should be covered with an occlusive dressing to prevent drying of the wound.

Zinc Chloride Paste. Causes coagulation over a denuded area. Zinc chloride paste is sometimes used after Mohs' micrographic surgery.

Tannic Acid. A powder made from an astringent plant, tannic acid is used occasionally on mucous membranes of the nose and throat to help stop capillary bleeding.

Thrombin. An enzyme extracted from bovine blood is used therapeutically as a topical hemostatic agent in 5000- or 10,000-unit solutions. Thrombin accelerates coagulation of blood and controls capillary bleeding. It unites rapidly with fibrinogen to form a clot. Topically it may be used as a dry powder to sprinkle on an oozing surface or as a solution, alone or to saturate a gelatin sponge. Topical thrombin may be sprayed on areas of capillary bleeding that do not lend themselves to other means of hemostasis, such as sealing a skin graft onto a denuded area. It should not be allowed to enter large vessels.

Thrombin is used for topical application only. It is never injected. It is recommended that thrombin be mixed just before use because it loses potency after 3 hours. Thrombin solution should be labeled with the name of the drug and the concentration and kept separate from any other solutions on the instrument table. The manufacturer's instructions should be followed for mixing solution. Thrombin is contraindicated if the patient is allergic to bovine products.

Sclerotherapy. A caustic sclerosing solution may be injected into veins, as in the mucosal lining of the esophagus or anus, to stop or prevent venous bleeding. The solution may be a mixture of equal parts of dehydrated alcohol, bacteriostatic saline, and sodium tetradecyl in a contrast medium base. Other sclerosants are mixtures of absolute ethanol or ethanolamine.

Embolization. A hemostatic agent can intentionally be placed inside a vessel to occlude the blood supply to a tumor. Several substances are used as embolic agents to thrombose a vessel. The embolization depends on the amount of thrombus formed within the substance of the hemostatic agent. Patients on anticoagulants may not form an adequate clot to embolize the desired area. In some circumstances, the embolized area can recannulate and become patent.

The hemostatic agent is delivered under fluoroscopy to the site via injection mixed as a suspension in contrast medium and sterile saline for intravascular use. Albumin or dextran can be used to create a more viscous suspension. A commonly used agent is polyvinyl alcohol foam fibers.

[3]www.z-medica.com.

Other "off label" materials used in embolization include the following:

- Gelfoam powder can be used as a slurry. The occlusion can last several weeks or months, depending on the physiology of the area to be embolized.
- Avitene provides quick embolization that lasts 2 to 3 months.
- Dehydrated alcohol can be used to embolize low-pressure venous lesions. It is mixed with contrast to perform the injection under fluoroscopic guidance.
- Ethiodol (oil-based) can be mixed with chemotherapeutic agents for hepatic chemoembolization. Ethiodol has contrast medium properties.

Other embolization devices such as coils can be placed via the endovascular route to an area of aneurysm by catheter technique. Some lesions can develop collateral circulation, and it may not be possible to repeat the procedure if the blood supply is persistent distal to the coil. Several coils can be placed at one time and may take varying amounts of time to be effective.

Silicone balloons can be deployed into a vessel that develops distal and proximal thrombus at each end of its structure. The balloon deflates over time because it is somewhat permeable, but the lasting thrombus maintains the desired occlusion. Latex balloons are less permeable, but pose a risk to latex-sensitive or allergic patients.

Mechanical Methods of Hemostasis

External Mechanical Methods. Mechanical hemostasis is achieved by occluding severed vessels until normal forces of blood have time to form a clot. During the surgical procedure the surgeon uses many mechanical devices to apply pressure or to create a mechanical barrier to the flow of blood. Pressure also is used prophylactically preoperatively and postoperatively to control the tone of blood vessels and aid venous return.

Mechanical external pressure devices may be applied before the patient arrives in the OR or after the patient is transferred to the operating bed. The intended purpose may be prophylactic to prevent venous stasis, deep vein thrombosis (DVT), or pulmonary embolus intraoperatively and postoperatively. Or the function may be therapeutic to control internal hemorrhage preoperatively or hematoma postoperatively. A bloodless surgical field also can be created by external pressure devices.

Antiembolic Stockings. Elastic stockings may be applied to the lower extremities to prevent thromboembolic phenomena. Static compression on the legs helps prevent venous stasis. Stockings are available in knee- or groin-length sizes. To apply, the circulating nurse rolls the stocking from top to toe. After being placed over the patient's toes, the stocking is gently unrolled over the leg from foot to ankle to calf.

Sequential Compression Device. Inflatable, double-walled vinyl or woven fabric leg wraps use alternating compression and relaxation to reduce the risk of DVT in the legs of high-risk patients undergoing general anesthesia or experiencing extremes of intraoperative positioning. The leg wraps may be used over antiembolic stockings on each leg, although the compression device alone is sufficient in the prevention of DVT. The patient's foot is not encased

within the wrap. The circulating nurse should measure the patient's thigh or calf for the correct size selection (i.e., small, medium, large, or extra large) for either full-leg (thigh-high) or knee-high leg wraps. Proper selection and application are essential for effective compression. Disposable leg wraps are commercially available.

A motorized pump, attached by tubing to each wrap, sequentially inflates leg wraps at the ankles, then at the calves, and then at the thighs for full-leg compression. The pressure of this wavelike action is greatest at the ankles. The leg wraps are divided into chambers so that pressure can be regulated by preset or adjustable gauges. Pressure between 40 and 50 mm Hg applied for 12 seconds and then released for 48 seconds empties blood from deep leg venous sinuses. The action prevents venous stasis and accumulation of clotting factors in deep veins. The pumping action is started before induction of anesthesia, because general anesthesia reduces venous return and causes vasodilation.

The circulating nurse should check operation of the pump regularly and periodically inspect the leg wraps and tubing. Care is taken to ensure that the patient is not lying on the tubing. The type of device, time started, pressure and cycle settings, and time discontinued must be documented on the intraoperative record. If the surgeon wants leg wraps to remain on the patient postoperatively, the device is transported to the postanesthesia care unit (PACU) or intensive care unit (ICU) with the patient. Frequently, sequential compression is continued for 24 hours postoperatively or until the patient is fully ambulatory after an abdominal, hip, or neurosurgical procedure.

MAST Pneumatic Counterpressure Device. Although the concept dates back to 1903, external counterpressure was not a popular medical device until the Vietnam War. There it was used to control hemorrhagic shock until definitive hemostasis became available to casualties. Circumferential pneumatic compression counteracts postural hypotension, maintains venous pressure, and controls hemorrhage. Several types of pneumatic antishock garments (PASGs) are used, primarily to treat hypovolemic shock.

The acronym MAST can refer to medical antishock trousers, military antishock trousers, or a military anti-gravity suit. An inflatable, waterproof garment is fastened around the patient from ankles to ribcage. The trouser chambers are inflated first, to prevent venous stasis in the legs. The entire suit or only specific chambers of it can be inflated from the feet up. Each chamber is inflated separately with a foot pump. By increasing pressure on vessel walls of the legs and abdomen, systemic vascular resistance of peripheral vessels increases blood flow to the heart, lungs, and brain. Compression of torn vessel walls reduces the size of the laceration and diminishes blood loss.

The MAST device may be in place when the trauma patient arrives in the operating room (OR). Deflation begins after induction of anesthesia, beginning with the abdominal chamber. Leg chambers may remain inflated for counterpressure if blood pressure remains unstable. Deflation must be slow and gradual. The MAST suit is never cut off the patient. Rapid deflation reduces cerebral and cardiopulmonary circulation, with resultant shock. Blood pressure is monitored; it should not drop more than 5 mm Hg.

Pneumatic counterpressure devices may be used to prevent air embolism during some head and neck procedures performed with the patient in a sitting position. The increased venous filling produced decreases the possibility of an air embolus. Also, these devices may be used postoperatively to reduce bleeding or to stabilize the patient after massive blood loss during the surgical procedure.

Tourniquets. A tourniquet is a device used to provide hemostasis by constricting the flow of blood in an extremity. It is frequently used on the proximal aspect of an extremity to keep the distal surgical site free of blood. A bloodless field makes dissection easier and less traumatic to tissues and reduces surgical time. Bleeding must be controlled before pressure is released.

Precautions for tourniquet application and use are observed. A tourniquet should not be used when circulation in an extremity is impaired or when an arteriovenous access fistula for dialysis is present. A tourniquet can cause tissue, nerve, and vascular injury. Paralysis may result from excessive pressure on nerves. Prolonged ischemia can cause gangrene and loss of the extremity. Tourniquet time should be kept to a minimum. Metabolic changes may be irreversible after 1 to $1\frac{1}{2}$ hours of tourniquet ischemia. Consideration for latex sensitivity may be an issue for some devices used as tourniquets. Rubber materials should be latex-free if the patient is sensitive to latex products.

A tourniquet is dangerous to apply, to leave on, and to remove. A tourniquet may be applied by the surgeon, first assistant, or the circulating nurse on the surgeon's orders.

Pneumatic Tourniquet. Similar to a blood pressure cuff, although heavier and more secure, the pneumatic cuff consists of a rubber bladder shielded by a plastic insert inside a fabric cover with a hook-and-loop (Velcro) closure. Many different types of cuffs are available. Some are straight and cylindric; others are contoured. A cuff of appropriate length and width must be used; various sizes are available. Cuffs are inflated automatically with compressed gas (air or oxygen) by means of tubing interconnected between the cuff and a pressure cartridge, piped-in system, or battery-powered unit. The desired pressure is uniformly maintained by a pressure valve and registered on a pressure gauge. The tourniquet console, a pressure regulator with a gauge, may be contained in a unit mounted on a portable stand or hung on an IV pole. An automated tourniquet with a computerized microprocessor control signals both audible alarms and visual indicators for deviations from preset pressure and for elapsed time of inflation.

Correct pressure is the minimum amount required to produce a bloodless field. The calculation of tourniquet cuff pressure is according to the systolic blood pressure. An exact pressure to which the cuff should be inflated has not been determined. In a healthy adult, upper extremity pressure 30 to 70 mm Hg higher than the systolic value of the blood pressure may be sufficient to suppress arterial circulation. Tourniquet pressure on an average adult arm usually ranges from 250 to 300 mm Hg (up to 6 pounds). In the lower extremity, cuff pressure should be higher than the systolic pressure by one half the value. This may require 350 mm Hg on the thigh. Thin adults and children require less pressure; muscular and obese extremities may require more. Inflation time should also be kept to a minimum. If needed

for more than 1 hour on an arm or $1\frac{1}{2}$ hours on a leg, the tourniquet may be deflated at intervals periodically at the discretion of the surgeon.

A pneumatic tourniquet should be used and maintained according to the manufacturer's written instructions. These and institutional policies and procedures should be available to users of this complex equipment. The cuff, tubing, connectors, gauges, and pressure source should be maintained in working order. Precautions to be taken when using a pneumatic tourniquet include the following:

1. Inspect and test the pneumatic tourniquet equipment before each use.
   a. Inspect the inflatable cuff, connectors, and tubing for cleanliness, integrity, and function.
   b. Ensure that the cuff and tubing are intact and that the connectors are securely fastened to the tourniquet pressure source.
   c. Check the pressure gauge for accuracy. An aneroid pressure gauge can be checked by comparing it with a mercury manometer. Pressure drifts can be detected by wrapping the cuff around a rigid cylinder, inflating it to 300 mm Hg, and observing for pressure variations.
2. Protect the patient's skin under the tourniquet cuff.
   a. Place wrinkle-free padding around the extremity. A length of stockinette or lint-free cotton sheet wadding may be used (Webril). Disposable padded covers are commercially available.
   b. Keep the padding and cuff dry. Antiseptic solutions and other fluids should not contact or accumulate under the cuff. Skin maceration or burns could result. Placing an impervious drape around the cuff prevents the pooling of fluids.
3. Position the cuff at the point of maximum circumference of the extremity.
   a. Avoid vulnerable neurovascular structures. Nerves and blood vessels may be compressed against bone when the cuff is inflated. Soft tissue provides padding for underlying structures. The cuff should be placed on the upper arm or proximal third of the thigh.
   b. Select a cuff of appropriate width for the size and shape of the extremity. A wide cuff occludes blood flow at a lower pressure than does a narrow cuff.
   c. Select a cuff with adequate length to overlap at least 3 inches (7.5 cm) but not more than 6 inches (15 cm).
   d. Apply the cuff smoothly and snugly over padding, if used, before prepping the extremity.
   e. Apply a sterile cuff, if used, after prepping and draping. A sterile cuff may be used for an immunocompromised patient.
4. Preset pressure gauges. The surgeon determines the pressure setting according to the patient's age, limb size, and systolic blood pressure and the width of the cuff to be used.
5. Exsanguination of the elevated extremity after prepping and draping, but before cuff inflation, to prolong the tourniquet time.
   a. Elevate the arm or leg for 2 minutes to encourage venous drainage.

b. Wrap a rubber Esmarch bandage around the extremity to compress superficial vessels. Non-latex varieties are commercially available.

c. Deflate the cuff completely and exsanguinate again if the cuff inflates either excessively or insufficiently. Reinflation over blood-filled vessels may cause intravascular thrombosis.

6. Inflate the cuff rapidly to occlude arteries and veins simultaneously to predetermined minimum pressure.

7. Monitor safety parameters during use of the pneumatic tourniquet.

   a. Monitor the pressure gauge to detect pressure fluctuations within the bladder of the cuff.

   b. Monitor the duration of inflation. Inform the surgeon when the cuff has been inflated for 1 hour and every 15 minutes thereafter. In some ORs the circulating nurse posts the tourniquet time on a tally board in view of the surgeon.

8. Document the use of a tourniquet on the intraoperative record.

   a. Record the times the tourniquet is applied, inflated, deflated, and removed. The anesthesia provider also records the inflation time on the anesthesia sheet when a tourniquet is used with a Bier block for regional anesthesia.

   b. Record the location of the cuff, who placed it, and the pressure setting.

   c. Record the model and serial number of the tourniquet used.

   d. Document assessment of the skin condition of the extremity preoperatively and evaluation of skin and tissue integrity after removal of the cuff.

9. Clean and inspect the pneumatic tourniquet after each patient use.

   a. Wash the reusable cuff and bladder according to the manufacturer's instructions. An enzymatic detergent should be used if blood or body fluid came in contact with the cuff. A disposable cuff cover facilitates cleaning.

   b. Rinse and dry the cuff and bladder. Water droplets inside the bladder can damage the pressure mechanism if forced backward during subsequent deflation. Care should be taken to prevent water from getting into the bladder during washing.

   c. Wipe the connecting tubing with a disinfectant.

   d. Test the cuff, tubing, connectors, and gauges before storage between uses. A malfunctioning device must be removed from service until repaired and tested by appropriate personnel.

A pneumatic tourniquet is used most frequently to produce a bloodless surgical field. Other types of tourniquets include the following:

• *Blood pressure cuff:* The cuff is inflated with ambient air. The surgeon determines the amount of pressure to be sustained. The regulator valve is tightened. The pressure gauge or sphygmomanometer must be monitored for pressure deviations.

• *Rubber band:* This may be used as a tourniquet for a finger or toe. The surgeon will put a sterile rubber band on the digit after draping. This method is not used for latex-sensitive patients.

• *Rubber bandage (Esmarch bandage):* Friedrich von Esmarch, a German military surgeon, introduced an elastic bandage for the control of hemorrhage on the battlefield in 1869. Known today as the Esmarch bandage, a 3-inch (7.5-cm) latex rubber roller bandage is used to compress superficial vessels to force blood out of an extremity.

An Esmarch bandage is not used, however, to empty vessels of blood preoperatively in a patient who has sustained traumatic injury or if the patient has been in a cast. Danger exists that thrombi might be present in vessels because of injury or stasis of blood. These could become dislodged and result in emboli. An extremity with active infection or a malignant tumor also is not wrapped with an Esmarch bandage.

Starting at the distal end of the extremity, the surgeon wraps a sterile Esmarch bandage tightly, overlapping it spirally, to the level of the blood pressure cuff or a pneumatic tourniquet. (An elastic Ace bandage may be used.) The circulating nurse tightens the tourniquet. Then the rubber bandage is removed. Or, starting from the distal end of the extremity, the rubber bandage can be partially removed, leaving the last three rounds, which constitute a tourniquet.

After terminal cleaning of a reusable Esmarch bandage, a layer of gauze bandage is rolled between layers of the rubber bandage to ensure sterilization of all surfaces. The gauze must be removed and the bandage rerolled before use. Disposable sterile Esmarch bandages are commercially available.

• *Rubber tubing:* When an intravenous (IV) infusion is started, a small length of rubber tubing is tied around the extremity, usually an arm, while the needle is being inserted. This stops venous return and makes the vein more visible for venipuncture. A Penrose drain is commonly used as a tourniquet.

Pressure Dressings. Pressure on the wound in the immediate postoperative period can minimize the accumulation of intercellular fluid and decrease bleeding by eliminating dead space. Pressure dressings are used on some extensive wounds to decrease edema and potential hematoma or seroma formation. They may be used as an adjunct to wound drainage to distribute pressure evenly over the wound.

Packing. Packing is used with or without pressure to achieve hemostasis and to eliminate dead space in an area where mucosal tissues need support, such as the vagina, rectum, or nose. Packing impregnated with an antiseptic agent, such as iodoform gauze, may be used to ensure closure of an incision from the wound base toward the outside (i.e., healing by second intention), as in a large abscess cavity. The surgeon inserts sterile packing as the final stage of the surgical procedure. It is usually removed in 24 to 48 hours. The intraoperative record and patient's chart should reflect the type, amount, and location of packing.

Internal Mechanical Methods.
Meticulous hemostasis during the surgical procedure is essential to control bleeding and to minimize blood loss. The surgeon uses many mechanical tools to achieve hemostasis.

Hemostatic Clamps. Clamps for occluding vessels are used to compress blood vessels and to grasp or hold a small amount of tissue. The hemostat is the most frequently used surgical instrument and the most commonly used method of hemostasis. This instrument has either straight or curved jaws that narrow to a fine point. Often the pressure of clamping an instrument is sufficient to constrict and seal a vessel with minimal trauma or adjacent tissue necrosis. A wide variety of hemostatic clamps are used for vessel occlusion, including noncrushing vascular clamps that do not damage large vessels.

Ligating Clips. When placed on a blood vessel and pinched shut, clips occlude the lumen and stop the bleeding from the vessel. Metallic clips, such as stainless steel or titanium clips, are small pieces of thin, serrated wire that are bent in the center to an oblique angle. Absorbable polymer clips are similar in configuration. Clips are most frequently used on large vessels or those in anatomic locations difficult to ligate by other means. Many surgeons use clips for ligating vessels, nerves, and other small structures. A specific forceps is required for the application of each type available. Single clips may be mounted in a sterile plastic cartridge that can be secured in a heavy stainless steel base to facilitate loading the applier forceps. Disposable manual and powered appliers preloaded with multiple clips also are available. Some disposable clip appliers ligate as they apply the clip to a vessel.

Ligating clips were devised in 1917 by Dr. Harvey Cushing for use in brain surgery. Cushing clips are made of silver. Titanium clips are more common today, because they cause less interference with computed tomography (CT) and magnetic resonance imaging (MRI) examinations. The serrations across the wire prevent their slipping off the vessels. Polymeric clips have a locking device to secure them on vessels.

Metallic clips also may be used to mark a biopsy site or other anatomic areas to permit radiographic visualization and thus detect postoperative complications. For example, migration of a marker clip could indicate the presence of a hematoma in the wound. The artifacts (i.e., distortion) caused by stainless steel clips may be a disadvantage in future radiologic studies or MRI. Titanium and absorbable polymeric clips are preferred to eliminate or decrease image distortion of CT and MRI scans.

Ligatures. A ligature, commonly called a tie, is a strand of material that is tied around a blood vessel to manually occlude the lumen and prevent bleeding. Frequently the ligature is tied around a hemostat and slipped off the point onto the vessel and pulled taut to effect hemostasis. Vessels are ligated with the smallest-size strand possible and include the smallest amount of surrounding tissue possible. Ends are cut as near the knot as possible.

Large and pulsating vessels may require a transfixion suture. A ligature on a needle (stick tie) is placed through a "bite" of tissue and brought around the end of the vessel. This eliminates any possibility of its slipping off the vessel. All bleeding points should be ligated before the next layer of tissue is incised.

Pledgets. Small pieces of Teflon felt are used as a buttress under sutures when bleeding might occur through the needle hole in a major vessel or when friable tissue might tear, such as cardiac muscle during cardiomyotomy. Placed over an arteriotomy site, they exert pressure to seal off bleeding. Pledgets are used most frequently in cardiovascular surgery and remain in place as part of the suture.

Packs. Packs are used to sustain pressure on raw wound surfaces and keep viscera from becoming injured during a procedure. The application of sponges or laparotomy tapes effectively controls capillary ooze by occluding the capillaries. The surgeon usually wants these moistened, often with room-temperature but sometimes with warm normal saline solution. Warm packs promote hemostasis by accelerating the coagulation mechanism.

Compressed Absorbent Patties. Compressed absorbent radiopaque patties (cottonoids) are used for hemostasis when placed on the surface of brain tissue and to absorb blood and fluids around the spinal cord or nerves. These patties are available in an assortment of sizes. Before use, the scrub person counts and moistens them with normal saline solution, presses out excess solution, and keeps them flat. Some surgeons prefer an antibiotic, thrombin, or epinephrine solution to moisten the patties for hemostasis.

Bone Wax. Composed of a sterile nonabsorbable mixture of beeswax, isopropyl palmitate, and a softening agent, bone wax provides a mechanical tamponade barrier to stop oozing from cut bone surfaces. Each packet contains 2.5 g of wax and is opened just before use to minimize drying. The scrub person can warm wax to the desired consistency by manipulating it with the fingers or by immersing the unopened packet in warm solution. Small pieces can be rolled into 1-cm balls and placed around the rim of a medicine cup. When needed, the cup can be presented to the surgeon.

Bone wax is used in some orthopedic and neurosurgical procedures and when the sternum is split (sternotomy) for cardiothoracic procedures. Bone wax should be used sparingly and is contraindicated when rapid bone regeneration is desired. The wax is a mechanical barrier and may impede ossification as a foreign body reaction. It is contraindicated in the presence of infection.

The product is cobalt sterilized, and the expiration date should be checked before use. It should not be stored in areas that exceed 77° F (25° C).

Bone Wax Alternatives. Biodegradable, water-soluble material that looks and feels like bone wax is a physical, mechanical barrier on cut bone edges and is intended to be used sparingly. One type, Ostene,[4] is an inert alkylene oxide copolymer, derived from ethylene oxide and propylene oxide.

Bone wax alternative is sterilized by irradiation and cannot be reprocessed. It should be warmed and worked into soft 1-cm balls just like bone wax. It has no biophysical cellular action and its presence in the wound does not impair osteogenesis. It is contraindicated in the presence of infection.

Digital Compression. When digital pressure is applied to an artery proximal to the area of bleeding, such as in traumatic injury, hemorrhage is controlled. The main disadvantage of digital pressure is that it cannot be applied permanently. Firm pressure is applied on the skin on both sides as the skin incision is made, to help control subcutaneous bleeding until vessels can be clamped, ligated, or cauterized. Pressure is applied while the surgical area is sponged to locate a bleeding vessel.

---

[4]www.ostene.com.

Suction. Suction is the application of pressure less than atmospheric, either continuously or intermittently. It is used during surgical procedures for removal of blood and tissue fluids from the surgical field, primarily to enhance visibility. An appropriate diameter and style of tip for locating bleeding is attached to sterile disposable suction tubing. The scrub person hands the end of the tubing to the circulating nurse, who attaches it to a suction collection container.

A powered suction/irrigation system may be used to simultaneously irrigate the wound and evacuate solution. The irrigation may be pulsed (i.e., intermittent to remove debris and clots) or continuous with gravity flow. The surgeon adjusts the flow of irrigation and suction with controls on the disposable tip assembly. Spatter screens that fit around the tip of the irrigator like a cone to minimize splashes and aerosolization are commercially available.

Drains. Postoperatively, drains aid in removal of blood, fluid, and air from the surgical site to obliterate dead spaces and to enhance approximation of tissues, thus preventing hematoma and seroma formation. Drains usually are placed through a stab wound in the skin adjacent to the primary incision.

Thermal Methods of Hemostasis

Hemostasis may be achieved or enhanced by application of either cold or heat to body tissues.

Cold Methods

Cryosurgery. Cryosurgery is performed with the aid of special instruments for local freezing of diseased tissue without harm to normal adjacent structures. Extreme cold causes intracapillary thrombosis and tissue necrosis in the frozen area. Frozen tissue may be removed without significant bleeding during or after the surgical procedure. Cryosurgery is also used to alter cell function without removing tissue. It tends to be hemostatic and lymphostatic, particularly in highly vascular areas.

Extreme cold is delivered to extract heat from a small volume of tissue in a rapid manner. Liquid nitrogen is the most commonly used refrigerant; however, carbon dioxide gas may be used. The liquid or gas is in a vacuum container and comes through an insulated vacuum tube to a probe. All but the tip of the probe is insulated. Freezing of tissue at this tip is a result of the liquid nitrogen at the lowest temperature of $-320°$ F ($-196°$ C) becoming gaseous. In the process, heat is removed from the tissue. A ball of frozen tissue gradually forms around the uninsulated tip. The extent of tissue destruction is controlled by raising or lowering the temperature of cells surrounding the lesion to $-4°$ to $->6°$ F ($-20°$ to $-60°$ C).

The machines vary in range of temperatures obtained according to their design and type of refrigerant used. Some are nonelectric with foot switch–operated probes. Special miniature, presterilized, disposable models for single-patient use are particularly suitable for ophthalmic applications.

Because the process is rapid, involves less trauma to destroy or remove tissue, controls bleeding, and minimizes local pain, cryosurgery is used to alter the function of nerve cells and to destroy otherwise unapproachable brain tumors. Other techniques for which it is used include removal of superficial tumors in the nasopharynx and the skin, destruction of the prostate gland, removal of highly vascular tumors and some otherwise nonresectable liver tumors, removal of lesions from the cervix and anus, cataract extraction, and retinal detachment. The amount of tissue destroyed is influenced by the size of the tip of the probe, temperature used, duration of use, kind of tissue and its vascularity, and skill of the surgeon.

Hypothermia. Cooling of body tissues to a temperature as low as 78.8° F (26° C) in adults and large children and 68° F (20° C) in infants and small children, well below normal limits, decreases cellular metabolism and thereby decreases the need for oxygen by tissues. The decreased requirement for oxygen decreases bleeding. Hypothermia lowers blood pressure to slow the circulation and increases the viscosity of blood. This process results in hemoconcentration, which contributes to capillary occlusion and microcirculatory stasis to provide an essentially dry field for the surgeon. Hypothermia may be localized or generalized (systemic). Hypothermia is used as an adjunct to anesthesia, particularly during heart, brain, or liver procedures.

Hot Methods

Diathermy. Oscillating, high-frequency electric current generates enough heat to coagulate and destroy body tissues. Heat is generated by resistance of tissues to passage of alternating electric current. A short-wave diathermy machine produces a high frequency of 10 to 100 million cycles per second. The machine should not be activated until the surgeon is ready to deliver this current. Diathermy is useful in stopping bleeding from small blood vessels. It is used primarily to repair a detached retina and to cauterize small warts, polyps, and other small, superficial lesions.

Electrocautery. A small, battery-operated pencil with a tiny, thin wire loop heated by a steady, direct electric current to red heat will coagulate or destroy tissue on contact. Heat is transferred to tissue from the preheated wire. These cautery pencils are commonly used for plastic surgery, eye procedures, and vasectomies. The hot point of the cautery should be at least 24 inches (60 cm) from the anesthesia machine and patient's oxygen source (face mask or endotracheal tube), which is an oxygen-rich environment. Cautery should not be used in the mouth, around the head, or in the pleural cavity. Cautery should not be used when any flammable agent is present. To prevent fire, only moist sponges should be permitted on the field while any cautery is in use.

Electrosurgery. High-frequency electric current provided from an electrosurgical unit (ESU) frequently is used to cut tissue and to coagulate bleeding points. The concentration and flow of current generate heat as it meets resistance in passage through tissue. Because air has low electrical conductivity, an active electrode tip delivering radiofrequency energy must be in direct contact with tissue. Both cutting and coagulating currents are used in many open and minimally invasive surgical procedures. Some surgeons prefer electrosurgery to other methods of cutting and ligating vessels.

Coagulated tissue is devitalized and causes a foreign body reaction that must be resorbed by the body during healing. If a large amount of coagulated tissue is present, sloughing may result, so the wound may not be sutured and heal by primary intention. Because the high-frequency electric current goes through tissues, a dispersive return electrode is applied to the patient and plugged into the grounded generator. Smoke, or plume, from use of the ESU should be removed from the air with a smoke evacuator. ESUs are described in detail in Chapter 20.

Fulguration. Sparks of high-voltage electric current char the surface of tissue, producing a thin, coagulated crust (eschar) without damaging underlying tissues. Fulguration uses a spark-gap generator that emits a higher-frequency current than does electrocoagulation from an ESU. This high-voltage arcing, described as spray coagulation, is used primarily for transurethral bladder and prostate procedures. A dispersive electrode pad is used on the patient.

Argon Beam Coagulator. Argon gas in combination with an ESU pencil effectively delivers radiofrequency energy to tissue in a coaxial, noncontact, white-light beam for the purpose of rapid hemostasis by coagulation. The argon beam coagulator directs a gentle flow of ionized argon gas from a generator to a pencil-shaped handpiece. The nonflammable gas flow over tissues clears blood and fluid from the target site and allows creation of a superficial eschar directly on tissue by the ESU pencil. Less necrotic tissue is produced than with the high-current density of electrocoagulation because the temperature never exceeds 230° F (110° C), and penetration is approximately half the depth, which minimizes tissue destruction.

The depth of penetration depends on the power, duration of application, and electrical characteristics of the tissue. Coagulation occurs through the arcing effect of electrical energy, not through the action of the argon gas. The coaxial flow of gas delivers monopolar current that coagulates the surface with practically no smoke or odor. A dispersive return electrode is applied to the patient to complete the electrical circuit.

The argon beam coagulator is used to control hemorrhage from vascular structures, surface bleeding of an organ such as the liver, and diffuse oozing and to achieve hemostasis of bone marrow. Handpieces and electrodes are available for use through endoscopes, but they are not used in fluid environments, such as joints.

Hemostatic Scalpel. The sharp steel blade of the hemostatic scalpel seals blood vessels as it cuts through tissue. The disposable blade, size No. 10, 11, or 15, has a heating and sensing microcircuitry between the steel and a layer of copper coated with electrical insulation and a nonstick surface. The blade fits into a reusable handle that contains control switches. The scrub person hands the end of the electrical cord attached to the handle to the circulating nurse, who plugs it into the controller unit. When the surgeon activates it at the handle, the blade transfers thermal energy to tissues as the sharp edge cuts through them. An audible sound is emitted to signal the activation of the device. The temperature can be adjusted between 230° and 518° F (110° and 270° C). The surgeon can raise or lower the temperature in increments of 50° F (10° C). After use, it remains hot to the touch for 30 to 40 seconds. The blade also can be used cold, like any other scalpel.

The hemostatic scalpel can be used to incise skin, soft tissues, and muscle in a long, smooth stroke. This is particularly advantageous in vascular areas, such as the scalp, head and neck, and breast. The blade is kept clean by wiping with a damp surgical sponge. Scraping the surface of the blade on a tip polisher will decrease its efficiency. Care is taken not to touch the hemostatic scalpel blade to an active ESU tip; the circuitry will be damaged.

This scalpel may be used to debride burns. Blood flow into the incised area is minimal, providing the surgeon with a clear, dry field, thus shortening surgical time. The rapid hemostasis with minimal tissue damage promotes wound healing and may eliminate a need for blood replacement. It is not effective in a bloody field or for vessels larger than 1.5 mm. Because electric current from the microcircuitry does not pass through tissue, a grounding pad or dispersive electrode is not required. This also prevents muscle contractions.

Plasma Scalpel. The plasma scalpel vaporizes tissues and stops bleeding as it simultaneously cuts and coagulates tissue. Within the instrument, which looks like a large ballpoint pen, argon or helium gas passes through an electric arc that ionizes it into a high thermal state. These gases are inert and noncombustible. As the instrument moves over tissue, the gas that flows from the tip is visible, allowing the surgeon to see the depth and extent of the incision. Tissue damage, with resultant inflammatory response during wound healing, is greater than that caused by a steel knife blade but less than that caused by other electrosurgical instruments and lasers. Because it will coagulate blood vessels up to 3 mm in diameter, the plasma scalpel is useful in highly vascular areas.

Ultrasonic Scalpel. The titanium blade of the scalpel moves by a rapid ultrasonic motion that cuts and coagulates tissue simultaneously. The portable generator, a microprocessor with piezoelectric disks, converts electrical energy into mechanical energy. This energy is transmitted through a handpiece to a single-use blade. All three parts of the system lock into a frequency of 55,500 movements per second. When this happens, the system is said to be in harmony, thus the name harmonic scalpel. The scalpel can be used for sharp or blunt dissection without damage to adjacent tissues. Vibrations from the blade denature protein molecules as it cuts through tissue, producing a coagulum that seals bleeding vessels. The continuous vibration of the denatured protein generates heat within the tissue to cause deeper coagulation. This action does not raise tissue temperature above 176° F (80° C), so that char or smoke is not produced. A fatty particulate mist may be generated. The vibrating blade also produces a cavitation effect (as it cuts through tissue with high water content) that disrupts cell walls and separates tissue, which aids in dissection.

The ultrasonic scalpel is used primarily for laparoscopic and thoracoscopic procedures. Blades and accessories for open procedures make this technology available to all surgical specialties. Because electricity is not required for effects on tissue, a grounding pad is not necessary.

Laser. Laser light is used for control of bleeding or for ablation and excision of tissues in organs that can be exposed or are accessible endoscopically. The laser furnishes an intense and concentrated light beam of a single wavelength from a monochromatic source of nonionizing radiation. Thermal energy of this beam may simultaneously cut, coagulate, and/or vaporize tissue. The laser wound is characterized by minimal bleeding and no visible postoperative edema. The amount of tissue destruction is predictable by adjusting the width and focus of the beam. Different lasers have selective uses. Lasers are described in detail in Chapter 20.

Photocoagulation. The photocoagulator uses an intense multi-wavelength light furnished by a xenon tube to coagulate tissue. Its use is limited to ophthalmology.

WOUND CLOSURE

Closure of a surgical site or other wound is performed after necessary hemostasis has been achieved. Wounds include deep and superficial structures. Methods of wound closure include sutures, staples, clips, tapes, and glues.

Sutures

The noun suture is used for any strand of material used for ligating or approximating tissue; it is also synonymous with stitch. The verb to suture denotes the act of sewing by bringing tissues together and holding them until healing has taken place.

If the material is tied around a blood vessel to occlude the lumen, it is called a ligature or tie. A suture attached to a needle for a single stitch for hemostasis is referred to as a stick tie or suture ligature. A free tie is a single strand of material handed to the surgeon or assistant to ligate a vessel. A tie handed to the surgeon in the tip of a forceps is referred to as a "tie on a passer."

Suturing Techniques

Halsted Suture Technique. The education a physician receives during postgraduate surgical training exerts a lasting influence on his or her surgical techniques. The classic example of the influence of a professor on his students is that of Dr. William Stewart Halsted (1852-1922). Halsted, a professor of surgery at Johns Hopkins Hospital in Baltimore from 1893 to 1922, perfected and brought into use the fine-pointed hemostat for occluding vessels, the Penrose drain, and rubber gloves. He is best known for his principles of gentle tissue handling. The silk suture technique he initiated in 1883, or a modification of it, is in use today. Its features are as follows:

1. Interrupted individual sutures are used for greater strength along the wound. Each stitch is taken and tied separately. If one knot slips, all the others hold. Halsted also believed that interrupted sutures were a barrier to infection, for he thought that if one area of a wound became infected, the microorganisms traveled along a continuous suture to infect the entire wound.
2. Sutures are as fine as is consistent with security. A suture stronger than the tissue it holds is not necessary.
3. Sutures are cut close to the knots. Long ends cause irritation and increase inflammation.
4. A separate needle is used for each skin stitch.
5. Dead space in the wound is eliminated. Dead space is that space caused by separation of wound edges that have not been closely approximated by sutures. Serum or blood clots may collect in a dead space and prevent healing by keeping the cut edges of tissue separated.
6. Two fine sutures are used in situations usually requiring one large one.
7. Silk is not used in the presence of infection. The interstices (braid pattern) can harbor microorganisms.
8. Tension is not placed on tissue. Approximation versus strangulation preserves the blood supply.

Halsted's principles were based on use of the only suture materials available to him: silk and surgical gut. With the advent of less reactive synthetic materials, wound closure may be safely and more quickly performed with different techniques without complications.

Principles of Suturing. The strength of the wound is related to the condition of the tissue and the number of stitches in the edges. Care is taken not to place more sutures than necessary to approximate the edges. The amount of tissue incorporated into each stitch directly influences the rate of healing. The adequacy of the blood supply to the tissue needs to be preserved for healing to take place.

Methods of Suturing. The edges of the wound are intentionally directed by the placement of sutures during closure. Suturing techniques are depicted in Figure 28-2. Examples of suturing techniques that direct the wound edges for specific healing mechanisms include but are not limited to the following:

1. *Everting sutures:* These interrupted (individual stitches) or continuous (running stitch) sutures are used for skin edges.
    a. *Simple continuous (running):* This suture can be used to close multiple layers with one suture. The suture is not cut until the full length is incorporated into the tissue (see Fig. 28-2, *A*).
    b. *Continuous running/locking (blanket stitch):* A single suture is passed in and out of the tissue layers and looped through the free end before the needle is passed through the tissue for another stitch. Each new stitch locks the previous stitch in place (see Fig. 28-2, *B*).

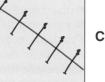
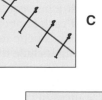
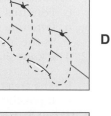
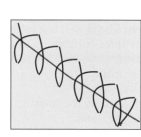
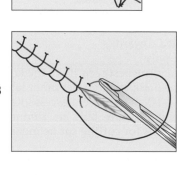
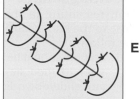

FIG. 28-2 Examples of suturing techniques. **A,** Simple continuous. **B,** Continuous locking. **C,** Simple interrupted. **D,** Horizontal mattress. **E,** Vertical mattress.

c. *Simple interrupted:* Each individual stitch is placed, tied, and cut in succession from one suture (see Fig. 28-2, *C*).

d. *Horizontal mattress:* Stitches are placed parallel to wound edges. Each single bite takes the place of two interrupted stitches (see Fig. 28-2, *D*).

e. *Vertical mattress:* This suture uses deep and superficial bites, with each stitch crossing the wound at right angles. It works well for deep wounds. Edges approximate well (see Fig. 28-2, *E*).

2. *Inverting sutures:* These sutures are commonly used for two-layer anastomosis of hollow internal organs, such as the bowel and stomach. Placing two layers prevents passing suture through the lumen of the organ and creating a path for infection. A single layer is placed for other structures, such as the trachea, bronchus, and ureter. The edges are turned in toward the lumen to prevent serosal and mucosal adhesions. The number of layers is proportional to the quality of the blood supply. Stitches can be interrupted or continuous.

a. *Halsted suture:* A two-layer modification of the horizontal mattress suture used for friable tissue.

b. *Connell suture:* A continuous single-layer suture of gut used for hemostasis in the inner layer of bowel with a separate outer inverting layer of alternating horizontal and vertical mattress sutures.

c. *Cushing suture:* A continuous vertical mattress suture that unites one half of the lumen followed by a second continuous vertical mattress suture that completes the second half of the circumference.

d. *Grey-Turner suture:* A series of inverted interrupted horizontal or vertical mattress stitches.

e. *Pursestring suture:* A continuous stitch that encircles and closes a lumen while inverting the edges.

Knot Placement. Each suture placed in tissue usually requires the placement of a knot to secure the ends. Interrupted stitches require individual knots, and therefore placement of each knot can influence how well the wound heals and the cosmetic result. Principles concerning knots and knot tying include the following:

1. The knot should be tied away from:
   a. Vital structures, such as the eye
   b. Sources of contamination, such as the mouth
   c. Potential irritants, such as the nares
   d. Potential sources of increased inflammation, such as the incision line

2. The knot should be tied toward:
   a. The better blood supply
   b. The area that provides the best security of the knot
   c. If possible, where the mark would be less noticeable

Cutting Sutures. Care is taken to prevent excess suture from remaining in the wound. Suture tails are trimmed close to the knot. Considerations for cutting suture include the following:

1. Scissors should be stabilized by the index finger on the screw (tripod stance), the blades are angled slightly and slide down to the area just above the knot, and the suture is cut with the tips of the scissors.

2. The tips of the scissors must be visible to ensure that other structures are not injured by the cutting motion.

3. A hemostat and/or a second suture should be available in the event that the knot is inadvertently cut, releasing the sutured tissue.

4. A hemostat may be placed on one of the suture ends to stabilize the suture to be cut.

5. If removing a suture, a forceps is used to grasp the suture at the knot. Cut the suture between the knot and the skin. Extract the cut suture with the forceps.

Retention Sutures. Interrupted nonabsorbable sutures are placed through tissue on each side of the primary suture line, a short distance from it, to relieve tension on it. Heavy strands are used in sizes ranging from 0 through 5. The tissue through which retention sutures are passed includes skin, subcutaneous tissue, and fascia and may include rectus muscle and peritoneum of an abdominal incision.

After abdominal surgical procedures, retention sutures are used frequently in patients in whom slow healing is expected because of malnutrition, obesity, carcinoma, or infection; in geriatric patients; in patients receiving cortisone; and in patients with respiratory problems. Retention sutures may be used as a precautionary measure to prevent wound disruption when postoperative stress on the primary suture line from distention, vomiting, or coughing is anticipated. Retention sutures should be removed as soon as the danger of sudden increases in intraabdominal pressure is over, usually on the fourth or fifth postoperative day. Retention sutures are also used to support wounds for healing by second intention and for secondary closure after wound disruption for healing by third intention.

Retention Bridges, Bolsters, and Bumpers. To prevent heavy retention suture from cutting into skin, several different types of bridges, bolsters, or bumpers are used:

• Bridges are plastic devices placed on the skin to span the incision. The retention suture is brought through the skin on both sides of the incision and through holes on each side of the bridge and is fastened over the bridge. One type allows adjustment of tension on the edges of the incision during the postoperative healing period.

• Bumpers are segments of plastic or rubber tubing. One end of the suture is threaded through the tubing before the suture is tied. It covers the entire retention suture strand that is on the skin surface to prevent irritation (Fig. 28-3, *F*). Compression bolsters are made from polyethylene foam held in place with malleable aluminum buttons to secure and distribute tension of retention sutures.

• Buttons and beads are used as bolsters and bumpers to prevent the suture from retracting or cutting into skin or friable tissue. The suture is pulled through holes and tied over a button (e.g., with pull-out tendon sutures). Beads may be placed on the ends of pull-out subcuticular skin sutures. The devices are used most frequently in plastic and orthopedic surgery.

Traction Suture. A traction suture may be used to retract tissue to the side or out of the way, such as the tongue in a surgical procedure in the mouth. Usually a nonabsorbable suture is placed through the part. Other materials may be used to retract or ligate vessels, including the following:

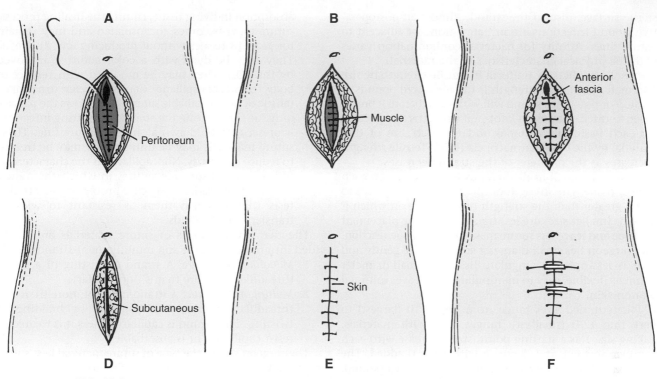

FIG. 28-3 Suturing incised tissue layers. **A,** Peritoneum (continuous stitch, taper-point needle). **B,** Muscle (interrupted stitch). **C,** Anterior fascia (interrupted stitch, cutting needle). **D,** Subcutaneous (not always sutured, taper-point needle). **E,** Skin (interrupted stitch, cutting needle). **F,** Retention sutures. Note bumpers to protect skin.

- *Umbilical tape:* Aside from its original use for tying the umbilical cord on a newborn, umbilical tape may be used as a heavy tie or as a traction suture. It may be placed around a portion of bowel or a great vessel to retract it. These should be counted and accounted for at the end of the procedure.
- *Vessel loop:* A length of flat silicone can be placed around a vessel, nerve, or other tubular structure for retraction. It can be tightened around a blood vessel for temporary vascular occlusion. These should be counted and accounted for at the end of the procedure.
- *Aneurysm needle:* An aneurysm needle is an instrument with a blunt needle on the end for passing suture. The eye is on the distal end of the needle. The needle forms a right or oblique angle to the handle, which is one continuous unit with the needle. The needles are made in symmetric pairs right and left. The surgeon uses them to place a ligature around a deep, large vessel, such as in a thyroidectomy or in thoracic surgery. They can be used to pass a suture tape around and incompetent cervix to perform cerclage. These should be counted and accounted for at the end of the procedure. (Refer to Figure 34-16 in Chapter 34.)

Endoscopic Suturing. Endoscopic sutures are available as ligatures and preknotted loops or with curved or straight, permanently swaged needles for use through an endoscope. The ligatures are fashioned into loosely knotted loops before being passed through the endoscope to tie off vessels and tissue pedicles. After the loop is placed around the target site, the knot is slid into position and tightened. The ends are cut with endoscopic scissors and removed through the endoscope. Suture with a permanently swaged needle is placed through either a 3-mm suture introducer for a straight needle or an 8-mm suture introducer for a curved needle. Used to suture vessels, reconstruct organs, approximate opposing tissue surfaces, and anastomose tubular structures, the technique varies according to the method used for knot tying. The methods of endoscopic knot tying are as follows:

- *Extracorporeal method:* The swaged needle and both ends of the suture are brought outside the body through the trocar. The needle is cut off, and the knot is loosely fashioned. The knot is reintroduced into the body through the trocar by means of a knot-sliding cannula. It is snugged into position and tightened against the tissue. The ends of the suture are cut close to the knot with endoscopic scissors. Excess suture ends are removed through the endoscope.
- *Intracorporeal method:* The needle and suture are passed through the tissue with an endoscopic needle holder. Endoscopic instruments are used to tie the knot and cut the suture inside the body.

Specifications for Suture Material
- It must be sterile when placed in tissue. Sterile techniques must be rigidly followed in handling suture material. For example, if the end of a strand drops over the side of any

sterile surface, discard the strand. Almost all postoperative wound infections are initiated along or adjacent to suture lines. Affinity for bacterial contamination varies with the physical characteristics of the material.

- It must be predictably uniform in tensile strength by size and material. Tensile strength is the measured pounds of tension or pull that a strand will withstand before it breaks when knotted. Minimum knot-pull strengths are specified for each basic raw material and for each size of that material by the U.S. Pharmacopeia (USP). Tensile strength decreases as the diameter of the strand decreases.
- It must be as small in diameter as is safe to use on each type of tissue. The strength of the suture usually needs to be no greater than the strength of the tissue on which it is used. Smaller sizes are less traumatic during placement in tissue and leave less suture mass to cause tissue reaction. The surgeon ties small-diameter sutures more gently and thus is less apt to strangulate tissue. A small-diameter suture is flexible, easy to manipulate, and leaves minimal scar on skin.
- USP-determined sizes range from heavy 10 (largest) to very fine 12-0 (smallest); ranges vary with materials. Taking size 1 as a starting point, sizes increase with each number above 1 and decrease with each 0 added. The more 0s in the number, the smaller the size of the strand. As the number of 0s increases, the size of the strand decreases. In addition to this system of size designation, the manufacturer's labels on boxes and packets may include metric measures for suture diameters. These metric equivalents vary slightly by types of materials. Box 28-1 shows how suture gauge is measured in numeric descriptions from smallest to largest.
- It must have knot security, remain tied, and give support to tissue during the healing process. However, sutures in the skin are always removed 3 to 10 days postoperatively, depending on the site of incision and cosmetic result desired. Because they are exposed to the external environment, skin sutures can be a source of microbial contamination of the wound that inhibits healing by first intention.
- It must cause as little foreign body tissue reaction as possible. All suture materials are foreign bodies, but some are more inert (less reactive) than others.

Choice of Suture Material.

Surgical sutures are classified as either absorbable or nonabsorbable:

1. *Absorbable sutures:* Sterile strands prepared from collagen derived from healthy mammals or from a synthetic polymer. They are capable of being absorbed by living mammalian tissue but may be treated to modify resistance to absorption. They may be colored by a dye approved by the U.S. Food and Drug Administration (FDA).
2. *Nonabsorbable sutures:* Strands of natural or synthetic material that effectively resist enzymatic digestion or absorption in living tissue. During the healing process, suture mass becomes encapsulated and may remain for years in tissues without producing any ill effects. They may be dyed with a color additive approved by the FDA. They may be modified with respect to body, texture, or capillarity. Capillarity refers to a characteristic of nonabsorbable sutures that allows the passage of tissue fluids along the strand, permitting infection, if present, to be drawn along the suture line. These suture materials may be untreated or may be treated to reduce capillarity. Noncapillarity is the characteristic of some nonabsorbable sutures in which the nature of the raw material or specific processing meets USP tests that establish them as resistant to wicking transfer of body fluids.

The two classifications of suture materials are subdivided into monofilament and multifilament strands:

1. *Monofilament suture:* A strand consisting of a single threadlike structure that is noncapillary.
2. *Multifilament suture:* A strand made of more than one threadlike structure held together by braiding or twisting. This strand is capillary unless it is treated to resist capillarity or is absorbable.

The surgeon selects the type of suture material best suited to promote healing. Factors that influence choice include the following:

- Biologic characteristics of the material in tissue (e.g., absorbable vs. nonabsorbable, capillary vs. noncapillary, or inertness).
- Healing characteristics of tissue. Tissues that normally heal slowly, such as skin, fascia, and tendons, usually are closed with nonabsorbable sutures. Absorbable suture placed through the skin may cause a stitch abscess to develop because it is inclined to act as a culture medium for microorganisms in the pores of the skin. Tissues that heal rapidly, such as stomach, colon, and bladder, may be closed with absorbable sutures.
- Location and length of the incision. Cosmetic results desired may be an influencing factor.
- Presence or absence of infection, contamination, and/or drainage. If infection is present, sutures may be the origin of granuloma formation with subsequent discharge of suture and sinus formation. Foreign bodies in potentially contaminated tissues may convert contamination to infection. Foreign bodies in the presence of some body fluids may cause stone formation, as in the urinary or biliary tract.
- Patient problems such as obesity, debility, advanced age, and diseases, which influence the rate of healing and time desired for wound support.
- Physical characteristics of the material such as ease of passage through tissue, knot tying, and other personal preferences of the surgeon.

BOX 28-1	**Suture Gauge Diagram**

Smaller Gauge										Zero									Larger Gauge		
12-0	11-0	10-0	9-0	8-0	7-0	6-0	5-0	4-0	3-0	2-0	0	1	2	3	4	5	6	7	8	9	10

Absorbable Sutures

Surgical Gut. Surgical gut is collagen derived from the submucosa of sheep intestine or serosa of beef intestine. The intestines from these freshly slaughtered animals are sent to processing plants. There they undergo many elaborate mechanical and chemical cleaning processes before intestinal ribbons of collagen are spun into strands of various sizes, ranging from the heaviest (size 3) to the finest (size 7-0). Although the larger sizes are made from two or more ribbons, the behavior of surgical gut is that of a monofilament suture.

Surgical gut is digested by body enzymes and absorbed by tissue so that no permanent foreign body remains. The rate of absorption is influenced by the following:

- *Type of tissue:* Surgical gut is absorbed much more rapidly in serous or mucous membrane. It is absorbed slowly in subcutaneous fat.
- *Condition of tissue:* Surgical gut can be used in the presence of infection; even knots are absorbed. However, absorption takes place much more rapidly in the presence of infection.
- *General health status of the patient:* Surgical gut may be absorbed more rapidly in undernourished or diseased tissue, but in geriatric or debilitated patients it may remain for a long time.
- *Type of surgical gut:* Plain gut is untreated, but chromic gut is treated to provide greater resistance to absorption. Surgical gut may be made pliable to enhance its handling characteristics, but the process significantly reduces tensile strength.

Plain Surgical Gut. Plain surgical gut loses tensile strength relatively quickly, usually in 5 to 10 days, and is digested within 70 days because collagen strands are not treated to resist absorption. Plain surgical gut is used to ligate small vessels and to suture subcutaneous fat. It is not used to suture any layers of tissue likely to be subjected to tension during healing. It is available in sizes 3 through 6-0. Generally used in its natural yellow-tan color, it may be dyed blue or black.

Fast-absorbing plain surgical gut is specially treated to speed absorption and tensile strength loss. It may be used for epidermal suturing where sutures are needed for no more than a week. These sutures are used only externally on skin, not internally, particularly for facial cosmetic surgery.

Chromic Surgical Gut. Chromic surgical gut is treated in a chromium salt solution to resist absorption by tissues for varying lengths of time, depending on the strength of the solution and duration and method of the process. The chromicizing process either bathes each ribbon of collagen before it is spun into strands or applies solution to the finished strand. This treatment changes the color from the yellow-tan shade of plain surgical gut to a dark shade of brown. Chromic surgical gut is used for ligation of larger vessels and for suture of tissues in which nonabsorbable materials are not usually recommended because they may act as a nidus for stone formation, as in the urinary or biliary tracts. In closure of muscle or fascia, it has the disadvantage of rapidly declining tensile strength. If the absorption rate is normal, chromic surgical gut will support the wound for about 14 days, with some strength up to 21 days, and will be completely absorbed within 90 days. Sizes range from 3 through 7-0. Chromic surgical gut may be dyed blue or black.

Collagen Sutures. Collagen sutures are extruded from a homogeneous dispersion of pure collagen fibrils from the flexor tendons of beef. Both plain and chromic types are similar in appearance to surgical gut and may be dyed blue. Sizes range from 4-0 through 8-0. These sutures are used primarily in ophthalmic surgery.

Handling Characteristics of Surgical Gut and Collagen

1. Most surgical gut and collagen sutures are sealed in packets that contain fluid to keep the material pliable. This fluid is chiefly alcohol and water but may be irritating to ophthalmic tissues. Hold the packet over a basin and open carefully to avoid spilling fluid on the sterile field or splashing it into your own eyes. Rinsing is necessary only for surgical gut or collagen sutures to be implanted into the eye.
2. Surgical gut and collagen sutures should be used immediately after removal from their packets. When the material is removed and not used at once, the alcohol evaporates and the strand loses pliability. Many surgeons prefer that the scrub person quickly dip the strand into water or normal saline solution to soften it slightly. Do not soak. Excessive exposure to water will reduce the tensile strength. Before unwinding, the strand can be dipped momentarily in water or normal saline solution at room temperature; heat will coagulate the protein.
3. Unwind the strand carefully. Handle it as little as possible. Never jerk or stretch surgical gut; this weakens it. Do not straighten suture by running fingers down the length of the strand; excessive handling with rubber gloves can cause fraying. Grasp the ends and tug gently to straighten.

Synthetic Absorbable Polymers. Polymers, either dyed or undyed, are extruded into absorbable suture strands. These synthetic sutures are absorbed by a slow hydrolysis process in the presence of tissue fluids. They are used for ligating or suturing except when extended approximation of tissues under stress is required. They are inert, nonantigenic, and nonpyrogenic and produce only a mild tissue reaction during absorption. They may be monofilament or multifilament, coated or uncoated.

Polydioxanone Suture (PDS). Monofilaments extruded from polyester poly (p)-dioxanone (polydioxanone) suture (PDS) and PDS II are particularly useful in tissues in which slow healing is anticipated, as in the fascia, or where extended wound support is desirable, as in geriatric patients, but an absorbable suture is preferable. These sutures may be used in the presence of infection; they will not harbor bacterial growth because of their chemical and monofilament construction. PDS II is more pliable than PDS. Absorption is minimal for about 90 days and then complete within 6 months. Approximately 50% of the tensile strength is retained for 4 weeks, and 25% is retained for 6 weeks. PDS retains its breaking strength longer than any other synthetic absorbable suture. Violet PDS is available in sizes 2 through 9-0, blue PDS is available in sizes 7-0 through 10-0 for ophthalmic tissues, and clear PDS is available in sizes 1 through 7-0.

Poliglecaprone 25 (Monocryl Suture). Prepared from a copolymer of glycolide and epsilon-caprolactone, Monocryl suture is the most pliable of the monofilament synthetic sutures. It retains approximately 50% to 60% of its tensile strength in tissue for 7 days, retains approximately 20% to 30% at 14 days, and loses all tensile strength by 21 days. Absorption is essentially complete between 91 and 119 days. Because of its strength retention and absorption profiles, it is indicated for use in all types of soft tissue approximation and/or ligation, especially in general, gynecologic, urologic, and plastic surgery, but it is not indicated for use in cardiovascular, neural, or ophthalmic tissues. Undyed and natural golden in color, it is available in sizes 2 through 6-0.

Polyglyconate (Maxon Suture). A monofilament is prepared from a copolymer of glycolic acid and trimethylene carbonate. It is indicated for approximation of soft tissue except in cardiovascular, neural, and ophthalmic tissues. Absorption is minimal for about 60 days and then is complete within 6 months. Approximately 70% of tensile strength remains at 2 weeks, and 55% remains at 3 weeks. Clear or dyed green, this suture is available in sizes 2 through 7-0. Maxon CV monofilament absorbable suture is available for pediatric cardiovascular and peripheral vascular procedures.

Polyglactin 910 (Vicryl Suture). The precisely controlled combination of glycolide and lactide results in a copolymer with a molecular structure that maintains tensile strength longer than surgical gut but not as long as polydioxanone. Approximately 30% of original strength is retained at 3 weeks. Absorption is minimal for about 40 days; then it absorbs rapidly within 90 days. The acids of both glycolide and lactide exist naturally in the body and are readily excreted in urine. Polyglactin 910 braided sutures are available in two forms: uncoated and coated:

1. Uncoated polyglactin 910 (Vicryl suture) is available dyed violet in sizes 9-0 and 10-0 for ophthalmic procedures.
2. Coated polyglactin 910 (coated Vicryl suture) is a braided strand coated with a mixture of equal parts of a copolymer of glycolide and lactide (polyglactin 370) and calcium stearate. The coating provides a nonflaking lubricant for smooth passage through tissue and precise knot placement. This absorbable coating does not affect the absorption rate or tensile strength of the suture. It absorbs with the suture. Coated Vicryl suture is available dyed violet in sizes 2 through 9-0 and undyed in sizes 1 through 8-0.

Polyglycolic Acid (Dexon Suture). The homopolymer of glycolic acid loses tensile strength more rapidly and absorbs significantly more slowly than polyglactin 910. Strands are smaller in diameter than is surgical gut of equivalent tensile strength. Polyglycolic acid suture loses approximately 45% of its tensile strength by 14 days and absorbs significantly by 30 days. It is a braided suture material available in two forms, uncoated and coated:

1. Uncoated polyglycolic acid (Dexon suture) is available dyed green in sizes 2 through 8-0 and undyed natural beige in sizes 2 through 7-0. (A 9-0 monofilament suture, dyed green, is also available.)
2. Coated polyglycolic acid (Dexon Plus suture) has a surfactant, poloxamer 188, on the surface that becomes slick in contact with body fluids for smooth passage through tissue. This suture requires two or three extra throws in knot tying, and the ends must be cut

longer than for uncoated material. The coating virtually disappears from the suture site within a few hours, which may strengthen knot security. Sutures are available in the same sizes as uncoated polyglycolic acid sutures.

Handling Characteristics of Synthetic Absorbable Polymers

- Synthetic absorbable sutures have an expiration date on the package. Therefore rotate stock. "First in, first out" is a good rule to follow.
- Sutures are packaged and used dry. Do not soak or dip in water or normal saline solution. The material hydrolyzes in water, so excessive exposure to moisture will reduce the tensile strength. It is smooth and soft and will retain its pliability.

Nonabsorbable Sutures

Surgical Silk. Surgical silk is an animal product made from the fiber spun by silkworm larvae in making their cocoons. From the raw state, each fiber is processed to remove natural waxes and gums. Fibers are braided or twisted together to form a multifilament suture strand. The braided type is used more frequently because surgeons prefer its high tensile strength and better handling qualities. Surgical silk is treated to render it noncapillary. It also is dyed, most commonly black, but it is available also in white. Sizes range from 5 through 9-0. Silk sutures are used dry. They lose tensile strength if wet. Therefore they should not be moistened before use.

Silk is not a truly nonabsorbable material. It loses much of its tensile strength after about 1 year and usually disappears within 2 years. It gives good support to wounds during early ambulation and generally promotes rapid healing. It causes less tissue reaction than does surgical gut, but it is not as inert as most of the other nonabsorbable materials. It is used frequently in the serosa of the gastrointestinal tract and to close fascia in the absence of infection.

Virgin Silk. Virgin silk suture consists of several natural silk filaments drawn together and twisted to form 8-0 and 9-0 strands for tissue approximation of delicate structures, primarily in ophthalmic surgery. It is white or dyed black.

Dermal Silk. Dermal silk suture is a strand of twisted silk fibers encased in a nonabsorbing coating of tanned gelatin or other protein substance. This coating prevents ingrowth of tissue cells and facilitates removal after use as a skin suture. Because of its unusual strength, it is used for suturing skin, particularly in areas of tension. It is black and comes in sizes 0 through 5-0.

Surgical Cotton. Cotton is a natural cellulose fiber. Suture is made from individual, long-staple cotton fibers that are cleaned, combed, aligned, and twisted into a smooth multifilament strand. Sizes range from 1 through 5-0. Usually white, it may be dyed blue or pink.

Cotton is one of the weakest of the nonabsorbable materials; however, it gains tensile strength when wet. It should be moistened before it is handed to the surgeon. Tensile strength is increased 10% by moisture. Also, moisture prevents clinging to the surgeon's gloves. Like silk, cotton suture may be used in most body tissues for ligating and suturing, but it offers no advantages over silk. It is rarely used, with the exception of umbilical tape. When left in body tissue, there is much tissue reaction.

Surgical Stainless Steel. Stainless steel sutures are drawn from 316L-SS (L for low carbon) iron alloy wire. This is the same metal formula used in the manufacture of surgical stainless steel implants and prostheses.

Two different kinds of metal should not be embedded in the tissues simultaneously. Such a combination creates an unfavorable electrolytic reaction. Some implants and prostheses are made of Vitallium, titanium, or tantalum. Suture material in the wound must be compatible with these metals.

Before the availability of surgical stainless steel from suture manufacturers, commercial steel was purchased by weight, using the Brown and Sharpe (B&S) scale for diameter variations. Many surgeons still refer to surgical stainless steel size by the B&S gauge, from 18 (the largest diameter) to 40 (the smallest). One manufacturer labels surgical stainless steel with both B&S gauge and equivalent USP diameter classifications from 7 through 6-0. Both monofilament and twisted multifilament stainless steel strands are available.

Surgical stainless steel is inert in tissue and has high tensile strength. It gives the greatest strength of any suture material to a wound before healing begins and supports a wound indefinitely. Some surgeons use stainless steel for abdominal wall or sternal closure or for retention sutures to reduce the danger of wound disruption in the presence of contributing factors. It may be used in the presence of infection or in patients in whom slow healing is expected. It is used for secondary repair or resuturing after wound disruption.

Unlike most other suture materials, steel lacks elasticity. A suture tied too tightly may act as a knife and cut through tissue. Stainless steel sutures are harder to handle than any other suture material. A painstaking knot-tying and twisting technique is required. For most surgeons this disadvantage more than outweighs the advantages for routine use. However, in selected situations it fills an important need. It is used in the respiratory tract, in tendon repair, in orthopedics and neurosurgery, and for general wound closure. Wire suture is cut with wire scissors. Do not crimp it with a hemostat.

Handling Characteristics of Surgical Stainless Steel

1. Surgical stainless steel strands are malleable and kink rather easily. Kinks in the strand can make it practically useless. Therefore use care in handling to keep the strand straight.
2. Use wire scissors for cutting stainless steel sutures. Barbs on the end of a strand can tear gloves, puncture the skin, or traumatize tissue.
3. If surgical stainless steel must be threaded through a needle, some surgeons prefer one or two twists of the end around the strand just below the eye of the needle to prevent unthreading during suturing.

Synthetic Nonabsorbable Polymers. Although silk is the most frequently used nonabsorbable suture material, synthetic nonabsorbable materials are used because they offer unique advantages in many situations. They have higher tensile strength and elicit less tissue reaction than does silk. They retain their strength in tissue. Knot tying with most of these materials is more difficult than with silk. Additional throws are required to secure the knot. The surgeon may sacrifice some handling characteristics and ease of knot tying for strength, durability, and nonreactivity of the synthetics. These advantages may outweigh the disadvantages.

Surgical Nylon. Nylon is a polyamide polymer derived by chemical synthesis from coal, air, and water. It produces minimal tissue reaction. Nylon has high tensile strength, but it degrades by hydrolysis in tissue at a rate of about 15% to 20% per year. It may be used in all tissues where a nonabsorbable suture is acceptable, except when long-term support is critical. It is available in three forms: monofilament, uncoated multifilament, and coated multifilament:

1. *Monofilament nylon (Ethilon suture, Dermalon suture):* A smooth, single strand of noncapillary material, clear or dyed black, blue, or green. The smaller the diameter becomes, the stronger the strand becomes proportionately. Sizes range from 2 through 11-0; the latter is the smallest of all sutures manufactured for use in microsurgery. Monofilament nylon is also used frequently in ophthalmic surgery because it has a desirable degree of elasticity.

   Larger sizes are used for skin closure, particularly in plastic surgery where cosmetic results are important, and for retention sutures. Wet or damp monofilament nylon is more pliable and easier to handle than is dry nylon. A limited line of sutures is supplied in a moisturized state; most are supplied dry.
2. *Uncoated multifilament nylon (Nurolon suture):* Very tightly braided and treated to prevent capillary action. Usually dyed black but also available in white, nylon looks, feels, and handles similarly to silk, but it is stronger and elicits less tissue reaction. Sizes range from 1 through 7-0. It may be used in all tissues in which a multifilament nonabsorbable suture is acceptable.
3. *Coated multifilament nylon (Surgilon suture):* A braided strand of nylon treated with silicone to enhance its passage through tissue. Otherwise its characteristics are similar to silk and uncoated multifilament nylon.

Polyester Fiber. A polymer of terephthalic acid and polyethylene, Dacron polyester fiber is braided into a multifilament suture strand that is available in two forms: uncoated and coated fibers:

1. Uncoated polyester fiber suture (Mersilene suture, Dacron) is closely braided to provide a flexible, pliable strand that is relatively easy to handle. However, uncoated braided polyester fiber suture has a tendency to drag and exert a sawing or tearing effect when passed through tissue. It may be used in all tissues in which a multifilament nonabsorbable suture is indicated. It is especially useful in the respiratory tract and for some cardiovascular procedures. Available white or dyed green or blue, sizes range from 2 through 11-0.
2. Coated polyester fiber suture has a lubricated surface for smooth passage through tissue. It is widely used in cardiovascular surgery for vessel anastomosis and placement of prosthetic materials because it retains its strength indefinitely in tissues. Sutures are available with different coating materials:
   a. Polybutilate is the only coating developed specifically as a surgical lubricant. This polyester material adheres strongly to the braided polyester fiber.

Polyester fiber coated with polybutilate (Ethibond suture) provides a strand superior to any other braided material, coated or uncoated, in decreasing drag through tissue. Colored green or white, sizes range from 5 through 7-0.

b. Polytetrafluoroethylene, a commercial product of Du Pont named Teflon, is used as a coating bonded to the surface (Polydek suture) or impregnated into spaces in the braid of the polyester fiber strand (Tevdek suture). Minute particles of this coating can flake off the strand. Because these particles are insoluble and resistant to enzymes, foreign body granulomas may be produced. Sutures with this material on them are white or dyed green and are available in sizes 5 through 10-0.

c. Silicone, a commercial lubricant, provides a slippery coating but does not bond well to polyester fiber. It can become dislodged in tissues as the strand is tied. Sutures with this coating (Ti-Cron sutures) are available white or dyed blue in sizes 5 through 7-0.

Polybutester (Novafil Suture). A copolymer of poly (glycol)–terephthalate and poly (butylene)–terephthalate is extruded into a monofilament strand. It is more flexible and elastic than are other synthetic polymers, which may be a physiologic advantage in limited circumstances for apposing wound edges. It is available clear or dyed blue in sizes 2 through 10-0.

Polyethylene (Dermalene Suture). A long-chain polyethylene polymer is extruded into a monofilament strand. It is available dyed blue in sizes 0 through 6-0 for use in some situations in which a monofilament material is desirable.

Polypropylene (Prolene Suture, Surgilene Suture). A polymerized propylene is extruded into a monofilament strand. It is the most inert of the synthetic materials and almost as inert as stainless steel. Polypropylene is an acceptable substitute for stainless steel in situations in which strength and nonreactivity are required, and it is easier to handle. The suture may be left in place for prolonged healing. It can be used in the presence of infection. It has become the material of choice for many plastic surgery and cardiovascular procedures because of its smooth passage through tissues, as well as its strength and inertness. It is frequently used for continuous abdominal fascia closure, as a subcuticular pull-out suture, and for retention sutures. It is available dyed blue in sizes 2 through 10-0 and clear in sizes 4-0 through 6-0.

Hexafluoropropylene-VDF (Pronova Suture). Especially designed for cardiovascular and cardiac surgery. Pronova is structurally enhanced for strength and delicate performance.

Barbed Polydioxanone (Quill Suture, Contour Threads). This clear synthetic self-anchoring suture is approved for use by the FDA. It is used for dermal suturing without the need for knotted ends. The surface of the suture has raised barbs that are angled from the center to the ends in both directions. During closure the suture is placed with a slight reverse torque to anchor the barbs into the dermis from the center in one direction and then the reverse is performed in the opposite direction. The result is a well-approximated incision line.

Barbed sutures can be used to contour facial sagging for a lifted appearance without extreme incisions. The dermal and fascial tissue is lifted by the barbed attachments and is secured by its own barbed surface.[5]

Handling Characteristics of Synthetic Non-absorbable Polymers

1. Physical damage to suture materials can occur from the time the suture is removed from a packet if the strand is mishandled. Handle all sutures and needles as little as possible. Avoid pulling or stretching. Sutures should be handled without using instruments except when grasping the free end during an instrument tie. Clamping instruments, especially needle holders and forceps with serrations, on strands can crush, cut, and weaken them.

2. All synthetic materials require a specific knot-tying technique. Knot security requires additional flat and square ties. Multifilament materials are generally easier to tie than are monofilament sutures.

Surgical Needles

Except for simple ligating with free ties, surgical needles are needed to safely carry suture material through tissue with the least amount of trauma. The best surgical needles are made of high-quality tempered steel that is:

- Strong enough so that it does not break easily
- Rigid enough to prevent excessive bending, yet flexible enough to prevent breaking after bending
- Sharp enough to penetrate tissue with minimal resistance (yet it need not be stronger than the tissue it penetrates)
- Approximately the same diameter as the suture material it carries to minimize trauma in passage through tissue
- Appropriate in shape and size for the type, condition, and accessibility of the tissue to be sutured
- Free from corrosion and burrs to prevent infection and tissue trauma

Because needles are made of steel, theoretically they are detectable by radiograph if inadvertently lost in tissue. The location in tissue may preclude the needle from appearing on a radiograph. For example, the angle of the needle or its position behind bone may obstruct detection. The smaller the size of the needle, the more likely the image is to be obstructed. All needles should be accounted for so that they do not become foreign bodies in tissue.

Many shapes and sizes of surgical needles are available. Names vary from one manufacturer to another; general classification only, not nomenclature, is standardized. They may be straight like a sewing needle or curved. All surgical needles have three basic components: the point, the body (or shaft), and the eye. They are classified according to these three components.

Point of the Needle. Points of surgical needles are honed to the configuration and sharpness desired for specific types of tissue. The basic shapes are cutting, tapered, and blunt (Fig. 28-4).

---

[5]www.contourthreads.com.

Cutting Point. A razor-sharp, honed cutting point may be preferred when tissue is difficult to penetrate, such as skin, tendon, and tough tissues in the eye. These make a slight cut in tissue as they penetrate. The location and degree of sharpness of cutting edges vary.

Conventional Cutting Needles. Two opposing cutting edges form a triangular configuration with a third edge on the body of the needle. Cutting edges are on the inside curvature of a curved needle. Cutting edges may be honed to precision sharpness to ensure smooth passage through tissue and a minute needle path that heals quickly.

Reverse-Cutting Needles. A triangular configuration extends along the body of the needle. The edges near the point are sharpened or honed to precision points. The two opposing cutting edges are on the outer curvature of a curved needle.

Side-Cutting Needles. Relatively flat on the top and bottom, angulated cutting edges are on the sides. Used primarily in ophthalmic surgery, they will not penetrate underlying tissues. They split through layers of tissue.

Trocar Point. Sharp cutting tips are at the points of tapered needles. All three edges of the tip are sharpened to provide cutting action with the smallest possible hole in tissue as it penetrates.

Taper Point. These needles are used in soft tissues, such as intestine and peritoneum, which offer a small amount of resistance to the needle as it passes through. They tend to push the tissue aside as they go through, rather than cut it. The body tapers to a sharp point at the tip.

Blunt Point. These tapered needles are designed with a rounded blunt point at the tip. They are used primarily for suturing friable tissue, such as liver and kidney. Because the blunt point will not cut through tissue, it is less apt to puncture a vessel in these organs than is a sharp-pointed needle. Blunt needles also may be used in some tissues to reduce the potential for needlesticks, especially in general and gynecologic surgery.

Body of the Needle. The body, or shaft, varies in wire gauge, length, shape, and finish. The nature and location of tissue to be sutured influence the selection of needles with these variable features. Most manufacturers have designated a specific alphanumeric code to describe each needle they produce. Examples of alphanumeric codes for taper-point needles can be found in Table 28-1.

Considerations relating to the body of the needle are as follows:
1. Tough or fibrosed tissue requires a heavier-gauge needle than the fine-gauge diameter needed in microsurgery.
2. The depth of the bite (placement) through tissue determines the appropriate needle length.
3. The body of the needle may be round, oval, flat, or triangular. The point determines the shape: round or oval bodies have trocar, taper, or blunt points; flat or triangular bodies have cutting edges. The shape may also be straight or curved (Fig. 28-5).
   a. Straight needles are used in readily accessible tissue. They have cutting points for use in skin, which is their most frequent use, or tapered points for use in intestinal tissue.
   b. Curved needles are used to approximate most tissues, because quick needle turnout is an advantage. The curvature may be ¼, ⅜, ½, or ⅝ circle; half-curved with only the tip curved; or compound curved. Curved needles always are armed in a needle holder before being handed to the surgeon.
   c. J-shaped needles range from 15.5 cm to 17.5 cm in length. The width of the J bend at the tip is available in 7- to 9-mm curvature. They are used for 10- to 14-mm fascial incisions created for trocar use during laparoscopy. They are multiuse needles that can be threaded with the suture of the surgeon's choice at the point of use. Their unique shape enables the surgeon to close the deep layers of the wound

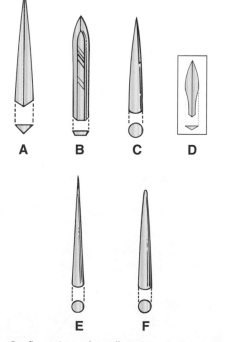

FIG. 28-4 Configurations of needle points. **A,** Conventional cutting and reverse cutting. **B,** Side cutting. **C,** Cutting edge at end of tapered body with, **D,** trocar point. **E,** Taper. **F,** Blunt.

TABLE 28-1	Select Examples of Common Taper-Point Needles (Alphanumeric Codes) and Representative Manufacturers		
Purpose	Ethicon	U.S. Surgical	Configuration
General closure	CT	GS 24	½ circle taper 40 mm
General closure	CT 1	GS 21	37 mm
Cardiovascular	RB	EV 23	17 mm
Gastrointestinal	SH	EV 20	25 mm
Multilayer closure	CTX	GS 25	48 mm
Cardiovascular	BB	CV 15	⅜ circle taper 17 mm
Urologic	UR 6	GU 46	⅜ circle taper 27 mm

without perforation of underlying organs while visualizing closure of the accessory ports with the laparoscopic camera.

4. Curved needles that have longitudinal ribbed depressions or grooves along the body on the inside and outside curvature can be cross-locked in the needle holder. This feature virtually eliminates twisting or turning of the needle in any position in the needle holder.
5. In all needles, the body must have a smooth finish. Many needles have a surface coating of microthin plastic or silicone to enhance smooth passage through tissue. Others have a black surface finish to enhance visibility at the surgical site.

Eye of the Needle. The eye is the segment of the needle where the suture strand is attached. Surgical needles are classified as eyed, French eye, or eyeless (also known as swaged or atraumatic) (Fig. 28-6).

Eyed Needle. The closed eye of an eyed surgical needle is like that of any household sewing needle. The shape of the enclosed eye may be round, oblong, or square. The end

of the suture strand is pulled 2 to 4 inches (5 to 10 cm) through the eye so that the short end is about one sixth the length of the long end.

French Eye Needle. Sometimes referred to as spring eye or split eye, a French eye needle has a slit from the inside of the eye to the end of the needle through which the suture strand is drawn. To thread a French eye after arming the needle in a needle holder, 2 to 3 inches (5 to 7.5 cm) of the strand is secured between the fingers holding the needle holder. The strand is pulled taut across the center of the V-shaped area above the eye and drawn down through the slit into the eye (Fig. 28-7). French eye needles as a general rule are used with pliable braided materials, primarily silk and cotton, of medium or fine size. These needles are not practical for surgical gut; the strand may fray, or the eye may break because the diameter is usually too large for the slit.

Handling of Eyed and French Eye Needles. Eyed and French eye needles have the following disadvantages for the scrub person, surgeon, and patient:

• Each needle must be carefully inspected by the scrub person before and after use for dull or burred points, corrosion, and defects in the eye.

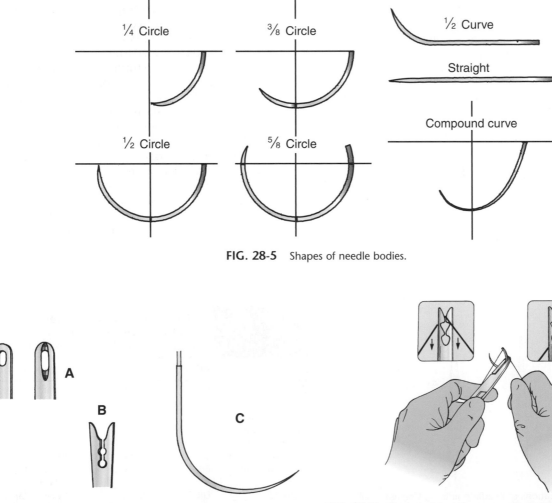

FIG. 28-5   Shapes of needle bodies.

FIG. 28-6   Eyes of needles. **A,** Oblong eyes. **B,** French eye. **C,** Eyeless (swaged).

FIG. 28-7   To thread French eye needle, pull strand taut across center of V-shaped area and draw down through slit into eye.

- Care must be taken to avoid puncturing gloves with the needle point when threading.
- If the scrub person must choose an appropriate needle to thread, the needle should be the same approximate diameter as the suture size requested by the surgeon.
- Needles can unthread prematurely. This is an annoyance to the surgeon and prolongs operating time for the patient. To avoid this, the surgeon may prefer the suture strand threaded double with both ends pulled the same length through the eye; the ends may be tied together in a knot, if desired. Or the scrub person may lock the suture strand by threading the short end through the eye twice in the same direction.
- Two strands of suture material are pulled through tissue when threaded needles are used. The bulk of the double strand through the eye creates a larger hole than the size of the needle or suture material, causing additional trauma to tissue.

Eyeless Needle. An eyeless needle is a continuous unit with the suture strand. The needle is swaged onto the end of the strand in the manufacturing process. This eliminates threading at the operating bed and minimizes tissue trauma, because a single strand of material is drawn through tissue (Fig. 28-8). The diameter of the needle matches the size of the strand as closely as possible. The surgeon uses a new sharp needle with every suture strand. Usually referred to as swaged needles, four types of eyeless needle-suture attachments are available.

Single-Armed Attachment. One needle is swaged to a suture strand.

Double-Armed Attachment. A needle is swaged to each end of the suture strand. The two needles are not necessarily the same size and shape. These are used when the surgeon wishes to place a suture and then continue to approximate surrounding tissue on both sides from a midpoint in the strand.

Permanently Swaged Needle Attachment. This attachment is secure, so the needle will not separate from the suture strand under normal use. The needle is separated by cutting it from the suture.

Controlled-Release Needle Attachment. This attachment is secure, so the suture strand will not separate from the needle inadvertently but it will release rapidly when pulled off intentionally. The surgeon grasps the suture strand just below the needle, pulling the strand taut, and releases the needle with a straight tug of the needle holder on the needle. This facilitates fast separation of the needle from the suture when desired. This type of needle is referred to as a pop-off needle.

Placement of the Needle in the Needle Holder. Needle holders have specially designed jaws to securely grasp surgical needles without damage if they are used correctly. The scrub person should observe the following principles in handling needles and needle holders:

1. Select a needle holder with appropriate-size jaws for the size of the needle to be used. An extremely small needle requires a needle holder with very-fine-tipped jaws. As the wire gauge of the needle increases, the jaws of the needle holder selected should be proportionately wider and heavier. Curved jaws or angulated handles may be needed for placement of the needle in tissues.
2. Select an appropriate-length needle holder for the area of tissue to be sutured. When the surgeon works deep inside the abdomen, chest, or pelvic cavity, a longer needle holder will be needed than is needed in superficial areas.
3. Clamp the body of the needle in an area one fourth to one half of the distance from the eye to the point (Fig. 28-9). Never clamp the needle holder over the swaged area. This is the weakest area of an eyeless needle because it is hollow before the suture strand is attached. Pressure on or near the needle-suture juncture may break the needle.
4. Place the needle securely in the tip of the needle holder jaws, and close the needle holder in the first or second ratchet. If the needle is held too tightly in the jaws or the needle holder is defective, the needle may be damaged or notched in such a manner that it will have a tendency to bend or break on successive passes through tissue.

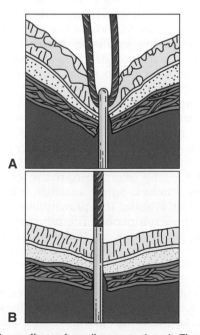

FIG. 28-8 Tissue effects of needle penetration. **A**, Threaded. **B**, Swaged atraumatic.

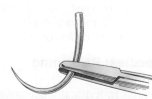

FIG. 28-9 Correct position of curved needle in needle holder, about one third down from swage or eye.

5. Pass the needle holder with the needle point up and directed toward the surgeon's thumb when grasped so that it is ready for use without readjustment. If a hand-free technique is preferred, place the needle holder on a tray or magnetic mat with the needle point down.

6. Hand the needle holder to the surgeon so that the suture strand is free and not entangled with the needle holder. Hold the free end of the suture in one hand while passing the needle holder with the other hand. Protect the end of the suture material from dragging across the sterile field. The assistant may take hold of the free end to keep the strand straight for the surgeon and to keep it from falling over the side of the sterile field.

7. Hand the needle holder to an assistant to pull the needle out through tissue. A hemostat or other tissue forceps is not used for this purpose because the instrument may be damaged or may damage the needle. The needle should be grasped as far back as possible to avoid damage to the taper point or cutting edges.

Considerations in the Choice of Needle and Suture

The surgeon chooses from available types and sizes of sutures and needles, the ones that best suit each purpose. In general, fine sizes are used for plastic, ophthalmic, pediatric, and vascular surgery; medium sizes are used for all other kinds of surgery; heavy sizes are used for retention and for anchoring bone. In general, cutting needles are used in tough tissue such as skin, fascia, tendon, and mucous membranes, including the cervix, palate, tongue, and nose. Medium tissue calls for round taper-point or cutting needles. Round taper-point needles generally are used for nerve, peritoneum, muscle, and other soft tissue, such as lung and intestine, subcutaneous tissue, and dura.

It is almost impossible to learn the needle-tissue-suture-surgeon combinations by memory alone because of the unlimited number of combinations. Learning the general classification of needles, sutures, and tissues is the first step; practical experience is necessary to remember the combinations. One should not feel discouraged by not being able to anticipate the surgeon's wishes and should not hesitate to ask if uncertain of the proper combination at the proper time.

The preference card usually lists the surgeon's usual suture-and-needle routine by tissue layer. Some cards list swaged sutures by order number. Others list sutures by size and materials and needles by size and shape. Suture and needle sizes are as variable as patient sizes. Therefore the surgeon may unexpectedly request a smaller or larger size out of routine for a particular patient's situation. Each manufacturer produces different needle styles. Most types have a comparable counterpart in another brand name. Table 28-1 describes cross-referencing of needle types by alphanumeric codes among different manufacturers.

Sutures and Needles: Packaging and Preparation

Most suture material is individually packaged and supplied sterile by the manufacturer. It is sterilized by cobalt-60 irradiation or ethylene oxide gas. A few materials can be steam sterilized, but most cannot. Protein in absorbable materials derived from animals will coagulate; synthetic absorbable materials are affected by moisture and heat. Only stainless steel can be repeatedly steam sterilized. Nylon, polyester fiber, and polypropylene can be steam sterilized a maximum of three times without loss of tensile strength. The manufacturer's recommendations should be followed for sterilization of nonsterile suture materials.

Swaged needles come in sterile packets with the suture material. They eliminate the labor and expense of cleaning, packaging, and sterilizing needles. Disposable eyed and French eye needles are packaged and sterilized by the manufacturer. Needles are counted when dispensed to the sterile field.

Preparation of Reusable Needles. Standard sets of reusable eyed and French eye needles may be prepared for each surgical procedure. This necessitates preparing many more needles in a set than any one surgeon uses if each surgeon's preferences are to be accommodated. An alternative may be to choose needles for each procedure on the surgical schedule according to each surgeon's preferences as listed on the preference card.

Eyed needles can be loaded on a metal rack with a spring to hold them. The rack can be steam sterilized with the instruments for that surgical procedure, or it may be wrapped, labeled, and sterilized separately. Needles are counted before and after use. Disposable needles are used more commonly than reusable varieties. Single-use needles ensure a sharper point with less tissue trauma.

Packaging of Suture Materials. A strand of sterile suture material is supplied with as many as four coverings.

Box. Each box contains one, two, or three dozen packets of sterile suture material. The label on the box may be color-coded by suture material (e.g., light blue for silk; yellow for plain surgical gut). Most boxes fit into a suture cabinet rack. Competing manufacturers frequently select similar colors as their competitors for box labels and suture material identification. Many synthetic sutures have expiration dates because the material degrades with time. Each box is provided with a lot number that corresponds to the lot number on the individual suture packets.

Overwrap. Each packet has a sealed outer overwrap. The overwrap is peeled back to expose the inner primary packet for sterile transfer to the sterile table. The circulating nurse must not contaminate the sterile inner primary packet as the overwrap is peeled apart and the packet is transferred onto the sterile table or presented to the scrub person.

Primary Packet. Suture material, with or without swaged needles, is sealed in a primary inner packet that is opened by the scrub person. The primary packet may be made of foil, paper, plastic, or combinations of these. Labels may be color-coded by material, the same as the box. If a swaged needle is enclosed, a silhouette of the needle is included on the label, along with the size and type of suture material. A single strand of material or multiple strands may be in the primary packet. The packet may be designed for dispensing individual strands from a multiple suture packet. Packaging configurations and considerations include the following:

1. Suture packets should be opened only as needed, to minimize waste.
2. Custom kits with multiple suture packets within a single package facilitate dispensing sutures to and organizing them on the sterile table. The kit may have appropriate sutures, with or without swaged needles, to meet the requirements of a particular surgeon or procedure. The packets are organized in order of use. The contents are listed on the cover of the package to facilitate counts.
3. Sterile suture packets are labeled "Do Not Resterilize." Component layers of the packaging materials cannot withstand exposure to the heat of steam sterilization without potential physical damage to the contents and packets. The manufacturer will not guarantee product stability or sterility for packets resterilized in the hospital or in secondary processors, or for strands removed from packets and sterilized.
4. Some suture materials have an expiration date stamped on the box and primary packet to indicate the stability of the material. Oldest sutures should be used first. Sutures should not be used past this expiration date because the chemical composition may have started to degrade, and the safety of the suture is in question.

Inner Dispenser. Suture material is contained within the primary packet in a manner that facilitates removing or dispensing it. This may be a folder, reel, organizer, or tube that may or may not be removed with the suture strands.

Preparation of Suture Material. The length of each strand of suture material within the primary packet varies; the shortest is 5 inches (approximately 13 cm), and the longest is 60 inches (150 cm). The most commonly used lengths range from 18 to 30 inches (45 to 75 cm). The length the surgeon prefers should be noted on the preference card. The scrub person may have to cut the strands to the desired length, depending on the lengths available.

Standard Length. The term standard length refers to a 60-inch (150-cm) strand of nonabsorbable material or a 54-inch (135-cm) strand of absorbable material without a swaged needle. It is never handed to the surgeon in this length. The scrub person may cut it into a half-length, third-length, or fourth-length for use as a free tie (suture

ligature) or thread it for a stick tie or suture, as shown in Figures 28-10 and 28-11.

Ligating Reels. Twelve-foot (approximately 4-m) lengths of nonabsorbable or 54-inch (135-cm) lengths of absorbable suture are wound on plastic reels. These reels are color-coded by material and have size identification. The surgeon keeps the reel in the palm of the hand for a series of free ties. The reel is radiopaque in case it is inadvertently dropped in a body cavity. If reels are not stocked, the surgeon may ask the scrub person to wind a standard length onto a rod or other device for this purpose.

Precut Lengths. Most suture materials are supplied in precut lengths of 12 to 18 inches and are ready for use as

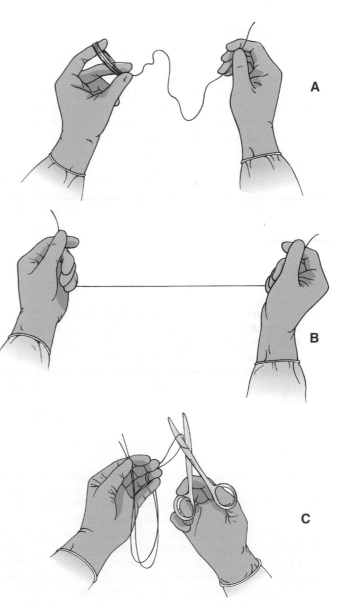

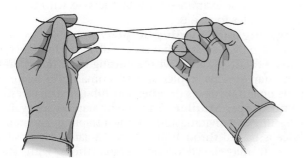

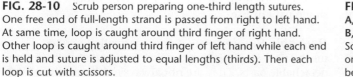

FIG. 28-10 Scrub person preparing one-third length sutures. One free end of full-length strand is passed from right to left hand. At same time, loop is caught around third finger of right hand. Other loop is caught around third finger of left hand while each end is held and suture is adjusted to equal lengths (thirds). Then each loop is cut with scissors.

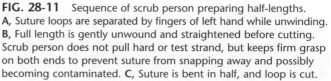

FIG. 28-11 Sequence of scrub person preparing half-lengths. **A,** Suture loops are separated by fingers of left hand while unwinding. **B,** Full length is gently unwound and straightened before cutting. Scrub person does not pull hard or test strand, but keeps firm grasp on both ends to prevent suture from snapping away and possibly becoming contaminated. **C,** Suture is bent in half, and loop is cut.

free ties or for threading. These facilitate handling for the scrub person. They are dispensed individually from some primary packets or may be removed and placed in a fold of the suture book. Packets contain from 3 to 17 strands, depending on the material.

Swaged Needle-Suture. The manufacturer predetermines lengths of sutures; however, the surgeon has a wide variety of choices to meet all suturing needs. The scrub person must remember that a strand can be shortened but not extended. An appropriate length for location of tissue must be handed to the surgeon. A packet may contain one suture strand armed with a single or double needle(s) or multiple strands with swaged needles. The needle may be armed in a needle holder and withdrawn from the inner dispenser of some packets.

Surgical Staples

Surgeons can join many tissues with staples. This involves inserting stainless steel or titanium staples through tissues with a stapler—a device specifically designed for this purpose. Some surgical procedures have become simplified or feasible since the advent of surgical stapling techniques. As Hültl recognized in 1908, for stapling to be successful, fine wire as the basic material must form a B shape. This shape allows blood to flow through tissues, preventing necrosis secondary to devascularization beyond the staple line. Sufficient pressure must be exerted, however, to provide hemostasis of cut tissues. The length and width of the staples must accommodate tissue being approximated or transected. The number of staples varies with the length of the staple line.

Advantages of Using Staples. Staples can be used safely in many types of tissues and have a wide range of applications:

- Stapling is a rapid method of ligating, anastomosing, and approximating tissues. The time saved, as compared with suturing techniques, reduces blood loss and the total operating and anesthesia time for the patient.
- Wound healing may be accelerated because of minimal trauma and the nonreactive nature of metallic staples.
- Staples produce an even surface and an airtight, leak-proof closure.
- Staples can be placed through an endoscope.

Stapling Instruments. Each stapler is designed for stapling specific tissues (i.e., skin, fascia, bronchus, gastrointestinal tract, vessels). The surgeon selects the correct instrument for the desired application. The consequences of an erroneous staple application, however, are much more difficult to correct than those of manually placed sutures. The surgeon must learn when and how to use each instrument. Whether the stapler is reusable or a single-use disposable, the basic technical mechanics of stapling are the same.

Staplers either fire a single staple or simultaneously fire straight or circular rows of staples. A different instrument must be used for each type of firing.

Skin Stapler. To approximate skin edges, the stapler fires a single staple with each squeeze of the trigger. Edges of both cuticular and subcuticular layers are aligned, with the edges slightly raised in an everted direction, as close to their original configuration on the horizontal plane as possible. The stapler is positioned over the line of incision so that the staple will be placed evenly on each side. The staple forms a rectangular shape over the incision. As many staples as needed are placed to close the incision.

Skin staplers are supplied preloaded with different quantities of staples in varying widths (i.e., crown span). The most appropriate stapler should be chosen for the selected use. For example, an average range of 28 to 35 staples is needed to close most abdominal incisions. More may be needed to close the chest; fewer may be needed for an inguinal herniorrhaphy.

Skin staples are removed 5 to 7 days postoperatively. Extractors are used for this purpose. As it heals, the skin flattens out to form an even surface with excellent cosmetic results if the staples have been properly placed lightly over the skin. Imbedded staples are difficult to remove, and results may be less than desired.

Linear Stapler. Two staggered or side-by-side straight double rows of staples are placed simultaneously in tissue with a linear stapler. This stapler is used throughout the alimentary tract and in thoracic surgery for transection and resection of internal tissues. The tissue is positioned in the straight jaws, of appropriate length, of the stapler. The gap between the jaws must be adequate for the thickness of tissues. A tissue-measuring device may be used for this determination in the gastrointestinal tract in conjunction with a disposable stapler so that the instrument can be adjusted to the appropriate settings for the desired staple height.

When formed, each staple is shaped like a capital B. This shape allows staples to hold tissues together without crushing so that tissue perfusion is maintained. The number of staples that will be fired depends on the length of the stapler jaws.

Intraluminal Circular Stapler. With the circular stapler, a double row of staggered staples is placed in a circle for intraluminal anastomosis of tubular hollow organs in the gastrointestinal tract. Because the diameter of the lumen of organs in the alimentary tract varies, the surgeon must choose a stapler with an appropriate head size. The number of staples the instrument fires depends on its head size. A circular knife within the head of the stapler trims tissue to produce a proper lumen as the stapler is fired. The result is a circular anastomosis and two distinct circles of tissue from the anastomosed region. These are sent as specimens to be examined for intactness. As with the linear stapler, staples form a B.

Ligating and Dividing Stapler. A double row of two staples each ligates tissue that is then divided simultaneously between the staple lines with a cutting knife incorporated in the stapler. This stapler is used primarily to ligate and divide omental vessels or other soft tubular structures.

Endoscopic Stapler. Endoscopic staplers are available for ligating and dividing and for linear stapling. The stapling device is passed through an 11- or 12-gauge laparoscopic trocar. It may be reloaded several times with staple cartridges for multiple firings. The stapler is discarded after single-patient use.

Reusable Staplers. Reusable, manually operated, heavy mechanical stapling instruments have many moving and detachable parts. They are not always mechanically reliable.

They must be precisely aligned to fire accurately. The scrub person is responsible for correctly assembling instruments. The manufacturer's instructions for use and care must be followed to avoid technical failures.

Reusable staplers are supplied with presterilized, disposable cartridges preloaded with staples. Quantities vary according to the stapler they fit. The number of cartridges needed varies with the procedure and/or design of the instrument. Cartridges are color-coded by the size of the staples.

Reusable staplers are disassembled, cleaned, and terminally sterilized before placing in an ultrasonic cleaner. They should be completely disassembled, wrapped, and steam sterilized before use in patient care, according to the manufacturer's recommendations.

Disposable Staplers. Preassembled, sterile disposable staplers eliminate assembling, cleaning, and sterilizing processes. These self-contained, lightweight instruments with integral or reloadable staple cartridges are discarded after single-patient use. To avoid unnecessary contamination of a sterile instrument, the package should not be opened until the surgeon determines the correct size for the intended use of the stapler. The number and size of staples in cartridges vary; the length of the linear jaws or the diameter of the circular head varies for internal use. Internal staplers are available with either stainless steel or titanium staples. The surgeon may prefer titanium, because it creates less distortion when CT and MRI scans are used.

Tissue Adhesives

Conventional suturing and stapling materials hold tissues in apposition during the healing process. Sutures and staples will not fuse or bond tissues. Ancient Egyptians used resins and gums to hold tissue surfaces together. Research is ongoing for an ideal tissue adhesive that will bond tissue, effect hemostasis, promote regeneration of cells, and serve as a barrier to microbes, fluid, and air. Biologic and synthetic tissue adhesives have extensive potential applications for wound closure and reconstruction.

Biologic Adhesives. Fibrin sealants, most commonly called fibrin glue, act as biologic adhesives and hemostatic agents. The components are fibrinogen, cryoprecipitate from human plasma; calcium chloride; and reconstituted thrombin of bovine origin. When applied directly to tissues, thrombin converts fibrinogen to fibrin to produce a clot. Fibrin sealants can be applied to deeper tissues as a liquid, gel, or aerosol spray to control bleeding and approximate tissues technically difficult to approximate by suturing, especially after resections or traumatic injuries of friable or highly vascular tissues, such as liver, spleen, and lung. Each component is applied simultaneously with separate syringes to prevent congealing before application to the tissue site. A sample formula and supplies for fibrin glue compound are found in Box 28-2.

Fibrin glue may also be used for microsurgical anastomoses of blood vessels, nerves, and other structures such as fallopian tubes; for reconstruction of the middle ear; to fix ocular implants; to close superficial lacerations and fistula tracts; and to secure some skin grafts. It may be used as a carrier for demineralized bone powder to promote osteoregeneration.

BOX 28-2	**Sample Fibrin Glue Compound and Supplies**

Sterile specimen cup
Two 2-mL disposable syringes
Two 14-gauge intravenous (IV) catheters
6 units thawed cryoprecipitate
1 ampule calcium chloride (CaCl) (10%, 1 g)
50,000 units thrombin

INSTRUCTIONS
Mix CaCl and thrombin in the specimen cup. Draw into the 20-mL syringe, and attach a 14-gauge IV catheter. Draw cryoprecipitate into the second syringe with a 14-gauge IV catheter on the end. Both syringes are discharged over the wound at the same time. The fibrin glue will form a clot over the wound.

In 1998 the FDA approved Tisseel, a fibrin glue produced by Baxter Healthcare Corporation. Tisseel is derived from the blood proteins fibrin and thrombin and is applied in the same manner as earlier forms of fibrin sealant.

Autologous or Homologous Plasma. Plasma collected from the patient (autologous) or a single donor (homologous) is processed into a cryoprecipitate containing clotting factor XIII to produce fibrinogen. Autologous plasma is obtained preoperatively and prepared either in the blood bank or in the OR. A single donor must be tested and found to be negative for human immunodeficiency virus (HIV) and hepatitis before plasma is processed.

Autologous or homologous fibrinogen is warmed to 98.6° F (37° C) immediately before use. Thrombin is reconstituted to 1000 units/mL. Equal volumes of fibrinogen and thrombin are applied simultaneously.

Pooled-Donor Plasma. Fibrin glue commercially prepared from pooled-donor plasma (i.e., blended from multiple donors) has significantly greater bonding strength than does autologous or single-donor plasma. The fibrinogen must undergo purification and viral inactivation, however, to prevent transmission of bloodborne pathogens. Used extensively in Europe, this product has not been approved by the FDA for use in the United States.

Synthetic Adhesives. Synthetic gluelike adhesive substances that polymerize in contact with body tissues effect hemostasis and hold tissues together.

Cyanoacrylate. Butyl cyanoacrylate and cyanoacrylate derivatives may be used for skin closure. Dermabond is a synthetic product for skin closure that is derived from cyanoacrylate and applied with an applicator along approximated, clean wound edges. The glue dries after $2\frac{1}{2}$ minutes and remains on the wound for 5 to 10 days. It is contraindicated in the presence of infection and for patients allergic to cyanoacrylate or formaldehyde. (Additional information is available at www.ethiconinc.com.)

Indermil is a tissue adhesive product of US Surgical Syneture division. The chemical makeup is n-butyl-2-cyanoacrylate monomer. (More information is available at www.syneture.com.)

Methyl Methacrylate. Methyl methacrylate is used to augment fixation of pathologic fractures and to stabilize prosthetic devices in bone. It is an acrylic, cement-like substance commonly referred to as bone cement. It is a drug supplied in two sterile components that must be mixed together immediately before use. One component is a colorless, highly volatile, flammable, liquid methyl methacrylate monomer in an ampule. This powerful lipid solvent must be handled carefully. The other component is a white powder mixture of polymethyl methacrylate, methyl methacrylate–styrene copolymer, and barium sulfate in a packet. The barium sulfate provides radiopacity to the substance. When the powder and liquid are mixed, an exothermic polymeric reaction forms a soft, pliable, doughlike mass. This reaction liberates heat as high as 230° F (110° C). As the reaction progresses, the substance becomes hard in a few minutes. The mixing and kneading of the entire contents of the liquid ampule and powder packet must be thorough and should continue for at least 4 minutes. The substance must be adequately soft and pliable for application to bone. The completion of polymerization occurs in the patient. After it hardens, it holds a prosthesis firmly in a fixed position.

A hazard to OR personnel has been reported in regard to the use of methyl methacrylate in the OR. Some personnel have experienced dizzy spells, difficulty breathing, and/or nausea and vomiting after mixing of methyl methacrylate. The fumes can cause severe eye irritation in people wearing contact lenses during the use of this chemical compound. The monomer and several of its ingredients are potent allergenic sensitizers when vapor is inhaled. A suitable means of local exhaust should be provided that will collect vapor at the source of mixing at the sterile field and will discharge it into outside air or absorb the monomer on activated charcoal.

Implantable Tissue Repair and Replacement Materials

Tissue deficiencies may require additional reinforcement or bridging material to obtain adequate wound healing. Sometimes edges of fascia, for example, cannot be brought together without excessive tension. In obese or older patients, the fascia cannot withstand this tension because of weakness caused by the infiltration of fat. Biologic or synthetic mesh materials are used to fill congenital, traumatic, or acquired defects in fascia or a body wall and to reinforce fascia, as in hernia repair.

Implants must be sterile and compatible with the recipient. Administrative controls concerning implantable materials include documentation of the source material, the lot number in case of a recall, and special preparatory handling. The circulating nurse dispenses the implant to the sterile field and the scrub person readies the material for use. Implants should not be handled excessively to prevent damage to the surface or contamination with particulate from the field. Examples of implant characteristics of implants include the following:

- Dimensional space-holding as in breast implants
- Load bearing as in orthopedic implants
- Passage creation as in a stent
- Bone integration for increased density
- Flexion with low friction as in hernia mesh

Implants can be permanent or temporary and composed of many materials. Some are mechanical. Any implant that is removed (explanted) is usually sent to the pathology lab for accession. Please refer to Table 28-2 for a collective comparison of implants for tissue repair and replacement.

Biologic Materials

Cargile Membrane. A thin membrane is obtained from the submucosal layer of cecum of the ox. Cargile membrane is rarely used, although it is still commercially available in a 4 × 6 inch (10 × 15 cm) sheet to cover peritoneum to prevent adhesions, for isolating ligations, as a covering for packing in submucous nasal resections, and as a dural substitute.

Fascia Lata. Strips of fascia lata are obtained from the fibrous connective tissue that covers thigh muscles of beef cattle. In lieu of commercial fascia lata (a heterogeneous graft), the surgeon may strip a piece of fascia from the patient's thigh (an autologous graft). Fascia lata also is obtained from cadavers and freeze-dried (an allograft). Fascia lata contains collagen. It increases the amount of tissue already present and becomes a living part of the tissue it supports. It is used to strengthen weakened fascial layers or to fill in defects in fascia.

Synthetic Meshes.
Synthetic meshes offer several advantages for reinforcing or bridging fascial or other tissue deficiencies:

1. They are easily cut to desired size for the defect.
2. They are easily sutured underneath the edges of tissue to create a smooth surface.
3. They are pliable to preclude erosion into major structures.
4. They are inert to avoid inflammatory response and to minimize foreign body tissue reaction.
5. They are porous to allow free drainage of exudate.
6. Fibrous tissue easily grows through openings to incorporate mesh into tissue to maximize tensile strength.

The manufacturer's instructions must be followed for each type of mesh product. Unused mesh should be discarded.

Polyester Fiber Mesh (Mersilene Mesh). Mesh remains soft and pliable in tissue but has limited elasticity. It is the least inert of the synthetic meshes. It is not preferred in the presence of infection or in contaminated wounds because of its multifilament construction. Polyester fibers are knitted by a process that interlocks each fiber juncture to prevent unraveling when cut. However, a minimum of $\frac{1}{4}$ inch (6.5 mm) of mesh should extend beyond the suture line. Sterile sheets are available in sizes $2\frac{1}{2}$ × $4\frac{1}{2}$ inches (6 × 11 cm) and 12 × 12 inches (30 × 30 cm).

Polyglactin 910 Mesh (Vicryl Mesh). Mesh is knitted fibers of undyed and uncoated polyglactin 910. Because it is absorbed by hydrolysis, this mesh is intended for use as a buttress to provide temporary support during healing. The mesh acts as a scaffold for ingrowth of connective tissue. It may be used to support a traumatized spleen, kidney, or abdominal wall and to support facial fascia. Absorption is essentially complete in 60 to 90 days. Sterile sheets are available in sizes $10\frac{1}{2}$ × $13\frac{1}{2}$ inches (26.5 × 34 cm) and 5 × $6\frac{1}{2}$ inches (13 ×17 cm).

TABLE 28-2	Implants: Tissue Repair and Replacement Materials						
Natural (Biologic)				**Synthetic**			
Autologous	**Allogeneic**	**Xenograft**	**Biomaterials**	**Chemical**	**Metallic**	**Polymer**	**Mechanical**
Skin	Bone	Porcine dermal collagen	Biodegradable fixation S-1 (CO_2 and H_2O)	Glial antibiotic disc	Plates/screws	Solid	Pacer
Cartilage	Tendon and ligament	Tricalcium phosphate	Hydroxyapatite ceramic	Bone cement	Rods	Expandable	Penile hydraulics
Bone	Cornea	Porcine heart valve	Bioengineered stent endothelial	Drug eluting stent	Stent	Shunts	Medication pump
Muscle	Alloderm	Bovine xenograft screws	Bovine collagen polyester graft	Conduit graft	Joint	Stents	Cochlear components
Gut	Tissue matrix: Periosteal Chondrium	Calcium alginate gel		Mesh graft	Grid	Thermoplastic polymer	Heart assist device
Hair follicles	Fascia	Coral			Clips and staples	Liquid	Internal defibrillator
Vessels	Saphenous veins	Bovine collagen dressing			**Metallic oxide, ceramic**	Polyethylene	Nerve stimulator
	Heart valve	Bovine collagen matrix			Zirconium oxide	Polyurethane	
	Ossicles	Porcine collagen matrix			Chromium oxide	Nonabsorbable ligating clip	
					Aluminum oxide		
					Dental ceramic		

Polypropylene Mesh (Prolene Mesh, Marlex Mesh). Knitted mesh of polypropylene has high tensile strength and good elasticity. However, Marlex mesh is stiffer and exhibits greater fiber fatigue than does Prolene mesh. Because polypropylene is inert, it may be used in the presence of infection or during healing by second intention. Mesh is used to span and reinforce traumatic abdominal wall defects, incisional ventral hernias, large inguinal hernias, and other fascial deficiencies. It stimulates rapid tissue ingrowth through interstices of mesh. Mesh remains soft and pliable in tissues. It will not unravel when cut. Sterile sheets are available in sizes $2\frac{1}{2} \times 4\frac{1}{2}$ inches (6 × 11 cm), 6 × 6 inches (15 × 15 cm), and 12 × 12 inches (30 × 30 cm).

Polytetrafluoroethylene (Gore-Tex Soft Tissue Patch). A sheet of expanded polytetrafluoroethylene (PTFE) may be used to repair hernias and tissue deficiencies that require prosthetic material. This material is flexible, soft, and porous to allow tissue ingrowth. It is not used in the presence of infection. It must be handled only with clean gloves or rubber-shod forceps. Nonsterile patches may be sterilized by steam or ethylene oxide gas according to the manufacturer's instructions.

Stainless Steel Mesh. Available in nonsterile sheets 6 × 12 inches (15 × 30 cm) and 12 × 12 inches (30 × 30 cm), steel is the most inflexible and difficult of the meshes to handle. The sharp edges may puncture gloves. Wire scissors, not dissecting scissors, should be used to cut it. Steel is opaque to x-rays, which may be a disadvantage for the patient in later life. Also, the mesh may fragment and cause patient discomfort.

Tissue Replacement Materials

For centuries surgeons have sought materials to replace parts of anatomy. Tissue may be absent or distorted because of congenital deformity, traumatic injury, degenerative disease, or surgical resection. Replacement or substitution of tissue may be possible with biologic dressings or implanted materials, or with synthetic prosthetic materials implanted in the body. An overview of the types of biologic and synthetic tissue replacement materials is given here. Their uses are referenced in other chapters by surgical specialty or procedure.

Biologic Wound Cover. A biologic dressing temporarily covers an open surface defect in skin and underlying soft tissues. Although defects are usually the result of trauma such as burns, vascular or pressure necrosis can cause skin ulcers. Open wounds quickly become contaminated. The dressing arrests loss of fluid, reduces or eliminates microbial growth, and minimizes scarring. It promotes production of granulation tissue and epithelialization before healing by second or third intention. A fibrin-elastin biologic bonding adheres the dressing to exposed surfaces. Biologic dressings are dermal replacements. The source determines the type of dressing.

Autograft. Skin is grafted from one part of the patient's body to another part.

Allograft. Human tissue obtained from one genetically dissimilar person (i.e., unmatched donor) is grafted to another person. This is referred to as an allograft. Negative HIV and hepatitis B virus (HBV) status of donor and recipient should be determined and documented before use. Any natural body tissue transferred from one human to another must be infection-free.

Cryopreserved Skin. Allograft skin provides a protective covering that initially acquires, and then eventually loses, vascular connection with underlying tissue. A cadaver usually is the source of skin for a dermal allograft. Cryopreservation maintains viability of skin during prolonged storage. Skin is frozen by cooling at a rate of 1.8° to 9° F (1° to 5° C) to –94° F (–70° C) until frozen and then stored in a liquid nitrogen freezer. Immediately before use, skin is warmed by immersion in sterile water at 107.6° F (42° C), the maximum compatible with cellular viability. Skin should be warmed at a rate of 90° to 126° F (50° to 70° C) per minute. (The patient's own skin can be cryopreserved for prolonged storage for later use as an autograft.) Allografts may be obtained from a skin bank.

For storage of allografts or autografts up to 14 days, skin may be placed in isotonic saline solution or tissue nutrient medium and refrigerated at 33.8° to 50° F (1° to 10° C).

Amniotic Membrane. Prepared from human placenta, amniotic membranes can be used as biologic dressings to promote the healing of burns, skin ulcers, and infected wounds and to cover defects such as spina bifida. The placenta has two loosely connected membranes: amnion is used for partial-thickness wounds; and chorion is used for full-thickness defects. Membranes are prepared by cleaning blood and clots from the placenta immediately after delivery, placing the placenta in an iodophor solution, and refrigerating it at 39° F (4° C). Membranes should be stripped from the placenta within 36 hours after delivery. Amnion can be used fresh or preserved frozen or dried. It may be obtained from a tissue bank that prepares and stores amniotic membranes.

Xenograft. Skin obtained from a dissimilar species may be placed on human tissue as a temporary dressing.

Porcine Dermis. Porcine (pig) skin is used to cover body surfaces denuded of full-thickness skin until permanent skin grafting can be accomplished. Vascularization does not occur, but the xenograft adheres tightly while reepithelialization proceeds underneath it. It may remain in place for as long as 2 weeks before it dries up and peels off spontaneously. Porcine biologic dressings are available in rolls or strips. They may be prepared fresh for refrigeration, fresh frozen, irradiated and then frozen, or dried. Some dressings are soaked in an iodophor and should not be placed on a patient allergic to iodine. Dressings must be prepared and used according to the manufacturer's instructions.

Artificial Skin. A skin substitute may be prepared from a layer of collagen obtained from the dermis of a calf or pig and coated with autologous epithelium obtained from the recipient. Another type is synthesized from a bilayered poly-meric membrane. The top layer is silicone elastomer. The bottom layer is a porous cross-linked network of collagen and glycosaminoglycan. This artificial skin is biodegradable, but it can be used as a temporary covering that is similar to porcine xenografts.

Biologic Materials. Autologous tissues may be grafted or transferred from one part of the patient's body to another. Allograft tissues or organs may be transplanted from another human. Xenograft biomaterials may be used to supplement tissues.

Standards are set by the American Association of Tissue Banks for screening donors and retrieving, processing, and preserving allogenic tissues, including skin, cartilage, bone, and blood vessels. Potential donors of allografts are tested for HIV and HBV. Excluded from donating are people who are HIV-positive, have a history of hepatitis, have an active infection, have an immune disorder, or have a suspected prion disease.

Bone Grafts. A bone graft affords structural support and a pattern for regrowth of bone within a skeletal defect. Cancellous bone is porous. Its porosity permits tissue fluid to reach deeper into it than into cortical bone, and thus most of the bone cells live. Cortical bone is used for bridging large skeletal defects, because it gives greater strength. It may be fixed in the recipient site by means of metallic suture or screws. Bone obtained from the crest of the ilium or a rib is cancellous and cortical bone; cortical bone is obtained from the tibia. The main purpose of a bone graft is to stimulate new bone growth.

Autologous bone, which is obtained from the patient, usually is taken from the ilium, tibia, or ribcage at the time of the surgical procedure. Calvarial bone from the frontal, parietal, or occipital cranial bones may be harvested for maxillofacial bone grafts. A free bone graft with its vascular pedicle, such as a free fibular graft, may be obtained for revascularization by microvascular anastomosis after removal of dead (avascular) bone. A separate, small sterile table may be prepared for the instrumentation required for the donor site. If the recipient area is potentially contaminated, the donor site must not be cross-contaminated from the recipient site.

Allogeneic bone, which is obtained from a cadaver, is dead bone. This bone is weaker than autologous bone, thus requiring a longer time of immobilization. Union occurs from bone regeneration in the recipient with this type of bone graft. It may be desirable, however, in order to spare the patient the added operating time and trauma of removing an autologous graft.

Composite bone grafts are freeze-dried allografts combined with autologous particulate cancellous bone and marrow. A crib formed from a cadaver bone (e.g., rib) is packed with the patient's bone particles and marrow. When implanted to reconstruct bony defects, the composite graft induces bone regeneration in the recipient site. The freeze-dried allograft is biodegradable by slow resorption. Eventually it is replaced by mature, functional bone.

Decalcified bone and demineralized bone chips or powder, prepared from homogenous bone, also are used to stimulate bone regeneration or to fill defects in bone. This material is sterilized and stored at room temperature. For use, it is soaked in Ringer's lactate solution. The powder then becomes a paste that can be used to fill a depressed area or to caulk an irregularity (e.g., in craniofacial reconstruction).

Bone Bank. Bone may be preserved and stored in a bone bank until needed. Autologous bone may be preserved after the surgical procedure by storage in a bone bank for subsequent grafting into the same patient. Bone such as a rib or femoral head may be salvaged from patients (i.e., living donors) who are free of malignancy or infection for an allogenic graft into another person. Bone may also be obtained from cadavers (i.e., nonliving donors).

Bone used for allografts must be clean and sterile. Immediately after removal, bone marrow, fat, and blood are rinsed out with sterile distilled water or normal saline solution. The bone may be put in sterile nested glass jars or double plastic or metal containers. If it is to be used for an allogenic graft, a small piece of bone is put into a sterile Petri dish and sent to the laboratory for culture tests. Bone should never be used until negative results of culture and serology are received. Several methods are used to preserve bone:

- ***Freezing*** is the most common method of preserving bone. Bone is quick-frozen in a freezer at –94° F (–70° C) or in liquid nitrogen. If bone will be used within 6 months, it can be stored in a refrigerator freezer at –4° to –5° F (–20° to –20.6° C). For prolonged storage of more than 6 months, the freezer temperature must be maintained below –4° F (–20° C) to avoid damage from a buildup of ice crystals. Bone frozen by liquid nitrogen is stored in vapor at about –238° F (–150° C). The container initially is placed on a shelf labeled "Not Ready for Use." It is labeled "Sterile" and moved to the freezer compartment labeled "Ready for Use" when negative results of culture and serology tests are recorded on the identification card. Bone is thawed rapidly immediately before grafting.
- ***Freeze-drying*** requires specialized equipment that removes moisture as the freezing process takes place in a condenser with a vacuum cycle.
- ***Ethylene oxide sterilization*** ensures safety of bone. It must be aerated for 72 hours before storage at room temperature or in a refrigerator. When protected from air and contamination, sterilized bone can be stored indefinitely, although a 1-year expiration date is recommended if bone is placed in a heat-sealed peel-apart package. In lieu of ethylene oxide sterilization, packaged bone may be shipped in dry ice to a center equipped to sterilize it by irradiation.
- ***Formaldehyde solution,*** 0.25% to 1% concentration, may have a bacteriostatic effect around the graft site in infected or contaminated wounds, such as in osteomyelitis. During storage, temperature is maintained at 35.6° to 39° F (2° to 4° C) in a refrigerator.

The container must be labeled with donor information and not used until laboratory reports are available. The donor must be seronegative for hepatitis B surface antigen and HIV. Bone from a living donor is quarantined for 90 days, awaiting results of a repeat test for HIV.

Xenograft Bone Implant. Coraline hydroxyapatite, which is composed of skeletons of sea coral, and collagen may be used to replace facial or cranial bone. This material has hardness, mineral content, and porosity similar to that of human bone. These implants stimulate bone growth into the porous architecture of the coral.

Organ Transplants. Some whole body organs can be transplanted from one human to another. This is done in an effort to sustain life by compensating for physiologic deficits or inadequate function of vital organs.

Tissue Transplants. Skin and blood vessels are frequently transplanted from one part of the body to another. These are referred to as autografts, because the patient is both donor and recipient. The transplanted tissue becomes a part of the living tissue in the recipient site.

Some tissues can be transplanted from one person to another to restore function, such as the cornea, or to provide support in structures, such as cartilage in nasal reconstruction. These are referred to as allografts. Some allografts are commercially prepared, such as lyophilized human dura mater and human umbilical cord vein graft.

Human Dura Mater. A trimmed and measured piece of cadaver dura mater is freeze-dried, sterilized by exposure to ethylene oxide, and stored in a vacuum container. It may be stored at room temperature indefinitely, provided that the vacuum is maintained. The graft is reconstituted by the addition of normal saline solution to the container for a minimum of 30 minutes. Most of these grafts are used for closure of dural defects, but they may be used also to repair abdominal and thoracic wall and diaphragmatic defects.

Neurologic tissue for transplant may harbor the prion responsible for the development of Creutzfeldt-Jakob disease (CJD). Routine sterilization does not render this material safe for use in the presence of CJD. Routine testing does not reveal CJD contamination.

Human Umbilical Cord Vein Graft. A glutaraldehyde tanning process converts an umbilical vein into an inert, antithrombogenic graft. A polyester mesh covering over the outer surface allows tissue ingrowth and provides added strength. Commercially supplied, an allograft modified human umbilical vein graft is an acceptable graft material for arterial reconstruction when an autologous saphenous vein is not available.

The glutaraldehyde is thoroughly rinsed from the graft with sterile heparinized saline or Ringer's lactate solution before implantation. A series of three basins filled with sterile solution of choice are used for the rinse process. The basins should be set up on a separate sterile surface away from the main sterile field and discarded after use.

After rinsing, the graft should remain in sterile heparinized saline solution to keep it moist until implanted. Only non-crushing clamps should be used to avoid damage to the graft during handling.

Xenograft Biomaterials. In addition to porcine skin used as biologic dressings, artificial skin derived from the collagen of a calf or pig, allogeneic bone, and other materials derived from animals are commercially prepared for tissue replacement. Some are supplied in glutaraldehyde solution and require rinsing as described above before use.

Arteriovenous Shunts. Enzymatically treated bovine carotid artery xenografts are used for blood access in patients on hemodialysis therapy who have poor blood vessels or in whom it is difficult to create either fistulas or shunts. Femoral arteriovenous bovine shunts can be punctured innumerable times with a low incidence of thrombus formation.

Collagen. Collagen is used in its natural form, such as a processed bovine graft and microfibrillar hemostatic powder, and restructured into membranes or films. It can be injected into middle to deep dermis to fill and smooth nasolabial furrows and facial creases. It is implanted to correct soft tissue defects and contours. The duration of effect is 4 to 6 months. Collagen can be altered by a variety of techniques to change its physical properties and duration of action in tissue.

Corium. Corium implants are prepared from porcine dermis to replace tissue loss or to support tissues. They can be used as a fascia lata substitute or dural replacement or to repair tympanic membrane, hernia, or bladder sling. Corium will form a collagen matrix to close a defect in soft tissues around teeth. Available in sterile sheets of several sizes, corium implant (ZenoDERM) is freeze-dried or air-dried before sterilization by gamma irradiation. It should not be resterilized.

Human Skin Equivalent. In 1998 the FDA approved a new bioengineered skin product referred to as Apligraf and derived from bovine collagen and human tissue taken from discarded foreskins of circumcised newborns. The mixture takes 5 days to generate and grow under sterile conditions in the laboratory. It is specially ordered for each patient and cannot be stored for additional uses. The cell culture mixture is applied to nonhealing wounds, such as venous stasis ulcers after debridement.

Synthetic Materials.

A prosthesis is a permanent or temporary replacement for a missing or malfunctioning structure. Some implants replace vital structures, such as diseased heart valves and blood vessels. Devices such as pacemakers assist the function of vital organs. Other materials are used to repair or replace defects. Prosthetic materials implanted into the body must:

- Be compatible with physiologic processes
- Produce no or minimal tissue reaction
- Be sterile so they will not cause infection or become a culture medium
- Be noncarcinogenic or other disease causative
- Have viable and adequate tissue coverage unless used as a biologic dressing over denuded skin surfaces
- Have adequate blood supply through or around them
- Be stable so that they will not degenerate or change shape if used for permanent function
- Contour or conform to normal tissue configuration as desired

Permanently implanted devices can provide support, restore function, and augment or restore body contour. Inorganic substances cannot unite with tissue, however. Their physiologic responses may be predictable. All synthetic materials implanted in contact with blood will activate coagulation and promote the process of thrombosis. The surface of some materials is less thrombogenic (i.e., less likely to form clots) than others.

The magnitude of the inflammatory response they stimulate varies in patients. An immune response may cause chronic inflammation from bacterial adhesion. Infection that develops around a prosthesis usually necessitates its removal. Most infections arise from microorganisms inoculated into the wound at the time of implantation. Therefore, meticulous sterile technique is mandatory.

Prosthetic implants should not be flash sterilized in steam. They must be sterilized in a standard cycle for the agent used (see Chapter 17). The cycle should be monitored with a biologic indicator, and a negative spore test result should be confirmed before the implant is used. Implants sterilized by the manufacturer are preferred because the sterilization controls are closely monitored. Biologic testing is imperative.

Carbon Fiber. Pure carbon fibers braided into a strip are used for ligament replacement and articular resurfacing. Inert in tissue, carbon fiber stimulates regrowth of connective tissue and cartilage. The fibers may be braided with polypropylene or coated with a resorbable gelatin or lyophilized dura. The prosthesis should be soaked in normal saline solution before implantation to facilitate handling.

Metal. Stainless steel, a cobalt alloy (with the trade name Vitallium), and titanium are manufactured into prosthetic implants. Used primarily for stabilization of bone, metal implants must be strong enough to withstand the stress of weight bearing or muscular action and must not corrode in body tissues. They are never reused because of the weakening that can occur with use.

Special care must be taken in handling metal implants to protect the surfaces. A simple scratch on a metal implant can lead to its corrosion in the body. The implant will be bathed continuously by weakly chloride body fluids. If corrosion begins, the implant may fail and have to be removed. It is very important, therefore, that all metal implants be protected from scratches. This can be accomplished by the following:

1. Wrapping each implant individually, or wrapping sets with each size implant in a separate compartment, for both storage and sterilization. Most prostheses come from the manufacturer in protective coverings or cases. Some of these are suitable for adequate sterilization, with subsequent placement in the sterile field to minimize handling before implantation.
2. Preventing implants from coming into contact with other hard surfaces of metal or glass, both during storage and sterilization and on the instrument table.
3. Not handling or transferring an unprotected implant with any type of forceps.

Implants of one metal should not come into contact with those of another metal because an electrochemical reaction occurs between metals. Two different metals are not implanted in the same patient for this reason. Instruments used for insertion also should be of the same metal as the implant (e.g., a stainless steel screwdriver and screw).

Methyl Methacrylate. A highly refined methyl methacrylate mixture can be molded and shaped to fit a defect in bone. When it hardens, this material looks and feels very much like bone. It is used to repair a skull.

Polyester Fiber. Polyester fibers (Dacron) woven or knitted into seamless cylinders are used to replace major arteries.

Polyethylene. Polyethylene tubing may be inserted into structures such as fallopian tubes or ureters to give support during healing or to bridge a defect in tissue continuity. Polyethylene may be combined with silicon to produce a thromboresistant coating for vascular grafts and artificial hearts.

A polyethylene sliding rail, as on a reclosable plastic bag, affixed to polypropylene mesh is used in the manufacture of a surgical zipper. A zipper may be used for temporary abdominal wound closure in the presence of extensive sepsis, to allow repeated access to the abdomen.

Implants of porous polyethylene are used for anatomic reconstruction, such as of the external ear. The porosity of the implant encourages both soft tissue and vascular ingrowth. Collagen deposited along the framework adds strength. Porous polyethylene is a strong, flexible material that can be molded or shaped to the desired configuration. When dipped into boiling normal saline solution, the material becomes pliable for molding by hand. An implant can be shaped by cutting with a scalpel blade. Glove powder, lint, and dust particles must not adhere to the implant, because they can cause a foreign body reaction around the implant.

Polytetrafluoroethylene (Teflon). Some prostheses or parts of prosthetic devices are made of the polymer PTFE. It may be woven into a fabric for arterial grafts, extruded into tubing for struts, or molded into a solid configuration for valves or joints. Its lubricity makes it a useful replacement for tissues when motion is desirable.

Silicone. Silicone is one of the most inert of the synthetic polymers used for implantation. It has a durable and non-thrombogenic surface. It is used in many forms: gel, sponge, film, tubing, liquid, and preformed molded anatomic structures. It may be coated with polyurethane or polyester or used as an elastomer to coat polyester. A medical-grade silicone elastomer (Silastic) in one form or another is used in virtually every surgical specialty for tissue reconstruction or replacement. Silicone may migrate from a ruptured or leaking gel- or liquid-filled implant and cause systemic illness.

Complete instructions for cleaning and sterilizing silicone implants before use are supplied by the manufacturer with each type of prosthesis. These instructions must be followed meticulously. Implants are not handled with bare hands, and care must be taken to ensure that they do not pick up lint and dust. Gloves worn during handling must be entirely free of powder. Skin oil, lint, dust, powder, and other surface contaminants can evoke foreign body reactions around the implant in tissue.

Skin Closure

In addition to sutures and staples, other materials may be used to hold skin edges in approximation.

Wound Zipper. Patients requiring multiple open abdominal procedures may benefit from a simple method of regaining entry to the peritoneal cavity. Commercially prepared sterile nylon wound zippers (Woundmate) are available from Wound Care International for repeated wound opening and closure. This method can be used for other body areas, such as facial wounds or extremities. The self-adherent zipper should be 2 to 4 cm longer than the surgical site and placed over clean, dry skin edges. Available sizes range from 4 to 50 cm. The zipper can be opened under sterile conditions for irrigation, repeated debridement, or additional tissue sampling.

The resultant scar is minimal, and cosmetic effects can be achieved. (More information is available from the manufacturer at [800] 361-4693.)

Skin Closure Strips. Adhesive-backed strips of microporous nylon (Proxi-Strip) or polypropylene (Steri-Strip) or rayon acetate are placed at intervals across the line of incision. They may be used to approximate skin edges of superficial lacerations, as the primary closure of skin in conjunction with subcuticular suture, or in conjunction with interrupted skin sutures or staples. Often they are used after early suture or staple removal to support the wound during healing. A skin tackifier, such as tincture of benzoin, may be recommended by the manufacturer for ensuring adhesion to skin.

Sterile strips are available in widths of $\frac{1}{8}$, $\frac{1}{4}$, and $\frac{1}{2}$ inch (3, 6, and 12.7 mm) and in lengths from $1\frac{1}{2}$ to 4 inches (3.7 to 10 cm). They are ethylene oxide gas–sterilized in peel-apart packets. Skin closure strips have the following advantages:

- They may be used in the emergency department on superficial lacerations to eliminate the need for sutures that would require local anesthesia for placement and subsequent return of the patient for suture removal.
- They eliminate foreign body tissue reaction of suture material in skin.
- They have enough porosity to permit adequate ventilation of clean or contaminated wounds.
- They permit removal of sutures within 32 to 48 hours postoperatively. Crosshatch scarring (referred to as railroad tracks) and the possibility of infection are reduced when sutures are removed early. Skin closure strips provide long-term wound reinforcement and support.
- They permit visibility of the healing wound so that the surgeon can see how well the wound edges have coated. Some strips are translucent; others have a color tone or opacity that does not afford this advantage.
- They minimize skin irritation, because they are hyporeactive.
- They can be applied and removed rapidly.
- They can be easily cut to meet exact length requirements.

The team should keep in mind that the external part of the closure is what the patient sees and on which an opinion of the entire surgical experience is based. The shape of the repaired site and scar formation can lead the patient to believe that surgery was unsuccessful. Proper closure and wound care can help minimize scarring and preserve the patient's self esteem.

Bibliography

Alam HB et al: Hemorrhage control in the battlefield: Role of new hemostatic agents, *Military Med* 170(1):63-69, 2005.
AORN (Association of periOperative Registered Nurses): *AORN standards, recommended practices, and guidelines,* Denver, 2006, The Association.
Brose S et al: Comparison of ultrasonic scalpel versus argon beam and conventional electrocautery for internal thoracic artery dissection, *Thorac Cardiovasc Surg* 50(2):71, 2002.
Carr BI: Hepatic artery chemoembolization for advanced stage HCC: experience of 650 patients, *Hepatogastroenterology* 49(43):79-86, 2002.
Chattar CD et al: Ultrasound guided thrombin injection of iatrogenic pseudoaneurysm at a community hospital, *Ann Vasc Surg* 16(3):294-296, 2002.

Eisle DW: The Shaw hemostatic scalpel in parotid surgery, *Arch Otolaryngol* 125(1):119, 1999.

Fahey C: Experience with a new human skin equivalent for healing venous leg ulcers, *J Vasc Nurs* 16(1):11-15, 1998.

Maddern BR: Electrosurgery for tonsillectomy, *Laryngoscope* 112(8 Pt 2):11-13, 2002.

Majewski J: Advances in general and vascular surgical care of Jehovah's Witnesses, *Int Surg* 85(3):257-265, 2000.

Mathias JM: Fibrin sealants likely to stick around, *OR Manager* 18(7):20-22, 2002.

Trott A: *Wounds and lacerations: emergency care and closure,* ed 2, St Louis, 1998, Mosby.

Chapter 29

Wound Healing

CHAPTER OBJECTIVES

After studying this chapter, the learner will be able to:
- Identify tissue layers specific to the anatomic site of a wound.
- List several factors that affect wound healing.
- Describe the process of wound healing.
- List three wound healing complications.
- Describe three dressing materials and their application.

CHAPTER OUTLINE

KEY TERMS AND DEFINITIONS

Adhesion Band of scar tissue that holds or unites surfaces or structures together that are normally separated.

Contracture Formation of extensive scar tissue over a joint.

Dead space Space caused by separation of wound edges or by air trapped between layers of tissue.

Debridement Removal of damaged tissue and cellular or other debris from a wound to promote healing and to prevent infection.

Dehiscence Partial or total splitting open or separation of the layers of a wound.

Edema Abnormal accumulation of fluid in interstitial spaces of tissues.

Evisceration Protrusion of viscera through an abdominal incision.

Extravasation Passage of blood, serum, or lymph into tissues.

Exudate Fluid, cells, or other substances that have been discharged from vessels or tissues. It contains white blood cells, lymphokines, and growth factors that stimulate healing.

Granulation tissue Formation of fibrous collagen to fill the gap between the edges of a wound healing by contraction (i.e., second intention).

Granuloma Inflammatory lesion that forms around a foreign substance, such as glove powder or a suture knot.

Hematoma Collection of extravasated blood in tissue.

Hemostasis Arrest of blood flow or hemorrhage; the mechanism is by coagulation (formation of a blood clot).

Incision Intentional cut through intact tissue (synonym: surgical incision).

Ischemia Decrease of blood supply to tissues.

Necrosis Death of tissue cells.

Scar Deposition of fibrous connective tissue to bridge separated wound edges and to restore continuity of tissues.

Seroma Collection of extravasated serum from interstitial tissue or a resolving hematoma in tissue.

Tensile strength Ability of tissues to resist rupture.

Tissue reaction Immune response of the body to tissue injury or foreign substances.

Wound disruption Separation of wound edges.

SUPPLEMENTAL MATERIAL ON EVOLVE WEBSITE — *evolve*

http://evolve.elsevier.com/BerryKohn
- Content Updates
- Glossary
- Full Set of Perioperative Flash Cards
- Interactive Key Term Flash Cards
- Student Activities
- WebLinks

HISTORICAL BACKGROUND

Historically, warfare has necessitated that there be some means of controlling hemorrhage, closing intentional and unintentional wounds, and promoting healing. Egyptian papyri dating back to 2100 BC describe how various injuries, including head injuries and fractures, were treated.

Wound management techniques improved slowly and sporadically. Two schools of surgical wound management taught clearly opposite theories and approaches. Fourteenth-century French surgeon Guy de Chauliac (1300-1368) and other followers of Galen's technique believed that a wound needed to suppurate, or generate laudable pus, before it could heal. Followers of Theodoric, such as Henri de Mondeville (1260-1320), stressed the need for clean wounds and healing by first intention.

Sixteenth-century French battle medic Ambroise Paré (1510-1590) found that treating gunshot wounds with a mixture of egg yolk, rose or lily oil, and turpentine was more beneficial than pouring boiling oil into the wound. His methods openly challenged the practices of his day yet eventually became the standard of care. He never attended medical school, but he taught that observation of the patient was more important than blind adherence to dogma. In his 1547 text, *The Method of Treatment for Wounds Caused by*

Firearms, he described how, when he ran out of boiling oil, he dressed the patient's wounds with lard. He observed that the patients treated with boiling oil were feverish and the ones treated with lard were afebrile.

Research in wound healing did not occur before the eighteenth century. John Hunter (1728-1793), a Scottish surgeon, recorded observations of inflammation and healing patterns for the first time. He differentiated healing by first intention from healing by second intention by calling the first type of healing adhesive inflammation and second type suppurative inflammation. He also distinguished between epithelialization and granulation in healing wounds. He was the first to demonstrate that inflammation could be the cause of wound infection but was also necessary for wound healing.

In the late nineteenth century, French physician Alexis Carrel (1873-1944) studied the growth of tissues for transplantation. He grew several types of tissues in laboratory flasks. His studies provided the groundwork for tissue and skin cell transplantation as it is today. He developed the triangulation method for anastomosis of blood vessels, for which he won the Nobel Prize in 1912.

ANATOMY AND PHYSIOLOGY OF BODY TISSUES
Structure and Function of Tissue

Tissue structure and function vary according to location in the body. Basic tissue types are described in Table 29-1.

Structure and Function of the Skin

The skin contributes to the health and well-being of the patient. Intact skin is an effective barrier to most harmful elements. Wounded, nonintact skin is an open avenue for microbial entry. Wounds occur intentionally or unintentionally. Most wounds, when treated properly, heal without incident. Unfavorable outcomes occur when wound healing is disrupted by poor circulation, infection, or immune dysfunction.

Skin is a multifunction body cover, and skin assessment is an important measurement of generalized wellness. Skin color, texture, and condition can be the best predictors of how well a surgical site will heal. The most intricate procedure can be done in deep tissue layers, but the superficial layers are what the patient sees and measures the outcome against. Durability and viability of the skin of the perioperative patient are influenced by many factors. Within reasonable limits, in the absence of hemorrhage and sepsis, wound healing is predictable. Disregard for the principles of tissue handling and wound management can lead to complications. The intent of this chapter is to provide an overview of body tissues, mechanisms of wounding, healing influences, and postoperative wound care.

The skin is the largest and heaviest organ of the body. The two main skin layers are the epidermis and the dermis. The thickness of the skin and its layers is determined by its location. The combined thickness of the epidermis and dermis ranges from 4 mm on the back to 1.5 mm of scalp. Figure 29-1 shows a cross section of the skin and its layers.

The two basic types of skin are glabrous skin and hairy skin. Glabrous, smooth skin is very thick and is found on the palms and soles. The surface is marked by ridges and sulci arranged in unique configurations referred to as dermatographics, or fingerprints. These ridges first appear in the fingertips during the thirteenth week of fetal life. Sweat glands are present in the dermal layer, but a marked absence of hair follicles and oil glands is characteristic of this tissue.

Hairy, thin skin has hair follicles, sweat glands, and oil glands. Other types of sweat glands are found in the axilla and groin.

Epidermis. The epidermis is the outermost layer. It is organized into five levels of stratified squamous epithelium and contains no organs, glands, nerve endings, or blood vessels. It renews itself every 15 to 30 days, depending on the body surface area, the age of the individual, and the individual's generalized condition. The basic anatomy and physiology of epidermal layers are as follows:
- *Stratum corneum:* Keratinized cells make up 75% of the epidermal thickness. Cells are shed from this level, which is referred to as the horny layer. It is thinner in hairy, thin-skinned areas.

TABLE 29-1	Four Basic Histologic Tissue Types	
Histologic Tissue Type	**Description**	**Implications to Surgical Team**
EPITHELIAL TISSUE		
A. Types		
1. Simple	Single layer of cells (endothelium) that lines the blood vessels, heart, and lymphatics	Delicate tissue that is easily damaged rough handling
2. Stratified	Several layers of cells that form the skin, gastrointestinal tract, genitourinary (GU) tract, reproductive tract, and oropharynx; lines area that serves as a passage; reduces friction with mucus; can convert into keratin	Superficial layer of body cover; surface modifications are performed here; forms hair and nails
3. Transitional	Combination of simple and stratified layers found in ureters and bladder	Encountered during GU reconstruction and neoconstruction
B. Cellular surface structure		
1. Squamous	Flat	
2. Columnar	Tall, cylindric	
3. Cuboidal	Square	

TABLE 29-1	Four Basic Histologic Tissue Types—cont'd	
Histologic Tissue Type	**Description**	**Implications to Surgical Team**
CONNECTIVE TISSUE		
A. Fluid	Blood, lymph, chyle, cerebrospinal fluid, synovium vitreous and aqueous, and mucinous material	Care with body substance isolation and provision of hemostasis
B. Fibrous		
1. Areolar	Loose network forming the frame for subcuticular tissue	Reorganized during liposuction and fat transplantation procedures
2. Adipose	Fat that fills the loose network; visible in fetus at 14 weeks' gestation; not found in eyelid, penis, scrotum, labia minorum, cranium, and lung tissue	
3. Reticular	Forms firmer framework for organs and vessels	
C. Supportive		
1. Cartilage	Avascular, no lymphatics or nerves	Structural integrity is altered during rhinoplasty and otoplasty; cartilage may be used as graft material; radical neck reconstruction may involve tracheal rings or laryngectomy for multidisciplinary treatment
a. Hyaline	Translucent, articular, and rubs against other articular surface; forms the epiphyseal line in long bone, portions of the nose, and trachaeal rings	
b. Costal elastic	Becomes fibrous with age; found in ribs, nose, trachea, and larynx	
c. White fibrocartilage	Forms circular menisci in joints and between vertebrae	
d. Yellow elastic	Found in auricle of ear, eustachian tubes, and epiglottis	
2. Erectile	Found in corpus cavernosa, clitoris, and nose	
D. Hard	Bony surfaces covered with periosteum except at articulations and cartilaginous areas of circulating nursey insertion points	Reconstruction requires framework of underlying bone or graft material; autologous bone may be harvested from graft site for neoconstruction; donor bone may be used as transplant material
1. Cancellous bone	Spaces are filled with red marrow; erythroblasts and smaller vessels	
2. Compact bone	Hollow center filled with yellow marrow (higher fat content) and larger vessels	
MUSCLE TISSUE		
A. Visceral	Smooth, involuntary muscle; hollow organs, vessels, glands, areola, scrotum, iris of eye	Skeletal muscle may be used to replace bulk lost to debridement; vascularized flaps replace radical tissue excisions
B. Skeletal	Cylindric, striated, voluntary cells	
C. Cardiac	Branching cells, nonnucleated, less fibrous connective tissue	
NERVE TISSUE		
A. Types		
1. Neuron	Cells generate and conduct nerve impulses; has multiple cytoplasmic fibers on one side (dendrites) and a single myelinated extension from the other side (axon)	Nerves may be injured during any procedure
2. Neuroglia	Insulate and support neurons in central nervous system	
B. Classification by activity type		
1. Afferent	Sensory	
2. Efferent	Motor	

From Fortunato NM, McCullough SM: *Plastic and reconstructive surgery,* St Louis, 1998, Mosby.

- *Stratum lucidum:* Cells are flattened. Organelles and nuclei are absent.
- *Stratum granulosum:* This level is arranged in three to five layers. Mitotic activity creates cells for renewal of epidermal layers.
- *Stratum spinosum:* This layer creates cells for renewal of epidermal layers.
- *Stratum basale:* A single cell layer that lies between the junction of the epidermis and the dermis. Intense mitosis in this layer in combination with the basal layer and

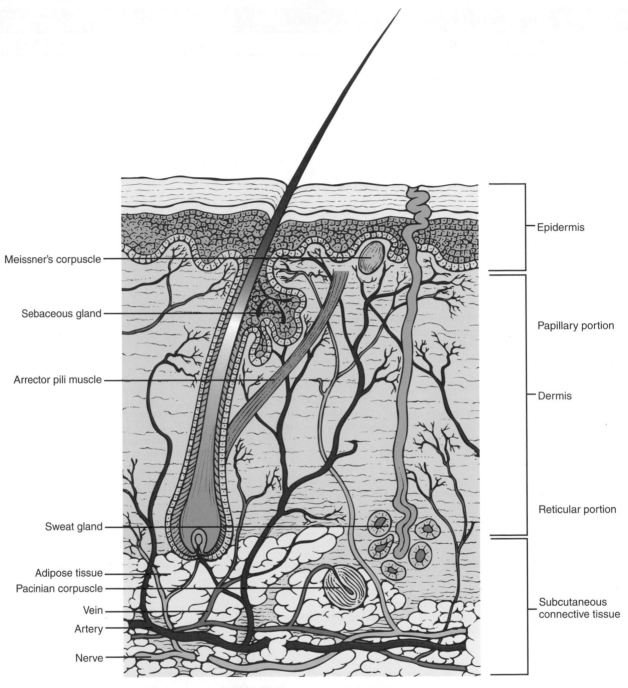

Meissner's corpuscle

Sebaceous gland

Arrector pili muscle

Sweat gland

Adipose tissue
Pacinian corpuscle

Vein

Artery

Nerve

Epidermis

Papillary portion

Dermis

Reticular portion

Subcutaneous
connective tissue

FIG. 29-1   Anatomy of the skin.

the spinosum causes epidermal regeneration. As cells are generated, they migrate upward, toward the surface. Melanocytes, located between basal cells and in hair follicles, create melanin, which causes skin pigmentation. Melanin enters and accumulates in keratocytes, causing superficial skin tone and providing ultraviolet protection. Exposure to sunlight causes darkening of existing melanin and accelerated generation of new melanin.

Each epithelial layer consists of keratin-producing cells (keratinocytes). Keratin is modified into functional components such as hair and fingernails on select body surfaces.

Overactivity of the spinosum and basal levels can increase epidermal thickness in normally thin areas, causing psoriasis.

Dermis.   The dermis is composed of papillary and reticular layers of flexible connective tissue. Superficially, the dermis has an irregular surface of papilla-like fingers that project into the strata basale of the epidermal layers. The dermis, regardless of location, is a loose areolar connective tissue that contains pain and touch receptors, glands, blood vessels, and lymphatics. It is the key layer in wound repair and tissue healing.

Glandular Structures and Ducts

Oil Glands (Sebaceous Glands). Sebaceous and sudoriferous glands are found within the dermal layers of the skin. Sebaceous glands are referred to as holocrine glands because the oily secretion sebum also carries cellular debris. The sebaceous duct empties into a hair follicle or, on nonhairy areas, directly onto the surface of the skin. Sebum is a lubricant with minor antibacterial and antifungal properties. The palms and soles lack sebaceous glands, but these glands are numerous on the scalp and face and around natural body orifices. Oily skin types sometimes have increased scar formation because the oil forms a mechanical barrier to healing.

Sweat Glands (Sudoriferous Glands). Sudoriferous glands are found on every area except the lips, nipples, and glans penis. Eccrine and apocrine glands are two types of sudoriferous glands. Eccrine glands are widely distributed over the entire surface of the body and are responsible for producing 700 to 900 g of sweat per 24 hours. These simple structures are embedded in the dermis and have a funnel-shaped exit path (pore) leading directly to the skin's surface. Secretions are produced in response to physical activity and cool the body by evaporation. These glands are most numerous on the palms, soles, and forehead.

Apocrine glands are located only in the axillary, perineal, and areolar areas in combination with eccrine glands. Apocrine glands are larger than eccrine glands and are embedded in subcutaneous tissue. These glands secrete a viscous fluid and have ducts that open into hair follicles. Initially the secretion is odorless, but it quickly develops an odor caused by bacterial decomposition. These glands secrete in response to stress or excitement. In animals, apocrine and sebaceous glands are thought to release pheromones, which are hormones thought to cause sexual attraction. Modified apocrine glands are found in the ear canals and secrete cerumen (earwax).

Blood Supply and Innervation. The dermis contains a rich blood and lymph supply. In some areas, arterial and venous communication is by direct shunting, without using a capillary mechanism. Arteriovenous shunts allow for thermoregulation and blood pressure control. Capillary networks are located in the papillary layer to nourish the epidermis. Effector innervation of the dermis is derived from postganglionic fibers of the sympathetic ganglia. Affector innervation is a superficial dermal network of free nerve endings, hair follicles, and encapsulated sensory organs.

Subcutaneous Adipose Layer. Below the dermis is a loose, fatty layer that is referred to as the subcutaneous layer. Beneath the subcutaneous tissue is a layer of striated muscle. The looseness of this structure allows for movement of the skin over supporting musculature. In males the distribution is through the nape of the neck, deltoids, triceps, abdomen, lumbosacral region, and buttocks. In females the fatty layer extends through the breasts, abdomen, buttocks, epitrochanteric area, and anterior thighs.

Fascia. The fascia is a fibrous areolar tissue that supports the superficial skin layers and encases the muscle. The superficial fascia is directly below the integument and is the point to which injection of a local anesthetic agent should extend for the best effect. Sensory nerve fibers run through this area, and an anesthetic agent is easily absorbed. Adipose cells occupy areolar spaces, rendering the fascia soft and pliable and permitting vessels, nerves, and lymphatics to pass through the layers.

The deep fascia is tough and less pliable. It runs the length of the muscle bundle and terminates in fibrous tendons that attach to bones beneath the periosteum. Incisions greater than 10 mm are sutured meticulously to prevent herniation of underlying structures. This includes laparoscopic trocar punctures.

Accessory Appendages to the Skin

Modifications in the epidermal layer cause varied degrees of keratin deposition. Thickness and durability are functionally related to the location of keratinization. Hair and fingernails are modified keratin.

Other skin appendages include glands, blood vessels, and sensory organs. Glands arise in the dermis, and some exit the body through ducts that penetrate the epidermis. Other glands empty into the superior segment of hair follicles.

Hair Follicles. Hair follicles are keratinized epidermal epithelium that terminates in the dermal layers. The follicle is nourished by a capillary bed. Loss of this blood supply results in death of the follicle. Small bundles of smooth muscle cells, referred to as arrector pili, form attachments to the surrounding connective tissue in a diagonal fashion. As arrector pili contract, the shaft of the hair is straightened to an upright position. This contraction causes the superficial skin to dimple and pucker, creating "goose bumps."

Nails (Ungues). The dorsal tip of each phalanx is tipped with a plate of specialized keratinized cells. Proximally, the nail root is covered by stratum corneum, which is referred to as the eponychium or cuticle. The nail plate rests on a bed of epidermis (nailbed). Nails are chemically similar to the surface epidermis. Peripheral blood supply may be assessed through the translucent nail plate but should not be the sole determinant of oxygenation of the patient.

MECHANISM OF WOUND HEALING

Interruption of tissue integrity, either intentionally or unintentionally, requires understanding of the mechanism and factors that cause wounding and influence wound healing. When tissue is cut, the body's inherent defense mechanisms respond immediately to begin repair. Three types of wound healing are recognized: first intention/primary union, second intention, and third intention/delayed primary closure (Fig. 29-2). Each has practical applications in making and closing incisions or traumatic wounds. The degree of contamination and the amount of viable tissues are factors in the determination of which method of healing is used.

First Intention/Primary Union

Healing by first intention is desired after primary union of an incised, aseptic, accurately approximated wound. Key elements of first-intention closure include the following:
- No tissue loss
- Well-approximated edges with suture, wound sealant, or wound-closure strips

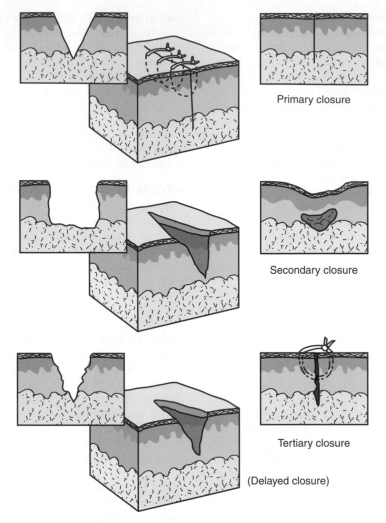

Primary closure

Secondary closure

Tertiary closure

(Delayed closure)

FIG. 29-2 Mechanisms of wound healing.
(From Trott AT: Wounds and lacerations: Emergency care and closure, ed 2, St. Louis, 1997, Mosby.)

- Minimal or no postoperative swelling
- No serous discharge or local infection
- No separation of wound edges
- Minimal scar formation

The rate and pattern of wound healing differ in various tissues. In general, first-intention wound healing consists of three distinct phases:

1. Lag phase of acute inflammatory response: Tissue fluids containing plasma, proteins, blood cells, fibrin, and antibodies exude from the tissues into the wound, depositing fibrin, which weakly holds the wound edges together for the first 5 days. Fibrin and serum protein dry out, forming a scab that seals the wound from further fluid loss and microbial invasion. At the same time, fibroblasts, fibrous tissue germ cells, and epithelial cells migrate from the general circulation. Subsequent adhesion of these cells, a process known as fibroplasia, holds the wound edges together. Leukocytes and other white blood cells produce proteolytic enzymes to dissolve and remove damaged tissue debris. Macrophages and neutrophils ingest foreign material, cellular debris, and bacteria.

2. Healing or proliferative phase of fibroplasia: After the fifth postoperative day, fibroblasts multiply rapidly, bridging wound edges and restoring the continuity of body structures. Collagen, a protein substance that is the chief constituent of connective tissue, is secreted from the fibroblasts and formed into fibers. Reepithelialization causes the rapid gain in tensile strength and pliability of the healing wound. Tensile strength is the ability of the tissues to resist rupture. The healing phase begins rapidly, diminishes progressively, and terminates on about the fourteenth day. It may continue for up to 20 days.

3. Maturation or differentiation phase: From the fourteenth postoperative day until the wound is fully healed, scar formation occurs by deposition of fibrous connective tissue. The collagen content remains constant, but the fiber pattern re-forms and crosslinks to increase the tensile strength. Wound contraction occurs over a period of weeks up to 6 months. As collagen density increases, vascularity decreases and the scar grows pale. The scar tissue is only 80% as strong as the original tissue.

Second Intention

The mechanism of second-intention healing is by granulation, eventual reepithelialization, and wound contraction rather than by suturing it closed by first intention. The wound will heal spontaneously if the dermal base is preserved. The following are considerations with this type of healing:

1. Infection, excessive trauma, loss of tissue, or poorly approximated tissue is common. Inflammatory response is exaggerated.
2. The wound is left open and allowed to heal from the inner toward the outer surface. Devitalized tissue is debrided, and the wound is packed with moist packing material.
3. Healing is delayed. The wound may need grafting.
4. Healing may produce a weak union, which may be conducive to incisional herniation (rupture) later.
5. The risk of secondary infection is proportional to the amount of necrotic tissue present in the wound and to compromised immune response in the patient. Repeated debridement may be necessary.
6. Scar formation is excessive.
7. Contracture of skin is pronounced. After healing is complete, the scar may need revision or release.

Third Intention/Delayed Primary Closure

Approximation and suturing is delayed or secondary for the purpose of walling off an area of gross infection or where extensive tissue was removed (e.g., in a debridement or by a traumatic injury). The edges are closed 4 to 6 days postoperatively after meticulous debridement. The following are considerations in healing by third intention:

1. The wound is cleaned and debrided.
2. The defect is packed with moist gauze to promote drainage and granulation.
3. Antibiotic therapy is implemented.
4. The wound may be an old traumatic or septic wound.
5. The area should not be devascularized, and deep sutures should be avoided. Granulomas can form.
6. Two clean surfaces of granulation tissue are brought together for later closure.
7. A deeper and wider scar usually results.

TYPES OF WOUNDS

A wound is an injury, either intentional or unintentional, that disrupts the continuity of body tissues with or without tissue loss. Wounds may be surgical, traumatic, incidental, or chronic.

Intentional Wounds

Surgical-Site Incision and/or Excision. An incision is a cut or an opening into intact tissue. An excision is removal of tissue. A sterile sharp scalpel, scissors, curette, or other cutting instrument may be used to separate skin and underlying tissues. Thermal instruments that both cut or vaporize tissue and coagulate surrounding blood vessels are used for incision and excision. The location, length, and depth of an incision must be planned.

The surgeon spreads the skin taut between the thumb and index finger in preparation for making the skin incision. With one stroke of evenly applied perpendicular pressure on the scalpel, a clean incision is made through the epidermis and dermis into the subcutaneous layers. A number of factors influence the ease with which a primary skin incision is made:

- Sharpness, shape, and size of the knife blade
- Resistance of self-adhering plastic drapes
- Toughness of skin or scar tissue
- Thickness of subcutaneous tissue

A clean stroke with a sterile surgical scalpel, followed by attention to all of the principles of sterile technique and tissue handling, is the best insurance for healing by first intention. The line of direction of the incision in relation to the natural lines of direction of the skin may be a factor in wound healing. Figure 29-3 depicts natural lines of skin tension (Langer lines). Excess tension on the healing wound can delay wound healing. Wounds heal side to side, not end to end.

Other Types of Intentional Wounds

Occlusion Banding. Hemorrhoid ligation results in ischemia and degeneration of a hemorrhoid. A Silastic band is placed around the hemorrhoid, using a special spring-loaded applicator. Other types of occlusion banding are performed on fallopian tubes with ligatures, Silastic bands, or plastic clips through a laparoscope. Portions of tissue distal to the occlusion point separate from perfused tissues, interrupting the continuity of the lumen of the part in the banding process.

Chemical Wounds. Chemicals can intentionally be applied to skin or other tissue surfaces to denude the area. These chemicals cause inflammation and reepithelialization of the surface. This procedure is common in facial peels used in plastic or dermatologic surgery.

Unintentional Wounds: Traumatic Injuries

After traumatic injury, preservation of life is the first critical concern. The patient's general condition is of prime consideration, and the plan of care is individualized to meet the patient's needs. Injuries are evaluated, and those that pose the greatest hazards to life or to return to normal function are cared for first.

The primary objective after life support is wound closure with minimal deformity and functional loss. Minor injuries are cared for in the emergency department. Patients with major injuries receive treatment in the emergency department before going to the operating room (OR) as quickly as their condition warrants it. Traumatic wounds can be considered closed or open, simple or complicated, clean or contaminated. Wound closure is predicated on the type, location, severity, and extent of injury.

Closed Wounds. Skin is intact in a closed wound, but underlying tissues are injured. A blister filled with serum or a hematoma of blood and serum may form under the epidermis. Torn ligaments and simple fractures are closed wounds.

Open Wounds. In open wounds, the skin is broken by abrasion, laceration, or penetration.

Simple Wounds. Continuity of skin is interrupted in simple wounds but without loss or destruction of tissue and without implantation of a foreign body. These lacerations

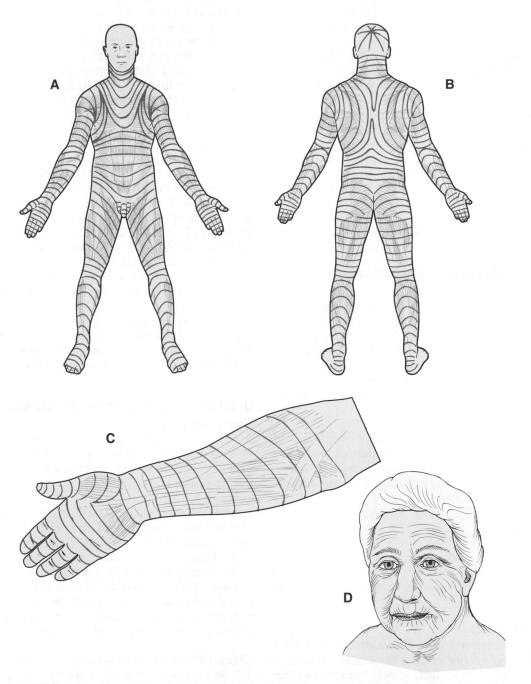

FIG. 29-3   Langer lines. **A,** Anterior view. **B,** Posterior view. **C,** Forearm. **D,** Relaxed skin tension lines of face. *(From Fortunato NM, McCullough SM: Plastic and reconstructive surgery, St. Louis, 1998, Mosby.)*

are usually caused by a sharp-edged object cutting or penetrating at a low velocity. These wounds can be closed by first intention unless underlying structures or organs have been injured.

Complicated Wounds. In complicated wounds, tissue is lost or destroyed by crush or burn or a foreign body is implanted by high-velocity penetration. If a penetrating wound was made by an object, such as a knife or bullet, this object is not removed until the surgeon explores the wound in the OR. The device should be stabilized to prevent additional injury. Movement of a foreign object may cause further trauma.

The depth of a penetrating wound is irrigated and may be excised. The wound may be closed by second or third intention. Skin grafting may be required if the dermis has been destroyed. Any object removed from the patient's wound may be forensic evidence. The hospital's policy and procedure manual should be consulted for guidance on handling potential police evidence.

Clean Wounds. Clean wounds will heal by first intention after closure of all tissue layers and wound edges. The cosmetic care of lacerated areas is important, as is treatment to provide normal function and satisfactory appearance of a part.

Contaminated Wounds. When dirty objects penetrate skin, microorganisms multiply rapidly. Within 6 hours, contamination can become infection. Debridement is performed to remove devitalized tissue, and the wound is irrigated. Devitalized tissue is removed because it acts as a culture medium. The wound may be left open to heal by second or third intention. Closure may be delayed for several days.

The patient's history should be assessed for tetanus bacillus immunization. Tetanus is most likely to occur in deep wounds contaminated by soil or animal feces. Adsorbed tetanus toxoid (0.5 mL) may be given as an initial immunizing dose or as a booster if the patient has been immunized within the previous 5 years. Tetanus immune globulin (human, 250 to 500 units) also should be given to any patient who has a severe wound or who has had the wound for more than 24 hours and has not been immunized within the previous 10 years.

Delayed Full-Thickness Injury. Industrial accidents commonly include crush injury or deep injection of substances, such as paint or printer's ink, beyond the level of the dermis. The full extent of the tissue damage may not be apparent for several days after the event as the effects of the injury cause increasing tissue loss. The patient may have occlusive dressings or casting for the initial apparent injuries but should be continually assessed for signs of increasing tissue necrosis or full-thickness tissue loss. Electrocution or lightning strikes act similarly by causing deep tissue necrosis several days after the initial wounding.

Incidental and Chronic Wounds

Pressure sores and decubitus ulcers may result from compromised circulation over bony prominences or other pressure points for extended periods. Positioning and padding considerations in the plan of care can help prevent incidental pressure-related injuries in the perioperative environment.

Ulcers. Venous stasis or arterial insufficiency in the legs may cause chronic skin ulcers. Tissue necrosis may occur after radiation therapy. These chronic wounds have tissue loss and usually have heavy bacterial contamination. Topical application of fibronectin (a platelet-derived wound-healing formula) or some other preparation of growth factors from the patient's own blood may help control infection and promote healing. Growth factors stimulate the growth of tissue, capillaries, and skin. If a wound fails to heal by second intention with formation of granulation tissue, debridement and skin grafting may be required.

FACTORS INFLUENCING WOUND HEALING

Each patient has internal and external forces that influence healing. Most wounds will progress to healing unless the closure is poor, an infection ensues, or the tissue is devitalized by other forces. Hemostatic and inflammatory responses must be intact for healing to take place.

The degree of wound contamination is evaluated, and the potential risk for postoperative wound infection is considered.

Surgical Wound Classification

The surgical site may be clean or contaminated when the surgeon makes the initial incision. A clean site may become contaminated depending on the type of wound, the pathologic findings or circumstances creating the need for the surgical procedure, the anatomic location, or the techniques of the OR team. After completion of wound closure, the circulating nurse should verify the wound classification with the surgeon. The wound class should not be assigned until the dressing is applied. This is documented in the patient's intraoperative records.

Surgical wounds are classified by the degree of microbial contamination or exposure that may predispose a patient to a postoperative wound infection. According to the Centers for Disease Control and Prevention (CDC), risk of infection increases in proportion to contamination of the incision and surrounding tissues exposed during the course of the surgical procedure. The true extent of risk cannot be evaluated until the procedure is completed. The wound is classified at the end of the surgical procedure as one of four types[1] (Box 29-1):

1. Clean
2. Clean-contaminated
3. Contaminated
4. Dirty and infected

Generalized Health Condition of the Patient

Chronic diseases alter normal physiology. Diseases such as diabetes, uremia, fibrocystic disease, cirrhosis, active alcoholism, and leukemia can delay wound healing.

Circulatory Status. Cardiovascular and respiratory insufficiency inhibit tissue perfusion. Oxygenation is essential to wound healing and to inhibit growth of anaerobic microorganisms.

[1]www.cdc.gov.

Classification of Surgical Wounds from the CDC

CLEAN WOUND
(EXPECTED INFECTION RATE: 1%-5%)
Elective procedure with wound made under ideal operating room conditions
Primary closure, wound not drained
No break in sterile technique during surgical procedure
No inflammation present
Alimentary, respiratory, and genitourinary tracts or oropharyngeal cavity not entered

CLEAN-CONTAMINATED WOUND
(INFECTION RATE: 8%-11%)
Primary closure, wound drained
Minor break in technique occurred
No inflammation or infection present
Alimentary, respiratory, and genitourinary tracts or oropharyngeal cavity entered under controlled conditions without significant spillage or unusual contamination

CONTAMINATED WOUND
(INFECTION RATE: 15%-20%)
Open, fresh traumatic wound of less than 4 hours' duration
Major break in technique occurred
Acute nonpurulent inflammation present
Gross spillage/contamination from gastrointestinal tract
Entrance into genitourinary or biliary tracts with infected urine or bile present

DIRTY AND INFECTED WOUND
(INFECTION RATE: 27%-40%)
Old traumatic wound of more than 4 hours' duration from dirty source or with retained necrotic tissue, foreign body, or fecal contamination
Organisms present in surgical field before procedure
Existing clinical infection: acute bacterial inflammation encountered, with or without purulence; incision to drain abscess
Perforated viscus

Smoking. Vasoconstriction caused by smoking decreases blood supply to the wound. Carbon monoxide in smoke binds with hemoglobin (forming carboxyhemoglobin) and further diminishes oxygenation. Smoking contributes to respiratory complications. This can cause forceful coughing that can raise intraabdominal pressure and create increased strain on an abdominal wound and impair healing.

Age. Loss of skin turgor and muscle tone and elasticity is a natural characteristic of the aging process. Thickened connective tissue, decreased subcutaneous fat, diminished capillary blood flow, and reduced vascularity are age-related factors that may delay wound healing. The tension of sutures on aged skin can further inhibit tissue perfusion. Sutures or skin staples should be reinforced with wound-closure strips. Newborn infants, especially those who are preterm, and geriatric patients are especially prone to infection.

Nutritional Status. Wound healing is impaired by deficiencies in proteins, carbohydrates, zinc, and vitamins A, B, C, and K. Protein provides essential amino acids for new tissue construction. Carbohydrates are necessary energy sources for cells, preventing excessive metabolism of amino acids to meet caloric requirements. Vitamin B complex is necessary for carbohydrate, protein, and fat metabolism. Vitamin C permits collagen formation. Although vitamin A and zinc are known to be important in collagen synthesis, their mechanism in wound healing is not well understood. Vitamin K is involved in the synthesis of prothrombin and other clotting factors. Copper and iron assist in collagen synthesis. Calcium and magnesium are important in protein synthesis. Manganese serves as an enzyme activator.

Malnutrition, whether primary or secondary to disease, can be a major factor in wound healing and infection. Impairment of physiologic functions associated with a body weight loss that is greater than 10% and protein energy malnutrition increase the risk of postoperative complications. Liver function, skeletal and respiratory muscle function, overall physical and mental activity, and inflammatory response to wound healing are altered in the malnourished patient. Protein and fat deficiency is especially significant in patients with extensive burns or multiple injuries, who have greatly increased caloric requirements. Malnutrition caused by anorexia or cachexia has a deleterious effect on wound healing. Hyperalimentation with vitamin, trace element, and mineral supplements preoperatively and postoperatively usually is indicated for malnourished patients.

Obesity. The bulk and weight of adipose tissue cause difficulty in confining excess fat and securing good wound closure in obese patients. To minimize dead space, the surgeon may place drains and sutures in subcutaneous fat; both may actually potentiate infection. Of all tissues, fat is the most vulnerable to trauma and infection because of its poor vascularity. Many morbidly obese patients, more than 100 pounds (45.4 kg) over ideal body weight, have cardiac decompensation and respiratory insufficiency.

Fluid and Electrolyte Balance. The body's system for balancing fluids and electrolytes is extremely complex. As a result of illness, injury, or infection, the patient may not be able to maintain normal fluid and electrolyte balance. Fever associated with infection, for example, can raise fluid requirements as much as 15% for each 1.5° F (or 1° C) rise in body temperature. Body fluid is intracellular (ICF [within cells]) and extracellular (ECF [outside cells as intravascular plasma and interstitial fluid between cells]). The electrolyte content differs. ECF contains more sodium than does ICF; ICF has more potassium than does ECF. Changes in this balance can affect kidney function, cellular metabolism, oxygen concentration in the circulation, and hormonal function. Adequate ECF volume is necessary for circulation of blood to tissues.

Hematology. The presence of an abnormal or pathologic condition affecting the blood should be carefully evaluated preoperatively. A low hemoglobin level (low red blood cell count) associated with anemia can result in tissue hypoxia, which alters synthesis of collagen and epithelialization. A hematocrit value below 20% lowers oxygen tension in tissues, which disrupts cell regeneration. An elevated leukocyte level (white blood cell count) indicates the presence of infection in the body.

Inflammatory and Immune Responses. The body repairs tissues at the cellular level in response to injury or exposure to foreign substances. It triggers an inflammatory response to mobilize cellular components associated with healing. Some foreign materials cause more inflammatory reaction than do others. Extremes of inflammation may result in response to allergy, infection, or chronic irritation and may delay wound healing. Inflammation should not be confused with infection, which has a pathogenic microbe that is causing the complications. Patients with an impaired immune response have an altered inflammatory response and do not heal appropriately.

Allergic Response. Hypersensitivity to substances inhaled, ingested, injected, or in contact with skin causes an acute allergic reaction. The type of allergic response displayed by the patient should be considered. A localized response may appear as a rash or hives. A systemic response may be more severe and include signs of airway obstruction and cardiac dysrhythmias.

Immunosuppression. The patient's immunologic response may be deficient because of a congenital or acquired immunologic disease, drugs, or radiation therapy. Immunosuppressed patients are easily infected with potentially pathogenic flora within their own bodies. They may not present the usual signs and symptoms of infection, such as initial inflammatory response. Lack of integrity of the immune system, such as leukopenia or defective immunoglobulin synthesis, can be life threatening.

Drug Therapy. Wound healing occurs basically through collagen synthesis. Agents that interfere with cellular metabolism have a potentially deleterious effect on the healing process. Prolonged high dosage of steroids such as cortisone preoperatively inhibits fibroplasia and collagen formation. Some antineoplastic agents used as chemotherapeutic adjuvants to surgery also may delay systemic wound healing or cause localized tissue necrosis from extravasation at the site of injection. Immunosuppressants are given to transplant patients to prevent organ or tissue rejection. Leukopenia and susceptibility to infection are common sequelae to administration of these drugs. Other drugs that interfere with wound healing include anticoagulants, antiinflammatory agents, and colchicine.

Radiation Therapy. Healing is delayed if the patient has had radiation in large doses preoperatively. The blood supply in irradiated tissue is decreased. However, little change from the normal healing pattern occurs if radiation has been given in low doses and the surgical procedure is performed within 4 to 6 weeks of radiation.

Surgical Technique

Devitalized tissue caused by laser or electrosurgery cannot regenerate. Interruption of blood supply and innervation decreases circulation and prevents epithelialization. Excess tension on the suture line that inhibits tissue perfusion prolongs healing time.

Aseptic Technique. Healthy tissues can combat a certain amount of contamination. Microorganisms are normally present in skin and air. Devitalized tissues have little power of resistance. Infection may occur from any one of a variety of causes that result in a breakdown of the wound postoperatively. The surgeon gives meticulous attention to sterile technique throughout the surgical procedure to minimize contamination of the surgical site. The entire OR team carefully carries out aseptic and sterile techniques. In addition, many precautions are taken by all OR personnel. Strict adherence to housekeeping techniques, air engineering, sterilization procedures, and all of the principles of aseptic technique is necessary. Infection may be caused by a break in the chain of asepsis.

Method of Hemostasis. Complete hemostasis must be achieved to prevent loss of blood and prevent hematoma (blood clot) formation. Blood loss is caused by tissue trauma. The method of dissection and coagulation of bleeders can cause devitalization of tissue. Devitalized tissue cannot heal; it only necroses. Delivery of oxygen to healing tissues is affected. Any condition that lowers circulating nursey flow and the delivery of oxygen to the tissues impairs healing.

Tissue Handling. All tissues should be handled very gently and as little as possible throughout the surgical procedure. The surgeon makes an incision that is just long enough to afford sufficient operating space. Careful consideration is given to underlying blood vessels and nerves to preserve as many as possible. Retractors are placed to provide exposure without causing undue pressure on tissues and organs or tension on muscles. Trauma to tissue in dissecting, handling with instruments, ligating, or suturing may cause edema and necrosis (death of tissue cells) with resultant slow healing. The body must rid itself of necrotic cells before the healing phase of fibroplasia takes place.

Tissue Approximation. Tissue edges are brought together with precision, avoiding strangulation and eliminating dead space, to promote wound healing. A closure that is too tight or closure under tension causes ischemia, a decrease of blood supply to tissues.

Dead space is caused by separation of wound edges that have not been closely approximated or by air trapped between layers of tissue. Serum or blood may collect in a dead space and prevent healing by keeping cut edges separated. Wound edges not in close contact cannot heal. A drain may be inserted to aid in removal of fluid or air from the surgical site postoperatively, or a pressure dressing may be applied over a closed wound to help obliterate dead space.

The choice of wound-closure materials and the techniques of the surgeon are prime factors in the restoration of tensile strength to the wound during the healing process.

Wound Security. The quality of approximated tissue and the type of closure material are two factors that determine the strength of the wound. Tensile strength of the tissues themselves varies; some are more friable than others. Drains or catheters may be placed in the wound to evacuate serum or fluid and prevent it from accumulating in the dead space postoperatively. Drainage tubes may cause a weak spot in the incision, and underlying tissue may protrude. Also, drains may provide an inlet for microorganisms, as well as an outlet for drainage. When possible, drains are placed through a stab wound in the skin rather than through the surgical incision.

When sutures are used, the suture material provides all of the strength of the wound immediately after closure. Closely spaced sutures give a stronger suture line. The strength of a suture should not be greater than the strength of the tissue in which it is placed. To minimize tissue reaction to sutures, the fewest and the smallest sutures consistent with the holding power of the tissues should be used. Inert surgical staples are used to approximate some tissues.

Immediately after closure, tissue along the incision is at about 40% of its original strength. It reaches its greatest strength in 7 to 15 days. The wound is about one third healed on the sixth postoperative day and two thirds healed on the eighth day. The condition of the patient, the type of surgical procedure, and many other factors may cause variance from the average patient response. As tensile strength of the wound increases, reliance on other support for wound security gradually lessens.

Postoperative Complications

Edema, vomiting, or coughing can place stress on the healing wound before fibroplasia takes place. Complications in other parts of the body, far from the surgical site, such as pneumonia, thrombus, or embolus, can inhibit oxygen supply to the wound site. Collagen synthesis is partly a function of the oxygenation of tissues. Therefore oxygen perfusion to tissues contributes to the rate of healing, tensile strength of the wound, and resistance to infection. This is particularly important in arterialized and microvascular tissue grafts and flaps used to cover soft tissue defects and in organ transplantation. Ischemic tissue is more susceptible to infection than is well-vascularized tissue.

Physical Activity

Early ambulation postoperatively is one of the most important factors in recovery for the surgical patient. Ambulation may be started immediately after recovery from anesthesia if the patient's condition does not contraindicate it. Some surgeons exempt only the patient whose blood pressure is not stable, the patient who has a cardiac problem, or the patient whose general condition is poor. If the patient's physical condition does not safely permit ambulation, the surgeon orders otherwise.

Ambulation is started gradually, with the patient first turning onto one side. The patient then sits up with the feet over the side of the bed and then stands on the floor for a minute before returning to bed. After repeating this several times, the patient takes a few steps and finally increases the distance walked. Sitting in a chair for prolonged periods is discouraged because this contributes to stasis of blood. The patient must understand the value of early ambulation, which includes the following:

- Early ambulation improves circulation, which aids in the healing process and eliminates stasis of blood, which may result in thrombus and embolus formation.
- The patient is better able to cooperate in deep-breathing exercises to raise bronchial secretions; thus pulmonary complications are reduced.
- Early ambulation decreases gas pain, distention, and the tendency toward nausea and vomiting. It helps prevent constipation. Bodily functions return to normal more readily.
- Increased exercise aids digestion. Thus the patient's oral intake progresses sooner after the surgical procedure, so that less supplementary intravenous fluid is necessary for hydration and nutrition.
- Early ambulation eliminates the general muscle weakness that follows bed rest.
- Fewer pain-relieving drugs are necessary.
- It boosts patients' morale to know that they will be out of bed early after the surgical procedure, able to care for themselves, and soon ready to go home. This helps the mental outlook and, through it, the physical recovery.
- Early ambulation shortens hospitalization.

WOUND MANAGEMENT

Providing appropriate conditions for wound healing has been a quest through the ages. In ancient mythology the Greek god Hermes carried a staff entwined with two snakes. This signified the snake's ability to repeatedly shed and regenerate its skin. Although humans do not shed their skin, they can regenerate tissue cells if the wound is protected from accumulations of blood and serum, mechanical injury, impaired circulation, and infection.

Drains

The use of devices to drain fluids and pus from the body dates back to the writings of Hippocrates. He wrote of insertion of a hollow tin tube with flushings of wine and tepid oil to treat empyema (Fig. 29-4). This was the first wound drainage system. In the nineteenth century, glass tubes, to be replaced by rubber catheters, were commonly used for gravity drainage. In 1897 Dr. Charles Penrose described a tubular drain made of gutta-percha, the coagulated latex from rubber trees, with a gauze wick inserted through the length of the lumen. This latex drain, which still bears his name, is in use today to maintain a vent for the escape of fluid or air or to wall off an area of exudate in the wound. Sump drains, commercially introduced in 1932, offered advantages, such as use with suction apparatus. Suction drainage has been used since 1947. Closed-wound drainage systems, first introduced in 1952, are used to enhance wound healing.

The use of gravity drainage through various types of tubes versus capillary drainage through wicking devices historically has been a controversial issue. Even today, surgeons

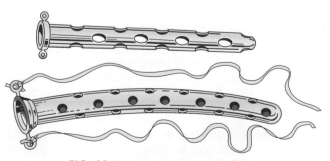

FIG. 29-4 Early reusable metal drains.

do not universally agree on the use of systems currently available. The location and purpose of the drain determine the surgeon's selection from the many types available. Drains may be used prophylactically or therapeutically during the surgical procedure and/or postoperatively. Drains and drainage reservoirs are not reprocessed. They are disposed of.

Intraoperative Drainage. Used prophylactically to evacuate gastric contents, intestinal fluids, or urine, intraoperative drainage and decompression help prevent tissue trauma and restore organs to normal function.

Gastrointestinal Decompression. A plastic or rubber nasogastric tube inserted through a nostril down into the stomach or small intestine removes flatus, fluids, or other contents. The tube has holes in several locations near the tip to permit withdrawal of the contents. Several types of nasogastric tubes are used; the most common are the Levin tube into the stomach and the Miller-Abbott tube into the small intestine. A vented tube, such as the Salem sump tube, is preferable for use with nasogastric suction.

To prevent aspiration of stomach contents, the anesthesia provider may insert a nasogastric tube preoperatively to empty the stomach before an emergency surgical procedure. The surgeon may ask the anesthesia provider to insert a tube during an intraabdominal procedure for one of the following purposes:

* Decompression of the gastrointestinal tract
* Relief of distention that obstructs the view of the surgical site
* Measurement of blood loss from gastric hemorrhage
* Evacuation of gastric secretions during intestinal anastomosis

The nasogastric tube may remain in place postoperatively to prevent vomiting and distention caused by decreased peristalsis after anesthesia, manipulation of the viscera during the surgical procedure, or obstruction from edema of tissues at the surgical site. For this purpose the tube is connected to a suction apparatus. The tube also may be used for nasogastric feeding during the healing process after a surgical procedure on the upper alimentary canal.

Urinary Drainage. Urethral or ureteral catheters inserted preoperatively provide constant drainage from the bladder or kidneys during the surgical procedure. The purpose may be to keep the bladder decompressed or to prevent extravasation of urine into the tissues around the surgical site during and after genitourinary procedures. Postoperatively the inflated balloon of an indwelling Foley catheter maintains an even pressure on the bladder neck, which may help control bleeding after prostatectomy, for example. An indwelling Foley catheter may be connected to a bladder irrigation or gravity drainage system until the bladder resumes normal function postoperatively.

Postoperative Drainage. Drains are used therapeutically in the presence of purulent or necrotic material. Prophylactically they may be inserted to evacuate fluids, including blood, or air from a wound or body cavity postoperatively. Drains are usually placed in a separate small stab wound adjacent to the surgical incision and secured with a nonabsorbable monofilament suture. Drains can stimulate a walling-off process around a surgical site in which subsequent drainage may accumulate. This enhances wound healing by the following:

* Eliminating fluid accumulation
* Obliterating dead space
* Allowing apposition of tissues
* Preventing formation of hematomas or seromas
* Preventing tissue devitalization or wound margin necrosis
* Minimizing a potential source of wound contamination
* Decreasing postoperative pain
* Minimizing scarring

The action of drains may be either passive or active.

Passive Drains. Passive drains provide the path of least resistance to the outside. They function by overflow and capillary action through the drain to the absorbent dressing. They are influenced by pressure differentials and may be assisted by gravity.

Penrose Drain. A Penrose drain is a thin-walled cylinder of radiopaque latex. The diameter may be $\frac{1}{4}$ to 2 inches (6 mm to 5 cm), depending on the surgeon's preference. The drain is usually supplied to the sterile field in a 6- to 12-inch (15- to 30-cm) length for the surgeon to cut as desired. Penrose drains are commercially available prepackaged and sterilized. However, if they are prepared for onsite steam sterilization, a gauze wick is inserted to permit steam penetration of the lumen.

Although Penrose drains generally are used without a wick, the surgeon may prefer that the wick of gauze packing be left in the lumen to absorb drainage from the wound. This is referred to as a cigarette drain. For use without a wick, the drain is moistened in normal saline solution before it is handed to the surgeon. After it is placed into the surgical area and brought out through a stab wound in the skin, the drain is secured with a skin suture, or a sterile safety pin is attached on the outside close to the skin to keep the drain from retracting into the wound. The head of the safety pin should be crimped closed with a large forceps to prevent it from opening and piercing the patient.

Constant Gravity Drainage. A drain may be inserted for drainage by gravity flow from the gallbladder, bladder, or kidney. Each OR suite has a supply of sterile rubber and/or silicone tubes and catheters. Those used for drains, such as a T-tube, should be radiopaque. Some have inflatable balloons (e.g., Foley catheters) or enlarged bulbous ends (e.g., mushroom, Malecot, Pezzer catheters) to help hold them in place.

A closed or semiclosed system is used to collect drainage. The scrub person keeps the end of the tube or catheter sterile until it is connected to the sterile end of the constant drainage tubing. Tubing should be connected or clamped as soon as the drain is brought through a stab wound in the skin or a tube or catheter is inserted into an organ. The circulating nurse connects tubing to a drainage bag. Constant drainage bags are marked in gradations from 500 to 2000 mL. The bag must be in a dependent position, lower than the site of the drain, to avoid retrograde reflux.

Active Drains. Active drains are attached to an external source of vacuum to create suction in the wound. A constant, gentle, negative-pressure vacuum evacuates tissue fluid, blood, and air through a silicone, polyvinyl chloride, or polyurethane drain. Suction levels vary, depending on the system, to create the negative pressure (less than atmospheric).

Closed Wound Suction Systems. These systems are used when it is necessary to apply suction to an uninfected closed-wound site in the chest wall (e.g., after mastectomy), in the upper part of the abdomen, and in areas of joint replacement. They also are placed under large tissue flaps or in subcutaneous spaces in obese patients to eliminate dead space and to hold tissues in apposition.

The sterile plastic drain with tubing connected to a stainless steel trocar is placed in the surgical area. The trocar makes a small stab wound in the skin as it is brought through the underlying tissues. The drain, either round or flat, has several perforations along the length placed in tissues. It also is radiopaque or has radiopaque markings to aid in checking its location on a radiograph, if desired. The tubing is connected to a sterile, self-contained disposable reservoir. Several different units are available with reservoirs of different capacities, as well as sizes of tubings. Calibrations on the side of the container measure the drainage, and a line designates when it should be emptied or changed. These units are made entirely or partially of clear plastic so that the surgeon can inspect drainage.

The drainage reservoir can be attached immediately after placement of the tubing or after wound closure; then the vacuum is activated. Directions printed on each unit must be followed to activate the vacuum. The amount of suction in these systems varies depending on the method of creating the vacuum. Manually activated, spring-loaded devices (Hemovac) and grenade-type or bulb evacuators (Relia-Vac, Jackson Pratt) have variable preset suction levels between 30 and 125 mm Hg (Fig. 29-5).

A portable, battery-powered device (VariDyne) can provide a constant and continuous vacuum at any setting between 10 and 350 mm Hg. With the latter system, the surgeon can determine the suction level on the basis of the material and area to be evacuated. With closed-wound suction systems, the drainage container does not need to be in a dependent position. An antireflux valve guards against backflow of fluids.

Sump Drains. Sump drains may be used for aspiration, irrigation, or introduction of medication. Either flat or round, a sump drain has a double or triple lumen. Usually made of radiopaque silicone, it has large lateral openings to minimize clogging. The drain is brought out through a separate stab wound. Sump drains create equalized negative pressure at the site to be drained, usually in the abdomen. They are connected to a constant drainage system, with or without suction. Irrigation of the surgical site and connection to suction as soon as possible enhance function. Levels of suction between 80 and 120 mm Hg are desirable. The tubing may be attached to a piped-in (wall) or portable vacuum system. The drain must be clamped when not attached to suction or connected to a closed container. It functions as a passive drain if suction is not used and must be in a dependent position.

Chest Drainage. Drainage of the pleural cavity ensures complete expansion of the lungs postoperatively. Air and fluid must be evacuated from the pleural space after surgical procedures within the chest cavity. One or more chest

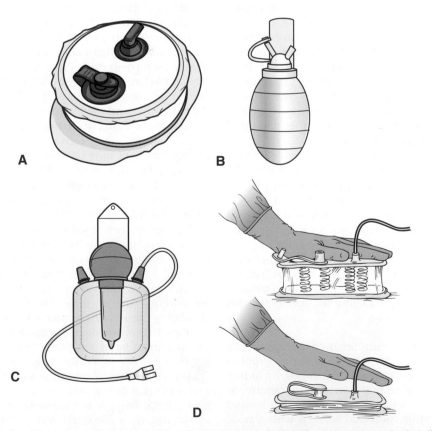

FIG. 29-5   Closed system drainage. **A,** Hemovac drain reservoir. **B,** Bulb vacuum reservoir. **C,** Balloon pump hard canister reservoir. **D,** Activating a Hemovac drain reservoir.

tubes are inserted. If the surgeon inserts two, the upper tube evacuates air and the lower tube drains fluid. After the chest tube is inserted during closure, the end is covered with sterile gauze until it can be connected to a sterile closed water-seal drainage system. The drainage system must prevent outside air from being drawn into the pleural space during expiration. Water in the collection unit seals off outside air to maintain a negative pressure within the pleural cavity (Fig. 29-6).

Two tubes vent the leak-proof top of the collection unit. A short air-outlet tube extends 1 inch (2.5 cm) or more above the stopper to about 3 inches (7.5 cm) below it into the collection unit. The long inlet tube extends from above the stopper, through it, to about 1 inch (2.5 cm) from the bottom of the collection unit. Sterile water is poured into the collection unit to a level 1 to 2 inches (2.5 to 5 cm) above the end of the long inlet tube. Clear sterile tubing connects the inlet tube to the tube placed into the pleural space. On the patient's initial expiration, water rises a short distance up into the inlet tube. With each subsequent inspiration-expiration, the water level in the tube fluctuates.

If the water level in the tube remains stationary, the chest tube or connecting tubing may be clogged or kinked. The collection unit must be kept well below chest level to prevent water from entering the chest and to keep the tubing free of kinks.

Fluid drains by gravity from the chest into the water. The collection unit should be calibrated so that drainage can be measured. Air bubbles through the water and escapes through the outlet tube.

If gravity drainage is not adequate for reexpansion of the lungs, suction may be applied at 15 to 20 cm water pressure to ensure evacuation of air and fluid. This requires the addition of one or two collection units to the system to act as a pressure regulator and the addition of a suction machine to maintain negative pressure. Disposable chest drainage units are available as a single unit or in a series of two or three. Some units have modifications based on the principle described for a closed water-seal system. The manufacturer's directions should be followed for use. The unit must be properly connected before the patient leaves the OR.

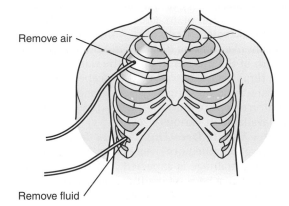

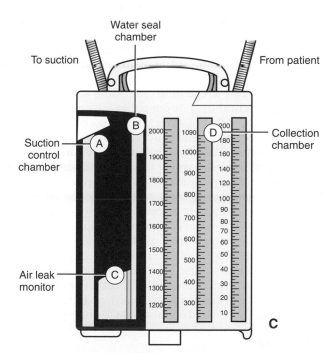

FIG. 29-6 Chest drainage. **A,** Placement of drains. **B,** Scrub person pours sterile water into the unit to create a water seal. **C,** Tubing attachment to three-chamber collection unit.

With some units the chest tube may be clamped during transportation as a safety measure. The surgeon should be consulted as to whether clamping is contraindicated. Indiscriminate clamping can create a mediastinal shift of the thoracic organs.

Patient Care Considerations. Drains, tubes, catheters, drainage tubing, and adapters are used for one patient only; they are never reused for another patient. If not properly handled by the scrub person and circulating nurse, a drain can be a source of wound contamination or irritation. When the surgeon inserts a drain, the following considerations should be kept in mind:

1. Drains, tubes, and catheters are kept sterile, ready for the circulating nurse to open if needed. They are available in many styles and sizes. They are patient charge items. Do not open until the surgeon specifies the style and size.
2. If the patient has a sensitivity to latex, do not use a drain, tube, or catheter with any latex components.
3. The scrub person keeps the end of the drain sterile until it is connected to the sterile end of the drainage tubing.
4. Tubing connections must be physically tight and secured. Do not completely obscure connections by wrapping tape around them.
5. The drain site is dressed separately from the incision site. A nonadherent dressing can be used as the contact layer around the drain. Gauze dressings can be slit in a Y shape to fit around the base of the drain.
6. Avoid tension on the drain and kinks in the drain and tubing. A gentle loop can be made and secured with tape at the time of dressing application.
7. Collection bags or containers connected to passive drains, including chest tubes, must be kept well below the level of the body cavity where the drain is inserted and below the level of the drainage tubing to prevent retrograde flow. The amount of drainage should be recorded.
8. The circulating nurse must check the suction level to be certain it is consistent with the surgeon's orders or should activate the suction as appropriate for the system being used.
9. A radiograph may be taken to verify placement of the drain or tube.
10. The type of drain and its location are documented on the intraoperative record and reported to the postanesthesia care unit (PACU) nurse.

Dressings

Most skin incisions and surgical wounds are covered with a sterile dressing for at least 24 to 48 hours to provide an optimal physiologic environment for wound healing. The dressing serves several functions:

- To keep the incision free of microorganisms, both exogenous and endogenous
- To protect the incision from outside injury, especially in children
- To absorb the drainage of exudates and secretions from the wound
- To maintain a moist environment that supports healing

- To give some support to the incision and surrounding skin, or to immobilize surrounding tissue
- To provide pressure to reduce edema or prevent hematoma
- To conceal the wound aesthetically

The function of a dressing is determined by its structure. The overall dressing should be:

- Large enough to cover and protect the wound site and tissue around it
- Permeable to gas and vapor, allowing circulation of air to the skin
- Secure to prevent slippage
- Comfortable for the patient

Types of Dressings. In considering the components to assemble for the dressing, the needs of the particular wound should be kept in mind. One wound may require a dressing that provides a function different from that needed for another type of wound. The dressing materials should be tailored to the location and condition of the wound site (Fig. 29-7).

One-Layer Dressing. A clean incision that is primarily closed with sutures, staples, or skin-closure tapes in which no or slight drainage is expected may be covered with an adhering occlusive dressing (e.g., Bioclusive, OpSite). These sterile, transparent, polyurethane film dressings are available in various sizes. The patient can bathe or shower with these in place. They usually are removed in 24 to 48 hours. Liquid collodion or an aerosol adhesive spray may be used.

Skin-Closure Dressing. A transparent plastic film with an adhesive backing (OpSite) can be placed over the entire length of the incision to hold the skin edges in apposition. The film is vented to allow the escape of exudate. An additional wound dressing may be overlaid to further splint and reinforce approximation of the skin edges. These dressings are available in various sizes.

Dry Sterile Dressing. A single-layered or multilayered dressing is applied dry over a clean incision from which no or slight drainage is expected. Dry gauze is not used on a denuded area because it adheres and acts as a foreign body. Granulation tissue will grow into it; bleeding can be reactivated when it is removed. A dry sterile dressing can be applied over a dry wound. It is secured with adhesive tape. A circumferential wrap may be preferred on an extremity, but it must not compromise circulation.

Three-Layer Dressing. When moderate to heavy drainage is expected, a complete dressing consists of at least three layers.

Contact Layer. The contact layer acts as a passageway for the secretion and exudates that emanate from a draining wound. It has a wicking action to help reduce the risk of infection and skin maceration. It must conform to body contours regardless of the site and extent of the wound and must stay in intimate contact with the wound surface for at least 48 hours yet be nonadherent for painless removal. The contact layer may be:

- *Nonocclusive:* Nonadherent materials, such as gauze sponges or compressed material on a thin plastic or aluminum film, draw secretions from the wound but remain air-permeable. The looser the weave of the material, the more nonocclusive it is.

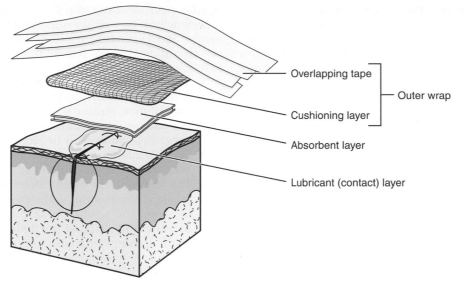

FIG. 29-7   Anatomy of a dressing.

- *Semiocclusive:* Hydroactive materials, such as foams, hydrogels, and hydrocolloids, provide a mechanical surface with permeability properties. Some of these agents actually help debride the wound.
- *Occlusive:* An airtight seal prevents drying of the wound. The dressing is impermeable to air and water but allows passage of exudates. This is usually a fine mesh gauze dressing impregnated with an oil emulsion, such as petrolatum, Xeroform, iodophor, antibiotic ointment, or scarlet red. It is nonadherent to the skin or wound.

Intermediate Layer. This layer absorbs secretions passing through the contact layer. To provide adequate capacity, it should be layered (e.g., with gauze sponges) to the thickness required by the particular wound. It should not be excessively bulky. It must not unnecessarily apply pressure that could compromise circulation.

Outer Layer. This layer holds the contact and intermediate layers in proper position. It should be conforming, stretchable to avoid constriction if edema develops, and capable of clinging to itself so that it will stay in position without telescoping if mobility is desired. The following materials are used for this purpose:

1. Nonallergenic tape is used most frequently.
2. An elastic bandage provides gentle, even pressure to hold bulky dressings in place or to bind a splint onto an extremity. It stretches to conform to body contours, does not constrict, yet gives firm support. The types available include the following:
   a. Four-ply crinkled-gauze bandage
   b. Cotton elastic bandage
   c. Cotton elastic bandage with adhesive on one side, which is especially useful in holding dressings on the chest because it is firm yet permits chest expansion
3. Montgomery straps are used to hold bulky dressings that require frequent changes or wound inspections. These are pairs of adhesive straps in assorted widths with strings attached to one folded end of each strap. The other end of each strap is secured to the skin on each side of the dressing. The strings are tied across the dressing to hold it in place, usually on the abdomen.
4. Stockinette is put over the dressing on an extremity before application of a rigid cast used for immobilization. Available in several widths, stockinette is a seamless tubing of stretchable knitted cotton.

Pressure Dressing. Bulky dressings are added to the intermediate layer of a three-layer dressing after many extensive surgical procedures, especially in plastic surgery and surgical procedures on the knee or breast. Pressure dressings are used for the following purposes:

- To eliminate dead space and prevent edema or hematoma
- To distribute pressure evenly
- To absorb extensive drainage
- To encourage wound healing and minimize scarring by influencing wound tension
- To immobilize a body area or support soft tissues when muscles are moved
- To help provide comfort to the patient postoperatively

Materials used for pressure dressings include the following:

- Fluffed gauze
- Combine pads, which are gauze-covered absorbent cellulose
- Single-piece bulk dressings, which are available for use on the trunk and extremities and save time in application
- Cotton rolls, which are used, for example, to apply pressure on each side of a knee after a surgical procedure on that joint
- Foam rubber

Stent Dressing. Stent fixation is a method of applying pressure and stabilizing tissues when it is impossible to dress an area, such as the face or neck. A form-fitting mold may be taped over the nose. Long suture ends can be crisscrossed over a small dressing and tied.

Bolster/Tie-Over Dressing. Dressing materials may be sutured in place to exert an even pressure over autografted wounds to prevent hematoma or seroma formation. Sterile gauze may be rolled into a tubular shape and tied with the ends of the wound closure suture (Fig. 29-8).

Wet-to-Dry Dressing. Dressing materials soaked in sterile normal saline solution are applied to the wound and allowed to dry thoroughly. The dried dressing is then removed, taking adhering tissue layers with it. This process is used to facilitate new tissue growth and is commonly used on burn wounds. Because this method of debridement is extremely painful, it is frequently performed in the OR with the patient under general anesthesia.

Wet-to-Wet Dressing. Dressing materials are soaked in sterile normal saline solution or other medicated solution and applied wet. This method provides little mechanical debridement and is less painful for the patient. The dressing material may be changed in the OR or under sterile conditions on the patient care unit.

Silicone Dressing. Silicone dressings are used as a measure of scar reduction and prevention. The sheet of silicone can be cut to fit and is snugly adherent to the wound preventing overgrowth of the cicatrix. Conventional dressing tape can be used, but is not usually necessary. The dressing can be rinsed off and reapplied by the patient during the healing period. The sheets should be worn a minimum of 6 hours per day and are replaced once per week.

The natural tackiness of the silicone sometimes causes difficulty when wearing gloves for placement of the sheet. Plastic surgeons use this material frequently.

Negative Pressure Dressing. This is an active dressing that provides a barrier while augmenting even pressure over the site. Negative pressure dressings are multilayer wound covers attached to a suction unit for even pressure maintenance. The dressing consists of a fenestrated nonadherent piece of plastic with encapsulated foam, which is placed over the wound then covered with a sheet of foam material. This multilayer wound cover is sealed with a plastic adherent sheet that is connected to negative pressure.

Application of Dressings. Applying sterile dressings is regarded as part of the surgical procedure. The scrub person and circulating nurse assist the surgeon or first assistant in dressing the wound properly. The procedure is as follows:

1. The circulating nurse opens sterile dressings after the final sponge count is completed. Radiopaque sponges are not used because they could distort a postoperative radiograph or cause an incorrect count if the patient's incision must be reopened.
2. Skin surrounding the incision is cleaned of blood with a sterile saline–dampened sponge.
3. The incision and wound drainage sites are dressed separately unless the drain comes out through the incision. The scrub person cuts a Y-shaped slit in dressings to go around the drain.
4. Sterile dressings are applied before drapes are removed.
5. Benzoin or some other adhesive substance may be applied on the skin around the intermediate layer before adhesive tape is applied, to increase its adhesion.
6. The circulating nurse applies tape or Montgomery straps firmly but not tightly to avoid wrinkling and traction on skin. Traction and wrinkling can cause skin irritation. If a patient has a known sensitivity to regular adhesive tape, hypoallergenic tape should be used. It is lightweight, yet strong, sticks well, is porous, and allows skin to breathe.
7. The surgeon or first assistant applies elastic bandages, pressure dressings, stockinette and casts, and splints. The circulating nurse provides the necessary supplies and assists as appropriate. A patient care assistant may help hold the patient's torso or extremity during application of an elastic bandage or cast.

COMPLICATIONS OF WOUND HEALING

The surgeon gives meticulous attention to sterile technique, hemostasis, tissue handling and approximation, and selection of wound-closure materials, including drains and dressings. The entire OR team carries out strict aseptic and sterile techniques to prevent infection and other possible complications of wound healing.

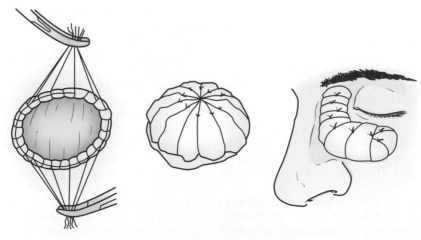

FIG. 29-8   Bolster/tie-over dressing.

Hematoma/Seroma

Collections of blood or serum in a wound can act as a mechanical barrier to margination of the wound. Circulation can be interrupted, and neovascularization cannot take place. Studies have shown that biochemical action of the collection causes tissue destruction and promotes bacterial growth. Hematomas in deep tissue can lead to abscess formation.

Scar/Surgical Cicatrix

After the natural process of wound healing, a scar (cicatrix) will remain on the skin surface. To achieve a cosmetically acceptable scar, the surgeon attempts to make the surgical incision along natural creases or within natural skin folds or hairlines. The location and direction of the incision affect scarring. Tension needed for approximation of wound edges during closure and subsequent movement of underlying tissues can affect wound healing and scar formation. Wounds in mobile skin will contract, resulting in a smaller scar.

Hypertrophic scars, which are a result of excessive fibrin formation within the borders of the scar, can develop from too much tension on the wound, poor approximation of wound edges, or infection. Some suture materials may contribute to hypertrophy. Burn wounds are also conducive to excessive scarring. The patient may wish to have an unsightly scar revised at a future time.

Keloids develop when the inflammatory response and fibroblast proliferation are overactive during wound healing (Fig. 29-9). This is an inherited trait, most common among Africans, Asians, and people with dark skin tones or those who freckle. Keloids extend beyond the borders of the scar and can continue to grow and become very large over a prolonged period after the surgical procedure.

A keloid may be painful, itchy, and prone to bleeding. They can be excised, leaving a small border of scar tissue. The edges are approximated using skin staples or fine monofilament nonabsorbable suture. If a patient is known to form keloids, an antiinflammatory agent may be injected into tissue before closure. A pressure dressing is useful in minimizing keloid formation. Application of silicone gel sheeting placed over healed bulky tissue scars for 24 hours over a period of 2 weeks can reduce the size of the scar.

Nodules and granulomas may form in the scar if excess suture material is used. Scar tissue hypertrophies around the suture, particularly the knot. Some patients will extrude

suture pieces through their incision line for several months or years postoperatively. This may represent a sensitivity to the suture material.

Adhesions

An adhesion is a fibrous scar band that binds together two surfaces or structures that normally are separate. Fibrous bands that develop in the peritoneal cavity can hold viscera together, sometimes causing bowel obstruction or female infertility. The most common cause is previous abdominal or pelvic surgery, but acute appendicitis or peritonitis can cause adhesion formation. Serosal injury caused by abrasion from sponges or gloves, tissue handling, infection, and tissue ischemia may be precipitating factors. Other substances, such as blood and biologic debris, can contribute to adhesion formation. Granulomas that form from powder on gloves, lint on sponges, or other foreign material left in the wound also predispose the patient to adhesion formation.

Techniques to prevent peritoneal adhesions include gentle tissue handling, careful irrigation with sterile saline or Ringer's lactate solution, and prevention of foreign body introduction, such as glove powder and lint. Placing a flap of omentum over the affected organ before closure is another acceptable method.

A single-layer, knitted, absorbable adhesion barrier sheet, such as Interceed (TC7), can be placed over abdominal organs after attaining hemostasis and before closure. It is composed of oxidized regenerated cellulose and absorbs in about 4 weeks. This product is contraindicated in the presence of known infection. One type of barrier sheet, composed of sodium hyaluronate and carboxymethylcellulose (HA/CMC), can be used over organs at risk for adhesion formation. Once moistened, it adheres to the surface of the organ. No suturing is necessary. It converts to a gel form and is absorbed by the body in 7 days.

Postoperative Wound Disruption

Failure of a wound to heal or closure material to secure it during the healing process leads to wound disruption—a separation of wound edges. Disruption usually occurs between the fifth and tenth postoperative days. This is the lag period in healing, the time when the wound is not yet strong. Wound disruption is caused not by a single factor but by a combination of predisposing factors that influence healing.

Although it may occur in any body area, acute wound disruption most frequently follows abdominal laparotomy, surgical incision into the peritoneal cavity. It starts with a small opening in the peritoneum, which allows a wedge of omentum to slip through it. This omentum becomes edematous and extends the opening along the line of incision and upward through other layers of the abdominal wall. Disruption is usually precipitated by distention or a sudden strain, such as vomiting, coughing, or sneezing. Terms used to describe abdominal wound disruption include the following:

- *Dehiscence:* Partial or total separation of the superficial layers of the wound. The strength of the tissues and extent of separation determine whether or not the wound must be reclosed. Strangulated sutures can cause devitalized wound edges that may fail to heal. Wound infection can cause dehiscence.

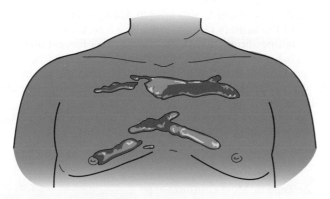

FIG. 29-9 Keloid scars can form over chest and neck of susceptible patients as a complication of wound healing.

- *Evisceration:* Protrusion of viscera through the full thickness of the abdominal incision. Although wound disruption of any degree calls for emergency care, an evisceration requires immediate replacement of viscera and reclosure of the incision.
- *Herniation:* The surface layers remain intact, but the deep layers separate, permitting the underlying muscles or organs to bulge.
- *Fistula:* Draining tunnels may form between two organs, such as between loops of bowel and the bladder.
- *Sinus tract:* An abscess may form in deeper tissues and form a tunnel to the outside of the body.

Symptoms. Patients who subsequently experience wound disruption often do not have a smooth course immediately after surgery. They may have undue pain, discomfort, nausea, drainage, slight fever, vomiting, or hiccups. Acute symptoms of wound disruption include the following:
- Tachycardia
- Vomiting
- Abnormal serosanguineous discharge
- Change in contour of the wound
- Sudden pulling pain during straining (the patient feels something "give")

Any seepage of serosanguineous fluid is suspicious and should be sent for culture and sensitivity. A swab culture for both aerobic and anaerobic microorganisms should be obtained. If the patient has had antibiotic therapy, this should be noted on the laboratory request. The patient's wound, rather than the eschar, should be swabbed. Gloves should be worn when culturing a patient's wound or handling dressing material.

Any of these symptoms should be investigated at once. Examination of the wound may show it gaping somewhat, or viscera may appear at the skin surface.

Treatment at the Bedside
1. Place an emergency call for the surgeon. Have a nasogastric tube ready for insertion to relieve distention.
2. Reassure the patient.
3. Apply sterile, moist saline dressings over the wound and a loose binder.
4. Give drugs according to the surgeon's order.
5. Do not give the patient anything by mouth.
6. Prepare the patient for return to the OR. Treatment in the OR consists of secondary wound closure. Grossly infected wounds may require delayed primary closure.

Compartment Syndrome

Extreme inflammation can cause swelling between the fascial layers in any plane of the body. Compartment syndrome is frequently seen in limbs, although it can happen in any area of the body where skeletal muscle is encapsulated with fascia. Fluids, exudates, and transudates build up between the tissue layers causing tissue ischemia and destruction of cells.

Compartment syndrome is a surgical emergency requiring linear incisions to release the pressure within the capsule. Fasciotomy is performed to save the tissue from necrosis. The fascial incisions are left open to drain for weeks or months. Primary closure is complex after repeated debridement. Scarring is deep and disfiguring because much vital tissue is lost.

POSTOPERATIVE WOUND INFECTIONS

Wound healing can be interrupted by infection at almost any phase. Infection results from introduction of virulent microorganisms into the receptive wound of a susceptible host. Moisture and warmth in the wound create an environment conducive to bacterial growth. Wound infections warrant special attention, because many occur in clean wounds as a result of microorganisms introduced at the time of the surgical procedure. Secondary contamination is uncommon, because fibrin seals the wound within hours after the surgical procedure.

A postoperative wound infection may occur in the incision or in deep structures that were entered or exposed. Its nature and severity vary because of local, systemic, technical, or environmental factors. Each factor is important; all are interrelated in clinical infection. Usually a postoperative infection is localized, but severe systemic reaction is possible. The specific pathogen and site of infection determine its gravity. Postoperative wound infections are classified as follows:
- *Incisional infection:* An infection occurs at the site of the incision within 30 postoperative days. It involves skin, subcutaneous tissue, or muscle. The incisional area is usually inflamed and sore. Purulent drainage or an organism identified by culture is present. The surgeon usually must open and drain the wound.
- *Deep wound infection:* An infection occurs at the surgical site within 30 postoperative days if a prosthesis was not implanted or within 1 year around the site of an implant. The infection involves tissues or spaces at or beneath the fascia. Pus may be present. The wound may spontaneously dehisce. The surgeon may need to open and drain the wound or remove an implant. Infection involving an implant or gross necrotic tissue is prone to serious sequelae.

Compromised patients and geriatric patients are highly likely to develop endogenous infection. Procedures on potentially contaminated areas, such as the gastrointestinal tract, are more apt to result in postoperative infections. Wound infections can progress to septicemia and multisystem organ failure.

Necrotizing Fasciitis

Necrotizing fasciitis is also known as flesh-eating bacteria. Signs of the acutely rapidly spreading infectious condition are swelling, bright red surface, pain, and fever. Mortality is high because the toxic effects of the necrosis become system rapid destruction of organ systems. Surgical treatment requires wide debridement of muscle and fascia. There are three types of necrotizing fasciitis:
1. Type I: Aerobic (gram negative) and anaerobic (gram positive) microorganisms
   a. Streptococci other than group A
   b. *Escherichia, Enterobacter, Klebsiella,* and *Proteus*
   c. *Cornybacterium*
2. Type II: Most common type
   a. Beta hemolytic *Streptococcus*
   b. *Staphylococcus aureus* (less common)

3. Type III: Water-borne microorganisms from fish or insects
   a. *Vibrio*

Prevention of Wound Infections

Prevention of wound infection and a successful outcome of surgical intervention are goals of the team administering perioperative care to surgical patients. In summary, preventive measures should focus on the following:

- Adherence to aseptic and sterile techniques and standard precautions with all patients
- Control of endogenous infection
- Meticulous surgical technique and wound closure
- Reduction of exogenous or environmental sources of contamination, such as airborne microorganisms
- Thorough, prompt cleansing and debridement of traumatic wounds
- Prevention of intraoperative contamination of a wound
- Appropriate use of prophylactic antibiotics
- Frequent handwashing
- Sterile technique for dressing changes

Serious sequelae, such as wound disruption or septicemia, may follow wound infection. Therefore they must be assiduously prevented so that wound healing can occur naturally.

WOUND ASSESSMENT

The stages of wound healing will vary among individuals according to generalized health and age. Other factors influence the mechanism and should be considered when assessing the progress of healing postoperatively. (More information about wounds and wound management can be found at www.worldwidewounds.com.)

Objective Inspection of the Postoperative Wound

The perioperative nurse should inspect the patient's wound and document its condition. The nurse should have a basic understanding of the mechanism of the injury or the source of the wound, such as a surgical incision, and should be able to assess the wound for complications. All complaints of pain should be investigated and referred to the physician. Gloves should be worn during wound assessment. Sterility should be maintained as appropriate. Assessment of the wound should include the following:

1. Location of single or multiple sites.
   a. Laparoscopy can yield multiple puncture sites.
   b. Trauma can cause multiple wounds varying in type.
   c. Some injuries are not immediately visible, such as organ trauma.
   d. Incidental wounds, such as pressure sores, may not be obvious for several days postoperatively.
2. Color of the wound and surrounding tissue. It may be a combination of one or all colors. Estimate the volume of each color in percentages of the total wound.
   a. A red wound bed indicates healing, granulating tissue. Pink indicates epithelialization.
   b. Yellow to yellow-white indicates exudate caused by microorganisms. The color can range from greenish to beige, depending on which organism is present and if antibiotic therapy is in place.
   c. Black indicates necrotic tissue that can interfere with healing and supports the growth of microorganisms.
   d. Redness combined with swelling surrounding the edges of the wound may indicate infection.
   e. Macerated tissue around a wound may indicate the need for thicker dressing material or a pouch to collect drainage.
3. Perfusion of the patient's tissues.
   a. Capillary refill should be assessed.
   b. Blanching of surrounding tissues may indicate lack of blood flow.
4. Size in length, width, and depth.
   a. The wound should be measured in centimeters.
   b. The depth can be measured with a sterile cotton-tipped swab.
   c. Tunneling should be noted for direction and depth.
   d. Anatomic description pertaining to lines of direction should be described like the face of a clock. The direction of the patient's head should be considered as 12 o'clock.
5. Temperature of the site(s) and the patient.
   a. Hot to warm tissue surrounding the wound may indicate infection.
   b. Elevated body temperature may indicate systemic sepsis.
6. Dressing type and condition.
   a. Is the dressing wet or dry?
   b. Is the dressing constrictive?
   c. Is the dressing effective for its intended purpose?
7. Drainage and/or drainage device.
   a. Odors usually indicate drainage and infection.
   b. The presence of embedded material may become obvious as the wound bed sloughs. Traumatic or industrial wounds may entrap foreign material that could be extruded in exudate.
   c. Drainage of more than 50 mL/day should be pouched for collection.
   d. Gastrointestinal contents, such as bile, stool, or pancreatic enzymes, should not be permitted to contact surrounding skin. An ostomy appliance should be used.

BASIC WOUND CARE

Gloves are worn for all dressing change procedures. Eye protection or full face shields should be worn if syringes are used for irrigation. The wound should be cleansed before replacing the dressing. Rinsing with sterile normal saline provides a moist environment for healing and promotes granulation formation. Some antiseptics, such as povidone-iodine, hydrogen peroxide, or acetic acid, can cause tissue injury and delay wound healing. The wound should be cleaned before the surrounding area is cleaned, to prevent contamination of the open site. Gauze used for cleansing surrounding tissue should not drag across the open wound.

Debridement may be necessary. Nonsurgical methods of debridement include chemical autolysis and mechanical packing materials. Autolysis involves placing proteolytic enzymes in the wound to break down necrotic tissue. The viable tissue is unaffected. Mechanical debridement is accomplished by the use of wet-to-dry dressings. The results of debridement are fresh granulation tissue and a clean wound bed. Surgical debridement may be performed with dissection instruments, such as scissors or a scalpel. A laser is sometimes used, although it can cause devitalization of tissue by charring.

Dressing material and wound care products are determined by physicians' orders. Types, advantages, and disadvantages of various wound care materials can be found in Table 29-2.

TABLE 29-2	Wound Care Materials				
Dressing Material	Composition and Properties	Indications for Use	Advantages	Disadvantages	Notes
Alginate	Originates from brown seaweed; highly absorbent; becomes a gel when exposed to exudate, creating a moist environment	Used for infected and noninfected wounds with moderate to heavy drainage; some are used for tunneling wounds	Can absorb 20 times its own weight in fluid; rehydrates wound and facilitates debridement; requires secondary dressing cover	Contraindicated for use with light exudate or dry eschar; can promote bacterial growth if used with occlusive dressing cover; not used with third-degree burns	Packaged as ropelike fibers or pad; do not use with alkaline solutions; packaged sterile; remains in place 2 to 4 days
Composite	Composed of two or more moisture-enhancing materials in combination with absorbent material	Used for partial- or full-thickness wounds with moderate to heavy exudate; can also be used over fresh granulation or necrotic tissue	Facilitates debridement and allows for moisture/vapor exchange; safe for use over healthy or infected tissue; easy to apply and remove	Should be placed in area with border of healthy intact tissue for anchoring; should not be used for light exudate; may cause excess moisture loss; can become very adherent	Check manufacturer's recommendations about use with adjunct topical medications
Exudate absorber	Added to wound surface to eliminate dead space and absorb exudate; minimizes odors	Used for full-thickness wounds with moderate to heavy exudate; can be used with necrotic wounds; some can be used as lining material before packing and surface dressing	Can absorb five times its own weight in fluid; rehydrates wound and facilitates debridement; requires secondary dressing cover	Contraindicated for use with light exudate or dry eschar	Supplied in bottles or packets; clean wound and irrigate before use; fill the wound cavity to eliminate dead space and line the defect
Foam	Semipermeable, either hydrophilic or hydrophobic	Creates a moist environment and affords thermal insulation	Nonadherent; repels contaminants and is easy to apply and remove; absorbs light to moderate exudate; can be used with compression dressings; requires secondary dressing cover	Not used for dry wounds; can cause maceration of adjacent skin	Some erythema or itching may occur during the first 24 hours; not used with occlusive dressings; change more frequently if exudate is heavy
Gauze	Composed of woven or nonwoven materials; can be impregnated; used as primary or secondary dressing; can be natural or synthetic material; nonocclusive	Used for wound protection, wicking, and absorption; can be used wet or dry; packaged in rolls, pads, or strips	Moderately absorbent; less expensive to use and can be used in combination with other material; can be used as packing	Needs to be changed frequently; can leak or strike through; can dry out, causing injury to healing tissue	If applied wet and allowed to dry, gauze can be used as debridement agent; may be saturated with oils, iodophor, bismuth, petroleum jelly, scarlet red

TABLE 29-2	Wound Care Materials—cont'd				
Dressing Material	**Composition and Properties**	**Indications for Use**	**Advantages**	**Disadvantages**	**Notes**
Hydrocolloid	Occlusive, adhesive wafer; the contact layer may differ in composition; creates a moist environment; supplied in packets, tubes (paste), oral disks, and wafers; can be cut to fit	Clean wounds will granulate, and necrotic wounds will debride autolytically	Impermeable to contaminants; self-adhesive and can remain in place for 3 to 5 days without tissue damage; slight to moderate absorption	Not used with heavy exudate, sinus tracts, or infection; not intended for full-thickness wounds exposing bone; unable to visualize the wound; occlusive properties inhibit air exchange; can injure fragile tissue at wound edges	Safe to use under compression devices and wraps; can be used at ostomy sites or areas affected by incontinence
Hydrogel	Water- or glycerin-based gel, gauze, or sheet dressing that has high moisture content; supplied in tubes, packets, spray, liquid	Used for partial- and full-thickness wounds; good for burns, necrosis, and radiated tissue	Very soothing; can rehydrate dried tissues; used to fill dead space and facilitate debridement	Not used for absorption of exudate because of inherent moisture content; can dry out easily; not a bacterial barrier; may be difficult to secure to wound	Keep covered after application to prevent evaporation of the gel
Transparent film	Adhesive, semipermeable membrane; bacterial and water barrier, permeable to oxygen	Waterproof, but permeable to air and moisture vapors; bacterial barrier	Promotes a moist environment for new granulation and autolysis of necrotic tissue	Not used for infected wounds; periphery of wound needs to be intact to apply the film; may be hard to apply	Used for superficial and partial-thickness wounds with minimal exudate
Skin sealant	Barrier film applied in liquid form that dries to form a plastic-like barrier coating; supplied in liquid form and individual wipes	Used on intact skin surrounding a wound, ostomy site, or over a surgical incision closed by primary intention	Waterproof barrier	Can sting raw skin when applied; has alcohol base to cause drying by evaporation	Some have vapors that may be harmful to inhale as product evaporates

Bibliography

Alexander LN, Jarvis WR: Surveillance and control of surgical site infections in the era of managed care, *SSM* 6(3):15-20, 2000.

Barnard BM: Fighting surgical site infections, *Infect Control Today* 6(4):26-28, 2002.

Dix K: Immunocompromised patients present a special challenge to infection control, *Infect Control Today* 6(11):20-24, 2002.

Fortunato NM, McCullough SM: *Plastic and reconstructive surgery*, St Louis, 1998, Mosby.

Gardener SE et al: Diabetes and inflammation in infected chronic wounds, *Wounds* 17(8):203-205, 2005.

Huljev D, Kuclsec-Tepes N: Necrotizing fasciitis of the abdominal wall as a post-surgical complication: A case report, *Wounds* 17(7):169-177, 2005.

Kaimal AJ et al: How much pressure does a pressure dressing press? *Wounds* 18(3):51-53, 2006.

Pray WS: Caring for minor wounds, *US Pharmacist* 13(4):16-23, 2006.

Ramazi O et al: Negative pressure dressings: An alternative to free tissue transfers? *Wounds* 17(8):206-212, 2005.

Roark J: Essentials of wound and burn care, *Infect Control Today* 9(4):18-26, 2005.

Worley CA: So, what do I put on this wound? *Dermatol Nurs* 17(4):299-300, 2005.

Chapter **30**

Postoperative Patient Care

CHAPTER OBJECTIVES

After studying this chapter, the learner will be able to:
- List several functions of a postanesthesia recovery unit.
- Discuss the role of the perianesthesia nurse.
- Define the differences in postanesthesia phases as compared with patient condition.

CHAPTER OUTLINE

KEY TERMS AND DEFINITIONS

Dermatome Unilateral segment of skin and subcutaneous tissue supplied by a single sensory nerve root. Level is named for the area of the spine from which the afferent nerve originates.

Dermatome map Topographic outline of bilateral sensory nerve root distribution beginning with the cervical spinal nerves and ending at the sacral spinal nerves.

Perianesthesia nursing Providing patient care before and after the administration of anesthesia for a surgical procedure.

SUPPLEMENTAL MATERIAL ON EVOLVE WEBSITE *evolve*

http://evolve.elsevier.com/BerryKohn
- Content Updates
- Glossary
- Full Set of Perioperative Flash Cards
- Interactive Key Term Flash Cards
- Student Activities
- WebLinks

HISTORICAL BACKGROUND

The concept of a postanesthesia care unit (PACU; formerly referred to as a postanesthesia recovery room) has been popular since the early 1940s, when postoperative mortality and morbidity studies demonstrated that appropriate observation and monitoring could have prevented death in a significant number of postsurgical patients. Before this, patients were sent to various patient care areas and did not have the benefit of appropriate monitoring. Causes of death documented within the first 24 hours of anesthetic administration and surgical procedure were obstruction of airway, laryngospasm, hemorrhage, cardiac arrest, and inappropriate administration of medication. Contributing factors included inadequate postoperative patient care, a lack of standardized observation parameters, and an absence of medical supervision. Postoperative patient care was inconsistent and inefficient. The need for postoperative care performed by appropriately educated registered nurses in a controlled environment was identified in these studies.

The 1950s were years of great progress in postanesthesia recovery. Blood pressure monitoring and mechanical respirators improved quality of care. Many facilities expanded to include specialized departments designed to accommodate patient admission directly from the operating room (OR). By 1960, most hospitals had a recovery room near the OR suite.

Instrumentation and monitoring equipment increased the efficiency of postoperative recovery during the 1970s. Many surgical procedures required prolonged intensive recovery. Personnel hours increased, and recovery room activities extended beyond an 8-hour shift. Disposable supplies were more readily available and made the job much easier. By the 1980s, the use of computerized equipment was becoming the standard of care. Ambulatory surgery was more common, and the average length of stay in recovery was 1 hour.

The PACU of the 2000s has increased the capability for invasive and noninvasive monitoring. Patient care standards are integral to perianesthesia care. The outcomes are more readily evaluated when all perioperative caregivers participate in the plan of care.

POSTANESTHESIA CARE

Surgical procedures are performed in many diverse settings, including surgeons' offices, ambulatory surgery centers, and hospital-based surgical suites and specialty units. In general, the selection of the surgical setting is influenced by the anticipated complexity of the procedure, the patient's health status, available technology, and financial resources. Regardless of the surgical setting or procedure, the patient should be observed and monitored postoperatively for physiologic condition in a controlled postsurgical/postanesthesia environment before being transferred to a patient care unit or discharged from the facility.

The postoperative phase of the surgical patient's perioperative experience begins after the surgical procedure is completed and the patient is admitted to a postprocedure area (usually a PACU or an intensive care unit [ICU]) or discharged to home.

Ideally, an area is designated for the care of postoperative/postprocedure patients. The area may vary in name or location according to its specific function within the health care facility. In some settings in which only local anesthetics are used, the patient has a brief postoperative observation period in the room where the procedure was performed. When determined to be physiologically stable, the patient is discharged from the facility. Dental, podiatric, and dermatologic offices often function in this capacity.

Immediate postoperative patient care is usually provided in a designated area of the hospital or ambulatory care facility. This area may be called the recovery room (RR) or postanesthesia recovery unit (PAR). In this text the term *postanesthesia care unit* is used to describe a specialized area for patient care during recovery from anesthesia. Institutional policies and procedures guide patient care activities in PACU according to protocol established by the anesthesia and surgical services departments. The American Society of Anesthesiologists (ASA) has devised a scale of physical assessment ratings by which patients are categorized by perioperative/perianesthesia risk and outcome (Table 30-1).

Organized in 1980, the American Society of PeriAnesthesia Nurses (ASPAN), formerly known as the American Society of Post Anesthesia Nurses, has established standards of practice for the postoperative care of diverse populations, such as pediatric, adult, and geriatric patients. ASPAN has identified specific phases of care:

- *Preanesthesia phase:* Focuses on the emotional and physical preparation of the patient before a surgical

procedure. The patient is assessed to establish the nursing diagnoses for the perianesthesia period.
- *Postanesthesia phase I:* Focuses on providing immediate postoperative care from an anesthetized state to a condition requiring less acute intervention. The patient may be ASA III or IV. Nurses in this realm of care should be certified in advanced cardiac life support (ACLS) or have equivalent education. Registered nurses who care primarily for pediatric patients should be certified in pediatric advanced life support (PALS).
- *Postanesthesia phase II:* Focuses on preparing the patient for self-care or care in an extended-care setting.
- *Remote postanesthesia phase III:* Focuses on the patient who is preparing for discharge.

The goal of postanesthesia/postprocedure care is to assist the patient in returning to a safe physiologic level after having received an anesthetic agent or after having undergone a surgical procedure. In some settings, perianesthesia nurses follow the patient to phase III, with a phone call to the patient's home within 24 to 48 hours of discharge. (More information about ASPAN position statements concerning patient care is available at www.aspan.org.)

Postanesthesia Care Unit

Located in proximity to the operating room (OR), the basic PACU design consists of a large room (approximately 80 square feet) divided into a series of individual cubicles that are separated by privacy curtains. The beds should be a minimum of 4 feet apart, and there should be equivalent spacing between the bedside tables and walls. Each cubicle has a cardiac monitor, pulse oximeter, blood pressure measurement device, suction apparatus, and oxygen administration equipment.

Additional supplies that are available include warming devices, airway management equipment, intravenous fluids and administration sets, dressing reinforcement materials, medications, indwelling Foley catheters and drainage systems, emesis basins, and bedpans. Lead screens should be available when radiographs are taken.

Other equipment, including crash carts with defibrillators, should be positioned strategically throughout the room for easy accessibility when needed. More than one emergency setup should be immediately available in case the other is in use. Foot- or elbow-controlled handwashing stations should be in proximity to patient care areas.

Some facilities include isolation rooms for patients who are highly contagious or highly susceptible to infection. If the PACU does not have a partitioned isolation area, these patients may be placed at one end of the room and separated from other patients by screens or curtains. Isolation procedures should be used in handling bedding and equipment per institutional policy. All patients have the right to receive the same level of care regardless of extenuating circumstances.

Ideally, the amount of cubicle space is allotted according to the number of ORs in the OR suite. This allotment may vary between one and one half to two cubicles per OR and is based on the caseload, duration of surgical procedures, and room turnover time in the OR. A rapid succession of short procedures could easily fill the PACU and leave no vacancy for additional postoperative patients. This scenario

TABLE 30-1	American Society of Anesthesiologists Physical (P) Status Classification
Status*	Definition
P1	A normal healthy patient
P2	Mild systemic disease without functional limitations
P3	Severe systemic disease associated with definite functional limitations
P4	Severe systemic disease that is an ongoing threat to life
P5	Patient is unlikely to survive 24 hours without the surgical procedure
P6	Patient is brain dead and being prepared as an organ donor

*With P2, P3, and P4, the systemic disease may or may not be related to the cause for surgery. If a patient (P1-P5) requires emergency surgery, an E is added to the physical status (e.g., P1E, P2E). ASA 1 through ASA 6 or I-VI is often used for physical status.
From American Society of Anesthesiologists: *Manual for anesthesia departments*, Park Ridge, Ill, 1997, the Society.

is more common in facilities in which the PACU doubles as a special procedure care unit for ambulatory patients who are receiving nerve blocks for pain therapy.

Some institutions allow an uncomplicated endoscopy to be performed in the PACU. The rationale behind this practice is that patients having special procedures need to be monitored by experienced personnel for a short time after a treatment or test. For some procedures the PACU nurse monitors a patient receiving intravenous conscious sedation and may assist the physician, thus depleting the staff available for postoperative care.

In larger institutions in which prolonged and complex surgical procedures are performed (e.g., transplantation, multiple trauma), postoperative patients may remain in the PACU for more than 24 hours because of the potential need to return to the OR for an additional surgical procedure. In such cases, the PACU doubles as a surgical ICU.

Increased patient load and acuity increase the need for adequate staffing, space allocation, education of personnel, and management of resources. The consolidation of facilities and personnel should not jeopardize the delivery of safe postoperative patient care. Use of the PACU as an overflow ICU depletes the resources intended for the adequate care of postsurgical patients.

Postoperative Observation of the Patient

The duration and type of postoperative observation and care will vary according to the following:

- Patient's condition (e.g., alert and oriented vs. unresponsive)
- Need for physiologic support (e.g., ventilator-dependent vs. awake and extubated)
- Complexity of the surgical procedure (e.g., open laparotomy vs. laparoscopy)
- Type of anesthetic agent administered (e.g., a general inhalation agent vs. local infiltration)
- Need for pain therapy (e.g., intermittent analgesic administration vs. continuous epidural infusion)
- Prescribed period for monitoring parameters to evaluate physiologic status (e.g., stable vs. unstable vital signs)

Perianesthesia Patient Care Personnel

Adequate numbers of personnel should be available to monitor patients and to provide appropriate care as needed. The education and training of PACU nurses should include knowledge of the following:

- Airway management techniques, including positioning, chin lift, jaw thrust, suctioning, bagging, and placement of an airway
- Circulatory assessment, including hemodynamics, neurovascular condition, and renal function
- Neurologic condition, such as level of consciousness or dermatome level associated with epidural infusion (Box 30-1 and Fig. 30-1)
- Anesthetic agents and their actions (e.g., physiologic depression associated with general anesthesia)
- Medications and their actions (e.g., narcotics, tranquilizers)
- Most invasive and minimally invasive surgical procedures (e.g., open laparotomy, laparoscopy)

BOX 30-1	Dermatome Sensory Somatic Landmarks		
C2	Occiput	L1	Groin to dorsum of
C5	Shoulder	L5	foot
T1	Little finger	S1	Dorsum of foot
T4	Nipple line	S3	Heel, lateral foot to sole
T6	Xiphoid process	S5	of foot
T12	Iliac crest		Genitalia
			Perianal area

PACU nurses should demonstrate competency in the following:

- Physical assessment (e.g., heart, lung sounds)
- Recognition of physiologic complications (e.g., airway obstruction, hypothermia, malignant hyperthermia, pain, nausea or vomiting, and/or oropharyngeal aspiration)
- Management of physiologic emergencies (e.g., airway obstruction, hemorrhage, cardiac arrest)
- Interpretation of monitoring data from electrocardiogram (ECG) and oximetry devices

Additional competencies should include certification in cardiopulmonary resuscitation (CPR)—both basic cardiac life support (BCLS) and ACLS. If pediatric patients are involved, credentials should include PALS.

Professional Activities. In 1986, ASPAN developed specialty certification for perianesthesia nurses. Eligibility for certification includes current licensure as a registered nurse and 1800 hours of perianesthesia nursing experience as a caregiver, manager, educator, or researcher. A nurse specializing in the care of phase I postanesthesia patients in hospital-based or extended-recovery care facilities may attain certification as a certified postanesthesia care nurse (CPAN) by taking and passing a written examination. In ambulatory surgery settings, nurses who specialize in the postanesthesia care of patients who move rapidly from phase I to phase II to phase III can attain certification in ambulatory postanesthesia care (CAPA).

The certification for both CAPAs and CPANs is valid for 3 years and can be renewed by passing a written examination or by obtaining 90 contact hours of continuing education credits. ASPAN has produced a core curriculum as an additional reference for perianesthesia nurses who plan to take the certification examination.

Other personnel in the PACU may include licensed practical/vocational nurses (LPNs/LVNs) and other unlicensed patient care personnel. These caregivers are supervised by a registered nurse, who is responsible for their training and assignments within the PACU. Their duties vary according to the needs of the department.

ADMISSION TO THE POSTANESTHESIA CARE UNIT

Before the phase I or phase II patient leaves the OR, the circulating nurse should call the PACU nurse to give the estimated time of arrival in the PACU and to advise of a

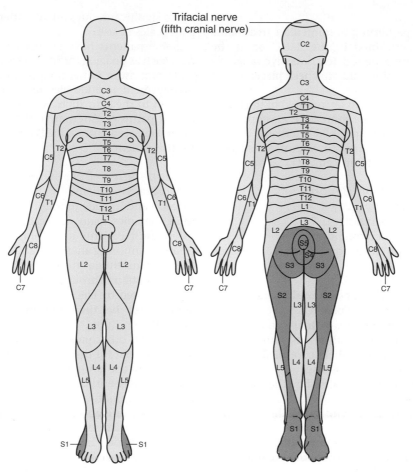

Trifacial nerve
(fifth cranial nerve)

FIG. 30-1 Dermatome levels.

need to have special life support equipment on standby for immediate use. As the patient enters the PACU, his or her immediate physiologic and psychologic status is reported to the PACU nurse by the accompanying personnel (usually the circulating nurse, first assistant, or resident). This reporting is referred to as the "hand-off" report. Any necessary life support equipment, such as a ventilator, is connected. The PACU nurse connects the ECG electrodes, attaches a pulse oximeter lead, and places a blood pressure cuff on the patient.

Many PACUs are supplied with automatic or computerized equipment that provides an immediate display of vital signs and physiologic data from monitors attached to the patient in to OR and that remain on the patient during transport. The PACU nurse simultaneously assesses the patient and assimilates the data. The flow of activity is fast paced but directed toward the immediate physiologic needs and support of the patient.

Postoperative Report

The postoperative report provides information from the anesthesia provider (if one was in attendance), the surgeon (or appropriate designee, such as the first assistant), and the circulating nurse. Much of the report is delivered verbally, but postoperative orders and pertinent information regarding the patient's condition and intraoperative care are rein-

forced in writing. If the surgeon gives a verbal order, he or she should co-sign the chart within 24 hours. The content of the postoperative report to the PACU nurse should include but is not limited to the information discussed in the following sections.

Anesthesia Provider's Report

- Patient's name, gender, age, preoperative and postoperative diagnosis, surgical procedure, and surgeon
- Type of anesthesia and the patient's response(s)
- Baseline preoperative vital signs and summary of vital sign flow during the surgical procedure up to the point of discharge from the OR
- Allergies and reaction to allergen
- Any physiologic changes or existing conditions and interventions to counteract them (e.g., diabetes, chronic obstructive pulmonary disease, previous myocardial infarction, hypertension)
- Medications administered preoperatively, intraoperatively, and postoperatively (e.g., preoperative sedation, intraoperative antibiotic, continuous infusion of medication)
- Intravenous fluid administration and body fluid output (e.g., blood products, urine, gastric contents)
- Specific patient care orders to be performed in the PACU or in the immediate postoperative period (e.g., aerosol or mist mask)

Surgeon's Report

- Postoperative orders pertaining to immediate treatments or therapies to be performed in the PACU or in the immediate postoperative period (e.g., passive-range-of-motion device, radiographic study to check placement of central line catheter)
- Serial diagnostic tests that are to be initiated in the PACU and continued through the immediate postoperative period (e.g., blood counts at specified intervals)
- Specific interventions pertaining to care of the surgical site (e.g., dressing change, reinforcement)

Circulating Nurse's Hand-off Report

- Baseline assessment data
- Positioning and skin preparation
- Condition of dispersive electrode site
- Use of specialized surgical equipment (e.g., laser, endoscope)
- Intraoperative irrigation fluids
- Administration of medication or dyes in the surgical field
- Any implants, transplants, or explants
- Type of dressings and the presence of drains and/or stents
- Intraoperative urinary catheterization and output
- Patient's indication of pain (verbal score of 0 to 10 or nonverbal grimace, crying, restlessness)
- Any pertinent information not reported by the anesthesia provider or surgeon
- Location of family member or significant other who may be waiting

The postoperative report will vary according to the type of anesthesia and the surgical procedure, the preferences of the anesthesia provider and surgeon, and institutional policy and procedure. The main emphasis is the patient's needs in the immediate postoperative period. This continues until the patient is discharged from the PACU.

Patient Care Activities

The application of physiologic and psychosocial knowledge, principles of asepsis, and technical knowledge and skills is necessary to promote, restore, and maintain the patient's physiologic processes in a safe, comfortable, and effective environment. Particular attention is given to monitoring oxygenation, ventilation, and circulation. PACU care includes maintaining adequate ventilation, alleviating nausea and vomiting, preventing shock, and alleviating pain.

Patient Assessment for Pain.
Patients are assessed for vital signs and level of discomfort. Pain is referred to as the fifth vital sign. Pain has been described as both physiologic and psychologic. The adult patient is offered an opportunity to describe pain according to a numbered scale of 0 to 10. The patient's ethnicity and sex can influence the expression of pain. Some groups consider demonstrating pain is a form of weakness.

The perianesthesia nurse should be aware that the patient's demeanor may not adequately relate to the patient's comfort level. Pediatric patients may better describe pain according to the FACES scale (refer to Fig. 8-2). Before administering medication for pain, the patient's communication level should be determined regardless of age. Assessing for speech, language, and hearing can give the perianesthesia nurse significant clues about patient understanding of the pain scales in use.

Some patients have alternative methods for managing pain such as imaging, breathing exercises, meditation, Reiki,[1] and acupressure. Other nonpharmacologic methods of pain management include electronic nerve stimulators[2] either applied to the skin such as TENS or implanted within the neural pathway. Alternative therapies should not be considered replacements for medications when providing comfort for the patient.

Postoperative Care Orders.
Postoperative medical orders are coordinated by the anesthesia provider and the surgeon and include monitoring requirements, oxygen and fluid therapies, pain medications, and other special considerations. Patients are evaluated continually by appropriate monitoring methods and frequent observations by the perianesthesia nurses. Clinical evaluation of each patient's status through listening, watching, and feeling is augmented by electronic monitoring devices. Machines should not be the only method of determining the patient's condition.

As in all other patient care areas, standard precautions are carried out for the disposal of needles and the handling of any item contaminated by blood and body fluids. Handwashing is essential after each patient contact to prevent cross-contamination.

Family members are notified when a patient is admitted to the PACU. This lets them know the surgical procedure is complete, which helps to relieve the anxiety experienced during the hours of waiting. Depending on institutional policy, some facilities allow parents or other visitors in the PACU. No special attire is required.

Postsurgical Overflow Considerations

PACU nurses are very knowledgeable and skilled in the care of critically ill patients. This measure of versatility sometimes places the PACU nurses in the position of keeping and monitoring patients that should be housed in ICU. Sometimes ICU does not have a readily available bed space for the critical postoperative patient, and therefore the PACU nurse provides this care. In some circumstances, general perioperative patient population is maintained in PACU when space is not immediately available on the patient care floors. Some facilities have developed a specialty float pool to work in combination with the PACU team to manage the patient load.

Patients who would normally be discharged to the patient care unit from PACU can be consolidated with float pool nurses to relieve the PACU nurses for more postprocedure or postoperative patient care. Consideration must be given at all times to the availability of appropriate qualified staff

---

[1]Reiki is a Japanese technique for stress reduction and relaxation. It is administered by "laying on hands." More information can be found at www.reiki.org.

[2]Electronic stimulation of nerves can stop the pain signal from being carried to the brain, blocking pain perception. Natural body chemicals referred to as endorphins are released in the brain to act as analgesia.

and bed space for care of immediate postanesthesia patients, despite the extra load of patients who should be housed elsewhere.

Documentation

Institutional policies and procedures should be followed in documenting PACU care. Observations of respiratory and circulatory functions and level of consciousness are recorded at frequent intervals. Postoperative physiologic and psychologic status are documented at the time of any significant event (e.g., the administration of medication), as well as routinely at 5- to 7-minute intervals for the first hour and at 15- to 30-minute intervals for the second hour and thereafter. Pertinent observations are recorded as appropriate or necessary.

DISCHARGE FROM THE POSTANESTHESIA CARE UNIT

Most patients remain in the PACU at least 1 hour or until they have sufficiently recovered from anesthesia so that their vital signs have stabilized and they are capable of reasonable self-care. The patient's condition is scored using a postanesthesia scoring system according to vital signs, activity level, and consciousness; several standardized formats are available for this purpose. The anesthesia provider assesses the patient as necessary and may determine when the patient is stable enough for discharge from PACU. After discharge from PACU, the patient is transported to a patient care unit or an ICU or is released from the ambulatory care facility.

A physician is responsible for the patient's discharge from the PACU. The anesthesia department staff and medical staff may approve discharge criteria for the PACU nurse to use in determining readiness for discharge. These criteria should be consistent with the standards of the ASA and the accreditation standards of the Joint Commission on Accreditation of Healthcare Organizations (JCAHO) and/or the Accreditation Association for Ambulatory Health Care (AAAHC).

Postoperative Evaluation of Expected Outcomes

Ideally, the perioperative nurse who preoperatively assessed the patient and intraoperatively developed and implemented the plan of care will have the opportunity to assess and/or interview the patient postoperatively and evaluate patient care outcomes. An assessment is performed in person if possible, or the patient may be interviewed by a follow-up telephone call within 24 to 48 hours of discharge.

The plan of care should be evaluated in terms of the attainment of expected outcomes. The identification of influencing factors provides a foundation for ongoing improvement of perioperative patient care services. Considerations for the design of the postoperative evaluation include but are not limited to the following:

1. Was a preoperative visit made, and was it helpful to the patient?
2. Were the patient and family adequately prepared for the surgical procedure physically, psychologically, emotionally, and spiritually? Did the patient receive written preoperative instructions?
3. What could have been improved?
4. Were all pertinent patient needs, problems, or health status considerations identified in the nursing diagnoses?
5. Did the plan of care address the nursing diagnoses?
6. Did the patient experience any complications?
7. Was preoperative teaching used? Was it adequate and helpful?
8. What were the patient's perceptions of the surgical experience?
9. Were the expected outcomes achieved to the patient's satisfaction?
10. To what degree do the patient's observable physiologic and psychosocial responses indicate the attainment of expected outcomes?
11. Was the patient given a postage-paid, follow-up survey of satisfaction to complete and return to the department?

The evaluation of patient outcomes helps identify environmental influences and procedural activities that may need to be modified by the OR staff. For example, if the patient has developed a reddened pressure area over a bony prominence, was the positioning equipment at fault or was the area unpadded? A reevaluation of products currently being used may be indicated. Injury to skin may be caused by the pooling of prep solutions under the patient, inadequate padding of body prominences, or faulty electrical equipment.

The subjective data received from the patient will help evaluate how much discomfort the patient is experiencing, especially paresthesia (a numb, tingling sensation). Neurovascular injuries may be related to positioning on the operating bed. The perioperative nurse may suggest comfort measures to help this patient, but an adverse outcome indicates a need to improve positioning procedures for subsequent patients.

The postoperative assessment or follow-up telephone call terminates the direct perioperative nurse–patient relationship. The evaluation of the degree of attainment of expected outcomes completes the perioperative nursing process.

To be successful, a postoperative evaluation program requires the cooperative effort of and input from all personnel involved with patient care, including registered nurses, technicians, and physicians. Administrative personnel may seek specific information and should be consulted for input. They should participate in structuring the program at its inception to avoid duplication of action and to promote a collegial effort. Postoperative evaluation data may be collected through the following measures:

- Interview and assessment of the patient
- Conferences with physicians, nurses, and other caregivers
- Review of responses on the patient evaluation form

The postoperative evaluation program should be reviewed periodically and revised as necessary. An interdisciplinary conference is an effective medium for the accomplishment of these objectives. An effective perioperative evaluation program and positive patient experiences promote good public relations and demonstrate a caring image to the public it serves.

Bibliography

American Society of Anesthesiologists: *Standards for postanesthesia care*, Park Ridge, Ill, 1988 (date of adoption), the Society.

American Society of PeriAnesthesia Nurses: ASPAN pain and comfort clinical guideline, *J Perianesth Nurs* 18(4):232-236, 2003.

Barnes S: Are you watching the clock? Let criteria define discharge readiness, *J Perianesth Nurs* 15(3):174-175, 2000.

Burden N, Saufel N: PeriAnesthesia standards for ethical practice, *J Perianesth Nurs* 16(1):2-5, 2001.

Harper JP: Post anesthesia care unit nurse's knowledge of pulse oximetry, *J Nurs Staff Devel* 20(4):177-180, 2004.

Hegedus MB: Taking the fear out of postanesthesia care in the intensive care unit, *Dimens Crit Care Nurs* 22(3):237-246, 2003.

Keita H et al: Predictive factors of early postoperative urinary retention in the postanesthesia care unit, *Anesth Analg* 101(2):592-596, 2005.

Knoerl DV et al: Evaluation of orthostatic blood pressure testing as a discharge criterion from PACU after spinal anesthesia, *J Perianesth Nurs* 16(1):11-18, 2001.

Mamaril M: The official ASPAN position: ICU overflow patients in the PACU, *J Perianesth Nurs* 16(4):274-277, 2001.

Manias E et al: Nurse's strategies for managing pain in the postoperative environment, *Pain Manage Nurs* 5(1):18-29, 2005.

Panagiotis K et al: Is postanesthesia care unit length of stay increased in hypothermic patients? *AORN J* 81(2):379-388, 2005.

Pasero C, Belden J: Evidence-based perianesthesia care: Accelerated postoperative recovery programs, *J Perianesth Nurs* 21(3):168-176, 2006.

Sullivan EE: General surgery overflow: A new challenge for the PACU, *J Perianesth Nurs* 17(1):43-45, 2002.

Wilson L, Kolcaba K: Practical application of comfort theory in the perianesthesia setting, *J Perianesth Nurs* 19(3):164-170, 2004.

Chapter 31

Potential Perioperative Complications

CHAPTER OBJECTIVES

After studying this chapter, the learner will be able to:
- Describe several respiratory complications that are possible in the perioperative period.
- Identify three potential dysrhythmias that may complicate the patient's perioperative course.
- Demonstrate the procedure for weighing surgical sponges in the operating room.
- List the primary drugs used in the management of an acute malignant hyperthermic crisis.
- Identify three methods for preventing hypothermia in the perioperative patient.

CHAPTER OUTLINE

KEY TERMS AND DEFINITIONS

Anemia   Reduction of the number of functioning red blood cells capable of containing enough hemoglobin to transport oxygen.

Anoxia   Absence of oxygen. (Not synonymous with hypoxia.)

Aspiration   Entry of gastric, oropharyngeal, or other substance into the lungs.

Atelectasis   Collapsed or airless lung.

Cardiotonic   Drug that increases the tone of the heart, such as digitalis.

Dysrhythmia   Abnormal, disordered, disturbed rhythm.

Embolus   A blood clot or other substance, such as plaque or fat that occludes a segment of the cardiovascular system.

Hemoglobinopathy   Any one of a group of blood diseases that are characterized by abnormal forms of hemoglobin in the blood.

Hemorrhage   Abnormal internal or external loss of blood from an arterial, venous, or capillary source.

Hypertension   Elevated blood pressure. If on several occasions the systolic pressure is above 140 or the diastolic pressure is above 90, the patient is considered hypertensive.

Hypotension   Low blood pressure. If on several occasions the systolic pressure is lower than 100, the patient is considered hypotensive. This should be compared with other assessment parameters.

Hypoventilation   Reduced rate and depth of breathing that causes an increase in carbon dioxide.

Hypoxia   Decreased concentration of oxygen.

Metabolic crisis   Physical and chemical changes that cause catabolic or anabolic activity that may be life threatening:
- **Anabolism**   Buildup of tissues or properties.
- **Catabolism**   Breakdown of tissues or properties.

Thrombus   A blood clot within a blood vessel.

Vasoconstrictor   A drug that causes narrowing of a blood vessel.

Vasodilator   A drug that causes relaxation of a blood vessel or causes opening (dilation).

SUPPLEMENTAL MATERIAL ON EVOLVE WEBSITE   *evolve*

http://evolve.elsevier.com/BerryKohn
- Content Updates
- Glossary
- Full Set of Perioperative Flash Cards
- Interactive Key Term Flash Cards
- Student Activities
- WebLinks

HISTORICAL BACKGROUND

From early times, it was known that loss of blood meant loss of life, although the circulation of blood was not clearly understood. The writings of Aristotle (384-322 BC) reveal that veins were thought to contain all or most of the blood. Arteries were thought to contain air, with only a small amount of blood. This doctrine continued until the physiologist Galen (AD 130-200) demonstrated that arteries, like veins, contain blood, which he believed just ebbed and flowed. This theory held for about 1500 years, until William Harvey (1578-1657), an English anatomist, realized that blood circulated and could flow only in one direction. His hypothesis that it passed from arteries to veins through capillaries was proved under the microscope in 1661 by Marcello Malpighi (1628-1694), an Italian anatomist.

Before the advent of anesthesia in 1846, surgical skill was based on speed. Most surgical procedures were done for major injuries or life-threatening conditions, such as gangrene or infection in an extremity. Amputations were swift and guillotine-style. Blood dripped onto the floor or into a box of sawdust. Loss of blood was one of the most dangerous complications of surgery.

The first attempt to transfuse blood in humans occurred in 1818 when English physician James Blundell transfused blood by syringe from a husband to his wife, who was dying of postpartum hemorrhage. He developed transfusion instrumentation and successfully performed this procedure on five other patients between 1825 and 1830. American physicians attempted volume expansion between 1873 and 1880 using cow, goat, and human milk, with many adverse reactions. Later in the century saline was used for this purpose, and in 1886 John Duncan transfused autologous blood directly from the surgical field into a trauma patient by femoral injection.

In 1901 Karl Landsteiner (1868-1943), an Austrian-American pathologist, discovered the blood groups A, B, and O. Other researchers discovered group AB the following year. In 1930 Landsteiner was awarded the Nobel Prize for his work in transfusion research. The knowledge of blood groups led to the feasibility of donor (allogenic) blood transfusions. Plasma was first used during World War I to combat shock.

The development of blood banking superseded previous attempts at autotransfusion. The first blood bank was established in 1936 at the Mayo Clinic in Rochester, Minnesota. Interest in allogenic blood prospered during World War II, because a large donor pool collected by the Red Cross, along with improved methods of typing and crossmatching, made banked blood easier to obtain and safer to use. Resurgence of interest in autologous blood occurred, however, with direct salvage devices during the Vietnam War. The first technically safe commercial autologous blood recovery equipment was marketed in 1971.

Although blood loss is a serious concern for the surgical patient, other systemic complications can cause problems with other vital functions. The perioperative caregiver should be aware of the potential for respiratory, cardiac, vascular, and metabolic complications and be prepared to assist in supportive care.

POTENTIAL FOR COMPLICATIONS DURING AND AFTER SURGERY

Many facilities use scoring systems as guidelines to predict the potential for complications during the perioperative care period. The patient receives care from a multidisciplinary team that plans for his or her safety by assessing risks and benefits of the surgical procedure. Preoperatively, the patient is assessed by the anesthesia provider using the American Society of Anesthesiologists (ASA) scoring system. Intraoperatively, the patient's risk for infection is assessed using the Centers for Disease Control and Prevention (CDC) wound classification scheme. In the postanesthesia care area, the patient's readiness for discharge is scored according to one of several predictive indicator grids based on his or her physiology. All of the scoring systems add up to a number that is used in decision making concerning the plan of care and progression toward wellness.

The purpose of this chapter is to acquaint the caregiver with the potential complications that patients experience during and after surgery. A satisfactory score in one care period is not always a predictor of how the patient will do in subsequent phases of care after the physical changes associated with surgery. Each organ system interacts with other organ systems to produce homeostasis in the patient. An alteration in one organ system will affect all of the others, causing the potential for a poor outcome. Morbidity and mortality can be minimized with prompt detection and precise intervention.

RESPIRATORY COMPLICATIONS

One of the primary areas of postoperative complications is the respiratory system. The patient's potential for developing pulmonary problems depends on several factors. Any pre-existing lung disease, such as emphysema, infection, or asthma, predisposes the patient. Smokers have the highest risk of succumbing to postoperative pulmonary problems because of chronic irritation of the respiratory tract with consequent production of excess mucus. Chest wall deformities, obesity, and extremes of age are other pertinent preoperative influences. Intraoperative factors include the following:

- Type of preoperative medications
- Type and duration of anesthesia
- Type and duration of assisted ventilation
- Position of the patient during the surgical procedure
- Extent of the surgical procedure

Postoperatively, one of the most critical factors is the patient's ability to mobilize secretions by deep breathing, coughing, and ambulation. Patients undergoing chest and abdominal surgery are likely to breathe shallowly because of pain and therefore may not adequately raise accumulated secretions. Development of one pulmonary complication often predisposes the patient to development of another. Acute respiratory distress syndrome (ARDS), also known as progressive pulmonary insufficiency or shock lung, may develop in the first 24 to 48 hours after a traumatic injury.

Aspiration

Aspiration of gastric contents into the lungs may occur because of decreased throat reflexes when the patient is unconscious or is conscious with the throat anesthetized, as for bronchoscopy. Residual effects impede lung function and blood-gas exchange. A chemical pneumonitis results from aspiration of highly acidic gastric juices. Edema forms, alveoli collapse, ventilation-perfusion mismatch occurs, and hypoxemia results. Aspiration of solids in emesis results in edema, severe hypoxia, and respiratory obstruction. Bronchospasm and atelectasis may be followed by pneumonitis or bronchopneumonia. Most aspirate is irritating, but it can be infectious if nasopharyngeal or gastric flora are aspirated. Pneumonia or lung abscess may result with necrosis of the pulmonary parenchyma.

Etiology. Every patient who has food in the stomach is a poor risk for anesthesia. Increased intragastric pressure is an aspiration hazard and may result from conditions such as diaphragmatic hernia, gastrointestinal bleeding, intestinal obstruction, or gas forced into the stomach by application of positive pressure ventilation without use of a cuffed endotracheal tube.

Signs and Symptoms. Signs and symptoms include central cyanosis, dyspnea, gasping, and tachycardia, followed by cardiac embarrassment, lung collapse, and consolidation.

Treatment. Most effective treatment occurs during the first minutes after aspiration. The strategy is to remove as much aspirate as possible and limit the spread of what is left in the lung. The head of the operating bed is lowered with a right lateral tilt for postural drainage; the right mainstem bronchus bifurcates slightly higher than the left mainstem bronchus. The oropharynx and tracheobronchial tree are suctioned. If the patient has aspirated particulate matter that causes obstruction of the airways, bronchoscopy must be performed to remove it. Suctioning must be interrupted every 10 to 15 seconds to administer oxygen. Oxygenation and carbon dioxide removal are high priorities.

Aspiration of acid gastric content injures the alveolar capillary interface, resulting in intrapulmonary shunting and pulmonary edema. Intensive pulmonary care is aimed at improving ventilation-perfusion ratios and decreasing abnormal gas exchange. This may require endotracheal intubation for mechanical ventilation with continuous positive pressure. Most cases of severe hypoxemia occur rapidly within the first 30 to 60 minutes after aspiration. Careful cardiovascular monitoring and frequent blood-gas and acid-base determinations guide therapeutic measures to maintain intravascular volume. Prophylactic antibiotics may be given for aspiration of bowel-contaminated fluid to prevent infection, and a bronchodilator may be used to treat spasm. Most cases of permanent injury or death result from the initial hypoxemia.

Prevention. Prevention involves adequate preoperative preparation (withholding oral intake 8 to 10 hours before induction) and careful administration of anesthetic agents. The anesthetic is decreased near the end of the surgical procedure, hastening the return of throat reflexes. All trauma and obstetric patients receiving general anesthesia should be treated as if they have full stomachs and should be intubated using cricoid pressure. The cricoid pressure should be released after verification of endotracheal tube placement. Gastric evacuation is delayed during labor and by analgesic medications. A nasogastric tube may be inserted preoperatively or intraoperatively.

Laryngospasm and Bronchospasm

Laryngospasm is a partial or complete closure of the vocal cords as an involuntary reflex action. Bronchospasm is contraction of smooth muscle in the walls of the bronchi and bronchioles, causing narrowing of the lumen. Spasms or abnormal narrowing is produced by a marked increase in smooth muscle tone of the airway walls. Marked elevation of airway resistance profoundly alters gas flow into and out of the lungs. Accompanying changes result in a decreased ventilation-perfusion ratio with a subsequent reduction in Pao_2 and rise in $Paco_2$. Many factors can precipitate spasm.

Etiology. Etiologic factors include mechanical airway obstruction, use of certain anesthetics and drugs, allergic conditions such as asthma, vagal reflex, stimulation of the pharynx and larynx with the patient under light anesthesia, traction on the peritoneum, foreign material in the tracheobronchial tree, movement of the head or neck or traction on the carotid sinus, and painful peripheral stimuli. The degree of spasm varies from mild to severe.

Symptoms. Symptoms include wheezing respirations or stridor, reduced compliance, central cyanosis, and respiratory obstruction.

Treatment. Treatment depends on the precipitating factor. Methods generally used include positive pressure ventilation, oxygen, tracheal intubation, and neuromuscular blockers for relaxation. Bronchodilator drugs such as aminophylline, isoetharine, and metaproterenol are given with caution because they act as cardiac stimulators and, in the presence of hypoxia, may contribute to cardiac dysrhythmia and cardiac arrest. Patients may be refractory (unresponsive) to bronchodilators because of acid-base abnormalities. Correction can reduce the side effects and augment the beneficial effects of bronchodilators. If the etiologic factor is an allergy, steroids and antihistamines may be given. Vagal reflexes are inhibited by atropine. If reflex is the cause, anesthesia is deepened. Drying agents are given for excessive secretions. Immediate effective treatment is mandatory to counteract hypoxia and prevent cardiac arrest.

Prevention. Prevention involves maintenance of a patent airway, appropriate premedication such as glycopyrrolate, avoidance of factors stimulating the vagal reflex, and treatment of the predisposing pulmonary condition.

Airway and Respiratory Obstruction

An airway is maintained with an oral airway or endotracheal tube. Airway obstruction is the most frequent cause of respiratory difficulty in the immediate postoperative period. The patient may exhibit paradoxical respiration (i.e., downward movement of the diaphragm occurring with contraction rather than expansion of the chest), resulting in hypoxia and carbon dioxide retention. As the condition worsens, the patient becomes restless, diaphoretic, cyanotic, and finally unconscious. If not relieved within seconds, this serious complication may lead to cardiac arrest.

Etiology. Etiologic factors include blocking of the airway by the tongue, soft tissue, excessive secretions, or a foreign body; laryngospasm or bronchospasm; or positioning of the head with the chin down.

Symptoms. Symptoms of respiratory obstruction include increased respiratory effort with inadequate ventilatory exchange, visible use of accessory muscles, and respiratory motion of the chest and abdomen without audible air movement at the airway. If the airway is totally obstructed, breath sounds will be absent; if it is partially obstructed, a snoring sound will be elicited. The pulse is rapid and thready.

Assessment of oxygenation is essential if the patient's airway patency is in question. Visual inspection of the patient may reveal *peripheral cyanosis* (i.e., pallor, duskiness, or bluish color of the nailbeds and extremities). This is caused by a decrease in capillary oxygen levels. Peripheral cyanosis is not always indicative of impending danger to the patient. It can be caused by hypothermia, stress, medications, or other physiologic factors that cause peripheral vasoconstriction.

If the patient is in an arterial hypoxemic state, he or she will exhibit *central cyanosis*—pallor, duskiness, or bluish color of the lips, face, and generalized body surface. Central cyanosis is a serious sign that requires immediate airway and ventilatory assessment followed by emergent treatment. Central cyanosis may develop more slowly if the patient has been breathing a high concentration of oxygen.

Treatment. Suctioning blood, mucus, or emesis, gently hyperextending the neck, and elevating the chin may eliminate the cause of obstruction. Oxygen is administered by positive pressure; a nasal airway or endotracheal intubation may be necessary. If the anesthesia provider has been unable to manually ventilate or intubate the patient in two or three attempts, it may be necessary to establish an indirect airway by opening the patient's anterior neck; a needle is inserted through the cricoid cartilage for a cricothyrotomy or, if time permits, a tracheotomy.

Hypoventilation

The ability to oxygenate depends on the condition of the lungs, hemoglobin concentration, cardiac output, and oxygen saturation. Inadequate or reduced alveolar ventilation can cause a deficit in oxygenation. This can lead to hypoxia (a decreased level of oxygen in arterial blood and tissues), hypoxemia (a decreased level of oxygen in arterial blood), and hypercapnia, also known as hypercarbia (an elevated level of carbon dioxide in arterial blood).

The body compensates for mild hypoxia with increased heart and respiratory rates, bringing oxygen to the blood and tissues at a faster rate. If hypoxia progresses, this compensation is inadequate. If hypoxia is prolonged, cardiac dysrhythmias or irreversible brain, liver, kidney, and heart damage result. Retention of carbon dioxide also leads to acidosis.

Etiology. Contributing factors to hypoventilation include alveolar impairment, pain, faulty positioning, a full bladder, or a short, thick neck. Inadequate pulmonary ventilation from depression of the medullary center in the brain by narcotics or anesthetics, neurologic effects of spinal or epidural drug administration, reduced cardiac output, severe blood loss, obstruction to the respiratory passages, or abnormality of the ventilation-perfusion ratio also can contribute to hypoxia and hypercapnia.

Symptoms. Symptoms of hypoventilation and hypoxia include an increased pulse rate; pallor or central cyanosis from hypoxia or a flushed or reddened appearance from hypercapnia; decreased volume of respirations; stertorous or labored respirations; and dark blood in the surgical field. The acid-base balance can be affected.

Treatment. The immediate administration of oxygen in the proper dosage is the treatment of choice for hypoventilation and hypoxia. Oxygen is a medication requiring proper dosage for safe, effective administration. In the healthy patient, changes in the concentration of carbon dioxide in the blood stimulate the primary central chemoreceptor (respiratory center) in the medulla of the brain. In response to this stimulation, the patient takes a breath to increase oxygenation. Patients with chronic obstructive pulmonary disease (COPD) have higher than normal levels of circulating carbon dioxide and have a decreased primary chemoreceptor

response. They rely on secondary chemoreceptors in the carotid and aortic bodies to sense the changes in carbon dioxide levels in the blood. High concentrations of oxygen decrease the sensitivity of the secondary chemoreceptors in patients with COPD, causing respiratory depression known as carbon dioxide narcosis.

To minimize the risk for respiratory arrest in these patients, a 2- to 3-liter per minute (L/min) flow of oxygen per nasal cannula is recommended postoperatively. An endotracheal tube may be left in place postoperatively to support assisted ventilation in select patients.

Patients are encouraged to cough and breathe deeply postoperatively. If a patient received naloxone hydrochloride (Narcan) to reverse the respiratory depressant effect of a narcotic, the patient may awaken rapidly and cough, inadvertently causing extubation. The patient must be watched closely during recovery.

Prevention. A patent airway, appropriate oxygenation, and proper positioning help prevent hypoventilation. Intraoperative measurements of arterial pH, Pco_2, and Po_2 enable the anesthesia provider to evaluate oxygenation and carbon dioxide gas exchange. To prevent hypoventilation and hypoxia, patients may be given oxygen and assisted ventilation during transport to the recovery area.

Pulmonary Embolism

Pulmonary embolism is a major cause of death during a surgical procedure and in the immediate postoperative period. Some intraoperative problems may extend into postoperative recovery.

Pulmonary embolism is an obstruction of the pulmonary artery or one of its branches by an embolus, most often a blood clot, but can be fat or other material. The most important factor leading to pulmonary emboli is stasis of blood, particularly in the low-pressure regions such as deep veins of the legs and pelvis, where the majority of thrombi arise. These become detached and are carried to the lungs. Changes in vessel walls and coagulative changes in blood also are important factors. A prolonged period on the operating bed may decrease blood flow to the lower extremities by more than 50%. Blood flow is impaired further if the knees are raised on a hard rolled towel, putting occlusive pressure on the vessels.

Venous stasis also is correlated with obesity, dehydration, congestive heart failure, and atrial fibrillation. Local trauma to a vein or venous disease enhances the chance of thrombus formation. Hypercoagulability may coexist with conditions such as pregnancy, fever, myocardial infarction, and some malignancies and after abrupt cessation of anticoagulant therapy. Prevention consists of a regimen of prophylactic anticoagulants or antiplatelets for high-risk patients and routine measures to prevent venous stasis, such as intermittent compression or antiembolic stockings.

Because of the origin of thrombi in deep veins, it is important to observe the patient postoperatively for thrombophlebitis, evidenced by heat, edema, redness, pain in the calf, or a positive Homans' sign, which is pain in the calf on forceful dorsiflexion of the foot.

Nonspecific symptoms depend on whether the embolism is mild or massive. The patient may have dyspnea, pleural pain, hemoptysis, tachypnea, crackles, tachycardia, mild fever, or persistent cough. Patients with massive emboli have air hunger, hypotension, shock, and central cyanosis. Treatment of pulmonary emboli consists of bed rest, oxygen therapy, anticoagulant therapy, thrombolytic agents, and sometimes a surgical procedure to remove the emboli or to place a vena cava filter to prevent additional clots from reaching the lungs.

Fat embolism occurs primarily after fracture of a long bone, pelvis, or ribs. However, it sometimes occurs after a blood transfusion, cardiopulmonary bypass, or renal transplant. Fat globules enter a venous sinus and become bloodborne. Symptoms develop when globules block pulmonary capillaries, causing interstitial edema and hemorrhage.

Frequently, ARDS ensues 24 to 48 hours after injury, with hypoxia and decreased surfactant production, resulting in collapse of the alveolar membrane and microatelectasis. The syndrome develops most frequently in patients older than 10 years, especially those who have traveled long distances with an immobilized fracture. Symptoms include disorientation, increased pulse rate, elevated temperature, tachypnea, dyspnea, crackles, and pleuritic chest pain. Other significant signs are fat in the sputum and urine and a petechial rash on the anterior chest. Treatment is supportive. Mortality is high.

Air embolism may follow incidental injection of air into a body cavity or a bolus of air in an intravenous (IV) or intraarterial infusion. Another means of entry is during transection of large veins with the patient in a sitting or prone position. The pull of gravity on the venous drainage exerts a significant negative pressure that sucks air into the veins and into the right atrium of the heart. The air embolus blocks the tricuspid valve. This can be a complication in handling central venous catheters and using syringes to obtain blood for gas analysis.

Immediate treatment of air embolus is to place the patient into Trendelenburg's position with the right side slightly elevated. The anesthesia provider can place a venous catheter into the patient's jugular and slide it into the right atrium to evacuate the air.

Intrauterine fetal death, abruptio placentae, or placenta previa may precipitate an embolism of amniotic fluid. Also, tumors may cause emboli from primary or metastatic sites. Other material such as plaque or hemostatic material can embolize, causing injury or death to the patient.

Pneumothorax

Although it is rare, insertion of a needle into the thoracic cage can occur during a nerve block or subclavian catheter insertion. Excision of a breast mass close to the chest wall can precipitate pneumothorax. The primary symptoms are pain and shortness of breath. Confirmation is made by radiograph. If the pneumothorax is extensive and the lung fails to reexpand, a chest tube with an underwater seal is required.

Intercostal Muscle Spasm

A "rigid chest" may occur after large doses of IV fentanyl or on emergence from general anesthesia. It may reverse itself, or neuromuscular blockers may be needed.

Atelectasis (Pulmonary Collapse)

Partial collapse of a lung is one of the most common postoperative problems. If mucus obstructs a bronchus, air in the alveoli distal to the obstruction is resorbed. That segment of lung then collapses and consolidates. Retained mucus becomes contaminated by inhaled bacteria; the patient may develop bronchopneumonia.

Etiology. Factors that promote increased production of mucus, such as certain irritating anesthetics, and decreased mobilization of mucus, such as from a tight abdominal dressing, predispose the patient to pulmonary collapse. Furthermore, normal respiration includes a deep sigh several times an hour to help keep the lungs expanded. This natural sigh is inhibited by anesthetics, narcotics, and sedatives. Oxygen and carbon dioxide are absorbed into the pulmonary blood flow, and the alveoli collapse. Low tidal volume intensifies the problem. High concentrations of oxygen remove nitrogen from the lungs, leaving oxygen, carbon dioxide, and water in the alveoli.

Symptoms. Atelectasis increases the temperature, pulse, and respiratory rate. The patient may appear cyanotic and uncomfortable, with shallow respirations and pain on coughing. Breath sounds are diminished, with fine crackles. Chest radiograph reveals collapsed areas of the lungs as patch opacities, generally involving the lung bases.

Treatment and Prevention. Measures to help prevent or treat atelectasis are abstention from smoking, a regimen of coughing and deep breathing, and early ambulation. An upright position allows for better lung expansion. Medication for pain, when appropriate, before breathing exercises or ambulation improves the ability to breathe deeply and cough effectively. Splinting the thoracic or abdominal incision with a pillow also helps decrease the pain of coughing. Repeated vigorous coughing is contraindicated in some patients (e.g., after cataract extraction, craniotomy, herniorrhaphy).

Pulmonary Edema

Pulmonary edema may be defined as an abnormal accumulation of water in extravascular portions of the lungs, including both alveolar and interstitial spaces. In surgical patients the most probable cause is increased microvascular pulmonary capillary permeability or capillary endothelial injury. Blood stagnates in the pulmonary circulation. Fluid exudes from capillaries into the alveoli and interstitial spaces. Reduction of capillary membrane perfusion leads to hypoxia. Symptoms, usually seen postoperatively in the postanesthesia care unit (PACU) or intensive care unit (ICU), may include a bounding, rapid pulse; crackles; dyspnea; and engorged peripheral veins.

CARDIOVASCULAR COMPLICATIONS

The emotional and physical stresses to which a surgical patient is subjected may lead to cardiovascular complications. The patient who fears dying while under anesthesia runs a greater risk of cardiac arrest on the operating bed than do patients with known cardiac disease. Psychologic stress can have physiologic manifestations. Extreme preoperative anxiety predisposes the patient to a difficult induction and intraoperative period and to postoperative discomfort.

Patients with a history of cardiovascular problems are prone to develop complications. These may include dysrhythmias, hypotension, thromboembolism and/or thrombophlebitis, myocardial infarction, or congestive heart failure. Cerebral thrombosis or embolism may result in prolonged coma. Patients must be closely monitored for symptoms of cardiovascular complications. Anoxia, the complete or almost total absence of oxygen from inspired gases, arterial blood, or tissues, is a precursor to cardiovascular collapse. Cardiac arrest can result in death in the operating room (OR).

Hypotension

Reduced blood pressure, with resultant inadequate circulation, may accompany depression of the myocardium, depression of the vasomotor center in the brain, a decline in cardiac output, or dilation of the peripheral vessels. Hypotension may occur also when positive pressure is applied to the airway. Progressive deepening of general anesthesia usually produces peripheral vasodilation and diminished myocardial contractility. Adequate blood flow to the brain and heart, the two most vulnerable vascular beds because of their high metabolic demand, must be maintained. If arterial hypotension is uncontrolled, it may cause a cerebrovascular accident, myocardial infarction, or death.

Etiology. Overdosage of general anesthetic agents or rapid vascular absorption of local agents may result from the patient's receiving an amount of the agent that exceeds his or her tolerance. Tendency for overdosage occurs during prolonged anesthesia with large amounts of drugs absorbed, in age-extreme patients, or with unrecognized hypothermia during lengthy abdominal or thoracic procedures. Circulatory effects of spinal or epidural anesthesia, such as diminished cardiac output or reduced peripheral resistance, also produce hypotension.

Other causes of hypotension include the following:
- Volume depletion and/or hemorrhage
- Circulatory abnormalities (e.g., cardiac tamponade, heart failure)
- Cerebral or pulmonary embolism (fat embolism from fracture sites, amniotic fluid emboli during delivery, or air emboli from introduction of air into the circulation during an infusion or procedure)
- Myocardial ischemia or infarction
- Changes in position, especially if executed rapidly or roughly
- Excessive preanesthetic medication (postural hypotension may follow narcotic administration)
- Epidural or spinal anesthesia above the level of T6 (sympathetic block)
- Potent therapeutic drugs (e.g., tranquilizers, adrenal steroids, antihypertensives) given before the anesthetic
- Hypoxia

Surgical manipulation may mechanically induce hypotension by obstructing venous return to the heart with packs, retractors, or body rests, or hypotension and bradycardia may result from a vagal-induced reflex precipitated by intraperitoneal traction, manipulation in the chest or neck area, rapid release of either increased intraabdominal pressure or overdistention of the bladder, anorectal stimulation, or stimulation of the periosteum or joint cavities. Other causes are transfusion reaction (suggested by accompanying cyanosis and oozing at the surgical site), septic shock, severe hyperthermia, and anaphylactic reaction.

Symptoms. Early reversible shock is accompanied by unstable blood pressure, vasoconstriction, elevated serum pH, and elevated catecholamine levels. Late manifestations are pallor or central cyanosis, clammy skin, dilated pupils, decreased urinary output, tachycardia, decreased bleeding in the surgical field or pallor of organs caused by compensatory vasoconstriction, nausea, vomiting, sighing respirations, or air hunger in conscious patients.

Diagnosis. Determination of arterial blood pressure and pulse rate and estimation of pulse volume are indicative of the volume of cardiac ejection. Arbitrary figures of measured blood pressure are not as important as individual circulatory status. A specific measurement in a healthy adult may be relatively insignificant, whereas the same figure in a geriatric patient could be hazardous. In critically ill patients, direct arterial pressure, central venous pressure (CVP), and urinary output are monitored.

Treatment. Treatment must be prompt to avoid circulatory collapse. The aim is to increase perfusion of the vital organs and to treat any specific cause while giving general supportive therapy. Supportive measures include oxygen by mask with assisted respiration; elevation of the legs to increase blood pressure by draining pooled blood, especially after sympathetic blockade; and rapid IV fluid therapy to increase blood volume. Because the volume of fluid is more vital than its composition, various solutions are applicable for early treatment in an emergency. If whole blood is not available, crystalloid solutions (e.g., Ringer's lactate), 5% dextrose in water, physiologic saline solution, plasma or serum albumin, or 6% dextran (plasma expander) may be given. Rapid infusion under pressure may be necessary. Vasoactive drugs are given as necessary; these are usually vasopressors to constrict arterioles and veins while increasing the myocardial contractile force. Blood gases should be monitored.

Prevention. The causes must be reversed or avoided. Therefore the patient should be observed constantly throughout anesthesia; in suspected individuals, the cardiovascular response to the desired surgical position should be tested before induction. Overdosage of premedication and anesthetic drugs is avoided. The patient's position is changed slowly, tissue is manipulated gently, and blood and fluid loss are replaced promptly. The anesthesia provider administers a minimal amount of the anesthetic and takes adequate time to induce and deepen anesthesia so as not to raise the blood level of the anesthetic too rapidly. Positive pressure is applied to the airway prudently.

Some narcotics and anesthetic agents, surgical trauma, anoxia, and blood loss can lead to postoperative hypotension. When combined, these factors interfere with the complex physiologic mechanisms that support blood pressure. Peripheral vessels dilate. A degree of cardiovascular collapse ensues. Vasoconstriction reduces renal blood flow, causing decrease or failure of kidney function. Patients must be monitored postoperatively for sudden drops in blood pressure or other signs of shock. Vasoactive drugs and oxygen may be administered. To avoid hypotension, fluid management is critical to renal function after restoration of systemic blood pressure.

Hypertension

Abnormal elevation of the blood pressure may occur, especially in a hypertensive or arteriosclerotic patient. Even mildly hypertensive patients are prone to myocardial ischemia (inadequate blood flow to the heart) during induction of and emergence from anesthesia. Intubation stimulates the sympathetic nervous system. Other predisposing factors include pain, shivering, hypoxia, hypercapnia, effects of vasopressor drugs, or hypervolemia from excessive replacement of fluid losses. Treatment consists of administration of oxygen, diuretics, and antihypertensive beta-blocker drugs as indicated. If not controlled, hypertension may precipitate a cerebrovascular accident or myocardial infarction. It may cause bleeding from the surgical site or may threaten the integrity of a vascular bypass.

Venospasm

If caused by cold IV fluid infusion, venospasm may manifest as very slow flow. It may result from pressure infusion or extravasation. IV procaine relieves spasm. Thrombophlebitis may follow venospasm.

Coronary Thrombosis

Coronary thrombosis can occur from severe hypoxia and lack of oxygen to coronary vessels. Sometimes its occurrence is the reason for a patient's never regaining consciousness after a surgical procedure.

Air Embolism

Air embolism may occur intraoperatively with the patient in a sitting position for a craniotomy or posterior cervical operation. Cerebral diploic veins are noncollapsible; venous sinuses in the skull remain open. Air entering a vein is carried rapidly to the right side of the heart and pulmonary circulation, obstructing ventricular flow. Cardiac dysrhythmias and unexplained hypotension are prime signs and symptoms. A characteristic heart murmur may be audible with a precordial stethoscope or Doppler device. Air embolism also may occur during cardiopulmonary bypass, thyroidectomy, or laparoscopy.

Preoperative placement of a central venous catheter allows immediate aspiration of air. To relieve ventricular obstruction if no catheter is in place, the patient is placed in a steep head-down position with the right side up. A catheter is placed in the right atrium to remove the air. If cardiac arrest occurs, cardiopulmonary resuscitation (CPR) is begun. Closed heart massage may move an embolus obstructing the coronary artery.

Venous Stasis

Venous return of blood from the lower extremities can be slowed by the effects of general or spinal anesthesia and by the position of the legs during prolonged surgical procedures. The venous stasis that develops in most patients during a surgical procedure can be effectively counteracted.

To prevent thrombophlebitis and thrombosis in patients with thromboembolic disease, anticoagulants may be administered. Antiembolic stockings, with or without a sequential pneumatic compression device, augment venous flow from the legs. Elevation of the legs as little as 15% above horizontal can assist in venous return.

Postoperatively the patient may be placed in Trendelenburg's position with the legs elevated. Flexion and extension of the legs and feet, frequent turning, and early ambulation, unless contraindicated, aid circulation.

Deep Vein Thrombosis

Venous stasis, changes in clotting factors in the blood, and damage to vessel walls are the primary causes of deep vein thrombosis (DVT) in the lower extremities. Age, obesity, immobility, and a history of thromboembolic or other cardiovascular disease are predisposing factors. The type, location, and extent of the surgical procedure can contribute also. Preoperative prophylactic interventions, including anticoagulants, sequential compression devices, or antiembolic stockings, can reduce the risk of postoperative pulmonary embolism, which is a life-threatening complication of DVT.

Disseminated Intravascular Coagulation

Although it occurs rarely, disseminated intravascular coagulation (DIC) is a life-threatening syndrome. It is a complex derangement of clotting factors. The hemostatic process involves vasoconstriction with platelet aggregation and clotting. In DIC the normal clotting mechanisms do not function. Instead, a repetitive, overactive cycle of clot formation and simultaneous clot breakdown (fibrinolysis) occurs. This leads to consumption of platelets and coagulation factors and release of fibrin degradation products that act as potent anticoagulants.

DIC can follow hemorrhage, thrombi, emboli, infection, or allergic reaction to an incompatible blood transfusion. It may be precipitated by septic shock, abruptio placentae during pregnancy, or massive soft tissue damage of extensive trauma or burns. As blood becomes depleted of platelets and major clotting factors, coagulation is initiated throughout the bloodstream, especially in microcirculation. Prolonged bleeding may be noted; hematomas and cutaneous petechiae may appear. Massive hemorrhage and ischemia of vital organs may ensue. Bleeding may be noted from various sites, such as through the nasogastric tube.

The patient may have hypotension and oliguria. Postoperatively the patient may have nausea and vomiting, severe muscular pain, and convulsions and may lapse into a coma. Diagnosis is based on laboratory blood studies. Treatment begins with control of the primary condition. Blood, plasma, and dextran can be administered IV. Heparin and clotting factors, if given early, may prevent hemorrhage.

Cardiac Dysrhythmias

An alteration of normal cardiac rhythm may decrease cardiac output, exhaust the myocardium, and lead to ventricular fibrillation or cardiac arrest. Bradycardia is the slowing of the heart or pulse rate. Tachycardia is an excessive rapidity of the heart's action. Ventricular tachycardia and ventricular fibrillation are the dysrhythmias of most serious consequence and thus most feared.

Etiology. Etiologic factors include hypoxia; hypercapnia; acidosis; electrolyte imbalance; coronary disease; myocardial infarction; vagal reflexes; anesthetic agents; toxic doses of digitalis, epinephrine, or other drugs; and laryngospasm and coughing initiated by the presence of secretions in the airway after induction. Other causes may be hypotension, hemorrhage, hypovolemia, pneumothorax, and mechanical injuries.

Ventricular Dysrhythmias. An impulse originating in the ventricles must travel to the rest of the myocardium from one ventricle, then proceeding to the other. Because the impulse does not travel via the rapid, specialized conduction system, depolarization of both ventricles takes longer and is not simultaneous. The complexes of dysrhythmias have an abnormal appearance on an electrocardiogram (ECG) as compared with normally initiated and conducted impulses.

Premature Ventricular Contraction. An ectopic focus in the ventricles stimulates the heart to contract or beat prematurely before the regularly scheduled sinoatrial impulse arrives (Fig. 31-1). Primary precipitating factors are electrolyte or acid-base imbalance, myocardial infarction, digitalis toxicity, and caffeine. The premature ventricular contraction (PVC) must be distinguished from a premature atrial contraction (PAC). Isolated PVCs may not require treatment, but those occurring in clusters of two or more or more than five or six per minute require therapy. The aim is to quiet the irritable myocardium and restore adequate cardiac output.

Treatment consists of a lidocaine bolus followed by a continuous drip by infusion, correction of the cause (e.g., hypoxia), and other antidysrhythmic drugs if indicated (e.g., procainamide, quinidine). Temporary pacing may be used for severe bradycardia. Paired PVCs pose an increased danger of ventricular tachycardia.

Ventricular Tachycardia. A rapid heart rate (100 to 220 beats per minute) may be caused by ventricular ischemia or irritability, anoxia, or digitalis intoxication. The heart rate does not allow time for ventricular filling (Fig. 31-2). The resultant reduced cardiac output predisposes the patient to ventricular fibrillation or cardiac failure. Ventricular tachycardia is treated by prompt IV administration of lidocaine or procainamide, or intramuscular quinidine.

Synchronized cardioversion of 10 to 200 joules may be used if the blood pressure is palpable. This is the application of a high-intensity, short-duration electric shock to the chest wall over the heart to produce total cardiac depolarization. This countershock is timed to interrupt an abnormal rhythm in the cardiac cycle, thereby permitting resumption of a normal one. Cardioversion is usually applied in instances of nonarrest for a dangerous ventricular tachycardia. It may be an elective or emergency treatment. Asynchronous cardioversion is used if the patient is pulseless. Treatment includes correction of the underlying cause.

Ventricular Flutter. Often called fine ventricular fibrillation, the flutter appears as a transient state between ventricular tachycardia and ventricular fibrillation. The patient will show signs of poor cardiac output.

Ventricular Fibrillation. The most serious of all dysrhythmias, fibrillation is characterized by total disorganization of ventricular activity (Fig. 31-3). There are rapid and irregular, uncoordinated, random contractions of small myocardial groups without effective ventricular contraction or cardiac output. Circulation ceases. The patient in fibrillation is unconscious and possibly convulsing from cerebral hypoxia.

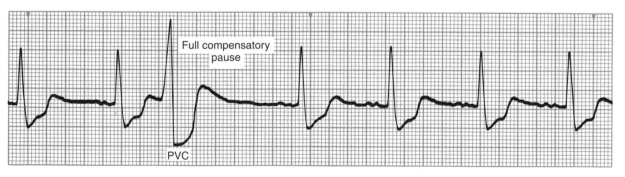

FIG. 31-1   Premature ventricular contractions.

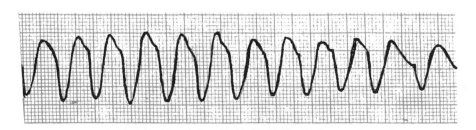

FIG. 31-2   Ventricular tachycardia.

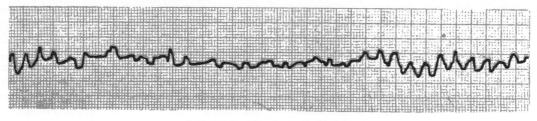

FIG. 31-3 Ventricular fibrillation.

Treatment. Because respiratory and cardiac arrest quickly follow, ventricular fibrillation is rapidly fatal unless successful defibrillation is effected as follows:

1. *Precordial thump:* In a monitored patient a fast, sharp, single blow to the midportion of the sternum (using the nipple line as a landmark) may be delivered with the bottom fleshy part of a closed fist struck from 8 to 12 inches (20 to 30 cm) above the chest. The blow generates a small electrical stimulus in a heart that is reactive. It may be effective in restoring a beat in cases of asystole or recent onset of dysrhythmia.
2. *Asynchronous cardioversion:* Prompt defibrillation by short-duration electric shock to the heart produces simultaneous depolarization of all muscle fiber bundles, after which spontaneous beating (conversion to spontaneous normal sinus rhythm) may resume if the myocardium is oxygenated and not acidotic. Defibrillation of an anoxic myocardium is difficult. The time that fibrillation is started should be noted. The electric shock is coordinated with controlled ventilation and cardiac compression. CPR begins as soon as fibrillation is identified. Many variables may affect defibrillation, such as body weight, paddle position, electrical waveform, and resistance to electric current flow. Procedures follow an established protocol.
3. *Adjunct drug therapy:* Drugs are given as necessary: vasopressor, cardiotonic, and myocardial stimulant drugs to maintain a useful heartbeat; vasodilator or antidysrhythmic drugs to prevent recurrence; and sodium bicarbonate to combat acidosis. Continuous monitoring of the heart and laboratory analysis of arterial blood gases is essential.

Defibrillation: Equipment and Technique. Necessary equipment for defibrillation includes a defibrillator machine and two paddle electrodes. Defibrillators use direct electric current. Most have integrated monitors; monitor and defibrillator switches may be separate or combined. An operational monitor does not always indicate that the fibrillation power is on. Many monitor-defibrillator units can monitor the ECG from the paddle electrodes, as well as from separate patient leads. These paddles and patient leads cannot operate simultaneously, however. Depending on the type of defibrillator, the electrical cord must be plugged in or batteries charged. All defibrillators should be checked regularly with suitable test equipment. Paddles must be cleaned immediately and prepared for reuse. This is emergency equipment and must be available at all times.

External Defibrillation. External defibrillation of the heart is used unless the chest is already open, as for intrathoracic surgery. Standard electrode paste or jelly or saline-soaked 4 × 4–inch gauze pads reduce the resistance of the skin to passage of the electric current. If paste is used on paddles, it should not extend beyond the electrodes or onto any part of the handles. Gel pads between the paddles and the patient's skin provide the advantage that if external cardiac compression is resumed after defibrillation, hands will not slip on the chest. The large diameter of the paddles increases the area of skin contact, thus reducing the possibility of skin burns by spreading of the current. The paddles must be held flat against the skin and more than 2 inches (5 cm) apart to prevent electrical arcing. They must be kept scrupulously clean because foreign material reduces the uniformity of the shock. The electrodes must be pressed firmly against the chest wall for good contact. One of two external paddle positions may be used:

1. *Standard position:* One electrode is placed just to the right of the upper sternum below the clavicle. The other is positioned to the left of the cardiac apex (i.e., left of the nipple at the fifth intercostal space along the left midaxillary line). The delivered current flows through the long axis of the heart.
2. *Anterior-posterior position:* One electrode is placed anteriorly over the precordium between the left nipple and the sternum. The other is positioned posteriorly behind the heart immediately below the left scapula, avoiding the spinal column. This allows for more energy passage through the heart, but placement is more difficult.

Internal Defibrillation. For internal defibrillation, sterile electrodes are placed on the myocardium—one over the right atrium, the other over the left ventricle. If these electrodes are gauze covered, they are dipped in sterile saline solution before use. Minimal current is needed when paddles are placed directly on the heart.

Perioperative team members must understand the functioning of the defibrillator for the patient's safety and their own. The person holding the electrode paddles delivers the electric charge by pressing a switch on the handle or a foot switch. The safest method is to activate both paddles simultaneously for discharge of electrical energy. The operator should have dry hands and stand on a dry floor. To avoid possible self-electrocution when using a defibrillator, neither the person holding the electrodes nor anyone else should touch the metal frame of the operating bed or the patient while the current is being applied. No part of the operator's body should touch the paste or the uninsulated electrodes. Loud verbal warning is given before discharge. Countershock is repeated at intervals if fibrillation persists. Transthoracic impedance falls with repetitive, closely spaced electrical discharges. After each countershock, the ECG and pulse should be reassessed.

Myocardial damage resulting from defibrillation efforts are in direct proportion to the energy used; therefore maximal settings, when not required, may increasingly impair an already damaged myocardium. The energy level delivered through a specific ohm load should be indicated on the front panel of the defibrillator. Delivery output ranges vary among machines. The strength of the countershock is expressed in energy as joules or watt-seconds—the product of power and duration. If the patient's chest muscles do not contract, no current has reached the patient. The defibrillator's connection to the electrical source and the "off" button to the synchronizer circuit should be checked. If the machine is battery operated, the battery must be charged enough to energize the capacitor. Personnel must be familiar with and follow operating instructions for the defibrillator in use.

Prevention. Appropriate preoperative sedation and skillfully administered anesthetic help prevent hazardous cardiovascular reflexes. Because PVCs are precursors to ventricular fibrillation, in itself a precursor to cardiac arrest, any cardiopulmonary emergency in a prearrest phase requires the following:

1. *Monitoring of the heart rhythm and rate:* The ability to recognize the rhythms that precede arrest permits intervention that may prevent arrest. If the cardiac status is not under constant monitoring, hypoxia and acidosis may be present and require correction before other therapeutic modalities can be used effectively.

2. *Establishment of an IV lifeline:* Venous cannulation provides access to peripheral and central venous circulation for administering drugs and fluids, obtaining venous blood specimens for laboratory analysis, and inserting catheters into the right side of the heart and pulmonary arteries for physiologic monitoring and electrical pacing. If cardiac arrest appears imminent or has occurred, cannulation of a peripheral or femoral vein should be attempted first so as not to interrupt CPR. To keep the infusion open, the rate should be kept slow. The usual complications to all IV techniques should be guarded against.

Cardiac Arrest

In cardiac arrest there is cessation of circulatory action; the pumping mechanism of the heart ceases. Cardiac standstill represents total absence of electrical cardiac activity (asystole), reflected as a straight line on an ECG rhythm strip. It may occur as primary cardiac failure or secondary to failure of pulmonary ventilation. The types of circulatory arrest are profound cardiovascular collapse, electromechanical dissociation, ventricular fibrillation, and ventricular asystole or standstill. Cardiac arrest may precede or follow failure of the respiratory system, because the systems are interrelated.

Incidence. Arrest may occur during induction of anesthesia, intraoperatively, or postoperatively. Occurrence during cardiac surgery or after massive hemorrhage is not uncommon. Patients more prone to arrest include those at age extremes and those with previously diagnosed paroxysmal dysrhythmias, primary cardiovascular abnormalities, myocarditis, heart block, or digitalis toxicity. An unexpected arrest is one that happens in a patient of general good health who is undergoing a low-risk or relatively routine procedure. These arrests are associated with major morbidity and mortality.

Etiology. A single factor or combination of factors may precipitate arrest, but the general cause is inadequate coronary arterial blood flow. Defective respiratory function produces systemic hypoxemia, causing myocardial hypoxia and depression. It also increases myocardial irritability and the heart's susceptibility to vagal reflexes. Some of the specific precipitating factors are dysrhythmias, emboli, extreme hypotension or hypovolemia, respiratory obstruction, aspiration, effects of drugs, anesthetic overdosage, excessively rapid or unsmooth induction, sepsis, pharyngeal stimulation, metabolic abnormalities (acidosis, toxemia, electrolyte imbalance), poor cardiac filling caused by positioning, manipulation of the heart, central nervous system trauma, anaphylaxis, and electric shock from ungrounded or faulty electrical equipment.

Symptoms. Symptoms include loss of heartbeat and blood pressure; sudden fixed, dilated pupils; sudden pallor or cyanosis; cold, clammy skin; absence of reflexes; unconsciousness or convulsions in a previously conscious patient; respiratory standstill; and dark blood or absence of bleeding in the surgical field.

Diagnosis. The ECG monitor readily detects arrest during anesthesia, with absence of blood pressure and precordial heart sounds and the lack of a palpable carotid pulse. The onset of pupillary dilation is within 45 seconds after cerebral anoxia; full dilation is reached about 90 to 110 seconds after cessation of cerebral circulation.

Treatment. CPR is initiated immediately to restore oxygenation to vital organs. Defibrillation may be needed for ventricular fibrillation. IV drugs generally are used to improve cardiopulmonary status.

Prevention. Optimal psychologic preoperative assessment to identify the level of anxiety and testing for abnormalities and sensitivities are important preoperative preparations. Intraoperative precautions include the following:

- ECG and temperature monitoring
- No stimulation during induction
- Maintenance of an adequate airway
- Oxygen and carbon dioxide monitoring
- Arterial blood pressure monitoring
- Medications
- Appropriate positioning and slow position changes with the patient under anesthesia; no weight on the patient
- Gentle handling of tissues with minimal traction and manipulation
- Skillful anesthetic administration

INTRAVENOUS CARDIOVASCULAR DRUGS

An important factor in optimal anesthesia management is prompt recognition of the causes of hypotension, shock, and other complications that could lead to cardiac arrest. Prompt correction of reversible precipitants is critical. Many IV drugs are used to correct hypoxia and metabolic acidosis, manipulate cardiovascular variables, or treat pulmonary edema.

Pharmacodynamics

Uptake, movement, binding, and interactions of drugs vary at the tissue site of their biochemical and physiologic actions. Drug action is determined by how the drug interacts in the body. Some drugs alter body fluids; others, such as anesthetics, interact with cell membranes; most act through receptor mechanisms.

Receptor Mechanisms. Most drugs mimic naturally occurring compounds and interact with specific biologic molecules to produce biologic responses. For example, some cardiovascular drugs are sympathomimetics. They evoke physiologic responses similar to those produced by the sympathetic nervous system. A receptor is a structural protein molecule on a cell surface or within cytoplasm that binds with a drug to produce a biologic response. Three types of receptors are noteworthy in understanding the drugs used to counteract complications that may occur during anesthesia.

Adrenergic Receptors. Adrenergic receptors are innervated by sympathetic nerve fibers and activated by epinephrine or norepinephrine secreted at the postganglionic nerve endings. These receptors are classified as alpha or beta, depending on their sensitivity to specific adrenergic activating and blocking drugs. Alpha$_1$ and alpha$_2$ receptors are located primarily in peripheral and renal arteriolar muscles; beta$_1$ receptors predominate in the heart; beta$_2$ receptors are primarily in smooth muscle of the lungs and blood vessels.

Cholinergic Receptors. Cholinergic receptors are sites where acetylcholine exerts action to transmit nerve impulses through the parasympathetic nervous system to regulate the heart rate and respirations.

Opiate Receptors. Opiate receptors are regions in the brain capable of binding morphine in areas related to pain.

Drug Interactions. No drug has a single action. Each modifies existing functions within the body by interactions to stimulate or inhibit responses. The desired action may be accompanied by side effects or an exaggerated response. An allergic reaction may occur immediately after exposure or may be delayed.

Anaphylaxis is a life-threatening, acute allergic reaction in which cells release histamine or a histamine-like substance. Anaphylaxis, a form of vasogenic shock, causes vasodilation, hypotension, and bronchial constriction. Within seconds, the patient will exhibit edema, wheezing, cyanosis, and dyspnea. Treatment includes epinephrine and antihistamines to control brochospasm. Isoproterenol, vasopressors, corticosteroids, and aminophylline also may be administered.

In combination with local, regional, or general anesthetics, drugs must be carefully administered and monitored. The action of one drug may counteract the action of another drug. Patients who do not respond to one drug (e.g., a catecholamine) may respond to another. Physicians do not always agree on the use of potent drugs. For example, a vasoconstrictor used to treat hypotension may possibly cause ischemic damage to organs. The physician's orders should be followed for all drugs.

Intravenous Administration. The speed of administration and dosage will depend on the drug and its intended action. Dosages given in this text vary according to individual patient circumstances. The technique of IV administration also varies.

Continuous Intravenous Drip. The drug is diluted in a volume of dextrose or normal saline solution. The rate of administration is regulated by adjusting the number of drops per minute from the solution container into the IV tubing. A drug that might be absorbed by plastic should not be added to solution in a plastic infusion bag.

Bolus. A bolus is a single rapid injection of the full dosage of a drug that cannot be diluted. It is usually given through an existing IV line, and it may be injected directly into a vein or an intrathecal catheter. Some drugs can be given via an endotracheal tube for absorption through the alveoli or mucous membranes. The drug quickly reaches peak level in the bloodstream.

Intravenous Push. A drug may be injected slowly into an IV line or through an intermittent infusion pump over a period of minutes. The total dose may be diluted and given in repeated doses over a period of hours. An infusion pump may be used to control the rate of delivery precisely.

Titration. Dosage is calculated on the basis of body surface area (BSA) and hemodynamic parameters. Cardiac output is evaluated in terms of BSA. This may be determined by the ratio of the patient's height and weight on the BSA scale or by thermodilution. The patient's physiologic responses also will determine total dosage.

Considerations for Drug Administration. Some drugs are inactivated by others. The IV tubing should be flushed or changed to avoid precipitation, such as can occur with sodium bicarbonate. Many potent drugs should be infused through an IV catheter, which is safer than a needle to prevent extravasation. If a drug extravasates at the site of injection, the area must be promptly infiltrated with phentolamine (Regitine) to prevent the necrosis that can result from some vasoactive drugs.

Drugs by Classification

Pharmacokinetics includes the mechanisms of absorption, distribution, and metabolism of drugs in the body and elimination from the body. Nurses must have knowledge of drug actions and of how to prepare and administer drugs. The following drugs are classified by their pharmacodynamics to counteract adverse cardiovascular and pulmonary status.

Sympathomimetics are used most often for the following purposes:

- To increase force (inotropic effect), maintain contractility (noninotropic effect), or decrease the stroke volume of myocardial contractions
- To increase the pulse rate
- To increase or decrease arterial blood pressure

- To correct dysrhythmias
- To increase renal blood flow
- To stimulate the central nervous system
- To treat bronchospasm
- To prolong the effect of local anesthetics
- To manage life-threatening emergencies

Patients receiving any of the following drugs must be carefully monitored.

Antidysrhythmics.
Antidysrhythmics control the heart rate and rhythm. They may induce a decreased rate and cardiac output. They may reduce cardiac conduction and increase dilation of peripheral vessels.

Lidocaine (Xylocaine). Lidocaine increases the threshold for ventricular irritability by exerting a focal anesthetic effect on the myocardial cell membrane. It is used for ventricular tachycardia and fibrillation, especially if resistance to defibrillation effort occurs. It can be given IV, intrathecally, or by endotracheal tube. DOSAGE: 1 mg/kg or 75 to 100 mg by IV push over 30 to 60 seconds, followed by half the initial dose every 8 to 10 minutes to a total of 3 mg/kg if ectopic heartbeats continue. After conversion, a maintenance dose of 2 to 4 mg/min can be given by IV drip. Half these dosages are used to treat shock or pulmonary edema.

Bretylium (Bretylol). Bretylium lowers the defibrillation threshold, permitting otherwise refractory rhythms to be electrically converted. It is indicated for ventricular tachycardia and fibrillation unresponsive to other therapy. DOSAGE: 5 mg/kg by rapid IV bolus, followed by defibrillation. If fibrillation continues, the dose can be doubled and repeated as necessary. For ventricular fibrillation, 300 to 600 mg may be required. The drug may be diluted for continuous IV drip at a dosage of 1 to 2 mg/min for ventricular tachycardia and to prevent fibrillation. Some degree of hypotension may occur.

Procainamide (Pronestyl). Procainamide suppresses PVCs and recurrent tachycardia. This drug may be used if lidocaine is contraindicated or has not controlled ventricular tachycardia. DOSAGE: 100 mg by IV push every 5 minutes until dysrhythmia ceases, or to a total of 1 g. Maintenance IV drip is 1 to 4 mg/min. Marked hypotension may occur if infusion is too rapid.

Adenosine (Adenocard). Adenosine slows atrioventricular (AV) node conduction. This action converts supraventricular tachycardia to normal sinus rhythm. DOSAGE: 6 to 12 mg by IV bolus followed immediately by a saline bolus. Incremental doses of 0.05 mg/kg can be given as necessary. This drug is contraindicated for patients with asthma.

Verapamil (Isoptin, Calan). A calcium channel blocker, verapamil inhibits calcium ions to slow myocardial contractility, the heart rate, and the demand for oxygen. It is used as an antidysrhythmic to treat paroxysmal supraventricular tachycardia, acute atrial flutter, and atrial fibrillation. DOSAGE: 5 to 10 mg (0.075 to 0.15 mg/kg adult body weight) by slow IV push over 2 minutes; may be repeated after 30 minutes. This drug is not given to patients with severe hypotension or cardiogenic shock, nor is it given concurrently with an IV beta-adrenergic blocker, such as propranolol.

Propranolol (Inderal). A beta-adrenergic receptor blocking agent, propranolol is used to control supraventricular dysrhythmias and to treat hypertension. It reduces myocar-dial oxygen consumption by blocking catecholamine-induced increases in the heart rate, blood pressure, and cardiac contractions. It may be used if control of ventricular fibrillation is not achieved with lidocaine or other drugs. DOSAGE: 1 to 3 mg by IV push, not to exceed 1 mg/min, titrated for heart rate and rhythm. This drug is contraindicated for patients with asthma, bronchospasm, or cardiac depression.

Isoproterenol (Isuprel). A beta-adrenergic receptor stimulant, isoproterenol stimulates the sympathetic tone, rate, and strength of myocardial contractions and cardiac output. It increases the myocardial demand for oxygen. It may be used for ventricular dysrhythmias, but it may produce tachycardia or dysrhythmia. It is indicated to control hemodynamically significant bradycardia in a patient who has a pulse but who is unresponsive to atropine. It is a vasodilator and bronchodilator. DOSAGE: IV drip of 1 mg to 500 mL of dextrose or saline solution at the rate of 1.25 mL/min, titrated according to the heart rate and rhythm.

Antimuscarinics/Anticholinergics.
Antimuscarinics/anticholinergics block passage of impulses through the parasympathetic nerves to the heart and smooth muscles. When both the sympathetic and parasympathetic components of the autonomic nervous system are stimulated, the parasympathetic dominates to slow the heartbeat and respirations. An anticholinergic allows desired sympathetic action.

Atropine. Atropine reduces cardiac vagal tone, enhances AV conduction, and increases cardiac output. It accelerates the cardiac rate in sinus bradycardia with severe hypotension or in bradycardia associated with hypoxia and reduced cardiac output. It may restore cardiac rhythm in AV block or ventricular asystole. It is a primary drug used in cardiopulmonary arrest. Atropine may be given IV, intrathecally, or via an endotracheal tube. DOSAGE: 1 mg by IV bolus for asystole, 0.5 mg for bradycardia, at 5-minute intervals until the desired rate is achieved or to a total dose of 2 mg. Full vagal blockage could result from overdosage.

Vasodilators.
Vasodilators are noninotropic drugs that relax smooth muscle in the capillaries and cause peripheral dilation. They dilate arteries and veins almost equally without increasing myocardial contractility. This reduces venous return to heart. They are used to alter blood flow and lower blood pressure in patients who have severely reduced cardiac output or who are in hypertensive crisis.

Sodium Nitroprusside (Nipride, Nitropress). Sodium nitroprusside acts rapidly as a direct peripheral vasodilator to increase cardiac output and redistribute cardiac work in patients with pump failure. It increases tissue perfusion without reflex tachycardia. DOSAGE: IV drip, not to exceed 10 mcg/kg/min, of 50 mg dissolved in 2 to 3 mL of dextrose added to 250 to 1000 mL of 5% dextrose in water for infusion. An infusion pump or microdrip-regulating system ensures a precise flow rate. The solution deteriorates in light, so it must be protected by opaque material such as aluminum foil. No other drug should be injected into the IV line while sodium nitroprusside is infusing.

Nitroglycerin (Nitrostat IV, Nitrol IV, Tridil). Nitroglycerin decreases venous return to the heart and reduces preload and afterload, thus lowering myocardial oxygen demands. It is used for control of blood pressure in hypertension associated with cardiovascular procedures or endotracheal intubation, or in the immediate postoperative period. DOSAGE: Up to 50 mcg/min by IV push. The drug should be titrated to increase the dose, and the time intervals between infusions should be adjusted, depending on lowering of the blood pressure. This potent drug must be diluted in dextrose or saline solution. It is absorbed by polyvinyl chloride (PVC) plastic, so glass solution bottles and tubing that is not made of PVC should be used. The drug is also light sensitive.

Trimethaphan (Arfonad). A ganglionic blocking agent, trimethaphan is used to produce controlled hypotension during surgical procedures and to lower blood pressure in patients with hypertension or in patients with an acute hypertensive crisis. DOSAGE: 500 mg diluted in 500 mL of 5% dextrose in water (1 mg/ mL) IV drip. Initially the drug is infused slowly at the rate of 1 to 2 mg/min and increased gradually to an average dose range of 3 to 6 mg/min.

Cardiotonics. Cardiotonics combine inotropic effect on the contractility of muscle with vasodilation of blood vessels. They stimulate myocardial function. Vasodilation reduces cardiac afterload, thereby improving cardiac performance and correcting peripheral vascular compensations.

Inamrinone (Inocor). Inamrinone possesses significant vasodilator activity to improve tissue perfusion, especially to the kidneys, and to improve cardiac output. It is used for short-term effect in patients with ischemic heart disease and severe heart failure. The blood pressure and heart rate remain unchanged, whereas peripheral arteriolar resistance falls. DOSAGE: 0.5 to 3.5 mg/kg by IV bolus followed by IV drip of 5 to 10 g/kg/min. Titrated to hemodynamic response, a second bolus can be given after 30 minutes.

Dobutamine (Dobutrex). A synthetic derivative of dopamine, dobutamine increases myocardial contractility while producing little systemic arterial constriction. It is used for short-term treatment of refractory heart failure, cardiogenic shock, and hemodynamically significant hypotension. DOSAGE: 2.5 to 10 mcg/kg/min IV drip. Tachycardia or dysrhythmia may result from a larger dose. It is incompatible with alkaline solutions and drugs such as sodium bicarbonate.

Catecholamines. Catecholamines are vasoconstrictors that improve tissue perfusion by maintaining perfusion pressure, preventing or diminishing blood loss, decreasing tissue vascularity, and improving coronary blood flow. Among indications for their use are anesthetic overdose, hypotension associated with blood loss, and adrenergic insufficiency. They raise the blood pressure. They are antispasmodic.

Epinephrine (Adrenalin). An endogenous catecholamine and alpha-adrenergic receptor stimulant, epinephrine plays an essential role in restoration of spontaneous circulation in asystole; therefore it is the first drug administered in cardiac arrest. By increasing systemic vascular resistance, it improves coronary perfusion pressure and cardiac output produced by cardiac compression during CPR. It improves myocardial contractility and tone and causes

vasoconstriction of arteries. It may be given IV, intrathecally, via endotracheal tube, or by intracardiac injection. DOSAGE: 0.5 to 1 mg by IV bolus, repeated every 5 minutes as necessary. It is available in preloaded syringes of 1:10,000 dilution (1 mg/10 mL). It may be added to an IV infusion of 250 mL of 5% dextrose in water. It is inactivated by alkaline solutions. Continuous infusion may increase the heart rate, blood pressure, and cardiac output. Side effects include elevated myocardial oxygen demand and possible PVCs or ventricular fibrillation.

Norepinephrine (Levophed). An endogenous catecholamine, norepinephrine restores and maintains blood pressure. It may be given after peripheral vascular collapse as a result of severe hypotension or cardiogenic shock. It constricts renal and mesenteric vessels and may cause severe peripheral vasoconstriction. DOSAGE: 16 mg/L administered at the rate of 0.5 to 1 mcg/min and titrated up to 30 mcg/min IV drip in 5% dextrose in water, titrated to the desired blood pressure; average dose range is 2 to 4 mg/min. The drug is toxic if extravasation occurs. Hypotension from hypovolemia is a contraindication.

Diuretics. Diuretics increase the amount of urine excreted. Potent diuretics are used to treat pulmonary edema and postarrest cerebral edema. They inhibit resorption of sodium. They are used with caution because they may have a direct vasodilating effect or may lead to fluid and electrolyte depletion. The most commonly used diuretics are the following:

- Furosemide (Lasix), 0.5 to 2 mg/kg injected slowly over 1 to 2 minutes by IV push; the dose can be repeated in 2 hours
- Ethacrynate sodium (Sodium Edecrin), 40 to 50 mg or 0.5 to 1.0 mg/kg injected slowly by IV push

Vasopressors. Vasopressors exert an inotropic vasoconstriction action on arterioles and veins through stimulation of alpha-adrenergic receptors, and they increase the heart rate, blood pressure, and myocardial contractility by activation of beta-adrenergic receptors. These drugs cause vasomotor depression of the peripheral circulation but increase coronary flow. They may increase ventricular contractile force, alter sinoatrial nodal activity, constrict smooth muscles, and dilate renal and mesenteric blood vessels. They may produce ventricular dysrhythmia, which can be intensified by hypoxia or hypercapnia. Drug effectiveness is reduced in the presence of respiratory or metabolic acidosis.

Dopamine (Intropin). In high dosages (greater than 10 mcg/kg/min IV drip), dopamine causes peripheral vasoconstriction to increase cardiac output and blood pressure. It may be used during cardiogenic shock, severe hypotension, and asystole and then be titrated to the desired blood pressure. Discontinuance should be gradual. A low dose, 1 to 5 mcg/kg/min IV drip, dilates renal and mesenteric blood vessels to maintain urinary output but may not increase the heart rate or blood pressure. The drip rate may be increased until organ perfusion is evidenced by the blood pressure and urinary output. Tachydysrhythmias are an indication for reduction in dose or discontinuation. Dopamine is inactivated in alkaline solution and by sodium bicarbonate. It is caustic if it extravasates. It should be diluted immediately

Metaraminol (Aramine). Metaraminol produces marked vasoconstriction and increases cardiac output and blood pressure, which may be useful to treat severe hypotension. It may be given IV or via endotracheal tube. DOSAGE: 0.4 mg/min IV drip in 5% dextrose in water.

Other Vasopressors. These drugs have various actions. Selection will depend on the action needed. Drugs that may be used include the following:
- Isoproterenol (Isuprel)
- Methoxamine (Vasoxyl)
- Mephentermine (Wyamine)
- Norepinephrine (Levophed)
- Phenylephrine (Neo-Synephrine)

Other Drugs. The foregoing list is not intended to be all-inclusive. Other drugs are used for specific problems. Life-threatening acid-base or electrolyte imbalances associated with cardiovascular or pulmonary complications may need to be corrected (e.g., after CPR). The following two drugs may be used with caution; they are not recommended for routine administration at the onset of CPR.

Calcium Salts. Calcium should be avoided unless the patient has hyperkalemia, hypocalcemia, or calcium channel blocker toxicity. It may be administered by IV bolus as calcium chloride, 2 mL of 10% (1 g/10 mL) solution repeated as necessary at 10-minute intervals; calcium gluconate, 5 to 8 mL; or calcium glucaptate, 5 to 7 mL.

Sodium Bicarbonate. Metabolic acidosis secondary to accumulation of lactic acid produced by respiratory metabolism may need to be corrected. Bicarbonate binds with hydrogen ion from lactic acid to produce carbonic acid that breaks down into carbon dioxide and water. Sodium bicarbonate may be given after other resuscitation measures to reverse acidosis. DOSAGE: 1 mEq/kg by IV bolus initially, titrated according to blood gas analyses for subsequent doses, usually no more than 0.5 mEq/kg at 10- to 15-minute intervals. An excessive dose can produce metabolic alkalosis. Sodium bicarbonate should not be mixed in an IV line with any other drug; it will precipitate calcium salts and inactivate catecholamines.

CARDIOPULMONARY RESUSCITATION

CPR is aimed at rapidly restoring oxygen delivery to vital organs to reverse the processes that lead to death. CPR is an emergency procedure requiring special training to recognize cardiac or respiratory arrest and to perform artificial ventilation and circulation. To prevent irreversible brain damage, resuscitative measures must be instituted immediately, within 3 to 5 minutes after the arrest. The combination of anoxia and acidosis can make restoration of normal function impossible.

Resuscitation is not a one-person job. The team must be completely familiar with the preplanned routine before the necessity for its use arises. Success depends on prompt diagnosis and immediate effective treatment. Outcome is directly related to the rapidity with which a functional, spontaneous heart rhythm can be restored. Patients who experience arrest in an OR may be on monitors with an IV line already in place and resuscitation equipment on hand. These arrests are referred to as witnessed arrests. The time of onset of arrest should be noted and the time-elapsed clock started. Basic life support is instituted at once to reestablish oxygenation and restore the heartbeat.

Basic Life Support

Basic life support (BLS) is that particular phase of emergency cardiac care that either prevents circulatory or respiratory arrest or insufficiency through prompt recognition and intervention or externally supports circulation and respiration of a victim of cardiac or respiratory arrest through CPR. BLS can and should be initiated by any person present when cardiac arrest occurs.

The ABCs of resuscitation are as follows:
- Airway: patent and free of secretions or foreign body for effective pulmonary ventilation
- Breathing: prompt restoration and maintenance of oxygenation through artificial ventilation
- Circulation: provision of oxygen to vital tissues by means of cardiac compression (artificial circulation)

These steps should be started immediately and performed in the order given except when the patient is already intubated. Advanced cardiac life support should be instituted without delay to restore circulation. Resuscitation continues until the patient can resume normal, spontaneous respiration and circulation or until its discontinuation is warranted by diagnosis of brain death.

When the arrested patient is in the OR, anesthesia providers and other team members are present. In a witnessed arrest, the carotid pulse is palpated. The carotid artery is located in the groove between the trachea and muscles of the side of the neck. Palpation of the femoral artery is an acceptable option. If the patient has respiratory arrest, two quick, full lung inflations are given without allowing for full lung deflation between breaths. Maintenance of positive pressure in the lungs more effectively fills, ventilates, and prevents collapse of alveoli. If pulse and breathing are not immediately restored, CPR is begun.

If ventricular fibrillation or tachycardia without a pulse is evident, countershock is delivered as soon as possible (DC 200 to 300 joules delivered energy in an adult; 2 joules/kg or 1 joule/lb in an infant or child). If this is unsuccessful, additional countershocks and medications are given as ordered or per written protocol. In open heart defibrillation, between 5 and 40 joules is delivered, beginning with lower energy levels.

In infants and small children, a hand is placed over the precordium to feel the apical beat or the brachial pulse is checked in lieu of a carotid pulse. The brachial pulse is on the inside of the upper arm midway between the elbow and the shoulder. The index and middle fingers are used. A precordial thump is not given to an infant or child. In infants and children, bradydysrhythmias and heart block lead to cardiac arrest more commonly than does ventricular fibrillation.

Ventilation. Immediate opening of the airway is mandatory to combat respiratory failure. If respiratory obstruction is present, it must be cleared. During general anesthesia either an oropharyngeal or nasopharyngeal airway or endotracheal tube may be in place to maintain a patent air passage. Oxygen (100%) can be delivered at once under positive pressure by manual ventilation. Otherwise, ventilation by other means, such as an esophageal obturator airway or expired-air technique, should be initiated to sustain oxygenation, followed by tracheal intubation as soon as possible.

A cuffed endotracheal tube permits continuous delivery of high oxygen concentration without the hazard of stomach distention or aspiration. It facilitates adequate ventilation because with its use interposed breaths are not necessary, thereby permitting a faster, uninterrupted cardiac compression rate of 80 beats per minute. When a tube or airway is lacking, the most rapid means of reestablishing oxygenation is by an expired-air technique or mouth-to-mouth or mouth-to-nose artificial ventilation. When artificial ventilation is combined with cardiac compression, tissues receive oxygen. In the OR the anesthesia provider manages artificial ventilation. The following principles apply to artificial respiration:

1. If attempts to ventilate the patient are unsuccessful despite proper opening of the airway, further attempts to remove the obstruction should be made. Laryngoscopy, cricothyrotomy, or tracheotomy may be indicated.
2. Tracheal suctioning should last no longer than 5 seconds at a time without ventilation, to prevent hypoxia.
3. If spinal injury is suspected or present, extension of the neck is avoided and a modified jaw-thrust technique is employed. The head, neck, and chest are kept aligned.
4. Ventilation is assessed by seeing the chest rise and fall and hearing and feeling air escape during the patient's exhalation.

Circulation. Cardiac compression must accompany ventilation in a pulseless patient to maintain adequate blood pressure and circulation, thereby keeping tissues viable, preserving cardiac tone and reflexes, and preventing intravascular clotting. This may be accomplished by external closed-chest cardiac compression—the rhythmic application of pressure over the lower half of the sternum above the xiphoid process (Figs. 31-4 and 31-5). Because the heart occupies most of the space between the sternum and the thoracic spine, intermittent sternal compression 1½ to 2 inches raises intrathoracic pressure and produces cardiac output (Fig. 31-6). Blood is forced from the heart into the pulmonary artery and aorta. During relaxation of pressure, negative intrathoracic pressure causes venous blood to flow back into the heart from the pulmonary and systemic circulatory

systems (Fig. 31-7). Blood moves in the arterial direction through the heart valves. Carotid artery blood flow from this technique usually is only one quarter to one third of normal (mean blood pressure 40 mm Hg), although systolic blood pressure is raised. It may peak at 100 mm Hg, but diastolic pressure is low.

Artificial ventilation is always required when external cardiac compression is employed because oxygenation of the circulating blood is inadequate. The brain and myocardium must be perfused effectively for survival. External cardiac compression must be instituted immediately on cessation of circulation. Any interruption in compression causes cessation of blood flow and a drop in blood pressure.

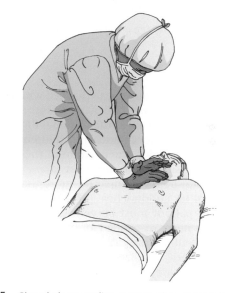

FIG. 31-5 Closed-chest cardiac compression. Patient is supine on hard, flat surface. Resuscitator places heel of one hand over lower half of sternum with heel of other hand on top. Fingers are arched upward to avoid exerting force on ribs. Elbows are straight and locked, with shoulders straight over hands.

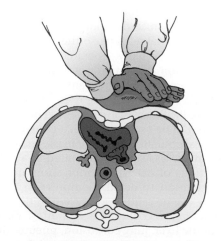

FIG. 31-6 Manual depression of sternum raises intrathoracic pressure and produces cardiac output. Blood is sent from heart into pulmonary artery and aorta.

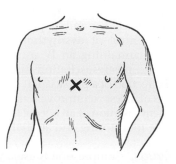

FIG. 31-4 Cross indicates correct spot to place hands for performing closed-chest cardiac compression: over lower half of sternum and above xiphoid process.

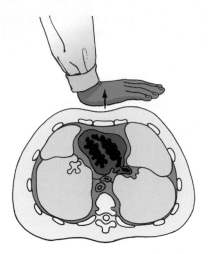

FIG. 31-7   Releasing pressure on sternum allows heart to fill with venous blood.

Cardiac compression must be performed with knowledge and care. All physicians and patient care personnel must be trained and certified in CPR at the minimal BLS level. Basic principles are the same for infants and children. Differences in technique are related to the position of the heart in the chest, small chest size, and faster heart rate.

BLS should not be interrupted for more than 5 seconds at a time except for endotracheal intubation. If intubation is difficult, the patient must be ventilated between short attempts. CPR is never suspended for more than 30 seconds, such as during defibrillation. Preferably, the patient should not be moved until stabilized and ready for transport or until arrangements are made for uninterrupted CPR during movement.

Elevation of the legs to a 60-degree angle with the trunk aids venous return and augments artificial circulation. Cardiac compression is successful only if the heart fills with blood between compressions and the resuscitator can move an adequate volume of oxygenated blood. The carotid or femoral pulse is checked every few minutes to indicate compression effectiveness or return of a spontaneous, effective heartbeat.

Manual external cardiac compression causes fatigue, leading to variation in cardiac output; therefore, it is advisable to have additional relief personnel available. Commercially available, manually operated mechanical chest compressors or automatic compressor-ventilators that provide simultaneous compression and ventilation eliminate this problem. When such devices are used, compression must always be started with the manual method first. Compressor-ventilators should be used only with a cuffed endotracheal tube, esophageal obturator airway, or mask, and only by experienced operators. Use should be limited to adult patients.

Complications of external compression are minimized by careful attention to detail. Compression must be performed with extreme caution to prevent injuries such as rib or sternal fracture, costochondral separation, fat embolism, laceration of the liver, lung contusion, pneumothorax, and hemothorax. To prevent fractures, the xiphoid process at the tip of the sternum is never compressed and pressure is never exerted on the ribs.

Internal Cardiac Compression.   Internal cardiac compression is instituted if the patient's chest is already open, such as during a cardiothoracic procedure. Thoracotomy may be performed and internal compression administered in instances where external compression may be ineffective (e.g., internal thoracic injuries, such as penetrating wounds of the heart; flail chest; pericardial tamponade caused by hemorrhage; chest or spinal deformities). The advantages of internal compression are (1) more complete ventricular emptying with greater outflow of blood into the circulation and (2) rapid diastolic filling for a faster stroke rate than with external compression. Less blood flows in a retrograde manner. The disadvantages are (1) delay in compression, (2) potential trauma to the lungs and myocardium, and (3) possible infection.

If the chest is not open, the incision is made through the left fifth or sixth intercostal space. The pericardial sac is opened for direct manual compression of the myocardium. A rib spreader is placed to avoid strangulation of the operator's hands. By cradling the heart in both hands, the operator compresses the ventricles between the thumb and fingers of one hand, or the fingers of both hands, 80 times per minute. Venous filling is necessary for adequate ventricular stroke volume.

Checking the Effectiveness of Cardiopulmonary Resuscitation.

Signs suggestive of effective compression are constricted, reactive pupils; a palpable peripheral pulse; an audible heartbeat; and improvement in color of the mucous membranes, skin, and blood. Additional signs indicative of potential recovery are prompt return of spontaneous respiration and consciousness. Continuous compression is stopped when arterial blood pressure remains above 70 to 90 mm Hg and a strong spontaneous pulse is resumed. CPR may be performed intermittently as necessary to assist the restored heart.

Persistent dilation of the pupils and lack of reaction to light are ominous signs usually indicative of brain damage. Cell destruction is also manifested by convulsions, hyperpyrexia, and persistent coma. Survival in relation to these symptoms is usually accompanied by tragic consequences such as decerebration or paralysis.

Advanced Cardiac Life Support

Advanced cardiac life support (ACLS) consists of definitive therapy intended to reinstitute spontaneous oxygenation. It includes BLS; use of adjunctive equipment and special techniques for establishing and maintaining effective ventilation and circulation; cardiac and supplemental monitoring; recognition and control of dysrhythmias; defibrillation; establishing and maintaining an IV infusion route; drug administration; and postresuscitation care. It requires the supervision and direction of a physician. It should be initiated within 8 minutes of arrest to improve long-term functional survival. Subsequent insertion of an arterial line supplies access for direct pressure monitoring and arterial blood gases.

Intravenous Drugs.

Compression is usually accompanied or followed by judicious use of drugs, administered IV, to manipulate cardiovascular variables, such as hypoxia and acidosis. These drugs may improve the patient's cardiopulmonary status by increasing the perfusion pressure during cardiac compression, stimulating spontaneous or more forceful myocardial contractions, accelerating the cardiac rate, and suppressing abnormal ventricular activity.

Oxygen, epinephrine, and atropine are the mainstays of pharmacologic management in CPR. Used in combination with basic life support, lidocaine, and defibrillation, they correct most CPR oxygen-delivery problems. Each additional drug serves as a vital adjunct in definitive therapy and postresuscitation care.

Crash Cart

An emergency arrest cart should be available at all times in all critical care areas (i.e., OR, emergency department [ED], PACU, and ICU). Specific drugs and equipment vary, depending on how well equipped the anesthesia provider is for emergencies. Equipment on a portable cart usually includes the following:

- Oxygen and resuscitation equipment, including oxygen cylinder, tubing, mask, Ambu bag, or bag-valve-mask
- Laryngoscope tray, blades, endotracheal equipment and tubes, assorted airways (oral and nasal), stylet, padded tongue blades
- Tracheotomy tray
- Sterile gloves, sterile gauze sponges, prep swabs or spray, adhesive tape, tourniquets, sutures, armboard, drapes
- Suction machine, catheters and suction tips
- IV infusion solutions and sets, IV needles and catheters (14 and 16 gauge), tubing stopcocks, infusion pump, additive labels
- Cutdown tray, venous cannulas, wire-guided catheters
- Assorted sterile syringes: 3, 5, 10, 20, and 50 mL
- Assorted sterile needles: 25 gauge × ⅝ inch; 20 gauge × 1½ inches; 18 gauge × 1½ inches; 20 gauge × 3 inches (intracardiac); spinal needles
- Arterial blood sampling kit with needles, heparinized syringes; arterial line tray
- Disposable scalpels, hemostats
- Emergency thoracotomy set, including scalpel with No. 20 blade, rib retractor, self-retaining retractor
- ECG monitor, leads, recording sheets
- Cardiac arrest board
- Defibrillator with paddles (adult, pediatric, external, internal), electrode jelly or paste, saline pads
- Cardiac arrest record for treatment documentation/flow sheets
- Cardiac pacemaker
- Drugs—mainly vasoconstrictors, cardiotonics, vasopressors, cardiac depressants, anticholinergics, cerebral dehydrating agents, pulmonary dehydrating agents (many frequently used emergency drugs are available in sterile, commercially prefilled syringes to avoid delay in preparation; they are routinely checked for expiration dates)
- CVP manometer
- Nasogastric tube and bulb syringe
- Flashlight and batteries for checking pupils

Personnel Responsibilities

During CPR, team members must remain calm but react quickly and act efficiently. Cardiac arrest in OR during business hours may be more easily managed because more personnel may be on the premises. Codes after business hours are more complex and may involve minimal personnel who are required to perform multiple functions. The following outline is a suggestion of expected behaviors of team members during a code situation:

1. *Director of the code:* One person, the most knowledgeable in resuscitation efforts and patient physiology, usually the anesthesia provider, commands resuscitation efforts. He or she is assisted by surgeons, nurses, surgical technologists, and other available personnel. A cardiologist is usually summoned (if available). Resuscitation teams are multidisciplinary.

   The person in charge directs lifesaving interventions that entail minute-to-minute decisions such as medications and defibrillation. To avoid confusion, the director of the code issues orders for others to follow. Every circulating nurse should be qualified and prepared to organize and assign tasks to members of the support staff in the event of cardiac arrest on the off-shifts.
2. *Circulating nurse:* Initiate the code and summon help.
   a. Start the time-elapsed clock (if available), and record the time of arrest.
      (1) Remain calm and support calmness in the team.
      (2) Documentation is performed according to facility policy. Most have preprinted code sheets.
   b. Activate the emergency alarm to alert the OR manager and summon assistance.
      (1) Several physicians and registered nurses should respond to form the code team.
      (2) Support staff should respond to become runners.
   c. Help reposition the patient as necessary into the supine position for CPR. Lower the operating bed and provide the resuscitator with a standing platform to facilitate cardiac compression. The circulating nurse must be able to perform chest compressions if an additional resuscitator is not immediately available.
      (1) Prone patient's transport cart should be immediately available.
      (2) A firm surface should be placed under patient's back.
      (3) If patient is on an irregular surface (i.e. fracture table) compressions may be difficult.
   d. Send a runner for the crash cart. Prepare necessary equipment from the crash cart, such as medications, the defibrillator, and the ECG if it is not already in use.
      (1) On the off-shift the scrub person may have to break scrub and become the runner.
      (2) The circulating nurse remains in the room to assist the director of the code.
      (3) Record drugs, times, routes if a recorder has not been assigned.
   e. Control traffic. Exclude unauthorized personnel from the room. Students should either be instructed to stand back or enlisted to obtain supplies as able. Provide an optimal environment for successful resuscitation.
   f. Help with and observe IV and monitoring lines, such as an arterial line. Assist in collection of blood samples.

g. Maintain accuracy of sponge, needle, and instrument counts and sterility to best of ability if wound closure progresses (but sterility is secondary to resuscitation efforts).

(1) Counts may be aborted, but accountability remains important.

(2) Radiographs may be taken as patient condition permits.

h. Document all medications given, the time and amount, and the sequence of procedures performed. Documentation is important in guiding therapy and providing legal protection.

i. Supervise termination of the procedure as necessary.

(1) Arrange for crash cart replacement.

j. In unsuccessful resuscitation, follow protocol regarding notification of family, care of the deceased, specimens to be saved, and forms to be filled out after a death in the OR.

(1) Observe respect for the patient's dignity as possible.

3. *Scrub person*

a. Remain sterile and keep the tables sterile if possible. If arrest occurs during a noncardiac surgical procedure, when the chest is not open, the surgical site is packed with saline-soaked sponges and covered with sterile drape, and the patient is repositioned as necessary for CPR. If the surgical site is in an area that can be closed rapidly during resuscitation, this may be done.

(1) During regular business hours support staff should be the runners.

(2) Off-shift times the support staff is minimal, it is necessary to break scrub and be the runner.

(3) Obtain the crash cart

b. Keep track of sponges, needles, and instruments. Counts are completed as possible, and the surgical site is closed as soon as possible despite the outcome. In a life-threatening emergency, the surgeon may order that counts be aborted. Follow the written institutional policy and procedure for counts during emergency situations.

(1) Keep all unnecessary instruments and supplies off the field.

(2) Push back table off to the side of the room. Move the Mayo stand away from the patient.

c. Give attention to the field and the surgeon's needs. If the patient is hemorrhaging, keep suction tubing clear and tapes available.

d. If the circulating nurse is performing chest compressions and no other support personnel are available, assist as required.

4. *OR manager* (on duty during business hours)

a. Assign professional and assistive support personnel to augment the team (e.g., an extra circulating nurse, medication nurse, runners [personnel to obtain supplies or handle laboratory samples]).

b. Notify the attending physician, if not present, and appropriate administrative personnel.

c. Alert the ICU of a potential patient admission.

d. Reassign subsequent patients' scheduling.

e. Keep track of resuscitation progress.

f. Evaluate the arrest procedure and emergency equipment; verify the documentation.

g. Support the team as necessary. Keep the surgical suite running smoothly during the emergency.

Duration of Cardiopulmonary Resuscitation. CPR may be done as long as necessary to restore circulatory function if adequate ventilation and a good peripheral pulse have been restored. It is not uncommon for a second arrest to occur after successful resuscitation. The time frame for survival is shortened drastically if the arrest is unwitnessed. When the patient's condition is adequately stabilized and the surgical site is closed, he or she is transferred to the ICU.

The decision to discontinue resuscitative efforts in the OR is made by a physician. The decision is based on assessment of cerebral and cardiovascular status. The end point of cardiovascular unresponsiveness is suggested as the most reliable basis for this decision.

Appropriate administrative personnel and services, such as the nursing unit, ICU, and clergy, as well as the patient's family, are notified of the cardiac arrest as required. In case of death, the surgeon notifies the family.

Postresuscitation Care. Postarrest supportive therapy depends on the cause and duration of arrest. Care centers on cardiac and cerebral preservation, maintaining circulation and ventilation, and minimizing sequelae such as cerebral edema. The patient must be carefully monitored and closely observed for 48 to 72 hours postarrest. In select patients, hypothermia may be used to reduce oxygen needs. Vital signs, acid-base and electrolyte balances, and urinary output are closely watched. Seizures should be controlled to prevent further anoxia. The patient is observed for signs of embolism, pulmonary edema, fractured ribs caused by chest compressions, and hemopericardium. A chest radiograph is taken as soon as feasible after the arrest. An IV fluid lifeline must be left in place. If cerebral damage is evident, the prognosis is guarded.

Staff Education. Practice sessions of a cardiac arrest emergency and CPR with subsequent evaluation and revision are valuable to review the protocol and prepare the OR staff before need for implementation. Current CPR/BLS certification is required of all OR personnel. Many ORs require yearly BLS review, with recertification every 2 years. ICU personnel are required to be ACLS-certified.

FLUID AND ELECTROLYTE IMBALANCES

Fluid and electrolyte imbalances may be caused by many different factors and may be manifested by numerous symptoms. Maintenance of correct balance, which greatly influences the outcome of surgical intervention, is a very relevant aspect of intraoperative and postoperative care.

Fluid loss is replaced by IV infusion. Usually normal saline or dextrose (5% or 10% in water or saline) solution is started initially. Electrolytes may be added to the solution as needed. Two other IV solutions are commonly used to maintain balance:

1. Mannitol: An osmotic diuretic agent, has an effect on renal vascular resistance. Depending on the percentage

of drug in solution, it can either increase or decrease renal blood flow. It may be given prophylactically to prevent renal failure. It is used also to decrease intracranial and intraocular pressure. It is rapidly excreted by the kidneys.

2. Ringer's lactate solution: A physiologic salt solution, may be infused when the body's supply of sodium, calcium, and potassium has been depleted or for improvement of circulation and stimulation of renal activity. Its electrolyte content is similar to that of plasma.

Changes in fluid and electrolyte balances affect renal function, cellular metabolism, and oxygen concentration in the circulation.

Acid-Base Balance

For enzyme systems to function, a normal balance must be maintained between acidity and alkalinity of body fluids located within intracellular and extracellular compartments. The symbol pH represents the hydrogen ion concentration that determines acidity or alkalinity of a solution; neutral pH is 7, below 7 is acid, and above 7 is alkaline. Urine is usually acid, with a pH range between 4.6 and 8. Normal serum pH is 7.40, within a range of 7.35 to 7.45.

Hydrogen ions do not exist as separate electrolytes in body fluids but are maintained in balance with other electrolytes to ensure neutrality. Because most metabolic processes produce acids, chemical buffers interact with hydrogen ions. Carbonic acid and a hydrogen ion form bicarbonate (HCO_3)—the most important buffer. The kidneys and lungs regulate this system by excreting or retaining needed ions in body fluids. Abnormal acid-base balance results from the following:

1. Respiratory malfunction in handling carbon dioxide produced from carbonic acid
   a. Acidosis: pH less than 7.35 with carbon dioxide above 45 torr
   b. Alkalosis: pH more than 7.45 with carbon dioxide below 35 torr
2. Metabolic abnormality in balance between hydrogen and serum HCO_3
   a. Acidosis: pH less than 7.35 with HCO_3 less than 22 mEq/L
   b. Alkalosis: pH more than 7.45 with HCO_3 more than 26 mEq/L

Electrolytes

Compounds that separate into ions, which are charged particles capable of conducting electrical impulses, are essential in maintaining fluid and acid-base balance and in regulating cell functions. The primary electrolytes in the body (Table 31-1) are as follows:

1. *Sodium:* A key regulator in water balance, sodium is necessary to the normal function of muscles and nerves. Large amounts are in extracellular fluid in concentrations of 136 to 145 mEq/L; intracellular concentration is 10 mEq/L. This balance is necessary for normal metabolism.
   a. Hyponatremia (insufficient serum sodium) usually accompanies excessive fluid loss or adrenal insufficiency. Muscle twitching, hypovolemia, hypotension, and tachycardia may be symptoms.

TABLE 31-1	Normal Blood Chemistry Laboratory Values
Parameter	**Normal Values for Adult**
Alanine aminotransferase (ALT)	10-35 international units/L
Aspartate aminotransferase (AST)	4-36 international units/L
Base excess of blood	0 ± 2 mmol/L
Bicarbonate (HCO_3)	22-26 mEq/L
Bilirubin (total)	0.1-1 mg/dL
Blood urea nitrogen (BUN)	5-20 mg/dL
Calcium (Ca)	9-10.5 mg/dL
Carbon dioxide (CO_2) in serum	23-30 mEq/L
Chloride (Cl)	90-110 mEq/L
Creatinine	0.7-1.5 mg/dL
Creatine phosphokinase (CPK)	12-80 units/L
Glucose	70-115 mg/dL
Magnesium (Mg)	1.6-3 mEq/L
pH of serum	7.35-7.45
Phosphate (P)	2.5-4.5 mg/dL
Potassium (K)	3.5-5 mEq/L
Sodium (Na)	136-145 mEq/L

b. Hypernatremia (elevated serum sodium) may be caused by hyperglycemia or administration of mannitol. Diaphoresis (sweating) may be the only obvious symptom. Convulsions can occur.

2. *Chloride:* Essential to electrochemical reactions for acid-base regulation, chloride is in extracellular fluids in large amounts. Chlorides are retained or excreted by the kidneys to offset HCO_3 excretion. Sodium tends to carry chloride with it.
   a. Hypochloremia (loss of chloride) may occur from vomiting, suctioning, sweating, and diuresis. It produces symptoms of metabolic alkalosis: slow, shallow respirations and muscle tightening.
   b. Hyperchloremia (excessive chloride) can result in renal failure. Acidosis develops, and breathing becomes labored.

3. *Potassium:* One of the main constituents of cell protoplasm, potassium is primarily (98%) in intracellular fluid. It is essential for electrochemical reactions for cellular functions.
   a. Hypokalemia (shift of potassium from the blood to the cells or depletion of potassium from the body) can be associated with metabolic alkalosis. Cardiac dysrhythmias can occur when the serum potassium level falls.
   b. Hyperkalemia (increase in serum potassium) may be caused by renal failure and may lead to respiratory and/or cardiac arrest. Metabolic or respiratory acidosis can occur.

4. *Calcium:* Essential to normal muscle physiology, calcium also is an integral part of the blood-clotting mechanism.
   a. Hypocalcemia (decreased calcium intake or absorption) may be a result of increased excretion. This can cause cardiac dysrhythmias.
   b. Hypercalcemia (increased serum calcium) may be a result of a shift of calcium from the bones to plasma,

decreased excretion, or increased uptake and absorption. It causes neuromuscular depression and cardiac dysrhythmias.

5. *Magnesium:* Essential to electrochemical reactions for normal body functions, magnesium is primarily in intracellular fluid. An imbalance may be accompanied by calcium and/or potassium imbalances.

   a. Hypomagnesemia (low magnesium level) usually is associated with hypokalemia. This may be the most undiagnosed electrolyte deficiency in geriatric patients or in patients who have illnesses associated with malabsorption in the intestine or kidneys. It may cause cardiac dysrhythmias and nervous system and muscular irritability, and it may exaggerate drug toxicities.

   b. Hypermagnesemia (elevated serum magnesium) can inhibit nerve and muscle responses. It may lead to respiratory depression and cardiac arrest.

6. *Phosphate:* Normally in intracellular fluid, phosphate allows electrochemical reactions for metabolic functions. Phosphate and calcium vary inversely; thus phosphate will buffer acidosis from a rising calcium level.

   a. Hypophosphatemia (low serum phosphate level) may produce tissue hypoxia.

   b. Hyperphosphatemia (increase in phosphate) usually occurs in renal failure. It is associated with hypocalcemia.

Disturbances in fluid and electrolyte balance can result from the following:

- *Acid-base imbalances associated with chronic disease or organ dysfunction:* Acidosis increases serum chloride, potassium, and calcium; alkalosis decreases chloride, potassium, calcium, and phosphate.
- *Cell destruction leading to hyperkalemia:* Cellular potassium is depleted, with serum potassium increase.
- *Shift of potassium from blood into cells, causing hypokalemia:* This may be caused by the effects of epinephrine, insulin, bicarbonate, hypothermia, or cardiopulmonary bypass.
- *Changes in blood lipids:* Calcium and magnesium are depleted by poor absorption.
- *Fever:* Metabolic rate is increased; water and electrolytes are lost.
- *Stress:* Glucose tolerance is diminished, and blood glucose and serum potassium levels are increased.
- *Gastric drainage:* Sodium and chlorides are lost.
- *Fluid loss from drainage tubes, diaphoresis, vomiting, or diarrhea:* Sodium, chloride, and potassium are lost.
- *Maxillofacial injury:* Oral intake is inhibited.
- *Radiation enteritis:* Magnesium and potassium are diminished.
- *Disease of the bowel, liver, or biliary tract; intestinal tract obstruction; or gastrointestinal fistula:* Calcium and phosphate are poorly absorbed.
- *Loss of muscle mass as a result of preoperative malnutrition:* Nitrogen loss is increased.
- *Drugs:* Metabolic balance can be adversely affected; losses of potassium, magnesium, and chloride from diuretics are examples.
- *Inadequate oxygen/carbon dioxide exchange:* Acid-base balance is disrupted.

Hypovolemia

Hypovolemia is a decreased circulating blood volume from loss of blood and plasma or a deficit of extracellular fluid volume commonly referred to as dehydration. When excessive fluid loss is greater than absorption of interstitial fluid into the circulation, the patient may go into hypovolemic shock.

Etiology. Etiologic factors include reduced fluid intake; hemorrhage; plasma loss (e.g., through extensive burns, wound drainage); and dehydration from loss of gastrointestinal fluids (e.g., by vomiting), from diaphoresis caused by fever, from diuresis). Impaired renal function and metabolic acidosis are predisposing factors. Prolonged cardiopulmonary bypass can cause hypovolemic shock.

Signs and Symptoms. Signs and symptoms include dry skin and mucous membranes, depressed blood pressure, elevated pulse, oliguria, decreasing CVP and blood volume determinations, and deep, rapid respirations.

Treatment. Hypovolemic shock resulting from hemorrhage or underestimated blood loss is most often seen in the OR. This is usually reversed by prompt restoration of circulating blood volume. The extent of hypovolemia will determine treatment:

1. *Fluid volume replacement:* Whole blood, plasma expander, or infusion of Ringer's lactate or other IV fluid is indicated to increase blood volume. Hypervolemia must be avoided in replacement.
2. *Position:* Elevation of the legs may aid venous return and cardiac output except in severe oligemia (low total blood volume [TBV]).
3. *Temperature:* The patient is kept warm but not overheated. Perspiration increases fluid loss. Shivering can cause hypothermia.
4. *Oxygen:* Oxygen is administered when Po_2 is low because the circulation is not delivering enough oxygen to tissues.
5. *Drugs:* Drugs are administered as needed to maintain blood pressure, correct acidosis, or protect the kidneys from failure.

Prevention. Decreased blood volume, if present preoperatively, increases surgical risk and morbidity. It should be treated, and the electrolyte imbalance should be corrected. Fluids, blood gases, and blood loss must be monitored intraoperatively.

Hypervolemia

Hypervolemia is an excess of extracellular fluid in the blood, commonly referred to as edema. IV infusions given too rapidly or in excessive amounts, especially isotonic saline solution, can cause hypervolemia. Prolonged administration of adrenocorticosteroids is also a predisposing factor. Hypervolemia may progress to pulmonary edema.

Dyspnea, coarse crackles, an elevated pulse and respiratory rate, and diminished urinary output are symptomatic of hypervolemia. Increasing CVP may indicate fluid overload with venous distention. Diuretics and fluid restriction ameliorate hypervolemia and prevent pulmonary edema.

BLOOD VOLUME COMPLICATIONS

Blood Loss Considerations

Some blood loss is inevitable whenever tissues are severed by intent or traumatic injury. Blood loss is computed as a percentage of TBV. TBV averages from 6% to 8% of total body weight. This equals about 75 mL/kg in the average healthy adult man and 60 to 70 mL/kg in the average woman. Calculation of TBV depends on the venous hematocrit value. Normal hematocrit, the volume of red blood cells expressed as a percentage of the volume of whole blood, is 42% to 52% in men and 37% to 47% in women. An infant reaches these blood volume levels at approximately 3 months of age.

An increase in hematocrit indicates a decrease in plasma volume, normally by dehydration and loss of sodium. A decrease in hematocrit indicates a decrease in the number of red blood cells, but this does not necessarily reflect blood loss; it may be caused by overhydration. Fluid and electrolyte balance is important for maintenance of blood volume. Inadequate fluid replacement can lead to a decrease in cardiac output and cardiovascular collapse.

A decrease in red blood cells (erythrocytes) and in hemoglobin, the chief oxygen-carrying component of these cells, causes hypoxia if values fall below normal (Table 31-2). Therefore, determination of intraoperative blood loss may be critical to physiologic functions. The extent of blood loss will depend on the location and magnitude of the surgical procedure. Blood loss can be categorized as follows:

- *Minor:* Loss of 500 to 700 mL is about 15% of TBV.
- *Moderate:* Loss of 750 to 1500 mL is about 15% to 30% of TBV. A resultant decrease in pulse pressure and slight tachycardia (rapid heart rate) may progress to tachycardia, tachypnea (rapid breathing), and postural hypotension (reduced blood pressure on position change).
- *Major:* Loss of 1500 to 2250 mL is about 30% to 45% of TBV. The blood pressure drops, the skin becomes cold and clammy, and urinary output decreases.
- *Catastrophic:* Loss of more than 2250 mL is greater than 45% of TBV. Hypoxia (decrease in oxygen level) develops from loss of hemoglobin (red blood cells). Prolonged hypoxia leads to irreversible heart, brain, liver, and kidney damage.

Hemorrhage

Severe bleeding into or from a wound is a major contributing factor to intraoperative and postoperative morbidity and mortality. If bleeding is uncontrolled, exsanguination can occur. Massive hemorrhage may cause hypovolemic shock, ventricular fibrillation, or death as a result of marked decrease in cardiac output. Common symptoms are arterial hypotension, pale or cyanotic moist skin, oliguria, bradycardia from hypoxia or tachycardia after moderate to marked blood loss, restlessness, and thirst in the conscious patient.

In the OR, hemorrhage is readily visible. Meticulous hemostasis during every step of the surgical procedure and good nutritional status of the patient preoperatively are crucial to prevention. Preoperative evaluation of the patient's clotting time and history of bleeding (personal and familial), type and crossmatch of blood, and insertion of an IV line before incision are necessary precautions.

In treating hemorrhage, the surgeon locates the source of bleeding and applies digital compression to severed or traumatized blood vessels until noncrushing vascular clamps can be placed to occlude the vessel proximal and distal to the site of bleeding. The vessel is then ligated, clipped, electrocoagulated, or sutured. Circulating blood volume must be restored promptly.

If allogenic blood is transfused, it must be fresh and warmed to limit electrolytic changes. Sodium bicarbonate may be given IV to reduce acidosis. Multiple IV infusion routes can be used, by cutdown if necessary, to infuse blood under pressure. Ringer's lactate solution or other plasma expanders are used when blood is contraindicated (e.g., for religious reasons). Oxygen is administered to combat hypoxia. Accurate measurement of blood and fluid losses intraoperatively, followed by adequate replacement, will help prevent hypovolemic shock. Autotransfusion may be feasible.

Hemorrhage can be detected postoperatively by observation of blood-soaked dressings. The patient must be checked frequently for both observable and nonobservable symptoms of hemorrhage. Slipping or sloughing of a ligature or the passage of clots from ligated or coagulated vessels can cause internal bleeding.

Estimation of Blood Loss

An accurate determination of TBV involves measuring plasma and red blood cell volumes separately and then adding these values together. This may be done rapidly by an electronic counting device. In lieu of this, blood loss is estimated in all surgical procedures in which a major loss is anticipated. This can be done by the following:

- Visual inspection of blood on drapes and the floor by the anesthesia provider.
- Estimation of blood in the suction container. Allowance must be made for the presence of other body fluids and irrigating solution, if used. The scrub person must estimate the amount of solution suctioned into the

TABLE 31-2	Normal Values of Blood*		
	Males	**Females**	**Children**
Red blood cells (RBCs)	4.7-6.1 million/mm³	4.2-5.4 million/mm³	3.8-5.5 million/mm³
Hemoglobin (Hgb)	14-18 g/dL	12-16 g/dL	11-16 g/dL
Hematocrit (Hct)	42%-52%	37%-47%	31%-43%
Prothrombin time (PT)	11.0-12.5 seconds	Same	Same
Platelets	150,000-4000,000/mm³	Same	Same after 1 week of age
Partial thromboplastin time (PTT)	30-40 seconds	Same	25-35 seconds

*Values vary depending on calibration of testing equipment in the laboratory that services the health care facility.

container through irrigation of the wound and/or tubing. This can be done by knowing the capacity of the irrigation syringe in use and keeping track of the number of times it is used. The circulating nurse subtracts these amounts to estimate the volume of blood in the container.

- Visual inspection of blood in sponges by the anesthesia provider.
- Measurement of blood in sponges by weighing them. Sponges are weighed after use as they are discarded from the surgical field.

Weighing Sponges. Some anesthesia providers and surgeons prefer to have sponges weighed to determine blood loss rather than visually estimating the loss (Box 31-1). A scale calibrated in grams is used. The dry and wet weights of each type of sponge must be known. Wet weight is that of a sponge soaked in normal saline solution and wrung out until almost dry. A chart of these weights should be available; often it is attached to the scale. The number of sponges being weighed is multiplied by the appropriate dry or wet weight.

BOX 31-1　Weighing Surgical Sponges

Use a scale that measures in grams. Always wear personal protective equipment (PPE). This method helps to subtract the weight of the actual sponges and the container they are weighed in.

WEIGHING DRY SPONGES:

1. Obtain a small plastic sponge basin and one pack of each type of sponges used for the procedure.
2. Weigh a complete unwrapped complement of each type of sponge in the plastic sponge basin (e.g., 10 unwrapped Raytec, 5 unwrapped laparotomy sponges of the correct size).
   - Raytec: Place the open pack of dry Raytec in the plastic sponge basin on the scale and set the dial to zero. This will account for the weight of the sponges and the basin without the blood.
     - Remove the dry sponges from the plastic basin and set aside.
     - Place the counted bloody sponges into basin.
     - Take the weight reading. The number of grams of weight is recorded.
   - Laparotomy sponges: Place the open pack of dry laparotomy sponges in the plastic sponge basin on the scale and set the dial to zero. This will account for the weight of the sponges and the basin without the blood.
     - Remove the dry sponges from the plastic basin and set aside.
     - Place the counted bloody sponges into basin.
     - Take the weight reading. The number of grams of weight is recorded.

WEIGHING SPONGES PREMOISTENED WITH SALINE:

Repeat the above steps with the following changes:

1. Dip the complete set of dry Raytec or laparotomy sponges into water and wring out all excess liquid. This will simulate the dampening of the sponges with the sterile saline.
2. Place the damp set into the plastic basin and set the dial on the scale to zero. This accounts for the weight of the damp sponges and the container.
3. Remove the moist sponges and replace them with the same number and type of bloody sponges.

Each type must be weighed separately, with the dry sponges separated from the wet ones. To allow for (i.e., by subtracting) dry or wet weights and the weight of a moisture-proof cover on the scale platform or a container, the scale is adjusted to register at zero. When blood-soaked sponges are weighed, the reading on the scale equals the blood loss; 1 g equals 1 mL. The scale is checked at each use for readjustment to zero. Some scales are controlled by a microprocessor that automatically makes calculations.

The circulating nurse must weigh sponges before they dry out. Blood loss is recorded each time sponges are weighed, adding new weight to previous ones to keep a current total. A tally board for this purpose may be mounted on the wall where the anesthesia provider and surgeon can read it. The estimated blood in the suction container can be recorded here also. Irrigation solutions used for moistening sponges should be carefully measured and documented.

Reduction of Blood Loss

When significant bleeding can be anticipated, several techniques are used to reduce red blood cell loss during the surgical procedure or to eliminate blood transfusion requirements.

Hemodilution. Acute normovolemic or isovolemic hemodilution reduces red blood cells but maintains normal or equal blood volume. After induction of anesthesia, a physician, usually the anesthesia provider, withdraws blood through an arterial or venous catheter. The blood is drawn into bags containing anticoagulant, usually citrate. Citrate metabolizes rapidly, thus minimizing the risk of systemic anticoagulation when blood is reinfused. The amount withdrawn depends on the anticipated blood loss and the patient's estimated TBV and hematocrit. A plasma volume expander is given by IV infusion while blood is removed, to restore blood volume. This hemodilution technique reduces red blood cell loss during the surgical procedure because the hematocrit has been lowered. The surgical procedure begins when the hematocrit is between 27% and 30%. Adequate intravascular volume and oxygenation are maintained. Urinary output must be measured.

Each bag of blood must be labeled with the patient's name and identifying number and the time of withdrawal. Blood may be stored at room temperature for 6 hours or in a refrigerator for 24 hours. At the conclusion of the surgical procedure, or sooner if indicated, the blood is reinfused IV to raise the hematocrit back to the preoperative level. Units are reinfused in reverse order of withdrawal (i.e., last one first) so that the unit with the highest concentration of red blood cells and coagulation factors is infused last. (More information is available at the website of the American Association of Blood Banks, www.aabb.org.)

Blood Volume Expanders. Crystalloid or colloid solutions are administered IV for fluid replacement and plasma volume expansion. They are not sole replacements for blood loss. They must be used with caution. The following are the most commonly used plasma volume expanders:

- *Dextran:* This crystalloid polymer of glucose acts by drawing fluid from tissues to decrease blood viscosity. It remains in circulation for several hours. It interferes with the crossmatching of blood; thus a blood sample for this purpose must be drawn before dextran is infused. It may be used until blood or blood products are available or for hemodilution. As a 6% or 10% solution, it may be mixed in water with glucose or sodium chloride.

- *Ringer's lactate solution:* This crystalloid physiologic salt solution is infused for the improvement of circulation and stimulation of renal activity and in patients in whom the body's supply of sodium, calcium, and potassium has been depleted.

- *Hetastarch (Hespan):* This colloid polymer expands plasma volume slightly in excess of the volume infused. It approximates the action of serum albumin. Large volumes may alter coagulation factors. It can be used for hemodilution.

Pharmacologic Agents. The action of specific pharmacologic agents either stimulates or retards the coagulation mechanism. This action may reduce blood loss and help provide hemostasis in patients with hematologic disorders. Some of these disorders are associated with cardiovascular disease or end-stage renal disease. Others are congenital or acquired coagulopathies. Three types of agents affect bleeding.

Desmopressin Acetate. Desmopressin promotes hemostasis in patients with von Willebrand disease and shortens the bleeding time in patients with uremia. When given prophylactically, this synthetic vasopressin analog can decrease surgical blood loss in patients undergoing spinal surgery and reduce blood loss after cardiac surgery.

Vasodilators. Vasodilators lower systemic blood pressure, thus decreasing bleeding. Sodium nitroprusside, nitroglycerin, and trimethaphan are the most commonly used.

Anticoagulants. Anticoagulants minimize the tendency of blood to clot yet do not lead to excessive bleeding during or after the surgical procedure. These agents provide adequate anticoagulation with a minimum of hemorrhagic complications. They help prevent venous stasis to reduce the incidence of DVT and pulmonary embolus. They may be given orally, subcutaneously (subQ), or IV, beginning preoperatively, especially in patients who have a history of thromboembolic disease. The action of each anticoagulant is different and is described as follows:

- Heparin acts to inhibit conversion of prothrombin to thrombin. This prolongs clotting time. It may be administered subQ to keep activated partial thromboplastin time in the high-normal range between 30 and 40 seconds. Given IV, heparin is effective immediately. It may be used as a flush to keep IV lines open or to flush the lumen of a blood vessel (1 mL of heparin in 100 mL of normal saline solution). Heparin does not dissolve a thrombus, but it will prevent a clot from becoming larger.

- Coumarin derivatives depress blood prothrombin and decrease the tendency of blood platelets to cling together, thus decreasing the normal tendency of blood to clot. They also interfere with action of vitamin K to prevent the synthesis of prothrombin and fibrinogen. Warfarin sodium is the most commonly used coumarin derivative.

- Low-molecular-weight dextran reduces platelet adhesiveness and aggregation to prevent sludge from forming in the bloodstream. It coats blood platelets to keep them from massing together.

- Aspirin diminishes clumping of platelets by inhibiting the release reaction of platelet factors and action of vitamin K.

Vitamin K enables the liver to produce clotting factors in blood, including prothrombin. To reduce the possibility of intraoperative hemorrhage, patients who have been receiving anticoagulant therapy and those who have faulty metabolism or absorption of vitamin K are given it preoperatively. It also is given to geriatric or debilitated patients before intraocular surgery, to newborns preoperatively, and to mothers just before delivery. The latter helps prevent postdelivery hemorrhage and ensures that the baby has an adequate prothrombin level until a sufficient amount is produced by the liver.

Hypotensive Anesthesia. In selected situations when excessive blood loss is anticipated or encountered, arterial blood pressure may be deliberately lowered to produce an essentially bloodless field. When induced, hypotension is carefully controlled by the anesthesia provider.

Hematologic Disorders

Some hemolytic and hemorrhagic disorders require special consideration during perioperative care to minimize risks of surgical intervention. Concern is for the maintenance of adequate tissue perfusion and oxygenation and for hemostasis and coagulation in patients at risk. Patients at risk for intraoperative bleeding or who have a known hematologic disorder should have a complete blood count, sequential multichannel autoanalyzer (SMA)–18 test, and urinalysis done preoperatively. Hemoglobin, hematocrit, and red blood cell counts are critical determinants for blood replacement requirements preoperatively and intraoperatively. Precautions can be taken to minimize the risks of surgical intervention with adequate blood replacement.

Anemia. Anemia is a symptom of a deficiency in either the quantity or quality of red blood cells (erythrocytes). Hemoglobin, the chief component of these cells, delivers oxygen to tissues. Normal hemoglobin values are 14 to 18 g/dL of blood in males, 12 to 16 g/dL in females, and 11 to 16 g/dL in children. These values are lower in anemic patients. Thus anemia may result in tissue hypoxia. The various types of this disorder may be caused by the following:

- *Blood loss from massive bleeding (e.g., from a traumatic injury) or chronic blood loss (e.g., from a gastric or intestinal ulcer):* This blood loss can be replaced by transfusion of blood products.

- *Dietary deficiency of sufficient iron, protein, vitamins, and minerals to form red blood cells or produce hemoglobin:* Dietary supplements are given to correct the deficiency.

- *Diseases or drugs that inhibit the bone marrow from producing blood cells, such as tumors or chronic renal disease:* The cause must be diagnosed and treated.

- *Destruction of red blood cells by an overactive reticuloendothelial system in the spleen or liver:* A splenectomy may be indicated for hypersplenism or hereditary spherocytosis, for example.

- *Destruction of red blood cells by foreign substances entering the circulatory system (e.g., through an incompatible blood transfusion):* Neonatal anemia may necessitate an exchange transfusion.

• *Abnormal blood cells produced by the bone marrow:* These are usually caused by genetic or hereditary factors.

The average normal life span of red blood cells is 120 days. In patients with any one of the many forms of hemolytic anemia, red blood cells have a shortened life span. Hemolytic anemias may be acquired or inherited. All must be adequately assessed preoperatively.

Sickle Cell Hemoglobinopathies. A severe, chronic, inherited hemolytic disorder, sickle cell anemia is most prevalent among blacks of African descent. It may be found in other ethnic groups, particularly people of Mediterranean descent. Pairing of identical abnormal recessive genes causes substitution of a single amino acid for glutamic acid in the polypeptide chain, which alters the hemoglobin. These abnormal cells, known as hemoglobin S, become distorted in shape when exposed to low oxygen tension in the venous circulation. Dehydration, cold, infection, and physical or emotional stress may precipitate crisis periods that vary in duration and intensity when sickling occurs.

A crisis may also occur spontaneously without apparent cause. The resultant sickle-shaped red blood cells occlude the microcirculation through the capillaries, arterioles, and venules. Occlusion results in blood stasis, hypoxia, vasospasm, ischemia, and necrosis, which cause pain and ultimately permanent damage to tissues and organs. Stasis ulcers and biliary tract disease are common complications that may require surgical intervention. Elective surgical procedures are performed when the patient is not in crisis, but these patients are always at risk of crisis.

Sickle cell trait is present when one abnormal gene is inherited. The red blood cells have both hemoglobin A (normal) and hemoglobin S (sickle cell). People with this trait usually are asymptomatic and tolerate routine anesthesia and surgical intervention well. However, when they are stressed by hypothermia, acidosis, or hypoxemia, local or regional sickling can occur during the surgical procedure.

Sickle cells have a life span of 15 to 30 days. The severity of the hemolytic process is proportional to the amount of hemoglobin S in the blood. Hemoglobin in patients with sickle cell anemia usually ranges from 6 to 9 g, with a hematocrit of 25% to 30%. Patients of African descent and other susceptible people should be tested preoperatively. Electrophoresis is the standard laboratory test for hemoglobin S. Consideration must then be given to the following in the perioperative management of patients with sickle cell anemia or sickle cell trait:

1. Transfusion of whole blood, packed cells, or low-molecular-weight dextran may be administered preoperatively, especially if the patient's hemoglobin is 5 g or less.
2. Urea may be given orally or IV prophylactically to prevent a sickle cell crisis. It may also be used to reverse a crisis.
3. Systemic antibiotics are initiated preoperatively, because these patients are susceptible to postoperative infection.
4. Normal body temperature must be maintained. Any lowering increases the requirement for oxygen. The patient must be kept warm to avoid hypothermia.
   a. Add extra blankets during transport to the OR suite.
   b. Avoid drafts from the air-conditioning system in the holding area, OR, and PACU.
   c. Cover the patient's head for warmth.
   d. Raise the temperature in the OR to 80° to 85° F (27° to 29° C).
   e. Place the patient on a hyperthermia blanket on the operating bed.
   f. Monitor the patient's temperature intraoperatively with an electronic probe.
   g. Place warm blankets over the patient before transfer to the PACU.
5. Oxygen is administered during induction of anesthesia, intraoperatively, and after extubation to prevent deoxygenation of the sickle cells and subsequent ischemic infarction in tissues.
6. Blood gases are monitored to avoid hypoxia, acidosis, hypotension, and hypovolemia. Fluid and blood replacement intraoperatively reduces the risk of crisis from dehydration.
7. Scheduling an elective surgical procedure early in the morning minimizes dehydration after a period of nothing by mouth (NPO).

Hemorrhagic Disorders. Patients with a disorder in the mechanism of blood coagulation have abnormal bleeding tendencies. These may be related to the following:

• Hemorrhagic diseases, such as a type of purpura in which spontaneous bleeding occurs under the skin, through mucous membranes, or in the gastrointestinal tract, that is idiopathic (cause unknown) or secondary to a systemic or an infectious disease or to exposure to chemical agents
• Platelet deficiency in the blood, such as thrombocytopenia as a result of decreased production of platelets by bone marrow or excessive destruction of platelets in the peripheral circulation
• Abnormal clotting factors, such as in hemophilia and von Willebrand disease, which are inherited genetic disorders

A baseline of blood values should be established preoperatively. The baseline consists of a complete blood count, including platelets, plasma clotting time, bleeding time, prothrombin time, and partial thromboplastin time. Adequate blood replacement of the deficient factors must be available during the surgical procedure and postoperatively.

Hemophilia. The term *hemophilia* refers to a group of genetic bleeding disorders characterized by abnormal clotting factors.

Hemophilia A, the classic disorder, is caused by a deficiency of functional factor VIII, the antihemophilic globulin in plasma. Hemophilia B, also known as Christmas disease, is caused by a lack of functional factor IX—the plasma thromboplastic cofactor. A carrier mother transmits to her son this sex-linked recessive trait of the specific clotting factor. Hemophilia occurs most commonly in males of Russian-Jewish descent.

The severity of the disorder depends on the percentage of functional versus nonfunctional factor in the blood. Partial thromboplastin times or thromboplastin generation times are the standard tests for this determination. These patients have normal vasculature and platelets (150,000 to 400,000/mm³ of blood); thus bleeding time (1 to 3 minutes by the Duke method) and prothrombin time (11 to 12.5 seconds) test results are normal.

Severely affected hemophiliacs have spontaneous bleeding episodes into the skin, muscles, and joints, most commonly the ankles, knees, wrists, and elbows. If untreated, joint deformities can result. Bleeding will be excessive from even a minor wound such as a bruise or cut.

For hemostasis during a severe bleeding episode, replacement therapy must be initiated to raise the clotting factor to between 60% and 100% (normal individuals have clotting factor levels of 60% to 120%). In hemophiliacs, fibrin clots do not form, and bleeding continues. The missing clotting factor must be raised temporarily to control hemorrhage. This is started preoperatively for elective surgery. Concentrates available for replacement therapy include the following:

1. Factor VIII for hemophilia A
   a. Lyophilized concentrate products, such as Hemofil CT and Koate HT or HS reconstituted with diluent provided by the manufacturer
   b. Cryoprecipitate
   c. Fresh frozen plasma or concentrate
2. Factor IX for hemophilia B
   a. Lyophilized concentrate products, such as Konyne and Profilnine reconstituted with diluent provided by the manufacturer
   b. Fresh frozen plasma
3. Lyophilized concentrate with inhibitors to neutralize the antibody that prevents clotting

Lyophilized concentrates are made from pooled normal human plasma obtained by plasmapheresis, a process of separating red blood cells by centrifugation. The circulating nurse should obtain factor concentrate from the blood bank and must be familiar with how to prepare it. The dosage for factor deficiency is calculated on the basis of the plasma volume, half-life of the factor, and percentage of the deficit. It is given by IV infusion intraoperatively and postoperatively.

Blood Loss Replacement

Despite meticulous hemostasis and methods to reduce blood loss, blood replacement is necessary during many extensive surgical procedures, particularly cardiovascular, orthopedic, organ transplantation, and trauma surgery. Surgeons limit the use of transfused blood whenever possible. However, to compensate for blood loss of more than 1200 mL or a hematocrit value below 30% and to prevent shock, transfusions of whole blood, fresh frozen plasma, packed red blood cells, platelets, serum albumin, or blood substitutes must be carried out according to policy. Transfusions may be allogenic, autologous, or a blood substitute. Informed consent should be obtained before blood loss replacement methods are selected.

Allogenic Blood. Allogenic blood is that drawn from one individual for transfusion into another. It must be compatible (i.e., not cause a reaction). Therefore, blood typing and crossmatching are essential to determine compatibility between donor and recipient. The four main blood types are A, B, O, and AB. In addition, many subgroups of antigens

exist in red blood cells. Also, agglutinogens, known as Rh factor, may be present (i.e., Rh positive or negative). If these are not present in red blood cells, the blood is Rh negative. A recipient must receive donor blood of the same type and Rh factor. In extreme emergency situations, O-negative blood, referred to as universal donor blood, may be given until the patient's blood can be typed and crossmatched or until compatible blood can be obtained. Conversely, type AB is considered to be the universal recipient, being compatible with A, B, O, and AB.

A transfusion of the wrong blood type can be fatal. Transmission of hepatitis B or C, human immunodeficiency virus (HIV), and other viruses and infections is a potential danger, even with current testing of all donor blood. According to the American Association of Blood Banks, in 1998 the Transmissible Spongiform Encephalopathy Advisory Committee of the U.S. Food and Drug Administration (FDA) recommended deferral of potential donors who have traveled to or resided in the United Kingdom. This exclusion is intended to prevent the risk of new-variant Creutzfeldt-Jakob disease (nvCJD) transmission. Other diseases that require deferral of blood donation include the following:

- Syphilis
- Hepatitis B, C
- HIV
- Human T-lymphotropic virus (HTLV) 1 and 2
- Cytomegalovirus (CMV)
- Malaria
- Babesiosis
- Toxoplasmosis
- Chagas' disease
- Lyme disease
- Creutzfeldt-Jakob disease (and patients who have had injections of human pituitary hormone or human dura mater tissue implants)

Consequently, because of many transmissible disease issues, many patients prefer "directed donors." When blood replacement is anticipated before a surgical procedure, a family member or friend with a compatible blood type can be asked to donate blood to be held in the blood bank for the patient. Directed donations are not necessarily safer than nondirected voluntary donations supplied from the blood bank, however. When multiple units of blood must be transfused, packed cells, fresh frozen plasma, and platelets usually are given to supplement units of whole blood. These components are not part of whole blood replacement.

All established measures must be strictly observed for the patient's safety. The following basic rules apply to the transfusion of all allogenic blood products:

1. Blood products are obtained from the blood bank by a person responsible for signing them out to a specific patient.
2. To have blood nearby, a refrigerator with controlled temperature may be installed in the OR suite. Blood products for transfusion are kept at a constant temperature between 34° and 43° F (1° and 6° C), verified by a recording thermometer on the outside and a standard one inside. Both audible and visible alarms are activated if a dangerous temperature is reached. Fluctuations in temperature cause red blood cells to deteriorate. Microorganisms can multiply in unrefrigerated blood.

If blood is brought into the OR and not needed, it should be returned to the refrigerator in the suite or blood bank immediately. Do not allow whole blood or its derivatives to stand unrefrigerated in the OR. Before use, each blood product should be checked for the expiration date. Each product has a specific shelf life (Table 31-3).

3. Blood products are administered by a physician or nurse after a careful comparison of the label on the bag with the identity of the patient. A second professional person confirms the data. The label stays on the container while the blood product is being transfused.

4. Cold, refrigerated blood may induce hypothermia. Blood should be warmed as it is transfused by immersion of administration tubing in a controlled water bath or through coils in a temperature-modifying device. The temperature must be maintained between 89° and 105° F (32° and 41° C). Hemolysis may occur if the temperature exceeds 110° F (43° C).

5. Another solution may be infused immediately before a blood product is administered. In changing to the blood product, avoid the possibility of air entering tubing. A blood filter must be used for transfusion. The filter should be changed after the second or third unit of whole blood, because the filter can become clogged with microaggregates.

6. The anesthesia provider records on the anesthesia record the following information for each unit transfused:
   a. The name of the person who started the transfusion.
   b. The type and amount of product transfused (i.e., whole blood, plasma, packed cells, platelets, albumin).
   c. The time started and drops per minute.
   d. Information on the label, including the blood group, Rh factor, and number.

7. The patient is observed closely for any type of reaction. This probability increases in direct proportion to the number of units transfused. The most common type of reaction is allergic; febrile is almost as common, and hemolytic reactions are possible. Transfusion reactions with the patient under anesthesia may be accompanied by profound hypotension, temperature change, blood in urine, and/or skin rash. The common physical reactions and chills are not seen in an anesthetized patient. If any suspicious reactions occur:

a. Stop the transfusion. Keep the IV line patent with IV solution as directed by the physician.
b. Return unused blood to the blood bank along with a sample of the patient's blood.
c. Send a urine sample to the laboratory as soon as possible.
d. Take vital signs (temperature, pulse, respirations, blood pressure) every 5 to 10 minutes until the patient is stable.
e. Have emergency medications and resuscitation equipment available.
f. Document on the patient's chart the type of reaction, action taken, patient's response, and other documentation as required by the institution.

Autologous Blood. Autologous blood is blood recovered from the patient and reinfused. Referred to as autotransfusion, this process is the preferred method of replacement for either elective or emergency procedures. The patient's own blood is the safest form of transfusion; it eliminates concerns about compatibility/reactions and transmission of exogenous organisms. Autologous blood is equal or superior in quality to allogenic blood. It may be obtained preoperatively from patients and returned to them intraoperatively or postoperatively as needed.

Some patients who, because of religious beliefs, will not accept allogenic blood may accept autotransfusion in the form of cell salvage, red cell fractions, plasma fractions, white cell fractions, or platelet fractions. Jehovah's Witnesses,[1] for example, believe that receiving blood or blood products violates a biblical prohibition against consumption of blood. They have the right to refuse transfusion that should not be interpreted as a death wish. Some will accept blood fractions as a personal decision. Written informed consent should be obtained from all patients for whom autotransfusion or administration of blood fractions is contemplated.

Preoperative Blood Donation. One or more units of whole blood or blood components can be obtained by phlebotomy from the patient preoperatively and stored in the blood bank. Blood may be donated as often as every seventh day for a period of 6 weeks if the hemoglobin remains at least 11 g/dL or the hematocrit is 33%, with the final unit donated no less than 72 hours before the scheduled surgical procedure. If two or more units are donated, an oral or intramuscular iron supplement may be prescribed because as much as 10% of iron stores are lost with each donation. Epoetin alfa, a glycoprotein, can be administered subQ or IV for up to 6 weeks preoperatively to stimulate red blood cell production. Red blood cell stimulation can be continued postoperatively and is effective if iron stores are adequate. The patient's body replenishes the fluid lost in donation within 24 hours.

Autologous blood is usually stored in a liquid state as whole blood or packed red blood cells. Whole blood with anticoagulant can be stored for 35 days, and red blood cells with preservative for 42 days. Red blood cells and plasma

TABLE 31-3	**Shelf Life of Blood Products According to the American Association of Blood Banks**
Blood Products	**Shelf Life**
Red blood cells	42 days refrigerated
Frozen red blood cells	10 years
Platelets	5 days at room temperature
Fresh frozen plasma	1 year
Cryoprecipitated antihemophiliac factor	Frozen 1 year
Granulocytes	Transfuse within 24 hours of collection

---

[1] Genesis 9:3, 4: Leviticus 17:13, 14; Acts 15:19, 20. *New World translation of the Holy Scriptures*, 1970 C.E. Watch Tower Bible & Tract Society of Pennsylvania, USA.

can be frozen for prolonged storage. The same protocol is used in the OR for reinfusing autologous blood as described for allogenic transfusions. If the patient does not need reinfusion, the blood is discarded. It is not given to another patient.

Intraoperative Autotransfusion. Recovery of blood as it is lost requires sterile equipment that suctions blood from the surgical site, filters and anticoagulates it, and contains it for IV reinfusion to the patient with minimal damage to cells. Intraoperative blood salvage is widely used when potential blood loss may exceed 20% of the patient's blood volume. Blood can be suctioned directly from a body cavity or the wound. Any plastic devices, including suction tubing and pouches, used for blood recovery must be approved by the FDA.

Blood is not salvaged if microfibrillar collagen (Avitene) has been used for hemostasis. This may not wash out when red blood cells are processed and can predispose the patient to DIC or ARDS. Also, blood contaminated with enteric organisms or amniotic fluid is not salvaged. If a malignant tumor can be resected intact, autotransfusion may benefit the patient with cancer. Most cancer cells will filter out of processed blood. Autologous blood is not collected from patients with known systemic infections or from open traumatic wounds. Other patients, of all ages, are candidates for autotransfusion.

The autotransfusion unit must be easily and quickly assembled because it may be lifesaving for a trauma patient in an emergency situation. All fluid paths should be disposable and must be sterile. Three basic systems are used for intraoperative autotransfusion:

1. *Automated cell salvage processor:* Blood is suctioned through double-lumen tubing. An anticoagulant solution of heparinized saline or citrated dextrose mixes with blood at the tip end of the tubing. The aspirate passes through a 140-mm filter before entering the collection reservoir. This filter removes fat and debris. When a sufficient quantity to be processed has accumulated, the blood is pumped into a centrifuge bowl. The centrifugal force separates red blood cells from plasma, platelets, white blood cells, and other debris, including anticoagulant. These red blood cells are washed with normal saline solution. A suspension of red blood cells in saline solution is pumped into a reinfusion bag. Each bag contains about 250 mL of washed packed red blood cells with a hematocrit of 50% to 55%, ready for IV reinfusion. The entire cycle takes 3 to 7 minutes. Some autotransfusion units have automatic, programmed cycles, including process air and foam detectors; others operate manually. Platelet-rich plasma suitable for autotransfusion can be sequestered from some units.
2. *Canister collection method:* Blood is suctioned and anticoagulated as described for the cell processor. From the tubing, the blood collects in a reservoir with a disposable liner. When the reservoir becomes full, or at the end of the surgical procedure, the liner is removed. The contents are washed in a standard red blood cell washer before being reinfused. This equipment may be located in the blood bank. The liner must be labeled with the patient's name and identifying number if it leaves the OR for washing. Autologous blood obtained using this technique has a high hematocrit level and is almost free of protein, anticoagulant, and debris.
3. *Salvage collection bag:* An anticoagulant, usually citrate, is added to blood collected directly into a single-use, self-contained transfusion bag. The blood is not washed. It is reinfused through a blood filter. This simple method is most appropriate when profuse bleeding occurs in areas that form pools that can be easily suctioned, such as the abdominal or chest cavities.

All three methods are safe when used according to the manufacturer's instructions. The automated cell salvage devices are the most sophisticated and complex. Only properly trained personnel should operate them. OR personnel may be trained to set up the sterile suction and containers.

Postoperative Autotransfusion. Autologous blood may be collected, processed, and bagged during a surgical procedure for reinfusion postoperatively. Bags must be labeled with the name and identifying number of the patient and the time of processing. Autologous blood also can be salvaged postoperatively from a drainage tube placed into the surgical wound, most commonly a chest tube. The tube may be connected to a cell washer in a portable unit that attaches to wall suction in the PACU or ICU. Another method collects wound drainage by suctioning it directly into a filtered collection bag. With both of these methods, blood is anticoagulated. It may be collected for a maximum of 6 hours. The concentrated red blood cells, either washed or unwashed, are reinfused IV. Whether obtained intraoperatively or postoperatively, unwashed blood can be kept at room temperature for 4 hours, and washed blood can be kept for 6 hours at room temperature or refrigerated for 24 hours at 39.2° F (4° C).

Blood Substitutes. Oxygen-carrying blood substitutes offer another alternative for transporting oxygen. Oxygenation of body tissues is a serious issue when the patient's blood volume or hemoglobin level is decreased because of blood loss. These substitutes may be used in anemic patients, in people who refuse blood or blood products for religious reasons, or when compatible allogenic blood is not available. Examples of blood substitutes under investigation include:

- *Fluorovent:* Oxygen-carrying perfluorocarbon (PFC) can be used for preterm infants with underdeveloped lungs and in both adults and children with ARDS. It is a liquid instilled directly into the lungs to act as a surfactant. It encourages the exchange of oxygen and carbon dioxide. Patients with COPD may benefit from its use as well.
- *Oxycyte:* This IV form of PFC carries five times the amount of oxygen carried in hemoglobin. The oxygen-hemoglobin exchange ratio is extremely efficient, because the molecules are $\frac{1}{70}$ the size of a red blood cell and can reach tiny capillary surfaces. It can be stored at room temperature and requires no crossmatching.
- *Hemopure:* This bovine hemoglobin–based polymer solution has been used in clinical trials in the United States and Europe. It is stable for 2 years at room temperature and requires no crossmatching. It is given by IV infusion and is compatible with all blood types.

- *PolyHeme:* Human polymerized hemoglobin is processed from outdated human red blood cells. The product is screened for infectious disease, pasteurized, and polymerized. It is safe for use with any blood type. The shelf life is 12 months.
- *Oxyglobin:* This red blood cell alternative for veterinary services is compatible with all blood types.

Complications of Blood Loss or Replacement

The patient is constantly monitored to detect any complications that might be developing as a result of blood loss or replacement or as a compromise of the cardiovascular system. Hemorrhage can cause shock and DIC. Earlier PFC emulsions caused pulmonary complications, such as hyperinflated, noncollapsible lungs. Traces of older PFC emulsions can persist systemically and cause the threat of accumulation in fatty tissue. Accumulation could compromise developing neonatal nervous tissue, which has a high fatty content. Newer PFCs have been refined to have a shorter persistence period.

Early blood substitute products have been associated with gastrointestinal problems, coagulopathies, kidney and liver dysfunction, fever, and vasoconstriction. (More information is available at www.biopure.com or at www.sybd.com.)

SHOCK

Shock is a state of inadequate blood perfusion to parts of the body. If untreated, it will become irreversible and result in death. All forms of shock carry high mortality.

Hemorrhagic shock results from a decrease in circulating blood volume caused by loss of blood, plasma, or extracellular fluid. Fluid loss is excessive when it is greater than compensatory absorption of interstitial fluid into the circulation. Shock resulting from hemorrhage or inadequate blood volume replacement, as seen in the OR and PACU, usually is reversed by prompt restoration of circulating blood volume.

Shock is a complex phenomenon, a life-threatening condition in which circulation fails for one or several reasons. Loss of circulating blood volume, loss of the pumping power of the heart, or loss of peripheral resistance can result in insufficient flow of blood for adequate tissue perfusion or oxygenation. If it is prolonged, inadequate organ blood flow with deficient microcirculation profoundly depresses vital processes. Because the objective of circulation is achieved in the capillaries, defective cellular metabolism derived from shock interferes further with the body's inherent defenses, and metabolic acidosis occurs. Normal defense mechanisms are reflex vasoconstriction and increased pulse rate, which tend to redistribute the flow of blood to the heart and brain at the expense of the other vital organs. If shock is promptly recognized, treated, and reversed, permanent damage is avoided. If it progresses to irreversibility, death ensues from cellular dysfunction and organ hypoperfusion.

Multiple types and causes of shock present problems in relationships among the heart, circulatory system, and blood volume. Circulatory inadequacy may originate from a marked decrease in cardiac output, venous return to the heart, or peripheral vascular resistance. All forms of shock carry high mortality rates. The best treatment is prevention. Shock is classified according to the cause of inadequate tissue perfusion.

Hypovolemic Shock

Fluid loss is greater than compensatory absorption of interstitial fluid into the circulation.

Hemorrhagic Shock

Shock results from hemorrhage or inadequate blood volume replacement.

Cardiogenic Shock

The pumping action of the left ventricle is insufficient to pump enough blood to vital organs. Cardiogenic shock may be precipitated by congestive heart failure, myocardial contusion or infarction, coronary air embolism, mechanical venous obstruction, or hypothermia. In addition to drugs, various mechanical devices may be used, such as an auxiliary ventricle or counterpulsation with an intraaortic balloon pump (IABP) to temporarily increase left ventricular function.

Neurogenic Shock

Loss of vasomotor tone in peripheral blood vessels leads to sudden vasodilation and pooling of blood. Vasodilation produces hypotension. Peripheral resistance is too great for compensation by increased cardiac output, increasing the risk for congestive heart failure and pulmonary edema. Causes may be brain damage, deep anesthesia, emotional trauma, vagal reflex from pain or surgical manipulation, or spinal cord injury.

Traumatic Shock

Damage to the capillaries caused by soft tissue trauma increases capillary permeability, with loss of blood volume into the tissues. This state is aggravated by pain, which inhibits the vasomotor center, leading to vasodilation and hypovolemia. Toxic factors associated with intravascular coagulation lead to pulmonary, renal, and/or multiple organ failure.

Vasogenic Shock

Anaphylaxis and septic shock are the most common types of vasogenic shock.

METABOLIC CRISES
Convulsions

Convulsions occur most often in patients with a hyperactive metabolic rate, especially in dehydrated or febrile children. Anoxia and death can occur.

Etiology. Etiologic factors include severe hypoxia and carbon dioxide retention, hypernatremia, hyperthermia, overdose of regional anesthetic drugs, air embolism, and epilepsy.

Symptoms. Symptoms include muscular twitching, dilated pupils, rapid snorting respirations, rapid pulse, grimacing, and cyanosis.

Treatment. Oxygen is administered to maintain respiration, and diazepam, a rapid-acting barbiturate, or a neuromuscular blocker is given to stop muscular activity. Mechanical ventilation may be needed for apnea or to support circulation.

Prevention. Metabolic crises are prevented by maintaining normal body temperature and fluid and electrolyte balance.

Inadvertent Hypothermia

A decrease in the patient's core body temperature to below 96° F (35° C) can affect vasoconstriction and vasodilation, cardiac output, and renal function. Depending on the degree of body heat loss, hypothermia is categorized as follows:

- Mild (down to 90° F [32° C])
- Moderate (down to 85° F [30° C])
- Deep (down to 80° F [27° C])

If core temperature falls below 68° F (20° C), brain activity ceases. Patients can emerge from anesthesia with a body temperature below normal. Inadvertent hypothermia occurs spontaneously intraoperatively; it is not to be confused with induced hypothermia. Age-extreme, thin, and debilitated patients are most susceptible, as are patients undergoing neurosurgical, cardiovascular, thoracic, and abdominal procedures.

Etiology. Anesthesia inhibits the protective reflexes that generate body heat (i.e., shivering). It also depresses the thermoregulatory center in the hypothalamus, decreases the basal metabolic rate, and increases vasodilation for heat loss by radiation and conduction. Core body heat is lost by exposure to a cool external environment (e.g., during skin preparation) and through the surgical incision. Other factors include preoperative sedation, use of general versus regional anesthesia, adjunctive drugs, the length of the surgical procedure, blood and fluid loss and replacement, the room temperature, and evaporative loss through the skin and respiratory tract.

General anesthesia commonly causes a 1° to 1.5° F decrease in core temperature during the first hour, extending the action of propofol by 30%. The greatest risk for hypothermia is in the patient who has had combined general and epidural anesthesia. Protective central inhibition of the thermoregulatory center in the hypothalamus and peripheral nervous system is delayed.

Symptoms. Hypothermia can cause adverse cardiovascular, hematologic, immunologic, metabolic, and neurologic effects. Cardiac dysrhythmias, hypoxia, metabolic acidosis, hyperglycemia, and dilated pupils may be a result. A depressed central nervous system, which can lead to coma, may not be evident until the postoperative period. Shivering, impaired speech, muscle rigidity, peripheral or central cyanosis, a weak pulse, falling blood pressure, and dysrhythmias seen in the PACU may be symptoms of hypothermia. The incidence of ventricular tachycardia is doubled, causing an increased incidence of postoperative myocardial infarction.

Treatment. The hypothermic patient must be rewarmed as soon as possible. However, postanesthesia shivering during the rewarming process can be hazardous. Shivering is an involuntary rhythmic contraction of muscle groups with irregular and intermittent relaxation. This physiologic response to cold is activated when the hypothalamus senses that the core temperature has dropped. Some postanesthesia shivering is caused by anesthetic agents. Untreated shivering leads to increased oxygen consumption as a result of muscular activity and to increased cardiac stress as a result of hypoxia.

In the PACU a forced-air skin surface warmer (Bair Hugger) or an ultraviolet or infrared heat lamp directed at the lightly covered patient are effective means for raising the body temperature. A temperature-regulating hypothermia/hyperthermia machine, set at 104° to 107° F (40° to 42° C), may be used with a heated blanket beneath the patient. If warmers are not available, warm blankets placed over and underneath the patient should be changed at 15-minute intervals. Blankets can be heated to 105° F (40.5° C) for an adult or 100° F (38° C) for a small child or infant. The patient should wear a cap. Warmed humidified oxygen and IV fluid should be administered. Coniine (an alpha$_2$-adrenergic agonist) or analgesics such as meperidine or morphine derivative may suppress shivering.

Prevention. Prevention of hypothermia is the best treatment. Prevention begins before the patient arrives in the OR and continues during the procedure:

1. Place a hypothermia/hyperthermia mattress or reflective blanket on the operating bed. A radiant heat source can be placed over an infant.
2. Check the room temperature and humidity.
3. Apply warmed blankets as soon as the patient arrives in the OR and immediately after drapes are removed. A warm blanket can be put on the stretcher under the patient.
4. Limit skin exposure during positioning and skin preparation (i.e., keep the patient covered as much as possible).
5. Minimize the time of exposure between skin antisepsis and draping.
6. Keep the sheet under and the drapes over the patient and around the surgical site dry to provide insulation, prevent heat loss, and maintain asepsis. Dry the area after skin preparation.
7. Warm antiseptic, irrigating, and IV solutions, including blood, before administration. Anesthetic gases, including oxygen, can be warmed also.
8. Monitor body temperature.
9. Leave a cap on the patient; a plastic head covering retains more heat than do other materials.

Malignant Hyperthermia

Malignant hyperthermia (MH) is a hypermetabolic crisis in susceptible people. It is triggered by potent halogenated anesthetic agents and depolarizing skeletal muscle relaxants. MH, a potentially fatal complication of anesthesia, is characterized by uncontrolled acceleration of muscle metabolism accompanied by tremendous oxygen consumption and production of heat and carbon dioxide. The body temperature can rapidly rise at a rate of 1.8° F (1° C) every 5 minutes if MH is untreated. A temperature as high as 117° F (47° C) has been recorded, but 111.2° F (44° C) is probably highest with survival. The survival rate with appropriate treatment is between 80% and 90%. The mortality rate without appropriate treatment is around 90%; thus MH is of significant concern.

Etiology. The exact cause of MH is unknown. It is understood that certain patients are susceptible, and some anesthetic agents may trigger this crisis.

Susceptible Patients. A familial genetic transmission exists as an autosomal dominant trait with variable multifactor inheritance patterns. The genetic defect manifests by increasing calcium levels in skeletal muscles. The crisis results from a hereditary inability of the sarcoplasmic reticulum, a skeletal muscle cell membrane, to control intramyoplasmic levels of calcium. Skeletal muscle undergoes contraction as a result of release of calcium ions in response to drugs or stress. A rapid increase of calcium in muscle fiber leads to generalized catabolism. As biochemical reactions occur, the body produces heat and carbon dioxide.

Susceptible patients also include those with any type of myopathy or acquired muscle disease, such as ptosis, strabismus, hernia, muscle weakness or hypertrophy, or muscular dystrophy. The incidence of MH is higher in children than in adults. Patients, especially children, with rheumatoid arthritis are particularly susceptible to MH. MH may occur in a patient's first exposure to anesthesia or in a later one; one third of reported cases of MH have occurred in a second or subsequent anesthesia.

Triggers. Several agents may trigger this abnormal hypermetabolic response in susceptible individuals. Succinylcholine, halothane, enflurane, desflurane, and isoflurane are the main triggers of MH.

Symptoms. Clinical signs and symptoms occur according to the swiftness of onset. The onset may be rapid, occurring immediately after induction, or may occur after several hours of general anesthesia or even in the postoperative recovery period.

Spasm of the jaw muscles with rigidity of the masseter muscles (trismus) or severe fasciculation after succinylcholine administration may suggest MH development to the anesthesia provider, although this activity is not uncommon in pediatric patients.

The most common presenting sign of MH is unexplained ventricular dysrhythmia, primarily tachycardia or PVCs. This is associated with an unexplained increase in end-tidal carbon dioxide, tachypnea, cyanosis, skin mottling, and unstable blood pressure. Blood in the surgical field may appear dark as a result of central venous desaturation.

When a sudden, generalized hypermetabolic state is produced, the temperature rises rapidly as more heat is produced than the body can eliminate. This is not a first sign. Elevated temperature may be a late sign or may be absent in MH syndrome. Fever, hot skin or tissues, and diaphoresis are symptoms of heat buildup. A favorable prognosis decreases when excessive heat in the tissues is noted through the surgeon's gloves or when the anesthesia provider senses heat in the reservoir bag or soda lime canister on the anesthesia machine. The body tries to adjust by vasodilation and increased cardiac output.

If rapidly increasing tissue demands are not met, hypoxia, central venous hypercapnia, and severe respiratory and metabolic acidosis occur, progressing to cardiovascular collapse. Blood tests will reveal increased serum levels of potassium, magnesium, creatine phosphokinase (CPK), and myoglobin. Excessive myoglobin release caused by rapid muscle destruction (rhabdomyolysis) can cause renal failure and lead to anuria.

Late clinical findings include hyperkalemia; acute renal failure; left-sided heart failure; DIC; skeletal muscle swelling or necrosis from hypoxia and acidosis; pulmonary edema; neurologic sequelae, including paraplegia and decerebration; and coma from ischemia secondary to hypoxia. Recurrence of MH crisis can occur 24 to 72 hours postoperatively.

Monitoring. Parameters and studies to be monitored routinely in patients at risk for MH who undergo general anesthesia are heart rate and rhythm, blood pressure, core temperature by esophageal probe, pulse oximetry, capnometry, nerve stimulation to measure the level of muscle relaxation, and precordial stethoscopy. A rise in temperature greater than 0.5° F per hour should raise suspicion of MH.

Treatment. Success is contingent on complete preparedness (preplanned action, written protocol, immediate equipment supply), early diagnosis, and vigorous therapy. The following treatment outline is the suggested protocol established by the Malignant Hyperthermia Association of the United States (MHAUS). (Emergency therapy wall charts can be ordered from the organization by calling the nonemergency telephone number [800] 986-4287 or online at www.mhaus.org.) Institutional policies and procedures should be in place as follows to guide the perioperative team in caring for a patient in MH crisis:

1. Discontinue inhalant anesthesia and stop the surgical procedure immediately. The anesthesia provider immediately institutes hyperventilation with 100% oxygen at a high flow rate of at least 10 L/min. Research has shown that the breathing circuit and anesthesia delivery machine need not be changed because the high concentration of oxygen delivery clears the machine of anesthetic gases very rapidly. If the surgical procedure cannot be interrupted, safe agents may be employed to maintain anesthesia during the stabilization period.
2. Immediately start drug therapy. Administer:
   a. Dantrolene sodium (Dantrium IV), 2 to 3 mg/kg in an initial IV bolus and repeat every 5 to 10 minutes until the maximum dose of 10 mg/kg is given or the MH episode is controlled. Patients generally respond to the drug quickly. The onset of action is usually 2 to 3 minutes. Occasionally doses higher than 10 to 20 mg/kg are needed.

   Dantrolene is a specific drug for treatment of MH. It directly blocks accumulation of calcium within the muscles by preventing its release from the sarcoplasmic reticulum and by uncoupling excitation-contraction, thus relaxing skeletal muscle. It has no effect on cardiovascular or respiratory functions. Calcium channel blockers may not be given with dantrolene because they may cause hyperkalemia, myocardial depression, and cardiovascular collapse. Verapamil is contraindicated.

   Given IV, dantrolene is supplied in 70-mL vials as a sterile, lyophilized powder that contains 20 mg of dantrolene and 3 g of mannitol. Each vial must be reconstituted before use with 60 mL of sterile water for injection without a preservative agent. The large quantities of sterile water that are needed would contain the preservative agent in toxic amounts. A semiautomatic fluid-dispensing syringe expedites mixing. If this is not available, additional personnel should help with the reconstitution process because large quantities of the diluted drug will be needed and each vial will require vigorous shaking to mix. The solution will be yellow-orange when mixed. In extreme circumstances the drug may be given through a filter to remove particulate from the solution. Once reconstituted, dantrolene must be used within 6 hours and must be protected from exposure to light.

If other IV solutions have been running, the line should be flushed with sterile water before dantrolene is injected; this will prevent precipitation. Do not use Ringer's lactate solution, because it will increase the level of acidosis. An additional IV site should be established to infuse iced normal saline solution at the rate of 15 mL/kg every 15 minutes for at least 45 minutes.

Dantrolene is continued postoperatively at a minimum of 1 mg/kg every 6 hours for 24 to 72 hours postepisode. After the initial 48 hours, 1 mg/kg every 6 hours may be given orally for 24 hours. No serious side effects have been reported with short-term use, but muscle weakness may be evident for 24 to 48 hours after administration. A few isolated reports of nausea, vomiting, and fatigue have been documented. Prolonged administration may lead to hepatotoxicity.

b. Procainamide (Pronestyl), 15 mg/kg diluted in 500 mL physiologic saline solution IV over 60 minutes. Procainamide treats cardiac dysrhythmia if required.

c. Sodium bicarbonate, 1 to 2 mEq/kg IV stat and repeat as guided by blood gas analysis. An alkali, sodium bicarbonate raises pH temporarily. It combats acidosis and antagonizes hyperkalemia by lowering the plasma potassium level. It can cause rebound acidosis. Monitoring of arterial pH and Pco_2 is necessary to determine subsequent doses.

d. Regular insulin, 10 units in 50 mL of 50% dextrose in water IV. Insulin offsets the high glucose metabolic demands and improves glucose uptake. It shifts potassium back into the cells to help treat hyperkalemia. Blood glucose and potassium levels must be monitored.

e. Calcium chloride, 2.5 mg/kg, to treat severe cardiac toxicity caused by hyperkalemia.

f. Mannitol, 0.25 g/kg IV, and furosemide (Lasix), 1 mg/kg IV, up to four doses each. These drugs dislodge myoglobin from the renal tubules and sustain urinary flow. Urinary output greater than 2 mL/kg/hr must be maintained to prevent renal failure. The dose is calculated in consideration of the mannitol contained in the dantrolene solution.

3. Begin active cooling. Administer refrigerated or iced normal saline IV. Lavage the stomach and rectum. Avoid irrigating the bladder if at all possible, because accurate measurement of urinary output and urinalysis is important. If the peritoneal or thoracic cavity is open, cool sterile saline may be poured into the opening. Cool the body surface by placing the patient on a plastic sheet and applying ice bags and ice water, or use a hypothermia blanket. If readily available, use extracorporeal perfusion apparatus for partial (femoral-to-femoral) cardiopulmonary bypass to cool the viscera. Body temperature must be carefully monitored to avoid accidental cooling to dysrhythmic levels. Medication may be given to limit shivering, normally a heat-retaining mechanism that also increases oxygen consumption. Surface cooling is considered more effective in children because of their high ratio of surface area to body volume. Cooling that is too vigorous can result in inadvertent hypothermia and cardiac arrest. To avoid hypothermia, cooling should be discontinued when the core temperature reaches 100° F (38° C).

4. Correct the electrolyte imbalance on the basis of blood sampling of electrolytes, pH, and blood gases. After the presumed onset of MH, an arterial line must be established if one is not already in place. Blood samples are taken at 10-minute intervals for pH, Pco_2, Po_2, sodium, potassium, chlorides, calcium, magnesium, and phosphate. Hypocalcemia and hyperkalemia followed by hypokalemia may be expected.

Also measured are CPK, aspartate aminotransferase (AST, formerly serum glutamic-oxaloacetic transaminase [SGOT]), alkaline phosphatase, and lactate dehydrogenase for indication of muscle destruction. Blood urea nitrogen (BUN) for kidney function, bilirubin for liver function, coagulation studies, blood lactate and pyruvate, and serum thyroxine levels may be ordered.

5. CVP should be monitored. A CVP line may need to be inserted if one is not already in place.

6. Urinary output is monitored via an indwelling Foley catheter. In addition to the measurement of volume, urine is sampled for hemoglobin and myoglobin. The urine may be brown as the amount of hemoglobin and myoglobin increases.

Supplies for Malignant Hyperthermia. Supplies should be kept in a specific location and must be immediately available for both adult and pediatric patients. A cart marked for use in MH is convenient. Supplies that may be needed include the following:

1. Monitors, including ECG, electronic temperature probes, recorder

2. IV equipment, including blood administration sets and pumps; CVP line setup; IV solutions—12 bags, 1000 mL each, of physiologic saline kept in a refrigerator

3. Arterial line setup

4. Intubation equipment

5. Ice chips and plastic bags, hypothermia blankets

6. Gastric lavage set, three-way indwelling catheter for insertion into the rectum, 50-mL syringes

7. Blood sampling and arterial blood gas equipment

8. Indwelling Foley catheter, urometer bag

9. Drugs:

   a. Thirty-six 20-mg vials of dantrolene sodium (the quantity needed to treat and stabilize a 70-kg adult)

   b. Thirty-six 60-mL vials of sterile water without a preservative agent to reconstitute dantrolene (the quantity needed for a 70-kg adult is 2100 mL)

   c. Five 100-mL prefilled syringes of sodium bicarbonate 5%

   d. Six 1-g ampules of procainamide

  e. Ten 50-mL vials of 20% mannitol
  f. Four 2-mL (20-mg) prefilled syringes of furosemide
  g. One 100-unit vial of regular insulin
  h. Two 50-mL vials of 50% dextrose in water
  i. Three 1000-unit vials of heparin
  j. Ten 250-mg vials of hydrocortisone sodium succinate (Solu-Cortef)
10. Associated needles and syringes
11. Extracorporeal perfusion apparatus if available
12. Defibrillator machine and electrodes

Prevention. Identification of susceptible patients is the best prevention. The preoperative history should routinely include questions about the patient's previous anesthesia experiences, unexplained incidents or death of family members who underwent anesthesia, and known muscular abnormalities or episodes of heatstroke in the patient or relatives. Hereditary predisposition has been detected in three generations; however, the patient's family history frequently is not known.

The most prominent clue to identification of a patient susceptible to MH is a family history of unexplained death while under general anesthesia. Genetic counseling of the patient and family is advised. Although the crisis usually occurs when the patient is under general anesthesia, it can occur during periods of emotional or physical stress. Susceptible people should wear a Medic-Alert bracelet or tag.

Diagnosis of susceptibility to MH can be accomplished by preoperative muscle biopsy. A 1-g specimen of skeletal muscle is excised from the thigh with the patient under local anesthesia. The specimen is removed from the muscle as a strip and outstretched between the prongs of a double-tipped clamp. Evaluation of the muscle response to caffeine-induced contracture during exposure to halothane reveals sensitivity. Although a local anesthetic is used to obtain the muscle biopsy, dantrolene should be readily available in the unlikely event of an episode of MH.

The blood CPK level may be elevated in susceptible patients, but it can also be influenced by alcohol consumption or strenuous exercise. A normal CPK level does not ensure absence of the MH trait. Nuclear magnetic resonance imaging using phosphorus also may detect susceptibility, but it is not always a reliable indicator.

Prophylaxis. Dantrolene may be given preoperatively to susceptible patients. The suggested dose is 1-mg/kg increments every 4 to 6 hours orally up to a total dose of 4 mg/kg, followed by 2.5 mg/kg IV 30 minutes before induction of general anesthesia. Intraoperative monitoring is mandatory. When nontriggering anesthetic agents are used, prophylactic dantrolene therapy may be unnecessary. Each patient should be evaluated individually. Some indications for dantrolene prophylaxis may include the following:

• Previous history of suspected MH episode
• Family history of MH (actual or suspected)
• Known MH susceptibility
• Prolonged procedure anticipated in an MH-susceptible patient
• Underlying disease or physiology causing suspicion of MH susceptibility

Nontriggering anesthetic agents should be administered to MH-susceptible individuals. Barbiturates, benzodiazepines, and narcotics are considered safe. Nitrous oxide by inhalation or IV propofol or ketamine hydrochloride can be administered for general anesthesia. Most of the synthetic nondepolarizing neuromuscular blockers are safe muscle relaxants. Amino amide and ester agents can be used safely for local anesthesia.

Postoperatively the patient should be continuously monitored in the ICU for 24 to 48 hours. If the vital signs remain stable during this time, the patient may be discharged. (More information is available from MHAUS at www.mhaus.org.)

PHYSIOLOGIC INJURY

Physiologic injuries are many and varied. The anesthesia provider may inadvertently loosen teeth or damage dental work during endotracheal intubation. Nerves can be injured from faulty positioning, such as hyperabduction or extension of the arm. Pressure sores may develop on poorly padded areas. Fingers and body parts can be pinched in table flexures. Careless handling of an anesthetized patient can result in paralysis, fractures, or postoperative pain.

Eyes can be injured from irritating anesthetics or face masks or from drying or scratching of the cornea if the eyelids are not closed. Patients with protruding eyes, faces covered by drapes, or those in prone positions are at high risk for eye injury. Use of an ocular lubricant protects the cornea from drying, and taped eyelids prevent corneal abrasions.

Extravasation, thrombophlebitis, and air emboli are associated with IV infusions. IV cannulas should be visible and not entirely hidden beneath drapes; infusions should be checked frequently. Precaution is the best prevention of injuries.

Bibliography

Chavez J, Brewer C: Stopping the shock slide, *RN* 65(9):30-35, 2002.
Fowler R, Pepe PE: Fluid resuscitation of the patient with major trauma, *Curr Opin Anesthesiol* 15(2):173-178, 2002.
Gannon CJ, Napolitano LM: Severe anemia after gastrointestinal hemorrhage in a Jehovah's Witness: New treatment strategies, *Crit Care Med* 30(8):1893-1895, 2002.
Hariharan S, Zbar A: Risk scoring in perioperative and surgical intensive care patients: A review. *Curr Surg* 63(3):226-236, 2006.
Haslego SS: Malignant hyperthermia: how to spot it early, RN 65(7):31-36, 2002.
Kasai T et al: Preoperative risk factors of intraoperative hypothermia in major surgery under general anesthesia, *Anesth Analg* 95(5):1381-1383, 2002.
Kehlet H, Wimore DW: Multimodal strategies to improve surgical outcome, *Am J Surg* 183(6):630-641, 2002.
Marcario A, Dexter F: What are the most important risk factors for a patient's developing intraoperative hypothermia? *Anesth Analg* 94(1):215-220, 2002.
Menon V, Hochman J: Management of cardiogenic shock complicating acute myocardial infarction, *Heart* 88(5):531-537, 2002.
Moss R: Inadvertent perioperative hypothermia, *AORN J* 67(2):460, 462-463, 1998.
Phillips N: Malignant hyperthermia: update 2000, *Crit Care Nurs Clin North Am* 12(2):199-210, 2000.
Sprung J et al: The use of bovine hemoglobin glutamer-250 in surgical patients, *Anesth Analg* 94(4):799-808, 2002.
Strong RM, Chance N: Building a bloodless medicine and surgery program, *SSM* 6(2):38-42, 2000.
Tarrac SE: A description of intraoperative and postoperative complication rates, *J Perianesth Nurs* 21(2):88-96, 2006.
Traber DL: Fluid resuscitation after hypovolemia, *Crit Care Med* 30(8):1922, 2002.
Trovarelli T et al: Transfusion-free surgery is a treatment plan for all patients, *AORN J* 68(5):773-776, 778, 780-784, 1998.

Endoscopy and Robotic-Assisted Surgery

CHAPTER OBJECTIVES

After studying this chapter, the learner will be able to:
- Describe the difference between rigid and flexible endoscopy.
- List the eight essential elements necessary for all endoscopy.
- Identify three potential hazards of puncture endoscopy.
- List three considerations for patient safety during endoscopy.

CHAPTER OUTLINE

KEY TERMS AND DEFINITIONS

Endoscopy   Examination of a body part or cavity with an optical system in a tubular structure.
Insufflation   Act of filling with gas. Laparoscopy is performed with carbon dioxide.
Laparoscopy   Endoscopic examination of the peritoneal body cavity through a percutaneous access portal, placement of expansion medium to create a working space, and manipulation of intraabdominal organs.
Pelviscopy   Laparoscopy of the pelvis.
Percutaneous   Puncture through the skin.
Pneumoperitoneum   The peritoneal cavity is filled with gas.
Trocar   Surgical instrument that consists of a sheath with a sharp obturator used to puncture or penetrate multiple layers of tissue. The sheath remains in place as the obturator is removed. Additional instrumentation is passed through the sheath. Blunt styles are available.
Veress needle   Spring-loaded needle that delivers CO_2 for the creation of a pneumoperitoneum.

SUPPLEMENTAL MATERIAL ON EVOLVE WEBSITE

evolve

http://evolve.elsevier.com/BerryKohn
- Content Updates
- Glossary
- Full Set of Perioperative Flash Cards
- Interactive Key Term Flash Cards
- Tips for the Scrub Person and Circulating Nurse: Flexible, Rigid, Laparoscopy
- Student Activities
- WebLinks

HISTORICAL BACKGROUND

Although physicians sought to visualize the interior of body organs, development of endoscopy was slow. Early scopes were used as specula for natural body orifices. Hippocrates described the use of a rectal speculum, and his contemporaries were using vaginal specula. Archigenes from Syria developed a vaginal speculum and wrote instructions about patient positioning for best use of the instrument. This concept was embellished when Arabian physician Abulkasim (AD 936-1013) used a series of mirrors to enhance illumination.

Endoscopy began to take on new meaning in the early 1800s when Philip Bozzini (1773-1809) developed the Lichtleiter, which was a modified light conductor made of mirrors, tin, and leather. The illumination source was a candle. It was the forerunner of the modern endoscope. Around 1853 Antonin Desormeaux (1815-1881) introduced a cystoscope that burned alcohol and turpentine for illumination. He had considered electricity but thought the fuel-burning model was more portable. A few years later, Julius Bruck, a dentist, developed the first internal light source made of looped platinum wire heated to glowing brightness by electricity. The risks were inherent because surrounding structures were frequently burned by the intense heat. He did develop a series of water-cooling covers, but these increased the size of the device and made it awkward to handle.

It was not until the early nineteenth century that Austrian urologist Maximilian Nitze (1848-1906) developed a urologic instrument that became the basis of modern endoscopy.

He used the light source model developed by Bruck and, with the help of an optician, fashioned a tri-lensed endoscope that allowed a greater field of vision with an internal illumination source. By 1880 medical catalogs featured his cystoscope. Thomas Edison's invention of the incandescent lightbulb revolutionized the whole concept of internal illumination for endoscopy, and by 1886 miniature lightbulbs were placed in cystoscopes for use in internal bladder inspection.

Dr. Chevalier Jackson of Philadelphia further enhanced endoscopy by developing a laryngoscope and bronchoscope. Endoscopic inspection of the human abdominal cavity, introduced in 1902, was augmented in 1910 by Swedish surgeon Hans Christian Jacobaeus (1879-1937) when he introduced the concept of creating a working space by insufflating air into the peritoneum and viewed the abdominal contents with a Nitze cystoscope.

The first use of carbon dioxide (CO_2) as a means of creating a working space was described around 1924 by Richard Zollikofer of Switzerland. He demonstrated that CO_2 was not explosive in the abdomen and was readily absorbed without event. This was later supported in the literature by German surgeon Roger Korbsh. He found that the intraabdominal pressure should be kept at 15 cm H_2O or lower to avoid physiologic complications associated with pressure on the diaphragm. The delivery of CO_2 into the peritoneal cavity was initially done via the sheath for the cystoscope. However, around 1938 a spring-loaded needle, which had been developed by Hungarian surgeon Janos Veress for the purpose of draining ascites, was used. This needle, referred to as the Veress needle, is still the preferred method of insufflation. Because CO_2 is nonflammable, tubal sterilization by electrocoagulation was possible in the 1950s and was made popular by gynecologic surgeons Raoul Palmer from France and Frangenheim from Germany.

In the 1960s Professor Harold Hopkins developed the rod-lens system of rigid scopes in England. He went to Germany to work with Karl Storz on his prototype, and the fiberoptic system for illumination was born. Color photography of the body's internal surface could now be performed clearly.

EIGHT ESSENTIAL ELEMENTS OF ENDOSCOPY

Endoscopic technology, regardless of whether it is performed with a rigid scope or a flexible scope, has eight elements in common: access portal, working space, illumination, vision, manipulation, capture, evacuation, and closure (Box 32-1). These essentials of endoscopy are described in more detail as follows:

Access Portal into the Body

1. Natural orifice or functional stoma.
   a. Oral, nasal, vaginal, anal, urethral. Some rigid scopes have an obturator (a blunt-tipped rod placed through the lumen) to permit smooth insertion of the instrument, such as into the anus.
   b. Ear canal.
2. Puncture or incision: Placement of the initial devices to introduce the expansion medium for creation of the working space requires interruption of the body's intact surface.

BOX 32-1	Eight Essentials of Endoscopy
Access portal	Natural orifice or percutaneous puncture
Working space	Fluid, gas, or positional expansion to accommodate instrumentation
Illumination	Fiberoptics or incandescent bulb
Vision	Direct or indirect viewing with lens or camera
Manipulation	Tissue grasping, debulking, and dissection
Capture	Collection of specimens
Evacuation	Remove gases, plume, or fluid
Closure	Suturing, stapling, or minimizing the access portal

a. Multiple sites based on the type of cavity or space and the location of landmarks and blood supply.
   (1) Open method: An incision is made into the skin and a 5- to 10-mm blunt Hasson trocar and sheath are placed into the cavity or space. Expansion medium can be placed through a port into the cavity or space. This procedure may be used for the patient who has many adhesions or has had multiple previous surgeries.
   (2) Closed method: A tiny nick is incised into the skin, and a Veress spring-loaded needle is placed through the skin into the cavity for the delivery of an expansion medium such as a fluid or gas.
b. Access devices for insufflation and creation of a working space.
   (1) Veress needle: A tiny 1- to 2-mm nick is made with the scalpel at the inferior edge of the umbilicus. The Veress needle is inserted by blind puncture through the skin into the abdominal cavity. This needle has an exterior sharp bevel and an interior spring-loaded obturator that displaces as it passes through tissue. The valve key on the top should be closed for insertion. As the sharp bevel passes through the tissue layers, the rounded obturator snaps forward to guard against inadvertent punctures of nontarget tissue. Slight popping noises are made by the needle and spring mechanism as the needle passes through each layer. The last sound is the peritoneal perforation.
      Some surgeons test intraabdominal placement of the Veress needle by placing a drop of saline onto the Luer-Lok and opening the valve key. The saline is sucked into the aperture of the needle by the negative force of the closed peritoneal cavity. The CO_2 tubing can be connected for insufflation of a working space when the surgeon is reasonably assured that the Veress needle tip is in the correct space.
      (a) One-hand placement: The surgeon grasps and lifts the lower abdominal segment midway between the umbilicus and the superior margin of the pubis. As the abdomen is raised, the surgeon directs the Veress needle through the tissue layers.
      (b) Two-hand placement: The surgeon and the first assistant grasp the abdominal tissue on either side of the umbilicus and lift. The

surgeon introduces the Veress needle through the abdominal wall into the peritoneal cavity.

  (2) Trocar and sheath (sleeve): A trocar consists of a sharp or blunt obturator and a sheath or sleeve. Some sheaths have ports with key valves for instillation of fluids or gases. The trocars are inserted with the key valve closed.

    (a) Sharp trocar

      (1) Pyramidal or conical tip: Describes the configuration of the tip.

      (2) Shielded: A spring-loaded shield drops down and protects the sharp tip of the trocar when it is not actively cutting through tissue. Studies have shown that this mechanism does not necessarily reduce the incidence of trocar-induced punctures.

    (b) Blunt trocar: The trocar is rounded. The trocar and sheath are introduced through a small infraumbilical incision. The sheath has graduated threads that permit the device to create a seal when placed through the abdominal layers. Insufflation for creation of a working space is performed through the key valve. A Veress needle is not used.

    (c) Dilating sleeve: The initial trocar/obturator and primary sleeve are small diameter (between 1.9 and 2.1 mm) and are introduced through a small nick in the inferior aspect of the umbilicus. The trocar is rigid, and the sheath is a flexible plastic meshwork with a stopcock for insufflation of the pneumoperitoneum.

      As the initial trocar is removed, larger-diameter instrumentation can be introduced through the radially dilating sleeve, causing it to dilate or "step up." The texture of the sleeve expands to accommodate larger diameters. The skin puncture stretches and forms a seal around the access portal, anchoring it in position. The fascial puncture can be stretched to accommodate 12-mm instrumentation. The wounds measure around 4 mm when the sleeve is withdrawn and rarely need closure with suture.

  c. Secondary insertion of accessory trocars for manipulation within the working space. Additional trocars and sleeves may be used in a triangular position around the umbilicus or primary trocar. Instrumentation for manipulation and capture is placed though these ports.

Working Space Within the Body

1. Structural working space.

  a. Abdominal lift device for creation of a gasless working space. No expansion media used. The working space is somewhat smaller than that created from gas insufflation. The bowel is not compressed and may be distended. Care is taken when placing the abdominal lift hooks so as not to snare the omentum or bowel. The lift devices are sometimes difficult to remove without ensnaring abdominal contents. Trocar insertion is sometimes difficult because there is no back pressure or resistance to the force of placement. Blind puncture is not commonly used.

An expandable balloon can be used to bluntly dissect and separate the abdominal wall from the abdominal contents for instrumentation placement. It takes some of the pressure off the actual lift device as it pulls upward on the abdominal wall.

    (1) Linear lift requires a frame such as an arc above the patient that attaches to a cable system placed through the patient's abdominal wall. The shape of the working space may be irregular.

    (2) Planar lift uses a corkscrew-like hook or a fanlike retractor that is placed through the abdominal wall and suspended from an articulating arm attached to a frame on the operating bed. The shape of the working space is more trapezoid than domed like a pneumoperitoneum.

  b. Physiologic muscularity or structural framework, such as cartilage in the trachea and bronchus.

  c. Speculum support between muscular layers such as the vaginal speculum or anoscope.

2. Expansion media.

  a. Fluid: The bladder, uterus, and joint spaces can be expanded with fluid to create a working space.

  b. Gas: The peritoneal cavity is filled with CO_2 gas, creating a gas lake called a pneumoperitoneum, before a laparoscope is inserted through the abdominal wall. The pneumoperitoneum expands the abdomen and provides a working space (Fig. 32-1). With the tip of a scalpel, a small incision (1 to 2 mm) is made into the abdominal wall at the infraumbilical margin. A special spring-loaded Veress needle measuring 120 to 150 cm is inserted through the tiny incision at the thinnest portion of the abdominal wall. The CO_2 is delivered by an insufflator, which is a specially designed machine that allows a metered flow between 6 and 9.9 L/min of gas at a controlled pressure of between 12 and 18 mm Hg.

    The gas passes through sterile disposable tubing with an inline, single-use hydrophobic filter that prevents particulate matter and condensation from entering the abdominal cavity. It filters particulate as small as 0.2 micron. The insufflator should be positioned higher than the patient's abdomen for maximum performance. If the cylinder is placed below the level of the patient, the pressure gradient on the patient's side increases, causing a backflow of biologic contaminants into the insufflator. As a result, the internal aspect of the insufflation machine can become biologically contaminated. This can be the source of cross-contamination between patients.

    The gas itself is not sterile and is delivered to the body cold, around 23° C when not passed through a heating and humidifying element. Studies have shown less hypothermia in patients when the gas is delivered at temperatures between 86° F and 95° (30° and 30.5° C). The patient is at risk for hypothermia if core body temperature is less than 36° C. Studies have shown a decrease of 32° F (0.3° C) body temperature for each 50 L of CO_2 cycled through the patient.

    Once the pneumoperitoneum is established, a 10- or 12-mm trocar is inserted and the insufflation

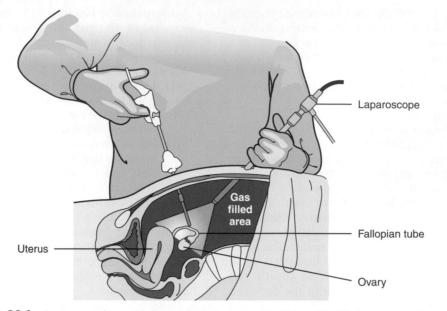

FIG. 32-1   Surgeon working with laparoscopic instruments within a CO_2-filled pneumoperitoneum.

tubing is attached to a port on the side of the trocar sleeve. A secondary 5- or 7-mm trocar with a gas port will be inserted.

c. Air: Ambient room air can be delivered into a natural body orifice by a hand pump bulb or machine to expand the lumen of the bowel for sigmoidoscopy or colonoscopy.

d. Balloon expansion between tissue planes: A balloon device can be inserted between tissue layers and expanded with saline to separate and bluntly open the preperitoneal plane of dissection. After blunt dissection and expansion, the balloon is deflated and withdrawn. The space is then insufflated. This is useful for laparoscopic hernia repair procedures. Saphenous vein harvests and spinal surgery can be performed using this method (Fig. 32-2).

Illumination of the Working Space

Illumination within the body cavity is essential for visual acuity. The light source may be through a fiberoptic bundle or, rarely, from an incandescent lightbulb. The light carrier may be an integral part of the viewing sheath, as in flexible scopes and rigid telescopes, or it may be a separate light carrier accessory to a hollow rigid scope. The power source is usually electricity, but some handheld rigid scopes can use batteries.

1. Fiberoptic light: With fiberoptic lighting, an intense cool light illuminates body cavities, including those that cannot be seen with other light sources. Light is conducted through a bundle of thousands of coated glass fibers encased in a plastic sheath attached to a light source generator. Each fiber is drawn from optical glass into a strand 10 to 70 mm in diameter that is coated to minimize loss of light by reflection. Light entering one end of the fiber is transmitted by refraction through its entire length.

    The light produced through the bundle of fibers is nonglaring and evenly distributed on the area to be visualized. Although it is of high intensity, the light is cool. A minimal rise of temperature in the tissues exposed to it may occur. Although the light inside the patient is cool, the cable should not be allowed to lie on the drapes because it is a potential source of ignition.

    Both ends of the fiberoptic cable must have the correct fittings to attach to the lamp and to the scope or removable light carrier. The diameter of the cable varies from 2 to 5.5 mm to be compatible with the aperture for the light source. Cable lengths also vary from 6 feet (180 cm) to 9 feet (275 cm), so the projection lamp can be positioned at a distance from a sterile field. Before use, the fiberoptic cable should be checked for damage. One end of the cable is held toward a low-power light, such as the overhead operating light. With a magnifying glass, the opposite end is examined. Broken fibers in the cable will appear as dark spots, even to the naked eye. The cable should be replaced if more than 20% of the area appears dark.

    A xenon, quartz-halogen, or halide lightbulb provides an intense light source for transmission of light through a fiberoptic bundle to the distal end of the scope. Usually a portable, compact, self-contained unit, the light has an intensity that may be regulated from 400 foot-candles to as much as 5200 foot-candles, and up to 5500 Kelvin daylight in some illuminators.

2. Other.

    a. Incandescent bulbs screw into the fitting either at the end of a removable light carrier or at the end of a built-in lens system. Electric current is conducted through a single-filament wire to illuminate the tiny incandescent lightbulb. Very few instruments use this lighting system. Older-model rigid laryngoscopes are an example.

    b. Indirect lighting is used with specula, such as vaginal, nasal, or anal.

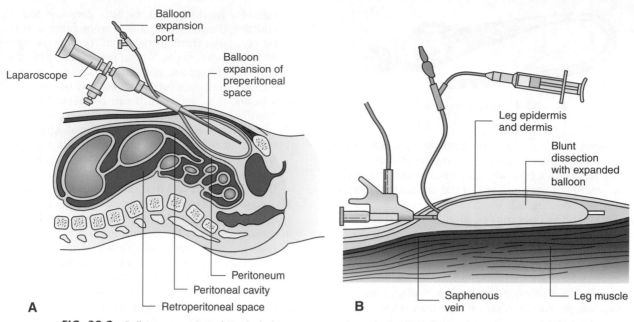

FIG. 32-2   Balloon expansion of surgical planes. **A,** Preperitoneal expansion. **B,** Saphenous vein harvest using balloon dissection technique.

Vision Within the Working Space

1. *Scope:* The length of the scope varies but is appropriate to reach the desired structure. The surgeon views anatomic structures through a telescopic lens. The diameter of the scope varies from the 1.7-mm needle fetoscope to the 5 mm or less of the arthroscope to the 10 to 12 mm of a laparoscope.

   a. *Rigid:* A rigid scope is a telescopic rod-lens system that permits viewing in a variety of directions, such as a cystoscope. Laparoscopes are made in two styles—diagnostic and operative. The diagnostic laparoscope is a single telescopic rod-lens with no accessory ports (Fig. 32-3, *A*). The operating laparoscope has the rod-lens system with a working channel (Fig. 32-3, *B*). Rigid telescopes are metal and use fiberoptic illumination. Disposable models are available. The rigid telescope used in laparoscopy is placed into the body through a sheath referred to as a trocar.

   b. *Rigid hollow:* Disposable plastic sigmoidoscopes, anoscopes, and otoscopes are available. Illumination is from a separate light carrier rod. Rigid bronchoscopes have additional side ports for administration of oxygen or anesthetics.

   c. *Flexible:* Flexible scopes have a directional adjuster dial that contours the lensed tip into and around anatomic curvatures to permit visualization of all surfaces of the wall of a hollow structure, such as the upper and lower gastrointestinal tract (Fig. 32-4). The user can look directly into the eyepiece, or an attachment can be placed over the eyepiece to project the image onto a video screen. Flexible endoscopes have working channels that permit the manipulation of flexible biopsy forceps and laser fibers. A separate suction channel is on the opposite side. Two trumpet valves located near the eyepiece control suction and insufflation with air

to create a viewing and working space. The covering of flexible endoscopes is made of silicone-plastic material and is usually latex-free.

2. *Camera:* A camera can be mounted to the eyepiece of the endoscope. Some cameras are used sterile, and others are

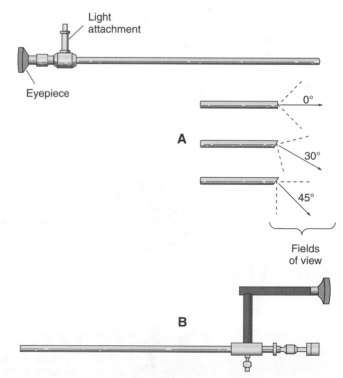

FIG. 32-3   Basic rigid endoscopes. **A,** Standard rigid endoscope. **B,** Single-puncture laparoscope with working channel.

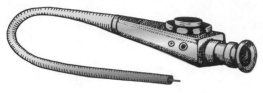

FIG. 32-4   Flexible endoscope.

high-level disinfected and covered with a sterile camera drape. The camera consists of a coupler that attaches to the eyepiece of the endoscope, a camera head, a connecting cable, and a connector to attach the camera to the camera controller box (Fig. 32-5).

a. *Video:* Endoscopes may be attached to a still or video camera so that organs or lesions can be photographed during a procedure. Video cameras with recorder/player/printer equipment require high-powered light sources for photographic applications and video documentation. By viewing high-resolution monitor(s), the endoscopist can manipulate instruments for diagnostic examination or to perform a therapeutic procedure. Video documentation can be obtained by recording the examination or procedure on videotape or to a CD. Microcomputer imaging systems with a printer can reproduce these images into still photographs. This equipment is either kept on a mobile cart or permanently placed in ceiling-mounted articulated booms (Fig. 32-6).

b. *Monitor:* More than one video monitor is recommended for ease of viewing the image transmitted by the endoscope by the entire team. Placement of the monitors in the direct line of vision of the surgeon and the first assistant eliminates the need to turn the head away from the field and prevents stiff neck and fatigue. Newer flat-panel monitors can be suspended from the ceiling on articulated arms that permit the user to place the viewing plane in a position of function.

c. *Wireless capsule endoscopy:* Endoscopic camera can be ingested to visualize the small bowel. The camera weighs around 4 g and measures 11 mm—about the size of a jellybean. The capsule contains four light-emitting diodes (LEDs) and a color camera. It travels by peristalsis through the small bowel, taking up to 50,000 images over an 8-hour period. The patient wears adhesive reception pads that transmit to a small receiver worn on a belt. No food may be consumed for 4 hours; however, liquids can be taken 2 hours after swallowing the capsule. The capsule is excreted naturally in the feces after a few days. The diagnostic capabilities have proven effective even when a negative finding was noted by other means. This method of video endoscopy is useful for patients who weigh more than 20 kg and children older than 10 years.

3. *Microscopic attachments:* The optical system of some endoscopes can be attached to a specially designed operating microscope such as the colpomicroscope. The illumination of the endoscope and binocular magnification of the microscope permit study of abnormal tissues and/or therapeutic procedures in areas otherwise inaccessible without an open surgical procedure. Many microscopes have manipulators or "joysticks" that permit the use of laser during the procedure.

4. *Ultrasound probes:* A high-frequency ultrasound transducer at the end of a fiberoptic endoscope provides visualization of the heart, liver, pancreas, spleen, and kidneys.

5. *Radiographic assisted:* Fluoroscopy may be preferred to video images for visualization of certain procedures such as radioactive implantation.

   a. *Contrast media:* Radiopaque dye can be injected into the lumen of the biliary system or other structure to observe for patency or obstruction.

   b. *Radioisotopes:* Radioisotopes can be injected and traced with sensitive detector probes.

Manipulation and Maneuverability within the Working Space

For puncture endoscopy, one or more additional 5- to 12-mm trocars are inserted through the abdominal wall under direct video visualization at strategic points. This is to create working access portals for graspers, cutters, dissectors, staplers, and suturing devices for tissue manipulation. These accessories can be passed through channels in the endoscope to, for

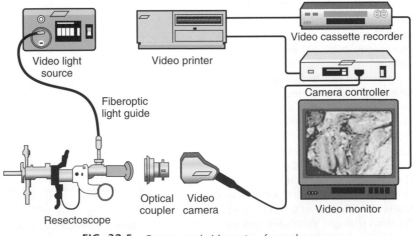

FIG. 32-5   Camera and video setup for endoscopy.

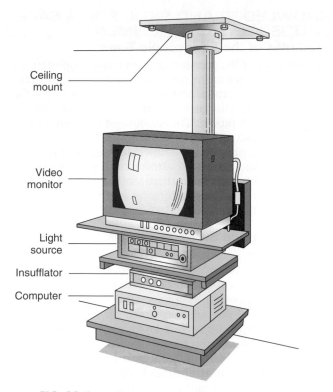

FIG. 32-6   Ceiling-mounted endoscopic equipment.

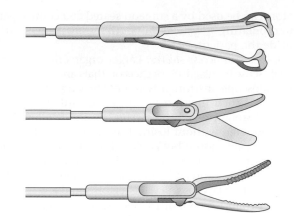

FIG. 32-7   Examples of instrumentation used in endoscopes.

example, remove fluid or tissue, coagulate or ligate bleeding vessels, or inject fluid or dye to distend cavities. The accessories will be determined by the type of endoscope and purpose of the procedure.

1. *Instrumentation:* Dissectors, graspers, hooks, clamps, needle holders, and probes are available for tissue manipulation through the endoscope (Fig. 32-7). The length and diameter are appropriate to the type of endoscope in use. The handle and shaft of the instrument can be rigid or flexible for procedure-specific maneuverability.

2. *Functional energy-driven devices (laser, ultrasonics, suction, irrigation, electrosurgery):* A laser beam can be focused through some endoscopes. Argon, holmium:yttrium aluminum garnet (Ho:YAG), and neodymium (Nd):YAG lasers will pass light through a fiber. The CO_2 laser can be directed through a rigid endoscope or the interior mirror system of a multiarticulated arm of the operating microscope. The beam is then focused through the endoscope, which is usually held in a self-retaining device. A distal smoke-evacuation suction device clears plume to maintain visibility through the scope and at the site of lasing. The endoscopes are specifically designed for adaptation to the articulated arm of the CO_2 laser (e.g., the CO_2 laser laparoscope and CO_2 laser bronchoscope).

   Ultrasonic waves can be used through an endoscope to disassociate tissue or materials such as stones for removal from the body via suction or retrieval devices. Other forms of ultrasonic dissection are found in the harmonic scalpel, which moves at more than 50,000 vibrations per second to denature protein without heat. It seals small vessels by coagulation as it incises.

An active electrode connected to a monopolar electrosurgical unit (ESU) may be used through an endoscope for surgical procedures or a resectoscope for transurethral surgery in urology. A variety of electrodes, both disposable and reusable, are available in many lengths and configurations. They must have adequate insulation and be inspected before use for any defect. Electrical energy transfers by capacitance from the activated electrode through intact insulation into other nearby conductive materials. Unless a safe path is provided for current to return to ground, the current induced by capacitance might cause an unintentional burn on non-targeted tissue. Direct coupling occurs when the activated electrode touches other metal instruments, particularly the laparoscope. An all-metal trocar/cannula system allows accidental contact to dissipate through the abdominal wall. The surgeon should avoid activating the electrode unless it is in direct contact with the tissue. A shielding and monitoring system is commercially available for monopolar endoscopic electrosurgical electrodes. Bipolar instruments, including dissectors, scissors, and graspers, eliminate the potential hazard of stray currents with monopolar electrodes.

3. *Adjunct organ displacement:* A uterine manipulator such as a tenaculum can be placed through the vagina to the inside of the uterus or attached to the cervix. This manipulator can be reusable or disposable and may have a channel for the instillation of dye for chromopertubation or radiopaque contrast medium to observe for uterine configuration and tubal patency by radiograph. The uterus can be displaced into the desired position by moving the exterior portion of the device cephalad, laterally, anteverted, or retroverted to view the pelvic structures. Some devices have a disposable patient intrauterine cannula with a reusable handgrip.

   Retractors can be placed through the laparoscope to provide additional exposure or displacement of organs in the endoscopic field.

4. *Robotics:* A voice-actuated articulated arm can be used as a steady camera-holding device. The surgeon uses a programmed voice card to instruct the arm where to position and reposition the camera. Adjunct robotic manipu-

lators can be used by a surgeon seated at a control panel manipulating joysticks to activate instrumentation inside the patient.

5. *Hand-assisted access sleeves:* Larger organs may require a tactile sense for diagnosis or excision that cannot be attained by endoscopic instruments alone. The surgeon can make a small 3-inch incision and insert an inflatable or gel sleeve through which he or she can insert a hand into the abdomen without losing the pressurized field.

After sleeve assembly is placed in the incision, pneumoperitoneum can be established. Organs can be palpated or grasped by hand and removed. This method is particularly good for laparoscopic splenectomy and any specimen greater than 5 to 8 cm. Darker gloves are suggested for less light reflection on the video monitor.

Capture of Specimens within the Working Space

1. Graspers and snares can be used through an endoscope to remove tissue specimens through the same access portals as the trocars. Instrumentation used in tissue capture can be used through all forms of endoscopes. Some instruments of this type have electrosurgical capabilities to provide hemostasis in the process.
2. Pouches can be introduced through the trocar to capture an entire specimen for delivery to the surface via the access portals created for the trocars. These are available in many sizes and are commonly used in laparoscopy.

Evacuation of Gases, Fluids, and Solids from the Body

1. Gases, fluids, and solids can be evacuated through an endoscope. Suction irrigators are commonly used. Ultrasonic dissectors use this principle for the evacuation of tissue through the suction port on the endoscopic instrument. The substances are biohazardous because they contain blood and body fluids.
2. Containment is used when evacuating CO_2 after the procedure is completed. The gas should not be evacuated into the room air, because it contains biologic particles.

Closure or Minimizing of the Access Portal(s)

1. Closure of target internal organs with suture or other media such as staples and clips can be performed through the endoscope. Intraabdominal ligation is achieved with loops of chromic or plain surgical gut (Endoloop ligatures). After the applicator is passed through the scope, the loop is placed around the tissue and pulled taut. An endoscopic swaged needle-suture is passed in a needle holder for suturing. Intracorporeal (inside body) and extracorporeal (outside body) knotting techniques are used to secure sutures. Endoscopic ligating clips and staples also are used for ligation and tissue approximation.
2. External punctures and incisions are closed. In adults, incisions of 5 mm are closed at the subcutaneous level; however, 10-mm incisions are closed at the fascial level to prevent herniation. In pediatric patients, 5-mm incisions are closed at the fascial level proportionate to body size.
3. Natural closure by physiologic structures such as muscular sphincters requires no intervention by the surgeon. Rigid tubular anatomy, such as bronchi, is unaffected and requires no specific closure.

KNOWLEDGE AND SKILL FOR A SAFE ENDOSCOPIC ENVIRONMENT

Attributes of the Endoscopic Team

Each member of the endoscopic team has an important role in the performance of the surgical procedure. The intricacies of the instrumentation and the limits of the visual field require strict attention to detail and awareness of each step in the endoscopic process. The attributes of the team members complement each other within their own scope of practice. Together, they provide the knowledge and skill necessary for the safe and effective performance of an endoscopic procedure. Each member anticipates the needs of the other and is prepared to convert to an open procedure at a moment's notice.

Attributes of the Surgeon

The surgeon must have an expert knowledge of anatomy and physiology. Landmarks can look distorted and unusual through an endoscope. An inexperienced person would not be able to recognize physiologic structures in this visual context. Manual dexterity is critical for all phases of the procedure. During a puncture laparoscopy, major vascular and digestive structures are in significant jeopardy if an insufflation needle is blindly placed or if a trocar is aimed in the wrong trajectory. Eye-hand coordination is essential for specimen capture and tissue suturing. The inability to directly view target structures with the naked eye may present some distortion of the field. Working from a monitor screen instead of using direct vision can be awkward because the eyes are not directed to the area of manipulation.

TYPES OF ENDOSCOPIC PROCEDURES

Not all endoscopic procedures are performed as sterile procedures; some are aseptic (high-level disinfection). An endoscope is introduced into the gastrointestinal tract through the mouth or anus. It touches only mucous membranes. The gastrointestinal tract normally harbors resident and transient microorganisms. Although the procedure is not considered sterile, patients and personnel are protected from cross-contamination. Endoscopes and their accessories are thoroughly cleaned and terminally sterilized or undergo high-level disinfection after use. Sterility is not maintained between and during patient uses. Instruments should be stored according to the manufacturer's recommendations. Many endoscopic procedures are performed in an endoscopy unit rather than in the operating room (OR).

Endoscopy is performed as a sterile procedure if body tissue will be incised or excised or if a normally sterile organ or body cavity is entered, such as the bladder or uterus. Ideally, the endoscope and all accessories should be sterile regardless of the point of entry. It may not be feasible to sterilize some heat-sensitive parts, such as a lensed telescope, between patient uses when several procedures are scheduled in succession. Control of scheduling endoscopic procedures and adequate instrumentation will help provide sterile endoscopes for every patient. Written policies and procedures must specify accepted practices for patient care and infection control. AORN has developed recommended practices for the use and care of endoscopes to be used as a guide in establishing processing procedures.

Only sterile endoscopes and accessories should be used on patients with suppressed immune systems, such as from chemotherapy or steroid therapy or human immunodeficiency virus (HIV)–related diseases.

Routine practices should be established to reduce the risk of potential patient injuries and complications. These practices include but are not limited to the following:

- Training for and demonstrating competence in the use and care of endoscopic equipment by surgeons and perioperative personnel
- Providing complete sets of properly prepared, functional instruments
- Monitoring the patient for changes in physiologic status (e.g., development of hypercapnia and/or hypothermia can be caused by CO_2 insufflation)

All patients should be prepped and draped for conversion to an open procedure when warranted because of recognized or potential complications. Instrumentation and supplies for an open procedure should be precounted and readily available. The surgeon should inform the patient preoperatively of this possibility and should obtain an informed consent.

LAPAROSCOPIC PROCEDURE

After the patient has been anesthetized, intubated, prepped, catheterized, and draped, the operating bed may remain flat or be tilted approximately 5 to 10 degrees into a slight Trendelenburg position. A Veress insufflation needle or blunt Hasson trocar is inserted into the peritoneal cavity through a small infraumbilical incision. The anterior abdominal wall is thinnest at the lower edge of the umbilicus, along the linea alba, which makes this area easiest for penetration of a single layer of fascia and peritoneum with minimal interruption of skin and dermal blood vessels.

The peritoneal cavity is insufflated with CO_2 to an intraoperative pressure of 12 to 15 mm Hg. The circulating nurse monitors this pressure during insufflation; it should not fall below 8 mm Hg. After sufficient pneumoperitoneum is established, the patient is placed in a slight reverse Trendelenburg's position for upper gastrointestinal procedures. A padded footboard should be in place to prevent the patient from sliding downward on the operating bed. Moderate Trendelenburg position is used for lower pelvic procedures.

If an insufflation needle is used to fill the peritoneal cavity with carbon dioxide gas, then it is replaced by a trocar and sheath, which is inserted straight into the peritoneal cavity. The sharp obturator is then removed from the trocar sheath. A rigid laparoscope is introduced into the abdomen through the trocar sheath. The sheath matches the size of the laparoscope. A 7- or 10-mm, 0-degree telescope is inserted through the sheath for direct visualization within the peritoneal cavity.

Secondary 5-, 7-, or 10-mm trocars are inserted through the abdominal wall under direct vision through the laparoscope. If 10-mm trocars are used, sizing caps or lumen reducers can be used to reduce the opening of the sheath for the use of smaller endoscopic instruments and probes. The use of size-reducing caps prevents the escape of pneumoperitoneum. A sterile camera attached to the laparoscope transmits images on video monitor(s). Two monitors, one on each side of the operating bed, generally are used. Without straining their necks, the surgeon and the team can view the manipulation of instruments inserted through secondary ports in the direct line of vision.

At the conclusion of the procedure, the carbon dioxide should be evacuated through the suction port on the trocar into the vacuum system and not expelled directly into the room air. The expelled gas contains plume, blood, and body fluids that cause airborne contamination. Personal protective equipment, such as masks and eyewear, should be worn by all personnel in the room.

Some surgeons prefer to use a gasless method for displacing and expanding the abdomen during laparoscopy. A device referred to as an abdominal lift can be used to elevate the abdominal wall for minimal access procedures without the use of CO_2. Shorter instrumentation can be used, because the internal organs are closer to the surface.

Pediatric Endoscopy

Pediatric endoscopy is gaining favor as a method of diagnosis and treatment. Procedures such as appendectomy, pyloromyotomy, fundoplication, and cancer staging are examples of endoscopic surgery performed successfully in children.

Procedural Considerations for Laparoscopy in Children. Anatomic differences between children and adults are most pronounced between the ages of birth to 8 years. Infants have large umbilical vessels that are easily damaged and may even be permeable to CO_2. The processus vaginalis at the inguinal ring may be weak and easily inadvertently opened by a pneumoperitoneum. The aortoiliac axis is nearer the surface and may be punctured by the trocars or instrumentation. The left epigastrium or the right hypochondrium is a good site for initial insufflation. Smaller instruments and scopes should be used. The visual field is limited by the small size of the child, sometimes as small as 4 to 5 mm. Hasson trocars and sheaths may be preferred to other methods if CO_2 insufflation must be used. In some circumstances, abdominal wall lift devices are more appropriate for a safe and effective procedure.

General anesthesia is used, and the child should have an empty bladder. A Foley catheter and a nasogastric tube are useful for decompression of internal structures before a laparoscopy. After the skin prep and sterile draping, the infraumbilical incision is made. A mosquito hemostat is inserted into the incision and opened to stretch the wound slightly. Some surgeons prefer to use an open laparoscopic method as opposed to a blind puncture. A radial dilating trocar can be placed in the tiny incision and can be sequentially enlarged with instrumentation to the desired size. It can be secured with suture to prevent dislodgment. Pneumoperitoneum is established with CO_2 insufflation at 8 mm Hg to the desired level. Pressure should not exceed 8 cm H_2O for infants and 12 cm H_2O in children to 8 years of age. Smaller telescopes are usually adequate with a 0- to 30-degree viewing angle. Secondary trocars are inserted sharply under direct vision of the laparoscope.

HAZARDS OF ENDOSCOPY

Endoscopy is not without its hazards. Minimally invasive surgery requires appropriate credentialing. Surgeons who wish to perform laparoscopy and other endoscopic techniques should be credentialed through the medical staff department. Personnel who are responsible for scheduling endoscopic procedures should confirm the surgeon's practice privileges. Serious complications of endoscopy include the following:

1. *Perforation:* Perforation of a major organ or vessel is a constant cause for concern when sharp trocars and rigid scopes are used. Flexible fiberoptic endoscopes have decreased this danger, but it remains a potential complication. Patient positioning from supine to the Trendelenburg position shifts the intraabdominal anatomy, causing elevation of the major vessels of the lower abdominal cavity. Care is taken to prevent inadvertent injury to these structures while holding cameras or other devices situated in intraabdominal trocar sleeves during repositioning of the operating bed.

    The sharp obturator should be examined briefly after it is withdrawn from the trocar sleeve. The presence of gross blood, stool, bile, or other unidentified substance may indicate perforation of an intraabdominal organ.

2. *Bleeding:* Bleeding can occur from a biopsy site, pedicle of a polyp, or other area where tissue has been cut. Endoscopic sutures or clips can become dislodged. Care is taken to observe for pooling of blood in the body cavity that may indicate venous oozing or other vessel disruption.

3. *Hypothermia:* Carbon dioxide gas is colder than body temperature. The patient may experience moderate to severe hypothermia if other warming measures, such as forced-air warming or heating blankets, are not used. Hypothermia can alter the effects of propofol and increase the incidence of hypothermic coagulopathy.

Electrical systems used with endoscopy must conform with the standards and be subjected to the routine maintenance procedures prescribed by the National Fire Protection Association code for electrical safety. Two major electrical hazards associated with endoscopy are as follows:

1. *Improperly grounded electrical equipment:* If the surgeon will be using a monopolar ESU, place the dispersive electrode on the patient with adequate skin contact to allow return of electric current. Only solid-state generators, and preferably bipolar active electrodes, should be used, to avoid variances in voltage. A new dispersive electrode should be placed if the patient is repositioned from lithotomy to supine position for an open abdominal procedure. The dispersive electrode may gape and lose sufficient contact with the skin when the legs are moved. Pads should not be removed and repositioned. The adhesive may have weakened after the first application.

2. *Unsuspected current leaks:* Corrosion or accumulation of organic material can inhibit flow of current across the screw fitting between the light carrier and the bulb. Current can leak through the instrument to the patient. Ideally, endoscopes should not contain electrically conductive elements or metals that can corrode. Corrosion can be caused by repeated exposure to body fluids, hard water, or chemical agents.

Microorganisms, such as *Mycobacterium tuberculosis,* can be transmitted from one patient to another via a bronchoscope. *Streptococcus pneumoniae, Pseudomonas aeruginosa, Clostridium* organisms, and bloodborne pathogens also present potential hazards of cross-contamination. Personnel are exposed to potentially infectious body fluids and blood from aerosols, splashes, and contact with contaminated instrumentation. Gloves, masks, protective eyewear, gowns, and/or aprons are worn during endoscopic procedures and cleaning of equipment. Personnel should use standard precautions during endoscopic procedures and when handling and processing contaminated endoscopes and accessories.

CARE OF ENDOSCOPES

Endoscopes are delicate and expensive instruments. Rough handling, jarring, or bending of parts should be avoided. They should never be piled on top of each other or mixed with other instruments.

All parts of endoscopes and accessories are thoroughly disassembled, mechanically cleaned, and terminally sterilized or subjected to high-level disinfection after use. The primary causes of infection, such as herpes, hepatitis, or condylomata transmitted endoscopically, are inadequate cleaning and disinfection or sterilization of endoscopic equipment.

Cleaning

All parts of the endoscope should be cleaned as soon as possible after use while organic debris is still moist. Mucus, blood, feces, and protein-type residue can become trapped in the channels of the scope. This material is difficult to remove if it dries and may render the scope useless.

Endoscopes should be washed in warm, never hot, water and a neutral, nonresidue liquid-detergent solution. A pipe cleaner or small brush may be used to clean inside the lumens of all channels. The stopcocks on some scopes should be thoroughly disassembled for cleaning, too, because dirty valves will stick. Stopcocks are opened for cleaning; they should never be forced but can be loosened with a drop of solvent or lubricant.

Particular attention should be paid to lens cleanliness, or viewing will be obstructed. Debris can be carefully removed from around the lens with a fine toothpick. Special lens paper is used on the lens itself. Lensed instruments should not be cleaned with any substance that could dissolve cement around the lens. Consult the manufacturer's recommendations.

The endoscope is rinsed thoroughly and dried well. If scopes are to be sterilized in ethylene oxide gas, they must be thoroughly dry. Gas combines with water on items that are damp, to form ethylene glycol. Alcohol on cotton can be used on a wire stylet or a pipe cleaner to dry insertion tubes. Air can be forced through channels to dry inside them. Because organisms will multiply in a moist environment, all parts should be dry during the interval before further processing or storage.

An endoscope processor is available to clean long, flexible fiberoptic scopes, such as a colonoscope. It has two modes of operation to process the scope and its channels: a wash-and-dry cycle and a cycle of wash, disinfectant soak with activated glutaraldehyde solution, rinse, and dry. This equipment is an automated washer/disinfector.

Accessories are scrupulously cleaned. All debris is removed to ensure adequate steam sterilization. Disposable, single-use biopsy forceps and cytology brushes are recommended because the configurations of these accessories are particularly difficult to clean. Some trocars, scissors, and forceps have disposable or replaceable points or tips on reusable shafts or handles. These combination instruments facilitate cleaning and ensure a sharp cutting edge with each use.

Scopes and accessories should be inspected for damage after cleaning. Preferably, all endoscopic equipment should be terminally sterilized; otherwise it should be high-level disinfected after thorough mechanical cleaning.

Sterilization

After cleaning and drying, each endoscope with all of its parts disassembled is placed in a well-padded perforated tray of convenient size. Some endoscopes, such as an arthroscope, are supplied in a perforated case lined with foam cut to fit each disassembled part. The tray or fitted case is wrapped for sterilization. Instruments should be wrapped and sterilized by the method recommended by the manufacturer.

Some parts of endoscopes can be safely steam sterilized and therefore should be. Hollow, rigid metal sheaths, such as a sigmoidoscope, can be terminally steam sterilized after use but then may be stored to keep clean rather than sterile for a surgically clean procedure. Some fiberoptic cables also can be steam sterilized. Reusable biopsy forceps should be steam sterilized.

Parts with lenses and some fiberoptic carriers, such as a colonoscope, cannot be steam sterilized. High temperature and moisture will soften the cement holding lenses or fiberoptic fibers in place. The flexible shafts of some accessory instruments may erode when steam sterilized. These parts should be sterilized in ethylene oxide gas, hydrogen peroxide plasma, or formaldehyde gas or soaked in a chemical sterilant solution if ethylene oxide or hydrogen peroxide is not available.

The manufacturer may recommend that the pressure not exceed 5 pounds during ethylene oxide sterilization of a fiberoptic lighting system. The manufacturer's instructions for handling, using, cleaning, and sterilizing these items should be followed. Aeration is necessary after ethylene oxide sterilization. Ethylene oxide is a vesicant if it comes into contact with skin. It also can cause eye irritation.

If endoscopes and accessories are immersed in activated glutaraldehyde, acetic acid, or formaldehyde solution, a plastic tray should be used without a towel in the bottom. Prolonged use of a stainless steel tray may create an electrolytic action between the metals and can cause metallic deposits on instruments. Scopes and all accessories should be well rinsed in sterile distilled water before they are used, to prevent tissue irritation from solution.

Peracetic acid, another chemical sterilant in solution, is commercially available for sterilizing endoscopes for immediate patient use. The STERIS system has specialized tray assemblies for endoscope processing. These tray assemblies are not intended for long-term storage of sterilized instruments, but for immediate patient use.

Storage

If endoscopes are not wrapped for sterilization and storage, they are terminally sterilized by chemical means or at least undergo high-level disinfection before being returned to their respective storage cabinets. Clean, dry, unwrapped rigid instruments should be stored on a soft material such as plastic sheeting or foam. Towels hold a residue of laundry detergent that can tarnish metal. Flexible endoscopes with detachable parts should be stored disassembled, hung in a vertical position with the distal end pointed downward. Accessories also may be hung. The lumens should be flushed with alcohol to facilitate fluid evaporation.

The scope should be subjected to high-level disinfection or peracetic acid sterilization before use in patient care.

CONSIDERATIONS FOR PATIENT SAFETY

Endoscopy through a natural body orifice is usually performed on a patient who is not under general anesthesia. The following considerations should be included in the plan of care:

1. The patient should be monitored for signs and symptoms of reaction to drugs. Endoscopy is frequently performed with the use of sedatives and a topical or local anesthetic agent or with no anesthetic at all. The patient is awake during these procedures. Drugs such as midazolam (Versed) and diazepam (Valium) and narcotics such as meperidine hydrochloride (Demerol) may be administered intravenously as an adjunct to other preoperative sedation to produce relaxation and cooperation during the procedure and amnesia afterward. Respiratory depression and transient hypotension can occur. Antagonistic drugs should be available to reverse narcotic depression. Emergency resuscitation equipment should also be available.
2. A topical agent is frequently applied to nasal or oral and pharyngeal mucosa before introduction of an endoscope into the tracheobronchial tree or gastrointestinal tract. A topical agent may be instilled into the urethra before introduction of a cystoscope.
3. The teeth, gums, and lips are protected if the endoscope is introduced through the mouth. Dentures are removed. A mouthpiece is inserted.
4. Hydrogen and methane gases are normally present in the colon. These gases are flushed out with carbon dioxide before laser surgery or electrosurgery through the colonoscope to avoid the possibility of explosion within the colon.
5. Power sources and lights should be tested before each use and after cleaning. They should be kept in working order.
6. The heat generated from the projection lamp of a fiberoptic illuminator is dissipated. It should not be enclosed in drapes because the heat could set them on fire. If the unit contains a fan for heat regulation, the direction of airflow should be away from the patient and the sterile field to minimize airborne contamination.
7. Endoscopes should be smooth, with no nicks on the surface. A scratch on the sheath could injure tissue or the mucous membrane lining of an orifice. Metal endoscopes should be individually wrapped and sterilized to prevent surface scratches from contact with other metallic instruments. Metallic endoscopes should be handled only with the gloved hands.

8. Extreme care should be taken to observe patients after endoscopic procedures for effects of respiratory or circulatory system distress caused by gas absorption, trauma, or medication. Many flexible endoscopic procedures are performed on ambulatory outpatients. The patients must not leave the facility until vital signs are stable and side effects have passed. Follow-up phone calls are suggested within 24 to 48 hours to monitor patient progress and answer questions. Any patient concerns should be directed to the surgeon. Additional follow-up phone calls may be necessary.

DUTIES OF THE ASSISTANT FOR FLEXIBLE ENDOSCOPY

Often only a circulating nurse assists the surgeon with a minimally invasive procedure. The assistant's duties are as follows:

1. Set up the supplies and equipment as much as possible before the patient and surgeon arrive. Consult the procedure book. Remember that sterility must be maintained for a sterile procedure.
2. Explain the steps of the procedure to the patient as appropriate. It is important that the patient know the reasons for any discomfort that may be experienced so that symptoms of discomfort will be recognized as normal.
3. Explain the position and need for it before positioning the patient. The position the patient must assume during the procedure is often uncomfortable.
4. Drape the patient properly to prevent unnecessary exposure.
5. Adjust room lighting. The surgeon may want the room in semidarkness. A dimmer on the room light is helpful, but if one is unavailable, the x-ray viewboxes may be illuminated to provide indirect lighting.
6. Divert the patient's attention as much as possible during the procedure. The patient may complain of pain more than is justified as a way of expressing displeasure at the invasion of the endoscope or the position required during the procedure. The circulating nurse should stay with the patient to offer reassurance and emotional support. Suggest that slow, deep breaths may help relaxation and lessen the discomfort. Soft music may help the patient relax. The surgeon may allow the patient to watch the procedure through a viewing attachment on the endoscope or on a video monitor.
7. Evaluate the patient's level of discomfort, and inform the surgeon of unusual reactions. The circulating nurse also monitors the patient's respiratory status, blood pressure, and pulse. Pulse oximeter and automated blood pressure devices may be used routinely. Vital signs should be documented before the procedure begins, every 15 minutes during the procedure, and again at the conclusion. Additional vital signs should be recorded when medication is given or tissue samples are excised.
8. Know how to assemble the different scopes and their accessories and how to operate them. When passing the suction tube or biopsy forceps, place the tip directly at the lumen of the scope so that the surgeon can grasp the shaft and insert it without moving his or her eyes from the scope.
9. Care for surgical specimens as appropriate.
10. Take care not to drop endoscopic instruments; they are delicate and expensive. Fiberoptic bundles are glass; do not kink or bend them.

Endoscopic procedures are considered minimally invasive except for ophthalmoscopy, because the scope is placed into a body orifice or cavity. Many require one or more small skin incisions for insertion of the scope and accessories. Endoscopy is used for many diagnostic and surgical procedures.

The Association of periOperative Registered Nurses (AORN) has developed recommended practices for endoscopic minimally invasive surgery.

ROBOTIC-ASSISTED ENDOSCOPY AND TELEMEDICINE

The first robotic system available in the United States AESOP (Automated Endoscopic System for Optimal Positioning) was developed by Computer Motion[1] to provide a stable laparoscopic telescope/camera holder with a bed-mounted articulated arm controlled by a voice-actuated computer. The device was voice actuated by the surgeon who wore a microphone headset during the procedure to verbally direct the aim and direction of the laparoscope. The robot was able to discern verbal commands because a voice card trained with the surgeon's spoken word was inserted into a microprocessor housed in the base of the unit. Each command caused the sterile-draped articulated arm to respond by assuming the exact position requested by the surgeon.

Intuitive Surgical later developed Navigator to hold the laparoscope/camera assembly steady and to change the visual field from micro to macro without causing the sensation of "seasickness" in the team as they visualize the surgical site on the monitor. The Navigator regulates the temperature of the laparoscope to prevent fogging.

Intuitive Surgical and Computer Motion merged intellectual properties in 2003 to develop high-technologic robotic units combining aspects of both systems. Computer Motion Zeus robots are no longer manufactured; however, Intuitive Surgical continues to support repairs, upgrades, and trade-ins toward the latest Intuitive Surgical robotics on the market. The names of the current older models have not been changed.

Robotic technology has revolutionized the endoscopic approach to surgery. The devices currently found in operating rooms around the world range from simple camera holders to full room control at the command of the surgeon. Examples of contemporary robotic-integrated components include the following:

- Environmental control computer platform
- Functional peripheral equipment
- Instrument manipulating robot
- Master control console

---

[1]Currently merged with Intuitive Surgical (formerly known as Integrated Surgical Systems).

Environmental Control by Robotics

Environmental control robotic systems are built into a computer-directed platform wherein the surgeon verbally controls other computer-generated activities such as lights, bed motion, and other devices during the surgical procedure.

HERMES by Computer Motion and EndoALPHA by Olympus are environmental control systems by which peripheral equipment such as the ESU, lights, OR bed, insufflator, light source, and other mechanized devices in the OR are voice controlled by the surgeon. The surgeon can address the system through his or her headset and request a preloaded computed tomography (CT) scan to appear on a computer monitor.

Real-time verbal and video documentation is recorded for the permanent record. The surgical report is generated by electronic media, and a hard copy is printed simultaneously. Many companies such as STERIS, SKYTRON, Stryker, STORZ, Olympus, Medtronic, Ethicon Endosurgery, ConMed, and Berchtold have coordinated with Intuitive Surgical Corporation to develop HERMES- and EndoALPHA-compatible devices.

Functional Peripheral Equipment

Machines used during the surgical procedure can be controlled by the environmental control computer platform. All the endoscopic equipment such as light source, insufflator, electrosurgery unit, irrigator, aspirator, image recorder, and video monitor can be activated, adjusted, and directed by the surgeon's touch on a foot pedal or command into his or her headset. Other devices in the room such as the spotlights and operating bed respond in kind to the direction given by the surgeon. Casual conversation is ignored by the computer.

Instrument Manipulating Robot and the Master Console

Surgical robotic examples include ZEUS (originally from Computer Motion) and da Vinci (Intuitive Surgical), which are hands-free systems wherein the surgeon sits at a master console several feet away from the field (Fig. 32-8). He or she can remotely manipulate three to four articulated arms with joysticks while observing each precision action with a 3-D laparoscope and a 3-chip digital camera on a 3-D video screen with full depth of field (Fig. 32-9). The da Vinci camera system can work with low levels of light. The latest model, da Vinci S, offers the surgeon a multi-image viewer that can tile the images for comparative views.

The surgeon has one cubic foot of comfortable space wherein to work the controls and switch views in real-time action. The da Vinci robot will not operate if the surgeon's head is not seated inside the face port viewer. The unit will lock and remain immobile until the surgeon's head is again placed in the correct position (Fig. 32-10).

The backup battery will run for 20 minutes in the event of a power failure. Each instrument is specially designed with a microchip that communicates with the computer to log each use. The computer tracks the function of the instrument and reports when it needs to be changed or repaired. Only instruments made by Intuitive Surgical work with the da Vinci robot.

The system is voice actuated and may be controlled by a surgeon who is many miles away by telecollaboration.

Many cardiac, prostatic, gynecologic, and general surgery procedures have been successfully performed by the surgeon using robotic technology. The articulated arms perform the procedure using a three- or four-arm laparoscopic system that offers a circumferential 360-degree wristlike[2] movement for precision grasping, manipulation, dissection, clamping, and suturing of tissues. Hand tremor is eliminated and ambidextrous movement is facilitated with natural hand-wrist motion.

Motions are described in geometric terms aligned with 7 degrees of freedom in human wrist- and arm-articulated motion.[3] These motions are described as:

* Roll—rotation or circumduction
* Pitch—up and down
* Yaw—side to side
* Grip—open and close
* Insertion—back and forth
* Clockwise
* Counterclockwise

The newest telemedicine module is Socrates. This computerized telecollaboration system originally created by Computer Motion permits more than one surgeon to have shared control of the field—even when the surgeons are miles apart. The implications include the facilitation of learning new procedures under the guidance of a mentor. Distance can be an issue if the signal is delayed or interrupted between surgeons.[4] Other interference such as signal strength and speed can be factors. This unit does not interface with the da Vinci system at this time.

Specialty services such as orthopedics and neurosurgery have used robotics such as ROBODOC, ORTHODOC, and Neuromate by Intuitive Surgical. ROBODOC is a computer-controlled robot that drills bones for prosthetic implants and can remove old bone cement. ORTHODOC displays CT images for preoperative planning for hip arthroplasty. Neuromate is a surgical robot to assist with stereotactic brain surgery.

PROBOT assists with urologic surgery for prostatectomy. Instrumentation used through the access portals includes monopolar and bipolar electrodes, ultrasonics, sharp and blunt dissectors, graspers, clip appliers, and needle holders.

Virtual Reality

Research is being done to develop virtual reality training for surgeons and operators of complex technologic equipment. Virtual reality is the computer science of simulating real-life motion, time, and space. Computer-generated images mimic real-life situations. The surgeon-in-training practices a procedure without touching a real patient. The surgeon dons a specialized headset/visor and sensor gloves and selects the training scenario to be practiced. The computer displays a 3-D video of human anatomy in the headset/visor. The sensor gloves signal motion, direction, and pressure to a

---

[2]EndoWrist from Intuitive and MicroWrist from Computer Motion.
[3]www.bhj.org/journal/2002_4402_apr/endo_208.htm.
[4] The mean time delay between New York and France was 155 milliseconds. The commands took 0.1 second to take place according to the U.S. Food and Drug Administration (FDA) records. The procedure studied was a cholecystectomy. The robot took 15 minutes to set up and the procedure took 54 minutes.

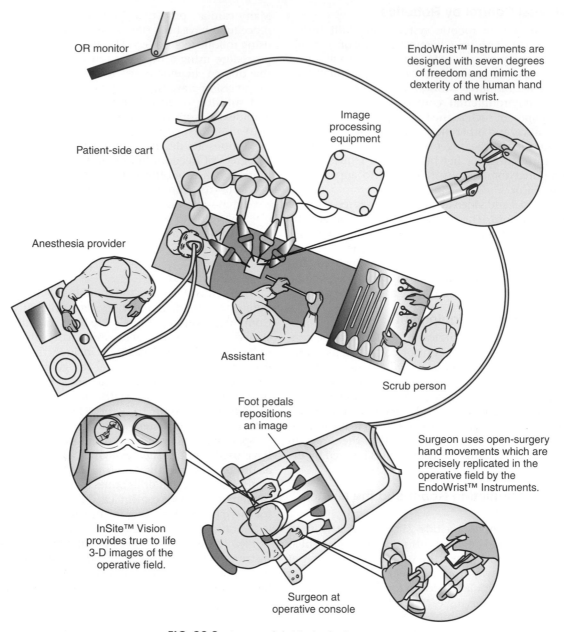

OR monitor

EndoWrist™ Instruments are designed with seven degrees of freedom and mimic the dexterity of the human hand and wrist.

Image processing equipment

Patient-side cart

Anesthesia provider

Assistant

Scrub person

Foot pedals repositions an image

Surgeon uses open-surgery hand movements which are precisely replicated in the operative field by the EndoWrist™ Instruments.

InSite™ Vision provides true to life 3-D images of the operative field.

Surgeon at operative console

FIG. 32-8   Layout of da Vinci robotic system.

computer and in turn create a sensation of touch for the surgeon. The entire activity looks, feels, and responds as if the surgeon were performing surgery on an actual patient. This investigative technology can allow for "practice surgery" while evaluating the skill and dexterity of the surgeon.

The possibilities for integrating advanced technologies to simplify surgery and make it less painful and safer for patients seem endless as surgeons develop and refine innovative techniques. The challenges for all members of the OR team are to learn about technologic advances and to monitor the quality of patient care in their application. Engineering performance (i.e., clinical application of biotechnology) is measured by reliability, safety, maintenance, and effectiveness of equipment. Clinical performance is

measured by the skills of users to achieve desired results—a successful outcome for the patient.

Human Intervention During Robotic-Assisted Procedures

A sterile team is at the sterile field to guide tiny 1- to 2-cm incisions through the skin, place the Veress needle or trocars, and perform typical activities, such as draping, sponging, and dressing the surgical site.

The FDA requires the manufacturers to provide training for surgeons. Facilities using robotics require credentialing before the surgeon can schedule procedures. The surgeon should be mentored for 15 or more procedures before operating solo.

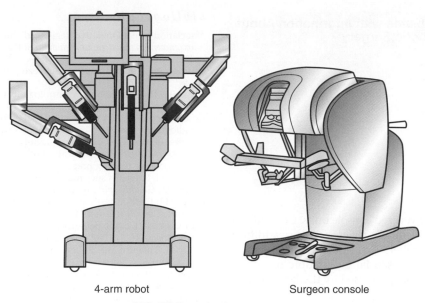

4-arm robot   Surgeon console

FIG. 32-9   Robotic components.

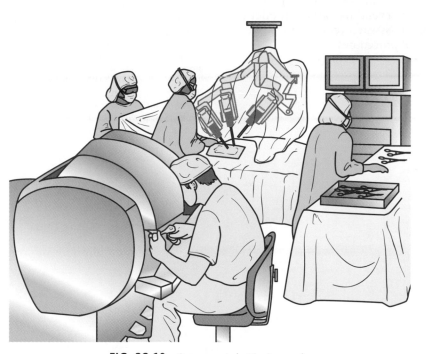

FIG. 32-10   Surgeon at da Vinci console.

Although referred to as "robotic," the procedures performed using machines like da Vinci require the surgeon's hands to manipulate the joysticks so the articulated arms and tips can mimic his or her motions on a microscopic level. None of these devices have the power of decision making and cannot run without human intervention.

Advantages and Disadvantages of Robotic-Assisted Surgery

Advantages of robotic-assisted techniques include greater precision than the human hand can provide alone with greater freedom of motion without the tremor and fatigue associated with maintaining a position for a long period.

Disadvantages of the computerized systems include startup costs,[5] the learning curve, and time in training. Long-term studies need to be done to establish the full range of uses and efficacy. Many standardized procedures will need revision in order to be suited to the new technology. Additional consideration should be given to the size and positioning

---

[5]Zeus costs about $975,000; da Vinci is around $1 million.

BOX 32-2	Websites with Information About Robotic Surgery

www.intuitivesurgical.com
www.computermotion.com
www.robodoc.com
www.maquet.com
www.fda.gov
www.techreview.com
www.thetrocar.net

of the robotic arms and oversized console units. Computerized technology requires adequate space for the additional machinery and team members. Ceiling-mounted booms may provide consolidation of essential endoscopic machinery, thereby reducing the floor space used by the large pieces of equipment.

Some surgeon state that the "haptic sense" is lacking, meaning that the tactile sense, or touch, of tissues is not as sensitive as working inside an open patient for some procedures. Box 32-2 lists several websites that offer more information about robotic-assisted procedures. Some sites have video clips of actual procedures.

Bibliography

Association of periOperative Registered Nurses: *AORN standards, recommended practices, and guidelines,* Denver, CO, 2006, The Association.

Berlinger NT: Robotic surgery—Squeezing into tight places, *N Engl J Med* 354(20):20992101, 2006.

Camarillo DB et al: Robotic technology in surgery: Past, present, and future, *Am J Surg* 188(10):2-15, 2004.

Costamagna G et al: A prospective trial comparing small bowel radiographs and video capsule endoscopy for suspected small bowel disease, *Gastroenterology* 123(4):999-1005, 2002.

Francis P, Winfield HN: Medical robotics: The impact on perioperative nursing practice, *Urol Nurs* 26(2):99-108, 2006.

Freeman G: Surgeons sues maker of trocar shield after death of patient, *Laparoscopic Surg Update* 8(9):97-99, 2000.

Gilger MA: Gastrointestinal endoscopy in children, past, present and future, *Curr Opin Pediatr* 13(5):429-434, 2001.

Gutt CN et al: Early experiences of robotic surgery in children, *Surg Endosc* 16(2):1083-1086, 2002.

Hanly EJ, Talamini MA: Robotic abdominal surgery, *Am J Surg* 188(10):19-26, 2004.

Jirecek S et al: Direct visual or blind insertion of the primary trocar, *Surg Endosc* 16(4):626-629, 2002.

Lafranco AR et al: Robotic surgery: A current perspective, *Ann Surg* 239(1):14-21, 2004.

Lafullarde T, Guys T: Risk factors and the prevalence of trocar site herniation after laparoscopic fundoplication, *Surg Endosc* 16(7):1115-1116, 2002.

Lobritto SJ: Endoscopic considerations in children, *Gastrointest Endosc Clin North Am* 11(1):93-109, 2001.

Mariano ER et al: Anesthetic concerns for robot-assisted laparoscopy in an infant, *Anesth Analg* 99(6):1665-1667, 2004.

Rovario GC et al: Major vascular injuries in laparoscopic surgery, *Surg Endosc* 16(8):1192-1196, 2002.

Thomson M: Colonoscopy and endoscopy, *Gastrointest Endosc Clin North Am* 11(4):603-609, 2001.

Wolf JS Jr: Devices for hand-assisted laparoscopic surgery, *Expert Rev Med Devices* 2(6):725-730, 2005.

Chapter 33

General Surgery

CHAPTER OBJECTIVES

After studying this chapter, the learner will be able to:
- Identify the pertinent anatomy of the abdominal organs within the peritoneal cavity.
- List six common surgical incisions used in general surgery.
- Describe the method of preparing a patient for an abdominal procedure.
- Discuss the importance of surgical landmarks.

CHAPTER OUTLINE

KEY TERMS AND DEFINITIONS

Chevron Multiangle oblique subcostal.
Femoral Right or left side.
Horizontal flank Right or left side.
Inguinal Right or left side.
Landmark Location on the surface of the body or at organ level that provides orientation for the surgical incision.
Laparostomy Surgically opening the abdomen for an exploratory laparotomy and finding it necessary to leave the abdomen open and planning delayed primary closure for several days later.
McBurney Right side.
Midline/longitudinal Centered above or below umbilicus.
Paramedian Right or left of umbilicus, above or below umbilicus.
Pfannenstiel Langer line just above pubis.
Puncture/stab Can become round or oblique.
Subcostal/oblique (Kocher) Above umbilicus.
Transverse Above or below umbilicus.
Umbilical (supraumbilical or infraumbilical) Above or below umbilicus.

SUPPLEMENTAL MATERIAL ON EVOLVE WEBSITE *evolve*

http://evolve.elsevier.com/BerryKohn
- Content Updates
- Glossary
- Full Set of Perioperative Flash Cards
- Interactive Key Term Flash Cards
- Tips for the Scrub Person and Circulating Nurse: Hernia, Mastectomy
- Student Activities
- WebLinks

HISTORICAL BACKGROUND

The earliest time in which surgical procedures were performed is not exactly known. Artifacts documenting brain and bone surgery have been found in archeologic excavations of ancient civilizations. The Egyptians had extensive knowledge of surgical anatomy that they acquired through the art of embalming and preserving abdominal organs. This practice allowed them to observe the position and natural appearance of the internal organs. The cases of earliest human dissection were performed by Egyptian priests, who later translated these acts into surgical procedures on the living. Organ structures became part of the written hieroglyphic language.

Documented historic surgical procedures include those performed in the sixteenth century by Ambroise Paré (1510-1590), a French barber turned military surgeon. He used ligatures instead of boiling oil to stop bleeding and was called a "Master Barber-Surgeon" in 1541. Paré was a very religious man who used the phrase "I dressed the wound, but God healed him" to describe his work. The seventeenth century saw the 1597 publication of *A Discourse in the Whole Art of Chirurgie* by Scottish surgeon Peter Lowe (1550-1610)—the first surgical textbook written in English, which was without illustrations and followed the format of a discussion between a surgeon and his student. (In this era, all books for physicians were written in Latin.) Lowe was highly influenced by Paré and included wound dressings of balm of Hypericum, turpentine, egg yolk, and rose oil. Editions published after 1610 had hand-drawn illustrations by subsequent editors, some of which were excerpted from Paré's works.

Strides in the eighteenth century included the addition of pathologic study associated with the art of surgery. Scottish anatomist John Hunter (1728-1793) was considered the "Father of Experimental Surgery" because he emphasized that surgical wounds would not heal without the inflammatory process. Hunter was commissioned as an English Army surgeon in 1763 and studied the management of war wounds. He became the surgeon general in 1789. Two of his famous students were Edward Jenner (1749-1823), who discovered the smallpox vaccine, and Sir Astley Cooper (1768-1841), for whom the suspensory ligaments of the breast are named.

Records indicate the removal of a 20-pound ovarian tumor by American surgeon Ephraim McDowell in 1809. The procedure was performed by candlelight in 25 minutes with rudimentary instruments and no anesthesia. Crowds gathered outside the patient's home in Kentucky where the surgical procedure was taking place, and they threatened to hang the physician if he failed in his task. Fortunately, the patient survived to get up and make her own bed after 5 days and take a cross-country trip at postoperative day 25. Although he never completed his medical degree, he was sought after by private medical students for his expertise in ovarian tumors.

The first recorded successful appendectomy was performed in 1885 by William West Grant, an American surgeon. He was the first to open the abdomen specifically to isolate the cecum and amputate the appendix. The patient, a 22-year-old woman from Iowa, survived the procedure without any serious complications. Most surgeons of this time considered the abdomen an area not to be opened unless by accident. The most famous recorded appendix-related procedure was on soon-to-be-crowned King Edward VII in 1902. Two weeks before his coronation he suffered acute appendicitis. English surgeon Frederick Treves (1853-1923) was called to perform the operation for appendicitis, which he termed *perityphlitis*. At first the young king refused surgery, but he later permitted the procedure when he was told he would certainly die without it. An appendiceal abscess was drained without removing the appendix. The procedure was performed at the palace and took less than an hour. The coronation took place as planned.

The nineteenth century did not see an increase in the number of surgical procedures until developments in anesthesia permitted surgeons to operate with greater precision on anesthetized patients. Although complex surgical procedures were becoming increasingly common, fewer procedures were performed in 1 year in past history than are currently performed in 1 day at any given facility today.

SPECIAL CONSIDERATIONS FOR GENERAL SURGERY

The discipline of general surgery provides the fundamentals for surgical practice, education, and research. The definition of general surgery agreed on by the American Board of Surgery and the Residency Review Committee for Surgery serves as the basis of graduate education and certification as a specialist in surgery. The following principles are inherent in general surgery:

- A central core of knowledge and skills common to all surgical specialties (e.g., anatomy, physiology, metabolism, pathology, immunology, wound healing, shock and resuscitation, neoplasia, and nutrition)
- The diagnosis and preoperative, intraoperative, and postoperative care of patients with diseases of the alimentary tract; the abdomen and its contents; breast; head and neck; endocrine system; and vascular system (excluding intracranial vessels, the heart, and vessels intrinsic and immediately adjacent thereto)
- Responsibility for the comprehensive management of trauma and critically ill patients with underlying surgical conditions

In a community hospital, the practice of general surgery usually encompasses many aspects of surgical care. In larger teaching facilities, general surgery services are commonly specialized (e.g., breast, biliary tract, gastrointestinal, or colon and rectal surgery). The introduction of surgical specialties was the outgrowth of increased knowledge of the etiology of disease and specialized treatment of all parts of the body. General surgery, the basis for all specialties, has decreased in breadth as specialization has increased. The anatomic parts not specifically delegated to specialists have remained in the realm of the general surgeon. Other surgical disciplines depend on general surgeons for clinical collaboration in reconstruction involving the gastrointestinal and vascular systems. The scope of this chapter focuses on procedures commonly categorized as general surgery.

Technologic advances characterize many aspects of surgical practice. The general surgery team of today should be familiar with endoscopic techniques for diagnosis and treatment. Electrosurgery, lasers, and surgical staplers are part of the setup for standard general surgery. Patients are best cared for when the entire perioperative team understands the principles of available technologies and has clinical experience in the safe use of these technologies. The following are examples of technologic applications and the associated aspects of patient care:

1. Malignant lesions, especially those of the breast, thyroid, and gastrointestinal tract, account for a large percentage of surgical interventions. The extent of the surgical excision of a lesion may be determined only after thorough exploration during a surgical procedure, sometimes scheduled as a diagnostic laparoscopy or as a biopsy and frozen section.
   a. Although the patient has been informed preoperatively of an anticipated procedure, the unknown factor is cause for apprehension. The circulating nurse should provide comfort while the patient is awake. A biopsy or endoscopic procedure may be performed with the patient under local anesthesia and with or without moderate sedation.
   b. A definitive open or laparoscopic surgical procedure may be performed on the basis of results of the biopsy and frozen section or endoscopic examination while the patient is under anesthesia. The scrub person should be prepared with two draping and instrument setups, depending on the diagnosis established and the surgeon's plan for the surgical procedure. Anticipated equipment and supplies should be available without delay.
2. The types of anesthesia administered are as varied as the types of surgical procedures. Blood pressure,

pulse, respiration, electrocardiogram (ECG), and pulse oximetry should be monitored for all patients, regardless of the anesthetic used. Personnel responsible for monitoring patients should be qualified to interpret data, assess the patient, and effect corrective action in the event of an untoward reaction.

3. Patients are placed in the supine position for many general surgical procedures. Extra padding and accessory positioning aids should be available for other positions.

4. Draping for abdominal incisions is usually standardized. Modifications are necessary for other sites, such as the breast or neck.

5. Instrumentation is quite varied and suited to function in a specific anatomic area. For example, gastrointestinal procedures require crushing clamps (e.g., Pean clamps to occlude the intestinal lumen before resection) and atraumatic clamps (e.g., Bainbridge clamps to protect delicate tissues). Included in all procedures are instruments for exposing, dissecting, grasping, clamping, suctioning, and suturing. For atraumatic retraction, various lengths of umbilical tape, hernia tape, or vessel loops may be placed around vessels or other structures to retract them. These materials should be included in the count.

6. Some procedures require minimal access and are adaptable to ambulatory surgery; others are extremely extensive. More complex procedures, such as colectomy and cholecystectomy, are often performed endoscopically and require less in-house hospitalization.

7. The electrosurgical unit (ESU), argon beam coagulator, laser, endoscope, laparoscope, and/or ultrasound transducer may be used during the procedure.

8. In complex open and laparoscopic abdominal and pelvic procedures, the following should be noted:
   a. Indwelling Foley or ureteral catheters may be inserted preoperatively.
   b. Nasogastric tubes may be passed before or during the surgical procedure.
   c. After the abdominal cavity is entered, single, free 4 × 4 sponges should be removed from the field. They are used only while folded and secured on a sponge stick. Wet or dry tapes (laparotomy packs) are used in the abdominal cavity. A small dissector (peanut or Kitner) is always clamped in a forceps before being handed to the surgeon.
   d. Before the peritoneum is incised, suction should be available and ready for immediate use, especially in biliary or intestinal procedures or when fluid or blood may be anticipated in the peritoneal cavity.
   e. Drains may be exteriorized through a stab wound in the adjacent abdominal wall before closure.
   f. Contaminated items, such as those used to anastomose intestinal segments, are isolated in a basin on the back table.
   g. Before closure, the wound is irrigated with warm, sterile, normal saline solution to remove blood and debris.
   h. Retention sutures may be used to give additional strength to wound closure.

9. Assorted sizes of drains, tubes, drainage bags, and wound suction systems should be available. Care is taken to ensure that the patient is not latex sensitive.

10. Irrigating solutions should be at body temperature when they are used. All radiopaque dyes, anticoagulants, and solutions on the instrument table are clearly labeled to avoid any error in administration.

11. Blood loss and urinary output are recorded on the perioperative record.

BREAST PROCEDURES

The mammary glands are bilateral organs (modified sweat glands) lying in the superficial fascia of the pectoral area (Fig. 33-1). They are attached to the underlying muscles by loose areolar tissue and suspended by Cooper ligaments. The breasts extend from the border of the sternum to the anterior axillary line (tail of Spence) and from approximately the first to the seventh rib. The breasts are highly vascular. The blood supply is derived laterally from the thoracic branches of the axillary, intercostal, and internal mammary arteries (Fig. 33-2). Venous drainage forms an anastomotic circle around the base of the nipple, with branches draining the circumference of the gland into the axillary and internal mammary veins. Lymphatic drainage follows the same path as the venous system and empties into the thoracoabdominal and lateral thoracic vessels. Innervation arises from the anterior and lateral cutaneous nerves of the thorax.

General surgery on the breast for males and females includes diagnostic procedures and those performed for known pathologic disease, such as cancer. Diagnostic techniques include mammography, xeroradiography, ultrasonography, and thermography, as well as the traditional tissue biopsy.

The desired surgical procedure should be determined on an individual basis after careful diagnostic studies and histologic diagnosis. Size, location, and type of diseased tissue and stage of malignancy are important considerations. No single surgical procedure is suitable for all patients.

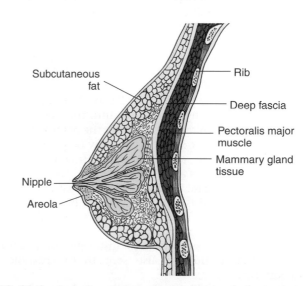

FIG. 33-1 Sagittal section of normal breast in relation to chest wall and ribcage.

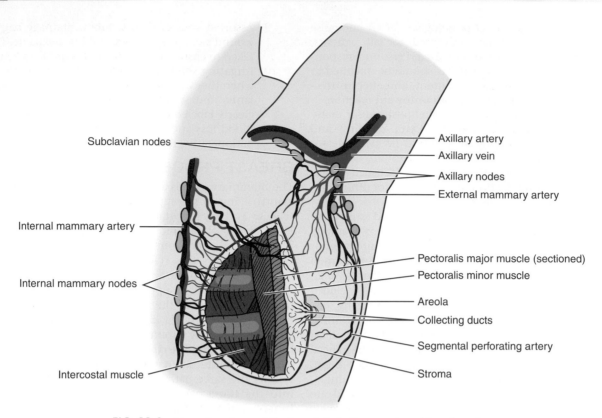

Subclavian nodes

Axillary artery

Axillary vein

Axillary nodes

External mammary artery

Internal mammary artery

Internal mammary nodes

Pectoralis major muscle (sectioned)

Pectoralis minor muscle

Areola

Collecting ducts

Segmental perforating artery

Intercostal muscle

Stroma

FIG. 33-2 Normal anatomy of the breast, including vessels and lymph nodes.

Incision and Drainage

Surgical opening of an inflamed and suppurative area is most often carried out because of infections in the lactating breast. The cavity is usually irrigated, and the wound is packed and allowed to heal by granulation. The causative organism is often *Staphylococcus*.

Breast Biopsy

The average size of lumps found by women who do and do not practice breast self-examination (BSE) is illustrated in Chapter 22 (see Fig. 22-3). All breast masses are considered malignant until proved benign. To determine the exact nature of a mass in the breast, tissue is removed for pathologic examination. The size and location (Fig. 33-3) of the lesion influence the type of biopsy:

- *Fine-needle aspiration (FNA).* A 22- or 25-gauge needle attached to a syringe is inserted into the tumor mass. A few cells are aspirated and sent to the pathology laboratory for cytologic studies. This may be performed in conjunction with a mammogram (mammographic breast biopsy) or as an office procedure. FNA also may be used to evacuate fluid from benign cysts.
- *Core biopsy.* For this type of incisional biopsy, a large-bore trocar needle, such as a Tru-Cut or Vim-Silverman biopsy needle, is inserted into the mass. A core of suspected tissue is withdrawn for histologic examination. Any retrieved fluid is also sent to the pathology laboratory.
- *Stereotactic breast biopsy.* The patient is placed prone on a special radiographic table, and her breast is placed in

an opening in the table. A computer-guided system is used to digitally locate and pinpoint nonpalpable breast lesions. The biopsy is obtained with a vacuum-assisted Mammotome while the patient is under local anesthesia.

- *Incisional biopsy.* The mass is incised, and a portion is removed for histologic examination.
- *Excisional biopsy.* The entire mass is removed for pathologic study.

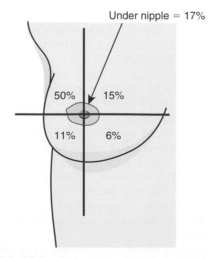

Under nipple = 17%

50%   15%

11%   6%

FIG. 33-3 Breast cancer location by quadrant.

- *Sentinel node biopsy.* The breast mass is injected with a radioisotope (technetium) in the radiology department several hours before the planned surgical procedure. In the OR, the tumor is injected with a dye containing isosulfan blue that is taken up by the lymph nodes of the breast. The nodes are excised before the primary mass. A sterile Geiger counter probe is used on the field to locate the areas of radioactivity. The specimens are sent to pathology for immunohistochemical staining. Lead containers are used to house the specimens for 24 hours before the pathologist examines them.
- *J-wire or needle localization in radiology department.* The mass is identified on mammography and the patient undergoes the insertion of a wire into the mass in the radiology department under fluoroscopy (Fig. 33-4, *A, B*). The wire remains taped in place as the patient is taken to the OR. The mass is excised with the wire intact (Fig. 33-5, *A-C*). The specimen is taken back to the radiology department to be radiographed as a confirmation that the wire is still in the mass. After the radiograph the specimen is taken to pathology.
- *Fiberoptic ductoscopy.* A flexible 0.9-mm scope with a 0.2-mm working channel is used in the ductal lumens of the breast. Studies have shown that 85% of breast cancer originates in the ductal system in the epithelial lining. The image is enlarged to 200 times by magnification. The scopes are approved for 10 uses each by the U.S Food and Drug Administration (FDA). The ducts may need to be dilated with lacrimal probes before inserting the scope. Specimens can be obtained by this method, and ductal lavage can be performed for cell studies.

Preoperatively, the surgeon discusses with the patient possible findings and treatment options. The patient may agree to an immediate definitive surgical procedure if warranted by the biopsy and frozen section results. Two separate prepping, draping, and instrument sets are necessary.

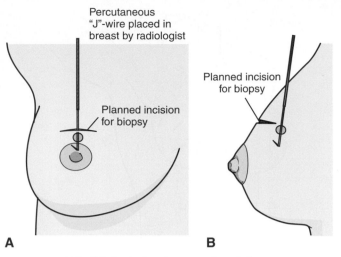

FIG. 33-4   J-wire placement in radiology.

To minimize disfigurement, many women with early operable breast cancer (a mass less than 5 cm) opt for limited resection followed by radiation and chemotherapy (Fig. 33-6). The difference between tumor and deep tumor-free resection margin remains an important consideration in determining the most appropriate type of mastectomy incision (Table 33-1).

Lumpectomy

Lumpectomy, a partial mastectomy, consists of removal of the entire tumor mass along with at least 1 to 2 cm of surrounding nondiseased tissue. This procedure is recommended for peripherally located tumors that measure less than 5 cm. Lumpectomy is contraindicated if breast size precludes postoperative radiation or if negative margins around the tumor cannot be obtained. Compared with mastectomy, the lumpectomy incisions are less disfiguring.

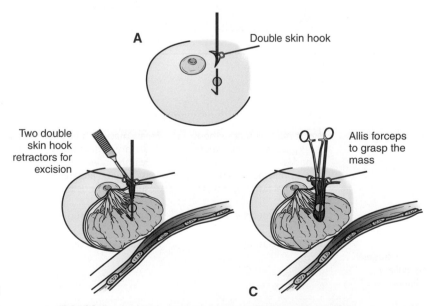

FIG. 33-5   Excision of breast mass in OR with J-wire in place.

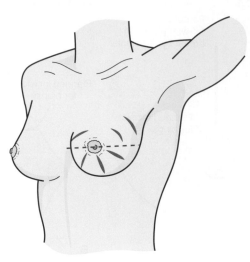

FIG. 33-6 Common conservative breast incisions followed by radiation therapy.

Breast conservation, the surgical treatment of choice for many women with breast cancer, includes a lumpectomy to excise a primary tumor and axillary node dissection followed by radiation therapy. This approach maintains the appearance and function of the breast (Fig. 33-7). The surgeon may prefer to perform the lumpectomy first, followed by axillary dissection (Fig. 33-8). The patient should be reprepped and redraped between procedures. A separate set of instruments is used for each procedure to avoid possible tumor cell implantation in the axilla. A transverse incision for axillary dissection, approximately 1 cm below the axillary hairline, extends from the pectoralis major muscle anteriorly to the latissimus dorsi muscle posteriorly. Lymphoareolar tissue between these muscles is removed—usually at least 10 lymph nodes.

Segmental Mastectomy

In a segmental mastectomy, a wedge or quadrant (quadrantectomy) of breast tissue is removed; this wedge includes the tumor mass and the lobe in which it is growing. Some surgeons explore the axilla and take a few lymph nodes for histologic studies.

Simple Mastectomy (Total Mastectomy)

In a simple mastectomy, the entire breast is removed without lymph node dissection. A simple mastectomy may be performed for a malignancy that is confined to breast tissue with negative nodes, as a palliative measure for an advanced ulcerated malignant tumor, or for the removal of extensive benign disease. Skin grafting may be necessary if the primary closure of skin flaps would create unacceptable tension. Skin flaps are then loosely approximated, and grafts taken from the thigh are applied to the remaining defect. A latissimus dorsi or rectus abdominis myocutaneous flap may be preferred for reconstruction.

A subcutaneous mastectomy may be performed for patients with chronic cystic mastitis who have had multiple previous biopsies, for patients with multiple fibroadenomas or hyperplastic duct changes, and for patients with central tumors that are noninvasive in origin. All breast tissue is removed, but the overlying skin and nipple remain intact. A prosthesis may be inserted at the time of the surgical procedure, depending on the surgeon's decision and the patient's wishes.

Modified Radical Mastectomy

A modified radical mastectomy is usually performed for infiltrating ductal and localized small malignant lesions. The term modified encompasses various techniques, but all include removal of the entire breast (total mastectomy). In addition, all axillary lymph nodes are resected. The underlying pectoralis major muscle is left in place; the pectoralis

TABLE 33-1	Stages of Breast Cancer		
Stage I	Stage II	Stage III	Stage IV
SIZE			
≤1-2 cm	2-5 cm	≥5 cm	Large and fully integrated with surrounding tissue
LOCATION			
Confined to breast	Breast mass with or without suspicious axillary lymph nodes	Breast mass with palpable, fixed axillary and/or subclavicular lymph nodes	Distant metastasis; extension to skin
	May or may not extend to pectoral fascia or muscle	Mass may be adherent to surrounding tissue	Lymphedema above or below the clavicle
	No distant metastasis	No distant metastasis	
SURGICAL OPTIONS			
Segmental mastectomy	Total mastectomy	Modified or radical mastectomy	Radical or extended radical mastectomy
Breast conservation surgery for stages I and II lumpectomy with axillary node dissection and radiation therapy			

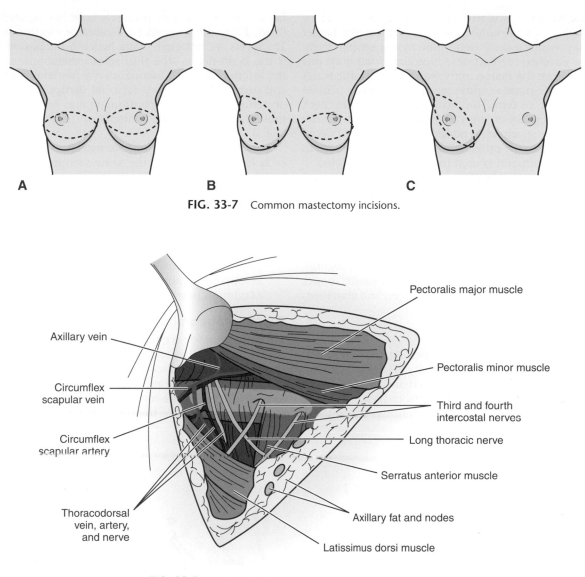

A   **B**   **C**

FIG. 33-7 Common mastectomy incisions.

Axillary vein

Circumflex
scapular vein

Circumflex
scapular artery

Thoracodorsal
vein, artery,
and nerve

Pectoralis major muscle

Pectoralis minor muscle

Third and fourth
intercostal nerves

Long thoracic nerve

Serratus anterior muscle

Axillary fat and nodes

Latissimus dorsi muscle

FIG. 33-8 Axillary lymph node dissection for breast cancer.

minor muscle may or may not be removed. In patients with small lesions and no metastases, breast reconstruction may be performed immediately or a few days after the procedure.

Radical Mastectomy

A radical mastectomy is performed to control the spread of malignant disease from large infiltrating cancers. After a positive finding on the tissue biopsy, the entire involved breast is removed along with the axillary lymph nodes, the pectoral muscles, and all adjacent tissues. During the surgical procedure, skin flaps and extensive exposed tissue are covered with moist packs for protection. The chest wall and axilla are irrigated before closure.

Extended Radical Mastectomy

Cancer is a disease that grows both deeply and laterally. An extended radical mastectomy is indicated when malignant disease is present in the medial quadrant or subareolar tissue because it tends to spread to the internal mammary lymph nodes. The involved breast is removed en bloc along with the underlying pectoral muscles, axillary contents, and upper internal mammary (mediastinal) lymph node chain. This procedure is more difficult than a classic radical mastectomy.

Considerations for Female Breast Procedures

For a breast procedure, the patient is placed in the supine position; the involved side is positioned close to the edge of the operating bed, and the arm on the affected side is extended on an armboard. The affected side is elevated with a small pillow. The anterior part of the chest is prepped from the chin to the umbilicus and from the axilla on the affected side to the nipple line of the opposite breast. The entire arm on the affected side is included in this preparation. General anesthesia is usually preferred for a mastectomy, because local infiltrate may obscure a tumor.

Because of the vascularity of breast tissue, a laser or electrosurgery is commonly used for hemostasis. Larger vessels may require a tie. Patients undergoing a mastectomy should be watched for excessive bleeding. Some surgeons prefer to irrigate the mastectomy wound with sterile water instead of sterile normal saline solution to crenate (shrivel or shrink) cancerous cells. The circulating nurse should check with the surgeon about the care of the specimen for the pathologist. The specimen is placed in sterile normal saline solution if estrogen or progesterone receptor studies are to be performed. Formalin is used for permanent sections.

A bulky compression dressing and Surgi-Bra may be applied in the OR. Depending on the amount of tissue resected, a closed-wound suction system may be inserted to remove extravasation of blood and serum and to prevent pressure necrosis of skin flaps.

Patients who have undergone a mastectomy are often referred to the Reach to Recovery rehabilitative program. In this program, volunteers who have had mastectomies visit patients, share information with them, and give them encouragement.

ABDOMINAL SURGERY

A laparotomy involves surgically opening the abdominal wall and entering the peritoneal cavity (Fig. 33-9). In this procedure, the skin and subcutaneous tissue are incised and the blood vessels are ligated or electrocoagulated. Fascia covers the muscles anteriorly and posteriorly. The anterior fascia is incised, and each muscle layer is separated and/or divided; bleeding vessels are ligated or electrocoagulated. The layers are retracted. Lying beneath the posterior fascia is the peritoneum—the thin serous membrane that lines the interior of the abdominal cavity (parietal peritoneum) and surrounds the organs (visceral peritoneum). Both the posterior fascia and the peritoneum may be cut at the same time, thus exposing the contents of the abdominal cavity (Fig. 33-10).

Various types of incisions are used in a laparotomy, but each follows essentially the same technique (Fig. 33-11). Before the procedure begins, the surgeon chooses the most suitable incision for the procedure being performed. All incisions incorporate, with varying degrees of success, certain characteristics that include the following:

- Ease and speed of entry into the abdominal cavity
- Maximum exposure
- Minimum trauma
- Least postoperative discomfort
- Maximum postoperative wound strength

Types of Abdominal Incisions

The primary reference point for abdominal incisions is the umbilicus. Secondary surface landmarks include the xyphoid, the pubis, and the iliac crests. Incisions may be vertical, horizontal, or oblique and may occur in various areas of the torso (Fig. 33-12). The incisions discussed in the following sections are applicable to open abdominal or pelvic proce-

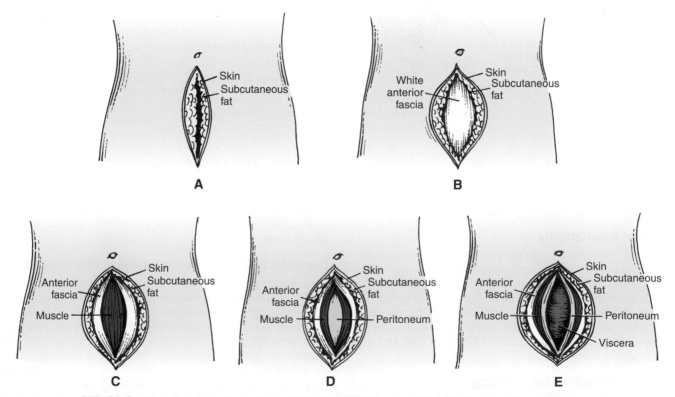

FIG. 33-9   Dissecting tissue layers of the abdomen. **A,** Subcutaneous fat (yellow). **B,** Anterior fascia (white). **C,** Muscle (red). **D,** Skin through muscle dissected. Thin white peritoneum is shown for dissection. **E,** Open peritoneum with viscera beneath.

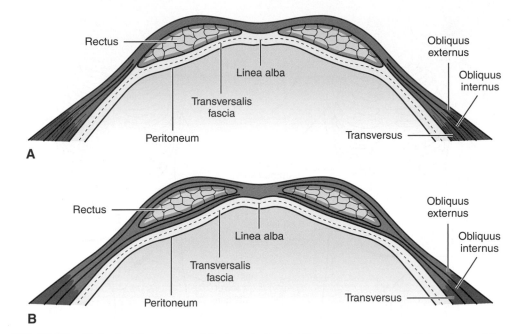

FIG. 33-10 Abdominal tissue layers at the arcuate line. **A,** Above the umbilicus. **B,** Below the umbilicus.

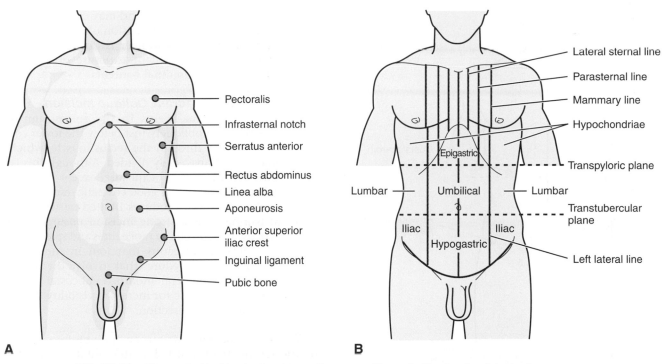

FIG. 33-11 The surgical incision is placed according to specific surgical landmarks of the body. **A,** Surface anatomy. **B,** Topographic landmarks.

dures for specific organs or organ systems (Fig. 33-13). Laparoscopy is performed through multiple (usually two to five) incisions that are smaller (usually 5 to 10 mm), separate, and distinct.

Paramedian Incision. The paramedian incision is a vertical incision made approximately 4 cm (approximately 2 inches) lateral to the midline on either side in the upper or lower abdomen. After the skin and subcutaneous tissue are incised, the rectus sheath is split vertically and the muscle is retracted laterally. This incision allows quick entry into and excellent exposure of the abdominal cavity. It limits trauma, avoids nerve injury, is easily extended, and gives a firm closure. Examples of use include access to the biliary tract or pancreas in the right upper quadrant and access to the left lower quadrant for resection of the sigmoid colon.

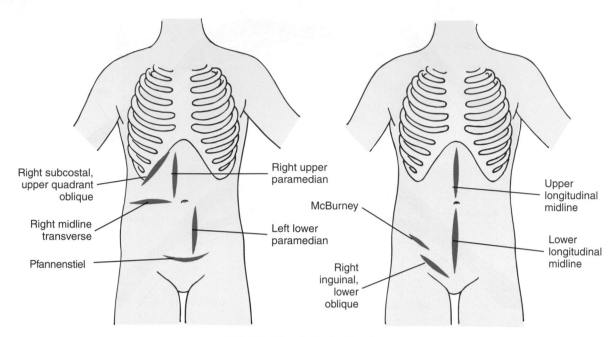

FIG. 33-12   Abdominal incisions.

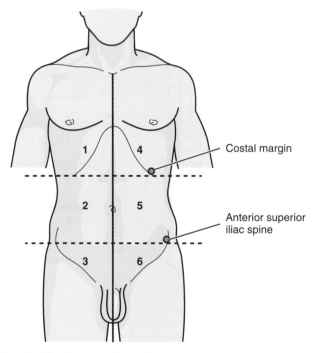

FIG. 33-13   Determination of incision placement by organ position. *1,* Liver, gallbladder, pancreas, stomach; *2,* right kidney, retroperitoneal mass, colon, aortic aneurysm, jejunum, ileum, appendix; *3,* cecum, terminal ileum, ovary, fallopian tube, uterus, ureter; *4,* spleen, splenic artery aneurysm, pancreas, stomach; *5,* left kidney, colon, aortic aneurysm, jejunum; *6,* sigmoid colon, ovary, fallopian tube, uterus, ureter.

Longitudinal Midline Incision. A longitudinal midline incision can be upper abdominal, lower abdominal, or a combination of both going around the umbilicus. Depending on the length of the incision, it begins in the epigastrium at

the level of the xiphoid process and may extend vertically to the suprapubic region. After incision of the peritoneum, the falciform ligament of the liver is divided. An upper midline incision offers excellent exposure of and rapid entry into the upper abdominal contents.

Subcostal Upper Quadrant Oblique Incision. A right or left oblique incision begins in the epigastrium and extends laterally and obliquely just below the lower costal margin. It continues through the rectus muscle, which is either retracted or transversely divided. Although this type of incision affords limited exposure except for upper abdominal viscera, it provides good cosmetic results because it follows skin lines and produces limited nerve damage. Although painful, it is a strong incision postoperatively. Examples of use include biliary procedures and splenectomy.

Bilateral subcostal incisions that join in the midline may be preferred for procedures that involve the stomach and/or pancreas. A bilateral modified subcostal incision (chevron incision) is made for increased visibility during a liver transplantation or resection.

McBurney's Incision. McBurney's point is located in the right lower quadrant, just below the umbilicus and 4 cm (approximately 2 inches) medial from the anterior superior iliac spine. McBurney's incision involves a muscle-splitting incision that extends through the fibers of the external oblique muscle. The incision is deepened, the internal oblique and transversalis muscles are split and retracted, and the peritoneum is entered. This is a fast, easy incision, but exposure is limited. Its primary use is for appendectomy.

Thoracoabdominal Incision. For a thoracoabdominal incision, the patient is placed in a lateral position. Either a right or a left incision begins at a point midway between the xiphoid process and umbilicus and extends across the abdomen to the seventh or eighth costal interspace and along the interspace into the thorax. The rectus, oblique, serratus, and intercostal muscles are divided in the line of incision down to the peritoneum and pleura. This converts the pleural and peritoneal cavities into one main cavity, thus allowing excellent exposure for the upper end of the stomach and lower end of the esophagus. Examples of use include esophageal varices and the repair of a hiatal hernia.

Midabdominal Transverse Incision. The midabdominal transverse incision starts on either the right or left side and slightly above or below the umbilicus. It may be carried laterally to the lumbar region between the ribs and crest of the ilium. The intercostal nerves are protected by cutting the posterior rectus sheath and peritoneum in the direction of the divided muscle fibers. The advantages are rapid incision, easy extension, a provision for retroperitoneal approach, and a secure postoperative wound. Examples of use include choledochojejunostomy and transverse colostomy.

Pfannenstiel Incision. A Pfannenstiel incision is a curved transverse incision across the lower abdomen and within or superior to the hairline of the pubis. The incision follows the Langer lines of the natural skinfolds. The rectus fascia is incised transversely, and the muscles are separated.

The peritoneum is incised vertically in the midline. This lower transverse incision provides good exposure and strong closure for pelvic procedures. Its primary use is for an abdominal hysterectomy and cesarean section.

Inguinal Incision (Lower Oblique). An oblique incision of the right or left inguinal region extends from the pubic tubercle to the anterior crest of the ilium, slightly above and parallel to the inguinal crease. Incision of the external oblique fascia provides access to the cremaster muscle, inguinal canal, and cord structures. Its primary use is for inguinal herniorrhaphy.

BILIARY TRACT PROCEDURES

The gallbladder is located in the right upper quadrant in a fossa under and immediately adjacent to the right lobe of the liver (Fig. 33-14). The gallbladder is a thin-walled sac and has a normal capacity of 50 to 75 mL of bile. Bile secreted by the hepatic cells enters the intrahepatic bile ducts and progresses to the common bile duct. When not needed for digestion, bile is diverted through the cystic duct into the gallbladder, where it is stored. When bile is needed, the gallbladder contracts and empties bile into the cystic duct; the bile flows into and through the common duct into the duodenum.

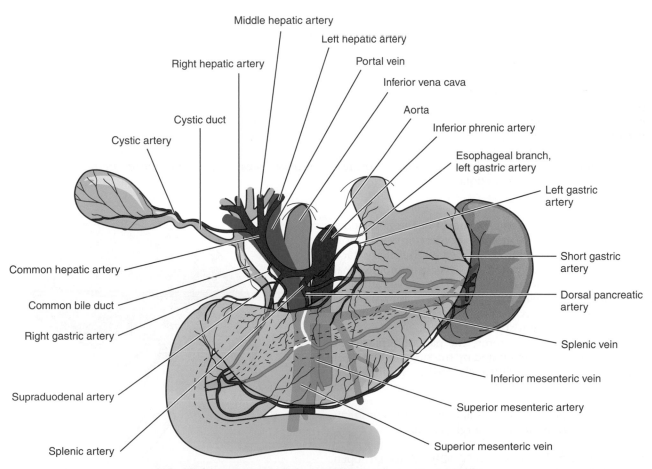

FIG. 33-14 Normal anatomy of the biliary system and portal system.

Gallstones are concretions of elements of bile, particularly cholesterol (about 50%), and may be found in the gallbladder or in any portion of the extrahepatic biliary duct system. Brown stones are usually fatty acids, and black stones comprise inorganic salts. The incidence of stones, referred to as cholelithiasis, increases with age and is more prevalent in women and in people who are obese. Acute or chronic inflammation of the gallbladder, common duct stones (choledocholithiasis), carcinoma, and the congenital absence of bile ducts (biliary atresia) are the most common indications for a surgical procedure. Obstructive jaundice, which is potentially fatal, may be a sign of ductal cholelithiasis or the presence of a neoplasm. The cause of jaundice should be determined and the condition relieved to spare the patient irreversible progressive liver damage. Biliary stones are sent as dry specimens if removed separately.

The greatest hazards of biliary tract surgery are associated with the anatomic relationships of the ducts and the cystic artery (see Fig. 33-14) and with pathologic changes in the gallbladder. Complications include hemorrhage and injury to the extrahepatic biliary duct system. Spilled bile can cause peritonitis postoperatively.

Ultrasonography, nuclear imaging such as hepatic intraductal assay (HIDA) scan, and computed tomography (CT) scanning are used for the diagnosis of gallbladder disease. Oral and intravenous (IV) cholecystography may be used for visualization of the gallbladder in the initial evaluation of patients with biliary symptoms. Endoscopic retrograde cholangiopancreatography also may be performed, usually by a gastroenterologist, to identify stones, tumors, inflammatory lesions, or an obstruction. A flexible fiberoptic duodenoscope is introduced with the patient under IV sedation and with the use of a topical anesthetic to control the gag reflex.

Dye is injected to opacify the entire biliary tract and pancreatic duct under fluoroscopy. Some definitive therapy is possible during this procedure, such as stone retrieval (endoscopic papillotomy), stent insertion, and sphincterotomy. A percutaneous transhepatic puncture is used to biopsy tumors, dilate strictures, place stents in the bile duct, and establish temporary drainage through ducts. A contrast medium can be injected for a cholangiogram.

Cholecystectomy

Gallbladder disease is cured by removal of the gallbladder in a procedure referred to as a cholecystectomy—the most common surgical procedure performed on the biliary tract. A cholecystectomy is performed to relieve the gastrointestinal distress common in patients with acute or chronic cholecystitis (with or without gallstones); it also removes a source of recurrent sepsis. Persistent infection in the biliary tract may cause recurrent stones.

For an open cholecystectomy, the patient is placed in the supine position. As requested by the surgeon, the right upper quadrant may be slightly elevated on a gallbladder rest or pillow after the induction of general anesthesia. The operating bed may be tilted slightly into a reverse Trendelenburg's position so the abdominal viscera gravitate downward, away from the surgical area.

Open Abdominal Cholecystectomy. With an open abdominal cholecystectomy, the gallbladder is usually exposed through a right subcostal incision (Kocher incision) that may be extended over to the midline at the level of the xiphoid. The incision should be adequate for good exposure of the gallbladder and bile ducts. After exploration of the abdominal cavity, laparotomy packs are used to wall off the surrounding organs for exposure. The bilious contents of the gallbladder may be aspirated to prevent bile from spilling into the peritoneal cavity—a potential source of peritonitis, especially if the gallbladder is inflamed and tightly distended. The cystic duct, cystic artery, hepatic ducts, and common bile duct are accurately identified.

After palpation of the ducts for stones, the cystic duct and artery are ligated with hemostatic clips and divided. Using blunt dissection, the gallbladder is freed and removed from the liver and its fossa (Fig. 33-15). Some surgeons use ESU and/or neodymium:yttrium aluminum garnet (Nd:YAG) or holmium (Ho):YAG laser for sharp dissection and coagulation. Stones removed as part of the specimen should be sent to the pathology department for analysis and documentation. If bile leakage or hemorrhage has been excessive, a sump drain or closed-wound suction drain may be placed in the subhepatic space and brought out through a stab wound after intraabdominal irrigation.

Laparoscopic Cholecystectomy. With a laparoscopic cholecystectomy the patient is supine in a slight to moderate reverse Trendelenburg's position. A rigid fiberoptic laparoscope is inserted through a sheath into the peritoneal cavity. Trocars are inserted through three or four puncture triangulated wounds in the right upper quadrant: one or two just right of midline, with the uppermost trocar slightly below the xiphoid and costal margin and the other midway to the umbilicus; one laterally in an anterior axillary line above the iliac crest at the costal margin; and another in a midclavicular line slightly above the level of the umbilicus and 2 cm below the rib. The location of puncture sites will vary according to patient size and surgeon preference (Fig. 33-16).

A camera attached to the laparoscope allows the surgeon to view the manipulation of instruments through the sheaths of these trocars. Viewing monitors are positioned on each

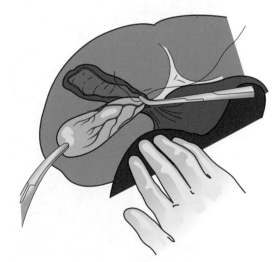

FIG. 33-15 The gallbladder is dissected from the liver bed.

side of the head of the operating bed (Fig. 33-17). With this procedure, the fundus of the gallbladder is grasped through lateral port(s) and held by the assistant. After careful dissection, the surgeon ligates and divides the cystic duct and artery with suture loops or clips. A laser, an ESU, or microscissors may be used to transect these structures. The gallbladder is freed, most often by using an ESU or by using argon, potassium titanyl phosphate (KTP), contact Nd:YAG, or Ho:YAG laser. The gallbladder is usually aspirated to remove bile and collapse the sac. It may then be removed

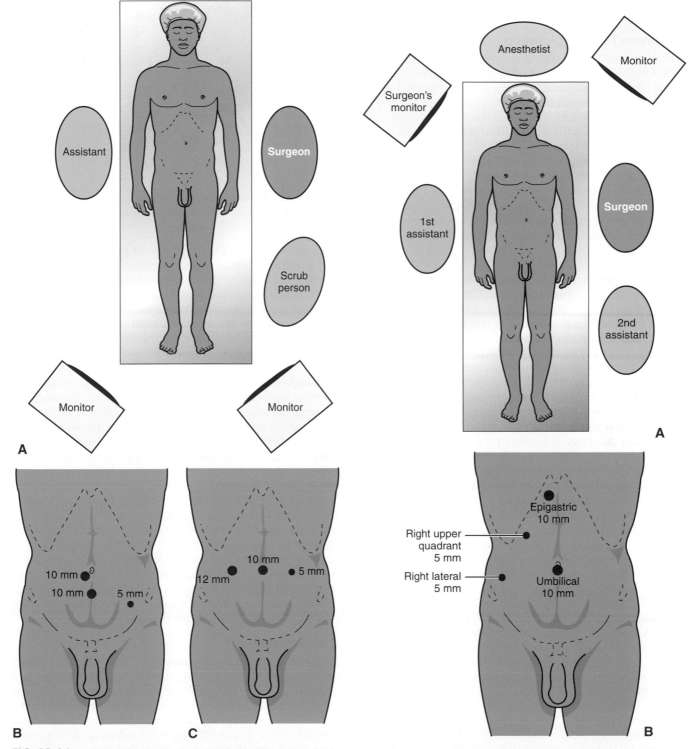

FIG. 33-16   Laparoscopic setup. **A,** Position of personnel for a basic laparoscopy. **B,** Trocar placement will be determined by the target organ position. **C,** Trocars used will vary in size according to position of function for dissection and hemostasis.

FIG. 33-17   Laparoscopic cholecystectomy. **A,** Placement of personnel and monitors for gallbladder removal. **B,** Trocar placement for gallbladder removal.

in one piece or cut into sections and withdrawn through the periumbilical incision.

The perioperative team must be ready to convert from laparoscopic to an open procedure in the event of bleeding or other difficulty during the procedure. Supplies and instrumentation should be immediately available. It is advantageous to have precounted sets in the room during these procedures.

Common Duct Exploration

Concomitant exploration of the common duct is often but not routinely performed during cholecystectomy. Curved stone forceps, small malleable scoops, dilators of various sizes, balloon catheters, stone baskets, and nylon brushes are useful in clearing the hepatic and biliary ducts of stones to prevent them from lodging in the duct and causing subsequent obstructive jaundice.

Palpable stones, jaundice with cholangitis, and dilation of the common bile duct are indications for exploration. A T-tube drain may be inserted to stent the duct and provide postoperative drainage. The surgeon may choose other intraoperative techniques to identify unsuspected stones, pathologic conditions, or anatomic variations in the hepatic duct system.

Intraoperative Cholangiograms. Radiographs are obtained during either open abdominal or laparoscopic procedures. The radiology department is notified in advance if a cholangiogram is anticipated. To check for patient position, scout films should be obtained when the patient is initially positioned on the operating bed—before the procedure is started. The circulating nurse should assess the patient for allergies or sensitivities to contrast media and should ensure that the operating bed has a radiographic top or can be equipped for radiographs or fluoroscopy.

The radiology technician returns to the operating room (OR) when the surgeon is ready for films. Cholangiograms may be obtained after the gallbladder is removed or before the cystic duct and artery are ligated. A radiopaque contrast medium, usually diatrizoate sodium (Hypaque or Renografin), is injected into the cystic duct or common bile duct with a 50-mL syringe. Unless fluoroscopy is used, a series of three or four radiographs are obtained and displayed in digital format. Before each exposure, the surgeon injects dye through a Cholangiocath (a plastic catheter inserted into cystic or common duct), cannula, or direct needle puncture in the common duct (Fig. 33-18). Instruments are removed from the field to the extent possible to minimize the obstruction of structures on the radiographs. The field is covered with a sterile barrier before the radiograph machine or C-arm is positioned over the patient. Sterile radiograph tube and C-arm covers are commercially available. All other radiologic precautions for patient and personnel safety should be observed.

Ultrasonography. Ultrasonography, a noninvasive technique, takes less time and does not have the radiation hazards of intraoperative cholangiograms. A sterile ultrasound probe is manipulated along the common bile duct from the liver to the duodenum. The probe transmits high-frequency sound waves back to the ultrasound unit in the

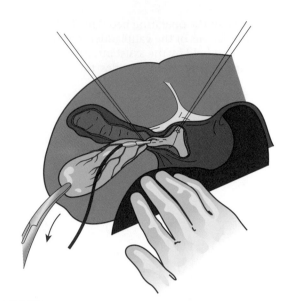

FIG. 33-18 The cystic duct is dissected free, and a cholangiogram catheter is inserted. Radiographs are taken, and the duct is ligated.

form of echoes, which are displayed on a screen as black-and-white real-time images. To enhance the transmission of ultrasound waves, the abdominal cavity is irrigated with warm normal saline solution. Density in tissue causes sound waves to echo in altered patterns and directions. Gallstones appear as bright echoes, often with an acoustic shadow. Photographs or a videotape can be obtained to document the findings of ultrasonography.

Choledochoscopy. Intraoperative biliary endoscopy provides image transmission and illumination, thus allowing the surgeon visual guidance in exploring the biliary system. Intrahepatic and extrahepatic bile ducts can be visualized with a flexible fiberoptic choledochoscope introduced into the common duct. To provide distention of the biliary tract, normal saline solution must continuously flow through the irrigation channel.

Stones are easily seen and are usually free-floating under the pressure of the irrigating solution. A flexible stone forceps or a basket or a balloon-tipped biliary catheter may be inserted through the instrument channel of either a rigid or flexible scope to allow manipulation of a stone under direct vision. A biopsy forceps may be inserted to obtain a tissue sample. An Nd:YAG laser fiber may be used through the choledochoscope to crush bilirubin stones in the distal common hepatic duct; this allows easy removal of the stones.

Cholelithotripsy

Cholelithotripsy is a noninvasive procedure in which high-energy shock waves are used to fragment cholesterol gallstones. The procedure is performed under IV sedation or general anesthesia. The patient is usually placed in the prone position but may also be in the supine or lateral position, on a lithotripter table, or submerged in a water bath. Spark-gap shock waves generated from an electrode pass through a fluid medium into the body until they reach the stone, which is focused with an ultrasound probe and computer. The shock waves are synchronized with the

R waves of the patient's cardiac rhythm, which is monitored by ECG to avoid dysrhythmias. Each shock pulverizes the stone(s) into small fragments, which then pass through the bile duct. This passage may be aided by oral administration of deoxycholic acid (ursodiol) taken daily after lithotripsy to dissolve the fragments.

Choledochostomy and Choledochotomy

With choledochostomy, a T-tube is used to drain the common bile duct through the abdominal wall. A choledochotomy is the incision of the common bile duct for the exploration and removal of stones. Intraoperative cholangiography may be performed before and after exploration and/or stone removal. The duct is irrigated after calculi are removed. Patency of the duct and of the ampulla of Vater is investigated, often through a choledochoscope. If a neoplasm is found during exploration, resectability is determined; many tumors of the liver or pancreas are inoperable.

Cholecystoduodenostomy and Cholecystojejunostomy

Either a cholecystoduodenostomy or cholecystojejunostomy is performed to relieve an obstruction in the distal end of the common duct. Through anastomosis, these procedures establish continuity between the gallbladder and either the duodenum or jejunum. Careful evaluation precedes the surgical procedure. Cholecystoduodenostomy and cholecystojejunostomy are bypass procedures to avoid further obstructive jaundice, but they do not solve the problem. Common causes of the obstruction are calculi, stricture of the duct, or neoplasms of the duct, ampulla of Vater, or pancreas.

Choledochoduodenostomy and Choledochojejunostomy

Choledochoduodenostomy and choledochojejunostomy are side-to-side anastomoses between the duodenum or jejunum and the common duct. These procedures are carried out for difficult or recurrent biliary or pancreatic obstruction as a result of benign or malignant disease.

LIVER PROCEDURES

The liver, the largest gland in the body, is divided into left and right segments (or lobes) and is located in the upper right abdominal cavity beneath the diaphragm (Figs. 33-19 and 33-20). Part of the stomach and duodenum and the hepatic flexure of the colon lie directly beneath the liver. A tough fibrous sheath, Glisson capsule, completely covers the organ; the tissue within this capsule is very friable and vascular. The hepatic artery, a branch of the celiac axis, maintains the arterial supply. Blood from the stomach, intestine, spleen, and pancreas is carried to the liver by the portal vein and its branches.

The many functions of the liver include forming and secreting bile, which aids digestion; transforming glucose into glycogen, which it stores; and helping to regulate blood volume. The liver is vital for the metabolic functioning of the body. It metabolizes fats, proteins, and carbohydrates; synthesizes cholesterol; excretes bilirubin; and secretes hormones. This organ has remarkable regenerative capacity, and up to 80% of it may be resected with little or no alteration in hepatic function. Liver function tests are used

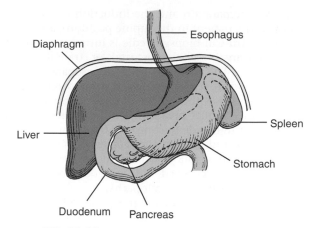

FIG. 33-19 Organs in upper abdominal cavity.

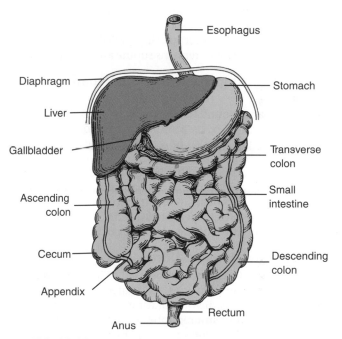

FIG. 33-20 Abdominal organs within peritoneal cavity.

to assess the degree of functional impairment and to evaluate liver activity and reserve. Most of these tests involve taking a series of blood samples from the patient for specific studies. Ascites may result from impaired liver function.

Liver Needle Biopsy

A percutaneous needle biopsy may help establish a diagnosis of liver disease. Because the procedure is performed with the patient under local anesthesia, moderate sedation, or monitored anesthesia care (MAC), the patient should be instructed to take several deep breaths and then hold the breath and remain absolutely still while the needle is inserted. Failure of the patient to cooperate can cause needle penetration of the diaphragm or hepatic injury and result in hemorrhage, a serious complication. Leakage of bile into the abdominal cavity may produce chemical peritonitis, an additional hazard.

After skin preparation and the induction of local anesthesia (with the patient in the supine position), a Franklin-Silverman or Tru-Cut biopsy needle is introduced into the liver via a transthoracic intercostal or transabdominal subcostal route. The needle is rotated to separate a small core of tissue, and it is then withdrawn to remove the specimen. As soon as the needle is removed, the patient is told to resume normal breathing and is assisted to turn onto his or her right side to compress the chest wall at the penetration site and prevent the seepage of bile or blood. Slight bleeding may follow a liver biopsy; the patient's prothrombin time is checked. This method of biopsy is not used if the patient has a coagulopathy.

In certain patients under local anesthesia, a laparoscopic-assisted approach may be used to enhance visualization of the biopsy site. The anterior abdominal wall is elevated with a low volume of carbon dioxide insufflation or a planar lift device without insufflation. The biopsy needle is inserted through the abdominal wall as described previously. A topical hemostatic gelatin sponge or other topical chemical hemostatic agent is laparoscopically applied to the biopsy site on the liver. The patient remains supine after this procedure.

Drainage of Subphrenic and Subhepatic Abscesses

Abscesses in and around the liver may be caused by a variety of microorganisms or as a result of secondary infections from abdominal organs. In general, these abscesses are treated by incision and drainage. A catheter may be introduced into the abscess cavity, which has been localized on a CT scan. The location of the abscess determines the percutaneous approach (i.e., transpleural, subpleural, transperitoneal, or retroperitoneal). Care must be taken to avoid contamination of the pleural or peritoneal cavity.

Intraoperative Hepatic Ultrasound

Intraoperative ultrasound can be used to identify anatomic structures or liver densities associated with a primary tumor or metastasis. Before rotating the liver forward and excising diseased or injured lobes or segments, it is necessary to divide the appropriate ligamentous attachments and to ligate the veins and arteries. Lesions not accessible for resection may be treated with cryosurgery or a Cavitron ultrasonic aspirator. These techniques may also be used in conjunction with resection. An ultrasonic aspirator permits the precise removal of tissue and controls bleeding during resection.

Hepatic Resection

The standard anatomic resections of the liver are right or left lobectomy, right or left trisegmentectomy, and left lateral segmentectomy. Because it is a vital organ, the entire liver cannot be removed without liver transplantation. Lobectomy or segmental resection is indicated for cysts, benign or malignant tumors, or severe penetrating or blunt trauma. Depending on the location of the lesion to be resected, a right or bilateral subcostal incision or an upper midline incision is made and can be extended as needed for exposure and exploration. The liver is the most commonly injured abdominal organ. Hepatic parenchymal injuries usually cause intraperitoneal hemorrhage and shock.

Liver tissue is very friable. The prevention or arrest of hemorrhage is a prime concern. Omental flaps, falciform ligament, or a Gerota fascia flap may be used for coverage and tamponade of bleeding surfaces in conjunction with local hemostatic substances. Microfibrillar collagen or oxidized cellulose is often used to control bleeding. Large, blunt, noncutting needles are used to suture the liver. Drains are usually placed in the wound and brought out through stab wounds. Equipment for blood replacement, portal pressure measurement, and chest drainage should be available.

Portosystemic Shunts

Portal hypertension, bleeding esophageal varices, or massive gastrointestinal hemorrhage may necessitate an emergency surgical procedure for decompression of the portal venous system. Often the patient is alcoholic, with cirrhosis, poor nutrition, and unstable blood volume, or generally is a poor surgical risk. A portosystemic shunt is a vascular anastomosis between the portal and systemic venous systems. The surgeon may select one of several techniques for a portacaval or mesocaval shunt. In patients with portal hypertension and hypersplenism, a splenorenal shunt may be performed in conjunction with a splenectomy for portal decompression.

SPLENIC PROCEDURES

The highly vascular spleen is located in the upper left abdominal cavity and lies beneath the dome of the diaphragm; it is protected by the lower portion of the ribcage (see Fig. 33-19). The capsule of the spleen is covered with peritoneum and is held in place by numerous suspensory ligaments. The splenic artery furnishes the arterial blood supply, and the splenic vein drains into the portal system. As the largest lymphatic organ of the body, the spleen has an intimate role in the immunologic defenses of the body and acts as a blood reservoir. The main functions of the spleen involve the formation of blood elements. Radionuclide scanning and other radiographic studies provide information for analysis.

Splenectomy

The most common reason for removal of the spleen is hypersplenism—overactivity that causes a reduction in the circulating quantity of red cells, white cells, platelets, or a combination of them. Splenectomies are often scheduled at specific times because patients often require the administration of whole blood immediately before a surgical procedure. Often these patients are also receiving steroid treatment, and provisions are made to maintain therapy during the surgical procedure and postoperatively. Hematologic disorders, tumors, or accessory spleens may also necessitate surgical intervention. A splenic rupture requires an immediate surgical procedure to prevent fatal hemorrhage and may require a splenectomy. In certain patients with benign disease, a laparoscopic approach has been successfully used for splenectomy.

In performing a splenectomy, a left rectus paramedian, midline, or subcostal incision is used to enter the peritoneal cavity, and the spleen is displaced medially by careful manual manipulation. The splenorenal, splenocolic, and gastrosplenic ligaments are ligated and divided. Great care should be exercised in ligating the splenic artery and vein because these vessels are often friable. Hemorrhage is the principal intraoperative hazard. After removal of the spleen and before closure, careful inspection for bleeding from the splenic pedicle and retroperitoneal space is essential.

Splenorrhaphy

After a splenectomy, patients—especially children—are immunologically impaired (i.e., more susceptible to infection), which sometimes can produce catastrophic results. To protect the patient's immune competence, surgeons attempt to salvage splenic tissue after splenic trauma. Splenorrhaphy, or splenic repair, can be accomplished in several ways. Once the spleen is mobilized, actively bleeding vessels are ligated and devitalized tissues are debrided. The spleen can then be sutured or stapled along the edge of a partial splenectomy. Microfibrillar collagen or absorbable gelatin sponges can be placed over a small laceration or capsular tear to effect hemostasis. The splenic artery may be ligated.

The spleen may be wrapped in omentum or synthetic mesh. Segments can be reimplanted into an omental pouch in the intraperitoneal space to preserve splenic function. In patients with extensive trauma, a drain that is exteriorized through a stab wound may be inserted into the left subdiaphragmatic space.

PANCREATIC PROCEDURES

The pancreas is both an endocrine gland and an exocrine gland. The islets of Langerhans form the endocrine division and secrete the hormones insulin and glucagon, both of which are essential to the metabolism of carbohydrates and the storage of calories. Acini and the ducts leading from them constitute the exocrine portion, which secretes pancreatic juice into the duodenum. Pancreatic juice neutralizes stomach acid; the loss of pancreatic juice results in severe impairment in the digestion and absorption of food.

The pancreas lies transversely across the posterior wall of the upper abdomen behind the stomach. The head, or right extremity of the pancreas, is attached to the duodenum; the tail, or left extremity of the pancreas, is in proximity to the spleen (Fig. 33-21).

Disorders of the pancreas generally include acute and chronic inflammation, cysts, and tumors. The head of the

pancreas is the most common site of a malignant pancreatic tumor. Accuracy in the diagnosis of pancreatic problems is difficult, but evaluation by ultrasonography, endoscopic retrograde cholangiopancreatography, and scanning has led to significant improvements in planning surgical treatment. An exploratory laparotomy is the most reliable means of diagnosing and evaluating pancreatic trauma. Pancreatitis is associated most often with pancreatic duct stones, gallstones, or alcoholism. Corrective biliary tract procedures usually alleviate gallstone pancreatitis.

Pancreaticojejunostomy

Pancreaticojejunostomy may be performed for relief of pain associated with chronic alcoholic pancreatitis and pseudocysts of the pancreas. There are several types of procedures for the drainage of obstructed ducts or pseudocysts. These methods involve anastomosing a loop of the jejunum (Roux-en-Y loop) to the pancreatic duct. Hemorrhage and leakage of bile are complications to be avoided.

Pancreaticoduodenectomy (Whipple Procedure)

Pancreaticoduodenectomy is an extensive procedure performed on patients with carcinoma of the head of the pancreas or the ampulla of Vater. A gastrointestinal setup is used for this procedure. The abdominal cavity is exposed through one of several possible anterior incisions, but a long right paramedian incision is usually made. The abdominal and pelvic cavities are explored for distant metastases. Because many vital structures and organs are involved in resecting the diseased proximal portion of the pancreas, careful dissection of vessels is necessary to prevent hemorrhage, which complicates the procedure. Resection includes the distal stomach, the duodenum distal to the pylorus, the distal end of the common bile duct, and all but the tail of the pancreas.

Several methods of reconstructing the digestive tract are possible, but all include anastomosis of the pancreatic duct, common bile duct, stomach, and jejunum. Most surgeons reestablish biliary-intestinal continuity by end-to-side choledochojejunostomy (see Fig. 33-21). The stomach and pylorus may be preserved in patients with benign disease or localized, small tumors. After pancreatic and biliary reconstruction, the divided end of the duodenum is anastomosed to the side of the jejunal limb used for the reconstruction. A watertight seal of all anastomoses is essential to prevent peritonitis or pancreatitis. Drains are inserted.

Improvements in preoperative and postoperative care and the refinement of technical details have increased the survival rate of patients who undergo this potentially hazardous radical surgical procedure. The most common postoperative complications of pancreaticoduodenectomy are shock, hemorrhage, renal failure, and pancreatic or biliary fistula. If a fistula should occur, wound suction is continued until the fistula closes. In general, the fistula will close spontaneously if adequate nutrition and electrolyte balance are maintained.

Pancreatectomy

Subtotal distal pancreatectomy is usually performed to resect a benign tumor or for chronic pancreatitis. The distal tail is resected to the head of the pancreas. A splenectomy

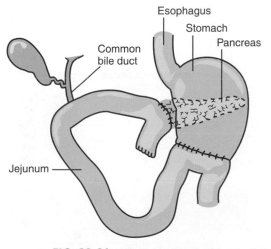

FIG. 33-21 Whipple procedure.

is usually performed with this procedure because the blood supply to the tail of the pancreas comes from splenic vessels that are sacrificed.

A total pancreatectomy allows a wide resection of a primary malignant tumor and its multifocal sites in the pancreas. A patient who has undergone a total pancreatectomy will have some endocrine and pancreatic insufficiency.

Pancreaticoduodenal Trauma

Combined injuries of the pancreas and duodenum from penetrating wounds or blunt trauma are among the most complicated to treat. A midline incision is used to explore the abdomen. Suturing to control bleeding, debriding of devitalized tissue, and draining are the initial therapies. Pancreatic fistulas and abscesses are potential complications. Extensive injury of the head of the pancreas and duodenum may require pancreaticoduodenal resection with gastrojejunostomy.

ESOPHAGEAL PROCEDURES

The esophagus is the 25- to 30-cm-long musculomembranous tube between the pharynx in the throat and the stomach in the abdomen. It is composed distally of striated skeletal muscle and proximally of smooth muscle. It passes through the thoracic cavity and enters the abdominal cavity through the esophageal hiatus (opening) in the right crus of the diaphragm; it joins the right medial surface of the stomach. The esophagus propels food by peristalsis. Within the abdominal cavity, the esophagus is bordered by the liver anteriorly and the aorta posteriorly and slightly to the left (with the spleen on the left), and between the right and left branches of the vagus nerve (see Figs. 33-19 and 33-20). The blood supply is derived from the inferior thyroid arteries, the bronchial, gastric, and phrenic branches directly off the aorta.

Patients with long-standing (more than 5 years) gastroesophageal reflux with erosive esophagitis can develop Barrett esophagus. This can happen when the cellular structure at the gastroesophageal junction has changed from squamous cells to columnar cells. Although there is no cure, further damage can be prevented with appropriate medical treatment. If strictures form, frequent dilation with bougie (pronounced *boogee*) instrumentation may be necessary. The bougies range in size from 16 to 60 French (Fr). The risk for developing cancer is between 5% and 10%, and patients with Barrett esophagus are frequently assessed and screened by esophagoscopy and biopsy.

Diverticula (pouches or pockets) can be present at the distal end of the esophagus near the dorsal aspect of the throat at the level of C5-C6. These pockets can herniate and collect food and can progressively become larger. These pockets are referred to as Zenker diverticula, which account for 65% of all diverticula in the esophagus. They can become infected and necrotic or engorged to the point of rupture, which then becomes a surgical emergency. Some texts refer to the hernia as a Killian dehiscence.

Esophageal Hiatal Herniorrhaphy

When intraabdominal pressure exceeds pressure in the chest, the abdominal esophagus and a portion of the stomach may slide through the esophageal hiatus and into the thoracic cavity. Although this condition (referred to as hiatal or diaphragmatic hernia) is quite common, a surgical procedure is indicated when the resultant esophagitis causes ulceration, bleeding, stenosis, or chest and back symptoms. Reflux esophagitis and sphincter incompetence also may have other causes that necessitate a surgical procedure.

The abdominal approach to correct the problem involves a midline or left subcostal incision. Because visualization of the hiatal area may be difficult, the incision may be extended over the lower ribcage. The patient may be placed in a slight reverse Trendelenburg's position. Organs and vital structures should be protected with moist tapes and gently retracted to expose the hiatus. Long-handled clamps are needed. After mobilization, the hiatus is narrowed with heavy sutures and the fundus of the stomach is anchored against the diaphragm to prevent recurrent herniation and gastroesophageal reflux.

Prevention of reflux is one of the prime objectives of fundoplication, because it was the cause of the patient's previous esophagitis. Lengthening the intraabdominal esophagus and increasing pressure on the lower esophageal sphincter also help control reflux. The esophagus is secured by wrapping the proximal stomach (fundus) around the gastroesophageal junction in one of two ways: either by a total 360-degree wrap (Nissen fundoplication); or by a 180- to 200-degree wrap (Toupet partial fundoplication) (Fig. 33-22). The fundus of the stomach acts as a flap valve to create pressure around the distal esophagus, thus decreasing reflux. As an alternative to fundoplication, some surgeons insert an antireflux collar-like prosthesis around the esophagus just above the gastroesophageal junction.

A laparoscopic fundoplication, which may be performed in select patients, has similar advantages to laparoscopic cholecystectomy. The procedure involves mobilizing the esophagogastric junction and repairing the hiatal defect with a continuous suture technique. This is followed by a total fundoplication to fix the anterior margin of the diaphragmatic hiatus proximally and the esophagogastric junction distally. The laparoscopic approach has been successful in treating gastroesophageal reflux as a minimally invasive procedure.

Esophagogastrectomy

Removal of the lower portion of the esophagus and proximal stomach may be indicated to resect malignant tumors,

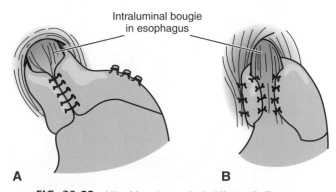

FIG. 33-22   Hiatal hernia repair. **A,** Nissen. **B,** Toupet.

benign strictures, or perforations at or near the esophagogastric junction. A left thoracoabdominal or upper midline incision is made. After the esophagus and stomach are mobilized and divided, an end-to-end esophagogastric anastomosis may be completed with staples and/or sutures. An end-to-side anastomosis with plication of the stomach around the distal part of the esophagus may be preferred. Depending on the extent of esophageal resection, other options for restoring continuity of the alimentary tract may be necessary.

Surgical Procedures for Esophageal Varices

Esophageal varices are tortuous, dilated veins in the submucosa of the lower esophagus that may extend up into the esophagus or down into the stomach. This condition is caused by portal hypertension and is usually associated with obstruction within a cirrhotic liver. The rupture of esophageal varices can cause massive hemorrhage. The patient may come to the OR with a Sengstaken-Blakemore tube in place to control bleeding by the use of pressure from the inflated balloon in the tube.

During the surgical procedure, varices may be sclerosed through an esophagoscope. A sclerosant is injected via a needle puncture into each varix. Several injections may be necessary to achieve complete hemostasis. Sclerotherapy is usually attempted before more radical procedures are performed. The lower esophagus may be transected and the distal segment anastomosed with a circular stapler just proximal to the stomach. A portosystemic shunt procedure may be performed for portal decompression.

GASTROINTESTINAL SURGERY

Advances in the surgical management of patients with gastrointestinal problems have lessened the mortality rate. Interference with the gastrointestinal tract affects its functioning; specific deficiencies may result from gastrointestinal surgery depending on the site and extent of the surgical procedure. Massive resection of the small intestine can produce long-term nutritional problems such as weight loss and malabsorption of most nutrients. Metabolic bone disease may follow gastric surgery because of poor absorption of calcium and vitamin D. Patients who have undergone extensive gastrointestinal procedures should have a periodic nutritional evaluation. Biochemical tests monitor nutritional status and include serum proteins, albumin-globulin ratio, and blood urea nitrogen (BUN). Body weight is also significant. If caloric intake is inadequate, protein is converted to carbohydrates for energy and, as a result, protein synthesis suffers.

Considerations for Gastrointestinal Surgery

The separation of instruments used for resection and anastomosis and for abdominal closure is a matter of preference of the surgeon and institution. Two distinct setups may be used, but the single setup is most commonly used. The single setup consists of identifying and using only selected instruments and supplies for resection, anastomosis, and abdominal closure and discarding contaminated instruments and equipment from the field after use. Acid secretions from the gastric resection site are very irritating and may cause peritonitis. In addition, the intestinal tract harbors many microorganisms. Leakage into the peritoneal cavity can be a source of generalized peritoneal sepsis. Gloves should be changed after anastomosis is completed; gowns also may be changed.

A nasogastric tube is often inserted for the aspiration of gastric contents or for decompression of the intestinal tract. A variety of gastrointestinal tubes should be available for aspiration and irrigation.

Normal saline solution, not sterile water, should be used in abdominal procedures to moisten laparotomy packs. Normal saline is an isotonic solution and has the same osmotic pressure as blood serum and interstitial fluid. It will not alter sodium, chloride, or fluid balance because it does not cross cell membranes. (Hypotonic solutions cause cells to swell; hypertonic solutions cause them to shrink.) Normal saline is used for intraperitoneal irrigation unless the surgeon prefers to use a solution such as Ringer's lactate. Antibiotic solutions also may be needed for irrigation.

ESUs are used routinely by many surgeons for electrocoagulation of bleeding vessels in the abdominal wall, omentum, and mesentery. Ligating clips or suture ligatures are used for large vessels. To reduce tissue trauma, the jaws of intestinal forceps should be protected with soft covers made of rubber or fabric. Stapling devices are preferred by most surgeons for mechanical organ anastomosis. An intraluminal circular stapler can be used for end-to-end, end-to-side, or side-to-side anastomoses from the esophagus to the rectum. A straight linear stapler may be preferred for some gastrointestinal anastomoses and resections. Because the size of the lumen varies in different organs of the gastrointestinal tract, the circulating nurse should not open a sterile disposable stapler until the surgeon determines the appropriate head size or cartridge length for the instrument to be used.

The technical principles that guide the surgeon for all gastrointestinal anastomoses include:
- Good blood supply
- No tension
- Adequate lumen
- Watertight and leak-proof
- No distal obstruction

A sutured anastomosis produces an inverted suture line with serosa-to-serosa approximation. A stapled anastomosis results in anastomosed mucosa-to-mucosa apposition.

GASTRIC PROCEDURES

The stomach, a hollow muscular organ, is situated in the upper left abdomen between the esophagus and duodenum (see Figs. 33-19 and 33-20). Anatomically, it is divided into the fundus, body, and pyloric antrum. The two borders of the stomach, the lesser and greater curvatures, are important surgically because of their relation to the major vascular and lymphatic systems that supply the stomach. The blood supply is derived from the celiac axis. The gastroduodenal artery and the right and left gastric arteries are the main tributaries. The splenic artery gives rise to the gastroepiploic arteries that are located at the greater curvature. The venous drainage follows the arterial supply but empties into the portal circulation of the liver. The lymphatics empty into the pancreaticosplenic nodes and into the cisterna chyli via the celiac group. Omentum, a double fold of peritoneum attached to the lesser and greater curvatures, loosely covers the stomach and small intestine.

The innervation is both sympathetic and parasympathetic. The vagus nerve controls the reflex activities of movement and the secretions of the alimentary canal and is significant in rhythmic relaxation of the pyloric sphincter.

Food entering the stomach is reduced to chyme, a semiliquid, and then passes through the duodenum and small intestine. The chyme is absorbed through the lacteals of the intestine into the lymphatics, where it is converted to a milky white chyle. The chyle flows into the cisterna chyli and into the thoracic duct.

The main functions of the stomach are motor, secretory, and endocrine. The motor aspect moves the food along. The secretory actions cause the food to break down. The endocrine component is responsible for the release of gastrin and somatostatin. Gastrin causes the release of acid, and somatostatin inhibits the release of gastrin.

The interference of gastric motor activity or muscular contractions results in gastrointestinal complaints of abdominal pain, nausea, vomiting, hemorrhage, and dyspepsia. Some diseases, such as cancer, may not produce symptoms until the condition is far advanced. A surgical procedure is indicated when the presence of disease is established after laboratory tests such as gastric analysis, gastroscopy, and/or radiographic studies.

After gastric surgery, dumping syndrome may be experienced by patients shortly after eating. This complication occurs when food and fluids empty rapidly into the jejunum. It is characterized by nausea, vomiting, weakness, dizziness, pallor, sweating, palpitations, and diarrhea, and it may persist for 6 months to 1 year.

Gastroscopy

Gastroscopy involves the passage of a flexible fiberoptic gastroscope. This procedure is usually performed while the patient is sedated, with a topical anesthetic applied in the oropharynx to control the gag reflex. The operator visually inspects the mucosal walls of the stomach, and tissue specimens are sometimes obtained. Bleeding points may be coagulated with a laser beam, electrocoagulation, or a sclerosing agent.

Gastrostomy

Establishment of a temporary or permanent opening in the stomach may be indicated for gastrointestinal decompression or to provide alimentation for a prolonged period when nutrition cannot be maintained by other means. A gastrostomy tube eliminates the incidence of aspiration that may occur around a nasogastric tube. Often the patient is too debilitated to tolerate a major surgical procedure or may have an inoperable esophageal tumor or oropharyngeal trauma. A Foley, Malecot, Pezzer, or mushroom catheter may be inserted percutaneously into the stomach.

Simple Gastrostomy. With the patient under general anesthesia, the stomach is exposed through a small upper left abdominal or midline incision. The catheter is inserted into the anterior gastric wall and is held in place with pursestring sutures; it is brought out through a separate stab wound in the left upper quadrant. The stomach is sutured

to the abdominal wall at the exit site of the catheter. After an abdominal procedure on a critically ill patient, the surgeon may prefer to place a small-bore catheter into the jejunum rather than the stomach for enteral hyperalimentation.

Percutaneous Endoscopic Gastrostomy. With percutaneous endoscopic gastrostomy, the patient is placed under IV sedation and an endoscopist introduces a fiberoptic gastroscope and insufflates the stomach with air to create a working space and a turgid surface to the stomach. Light from the scope is directed anteriorly for transillumination through the abdominal wall. The surgeon infiltrates the skin with a local anesthetic at a selected gastrostomy site, usually approximately one third of the distance along the left costal margin at the midclavicular line. The gastrostomy tube is introduced through a percutaneous puncture and secured with sutures.

Gastric Resections

The stomach may be totally or partially resected for removal of a malignant tumor or for benign chronic ulcer disease. Although surgical resection is the only cure, gastric carcinomas are often inoperable because of metastases to the liver or extension into surrounding tissues. In such cases, palliative procedures may be performed. The appropriate procedure is determined after thorough exploration of the abdominal cavity by the surgeon. Circular staplers are commonly used for anastomosis after resection. Leakage at the site of anastomosis leads to peritonitis. Some surgeons oversew the staple line (Fig. 33-23).

Total Gastrectomy. With a total gastrectomy, the entire stomach is excised for malignant lesions through a bilateral subcostal, long transrectus, or thoracoabdominal incision. A total gastrectomy necessitates reconstruction of esophagointestinal continuity by establishing an anastomosis between a loop of jejunum and the esophagus. This anastomosis may be end-to-side with a lateral jejunojejunostomy or end-to-end with a Roux-en-Y jejunojejunostomy. The purpose of the jejunojejunostomy is to prevent the reflux of bile and pancreatic fluids into the esophagus. Some surgeons create a jejunal pouch for this purpose.

Subtotal Gastrectomy. Partial resections of the stomach, originally described by Theodor Billroth (1829-1894), are often referred to as Billroth procedures. A benign lesion (usually an ulcer) or a malignant lesion located in the pyloric half of the stomach requires removal of the lower half to two thirds of the stomach. In a patient with a gastric or duodenal ulcer, a partial resection limits gastric acidity and relieves pain, bleeding, vomiting, and weight loss.

In this procedure, the peritoneal cavity is entered through a right paramedian or upper midline abdominal incision. A variety of surgical procedures may be used to reestablish gastrointestinal continuity. Anastomosis of the remaining portion of the stomach to the duodenum (gastroduodenostomy, antrectomy, or Billroth I, Fig. 33-24) or to a loop of the jejunum (gastrojejunostomy, or Billroth II, Fig. 33-25) is often performed. A truncal vagotomy, which is discussed in the following section, is performed to eliminate the possibility of postoperative peptic ulceration.

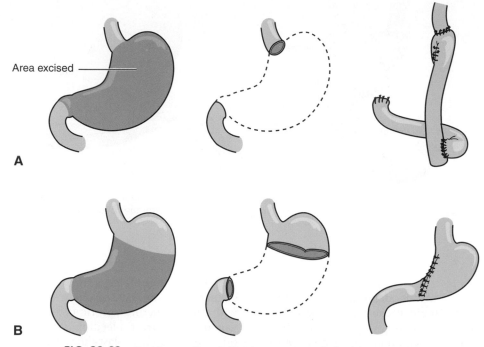

FIG. 33-23 Gastric resection. **A,** Total gastrectomy. **B,** Partial gastrectomy.

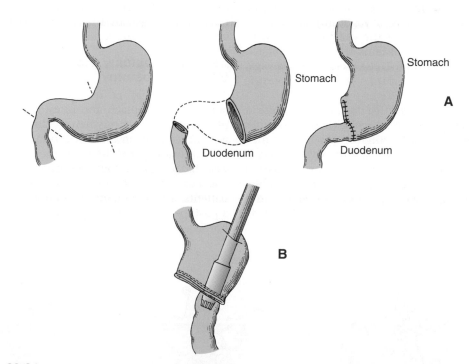

FIG. 33-24 Billroth I gastroduodenostomy. End-to-end anastomosis of duodenum to stomach may be sutured (**A**) or stapled with an intraluminal circular stapler (**B**).

Common modifications of the Billroth I procedure are the Schoemaker and von Haberer–Finney techniques. The Schoemaker procedure involves end-to-end anastomosis of the stomach and duodenum after the lesser curvature of the stomach is sutured to make the anastomosis site the same size as the duodenum. With the von Haberer–Finney method, the lateral wall of the duodenum is brought up to the stomach so that the entire end of the stomach is open for direct anastomosis.

Popular modifications of the Billroth II procedure include the Polya and Hofmeister techniques, both of which involve variations of end-to-side gastrojejunostomy.

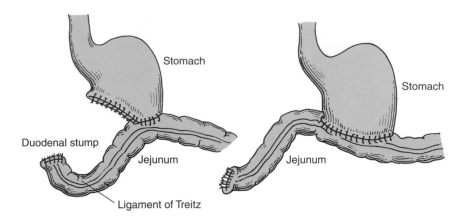

FIG. 33-25   Billroth II gastrojejunostomy with end-to-side sutured anastomosis of stomach to loop of jejunum.

Vagotomy

Chronic gastric, pyloric, and duodenal ulcers that do not respond to medical treatment cause patients severe pain and difficulty in eating and sleeping. Vagotomy, the division of the vagus nerves, may be recommended to interrupt vagal nerve impulses, thus lowering the production of gastric hydrochloric acid and hastening gastric emptying. Vagotomy can be performed at several different locations along its course (Fig. 33-26). Proximal gastric vagotomy, also known as parietal cell vagotomy, divides the vagal nerve fibers to the proximal stomach but maintains the entire stomach and vagal nerves to the antrum. These sections of the vagal nerve inhibit the release of gastrin, a stimulant of gastric secretion.

Truncal vagotomy and selective vagotomy require a concomitant drainage procedure, because these procedures denervate the stomach. A gastroenterostomy is performed with a truncal vagotomy, which divides the vagal trunks at the distal esophagus. An antrectomy is performed with a selective vagotomy, which transects the gastric branches. Vagotomy with drainage is a compromise procedure and is restricted to high-risk patients or those with severe duodenal deformity.

Pyloroplasty, enlarging the pyloric opening between the stomach and duodenum, may be performed in patients with an obstructing pyloric ulcer or in conjunction with vagotomy to treat bleeding duodenal ulcers. Duodenal dilation or duodenoplasty may be indicated.

Vagotomy procedures, which are conservative surgical therapies compared with gastrectomy, decrease the surgical risk for select patients with chronic ulcers. It is now known that ulcers caused by the *Helicobacter pylori* organism can be cured with antibiotics.

Gastrojejunostomy (Roux-en-Y Gastroenterostomy)

A procedure may be necessary to reestablish continuity between the stomach and intestinal tract, such as after a partial gastrectomy or when the lower end of the stomach is obstructed by an ulcer or a nonresectable tumor. A gastrojejunostomy may be performed to treat alkaline reflux gastritis, postgastrectomy syndromes such as postvagotomy diarrhea, and dumping syndromes. Except in geriatric patients, a concomitant vagotomy is necessary to prevent a postoperative gastrojejunal ulcer when the acid-forming portion of the stomach is not resected.

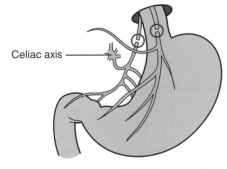
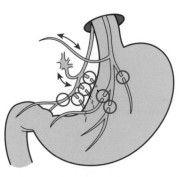
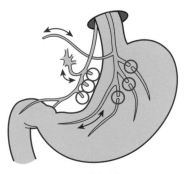

Celiac axis

Truncal

Selective
or
gastric

Highly selective
or
parietal cell vagotomy

FIG. 33-26   Vagotomy.

In this procedure, a loop of jejunum may be anastomosed to either the anterior or the posterior wall of the stomach; both approaches have advantages and disadvantages. In a Roux-en-Y gastrojejunostomy, the jejunum is divided. The distal end is anastomosed to the side of the stomach, and the proximal end is anastomosed to the side of the jejunum at a lower level. The result is a Y-shaped double anastomosis that diverts the flow of bile and pancreatic enzymes directly into the jejunum, bypassing the created gastric stoma. An adaptation of a Roux-en-Y anastomosis is also used to drain the biliary tract or other organs, such as the pancreas or esophagus, directly into the jejunum to bypass the stomach and prevent the reflux of intestinal contents.

Bariatric Surgery

An interest in the study of morbid obesity, or bariatrics, has led to the development of a subspecialization in general surgery—bariatric surgery. AORN has published guidelines for the safe care of patients undergoing bariatric procedures.

Bariatric surgery can be performed as an open abdominal surgery or as a five-trocar laparoscopic procedure (Fig. 33-27). The surgical landmarks are altered in obese patients because the body habitus is large and extends beyond the borders of the average-sized patient. The umbilicus, for example, lies several inches lower on a pendulous abdomen. Using the umbilical area of the patient as a trocar site could cause injury to nontarget organs.

Bariatric procedures produce three types of results:
1. Restricted intake caused by an inflatable Silastic band (Fig. 33-28)
2. Bypass the food and decrease absorption (Fig. 33-29)
3. Bypass absorption and restrict intake

People who have a body mass index (BMI) of 40 and more and weigh 100 pounds (45.4 kg) more than their ideal weight and who have failed to lose weight despite years of medical treatment are potential candidates for bariatric surgery. Patients with a BMI of 35 to 40 and have serious comorbid disease, such as obstructive sleep apnea, cardiomyopathy, and uncontrolled diabetes, may be candidates after careful screening. The plan of care requires the patient to have psychological and physiologic support during the process or the procedure could be a failure. Some facilities have extended the procedure to obese adolescents ages 15 years and older, with varying degrees of success.

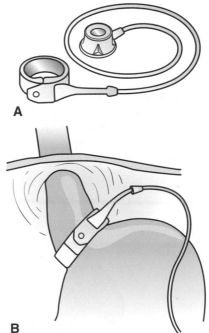

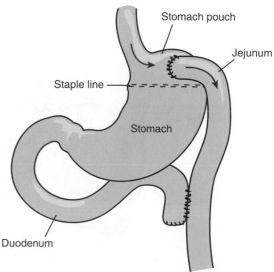

FIG. 33-28 Gastric banding. **A,** Gastric band with port. **B,** Gastric band in place.

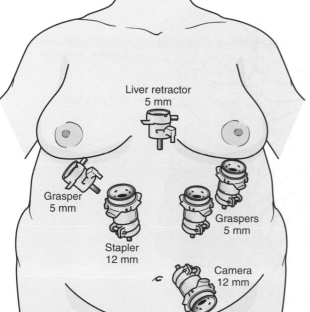

FIG. 33-27 Laparoscopic ports for a bariatric procedure. Note the displacement of the umbilical landmark.

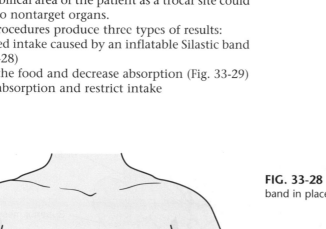

FIG. 33-29 Gastric bypass for a bariatric procedure.

The physical size of a patient who is obese presents special needs with respect to transporting and positioning, selecting instrumentation, and providing psychological and physiologic support. Many morbidly obese patients have medical complications such as hypertension, peripheral vascular disease, cardiac disease, degenerative arthritis, gallbladder disease, or diabetes mellitus.

The plan of care for obese patients usually includes the application of antiembolic stockings and the insertion of a nasogastric tube, a Foley catheter, IV, arterial lines and CVP. Because respiratory distress is a potential complication during the induction of anesthesia, intubation while the patient is awake may be the technique of choice. Bariatric procedures for gastric restriction are not without risks. Nutritional deficiencies, anemia, wound infection, and a failure of staple lines have occurred postoperatively. The capacity of the stomach is reduced to approximately 30 mL to restrict food absorption or intake. Most patients lose at least 50% of their excess body fat.

Gastroplasty. In gastroplasty, which is usually referred to as a vertical banded gastroplasty, four linear staple lines are placed vertically on the lesser curvature side of the stomach just left of the gastroesophageal junction in addition to a gastric band to cause restriction of intake. This creates a small channel for the passage of gastric contents from the proximal to the distal segments. The total intake at any given time is about 1 ounce. The stomach is divided between staple lines and oversewn with sutures.

To prevent dilation, the outlet at the end of the staple line is usually reinforced with a Silastic band. This method does not have the same restricted absorption as gastric bypass. Some patients do not lose satisfactory amounts of weight because they take in excess high-calorie liquids and sugary foods.

Gastric Bypass. In a gastric bypass procedure, the capacity of the stomach is restricted by creating a small pouch in the fundus (the proximal segment of the stomach) and bypassing portions of the small intestines to decrease the absorptive qualities of the gastrointestinal tract (see Fig. 33-29). The stomach is transected horizontally with a linear stapler, and the proximal jejunum is divided. A Roux-en-Y gastrojejunostomy is constructed between the 1-ounce-sized pouch, vertically oriented stomach pouch, and the jejunum, bypassing the remainder of stomach to establish intestinal continuity for the passage of gastric contents. The proximal jejunal segment is anastomosed end-to-side to the distal segment for drainage of gastric, biliary, and pancreatic fluids.

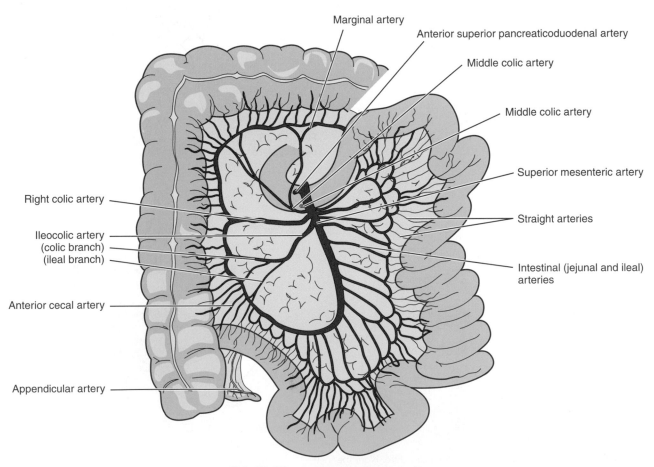

FIG. 33-30 Small bowel blood supply.

Patients are advised not to eat concentrated sugars because it stimulates dumping syndrome. Nutrient supplements, such as vitamins, iron, and calcium, are necessary to prevent anemia and osteoporosis

INTESTINAL PROCEDURES

Anatomically, the intestines are divided into the small (upper) and large (lower) intestine, and there are subdivisions of each.

The small intestine extends from the pylorus to the ileocecal valve. The three sections include the duodenum (proximal portion), the jejunum (middle section), and the ileum (distal portion that joins the large intestine). The ileocecal valve, a sphincter muscle, lessens the backflow of material that has been discharged to the large intestine. The blood supply to the small bowel is divided into arcades with several subdivisions (Fig. 33-30).

The large intestine, or colon, extends from the ileum to the rectum and is generally divided into the ascending, transverse, descending, and sigmoid colon. The cecum is the pouch formed where the large intestine joins the small intestine. The blood supply to the large bowel is united on the mesenteric border by the marginal artery of Drummond with widely dispersed arcades of vessels (Fig. 33-31).

The mesentery, a peritoneal fold, attaches the small and large intestines to the posterior abdominal wall and contains the arteries, veins, and lymph nodes that supply the intestines.

Inflammation, intestinal obstruction, and disruption in absorption and motility are disorders that may lead to surgical intervention. Etiologic factors determine the surgical procedure. Segments of bowel can be removed and the continuity can be reestablished by anastomosis (Fig. 33-32).

Resection of the Small Intestine

Tumors, as well as strangulation from adhesions, volvulus, obstruction, and regional ileitis, usually are treated by resection of the involved segment. An abdominal incision is made over the suspected or known site of disease. After exposure, clamps are placed above and below the diseased segment of the bowel and mesentery to avoid spillage. The involved area is resected, and an end-to-end, end-to-side, or side-to-side anastomosis is performed to restore continuity. Variations of this technique are used for other related problems of the small intestine, such as extensive perforation. Bowel strangulation and obstruction necessitate an immediate surgical procedure to prevent necrosis, peritonitis, and death.

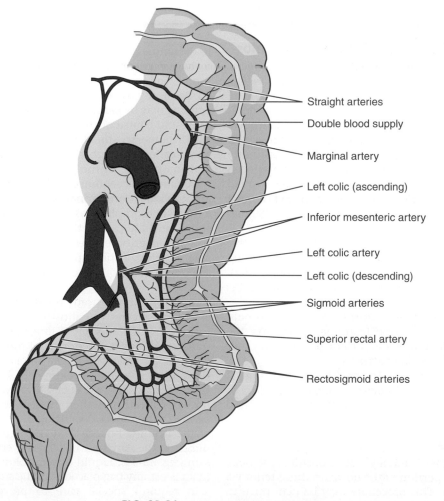

Straight arteries
Double blood supply
Marginal artery
Left colic (ascending)
Inferior mesenteric artery
Left colic artery
Left colic (descending)
Sigmoid arteries
Superior rectal artery
Rectosigmoid arteries

FIG. 33-31 Large bowel blood supply.

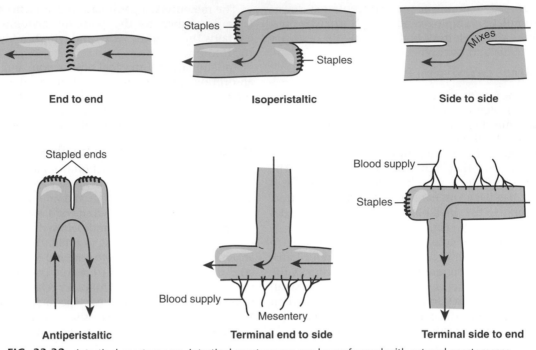

FIG. 33-32   Intestinal anastomoses. Intestinal anastomoses can be performed with sutured anastomoses or with circular or linear staplers, as shown here.

Hemicolectomy, Transverse Colectomy, Anterior Resection, and Total Colectomy

Colitis, diverticulitis, obstruction, and neoplasms are the most common reasons for surgical intervention to remove a diseased segment of the colon. Most surgical procedures involve opening the abdomen, walling off the peritoneal cavity, incising and clamping at the points where resection is to be carried out, and, finally, reestablishing continuity by anastomosis. In select patients, a laparoscopic approach may be used to mobilize the segment of the large or small bowel to be resected. The resected bowel is removed through a small minimal-access incision in the abdominal wall. Stomas can also be created with the laparoscopic technique.

The perioperative plan of care includes preoperative administration of intestinal antibiotics, bowel-cleansing methods, and diet restrictions (e.g., a clear liquid diet). Bowel cleansing can cause depletion of electrolytes and is performed only as necessary.

Intraoperatively, separate instrument technique should be used during the procedure. Instruments used on the interior aspect of the bowel should not be used on other tissues and should be isolated after use.

A nasogastric tube may be inserted before the surgical procedure and may remain in place until partial healing of anastomosis occurs and effective peristalsis returns. Fluid and electrolyte balance is maintained.

Intestinal Stomas

An intestinal ostomy is a surgically created opening, or stoma, that extends from a portion of the bowel to the exterior via the abdominal wall. This procedure may be performed to divert intestinal contents so that inflamed bowel can heal, to decompress pressure caused by an obstructive lesion, or to bypass an obstruction such as a benign or malignant tumor. The type and level of the lesion determine whether an ileostomy, cecostomy, or colostomy is indicated. The opening may be permanent or temporary, depending on the cause and course of the disease or obstruction. In patients with a temporary stoma, intestinal continuity is reestablished after healing, through closure of the opening in the bowel, and anastomosis of the previously separated ends.

A patient's acceptance of these procedures is as varied as an individual's emotional reactions. Each patient requires a rehabilitation plan based on personal needs. These plans should include care of the pouching system, maintenance of skin integrity, proper diet, odor control, and comfortable clothing. Patient participation is an integral part of the preparation for self-care and enhances self-confidence.

Ileostomy.   An ileostomy is performed for conditions such as chronic ulcerative colitis or after removal of the colon (colectomy). In this procedure the proximal end of the transected ileum is exteriorized through the abdominal wall (Fig. 33-33). The usual stoma site is the midportion of the right rectus sheath, approximately 3 cm below the level of the umbilicus. First, a disk of skin is excised. The anterior and posterior sheaths are then incised, and the rectus sheath is divided with a muscle-splitting incision. The proximal end of the ileum is brought out through the peritoneum and muscle to the skin; here the end is everted and sutured to the skin (Fig. 33-34). Liquid or semisolid discharge is collected in an ileostomy bag placed over the stoma. The surrounding skin requires special care to prevent excoriation and irritation.

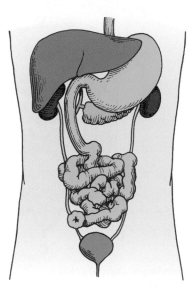

FIG. 33-33 Ileostomy. Proximal end of transected ileum is brought out through peritoneum and muscle. The end is everted and sutured to skin. Stoma site is in midportion of right rectus sheath below level of umbilicus.

The entire cecum and colon, as well as the rectal mucosa (mucosal proctectomy), are resected in the endorectal-ileoanal pull through procedure. The ileum is anastomosed to the anus, and the rectal and anal muscles are preserved for anal continence. A pouch is constructed from the terminal ileum proximal to the anal anastomosis to serve as a reservoir for intestinal contents. A temporary diverting loop or double-barreled ileostomy is brought to the skin for drainage during the healing of the anastomoses; after the anastomoses have healed, this stoma is closed. Although not without complications, these procedures offer acceptable alternatives to a permanent ileostomy stoma, especially in children and young adults.

In the Kock pouch procedure, a nipple valve is created by inverting an intestinal stoma to maintain continence. The patient intubates the valve regularly through the stomal nipple valve to empty the bowel of mucus and fecal matter.

Cecostomy. With a cecostomy, an opening is created in the cecum and a tube is inserted for decompression of the massive distention caused by colonic obstruction. The tube is placed into the cecum through the lower right side of the abdomen. Less severe distention may be relieved by suction and irrigation through a colonoscope and the insertion of an intestinal tube through the anus to the cecum. Cecostomy or colonoscopic decompression may precede subsequent colon resection.

Colostomy. An opening anywhere along the length of the colon to the exterior skin surface creates an artificial anus (Fig. 33-35). The section of colon to be exteriorized depends on the location of the lesion to be resected or treated. For example, a low anterior bowel resection necessitates a sigmoid colostomy. A permanent colostomy in the sigmoid colon forms an artificial anus after a combined abdominoperineal resection for rectal carcinoma (see Fig. 33-35, *A*). The rectum is removed. A collection device for fecal material is not needed after a patient's bowel evacuation becomes regulated. Most patients wear a stoma cap even when they are in the process of regulation.

Either a double-barreled or a loop colostomy may be performed as a temporary measure. In a double-barreled colostomy (see Fig. 33-35, *B*), the transverse colon is divided and both ends are brought out to the margins of the skin incision. The proximal stoma serves as an outlet for feces, and the distal opening leads to the nonfunctioning bowel. In a loop colostomy (see Fig. 33-35, *C*), a loop of colon is brought out onto the abdominal wall. A plastic rod or ostomy bridge is placed under the loop to hold it out on the exterior abdominal wall. The peritoneum is closed, and the wound around the colostomy is sutured.

Appendectomy

Appendicitis can occur at any age but is seen most often in adolescents and young adults. It may imitate other conditions such as a ruptured ovarian cyst or ureteral calculus.

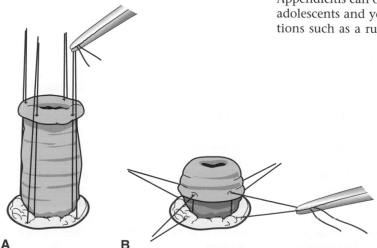

A   **B**

FIG. 33-34 Ileostomy stoma is brought through an opening in the skin and sutured into place. **A,** The edges of the intestinal mucosa are aligned with subcuticular tissues by sutures. **B,** The stoma is formed by everting the mucosa and tying the sutures.

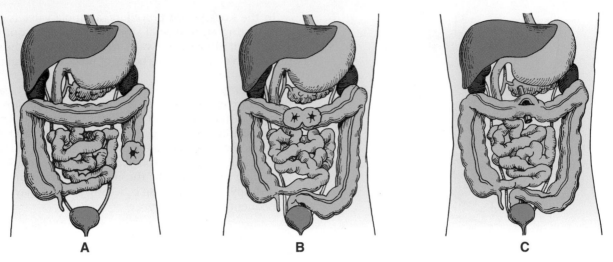

FIG. 33-35   Colostomy. **A,** Permanent colostomy. Terminal end of descending or sigmoid colon is brought out through the peritoneum and muscle and sutured to skin. **B,** Double-barreled colostomy. Both ends of transected colon are brought out to skin. **C,** Loop colostomy. Loop of colon is exteriorized over plastic rod for temporary fecal diversion.

Some appendices are retrocecal, which makes diagnosis and excision more difficult (Fig. 33-36). Classic symptoms of early appendicitis include pain in the right lower quadrant, rebound tenderness, nausea, and moderate elevations in temperature and white blood cell count.

An emergency appendectomy is necessary to prevent a progression to gangrene and the perforation of friable tissue, with subsequent peritonitis. The open abdominal approach involves a muscle-splitting incision in the right lower quadrant, over McBurney point. The blood supply to the appendix is ligated and severed. A crushing clamp is applied to the appendiceal base, which is then ligated and severed from the cecum. After amputation, the surgeon may elect to cauterize the stump with phenol and alcohol or wipe it with a sponge soaked with an iodophor (Betadine) to reduce contamination. The stump is then inverted into the cecum as a pursestring suture is tightened around the stump (Fig. 33-37).

Drainage is indicated in the presence of an abscess, appendix rupture, or any gross contamination of the wound. An appendectomy is usually an uncomplicated procedure with rapid convalescence unless life-threatening peritonitis results.

Laparoscopic Appendectomy.   After creation of a peritoneal working space with carbon dioxide (CO_2) trocars are placed and the laparoscope is inserted through the infraumbilical incision, the patient is placed in steep Trendelenburg's position. Secondary trocars are inserted in the suprapubic area and left lower quadrant for placement of graspers and dissectors. The appendix is located and hemostatically dissected from the mesoappendix with endoscopic clips or staples. Endoloop ligatures are placed at the base of the appendix, and endoscopic scissors are used to transect it. Grasping forceps are used to place the appendix into an endopouch collection reservoir to prevent the extrusion of contents during withdrawal through the infraumbilical trocar.

COLORECTAL PROCEDURES

Colorectal carcinoma is one of the most common abdominal malignancies, with the highest incidence in people older than 60 years. Resection of the carcinoma is the surgical procedure of choice; radiation and chemotherapy are adjuvant therapies or palliative therapies for advanced disease. Early diagnosis and prompt treatment of asymptomatic carcinoma improve the survival rates.

Diagnostic procedures are routinely performed in patients with bowel or rectal bleeding, chronic diarrhea, or a history of intestinal polyps and/or carcinoma of the colon. Serial guaiac stool tests may detect the presence of occult blood. A barium enema provides a complete radiographic study of the colon; an endoscopic examination is routine. Some therapeutic procedures may be accomplished with laser or electrocoagulation through endoscopes.

Sigmoidoscopy

Sigmoidoscopy is direct visual inspection of the sigmoid and rectal lumens by means of a flexible fiberoptic or rigid lighted sigmoidoscope. The flexible scope is more comfortable for the patient and gives the surgeon better visualization of the mucosal surface to evaluate the left colon and rectosigmoid. It may be used intraoperatively to check an anastomosis or for preoperative diagnosis. Water-soluble lubricant is used to help ease insertion of the scope.

The patient is prepared preoperatively with enemas and colon cleansing. Placing the patient in the left lateral position allows for anatomic positioning of the sigmoid colon. The knee-chest or Kraske position allows the sigmoid colon to fall forward into the abdomen. The Sims or lithotomy position may be used for an extremely obese or extremely ill patient.

The surgeon may inflate room air into the colon with a hand-pumped bulb to create a working space during insertion of the well-lubricated scope to better visualize the mucosal

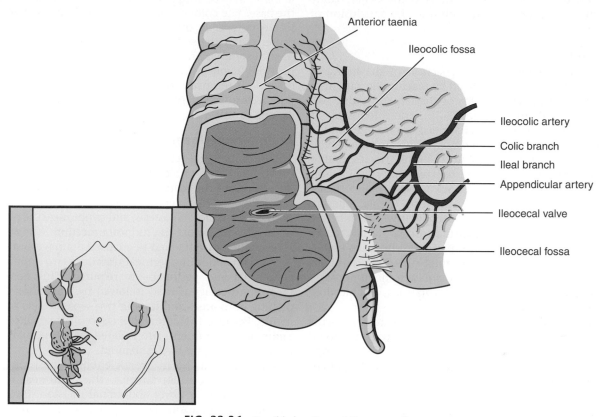

FIG. 33-36 Possible locations of the appendix.

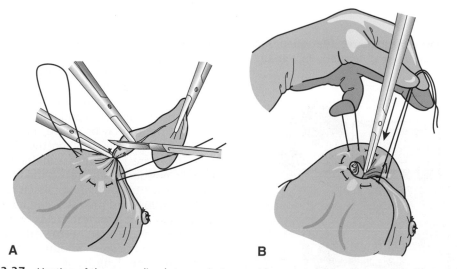

A   B

FIG. 33-37 Ligation of the appendiceal stump. **A,** A pursestring suture is placed around the base of the appendix. It is double-clamped and dissected with a scalpel. **B,** The appendiceal stump is inverted into the circumference of the pursestring suture. The suture is tightened as the stump buried within.

walls and folds. This insufflation stimulates the stretch receptors of the bowel, causing a feeling of desire to defecate, which necessitates reassurance of the patient. Have the suction handy for evacuation of air from the colon at the conclusion of the procedure.

Colonoscopy

Colonoscopy provides visual inspection of the lining of the entire colon. This is facilitated by placing the patient in left lateral position so the folds of the large intestine will be in anatomic alignment (Fig. 33-38). The colonoscope is flexible and consists of two channels: one for suctioning and irrigating and one for operating. Its greatest uses are to examine the lumen of the colon, to biopsy tissues, and to search for and excise or ablate polyps. Other indications are for the study of inflammatory bowel or diverticular disease, the passage of blood in the feces (hematochezia), or a change in bowel habits; as a preoperative screen before colostomy closure; for confirmation of radiographic findings; and as a follow-up for patients who have undergone intestinal procedures. Argon and Nd:YAG lasers or ESUs are used through a colonoscope to ablate some tumors and to treat polyps, arteriovenous malformations, and bleeding disorders.

Because the presence of stool in the rectum prevents adequate examination with the scope, the patient should have a preoperative bowel evacuation prep. Colonoscopy without moderate sedation is contraindicated if the patient is uncooperative. Relative contraindications may include acute, severe, or radiation-caused inflammatory disease or complete obstruction. Perforation can occur. Vital signs should be monitored during the procedure.

Complications of colonoscopy include electrical burn during polypectomy, tearing or perforation of the colon by tip pressure, tearing of the liver or spleen by air pressure, and tearing of diverticula resulting from the introduction of air into them.

Polypectomy

Most surgeons and pathologists agree that adenomatous mucosal polyps in the colon are potentially malignant and should be removed. A polypectomy is usually performed through a fiberoptic colonoscope. Polyps, which are often familial, may be single or multiple and are easily excised at the base. The colonoscope may be used intraoperatively to locate polyps. If the polyps are pedunculated, they are cauterized at the stalk and retrieved by a snare for microscopic examination. Electrocoagulation or lasing of the base provides hemostasis. Some polyps or the involved segment of colon is removed by laparotomy or laparoscopy. After a polypectomy, patients should have annual colonoscopic examinations.

Abdominoperineal Resection

Abdominoperineal resection is an extensive procedure for carcinoma. This procedure is performed mainly in the lower third of the rectum, but it may extend into the anal canal. Preoperative preparation is meticulous to verify diagnosis, to search for metastasis, and to optimize the condition of the patient. Before the surgical procedure, an indwelling Foley catheter is attached to a closed drainage system.

With an abdominoperineal resection, two approaches—abdominal and perineal—are required. This necessitates prepping (perineum first, followed by the abdomen) and draping both areas and having two separate sets of instruments. Because the colon is a reservoir for bacteria, contaminated instruments are isolated from the main sterile field after resection of the sigmoid.

With the patient in Trendelenburg's position in low lithotomy using Allen stirrups, the peritoneal cavity is entered through a lower abdominal incision. Preliminary exploration is performed to seek metastases. If the tumor is resectable, the sigmoid colon is mobilized, clamped, and divided. The proximal end of the sigmoid is exteriorized through a stab wound in the left lower quadrant to create a permanent colostomy. The mesentery may be sutured to the abdominal wall to prevent internal hernias. The distal end of the sigmoid is tied to prevent contamination and is placed deep in the presacral space for removal at the end of the procedure. The pelvic floor is reperitonealized, and the abdomen is closed. Dressings are placed on the abdominal incision and on the colostomy.

The second phase of the surgical procedure is closure of the anus with a pursestring suture, to prevent contamination, and removal of the anus, rectum, rectosigmoid, and surrounding nodes and lymphatics through a perineal incision. Drains may be placed, and the perineum is closed.

Two teams are used when the abdominal and perineal procedures are performed simultaneously. The patient is initially positioned supine in a modified lithotomy position using Allen stirrups. This approach reduces operating time and blood loss and provides simultaneous exposure of the abdominal and perineal fields. Sequential compression devices should be used on the patient's legs.

Because of the great amount of blood loss from vascular areas and the length of the procedure, patients are carefully monitored to prevent hypovolemic shock.

Low Anterior Colon Resection

The sigmoid colon and rectum lie within the bony pelvis, which makes the resection of tumors in the lower sigmoid colon, rectosigmoid, and rectum technically difficult. The

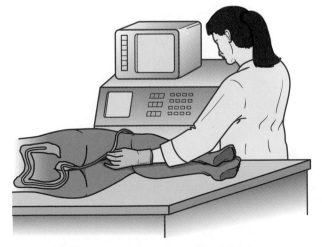

FIG. 33-38   Correct anatomic position for colonoscopy.

objective is to achieve wide local excision with en bloc resection of the lymphatics and perirectal mesentery. Intraluminal and linear staplers facilitate colorectal anastomosis in a low anterior colon resection. The distal colon is transected after closure with a linear stapler. The intraluminal stapler, with the anvil removed, is introduced through the anus and rectal stump either through or adjacent to the linear staple line. After the anvil is replaced, an intraluminal end-to-end or end-to-side anastomosis with the proximal segment of colon is completed.

Total excision of the mesorectum is necessary to prevent recurrence of the tumor in the pelvis or at the staple line; a distal tumor clearance of at least 2 cm is necessary. With this technique for low anterior colorectal anastomosis, colorectal continuity is restored and anal sphincter control is maintained without necessitating a permanent colostomy; with an abdominoperineal resection, a permanent colostomy is necessary.

The surgeon may check the colorectal anastomosis with a sigmoidoscope at the completion of the surgery before closing the abdomen. The sigmoidoscope will be placed in the rectum, and room air will be used to insufflate and expand the anastomosed segment. The abdomen will be simultaneously filled with warm irrigation. The anastomotic line will be observed for air leak. If a leak is present, air bubbles will rise up to the surface of the irrigation solution. If no leak is present, the irrigation is suctioned out of the abdomen using a Poole tip with a guard. The sigmoidoscope is withdrawn, and the air is permitted to escape.

ABDOMINAL TRAUMA

Trauma is the major cause of death in people younger than 40 years.[1] Bleeding from the disruption of solid organs or major vessels in the abdomen (including the pelvis) and infection from perforation of a hollow viscus are life-threatening injuries.

Abdominal trauma is usually caused by one of the following:
- Blunt trauma caused by direct impact, rapid deceleration, shearing forces, and/or increased intraluminal pressure can rupture or sever multiple structures, including those that are retroperitoneal.
- Penetrating injuries involve structures within the path of the weapon; gunshot wounds may also injure adjacent structures through the blast effect or cavitation. A stab or gunshot wound of the abdomen can penetrate across the diaphragm into the chest or vice versa.

Planning Perioperative Care for Abdominal Trauma Patients

Many patients have multiple injuries that affect more than one body system. These patients require a comprehensive approach to diagnosis and treatment by a multidisciplinary team. The philosophy of trauma management has changed from that of an individual surgeon treating an injured patient in the emergency department and OR to a system that begins at the site of the accident with stabilization by

[1]www.trauma.org is a good resource for trauma information. The site has a good image gallery that depicts the types of injuries discussed in this chapter.

trained personnel and continues with definitive care, including rapid surgical intervention and rehabilitation. This section will concentrate on abdominal trauma and the surgical evaluation and treatment.

Systematic Approach to Evaluation

When dealing with abdominal trauma patients the first thought is hemorrhage or fecal spill. Other injuries such as biliary or pancreatic spillage are less common. Severe penetrating trauma can be complicated by evisceration.

Ultrasonography, radiographs, and CT scan are useful presurgical diagnostic tests to assess the extent of abdominal injuries and to determine indications for surgical intervention. Free air in the abdomen generally indicates a ruptured organ, such as the bowel. This necessitates immediate laparotomy to locate the torn organ and control seepage of bowel contents. CT scan and ultrasonography provide additional assessment data.

Peritoneal Lavage. The patient who is hypotensive with left upper quadrant pain requires a peritoneal lavage to determine active intraabdominal bleeding. Before the procedure, the patient is positioned supine and a nasogastric tube placed to decompress the stomach and observe contents (if not contraindicated by upper body or facial injury). A Foley catheter should be inserted to decompress the bladder and observe the urine.

The peritoneal lavage procedure is done under local anesthesia by creating a 2-cm midline incision in one of two planes: infraumbilical or supraumbilical (if the patient is pregnant or has a fractured pelvis). The incision extends to the peritoneal membrane, which is anesthetized and grasped with hemostats. The peritoneum is incised only under direct vision. If blood is seen immediately rushing from the peritoneal incision, a rapid sequence induction is performed by the anesthesia provider and an immediate exploratory laparotomy is performed.

If no immediate hemorrhage is seen, proceed by instilling body temperature Ringer's lactate or sterile normal saline 10 mL/kg. The circulating nurse and anesthesia provider document all fluids in or out of the patient's abdomen. Allow the solution to sit in the abdomen for a few moments. The organs can be slightly agitated by hand and the solution drained into a basin or container with a lid. The circulating nurse labels the irrigant and sends it to the lab for a rush cell count. The lab personnel look for blood cells, stool, vegetable matter, or any other indicator of intraabdominal injury. Negative findings mean that the patient needs no further intraabdominal surgery at that time, but will be monitored closely for any change in condition.

Keep in mind that retroperitoneal bleeding may not be diagnosed with peritoneal lavage. Many major structures such as the great vessels and kidneys are retroperitoneal. Injuries to the great vessels require an immediate surgical procedure to control bleeding and restore vascular continuity. Major organ injuries mandate an open laparotomy for repair or reconstruction or to resect severely damaged tissues.

Emergency Exploratory Laparotomy

The patient is positioned supine and prepped from chin to groin. A nasogastric tube is placed and a Foley catheter

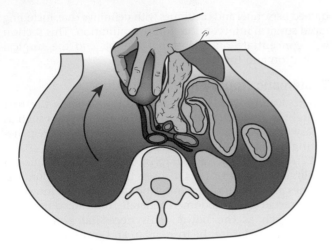

FIG. 33-39   Displacing organs during exploratory laparotomy.

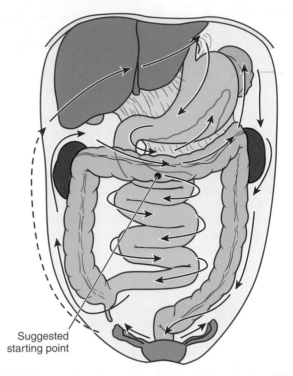

Suggested
starting point

FIG. 33-40   Direction for running the bowel. Examination of the bowel for injury after trauma.

inserted. The surgeon makes a midline incision from xyphoid to pubis in some cases. The surgeon carefully displaces the abdominal contents laterally to examine each angle of the individual organs (Fig. 33-39). After careful inspection of the viscera, the surgeon manually palpates the entire length of the bowel, starting at the duodenum and ending at the sigmoid flexure. This process is referred to as "running the bowel" (Fig. 33-40).

After the exploration any injuries to the organs caused by the trauma are repaired and the patient is closed. If the exploratory procedure was extensive, the patient's tissue may be extremely edematous and might not approximate without undue tension. The patient's abdomen may have to remain open for several days and the patient brought back to the OR for a delayed primary closure.

Each surgeon has a routine for protecting the patient's open incision (referred to as laparostomy) until the edges can be approximated. Some surgeons use sterile Silastic sheeting circumferentially stapled to the wound edges to form a temporary cover. Other surgeons have used sterile, 3000-mL IV bags that have been cut to fit like a patch (referred to as a bogata or silo bag). A bulky dressing is placed over the area, and the patient is transferred to intensive care for stabilization and monitoring.

Great care is taken to count and be accountable for instruments, sharps, and items used in the emergency procedure. The organized team works in concert to perform counts as possible based on the patient's condition. Some surgeons do a routine radiograph of the patient's abdomen before transfer to the unit. If laparotomy tapes or towels must be left inside the patient as visceral retainers, the circulating nurse documents the exact number placed inside the patient and communicates the same information to the surgeon and the intensive care nurse in the hand-off report. This information could be valuable if the patient crashes in the unit and some of the tapes must be removed outside the OR. Non-OR personnel may accidentally discard the sponges by not realizing that they are counted items. When the patient is brought back to the OR for closure, the sponges are to be accounted for in their entirety and documented as being retrieved. Care again is taken not to mix the removed sponges with the sponges used for the closure procedure.

COMPLICATIONS OF ABDOMINAL SURGERY

Patients are particularly prone to pulmonary complications after abdominal surgery. They are also subject to a variety of fluid and electrolyte imbalances because they generally have a nothing-by-mouth (NPO) status postoperatively. They may also lose sodium, potassium, chloride, and water through nasogastric suction. If great quantities of alkalotic pancreatic secretions are lost through decompression of the small bowel, metabolic acidosis may result. The loss of acidic stomach secretions may lead to metabolic alkalosis.

Peritonitis and wound infection may result after gastrointestinal surgery because of spillage of contaminants from the lumen of the gastrointestinal tract. *Escherichia coli* and *Bacteroides fragilis* are the most common organisms; *Clostridium perfringens*, the chief cause of gas gangrene, can be found in the intestinal tract. Wound infection can cause wound disruption and/or the formation of scar tissue; the latter is enhanced by peritonitis or postoperative radiation therapy. Even years after an abdominal procedure, increased intraabdominal pressure may induce an incisional hernia through an old scar that has weakened.

Adhesions are the most common cause of postoperative intestinal obstruction. They are caused by an outpouring of fibrin from traumatized tissues, which causes intestinal surfaces to stick together and thus limits mobility. Foreign bodies in the peritoneal cavity can produce granulomas that stimulate fibrin. Glove powder, lint from sponges, and some powerful antibiotics also can produce granulomas. Some patients must return to the OR for lysis of adhesions. Adhesions may present a contraindication for future laparoscopic surgery.

ANORECTAL PROCEDURES

Hemorrhoids, abscesses, fissures, and fistulas are often indications for surgical intervention. The anal region is well supplied with nerves, and these procedures often cause much discomfort. Patients are also sensitive and embarrassed because of the surgical site. After rectal surgery, patients may have an initial difficulty voiding and usually experience considerable pain, which requires medication and sitz baths.

Anoscopy, Proctoscopy, and Sigmoidoscopy

Endoscopic diagnostic procedures such as anoscopy, proctoscopy, and sigmoidoscopy are used for visual examination of the mucosa of the anus, rectum, and sigmoid. Sigmoidoscopy is routinely performed before rectal surgery. Some surgeons prefer a sigmoidoscope setup to be available for all colorectal procedures for periodic anastomosis checks. Fiberoptic equipment has aided in the early detection and treatment of tumors, polyps, and ulcerations.

Hemorrhoidectomy

Hemorrhoidectomy is the surgical removal of varicosities of veins or prolapsed mucosa of the anus and rectum that do not respond to conservative treatment. Hemorrhoids are classified as internal (occurring above the internal sphincter and covered with columnar mucosa), or external (appearing outside the external sphincter and covered with skin). Often both types are present in the patient. External hemorrhoids cause pruritus and pain, whereas the internal type often bleed and may become thrombosed and edematous. Rectal bleeding cannot be assumed to be a result of hemorrhoids; a thorough investigation is required to rule out gastrointestinal disease.

The usual procedure for a hemorrhoidectomy consists of dilating the sphincter, ligating the hemorrhoidal pedicle with suture ligatures or Silastic bands, and excising each hemorrhoidal mass with a sharp dissection, laser, ESU, or cryosurgical unit. The Kraske position generally is used, with the patient's buttocks retracted by wide adhesive strips that are fastened to the edges of the operating bed (Fig. 33-41).

Some surgeons prefer to position female patients in the lithotomy position to avoid contamination of the vagina with bloody anal fluid. When lithotomy is used for males, the scrotum gets in the way and may need to be retracted

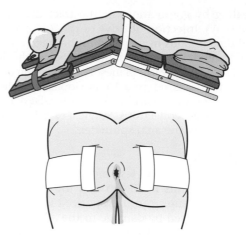

FIG. 33-41   Patient positioning for hemorrhoidectomy.

with temporary stay sutures or superficial skin staples. Petrolatum gauze packing may be inserted in the anal canal, or a compression dressing and perineal binder are applied at completion of the surgical procedure. Some surgeons insert a belladonna suppository to suppress peristalsis during the healing period.

As an alternative to a surgical procedure, McGivney rubber-band ligation of internal hemorrhoids is a common office procedure. After infiltration of a local anesthetic, the hemorrhoid is visualized with an anoscope and grasped with the McGivney ligating instruments (Fig. 33-42). Two bands are placed around the base of each hemorrhoid. Sloughing of the avascular hemorrhoid occurs in 7 to 10 days.

Incision and Drainage of an Anal Abscess

Localized infection in tissues around the anus results in abscess formation. Early incision and drainage are essential to prevent spreading of the infection.

Fistulotomy and Fistulectomy

An anal fistula often develops after incision and drainage or the spontaneous drainage of an anorectal abscess. A fistulous tract may be opened (fistulotomy) to allow drainage

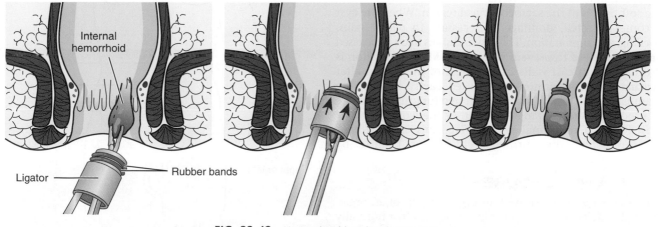

FIG. 33-42   Hemorrhoid banding instrument.

and healing by granulation, or the tract may be excised (fistulectomy). Injection of a dye or the use of a probe and grooved director aids in identifying the tract.

Fistulas tend to follow a predictable path along the ischiorectal or supralevator planes. The prediction of the path (origin and exit) is referred to as Goodsall's rule of anal fistulae. A Seton drain can be placed to assist drainage and healing of abscess collections. Surgical excision is staged to prevent injury to the anal sphincter.

Fissurectomy

When a benign ulcerative lesion occurs in the lining of the anal canal, the anus is dilated and the infected tissue is excised. Some fissures can be vaporized with a laser. Fecal incontinence caused by damage to the anal sphincter is a potential complication that the surgeon tries to avoid.

Treatment of Rectal Tumors

Surgeons prefer to resect a small rectal cancer instead of performing a radical surgical procedure. Many cancers within 20 cm of the anal verge are amenable to local treatment with endoscopic, laser, or cryosurgical techniques. Electrosurgical cutting and coagulating can be combined to remove superficial anorectal and pararectal lesions. For electrosection, the lesion should be small, mobile, and polypoid, with no palpable lymph nodes. The procedure may be performed for palliation to relieve bleeding, painful sphincter spasms (tenesmus), or severe constipation. Interstitial radiation therapy is sometimes used for small anorectal squamous cell carcinomas. The protocol may include external radiation, but bleeding lesions do not respond well to radiation.

In a procedure called transanal endoscopic microsurgery (TEM), tumors in the upper half of the rectum may be excised through an operating rectoscope. This long, tubular instrument improves the surgeon's visual image by incorporating a binocular stereoscope. With TEM, carbon dioxide is insufflated to hold open the walls of the rectum. Tissue graspers, a high-frequency knife, suction, needle holders, and other instruments can be inserted through ports in the airtight eyepiece on the rectoscope. TEM may be used to remove benign lesions and some malignant tumors.

EXCISION OF PILONIDAL CYSTS AND SINUSES

A painful draining cyst with fistulous tract(s) may occur in the soft tissues of the sacrococcygeal region. When the cyst becomes infected, drainage is necessary to relieve pain, swelling, and suppuration. The cyst and sinus tracts are excised or marsupialized to prevent recurrence. Marsupialization is the suturing of cyst walls to the edges of the wound after evacuation; this permits the packed cavity to close by granulation. A Z-plasty may be preferred for primary closure to produce a strong transverse scar, or the wound may be closed with a rotational pedicle flap. Surgical judgment determines whether primary closure or healing by granulation is chosen.

HERNIA PROCEDURES

A hernia is the protrusion of an organ or part of an organ through a defect in the supporting structures that normally contain it. A hernia may be congenital, acquired, or trau-

matic. Most occur in the inguinal or femoral region, but umbilical, ventral, and hiatal hernias also occur (Fig. 33-43). A hernia is usually composed of a sac (covering), hernial contents, and an aperture (opening), but in some locations the sac is absent.

A hernia is called reducible when the hernial contents can be returned to the normal cavity by manipulation. If this cannot be done, the hernia is called irreducible or incarcerated. Bowel present in an incarcerated hernia not only may lack adequate blood supply but also may become obstructed. This is referred to as a strangulated hernia, and an immediate surgical procedure is necessary to prevent necrosis and gangrene of the strangulated bowel.

Inguinal Herniorrhaphy

An inguinal hernia is often repaired with the patient under local anesthesia. An oblique inguinal incision on the affected side is extended through external oblique aponeurosis. The hernia sac is emptied of its contents, ligated, and excised, and the floor of the inguinal canal is reconstructed. Prosthetic mesh is sometimes needed to reinforce a large or recurrent defect.

Repair depends on whether the inguinal hernia is direct or indirect. In both types of inguinal herniorrhaphy in male patients, the spermatic cord and blood supply to the testis are protected from injury. The spermatic cord is retracted with a Penrose drain moistened with saline. Infarction of a testis can occur if the blood supply is compromised. The female round ligament, the homolog of the spermatic cord, passes through the inguinal ring.

Direct Hernia. A direct hernia protrudes through a weakness in the abdominal wall in the region between the rectus abdominis muscle, inguinal ligament, and medial to the

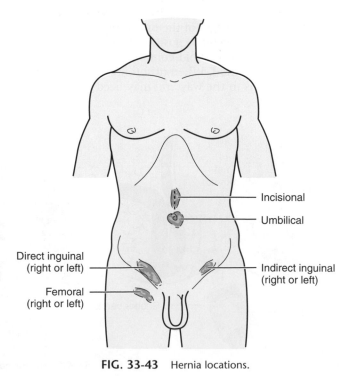

FIG. 33-43   Hernia locations.

inferior epigastric artery. This area is a surgical landmark referred to as the Hesselbach triangle. This hernia is the most difficult type to repair and is more common in men. An acquired weakness of the lower abdominal wall, a direct inguinal hernia often results from straining, such as heavy lifting, chronic coughing, or straining to urinate or defecate. Prompt surgical repair prevents possible discomfort and the threat of later complications.

Indirect Hernia. With an indirect hernia, the peritoneal sac containing intestine protrudes through the internal inguinal ring and passes down the inguinal canal outside Hesselbach's triangle. It directs lateral to the inferior epigastric vessels. It may descend all the way into the scrotum. An indirect inguinal hernia, more common in male patients but can be present in females, originates from a congenital defect in the fascial floor of the inguinal canal. Most inguinal hernias are indirect.

Laparoscopic Repair. A laparoscopic procedure may be used to repair either an indirect or a direct reducible inguinal hernia using mesh behind the hernial defect. This procedure is particularly advantageous for repairing bilateral or recurrent hernias. A transabdominal preperitoneal (TAPP) or intraperitoneal approach may be used, or a trans-extraperitoneal procedure (TEPP) can be performed. Polypropylene mesh is inserted to reinforce the wall of the inguinal canal; this is stapled in place.

Femoral Herniorrhaphy

Femoral herniorrhaphy involves repairing the defect in the transversalis fascia below the inguinal ligament, as well as removing the peritoneal sac protruding through the femoral ring. The transversalis fascia is normally attached to Cooper's ligament, which prevents the peritoneum from reaching the femoral ring. To repair this defect it is necessary to reconstruct the posterior wall and close the femoral ring. These hernias are more common in women.

Umbilical Herniorrhaphy

Repair of an umbilical hernia consists of closing the peritoneal opening and uniting the fasciae above and below the defect to reconstruct the abdominal wall surrounding the umbilicus. This type of hernia is seen most often in children and represents a congenital defect of protrusion of the peritoneum through the umbilical ring. It may also be acquired by women after childbirth.

Ventral (Incisional) Herniorrhaphy

Impaired healing of a previous surgical incision, usually a vertical abdominal incision, may cause an incisional hernia. Often the result of a weakening of abdominal fasciae, projections of peritoneum carrying segments of bowel protrude through fascial perforations. It is necessary to reunite the tissue layers to close the defect. After excising the old scar, the peritoneal sac is opened, the hernia is reduced, and the layers are firmly closed. If existing tissue is not sufficient for repair, synthetic mesh may be used to reinforce the repair. Incisional hernias are sometimes the aftermath of postoperative hematoma, infection, or undue strain.

Ventral hernias have a high recurrence rate when mesh is placed on the outside of a large repair. Through an intraabdominal laparoscopic approach, omentum can be placed over the mesh, or the peritoneum can be put back over the mesh.

Hiatal (Diaphragmatic) Herniorrhaphy

A hiatal hernia results when a portion of the stomach protrudes through the hiatus of the diaphragm. Ten percent of the population has this condition, but not all are symptomatic. The hiatus is the opening for the esophagus through the diaphragm, the chief muscle of respiration. A weakening in the hiatus permits violation of the muscular partition between the abdomen and the chest.

Symptoms are caused mainly by inflammation and ulceration of the adjacent esophagus, which results from the reflux of gastric juices from the herniated stomach. Symptoms include pain, blood loss, and difficulty in swallowing (dysphagia). Diagnosis is made by radiologic and endoscopic studies. This is not the cause of gastroesophageal reflux.

Surgical treatment is appropriate when medical therapy fails to alleviate the problem. The surgical approach may be thoracoabdominal or via the abdomen or chest; each approach offers certain advantages. The abdominal approach is generally preferred, but opening the chest may provide a better view of the hiatal region and thus may be preferred.

AMPUTATION OF EXTREMITIES

Amputation is the total or partial removal of any extremity. The need for amputation is associated most often with massive trauma, a malignant tumor, extensive infection, and vascular insufficiency. Orthopedic or vascular surgeons may perform these procedures.

In preparing the patient for a lower extremity amputation, the patient's chart is checked and both legs are exposed for comparison before skin preparation. It must be made absolutely certain that the correct leg is prepared. The surgeon must initial the correct surgical site. During the timeout phase of incision, the limb is confirmed again for correctness.

Many lower extremity amputations are performed with the patient under spinal anesthesia. It must be ensured that the specimen is *never* within the patient's sight. Policy is followed in regard to the patient's permission for disposal of an extremity.

In general, two types of amputation are performed: open (guillotine) and closed. The guillotine procedure is regarded as an emergency procedure and is rarely performed. Patients who are severely ill or toxic or who experience severe trauma (e.g., an extremity caught under an immovable object) are candidates for this procedure. In the guillotine procedure, tissues are cut circularly with the bone transected higher to allow soft tissues to cover the bone end. Blood vessels and nerve endings are ligated, but the wound is left open. The surgical procedure is often followed by prolonged drainage and healing, muscle and skin retraction, and excessive granulation tissue. A second procedure is often required for final repair.

The conventional flap or closed type of amputation is more desirable. Fashioning curved skin and fascial flaps before amputation of the bone allows deep and superficial fasciae to be approximated over the bone end before closure of the loose skin. Drainage by catheter or suction apparatus may be required. The wound usually heals in approximately 2 weeks.

Amputations of the Lower Extremity

Amputations of the lower extremity are classified as above-knee (AK), below-knee (BK), toe, transphalangeal, transmetatarsal, or the Syme amputation. The level of amputation is determined by the patient's general health, vascular status, and potential for rehabilitation.

Above-Knee Amputation. Amputation at the lower third of the thigh is selected when gangrene or arterial insufficiency extends above the level of the malleoli. A midthigh amputation involves making a circular incision over the distal femur, creating large anterior and posterior skin flaps, and transecting fasciae and muscles. Vessels and nerves such as the femoral and sciatic nerves, respectively, are ligated and severed. Sharp bone edges of the stump are smoothed and debulked with a rasp. The wound is irrigated with sterile normal saline solution before closure of tissue layers. Hemostasis is important to prevent massive hemorrhage or painful hematoma. Drains may be used depending on the surgeon's preference. A noncompressive dressing is applied. AK amputation is a more extensive procedure than BK amputation, and thus a longer time is required for rehabilitation. In general, a prosthesis is fitted 4 to 6 weeks after amputation.

Below-Knee Amputation. Amputation at the middle third of the leg provides for more functional prosthesis fitting and the reduction of phantom limb pain; it also permits a more natural gait (Fig. 33-44). An immediate postoperative prosthesis (IPOP) can be applied in the OR. The IPOP dressing requires a stump sock, felt and lamb's wool for padding, twill Y-straps that are attached to a fitted corset, and a rigid plaster dressing. This dressing not only protects the stump but also aids in controlling the weight placed on it. The prosthesis is metal and provides a pull on the stump. The pylon (foot) may be attached before the patient returns to the unit. If the patient is obese or debilitated, weight bearing may be delayed for several days.

Toe and Transmetatarsal Amputations. Toe and partial foot amputations are generally performed for gangrene and osteomyelitis.

Syme Amputation. A Syme amputation is usually performed for trauma and involves the distal part of the foot. The amputation is above the ankle joint. The skin of the heel is used for the flap (Fig. 33-45).

Hip Disarticulation and Hemipelvectomy. Hip disarticulation and hemipelvectomy involve total removal of the right or left pelvis, including the innominate hipbone, along the ipsilateral lower extremity. A multidisciplinary team of orthpedists and general surgeons perform the procedure because it involves massive soft tissue resection and bony excision.

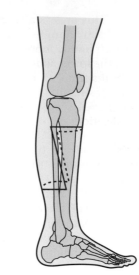

FIG. 33-44   Below-the-knee (BK) amputation.

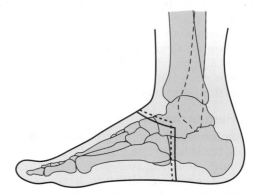

FIG. 33-45   Syme amputation of the foot.

The division of bone may be carried through the sacroiliac joint, or a portion of iliac bone and crest may be preserved. An internal hemipelvectomy includes the removal of innominate bone with adjacent muscles. The large defect created may be covered by a myocutaneous flap of the quadriceps femoris muscle and the overlying skin and subcutaneous tissue. The neck of the femur rests against the soft tissues. These radical procedures are indicated for malignant bone or soft tissue tumors and extensive traumatic injuries. Specialized prosthetic devices are available to permit ambulation.

Amputations of the Upper Extremity

Amputations of the Hand. Hand amputations usually result from trauma and include part or all of the distal phalanges of the digits. Attention is directed to keeping the hand as a working unit when one or more fingers are removed. Every effort should be made to save the thumb; the smallest stump is better than a prosthesis.

Forearm and Forequarter Amputation. Wrist, elbow, and humerus disarticulations are radical procedures performed for malignant tumors or extensive trauma.

Rehabilitation

Postoperative considerations for any amputation include control of bleeding and phantom limb sensations, stump care, immediate fitting of a functional terminal prosthesis, exercises to prevent flexion contractures, and ambulation or use of a hand or arm.

The loss of an extremity involves major psychological and physical adjustments. The rehabilitative process is very important and is often affected by the emotional reactions of the patient. Patients with an early postoperative prosthesis have a more positive outlook about their loss. Morale is boosted by being able to walk the first postoperative day or soon thereafter (which, in the case of a leg amputation, depends on the surgeon's orders for the weight-bearing program). This in turn aids in ambulation.

Phantom limb pain is particularly distressing to many patients. The nerves have been severed, but the patient has the sensation that the amputated part is still present. This sensation is often associated with painful paresthesia (i.e., tingling, prickling, tickling, burning). The pain is real. It usually responds to aspirin, acetaminophen (Tylenol), or a similar agent, but narcotics may be necessary to control pain. The combined efforts of the patient, family, and interdisciplinary professional personnel are needed for successful rehabilitation.

Bibliography

AORN (Association of periOperative Registered Nurses): *AORN standards, recommended practices, and guidelines,* Denver, 2006, The Association.

Barrow CL: Roux-en-Y gastric bypass for morbid obesity, *AORN J* 76(4):593-604, 2002.

Bittner R et al: Laparoscopic transperitoneal procedure for routine repair of groin hernia, *Br J Surg* 89(8):1062-1066, 2002.

Cox JA et al: Treating benign colon disorders using laparoscopic colectomy, *AORN J* 73(2):377-398, 2001.

Gavaghan M: The pancreas—Hermit of the abdomen, *AORN J* 75(6):1110-1130, 2002.

Goldberg S et al: Vertical banded gastroplasty: A treatment for morbid obesity, *AORN J* 72(6):988-1003, 2000.

Hofstetter W et al: Treatment outcomes of resected esophageal cancer, *Ann Surg* 236(3):376-385, 2002.

Kellar SJ: Sentinel lymph node biopsy for breast cancer, *AORN J* 74(2):197-201, 2001.

Madick S: Perioperative care of the patient with Zenker's diverticulum, *AORN J* 37(5):904-913, 2001.

Sparks CA: Using ductoscopy to detect breast mass at an early stage, *AORN J* 76(5):851-854, 2002.

Todd S et al: Outpatient Nissen laparoscopic fundoplication, *AORN J* 75(5):956-979, 2002.

World Health Organization: *Guidelines for essential trauma care,* Geneva, 2004, The Organization.

Chapter 34

Gynecologic and Obstetric Surgery

CHAPTER OBJECTIVES

After studying this chapter, the learner will be able to:
- Identify the organs of the female genitourinary system.
- Describe the physiology of the female reproductive system.
- Differentiate between adolescent and adult gynecologic health
- Describe the pertinent considerations when caring for a pregnant patient.

CHAPTER OUTLINE

KEY TERMS AND DEFINITIONS

Abortion   Termination of pregnancy. Several descriptions are as follows:

Elective voluntary surgical ending of pregnancy   *First trimester:* pregnancy is terminated during first 3 months of gestation; *Second trimester:* pregnancy is terminated during second 3 months of gestation; *Late:* pregnancy is terminated after the second trimester has ended.

Incomplete natural termination of pregnancy before the age of viability   Products of conception are partially retained and may need surgical removal to prevent sepsis in the mother.

Missed   Natural termination of gestation before the age of viability. Products of conception must be surgically removed to prevent sepsis in the mother.

Spontaneous   Natural termination of pregnancy before age of viability. Products of conception are expelled without surgical intervention.

Threatened   Pregnancy is diagnosed at risk for natural termination before the age of viability. Medical and/or surgical management may be attempted to prevent full natural termination.

Amenorrhea   Absence of menstrual periods.

Cesarean birth   Surgical delivery of a fetus through an abdominal incision. Also known as cesarean section.

Chromopertubation   Instillation of dye through the fallopian tubes as a test of patency.

Dilation and curettage (D&C)   Opening of the uterine cervix is progressively enlarged to permit instrumentation for debulking the endometrium and other surgical procedures.

Endometrium   Lining of the uterus that is normally shed during menstruation.

Fundus   The round top or dome of uterus.

Leiomyofibroma   Term for fibroid tumors. Also known as myoma (e.g., uterine muscle tumor).

Graafian follicle   Mature ovum.

Gravid   Pregnant.

Menarche   Beginning of menstruation.

Menometrorrhagia   Bleeding between menstrual periods in a premenopausal woman that is surgically treated by dilation and curettage, endometrial ablation, or hysterectomy.

Menorrhagia   Excessive bleeding at menstruation that is surgically treated by dilation and curettage, endometrial ablation, or hysterectomy.

Menstruation   The shedding of the endometrium during periodic hormonal cycles.

Neoplasia   New tissue overgrowth. Potentially cancerous.

Retained secundus   Products of conception are retained either at delivery of a viable fetus or at the time of incomplete abortion. Placental remnants.

Tanner's stages   Incremental measurement of sexual development from first signs of puberty to maturity in both sexes.

Thelarche   The beginning of breast development that is measured in stages.

SUPPLEMENTAL MATERIAL ON EVOLVE WEBSITE   *evolve*

http://evolve.elsevier.com/BerryKohn
- Content Updates
- Glossary
- Full Set of Perioperative Flash Cards
- Interactive Key Term Flash Cards
- Tips for the Scrub Person and Circulating Nurse: Dilation and Curettage, Abdominal Hysterectomy, Anterior and Posterior Colporrhaphy
- Student Activities
- WebLinks

HISTORICAL BACKGROUND

From its inception in 1930, the American Board of Obstetrics and Gynecology has emphasized the inseparability of gynecology and obstetrics because of their anatomic and physiologic relationships. Gynecology (commonly referred to as GYN) is the science of health and diseases of the female reproductive organs. Gynecologic surgery includes correction of certain problems of the female genitourinary tract. Obstetrics (OB) concerns the care of women during pregnancy, labor, and the puerperium (period from delivery to the time the uterus regains normal size, usually about 6 weeks).

Although all surgeons certified by the American Board of Obstetrics and Gynecology are competent in both disciplines, some limit their practice to either obstetrics or gynecology. Specialty certification boards have also been established in gynecologic oncology, endocrinology and infertility, and perinatal medicine. This text limits discussion to the most common surgical procedures performed by gynecologists and/or obstetricians in the perioperative environment.

Obstetric care, left to the mother herself or to a midwife, was neglected until the Renaissance. In prehistoric cultures the woman squatted on a bed of leaves, delivered, chewed off or cut the umbilical cord, bathed the infant in a stream, wrapped the infant in an animal hide, and resumed her "womanly duties" in the field. Up through the Dark Ages, based on the biblical decree, "In sorrow shalt thou bring forth children," it was believed that pregnant women should suffer. Some were attended by untrained midwives.

The first book on obstetric care was written by the German physician Eucharius Rösslin in 1513, but it was the treatise of François Mauriceau (1637-1709), published in Paris in 1668, that became the basis of obstetrics. Mauriceau's writings described how the mother's pelvic bones did not separate but remained intact during delivery. He is known as the "Founder of Modern Obstetrics and Gynecology."

The practice of gynecology was limited, bound by tradition, and even regressed during medieval times. New interest developed in the Renaissance. In 1663 the Dutch surgeon Hendrick von Roonhuyze (1622-1672) published the first book on surgical obstetrics and gynecology having modern connotations. He described extrauterine pregnancy, uterine rupture, and vesicovaginal fistula. He also performed cesarean sections.

In the eighteenth century, progress was made, particularly in England. Practitioners advocated the treatment of ovarian cysts. However, surgical gynecology did not become an independent specialty until the early nineteenth century. Early male gynecologists fought public prejudice against exposure of female organs, even for examination. Clergy, midwives, and physicians attempted to deter their practice. Opposition to the progress of surgery in general eventually was overcome.

In 1809 Ephraim McDowell of Kentucky successfully removed an ovarian cyst by an abdominal approach without benefit of modern anesthesia or aseptic techniques. The 22-year-old patient survived without complication. A limited variety of gynecologic procedures, such as oophorectomy and salpingectomy, were developed by succeeding pioneers. The first successful vaginal hysterectomy was performed in 1818. Use of the speculum was a notable advance for gynecologists.

The practice of dilating the cervix for a variety of purposes was known since the days of Hippocrates. Many instruments were used. In 1879 Alfred Hegar (1830-1914) developed graduated metal cervical dilators that bear his name and are still commonly used. Softening of the lower uterine segment is a recognized sign of early pregnancy that was named for him.

ANATOMY AND PHYSIOLOGY OF THE FEMALE REPRODUCTIVE SYSTEM

The female genitourinary system comprises the organs, glands, secretions, and other elements of reproduction referred to as the pudendum. Components of the female reproductive system are both external and internal organs.

Female External Genitalia

The term *vulva* is used collectively for the female external genitalia (Fig. 34-1). This sensitive, delicate area is highly vascular, with an extensive superficial and deep lymph supply and rich cutaneous sensory innervation. It includes the following:

Labia Majora. The labia majora are two large folds, or lips, containing sebaceous and sweat glands embedded in fatty tissue covered by hair-bearing skin. They join anteriorly in a fatty pad, the mons veneris, which overlies the pubic bone (symphysis pubis). In the adult female this area is covered with a triangular pattern of hair. Sebaceous secretions of the labia lubricate the proximal area. The labia majora atrophy and hair follicles decrease in number after menopause, making the labia minora more prominent.

Labia Minora. The labia minora, or small lips, lying within the labia majora, are flat folds of connective tissue containing sebaceous glands. Anteriorly these labia split into two parts. One part passes anteriorly over the clitoris to

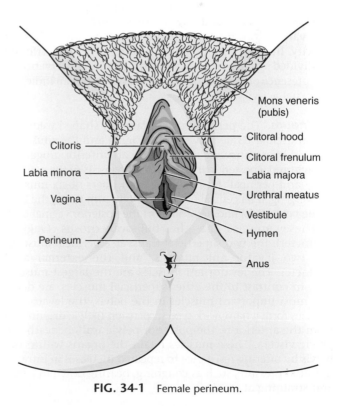

FIG. 34-1   Female perineum.

form a protective prepuce, or foreskin. The other passes behind the clitoris to shape a frenulum, a fold of mucous membrane. Posteriorly they join across the midline behind the vagina to form the fourchette, or fold of skin just inside the posterior vulvar commissure.

Clitoris. The clitoris, a 1-inch erectile organ composed of bilateral cavernosa and a glans, is the female homologe of the penis. It is attached by ischiocavernosus musculature to the pubic rami by a suspensory ligament. It is located at the apex of the labia minora, which form a prepuce, or hood-like covering. The mucous membrane covering the glans contains many nerve endings and is a source of sexual stimulation for the female. The blood supply is derived from a terminal branch of the pudendal artery, which is a terminal division of the internal iliac artery. The venous drainage is continuous with the labial plexae. Innervation is from the sacral plexus.

Vestibule. The vestibule is the space, or shallow elliptic depression posterior to the clitoris, enclosed by the labia minora. The urethral opening is located in this region posterior to the clitoris and anterior to the vagina. The fourchette forms the posterior boundary.

Bartholin Glands. Small bilateral Bartholin glands lie deep in the posterior third of the labia majora, within the bulbocavernosus muscle. The mucus secretion is a vaginal lubricant. These glands can become inflamed and infected, causing pain and discomfort.

Hymen. The hymen is a thin, vascularized connective tissue membrane that surrounds and may partially or completely occlude the vaginal orifice. It varies among individuals in thickness and elasticity. The central aperture permits passage of menstrual flow and vaginal secretions. This structure will vary according to individual anatomy and physical activity. In some patients the aperture may be imperforate or divided by a septum, requiring surgical intervention. The presence or absence of a hymenal ring is not an indicator of sexual activity.

Perineum. The perineum is a diamond-shaped wedge of fibromuscular tissue between the vagina and the anus. It is divided by a transverse septum into an anterior urogenital triangle and a posterior anal triangle. It consists of the perineal body and perineal musculature. With fibers of six muscles converging at its central point, the perineum forms the base of the pelvic floor and helps support the posterior vaginal wall.

These muscles are the bulbocavernosus (vaginal sphincter), the two superficial transverse perineal muscles, the two levator ani muscles, and the external anal sphincter. The levator ani muscles are the largest muscles and, in contrast to the other superficial muscles, are deep. The most important muscles in the pelvis, the levator ani muscles form a hammock-type suspension (pelvic diaphragm) from the anterior to the posterior pelvic wall, beneath the pelvic viscera. These muscles retain the organs within the pelvis by offering resistance to repeated increases in intraabdominal pressure, such as coughing, bearing down in labor, and straining at stool.

Internal Female Reproductive Organs

The internal female reproductive organs (Fig. 34-2) lie within the pelvic cavity, protected by the bony pelvis. Bones and ligaments form the pelvic outlet. The dilated cervix of the uterus and the vagina constitute the birth canal.

Vagina. The vagina is a thin-walled, 8-cm fibromuscular tube extending from the vestibule obliquely backward and upward to the uterus, where the cervix projects into the top of the anterior wall. The vagina is elastic and capable of distention during intercourse and parturition. The bladder lies anteriorly to it; the rectum lies posteriorly to it. It is lined with mucous membrane and contains glands that produce a cleansing acid secretion.

The anterior vaginal wall is shorter than the posterior wall. The upper third of the posterior wall is covered by peritoneum reflected onto the rectum. Normally the anterior and posterior walls relax and are in contact. However, the lateral walls remain rigid because of the pull of the muscles and therefore are in close contact with pelvic tissues.

A rich venous plexus in the muscular walls makes the vagina highly vascular. Uterine and vaginal arteries supplying the area are branches of the internal iliac artery. Branches of the vaginal artery extend to the external genitalia and the adjacent bladder and rectum. Lymphatic drainage is extensive. The upper two thirds of the vagina drain into the external and internal iliac nodes; the lower third drains into the superficial inguinal nodes.

The vault (upper part of the vagina) is divided into four fornices, or arches (Fig. 34-3). During digital pelvic examination, pelvic organs can be palpated through the thin walls of the vault. The anterior fornix, in front of the cervix, is adjacent to the base of the bladder and distal ends of the ureters.

The pouch of Douglas (retrouterine cul-de-sac) directly behind the larger posterior fornix lies behind the cervix. This pouch separates the back of the uterus from the rectum: anteriorly by the uterine peritoneal covering, which continues down to cap the posterior vaginal fornix; and posteriorly by the anterior wall of the rectum. Lateral uterosacral ligaments embrace the lower third of the rectum. The floor of the pouch, about 7 cm above the anus, is formed by

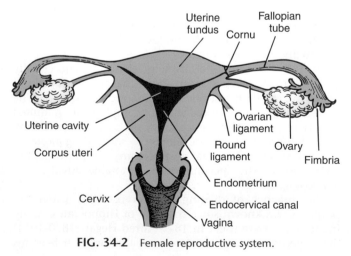

FIG. 34-2   Female reproductive system.

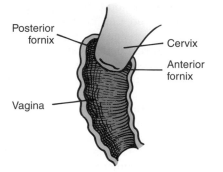

FIG. 34-3   Cervix in vaginal vault.

reflection of the peritoneum from the rectum to the upper vagina and uterus. The posterior cul-de-sac is the route of entry for a number of diagnostic or surgical procedures, because the pouch of Douglas (the lowest part of the peritoneal cavity) is separated from the vagina only by the thin vaginal wall and peritoneum.

The lateral fornices lie on either side of the cervix, in contact with anterior and posterior sheets of the broad ligaments surrounding the uterus. Proximal structures are the uterine artery, ureters, fallopian tubes, ovaries, and sigmoid colon.

Uterus. The uterus is the female organ of gestation. It receives and holds the fertilized ovum during development of the fetus and expels it during childbirth. Resembling an inverted pear in shape, this hollow muscular retroperitoneal organ is situated in the bony pelvis. It lies between the bladder anteriorly and the sigmoid colon posteriorly. The uterus is divided transversely by a slight constriction into a wider upper part (the body or corpus uteri) and a narrower lower part (the 2- to 3-cm cervix uteri or ectocervix that protrudes into the vagina). The corpus meets the cervix at the internal os. Peritoneum covers the corpus externally; the endometrium, ranging in thickness from 2 to 10 mm, lines it internally. This mucous membrane is uniquely adapted to receive and sustain the fertilized ovum. The fundus, or rounded top portion of the uterus, lies above the uterine cavity.

The shape of the uterine cavity (endometrial cavity), flattened from front to back, is roughly triangular in the nonpregnant female. The upper lateral angles extend out toward openings of the fallopian tubes, which enter bilaterally through the uterine walls at the cornua. The apex of the triangle is directed downward to the cervix. The cavity within the cervix, the endocervical canal, narrows to a slit at the distal orifice, where the cervix communicates with the vagina via the external os. The endocervix is the glandular mucous membrane of the cervix. The corpus of the uterus and the cervix are considered individually in relation to disease and therapy because they differ in structure and function.

The uterus is capable of expansion to accommodate a growing fetus. Much of the bulk of the corpus consists of involuntary muscle, the myometrium, composed of three layers. The inner layer prevents reflux of menstrual flow into the tubes and peritoneal cavity, which could result in

endometriosis. It also contributes to the competency of the internal os sphincter to prevent premature expulsion of the fetus. The middle layer encloses large blood vessels. These muscle fibers act as living ligatures for hemostasis after delivery. The outer layer has expulsive action, ejecting menstrual flow and clots, an aborted embryo, or the fetus at term.

Usually the uterus lies forward at a right angle to the vagina and rests on the bladder. Although the cervix is anchored laterally by ligaments, the fundus may pivot about the cardinal ligaments widely in an anteroposterior plane. Mobility rather than position is the criterion for normality.

Fallopian Tubes (Salpinges). The fallopian tubes (small, hollow musculomembranous tubes, sometimes called oviducts or uterine tubes) run bilaterally like arms from each side of the upper part of the uterus to the ovaries. Near each ovary, the open end of each tube expands into the infundibulum, which divides into fimbriae—fingerlike projections that sweep up the ovum (the female reproductive cell) as it is expelled from the ovary. Ciliated cells move the ovum toward the uterus.

The lumen of the tube becomes very narrow where it penetrates the uterine wall to reach the uterine cavity. Contractions in the muscular walls change the shape and position of the tubes. At ovulation they move the fimbriated ends into close apposition with ovarian surfaces. The fallopian tubes serve as a continuous passage from the external environment into the abdominal cavity via the vagina, cervix, and uterine body. Infectious diseases and other substances can enter the peritoneal cavity through this route.

Ovaries. The ovaries are oval glandular gonads located in shallow peritoneal fossae on the lateral pelvic walls, from which they are suspended by the infundibulopelvic ligaments. They are attached to the posterior layer of the broad ligament by the mesovarium (a peritoneal fold) and to the uterus by the ovarian ligament (a fibromuscular cord).

The ovaries, the counterpart of the male testes, contain ova. Each ovary measures 2 × 3 cm and consists of a center of cells and vessels surrounded by the cortex. This main portion contains the stroma or fibrous framework in which the ovarian follicles are embedded. Of the approximately 200,000 primordial follicles present at birth, fewer than 400 are likely to produce a mature ovum (graafian follicle) during the reproductive years. A serous covering derived from peritoneum surrounds the ovaries. In addition to protecting maturing ova, the ovaries, which atrophy after menopause, produce female sex hormones.

The ureters course along the retroperitoneum bilaterally and lie close to the ovarian blood supply just anterior to the common iliac arteries. The ovaries, when diseased, may be adherent to the ureters. Some surgeons will have a urologist place ureteral catheters to make the structural identification easier during dissection.

Muscles and Ligaments. Muscles and ligaments support and suspend the uterus and fallopian tubes in the normal position in the center of the pelvic cavity.

Broad Ligaments. Bilateral broad ligaments are composed of a broad double sheet of peritoneum extending from each lateral surface of the uterus outward to the pelvic wall. Between these two layers of peritoneum, the fallopian tubes are enclosed in the free upper borders (mesosalpinges), with the tubal ostia opening directly into the peritoneal cavity.

Round Ligaments. The round ligaments are fibromuscular bands that extend from the anterior surface of the lateral borders of the fundus to the labia majora. They run beneath the peritoneum and anterior sheet of the broad ligament down, outward, and forward through the inguinal canal to the labia.

Cardinal Ligaments. The lower portion of the broad ligaments, the cardinal ligaments are attached to the lateral vaginal fornices and supravaginal portion of the cervix. They act as a supportive pivot.

Uterosacral Ligaments. The uterosacral ligaments are peritoneal folds containing connective tissue and involuntary muscle. They arise on each side from the posterior wall of the uterus at the level of the internal os, pass backward around the rectum, and insert on the sacrum at the level of the second sacral vertebra. They pull on the cervix to keep the uterus anteverted and, through the cervix, the vagina in position as well.

Physiology

The function of the female reproductive organs is to conceive, nurture, and produce offspring. The development and function of these organs are influenced by the hormonal secretions of the ovaries and adrenal, thyroid, and pituitary glands. These hormonal relationships also affect primary and secondary sex characteristics.

The physiologic hormonal cycle prepares the uterus for the fertilized ovum. Hormone production stimulates the endometrium and breasts, resulting in thickening of tissue and increased blood supply.

Each month during the years from puberty to menopause, one (or both) of the ovaries matures a follicle from within. When the matured graafian follicle ruptures, it discharges the enclosed ovum, which enters the fallopian tube at the fimbriated end. The process of maturation and discharge of the egg is called ovulation, resulting in a fertile period that lasts several days. Changes in cervical mucus and vaginal epithelium also accompany ovulation.

Union of the ovum with a viable mature male germ cell (spermatozoon), which has ascended to the fallopian tube from the vagina, results in fertilization within 12 hours of ovulation. The union takes place in the outer third of the tube and travels toward the uterus over a period of 3 days. The fertilized ovum normally proceeds to the cornu of the uterus, where it enters to implant itself in the endometrium within 14 days of fertilization. By day 17, the blood supply of the fetal and maternal blood vessels is functional. The placental circulation is established. The ensuing pregnancy will last approximately 266 days, or 9 calendar months, if carried to full term.

The ovarian hormone estrogen, together with progesterone, causes a sequence of changes in the endometrial lining of the uterus to prepare for implantation of the fertilized ovum. Estrogen also produces the development of secondary sexual characteristics. Progesterone is responsible for maintaining pregnancy until hormones from the placenta assume this role.

Menstruation is the periodic discharge of blood, mucus, disintegrated ovum, and uterine mucosa formed during the hormonal cycle if pregnancy does not take place. The duration of the menstrual period varies but averages 3 to 5 days. The amount of blood lost varies greatly. The menstrual cycle, the time between the onset of each period, is approximately 28 days.

Regularity of menstruation can be disturbed by disease conditions and emotions, in addition to the onset of pregnancy. This physiologic cycle continually recurs throughout the reproductive life of the woman. Assessment of the female patient should include documentation of the age of menarche (first menses), the date of the last menstrual period (LMP), use of contraception, and sexual history.

The possibility of pregnancy should be considered if the female patient is within childbearing age, regardless of age, social status, or vocation. A surgical procedure and/or the administration of anesthetic agents could be hazardous to a developing embryo.

GYNECOLOGY: GENERAL CONSIDERATIONS

The emotional preparation of gynecologic patients presents a special challenge to the operating room (OR) team. Anticipation of physical exposure, potential loss of sexual function, infertility problems, or termination of pregnancy can create severe anxiety. Some surgical procedures terminate reproductive capability and produce menopause. Patients must be able to express concerns, ask questions, and receive reassurance and support.

Examination with the Patient Under Anesthesia (EUA)

Bimanual examination of the pelvis with the patient in the lithotomy position and relaxed from anesthesia usually precedes vaginal and abdominal gynecologic surgical procedures. This allows the surgeon to thoroughly assess the size, outline, consistency, position, and mobility of the uterus, fallopian tubes, and ovaries. This examination also helps the surgeon determine or confirm the approach for the procedure and whether a lesion is resectable. This is helpful in evaluating women experiencing pain or nervous tension or those who are obese. The vaginal vault and perineum are prepped and the examination is performed before prepping the abdomen for a diagnostic laparoscopy or exploratory laparotomy.

Special Features of Gynecologic Surgery

Diagnostic and surgical procedures may be carried out through a vaginal or an abdominal approach, or the two approaches may be combined. Each requires a different position and different preparation, drapes, and setup. Surgical techniques for general abdominal procedures apply to gynecologic surgery. Diagnostic and definitive surgical procedures are often combined and done in one surgical procedure.

The following apply to both vaginal and abdominopelvic procedures:

1. Spinal, epidural, or (more commonly) general anesthesia is used. An epidural catheter may be inserted preoperatively for postoperative pain control.

2. A Foley catheter may be inserted after the administration of the anesthetic agent, to prevent the bladder from becoming distended during the procedure and to record urinary output. The circulating nurse and the anesthesia provider should check the urinary drainage bag frequently and report urine volume or evidence of blood. This could indicate injury to the bladder or ureters. Percutaneous insertion of a cannula directly into the bladder through the abdominal wall (suprapubic cystostomy) provides an alternative indwelling urinary drainage system in select patients.

3. An electrosurgical unit (ESU), with either monopolar or bipolar electrodes, is frequently employed.

4. Argon, CO_2, and neodymium:yttrium aluminum garnet (Nd:YAG) lasers are used, generally in conjunction with a colposcope or laparoscope and the operating microscope for some procedures.

5. Closed-wound suction drainage, or another type of drain, may be used to prevent hematoma or serum accumulation in the pelvis and/or the wound.

6. Prophylactic preoperative anticoagulation with subcutaneous heparin, antiembolic stockings, sequential compression devices, and early ambulation are especially important in pelvic surgery because of the potential for deep vein thrombosis (DVT) and subsequent pulmonary emboli (PE).

Vaginal Approach

1. The patient is in the lithotomy position.
2. Instrumentation must be of sufficient length for use within the vaginal canal and uterine cavity. In addition to retracting, cutting, holding, clamping, and suturing instruments, vaginal setups include dilation and curettage (D&C) instruments for intrauterine procedures (Table 34-1).
3. A laser, ESU, or cryosurgical unit may be used to remove hypertrophied tissue or certain benign neoplasms.
4. A suction system, including a Poole suction tip with guard, tubing, and collection canister, is part of the setup.

5. Raytec sponges are rolled and secured on sponge forceps in deep areas (also referred to as sponge sticks). Long, narrow, 4 × 18–inch sponges with radiopaque markers on the end are used for packing off abdominal viscera in vaginal procedures. All counts are very important in these procedures.

6. Vaginal packing is inserted after certain procedures for hemostasis and/or therapeutic purposes. Antibiotic or hormone cream may be applied to the packing during insertion. Impregnated vaginal packing is commercially available. The packing should be recorded on the patient's chart and removed at the surgeon's order.

7. At the completion of the surgical procedure, a sanitary pad is placed against the perineum between the patient's legs.

Abdominal Approach

1. The supine or Trendelenburg's position is used for abdominopelvic procedures to displace pelvic organs cephalad. Preparation and drapes are the same as for abdominal laparotomy. Abdominal incisions commonly used in gynecologic open procedures are shown in Fig. 34-4.
2. When a large abdominal mass is present or the pelvic organs are pushed from their normal relationships, ureteral catheters may be inserted via cystoscopy before the surgical procedure to facilitate identification of the ureters to prevent inadvertent dissection. Severing of the ureters during the procedure greatly increases postoperative morbidity and mortality if the injury is not immediately detected and corrected.
3. Instrumentation includes the basic laparotomy setup with the addition of long instruments for deep manipulations within the pelvis; uterine graspers, such as a Somer uterine elevator.

TABLE 34-1	Instruments for Dilation and Curettage
Purpose	**Instruments**
To expose	Vaginal speculum
	Posterior retractor
	Weighted posterior retractor
	Narrow lateral Heaney retractors
To grasp and hold	Single- and double-toothed tenaculums
To measure uterine cavity	Uterine sound (graduated probe)
To dilate cervix	Graduated dilators
	Goodell dilator
To scrape tissue	Sharp and blunt, large and small uterine curettes
To obtain specimen	Endometrial biopsy suction curette
To carry sponges	Sponge forceps
To remove polyps and biopsy tissue	Polyp and biopsy forceps
To insert packing	Uterine dressing forceps

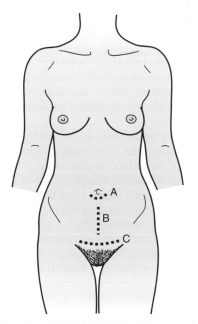

FIG. 34-4 Common abdominal incisions for gynecologic surgery. *A,* Infraumbilical incision. *B,* Lower midline incision. *C,* Pfannenstiel incision.

Abdominal Complications. Injuries to ureters, which can lead to loss of renal function if unrecognized, can occur during the surgical procedure because of their relationship to pelvic structures. The surgeon must identify and isolate the ureter(s) on the affected side(s) to prevent accidental crushing or kinking.

Adhesions after pelvic surgery can cause infertility, intestinal obstruction, and/or chronic abdominal pain. The surgeon may place a biodegradable fabric (Interceed Absorbable Adhesion Barrier) over tissues and pelvic organs before closing the peritoneal cavity. This satin-like knitted fabric acts as a physical barrier to prevent adhesion formation during the healing process. Within 8 hours the fabric becomes a gelatinous protective coating. This is completely absorbed within 28 days.

Combined Vaginal-Abdominal Approach. If vaginal and abdominal surgery is indicated, a combined procedure is planned. For example, the patient may be scheduled for a total abdominal hysterectomy with anterior vaginal colporrhaphy. In such instances the vaginal procedure is performed first. The patient is then removed from the lithotomy position and repositioned in the supine position, and the abdominal preparation and surgical procedure are carried out. Care is taken to ensure that the dispersive electrode has not been displaced, and a new one should be applied when the patient is repositioned.

The following considerations apply:
1. Because of the possibility of infection, separate sterile setups are used for vaginal and abdominal procedures performed concurrently.
2. Vaginal preparation precedes exploratory pelvic laparotomy in readiness for the unexpected or for a D&C scheduled to precede an abdominal procedure. A separate sterile prep table is used for the external genitalia and vagina. Another sterile setup is used for the abdominal preparation. The vaginal area is prepped first to prevent splashing up to a freshly prepped abdomen.

DIAGNOSTIC TECHNIQUES

The gynecologist employs both noninvasive and invasive diagnostic techniques. Some are performed as office or ambulatory procedures, especially those using the vaginal approach.

A pelvic examination includes inspection and palpation of the external genitalia; bimanual abdominovaginal and abdominorectal palpation of the uterus, fallopian tubes, and ovaries; and speculum examination of the vagina and cervix. This inspection is augmented by a cytologic study of smears of cervical and endocervical tissue obtained by scrapings. The Papanicolaou (Pap) smear has significantly facilitated diagnosis of cervical cancer and premalignant lesions. Characteristic cellular changes in cervical epithelial cells are identified. Cytologic aspiration from within the endocervical canal may reveal unsuspected carcinoma of the endometrium, fallopian tubes, or ovaries and occult cervical cancer.

The Schiller test involves staining the vaginal vault and cervical squamous epithelium with Lugol's solution. Glycogen in normal epithelium takes up the iodine. Abnormal tissues, with little or no glycogen, do not stain brown and thereby pinpoint sites for biopsy. Abnormal cytologic findings are an indication for further evaluation by histologic tissue study. Use of iodine products is contraindicated in patients with systemic iodine allergy.

Uterine cancer consists of two entities: cervical cancer and endometrial cancer. These differ by age-groups, types, and consequences. Cancer of the cervix appears most often in association with coitus at an early age, multiple partners, nonbarrier contraceptives, poor sexual hygiene, a chronically infected cervix, or a history of sexually transmitted diseases. These include infection with herpes simplex virus (HSV), human papillomavirus (HPV), cytomegalovirus (CMV), *Chlamydia trachomatis,* and *Trichomonas vaginalis.* A higher frequency of abnormal Pap smear findings is associated with these infections.

HPV produces condylomata (venereal or genital warts), which have been identified as a possible cause of cervical carcinoma. HPV screening is part of the routine gynecologic exam. HPV vaccination, a series of three injections given over a 6-month period, is recommended for all girls and women from 11 to 26 years of age as a cervical cancer preventive.[1] The Centers for Disease Control and Prevention (CDC) speculates that 50% of sexually active men and women will experience HPV infection (genital warts) during their lifetime.

Cancer of the endometrium, more common than cervical cancer, occurs primarily in postmenopausal women. It is often associated with obesity, low parity, late menopause, hypertension, and diabetes mellitus.

Biopsy of the Cervix
Cervical cancer may not present symptoms in the early stage and may progress to invasion before discovery. Spotting, postmenopausal bleeding, or chronic cervicitis may be the first visible sign. The condition may be suspected by results of cytologic examination or visual inspection, but diagnosis is made by biopsy.

Excisional Biopsy. In excisional biopsy an attempt is made to excise the entire cervical lesion by sharp dissection. Sutures or an ESU is used for hemostasis. Packing may be needed.

Incisional Biopsy. Incisional biopsy involves the use of a scalpel, punch biopsy, or other instrument to obtain tissue for diagnosis but not to remove the lesion. If a malignancy is diagnosed, additional evaluation and further treatment are carried out by additional surgery and/or radiation therapy.

Cone Biopsy. Patients diagnosed by Pap smear as having severe cervical dysplasia or intraepithelial carcinoma of the

---

[1]Immunization advisory panel of the CDC recommends vaccination as HPV prophylaxis as of 2006. The vaccine Gardasil was approved by the U.S. Food and Drug Administration (FDA) to protect women from 18 strains of the virus that is responsible for 70% of all cervical cancers and 90% of genital warts. The full benefit will not be apparent for at least 10 years.

cervix require conization to remove the lesion and rule out invasive carcinoma. The biopsy, obtained with a laser, scalpel, or cervitome (cold knife conization), includes the squamocolumnar junctions of the ectocervix (transformation zone) and is tapered to include the endocervical canal to the level of the internal os (Fig. 34-5). Most of the lesions categorized as cervical intraepithelial neoplasia (CIN), dysplasia, or carcinoma in situ are found in this area. Conization of the cervix provides the most comprehensive specimen to diagnose a premalignant or malignant lesion. Multiple blocks and sections are examined by the pathologist to determine the extent of invasive disease.

Complications include hemorrhage, infection, cervical stenosis, an incompetent cervix, and infertility. The CO_2 laser used for conization minimizes these risks. Hemostasis is secured with sutures as needed.

Cervical dysplasia can occur in sexually active females age 12 years and older; the peak incidence is between the ages of 25 and 35 years. Employed therapeutically for chronic inflammation and for premalignant lesions in women of childbearing age, conization may be performed by scalpel, electrosurgery, or laser. Laser conization is used to treat severe dysplasia and carcinoma in situ.

Loop electrosurgical excision procedures (LEEP) use a stainless steel or tungsten loop electrode to excise a central core of tissue from the transformation zone of the endocervical canal. Large loop excision of the transformation zone (LLETZ) is performed with minimal bleeding and few complications. These procedures may be performed in the OR or office setting with local anesthesia. Future childbearing is unaffected. Although the specimen is comparable in size to that obtained with cold knife conization, the specimen has superficial desiccation and may be inferior in quality. Wide conization may result in scarring and obstruction of the os.

Fractional Curettage. Tissue is obtained for histologic examination by scraping the uterine cavity. Fractional curettage differentiates specimens between the endocervix

and the endometrium in a series of two steps. A biopsy specimen may be taken from the cervix, if indicated by the Schiller test, in association with endocervical curettage. A small curette is introduced into the endocervical canal, which is scraped from the internal to the external os. The specimen is placed on a Telfa pad, and both are put into a container. This scraping precedes cervical dilation to avoid dislodging tissue from above the internal os.

After cervical dilation, a different curette is inserted into the uterine cavity for curettage of the endometrium. The endometrial specimen is placed in a separate container from the one used for the specimens obtained by endocervical curettage.

Colposcopy. Illumination and binocular magnification afforded by the colpomicroscope permit identification of abnormal epithelium to target for biopsy. The colposcope has a cool, intense white light that can be fitted with a green filter to improve visualization of the vascular pattern. With the colposcope positioned in front of the vulva, without touching the patient, the colposcopist can focus light through a speculum on the ectocervix, the lower part of the cervical canal, and the vaginal wall. The cervix is wiped with 3% acetic acid to eradicate mucus and to facilitate viewing the surface and vasculature. Biopsies are taken for histologic confirmation of the diagnosis. Endocervical curettage also may be performed. A video or still camera can be attached to a colposcope to photograph lesions.

Vaginal condylomata from the human papillomavirus (HPV) and adenoses, preinvasive lesions of the cervix, cervical dysplasia, CIN, and other vaginal and cervical lesions can be treated by laser with the colpomicroscope. Visualization, unobstructed by instruments, is excellent. Condylomata can incubate for 3 weeks to 6 months and will appear as white, raised areas when exposed to 3% to 5% acetic acid. Full-strength solutions will burn the patient's tissues. The CO_2 laser permits selective destruction of large areas of vaginal epithelium without vaginal or cervical stenosis. It cuts, coagulates, seals, and sterilizes simultaneously. This results in less blood loss, a shorter period of vaginal discharge after treatment of the cervix, and a lower incidence of infection than in other surgical treatment modalities.

Electrosurgery and cryosurgery are other options to ablate lesions. Care is taken to avoid contact with the plume from viral lesion ablation.

Culdocentesis and Colpotomy

Culdocentesis. In culdocentesis, blood, fluid, or pus in the cul-de-sac is aspirated by needle via the posterior vaginal fornix for suspected intraperitoneal bleeding, ectopic pregnancy, or tubo-ovarian abscess. Clear, straw-colored peritoneal fluid is a negative finding. Blood can indicate an ectopic pregnancy, trauma, or tumor. Bloody fluid should be sent to the laboratory in a heparinized specimen tube. A flat plate of the kidneys, ureters, and bladder (KUB) (radiographic examination without contrast medium) may show air under the diaphragm, which is indicative of a ruptured organ.

Posterior Colpotomy. In posterior colpotomy, a transverse incision is made through the posterior vaginal fornix into the posterior cul-de-sac to facilitate diagnosis by intraperi-

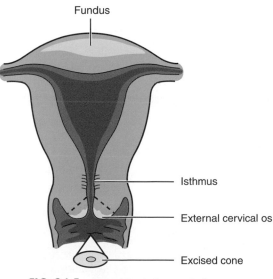

Fundus

Isthmus

External cervical os

Excised cone

FIG. 34-5 Cone biopsy for cervical cancer.

toneal palpation, inspection of the pelvic organs, or determination of free fluid, blood, or pus in the pouch of Douglas. Pus from a pelvic abscess or blood, possibly a sign of ectopic pregnancy or a ruptured ovarian cyst, is evacuated. Tubes and ovaries are inspected. If they are normal, the incision is closed. A drain may be inserted.

Some surgical procedures, such as aspiration of an ovarian cyst or reproductive sterilization by tubal ligation, can be performed through the incision, although exposure and visualization are limited. A tube or ovary is sometimes removed through the vagina.

Fallopian Tube Diagnostic Procedures

Tubal Perfusion. To test tubal patency, chromopertubation is performed. Methylene blue or indigo carmine dye in a solution of sterile normal saline is introduced into the uterine cavity via a 50-mL syringe or intravenous (IV) tubing attached to a cervical cannula. The surgeon views the ends of the fallopian tubes through a laparoscope. Dye seen coming from one or both tubes indicates patency.

Tubal Insufflation. Uterotubal insufflation may be used to test the patency of the fallopian tubes. It usually is done as an office procedure to study infertility. The test may be therapeutic in relieving minor obstructions. Contraindications include genital tract infection, possible pregnancy, and uterine bleeding.

A cannula with a seal (i.e., Kahn or Jarco) is inserted into the cervicouterine canal and connected to an insufflation apparatus. Carbon dioxide is introduced slowly under controlled flow. A relationship exists between tubal patency and the pressure required to force gas through the fallopian tubes into the peritoneal cavity. Resistance to flow (i.e., backpressure) is measured on a mercury manometer. To prevent gas embolism, the Rubin test is done before, never after, curettage. Intraabdominal irritation before total absorption of carbon dioxide from the peritoneal cavity causes referred pain in the shoulders. The patient may refer to the feeling as "gas pains."

Hysterosalpingography. Radiologic study of the uterus and tubes may afford further evaluation of infertility after repeated negative Rubin test findings. The patient is placed in the lithotomy position, and the vagina is prepped. The cervix is grasped with a single-tooth tenaculum. A cannula is inserted into the cervical canal, and 10 mL of a water-soluble radiopaque contrast medium is instilled with a syringe through the cannula (Fig. 34-6). This contrast medium ascends into the corpus uteri and fallopian tubes to yield information about structure and function. Serial radiographs may be taken to assess postprocedure tubal spillage. In some patients, tubal spasms prevent immediate passage of the contrast medium through the tubes. Iodine-based contrast medium is contraindicated in a patient with iodine allergy because of the risk of systemic absorption.

Pediatric and Adolescent Gynecology

Pelvic examination of an infant or child is rarely performed unless there is disease or trauma. The preadolescent has no hormonal stimulation and has not developed sexual characteristics such as rounded labia or pubic hair. In infants, the uterus regresses in size until the age of 6 years, when it regains the size it was at birth. The cervix is not palpable, and the uterine body is difficult to differentiate from surrounding tissues.

From the age of 7 years, the body begins to respond to estrogen stimulation. The mons thickens and the vagina begins to elongate. The uterus has a growth spurt at age 9 to 10 years and begins to have the pear shape of the adult uterus. The endometrium develops and proliferates. The vagina extends to its full length of 10 to 12 cm, and the external genitalia resemble those of an adult. Thelarche (first breast development) begins as nipple buds around age 10 years.

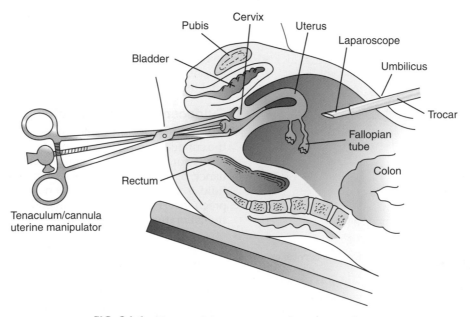

FIG. 34-6   Hysterosalpingogram cannula and tenaculum.

Menarche (first menstruation) is common between the ages of 12 and 14 years and averages 3 years from the onset of breast development and within 6 months of the appearance of axillary hair. The first routine gynecologic examination is recommended at age 16 years or when a girl becomes sexually active.[2] Routine exams will be individualized according to the needs and sexual activity of the girl. Sexually transmitted disease (STD) testing is performed. Females who have not developed secondary sex characteristics and menstruated by age 16 years should seek a gynecology consult.[3] Menarche can be delayed by anorexia nervosa or other dietary practices that diminish body fat stores below 17%.

Adolescent Pregnancy. According to the CDC the adolescent pregnancy rate is the lowest it has been in 60 years.[4] The 38% decline is in the 10- to 14-year-old group. Births to young mothers place them in high risk for problems during delivery resulting in preterm birth and cesarean section. Many of these young girls have had no prenatal care and are subject to preeclampsia (pregnancy-associated hypertension). Many of the babies are low birthweight and small for gestational age (SGA).

Gynecologic Pathology in Infants. The female infant should be thoroughly examined from a gynecologic standpoint at birth. Clitoral anomalies may be related to androgenic sexual hormones or a true genetic anomaly. If a vagina cannot be visualized, the hymen may be imperforate or there may be vaginal agenesis. Digital rectal examination is performed, and a slight central mass representing the rudimentary uterine cervix may be palpated. Ovaries are not large enough to be palpable unless a pathologic condition is present. Ultrasonography may need to be performed to differentiate anatomic structures.

Pelvic Endoscopy

Pelvic endoscopy is an established part of the gynecologist's diagnostic and therapeutic regimen. It permits detailed intraperitoneal inspection of the pelvic organs without laparotomy. These procedures are not without danger, however. Inadvertent perforation of vessels or a hollow viscus and/or infection are major potential hazards. Operator expertise, careful patient selection, adequate anesthesia, and safe equipment are essential. Pelvic endoscopy is a sterile procedure.

Vaginal and abdominal approaches are employed for direct visualization of pelvic organs and adjacent structures.

Culdoscopy. A culdoscope is introduced into the peritoneal cavity via the posterior vaginal fornix and pouch of Douglas. Some gynecologists prefer culdoscopy to investigate ovaries or posterior surfaces in the lower pelvis. Local or

[2]Recommended by the American College of Obstetricians and Gynecologists.
[3]Tanner stages of development indicate that menarche is typical by age 14 years or within 2 years of full breast development.
[4]www.CDC.gov/nchs: Trends and health outcomes: Births to 10- to 14-year-old mothers 1990-2002, 2004.

caudal anesthesia is used. The patient is placed in the knee-chest or lithotomy position. With the posterior lip of the cervix held by a tenaculum and retracted anteriorly, the uterus is elevated while counterpressure is applied to the posterior vaginal wall by the speculum. This maneuver stretches the posterior vaginal fornix while a trocar and cannula or sheath penetrate the thin wall and enter the pelvis between the uterosacral ligaments. When the trocar is removed with the cannula in place, air enters the cul-de-sac because of the negative intraabdominal pressure produced by the knee-chest position. Air displaces the bowel, and the scope may be inserted through the cannula.

At the completion of the procedure, the culdoscope is removed. Before the cannula is removed, the operating bed is straightened and the patient is flattened while as much air as possible is evacuated by hand pressure on the abdomen into low suction. Care is taken not to aerosolize body substances. Some surgeons place a suture in the puncture site.

Hysteroscopy. A rigid fiberoptic hysteroscope, introduced vaginally through the uterine cervix, provides direct inspection of the interior of the uterus to diagnose disease or treat conditions such as menorrhagia and uterine fibroids. The hysteroscope may also be used to identify and remove polyps, lost intrauterine devices (IUDs), or intrauterine adhesions. Adequate expansion of the uterine cavity is a prerequisite for viewing endometrial surfaces and tubal orifices. Fluid is instilled to expand the uterine cavity to create a working space. Hysteroscopy systems have been developed that use sterile normal saline as an expansion medium. The fluid should be delivered through a pressure-controlled infusion pump that tracks volume instilled. Intrauterine pressures should be maintained at or below the mean arterial pressure. Use of a continuous-flow pump makes it difficult to monitor intrauterine pressures.

The circulating nurse monitors inflow and outflow of the uterine expansion fluid medium and informs the surgeon and the anesthesia provider of any discrepancy in excess of 1500 mL. Visibility is further enhanced with a video camera and monitor screen. The procedure may be videotaped.

Hysteroscopy is used to perform endometrial ablation using a laser (Nd:YAG, argon, or potassium titanyl phosphate [KTP]) or ESU to stop or decrease uterine bleeding.

The Nd:YAG laser is the laser of choice for deep photocoagulation, causing endometrial destruction and scarring the uterine lining. The entire endometrial lining is treated from the fundus to about 4 cm above the external cervical os. The tip of the laser fiber can be held away from tissue (blanching technique) or in contact with endometrium (dragging technique). A specialized electrosurgical rollerball electrode is an alternative method to using a laser. This can provide relief from menorrhagia (i.e., excessively heavy menses). The destruction of the endometrium causes the woman to have amenorrhea, thereby causing sterility. Hormonal activity is unchanged.

Air or gas is not used for uterine insufflation or laser fiber cooling during hysteroscopy because of the risk of air or gas embolism. Also, 32% dextran 70 in dextrose (Hyskon) is not used as an irrigant or uterine expansion medium for endometrial laser ablation because of the systemic effects of fluid absorption through open capillaries. Precise measurements of intake and output are critical to patient safety and prevention of congestive heart failure. Hysteroscopy can be performed as an ambulatory surgery or office procedure.

Laparoscopy.

Procedures using a 10- or 12-mm fiberoptic laparoscope with a 0- or 30-degree-angle lens inserted into the peritoneal cavity permit direct observation of pelvic and abdominal organs and peritoneal surfaces. This endoscopic technique may be used to diagnose and treat ectopic pregnancy; inspect the ovaries for evidence of follicular activity and retrieve ova for in vitro fertilization; visualize and reduce pelvic masses; and determine the cause of infertility, endocrinopathies, or amenorrhea. Many pelvic diseases, such as endometriosis, adhesions, and ovarian cysts, may be identified and treated through the laparoscope and its accessory instrumentation. The gynecologist can perform myomectomy, salpingectomy, oophorectomy, hysterectomy, and other procedures such as tuboplasty and incidental appendectomy without the need for a large abdominal incision. Surgical procedures such as tubal sterilization by electrocoagulation with or without partial resection, placement of a clip or silicone ring on the tube, or biopsy can be performed.

Sterile laparoscopic equipment includes:
- D&C instrument tray, including uterine manipulator/cannula (Hulka tenaculum, Cohen/Jarcho cannula, HUMI or Kronner inflatable uterine cannula) (Fig. 34-7)
- 20-mL Luer-Lok syringe
- Endoscope (telescope)
- Veress needle: 120-mm needle for insufflation through a percutaneous abdominal puncture; 150-mm needle for insufflation in an obese patient; 150-mm needle can be used for insufflation through the cul-de-sac
- Appropriate-size trocars and insulated sheaths with sealing caps to prevent gas leakage. Reducer caps can be used to decrease the size of the sheath opening for the use of smaller diameter instrumentation.
- Insufflation tubing with an inline hydrophobic filter

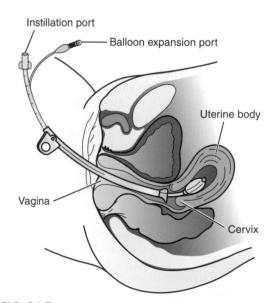

FIG. 34-7 Kronner uterine manipulator for laparoscopy.

- Aspiration cannula, biopsy forceps, and graduated probe. Most are insulated and compatible with a monopolar ESU
- Bipolar grasping forceps (Kleppinger forceps)
- Suction/irrigation tubing
- Endoscopic needle holders, sutures, clip appliers, and staplers. These may be needed for more complex procedures
- Electrosurgical probe or endocoagulator, and/or laser fiber

Nonsterile endoscopic equipment includes:
- Insufflator with full tank of carbon dioxide (CO_2)
- Fiberoptic light source
- Video camera and monitor(s)
- Laser and/or ESU

Usually a general anesthetic agent is administered. The patient is placed in a modified lithotomy position with the stirrups adjusted so that the legs are at 45-degree angles to the axis of the operating bed. The vaginal area is prepped, followed by the abdominal prep. The patient is straight-catheterized, or an indwelling Foley catheter is inserted. The patient is draped for a combined abdominovaginal procedure. The sterile drapes must provide two exposures (i.e., an abdominal opening and a perineal opening) and cover the legs.

A tenaculum is placed on the cervix. A cannula is inserted into the uterine cervix for instillation of dye and for manipulation of the uterus during the procedure to provide greater visibility. A D&C may be performed as part of the procedure after the injection of dye or contrast media.

Insertion of the scope is preceded by a pneumoperitoneum of CO_2 to produce a working space in the abdomen and pelvis. The infraumbilical midline area is most commonly used if no scars, with possible adherent viscera beneath, are present. This area is preferred because it has no abdominal wall vessels that might be injured. The firm attachment of the fascia to the peritoneum facilitates entry. Great care is taken to avoid injury to the great vessels or intraabdominal organs. Insufflation can be performed with a Veress needle or a blunt trocar, such as a Hasson.

The patient is placed in a 10-degree Trendelenburg's position to shift the abdominal organs cephalad. A small infraumbilical skin incision is made in the anterior abdominal wall. Through it a sharp trocar and sheath are introduced into the peritoneal cavity via blind puncture if a blunt Hasson is not used. Some sharp trocars and sheaths have spring-loaded end guards that cover the sharp tip and protect the underlying structures after penetration of abdominal tissue layers, although studies have not shown this to be an advantage. The trocar is removed, and a telescope of the same caliber is inserted through the trocar sheath, which remains in the cavity. Some sheaths have threads that are used to anchor it into position.

Additional secondary trocars and sheaths can be placed in the suprapubic hairline (see Fig. 34-12). These trocars may be inserted into the peritoneal cavity under direct vision through the endoscope, which offers good transillumination for the puncture when the room lights are dimmed, or visualization on the video monitor. A secondary trocar should have a gas port to which the CO_2 tubing can be attached to prevent the cold gas from causing the scope to fog. The suction/irrigation tubing is attached to a side port on the secondary sheath.

Before use, warming the tip of the telescope in a warm moist towel or normal saline solution can prevent fogging of the distal lens of the endoscope caused by the intraperitoneal temperature and moisture. (Sterile antifog solution is commercially available.) The telescope is connected to the light source by a fiberoptic cable. Because of the potential fire hazard to drapes, the light source is not activated until the cable is attached to the telescope. The video camera is draped and connected to the telescope.

At the completion of the surgical procedure, the carbon dioxide, video monitor, and light source are turned off, accessory instruments and sheaths are removed, and the patient is leveled into a flat supine position. Hemostasis is surveyed before the telescope is removed from the primary trocar site. The valve of its sheath closes as the telescope is withdrawn to prevent escape of CO_2 gas into the room air. The pneumoperitoneum contains aerosolized blood and body fluids and should be evacuated through the suction tubing into the suction canister. Electrosurgical plume also should be suctioned from the peritoneal cavity because it binds with hemoglobin and causes the arterial oxygenation to decrease. The patient can become hypoxic. The large fascial and skin incisions are sutured, and small dressings or adhesive bandages (Band-Aids or Steri-Strips) are applied.

The patient requires close monitoring by the anesthesia provider because increased intraabdominal pressure may lead to cardiovascular disturbances from vagal reflex. This reflex is caused by stretching of the peritoneum, retention of CO_2, or compression of the inferior vena cava.

Postoperative shoulder pain may follow the use of a pneumoperitoneum. This is referred pain caused by pressure on the diaphragm, which is somewhat displaced by CO_2 during the procedure. Slight elevation of the head after recovery from anesthesia relieves this pain. Although numerous complications have been reported, the most common are perforation of the intestine or major blood vessel, hemorrhage from a biopsy site, gas embolism from intravascular injection, and burns of the abdominal wall and bowel. Some injuries, such as viscus puncture or thermal damage, may not be immediately apparent. Symptoms may not be present until 48 to 72 hours postoperatively, when tissue necrosis or sloughing occurs.

VULVAR PROCEDURES

Benign growths on the vulva, although rare, consist mainly of fatty and fibrous tumors. These are excised if large. Suspicious lesions should be removed for pathologic examination. Cancerous lesions may be multicentric, with the majority found on the labia majora and a lesser percentage on the labia minora, vestibule, clitoris, and posterior commissure. Vaginal smears should be taken to determine the presence of metastatic growth to the vaginal wall. Treatment depends on the size of the primary lesion, involvement of nodes, and extent of metastasis. Mutilative procedures require emotional adjustment to permanent change.

Diseases of the Vulva

Wide local excision of a single well-localized area with no premalignant changes elsewhere may be done. Punch biopsies may be obtained. Leukoplakia and preinvasive lesions of the vulva may be treated with a laser or ultrasonic aspirator.

Simple Vulvectomy without Node Dissection. The labia majora and minora, part of the mons veneris, and the hymenal ring, including the clitoris, may be removed for premalignant lesions and early microinvasive cancer of limited penetration. The clitoris and perianal region are spared if the lesion is small. The incision must be wide to avoid local recurrence.

Total Vulvectomy. Basal cell carcinoma usually does not metastasize but is often locally extensive and prone to recur. Treatment consists of wide total vulvectomy, also without node dissection.

Radical Vulvectomy with Bilateral Inguinal-Femoral Lymphadenectomy. Radical vulvectomy is performed for invasive vulvar cancers or melanoma and is usually done in one stage. Resection lines may vary depending on the location and size of the lesion (Fig. 34-8). Because the procedure involves abdominal and perineal dissection, both areas, including the thighs to the knees, are prepped. Structures generally removed include all of those from the anterior surface of the pubis to the perianal region posteriorly, with wide lateral excision beyond the vulva, to fascial depth. More specifically, large areas of abdominal and groin skin, the labia majora and minora, the mons, the clitoris, Bartholin and periurethral glands, and bilateral inguinal lymph nodes are removed en bloc. Inguinal skin flaps are retained for closure. Deep pelvic node dissection is carried out if frozen sections determine that these nodes are cancerous. If the vagina, urethra, and/or anus are involved, they are removed also. Anal involvement may require a colostomy.

Lymphadenectomy is carried out with the patient in the supine position. Two teams may perform bilateral dissection. The patient is then placed in the lithotomy position for vulvectomy. Reconstruction of the pelvic floor and vaginal walls may be necessary. The legs are abducted for easier approximation of subcutaneous tissue during primary closure with sutures or staples. Closed-wound suction drainage is used postoperatively to avoid fluid collection beneath skin flaps. A pressure dressing is applied. (More information can be found at www.gyncancer.com.)

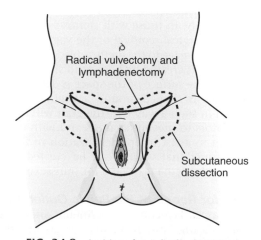

FIG. 34-8 Incisions for radical vulvectomy.

Bartholin Glands. Obstruction of the secretory duct of the Bartholin gland may be caused by inflammation. A cyst may be prone to secondary infection or abscess formation.

Marsupialization of Bartholin Cyst. A cyst enlarges as mucous secretions accumulate. Marsupialization establishes drainage from within the vagina by creation of a new, enlarged ductal opening. The cyst is incised linearly in the region of the normal opening and evacuated. The edges of the vaginal mucosa and cyst wall are sutured together to produce epithelialization so that the cyst cannot recur. An abscess may be drained.

VAGINAL PROCEDURES

The vaginal wall, cervix, and uterus may be approached with the patient in the lithotomy position. Tumors, benign or malignant, may be confined to any one of these structures or may involve adjacent tissues. Herniation or fistula formation may require repair of the vaginal wall and adjacent structures. Excision or repair may require a combined vaginal-abdominal procedure.

Vaginal Wall

Excision of a Vaginal Lesion. A biopsy taken from an epithelial tumor should be studied histologically to rule out adenocarcinoma. Vaginal adenosis and gross cervical abnormalities, as well as clear cell adenocarcinoma of the vagina, have occurred in female offspring of women who received diethylstilbestrol (DES) or similar synthetic estrogen during the first trimester of pregnancy to avoid spontaneous abortion. Adenosis may be treated with a laser.

Vaginectomy. Vaginectomy (partial or complete) is performed for carcinoma in situ or carcinoma of the vagina. Vaginoplasty is necessary for reconstruction. External radiation and radium implants, with possible eventual pelvic exenteration, is the treatment for advanced invasive malignancy. The proximity of the bladder and rectum makes therapy difficult.

Radical vaginal or abdominal hysterectomy and vaginectomy with extraperitoneal lymphadenectomy sometimes are combined for carcinoma of the upper and middle thirds of the vagina if the bladder or rectum is not involved.

Vaginoplasty. A vagina may be constructed in patients with congenital absence of the vagina (Rokitansky syndrome) or, more commonly, in those with stenosis after radiation therapy or after surgical removal of the vagina. Care must be taken to avoid damage to the urethra, bladder, and rectum. The vaginal space is created by blunt and sharp dissection. If a large part of the surface of the space is denuded, a skin or amnion graft is shaped around a vaginal mold. The mold is placed in such a way that the graft will take. With the use of dilators to prevent stenosis and with the use of estrogen cream to assist in epithelialization of the cavity, an adequate functional vagina can be created in many patients. A pseudovagina is created for transsexual surgery.

Procedures for Repair of the Pelvic Outlet. Injury to muscles and fascial layers of the perineum and/or genital tract, usually during childbirth, may result in extensive vaginal relaxation (Fig. 34-9). Manifestation of perineal

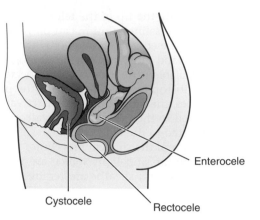

FIG. 34-9 Cystocele, rectocele, and enterocele.

hernias may be delayed until later years, when generalized loss of elastic tissue develops. Downward pressure is exerted on other structures, such as the bladder. Moderate to severe degrees of herniation of viscera require surgical intervention to restore pelvic floor integrity and sphincter competency. Vaginal plastic procedures for genital prolapse consist of narrowing and reconstructing the damaged pelvic floor. Vaginal repairs are referred to as vaginal plastic procedures.

Anterior Colporrhaphy (Kelly Procedure). Anterior colporrhaphy is performed for prolapse of the anterior vaginal wall to repair a urethrocystocele (herniation of the bladder into the vaginal canal). The wall is incised, and a strip of redundant vaginal mucosa is excised, the extent of which depends on the severity of the prolapse. The bladder is dissected free from the vaginal septum and returned to normal position by suturing the pubocervical ligaments beneath it. Approximation of the pubococcygeus muscles provides further suburethral support. The vaginal wall is closed with sutures.

By improving support to the bladder neck region, restoring the posterior urethrovesical angle, and narrowing the urethral opening, stress incontinence (urine leakage with coughing, sneezing, or laughter) is relieved. The surgical procedure also prevents voiding difficulty and the recurrent cystitis that accompanies retention of urine caused by a cystocele bulging below the bladder neck.

Posterior Colpoperineorrhaphy. Repair of the posterior vaginal wall for rectocele, a herniation of the rectum into the vagina, consists of a triangular excision of redundant vaginal mucosa and separation of the vagina from the rectum. Support is reestablished by suturing together rectovaginal fascia, as well as the levator ani, as high as possible. Perineal muscles are reconstructed to restore continuity of support. A lacerated perineum may also be sutured. The surgical procedure relieves fecal incontinence and/or constipation.

Repair of an Enterocele. An abnormally deep hernial sac may contain a segment of intestine, referred to as an enterocele or cul-de-sac hernia. Repair consists of opening the sac, reducing its contents, excising the sac, closing the aperture or weakness that allowed the sac to descend into the rectovaginal septum, and strengthening the normal anatomic coverings. Approximation of the uterosacral ligaments and levator ani in the midline removes the cul-de-sac defect.

Repair of a Prolapsed Uterus (Procidentia). Various surgical procedures correct and restore support of the prolapsed uterus (Fig. 34-10). Correction of prolapse anteverts the uterus and shortens an elongated cervix and cardinal ligaments. In a Manchester colpoperineorrhaphy, for example, the cervix is amputated and the cardinal ligaments are united in front of it. The anterior vaginal wall is plicated, and the posterior pelvic floor is reconstructed. Often cystocele and rectocele are present and are simultaneously repaired. In complete prolapse, both the cervix and the uterine body protrude through the vaginal aperture and the vaginal canal is inverted. Bleeding ulceration of exposed tissues may ensue. Vaginal hysterectomy is done for severe prolapse or prolapse accompanied by stress incontinence when child-bearing is no longer desired. A vaginal pessary to support a retrodisplaced or prolapsing uterus may be inserted in a woman who presents a poor surgical risk.

Repair of Vaginal Eversion. Outward protrusion of the vagina can occur after obstetric or surgical trauma or from inherent weakness in vaginal muscle tone, particularly in postmenopausal years. The fascia of the vagina is attached to the sacrospinous ligament, located within the coccygeus muscle. The resultant scarring and fibrosis fixate the vagina in a normal anatomic position.

Colpocleisis (Le Fort Procedure). Colpocleisis (obliteration of the vagina by denuding and approximating the anterior and posterior walls) is generally reserved for geriatric patients or those who present a poor surgical risk.

Procedures for Repair of Genital Fistulas. A genital fistula is an abnormal communication between a part of the genital canal and either the urinary or the intestinal tract. Various dye tests, cystoscopy, and pyelography help pinpoint a urinary tract fistula. Injury during parturition, surgical trauma (especially radical procedures for cancer), penetrating extension of cervical carcinoma, and radiation necrosis are common etiologic factors.

Repair of a Vesicovaginal Fistula. A vesicovaginal fistula, which develops between the bladder and vagina, is the most common type of genital fistula. A small opening permits seepage of urine, although the patient may void normally. Total incontinence may result from a large fistulous aperture and cause irritation of the vagina, vulva, and thighs. Through a vaginal approach, the anterior vaginal wall is dissected free. The fistula to the bladder is closed, and the

attachment of the bladder to the vagina is reestablished. The repair should be made with at least three layers of tissue. The bladder should be decompressed by an indwelling Foley catheter postoperatively. Antibiotics may be administered judiciously to prevent infection in the healing site.

If the vesicovaginal fistula is high in the vagina, a better result will be obtained by entering the bladder via suprapubic incision for direct repair rather than by using a vaginal approach. Care must be taken not to occlude ureteral orifices. This is accomplished by insertion of ureteral catheters, which can be removed after the procedure. Attention is given to excision of any infected tissue, closure with multiple layers, and bladder decompression by the Foley catheter.

Repair of a Rectovaginal Fistula. A fistula between the rectum and vagina may follow episiotomy or obstetric perineal lacerations, vaginal or rectal surgery, radiation therapy, trauma, or infection. Fecal incontinence and fecal material in the vagina are characteristic, although the anal sphincter is intact. Preoperative bowel preparation, including prophylactic antibiotic therapy, is important because of the contaminated surgical area. A temporary colostomy may be advisable before the surgical procedure to divert the fecal stream from the repair site. With a vaginal approach, a plastic repair of the perineum is done. Scar tissue and the fistulous tract are excised, and the edges of the perineal muscles and fascia are approximated.

Cervix

Surgical treatment of an abnormal cervix should be preceded by tests such as a Pap smear to rule out early malignant change.

Cauterization. The cervix may be cauterized by electrocautery to treat chronic inflammation and/or leukorrhea (i.e., vaginal discharge).

Trachelorrhaphy. Lacerations of the cervix may result from childbirth. Repair (i.e., trachelorrhaphy) involves reconstruction of the cervical canal as necessary. A vaginal plastic setup is used.

Trachelectomy. The cervix may be amputated to remove an intraepithelial cancer. Most surgeons prefer total hysterectomy to cervical amputation, because the remaining uterine component may become cancerous.

Removal of the uterine cervix in early-stage cancer with lymphadenectomy is a fertility-sparing option for some women.

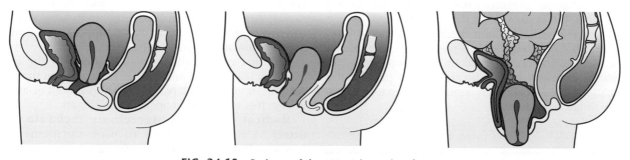

FIG. 34-10 Prolapse of the uterus, in varying degrees.

Studies in England between 1994 and 2005 demonstrated that 28 live births resulted from 55 pregnancies.[5] Cesarean birth was required for 26 of these mothers, and 13 were born preterm. Complications noted in the study included preterm labor and spontaneous abortion.

Uterus

Dilation and Curettage. The most frequently performed gynecologic procedure, D&C is done for diagnostic and/or therapeutic purposes. The main purpose of a D&C is to establish the cause of abnormal uterine bleeding so that the gynecologist can plan definitive treatment.

The procedure is performed for women with post-menopausal bleeding or symptoms suggestive of endometrial cancer, even when cytologic smear findings are negative. It may be performed in infertility studies or to confirm pre-operative diagnosis before amputation of the cervix or hysterectomy. D&C is performed therapeutically to relieve dysmenorrhea by cervical dilation only, to remove polyps or benign endometrial pathologic conditions, to remove residual tissue and arrest bleeding after incomplete abortion, or to perform voluntary abortion before the thirteenth week of pregnancy. A regional paracervical block or general anesthesia is required.

With the anterior lip of the cervix held in a tenaculum and the posterior vaginal wall retracted, a uterine sound is introduced into the uterus to determine the depth and direction of the intrauterine cavity. It is important that the surgeon know the shape and position of the uterus to avoid perforation. The cervical os is sequentially dilated with graduated metal probes. A small curette is introduced into the endocervical canal, which is scraped from the internal to the external os. Submucous fibroids are usually discernible as the curette passes over them. Exploration of the fundus with a polyp or placental forceps usually extracts any polyps present in the endometrium.

Intrauterine Thermal Balloon Ablation. A specialized electrically heated latex balloon probe can be introduced into the uterine cavity through the cervical os to treat menorrhagia (Fig. 34-11). The intrauterine probe is attached to a cable system controlled by a microprocessing unit that measures temperature, pressure, and time. The thermal balloon is expanded by the computer to fill the capacity of the uterine cavity and heated to 188.6° F (87° C). A depth of approximately 3 to 5 mm of endometrium is ablated within 8 minutes of contact. This procedure is suitable for patients who have regularly shaped uterine cavities with a capacity of less than 30 mL or 10 cm in depth. A larger or irregularly shaped uterine cavity would not evenly accommodate the expansion of the balloon.

Intrauterine thermal balloon therapy is contraindicated for women who wish to have future pregnancies. The thermal process destroys the endometrial lining that supports the placental attachment during pregnancy. As per all latex devices, use of a latex balloon is contraindicated for patients sensitive to latex products.

[5]*British Journal of Obstetrics and Gynecology*, June 2006.

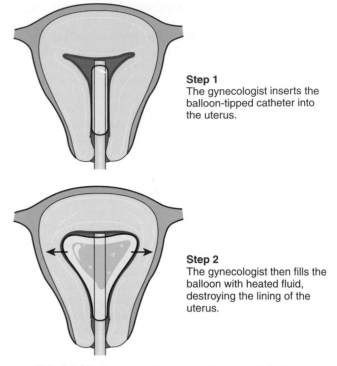

Step 1
The gynecologist inserts the balloon-tipped catheter into the uterus.

Step 2
The gynecologist then fills the balloon with heated fluid, destroying the lining of the uterus.

FIG. 34-11   Endometrial thermal ablation with balloon.

Vaginal Hysterectomy. Vaginal hysterectomy is performed for severe uterine prolapse or prolapse accompanied by stress incontinence and for patients with pelvic relaxation or a history of myomas, irregular uterine bleeding, or a treated premalignant lesion.

The uterus is removed through the vagina, with incision of the vaginal wall and the pelvic cavity. Urinary incontinence caused by an enterocele and/or a rectocele may be simultaneously repaired by anterior and posterior colporrhaphies and with reconstruction of the pelvic floor. Advantages of the procedure include restoration of normal anatomic relationship and preservation of vaginal function. The ovaries are not always removed. Contraindications are immobility of pelvic organs, a large uterus, a pathologic condition such as an ovarian mass, or pelvic cancer.

The vaginal wall is incised anteriorly, and the bladder is separated from the cervix. The incision is continued around the cervix. The peritoneal cavity is entered through the posterior cul-de-sac and the anterior uterovesical pouch. Ligaments supporting the uterus and uterine vessels are ligated and cut. The fundus is delivered, the upper pedicles are sutured, the uterus is removed, and the peritoneum is closed. Suturing the cardinal and uterosacral ligaments together and to the vaginal vault supports the vault and prevents prolapse of the vagina.

Potential complications include injury to the ureters, bowel, or bladder and massive hemorrhage from the uterine vessels. An unopened laparotomy setup should be available in case it is necessary to open the abdomen.

Radical Vaginal Hysterectomy (Schauta Procedure). A surgical approach to early carcinoma of the cervix, radical vaginal hysterectomy does not permit pelvic lymph node dissection but is useful in select patients (e.g., obese patients). It includes vaginal removal of the uterus, upper third of vagina, fallopian tubes, and ovaries. Damage to the ureters or bladder is a potential complication.

Laparoscopic-Assisted Vaginal Hysterectomy. In laparoscopic-assisted vaginal hysterectomy (LAVH), an abdominal endoscopic approach is used to dissect the uterus from its supporting ligaments and vasculature. Trocar placement is depicted in Fig. 34-12. Endoscopic clips, linear staplers, sutures, electrosurgery, or a laser may be used to enhance hemostasis. Once the intraperitoneal attachments of the uterus are ligated and divided, a vaginal approach is used to separate the bladder from the anterior aspect of the uterus as in a standard vaginal hysterectomy. Direct visualization of the bladder flap dissection through the endoscope from above enables the surgeon to avoid damage to adjacent structures (Fig. 34-13). The uterine vascular pedicles are ligated vaginally. In the Heaney technique the uterus is inverted and removed fundus-first through a posterior colpotomy. The uterosacral ligaments are sutured to the posterior aspect of the vaginal cuff, and the colpotomy is closed.

This method is used in moderate prolapse of the uterus. In the Döderlein technique a nonprolapsed uterus is inverted and removed fundus-first through an anterior colpotomy. This technique provides greater visibility of the uterine vessels and a more effective vaginal suspension. LAVH is the procedure of choice when a minimally invasive procedure is desired, when salpingo-oophorectomy may be necessary, and when the uterus is only moderately enlarged.

ABDOMINAL PROCEDURES

The open abdominal approach may be used for a fixed or enlarged uterus, exploration, inflammatory disease, and most malignant lesions of the uterus, fallopian tubes, and ovaries. This approach permits inspection of pelvic and abdominal organs and lymph glands for biopsy or treatment. Open laparotomy or minimally invasive endoscopic procedures are performed as appropriate to achieve desired outcomes.

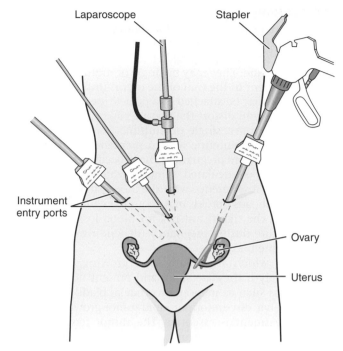

FIG. 34-12 Access portals for laparoscopically assisted vaginal hysterectomy.

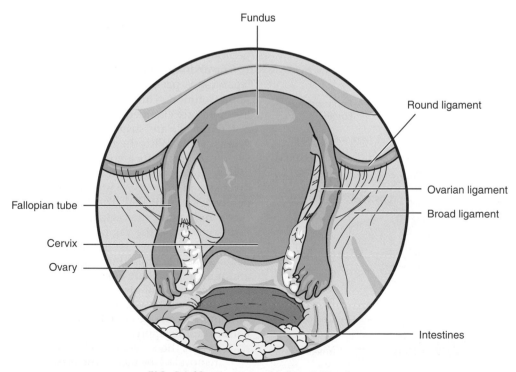

FIG. 34-13 Laparoscopic view of the uterus.

Myomectomy

The most frequent indication for abdominal hysterectomy is leiomyofibroma, commonly known as benign fibroids or myomas. Fibroids are composed of coiled muscle and fibrous connective tissue. They may be single or multiple and most often are present in the wall of the uterus (intramural) (Fig. 34-14). Some may be attached by a pedicle (pedunculated) or protrude into and distort the uterine cavity (submucous).

In myomectomy, single or multiple fibroid tumors are removed from the uterine wall in premenopausal women who may still desire pregnancy. The procedure is especially adaptable to pedunculated tumors, which may become necrotic from interference with the blood supply. Removal of large submucous fibroids may require opening the uterus, which poses the significant risk for blood loss and potential for rupture during pregnancy (depending on location on the uterine body).

Fibroids, which are usually slow growing, are treated conservatively if they are small and present no problems. If symptoms such as menometrorrhagia, bladder or bowel pressure, pelvic discomfort, or rapid tumor growth develop, surgical treatment is essential. The tumor has no active growth during pregnancy and after menopause because of hormonal changes.

Fibroid Embolization Through the Uterine Artery.

Symptomatic uterine fibroids are sometimes treated with occlusion of the arterial blood supply causing the substance of the fibroid to diminish. An intravascular placement of guidewires and catheters in an interventional radiology suite facilitates delivery of embolization materials, such as hemostatic gelatin particles or sclerosing solution. The location of the target fibroid and its direct blood supply are carefully located radiographically during the procedure.

Decreasing the uterine blood supply can impair future childbearing, and other fibroid management options should be explored before uterine artery embolization is performed.

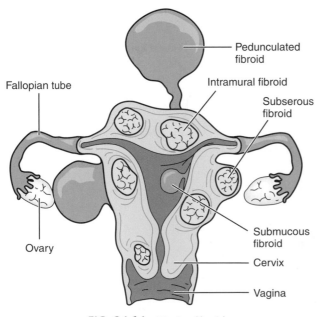

FIG. 34-14 Uterine fibroids.

Embolizing submucous fibroids can cause endometrial sloughing, infection, fever, and sepsis. Pedunculated submucous fibroids should be removed hysterscopically.

Abdominal Hysterectomy

Medical, psychosocial, and sexual ramifications must be considered when contemplating hysterectomy (removal of the uterus). Medically, the procedure may be lifesaving in patients with a malignant lesion or severe hemorrhage. However, the gynecologist has an obligation to consider the individual patient's attitudes when another mode of therapy is available as an alternative to hysterectomy. Because it signals the end of the patient's reproductive potential, a hysterectomy may cause psychologic stress and a sense of incompleteness, even though sexual responsiveness is not dependent on the uterus. Patients whose families are complete, however, may welcome reproductive sterilization.

The uterus is removed through an abdominal incision and opening of the peritoneal cavity.

Differential diagnoses include dysfunctional uterine bleeding caused by disturbed endocrine function, tubal or ovarian masses, and pelvic cancer. In addition to these indications, hysterectomy is performed for uterine prolapse, extensive endometriosis, and cervical or uterine cancer. Various types of hysterectomy are performed.

Total Abdominal Hysterectomy.

The entire uterus, including the cervix, is resected. Normal ovaries are preserved for hormone production whenever possible in women younger than 45 years. Studies have shown that after hysterectomy, women have a 20% increased risk for ovarian cysts within 5 years of the surgical procedure. Bilateral oophorectomy followed by hormone replacement therapy has eliminated the need for subsequent surgery for ovarian pathologic conditions.

The abdominal peritoneal cavity is entered through a vertical midline or a transverse Pfannenstiel incision. Vertical incision facilitates exploration. The patient is placed in a deep Trendelenburg's position. Incision through the uterine peritoneum is carried out laterally.

The abdominal organs are retracted and protected with laparotomy packs moistened with warm sterile normal saline solution. The fallopian tubes and round and broad ligaments are clamped, cut, and ligated. The ovaries, when not removed, are suspended to avoid adherence to the vaginal vault. With the uterus forward, posterior sheets of the broad ligaments are incised, the ureters are identified, and the uterine vessels and uterosacral ligaments are clamped, divided, and sutured. All uterine-supporting ligaments must be divided and ligated. The bladder is mobilized from the cervix and vagina, the vaginal vault is incised, and the cervix is dissected from the vagina.

After the uterus is removed, the connective tissue ligaments are anchored to the vagina. The vaginal mucosa and muscular wall are approximated by absorbable sutures or staples, and the bladder, vault, and rectum (i.e., pelvic floor) are reperitonealized (i.e., covered with peritoneum). Abdominal layers are closed as for laparotomy. The following considerations apply:

1. When the surgeon is closing the vaginal vault after removal of the uterus, the needle, suture, needle holder, or stapler and all instruments used on the cervix and

vagina are considered contaminated. Separate instruments may be used for abdominal closure.

2. Complications of hysterectomy include injury to the ureters with possible fistula formation or renal failure, injury to the bladder or bowel with fistula formation, or massive hemorrhage from damage to major vessels.

3. Some surgeons have a urologist place ureteral catheters before the hysterectomy begins so they are easily identified during the procedure. This is referred to a ureteral stenting and requires the use of a separate cystoscopy setup. The cystoscopy setup should remain sterile in the room after the stenting procedure in case an adjustment is necessary during the case. This saves creating another setup mid procedure.

Radical Hysterectomy with Pelvic Lymph Node Dissection (Radical Wertheim Procedure).

A radical Wertheim procedure may be performed for early stages of invasive cervical cancer and sometimes for endometrial cancer. It involves wide en bloc removal of paracervical and uterosacral tissues (uterus, tubes, ovaries, ligaments) and at least the upper third of the vaginal canal. Bilateral pelvic lymph nodes and channels surrounding the external iliac artery and vein, the hypogastric artery and vein, and the obturator fossae are also dissected and removed.

Some surgeons perform a modified Wertheim procedure for microinvasive carcinoma. This is somewhat less extensive than the radical procedure and may omit lymphadenectomy.

Because radical hysterectomy involves excision of paracervical and paravaginal tissue, bladder innervation is disrupted. This results in bladder dysfunction postoperatively, sometimes for as long as 6 months. Bladder complications are related to the extent of dissection.

Salpingo-oophorectomy.

Fallopian tubes and ovaries are removed along with the uterus. This procedure may be done for endometrial, tubal, or ovarian cancer; excessive vaginal bleeding; or large fibroids. In postmenopausal women for whom total hysterectomy is indicated, bilateral salpingo-oophorectomy is often performed to avoid future ovarian pathologic conditions.

Pelvic Exenteration

An ultraradical procedure for invasive, persistent carcinoma, exenteration is not performed for palliation but only when a possibility of cure exists. The extent of the disease determines the amount of exenteration. In anterior exenteration, the reproductive organs, the distal part of the ureters, the bladder, and the vagina are removed. This modification is performed for cancer of the cervix, vagina, or vulva with extension to the bladder. The ureters are diverted to an ileal conduit, whereas the bowel remains intact. Posterior exenteration removes the reproductive organs, sigmoid colon, and rectum. It is done for cervical carcinoma involving the rectum or advanced rectal carcinoma involving the uterus and posterior vaginal wall.

The urinary system remains intact; fecal diversion is by colostomy. Total or complete exenteration, rarely performed, involves en bloc dissection of the bladder, reproductive organs, perineum, rectum, and pelvic lymph nodes. Two setups are needed: abdominal and perineal. These procedures affect structure, function, body image, and sex life and should be preceded by intensive physical and psychologic preoperative preparation.

Numerous complications may occur involving any major system. Anesthesia and procedure times are long. Blood replacement and extensive monitoring are essential. Multiple stomas and gross pelvic defect with much dead space predispose the woman to infection; therefore several wound drains are used. Vascularized omental and myocutaneous flaps are used to fill pelvic defects.

Procedures Involving the Fallopian Tubes

The fallopian tubes are also referred to as the uterine tubes, oviducts, and salpinges.

Tubal Ligation for Reproductive Sterilization.

Tubal ligation should be considered a permanent method of reproductive sterilization, because reversal cannot be guaranteed. Thorough preoperative counseling of the patient and her husband or partner should preface this procedure.

A number of open surgical techniques can be used for tubal ligation. They are essentially similar, involving (1) removal of a portion of the middle part of the fallopian tube on each side for pathologic confirmation and (2) ligation of both the distal and proximal ends to prevent the cut ends from growing together. Frequently performed by laparoscopy, tubal ligation by open abdominal approach may be done alone, in conjunction with other abdominal surgery, immediately postpartum, or for patients in whom laparoscopic technique is contraindicated. Ligation may be performed through a small transverse incision in the pubic hairline area. An infraumbilical incision is used for postpartum patients. This is referred to as minilaparotomy. Tubal ligations are often performed immediately after cesarean delivery and closure of the uterine wall. No additional instruments are required other than those used for the cesarean section.

The Pomeroy technique of ligation is the most reliable, provides a surgical specimen of each tube, and causes minimal tubal destruction. The tube is tied with suture material, and a section is removed. The tube eventually pulls apart, destroying the passage between the ovary and uterus.

Sterilization may also be performed after vaginal delivery, on the first to third postpartum day, through an infraumbilical incision. In the cauterization technique the bipolar electrosurgical electrode transects and seals the ends of the fallopian tube or excises a section of the tube and seals the ends.

Laparoscopic application of a stretchable Silastic band (Fallope-Ring) or a ligating spring-loaded (Hulka or Filshie) clip may also produce occlusion. In some patients, however, the Pomeroy and other occlusion techniques may be reversible by a subsequent reparative procedure. An estimated 1% of sterilized women will seek reversal because of sterilization at an early age, remarriage, or death of a child.

Tuboplasty.

Removal of an obstruction may restore tubal patency to reverse infertility caused by diseased, damaged, or occluded tubes. Microsurgical techniques with fine suture materials and lasers have vastly improved results of tubal reconstructive procedures. Success depends on the extent of abnormal tissue or tubal destruction and/or the site of obstruction. The location of the previous ligation and normality of tissues at the severed ends of the tubes will influence the reversibility of a tubal ligation.

Although tubal patency may be restored, abnormal function may persist in tubes scarred by previous surgery, ectopic pregnancy or damaged by pelvic inflammatory disease (PID). The chance of successful uterine pregnancy may remain limited. The risk of a tubal pregnancy can increase after tuboplasty. Preoperative assessment may include a hysterosalpingogram to determine the length and patency of tubal segments and/or laparoscopy with tubal dye perfusion or ultrasound imaging with instillation of sterile normal saline solution to demonstrate patency. Contraindications for tuboplasty include active infection or disease and a tube that is less than 3 cm long.

Tuboplasties are microsurgical procedures performed through an abdominal incision. They include the options described in the following sections.

Salpingolysis.
Adhesions caused by an inflammatory process, such as a ruptured appendix or ovarian cyst, may surround the fallopian tubes. The tubes may function normally after lysis of adhesions.

Salpingostomy.
Tubal mucosa and/or fimbriae may become occluded secondary to PID or other infectious process. A salpingostomy creates an opening in a distally obstructed tube. A CO_2 laser may be used through the microscope to open fimbriated ends and to divide adhesions in blocked tubes. An incision in a tube also may be performed to evacuate an early small tubal pregnancy.

Tubal Anastomosis.
A proximal obstruction in the tube is resected. The remaining patent segment is then reimplanted into the uterus and anastomosed at the cornu. Salpingitis usually occludes the tube near the cornu, which may need to be shaved to reach healthy tissue. A previous sterilization procedure usually occludes the mid-isthmus. This anastomosis will be mid-tubal in the ampulla.

Salpingectomy and Salpingo-oophorectomy.
Salpingectomy (removal of a fallopian tube) is often performed in association with salpingo-oophorectomy (partial or total removal of the corresponding ovary). Procedures may be unilateral or bilateral. Indications are extensive damage from PID or endometriosis, cysts, primary adenocarcinoma of the tube, and ectopic pregnancy. Total abdominal hysterectomy and bilateral salpingo-oophorectomy may be performed for bilateral disease. Removal of a large tubo-ovarian abscess is essential to prevent rupture and dissemination of pus in the abdominal cavity.

Ovaries

Ovarian pain usually is referred to the lower abdomen just above either groin, making differential diagnosis from abdominal disease pertinent. Pelvic endoscopy, ultrasonography, and computed tomography (CT) scans assist diagnosis. An ovarian mass requires exploration for evaluation. The mass may be a cyst or a tumor. Ovarian tumors may be benign or malignant, cystic or solid. Epithelial ovarian cancer begins as a cystic intraovarian growth. It usually is asymptomatic until malignant cells have spread into the peritoneal cavity.

Ovarian cancer is usually confined to the peritoneal cavity and retroperitoneal lymph nodes, but advanced ovarian carcinoma can obstruct the urinary and intestinal tracts. Ovarian cancer is the leading cause of gynecologic cancer deaths in the United States.

Screening for Ovarian Cancer.
This disease is particularly deadly because 80% of symptomatic women present to their physician with advanced disease. Screening modalities include ultrasound, CT, pelvic ultrasound, serum CA125, and physical exam. Unfortunately, early diagnosis does not ensure a decrease in mortality.[6]

Benign cysts, more common than tumors, may arise from the graafian follicle, corpus luteum, or epithelium (dermoid). As they grow, ovarian cysts can cause menstrual disturbances, pain, and abnormal uterine bleeding. They may leak contents into the peritoneal cavity, causing irritation, or they may rupture, causing massive bleeding that necessitates immediate laparotomy.

Cysts or solid tumors, even if asymptomatic, should be removed as a precaution because they may degenerate into a malignant lesion, increase in size, or lead to twisting of the pedicle. The type of procedure depends on the type of cyst or tumor, the age of the patient, and the importance of childbearing potential.

Excision or Biopsy.
The surgeon examines the ovaries. If a cyst or tumor is found in one ovary, the surgeon inspects the other ovary to rule out a neoplasm. Pelvic washings may be obtained and tested for cancer cells. If ovarian cancer is highly suspected, the entire ovary is removed for tissue sampling to avoid dissemination of cancerous cells throughout the pelvis. Biopsy specimens may also be taken from paraaortic and pelvic lymph nodes.

Removal of an Ovarian Cyst.
A procedure to remove an ovarian cyst may be scheduled as an oophorocystectomy, cysto-oophorectomy, or ovarian cystectomy. Many benign ovarian cysts and tumors are treated by local excision with preservation of the ovary. A large cyst may be aspirated before removal. Immediately after removal, the surgeon incises the cyst for examination to determine its character, because gross appearance as well as frozen section is important. If there is reasonable assurance that the lesion is benign, removal of only the cyst or resection of a diseased portion (e.g., endometrioma) is justified, with preservation of normal tissue.

Oophorectomy.
The most frequent indications for oophorectomy (removal of an ovary) are benign ovarian

---

[6]Screening recommendation statement by U.S. Preventive Services Task Force does not encourage routine screening because evidence practice does not prove that early diagnosis reduces mortality. The task force did not determine if screening would be beneficial to high risk women. *Ann Fam Med* 2(3):260-262, 2004.

tumors. Many gynecologists believe that cystadenomas and all solid benign ovarian tumors should be treated by unilateral salpingo-oophorectomy because of the difficulty of clean dissection and the questionable assurance of their benign nature. In postmenopausal women, both ovaries, both tubes, and the uterus are removed to avoid future cancer.

If there is a strong probability or proof of malignancy in any ovarian cyst or mass, total hysterectomy and bilateral salpingo-oophorectomy are usually performed, regardless of age. Partial or complete omentectomy may be included because the rich blood supply of omentum contributes to rapid metastases. The extent of the surgical procedure is determined by the lesion. In malignant tumors, a differentiation is made between primary and metastatic ovarian cancer, which influences treatment. As much tumor as possible is removed, a procedure referred to as debulking, for management of advanced ovarian cancer. An ultrasonic aspirator may be used for debulking. The procedure may require resecting parts of small and large intestines and the urinary tract.

After debulking, most patients receive chemotherapy. This often is followed by a "second-look laparotomy" to reassess the peritoneal cavity for further palliative or therapeutic therapy.

Intraoperative Intraperitoneal Chemotherapy.
Ovarian cancer is primarily a peritoneal disease that is sensitive to chemotherapy. The goal of intraperitoneal instillation is to expose the greatest number of ovarian cancer cells with the least amount of systemic toxicity.[7] Earliest used agents include 5-fluorouracil and methotrexate in large quantities of irrigant to cover the greatest surface of the peritoneal cavity; however, cisplatin infusion is most commonly used today. The best results have been seen with minimal extensions of the disease, but it does seem to prolong life in advanced disease.

Great care is taken when handling chemotherapeutic agents.

Muscles and Ligaments of the Pelvic Floor
Urinary Stress Incontinence Procedures.
Urinary stress incontinence is the sudden, involuntary, and intermittent release of urine as a result of muscular changes around the proximal urethra, bladder neck, and bladder base. Differential diagnosis from fistulas, bladder neuropathies, and primary lesions is established by urethroscopy, a cystometrogram, and urodynamics. Surgical correction attempts to restore support. Three basic approaches are used. Anterior colporrhaphy with plication (i.e., reducing the size of the bladder neck) often is satisfactory. In a urethral sling procedure, a musculofascial sling is placed beneath the bladder neck and urethra; usually this is a combined vaginal and abdominal procedure.

Urethral suspension procedures reposition the urethra and bladder neck retropubically by suspending the urethra in a plane with the symphysis pubis through a transverse abdominal incision. Sometimes a combined abdominoperineal approach is necessary for urethral suspension.

Variations of these procedures have been devised, including an endoscopic suspension of the bladder neck.

Marshall-Marchetti-Krantz Vesicourethral Suspension.
After mobilization through an extraperitoneal abdominal approach into the prevesical space, the urethra and bladder neck are suspended to the posterior border of the symphysis pubis. Sutures are placed through the anterior vaginal wall on each side of the urethra and brought through the periosteum on the posterior surface of the symphysis pubis. Sutures may also be placed adjacent to the bladder neck and through the rectus muscle fascia to suspend the bladder neck.

This procedure may be performed in conjunction with other pelvic surgery. It is 85% effective in the treatment of stress incontinence in women. A suprapubic catheter may be used for bladder drainage for 48 to 72 hours postoperatively. Urinary retention is a common complication for up to 7 days.

PERIOPERATIVE OBSTETRICS

Diagnostic techniques such as ultrasonography, specialization in fertility problems, and techniques of fetal monitoring and management have brought significant changes in the field of reproductive biology. Perioperative personnel become involved in the care of obstetric patients, both in elective and emergency procedures, for both obstetric and nonobstetric procedures. The pregnant woman experiencing trauma or an acute surgical disease, such as appendicitis, presents challenges to the perioperative team. The well-being of the fetus depends on maternal physiologic factors. Anesthesia and positioning are especially critical concerns. The anatomic changes of pregnancy alter the appearance and location of commonly identified surgical landmarks. Laboratory values are altered as a result of the growing fetus within the mother's uterus (Table 34-2).

Planning care for the surgical obstetric patient includes determination of the expected date of confinement. The size of the uterus, competency of the placenta, and condition of the growing fetus are prime considerations.

Considerations for the Care of the Pregnant Patient

Oxygen consumption increases about 20% during pregnancy and as much as 100% above normal during labor in response to the increased metabolic demand. Hypoxia and hypercapnia develop rapidly. Fetal oxygenation varies in direct relation to that of the mother in normal and abnormal situations. In treating fetal distress, continuous 100% oxygen is administered to the mother until delivery or relief of the distress. Hypoventilation and hyperventilation are potentially harmful, because they induce hypoxemia and hypercapnia in both the mother and the fetus.

Maternal hypotension and hypovolemia diminish uterine blood flow and fetal perfusion. Hypoxia and acidosis threaten fetal well-being. The mother is safeguarded by appropriate anesthetic technique and selection of drugs. The fetus is protected by adequate uteroplacental perfusion and fetal monitoring by trained personnel. The patient should not be left alone in the holding area or OR. The fetal heart rate and uterine contractions are monitored continually. The procedure involves the care of two patients.

---

[7]The National Cancer Institute recommends intraperitoneal chemotherapy for ovarian cancer. *N Engl J Med* 354:34-43, 2006.

TABLE 34-2	Altered Laboratory Values of Pregnancy		
Test	Nonpregnant Female	Change in Pregnant Female	Gestational Timing
Hemoglobin (Hgb)	12-16 g/dL	↓1.5-2 g/dL	Drops to lowest point between 30th and 34th week, then stable
Hematocrit (Hct)	37%-47%	↓4%-7%	Drops to lowest point between 30th and 34th week, then stable
White blood cells (WBCs)	5000-10,000/cm^3	↑3.5 × 103	Gradual increase throughout pregnancy
Platelets	150,000-400,000/mm^3	↓Slightly	Gradual decrease throughout pregnancy
Fibrinogen	200-400 mg/dL	↑50%	Gradual increase throughout pregnancy
Calcium (Ca)	9-10.5 mg/dL	↓10%	Gradual decrease throughout pregnancy
Sodium (Na)	136-145 mEq/L	↓2-4 mEq/L	Decreases before 20th week, then stable
Chloride (Cl)	90-110 mEq/L	↑Slightly	Gradual rise, almost negligible
Potassium (K)	3.5-5 mEq/L	↓0.2-0.3 mEq/L	Decreases before 20th week, then stable
Creatinine clearance	95-125 mL/min	↑40%	Rises through 20th week, then stable
Blood urea nitrogen (BUN)	5-20 mg/dL	↓50%	Drops during first trimester, then stable
Glucose (fasting)	70-115 mg/dL	↓10%	Gradual decrease throughout pregnancy
Uric acid	2-6.6 mg/dL	↓33%	Decreases during first trimester, then stable
Albumin	3.2-4.5 g/dL	↓1 g/dL	Rapid drop before 20th week, then stable

Position. Uterine displacement to the left during transport and until after delivery is necessary to shift the uterus away from the large abdominal vessels. The positional effect on cardiac output is of major importance in avoiding maternal hypotension and maintaining fetal well-being. In the supine position the enlarged uterus compresses the inferior vena cava and aorta, resulting in diminished venous return to the heart, stroke volume, and cardiac output. The patient is positioned supine with the right side slightly elevated by a wedge or small roll to tilt the uterus to the left (Fig. 34-15). The operating bed may be tilted 30 degrees to the left. A slight Trendelenburg's position assists venous return.

Anesthesia. Anesthesia is selected on an individual basis. Regional anesthesia, such as spinal or epidural, is preferred, because it has a lesser effect on the physiology of the mother and her fetus. It is advantageous in patients with diabetes because of reduced metabolic expenditure, low incidence of vomiting, and earlier return to oral intake. General anesthetic is administered when the mother or fetus is in jeopardy and delivery is crucial, as in the presence of hemorrhage or severe fetal distress. The choice also depends on the reason for the surgical procedure, degree of urgency, and the patient's condition and preference. A cesarean section can be done with local anesthesia in an extreme emergency when an anesthesia provider is not immediately available. The anesthesia provider chooses the method safest for the mother and fetus. Gastric motility and emptying are inhibited by fear, pain, labor, and narcotic administration. Patients requiring emergency surgery may have eaten recently. A

pregnant patient should always be regarded as having a full stomach.

Spinal or epidural anesthesia allows the mother to see her newborn in the OR. It also reduces neonatal depression and risk of maternal aspiration. Hypotension is treated with IV fluid infusion and/or ephedrine given IV to increase blood pressure. Ephedrine, mephentermine (Wyamine), and metaraminol (Aramine) do not cause undesired uterine vasoconstriction. Other vasopressors can cause fetal hypoxia. Placentally transmitted drugs depressant to the fetus are avoided. A single injection of morphine may be given through the epidural catheter at the conclusion of the surgical procedure. With injection into the pain path, the drug significantly reduces postoperative pain for 24 to 36 hours with minimal side effects.

General anesthesia provides more rapid induction, less hypotension, greater cardiovascular stability, and better control of the airway and ventilation. Preoxygenation precedes induction. Rapid-sequence induction and intubation are used. Cricoid pressure during intubation occludes the esophagus to prevent regurgitation. Induction-to-delivery time is directly related to fetal hypoxia. Intervals greater than 3 minutes may lead to a lower pH of blood (metabolic acidosis) and respiratory depression of the infant from altered uteroplacental perfusion.

All efforts are made to deliver the newborn as rapidly as possible, consistent with safety, to minimize anesthesia and surgical time and to protect the fetus. With general anesthesia, all preparations, such as patient skin preparation, insertion of an indwelling Foley catheter, draping, gowning, and gloving, are done before induction of anesthesia.

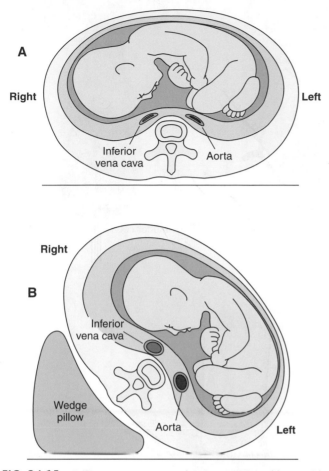

FIG. 34-15 **A,** Pressure on aorta and vena cava caused by gravid uterus. **B,** Pressure is relieved by placing a wedge under right hip.

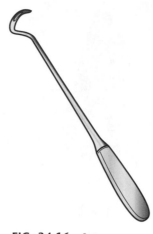

FIG. 34-16   Suture passer.

Threatened Abortion

Cerclage. Patients with painless dilation and effacement of the cervix during the second trimester may be at risk for preterm delivery caused by cervical incompetence. The pregnant patient at risk should be assessed for a history of previous preterm rupture of membranes or spontaneous abortion. The initial primipara cervical incompetence is rarely evident before 16 weeks' gestation. Diagnosis is commonly made between 18 and 26 weeks' gestation. Gestational ages appropriate for elective treatment of known cervical incompetence range between 12 and 16 weeks' gestation, before the cervix has dilated beyond 2 to 3 cm. Some patients may be suitable for this procedure up to 20 weeks' gestation. Cerclage is not usually performed after 26 weeks' gestation because the cervix is often too short to support suturing. Most cerclage is performed as an ambulatory procedure.

Occasionally, cerclage may be performed as an emergency procedure when the cervix is dilating and membranes are bulging, as long as the membranes have not ruptured or premature labor has not begun. The patient is placed in a deep Trendelenburg's position to take the uterine pressure off the cervix. No vaginal preparation is performed, to prevent accidental rupture of the membranes. It may be necessary to simultaneously perform transabdominal amniocentesis to decompress the membranes for the cerclage procedure.

General anesthesia is commonly used to provide relaxation of the uterine muscle. Cerclage is contraindicated in active infection, ruptured membranes, bleeding, or active labor. Cerclage is performed with ligature tape and a suture passer (Fig. 34-16).

Rarely, transabdominal cervicoisthmic cerclage (TCIC) may be performed as an open pelvic procedure for patients who have had severe cervical lacerations, congenital malformations of the cervix, or multiple failed cervical cerclage procedures. TCIC can be performed as early as 11 weeks' gestation after ultrasonographic documentation of a viable pregnancy. A 5-mm Mersilene tape is sutured around the cervical isthmus in an avascular plane. This procedure has been successful in preventing pregnancy loss characterized by painless cervical dilation and pregnancy loss during the third trimester.[8]

Shirodkar Procedure. A small incision is made in the anterior vaginal mucosa at the level of the bladder reflection and at the posterior cervix–cul-de-sac junction (Fig. 34-17). A tunnel under the cervical mucosa is then made to join the anterior and posterior incisions. A polyester (Mersilene) tape is drawn around the internal os and tied. The knot is secured posteriorly to prevent erosion into the bladder. The suture tail is cut long so that it can be located and released at 37 to 38 weeks' gestation or if active labor begins (before delivery). Mucosal incisions are closed. A cesarean section may be necessary at term.

McDonald Procedure. The polyester suture tape is placed around the cervix with a circumferential running stitch without mucosal dissection. Cervical scarring is less, and the procedure is quicker to perform. The tape can be removed at term for vaginal delivery.

Aborted Pregnancy

Termination of pregnancy may be spontaneous or induced. The procedure will depend on the gestational age of the fetus. Ultrasonography may be used to determine the stage of intrauterine pregnancy.

---

[8]Lotgering FK et al: Outcome after transabdominal cervicoisthmic cerclage, *ACOG* 107(4):779-784, 2006.

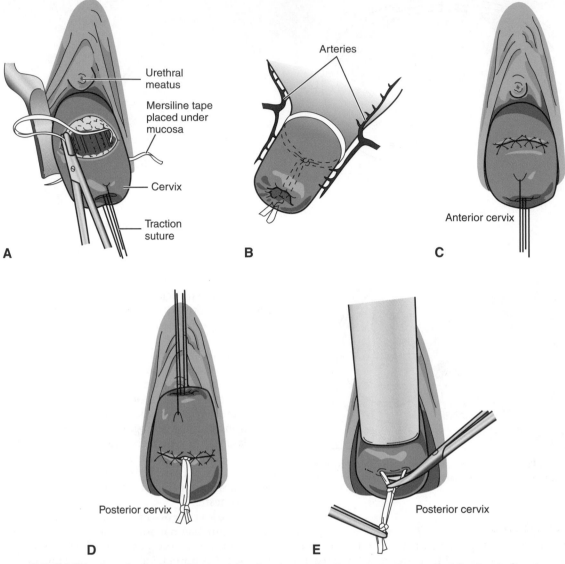

FIG. 34-17 Steps in the Shirodkar procedure for closure of an incompetent cervix. **A,** A ligature is placed below the mucosa circumferentially around the neck of the cervix. **B,** The uterine arteries are preserved and the ligature is tied on the posterior aspect of the cervix. **C,** The mucosal tissue is approximated with absorbable suture. **D,** A short length of ligature tape is left in place as a grasping tail. **E,** At term, the ligature tape is clipped to permit the cervix to open for the delivery of the fetus.

Some patients are psychologically repulsed by the word *abortion*. They may associate the word with elective termination regardless of natural causes or therapeutic need. Religious or personal beliefs may influence decision making about a pregnancy that cannot continue to full term. In some circumstances the patient may accept and understand the word *miscarriage* and feel freer to select appropriate treatment options without fear of reprisal or rejection. Consideration for the support of psychologic coping mechanisms of the patient in crisis is more important than using absolute words such as *abortion*. Females with RH-negative blood types are candidates for immune globulin (RhoGAM) injections to prevent sensitization from the potentially RH-positive fetus and complications with other pregnancies.

Suction Curettage. Intrauterine contents can be aspirated for voluntary pregnancy termination or for incomplete spontaneous abortion within the first 20 weeks of pregnancy.

Uterine Evacuation. A small, flexible plastic tip or cannula is inserted into the uterus in the first 8 weeks of pregnancy. Suction created by drawing back on the plunger of a large syringe attached to the cannula is sufficient to evacuate the contents of the uterus. Disposable equipment for suction curettage not requiring dilation or anesthesia is commercially available.

Dilation and Evacuation (D&E). For pregnancies of 8 to 16 weeks' duration, dilation and evacuation (D&E) must be performed. Cervical dilation is adjusted to the stage of pregnancy and the necessary cannula. A laminaria tent (i.e., a cone-shaped expansion plug) may be inserted preoperatively to gradually dilate the cervix, usually for 4 to 24 hours. Dilation with the laminaria, which is removed before the procedure, is gentler than instrument dilation, which can cause cervical tearing. Some instrument dilation may be necessary. A vacuum aspirator-cannula is inserted into the uterine cavity and connected by tubing to an adjustable electric vacuum pump. With gentle suction, the uterine contents are collected in a vacuum canister. Additional curettage with uterine curettes may be necessary to completely remove the uterine contents. The curetted contents are sent to the pathology department for gross examination.

After an incomplete spontaneous or missed abortion, it is vital to remove all retained products of conception to prevent infection, especially from anaerobic bacteria, which may progress to septic shock.

A D&C setup and suction curettage are used. The tissue is sent for culture and pathologic examination. Some patients may request baptism of an aborted fetus for religious reasons. Perioperative personnel may perform this function or request hospital clergy to assist. This has deep meaning for many patients.

Ectopic Pregnancy. A fertilized ovum may become implanted outside the uterine cavity. Referred to as an ectopic pregnancy, rarely does this fetus develop to full term. This type of pregnancy usually involves the fallopian tube (95%) but can develop in the uterine cervix, on the ovary, or intraabdominally (Fig. 34-18).

Symptoms of ectopic pregnancy are irregular growth patterns of the uterus, abdominal pain, and vaginal bleeding. Diagnosis is made by ultrasonography, by laparoscopy, or by detection of blood in the cul-de-sac by aspiration. Hemorrhage results from extensive trauma to the tube and mesosalpinx. The patient often goes into severe shock. Immediate surgical intervention is necessary.

Ruptured ectopic pregnancy is a true obstetric/gynecologic emergency. The affected tube is opened, and the products of conception are removed; hemostasis is attained; and the pelvic cavity is irrigated. The surgeon may attempt to repair

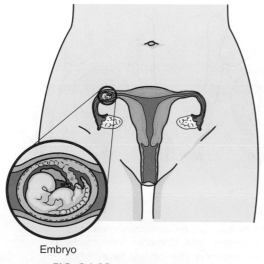

Embryo

FIG. 34-18 Ectopic pregnancy.

the affected tube. Removal of the associated tube and possibly the ovary depends on the extent of damage from the rupture.

If an ectopic pregnancy is diagnosed by ultrasound or laparoscopy before rupture, conservative surgery may be able to restore fertility. Tubal pregnancy can be removed through a linear salpingostomy or by segmental resection, followed by tuboplasty. Laparoscopic techniques may be used. Some ectopic pregnancies can be managed through a vaginal colpotomy incision or abdominal minilaparotomy.

Cesarean Birth

Commonly referred to as C-section, a cesarean section is a method of delivery by abdominal and uterine incisions. Cesarean delivery may take place in the labor and delivery department or in the OR. Pregnancy and labor produce many physiologic alterations. Both the mother and the newborn have specific needs requiring comprehensive care. To promote a positive experience, the perioperative team should be cognizant of these physiologic and psychologic needs and of the reasons for transabdominal delivery. A C-section is a significant family event. Partners or support persons may be permitted in the OR, and mothers are given regional anesthesia and are usually awake.

The frequency of cesarean delivery is attributed mainly to diagnosis and management of uterine dystocia (ineffective labor), failure to progress, and fetal distress detected by fetal monitoring. A C-section is performed when safe vaginal delivery is questionable or immediate delivery is crucial because the well-being of the mother or fetus is threatened. Indications may include hemorrhage, placenta previa, abruptio placentae, toxemia, fetal malpresentation, cephalopelvic disproportion (CPD), chorioamnionitis, genital herpes in the mother within 6 weeks of delivery, fetal distress, or prolapsed umbilical cord. The multiparous pregnant patient who has had previous cesarean delivery may attempt vaginal delivery or may elect to schedule a planned cesarean birth.

Severe, unanticipated complications, such as bleeding or fetal distress during late pregnancy or labor, adversely affect the mother and/or fetus, creating an emergency. For these patients, preparations for immediate delivery are rapid. The patient easily senses a loss of control, especially if she participated in a childbirth education program for vaginal delivery. She needs special support. Most mothers fear more for the survival of the fetus than for themselves.

An elective patient is admitted the morning of surgery. The patient is taken to the delivery suite. An emergency patient will go directly to the delivery room from the labor area. The pediatrician and neonatal personnel from the nursery are notified before the procedure so that they will be available to resuscitate and care for the infant in the delivery room. Sterile pediatric resuscitation equipment and supplies are made available.

Setup. Routine laparotomy skin preparation, draping, and setup are used for C-sections. Instruments are essentially those for a major gynecologic laparotomy with the addition of delivery forceps, a cord clamp, and a mucus aspiration bulb for infant suctioning on the field. A Foley catheter provides intraoperative bladder drainage. The patient is placed supine with the right side of the operating bed elevated or a small pillow under the right hip to displace the uterus from the inferior vena cava.

All preparations are made for the setup before the anesthetic is administered to the patient. If regional anesthesia is planned, the setup, counts, and preliminary routines can be performed simultaneously with the anesthesia procedures. The patient is prepped, catheterized, and draped after the anesthetic has taken effect. If general anesthesia is to be used, the setup, preparation, catheterization, and draping are performed before the anesthetic is administered to prevent prolonged depression of the fetus.

Incision and Delivery.
A low transverse Pfannenstiel or low midline vertical incision is made in the skin and underlying tissue layers. The length varies with the size of the fetus. Dissection is expeditious. The uterine incision is made by one of the following methods (Fig. 34-19):

- *Low transverse (Kerr incision).* The bladder is dissected off the uterus and retracted gently downward. The lower uterine segment is entered through a low horizontal curvilinear incision. This approach causes less intraoperative blood loss and decreased chance of rupture with subsequent pregnancies. Some patients will be able to have vaginal deliveries in future pregnancies.
- *Low vertical midline (Krohnig incision).* An 8-cm vertical incision is made in the lower uterine segment after the bladder is separated and retracted away. This incision is used when the fetus is small, preterm, and in the breech position. It is also used when cesarean hysterectomy may be performed after delivery.
- *Classic uterine incision.* The uterus is incised vertically above the attachment of the bladder. The bladder is not dissected off the lower uterine segment. This approach is rarely used but may be necessary for a fetus in transverse presentation or for multiple fetuses. It may be indicated for a low anterior placenta, varicosities of the lower uterine segment, or cervical cancer. A major disadvantage is the high incidence of rupture with subsequent pregnancy.

As the uterus is incised, the amniotic sac will be opened. The amniotic fluid will escape rapidly, requiring suction. Retractors are removed, and the fetal head or the presenting part is gently delivered as gentle pressure is applied to the fundus (Fig. 34-20).

Immediately on emergence of the head, the nares and mouth are aspirated with a bulb syringe to clear them of amniotic fluid. Newborns delivered by C-section have respiratory secretions. Delivery is completed, and the umbilical cord is double-clamped and cut between the clamps with sterile scissors. The newborn is transferred via a sterile sheet to the neonatal resuscitation team.

The circulating nurse or neonatal team member who receives the newborn should wear protective eyewear, a gown, and gloves until all blood and amniotic fluid are wiped off the infant. The risk of exposure to blood and amniotic fluid warrants the same adherence to standard precautions as with any other contact with blood and body fluids. The neonate is placed under a radiant warmer for resuscitation.

Oxytocin, 10 to 20 units, is administered IV to the mother to promote uterine contraction, minimize blood loss, and facilitate expulsion of the placenta and membranes. The placenta is delivered, visually inspected, and placed in a specimen basin. The uterine fundus is palpated for firmness and massaged as necessary to prevent hemorrhage from relaxation. Intrauterine injection of 10 units of oxytocin may be necessary to firm up an atonic uterus. The patient is returned to a horizontal supine position. The uterine incision is closed in layers with absorbable sutures, and hemostasis is ensured. Clots and excess intraperitoneal fluid are evacuated. After inspection of the pelvic organs and possible tubal ligation, the peritoneum and abdominal incision are closed.

Intraoperative assessment is the same as for any surgical patient. Sponges, tapes, and needles are counted before closure of the uterus and again before closure of the peritoneum, fascia, and skin.

Postpartum surveillance of the patient is essential. Lochia is observed. Abnormal bleeding, such as rapid saturation of the perineal pad, is immediately reported to the physician

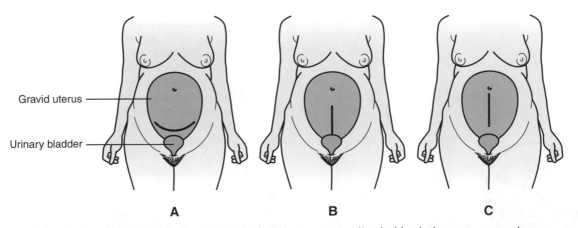

Gravid uterus

Urinary bladder

A   **B**   **C**

FIG. 34-19 Uterine incisions for cesarean birth. **A,** Low transverse Kerr incision is the most commonly used. **B,** Low midline Krohnig incision may be used for smaller or preterm fetus. **C,** Higher midline incision is referred to as a classic C-section and is only used in extreme circumstances. This method has a higher incidence of rupture in subsequent pregnancies.

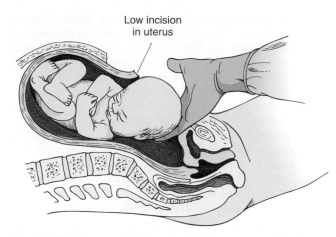

FIG. 34-20   Cesarean delivery after incising uterus and fetal membranes. As head is lifted through low uterine incision, pressure usually is applied to fundus of uterus through abdominal wall to help expel fetus.

and recorded. Nurses' notes should include the mother's contact with the infant, the mother's emotional reaction to the surgical procedure, and personnel in attendance, in addition to physical assessment data.

Neonate. Immediate postdelivery care is given in the OR by the neonatal team. The infant is taken to the nursery after careful examination by a pediatrician. The neonate traditionally has been evaluated by the Apgar score, acid-base status, and neurobehavioral examination. The Apgar score, first published by American anesthesiologist Virginia Apgar (1902-1974) in 1953, is an excellent screening tool for vital functions immediately (at 1- and 5-minute intervals) after birth, but the subtle effect of drugs may be overlooked.[9] The Neurologic and Adaptive Capacity Score does not use noxious stimuli but emphasizes neonatal tone. Drugs that will produce significant neurobehavioral changes in the newborn must be avoided during labor and delivery.

In the newborn the apical pulse is the most accurate. Oxygenation is extremely important. Hypoxia (too little oxygen) can lead to intracranial hemorrhage, brain damage, or necrotizing enterocolitis. Hyperoxia (too much oxygen), administered at a rate in excess of 40% concentration, can cause bronchopulmonary dysplasia or retrolental fibroplasia.

Father or Support Person in the Delivery Room. Paternal or support-person participation in the birthing process is well established for vaginal delivery to provide support to the mother, a family-centered birth, and immediate bonding with the infant. However, the presence of the father or support person in the OR during cesarean delivery is not universal and requires the surgeon's consent. Hospitals adopting this policy report favorable experiences. This person is informed of the conditions permitting and excluding his or her presence. Those who have attended a structured childbirth education course have more understanding of pregnancy and birth. In compliance with hospital policy,

donning of OR attire and supervised handwashing with an antimicrobial soap before entrance to the OR are stressed. The father or support person sits by the mother's head. He or she may accompany the infant to the newborn examining area after delivery. If the newborn and the mother's conditions permit, the father or support person may rejoin the mother in the OR for bonding.

Prenatal Testing

Potentially useful for management of some congenital developmental disorders or genetic defects, prenatal diagnostic studies are performed during pregnancy in select patients. Fetal anomalies are found in 2% of all women tested. Disorders in the fetus may be cause for induced abortion, elective cesarean delivery, or intrauterine fetal surgery.

Ultrasonography. Ultrasound is the standard tool for fetal imaging in utero. Ultrasonography, a noninvasive technique, permits accurate location of the placenta, determination of the gestational size of the fetus, assessment of fetal heart activity, and reliable diagnosis of structural defects (e.g., hydrocephalus, spina bifida). Other defects, such as missing limbs or conjoined twins, may be diagnosed.

Blood and Chorionic Villus Sampling. Ultrasound is also used for catheter or cannula guidance to obtain percutaneous umbilical blood samples or transcervical chorionic villus samples. Through direct fetal blood samples, anemia and some metabolic and chromosomal abnormalities can be diagnosed and treated in utero. Intravascular blood transfusions can be given to correct fetal anemia. Chorionic villi are a source of fetal genetic information. When obtained between the eighth and twelfth weeks of gestation, chorionic villi can aid in accurately diagnosing some enzymatic defects and in detecting the gender of the fetus.

Amniocentesis. Amniotic fluid is aspirated from the amniotic sac under ultrasound direction at 16 to 20 weeks' gestation for chromosomal analysis. This highly accurate test is indicated for known or suspected risk of chromosomal abnormality because of advanced maternal age, known parental translocation carrier, or a history of previous pregnancy with chromosomal defect in the fetus or infant. Maternal serum alpha-fetoprotein (AFP) measurement can predict neural tube disorders (e.g., myelomeningocele) or other defects in the fetus.

Fetoscopy. Fetoscopy permits direct visualization of the fetus. A fiberoptic needle scope (fetoscope) is inserted into the amniotic cavity to view fetal parts, to obtain a biopsy of skin, or to sample fetal blood. The fetoscope is 1.7 mm in diameter with a visual field of 70 degrees. To ensure an adequate volume of amniotic fluid, fetoscopy is done after 16 weeks of pregnancy. Because of the intent to view specific structures, the position of the fetus must first be determined and the procedure performed under sonographic-assisted visualization. Placental localization is important, especially in the area of umbilical cord insertion. Hemoglobinopathies and coagulation problems (e.g., hemophilia) may be rapidly diagnosed by aspiration of fetal blood from the placenta or umbilical cord. Congenital skin disorders

---

[9]www.neonatology.org.

and albinism may be detected by biopsy. Direct viewing of the fetus may reveal characteristic abnormalities of various congenital syndromes. The procedure is not without complications and should be performed only by trained physicians when genetic information is critical.

Intrauterine Fetal Surgery

Improvement and expansion in prenatal diagnosis have led to rapidly developing antenatal surgical intervention— intrauterine fetal surgery. Diagnostic screening by ultrasound, AFP, or some other method during gestation reveals abnormalities heretofore diagnosed after delivery. Some disorders can be treated in utero. Other conditions fall within the province of the surgeon. Prerequisites for fetal therapy include accurate diagnosis, known pathophysiology, workable treatment, and technical capability. Fetal surgery teams comprise radiologists, perinatologists, pediatric surgeons, anesthesia providers, obstetric nurses, perioperative nurses, and surgical technologists.

Most correctable malformations may be detected in utero but are best remedied by a surgical procedure after delivery at term. A full-term infant is a better surgical risk than is the fetus. Surgical treatment in utero is reserved for fetuses in whom continuing organ development could be normal if surgically treated (e.g., diaphragmatic hernia, spina bifida, tracheal stenosis, hydronephrosis caused by urinary tract obstruction).

Minimally invasive procedures facilitate the placement of shunts and catheters. Highly invasive procedures require hysterotomy (opening of the uterine wall) (Fig. 34-21). Preoperative preparation includes the administration of tocolytic drugs (indomethacin suppository) to prevent the onset of labor caused by uterine manipulation. An irritable uterus requires cancellation of the procedure.

The procedure is performed in the late second trimester with the patient under general anesthesia, using isoflurane because it is considered less hazardous to the fetus. The uterus is exposed through an abdominal incision, and a cannula is inserted through the uterine wall to decompress some of the amniotic fluid. The uterine anterior fundal incision is carefully extended down to the amnion. The sac is opened, and the edges are secured to the uterine edges with Raney clips. Meticulous hemostasis is necessary. ESU use is avoided. Small doses of fentanyl and pancuronium are administered to the fetus for anesthesia. A sterile pulse oximeter and electrocardiographic (ECG) leads are sutured to the fetus to monitor oxygenation and cardiac activity.

Great care is taken to avoid manipulation of the placenta or cord. Warmed sterile saline irrigation is continuously perfused through the amniotic cavity during the procedure. After the repairs are complete, a small, wireless transducer is placed in the fetal chest for continued postoperative monitoring of the fetus in utero. This transducer is removed after birth. If fetal repairs require thoracotomy and diaphragmatic patching, the pleural space is maintained with warmed Ringer's lactate solution to allow for continued lung growth.

On completion of the procedure, the amnion is sutured closed and fibrin glue is applied. The uterus is sutured, and the abdominal incision is stapled. The fetal wound healing is nearly scarless because of decreased inflammatory response and neotissue generation associated with continued fetal development. The pregnancy continues as long as possible after the open procedure, preferably to a minimum of 32 to 36 weeks' gestation. Lung maturity is the key issue for success. Preterm labor usually precipitates cesarean birth. Vaginal delivery is contraindicated because a classic uterine incision of the fundus is used for open intrauterine fetal surgery and may predispose the uterus to rupture during contractions.

ASSISTED REPRODUCTION

Infertility, the inability to conceive a child after a year or more of repeated attempts, can be emotionally devastating. Both partners undergo extensive testing to determine possible organic or functional causes. These may include a structural

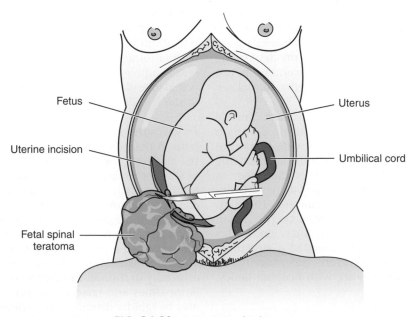

FIG. 34-21 Intrauterine fetal surgery.

defect in either partner, past or present infections, genetic and/or immunologic abnormalities, or an endocrine imbalance or deficit. In the woman, a hostile cervix, antibodies to sperm, endometriosis, or exposure to DES in utero may prevent conception. Tubal occlusion is the most frequent cause of infertility. A male partner may have an inadequate number, quality, or mobility of sperm or an absence of live spermatozoa in semen. When conventional infertility therapy has failed to produce a pregnancy, other options are available to assist in achieving pregnancy and birth of a mature, live infant.

In Vitro Fertilization

The term in vitro means "in glass." Fertilization literally takes place in a culture dish or test tube. In vitro fertilization (IVF) refers to removal of ova from the prospective mother via endoscopy, fertilization with the husband's or a donor's sperm, and incubation in the laboratory with subsequent embryo transfer to the uterus. Ovulation may be stimulated by administration of hormones. Multiple follicles may mature, and several ova are procured. The first documented birth from IVF and embryo transfer, performed by Dr. Robert Edwards and Dr. Patrick Steptoe, took place in England in 1978 by cesarean section. The first IVF clinic in the United States using the Edwards-Steptoe method was established in Virginia in 1980.

IVF is most successful in women younger than 30 years. In women younger than 34 years, the success rate is 30% to 40% for delivery per ovum retrieval. The success of this technology for pregnancy in women older than 42 years is less than 10%. However, reports of a live birth by this method to a woman 60 years of age are found in the literature.

Patient Selection. IVF is accepted therapy for women with severely damaged or nonfunctioning fallopian tubes, for men with scarce or absent sperm, or for infertility of unknown cause. Contraindications include a uterine myoma, single uterine cornu, or bicornate or septate uterus. The woman is evaluated preoperatively for a normal uterine cavity, an accessible ovary, and evidence of ovulation. These parameters are measured by pelvic ultrasonography and serum estrogen levels. A laparoscopy, endometrial biopsy, and hysterosalpingogram may be part of preoperative testing. Semen analysis is done to check the sperm condition and count of the male partner.

Some patients may be unable to provide an ovum, conceive, or carry a fetus to full term. In select situations, a surrogate mother will carry the developing fetus to term, surrendering the neonate at birth to the adoptive mother. Family members, such as a sister or other, may participate. Ethics and legal issues surround this event. Patient confidentiality is protected.

Induction of Ovulation. IVF is coordinated with timing of the ovulatory cycle. The medical protocol is prescribed for the individual couple. From day 2 or 3 of the menstrual cycle through day 6 or 7, the woman takes fertility drugs to stimulate growth and maturation of ovarian follicles. These drugs are a combination of clomiphene citrate (a synthetic hormone) and human luteinizing and follicle-stimulating hormones. Follicular growth is monitored daily, beginning about the eighth day, by ultrasonography and serum estrogen levels. The fluid-filled follicles on the surface of the ovaries contain ova (oocytes). When follicles reach a diameter of 15 to 20 mm, the woman is given human chorionic gonadotropin (HCG) intramuscularly to stimulate maturation of the ova.

Ovum Retrieval. The patient is scheduled for retrieval of mature ova about 35 hours after HCG injection. Ovum retrieval may be accomplished through ultrasound-assisted transvaginal, transvesical, or transabdominal approaches. The procedure is performed with the patient under general anesthesia or IV sedation. Transvaginal ovum retrieval is the procedure of choice, but the approach depends on accessibility to the ovary. With the patient in the lithotomy position, the ultrasound probe with an aspiration needle guide attached is advanced through the cervix, uterus, and fallopian tube to the ovary. The needle guide is directed toward the follicle, as seen on a monitoring screen. The follicle is punctured with a 14-inch × 17-gauge needle. Follicular fluid is aspirated into a 5-mL syringe. Ova procured from the graafian follicle are placed in sterile solution designated by the treating gynecologist.

Extensive scarring in tubes may make ovaries inaccessible via the transvaginal approach. For a transvesical approach, the ultrasound probe is inserted through the urethra and posterior bladder wall to the ovary. With the patient positioned supine, a retrieval probe can be inserted percutaneously through the abdominal wall to reach the ovary in the pelvic cavity.

Ova can be retrieved by laparoscopy. The surgeon visualizes the ovaries. The follicle is punctured with an 8-inch × 14-gauge needle and aspirated directly into a test tube through a catheter attached to the needle. All instruments and solutions used for retrieval are kept at a normal physiologic temperature of 98.6° F (37° C). After completion of aspiration, the syringe or test tube is carefully handed to the circulating nurse using aseptic technique.

To avoid contamination, fluid should not be exposed to the environment, including light. Dimmed room light also enhances the surgeon's view on the video monitor. The circulating nurse labels the specimen and sends it immediately to the laboratory for confirmation of ovum retrieval while instrumentation is still in place. If the report is negative, the search for another ovum continues until the laboratory gives a positive response of retrieval. The procedure may be repeated on the contralateral ovary. Many surgeons prefer to retrieve at least three to five ova for fertilization. Other women can be suitable volunteer donors for ova for women who have been unable to provide a suitable ovum.

Fertilization. The aspirated ova are placed in a culture dish containing a nutrient mixture similar to tubal secretions at midcycle, which prepares the ova for fertilization. Fresh semen obtained an hour or so before the woman undergoes ovum retrieval, or previously collected frozen sperm from a partner or donor, is added. Care is taken to confirm identification of the ovum and sperm to prevent error.

The culture dish is incubated for 40 to 48 hours for fertilization to take place. Cell division is detected by microscopic examination. When the embryo reaches the 4- to 8-cell stage of development, it is ready for transfer to the uterus.

Multiple oocytes can be fertilized, and embryos can be stored frozen for a period of up to 3 years for later implantation if desired. Embryos frozen at the 2-, 4-, 8-, or 16-cell stage, after thawing, have a viability rate of 60% to 80%. The embryo is transferred during a natural ovulatory cycle for the best results.

Embryo Transfer. Approximately 48 hours after retrieval, the woman returns for embryo transfer. She is placed in the knee-chest position. Anesthesia is unnecessary. A catheter prepared in the laboratory, containing the embryo in culture medium, is inserted into the uterus. The patient remains in the knee-chest position for at least an hour to allow the embryo to gravitate to the upper uterine fundus. Immediately after embryo transfer, an injection of progesterone is given. Necessary for implantation, injections are given daily for the next 12 to 15 days. Implantation is necessary for progression of the cell mass to an embryo. The woman's own ovarian function sustains early gestation, as confirmed by ultrasonography.

Failure to implant may result from escape of the embryo from the uterus with removal of the catheter, excess uterine contractility, inadequate luteal phase affecting the endometrium, mechanical disturbance of the endometrium, or encapsulation of the embryo in blood or mucus.

Gamete Intrafallopian Transfer

The procedure for gamete intrafallopian transfer (GIFT), developed in 1984, is similar to IVF but is always done laparoscopically. The woman must have at least one patent, functional fallopian tube. Ovulation is induced as described for IVF. Laparoscopy is scheduled 34 or 35 hours after injection of HCG. Fresh semen is obtained from the partner at least an hour before this procedure and is centrifuged and incubated at body temperature until use.

Ovum retrieval via laparoscope is accomplished as described for IVF. The follicular fluid is sent immediately to the laboratory, where an embryologist selects two or three ova. These and the sperm, along with the culture medium, are loaded into a catheter and sent back to the OR. The surgeon passes the catheter through the laparoscope and injects fluid into the ampulla of the fallopian tube. One or both tubes may receive an injection.

Other procedures, such as laser vaporization of endometriosis or lysis of adhesions, may be performed while the surgeon waits for the catheter. Additional ova may be inseminated and cryopreserved for IVF if GIFT is unsuccessful. Many implants may precede conception; it may never be successful.

Artificial Insemination

In vivo fertilization by artificial insemination of sperm may provide a reproductive option for a fertile woman. Homologous insemination deposits the partner's sperm into the upper vagina, cervical canal, or uterine cavity. Whole ejaculate is used when the man is unable to deposit sperm into the partner's vagina because of psychologic or physiologic factors. Washed sperm are used for intrauterine injection. Semen or sperm may be frozen and stored in a sperm bank for future use if reproductive capacity is threatened, such as by illness. Artificial insemination is coordinated with the recipient's ovulation for conception to occur.

Donor insemination involves the same techniques, but sperm are obtained from a donor. Donors are screened for sexually transmitted diseases, including infection with human immunodeficiency virus (HIV) and hepatitis B virus (HBV). Genetic screening also may be required. Donor sperm may be sought when the partner has a genetically transmitted disease or defect. The couple may have concerns about donor selection.

NONOBSTETRIC SURGICAL PROCEDURES AND THE PREGNANT PATIENT

The pregnant surgical patient who is brought to the OR for reasons other than childbirth presents a unique challenge to the perioperative team. The plan of care includes consideration for two patients: the mother and her developing fetus. The effects of surgical intervention can be disastrous to a pregnancy, but in some situations it is necessary to save the mother and/or the fetus. A developing fetus is intolerant of hypovolemia and hypoxemia. These considerations apply to all pregnant patients.

The average gestation, or duration of pregnancy, is 38 to 40 weeks, or 9 calendar months. This gestation period is divided into trimesters (3-month segments). Each trimester represents a specific developmental and viability concern (Box 34-1). Maternal anatomic and physiologic changes occur during each trimester of pregnancy (Table 34-3). Modifications to the plan of care vary according to these changes. Risks associated with surgical intervention may be specific to the fetus. During the first trimester, spontaneous abortion of the developing embryo (until the end of the eighth week) or fetus (from the eighth week) can occur. Preterm labor and/or delivery may be precipitated during the second and third trimesters. The surgeon and anesthesia provider should discuss the risks, benefits, and potential outcome with the patient and her family.

Nonobstetric surgical procedures on pregnant patients are usually performed for an urgent or emergent reason, such as cholecystitis, appendicitis, or trauma. Urgent surgical procedures are delayed until the second or third trimester if possible. Emergency procedures are performed immediately, regardless of gestational stage. If the maternal condition is critical, the primary concern is to save the mother. Elective surgical procedures should be deferred until after delivery of the neonate and the anatomic and physiologic changes of pregnancy have returned to normal.

Anesthesia Considerations in Pregnancy

The surgeon and anesthesia provider collaborate closely because the risks of anesthesia and surgical procedures are high for both the mother and the fetus. Perinatal morbidity and mortality are affected by maternal health, fetal viability, the type of anesthetic, and the surgical procedure. The incidence of preterm labor, low birthweight, and fetal death increases if a general anesthetic agent must be administered. The objectives of anesthesia management in the pregnant surgical patient include, but are not limited to, the following:

1. *Maternal safety.* The pregnant patient should always be treated as if she has a full stomach. Nausea and vomiting are common and place the patient at risk

BOX 34-1	Stages of Fetal Development and Viability Concerns

FIRST TRIMESTER (1-3 months, 1-12 weeks)
Zygote implants in uterine wall by 14 days.
Communication of venous sinus and arterial supply of maternal circulation is completed at 17 days.
Teratogens can impair organogenesis until 14th week.
Primitive placental system with umbilical cord is established by 7th week.
Heart rate is detectable on ultrasound at 10-12 weeks.
Facial features and external genitalia are present by 12th week.
Crown-to-rump length is 6-7 cm by 12th week.

SECOND TRIMESTER (4-7 months, 13-27 weeks)
Arms and trunk grow rapidly.
Little muscle tone.
Scalp hair, tiny nipples, and external ears develop by 20th week.
Meconium is present in intestine.
Body weight is 300 g.
Skeletal calcification is seen on radiograph.
Sucks thumb and moves freely at will.
Fetal heart rate is audible with fetoscope at 120-160 beats/min at 20th week.
Fingertip pressure causes ballottement (fetal rebound) in amniotic sac during 16th-32nd week.
Teratogens may cause minor structural and functional abnormalities, especially endocrine, brain, and special senses, from 10th week to term.
Body is covered with vernix (gray-white cheeselike substance) and lanugo (soft, downy hair).
Eyebrows and eyelashes are present.
Body weight is 454-630 g (1-1.4 pounds) by 24th week. May be viable.

THIRD TRIMESTER (7-9 months, 28-38 to 40 weeks)
Subcutaneous fat begins to develop.
Crown-to-rump length is 25 cm.
Testes are descended in male.
Body weight is 1100 g (2½ pounds).
Surfactant is present in alveoli of lungs by 28th week.
Increased chance of survival.
Body weight is 1361-1814 g (3-4 pounds) by 32nd week.
Body is fuller and rounded.
Muscle tone is good.
Less vernix and absence of lanugo by 36th week.
Body weight is 3402-3629 g (7½-8 pounds) by 38-40 weeks.
Crown-to-rump length is 36 cm.

for aspiration of regurgitated stomach contents during induction of anesthesia, intubation, and extubation. The condition of the mother directly affects the outcome of the pregnancy.

2. *Avoidance of teratogenic drugs.* Many anesthetic drugs cross the placenta and enter the fetus through the uteroplacental circulation. Some drugs that adversely affect the fetus during the first trimester are nitrous oxide, halogenated agents, sedatives, tranquilizers, antidepressants, and amphetamines.

Halogenated agents and nitrous oxide have been given without teratogenicity in emergency situations during the second and third trimesters. Only short-acting drugs should be used. The fetal liver is imma-

ture and metabolizes tranquilizers and other narcotics slowly. Neonatal respiratory depression is common if these drugs have been used.

Agents used in local and regional anesthesia have not shown teratogenicity in animal studies and may provide a safer anesthetic alternative than those agents used for general anesthesia when a surgical procedure must be performed.

3. *Prevention of fetal asphyxia.* Maternal hypoxia rapidly affects the oxygenation of the fetus. The oxygenation capability depends on the hemoglobin content and arterial oxygen tension of maternal blood and uteroplacental perfusion. Maternal hypotension and decreased uterine blood flow cause fetal hypoxia.

4. *Prevention of preterm labor.* Studies have shown no association of any single anesthetic agent with an increase or decrease in preterm labor. Manipulation of the gravid uterus can cause preterm labor. The use of halogenated agents in advanced pregnancy decreases uterine tone and prevents uterine contractions. Vasopressors and drugs used to reverse muscle relaxants may stimulate the uterus to contract and initiate preterm labor.

Special Considerations

Intraoperative Care of the Pregnant Patient. Both the mother and the fetus should be monitored during the surgical procedure. The mother's physiologic and psychologic condition rapidly affects the well-being of her fetus. Changes in the fetal condition may be the first indicators of a physiologic change in the mother. Intraoperative care and monitoring of the pregnant surgical patient include special considerations regarding the following objectives:

1. *Minimize the patient's time under anesthesia.* Skin preparation and draping should be done before induction of general anesthesia. Devices for electronic fetal and uterine monitoring should be in position and in proper working order.

2. *Monitor maternal oxygenation.* Pulse oximetry is useful for noninvasive measurement of oxygenation in hemoglobin. Readings should remain above 94% to prevent fetal hypoxia. Continuous oxygen is usually administered.

3. *Monitor the fetal heart rate.* An electronic fetal heart monitor (EFM) should be used by appropriately trained personnel for continuous monitoring. Fetal tachycardia may be the first indicator of maternal hypoxia. EFM is most effective after 16 weeks' gestation. Personnel qualified in EFM should be assigned this role.

4. *Monitor the uterine tone.* The uterus should be palpated frequently during the surgical procedure to detect contractions. Uterine manipulation, bladder stimulation, and several anesthetic drugs may cause preterm labor.

5. *Prevent aspiration.* Assist the anesthesia provider during intubation by providing cricoid pressure (Sellick's maneuver) as directed.

6. *Prevent maternal hypotension.* If the uterus is enlarged to the level of the umbilicus or above (17 to 20 weeks' gestation), place a small pad or folded sheet

under the right hip to laterally displace the uterus to the left. This redistributes the weight of the gravid uterus off the vena cava and abdominal aorta and facilitates a normotensive state. Renal perfusion is also improved.

7. *Monitor urinary output.* Minimum urinary output should be 25 mL/hr. Palpate the bladder every 30 minutes. Bladder distention can cause uterine irritability and preterm labor. The bladder is displaced above the pelvis during the second and third

TABLE 34-3	Maternal Anatomic and Physiologic Changes of Pregnancy		
System	First Trimester (1-3 Months, 1-12 Weeks)	Second Trimester (4-7 Months, 13-27 Weeks)	Third Trimester (7-9 Months, 28-38 to 40 Weeks)
Cardiovascular	Cardiac output begins to increase at 6th week.	Cardiac output increases 30%-50% by 16th week.	Cardiac output decreases slightly by 30th week.
	Plasma volume begins to increase.	Plasma volume continues to increase. Hypervolemic and hemodiluted.	Plasma volume increase peaks 50% at 32-36 weeks.
		Red blood cell (RBC) production increases 20%. White blood cell (WBC) production increases 30%-40%.	RBC increases, peaks at 33%.
	Breast veins dilate.	Capillary engorgement can cause epistaxis (nosebleeds) and epulis (bleeding gums).	May develop hemorrhoids and varicosities in leg veins. Increased risk for venous thrombosis.
	Vasculature increases to vulva and vagina.	Heart rate increases 15-20 beats/min.	Factors VII, IX, X increase causes hypercoagulative state. Plasma fibrinogen increases 40%-50%.
		Slight hypotension caused by decreased peripheral vascular resistance.	Normotensive by 26th week.
		Uterus presses on vena cava when supine.	Uterine circulation is 1 L/min by 38th-40th week.
		Physiologic anemia: hemoglobin, hematocrit, and platelets decrease.	
Pulmonary Lung compliance and pulmonary diffusion remain constant throughout pregnancy.	Vital capacity and partial pressure of oxygen (Po_2) are unchanged.	Diaphragm is displaced upward by rising fundus; thoracic circumference increases by 6 cm.	Diaphragm is displaced 4 cm by rising fundus. Thoracic breathing replaces abdominal breathing.
		Tidal volume increases 30%-40%.	Venous stasis increases risk for thrombus formation and pulmonary emboli.
		Respiratory rate increases 15% to accommodate increasing metabolism.	
		Mild dyspnea. Chronic state of compensated respiratory alkalosis.	
		Nasal congestion caused by estrogen-induced edema.	
Gastrointestinal	Nausea and vomiting. Constipation. Salivation increases.	Nausea and vomiting diminish. Incidence of cholecystitis is increased. Progesterone causes decreased gastrointestinal motility. Esophageal sphincter tone is decreased; at risk for gastric reflux.	Gastric emptying time is decreased. Gallbladder sluggish, frequently develop gallstones.
Neurologic	May feel some slight Braxton Hicks contractions starting at 8th week.	Intraocular pressure decreases. Some temporary visual changes develop; vision returns to prepregnant state after delivery.	Braxton Hicks contractions increase and become regular.
Endocrine	Human chorionic gonadotropin hormone secreted by corpus luteum of ovary is present in serum 9 days after conception. Progesterone production increases. Basal metabolic rate decreases. Blood glucose level decreases.	Protein binding causes increase in circulating hormones. Thyroid and adrenal hormone levels are elevated. Insulin production increases. Erythropoietin increases by 20th week. Metabolism increases.	Prolactin increases and peaks at delivery.

TABLE 34-3	Maternal Anatomic and Physiologic Changes of Pregnancy—cont'd		
System	First Trimester (1-3 Months, 1-12 Weeks)	Second Trimester (4-7 Months, 13-27 Weeks)	Third Trimester (7-9 Months, 28-40 Weeks)
Genitourinary Ureters and renal pelves and calyces dilate, increasing risk of urinary tract infection. Dilation is present throughout pregnancy.	Urinary frequency caused by uterine pressure on bladder.	Bladder pressure decreases as fundus elevates. Bladder is displaced superior to pelvis. Glomerular filtration rate increases 30%-50%. Drugs are excreted faster.	Lateral position facilitates renal blood flow and increases urinary output. Increased frequency as presenting part enters pelvis.
Integumentary	No appreciable change.	Striae gravidarum (stretch marks) appear on breasts and abdomen.	Dark line (linea nigra) appears between umbilicus and pubis. Increased pigmentation of face (chloasma).
Musculoskeletal	Feels fatigue. Weight loss first few weeks caused by nausea and vomiting. Average weight gain 2.2 pounds (1 kg) by 10-12 weeks.	Feels energetic. Weight gain 1 pound (0.45 kg) per week; desirable weight gain between 12th and 20th week is 8 pounds (3.62 kg). Gains 0.5-1 pound (0.24 kg-2.2 kg) per week between 20th and 38th week. Progressive lordosis to compensate for shifting center of gravity causes backache.	Energy declines. Ideal weight gain 25-30 pounds (11-13.6 kg) total for entire pregnancy. Increased lordosis as uterus expands and protrudes forward.
	Leg cramps.	Leg cramps increase by 24th week.	Pelvic joints relax and slight separation of symphysis pubis can be seen on radiograph.
Reproductive	Menstruation ceases.	Uterine fundus elevates halfway between symphysis pubis and umbilicus by 12th-16th week but rises above umbilicus by 24 weeks.	Uterine fundus elevates halfway between umbilicus and xyphoid process by 28th week and reaches xyphoid by 32nd week. Fundus decreases in height (caused by uterine weight) by 38th week. Uterine weight at term is 1100 g.
	Progesterone causes uterine lining to thicken. Estrogen causes uterine body to hypertrophy, anteflex, and become globular; by 3rd month fundus reaches pelvic brim.	Fetal movement is felt by 18th-20th week.	
	Cervix softens, and vulva and vagina appear blue (caused by increasing vascularity). Vaginal discharge increases.	Lower uterine segment elevates in pelvis.	
	Breast tissue enlarges and becomes sensitive.	Areolae darken.	Breasts feel full and tender. May secrete colostrum (precursor to milk).

trimesters and is easily injured. An indwelling Foley catheter should be inserted if the surgical procedure is anticipated to exceed 1 hour.

8. *Maintain a normothermic environment.* Warm the room to 75° F (24° C), and maintain a consistent temperature during the surgical procedure. Maternal hypothermia causes decreased uteroplacental perfu-sion and can cause fetal bradycardia. Use prewarmed blankets and irrigating solutions. Keep the mother's head covered.

9. *Prepare for emergency cesarean birth or preterm delivery.* In the event of untimely rupture of the membranes, preterm labor, or fetal distress, it may be necessary to perform a cesarean section or precipitous delivery

in an effort to save a viable fetus. A preterm fetus requiring immediate delivery after 24 weeks' gestation or 1 pound (500 g) weight may be considered viable. Fetal viability is individualized by measurement of lung maturity, body weight, and ability to sustain life after removal from the uterus.

10. *Protect the fetus from hazards in the environment.* The pregnant uterus at any stage of gestation should be shielded from ionizing radiation. During the first trimester, radiation may cause teratogenic damage. This may be unavoidable in trauma surgery.
11. *Reassure the mother.* Explain that she and her fetus will be monitored closely and that they will be carefully protected.

Intraoperative Risks.
The enlarging uterus displaces abdominal organs and distorts anatomic landmarks, making diagnoses of trauma or a pathologic condition complex. A motor vehicle accident is a common cause of abdominal trauma. A seat belt (lap belt) without a shoulder restraint can cause compression injury to the enlarged uterus. Spontaneous laceration and/or rupture can occur. Peritoneal lavage, if used to assess for intraabdominal bleeding, should be done through an incision above the umbilicus to avoid injuring the uterus.

Surgical procedures for reasons other than trauma, such as pathologic causes, require careful differential diagnosis. Anatomic and physiologic changes of pregnancy must be considered. For example, the appendix is displaced to the upper right quadrant and may mimic cholecystitis. In advanced pregnancy, chest drainage tubes should be inserted one or two intercostal spaces higher, if needed. Diagnosis is complicated, because laboratory tests are altered by the progressing pregnancy and results vary according to the gestational stage.[10]

Assessment of the patient's condition is difficult because compensatory mechanisms of pregnancy cause alterations in vital signs. The arterial blood pressure is lower than prepregnant values, and the pulse is elevated to accommodate an increase in circulatory volume. Decreased peripheral vascular resistance prevents overt physiologic signs of shock, such as cool, clammy skin.

Circulating blood volume can be reduced 30% to 35% before the patient shows any signs of hypovolemic shock, such as lowered blood pressure and increased pulse rate. In hypovolemic shock, blood is shunted away from the uteroplacental circulation at the expense of the fetus. The fetus becomes hypoxic. Fetal demise is 80% in maternal hypovolemic shock. An EFM can detect early signs of fetal hypoxia and uteroplacental insufficiency. Use of a fetal monitor is recommended during surgical procedures after 16 weeks' gestation. Personnel appropriately trained in fetal monitoring should perform this assessment throughout the perioperative period, including during the surgical procedure and postanesthesia recovery.

In the immediate postoperative period the pregnant patient must be assessed for uterine irritability, vaginal

bleeding, and/or ruptured membranes. Any combination of these signs may signal impending labor and possible preterm delivery and must be reported to the physician immediately. Bladder distention can cause uterine irritability and stimulate preterm labor. The bladder should be palpated frequently. A distended bladder is felt as a bulge above the symphysis pubis that is cooler than the surrounding skin.

Psychologic Considerations.
For most patients and their families, pregnancy is a time of joy and excitement. Their happiness is shattered when they are faced with the prospect of a surgical procedure and its inherent risks. In urgent and emergency situations, the family has little time to adjust to the pending procedure. The outcome is uncertain, and the risks to the mother and her fetus are great. The patient and family are also facing the possibility of a preterm delivery.

The perioperative team should consider the special needs of the pregnant patient and her family and provide as much reassurance as possible. Preterm emergent C-section after 25 weeks' gestation has a 45% fetal survival rate.

Perimortem C-section (at the death of the mother greater than 5 minutes) is not usually successful before 24 weeks' gestation and may be deemed by the surgeon to be futile. The team may feel emotional at the decision not to operate before the age of viability. The surgeon may elect to try to save the fetus by immediately cross-clamping the aorta (to conserve placental blood) and quickly opening the uterus for delivery.

Bibliography

Althuisius SM, Dekker GA: A five century evolution of cervical incompetence as a clinical entity, *Curr Pharm Des* 11(6):687-697, 2005.

Bhide A, Thilaganathan B: Recent advances in the management of placenta previa, *Curr Opin Obstet Gynecol* 16(6):447-451, 2004.

Bock K et al: Pathologic breast conditions in childhood and adolescence: Evaluation by sonographic diagnosis, *J Ultrasound Med* 24(10):1347-1357, 2005.

Boyle P et al: Cancer control in women, Update 2003, *Int J Gynaecol Obstet* 83 (Suppl 1):179-202, 2003.

Cass DL: Fetal surgery for congenital diaphragmatic hernia: The North American experience, *Semin Perinatol* 29(2):104-111, 2005.

Christensen ND: Emerging human papillomavirus vaccines, *Expert Opin Emerg Drugs* 10(1):5-19, 2005.

Forna F et al: Emergency peripartum hysterectomy: A comparison of cesarean and postpartum hysterectomy, *Am J Obstet Gynecol* 190(5):1440-1444, 2004.

Golombeck K et al: Maternal morbidity after maternal-fetal surgery, *Am J Obstet Gynecol* 194(3):834-839, 2006.

Hall, LF et al: Obesity and pregnancy, *Obstet Gynecol Surv* 60(4):253-260, 2005.

Harter P, du Bois A: The role of surgery in ovarian cancer with special emphasis on cytoreductive surgery for recurrence, *Curr Opin Oncol* 17(5):505-514, 2005.

Kobayashi Y et al: A case of successful pregnancy after treatment of invasive cervical cancer with systemic chemotherapy and conization, *Gynecologic Oncol* 100(1):213-215, 2006.

Lee, S et al: Fetal pain: A systematic multidisciplinary review of the evidence, *JAMA* 294(8):947-954, 2005.

Lim, AC et al: Pregnancy after uterine rupture: A report of 5 cases and a review of the literature, *Obstet Gynecol Surv* 60(9):613-617, 2005.

Lingman G: Management of pregnancy and labour in cases diagnosed with major fetal malformation, *Curr Opin Obstet Gynecol* 17(2):143-146, 2005.

Lo B: HPV vaccine and adolescents' sexual activity, *BMJ* 332(7550):1106-1107, 2006.

[10]Mattox KL, Goetzl L: Trauma in pregnancy, *Crit Care Med* 33(10):S385-389, 005.

Lotgering FK et al: Outcome after transabdominal cervicoisthmic cerclage, *Obst Gynecol* 107(4):779-784, 2006.

Mattox KL, Goetzl L: Trauma in pregnancy, *Crit Care Med* 33(10 Suppl):S385-S389, 2005.

McDonough PG: Evidence-based models for clinical care in pediatric and adolescent gynecology, *J Pediatr Adolesc Gynecol* 18(2):71-73, 2005.

Menon U: Ovarian cancer screening, *Can Med Assoc J* 171(4):323-324, 2004.

Minkoff H et al: Ethical dimensions of elective primary cesarean delivery, *Obstet Gynecol* 103(2):387-392, 2004.

Morrison J: Advances in the understanding and treatment of ovarian cancer, *J Brit Menopause Soc* 11(2):66-71, 2005.

Olshen E et al: Parental acceptance of the human papillomavirus vaccine, *J Adolesc Health* 37(3):248-251, 2005.

Quintero RA: Management of twin-twin transfusion syndrome in pregnancies with iatrogenic detachment of membranes following therapeutic amniocentesis and the role of interim amniopatch, *Ultrasound Obstet Gynecol* 26(6):628-633, 2005.

Robinson M: Frontiers in fetal surgery anesthesia, *Int Anesth Clin* 44(1):1-15, 2006.

Romero R et al: The role of cervical cerclage in obstetric practice: Can the patient who could benefit from this procedure be identified? *Am J Obstet Gynecol* 194(1):1-9, 2006.

Sanfilippo JS: How far reaching is pediatric adolescent gynecology? Just ask the Surgeon General, *J Pediatr Adolesc Gynecol* 17(1):1-2, 2004.

Santin A et al: Therapeutic vaccines for cervical cancer: Dendritic cell-based immunotherapy, *Curr Pharm Design* 11(27):3485-3500, 2005.

Shepherd JH: Uterus-conserving surgery for invasive cervical cancer, *Best Pract Res Clin Obstet Gynaecol* 19(4):577-590, 2005.

Spies JB et al: Recent advances in uterine fibroid embolization, *Curr Opin Obstet Gynecol* 17(6):562-567, 2005.

Sun S et al: Is sexual maturity occurring earlier among U.S. children? *J Adolesc Health* 37(5):345-355, 2005.

Tournigand C: Intraperitoneal chemotherapy in ovarian cancer: Who and when? *Curr Opin Obstet Gynecol* 17(1):83-86, 2005.

Vidaeff AC, Ramin SM: From concept to practice: The recent history of preterm delivery prevention. Part I: cervical competence, *Am J Perinatol* 23(1):3-13, 2006.

Chapter **35**

Urologic Surgery

CHAPTER OBJECTIVES

After studying this chapter, the learner will be able to:
- Identify the organs of the male genitourinary system.
- Compare the differences between male and female urinary systems.
- Describe the procedures performed for urinary incontinence.
- Describe the procedures performed for prostate cancer.

CHAPTER OUTLINE

KEY TERMS AND DEFINITIONS

Extraperitoneal   Outside the peritoneal cavity.
Hemolyze   Blood cells dissolve releasing hemoglobin.
Hyponatremia   Low salt concentration of the blood.
Impotence   Inability to have an erection.
Isosmotic   Solution having the same osmotic pressure as blood.
Litho-   Stone.
Meatotomy   Incising the meatus (distal opening) of the urethra.
Retroperitoneal   Behind the peritoneal cavity.
Transurethral   Through the urethral canal.

SUPPLEMENTAL MATERIAL ON EVOLVE WEBSITE   *evolve*

http://evolve.elsevier.com/BerryKohn
- Content Updates
- Glossary
- Full Set of Perioperative Flash Cards
- Interactive Key Term Flash Cards
- Tips for the Scrub Person and the Circulating Nurse: Hypospadius, Orchiopexy
- Student Activities
- WebLinks

HISTORICAL BACKGROUND

Writings from approximately 3000 BC tell of urinary diseases. The earliest known specimen of a bladder stone was found in an Egyptian grave that dates back to 4000 BC. People in India are known to have suffered from bladder stones around 2000 BC. Removal of a stone from the bladder through an incision is one of the earliest known surgical procedures. It was often performed by itinerant lithotomists, who flourished from the time of Hippocrates to the early eighteenth century. Hippocrates wrote that stone removal should be left to those trained for such work. For centuries this surgical procedure was not considered a part of medicine.

Although enlarged prostate glands were noted in the time of Hippocrates, attempts to remove part of them perineally or to tunnel through them with a sharp instrument were extremely dangerous.

Urethral sounds and bronze catheters have been found in the ruins of Pompeii, buried since AD 79. Metal catheters were used until the advent of rubber ones in the late nineteenth century.

The first urologists were mainly venereologists and instrumenteurs of the urethra. Urology advanced as a science with the invention of the microscope in the seventeenth century. Attempts to visualize the interior of the bladder were not made until the early nineteenth century, and the instruments and source of light were inadequate. In 1877 Maximilian Nitze (1848-1906), a German urologist, developed an electrically illuminated operating endoscope that is the basis of the modern cystoscope and urologic endoscopy. He systematically cauterized urinary tract tumors without using a fluid medium for bladder distention. He also authored an important monograph in 1889 that was dedicated to cystoscopy in patient care.

Urologists have contributed to the evolution of medicine in general. The use of antibacterial drugs by urologists freed internal medicine physicians from the time-consuming treatment of venereal disease. Urology has been and continues to be a supporting specialty within medicine and surgery and is interdependent with other specialties.

Urology is defined as that branch of medicine and surgery concerned with the study, diagnosis, and treatment of abnormalities and diseases of the urogenital tract of the male and the urinary tract of the female throughout the life span. Because of the shared responsibility in patient care with pediatricians, internists, nephrologists, endocrinologists, surgeons, plastic reconstructionists, and oncologists, close association with specialists in these disciplines is essential.

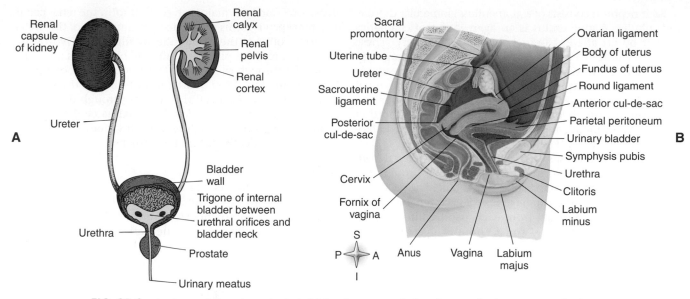

FIG. 35-1   Anatomy of the urinary tract. **A,** Male urinary tract. **B,** Female reproductive organs and urinary system.
*(**B,** From Thibodeau GA, Patton KT: Anatomy and physiology, ed 5, St. Louis, 2007, Mosby.)*

ANATOMY AND PHYSIOLOGY OF THE URINARY SYSTEM

The urinary system provides the vital life-sustaining functions of extracting waste products from the bloodstream and excreting them from the body. Organs of this system include bilateral kidneys and ureters, the bladder, and the urethra (Fig. 35-1). An obstruction to blood flow in the renal arteries or in any part of the urinary system can cause renal damage, which ultimately results in uremia (a biochemical imbalance) or renal failure if left undiagnosed and untreated. Vascular hypertension, tumors, infection, trauma, and other systemic or neurogenic disorders are of major concern to a urologist.

Kidneys

The kidneys are large, bean-shaped, glandular organs located bilaterally in the retroperitoneal space of the thoracolumbar region behind the abdominal cavity. The arterial blood supply (renal artery) of the kidney originates from the aorta and enters the hilum on the medial aspect. Venous drainage flows through the renal vein and into the inferior vena cava. The lymphatics drain into the lumbar nodes.

Each kidney is enclosed in a thin, fibrous capsule referred to as Gerota's fascia. The renal parenchyma, the substance of the kidney within the capsule, is composed of an external cortex and internal medulla. The medulla consists of conical segments called renal pyramids. Each pyramid and its surrounding cortex form a lobe. Within these pyramids are the essential components of renal function: the nephrons (Fig. 35-2). As the urine forms, it drips from the papillae at the tips of the pyramidal structures.

Ren is the Latin word for kidney—hence the adjective renal and combining forms of *ren-* and *reno-* in terms pertaining to the kidney as part of the renal system. The purposes of the kidney are as follows:

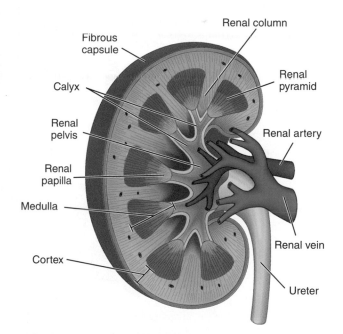

FIG. 35-2   Cross section of the kidney.
(From Thibodeau GA, Patton KT: Anatomy and physiology, ed 5, St. Louis, 2007, Mosby.)

- To remove metabolic waste, excess substances, and toxic substances from the blood
- To regulate and maintain body fluid and pH balance
- To help regulate and respond to blood pressure by producing the hormone renin
- To produce the hormone erythropoietin to control the rate red blood cells are produced by the bone marrow
- To assist in the production of water-soluble vitamin D, which is important for the metabolism of calcium

Each nephron consists of a glomerulus, glomerular capsule, and tubules. A glomerulus is an aggregation of capillaries formed by an afferent branch of the renal artery. These capillaries unite to form an efferent vessel. This capillary network is enclosed in a glomerular capsule (capsule of Bowman), which is the dilated beginning of the renal tubule. From the capsule, the tubule becomes tortuous and forms the proximal convoluted tubule. The distal portion forms the descending and ascending limbs of the medullary loop (loop of Henle) (Fig. 35-3).

Nitrogenous wastes, salts, toxins, and water filtered from the capillary network form urine, which flows through the medullary loop and into the collecting tubule. The collecting tubules converge at the papilla (apex) of each renal pyramid. Urine flows continuously from each papilla into a calyx. Each kidney has between 4 and 13 minor calyces that lead into 2 or 3 (rarely 4) major calyces that form the renal pelvis. The renal pelvis forms the dilated proximal end of the ureter.

Urine forms at the glomerulus by filtration. Hydrostatic pressure forces the plasma minus the blood cells and large molecules through the system. The amount of blood filtered is approximately 1700 quarts, from which is derived 200 quarts of filtrate. As this filtrate passes through the tubules, 99% of the water is resorbed and approximately 1 to 2 quarts of urine are produced. Failure of both kidneys to function is followed by death within a few weeks.

Ureters

The ureters are connecting tubes between the kidneys and bladder; they are 4 to 5 mm in diameter, have a 0.2- to 1-cm lumen, and are approximately 12 inches (25 to 30 cm) long. They lie bilaterally beneath the parietal peritoneum and

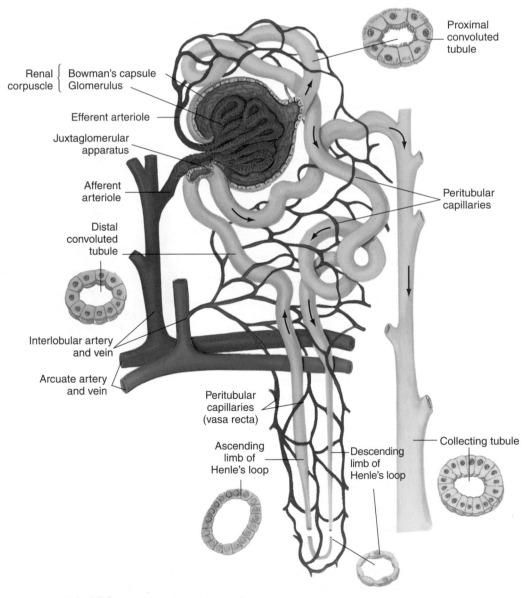

FIG. 35-3   Cross section of the nephron.
(From Thibodeau GA, Patton KT: Anatomy and physiology, *ed 5, St. Louis, 2007, Mosby.)*

descend along the posterior abdominal wall to the pelvic brim. From there, they pass along the lateral wall of the pelvis and curve downward, forward, and inward along the pelvic floor to the bladder. The wall of each ureter is continuous with the renal pelvis and is composed of mucous membrane, longitudinal and circular muscles, and an outer layer of fibrous and elastic tissue. Slow, rhythmic, peristaltic contractions carry urine from the kidneys to the bladder.

Urinary Bladder

The bladder is a hollow muscular reservoir lined with mucous membrane; it is located extraperitoneally in the anterior pelvic cavity behind the symphysis pubis. The ureters enter the bladder wall obliquely on each side. The triangular area between the ureteral and urethral orifices is called the trigone. Valves formed by folds of mucous membrane in the bladder wall prevent the backflow of urine into the ureters. Urine collects in the bladder until an autonomic nerve stimulus from the sacral reflex centers causes micturition (urination) through the urethra. This stimulus opens the muscle fibers that form an internal sphincter at the bladder neck, the vesicourethral junction.

The arterial supply of the urinary bladder is derived from the hypogastric arteries that branch from the internal iliac arteries. The venous drainage empties into the hypogastric veins. The lymphatics drain into the internal and common iliac nodes.

The autonomic innervation of the bladder controls filling and emptying of the bladder. The parasympathetic fibers from S3 to S5 promote emptying by contraction of the detrusor muscles. The sympathetic nerve fibers that originate from L1 to L2 cause relaxation of the detrusor muscles and closure of the internal urinary sphincter, allowing the bladder to fill. Somatic innervation of the external urinary sphincter responds to somatic fibers arising from S2 to S4 and is voluntarily controlled to contract the musculature. Spinal cord injury at or below the level of L5 can result in inability to empty the bladder.

Urethra

The male urethra is approximately 25 to 30 cm long and has a diameter of 7 to 10 mm. It consists of two segments (proximal and distal) that are further subdivided into three segments referred to as the prostatic, the membranous, and the cavernous urethral segments. The proximal (posterior) prostatic urethra passes from the bladder orifice, through the prostate gland, and to the pelvic floor. The membranous urethra passes from the pelvic floor to the base of the penis. The distal (anterior) segment consists of parts of the membranous, bulbous, and anterior urethral segments that pass through the penis to the external urethral orifice. The membranous and anterior urethras also serve as a passageway for secretions from the male reproductive system (see Fig. 35-1, *A*).

The female urethra is approximately 3 to 5 cm long and 6 to 8 mm in diameter. It is firmly embedded posterior to the clitoris and anterior to the vaginal opening. Females are predisposed to urinary tract infections because the urethra is anatomically located near the vagina and the anus, both of which have resident flora that can cause infection if introduced into the urethra. Mechanical injury during coitus

and the use of a pessary for vaginal support or diaphragm for contraception may be contributing factors to chronic urinary tract infection (see Fig. 35-1, *B*).

SPECIAL FEATURES OF UROLOGIC SURGERY
Urologic Endoscopy

Cystoscopic diagnostic procedures and some conservative urologic procedures approached through the urethra are performed in a specially designed and equipped area that is often referred to as the cysto room or suite. This area may be located within the operating room (OR) suite or in the urology clinic. Radiographic control booths and developing units are located adjacent to or within the area. Because radiographic procedures are often performed, the walls and doors of the room should be lined with lead and personnel remaining in the room with the patient during radiographs or fluoroscopy should wear lead aprons. Patients should be protected with gonadal and thyroid shields whenever feasible.

To protect the welfare of the patients and personnel, all safety regulations apply in the cysto room as they do elsewhere in the OR suite. All lighted instruments and electrical equipment should be checked for proper function before and after each use. Excess fluid should not be permitted to accumulate on the floor.

Proper OR attire is worn by all personnel entering the room. Personal protective equipment such as eyewear and masks should be worn if there is a possibility of splash or aerosolization. Many urologists don a water-repellant apron before scrubbing. It is recommended that the urologist wear a sterile gown and sterile gloves. Procedures performed in the cysto room should be performed as in a sterile field to prevent introducing microorganisms into the patient. Adherence to the principles of aseptic technique should be practiced to prevent urinary tract infection.

Urologic Bed

A urologic bed differs from the standard operating bed in that it provides a radiograph-compatible base, a drainage system, and lithotomy knee supports with safety belts (Fig. 35-4).

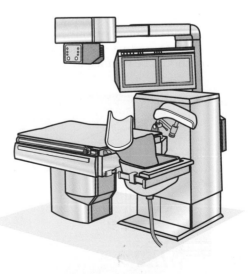

FIG. 35-4 Urologic bed.

Some urologic beds incorporate electrosurgical units (ESUs). Urologic radiographic studies use conventional radiographs, fluoroscopy and image intensification, and tomography. The imaging system is an integral part of the urologic bed. Some beds have a built-in automatic film-handling system, others have a film cassette holder, and others adapt to a C-arm.

The drainage system may have a drainage pan with tubing to drain port or single-use drainage bags. Under-knee/calf supports with gel pads and Velcro straps provide patient comfort in the lithotomy position (Fig. 35-5). Urologic beds are equipped with hydraulic or electric controls to adjust height and tilt. Some have tray attachments for the light source and auxiliary ESU, as well as hooks for irrigating solution bags.

Patient Preparation for a Cystoscopic Examination

1. Unless the procedure will be performed with the patient under general or regional anesthesia, the patient may be encouraged to drink fluids before coming to the cysto room. Fluids ensure rapid collection of a urine specimen from the kidneys. Some tests require the ability to void for bladder strength studies or while contrast medium passes through the urinary system. Electromyographic (EMG) data may be gathered during the process.
2. Intraurethral procedures are often performed with topical agents or local infiltration anesthetics. The patient should be reassured that the procedure usually can be performed with only mild discomfort. Respect the patient's modesty by providing appropriate drapes and keeping the cysto room door closed.
3. The patient is assisted into the lithotomy position with the knees resting in padded knee supports or stirrups. Gel pads behind the legs and knees help avoid undue pressure in popliteal spaces. Velcro straps are used to secure the patient's legs. Some cystoscopic procedures are performed with the male patient in the supine position.
4. The drainage pan is pulled out of the lower break of the urologic bed after the patient's legs have been positioned on knee supports and the foot of the bed has been lowered.
5. The pubic region, external genitalia, and perineum are mechanically and chemically cleansed with an antiseptic agent according to routine skin preparation procedure. The solution should be warmed according to the manu-

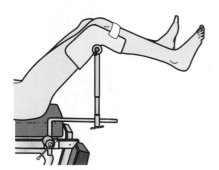

FIG. 35-5 Knee crutch stirrup commonly used with urologic table.

facturer's recommendations before it is applied to an unanesthetized patient. To prevent burns, the temperature of the solution should not exceed 110° F (44° C). Scrub soaps can be diluted with warmed sterile saline or water.

6. Topical anesthetic agents are instilled into the urethra at the end of the prep procedure. A viscous liquid or jelly preparation of lidocaine hydrochloride, 1% or 2%, may be used. This medium remains in the urethra rather than flowing into the bladder.
   a. For the female: The female urethra is most sensitive at the meatus. A small, sterile cotton-tipped applicator dipped into the anesthetic gel and placed in the meatus is sufficient anesthesia for local urethral procedures. The applicator is removed when the urologist is ready to introduce an instrument. Cone-shaped syringes are commercially available for intraurethral instillation of local lidocaine 2% jelly.
   b. For the male: A disposable cylinder with an acorn tip can be used for intraurethral insertion. The agent is injected into the urethra, and the penis is compressed with a penile clamp for a few minutes to retain the drug.
7. A sterile stainless steel filter screen is placed over the drainage pan. The patient is draped as for other perineal procedures in the lithotomy position. The urologist may need to have access to the rectum. The perineal sheet has two fenestrations: one exposes the genitalia, and the other fits over the screen on the drainage pan. A gauze filter is incorporated into this latter fenestration to capture resected tissue.

The urologist may prefer to wear a sterile disposable plastic apron over his or her gown. The apron is attached to the bed, which provides a sterile field from the urologic bed to the urologist's shoulders. A receptor kit that attaches to the apron eliminates the need for the drainage pan. Tissue specimens are collected as irrigating fluid passes through a collecting basket.

Urologic Endoscopes

Urologic endoscopic instruments and catheters are available in sizes to suit infants, children, and adults. The sizes of these instruments and catheters are measured on the French (Fr) scale: the diameter in millimeters (mm) multiplied by 3. The smallest ureteral catheter is 1 mm in diameter, or 3 Fr; the largest is 14 Fr.

Each type of procedure requires specific endoscopic equipment. All rigid urologic endoscopes have the same basic components, which are discussed in the following sections (Fig. 35-6).

Sheath. The hollow sheath, through which the urologic endoscope passes, may be concave, convex, or straight in configuration at the distal end (the end inserted into the urethra) (Fig. 35-7). The other end has a stopcock attachment for irrigation. Sheath sizes range from 11 Fr for infants to 30 Fr for adults. Space is provided within the sheath to accommodate instruments for work in the bladder or urethra. Other instruments and catheters can be inserted through the sheath into the ureters and/or kidneys for diagnostic or therapeutic procedures.

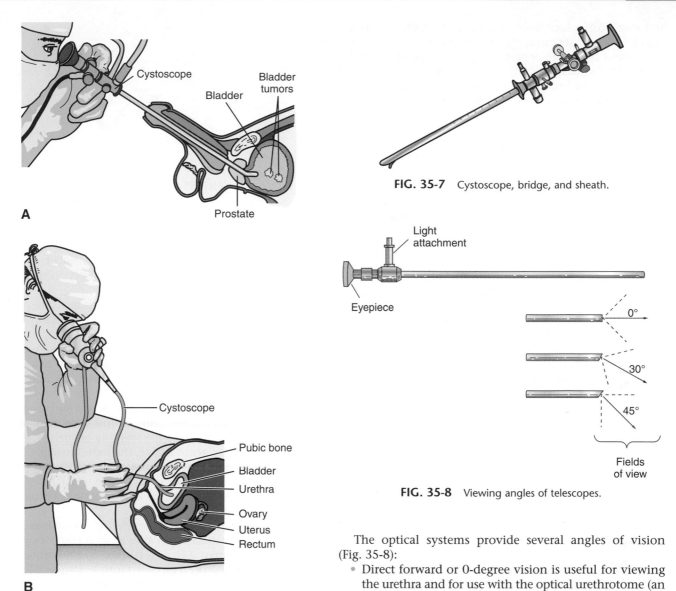

A

FIG. 35-7 Cystoscope, bridge, and sheath.

B

FIG. 35-6 **A,** Rigid cystoscopy. **B,** Flexible cystoscopy.

FIG. 35-8 Viewing angles of telescopes.

Obturator. The stainless steel obturator, which is inserted into the sheath, occludes the opening of the sheath and facilitates introduction into the urethra without trauma to the mucosal lining.

Telescope. Telescopes are complex precision optical systems; they are costly, delicate instruments that are handled gently at all times. Each telescope contains multiple, finely ground optical lenses that relay the image from the distal end inside the bladder or urethra to the ocular (eyepiece) used by the urologist to view internal structures. Additional rod-shaped elements (i.e., field lenses) are located between each pair of relay lenses. Properly spaced throughout the length of the telescope, the lenses provide undistorted and clear vision at the desired angle and with some magnification. All telescopes are stainless steel and have a Bakelite ocular. Some telescopes have operating or working elements incorporated into them.

The optical systems provide several angles of vision (Fig. 35-8):

• Direct forward or 0-degree vision is useful for viewing the urethra and for use with the optical urethrotome (an instrument for sharp resection of tissue in the urethra).
• Right-angle or 30-degree vision is most suitable for viewing the entire bladder and for insertion of ureteral catheters.
• Lateral, which deviates 70 degrees but includes an additional visual field at a right angle in the line of vision, is used for wide-angle viewing within the bladder.
• Foroblique, which is a forward vision with an oblique view somewhat in front of a right angle, is used to examine the urethra and for transurethral surgical procedures.
• Retrospective, which provides an approximate 55-degree angle of retrograde vision, is used to inspect the bladder neck.

Light Source. The light source is a fiberoptic bundle and may be an integral part of the sheath or the telescope. A cable connects the instrument to a fiberoptic light source.

Types of Urologic Endoscopes
Many different types of urologic endoscopes and accessories are used, including nephroscopes introduced into the kidney

and cystoscopes introduced through the urethra into the bladder. Before instrumentation is placed on the sterile instrument table, the preferred type and size of the endoscope for the examination and/or treatment should be verified with the urologist. The endoscopes and accessories most commonly used in the cysto room are described in the following sections.

Brown-Buerger Cystoscope. The stainless steel sheaths of the Brown-Buerger cystoscope range in size from 14 to 26 Fr. Used most often in adults is the size 21 Fr with a right-angle examination telescope for routine inspection of the bladder. Size 24 or 26 Fr is used to accommodate larger instruments and catheters that cannot be used through size 21 Fr. The sheath contains the light carrier.

A Brown-Buerger cystoscope set usually consists of two sheaths—one concave and one convex, each with its own obturator—and two or three right-angle telescopes. Along with the basic examination telescope, the set may have a combination operating and double catheterizing telescope (i.e., a convertible telescope), or the operating and double catheterizing functions may be in separate telescopes. The convertible operating and catheterizing telescopes have a small, deflectable lever on the distal end to aid in directing ureteral catheters or flexible stone baskets into the ureters. All corresponding parts of each set must be the same French size.

McCarthy Panendoscope. The stainless steel sheaths of the McCarthy panendoscope range in size from 14 to 30 Fr. These are used most often with the foreoblique telescope for viewing the urethra. Other telescopes are available for bladder visualization. The telescopes are interchangeable with all sizes of sheaths. A bridge assembly is required to fit the telescope properly to the sheath. The light is supplied through the telescope.

Wappler Cystourethroscope. The Wappler cystourethroscope combines the functions of the Brown-Buerger cystoscope and the McCarthy panendoscope. The stainless steel sheaths range in size from 17 to 24 Fr. The foreoblique and lateral telescopes, which also supply the light, are interchangeable with all sheaths. A visual obturator may be used to permit visualization and irrigation during the introduction of the sheath into the urethra.

Resectoscope. The resectoscope uses electric current to excise tissue from the bladder, urethra, or prostate (Fig. 35-9). Components of this instrument include the sheath, obturator, telescope, working element, and cutting electrode. The sheath, usually 24 to 28 Fr, is made of Bakelite or fiberglass to prevent a short circuit of the electric current. If the short beak post sheath is used with a wide-angle telescope, a Timberlake obturator is used to introduce the sheath into the urethra.

The working element of the resectoscope, which is inserted through the sheath, has a channel for the telescope and cutting electrode. The types of working elements differ by the method in which the cutting electrode moves:

- The Iglesias resectoscope uses a thumb control on a leaf spring–lock mechanism. The working element can

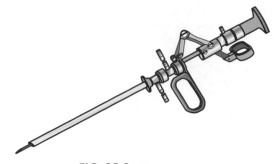

FIG. 35-9   Resectoscope.

be adapted for simultaneous irrigation and suction to control hydraulic pressure in the bladder.
- The Nesbit resectoscope uses a thumb control on a spring.
- The Baumrucker resectoscope uses finger control on a sliding mechanism.
- The Stern-McCarthy resectoscope uses a rack and pinion to move the loop forward and back. This requires two hands.

The cutting electrode is the most critical component of a resectoscope. Because it cuts and coagulates tissue, the electrode must be stabilized in the working element so it retracts properly into the sheath after each cut. The electrode has a cutting loop from which electric current is passed through tissue, an insulated fork, an insulated stem, and a contact that is inserted into the working element.

Several loop sizes are available; the stem is usually color-coded by size. Loop size corresponds to the French size of the sheath. The electrode is malleable and therefore is checked before use to be certain the insulation is intact and the loop is not broken.

Electric current is applied only when the loop is engaged in tissue, and it is inactivated after a cut is completed. The sheath can be charred if electric current is maintained after the cutting loop has been retracted into it. Disposable loop electrodes are commercially available and are preferred for use by most urologists.

Conductive lubricants may provide a pathway for electric current and therefore should never be used on the sheath. Cleanliness of the sheath and all other components is essential to proper function.

Endoscopic Accessories

Ureteral catheters, bougies, filiforms and followers, stone baskets, and sounds are commonly used by urologist-endoscopists. Other accessories, such as retractable baskets and graspers, are used to remove tissue or calculi (stones).

Electrodes. In addition to the cutting loops used with the resectoscope, primarily for transurethral resection (TUR), other types of electrodes with tips of various shapes are used in the bladder. One type, referred to as a Bugbee, is inserted through the operating telescope of the Brown-Buerger cystoscope or Wappler cystourethroscope. The Bugbee is used mainly for fulguration of bladder tumors, coagulation of bladder vessels to control bleeding after biopsy, and ureteral meatotomy. More electric current is needed when working in solution (as in the bladder) than when working in air.

A spark-gap generator is commonly used for transurethral resection and fulguration. A spark-gap ESU requires high-voltage arcing, which is described as spray coagulation. Spark-gap generator use requires the patient to be grounded with a grounding pad. The power control settings on the ESU should be as low as possible. Recommended practices as suggested by the Association of periOperative Registered Nurse (AORN) for the use and care of electrosurgical equipment (e.g., dispersive electrodes) apply also to urologic procedures. Additional information about electrosurgical units can be found in Chapter 20.

Lasers. Argon, neodymium:yttrium aluminum garnet (Nd:YAG), and holmium (Ho):YAG lasers can be adapted for use with urologic endoscopes. These are particularly useful for the ablation of hemangiomas and vascular tumors in the bladder and kidneys. The argon-pumped tunable dye laser is used for photodynamic therapy on solid bladder tumors. A flash lamp-pulsed dye laser will fragment a calculus in a ureter.

Lasers used through endoscopes require most of the same equipment as needed for standard urologic endoscopy. The bladder expansion medium can be either saline or water to create the working space because unlike with the ESU and electrodes, no ionic charge is emitted from the laser.

Irrigating Equipment. Continuous irrigation of the bladder is necessary during cystoscopy to do the following:
- Distend bladder walls so the urologist can visualize them
- Wash out blood, bits of resected tissue, or stone fragments to permit continuous visibility and collection of specimens

A sterile, disposable, and closed irrigating system is used because it prevents airborne contamination of the solution. The tubing is Y shaped (Fig. 35-10). Two or more liters of sterile irrigating solution may be needed for a single examination. Disposable tandem sets may be used to connect several containers together. Tandem sets allow for a continuous flow and for replacement of containers without interruption of flow.

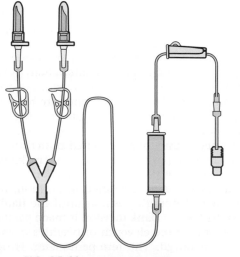

FIG. 35-10 Y-tubing for cystoscopy.

Sterile disposable irrigating tubing is connected to the irrigating solution container before it is hung on a hook on the urologic bed, in the ceiling, or on a stand placed beside the bed. The solution container should be at a level 2½ feet (0.75 m) above the bed; a lower level decreases flow, and a higher level increases hydraulic pressure with consequent fluid absorption by the tissues of the patient. Tubing should be filled with solution before being attached to the sheath of the cystoscope or resectoscope. The plastic tubing from the container to the instrument is for individual patient use only and is discarded after use.

Sterile isosmotic irrigating solutions that are nonhemolytic and nonelectrolytic are generally preferred by most urologists. Sterile distilled water may be used for visualization procedures and during resection or fulguration of bladder tumors with an ESU. Water may hemolyze red blood cells if a sufficient amount enters the circulation through open blood vessels. As much as 3 to 6 L of solution may be absorbed during a transurethral prostatectomy.

Saline is contraindicated for use with a monopolar ESU because the minerals in saline act as a conductor and disperse the current when the ESU is used.

Isosmotic solutions of 1.5% glycine (an amino acid) or sorbitol (an inert sugar) premixed in distilled water are commercially available in 1.5- and 3-L containers.

Glycine solution is sometimes used for TUR with an ESU; however, it can cause serious complications in some patients. Overabsorption of glycine can occur during TUR, causing water intoxication with resultant hyponatremia and acid-base imbalance (acidosis). This process has been called transurethral resection syndrome hallmarked by dilutional hyponatremia.

During a cystoscopy procedure, the flow of solution into the endoscope is controlled by the stopcock on the sheath where the tubing attaches. Rubber tips or sealing caps are used to seal other openings on the instrument to prevent solution from escaping during a procedure. The openings through which catheters or instruments are to be inserted are closed with rubber caps that have a central hole. The accessory can be inserted through this hole with the seal maintained. Silicone caps should be used instead of rubber caps if the patient or surgeon has a latex sensitivity.

The irrigating solution flows away from the instrument and into the drainage pan through the filter screen when the urologist needs to divert the flow. Solution drains from the pan, through the tubing, and into a collecting container that is emptied after each patient use. Some older cysto rooms have floor drains, which are a source of environmental contamination unless cleaned thoroughly. If large quantities of solution are used, the level of drainage into the container should be observed to prevent overflow onto the floor or around the foot pedal of the ESU, which can be an electrocution hazard.

Evacuators. Evacuators may be attached to the endoscope to irrigate the bladder and to aspirate stone fragments, blood clots, or resected tissue. Stone or tissue fragments collected in the evacuator are retrieved and sent to the pathology laboratory. The two most commonly used types are the Ellik evacuator and the Toomey evacuator:

- *Ellik evacuator.* The Ellik evacuator is a double bowl-shaped glass or firm disposable plastic receptacle (Fig. 35-11). It contains a trap for fragments so they cannot be washed back into the sheath of the endoscope during irrigation with pressure on the compression-bulb attachment.
- *Toomey evacuator.* The Toomey evacuator is a syringe-type evacuator with a wide opening into the barrel (Fig. 35-12). It may be used with any endoscope sheath. A metal adapter permits its use with a catheter.

Care and Preventive Maintenance of Urologic Endoscopes

1. Sterilization is preferred, although high-level disinfection with 2% glutaraldehyde is commonly used. Endoscopes and reusable accessories must be free of debris and residue for sterilization and/or high-level disinfection techniques to be effective.
   a. Disassemble all parts, and open all outlets.
   b. Clean all parts in an appropriate liquid detergent solution. Clean the interior of sheaths and openings with a soft brush.
   c. Rinse in clean water, and dry thoroughly.
   d. Wipe lenses gently with a soft, dry cloth.
2. After cleaning, place endoscopes on a towel to drain. With air, blow-dry the lumens. Moisture in the channels can dilute chemical sterilants and, if ethylene oxide is used, will form ethylene glycol, which is toxic to tissues.
3. Check the function of all moving parts, the clarity of vision through telescopes, and the patency of channels through instruments and catheters.
4. Keep sets of sounds, bougies, and filiforms and followers together so the urologist has a complete range of sizes readily accessible.
5. Wrap items for sterilization after cleaning. Flexible instruments should be protected by a rigid container.

6. Clean and dry stone baskets before sterilizing by low-temperature sterilization methods, such as plasma vapor, peracetic acid, or ethylene oxide. Retractable stone baskets are sterilized in the open position.
7. The principles and methods of sterilization apply to urologic endoscopy equipment.
8. Endoscopic processors and sterilizers, such as the STERIS unit, are useful for sterilizing instrumentation between patient uses. The instrumentation is used immediately after processing and is not stored in the processing tray.
9. If sterilization between patient uses is not feasible, high-level disinfection may be the method of choice for processing urologic endoscopic instruments.

SURGICAL PROCEDURES OF THE GENITOURINARY SYSTEM

Most patients commonly seen by urologists are in the preadolescent or older age-groups. Congenital and common pediatric problems are discussed in Chapter 8. This chapter focuses on adult problems, most of which occur in men older than 50 years who have prostatic disease and women who have urinary incontinence.

An open surgical procedure is performed only after conservative treatment fails or examination of the genitourinary (GU) tract confirms a condition that does not yield to treatment. Fortunately, most urologic conditions can be diagnosed and treated conservatively through a urologic endoscope and its accessories. Some laparoscopic procedures are performed to obtain lymph nodes for biopsy. When a congenital or acquired condition does not respond to conservative therapy, the urologist performs open surgical procedures to repair, revise, reconstruct, or remove organs.

Obstructive and neuromuscular disorders are common problems in the urinary tract. Renal calculus disease and tumors in the urinary tract are most commonly diagnosed in middle age. These conditions may cause obstruction and subsequent infection in the kidneys, ureter, or bladder.

Kidney

Definitive renal surgical procedures are justified for the management of renal neoplasms, large cystic lesions that compromise renal function and/or produce obstruction, inflammatory diseases that necessitate drainage, or renal vascular disease. Chronic degenerative disease or severe traumatic injury can produce irreparable damage to renal cells. Computed tomography (CT) and magnetic resonance imaging (MRI) identify the site, size, and extent of tumor involvement. Ultrasonography and intravenous (IV) urograms differentiate among solid tumors, stones, and cystic disease. A radionuclide scan may indicate renal function; arteriograms and venograms indicate the extent of renal vascular disease.

The kidney is usually approached posteriorly with the patient in a lateral position (Fig. 35-13). The kidney rest is raised, and the bed is flexed until the flank muscles become tense. After the patient is secured in position, the bed is tilted in Trendelenburg's position until the flank is horizontal to the floor. A flank incision is made parallel to and just below or over the eleventh or twelfth rib; the twelfth rib may be removed. The retroperitoneum is opened to expose the kidney.

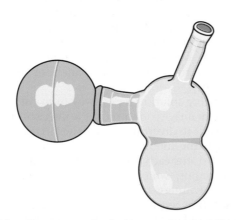

FIG. 35-11   Ellik evacuator for flushing prostate tissue from the bladder during transurethral resection of the prostate (TURP).

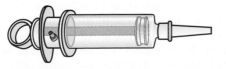

FIG. 35-12   Toomey irrigator.

The kidney can be approached anteriorly through a transverse, subcostal, or midline incision. A thoracoabdominal incision may be preferred in an obese patient or to reach a lesion in the upper pole of the kidney. These incisions, with the patient in the supine position, are often used for exposure of the aorta and vena cava for renovascular procedures. An anterior approach may be advantageous when prompt control of blood supply is important in renal trauma.

Nephrectomy. Removal of a lobe or the entire kidney is indicated when tumor, disease, or traumatic injury has resulted in the absence of renal function.

The entire kidney can be removed during a laparoscopic procedure. The organ is dissected, fragmented, and aspirated; vascular pedicles are stapled. This alternative technique is used primarily for benign renal disease.

Partial Nephrectomy or Heminephrectomy. Partial excision of the kidney may be sufficient when a lobe has been destroyed by localized disease or injury but the remainder of the kidney remains functional. The vascular supply to the segment to be removed must be identified, ligated, and divided. The parenchyma of the lobe is resected from the capsule by blunt dissection. The renal pelvis and remaining capsule are closed.

Radical Nephrectomy. In a radical nephrectomy, the renal vessels are dissected free, ligated, and divided. Prerenal fat and fascia are dissected to remove the kidney. The ureter is ligated and divided close to the bladder. The renal pedicle is ligated and divided, and the kidney is removed. Massive hemorrhage from the renal artery and veins is a potential complication, as is injury to adjacent structures (i.e., inferior vena cava, aorta, and duodenum on the right side or spleen on the left side).

A nephrectomy is performed in the OR on a living donor (unilateral) or on a cadaver donor (bilateral) to procure the kidney(s) for transplantation. Meticulous dissection is necessary to free the kidney, its blood vessels, and the ureter with minimal trauma. The ureter is dissected free and transected while the renal blood supply remains intact to ensure adequate urinary output. A kidney from a living-related donor may last longer than a kidney from a cadaver. Living donor kidney can be obtained by hand-assisted laparoscopy (HALS).

The left kidney is most commonly used for living related donor transplant because it is easier to access. The anatomy is more complex on the right side because of the renal vein structure and requires a longer surgical time, causing a longer scar. Studies are being conducted for right laparoscopic donor nephrectomy at the University of Alabama at Birmingham. Dr. Rizk El-Galley has developed a special angled clamp that permits HALS right nephrectomy by excising a cuff of vena cava with the renal vein for added length of the vessel.

Bilateral Nephrectomy. Removal of both kidneys may be indicated before transplantation in a patient maintained on chronic dialysis who has severe hypertension. If rejection is uncontrollable after kidney transplantation, the donor kidney may have to be explanted and the patient returned to chronic hemodialysis. This is less likely after transplantation from a live donor than from a cadaver.

Nephrostomy or Pyelostomy. An incision through the renal parenchyma or into the renal pelvis may be necessary to establish temporary or permanent drainage when an obstruction prevents the flow of urine from the kidney (Fig. 35-14). A tube placed in the kidney exits through the skin. A cutaneous nephrostomy tube may be used to drain a kidney postoperatively during healing after renal reconstruction or revascularization. Silastic tubes placed internally through a cystoscope via the ureter eliminate the need for an open surgical procedure for a temporary urinary diversion.

More commonly, temporary urinary diversion is performed percutaneously under fluoroscopic or ultrasound guidance by a radiologist and/or urologist. A plastic disc is applied to the skin to secure the catheter, which is attached to a drainage bag in a manner to prevent tension. The tubing may be connected to a leg bag to avoid tension on the catheter during ambulation.

Pyeloplasty. Revision or reconstruction of the renal pelvis is performed to relieve an anatomic obstruction in the flow of urine by creating a larger outlet from the renal pelvis into the ureter. This may be performed to repair or excise damaged tissue so that kidney function will be restored without a partial or total nephrectomy.

Either a rigid or a flexible fiberoptic nephroscope may be used to visually inspect the renal collecting system. A laser fiber may be used to ablate some tumors.

Renal Revascularization. Stenotic lesions of renal arteries are surgically correctable causes of hypertension. Renovascular reconstructive procedures (renal angioplasty) are designed either to improve blood flow through the stenotic area to the kidney or to bypass the stenotic area.

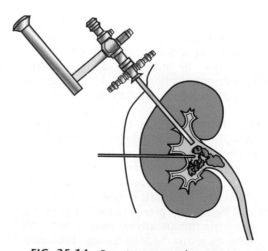

FIG. 35-14 Percutaneous nephrostomy.

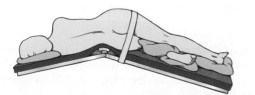

FIG. 35-13 Surgical position for open kidney procedure.

Revascularization procedures may have a dual purpose: to correct hypertension and to preserve renal function. The patient is placed in the supine position for these procedures because the renal arteries are approached through an abdominal incision.

In Situ Vascular Reconstructive Techniques. Obstruction of the renal artery most often occurs as a result of atherosclerotic stenosis at the origin of the artery or fibromuscular dysplasia (abnormal development) confined to the main renal artery. The obstruction is most often resected and replaced by an aortorenal saphenous vein bypass graft. A reversed segment of proximal saphenous vein, gently distended and irrigated, is anastomosed first to the aorta and then to the renal artery.

Prosthetic woven Dacron grafts may be used instead of an autogenous vein graft for renal artery bypass combined with distal aortic replacement. Segmental resection of diseased arterial segments with primary end-to-end anastomosis may be performed. Thromboendarterectomy is more often performed than is the latter procedure. All of these procedures may be performed bilaterally or as staged bilateral renal artery reconstructions. Percutaneous transluminal angioplasty may be preferred to these open procedures.

Ex Vivo Extracorporeal Kidney Surgery. When stenotic disease or another obstructive lesion extends into the branches of the renal artery, in situ reconstruction may be difficult, hazardous, or impossible. In these patients, a temporary nephrectomy with microvascular repair followed by autotransplantation of the kidney may be performed; this is referred to as workbench surgery. The kidney is completely mobilized from the retroperitoneal space. If one kidney is to be reconstructed, the ureter can remain intact and reconstruction is performed on a sterile bench (Mayo tray) placed over the patient's lower abdomen.

For a bilateral reconstruction, one kidney is detached from its ureter to permit complete removal from the abdomen. A second team works on the contralateral kidney in situ while the other kidney is reconstructed at an adjacent dissecting bench (table) ex vivo.

Extracorporeal perfusion is necessary for renal preservation during reconstruction. This may be accomplished either with perfusion of cold Ringer's lactate or other hyperosmolar solution by gravity flow or with a continuous hypothermic perfusion through a Belzer pump machine. A simple cold storage in saline slush may also be used for renal preservation. Dry ice is never used.

A kidney may be autotransplanted into the patient's pelvis for revascularization of the kidney, removal of renal tumors or calculi, or repair of ureteral injuries.

Traumatic Injury. Serious hemorrhage may result if a kidney is ruptured or injured by blunt trauma, a bullet, or a stab wound. This requires an immediate surgical procedure. The surgeon makes every effort to save kidney tissue and the ureter. A Foley catheter is inserted to keep an accurate record of urinary output and to check for the presence of hematuria preoperatively and postoperatively. Gross hematuria preoperatively usually indicates injury to the bladder or urethra. Kidney damage is diagnosed by the presence of blood seen microscopically.

Dialysis

End-stage renal disease and acute renal failure are potentially fatal conditions unless they can be controlled or reversed. Uremia and hypertension develop if renal failure is prolonged. Renal dialysis is the procedure of removing waste products and excess intravascular fluid from the body of a patient in acute or chronic renal failure by diffusion through a semipermeable membrane. This may be accomplished by either hemodialysis or peritoneal dialysis. The treatment modality alleviates the acute manifestations of uremia and controls many of the chronic long-term complications of end-stage renal disease.

Grossly undernourished and anemic patients with severe electrolyte imbalances must be adequately stabilized by dialysis before kidney transplantation. Some patients require dialysis for the remainder of their lives. Patients undergoing chronic dialysis must have a means of arterial-venous access established for long-term maintenance.

Patients with chronic renal failure can tolerate extensive surgical procedures with minimal complications. Their management in the OR must include strict attention to maintaining a patent hemodialysis access shunt, fistula, or catheter; careful monitoring of fluid and electrolyte balance; and the avoiding postoperative infections. After kidney transplantation, the patient may require postoperative dialysis; thus access must remain patent during and after the surgical procedure.

Hemodialysis. In hemodialysis, waste products are removed from the blood through the semipermeable membrane of a dialyzer (artificial kidney machine). An arteriovenous (AV) shunt or fistula is created subcutaneously in either an arm or a leg to provide access to the patient's circulation (Fig. 35-15). The Quinton-Scribner double-lumen shunt, developed in 1960, consists of two tips attached to tubing. One tip is placed in the artery and the other in a nearby vein. The tubing from each tip is exteriorized through a subcutaneous tunnel to form a loop. The arterial and venous blood mix in this shunt. Variations and modifications of this basic external shunt are used to create an AV conduit; some have self-sealing devices to minimize the potential problems of clotting and infection.

An anastomosis, usually between the radial artery and the cephalic vein in the forearm, creates an arterialized peripheral vein that permits dialyzer connections to be made by venipuncture. Needles are placed in the venous limb of the AV fistula for blood outflow and return (Fig. 35-16). The Brescia-Cimino radiocephalic AV fistula, first described in 1966, is easiest to construct and has the fewest complications. If creation of an AV fistula by direct anastomosis is not feasible, a biologic or synthetic graft may be interposed between the artery and the vein. Cryopreserved human vein, saphenous or other autologous vein, bovine carotid artery heterograft, and polytetrafluoroethylene (PTFE) grafts are used.

Peritoneal Dialysis. For acute, intermittent, or continuous peritoneal dialysis, a Tenckhoff silicone catheter is placed into the peritoneal cavity (Fig. 35-17). A paramedian incision generally is used to place a section of the catheter in subcutaneous tissue. The catheter has one or two

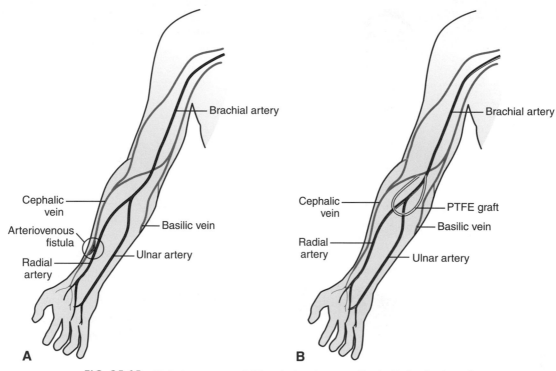

FIG. 35-15 Dialysis access modalities. **A,** Arteriovenous fistula. **B,** Synthetic graft.

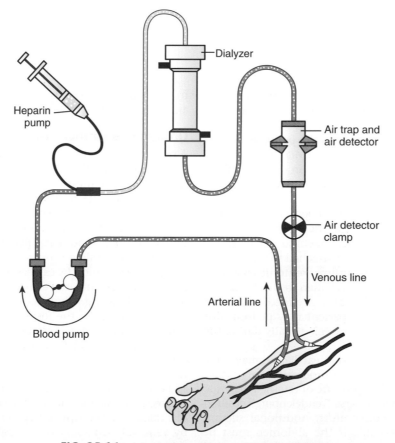

FIG. 35-16 Arteriovenous fistula and dialysis machine.

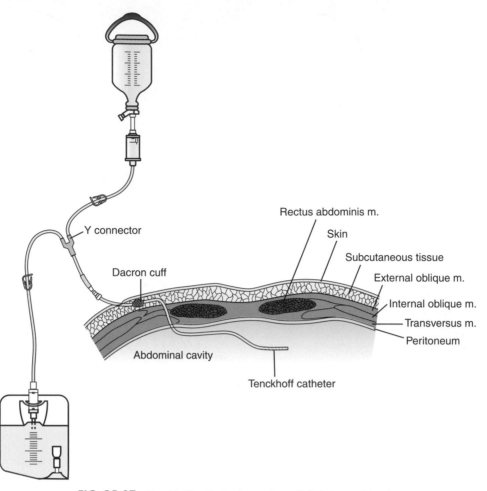

FIG. 35-17 Tenckhoff catheter for peritoneal dialysis. *m.,* Muscle.

synthetic fiber cuffs to anchor it in subcutaneous tissue and to block bacterial invasion along the catheter into the peritoneal cavity.

Dialysate is instilled over time into the peritoneal cavity to draw solutes from body fluids into the dialyzing solution across the peritoneal membrane. This process selectively removes electrolytes, metabolites, toxins, and water normally excreted by the kidneys.

Dialysate that has been warmed to body temperature is instilled, allowed to remain for a specified number of hours, and then withdrawn by a cycling machine or by gravity drainage. A Y-set disconnect system attached to the catheter allows separation of inflow and outflow. Peritonitis is always a potential complication. Infection is often treated by adding antibiotics to the dialysate. Heparin is added to prevent fibrin clots in the catheter. The patient may perform this routine at home several times per week, usually during the evening hours.

A patient being treated with peritoneal dialysis may come to the OR for an unrelated surgical procedure. Respiratory excursion may be impaired by pressure of retained dialysate under the diaphragm. A slight reverse Trendelenburg's position may alleviate respiratory discomfort. Additional suction containers should be available if the abdomen must be evacuated while the patient is in the OR. Fluid removed

from the peritoneal cavity is measured, and the appearance and volume are recorded on the intraoperative record.

Urolithiasis (Urinary Calculus)

A renal calculus (kidney stone) is a solid deposit or deposits of minerals and salts (Fig. 35-18). These deposits are called calculi and accumulate in the renal collecting system. Calculi can be the result of cystinuria (amino acid metabolic disorder), hypercalcemia (immobility or hyperparathyroidism), oxalate (oxalic and glycolic acid in urine), and uric acid (dietary purines). Renal colic is an intense pain caused when a calculus or fragments of calculi partially or completely obstruct the calyces or renal pelvis. Renal calculi often dislodge and move from the renal pelvis into the ureter. A nidus (e.g., an infection or an exposed suture postoperatively) can be the focal point for the formation of a calculus in the ureter. If calculi are small enough, they pass into the bladder and are voided. Those that remain lodged, causing obstruction to outflow from any part of the urinary tract, must be removed.

Preservation of renal function is the primary objective of surgical procedures for urolithiasis. Lithotomy is removal of a calculus. Lithotripsy is fragmentation of a stone followed by removal. Chemolysis is dissolution with a chemical substance. After removal from any location in the GU tract,

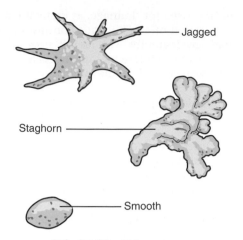

FIG. 35-18   Kidney stones.

urinary calculi should be placed in a dry container and sent to the pathology laboratory for chemical analysis.

Percutaneous Nephrostolithotomy or Nephrolithotripsy.
With percutaneous nephrostolithotomy or nephrolithotripsy, a guidewire inside a transluminal angioplasty needle is introduced, under fluoroscopy, through the flank into the renal pelvis. The access point is carefully closed. This procedure may be performed in the radiology department with the patient under local anesthesia. In the OR, dilators are placed over the guidewire to enlarge a nephrostomy tract for introduction of a nephrostomy tube or nephroscope. The patient is placed in a modified prone position to elevate the surgical side slightly.

Renal calculi may be removed with stone forceps or baskets, or they may be fragmented with a lithotriptor. Lithotripsy is necessary for large calculi such as a staghorn calculus, which branches from the renal pelvis into the calyces and may extend into the ureter. Size, density, composition, and location influence the urologist's choice of lithotripsy.

Ultrasonic Lithotripsy. With ultrasonic lithotripsy, ultrasonic waves are used to shatter the calculus into fragments. This procedure is usually performed with the patient under spinal or general anesthesia. Either a rigid or a flexible fiberoptic nephroscope is inserted percutaneously; a hollow, metal ultrasonic probe, which emits high-frequency sound waves, is inserted through the nephroscope. The probe is visually placed in contact with a calculus that is localized in the renal pelvis as identified radiographically or by fluoroscopy. The calculus fragments as the ultrasonic energy is absorbed, and the shattered particles are aspirated by suction through the probe. A nephrostomy tube may be placed in the renal pelvis for temporary drainage postoperatively; this tube is usually removed after 2 weeks.

Electrohydraulic Lithotripsy. With electrohydraulic lithotripsy, an electrohydraulic lithotriptor is used to create an electrical discharge in fluid and this discharge is transformed into a hydraulic shock wave. The calculus disintegrates when the probe is directed at it. Larger fragments may be removed with Randall stone forceps, and smaller ones are flushed out with irrigation. A tube is left in the nephros-

tomy tract for continued irrigation for several days after lithotripsy. This procedure may be performed with a local anesthetic with intravenous sedatives and analgesics.

Nephrolithotomy or Pyelolithotomy.
A large staghorn renal calculus that does not dislodge from the calyces or renal pelvis may need to be removed through an open incision. A nephroscope may be used during the surgical procedure for direct visual examination of the nephrons to locate and remove residual calculi. Ultrasound may also be used to identify retained fragments. Localized hypothermia provides the surgeon with a bloodless surgical field and lengthens the time in which the renal artery may be clamped safely without a loss of renal function during the search for and extraction of calculi.

Percutaneous Chemolysis.
Hemiacidrin may be instilled through a small nephrostomy tube to alkalinize cysteine and uric acid calculi and to dissolve any debris that remains after other lithotomy procedures.

Extracorporeal Shock-Wave Lithotripsy.
Many patients are scheduled for cystoscopy immediately before a noninvasive extracorporeal shock-wave lithotripsy (ESWL) procedure. A ureteral stent may be inserted to facilitate the passage of stone fragments. The ureteral stone may be manipulated back up into the renal pelvis. A radiograph may be obtained to check the location of the calculus.

Water Bag Lithotripsy. With a water bag lithotripsy, the patient first receives a continuous epidural or general anesthetic and then is positioned against a large fluid-filled pad on the operating bed. The calculus is visualized by fluoroscopy and approximately 1500 ultrasonic waves are generated over a period of 60 minutes by rapid high-voltage sparks that are discharged from the bottom of the operating bed and transmitted through the water bag to enter the body. The shock-wave energy is generated electromagnetically and focused with an acoustic lens. The impact of the sonic waves against the calculus causes fragmentation.

After each series of 150 to 200 waves, the focus on the calculus is rechecked by fluoroscopy. Each shock wave is synchronized with the patient's respirations and resting phase of the heartbeat; an electrocardiogram (ECG) monitors the patient's R waves to avoid disrupting the cardiac rhythm. A loud report sounds in the room each time a spark is fired, and therefore both the patient and personnel must wear protective earplugs.

Shock waves also may be produced by piezoelectric transducers activated by an electronic generator. These transducers are mounted on a bowl-shaped spherical dish; a soft, fluid membrane over this dish maintains contact with the patient's skin. Ultrasound images produced from an ultrasound localization system are used to position the stone at the focal point of the shock waves.

Ureters

The ureters are the vital anatomic structures for the flow of urine from the kidneys to the bladder. An obstruction to urinary flow must be either corrected or diverted. The ureters may be approached either through an endoscope or through an open incision.

Ureteroscopy. Both rigid and flexible, short and long, fiberoptic ureteroscopes allow direct visualization of the ureteral tumors, calculi, and strictures. These scopes are introduced percutaneously or cystoscopically. Biopsies of tumors can be performed, and strictures can be corrected by balloon dilation. Ureteral calculi can be extracted with stone baskets or forceps or fragmented using ultrasound or lasers.

Percutaneous endoscopic techniques can be used in conjunction with cystoscopy. A complete cystoscopy implies that the procedure extends beyond the bladder into the ureters. This procedure may be performed for the following:

- Drainage of the renal pelvis for differential diagnosis or renal function
- Insertion of ureteral catheters to provide constant drainage for one or both kidneys or to outline the ureters for a difficult pelvic surgical procedure
- Insertion of a ureteral stent for internal drainage of an obstructed ureter
- Transluminal dilation of a ureteral stricture
- Manipulation and removal of a calculus
- Ureteral meatotomy to enlarge the opening of one or both ureteral orifices into the bladder

Ureteral Catheters. Made of flexible woven nylon or other plastic material, ureteral catheters range in caliber from size 3 to 14 Fr and are approximately 30 inches (76 cm) in length. Sterile, prepackaged disposable catheters are available. Most are radiopaque so they can be visualized radiographically.

The urologist visualizes the ureteral orifice through the cystoscope. The catheter is inserted through the scope and introduced into the ureter.

The catheter has graduated markings in centimeters so the urologist can judge the distance that the catheter has been inserted. The urologist will request a size and style of catheter tip best suited for the intended purpose. The most common tips are shown in Figure 35-19.

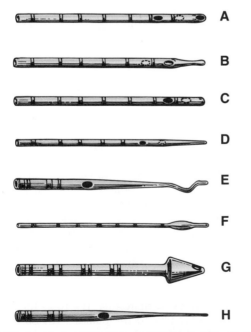

FIG. 35-19   Ureteral catheter tips. **A,** Whistle. **B,** Olive. **C,** Round. **D,** Flexible filiform. **E,** Blasucci curved. **F,** Braasch bulb. **G,** Acorn/cone. **H,** Garceau tapered.

- *Whistle tips.* Used for drainage, as ureteral markers, or for the injection of a radiopaque contrast medium for retrograde pyelography. The largest sizes are used to dilate ureters to facilitate passage of a calculus.
- *Olive tips.* May be used for the same purposes as whistle tips.
- *Round tips.* May be preferred for drainage.
- *Flexible filiform tips.* May be used to bypass an obstruction for drainage.
- *Blasucci curved tips.* May be used to bypass a ureteral stricture more easily than straight tips.
- *Braasch bulb with whistle tips.* Preferred to dilate the ureter or to inject contrast medium for a ureterogram.
- *Acorn or cone tips.* May be preferred for a ureterogram.
- *Garceau tapered tips.* Used to dilate ureters.

Ureteral catheters that are left indwelling to provide drainage must be attached to a sterile, closed urinary drainage system. Because ureteral catheters are smaller in diameter than standard urinary drainage catheters, an adapter is used. This adapter may be a small rubber tip or nipple placed on one end of a straight connector or on both ends of a Y-connector. The catheters are put through the hole in the tip(s).

The distal end of the connector is attached to a constant drainage system with a piece of sterile tubing. A separate drainage system for each catheter is usually desired by the urologist. Each drainage container is labeled to identify the right and left ureteral catheters.

Ureteral Stent. An indwelling ureteral stent is inserted for long-term drainage in a wide variety of benign and malignant diseases that cause ureteral obstruction.

A stent also may be indicated for temporary drainage or marking a ureter for abdominal surgery. Placement of ureteral stents requires a cystoscopy set up separate from the main surgical field. The table should be left intact for the duration of the abdominal procedure in the event a second cystoscopy is necessary.

Several types of stents are used. They can be made of durable and biocompatible silicone, polyurethane, or another copolymer. The stent may have a collar, a double-J configuration, a pigtail, or a coil to minimize migration up into the renal pelvis or down into the bladder. The stent is passed through the cystoscope and over a guidewire into the ureter, and it remains fixed for internal urinary drainage. As described for ureteral catheters, some types of stents are used to identify ureters and provide external drainage intraoperatively.

Percutaneous Ureterolithotomy. As described for percutaneous nephrolithotomy and lithotripsy, a calculus lodged in the renal pelvis or upper tract of the ureter can be extracted or fragmented through a ureteropyeloscope.

Transurethral Ureteroscopic Lithotripsy or Lithotomy. A urologic endoscope can be introduced transurethrally for direct visualization and lithotripsy or for extraction of a calculus that is obstructing a ureter (Fig. 35-20). Ultrasonic and electrohydraulic lithotripsy can be performed through a ureteroscope.

Laser Lithotripsy. The use of laser technology has improved the minimally invasive treatment of calculi. A flash lamp–pulsed dye laser beam is directed through a flexible fiberoptic ureteroscope to a calculus in the lower tract. The fine tip of the laser fiber probe extends beyond the end of the scope and is placed in direct contact with the calculi to produce fragmentation without ureteral injury. This pulsed laser has a green wavelength and is attracted to the yellow color of a calculus. The energy generated through the intermittent laser pulses fragments the yellow calculus by mechanical action without increasing its temperature to more than 50° F (10° C). This procedure may be performed with the patient under epidural or general anesthesia. Shattered calculi will pass with the patient's urine. An indwelling ureteral stent may be left in place for 48 hours and removed by the urologist in the office postoperatively.

Ureteral Stone Extraction. A flexible-shaft, basket-type stone-capture device (stone basket) is inserted into the ureter through a cystoscope in the bladder for extraction of a ureteral calculus. Several types of stone baskets are available, including the Dormia, Johnson, Levant, Pfister-Schwartz, and Lomac. These instruments have a fine wire or nylon basket that can be expanded through the shaft to ensnare a calculus located in the lower third of the ureter. Specialized stone baskets have a laser fiber port for calculus fragmentation. The basket is used to retrieve the central core after the exterior portion of the calculus is shattered.

Stone baskets must be cleaned promptly after use in a nonresidue liquid-detergent solution to remove debris. Removable parts must be disassembled. Debris should be brushed away from the junction of the basket and shaft with a small, soft brush. Inspection of the basket wires is critical during cleaning. If the wires are cracked or broken at the end closest to the shaft, the basket may be passed into the ureter but cannot be withdrawn without trauma.

Ureterolithotomy. If a calculus fails to pass spontaneously through the ureter or cannot be removed with a stone basket, an open surgical procedure may be necessary. If the calculus is high in the ureter near the kidney, the patient is positioned for a lateral flank incision below the twelfth rib. An abdominal incision is used to reach a calculus in the lower segment near the bladder. The exposed ureter will be dilated proximal to the calculus and collapsed distal to it. The surgeon makes a small incision directly over the calculus and extracts it from the ureter with a stone forceps.

Cystolithotomy and Litholapaxy. Calculi usually can be removed from the bladder through the urethra. Crushing a urinary calculus in the bladder is referred to as litholapaxy or lithotrity. If a litholapaxy is unsuccessful or contraindicated, the removal of a calculus by incision into the bladder may be necessary; this surgical procedure is a cystolithotomy. For a litholapaxy, a lithotrite (Fig. 35-21) is introduced into the bladder through the urethra and is used to pulverize and remove calculi. The instrument used may be a lithotrite with hinged jaws, an ultrasound lithotriptor, or an electrohydraulic lithotrite. The electrohydraulic lithotrite generates energy shock waves at the tip of a flexible probe inserted through a cystoscope by direct vision. The stone fragments are then irrigated from the bladder.

Ureteroneocystostomy. Implantation of the ureters into the bladder wall can be performed to relocate the ureters into a different site for correction of ureterovesical reflux, to reestablish urinary flow after temporary diversion or ureteral injury, or to establish urinary flow from a kidney transplant after bilateral nephrectomy and ureterectomy.

Ureteroureterostomy. Anastomosis of two segments of one ureter is usually performed to reestablish ureteral continuity after traumatic injury. A ureteral catheter may be inserted as a stent and the ureter sutured over it. This procedure, a transureteroureterostomy anastomosis, may be indicated to bypass a ureteral stricture or to eliminate ureteral reflux that may be the result of trauma. Injury to a ureter can occur as a complication of pelvic or abdominal surgical procedures, as well as from external penetrating wounds. Ideally, a transureteral anastomosis can be made 2 to 4 cm above the pelvic brim, because the ureters are close at this point and the recipient ureter has a straight course into the bladder.

Vesicopsoas Hitch Procedure. The loss of a large segment of a middle or distal ureter can result from trauma or ureteral resection for tumor or stricture. A vesicopsoas hitch may be the procedure of choice when the length of the remaining ureter is insufficient for ureteroneocystostomy or ureteroureterostomy. The bladder is mobilized through an extraperitoneal approach into the retroperitoneal space. It is attached (i.e., hitched) to the psoas muscle to reposition the bladder cephalad. The segment of proximal ureter is brought through and sutured to the bladder wall. The

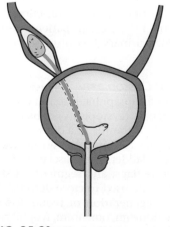

FIG. 35-20 Ureteral stone removal.

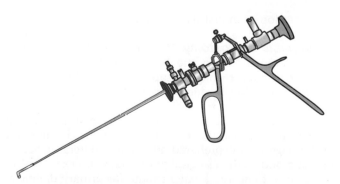

FIG. 35-21 Lithotrite for crushing bladder stones.

kidney also may be mobilized and attached to the psoas muscle if too much tension will be placed on the ureterovesical anastomosis.

Urinary Bladder

The bladder may be opened through a suprapubic incision when a neoplasm, calculus, obstruction of the bladder neck, or traumatic injury is not amenable to treatment through the cystoscope. Diagnosis is usually established through urodynamics (the study of bladder function) and direct visualization via a cystoscope.

Cystometrogram. A cystometrogram measures voiding pressure within the bladder to determine muscle tone and to check nerve supply. A calibrated recording tidal irrigator cystometer is used for this measurement. The patient should feel a desire to void when 350 mL of solution is put into the bladder. Carbon dioxide gas is used with some electronic transducers or radio pressure gauges. The normal maximum capacity of the bladder is 450 to 550 mL. Normal bladder pressure is 40 to 50 mL of water. If the problem is neurogenic, the cystometric findings are not higher than normal. If the problem is a hypertonic bladder, these measurements are higher than normal.

Cystoscopy. Cystoscopy is a visual examination of the interior walls and contents of the bladder. This term is used broadly because various concurrent procedures may be carried out by using specially designed instruments through the cystoscope. Complete cystoscopy and litholapaxy have been described. A plain cystoscopy is a routine examination of the bladder. In conjunction with plain cystoscopy, the following procedures also may be performed within the bladder:

- Biopsy of a tumor with a flexible-shaft biopsy forceps to obtain specimens
- Cystogram for diagnostic radiographs after injection of a contrast medium into the bladder
- Fulguration of a tumor by use of an electrode to destroy tissue
- Resection of or incision into a bladder neck obstruction with a resectoscope
- Coagulation of a hemangioma with an argon laser, vaporization of a superficial tumor of the bladder wall with an Nd:YAG laser, or photodynamic therapy to a solid tumor with argon-pumped tunable dye laser
- Removal of a foreign body with a flexible-shaft, foreign-body forceps
- Insertion of interstitial radionuclide seeds

Suprapubic Cystostomy. With a suprapubic cystostomy, urinary drainage from the bladder is established via a catheter inserted through a suprapubic incision or trocar puncture into the bladder (Fig. 35-22). If the bladder or urethra is injured by trauma associated with bony and soft tissue injuries of the pelvis, the bladder may be drained with a catheter placed above the pubic arch. This method of drainage is also preferred after some ureteral, bladder, prostatic, and urethral surgical procedures to decrease tension on sutures, to ensure a patent route for urinary drainage, and to minimize urinary retention.

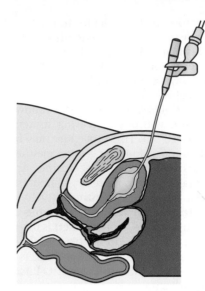

FIG. 35-22 Suprapubic cystostomy for urinary drainage.

A suprapubic catheter also can be used when the surgeon wants the patient to void some urine voluntarily via the urethra to maintain urethral function and tone, such as after bladder or vaginal repairs. Suprapubic catheters are connected to a sterile, closed, constant drainage system before the patient leaves the OR. The following are the most commonly used catheters for cystostomy drainage:

- Foley, 30-mL balloon, French sizes 20, 22, or 24
- Foley, 5-mL balloon, 24 Fr, three-way irrigating catheter (third lumen can be used for continuous irrigation)
- Bonanno suprapubic catheter

Cutaneous Vesicostomy. In a cutaneous vesicostomy, urinary drainage is established directly from the bladder into a collecting device affixed on the abdomen rather than through a suprapubic catheter. The bladder is opened through a transverse suprapubic incision, and a flap is raised at the dome. A skin flap is raised in the midline of the abdomen below the umbilicus. The bladder flap is sutured to the defect created in the skin and then covered with the skin flap. A transparent adhering skin dressing and collection device form a seal around the resultant bladder stoma. A cutaneous vesicostomy may preserve renal function and/or improve upper urinary tract structure in patients with a neurogenic or atonic bladder, urinary incontinence, or bladder outlet obstruction.

Cystotomy and Cystoplasty. An incision into the urinary bladder through a suprapubic incision (cystotomy) may be performed to repair (cystoplasty) a bladder laceration or rupture as a result of trauma or a defect in the bladder wall. Various techniques are used to restore the capacity and function of the bladder. Free fascial grafts, seromuscular grafts, myouterine flaps, and segments of stomach, ileum, or sigmoid colon are used to close defects.

To stimulate regeneration of tissue, the defect may be covered with peritoneum, omentum, lyophilized human dura, gelatin sponge, or a biodegradable or synthetic material.

The bladder is also incised to perform a Y-V–plasty to relieve a stricture or contracture of the bladder neck by broadening the outlet of the bladder into the urethra.

Cystectomy. In a cystectomy, the bladder is removed for invasive malignant disease. A radical total cystectomy with en bloc pelvic lymph node dissection is usually performed. The neurovascular bundle, which is required for penile erection, may be preserved in a male patient, or a penile prosthesis may be implanted during a subsequent surgical procedure.

A salvage or partial cystectomy with intraoperative radiation therapy may be an alternative to a total cystectomy. If a urinary diversion procedure (previously described) has not been performed before removal of the bladder, transplantation of the ureters into the skin or into the intestinal tract for urinary drainage is required at the time of cystectomy. A gastrocystoplasty may be the procedure of choice after a partial cystectomy, especially in a patient with impaired renal function.

Continent Urinary Diversion Procedures. The ureters may be permanently or temporarily transplanted to maintain the patency of urinary excretion from the body. The bladder may be bypassed or absent. Bilateral transplantation for permanent urinary diversion is performed when bladder function is impaired by neoplasm, chronic infection, congenital anomaly, trauma, or other cause.

The procedure follows completion of a total cystectomy (removal of the bladder), a radical cystoprostatectomy in a male patient, or radical hysterectomy with salpingo-oophorectomy and cystectomy in a female patient, with or without pelvic lymphadenectomy. The ureters may be implanted into the intestinal wall, but more commonly they are transplanted to an isolated loop or detubularized segment of intestine that becomes a reservoir for urine. Ideally, a urinary reservoir collects and stores urine and expels it under voluntary control (i.e., functions as the lower urinary tract).

The upper urinary tract should be protected from urine reflux, which can lead to kidney infection. Normal renal function and electrolyte balance also must be preserved. These objectives are not easily attained. Various procedures are used for urinary diversion.

With a continent reservoir, an intestinal pouch is created with bilateral antirefluxing ureteroenteric anastomoses. This high-capacity (up to 800 mL), low-pressure pouch provides an intraabdominal reservoir (neobladder) for the storage of urine. A one-way outflow valve provides continence (i.e., the ability to control function). A cutaneous stoma also may be created to empty the reservoir (Fig. 35-23). The procedure is performed through a low midline incision.

Several techniques are used to create the reservoir from a segment of ileum. Anastomoses may be stapled or sutured to reestablish intestinal continuity. Some types use the appendix as the external conduit. For some procedures, the umbilicus can be used as the stoma site. This is done for cosmesis, particularly in children.

Although creating a continent reservoir is a lengthy surgical procedure, the resultant quality of life for the patient makes this procedure, which prevents involuntary urinary leakage, the procedure of choice unless contraindi-

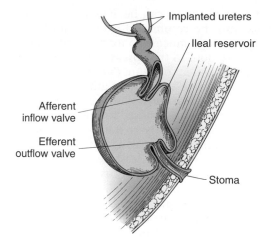

FIG. 35-23   Ileal reservoir created from segment of ileum with ureters implanted distal to inflow valve. Exteriorized stoma allows self-catheterization through continent outflow valve. A continent reservoir includes implanted ureters, afferent inflow valve, ileal reservoir, efferent outflow valve, and stoma.

cated by the patient's tolerance or pathologic condition. Two components are important to the creation of a continent reservoir: (1) a urinary collection reservoir is created from segments of bowel and (2) a catheterizable stoma is fashioned on the abdomen or in the umbilicus.

Indiana Pouch. The Indiana pouch, developed in 1987, is constructed by mobilizing a segment (6 to 8 inches [15 to 20 cm]) of terminal ileum, cecum, and ascending colon. The ureters are anastomosed to the colonic segment, inferiorly on each side of the pouch, to prevent reflux. The terminal ileum is exteriorized to form a continent stoma for self-catheterization. This is the most common form to date and demonstrates a 93% continence rate during the day.

Kock Pouch. With a Kock pouch, developed in 1982, a U-shaped pouch is created from a segment (28 to 32 inches [70 to 80 cm]) of ileum. Nipple valves are created on two sides by intussusception (i.e., a portion of ileum is ensheathed in another portion). The afferent inflow valve prevents reflux. The ureters are anastomosed end-to-side distally near this inflow valve. The efferent outflow valve provides continence.

Absorbable staples and/or mesh is used to help stabilize the valves. The reservoir will gradually increase in capacity to as much as 750 to 800 mL of urine. The patient does not wear a collection device but needs to use a catheter every 4 to 6 hours to empty the reservoir through the exteriorized cutaneous stoma. This form can have as high as a 25% failure rate.

Mainz Pouch. With a Mainz pouch, a reservoir is formed by mobilizing a segment (4 to 6 inches [10 to 15 cm]) of cecum and ascending colon and detubularizing two small segments of equal length of terminal ileum. The walls of the pouch are formed by anastomoses of the ascending colon and cecum with the ileal segments. The ureters are implanted into the ascending colon in an antirefluxive manner. To increase capacity, this pouch can be anastomosed to the urinary bladder remnant after partial cystectomy.

Continent diversion can be achieved by inverting the appendix into the cecum and exteriorizing the intussuscepted appendiceal mucosa to form a continent stoma for self-catheterization. In the absence of a healthy appendix, an additional segment of ileum (3 to 5 inches [8 to 12 cm]) can be used to create a continent umbilical stoma.

Ureterosigmoidostomy. With a ureterosigmoidostomy, the ureters may be anastomosed to a nonrefluxing segment of sigmoid colon. Urine diverted into the colon may cause physiologic complications, making this alternative for permanent urinary diversion the least desirable therapeutically. The transverse colon is commonly used. However, the patient does retain an intact body image.

Orthotopic Neobladder. Orthotopic neobladder is constructed from a segment of ileum or colon and anastomosed directly to the urethra. Care is taken to preserve the urethral musculature. To empty the bladder, the patient increases the abdominal pressure while relaxing the external sphincter.

Studer Pouch. First introduced in 1989, it is commonly used today as a neobladder that is anastomosed to the urethra. This type of pouch works well with short ureter segments.

Camey Pouch. An ileocystoplasty can be performed on a male patient if a U-shaped segment (approximately 16 inches [40 cm]) of ileum reaches the urethra at the pelvic floor without tension. The ureters are anastomosed through small enterostomies to the distal ends of the mobilized and divided ileum. A urethroileal anastomosis in the midsection of the ileal reservoir allows the patient to void through the urethra. Continence is maintained by spontaneous contraction around the outflow valve at the site of anastomosis. Micturition occurs by relaxation of the perineal muscles and a Valsalva maneuver (i.e., a forced expiratory effort).

Augmentation Bladder. Scientists in Germany have performed tests in pigs that demonstrate that bladder cells can be grown in a matrix of bovine collagen to create a new bladder. A segment of ileum is harvested and stripped of its mucosal layer. The epithelium-impregnated matrix acts as a scaffold for the growing cells, and blood vessels begin to form. The scientists believe that this is a step in augmenting a deficient bladder at this time but hope that this work will form the basis of total bladder replacement.

Transcutaneous Urinary Diversion

Ileal Conduit. In the creation of an ileal conduit, a procedure popularized by Bricker in the 1950s, both ureters are anastomosed to an isolated segment of the terminal ileum near its proximal end. The distal end is everted and sutured to a predetermined stomal site on the skin, usually on the right side of the abdomen below the waist.

A urinary collection appliance is secured over the stoma before the patient leaves the OR. An ileal conduit with an incontinent external stoma (Fig. 35-24) creates the psychological stress of an altered body image for the patient, but it may be the procedure of choice for the patient who will receive systemic chemotherapy after radical cystectomy. As a secondary procedure after chemotherapy, an incontinent ileal conduit may be converted to a continent ileal reservoir.

Cutaneous Ureterostomy. To create a cutaneous ureterostomy, the end of the ureter closest to the bladder is brought through the abdominal wall to the skin. This procedure can be performed unilaterally or bilaterally with

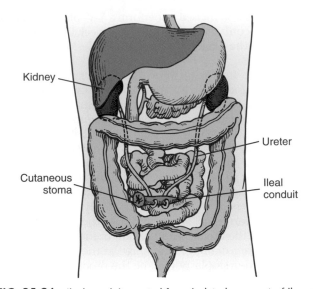

FIG. 35-24   Ileal conduit created from isolated segment of ileum with ureters anastomosed to segment between closed end and external stoma. Urinary collection device must be placed over incontinent stoma. Incontinent urinary diversion carries urine from kidneys through implanted ureters and ileal conduit to stoma.

a single cutaneous stoma or double-loop stoma. The patient must be fitted postoperatively with an appliance for collecting urine directly from the ureter to the exterior of the body. This procedure may be performed as a temporary emergency measure after trauma to the bladder, such as a ruptured bladder.

Urinary Incontinence. Involuntary, uncontrollable voiding may accompany congenital or acquired physiologic conditions, such as a loss of bladder control after spinal cord injury or neurogenic disease. Urinary incontinence may develop in males because of loss of sphincter control after prostatectomy and in females after obstetric injury, radiation therapy, or severe pelvic fractures. Surgical intervention is often necessary for stress incontinence—the intermittent leakage of urine as a result of a sudden increase in intraabdominal pressure (e.g., during coughing or sneezing) on weakened urethral sphincter muscles at the bladder neck. Various surgical procedures are performed as determined by urodynamics.

Gynecologists perform some bladder suspension procedures (e.g., Marshall-Marchetti-Krantz suprapubic vesicourethral suspension), and urologists perform other procedures. Laparoscopic approaches have been developed for bladder neck suspension with the use of synthetic mesh and titanium staples. Surgical procedures that suspend, support, or reposition the bladder can correct urinary incontinence or improve urinary continence.

Transvaginal Bladder Neck Suspension

Pereyra Procedure. In the Pereyra procedure, the bladder neck is elevated with sutures suspended from the anterior rectus fascia. The primary difference between this procedure and the Stamey procedure is that a Pereyra ligature carrier needle is passed blindly down through retropubic space and out into the vagina.

Both procedures relocate the proximal urethra and bladder neck into the zone of intraabdominal pressure without necessitating open pelvic surgery. The Pereyra procedure is used for uncomplicated recurrent urinary stress incontinence and is 80% effective for long-term resolution of urinary leakage.

Stamey Procedure. In the Stamey procedure, sutures are placed on both sides of the urethrovesical junction from the anterior rectus fascia into the vagina. The patient is positioned in a modified lithotomy position so the legs extend laterally to flatten the lower abdomen. Short suprapubic incisions, right and left of midline, are extended to the anterior rectus fascia. The vagina is incised transversely and dissected from the urethra to expose the trigone of the bladder. The urethrovesical junction is located by palpating the balloon of the Foley catheter inserted into the bladder. A straight or angled Stamey needle is passed through the rectus fascia, along the internal vesicle neck, and out through the vaginal incision.

The cystoscopic equipment should be set up on a separate sterile tabl, because contamination of the eyepiece is unavoidable. A cystoscope is inserted to ascertain correct needle placement without injury to the bladder. A heavy nylon suture threaded onto the needle is drawn from the vagina to the suprapubic incision; the needle is inserted again. The vaginal end of the suture is passed through a 1-cm length of polyester tubular graft before it is threaded onto the needle. When the suture is drawn to the abdominal wall, it establishes a suspending loop on one side of the bladder neck. The suture is tied over the anterior rectus fascia with enough tension to elevate the bladder neck by traction on the adjacent vaginal fascia. This procedure is repeated on the contralateral side.

Artificial Urinary Sphincter. A prosthesis may be implanted to apply pressure to the urethra to maintain continence between periods of voiding. The pressure-regulating mechanism has a balloon, a cuff, and a pump constructed of silicone rubber. A balloon with a desired predetermined pressure is positioned intraabdominally beside the bladder. Depending on the preferred surgical approach, the cuff encircles either the bladder neck or the bulbous urethra. The pump is placed in the subcutaneous tissue of the scrotum (in males) or labium (in females). A control assembly lies subcutaneously adjacent to the external inguinal ring; tubing connects the components. A radiopaque isotonic solution is used to fill the prosthesis. When a patient squeezes the pump, solution is transferred from the cuff into the balloon, thus releasing pressure on the urethra and permitting urine to flow.

Neurostimulation for Bladder Control. The detrusor muscle can be unstable and require electrostimulation. Electrostimulation simulates the signals from S2-S4 to mimic the autonomic activity necessary for bladder control. The patient is placed prone, and the leads are placed in the back through an incision. On completion of the lead placement, the patient is placed in a lateral position. A pocket is created in the flank for the small generator. Postoperatively the patient is taught to avoid metal detectors, theft devices in stores, and any large magnets. The patient is given a special magnet to turn the device on or off as needed.

Periurethral Injection of Bulking Agent. Collagen or Teflon may be injected into the tissues surrounding the urethra proximal to the external sphincter. The injection swells the tissue, narrowing the urethra sufficiently for sphincteric control. This procedure is performed in select patients with moderate to severe urinary incontinence, such as in a male after a transurethral resection or in a female in whom a suspension procedure has been unsuccessful. The injection is made transurethrally with a flexible syringe through a fiberoptic cystourethroscope. A suprapubic catheter is used for 3 to 5 days postoperatively to allow some voluntary passage of urine from the urethra. Postoperative complications include urinary retention, urethral fistulas, and infection.

Bladder Flap Urethroplasty. A bladder flap urethroplasty procedure is advisable when urodynamics show a resistance to urinary flow in a female with a neurogenic bladder. A lesion of the nervous system can cause bladder dysfunction.

Urethra

The urethra functions as the outlet for urine to pass from the bladder. Obstruction or dysfunction of the urethra may cause urinary retention or incontinence. Enlargement of the prostate may cause obstruction. Gonorrhea, other disease processes, or traumatic injury may cause a stricture.

Perineal Urethrostomy. When indwelling or intermittent urethral catheterization is contraindicated in a male patient with an obstructed or traumatized urethra, urinary drainage may be established through a perineal incision. An indwelling catheter is inserted into the bladder through an incision into the membranous urethra. Male patients may have a perineal urethrostomy after a total penectomy.

Urethral Dilation. Periodic dilation may be necessary for weeks to years after an infection or a trauma that has caused a urethral stricture. Either balloon dilators, woven filiforms and followers, bougies, or metal sounds are used. If the latter are preferred, curved metal Van Buren sounds (Fig. 35-25) are used to dilate a male urethra; straight sounds are used for a female urethra. A short urethral stent may be inserted.

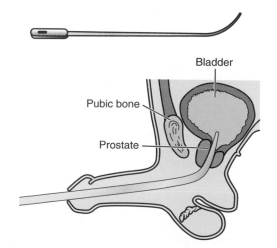

FIG. 35-25 Van Buren sound is curved for safe use in male urethral dilation.

Urethral Stent. To prevent collapse of the lumen caused by stricture, a spring-loaded stainless steel mesh stent can be placed into the male urethra via a cystoscope at a level proximal to the bulbar urethra and distal to the external urinary sphincter. The stricture is measured and dilated or incised by internal urethrotomy. To be effective, the stent selected should measure 1 cm greater than the length of the stricture. A special deployment applicator is used to place the stent in the urethra. The stent becomes a permanent urethral implant and is useful for males who have benign prostatic hypertrophy. It is contraindicated in bleeding disorders or for males who are receiving anticoagulation therapy. After the procedure, antibiotics are administered as a prophylactic measure.

Urethrotomy. An Otis urethrotome may be used to cut into a urethral stricture. After the instrument is passed into the urethra, the blade is released to cut the stricture. If a specimen of the urethra is taken for biopsy, a rigid biopsy forceps is used through a cystourethroscope. This scope also is used with a laser to open a urethral stricture.

Urethroplasty. Reestablishment of continuity without stricture is the ultimate objective after a traumatic urethral injury and is usually associated with pelvic fractures in males. Scrotal-inlay urethroplasty or another method of urethral reconstruction is usually delayed until the extent of injury can be fully evaluated by urethrograms. A suprapubic cystostomy catheter inserted as an emergency measure can maintain urinary drainage for several weeks to months.

Insertion of a urethral catheter into a ruptured urethra in the immediate posttraumatic period can produce periurethral infection, stricture, and other irreparable damage.

Perineum and Genital Surface Procedures

Ablation of Condylomata Acuminata. Condylomata are caused by a sexually transmitted human papillomavirus (HPV). Referred to as genital warts, this condition can affect the genitalia, perineum, perianal region, and mucous membranes of males and females. The incubation period is 1 to 2 months after exposure, but longer periods have been reported. HPV has been implicated in cervical cancer.

In the OR or office setting and with the patient under local anesthesia, condylomata are surgically ablated with a CO_2 laser. Before the procedure, acetic acid, 3% to 5%, is applied to the area to make the lesions visible by causing them to turn white and raised. As with all other laser procedures, laser precautions (e.g., appropriate eyewear for all persons in the room, proper instrumentation) are followed.

Viral mutation in laser plume has been documented, and personal protective equipment is required. Appropriate laser eyewear and masks should be worn by the staff and the patient to prevent contamination of respiratory and ocular mucosa with virus-laden plume. The eyewear also protects from laser light.

MALE REPRODUCTIVE ORGANS

The primary functions of the male reproductive organs are procreation, sexual gratification, and hormone secretion. These organs are both internal and external (Fig. 35-26).

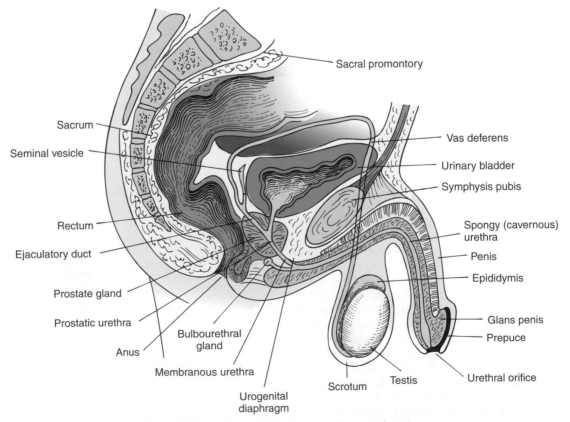

FIG. 35-26 Male reproductive organs in sagittal section.

Testes

The testes, or testicles, are both endocrine glands and male reproductive organs and are bilaterally suspended in the scrotum. They secrete hormones that influence growth and development, sexual activity, the production of spermatozoa, and the development of secondary sex characteristics. Disorders in or around one testis or both testes that inhibit sexual activity or reproductive capability or cause discomfort in the scrotum may necessitate a surgical procedure. If both testes are excised (a bilateral orchiectomy), the patient becomes sterile and deficient in male hormones.

Male patients should be instructed to perform a monthly testicular self-examination (TSE), which should be performed when the scrotum is relaxed (after a warm bath or shower). When performing a TSE, each testis is gently rolled between the thumb and forefingers. The testis should feel smooth and oval, should be without lumps or hardened areas, and should move freely within the scrotal sac. Palpation should be pain-free. Testicular cancer affects males in the 15- to 35-year age-range. Studies have shown that 63% of the males studied did not practice TSE.

Orchiectomy. A bilateral orchiectomy may be performed in patients with prostatic cancer to alter the hormonal environment. After this relatively simple procedure, control of the disease is attempted before the urologist considers other endocrine surgery, such as an adrenalectomy. Psychologic preparation is important to help the patient accept the sterilization and the other body changes, (e.g., breast enlargement) that may occur as a result of the alteration in the hormonal system.

In this procedure, bilateral oblique incisions in the inguinal canals extend into the upper anterior surface of the scrotum over the testes. The testes are removed from the scrotum after ligation of the spermatic cords at the external or internal inguinal rings. Silicone rubber prostheses may be implanted in the scrotal sac to improve aesthetic appearance, which helps with the psychologic rehabilitation of the patient.

The removal of one testis (unilateral orchiectomy) does not sterilize the patient. This procedure may be indicated after traumatic injury or infection, but it is more commonly performed to remove a tumor. Primary testicular tumors may be right- or left-sided; germ cell tumors may develop bilaterally. Accurate histologic findings and clinical evaluations of the type of tumor and stage of disease are mandatory for determining the appropriate therapy. CT and lymphangiography or lymphoscintigraphy are valuable diagnostic tools. Unilateral radical orchiectomy via an inguinal incision may be followed by radiation or chemotherapy and retroperitoneal lymph node dissection. The spermatic cord and vas deferens are ligated and divided separately at the internal ring so these structures can be identified if further dissection is needed for metastatic disease.

Retroperitoneal Lymphadenectomy. A transabdominal midline incision is made for exposure of the lymph nodes and sympathetic nerve fibers in the paraaortic plane, usually along the anterolateral aspect of the aorta in the retroperitoneal space. A unilateral lymphadenectomy usually is performed on the ipsilateral (same) side as the tumor unless regional metastases have spread via lymphatic invasion, in which case a bilateral dissection is indicated. If possible, the neurovascular bundles extending from the hypogastric plexus to the corporeal tissues of the penis are preserved. These nerve fibers are identified and placed in vessel loops before lymphadenectomy is carried out, thus preserving ejaculatory function.

Scrotal-Testicular Trauma. An injury may require exploration of the scrotum to ligate bleeding vessels or to insert a Penrose drain. Infection is likely to develop after a penetrating wound; therefore, extraperitoneal spaces in the scrotum must be drained thoroughly.

Testicular Torsion. The testicle can become twisted on the spermatic cord, causing extreme pain. Immediate correction is necessary or the testicle will become ischemic and tissue death will follow. Manual detorsion may be tried, but surgical intervention is indicated if reduction is not successful within 1 hour of onset.

Hydrocelectomy. A hydrocele is an accumulation of peritoneal fluid in the sac of the tunica vaginalis of the testis. Through an anterior incision into the scrotum, the hydrocele sac is dissected away from the testis and removed from the scrotum. There is a 5% incidence in newborns, most of which will resolve spontaneously. Hydrocele is more common in premature babies, because they may have been born before 32 to 38 weeks' gestation (the average gestational age at which closure vaginalis occurs). Hydrocele is also more common in children who have increased fluid in the peritoneum (i.e., ventriculoperitoneal shunt to drain hydrocephalus or peritoneal dialysis).

Spermatocelectomy. A small mass attached to the epididymis may be palpated in the scrotum superior to the testis. This painless cyst is a collection of testicular fluid and sperm cells. These cysts are repaired if they become annoying to the patient.

Varicocele Ligation. Dilation of the spermatic veins in the pampiniform plexus of the spermatic cord can cause a soft, elastic, often uncomfortable swelling in the scrotum. This condition, known as varicocele, occurs more often on the left side. It can cause a loss in testicular mass and a decrease of sperm density associated with male infertility caused by increased temperature. Ligation of the spermatic vein can improve sperm count if the testis has not atrophied.

The spermatic vein is ligated above the inguinal canal lateral to the inferior epigastric vessels or in the retroperitoneal space lateral to the iliac artery. In the latter approach, a transverse abdominal incision starts at the anterior superior iliac spine and extends toward the lateral aspect of the rectus abdominis muscle. The hemiscrotum must be manually emptied of all blood before the vein is ligated or the varicocele may persist postoperatively.

Laparoscopic approaches have been developed for spermatic vein ligation. In such a procedure, the internal inguinal ring is located laparoscopically and the spermatic cord and blood vessels are identified. The spermatic vein is dissected free, ligated with two endoscopic clips, and cut between the clips with endoscopic scissors. Most patients are able to return to work within 2 days of the procedure.

Vas Deferens

The vasa deferentia are the small fibromuscular excretory ducts that carry sperm upward through the spermatic cords from the epididymides (which lie along the upper portion of each testis) to the seminal vesicles, the pouchlike glands in front of the urinary bladder near the prostate gland. Interruption of or obstruction to a vas deferens inhibits normal spermatogenesis.

Vasectomy. Elective bilateral vasectomy is an established method of male sterilization and is usually performed as an ambulatory surgical procedure. In a vasectomy, a segment of each vas deferens is removed and sent to the pathology department in individually labeled specimen cups (Fig. 35-27). Depending on the preference of the urologist, the cut ends are either ligated with suture or clips or the endothelium of the lumen is coagulated with the ESU.

Techniques vary, but all patients should be informed that spontaneous regeneration of a severed vas deferens does occur in a small percentage of patients and that sterility is not immediate. Follow-up care includes semen testing for sperm count; repeat testing should continue until no sperm is found in the seminal fluid. Patient teaching includes instructions to use alternative birth control methods until the seminal fluid contains no sperm.

Vasovasostomy. Recannulization of the vas deferens for the restoration of fertility requires an unobstructed anastomosis. The vas deferens has a tough 2-mm outer diameter and an inner diameter of 1 mm or less at the distal end, as well as dilation at the proximal end. This makes precise anastomosis under the operating microscope preferable to nonmicrosurgical techniques, in which it is difficult to see the lumen of the vas deferens on the distal side. One-layer microscopic anastomosis and splinting techniques for a vasectomy reversal often result in a stricture caused by scarring within the lumen of the vas deferens, which inhibits the passage of sperm.

After a scrotal incision is made to expose the vas deferens above and below the site of previous ligation, the two ends are cut to excise scar tissue and to open the lumen. Under magnification of the operating microscope, interrupted sutures are placed in the mucosal lining of the lumen to create a fluid-tight anastomosis (Fig. 35-28). Muscularis is approximated separately. A carbon dioxide milliwatt laser may be used to weld tissue to overcome the scarring and stricture that may be associated with suturing. Sperm counts return to normal soon after the surgical procedure.

Male Infertility. Primary infertility is diagnosed after a failure to conceive during a period of 1 year of unprotected sexual intercourse. Causes of infertility include abnormality in the female and/or male reproductive systems. Male infertility can be the result of deficient sperm production, obstructed sperm passage, a mechanical inability to pass sperm, hormonal imbalance, testicular disease or injury, a low sperm count, and antibodies against sperm.

The history and physical examination should be concurrent with the female partner's gynecologic evaluation. Issues assessed should include sexual history, previous pregnancies, health history, the use of lubricants, drug use, radiation exposure, and timing and frequency of intercourse. Childhood illnesses such as high fevers and viral infections may be factors. A previous sexually transmitted disease can cause scarring that prevents the transport of sperm. Endocrine testing includes follicle-stimulating hormone, luteinizing hormone, testosterone, and prolactin levels. Urinalysis is performed to rule out infection and/or retrograde ejaculation.

The semen analysis includes determining ejaculate volume, sperm count and motility, morphology, and the presence or absence of white blood cells or red blood cells in the seminal fluid. The patient is advised to abstain from sexual intercourse for 2 to 3 days before the testing is performed.

Prostate Gland

The prostate gland, a musculoglandular organ in males, is encased in a fibrous capsule and surrounds the posterior urethra at the bladder neck. It is divided into five lobes. The normal function of this gland is to provide alkaline secretions to the seminal fluid for sperm mobility during ejaculation. The standard of care includes an annual digital prostate examination and prostate-specific antigen (PSA) testing after 40 years of age.

Although the prostate gland normally weighs 20 g, in most men it will enlarge to some degree by 50 years of age.

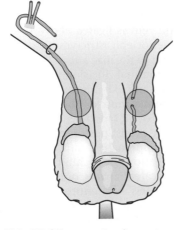

FIG. 35-27 Completed vasectomy.

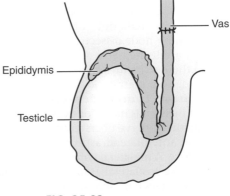

Epididymis

Testicle

Vas

FIG. 35-28 Vasovasostomy.

Fifty percent of all men older than 80 years will have prostatic cancer. Enlargement of the prostate gland can obstruct the urethra and interfere with voiding; this difficulty in voiding is what most often brings men with prostatic disease to a urologist. The urologist will examine the prostate and order a PSA blood test. If the tests indicate benign prostatic hypertrophy, surgery is not the first treatment method of choice. Conservative treatment for benign enlargement of the prostate includes administration of oral finasteride (Proscar). If the prostate does not respond to drug therapy by shrinking, then balloon dilation, stenting, or other surgical procedure may be indicated.

The entire prostate gland or one or more lobes can be resected from its capsule transurethrally. Prostatectomy can also be performed through a suprapubic or retropubic abdominal approach or a perineal incision. A radical prostatectomy, performed through a retropubic abdominal or perineal incision, includes extirpation of the prostate, periprostatic tissue, seminal vesicles, and vas ampullae en bloc. The approach and procedure depend on the urologist's preference for removing the type of pathologic condition.

Transrectal aspiration, core biopsies, or ultrasonography helps establish the correct diagnosis (Fig. 35-29). Prostatic carcinoma may be treated by surgical removal, interstitial and external beam radiation, chemotherapy, and/or hormonal therapy. Management depends on the stage of the disease and the age and condition of the patient. Carcinoma of the prostate is the second most common cause of cancer-related deaths in American men. Benign prostatic hypertrophy/hyperplasia (BPH) is a common indication for prostate intervention in men older than 50 years if the prostate symptoms do not respond to drug therapy. Men younger than 50 years may not qualify for definitive treatment if prostate enlargement is caused by prostatitis. Conservative antibiotic therapy is the treatment of choice. (More information about prostate health and patient teaching can be found at www.prostate.org.)

Balloon Dilation and Stenting of Prostatic Urethra. During cystoscopy, a balloon dilation probe can be inserted into the urethra and expanded to relieve obstruction caused by prostatic hypertrophy. One or more titanium stents can be deployed to maintain patency of the lumen. The stent remains in the lumen and becomes overgrown with urothelium. This procedure permanently relieves urinary retention (Fig. 35-30).

Transurethral Microwave Thermotherapy. With transurethral microwave thermotherapy (TUMT), ultrasound guidance is used to insert a microwave probe into the urethra to the level of the prostate blockage (Fig. 35-31). Microwaves are generated by a console and transmitted to the distal aspect of the probe. Heat generated by the microwave probe is absorbed by the urethral portion of the prostate for 1 hour. The probe is cooled with water circulation at 68° F (20° C) to protect nearby structures. A rectal probe is used to record rectal temperature. The heated tissue sloughs, which causes the urethral stricture to release. Most patients can void with ease, although a few patients require a Foley catheter for several days postoperatively.

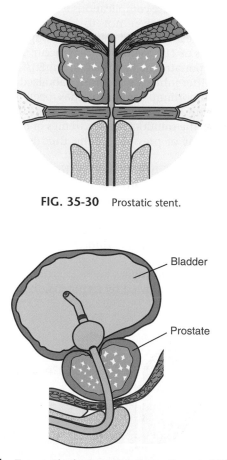

FIG. 35-30 Prostatic stent.

FIG. 35-31 Transurethral microwave thermotherapy (TUMT) probe delivers microwaves to the prostate tumor.

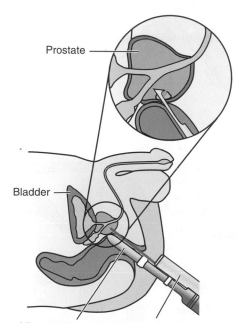

FIG. 35-29 Transrectal ultrasound-guided prostatic biopsy.

Prostate

Bladder

Ultrasound probe   Needle guide

Bladder

Prostate

Transurethral Needle Ablation. With transurethral needle ablation (TUNA), an ambulatory procedure, cystoscopic guidance is used to insert a probe into the urethra to the level of the prostate stricture. Two small needles are passed from the side of the telescopic probe into the hypertrophied prostatic tissue (Fig. 35-32). Radio waves are transmitted selectively into the tissue via the needles. Prostatic tissue in contact with the needles is ablated; nearby structures, such as nerves and vessels, are spared. Up to six select areas of stricture can be precisely ablated in the same procedure. Each application creates a defect in the prostate. The tissue reabsorbs over a period of 3 months, causing the stricture to release. The patient may complain of urinary retention or burning on urination for 24 to 96 hours after the procedure. The main side effect is the potential for retrograde ejaculation.

Transurethral Prostatectomy. Transurethral resection, also referred to as transurethral resection of the prostate (TURP), involves the removal of all or part of the glandular tissue within the prostatic capsule by electroresection through the urethra (Fig. 35-33). A resectoscope, via cystoscopy sheath, is introduced into the prostatic urethra. Using alternating currents from the ESU through the cutting loop electrode, the urologist resects tissue and coagulates bleeding vessels. The bladder is distended with solution to create a working space during resection. Nonconducting and non-hemolyzing, isosmotic glycine irrigating solution is commonly used; 10 to 12 L may be needed. Sterile water as an expansion medium can cause complications related to intravascular hemolysis. Care is taken not to permit the patient to absorb excessive amounts of solution through the prostatic venous sinuses or TUR syndrome may occur. This can cause dilutional hyponatremia less than 125 mEq/L. Glycine is a neurotransmitter inhibitor that is metabolized into glycolic acid and ammonium. Ammonia has been noted to be elevated during TUR syndrome. Risk factors include:

- Height of the solution bags (extremes of height increase the amount of pressure of the fluid as it enters the bladder)
- Deep resection (which allows for increased venous absorption of solution)
- Amount of tissue resected in excess of 45 g
- Duration of the procedure (risk increases when the procedure exceeds 90 minutes)

Signs of TUR syndrome include:
- Mental confusion
- Nausea and vomiting
- Hypertension followed by hypotension
- Symptoms of fluid overload and pulmonary edema
- Bradycardia and dysrhythmia
- Visual disturbances
- Seizures and twitching
- Coma

Treatment of TUR syndrome includes:
- Administration of IV hypertonic saline
- Monitoring of serum sodium levels
- Diuretics

Resected prostatic tissue is collected in an Ellik or other evacuator. After the surgical procedure, tissue fragments must be sent to the pathology department for analysis and weighing. The urologist may insert a three-way 30- or 50-mL Foley catheter for irrigation and hemostasis. The large inflated balloon compresses against the bladder neck fossa to form a tamponade to help control bleeding. Some urologists place the Foley catheter under direct tension by taping the catheter to the patient's leg or abdomen to increase the tamponade effect for hemostasis. The third lumen provides a means for continuous postoperative irrigation to prevent the formation of clots in the bladder.

Benign nodular hyperplasia of glands less than 50 g in size is the usual indication for TURP. This approach has the potential complications of impotence and urinary incontinence. The technique is one of the most difficult for a urologist to master. Although electroresection is used most commonly, transurethral incision of small prostate glands (less than 25 g), balloon dilation of the prostate, laser surgery, and cryosurgery are other invasive techniques for treating BPH. TURP may be performed for the diagnosis or treatment of localized cancer.

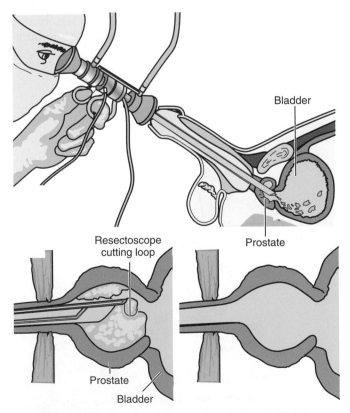

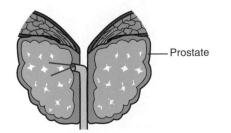

FIG. 35-32 Transurethral needle ablation (TUNA) probe delivers selective radiofrequencies to prostate via directed needles.

FIG. 35-33 Transurethral resection of prostate (TURP).

Suprapubic Prostatectomy. The suprapubic approach for prostatectomy is limited almost exclusively to the removal of a large, benign, hypertrophied gland weighing more than 50 g. Through a midline vertical incision above the symphysis pubis, the superior bladder wall is opened to expose the prostatic urethra (Fig. 35-34, *A*). The prostatic lobes are enucleated with a finger that is inserted through an incision into the mucosa of the urethra. This procedure may be termed transvesicocapsular prostatectomy, because the prostatic capsule is approached through the bladder. Hemostatic agents are usually packed into the extremely vascular prostatic fossa to help control bleeding. Pressure from the Foley catheter balloon inserted after closure of the urethra also helps obtain hemostasis. A suprapubic cystostomy tube is inserted to facilitate urinary drainage from the bladder during the healing process.

Retropubic Prostatectomy. In the retropubic approach, the prostate gland is exposed below the bladder neck through a vertical or transverse abdominal incision above the symphysis pubis. The bladder is not opened. The gland is removed through an incision in the prostatic capsule; this procedure is called a transcapsular prostatectomy. The periprostatic tissue, seminal vesicles, and vas ampullae also may be excised. This method is common for prostate glands larger than 50 g.

Radical Retropubic Prostatectomy. A limited pelvic lymph node dissection is performed for carcinoma with no evidence of spread beyond the prostatic capsule. This radical procedure may be carried out as initial curative therapy or after transurethral prostatectomy. After dissection of the lymph nodes, one of two approaches may be used to totally remove the prostate:

1. *Campbell technique.* An incision is made at the bladder neck, and the urethra is transected. The prostate and periprostatic tissue are widely dissected anterograde from the bladder. The bladder neck is reconstructed for the vesicourethral anastomosis. The patient will be impotent, because the nerves responsible for erection are transected. A penile prosthesis may be implanted.

2. *Walsh technique.* The prostate is resected retrograde beginning at the urethra, working back to the bladder neck. Dissection is carried out close to the prostatic capsule to preserve the neurovascular bundle and thus maintain potency. The vesicourethral anastomosis is completed.

Nerve-sparing procedures have been developed to preserve sexual potency. A device referred to as a CaverMap by UroMed Corporation can be used during the open prostatectomy procedure to locate nerves that control erection (Fig. 35-35). A sensor band is placed around the penis, and a handheld device with a nerve-stimulating probe is used to sense nerve impulses responsible for causing erection. Studies performed by the American Urological Association show that between 40% and 70% of radical prostatectomy patients experienced erectile dysfunction of varying degrees after the surgery. Some patients are unable to achieve erection until after 18 months postoperatively. The CaverMap helps to locate the nerves but does not ensure the ability to achieve erection postoperatively.

Perineal Prostatectomy. The perineum affords the most direct open surgical approach to the prostate through a relatively avascular field (Fig. 35-34, *B*). With the patient in an extreme lithotomy position, the perineum is incised between the scrotum and the anal sphincter (Fig. 35-36). The rectum is dissected from the posterior surface of the prostate, or dissection may be carried out between the external anal sphincter and the rectum. The perineal approach may be used to enucleate the prostate gland from its capsule or for radical cystoprostatectomy. This latter procedure includes removal of the entire prostate gland, its capsule, the seminal vesicles, and a portion of the bladder. The classic radical perineal prostatectomy with pelvic lymph node dissection may be the surgical procedure of choice to reduce the morbidity of prostatic carcinoma. Urinary incontinence and impotence are common outcomes with this procedure. Laparoscopic methods can be used to sample intraabdominal lymph nodes.

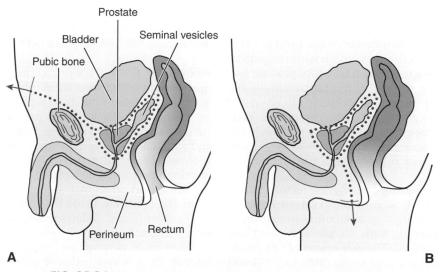

FIG. 35-34   A, Suprapubic prostatectomy. **B,** Perineal prostatectomy.

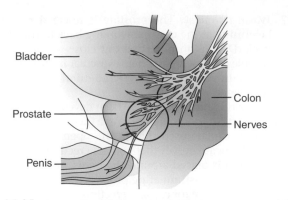

FIG. 35-35 Innervation of the male genitourinary organs and the relationship between prostatic and penile nerves.

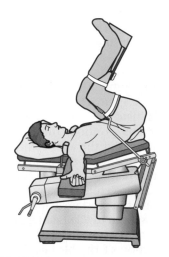

FIG. 35-36 High lithotomy position.

Robotic-Assisted Prostatectomy. The robotic-assisted laparoscopic approach used is dependent on the method used to dissect the seminal vesicles and the vas deferens away from rectum. Enucleation of the prostate is facilitated by traction on the Foley catheter.

Transperineal Prostatic Cryoablation. Transperineal prostatic cryoablation offers an alternative to radical prostatectomy in select patients with cancer of the prostate. This procedure is performed in the cysto room with the patient under general or spinal anesthesia. The entire prostate and periprostatic tissues are frozen. With the patient in the lithotomy position, an ultrasound probe is placed in the rectum for guidance in positioning five cryoprobes. Each cryoprobe is placed transperineally through a hollow sheath inserted in a small (18-gauge) needle puncture site. Liquid nitrogen is delivered to each probe from the cryosurgical device/console.

Care must be taken to avoid freezing the rectum. Warm water is run through a urethral catheter to keep the urethra warm to prevent tissue sloughing, a potential complication of transurethral cryosurgery. Both the prostate gland and the tumor cells are destroyed. The side effects of this procedure include a high risk for impotence (80% to 90%) and urinary incontinence (30%).

Pelvic Lymphadenectomy. A pelvic lymphadenectomy involves either a low abdominal incision into the extraperitoneal space or a laparoscopic approach. The lymph nodes are dissected bilaterally from the iliac vessels, obturator spaces, and hypogastric vessels. These nodes may be examined by frozen section to detect early and subtle metastases from prostatic carcinoma. If several nodes are positive for cancer, the patient is unlikely to benefit from a radical prostatectomy. If the nodes are negative, the urologist may proceed with a radical retropubic prostatectomy. Pelvic lymphadenectomy also may be performed as a staged procedure before radical perineal prostatectomy. If feasible, at least one neurovascular bundle is preserved.

Penis

The penis is the cylindric erectile male organ of copulation. Because it contains the urethra, a deviation or malformation in structure may affect normal urinary flow from the bladder. Circumcision or surgical procedures to repair congenital anomalies of the penis are usually performed during infancy and childhood. Penile anatomy consists of the glans at the distal section, the corpus spongiosum circumferentially the length of the urethra, and the corpus cavernosa bilaterally the length of the shaft (see Fig. 35-26). The distal portion where the urethra exits is referred to as the glans. In its natural state, the glans is covered by redundant skin, which is referred to as foreskin. Some cultures electively remove this skin covering from males in infancy by circumcision.

The arterial supply of the penis arises from the inferior pudendal arteries. Venous drainage is from the venules in the periphery of the corpora and the superior and deep dorsal veins into the cavernosal and pudendal plexae. Innervation is from both sympathetic and parasympathetic origin combined with autonomic reflexes.

The erection and ejaculatory responses are neurologically mediated by afferent and efferent pathways. Sacral efferent parasympathetic innervation causes both psychogenic and reflex erections. Destruction of these nerves during abdominal-perineal resection and radical prostatectomy will result in impotency in 70% to 100% of patients. At the level of the penis, innervation is from adrenergic nerves in the arteriolar smooth muscle. Complete transsection of the spinal cord can result in impotence. Reflex erections may be found in patients with lesions of the upper cord. An exact locus of impulses in the brain has not been identified.

Adult Male Circumcision. Difficulty in the retraction of the foreskin is referred to as phimosis. Paraphimosis is when the foreskin retracts to expose the glans and cannot be repositioned back. These conditions may necessitate circumcision or removal of the foreskin to prevent necrosis and gangrene. In some patients, a small cut in the foreskin, a dorsal slit, is sufficient to release the constriction. An erection that cannot be released because of tight foreskin is a medical and possibly a surgical emergency. Attempts to drain the penis are made by injecting vasodilators. Once the penis is flaccid, a determination is made as to surgical intervention.

Adult male circumcision requires more dissection and ligation than does a pediatric procedure (Fig. 35-37). The patient is placed in the supine position. The foreskin is

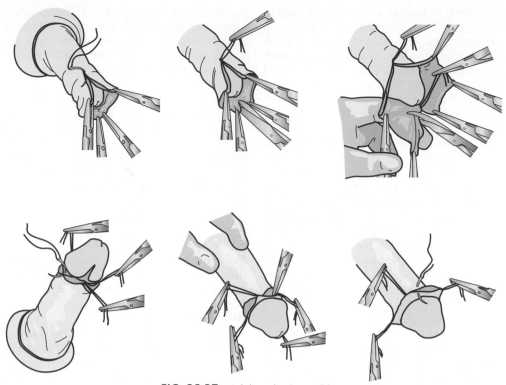

FIG. 35-37 Adult male circumcision.

retracted to prep the glans penis. ESU should be available; however, a small battery-operated cautery is usually sufficient to provide hemostasis for pinpoint bleeders. Some surgeons prefer fine absorbable free-ties. The tissue around the foreskin is dissected, incised, and trimmed away. The remaining edges are circumferentially sutured with fine interrupted absorbable sutures. Vaseline gauze is used as a dressing. A scrotal suspension strap may be used to hold the dressings in place and provide support.

Impotence. The cause of erectile dysfunction, or impotence, can be classified as organic or psychogenic. Patients are thoroughly evaluated by a urologist and properly selected for surgical therapy. Organic causes are confirmed by angiography, neurologic testing, and papaverine injection–induced erection studies. A test dose of sildenafil (Viagra) delineates vasculogenic causes from psychogenic causes. Viagra is ineffective if neurologic damage has occurred.

Studies of penile activities include the measurement of erections during the rapid eye movement (REM) phases of sleep. A small band attached to a pressure-sensitive machine is placed around the penis. Erections, referred to as nocturnal penile tumescence, are recorded during sleep. This helps rule out organic causes of impotence.

Psychogenic causes are suspected after organic causes have been ruled out. Some psychogenic causes may be attributed to a fear of sexual relations after a heart attack or surgical procedure. Antidepressants and psychologic counseling may be helpful.

Most procedures for the diagnosis and treatment of organic impotence are performed with the patient under regional anesthesia. Consideration for the patient's privacy should be included in the plan of care. (More information can be found at www.impotence.org.)

Dorsal Vein Ligation. A failed erection can be caused by inadequate filling or inadequate storage of blood in the erectile tissue of the corpus cavernosa of the penis. Some patients can achieve erection but cannot maintain it for more than a few minutes because of a cavernosal leak. The diagnosis is made by the dynamic infusion cavernosometry and cavernosography (DICC) procedure. In select patients with this condition, the urologist may elect to ligate the dorsal vein and several collateral vessels of the penis to delay the venous return from the erectile tissue and help sustain erection. This procedure is not always successful.

Penile Prosthesis. Implantation of a penile prosthesis as treatment for organic impotence can enable some men to achieve a satisfactory return of sexual activity within 4 to 6 weeks postoperatively. Complications include scar tissue formation and erosion of the implant through the penile tissue. Penile prosthetic implants are of three types: semirigid silicone, semiflexible silicone–braided silver, and an inflatable hydraulic device:
* The Small-Carrion semirigid prosthesis consists of two foam-filled silicone rods that are inserted into the corpus cavernosum on each side of the penis, usually through a vertical incision in the perineum underneath the scrotum. The suitable-size prosthesis is selected from available lengths. This prosthesis maintains a permanent semierection.

- The Finney Flexirod is similar to the Small-Carrion prosthesis except that it is hinged at the penoscrotal junction when implanted. This allows the penis to hang in a dependent position when an erection is not desired.
- The Jonas prosthesis is constructed of malleable braided silver and silicone. It is semiflexible.
- The Scott-Bradley inflatable hydraulic device is inserted through a midline incision that extends from the base of the penis to a point midway between the symphysis pubis and the umbilicus. Silicone cylinders are implanted into each corpus cavernosum (Fig. 35-38). Tubing connected to these cylinders at the base of the penis is brought into the left inguinal canal, the prevesical space, and the right inguinal canal, where it is connected to tubing from the pump-release mechanism placed in the scrotum. A reservoir filled with a radiopaque solution is sutured into the abdominal fascia of the prevesical space; the tubing from this reservoir is also connected to the pump-release mechanism. To achieve an erection, the patient squeezes the pump in the scrotum (Fig. 35-39).

Penectomy. Cancer of the penis is uncommon in the developed world. It accounts for 1.3% of all cancers occurring in men. Penile cancer is more commonly found in men between 50 and 70 years of age, although 22% are younger than 40 years. The common factor in the majority of penile cancer cases is an intact foreskin 3:1. Jewish males, who are circumcised at birth, rarely develop penile cancer. Any treated lesion of the glans that does not clear in 2 to 3 weeks should be investigated as a cancerous or precancerous lesion, especially in an uncircumcised man.

Approximately 78% of all penile cancers are located between the coronal sulcus and the distal aspect of the glans. Fewer than 2% are located on the shaft. Nearly 58% of males presenting with penile cancer have positive palpable inguinal lymphadenopathy on examination. Sentinel node biopsy can be used to guide inguinal node dissection. Diagnosis of superficial lesions can be done with Mohs microscopic mapping. A clear margin of 2 cm is desired. Treatment of penile cancer with chemotherapy has not been very successful.

The penis may be partially or completely resected because of neoplasm or trauma. A partial penectomy may allow the patient enough length for upright voiding. Cosmetic reconstruction may be possible in some patients. Invasive disease may necessitate a complete penectomy, including removal of the scrotum and testes. Reconstruction after a complete penectomy includes urethral diversion to the perineum. The plan of care should include consideration for psychologic counseling.

ENDOCRINE GLANDS

Two pairs of glands in the endocrine system are of primary interest to the urologist: the adrenal glands in both genders, and the testes in the male.

Adrenal Glands

The adrenal glands are located in the retroperitoneum on the superior margin of each kidney. The adrenal cortex is the outer covering and produces hormones, including glucocorticoids (cortisol) and mineralocorticoids (aldosterone), which control the body's metabolic processes and help regulate fluid and electrolyte balance. With low levels of cortisol or aldosterone, the body is not able to respond adequately under minimal physical or emotional stress, including change in temperature, exercise, or excitement. The adrenal medulla is the inner portion of the gland and secretes the stimulants epinephrine and norepinephrine and assists the body in coping with stress. The adrenal glands secrete hormones that stimulate the sexual organs.

An adrenalectomy may be indicated to remove a benign, malignant, or metastatic tumor within the adrenal medulla or to eliminate adrenal hormonal secretions. Pheochromocytoma, a tumor of the adrenal medulla, causes excessive amounts of these stimulants to be released, resulting in hypertension. Pheochromocytoma is most commonly found in younger patients. Only a small percentage of the lesions are malignant.

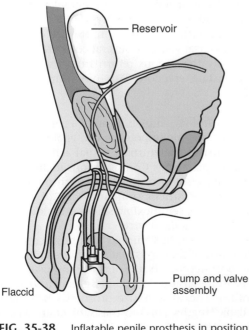
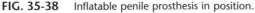

FIG. 35-38   Inflatable penile prosthesis in position.

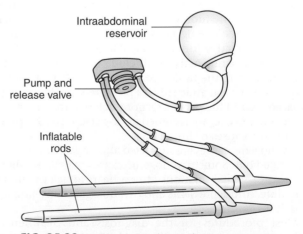

FIG. 35-39   Inflatable penile prosthesis components.

The adrenal glands are a rich source of estrogens, and estrogens may stimulate a recurrence or metastasis from prostatic or breast cancer. A bilateral adrenalectomy may be performed as a supplemental treatment of advanced prostatic or breast cancer to reduce the hormonal environment within the body.

For an open unilateral adrenalectomy, the adrenal gland is usually approached posteriorly through a lateral incision into the retroperitoneal space. The twelfth rib is usually resected on the right side because the adrenal gland lies above the kidney, behind the liver. The surgeon may also prefer a posterior approach for a bilateral adrenalectomy with the patient placed in a modified prone position for the bilateral incisions. Other surgeons prefer an anterior thoracoabdominal or transabdominal incision into the retroperitoneal space with the patient in the supine position.

The circulating nurse must verify with the surgeon the preferred position before the patient is positioned, prepped, and draped. Depending on the preoperative diagnosis, the thoracoabdominal incision may be preferred to extend the incision across the costal margin into the eighth or ninth intercostal space for exposure and exploration of the extra-adrenal paraganglion system. Laparoscopic methods are commonly employed by many surgeons with good results.

TRANSSEXUAL SURGERY (SEX REASSIGNMENT)

Transsexual surgery may be the only acceptable alternative for a patient who psychologically desires to become a member of the opposite sex—both physically and emotionally. Before having surgery, the patient is usually required to live in the desired sex role for a period of 1 year. This type of surgery presents challenges to both the urologic and the gynecologic teams.

Sex transformation requires a stable personality, psychiatric counseling for feasibility, and careful preparation and support. The patient changes legal identity and social status. The Harry Benjamin International Gender Dysphoria Association Standards of Care safeguards both transsexual people and the men and women who provide professional services for them. This set of standards divides the transition process into a series of discrete steps that enable the patient to progress at a livable pace during transition. These steps maximize the chance that the sex change process will be successful. The first step a transsexual should make is to locate a therapist who is familiar with the standards of care. It is also important to find a good support group.

Male to Female

Surgical techniques have been developed to eliminate the external genitalia of a male by dissecting the penile structures, shortening the urethra, and removing the testes. Preservation of the sensitive erogenous tissues was pioneered and perfected by Dr. Georges Borou, MD, in Morocco in the early 1960s. The patient undergoes counseling and feminization with female hormones (estrogen) preoperatively.

The patient is placed in the lithotomy position for the procedure. The process is performed in several steps as follows:

1. The perineum is dissected, and the penile shaft and scrotal skin are preserved for construction of a neovagina and labia.

2. A tissue tube is created from portions of the scrotal skin and sutured to the inverted penile skin for length.
3. A tunnel is created in the perineum between the urethra and the rectum at the space of Douglas and packed with lap tapes.
4. The corpus spongiosum is dissected, and the urethra is cut to length. A Foley is used to stent the urethral placement.
5. The dorsal vessels and nerves are spared as the glans is separated from the corpus cavernosa. The glans and a pedicle stalk are all that remain of the penile shaft. A clitoris is fashioned from the remaining glans and sutured into position. The lower abdomen is tunneled transversely and retracted superiorly so the pedicle of nerves and vessels can be nested into the retropubic space. Some procedures retain a thinly trimmed glans as a neocervix in an inverted penis-to-vagina transition.
6. The vaginal skin tube is placed inside the vaginal tunnel like a graft and sutured into place after removing the lap tapes. The neovagina is packed with vaginal packing to create equal pressure on the walls circumferentially.
7. The edges of the abdominal skin and dorsal penile tissue are pulled up and over the edge of the pubic bone and sutured into place as the anterior perineum. The remaining scrotal skin and perineal tissue are fashioned into the new posterior perineum and labia majora. The urethra is exteriorized and positioned by sutures. The apex at the superior margin is joined to form a clitoral hood and labia minora at a later procedure.
8. Drains are placed in the groins bilaterally, and the neovagina is packed.
9. The lateral edges of the left and right labia majora are approximated with temporary stay sutures to provide compression to the perineum to prevent dependent hematoma and loss of the vulvar flap. These sutures are removed several days postoperatively when the danger of hematoma is passed.

Breast implants are placed at a later date after enlargement with tissue expanders. Some patients prefer to have breast implants before the feminization procedure to make the transition preoperatively. Most patients have lived as a woman for several years before undergoing genitalia surgery. Suppression of beard and body hair, redistribution of adipose tissue, voice change, and removal of pronounced thyroid cartilage (Adam's apple) are gradual processes that are managed surgically or chemically over a period of time.

The prostate and seminal vesicles are retained so that clitoral orgasm with emission from the urethra is possible, although sperm are not produced. The actual success rate for orgasm potential is estimated at 25%. The resultant newly created vulva is realistic in form and function.

Female to Male

Female to male transsexual surgery is also possible in satisfactory candidates. Management of this change is complex. A treatment schedule of hormonal substitution (i.e., androgens [male hormones] in the female patient) is begun well in advance of the procedure.

In a one-stage procedure, a bilateral subcutaneous mastectomy or reduction, total abdominal hysterectomy, and bilateral salpingo-oophorectomy are performed. Three to five additional stages are necessary to complete the transformation:

1. Urethral elongation and reconstruction, to the tip of the enlarged clitoris. Some patients do not opt for urethral lengthening and maintain its natural position in the perineum.
2. Revision of the labia for penile lengthening and scrotal construction.
3. Flaps or grafts to create a penile shaft.
4. Placement of penile erection implants. Rigid implants are commonly used.
5. Prosthetic testicular implantation.

An understanding, nonjudgmental, unembarrassed attitude on the part of health care personnel can help the patient adjust psychologically, as well as recover physically, after the radical change. Consideration should be given to the patient's family and significant others, because they, too, must adjust. The patient may have married and produced children while in the role of his or her birth sex. In addition to confusion about parental roles, the patient may experience rejection or revulsion from offspring and other family members. Referral for family and individual counseling should be included in the plan of care.

POSTOPERATIVE COMPLICATIONS OF UROLOGIC SURGERY

Oliguria, the diminished capacity to form urine, is often seen after urologic surgery. Water and sodium are conserved by antidiuretic hormone, aldosterone, epinephrine, and norepinephrine secreted during stress; this decreases urinary output. Dehydration, shock, cardiac failure, renal failure, or third-space loss (e.g., edema, ascites) may contribute to oliguria. Because prolonged oliguria may result in renal failure, a urinary output of less than 30 mL an hour should be reported to the surgeon. Treatment depends on the cause.

Because of the introduction of the catheter and instruments, the patient should be watched for infection after all urinary tract procedures. Cloudy urine, dysuria, frequency, urgency, and pain or burning on urination are symptoms of urinary tract infections. Damage to bladder sphincters from instrumentation or urethral infection may lead to incontinence. Sharp abdominal pain after cystoscopy or the manipulation of a ureter to remove calculi may suggest peritonitis from bladder or ureteral perforation. Susceptibility to infection accompanies urinary diversion.

Bibliography

Beddhu S et al: The effects of comorbid conditions on the outcomes of patients undergoing peritoneal dialysis, *Am J Surg* 112(9):735-736, 2002.

Briganti A et al: Impact on sexual function of holmium laser enucleation versus transurethral resection of the prostate: Results of a prospective, 2-center, randomized trial, *J Urol* 175(5):1817-1821, 2006.

Burnett AL: Erectile dysfunction following radical prostatectomy, *JAMA* 293(21):2648-2653, 2005.

Byard RW et al: Glycine toxicity and unexpected intraoperative death, *J Forensic Sci* 46(5):1244-1246, 2001.

Chambers A: Transurethral resection syndrome—It does not have to be a mystery, *AORN J* 75(1):156-168, 2002.

Collins JW et al: Is using ethanol-glycine irrigating fluid monitoring and "good surgical practic" enough to prevent harmful absorption during transurethral resection of the prostate? *BJU Int* 97(6):1247-1251, 2006.

Fink KS et al: Adult circumcision outcomes study, *J Urol* 167(5):2113-2116, 2002.

Glassman DT, Docimo SG: Concealed umbilical stoma: long term evaluation of stomal stenosis, *J Urol* 166(3):1028-1030, 2001.

Hausberg M et al: Sympathetic nerve activity in end-stage renal disease, *Circulation* 106(15):1974-1979, 2002.

Lam JS et al: Treatment of proximal ureteral calculi: holmium: YAG laser ureterolithotripsy versus extracorporeal shock wave lithotripsy, *J Urol* 167(5):1972-1976, 2002.

Lin PH et al: Management of infected hemodialysis access grafts using cryopreserved human vein allografts, *Am J Surg* 184(1):31-36, 2002.

Mariela R et al: Cancer of the penis, *Cancer Control* 9(4):305-314, 2002.

Morley R, Nethercliffe J: Minimally invasive surgical techniques for stress incontinence surgery, *Best Pract Res Clin Obstet Gynaecol* 19(6):925-940, 2005.

Muntener M et al: Local anesthesia for transurethral manipulations: Is a transrectal periprostatic nerve block effective? *World J Urol* 23(5):349-352, 2005.

Overstreet DL, Sims TW: Robotic-assisted laparoscopic cystectomy with ileal conduit for urinary diversion, *Urol Nurs* 26(2):126-128, 2006.

Weizer AZ, Auge BK: Routine postoperative imaging is important after ureteroscopic stone manipulation, *J Urol* 168(1):46-50, 2002.

Wynd C: Testicular self-examination in young adult men, *J Nurs Scholarsh* 32(2):251-255, 2002.

Chapter 36

Orthopedic Surgery

CHAPTER OBJECTIVES

After studying this chapter, the learner will be able to:
- Identify the pertinent anatomy and physiology of the musculoskeletal system.
- Discuss several types of fractures and the stabilization of each.
- Describe several common specialty orthopedic instruments
- Discuss bone healing.
- Discuss the process for applying a cast.
- Describe the care of a patient undergoing orthopedic surgery.

CHAPTER OUTLINE

KEY TERMS AND DEFINITIONS

Arthrodesis Fusion of a joint.
Bi-valve cast Cut the cast into two parts—front and back for removal and reapplication.
Compartment syndrome Swelling between layers of fascia that causes damage to tissue.
Cast Material used to encase and stabilize a structure.
CR Closed reduction of a fracture without opening the skin.
Fasciotomy Emergency procedure to release pressure on region of compartment syndrome.
ORIF Open reduction and internal fixation of a fracture.

SUPPLEMENTAL MATERIAL ON EVOLVE WEBSITE *evolve*

http://evolve.elsevier.com/BerryKohn
- Content Updates
- Glossary
- Full Set of Perioperative Flash Cards
- Interactive Key Term Flash Cards
- Tips for the Scrub Person and Circulating Nurse: Arthroscopy, Total Joint Procedure
- Student Activities
- WebLinks

HISTORICAL BACKGROUND

Records tell of the treatment of fractures in Egypt 4500 years ago. Mummies have been found with splints still in place made from the bark of trees; others were strips of linen impregnated with a gluelike substance. Egyptian mummies and murals show evidence of crippling diseases. One Egyptian tomb drawing, from 2830 BC, shows a man using a crutch.

Hippocrates (460-370 BC) described scoliosis, congenital dislocation of the hip, and clubfoot. Many of the treatment methods he advocated date back before his time, demonstrating an ongoing, organized manner of medical study. Almost all of the principles of treating fractures currently followed are included in his book on fractures. Hippocrates discussed the use of traction, countertraction, bandages, splints, and treatment of compound fractures. He used mixtures of gelatinous substances and clay to coat bandages. He recognized the necessity of immobilizing a joint above and below a fracture. He described the proper position of fixing joints for the best possible future function. He wrote that exercise strengthens a part, but inactivity wastes it. He advocated mobilization of fractures as much as possible to prevent atrophy. For centuries, much of the wisdom in the books of Hippocrates was ignored or forgotten, and then rediscovered.

Galen (AD 129-199) is often referred to as the "Father of Sports Medicine." He was surgeon to the gladiators. Galen described nervous system control of muscles and their function as a motor system. He named and treated the spinal deformities known as lordosis, scoliosis, and kyphosis. His description of osteomyelitis, sequestration, and regeneration of bone was very accurate for his time.

Of the orthopedic surgeons in the late nineteenth century, no one contributed more to the development of the specialty than Charles Fayette Taylor (1827-1899). His investigations in kinesiatrics (movement therapy) and surgical mechanics contributed to the undertaking of exercise and rest in the treatment of musculoskeletal disorders.

The discovery of x-ray technology by German physicist Wilhelm Konrad Röntgen (1845-1923) in 1895 promoted orthopedics as a specialty. He won the Nobel Peace Prize in Physics in 1901. American surgeon Austin Moore (1889-1963) performed the first metallic hip replacement in 1942. In 1959 John Charnley (1911-1982) suggested in England that methyl methacrylate, used in dentistry, might be used to hold prosthetic components in place. Charnley introduced the low-friction torque prosthesis for total hip replacement in 1962. Modified versions of the Austin Moore and Charnley hip are still in use today. The principles of biomechanics have revolutionized orthopedic surgery.

THE ART AND SCIENCE OF ORTHOPEDIC SURGERY

The word *orthopedics* is derived from two Greek words: *orthos,* meaning "straight," and *paithee,* meaning "child." As the name implies, orthopedics began with the treatment of crippled children by means of rest, braces, and exercise. Degenerative diseases and disabilities affecting the musculoskeletal system cause loss of function and impair activity of the aged. Consequently, orthopedic surgeons treat a large number of geriatric and pediatric patients in comparison with other surgical populations.

Orthopedic patient care is individualized. As a branch of medicine and a contemporary surgical specialty, orthopedics is "concerned with the diagnosis, care, and treatment of musculoskeletal disorders—that is, injury to or disease of the body's system of bones, joints, ligaments, muscles, and tendons." Conservative, noninvasive medical and physical methods are used, if possible, to restore form and function.

Orthopedics depends on many disciplines to help evaluate and treat patients. Diagnostic imaging, bioengineering, electrobiology, genetics, microbiology, oncology, and transplantation are but a few of these. Professional registered nurses who specialize in orthopedic patient care are eligible for certification by examination through the Orthopaedic Nurses Certification Board (ONCB). Eligibility includes current unrestricted licensure in the United States or Canada and a minimum of 2 years' experience as a registered nurse with a minimum of 1000 hours of nursing practice in orthopedic patient care in the preceding 3 years. The certification period is 5 years and can be renewed through 100 contact hours of continuing education or by successful passage of the certification examination. (More information about certification and the National Association of Orthopaedic Nurses [NAON] is available at naon.inurse.com.)

ANATOMY AND PHYSIOLOGY OF THE MUSCULOSKELETAL SYSTEM

Structures that make up the musculoskeletal system provide bone shape, support, and stability; protect vital organs; and enable parts and the body as a whole to move. The musculoskeletal system includes bones, cartilage, joints, ligaments, muscles, and tendons. Orthopedic surgery is concerned primarily with these structures in the upper and lower extremities, including the shoulder and hip joints, and the vertebral column.

Bones

The human skeleton (Fig. 36-1) has 206 separate bones. The bony framework of the human body is divided into the axial skeleton, which consists of 80 bones that make up the skull, vertebrae, and ribcage, and the appendicular skeleton, which consists of 126 bones that make up the limbs. Each upper extremity is composed of 32 bones, and each lower extremity is composed of 31 bones. Bones are classified according to shape as long, short, flat, and irregular. The humerus in the upper arm, radius and ulna in the forearm, femur in the thigh, and tibia and fibula in the lower leg are long bones.

The end of a long bone is referred to as the epiphysis, and the shaft is referred to as the diaphysis. Thin plates of cartilage are found in the ends of long bones. In immature bone this is the area of growth and elongation. In mature bone these plates are ossified and do not grow (Fig. 36-2). The bones in the hand and foot are short bones. The scapula and patella are examples of flat bones. The vertebrae are irregular bones.

The cortex (outer layer) of bone is compact, hard connective tissue. This cortical osseous tissue surrounds porous, spongy, cancellous tissue. The innermost substance is bone marrow and is classified as either red or yellow according to its location and function (see Fig. 36-2).

The red marrow is found in the ends of long bones, in porosities of cancellous bone, and in flatter bones, such as the skull, sternum, and pelvic bones. This type of marrow is responsible for erythropoiesis, which is the formation of red blood cells and certain white blood cells. Yellow marrow is found in the medullary canals, or shafts of long bones, and has a higher adipose content.

Periosteum, a strong fibrous membrane, covers bone, except at joints. The blood supply and innervation penetrate periosteum and enter the bone through structures known as Volkmann canals. Lengthwise, lamellar structures, referred to as haversian canals, provide weight-bearing strength and passage for additional blood supply (Fig. 36-3). The inner aspect of bone is lined with endosteum, which is tissue similar to periosteum. In small children this layer contains osteoclasts that destroy bone to enlarge the marrow cavity for circumferential growth.

Bone Healing. Broken bones heal by a process referred to as union. Union of bones takes place in a series of steps (Fig. 36-4):

1. *Hematoma formation.* Blood accumulates in the area of break or injury. The inflammatory process ensues, and extravascular blood converts from liquid to a semisolid clot. Active phagocytosis removes necrotic tissue and debris.
2. *Callus formation.* Fibrin cells form a network around the injured area. The damaged periosteum is stimulated to generate osteoblasts, forming new bony substance referred to as osteoid. Minerals begin to accumulate in the network, forming a collagen callus. A callus is visible on radiograph within 1 to 2 weeks of injury.
3. *Calcification process.* Calcification begins and establishes support of the injury. Connective tissue proliferates across the site and is usually completely calcified within 6 weeks.
4. *Remodeling phase.* Excess cellular material is resorbed, and the bone resumes its preinjury strength and configuration. This remodeling phase is enhanced by stress and exercise. Depending on the site and severity of the injury, complete remodeling can take 6 months to 1 year to complete.

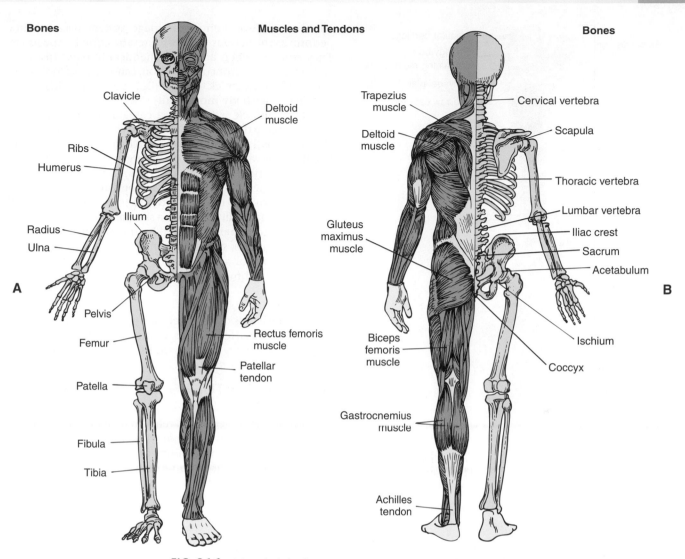

Bones   **Muscles and Tendons**   **Bones**

Clavicle

Deltoid
muscle

Ribs

Humerus

Radius

Ulna

Ilium

A

Pelvis

Femur

Patella

Fibula

Tibia

Trapezius
muscle

Deltoid
muscle

Gluteus
maximus
muscle

Biceps
femoris
muscle

Gastrocnemius
muscle

Achilles
tendon

Cervical vertebra

Scapula

Thoracic vertebra

Lumbar vertebra

Iliac crest

Sacrum

Acetabulum

Ischium

Coccyx

B

Rectus femoris
muscle

Patellar
tendon

FIG. 36-1   Musculoskeletal system. **A**, Anterior view. **B**, Posterior view.

Cartilage

Cartilage, a smooth, relatively firm, compressible connective tissue, cushions most articular surfaces at the ends of bones. It does not have a direct blood supply and is devoid of lymphatics and nerves. Cartilage derives its nutrition from synovial fluid and maintains a high water content except in pathologic states.

Joints

Bones give stability, but the body must bend and flex for locomotion. The ends of bones come together at joints. The articular cartilage and construction of the joint prevent bones from scraping against each other. Tough, fibrous connective tissue forms the outside capsule of the joint, and a finer membranous lining secretes synovium, which is similar to egg albumin. The synovial fluid contains macrophages and white blood cells that keep the joint free of debris and bacteria that could interfere with mobility.

Joints are classified by variations in structure that permit movement (Fig. 36-5). The hip and shoulder are ball-and-socket joints; the knee, ankle, elbow, and phalangeal joints

of the fingers are hinged; the wrist is a condyloid joint; and the thumb is a saddle joint. The proximal and distal bone ends are held securely in place by the joint capsule attached to both bone shafts and by ligaments.

Ligaments

Ligaments are bands of flexible, tough fibrous tissue that join the articular surfaces of bones and cartilage. They become strong when the parallel configuration of their collagen fiber is oriented against the forces applied to them (e.g., the cruciate ligaments stabilize the knee joint). Ligaments are avascular and heal slowly. They do not readily reattach to bone when torn and are prone to subsequent reinjury.

Muscles

The human body has hundreds of muscles. Muscles are all the contractile tissues of the body and are classified as smooth (involuntary), branching (cardiac), or striated skeletal (voluntary). Muscles have a rich arterial supply because they require oxygen to perform many functions, and they

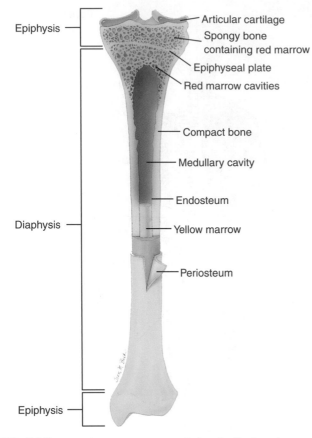

Epiphysis

- Articular cartilage
- Spongy bone containing red marrow
- Epiphyseal plate
- Red marrow cavities

Diaphysis

- Compact bone
- Medullary cavity
- Endosteum
- Yellow marrow
- Periosteum

Epiphysis

FIG. 36-2   Long bone structure seen in longitudinal section. *(From Thibodeau GA, Patton KT: Anatomy and physiology, ed 5, St. Louis, 2007, Mosby.)*

have a multilevel venous drainage system because they perform as the venous pumps for resaturation by the lungs. They contract when an electrochemical impulse from the brain crosses the myoneural junction, causing fibers to shorten. Groups of muscles work together (i.e., contract simultaneously to bring about body movement).

Skeletal muscle is the largest category of muscle tissue. There are more than 600 skeletal muscles in the human body. Skeletal muscle constitutes approximately 23% of small female body weight and 40% of larger male body weight. Each muscle fiber is a single cell that ranges in length from 0.04 to 3 inches (1 to 80 mm). The fibers are bound together into fascia-covered bundles referred to as fasciculi. Several fascia-bound fasciculi constitute a skeletal muscle and contract in response to signals mediated by the nervous system and neurotransmitters, such as acetylcholine.

The peripheral attachment is referred to as the origin. The distal attachment is referred to as the insertion.

Tendons

Tendons are bands of extremely strong, flexible fibrous tissue that attach muscle bundles to the periosteum of bones (see Fig. 36-1). They are encased in the synovial membrane sheath of movable joints.

SPECIAL FEATURES OF ORTHOPEDIC SURGERY

The orthopedic surgeon, also referred to as an orthopedist or orthopod, attempts to restore function of the musculoskeletal system lost as a result of injury or disease. Surgical procedures may be performed to repair traumatic injuries, such as fractures, dislocations, torn ligaments, or severed

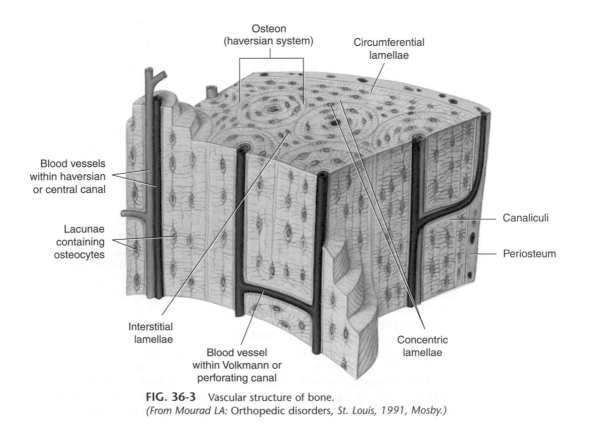

Osteon (haversian system)

Circumferential lamellae

Blood vessels within haversian or central canal

Lacunae containing osteocytes

Canaliculi

Periosteum

Interstitial lamellae

Blood vessel within Volkmann or perforating canal

Concentric lamellae

FIG. 36-3   Vascular structure of bone. *(From Mourad LA: Orthopedic disorders, St. Louis, 1991, Mosby.)*

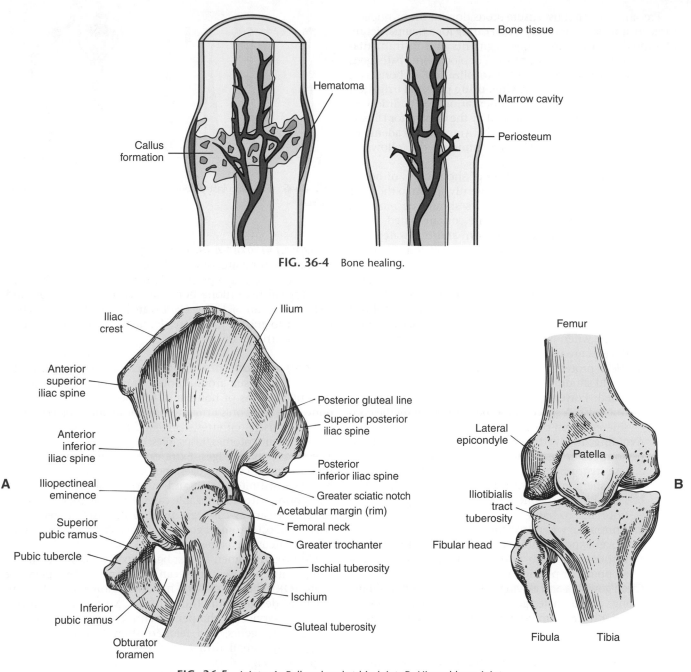

FIG. 36-4 Bone healing.

FIG. 36-5 Joints. **A,** Ball-and-socket hip joint. **B,** Hinged knee joint.

tendons. Other procedures reconstruct joints, eradicate a benign or malignant disease process, or correct postural disabilities.

In addition to conventional radiographs, computed tomography (CT), magnetic resonance imaging (MRI), and bone densitometers allow evaluation of conditions amenable to surgical correction. Arthroscopy enhances diagnosis and treatment of joint disorders, especially those caused by sports injuries. Highly sophisticated implants and instrumentation make many orthopedic procedures possible. A large percentage of orthopedic surgical procedures involve contaminated traumatic wounds or tissues highly susceptible to infection.

The occurrence of osteomyelitis (infection in bone) typically is after bone is injured in an accident or is involved in a surgical repair. Microorganisms may harbor in a hematoma or in soft tissues and spread directly to bone. Acute osteomyelitis may cause nonunion of fractures. Chronic infection may remain for life; it may cause loss of an extremity. Posttraumatic, postoperative, and health care–associated wound infections are leading causes of amputation. Chronic osteomyelitis is often associated with peripheral vascular disease. Meticulous attention to sterile technique is critical in all orthopedic procedures to prevent or at least minimize the devastating effects of infection. Sterility of implants and fixation devices is absolutely essential.

Precautions also must ensure protection for the orthopedic surgeon and team, especially when caring for a trauma victim. Manipulation of sharp bony fragments and instrumentation can be hazardous. Transmission of bloodborne pathogens is readily possible because of aerosolization of bone and debris during drilling and sawing, using powered irrigation units, and using heavy instrumentation. In addition to standard precautions recommended by the Centers for Disease Control and Prevention (CDC), the American Academy of Orthopaedic Surgeons (AAOS) recommends the following:

1. Wearing protective attire.
   a. Wear knee-high, waterproof shoe covers or boots. Blood and body fluids frequently splash to the floor and lower legs. Shoe covers should be removed and changed if they become contaminated.
   b. Wear a fluid-impervious gown and/or a waterproof apron under the gown. Copious irrigation frequently is used.
   c. Double-glove at all times, and/or have additional protection for fingers. Cloth gloves or glove liners of woven Kevlar may be worn between latex gloves in cases of trauma and major reconstructive procedures when sharp instruments and mechanical devices are used.
   d. Wear protective eyewear at all times. A full-face shield should be considered when splatter is anticipated. Powered bone instruments can produce a fine mist. A space suit–type helmet should be considered when powered bone instruments are used.
2. Avoiding inadvertent penetration of the skin of personnel during the surgical procedure.
   a. Use instrument ties and other nontouch suturing and sharp instrument techniques whenever possible.
   b. Pass sharp instruments on a tray or magnetic mat, not hand to hand.
   c. Announce when instruments are being passed.
   d. Cover exposed internal wires and pins that extend through the skin with appropriate tubing, cork stoppers, or plastic caps.
3. Clean gowning and gloving (i.e., the scrub person should change contaminated gloves before gowning and gloving another team member during the surgical procedure).

Instrumentation

Each orthopedic procedure must have the correct instrumentation for that particular bone, joint, tendon, or other structures the surgeon will encounter. An instrument used on a hip procedure is not appropriate for a hand procedure. Orthopedic instruments are heavy—often large and bulky, resembling carpentry tools—but also delicate. Each instrument has a specific purpose and requires special care and handling. Orthopedic instruments can be divided into categories by functional design.

Exposing Instruments. To expose a bone or joint, special retractors and elevators are used (Fig. 36-6). Retractors are contoured to fit around the bone or joint without cutting or tearing muscles. Periosteal elevators are semi-sharp instruments used to strip periosteum from bone without destroying its ability to regenerate new bone. They are used for blunt dissection.

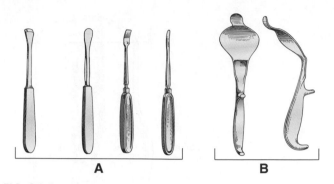

FIG. 36-6   Exposing instruments. **A,** Periosteal elevators. **B,** Bennett retractor.

Grasping Instruments. Grasping instruments are required to hold, manipulate, or retract bone. Bone-holding forceps should be selected appropriately for the size of the bone in the surgical field. Bone hooks are used for retraction and leverage (Fig. 36-7). Heavy clamps are needed to hold smaller bones or to grasp a joint capsule, such as a meniscus clamp for fibrocartilage in the knee.

Cutting Instruments. Cutting instruments are used to remove soft tissue around bone; to cut into, cut apart, or cut out portions of bone; and to smooth jagged edges of bone. The surgeon's armamentarium includes osteotomes, gouges, chisels, curettes, rongeurs, reamers, bone-cutting forceps, meniscotomes, rasps, files, drills, and saws (Fig. 36-8). These have sharp edges. Extra care should be taken not to nick or damage cutting edges; they should always be protected on the instrument table and during cleaning, sterilizing, and storing. Fitted sterilizable cases (Fig. 36-8, *E*), trays, foam towels, or canvas cases are used to keep sets together by sizes (e.g., osteotomes, gouges, chisels, curettes), as well as to protect cutting edges.

Cutting instruments must be sharp. Osteotomes, chisels, gouges, and meniscotomes can be sharpened by operating room (OR) personnel with handheld hones or a honing machine designed for this purpose. Most manufacturers provide a service for sharpening and repairing instruments. Curettes, rongeurs, and reamers should be returned for sharpening. Small drill bits and saw blades usually are disposable (Fig. 36-9).

Power-Driven Cutting Instruments. Instruments powered by electricity or compressed air or nitrogen offer precision in drilling, cutting, shaping, and beveling bone. The instrument may have rotary, reciprocating, or oscillating action. Rotary movement is used to drill holes or to insert screws, wires, or pins. Reciprocating movement, a cutting action from front to back, and oscillating cutting action from side to side are used to cut or remove bone.

Some instruments have a combination of movements and can be changed from one to another with hand controls. In some, the change may be made by adjusting the chuck forward or backward and locking it into the desired position. Powered instruments increase speed and decrease the fatigue caused by the use of manually driven drills, saws, and reamers. They also reduce blood loss from bone by packing tiny particles into cut surfaces.

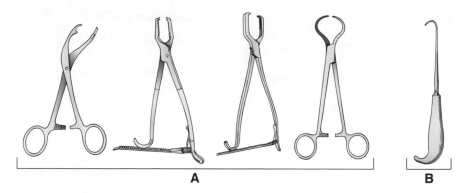

FIG. 36-7   Grasping instruments. **A,** Bone-holding forceps. **B,** Bone hook.

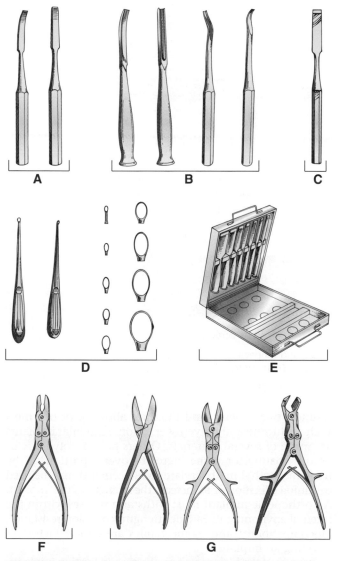

FIG. 36-8   Cutting instruments. **A,** Osteotome, curved or straight tapered blade. **B,** Gouge, curved, straight, or angled tip. **C,** Chisel, straight blade. **D,** Curette with assortment of sizes of cutting loops. **E,** Sterilizing case for set of osteotomes, gouges, chisels, or curettes. **F,** Rongeur. **G,** Bone cutter, straight or angled blade.

Measuring Devices. Rulers, calipers, depth gauges, and flexible devices for measuring angles are important for the appropriate sizing of implants and selective bone cutting. Measurements of bone diameter are performed when selecting a joint prosthesis (Fig. 36-10).

Implant-Related Instruments. Drivers, clamps, and retractors are used for inserting, securing, or removing fixation and prosthetic implants. Each type of implant requires its own instrumentation. Instruments used for insertion or extraction of metallic implants must be of the same metal as the implant to prevent galvanic reaction.

Items Used Frequently

The items to be discussed are handled frequently, although they are not used in every orthopedic procedure.

Bone Grafts. When necessary to provide structural support, a piece of bone from one part of the skeletal system may be obtained from the patient to reinforce another part of the skeletal system. Autogenous cancellous and cortical bone is obtained from the crest of the ilium, and cortical bone is obtained from the fibula. Free vascularized fibular grafts may be preferred to replace avascular (dead) bone or large segments of long bones after trauma or tumor resection. Autogenous bone may not have adequate shape or strength or may not be available in sufficient quantity, or the surgeon may deem it undesirable to subject the patient to a secondary incision or added operating time.

Allograft bone, coralline hydroxyapatite, or a bone graft substitute of tricalcium may be used. Donors, both living and cadaver, should be tested for human immunodeficiency virus (HIV) antibody before a graft is transplanted. Living donors should be retested 90 days after procurement if possible. People who are HIV positive, have any immune disorder or active infection, or have a history of hepatitis are excluded as donors. The probability of transmission of HIV in frozen or freeze-dried bone is remote. Secondary sterilization by ethylene oxide or ionizing radiation may increase the margin of safety but will reduce the biologic effectiveness of the graft.

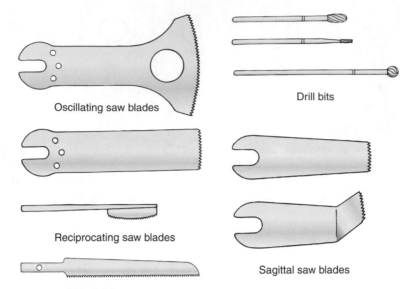

FIG. 36-9   Saw blades and drill bits.
(From Gregory B: Orthopaedic surgery, *St. Louis, 1994, Mosby.)*

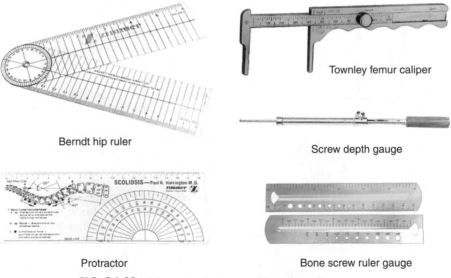

FIG. 36-10   Measuring devices used in orthopedics.
(From Gregory B: Orthopaedic surgery, *St. Louis, 1994, Mosby.)*

Soft Tissue Allografts. Cartilage, ligaments, and tendons obtained from cadavers may be frozen or freeze-dried for use to augment soft tissue repairs.

Fixation Devices. External and internal fixation devices are used to stabilize or immobilize bone, usually after skeletal injury. External devices provide temporary support during healing. Many types of screws, plates, and nails are used for temporary or permanent internal fixation of fractures or bone segments after a reconstructive procedure. Devices are also used to stabilize the vertebral column.

Prosthetic Implants. Prosthetic implants are used to permanently replace bone, joints, or tendons. They are made of nonmagnetic and electrolytically inert metals such as

stainless steel, cobalt, and titanium alloys or of polymers such as silicone and polyethylene. Some modular implants are made of several materials. Others have a polymeric or porous coating for tissue ingrowth over a portion of the implant. Methyl methacrylate (bone cement) may be used to reinforce fixation or to increase the strength of the implant. An orthopedic implant must withstand stresses within the internal environment. Fatigue strength, corrosion resistance, biocompatibility, and biomechanics are critical factors in selecting an implant.

Because of the high cost of prosthetic and fixation implants, the inventory is kept as low as possible, yet large enough to ensure availability when needed. These expensive implants are usually patient-charge items; they cannot be reused even if they are temporary. After measurements are taken, an implant of the correct size, shape, and design is selected from the sets available. Only the one to be used is handled, without the others being touched.

An infection around a fixation or prosthetic implant may require its removal, often resulting in permanent deformity or disability. Sterility at the time of implantation is imperative. Most implants are supplied sterile by the manufacturer. Others must be packaged and sterilized. Manufacturers may provide instructions for the recommended method of sterilization. Aeration time may be recommended after ethylene oxide sterilization.

Reprocessing is appropriate only if an implant has not been implanted or contaminated by blood or body fluids and if guidelines are provided by the manufacturer. Implants should not be flash-sterilized. Only standard cycles with appropriate biologic monitoring should be used. Some implants cannot withstand the heat of steam sterilization; ethylene oxide or some other appropriate method is used. The manufacturer's recommendations should be followed. Each sterilization cycle containing an implant(s) should be biologically tested and the implant(s) not used until a negative test result is known.

Implants made of or coated with polymers should be wrapped in an appropriate plastic or combination paper and plastic wrapper to prevent contamination with lint or other debris. A metal implant should not be removed from a package with an instrument. The surface could be scratched. An implant with a scratched or dented surface cannot be used because an electrolytic reaction will occur in the body. Powder-free gloves should be worn by team members who handle prosthetic implants.

Specifics about the device or prosthesis implanted must be recorded in the patient's intraoperative record. This includes the type, size, and other identifying information, such as the manufacturer's lot number. Lot numbers are recorded in the departmental lot number log as appropriate in case of recall.

Lasers. Although not used as commonly as in other surgical specialties, lasers are used in some orthopedic procedures. They are useful in confined areas (e.g., through an arthroscope) to minimize bleeding.

Carbon Dioxide Laser. Methyl methacrylate can be vaporized with a carbon dioxide (CO_2) laser to remove a cemented joint implant during a revision arthroplasty. Care is taken to use a smoke evacuator during the procedure. The CO_2 laser cannot be used in a fluid environment. A joint must be insufflated with gas; the distention medium is carbon dioxide. The vaporization of cellular water destroys soft tissue. The CO_2 laser is useful in arthroscopic surgery for sculpturing articular cartilage and for synovectomy. The joint is irrigated to remove charred tissue.

Holmium:YAG Laser. Used primarily in the knee, ankle, shoulder, and elbow, the holmium:yttrium aluminum garnet (Ho:YAG) laser is approved for all joints except the spine. The 2.1-mm wavelength with low penetration depth combined with pulsed high energy is delivered through a fine fiberoptic fiber. The Ho:YAG laser acts on water in cells without charring or damaging tissue extensively. It can ablate dense cartilage, bone, and soft tissue. It is used through an arthroscope to cut, shape, smooth, and sculpt cartilage and tissues in joints.

Neodymium:YAG Laser. The neodymium (Nd):YAG laser is used primarily in arthroscopy of the knee and shoulder joints on articular cartilage. It vaporizes protein and bonds collagen. It can be used for percutaneous disk procedures. Delivered fiberoptically, the Nd:YAG laser may have a reusable sapphire tip or a disposable, single-use ceramic contact tip. The Nd:YAG beam may be passed through a potassium titanyl phosphate (KTP) crystal, which has good cutting properties, to vaporize protein.

Bone Wax. Used for hemostasis in bone, bone wax is placed on the instrument table and opened as requested. The surgeon's preference card should be checked before the packet is opened.

Nerve Stimulator. A nerve stimulator is used occasionally to verify neural tissue during a partial nerve resection to control spastic muscles. When the popliteal nerve, for example, is given a slight shock with the nerve stimulator, the foot jerks. Both direct electric current and disposable battery-operated stimulators are available.

Sutures. Ligaments, tendons, periosteum, and joint capsules are fibrous tissues. They are primarily tough, stringy collagen and contain few cells or blood vessels. As a result, they heal more slowly than do vascular tissues. Nonabsorbable materials generally are used to suture ligaments, tendons, and muscles involved in movement of the bony skeleton. Absorbable suture is usually preferred to suture periosteum. The surgeon's preference card should be checked before the packet is opened.

Casts and Braces. A cast or brace is a means of obtaining external fixation of a fracture or a part after tendon repair, arthrodesis, or other surgical procedures. It is the means of putting a part at rest or attempting to correct an injury or abnormality. (More information about casting is located at the end of this chapter.)

Cast Room. Casts are applied in the cast room located outside of the OR suite, sometimes referred to as the plaster room. Many closed, noninvasive procedures are performed in the cast room. It keeps plaster dust from the perioperative environment—an important aspect of aseptic environmental control.

Ultraclean Air System. Special care must be used to carry out strict asepsis. Infection is the most serious, dreaded, and costly complication of orthopedic surgery. Some surgeons prefer to operate within an ultraclean air system, especially for total joint replacement procedures. Orthopedic surgeons use laminar airflow more frequently than do other surgical specialists.

A surgical isolation bubble system or patient isolation drape may be used to isolate the sterile field from personnel and equipment. Surgical helmets are available that isolate airborne contaminants from each team member. Hoses exhaust exhaled air. This system can be used independently or in conjunction with a laminar airflow system.

Isolation suits are fully contained gowns with acrylic plastic face shields and a battery-powered air filtration system. Because the suits retain heat, the OR may be kept at 70° F

(21° C) for the comfort of team members. The patient should be maintained in a normothermic state with forced-air warming or protected by some other warming method.

Orthopedic Table. An orthopedic table, often referred to as the fracture table, is used for many surgical procedures requiring traction, image intensification or conventional radiologic control, and/or cast application. The patient is anesthetized before he or she is positioned. The many available attachments make possible any desired position and traction on any part of the body. The table can be raised, tilted laterally, or put into Trendelenburg's or reverse Trendelenburg's position.

Attachments are designed not only for stabilizing the patient in the desired position but also for exerting traction to help reduce a fracture and for providing a means of evaluating the diagnosis or therapy by radiologic control. Bakelite or some other material that does not interfere with radiographic studies is used for attachments that might otherwise obscure the findings.

Essential standard component attachments on all models of orthopedic tables include three-section patient body supports, a lateral body brace, a sacral rest, and traction apparatus. Optional accessories are available to accommodate the types of procedures performed and the model of the table. When the orthopedic table is used, the following procedure is followed:

1. Consult the surgeon's preference card, procedure book, and manufacturer's manual for attachments needed for each desired position.
2. Check the patient's height and weight.
3. Assemble the necessary attachments. Pad all parts of the table and attachments to prevent pressure on joints, the sacrum, and the perineum.
4. Attach the standard components and accessories to the table frame so that all is in readiness for positioning the patient when the surgeon arrives.

Radiologic Control. Conventional radiographic equipment and fluoroscopy frequently are used during orthopedic procedures. Considerations for patient safety and personnel protection described in Chapter 13 apply to the use of radiologic control for invasive or noninvasive orthopedic procedures performed in the OR suite. Special positioning and draping techniques may be necessary, especially when C-arm fluoroscopy is used.

Often both anteroposterior (AP) and lateral views are necessary to assess the alignment of a bone or to determine the position of a fixation device or prosthetic implant. Radiographs or recorded fluoroscopic images document the work of the surgeon.

Special Considerations in Orthopedic Surgery

1. Unit beds are used to transport patients in traction apparatus. Beds, frames, and stretchers can be decontaminated in the vestibule/exchange area.
2. A cast should be removed preoperatively in the cast room. If the OR suite does not have a cast room, a cast may be bi-valved in the patient's room and then removed in the OR.
3. Positioning the patient intraoperatively and postoperatively should be directed by the surgeon. Immobilization

and good body alignment contribute to patient comfort and prevention of neurovascular injury. Pillows or other supports should not cause pain, impair function of unaffected muscles and joints, or compromise circulation.
4. Transcutaneous electrical nerve stimulation (TENS) may be used for postoperative analgesia. The electrode pads are affixed to the skin along the sides of the incision when a dressing is applied. Before application, the skin should be cleansed with water. (Saline is a conductor, so it cannot be used for cleansing.) The wires are connected to the stimulator in the postanesthesia care unit (PACU) or after recovery from anesthesia. The patient can be taught preoperatively how to use TENS for relief of pain postoperatively.
5. Electrostimulation promotes cellular responses in bone and ligaments. Mechanically stressed bone generates electrical potentials related to patterns of bone regeneration. If stimulated, healing may accelerate. Both internal direct-current stimulators and external pulsating electromagnetic field or electrical capacitor devices are used to stimulate bone and neural regeneration, revascularization, epiphyseal growth, and ligament maturation.

EXTREMITY PROCEDURES

Although instrumentation varies by procedure and the size of structures involved, basic techniques apply to handling both upper and lower extremities.

General Considerations

1. A sterile irrigating pan is placed under an extremity to catch solution if an open wound is to be cleansed, irrigated, and debrided, as for a compound fracture.
2. A pneumatic tourniquet generally is used for a surgical procedure on or below the elbow or knee to provide a blood-free field. The tourniquet cuff is applied before the extremity is prepped. It is not inflated until draping is completed. Always check the pressure setting with the surgeon before inflating a tourniquet. Ischemia time is a critical factor in patient safety. Notify the surgeon of the time lapse after the first hour and every 15 minutes thereafter throughout tourniquet inflation. Document the tourniquet location, time, pressure, and unit number.

   An Esmarch bandage is applied to the elevated extremity before the pneumatic tourniquet is inflated to exsanguinate the limb.
3. An extremity is always held up for skin preparation. See that the area under it is dry before draping. Prevent prep solution from running under the tourniquet cuff.
4. A self-adhering incise drape may be used as the first drape applied. It may be impossible to drape adequately with self-adhering plastic drapes or fenestrated sheets. If the extremity must be manipulated during the surgical procedure, the entire circumference must be draped. A limb or split sheet may be used. A sterile glove can be placed over the foot to protect the sterile field during lower limb surgery.
5. Stockinette may be used over a self-adhering plastic drape or to cover skin. This is cut with dressing scissors over the line of the incision. The cut edges may be secured over skin edges with skin clips if a plastic drape is not used. A medicine cup is a handy receptacle for these clips

after removal. The scrub person holds this at the field to receive clips as the surgeon removes them. They should be accounted for to prevent patient injury.

A self-adhering incise drape eliminates the need for either stockinette and metallic skin clips or towels and towel clips that might interfere with the interpretation of radiographs or image intensification.

6. A fluid-control drape collects blood and irrigating fluids in a pouch to prevent strike-through of and runoff from drapes. Fluids can be drained or suctioned for disposal. Blood may be suctioned for autotransfusion if blood loss is more than 400 mL, as in some hip procedures.

7. After a surgical procedure on a knee joint, a pressure dressing is usually applied to prevent serum accumulation. This may be a Robert Jones dressing, which includes a soft cotton batting roll, sheet wadding, and cotton elastic bandage. A cotton roll or other bulky material may be placed on each side of the knee and held in place with sheet wadding. A four-ply, crinkled-gauze bandage or cotton elastic bandage over this provides even, gentle pressure. Depending on the surgical procedure, a plaster splint or some other type of knee immobilizer may be preferred.

8. After a surgical procedure on a shoulder, the arm may be bound against the side of the chest for immobilization. An absorbent pad or a large piece of cotton or sheet wadding is placed under the arm to keep skin surfaces from touching, because they may macerate. The arm is held in a shoulder immobilizer that supports the humerus and wrist, or it may be bound firmly to the side of the chest with a cotton elastic bandage.

9. An extremity is elevated on a pillow placed lengthwise. This facilitates venous return, decreases swelling, and minimizes pressure on nerves. The hand should be elevated above the level of the heart; the toes must be higher than the nose.

Indications for Orthopedic Surgery

Preoperative assessment of an acute or a chronic disability affecting the musculoskeletal system of an extremity includes evaluation of the extent of bony or soft tissue involvement with or without concomitant neurovascular compromise. Assessment for signs and symptoms of neurovascular impairment in an extremity includes the six P's: Pallor, Pulses, Pain, Paresthesia, Puffiness, and Paralysis. The six P's are assessed postoperatively and monitored until support devices, such as castor splints, are removed from the surgical site.

Because they are the essence of adult orthopedic surgery and are caused either by trauma or by a degenerative disease process, procedures on the following major anatomic classifications of structures are discussed:
* Fracture of bones
* Reconstruction of joints
* Repair of tendons and ligaments

FRACTURES

Intact bones are essential to the stability and mobility of upper and lower extremities. A comminuted (splintered) or fractured (broken) bone can cause malfunction and pain. Fractures vary by cause, location, type of fracture line, and extent of injury. They are either traumatic or pathologic.

1. *Traumatic fracture.* The impact, forced twisting, or bending of an accidental injury can break one or more bones in the body. Traumatic fractures can occur when bone has become fatigued from overwork or has inadequate muscle support during exertion; a stress fracture may result (e.g., in the tibia or fibula of an athlete). Traumatic fractures are either closed or open.
   a. Closed fracture. Sometimes referred to as a simple fracture, broken fragments do not protrude through adjacent tissue to puncture the skin (Fig. 36-11, *A*).
   b. Open fracture. Also referred to as a compound fracture, either the proximal or distal end of bone, or both, protrude from the fracture site through adjacent tissues and skin (Fig. 36-11, *B*). Because of the risk of infection developing in the exposed bone, an open fracture is a surgical emergency
2. *Pathologic fracture.* Demineralization of bone (e.g., from osteoporosis or the aging process) and primary or metastatic malignant bone disease can spontaneously

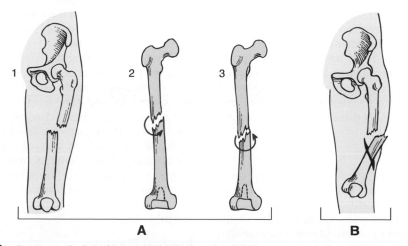

FIG. 36-11   Fractures of a long bone. **A,** Simple closed fractures. *1,* Transverse break runs across bone; *2,* oblique break runs in slanting direction across bone; *3,* spiral break coils around bone. **B,** Compound open fracture protrudes through skin.

fracture a bone without undue stress. Although they are technically simple fractures, pathologic fractures may require more than simple fixation of bone fragments.

Bone allografts or alloplastic grafts may be needed. Methyl methacrylate bone cement may be used to increase the strength of a fixation implant or as an adjunct to fill a bone defect (e.g., after removal of a tumor around a pathologic fracture). A compound made from collagen protein mixed with ceramic material may serve to stimulate creation of cartilage and osteoblasts (bone-forming cells).

Mechanical means are used to reduce a fracture and immobilize the parts, maintaining the fragments in proper alignment. Fractures must be handled gently with support above and below the site to prevent further trauma. A physician should assume responsibility for supporting the fracture site during transfer of the patient to or from a stretcher, bed, or table. Other personnel must be instructed regarding the special care needed to move a patient. The surgeon removes or directs removal of temporary splints, traction, or a pneumatic counterpressure device. An adequate number of personnel must be available so that the patient can be lifted gently. All lifters should be on the affected side, because this helps support the fracture during transfer.

In treating a fracture, the surgeon seeks to accomplish a solid union of bone in perfect alignment, to return joints and muscles to normal position, to prevent or repair vascular trauma, and to rehabilitate the patient as early as possible. Treatment of fractures usually includes three distinct phases: reduction, immobilization, and rehabilitation. The methods of treating fractures include:

* Closed reduction with immobilization
* Skeletal traction
* External fixation
* Internal fixation
* Electrostimulation

Closed Reduction

A fracture may be manipulated (set) to replace the bone in its proper alignment without opening the skin. This technique is referred to as a closed reduction. Many fractures of the lower leg or arm can be treated by closed reduction. When both lower leg bones are fractured, fibula fractures are generally disregarded and attention is directed to the tibia.

Often performed in the emergency department, closed reduction with the patient under anesthesia and application of a device for immobilization may be done in the cast room of the OR suite. A plaster, fiberglass, or other lightweight synthetic cast, cast-brace, or molded plastic fracture-brace may be used to hold the reduced fracture site in alignment during union.

Skeletal Traction

Traction is the pulling force exerted to maintain proper alignment or position. In skeletal traction the force is applied directly on the bone after insertion of pins, wires, or tongs placed through or into the bone. A small sterile setup is required. Traction is applied by means of pulleys and weights. Weights provide a constant force; pulleys help establish and maintain constant direction until the fractured bone reunites.

Forearm or Lower Leg. A Kirschner wire (K-wire), either plain or threaded, or a Steinmann pin is drilled through the bone (preferably cortical) distal to the fracture site. For forearm fractures the wire or pin must be strong enough to prevent side-to-side, angular, and rotary motion while the fracture is healing. A traction bow is attached to the protruding ends of the wire or pin. The pulleys are fastened to this bow. The ends of the wire or pin are covered with corks or plastic tips to protect the patient and personnel from the sharp ends.

Finger. A fine K-wire may be drilled through the distal phalanx. The ends may be attached to a banjo splint. Or a cast may be applied to the forearm with a loop of heavy wire incorporated in it that fans out beyond the fingers. The K-wire is fastened to this loop by a rubber band.

External Fixation

External fixation devices are used for the treatment of selected types of skeletal injuries, especially to the pelvis and extremities, with marked soft tissue loss and instability. Skeletal pins and connecting bars permit rigid fixation but with access to devitalized skin and soft tissue for wound management, especially for open injuries of the tibia. Fixation devices used for unstable pelvic fractures allow early ambulation.

Femur and Tibia. External fixation applies tension and compression forces to bone. Tension stimulates bone growth. Compression helps control infection and promotes union in fractures without bone loss. External fixators also can be used for correcting bone deformities and for lengthening the femur and tibia after osteotomy for limb length discrepancy. Several types of devices, used on the lower extremities, allow the patient to ambulate.

Stabilization Bar. Two or more pins or screws, parallel to each other, are inserted into the cortex of each fragmented section of bone. These may be connected to a metal bar, such as the dynamic axial fixator, that runs parallel to the bone on one side of the leg, or the pins may protrude through the leg and be clamped onto bars on both sides, such as with the Hoffman external fixation system.

Ilizarov Technique. Particularly useful for salvaging infected and nonunion fractures, the Ilizarov external fixator frame consists of a series of stainless steel rings connected by rods, nuts, and bolts. It can be assembled in various configurations and lengths. Wires are inserted percutaneously through the bone and connected under tension on both sides of the rings. Usually two wires are attached to each ring, at the proximal and distal levels, to stabilize bone fragments. The placement of wires is checked under C-arm fluoroscopy. Threaded rods are placed parallel to each other and in line with the longitudinal axis of the bone to connect and stabilize rings. The system has more than 120 interchangeable components, including wrenches, pliers, and wire cutters. Wire insertion is a sterile procedure. The frame is assembled on the sterile field. It weighs about 8 pounds (3.6 kg) when assembled.

Internal Fixation

Internal fixation is necessary for fractures that are not amenable to closed reduction and stabilization with cast or brace immobilization, skeletal traction, or external fixation methods. The fracture must be reduced to align fragments. Open reduction exposes the fracture site for realignment under direct visualization; closed reduction sometimes precedes the insertion of an internal fixation device. If vascular structures have been traumatized, internal fixation followed by vascular repair may be necessary to restore arterial tissue perfusion and adequate venous drainage.

The procedure may be performed with the patient under regional block anesthesia, especially in patients in poor physical condition, such as a geriatric patient or a patient who has suffered multiple trauma. Intravenous (IV) sedation may be given to dull the patient's awareness of the sound of drills and mallets.

Excellent results can be obtained with internal fixation of a fracture soon after it occurs. This method provides firm immobilization and close approximation of the fragments so that the gap between the ends is not too great for the callus to bridge. It reduces to a minimum the space between fragments and movement at the fracture site (Fig. 36-12). Healing seems to take place faster. The patient starts non–weight-bearing exercises and progresses to ambulation early, which reduces joint stiffness and muscle atrophy and prevents a long period of rehabilitation. Colles fracture of the radial bone in the wrist is sometimes surgically stabilized with plates and screws. (Fig. 36-13).

Screws, Plates, and Nails. Many types of rigid fixation implants are available. The surgeon chooses the type best suited to serve its purpose. The implant may remain permanently, or it may be removed after the fracture has healed, especially in a young person. For example, a plate can cause a stress fracture from the shielding forces exerted over time along its rigid edges on the less rigid underlying bone. If osteomyelitis develops, an implant must be removed.

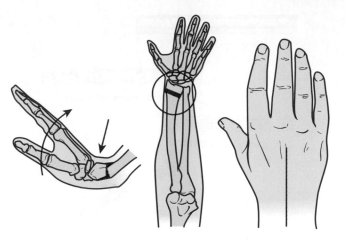

FIG. 36-13 Mechanism of Colles wrist fracture of distal radius and surgical incision for open repair.

Screws, plates, nails, rods, and pins are made of stainless steel 316 L, titanium, or cobalt alloys. These metals are nonmagnetic and electrolytically inert. Only one kind of metal is used in a patient. The instrumentation used to implant it must be of the same metal. Semirigid carbon fiber-reinforced plastic plates also are used in some situations. Biodegradable screws and rods provide stability during osteogenesis. A plate may be affixed to cortex of the bone, or an intramedullary rod can be inserted into the bone. The type and size of implant(s) must be documented in the patient's record and logged according to institution policy and procedure.

Screws. Screws alone may be used for fixation of an oblique or spiral fracture of a long bone. Screws must be long enough to penetrate both cortices. Hard cortical bone gives the best fixation, and two cortices generally hold better than one. Screws are available in various lengths and diameters. Not all screws have the same type of head (e.g., heads may be single slot, cross slot, concave cross slot, hexagon, or Phillips [Fig. 36-14]). The correct screwdriver must be used with each type of screw.

Compression Plates and Screws. Many fractures requiring open reduction are rigidly fixed through the compression method. Compression plates are heavy and strong. They are held in place by specially designed cortical lag screws. The threads of these screws are deeper than those on other types of screws and are farther apart, which allows a larger amount of bone between the threads. This construction gives maximum holding power and rigid fixation. A compression instrument may be used. It is connected to the end of the plate and then fastened to the bone with a short screw. When the nut on the compression instrument is tightened, the bone fragments are brought tightly together. The remaining screws are put into the plate, and the fracture is fixed. Screws alone are used only in selected situations. A cast may or may not be applied.

After open reduction of an acetabular fracture, a compression plate may be bent to conform to the contour of the acetabulum and secured with long cortical and cancellous lag screws.

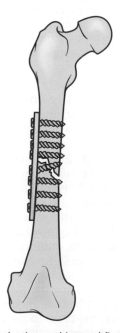

FIG. 36-12 Open reduction and internal fixation of femur with plates and screws. Note that one screw has been transfixed across the fracture line for stability.

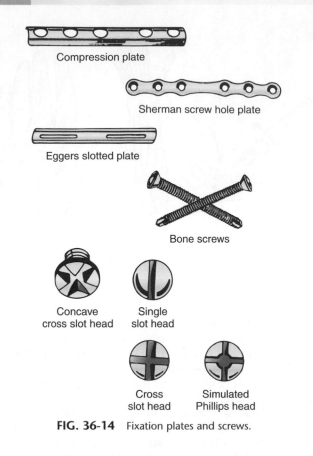

Compression plate

Sherman screw hole plate

Eggers slotted plate

Bone screws

Concave
cross slot head

Single
slot head

Cross
slot head

Simulated
Phillips head

FIG. 36-14   Fixation plates and screws.

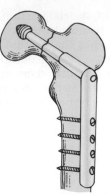

FIG. 36-15   Compression hip screw for fixation of fracture of femoral neck.

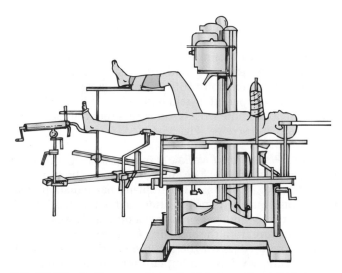

FIG. 36-16   Position on orthopedic table for nailing left hip. Note arm on affected side suspended from screen to remove it from surgical field. Note traction on affected leg and support under knee. Elevated right leg permits radiograph tube to be adjusted under it for lateral view.

Eggers Plate and Screws. The plate is slotted, which permits the muscle tone of the extremity to keep the ends of the fragments pressed closely together. The pressure stimulates osteogenesis.

Sherman Plate and Screws. The appropriate-size plate is fitted to the contour of the bone, by bending it slightly if necessary, before the screws are applied. With a drill guide, holes for the screws are drilled with an electric or air-powered drill in the center of the screw hole and perpendicularly to the plate. The drill bit should be slightly smaller than the screws. The screws should pass through both cortices of the bone.

Nails. An intertrochanteric or subtrochanteric fracture of the neck of the femur may be treated by inserting a nail, compression screw, or multiple pins through the neck into the head of the femur (Fig. 36-15). Many different types of nails are used. They are usually inserted over or alongside a guidewire. The nail may form a continuous angulated unit with a plate that fits on the outer lateral cortex of the femur, or the plate may be attached and the nail, screws, or pins inserted separately. Screws secure the plate to the shaft of the femur before or after the nail is inserted, depending on the design of the implant.

The patient is usually positioned on the orthopedic table. The surgeon and assistants assume responsibility for moving and positioning the patient. Figure 36-16 shows the position for nailing the left hip. If portable radiograph machines are used, one is on the unaffected side for an AP view, and one is at the foot of the table for a lateral view. The film for an AP view is placed on the cassette holder from the unaffected side. The procedure may be performed with C-arm fluoroscopic image intensification rather than conventional radiograph machines. All sterile tables are positioned on the affected side. The surgeon may sit to operate.

Intramedullary Nailing. An intramedullary nail, rod, or pin is driven into the medullary canal through the site of the fracture (Fig. 36-17). This brings the ends together for union, splints the fracture, and eases pain. It permits early return of function so that the patient can be ambulatory. Intramedullary implants also provide a method of holding fragments in alignment in comminuted fractures. Rigid implants generally are used for pathologic fractures or impending fracture of diseased bone. Flexible intramedullary rods may be preferred for some traumatic fractures, particularly femoral fractures. The length, size, and shape of the nail or pin depend on the bone to be splinted.

The patient with a femoral or tibial fracture is positioned on the orthopedic table. This permits traction as needed to maintain reduction. Figure 36-18 shows the position of the

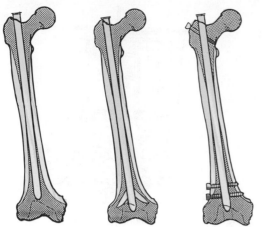

No lock   Cancellous lock   Cortical lock

FIG. 36-17   Examples of intramedullary nail and rod devices. *(From Gustilo RB et al: Fractures and dislocations, vol 1, St. Louis, 1993, Mosby.)*

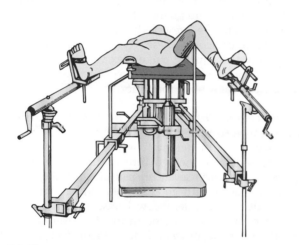

FIG. 36-18   Position on orthopedic table for intramedullary nailing of left tibia. Note left foot anchored to foot holder and knee resting on elevated curved knee rest. Right foot is anchored, and knee rest is adjusted for support of leg.

patient for intramedullary nailing of the left tibia. C-arm fluoroscopy is used for fluoroscopic control. The fracture may be reduced with visual exposure of the fracture site or by closed reduction. In some situations the medullary canal must be reshaped or enlarged before an implant is inserted. The implant may be removed after union at the fracture site has taken place, especially if it causes pain. If nonunion occurs, the implant may need to be removed.

Interlocking Nail Fixation. After closed reduction of the fracture, an intramedullary rod or nail is inserted the length of the shaft of a long bone without exposing the fracture site. This technique is called closed intramedullary nailing and may be used for transverse or short oblique fractures of the midshaft of the femur or tibia. An incision is made to expose the femoral trochanter or tibial tuberosity.

To stabilize more oblique, comminuted fractures and those beyond the midshaft region, transfixion screws are

also used with locking nails. These screws pass through the cortices of the bone and holes in the intramedullary nail. This method of closed interlocking nail fixation may be static or dynamic, depending on the location and configuration of the fracture. In the static method, screws are inserted in both the proximal and distal fragments; in the dynamic method, they are proximal or distal. Several types of interlocking nail systems are available, such as the Grosse-Kempf, Brooker-Wills, and Russell-Taylor systems. All systems prevent gliding and rotation of fragments, as well as shortening of the limb from bone loss.

JOINT PROCEDURES

Joint function depends on the quality of its structures. Articular cartilage covers the two ends of bone where they meet to form the joint. Bones are held securely in place at their articulation by ligaments and the joint capsule attached to both bone shafts. The synovial membrane lining the joint capsule secretes synovial fluid to lubricate the joint. When the joint is injured or altered by arthritis or some other degenerative disease, normal joint motion is impaired and/or painful.

Dislocations

Dislocation of one or more bones at a joint may occur with or without an associated fracture. Tendons, ligaments, and muscles are deranged. The articular surface of the bone is displaced from the joint capsule. The force of displacement damages the capsule and tears ligaments and surrounding tissues. Blood vessel and nerve damage can occur, impeding circulation and causing changes in sensation and muscle strength. Closed reduction, with or without skeletal traction, may be necessary at the time of an acute injury. If closed reduction fails to stabilize the joint and prevent recurrence, open reduction and internal fixation may be necessary. Surgical procedures to stabilize chronic recurrent dislocations are most frequently performed on the shoulder.

Arthrodesis

Fusion of a joint may be achieved by removing the articular surfaces and securing bony union or by inserting a fixation implant that inhibits motion. Arthrodesis may be performed after resection of a recurrent benign, potentially malignant, or malignant lesion that involves the ends of the bones and joint. After resection of the diseased portion of the bones, the joint may be stabilized with a bone graft or an intramedullary fixation implant.

This procedure is performed most frequently for lesions in the distal femur and proximal tibia around or including the knee joint. Arthrodesis may also be performed to relieve osteoarthritic pain or to stabilize a joint that does not respond to other methods of treatment after injury, such as instability of the thumb. Because arthrodesis limits motion, other joint reconstructive procedures are usually attempted first.

Triple arthrodesis of the ankle is performed to correct deformity or muscle imbalance of the foot. The subtalar, calcaneocuboid, and talonavicular tarsal joints are fused. Staples are sometimes used to hold bones together (Fig. 36-19).

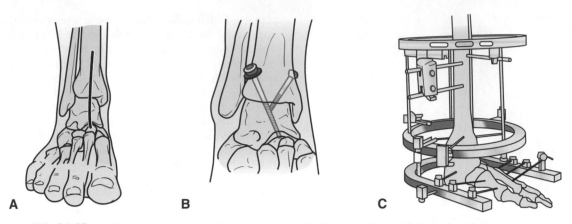

FIG. 36-19 Ankle arthrodesis. **A,** Incision for internal ankle fusion (arthrodesis). **B,** Fusion. **C,** External fixator during fusion.

Arthroplasty

Arthroplasty (reconstruction of a joint) may be necessary to restore or improve range of motion and stability or to relieve pain. This may be done by resurfacing, reshaping, or replacing the articular surfaces of the bones.

Femoral and Humeral Head Replacement. A metal prosthetic implant can replace the femoral or humeral head and neck (Fig. 36-20). These prostheses have a shaft that is driven into the medullary canal of the bone. The head of the bone is removed. The neck is shaped or removed as necessary for accurate placement of the prosthesis. A reamer may be used to enlarge the canal for insertion of the prosthesis. These prostheses are used for the following purposes:

- To mobilize the joint in arthritic patients
- To replace a comminuted fractured head when soft tissue attachments are destroyed
- To replace the head if avascular necrosis or nonunion occurs after reduction of fractures

A free vascularized fibular graft may be preferred to decompress the femoral head, provide structural stability,

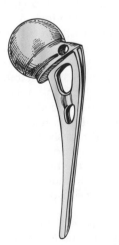

FIG. 36-20 Austin Moore prosthesis to replace femoral head and neck in hemiarthroplasty. Shaft is driven into medullary canal of femur.

and vascularize bone in an area of avascular necrosis. This procedure preserves the femoral head rather than replacing it with a prosthesis after removal of dead bone. The peroneal artery and vein are preserved with the graft. Under the operating microscope, these vessels are anastomosed to branches of the femoral circumflex vessels. Restoration of vascularization prevents progression of necrosis and stimulates osteogenesis (new bone formation).

Femoral Head Surface Replacement. As an alternative to femoral head replacement, a concentric metal shell is cemented over the femoral head. A high-density polyethylene shell is cemented into the acetabulum. Surface replacement to relieve severe hip pain and disability is reserved for young adults with good femoral and acetabular bone stock. Patients with sclerotic, well-vascularized subchondral bone of hypertrophic osteoarthritis, for example, may be candidates for this procedure. Resurfacing induces healing and reduces stress on the hip joint.

Total Joint Replacement. The surgeon's goal in total joint arthroplasty is to alleviate pain and to create functional mobility and stability. The prosthesis must maintain normal anatomic relationships and biologic fixation to bone. Correct alignment and fit of component parts are crucial aspects of their function. Although prosthetic implants for some joints have not been as well developed as those for others, total joint replacement is an accepted therapeutic modality, especially for the hip, knee, and elbow joints. Usually performed to improve mobility and relieve the pain of severe arthritic joints, total joint replacement may be indicated when other therapeutic measures have failed to correct a congenital defect, traumatic injury, or degenerative disease.

A functional design for a prosthesis must consider a combination of load bearing, strain-stress, and kinetics in association with the pathologic condition. Positioning of the prosthesis influences the distribution of stress and rate of wear.

The bones on both sides of the joints are replaced or resurfaced. Both component parts must be solidly anchored to avoid movement of the prosthesis and wear on surrounding tissue. All movement must be between the smooth articulating surfaces of the prosthesis. Various alloys, ceramics, and high-density polyethylene or silicone are used; component parts of many prostheses are made of more than one material.

Metal-to-plastic joints are self-lubricating. Natural synovial fluids help lubricate other types. The rate of wear on parts must be low so that the prosthesis will remain functional over a period of many years (the exact number is undetermined). The major complication of total joint arthroplasty is loosening of the prosthetic components over time, particularly in weight-bearing joints of obese and/or active patients. Configuration, surface features, and the method of fixation of component parts influence the mechanical stability of an "artificial" joint. The orthopedic surgeon must consider the following:

1. *Biomechanics.* Ideally, a prosthesis provides full range of motion. The support provided by cartilage, ligaments, and the articular capsule surrounding the prosthesis influences its stability. Prostheses may be constrained or nonconstrained.
   a. A constrained prosthesis provides a stable joint but restricts motion to a single plane or limits motion in all planes.
   b. A nonconstrained prosthesis allows gliding and shifting motions resembling normal range of motion, but it is inherently unstable.
2. *Biophysical components.* A total joint prosthesis has at least two components—one for each side of the articulation. To determine the size and shape of components to fit the patient, measurements of bones that form the joint may be obtained preoperatively by developing templates (i.e., patterns on grids) from the patient's radiographs. If templates have not been obtained, radiographs and measurements are taken at the surgical field. The surgeon also takes trial measurements at the site to verify the correct selection of the implant.
   a. Solid components have a predetermined configuration. The surgeon must select the most appropriate size from those available. Bone may need to be reshaped to accommodate the prosthesis.
   b. Modular systems have interchangeable components so that the surgeon can customize the prosthesis at the operating bed. For example, the width, depth, or length can be adjusted to the patient's anatomy. A quick-setting Silastic mold may be formed for precise matching in three dimensions. The mold is sent to a laboratory, where the prosthesis is customized with the use of a laser scanner and a computer-guided milling machine.
3. *Fixation.* The bone into which the component part is implanted and the surface of the prosthesis will determine the method of fixation.
   a. Press-fit fixation relies on direct bone-to-prosthesis contact. This can be achieved by a variety of methods, including reshaping the bone to the size and/or configuration of the implant and/or securing threads, pegs, or screws on the prosthesis into bone.
   b. Biofixation refers to a surface on the implant that allows tissue ingrowth for stability. Ingrowth is defined as the development of bony tissue in an empty

hole. A portion of the implant has a porous or rough surface. Bone grows into pores or interstices. Many types of coatings are used, such as tricalcium phosphate or coralline hydroxyapatite sprayed on the surface.

Others have a porous material, such as polysulfone bonded to metal. Surfaces that are porous enough for bone ingrowth without greatly expanding the surface area or weakening the implant are most desirable. These cementless prostheses require a precise fit in bones. They are particularly suited for young, active patients.

   c. Methyl methacrylate fixation uses self-curing thermoplastic acrylic cement to provide long-term fixation. Several different preparations of polymethyl methacrylate (PMMA), commonly referred to as bone cement, are available. The powder and liquid components are mixed at the instrument table immediately before insertion into the intramedullary canal of a long bone or socket of a joint. PMMA hardens in response to an exothermic reaction that reaches 140° F (60° C) and destroys surrounding cells.

The liquid portion is highly flammable and should not be placed in proximity to the pencil cautery. Use of appropriate venting devices during mixing provides an extra measure of safety for the team.

Bone cement is injected in a state of low viscosity under pressure to fill the interstices of bone. When the implant is placed, the cement fills the space around it for a secure fit. This is the method of choice for most patients older than 65 years because it allows early ambulation. Cement can crack or break and cause loosening of the prosthesis over time.

Physiologic responses to bone cement are varied. Some patients experience hypotension and can suffer an embolus or cardiac arrest during the cementing process. Close collaboration with the anesthesia provider during the use of bone cement affords the patient an additional measure of safety.

   d. Hybrid fixation refers to a combination of fixation methods. Some components are cemented; some are press-fitted or held by screws or some other noncemented technique.
   e. Bone grafts may be needed to replace bone loss around the joint. Either autologous or fresh frozen homologous bone may be used.

Total Hip Replacement. Total hip prostheses have greatly reduced the number of arthroplasty procedures previously described, especially in patients older than 50 years with degenerative hip disease. Several types and sizes of prostheses are available. Each has its own advantages and disadvantages. The surgeon must select the appropriate one for each patient's particular condition.

With the patient supine on the radiographic operating bed, an incision about 10 inches (25 cm) long is made along the lateral aspect of the thigh to remove the greater trochanter. Removal of the greater trochanter facilitates exposure to prepare sites for insertion of the prosthesis. However, its removal can cause abductor muscle weakness, instability, and other complications. Therefore some surgeons prefer an anterior approach to the hip joint with the patient supine; others prefer a posterior approach with the patient in a lateral position (Figs. 36-21 and 36-22).

With all approaches the femur is dislocated from the acetabulum. The femoral head is removed at the neck and replaced with a prosthesis. This may be a metal, usually titanium, head on a metallic stem that is seated into the medullary canal of the femur. Before the femoral prosthesis is inserted, the acetabulum is reamed to the configuration of the cup-shaped acetabular component (Fig. 36-23). This may be high-density polyethylene or metal with a smooth, rough, or porous outer surface. The inner surface is smooth polyethylene to articulate with the smooth finish on the head of the femoral prosthesis. The acetabular component is fixed in the socket. Then the femoral prosthesis is positioned. This sequence is reversed if a Silastic mold is made for a customized femoral component.

A computer-assisted surgical robot may be used to help the surgeon plan the surgical procedure, select the most appropriate type and size of hip prosthesis, and prepare the surface of the bone. A drill in the end of the robotic arm precisely drills the cavity in the femur to hold the implant stem.

Total Knee Replacement. Insertion of a total knee prosthesis may be indicated to provide for mechanical defi- ciencies in the function of the knee. The patient, usually older than 60 years, may have significant chronic pain and joint destruction as a result of arthritis, an inflammatory condition, or an autoimmune disorder. One or both knees may be affected. Bilateral total knee replacement can be performed safely in a patient who has the ability to actively participate in postoperative rehabilitation.

Selection of the appropriate prosthesis from among the types available depends on the deformity of the femorotibial articulation, patellofemoral articulation, and the structure of the cruciate and collateral ligaments. The prosthesis consists of a multiradius femoral component, a modular tibial compo- nent, and a patellar component (Fig. 36-24). The tibial and patellar components of high-density polyethylene articulate with the polished metallic surface of the femoral component.

With the patient supine on the operating bed, the knee is maintained in a flexed position (Fig. 36-25). Numerous commercial devices are available for this purpose. The pneu- matic tourniquet cuff is placed on the thigh before prepping and draping. A vertical midline incision is made over the front of the knee. After the distal femur and the proximal tibia are cut, a trial prosthesis is inserted. The knee is taken through a range of motion to assess alignment, ligament balance, and patellar positioning before the components are fixed in place. To achieve stability, permanent bone ingrowth

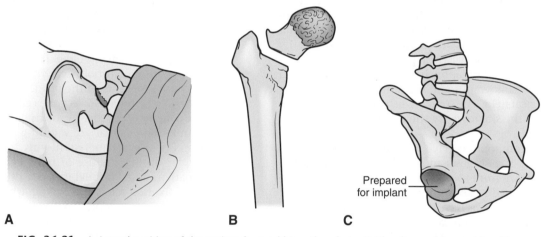

FIG. 36-21   **A,** Lateral position of the patient for total hip arthroplasty. **B,** The diseased femoral head is removed **C,** The diseased acetabulum is reamed to receive acetabular cup implant.

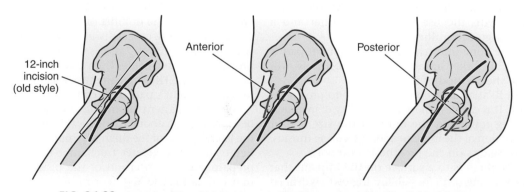

FIG. 36-22   Long traditional hip replacement incision compared with mini incisions.

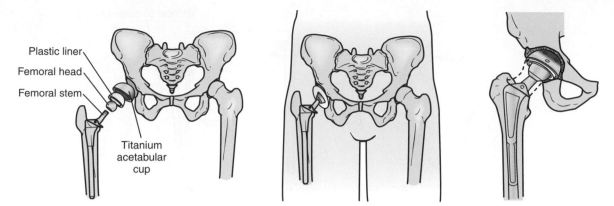

FIG. 36-23 Components of a total hip arthroplasty replacement prosthesis.

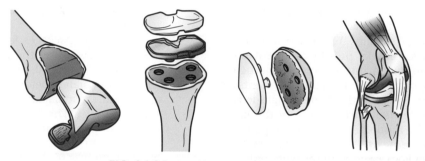

FIG. 36-24 Total knee joint replacement.

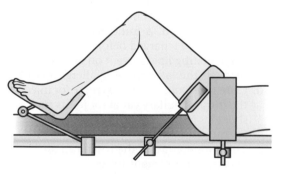

FIG. 36-25 Positioning device for knee surgery.

into a porous coated or rough-surface implant is desirable. Prostheses of this construction may not require bone cement for fixation. Hybrid fixation is used for others.

Total Ankle Replacement. Rheumatoid arthritis and posttraumatic osteoarthritis are the most common causes of ankle degeneration. Ankle joint replacement may be indicated as an alternative to arthrodesis in selected patients, usually older than 60 years, to relieve pain and secondarily to increase motion and provide stability in the tibiotalar joint. With the patient positioned supine, an anterior incision may be made from the base of the second metatarsal to the crest of the tibia. A posterior approach, with the patient positioned prone, may be preferred for wider exposure of anatomic structures. Procedures vary depending on the type of prosthesis to be implanted. The nonconstrained type allows normal dorsiflexion, plantar flexion, and rotation of the foot but is inherently unstable; the constrained type restricts motion to a single plane but is inherently more stable. The tibial components of both types are high-density polyethylene, and the talar components are metal. They are cemented in place.

Total Metatarsophalangeal Joint Replacement. Hallux rigidus and hallux abductus valgus deformities can lead to pain and altered gait. Through joint replacement, the deformity can be realigned with stability and motion. Several types of implants are available. The Silastic hinge toe, a double-stemmed silicone prosthesis with a hinge, is popular to restore motion of the great toe and lesser metatarsophalangeal joints.

Total Shoulder Replacement. Shoulder replacement may be indicated for severe destruction by disease or posttraumatic degeneration of the humeral articular surface with resultant loss of motion, instability, and pain. The prosthesis replaces the humeral head and resurfaces the glenoid cavity, the articular surface of the scapula (Fig. 36-26). Preferred if ligamentous or capsular support is sufficient, a nonconstrained prosthesis has a plastic component for the glenoid socket and a metal humeral head. Only the articular surfaces are replaced with these gliding metal-to-plastic components. A stable fixed-fulcrum, constrained prosthesis with interlocking components may be required to prevent dislocation. The patient is placed in a semi-Fowler position with the affected shoulder slightly off the edge of the operating bed for these surgical procedures.

Total Elbow Replacement. Prosthetic replacement may be indicated to correct intraarticular problems within

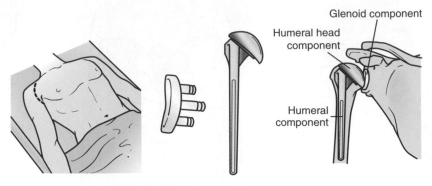

FIG. 36-26 Shoulder joint replacement.

the elbow joint, especially one with severe surface damage. Surface replacement with a nonarticulating, constrained prosthesis provides internal stability. A hinged or articulated, nonconstrained capitellocondylar prosthesis improves the functional range of motion in the humeroulnar articulation. Both the metallic humerus and ulnar components are cemented in place after shaping the bones. High-density polyethylene bushings facilitate articulation of the hinge assembly connecting the humoral and ulnar components.

Total Wrist Replacement. Silicone rubber implants are used to replace the radiocarpal joint in the wrist, primarily to improve function. A resection arthroplasty is done, usually from an anterior approach. The proximal row of carpal bones (i.e., scaphoid, lunate) and the trapezium are resected. Stems of the flexible, hinged implant are inserted into the intramedullary canals of the radius proximally and capitate carpal bone distally. A silicone cap is placed over the distal end of the ulna. Flexion and extension of the wrist are possible through free sliding of stems within the medullary canals. Some other types of prostheses have fixed stems.

Trapeziometacarpal Joint Replacement. A metal ball-to-plastic socket prosthesis restores function of the thumb. This prosthesis is cemented in place.

Metacarpophalangeal Joint Replacement. Known as implant replacement arthroplasty for small joints in the hands, the head of the affected metacarpal or proximal phalanx is removed. The silicone rubber implant bridges the excised joint. One stem fits into the medullary canal of the proximal metacarpal, and the other fits into the distal phalanx. The hinged body of the implant keeps the bones separated and mobile.

Patient Care Considerations in Arthroplasty. Patients of all ages have debilitating and painful arthritis; many are older than 65 years. Attention must be paid to support all joints during moving and positioning of these patients. Other unique aspects of joint replacement should be kept in mind:

1. The prosthesis must be handled carefully.
   a. Use only instruments specifically designed for implantation of the prosthesis.
   b. Avoid causing dents and scratches.
   c. Avoid glove powder and lint. Silicone implants should not be placed on fabrics; place the implant in a metal basin, or transfer it directly to the surgeon.
   d. Open sterile packages just before use, after the surgeon determines the size and style.
2. Bone cement, if needed, must be mixed by the scrub person immediately before use.
   a. Follow the manufacturer's instructions for handling this material. The scrub person should know by feel and appearance when the cement is of the correct consistency. A practice session is helpful before mixing for the first time during an actual surgical procedure.
   b. Avoid excessive exposure to vapors. In addition to causing irritation to the eyes, vapors may damage soft contact lenses if worn. A scavenging system should be used. A fume evacuator, if used, may need to be recharged before and after use.
   c. Avoid getting lipid solvent on gloves. It can diffuse through the latex to cause allergic dermatitis.
   d. Cement is poured into a syringe for injection into the intramedullary canal for joints such as hip or shoulder joints. Cement may be shaped manually for hinged joints.
   e. The temperature of the room can affect the time necessary for cement to set.
3. A Silastic mold, if used to customize the prosthesis, must be prepared at the sterile field. The scrub person mixes the catalyst and silicone quickly and thoroughly and then pours the mixture into the injector tube immediately before it is inserted into the bone. The customized prosthesis must be steam sterilized when it arrives from the laboratory. A standard sterilization cycle, not flash-sterilization, is used.
4. Air-powered drills, saws, and reamers must be properly connected with adequate pressure. Check the pressure in tanks of compressed air or nitrogen before the surgical procedure begins. It must be more than 500 pounds. Turn on the tank by turning the knob to the left. Turn off the tank by turning the knob to the right.
5. Suction tubing must be kept open and collection containers changed as necessary to maintain suction for irrigation during the surgical procedure.

6. Blood loss should be appropriately monitored. It can be extensive during total hip arthroplasty. Blood may be salvaged from the sterile field and processed (e.g., through a cell saver) for autotransfusion.

7. Closed-wound suction drainage generally is used, especially after hip, knee, and shoulder arthroplasty.

8. The exhaust system for personnel must be functioning properly if the surgical procedure is performed within an ultraclean air system.

9. Traffic through the OR should be restricted to minimize air turbulence. Infection is a major potential hazard of all bone and joint surgery. It can be both disabling and expensive.

10. The type of prosthesis used must be documented, including the manufacturer's identifying information. The label of a sterile implant can be affixed to the patient's record.

Arthroscopy

Arthroscopy, the visualization of the interior of a joint through an arthroscope, allows diagnosis and conservative treatment of some cartilaginous, ligamentous, synovial, and bony surface defects (Fig. 36-27). Most frequently used for definitive treatment of meniscal, articular cartilage, and ligamentous defects in the knee, an arthroscope may be used also in the shoulder, ankle, elbow, wrist, and hip. Fiberoptic arthroscopes have diameters ranging from 1.7 to 6 mm to accommodate the size of the joint. Angles of the viewing lenses also vary from 0 to 90 degrees.

Sterile irrigating solution, either Ringer's lactate or normal saline solution, at room temperature is necessary to distend the joint, although some arthroscopists prefer air or carbon dioxide. The solution is injected initially via a needle and syringe. Then through a small stab wound, a cannula is inserted into the medial aspect of the knee, for example, for inflow of irrigation. Outflow tubing is connected to the metal sheath of the arthroscope. It can be attached to suction or placed in a drainage bucket and allowed to drain by gravity.

The sheath (sleeve) over a sharp trocar is inserted through a stab wound in the skin at the selected site of entry for the arthroscope. When the trocar penetrates the capsule, the capsule and synovium form a tight seal around the sheath. The sharp trocar is replaced with a blunt obturator to advance the sheath into the joint. The obturator is removed, and the arthroscope is inserted through the sheath. The inflow and outflow irrigating tubes are connected to the stopcocks on the sheath.

An operating arthroscope may have a channel for passage of long, thin, manually operated instruments such as probes, hooks, scissors, knives, punches, and grasping forceps. Or these instruments may be manipulated through separate puncture sites (portals) into the joint under visualization through the scope. Power-driven shavers are also used to smooth rough articular cartilage or bony surfaces. A pulsed-energy Nd:YAG, Ho:YAG, or CO_2 laser may be adapted to some arthroscopes for use in a confined area and to minimize bleeding. A video camera attached to the eyepiece allows projection of the view to a closed-circuit television monitor so that the surgeon can manipulate instruments with precision (Fig. 36-28). Some cameras attach to the side of a beam splitter on the scope. Daylight film should be used with fiberoptic lighting.

Patient Care Considerations in Arthroscopy

1. All metal components of the arthroscope are steam sterilized. Some optical systems and fiberoptic cords can be steam sterilized; others require STERIS, STERRAD, or ethylene oxide (EO) gas sterilization. Protective sterilizing cases are recommended to protect the optics when the components are batch processed. Follow the manufacturer's recommendations for sterilization of the arthroscope and its component attachments.

2. The scrub person checks all sterile equipment and instruments while setting up.
   a. Check the arthroscope for clean lenses and unbroken optics.
   b. Check the patency of the inflow and outflow irrigation stopcocks and ports.
   c. All component parts must be the correct size; the optics, trocar, and obturator must fit securely into the sheath. Surgical instruments must pass through the channel. The fiberoptic cord must fit the arthroscope and projection lamp.
   d. Inspect the edges of cutting instruments, such as blades, burrs, knives, and scissors, under magnification. Blades must be sharp, set properly, and glide smoothly.
   e. Assemble power equipment. Rings must fit tightly. Forward and reverse rotating actions must function smoothly. Blades must be locked properly. The power source should be checked.

3. The circulating nurse checks all nonsterile equipment (i.e., fiberoptic projection lamp, video equipment, laser).

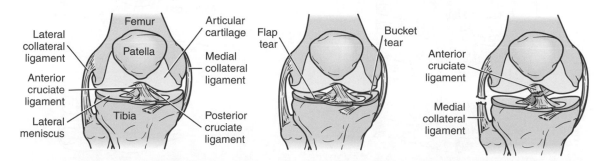

FIG. 36-27 Normal internal knee anatomy and typical sports injuries treated with surgery.

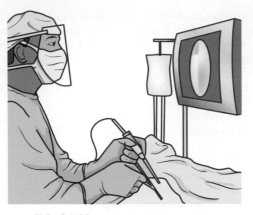

FIG. 36-28   Arthroscopic procedure.

4. The video camera and cable must be enclosed in a sterile cover unless the camera has been sterilized. The scrub person and circulating nurse coordinate draping.
5. The extremity must be firmly supported in a leg or arm holder that allows flexion of the joint (Fig. 36-29). A tourniquet is applied for arthroscopy of the knee, ankle, elbow, or wrist. Care is taken not to allow prep solution to run under the tourniquet cuff.
6. The patient is prepped and draped as for any sterile procedure on the extremity, with extra precautions to provide a waterproof barrier against contamination by irrigating solutions.
7. The circulating nurse hangs bags of sterile normal saline or Ringer's lactate irrigating solution on an IV pole at least 3 feet (1 m) above the joint to ensure adequate hydrostatic pressure to keep the joint distended and to maintain the flow of the irrigating solution. Some facilities use irrigation pumps. Two to four 3000-mL bags may be needed.

   The solution is maintained at room temperature to avoid hyperemia from warm solution, which may appear as inflammation of synovium, or blanching, which produces an avascular appearance from cold solution. Used solution should be disposed of per biologic waste protocol.
8. Equipment must be appropriately attached after the patient is draped.

a. The scrub person secures, for example, drainage tubes, fiberoptic cord, suction, and air-power cables to drapes in a location that will not impede movement of the extremity.
b. The circulating nurse attaches, for example, tubing to irrigating and suction systems and cords to power sources.

Arthrotomy

Arthrotomy (i.e., incision into a joint) may be necessary to remove bone or cartilage fragments or to repair a defect in the synovium or joint capsule. Synovectomy may be the procedure of choice for relief of pain and control of inflammation in a rheumatoid arthritic joint. If a joint is ankylosed (fused), fibrosed, or deranged, open arthrotomy rather than arthroscopy may be necessary. Occasionally during arthroscopy, an injury or disease process that cannot be adequately treated requires arthrotomy while the patient is anesthetized or it may be performed at a later time. In the knee, for example, potential neurovascular complications may preclude arthroscopic repair.

Bunionectomy

Hallux valgus, a lateral deviation in position of the great toe, increases the prominence of the adjoining metatarsal head. Pressure at the base of the first metatarsophalangeal joint causes inflammation that creates formation of an exostosis or bunion beneath the bursa and joint capsule. A bunionectomy is done to remove a painful exostosis and to functionally or cosmetically correct the deformity (Fig. 36-30). A capsulotomy must be performed to enter the first metatarsophalangeal joint. The procedure may be done with the patient under local infiltration anesthesia and IV sedation. A pneumatic tourniquet around the ankle provides hemostasis, unless contraindicated in a patient with a circulatory problem in the foot. One of several procedures may be selected.

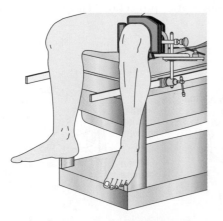

FIG. 36-29   Arthroscopy limb holder.

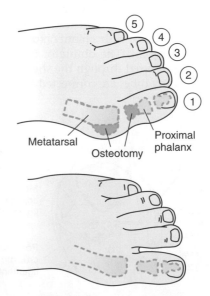

Metatarsal

Osteotomy

Proximal phalanx

FIG. 36-30   Bunionectomy.

- *Keller arthroplasty.* The proximal third of the proximal phalanx of the great toe is resected. A silicone implant may be placed in the intramedullary canal to stabilize the metatarsophalangeal joint.
- *Metatarsal osteotomy.* The metatarsal alignment is corrected by moving the metatarsal head laterally.
- *McBride operation.* The abductor tendon is fixed to the lateral portion of the metatarsal neck, and the sesamoid bone is excised.
- *Silver bunionectomy.* The medial aspect of the exostosis is removed from the first metatarsal head.

Bunionectomies are only one of many procedures performed by podiatrists, as well as orthopedic surgeons, in the treatment of foot-related disorders, including degenerative diseases and injuries of the foot and ankle.

Hammer Toes

A hammer toe is a deformity of the second, third, and/or fourth toes. The affected toe is bent at the middle joint and resembles a hammer. Hammer toes are flexible at first and can be corrected conservatively, but if they persist they can become fixed and require a surgical procedure, such as osteotomy to shorten the angle of the toe.

Hammer toe can form in the presence of bunions that cause walking in an unbalanced gait. Improperly fitted shoes cause the toes to bend. The external surface of the affected toes develops painful calluses and makes wearing shoes very painful.

Neurolysis

Neuropathy caused by entrapment of a nerve produces tingling, numbness, and a burning sensation with radiating pain and compromise of function. Known as a tunnel syndrome, this most frequently occurs in the wrist from entrapment of the median nerve (i.e., carpal tunnel syndrome). It may originate from compression of the radial nerve in the lower arm (i.e., radial tunnel syndrome) or from the posterior tibial nerve in the foot (i.e., tarsal tunnel syndrome).

The cause of formation of scar tissue or adhesions around the nerve may be related to repetitive stress, trauma, or inflammatory disease. Neurolysis, freeing of the nerve from the surrounding structures, relieves pain and restores sensation and function. For example, in the wrist, the transverse carpal ligament overriding the median nerve is incised. A segment may be excised and a synovectomy may be performed to relieve the symptoms of carpal tunnel syndrome. Release of the median nerve may also be accomplished endoscopically.

REPAIR OF TENDONS AND LIGAMENTS

Tendons and ligaments may be severed, torn, or ruptured. These injuries are frequently seen in athletes. Total or partial avulsion of the major ligaments and tendons torn from their attachments in or around an extremity joint requires repair to stabilize the joint.

Tendons can be lengthened, shortened, or transferred. When a surgical procedure is indicated, tendon repair is a meticulous but tedious procedure. Tenorrhaphy (close apposition of the cut ends of tendons, particularly extensor tendons) is imperative to successfully restore function. Tendons

heal slowly. Nonabsorbable or slow-absorbing suture is widely used in tendon repair because of its durability and lack of elasticity. A tendon may be wrapped in a silicone membrane to prevent adhesions after repair. Artificial tendons are made of a polyester center covered with silicone rubber. A double-velour polyester prosthesis is used for ligament repair of a shoulder separation.

Hand Surgery

Hand reconstruction has become a subspecialty of both orthopedics and plastic surgery. Tendon surgery is within the realm of orthopedic surgeons; however, many plastic surgeons also perform tendon repair and transfer for hand reconstruction. Restoration of function is the goal of the hand surgeon. The surgeon often manages surgical correction of fractures and rotational deformities of the fingers. Tenosynovectomy (excision of the tendon sheath) may be performed to release arthritic contractures.

Sports Medicine

Sports medicine deals with the anatomic, biochemical, physiologic, and psychological effects of motion, strength, and coordination on physical activity. Public awareness of and surgeons' concerns about athletic injuries have led to the development of sports medicine centers that emphasize physical conditioning, injury prevention, and rehabilitation of athletes. Sports medicine is a rapidly growing area of orthopedics, primarily as a result of interest in exercise among the general population. The intensity of a sports activity places physical demands on the musculoskeletal system that can result in injury. Most injuries involve ligaments, tendons, and muscles rather than broken bones. Most injuries, such as a strained muscle or tendon, do not require surgical intervention. MRI is a reliable method of assessing intraarticular injuries, either acute or chronic.

The knee, shoulder, and ankle are most prone to athletic injuries of ligaments and dislocations of joints. Arthroscopy is useful in the diagnosis and treatment of some injuries. Others require open surgical reconstruction to regain joint stability. For example, a complete ligament tear usually requires surgical repair. Some procedures combine arthroscopy and arthrotomy. Postoperative rehabilitation aims to restore range of motion, to minimize muscle atrophy, and to reestablish muscle endurance and joint position. The patient should commit to a long-term conditioning program to prevent reinjury.

Knee Injuries. The knee is the joint that is most vulnerable to both contact and noncontact sports injuries. Hyperextension, for example, can result from a noncontact activity. Contact sports can result in a combination of injuries to the cruciate and collateral ligaments, meniscus, and posterior capsule.

Anterior Cruciate Ligament. Knee stability is influenced by the dynamics of the anterior and posterior cruciate ligaments. Injuries to these ligaments are the most common and most serious types of knee injuries. The anterior cruciate ligament (ACL) can be partially or completely torn, ruptured, or avulsed. The extent of the injury determines the method of reconstruction. Arthroscopically, the ACL may be transferred into the posterior aspect of the lateral femoral condyle and secured with sutures, staples, or screws.

After an autograft is harvested through an open incision, the knee may be reconstructed through the arthroscope. One technique places a bone-patellar tendon-bone autograft and fixes it with cancellous or interference bone screws into tibial and femoral tunnels. In another method, a composite of autogenous semitendinosus muscle with a polypropylene ligament augmentation device sutured to it extends from the tibial attachment across the joint and is stapled to the distal femur. In the open Insall procedure, a bone-block graft with an iliotibial band of fascia lata is secured to the tibial tubercle.

Artificial ligamentous substitutes may be preferred for ACL reconstruction. These materials also are used to stabilize torn or ruptured ligaments in the ankle. Expanded polytetrafluoroethylene (PTFE) can be secured with screws. Allograft ligaments also are used. Woven bovine collagen, bovine and carbon fiber material, or a partially absorbable matrix of polylactic acid polymer and filamentous carbon may be used as a scaffold for new collagenous tissue ingrowth for disrupted ligaments. Concomitant partial meniscectomy or meniscal repair may be performed with ACL reconstruction.

Meniscus. Partial meniscectomy or repair of a meniscal tear may be done by open arthrotomy or closed arthroscopy. Neurovascular injury is a potential complication of these procedures. Patients selected for arthroscopy usually have a single vertical longitudinal tear that can be debrided. Localized synovium can be abraded. Sutures must be placed to reduce displacement and stabilize the meniscus.

Ankle Injuries. Ankle sprains are commonly caused by inversion injury. Ankle fractures are usually eversion injuries. Rupture of the Achilles tendon can occur spontaneously during a physical activity, such as basketball or racquet sports, usually from indirect trauma. A gap is palpable at the back of the ankle. Severed ends of the tendon may be brought together through an open or percutaneous repair with heavy (size No. 2) nonabsorbable suture.

Ankle arthroscopy may be the procedure of choice for placing internal fixation devices or for removing osteophytes (bony outgrowths) in the joint after healing of an ankle fracture.

Shoulder Injuries. Many anterior glenoid labrum and minor rotator cuff tears, the most common acute injuries, can be repaired arthroscopically. Some recurrent dislocations also can be stabilized with sutures, staples, or screws. For a major rotator cuff tear, an open Bankart repair usually is necessary to suture the labrum and reattach the glenohumeral ligament. An open Putti-Platt correction for recurrent dislocation will limit external rotation of the shoulder.

CAST APPLICATION

For closed reduction of fractures, traction, and postoperative applications, many orthopedic appliances must be available and at hand when needed. An orthopedic cart can provide the necessary items for these situations (Box 36-1). The items may vary somewhat at different hospitals, but many are universally used. The cart can be taken wherever needed in the OR suite. One shelf should be designated for sterile items.

BOX 36-1   Contents of an Orthopedic Cart

Suture removal supplies
Webril and soft roll
Assorted gauze dressings and bandages
Sterile and nonsterile gloves
Skin antiseptic agents
Disposable razors

NONSTERILE ITEMS ON ANOTHER SHELF
Pulleys and attachments for bed traction
Ropes, weights, and carriers
Felt padding and foam rubber
Arm and shoulder immobilizers
Pelvic slings and rods
Assorted sizes of gauze bandages and stockinette
Stapler
Safety pins
Cold cream and talcum powder
Disposable or reusable plaster bucket with plastic liner bag
Plastic bag for trash
Assorted sizes of plaster and/or fiberglass rolls and splints
Cast cutters, knives, scissors, spreaders, and bender

Casting supplies are commonly found on the orthopedic cart. A cast is a rigid form of dressing used to encase and support a part of the body. It supports and immobilizes the part in optimum position until healing takes place. A cast usually includes the joints above and below the affected area. It may suffice as a conservative mode of treatment (e.g., for fractures). It can be fitted to any body contour or position and can be worn for months. The following are requirements of a cast:

- It must fulfill its intended function of maintaining position of the desired parts.
- It must not be too tight and must have no pressure areas. Postapplication pain is an important symptom and must be promptly investigated because circulation may be impaired.
- It must not be too loose. It must be as light as possible, yet strong enough to withstand usage.
- It must be comfortable, with no binding or chafing.

Fiberglass Casts

A woven fiberglass tape impregnated with a water-activated polyurethane resin can be used for casting or bracing. Polypropylene stockinette is applied over the patient's skin. Polypropylene web wrap may be used for extra padding over bony prominences and pressure points. The person applying the cast must wear gloves or coat his or her hands with a silicone hand cream to facilitate smoothing and blending the layers of the fiberglass tape and to prevent resin pickup on the hands. The resin is activated by lukewarm water. The tape is applied in the same manner as plaster.

The fiberglass cast is lighter and thinner, yet stronger, than a plaster cast and is more porous, providing better ventilation. The outside may get wet without deterioration. X-rays penetrate synthetic materials better than they do plaster to evaluate the healing process. A combination of plaster and synthetic resin on a gauze backing produces a thinner, more waterproof cast that weighs less and is as strong as a plaster cast. Because of these advantages, casting tapes are preferred by many orthopedic surgeons for extremity casts.

Plaster Casts

Plaster is gypsum or anhydrous calcium sulfate. It is finely ground to break up the crystals and is then heated to drive out the water. When water is added again, recrystallization takes place and the plaster sets. It was first used as a method of splinting fractures in the nineteenth century.

Plaster bandages and splints are made of crinoline or some other fabric, with the plaster powder entrapped in the mesh. These are available in rolls or strips 2 to 8 inches (5 to 20 cm) wide. Plaster splints are either supplied precut or made from rolls as the need arises. Usually six or eight thicknesses of the desired length are used. To provide added strength, splints are applied over areas that may weaken from extra strain. Plaster bandages and splints are available with three types of plaster:

- *Slow-setting plaster* requires up to 18 minutes to set. It is used in large casts requiring more time to apply and mold. It permits blending of the layers.
- *Medium-setting plaster* requires up to 8 minutes to set. This type is used in average-size casts.
- *Fast-setting plaster* requires 4 to 5 minutes to set. It is advantageous for small casts on children who are difficult to keep in position. Many surgeons prefer using the fast-setting type in all kinds of casts; it is the most universally used type of plaster.

Application of Plaster

1. Spread a disposable plastic or nonwoven fabric sheet on the floor around the operating bed to catch drips.
2. Protect the table. If the orthopedic table is used, spread a sheet over table parts after the patient is suspended.
3. Protect the patient's hair with a cap.
4. Use a disposable plaster pail or a plastic liner bag in a plaster bucket.
5. Fill the bucket with water at room temperature. Water warmer than 70° to 75° F (21° to 24° C) will speed up the setting time and may cause excessive loss of plaster from the fabric. More important, plaster will get even hotter than its normal exothermic reaction if it is dipped in hot water. The patient could get burned.
6. Don nonsterile disposable gloves to protect the hands from irritation by lime content.
7. Remove the outer wrapping of the plaster roll. Start soaking the plaster only when the surgeon is ready to apply it. Keep just ahead in soaking it. Have the next roll ready when needed, but do not prepare several rolls ahead of time. They may harden and, if used, can produce an ineffective laminated cast. Avoid waste.
8. Hold the plaster roll under water in a vertical position to allow air bubbles to escape from the rolled ends. When air bubbles stop rising, the bandage is soaked through. Compress the ends between the fingers and palm of each hand to remove excess water. This procedure prevents telescoping during use.
9. Unroll the end about 1 inch (2.5 cm), and hand the roll to the surgeon.

10. Fan-fold a strip once toward the center, before soaking, leaving the ends free to grasp. When soaking, grasp an end in each hand, press the hands together, and submerge the strip in water for a few seconds; remove it, and pull the strip taut by the ends. It may seem drippy, but the layers blend together well when quite wet.
11. Ask the surgeon if another roll will be needed before soaking it when the cast appears near completion.
12. Handle the cast with flat, open hands, never fingers, and support the patient in such a way that he or she cannot attempt to bend an incorporated joint. Wet plaster has only one third to one half of its ultimate strength when dry. The person who supports an extremity while a cast is being applied takes care not to make finger-pressure areas in the plaster that will damage the tissue under it. Handle only with the palms of the hands.
13. Elevate an extremity on a pillow until the cast hardens. If it is laid on a hard surface, flat pressure areas may be pressed onto it.
14. Clean up as much as possible while the cast is being applied. Wipe plaster off equipment, as well as off the patient, before it dries. Plaster is easy to remove when still damp; after it dries, it must be scraped off. A cast dryer, if used, hastens drying.
15. Avoid splashing plaster on the furniture, walls, and floor.
16. Clean the equipment and table thoroughly. If the sink has a plaster trap, all plaster drip can be washed down the sink and the contents of the bucket poured into the sink. If there is no plaster trap, leave the bucket until the plaster in the bottom hardens; then empty the water and throw the plaster pail or plastic liner bag into the trash. Clean a reusable bucket as soon as you are finished with it.

Padding under Casts

Padding is usually placed under casts and serves several functions:

- It absorbs inevitable ooze from the wound after an open surgical procedure. Sterile padding is put on over the dressing before applying the cast.
- It protects the wound and the patient's skin.
- It protects bony prominences.

Materials used for padding include the following:

- *Stockinette.* A seamless tubing of knitted cotton 1 to 12 inches (2.5 to 30.4 cm) wide, stockinette stretches to fit any contour snugly.
- *Sheet wadding.* A glazed cotton bandage 2 to 8 inches (5 to 20 cm) wide is available as a sheeting. It is used over stockinette or in place of it.
- *Soft roll.* A soft roll of thin cotton batting has some stretch for smooth contour.
- *Felt.* Available in sheeting made of wool or blends of wool, cotton, or rayon in thicknesses ranging from $\frac{1}{8}$ to $\frac{1}{2}$ inch (3 to 13 mm), felt is cut into desired sizes to fit bony prominences. Felt pads are applied over sheet wadding. The plaster adheres to pads and prevents them from slipping.
- *Foam rubber.* Available in sheets $\frac{1}{4}$ to 1 inch (6.4 to 25 mm) in thickness, foam rubber may be used in place of felt.

- *Webril.* Webril is a soft lint-free cotton bandage. The surface is smooth but not glazed, so that each layer clings to the preceding one and the padding lies smoothly in place.

Common Cast Configurations

- *Cylinder.* A circular cast, made by wrapping the plaster bandages around an extremity, is used after closed or open reductions of fractures, after some surgical procedures for immobilization, or for the purpose of resting a part of an extremity (Fig. 36-31).
- *Walking cast.* A rubber walking heel or polyurethane sole is applied to the sole of a cylinder cast for ambulation. Use of a lower extremity helps maintain strength and muscle tone and helps prevent atrophy.
- *Hanging cast.* A cylinder is applied to the arm with the elbow flexed. It extends from the shoulder to over the hand, leaving the thumb and fingers free. A wire loop is incorporated at the wrist. A strap through this loop and around the neck suspends the arm. The weight of the cast provides needed traction on the humerus.
- *Shoulder spica.* Applied to the trunk, arm, and hand, leaving the fingers and thumb free, a spica cast is used after some surgical procedures on the shoulder or humerus or for a fracture of the humerus. The orthopedic table may be used for its application, or the patient may sit on a stool with the surgeon supporting the arm in the desired position.
- *Hip spica.* A hip spica cast is applied to the trunk and one or both legs after some hip procedures and fractures of the femur. The orthopedic table is used. The sacrum rests on a sacral rest. The perineal post provides counter-traction. Attachments may be used to support the legs of an adult.
- *Minerva jacket.* A Minerva jacket is applied from the hips to the head. If the head is to be completely immobilized, it is included in the jacket. The plaster is molded to fit around the face and lower jaw. A part of the plaster at the back of the head is cut out. It is used for fractures of the cervical or upper thoracic vertebrae. The orthopedic table is necessary.

- *Body jacket.* A body jacket extends from the axillae to the hips to immobilize vertebrae. Application of this cast usually requires the orthopedic or Risser table with the necessary attachments, although sometimes the patient may stand on the floor. Traction may be applied by an overhead sling. If an open surgical procedure is to be performed with the patient in a body cast, a cast cutter must be at hand in case of respiratory difficulty. However, a body cast is usually bi-valved before a patient is given an anesthetic.
  An opening is always made over the abdomen of a Minerva or body jacket to allow space for lung expansion and decompression of abdominal distention that normally occurs with ingestion of food. A folded towel may be placed over the abdomen before the stockinette is pulled over the body. This is removed when the opening is made in the cast to allow more space between the body and cast.
- *Plaster shell.* A body jacket is cut along each side, into anterior and posterior parts. The parts may be fastened together by heavy straps with buckles, or the patient may rest in one while the other is removed temporarily.
- *Wedge cast.* A wedge-shaped portion is cut from the cast. The edges are brought together and held with plaster reinforcement. This cast is used to overcome angulation in a fracture.
- *Plaster splint.* Six or more thicknesses of plaster of the desired width and length may be applied to the posterior part of an extremity and secured with gauze or a cotton elastic bandage. Excess water is pressed from the plaster splint after it is immersed in water. A splint may be used for immobilization of a fracture of the ulna or fibula. Inflatable air splints are commercially available.
- *Hairpin or sugar tong splint.* A splint twice as long as the lower arm and hand is used for a fracture of the ulna or radius. After the plaster is soaked, it may be covered with stockinette. Starting with one end on the back of the hand, the splint is placed around the flexed elbow. The palm of the hand and fingers rest on the other end of it. It is secured with a bandage.

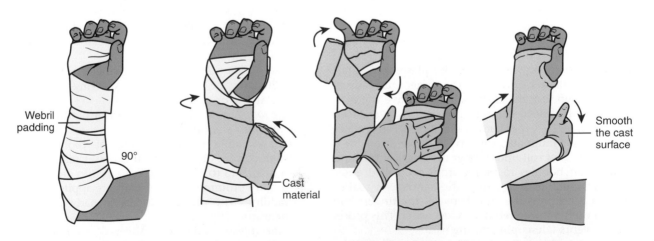

Webril padding

90°

Cast material

Smooth the cast surface

FIG. 36-31 Application of a short arm cast. Webril is applied as padding followed by the rolled casting material.

- *Abduction hip splint.* An abduction hip splint keeps hips in constant abduction. If desired for postoperative management, it is applied immediately after a hip procedure.
- *Plaster rope.* Plaster rope may support the arm in a shoulder spica or join legs in a bilateral hip spica. It is made by twisting a wet roll of plaster bandage into a rope as it is unwound, fan-folding to the desired length and drawing it through a cupped hand to blend the strands. A wooden splint may be incorporated into the rope for reinforcement.
- *Molds.* Molds are made as plaster patterns for removable metal or leather braces for the body, neck, or extremities.

Trimming, Removing, and Changing Casts

Rough edges of plaster are trimmed off and the edges of a cast are covered with stockinette or adhesive tape to protect the patient's skin. Instruments specifically designed for cutting through plaster must be used for trimming or removing casts. These include:

- Plaster knives, which have short, slightly curved blades.
- Plaster scissors, which are heavy bandage scissors.
- Electric cast cutter, which is an oscillating saw. It cuts the cast but not the stockinette or other padding under it because the padding moves with the oscillations. The patient's skin also moves somewhat and is not injured if touched lightly, although care should always be taken not to touch the skin. One model has a vacuum attached to pick up the plaster dust created by the saw (Fig. 36-32). A carbide steel blade is recommended for cutting a fiberglass cast. (A regular blade dulls quickly and can result in an inadvertent burn to the patient.)
- Cast spreader, which is a long-handled instrument that has thin, serrated jaws that can be inserted in the cutting line to pry open the cast.
- Cast bender, which is a heavy forceps-type instrument used to bend a small portion of the edge of a cast away from an area, such as a portion of a jacket away from the mouth and chin, to give freer movement.

Sharp plaster knives or scissors generally are used to trim casts. For large casts the electric cast cutter may be used, for example, to cut an opening over the abdomen of a body jacket. In a hip spica, adequate space is provided for use of the bedpan without soiling. If it is necessary to cut a "window" (i.e., a small opening in a cast to remove sutures or to inspect an area), it is put back in place and secured with a few turns of the plaster bandage. An opening in a cast encourages swelling of the tissues under it, known as window edema.

When the edema in a wound under a cast recedes, the cast does not furnish as much immobilization as may be desired. The cast is usually changed at this stage. A cast may be changed periodically during long-term immobilization because muscles atrophy with disuse. The cast becomes loose as muscle size decreases.

Skin sutures are removed at the time of a cast change if the cast was applied after a surgical procedure. A sterile suture removal tray should be ready for use when requested. Sterile sheet wadding may be needed to cover the wound after sutures are removed and before another cast is applied.

If the patient has been in a cast for some time, the skin is apt to be oily, somewhat soiled, and rough. If the surgeon wants the skin cleansed before applying another cast, only superficial dirt can be removed. Scrubbing off oily scales may cause irritation. Usually skin is not washed but, instead, rubbed with cold cream or powdered with talc before applying sheet wadding and a new cast.

A large plastic-lined trash container is used for disposal of the wrappings, trimmings, and removed cast during cast application and removal. The knives, scissors, cutter, spreader, and bender are washed promptly after use. Before instruments are put away, lubrication is applied to all instrument joints to prevent rust and corrosion.

COMPLICATIONS AFTER ORTHOPEDIC SURGERY

Thromboembolism is the most common postoperative complication of orthopedic surgery, particularly if the patient must be immobilized for an extended period. Pneumonia can be fatal for older patients. Urinary tract infection and skin breakdown also are potential problems, particularly in geriatric patients. As previously emphasized, wound infection can be devastating.

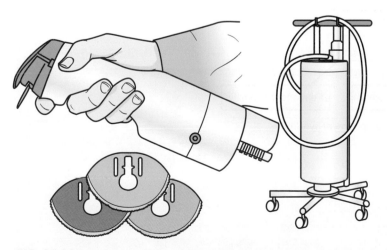

FIG. 36-32   Cast cutter and oscillating blades with vacuum attachment.

Embolus

Fat embolism is possible after fracture of a long bone or crush injury. The yellow bone marrow at the point of the fracture of the long bone releases adipose cells into the circulation. The fat emboli enter the pulmonary circulation and cause the release of fatty acids. The alveoli are damaged, and the lung surfactant is rendered ineffective.

Thromboemboli can result from deep vein thrombosis, causing pulmonary emboli. Any vessel wall injury can cause this event. Air can enter the lung, but gas exchange cannot take place because of vascular obstruction at the level of the pulmonary artery. A vena cava filter may be indicated.

Compartment Syndrome

Edema, hematoma, and seroma may form between tissue layers of the fascial plane, causing compartment syndrome. The pressure from the swelling results in further tissue destruction and necrosis that can lead to toxicity and death (Figure 36-33).

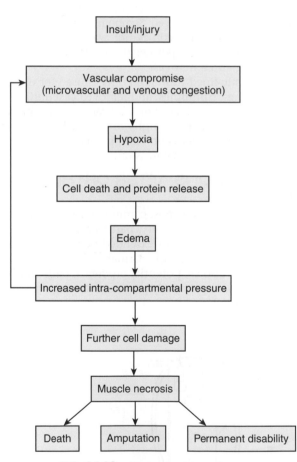

FIG. 36-33 Compartment syndrome.

The pressure is relieved by a series of longitudinal incisions that are left open to drain. Circulation cam be tenuous and the potential for nerve injury is great. Closure is not attempted for weeks or months. Healing is slow, with significant scar formation over the incision sites.

Bibliography

Altizer L: Compartment syndrome, *Orthop Nurs* 23(6):391-396, 2004.

Bach BR, Boonos CL: Anterior cruciate ligament repair, *AORN J* 74(2):152-164, 2001.

Burks JB, DeHeer PA: Triple arthrodesis, *Clin Podiatr Med Surg North Am* 21(2):203-226, 2004.

Calvo EG, Fernandez-Yruegas D: Criteria for arthroscopic treatment of anterior instability of the shoulder: a prospective study, *Br J Bone Joint Surg* 87(5):677-83, 2005.

Crowninshield RD et al: Changing demographics of patients with total joint replacement, *Clin Orthop Relat Res* 443:266-272, 2006.

Feldman MH, Rockwood J: Total ankle arthroplasty: A review of 11 current ankle implants, *Clin Podiatr Med Surg North Am* 21(3):393-406, vii, 2004.

Gartsman GM, Hasan SS: What's new in shoulder surgery? *J Bone Joint Surg Am* 83-A(1):145-151, 2001.

Kelly EW et al: Complications of elbow arthroscopy, *J Bone Joint Surg Am* 83(1):25-34, 2001.

Markel DC, Morris GD: Effect of external sequential compression devices on femoral venous blood flow, *J South Orthop Assoc* 11(1):2-8, 2002.

Melamed E, Robinson D: Effectiveness of external fixation and percutaneous pinning in maintaining distal radius fracture reduction over a 6-month period, *J Trauma Injury Infect Crit Care* 60(5):1150-1151, 2006.

Mosely JB et al: A controlled trial of arthroscopic surgery for osteoarthritis of the knee, *N Engl J Med* 347(2):81-88, 2002.

Nebelung W, Wuschech H: Thirty-five years of follow-up of anterior cruciate ligament-deficient knees in high-level athletes, *Arthroscopy* 21(6):696-702, 2005.

Olson SA, Rhorer AS: Orthopaedic trauma for the general orthopaedist: Avoiding problems and pitfalls in treatment, *Clin Orthop Relat Res* (433):30-37, 2005.

Pape HC et al: The timing of fracture treatment in polytrauma patients, *Am J Surg* 183(6):622-629, 2002.

Patt JC, Mauerhan DR: Outcomes research in total joint replacement: A critical review and commentary, *Am J Orthop* 34(4):167-172, 2005.

Prayson MJ: Baseline compartment pressure measurements in isolated lower extremity fractures without clinical compartment syndrome, *J Trauma Injury Infect Crit Care* 60(5):1037-1040, 2006.

Robinson AHN, Limbers J P: Modern concepts in the treatment of hallux valgus, *J Bone Joint Surg* 87(8):1038-1045, 2005.

Robinson CM et al: Implant-related fractures of the femur following hip fracture surgery, *J Bone Joint Surg Am* 84-A(7):1116-1122, 2002.

Chapter 37

Neurosurgery of the Brain and Peripheral Nerves

KEY TERMS AND DEFINITIONS

AVM Arteriovenous malformation. An abnormal collection of vessels that are not clearly defined as arterial or venous.

CNS Central nervous system.

Craniotomy Opening the skull.

Glioma Tumor that arises between the neurons in the connective tissue.

ICP Intracranial pressure.

PNS Peripheral nervous system.

Shunt Temporary or permanent bypass of a vascular or drainage system.

Stereotactic Using a computer imaging system to pinpoint the location of a tumor.

Subdural hematoma A collection of blood under the dural layer of meninges.

Trephine Create an opening into the skull (sometimes referred to as trepan).

Tumor A collection of cells that exhibit uncontrolled growth. Brain tumors are named for the type of cell that mutates or for the location of origin.
- **Malignant cancerous** Primary tumor began in the brain can spread to other CNS tissue.
- **Nonmalignant benign** Tumor that does not spread or invade local tissue. Can be injurious or fatal.
- **Secondary tumor** Spread to the brain from another area of the body. Metastatic cells from breast or lung form multiple brain tumors for example.

HISTORICAL BACKGROUND

Prehistoric skulls have been discovered that have evidence of successful craniotomy. Studies of trephined skulls have shown that new bony tissue regenerated around the skull perforation, demonstrating that the early patients frequently survived the procedure. Hippocrates (460-379 BC) described the use of a trephine to treat headache and postulated that the brain was the seat of intelligence. Herophilus (335-280 BC) described the ventricles of the brain. He believed that they were the seat of intelligence.

Early anatomists and physicians, such as Egyptian physician Marinus (AD first century), who identified cranial nerve X, began to realize that nerve pathways in the periphery led to the brain and cord. During his lifetime, seven pairs of cranial nerves were identified. English anatomist Thomas Willis (1621-1675) identified cranial nerve V and the communication of the cerebral vasculature known as the circle of Willis. By the eighteenth century the remainder of the 12 pairs of cranial nerves had been identified by German anatomist Samuel Soemmering (1755-1830).

Cranial surgery progressed slowly and until the early 1880s was limited to palliative treatment of hematoma or infection. English surgeon Sir Rickman Godlee is credited with the first surgical procedure for removal of a brain tumor in 1884. American surgeon William Keen (1837-1932) is credited with the first intracranial meningioma excision in the United States in 1888. He devised linear craniotomy, referred to as the Keen operation.

The recognized "Father of Modern Neurosurgery" is Harvey W. Cushing (1869-1939). Among his many accomplishments, Cushing described the relationship of intracranial pressure (ICP) to blood pressure in 1900, and in 1932 he described pituitary basophilism, commonly known as Cushing's disease. At Harvard he established the first school of neurosurgery, which led to the development of a discipline recognized throughout the world.

Application of increasing knowledge of neurophysiology and advances in diagnostic methods—such as those of American surgeon Walter E. Dandy (1886-1946), who performed ventriculography in 1918, and Portuguese neurologist Antonio Egas Moniz (1874-1955), who perfected cerebral arteriography—led to the success of intracranial and intraspinal procedures. He originated the frontal leucotomy (lobotomy). He was awarded the Nobel Peace Prize for Medicine in 1949.

English anatomist Sir Charles Sherrington (1857-1952) was a pioneer in the study of the physiology of the spinal cord. He originated the term *synapse* to denote the gaps between nerve fibers, identified the stretch receptors, and demonstrated that the cerebellum is responsible for proprioception and balance. He won the Nobel Peace Prize in 1932 for his work in the discovery of neuron function.

English neurosurgeon Sir Victor Horsley (1857-1916) developed a stereotropic brain stimulus—lesion locator in 1908. Stereotaxis led to the development of less destructive techniques to replace some extensive invasive procedures and to the treatment of some otherwise inoperable lesions. He used a modified bone wax made of seven parts beeswax and one part almond oil to control cranial bone bleeding.

The sophistication of physiologic monitoring techniques was enhanced by the development of the electroencephalogram in 1924 by German neurologist Hans Berger (1873-1941). Further developments in monitoring included evoked potentials in 1933 by Ralph Gerard.

The use of lasers has further enhanced neurosurgery. The operating microscope opened up a new field of microneurosurgery that has created interest in cerebral revascularization techniques previously unattempted and offers advantages in surgical management of many other pathologic lesions. The sophistication of physiologic monitoring techniques has facilitated these therapeutic modalities.

Neurosurgeons specialize in procedures associated with dysfunction, disease, or injury of the nervous system. The nervous system includes (1) the brain and spinal cord, also known as the neuraxis (or central nervous system [CNS]) and (2) the cranial, spinal, and autonomic peripheral nerves (the peripheral nervous system [PNS]). Neural tissues control motor and sensory functions throughout the body. Generalized cerebral function is manifested in overall behavior, level of consciousness, orientation, and intellectual performance. These functions may be altered by a metabolic disorder, a chromosomal defect, a disease process, or a traumatic injury. Assessment of neurologic deficits or changes in functional activity establishes the indications for neurosurgical intervention.

The scope of neurosurgery is broad and includes removal of pathologic lesions; relief of pain, spasm, or other neurophysiologic conditions; and repair of nerve injuries and tissue defects.

ANATOMY AND PHYSIOLOGY OF THE BRAIN

An understanding of basic anatomy and physiology is essential for preparing for the approach used to reach intracranial and spinal cord structures.

Cranium

The brain is enclosed within the bony vault of the cranium (skull). Eight bones form the cranium: the single frontal, sphenoid, and ethmoid bones anteriorly; the paired temporal and parietal bones forming the middle fossa; and the occipital bone posteriorly. Although these bones are fused together by synarthroses (nonmobile joints) referred to as sutures, the cranium is described as being divided into three areas: the anterior, middle, and posterior fossae. Galea (tough, highly vascular fascia-like tissue over the cranium) connects muscles of the temples, forehead, and base of the skull. The scalp (skin) covers the muscles and extracranial vessels and nerves in subcutaneous tissue.

Meninges

The membranous covering of the CNS, referred to as meninges, lines the cranium and covers the brain and spinal cord. The three distinct layers are the dura mater (in direct contact with the cranium), arachnoid (a weblike space), and pia mater (in direct contact with the surface of the brain).

Cranial dura mater, firmly attached to the inner aspect of the cranium, has two layers that separate in planes to form venous sinuses. The arachnoid, which lies under the dura mater, has weblike connections with the pia mater, which closely adheres to the gray matter of the brain. Cerebrospinal fluid (CSF) circulates through the arachnoid layer to bathe the brain. The pia mater follows the convolutions of the surface of the brain.

The dura is arranged in three large folds: the falx cerebri, which covers the hemispheres; the falx cerebelli, which separates the lobes of the cerebellum; and the tentorium cerebelli, which supports the temporal and occipital lobes. The tentorium is a surgical landmark denoting supratentorial structures and infratentorial structures, such as the brainstem and cerebellum.

Brain

The brain is divided into five main subdivisions composed of gray matter (neurons, cell bodies) and white matter (axons, dendrites, nerve fibers). The brain has three distinct anatomic units that consist of several subdivisions, as shown in Fig. 37-1. The cranial nerves (Table 37-1) originate from several locations in the brain and its subdivisions (Fig. 37-2).

The blood supply to the brain is derived from the carotid and vertebral arteries. The arterial component collectively joins at the circle of Willis (Fig. 37-3). The venous drainage is a series of valveless, bidirectional venous sinuses that communicate directly with the vertebral venous sinuses. The patterns of infectious spread and metastasis can be easily noted via the venous system ranging from the pelvis to the cranium.

Cerebrum. The right and left hemispheres of the cerebrum are connected centrally by the corpus callosum, a broad band of nerve fibers. The cerebrum, also known as the telen-

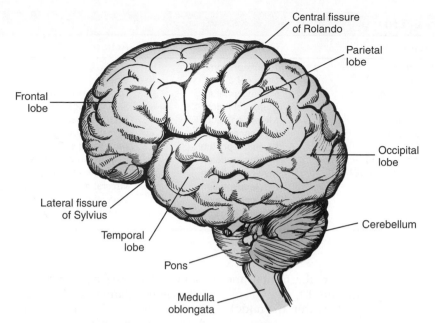

FIG. 37-1 Left lateral view of cerebral hemisphere.

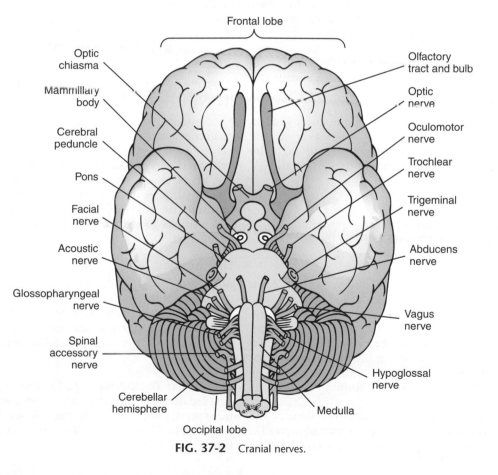

FIG. 37-2 Cranial nerves.

cephalon, occupies most of the area within the cranium and is arranged into superficial folds (called gyri) and furrows (called sulci), which are surgical anatomic landmarks. The outer cerebral cortex is the gray matter; the inner tissue is the white matter. Cranial nerve I originates here. Each

hemisphere of the brain is divided into four anatomic lobes:

1. The frontal lobe lies within the anterior fossa.
2. The parietal lobe lies in the superior and anterior portion of the middle fossa.

TABLE 37-1	Cranial Nerves		
Number	Name	Origin	Action
I	Olfactory	Telencephalon	Smell
II	Optic	Diencephalon	Vision
III	Oculomotor	Mesencephalon	Somatic motor for eyeballs, iris, and ciliary body
IV	Trochlear	Mesencephalon	Somatic motor for eyeballs
V	Trigeminal	Metencephalon	Motor and sensory
VI	Abducens	Myelencephalon	Somatic motor
VII	Facial	Myelencephalon	Motor and sensory
VIII	Vestibulocochlear	Myelencephalon	Hearing and balance
IX	Glossopharyngeal	Myelencephalon	Visceral motor and sensory, general sensory
X	Vagus	Myelencephalon	Visceral motor and sensory, general sensory
XI	Spinal accessory	Myelencephalon	Visceral motor
XII	Hypoglossal	Myelencephalon	Somatic motor

3. The temporal lobe lies inferior to the frontal and parietal lobes within the middle fossa.

4. The occipital lobe lies posteriorly within the middle fossa.

The hypothalamus and thalamus, referred to as the diencephalon, also lie within the cerebrum to form the floor and lateral walls of the third ventricle. All afferent impulses except smell pass through here to the cerebrum. The optic chiasma forms the anterior border. The diencephalon controls body temperature, emotion, hunger, thirst, sleep, and some hormones. Although it lies in the sella turcica outside the cerebrum, the pituitary body attaches to the inferior aspect of the hypothalamus.

The cerebral pedicles and the corpora quadrigemina form the midbrain, which is also referred to as the mesencephalon. The cerebral aqueduct runs through the full length of the structure. Cranial nerves III and IV originate here.

Brainstem

The brainstem lies anteriorly within the posterior fossa. It extends from the cerebral hemisphere to the base of the skull, where it merges with the spinal cord.

Pons and Cerebellum. The pons and cerebellum form the metencephalon. The pons is a bridge between the cerebrum and the medulla. It lies anterior to the bilobed cerebellum and is the origin of cranial nerves V, VI, VII, and VIII. The cerebellum lies below the occipital lobes of the cerebrum, posterior to the brainstem, within the posterior fossa. It is about one fifth the size of the cerebrum. The cerebellum controls motion and equilibrium.

Medulla. The medulla oblongata forms the floor of the fourth ventricle and contains the origin of cranial nerves IX, X, XI, and XII. It contains the vital centers, such as cardiac, vasomotor, and respiratory function.

Ventricles

Four spaces within the brain are referred to as ventricles (Fig. 37-4). The lateral ventricles, one lying in each hemisphere of the cerebrum, drain into the foramen of Monro. It opens into a central cavity, the third ventricle, which is connected by the aqueduct of Sylvius, with the fourth ventricle lying anterior to the cerebellum and posterior to the brainstem. CSF is a clear substance produced in the choroid plexuses, which are vascular extensions of the pia mater lining the ventricles. CSF is predominantly produced in the lateral ventricles and circulates through the subarachnoid space around the meninges covering the brain and spinal cord. The normal adult volume of circulating CSF is 125 to 150 mL. Obstruction of the CSF flow causes increased ICP.

SPECIAL CONSIDERATIONS IN NEUROSURGERY

Neurosurgical procedures are classified according to the anatomic location in the nervous system: brain and cranial nerves, spinal cord and nerve roots, or autonomic and somatic peripheral nerves. Regardless of the location of the surgical site, neural tissue is handled gently to minimize functional disability from surgical trauma. Hemostasis is a critical factor to sustain the vital functions of circulation and respiration. The visibility of structures in the surgical site also should be ensured.

Diagnostics

Magnetic Resonance Imaging (MRI). MRI provides a 3-D image of the complex structures of the brain, revealing tumors and aneurysms. Magnetic resonance spectroscopy is a variant of MRI that can differentiate necrotic tissue from vital tissue after the application of radiation to reduce tumor size.

Computed Tomography (CT). The computer creates a detailed image of the brain with or without contrast media; however, CT is not as accurate as MRI for diagnosis of brain tumor types. CT is useful for diagnosing trauma and bleeding into surrounding tissues. Sometimes CT is used to observe for tumor recurrence.

Positron Emission Tomography (PET). PET depicts the brain activity more than delineation of structure. It is used to distinguish living tissue from necrotic tissue and can be used to determine tumor grade after diagnosis. Interventional radiosurgery is facilitated by PET scan data.

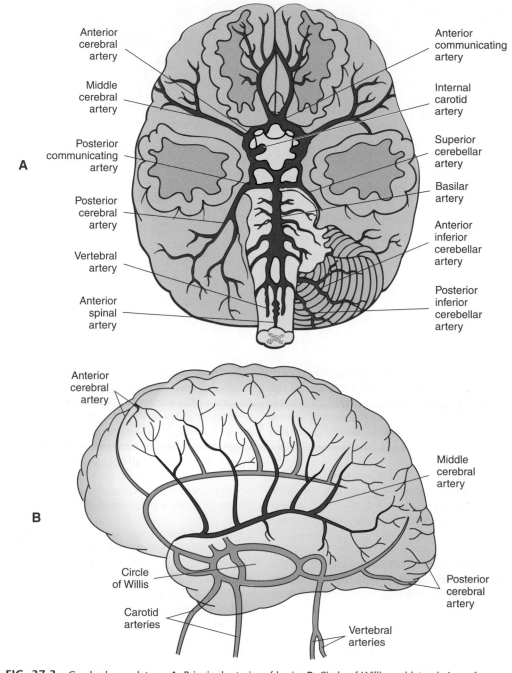

FIG. 37-3 Cerebral vasculature. **A,** Principal arteries of brain. **B,** Circle of Willis and lateral view of cerebral circulation.

Digital Holography. Three-dimensional mapping is done with holograms. This investigational technique is currently being studied for application in brain mapping and tumor diagnosis.

Prognostics

The survivability of a brain tumor is determined by several factors:

- Malignant or benign
- Cell type and location
- Duration of cell growth
- Surgically treatable
- Tumor grade (grades IV and V are the worst)
- Patient's age; age extremes have worse prognosis
- Ability to function
- Symptomatic conditions

Methods of Hemostasis

The hemostatic methods commonly used by the neurosurgeon for most procedures include the following.

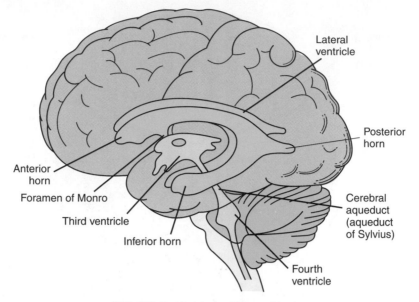

FIG. 37-4 Ventricular system of brain.

Scalp Clips. The scalp is highly vascular. Bleeding is controlled by Leroy or Raney clips placed over the edges of the wound with a special clip applier as the primary incision is made. These disposable clips are used as temporary wound pressure for hemostasis and are removed during closure of the wound.

Bone Wax. Bone wax is used on cranial and vertebral bones. The sterile wax is rolled into small 4- to 5-mm balls and placed on a smooth surface within reach of the neurosurgeon. Bone wax can act as a mechanical barrier to bone regrowth and healing.

Antibiotic Paste. Powdered antibiotic is mixed with saline or lactated Ringer's into a thick paste and smoothed over the cut ends of bones to seal off bleeders. Vancomycin powder is sometimes used in this way.

Compressed Absorbent Patties (Cottonoids). Compressed absorbent patties, made of rayon, cotton, or polyester, rather than gauze sponges are used on fragile, delicate neural tissues to absorb blood and fluids. They are also used for protection of wound edges and for hemostasis. Assorted sizes are moistened with normal saline, Ringer's lactate solution, or topical thrombin and pressed out flat on a smooth surface that is easily accessible to the neurosurgeon. Although they have no loose fibers, they could pick up lint if placed on a towel.

The standard for sponge counts includes counting these patties. They are retrieved before the surgical site is closed. Patties have a radiopaque thread securely attached to each one. This reminds the surgeon that they are in the wound and facilitates their removal. Care is taken not to suction patties into the suction tip. Some of the patties are as small as ¼ inch square. All patties are counted although they are detectable by radiograph. The strings should not be cut off.

Chemical Agents. Chemical hemostatic agents may be used after resection to control bleeding from large vessels, sinuses, or the surface of a tumor bed. The scrub person moistens a gelatin sponge with normal saline or topical thrombin before handing it to the neurosurgeon. Microfibrillar collagen, supplied in fibers or knitted sheet form, is applied dry. The tips of tissue forceps should be dry to prevent this substance from adhering to them. Oxidized cellulose also is applied dry but is removed after hemostasis has been attained, because it can interfere with wound healing.

Ligating Clips. Clips are applied on larger vessels where electrocoagulation would be insufficient or its thermal effect would be hazardous. Some permanent clips, such as intracranial aneurysm clips, are specifically designed only for neurosurgical use. Titanium is preferred because it is nonmagnetic and causes less interference with diagnostic cranial studies such as computed tomography (CT) or magnetic resonance imaging (MRI). Each type and size of clip requires a specific applier.

Electrosurgery. Monopolar ESU current is used to cut and coagulate tissue and small vessels of dermis and epidermis. Current is conducted through hemostatic forceps, fine smooth-tipped tissue forceps, or a metal suction tip to bleeding vessels. A combination suction-fulguration tip also may be used.

Bipolar current is frequently used for more precision in coagulation of tiny vessels without damage to surrounding tissue. The current does not travel through the patient's tissue to the dispersive electrode when bipolar ESU is used.

Lasers. Argon, carbon dioxide (CO_2), potassium titanyl phosphate (KTP), neodymium:yttrium aluminum garnet (Nd:YAG), and tunable dye lasers are selectively used in neurosurgery in conjunction with the operating microscope, endoscopes, and stereotaxis. Each type has benefits, but all have definite limitations. Depending on the type of laser and the location and type of tumor or vascular lesion, the laser may vaporize, shrink, or coagulate tissue. Precise hemostasis, minimal damage to contiguous structures, and visualization of effects are definite advantages of laser surgery for removal of brain and spinal cord tumors. Lasers are also used to assist in microvascular anastomoses.

Ultrasonic Aspiration. Although not technically a method of hemostasis, ultrasonic emulsification and aspiration devices fragment and remove tissue with minimal bleeding. The emulsification process assists in hemostasis of small vessels. The technique can be used to debulk or remove benign tumors in relatively inaccessible areas of the brain and intramedullary spinal cord. The high-frequency sound waves of the ultrasonic probe fragment the tumor while sparing adjacent structures, such as nerves and blood vessels. The tumor is emulsified and removed by suction. Various settings on the instrument allow the surgeon to adjust for removal of firm or calcified tumor or soft masses.

Interventional Neuroradiology. With fluoroscopy, a team consisting of a neurosurgeon and a neuroradiologist may insert a percutaneous transfemoral catheter into a strategic point in the intracranial circulation feeding an arteriovenous malformation, an aneurysm, or a vascular occlusion. A substance such as silicone or isobutyl 2-cyanoacrylate or a detachable microballoon or coil is injected to effectively embolize the lesion or its major deep-feeding arteries. This facilitates surgical resection of the lesion by minimizing potential hemorrhage. The intravascular procedure may be done preoperatively or intraoperatively.

Adjuncts to Visibility

Neural tissues should be as clean, dry, and visible as possible without damaging them. Visibility is enhanced by the following procedures.

Irrigation. Most wounds are irrigated frequently with normal saline or Ringer's lactate solution. The scrub person should keep a bulb syringe filled and ready for use. The solution should be maintained at close to body temperature or cooler to prevent vasodilation and excessive bleeding.

The tip of the bone drill burr should be irrigated during use to prevent overheating the tissues (Fig. 37-5).

Suction. Suction is necessary to evacuate blood, CSF, and irrigating fluid from the surgical site so that the neurosurgeon can identify structures. Necrotic tissue, pus, or cystic matter also may be aspirated. Usually a Frazier tip is used. Caution is taken to avoid applying vacuum directly on normal neural tissue, especially brain tissue. This tissue is protected by compressed absorbent patties. Suction should be available for all neurosurgical procedures.

Retractors. A variety of self-retaining retractors, such as Leyla or Greenberg bed-mounted styles, are used to retract scalp or skin and muscles. Dura mater is usually retracted with traction sutures. Blunt, malleable, flat, and spoon-shaped spatulas are used to retract brain tissue. Because visibility of structures is critical, retractors with a fiberoptic lighting

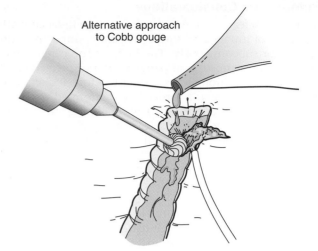

Alternative approach to Cobb gouge

FIG. 37-5 Irrigation at the tip of the drill is important to prevent overheating the tissues. Eye protection is needed to prevent splash of bone chips and solution.

system incorporated into them may be used, especially for intracranial procedures.

Headlight. A fiberoptic headlight is used by most neurosurgeons for supplemental lighting in the surgical site.

Endoscope. A side-viewing fiberoptic endoscope may be used to enhance visibility at obscure angles in otherwise visually inaccessible areas. This endoscope is particularly useful to identify lesions in the sella turcica, cerebral aneurysms, and intervertebral discs, for example. An endoscope may be used for placement of electrodes for stimulators or a catheter for radioisotopes.

The argon laser can be used through a ventriculoscope for intraventricular obliteration of the choroid plexuses and for intravascular treatment of lesions and neoplasms. The Nd:YAG laser can be used through a flexible or rigid neuroscope to vaporize a cyst. A straightforward, rigid, zero-degree scope may be used for electrocoagulation or laser obliteration of tissue and to obtain a CT-assisted stereotactic biopsy.

NeuroGuide Intraoperative Viewing System. The NeuroGuide intraoperative viewing system provides capabilities for viewing structures through a tiny opening in the brain for diagnostic and therapeutic procedures with minimal trauma to tissues.

Operating Microscope. The operating microscope provides an intense light as well as magnification for visualization of intracranial structures. Microsurgery permits removal of tumors and vascular lesions that are otherwise inaccessible or inoperable. The CO_2 laser may be used through a micromanipulator. The microscope also is used for some spinal procedures and peripheral nerve repair.

A fiberoptic camera attached to a microscope projects the surgical site onto a video monitor screen. This provides a clear view for the assistant and scrub person. In lieu of using the microscope, the surgeon may wear binocular loupes to magnify the surgical site.

Patient Care Considerations

The patient's fear of an inability to function independently as a result of intracranial surgery is paramount, either consciously or subconsciously. The brain is the core of one's being. Many neurosurgical patients are not premedicated, which allows neurologic assessment before induction of anesthesia or during a procedure performed with the patient under local anesthesia. The circulating nurse should be sensitive to the patient's fears and offer reassurance. Psychologic support is especially significant for an awake patient.

Explanation of what to expect is critical. The following considerations apply:

1. Preparation of the patient in the OR usually begins with clipping hair with electric clippers. Hair on the head is considered the patient's personal property. When all of it is removed, it is saved. Hair removal and its disposition are documented on the patient's chart.

2. The incision and the type of procedure determine the head holder that will be needed to position the patient. The basic unit of a neurosurgical headrest attaches in place of the headpiece on the standard operating bed. The head holder, either a headrest or a skull clamp, stabilizes and supports the head. The circulating nurse should be familiar with the desired neurosurgical positions and the headrests, skull clamps, and attachments for each.

   a. For the supine position, the configuration of the headrest contours to the back of the head. The supine position is used most commonly for approaches to the frontal, parietal, and temporal lobes within the anterior and middle fossae. A lateral position may be preferred for some of these surgical procedures, such as a unilateral approach to the right or left temporal lobe.

   b. For the prone position, a padded circular or horseshoe-shaped headrest equalizes weight distribution around the face. The eyes are lubricated and the lids are taped closed for protection. The prone position is used to reach the occipital lobe. It may also be used for a suboccipital approach; however, many neurosurgeons prefer a sitting position to approach the posterior fossa.

   The patient's transport cart should be immediately available in the event of the need for cardiac resuscitation. The patient would need to be placed supine in a rapid manner, and the nearby cart facilitates this maneuver.

   c. For the sitting position, the headrest is attached at the head end of the operating bed to support the back of the head for a unilateral or nasal approach. For a posterior approach, a head holder supports the forehead. The frame of the head holder is attached to side rails of the back section of the operating bed (Fig. 37-6) so that the patient's head can be lowered in the event of an air embolus. The sitting position allows greater torsion and flexion of the neck than either a lateral or the prone position and a more accessible approach to the cerebellopontine angle.

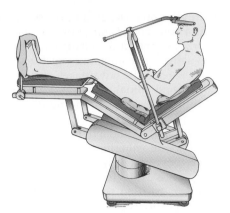

FIG. 37-6 Neurosurgical sitting position for posterior approach. Frame of head holder is attached to side rails of back section of operating bed. Note that legs are flexed at thighs and are approximately at level of heart. Feet are padded at right angles to legs. Subgluteal padding protects sciatic nerves.

   d. For rigid fixation of the skull, a skull clamp provides stability that is necessary for microsurgical procedures and is desirable during lengthy procedures. This eliminates the risk of pressure-related complications around the face or eyes with the patient prone or in a lateral position and minimizes the risk of air embolism with the patient sitting. Three pins on the clamp partially penetrate the outer table of the skull. Pins on one side may be spring-loaded, such as on the Mayfield skull clamp (Fig. 37-7), to join the skull and the clamp into one rigid mechanical unit. The skull clamp is attached to the operating bed with a frame that accommodates the desired position.

3. Infiltration of a local anesthetic agent with epinephrine beneath the scalp is desirable for many intracranial procedures. The scalp, extracranial arteries, and portions of the dura mater are the only structures covering the brain that are sensitive to pain. Epinephrine may be added to the agent to prolong its effectiveness and to constrict superficial blood vessels. The anesthetic may be injected before the patient is prepped and draped.

4. Administration of general anesthetic agents via an endotracheal tube may be preferred for extensive intracranial procedures, although the skull and brain are insensitive to pain. The patient is positioned after being anesthetized and before prepping and draping.

5. Anticipation of difficulty in achieving hemostasis by the methods previously discussed is not unusual in some procedures to remove vascular intracranial lesions. Controlled hypotension may be initiated by the anesthesia provider, with the concurrence of the neurosurgeon, to lower the blood pressure.

6. Prevention of cerebral edema during repair of cranial injuries may be accomplished with hypothermia. Hypothermia may also be used to decrease cerebral blood flow and venous pressure and to decrease brain volume and ICP. Patients are cooled to a core tem-

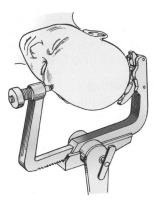

FIG. 37-7   Mayfield skull clamp stabilizes head for right frontotemporal craniotomy. Single pin on left and two spring-loaded pins on right penetrate outer table of skull.

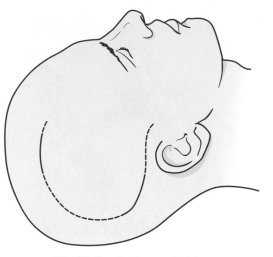

FIG. 37-8   Craniotomy incision.

perature between 57° and 68° F (14° and 20° C) by surface-induced hypothermia, bloodstream cooling, or a combination of both. Core body temperature can be monitored via a thermal probe placed in the esophagus or rectum or contained within the indwelling Foley catheter.

Hypothermia with elective circulatory arrest and extracorporeal cardiopulmonary bypass is an alternative when conventional approaches to the control of blood loss would be unsatisfactory. The desired core temperature before beginning extracorporeal cardiopulmonary bypass is 64° F (18° C). The cooling process may take 1 hour. An 18- to 24-French (Fr) arterial perfusion cannula is placed in the right femoral artery for oxygenated blood return, and a 28- or 32-Fr venous return cannula is placed in the left femoral vein for venous drainage.

Normally the brain cannot tolerate ischemia for more than a few minutes. This time is extended with lowering of body temperature. The average circulatory arrest time is between 12 and 45 minutes at 64° F (18° C). Hypothermia decreases cellular metabolism and therefore decreases oxygen consumption by the brain and heart during interruption of circulation. Intermittent administration of cold crystalloid cerebroplegia solution also may help protect the brain during cardiopulmonary bypass and profound hypothermia.

Blood viscosity increases as body temperature decreases. Two or three units of the patient's blood may be withdrawn and replaced with chilled normal saline solution. During rewarming, this blood is autotransfused. Crystalloid priming solution from the cardiopulmonary bypass machine also causes hemodilution.

7. Air embolism is a potential problem when a sitting position is used. The brain is higher than the heart in this position. Venous pressure may be lower than atmospheric and can allow for entry of air into the heart via an open venous channel. A pneumatic counterpressure device may be used. An antishock garment extends from the patient's rib margin to the ankles and is inflated if the patient becomes

hypotensive. In lieu of an antishock garment, antiembolic stockings or sequential compression stockings are worn. If a Gardner-Wells frame with pin fixation is used, antibiotic ointment is applied around each fixation pin to form an airtight seal. This reduces the risk of air embolism and infection. The anesthesia provider may need to place a right atrial catheter to remove an air embolus in the heart.

8. Reduction of ICP and brain volume may be accomplished by withdrawing spinal fluid. An intrathecal catheter or Touhy needle is inserted, before prepping and draping, for the anesthesia provider to remove CSF during the surgical procedure as desired by the neurosurgeon.

9. Demarcation of the desired outline for the incision may be made on the scalp after the skin preparation and before draping. A sterile disposable skin marker is available (Fig. 37-8).

10. Instrumentation is usually arranged on a Mayfield or Phalen table or on a double Mayo stand set up over the patient positioned supine or prone. The scrub person stands on a tiered platform to easily set up and reach the instruments as they are needed. The instrument table surface can be raised or lowered. The drapes over the head are attached to the table drapes. A one-piece sheet that provides a combined sterile table cover and the patient's cranial drape with a self-adhering incise area is available.

If the patient will be in a Fowler or a sitting position, the instrument table is placed above and lateral to drapes over the patient. The drapes form a tent on the side of the anesthesia provider so he or she can have access to the patient throughout the procedure.

The surgeon will incise the scalp along the predetermined line. The scalp edges are highly vascular and require careful hemostasis. Excessive use of the ESU would cause death of hair follicles so temporary plastic Raney clips are placed along the skin edges for hemostasis (Fig. 37-9). These clips are applied individually with great care (Fig. 37-10). Figure 37-11 shows the

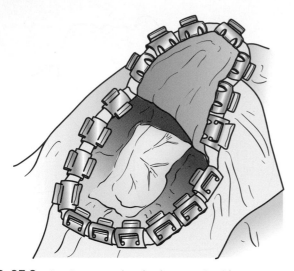

FIG. 37-9   Craniotomy scalp edge hemostasis with temporary plastic Raney clips.

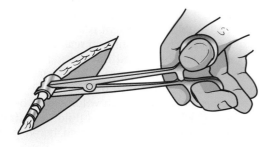

FIG. 37-10   Application of temporary plastic Raney clips.

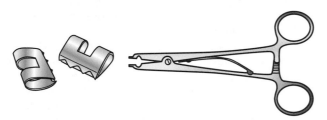

FIG. 37-11   Plastic Raney clips and clip applier.

clips and the special applier. This applier is used to remove the clips at the end of the procedure. The Raney clips are disposable. Other styles are available preloaded in 10s and 20s in an applier that resembles a skin stapler.

11. Prevention of sudden movement around the surgeon and of bumping the operating bed or microscope is crucial. A slip of the surgeon's hand under the operating microscope or in the cranial cavity could be fatal for the patient.

12. Prevention of peripheral nerve and circulatory damage requires that the circulating nurse check pressure points on the patient's body during prolonged procedures. Some microneurosurgical procedures

take 10 hours or longer to complete. Gel pads or a foam mattress similar in configuration to an egg crate should be used if the patient is supine or prone on the operating bed.

Physiologic Monitoring

Cerebral edema (brain swelling), cerebral arterial perfusion, and ICP can be safely controlled before, during, and after the surgical procedure. These parameters are continuously monitored. An intraarterial catheter is often inserted for continuous direct arterial blood pressure monitoring and for drawing samples for arterial blood gas analyses. A central venous pressure line may be established also. A pulmonary artery catheter may be inserted to measure fluid volume and to diagnose air embolism. Capnography is used routinely. Mass spectrometry is the most sensitive method of monitoring concentrations of inspired and expired gases. This sensitive device detects any type of gas, including nitrogen.

Doppler Ultrasound.   A precordial Doppler ultrasound transducer is secured over the precordium (i.e., over the right side of the heart to the right of the sternum between the third and sixth intercostal spaces). This is used primarily for continuous monitoring for gas entrapment or air embolism in the patient in a sitting position. An altered ultrasound response results if air is present in the right atrium. A catheter can be passed transarterially to evacuate air from the right atrium.

A sterile transcranial Doppler ultrasound transducer monitors changes in redistribution of cerebral blood flow, such as after obliteration of a large intracranial vascular malformation. This technique is also used to monitor cerebral vasospasm. Elevation of transcranial Doppler velocities precedes clinical signs of cerebral ischemia. The transducer can also be placed over the cerebral cortex to verify the location and depth of a tumor or cyst.

Evoked Potentials.   Somatosensory evoked potentials guide the anesthesia provider in handling arterial blood pressure, ventilation, inspired oxygen concentration, and patient positioning. Changes in cortical evoked potentials can indicate cerebral ischemia and systemic hypoxia. Both cortical and subcortical sensory evoked potentials can record surgical invasion of the spinal cord, peripheral nerve, nerve plexus, brainstem, or midbrain. To avert permanent injury to the patient, the surgeon may adjust retractors, alter the approach to a tumor, or perform a subtotal tumor resection on the basis of changes in evoked potentials. The anesthesia provider may adjust the depth of anesthesia.

Auditory brainstem evoked potentials, with a stimulus to the ear, may be used to monitor the eighth cranial nerve and brainstem during surgical procedures in the posterior fossa, if performed with the patient under local anesthesia.

Visual evoked potentials may be used during the surgical procedure for pituitary tumors, optic nerve decompression, aneurysms, and some other types of lesions. A strobe light flash is used to elicit responses. The light-emitting diodes are placed over closed eyelids and secured before the patient is prepped and draped.

Intracranial Pressure. ICP rises with an increase in volume of the brain, CSF, and/or cerebral blood supply or with decompensation (inability to compensate for pressure changes). In adults, normal ICP ranges from 10 to 20 mm Hg (or 13 to 27 cm H_2O). When an abnormal elevation is sustained, ICP prevents adequate perfusion of the cerebral cortex. The brain is deprived of its blood supply. Pressure monitoring is the only exact method to determine a rise in ICP and impending neurologic crisis during cranial procedures or after head injury. ICP monitoring is accomplished by implanting a ventricular catheter, subarachnoid screw, or epidural sensor.

A ventricular catheter is an invasive but the most accurate method of ICP monitoring. The cannula and reservoir are inserted into the ventricle through a burr hole or twist drill hole in the skull. Proper positioning of stopcocks is important, because incorrect placement may result in excessive CSF drainage with a sudden drop in ICP and possible brain herniation. This method evaluates volume/pressure responses and permits drainage of large amounts of CSF and instillation of contrast media and antibiotics. Catheter patency should be checked frequently. Postoperatively the patient is observed for signs of infection, such as meningitis or ventriculitis.

A hollow steel subarachnoid screw is placed in the subdural space via a twist drill hole in the skull and a small incision in the dura mater. Although this method measures ICP accurately and directly from CSF, it cannot be used to drain large amounts of fluid; it can provide access for CSF sampling. The screw may become occluded with blood or tissue. It should be checked frequently for patency.

A small epidural sensor is implanted in the epidural space of the brain through a small burr hole in the skull. The sensor is attached to a transducer, which converts CSF pressure to electrical impulses. The sensor cable is plugged into a monitor that produces a continuous readout. This is the least invasive method of ICP monitoring, but its accuracy is questionable.

Electroencephalogram. The function or organic activity of the brain may be monitored periodically throughout the surgical procedure by an electroencephalogram (EEG). Sterile subdermal needle electrodes may be used if surface scalp electrodes cannot be used.

SURGICAL PROCEDURES OF THE CRANIUM

Craniectomy

Craniectomy is the removal (-ectomy) of a portion of the bones of the skull (cranium). After the scalp incision, the bone is perforated or removed to approach the brain. This may be accomplished through one or more burr holes or twist drill holes. Each hole is drilled with an electrical or air-powered instrument or manually with a Hudson brace (Fig. 37-12). Burr holes are approximately ½ inch (13 mm) in diameter. Some diagnostic and therapeutic procedures are performed through them. Additional bone may be removed with a rongeur to increase exposure of the brain for more extensive procedures, such as an approach to the cranial nerves or tumors in the posterior fossa or suboccipital region.

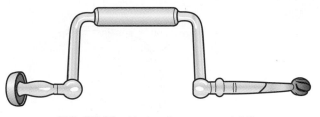

FIG. 37-12 Hudson brace manual drill.

The bone may be cut between the burr holes with a flexible multifilament wire (Gigli saw) or air-powered craniotome. A dura guard attachment protects the dura mater. A large area of bone is raised for temporary or permanent removal. Attached to the muscle, which acts as a hinge, the bone may be turned back to expose the underlying dura. This is referred to as raising a bone flap.

Burr holes may be plugged with a soft, pliable, silicone disc-shaped cover, with or without a channel for introduction of a hypodermic needle. The cover may be used to eliminate a cosmetically undesirable indentation of the scalp into the created bone defect. Postoperative access to the cranial cavity through the hole or channel in the cover can be used for drainage of fluid or instillation of chemotherapeutic drugs. ICP monitoring devices also can be attached. Other types of implantable infusion pumps also are inserted through a craniectomy.

Brain Pacemaker. Electrode plates of a brain pacemaker or cerebellar stimulator are implanted through small occipital and suboccipital craniectomies. Silicone-coated polyester fiber mesh plates, each with four pairs of platinum disc electrodes, are applied to the anterior and posterior surfaces of the cerebellum. One or two receivers, implanted just below the clavicle, are attached to the electrodes on the cerebellum by subcutaneously placed leads. Stimulation of the pacemaker electrodes is controlled by an external transmitter through an antenna placed on the skin over the subdermal receiver. This device is used to control muscular hypertonia and seizures related to cerebral palsy, epilepsy, stroke, or brain injury.

Craniotomy

Scalp, bone, and dural flaps are raised to expose a large area of the cerebrum for exploration, definitive treatment, or excision of lesions within the brain. Raney clips are applied to the galea and over the edge of the scalp flap. The bone flap is turned as described for craniectomy by drilling four or five burr holes along the edge of the proposed bone incision then cutting a line between the holes with a Gigli saw or a powered saw with a dural guard on the tip (Fig. 37-13). Moistened sponges protect both the scalp flap and the bone flap. The dural flap is protected with large compressed patties.

For wound closure, the thin but tough fibrous dural flap is laid over the brain. Usually it is sutured with many interrupted stitches to provide a tight seal that prevents leakage of CSF. The bone flap may be anchored with stainless steel sutures, silicone burr hole buttons, or plates and screws. Absorbable screws can be used for aesthetic appearance. The galea is closed with interrupted sutures before the scalp is sutured or approximated with staples.

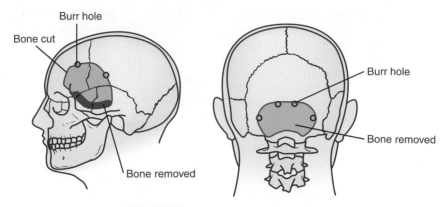

FIG. 37-13   Burr holes for craniotomy.

A silicone rubber suction drain may be placed in the subdural space to drain residual fluid from a subdural hematoma or the bed of a brain tumor or to remove red blood cells in CSF after a craniotomy.

Intracranial tumors can originate from the neural tissues of the brain, the meninges, glandular tissue, choroid plexuses, cranial nerves, blood vessels, embryonal defects, or metastatic lesions (Table 37-2). A craniotomy may be performed to remove a circumscribed, encapsulated, slow-growing, benign brain tumor. Some of these tumors, such as a meningioma, are highly vascular. Primary or secondary metastatic malignant tumors are broadly classified as gliomas. These have an unregulated cellular proliferation of rapidly growing cells, which invade surrounding brain tissue.

Glioblastoma multiforme, one of the most common brain tumors, is the most malignant type. Hemorrhagic and edematous effects of a rapidly growing tumor may be an indication for a lobectomy to give the brain an area for expansion and to impede mortality. The rigid characteristics of the skull prevent its expansion or contraction; however, the brain can expand or contract.

Subdural decompression by craniectomy to reduce ICP and papilledema may be the palliative procedure of choice. By anatomic location, some benign tumors are considered malignant because they cannot be safely removed without severe neurologic deficits or a threat to life-sustaining functions. Microneurosurgery and stereotaxis provide access to tumors in some anatomic locations that are otherwise impossible to reach, such as in third-ventricle and pineal regions.

Cranioplasty

Traumatic or surgically created skull defects are corrected with autogenous bone grafts or a synthetic or titanium prosthesis. Large defects in the anterior or middle fossae are covered for protection of the brain and for cosmetic effect. The bone flap may be removed after an intracranial procedure to allow cerebral decompression postoperatively. It is stored under sterile conditions in the bone bank until it can be placed in the skull.

Bone removed because of an extensively comminuted fracture or bone disease may be replaced with sterile methyl methacrylate. This material contours better than preformed titanium plates. Under sterile conditions the sterile resin powder is mixed with the sterile liquid polymer to form a doughy mass. This is placed in a sterile plastic bag and rolled to the thickness of the skull with a roller. While still pliable, it is molded to the contour of the head and the size of the defect. When hardened, it can be trimmed with a rongeur and the edges smoothed with a special small emery wheel mounted on the electric bone saw. The prosthesis is wired to the skull in several places. The brain expands to meet it and leaves no dead space between it and the dura.

Dural defects can be closed with autologous fascia graft, fibrin film, polyethylene film, synthetic absorbable mesh, or freeze-dried human cadaver dura mater grafts.

Intracranial Microneurosurgery

The magnification and lighting afforded by the operating microscope have refined intracranial microneurosurgical techniques and made possible approaches to many neurologic problems. A CO_2 laser may be adapted to the microscope for ablation of benign or malignant intracranial tumors. Discussions of some other microneurosurgical procedures follow.

Excision of an Acoustic Neuroma. Middle fossa or translabyrinthine approaches may be used by otologists for removal of small acoustic neuromas confined in the internal auditory canal. A neurosurgeon resects an acoustic neuroma that more commonly extends into the posterior fossa of the cranial cavity. An acoustic neuroma can grow progressively into the trigeminal, facial, and abducens nerves and into the cerebellopontine angle (the area between the pons, medulla oblongata, and cerebellum). Potentially life threatening, these involvements manifest symptoms of facial weakness, paresthesia, and dysphagia.

The suboccipital retrolabyrinthine approach is preferred by most neurosurgeons.

The patient is placed in a semi-Fowler or a sitting position, with pin fixation in the Gardner-Wells frame. This position provides good exposure but has the potential risk of air embolism. The operating microscope offers the potential for preservation of functional hearing. Particular caution is

TABLE 37-2	Intracranial Neoplasms		
Cell of Origin	**Site**	**Age and Gender**	**Degree of Malignancy**
ASTROCYTOMA—GRADES I AND II			
Astrocyte	Cerebrum	Young adults Equal between genders	Low malignancy; slow-growing tumor, becomes cystic, well-differentiated cell structure; average survival is 6 years Most common brain tumor
ASTROCYTOMA—GRADES III AND IV			
Astrocyte	Cerebrum, cerebellum and white matter	Middle age Males >females	Highly malignant, slow-growing tumor; poorly differentiated cell structure; 20% of all brain tumors are this type; average survival is 6 years
EPENDYMOMA			
Cells lining ventricular system of brain and central canal of the spinal cord; most common in fourth ventricle	Fourth ventricle and distal spinal cord	Children and young adults Equal between genders	Low malignancy; slow-growing tumor; variable differentiation of cell structure; may calcify; 10% of all brain tumors are this type; survival is measured in months according to location of tumor 30% of all spinal tumors
GLIOBLASTOMA MULTIFORME			
Glial cells	Cerebral hemispheres and corpus callosum	Middle age Equal between genders	Highly malignant; infiltrative, rapidly growing; highly cellular with many necrotic foci; 50% of all brain tumors are this type; average survival is 1 year
MEDULLOBLASTOMA			
Uncertain, primitive bipotential cells	Cerebellum, fourth ventricle, and subarachnoid space	Children Males >females	Moderate malignancy; rapidly growing tumor; moderate differentiation of cell structure; 10% of all brain tumors are this type; average survival is 15 months
MENINGIOMA			
Arachnoid cell	Parasagittal and lateral convexities, sphenoidal ridge, and thoracic spinal cord	Middle age Females >males	Usually benign; encapsulated and easily separated from nervous tissue
NEURILEMOMA (SCHWANNOMA)			
Schwann cells of cranial nerves and spinal nerve roots	Cranial nerve VIII in cerebellopontine angle and thoracic spinal cord	Middle age Equal between genders	Usually benign; pain and paresthesia are common
OLIGODENDROGLIOMA			
Oligodendrocyte	Cerebrum, white matter	Middle age Equal between genders	Low malignancy; slow-growing tumor; moderate differentiation of cells; 5% of all brain tumors are this type; average survival is 5 years

taken to obtain meticulous hemostasis, to spare the auditory artery if hearing is to be preserved, and to avoid trauma to or resection of the facial nerve. It is impossible to salvage facial nerve function in a percentage of patients. If the facial nerve is sacrificed, the patient may return for a facial-hypoglossal or facial-accessory nerve anastomosis 4 to 6 weeks postoperatively.

A retromastoid transtemporal approach with the patient in a lateral position or a subtemporal transtentorial approach with the patient supine may be preferred. The surgeon's decision to preserve or sacrifice the facial nerve and/or hearing will influence the approach to an acoustic neuroma. The ultrasonic aspirator and/or CO_2 laser may be used to remove the tumor.

Decompression of Cranial Nerves. Microvascular decompression relieves the severe and disabling symptoms of some cranial nerve disorders, such as trigeminal neuralgia (tic douloureux), glossopharyngeal neuralgia, acoustic nerve dysfunction, and hemifacial spasm. Initial symptoms of hyperactivity in a cranial nerve can progress to loss of function. Some disorders are caused by mechanical cross-compression, usually vascular, of the nerve root at the brainstem. Symptoms depend on sensory and/or motor functions of the nerve.

With the patient in a sitting position, a retromastoid craniectomy is performed to explore the cerebellopontine angle. A supracerebellar exposure is used for the trigeminal nerve, and an infracerebellar exposure is used for the remainder of the cranial nerves. An artery or vein compressing the nerve root may be mobilized away from the nerve. A tiny piece of Silastic sponge may be placed between the vessel and nerve to relieve the pulsating pressure on the nerve. A tissue sling may be created to lift the vessel off the nerve. Tumors that were not diagnosed preoperatively are excised. If vascular decompression or another pathologic condition is not evident, the nerve may be sectioned to relieve pain.

Cerebral Revascularization.

For cerebral revascularization, an extracranial artery is anastomosed to an intracranial artery for bypass of stenotic or occlusive vascular disease distal to the bifurcation of the common carotid artery. This provides an additional and significant source of blood to the cerebral circulation. An artery in the scalp, such as the superficial temporal or occipital artery or another branch of the external carotid artery, is anastomosed to a branch of the middle cerebral artery or to a cortical branch of the cerebral artery. Vessels must be 1 mm in diameter or larger for the anastomosis to work. The procedure is primarily prophylactic to prevent development of a major brain attack (stroke) in patients who have had transient ischemic attacks or minor strokes with temporary disruption of brain function caused by blockage of the cerebrovascular system.

The patient is positioned supine with the head turned or positioned laterally with the head stabilized flat on the operating bed for an approach through a temporal craniectomy. The anastomosis is made on the surface of the brain, either end-to-end, side-to-side, or end-to-side of the arteries.

In some patients, plaque can be removed from the middle cerebral artery rather than bypassing the occlusion. Cerebral embolectomy with a detachable balloon or other intravascular technique may be done to obliterate a carotid-cavernous fistula or arteriovenous malformation in conjunction with an extracranial-intracranial arterial bypass. Cranial bypass is the procedure of choice for cerebral revascularization in a patient who has a vascular lesion that cannot be treated by carotid endarterectomy.

Excision of an Arteriovenous Malformation.

An arteriovenous malformation (AVM) is an abnormal communication between the arterial and venous systems involving many dilated blood vessels (Fig. 37-14). As the fistulous connections gradually enlarge under pressure, blood is diverted from surrounding brain tissue, causing scarring and compression as a result of poor perfusion. This process is accelerated by multiple small hemorrhages from the thin, engorged vessels. Progressive neurologic deficits can cause seizures and life-threatening subarachnoid, intraventricular, or intraparenchymal hemorrhage.

A large, diffuse AVM involving multiple vessels and high-flow shunts can be difficult to excise. The strategy of the

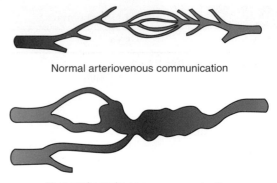

Normal arteriovenous communication

Abnormal arteriovenous communication

FIG. 37-14   Arteriovenous malformation.

neurosurgeon may be to perform a staged resection with intraoperative embolization initially to reduce the number of fistulous arteries and size of shunts. For embolization, small Silastic beads may be introduced into an AVM via a catheter placed into the internal carotid artery. This procedure usually is done a month before surgical resection.

Using the operating microscope, the surgeon carefully coagulates or clips the arteries as close to the AVM as possible. Normal arteries that perfuse the brain beyond the AVM are preserved. At least one vein must remain patent to drain the AVM until other vessels are occluded. Then this vein is occluded, and the AVM is removed.

Occlusion of Aneurysms.

Aneurysms of the cerebral and vertebral arteries vary from the size of a pea to the size of an orange. Most intracranial aneurysms are located near the basilar surface of the skull and arise from the internal carotid or middle cerebral arteries. Cerebral artery (berry) aneurysms are usually located on the circle of Willis at the base of the brain between the hemispheres of the cerebrum. Most aneurysms are associated with a congenital defect of the tunica media of the intracranial vessel wall. Hemodynamic forces of pulsatile pressure cause enlargement, outpouching, and thinning of the arterial wall, which eventually ruptures. This is the most common source of subarachnoid hemorrhage. Most aneurysms seal spontaneously, but a surgical procedure may be indicated to prevent rebleeding. If diagnosed, an unruptured asymptomatic aneurysm may be occluded with Guglielmi platinum coils by a minimally invasive endovascular approach before rupture.

For open treatment, the patient will be placed in a sitting position for suboccipital or subfrontal craniectomy and the aneurysm is exposed for occlusion. The neck (base) of the aneurysm is occluded with a low-pressure aneurysm clip or ligated if it can be isolated (Fig. 37-15). Micro coils can be placed in the aneurysm in the interventional radiation department to help prevent rupture (Fig. 37-16). If it cannot be isolated, the aneurysm and parent vessel may be wrapped in fine-mesh gauze and coated with methyl methacrylate, isobutyl 2-cyanoacrylate, or other epoxy resin to reinforce the wall. More commonly the aneurysm is coagulated with bipolar electrosurgery or a laser. Induced hypotension may be used to decrease blood flow in the artery feeding the

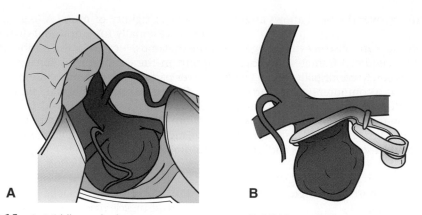

FIG. 37-15 **A,** Middle cerebral artery aneurysm exposure. **B,** Middle cerebral artery aneurysm with clip to prevent rupture.

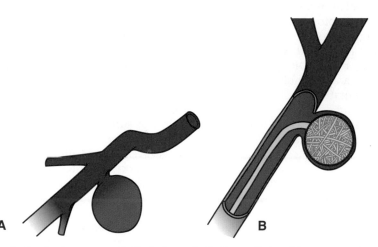

FIG. 37-16 **A,** Cerebral aneurysm. **B,** Occlusive embolization coil placed in aneurysm to prevent rupture.

aneurysm. This aids in dissection and occlusion. The operating microscope is used for delicate dissection of the arteries at the base of the brain.

Stereotaxis

Stereotaxis is the accurate location of a definite circumscribed area within the brain from external points or landmarks on the skull. It defines three-dimensional coordinates (planes) by which to approach deep structures without damaging overlying structures. The technique is used to create or ablate a lesion in otherwise inaccessible parts of the brain. By determination of specific reference points on a CT, PET, or MRI scan, the exact area for the target site of the lesion is calculated by computer. The computer, especially designed for stereotactic surgery, provides measurements for correct alignment of instrumentation and calculation of the depth of target tissue within the brain.

A stereoencephalotome, a specially designed mechanical apparatus, is attached to the skull with the patient in a sitting position. After this is in place, computerized data show localizers of the apparatus in relation to intracranial structures. The ventricular system provides the internal landmarks. Of the many models available, three basic types of stereoencephalotomes are used:

1. *Semicircle arc system.* Steel screws are tapped through each of four burr holes for fixation of the head to a ring supported from a table attachment or a pedestal on the floor (Fig. 37-17). The ring is secured to arc plates. The head is moved rather than the apparatus.
2. *Rectilinear system.* The apparatus can be moved back and forth and from side to side around the head to make adjustments.

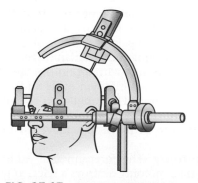

FIG. 37-17 Stereotactic head frame.

3. *Single arc system.* An arc over the head allows angular adjustments.

The stereoencephalotome can obstruct the surgeon's access for an intracranial procedure. A frameless stereotaxic system enables the neurosurgeon to continually interact with CT scans and MRI displays via a computer linkage throughout an intracranial procedure. Known as an interactive image-guided stereotactic neurosurgery system, the system incorporates three-dimensional images from cameras mounted over the operating bed, position-sensing probes and forceps, and a computer system.

With a stereoencephalotome in place, stereotactic surgery can be performed through a burr hole, rigid or flexible endoscope, or open craniotomy.

A lesion may be made or removed by laser, high-frequency or radiofrequency electrocoagulation, cryosurgery, ultrasound, radiation, hyperthermia, or mechanical curettage. Procedures are performed with the patient under local anesthesia when patient cooperation to test motor or sensory function may be needed during the surgical procedure. Various types of intracranial procedures are performed with computer-assisted stereotaxis. Operating room (OR) personnel are required to know how to sterilize and assemble the apparatus and prepare necessary instrumentation.

Aspiration. A needle or cannula is placed into target tissue to aspirate a cyst, abscess, or hematoma. Tissue may be obtained for biopsy.

Functional Neurosurgery. For functional neurosurgery, lesions are created in the brain to reduce intractable pain or to control tremors or psychotic behavior.

Electrostimulation. Intermittent electrostimulation of the brain by stereotactically implanted electrodes can control a variety of benign intractable pain problems. One electrode is placed in the somatosensory system to evaluate pain of central origin, and another is placed in the paraventricular gray matter to evaluate pain of peripheral origin. After postoperative evaluation of the effectiveness of electrical stimulation of each electrode, the patient returns to the OR to have a receiver placed under the skin on the anterior chest wall. A connecting wire is tunneled from the receiver to the electrode. An external transmitter and antenna placed over the receiver stimulate the electrode as desired by the patient.

Radiofrequency Retrogasserian Rhizotomy. Radiofrequency retrogasserian rhizotomy relieves the pain of trigeminal neuralgia, also known as tic douloureux. The fifth cranial (trigeminal) nerve carries sensory impulses for touch, pain, and external temperature from the face, scalp, and mucous membranes in the head. Trigeminal neuralgia is an intense paroxysmal pain in one side of the face. It can be controlled by damaging the gasserian (trigeminal) ganglion.

An insulated cannula with an uninsulated tip is placed through the cheek and foramen ovale and is advanced to the gasserian ganglion. The ganglion is coagulated when a radiofrequency generator activates the tip of the cannula. Several lesions can be made to achieve the desired extent of paresthesia.

Thalamotomy. The forerunner of other stereotactic procedures, thalamotomy destroys a selected portion of the thalamus for relief of pain, epileptic seizures, involuntary tremor or rigidity of muscles (e.g., in Parkinson's disease), and occasionally for emotional disturbances. Functionally, the thalamus, located in the midbrain, is the principal relay point in the cerebrum for sensory impulses passing from lower parts of the nervous system to the cerebral cortex.

Cingulotomy. Bilateral symmetric radiofrequency electrolytic lesions are placed to disrupt pathways of cingulum. The cingulum is a bundle of connecting fibers in the medial aspect of each cerebral hemisphere between the frontal and temporal lobes. Cingulotomies are performed for severe chronic pain, addiction, or some intractable psychoses that have not responded to other methods of treatment.

Pallidotomy. Stereotactic pallidotomy can be performed to decrease muscle rigidity associated with Parkinson's disease.

Psychosurgery. Intractable depression, obsessive-compulsive disorders, or chronic anxiety may be treated by cingulotomy as described or by frontal lobotomy. Under stereotaxic control, a probe is inserted into the white matter of the frontal lobe of the brain to create a lesion by cryosurgery or electrocoagulation. The lesion disrupts neural cortical/subcortical connections in the frontal lobe anterior to the lateral ventricles that control emotions.

Some surgeons implant fine electrodes that remain indwelling for weeks to months. These can be used for chronic stimulation of surrounding tissue or to create additional electrocoagulative lesions. Complications include epilepsy, indecisiveness, and altered personality. Studies have shown that memory and intellect are not impaired. Psychosurgery is performed only if other treatments, such as medication or psychotherapy, have failed to provide relief.

Intracranial Vascular Lesions. Some cerebral aneurysms or AVMs can be electrocoagulated, coagulated with an argon laser, vaporized with a CO_2 laser, or clipped through stereotactic instrumentation. Thrombosis of an aneurysm or embolization of an AVM may be performed for lesions that are otherwise inoperable or before a microneurosurgical procedure to control bleeding.

Intracranial Neoplasms. Computer-assisted stereotaxis helps locate and reach the margin of a deep-seated intracranial tumor either by open craniotomy or through an endoscope. Then a CO_2 or KTP laser beam or other agent can be directed to destroy the tumor while preserving normal cerebral tissue.

Cryohypophysectomy. Creation of cryogenic lesions may be the procedure of choice for treating growth hormone–producing pituitary adenomas with no suprasellar extension. The cryosurgical probe is introduced into the sella turcica through a frontal burr hole. During creation of the lesion, ocular movements and visual acuity are carefully monitored.

Interstitial Radiation. Radioactive substances may be stereotactically implanted into malignant brain tumors. Multiple catheters can be placed throughout the target volume. The catheters are afterloaded with radioactive iridium-192 or iodine-125 seeds. The catheters are inserted percutaneously through twist drill holes. For photoradiation therapy, a hematoporphyrin derivative may be injected preoperatively and activated by argon or a tunable dye laser to create a cytotoxic photochemical reaction in tumor cells.

Interstitial Hyperthermia. Catheters and remote sensors are implanted into the tumor volume. Sufficient heat is conducted through sensors to raise the temperature within the tumor to a degree that destroys its cells. This is effective against radioresistant hypoxic cells and poorly vascularized and metabolically inactive tumors.

Stereotactic Radiosurgery. Intense beams of high-energy gamma radiation or microwave-generated energy photons from a linear accelerator are directed to specific targets within the brain while sparing normal brain tissue. Gamma Knife stereotactic radiosurgery does not actually use a knife and is technically not surgery as the name implies. This noninvasive procedure uses stereotaxis to identify the location of an intracranial tumor or AVM. A specially designed helmet fits over the patient's head and the stereoencephalotome frame. A single high dose of cobalt-generated gamma radiation is directed through holes in the helmet. The beams are collimated and focused on the lesion. The gamma unit is a specific installation for this procedure. The treatment takes 5 to 30 minutes. It does not remove the lesion, but it can stop its growth and reduce its size.

Control of Epilepsy

Epilepsy, caused by erratic electrical rhythms in the brain, manifests in a variety of intermittent disabling behaviors—most commonly convulsive seizures. Epilepsy may result from a congenital anomaly within the brain or can develop after trauma, meningitis, or acute febrile illness. Patients with intractable seizures uncontrolled with medication may be candidates for surgery to remove the focal point of the seizures.

EEG monitoring and CT, PET, and MRI scans help identify the specific location of abnormal brain tissue, causing seizures. One of two invasive procedures may be necessary if these tests are inconclusive:

1. *Subdural grid implantation.* Via a frontotemporoparietal craniectomy, a Silastic grid with metal discs attached to stainless steel or platinum electrodes is placed on the cortex of the brain. The grid size varies depending on the area to be monitored. The grid is anchored to the dura mater. The electrodes are tunneled under the skin to an area outside the incision before the dura, bone, and skin flaps are closed.

    Subsequently, seizure activity coming from the surface of the brain is monitored for several days by an EEG monitor connected to the electrodes. The grid also maps the brain to locate areas of motor, sensory, visual, speech, and memory control. The patient returns to the OR for removal of the grid. Cortical resection also may be performed at this time.

2. *Stereotaxic depth electrode implantation.* By correlating CT, PET, and/or MRI images with reference points on the stereotactic frame, electrodes are implanted directly into the brain. These are connected to an EEG to determine the focus of seizures within specific areas of the brain. After weeks of monitoring, the patient returns to the OR for removal of the electrodes. The epileptic focus may be destroyed by creating a stereotactic lesion at this time.

    After an epileptic focus is identified, a definitive surgical procedure can be performed to stop or reduce seizure activity. The objective is to maintain cerebral capabilities for language, speech, memory, vision, movement, and other sensory and motor neurologic functions.

Cortical Resection. Epileptogenic tissue is resected from the cerebral cortex where the epileptic focus is localized. An anterior temporal lobectomy is most commonly performed. Frontal and other extratemporal sites may be resected if the epileptic focus does not interfere with neurologic functions.

Corpus Callosotomy. The corpus callosum (a fibrous band of neurons) or the anterior commissure connecting the two hemispheres in the midline of the brain is severed. This prevents passage of neuronal discharges from a focal seizure between the hemispheres, thereby preventing secondary generalized seizures.

Hemispherectomy. A hemisphere severely damaged by widespread, persistent, multifocal seizures may be removed. This radical procedure is usually performed only on children with unilateral pathologic foci, including infantile hemiplegia (palsy), hemiparesis (paralysis), and hemianopia (loss of vision). The hemisphere (i.e., half of the brain) is resected with preservation of the basal ganglia. If an abnormal hemisphere is removed at an early age, the normal half of the brain can take over much of the missing function.

Extracranial Procedures

The cranial procedures previously discussed include access to the surgical site through the skull. A few cranial neurosurgical procedures do not require craniectomy or intracranial incision.

External Occlusion of the Carotid Artery. When an internal carotid or middle cerebral artery aneurysm cannot be reached or controlled by other surgical techniques, a carotid clamp can be applied extracranially in the neck. Progressive turns on the clamp over several days cause it to occlude the carotid artery gradually until complete occlusion of the blood supply to the aneurysm is accomplished.

Endovascular Procedures. A thin catheter with a very fine guidewire can be advanced through a groin incision into a cerebral vessel to treat a problem within the brain. For example, under radiography, tiny platinum coils can be deployed or thrombotic material can be injected to seal off a cerebral aneurysm. Cerebral angioplasty uses a tiny balloon catheter to reopen the clogged or narrow lumen of a cerebral blood vessel. Stents can be placed to maintain patency.

Transsphenoidal Procedures. As a palliative surgical procedure, hypophysectomy (enucleation of the pituitary gland) may be performed for pain relief and endocrine ablation in patients with disseminated metastatic carcinoma of the breast or prostate gland or to relieve intractable pain from other types of disseminated carcinoma. The microsurgical transsphenoidal approach also is used for removal of intrapituitary tumors or other lesions within the region of the sella turcica, a cavity of the sphenoid bone. Visual loss and endocrinopathy are the main symptoms of a pituitary tumor.

Tumor tissue in the sella turcica is distinguished both by color and texture from the normal firm, yellowish anterior and red-gray posterior lobes of the pituitary.

The patient is placed in a semi-Fowler position with the head slightly flexed and tilted so that the patient's body is out of the way when the neurosurgeon sits in front of the face to work in the midsagittal plane. The image intensifier is positioned lateral to the patient's head with the horizontal beam centered on the sella turcica. A television monitor is placed behind and just above the patient's head so that the surgeon can look at the screen in line with the binocular of the microscope. Televised radiofluoroscopy is used as an aid in placing instruments and resecting tissue. The image intensifier is switched on and off, as needed, to minimize exposure to radiation.

The floor of the sella turcica is exposed through the sphenoid sinus. The procedure can be performed transnasally (Fig. 37-18) or through horizontal incision is made under the upper lip, at the junction of the gingiva, and carried deep to the maxilla. Soft tissues are elevated; bone and nasal cartilage are resected. The resected nasal cartilage is preserved on the instrument table for possible replacement. A specially designed nasal speculum is inserted in the oral incision to visualize the sphenoid sinus. This is opened wide until the floor of the sella turcica can be identified. The floor is opened with an air-powered drill. The microscope is brought into position for visualization of the pituitary and other structures and lesions inside and around the sella turcica.

Treatment of Head Injuries

A patient with severe head injury requires first a patent airway. A relaxed jaw and tongue should be raised; if necessary, suction should be applied through the mouth. An endotracheal tube may be inserted. Ultimately a tracheotomy may be necessary.

Vital signs, blood pressure, dilation of pupils, and level of consciousness are checked frequently. An intravenous (IV) osmotic dehydrating solution, such as mannitol, may be ordered to reduce cerebral edema if there is no evidence of intracranial hemorrhage. After these supportive

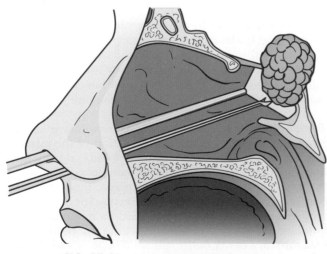

FIG. 37-18   Transnasal hypophysectomy.

measures have been carried out, definitive treatment is initiated:

1. Scalp lacerations are thoroughly cleansed, debrided, and sutured. Because the scalp is highly vascular, lacerations bleed profusely. Hypovolemic shock is rare but possible.
2. Simple linear or comminuted fractures usually require no treatment. A depressed skull fracture must be elevated when bone is pressed 5 mm or more into any part of the brain.
3. A compound fracture requires debridement. The extent of the surgical procedure depends on the specific extent of injury. Dura may need to be sutured. Some macerated brain tissue may have to be excised.
4. An intracranial hematoma may be present. Depending on the location, intracranial hemorrhage may require an immediate emergency surgical procedure.
   a. Epidural hematoma. Bleeding caused by rupture or tear of the middle meningeal artery (or its branches) forms a hematoma between the skull and the dura. Usually associated with a skull fracture, signs and symptoms of increased ICP caused by rapid compression of the brain may occur immediately or within a few hours. An arterial hemorrhage presents an extreme surgical emergency to evacuate the clot and clip or electrocoagulate the bleeding vessel through a burr hole or small craniectomy.
   b. Subdural hematoma. Bleeding between the dura mater and arachnoid is usually caused by laceration of veins that cross the subdural space. A large encapsulated collection of blood over one or both cerebral hemispheres produces increased ICP and other neurologic changes. The onset and extent of these changes depend on the cause, size, and rapidity of growth of the hematoma. Treatment may necessitate a burr hole. A bone flap may be raised if more extensive exploration is indicated. Subdural hematoma may be:
      (1) Acute. Usually caused by arterial bleeding, symptoms occur rapidly. The vessel is ligated with clips or electrocoagulated.
      (2) Subacute. Usually caused by venous bleeding, symptoms appear within 24-48 hours to 5 days after the injury.
      (3) Chronic. Symptoms do not appear until 6 or more months after the injury.
   c. Intracerebral hematoma. Tears in the brain substance at the point of greatest impact most commonly occur in the anterior temporal and frontal lobes. Although it is usually absorbed, a hematoma may require evacuation and debridement of necrotic tissue.

Complications of Cranial Surgery

All cranial procedures present risks of postoperative seizures and neurologic deficits. Paralysis, muscle weakness, gait disturbances, and ataxia may be temporary or permanent. Neurologic damage can follow hemorrhage, occlusion of cerebral circulation, and increased ICP.

Any sudden, sustained rise in ICP raises blood pressure to maintain the cerebral blood flow and elevates pulmonary vascular pressure. This can lead to acute neurogenic pulmonary edema. This is also a complication of venous air embolism. Both venous and arterial air embolisms can result in ventricular dysrhythmias and fibrillation. Infection is always a potential complication.

PERIPHERAL NERVE SURGERY

The PNS includes the cranial nerves, spinal nerves, and autonomic nervous system located outside the CNS. Ganglions, a group of nerve cell bodies also located outside the CNS, can transmit either autonomic (involuntary) or somatic (both reflex and voluntary) impulses. Somatic nerves supply voluntary muscles, skin, tendons, joints, and other structures controlling the musculoskeletal system. Afferent nerve fibers carry sensory impulses from the organs and muscles to the CNS. Efferent fibers transmit motor impulses from the CNS back to them. Peripheral nerve procedures are performed on both the autonomic and somatic nervous systems. The neurosurgeon may identify nerves and test function with a nerve stimulator before or after dissection or repair.

Autonomic Nervous System

The autonomic nervous system is an aggregation of ganglions, nerves, and plexuses through which the viscera, heart, blood vessels, smooth muscles, and glands receive motor innervation to function involuntarily. This system is divided into the following:

- *Sympathetic nervous system.* This thoracolumbar division, arising from the thoracic and first three lumbar segments of the spinal cord, includes the ganglionated trunk near the spinal cord, plexuses, and associated preganglionic and postganglionic nerve fibers. The efferent fibers transmit impulses that stimulate involuntary activity in the heart, blood vessels, smooth muscle of the viscera, and all of the glands in the body.
- *Parasympathetic nervous system.* This craniosacral division includes the preganglionic fibers that leave the CNS with cranial nerves III (oculomotor), VII (facial), IX (glossopharyngeal), and X (vagus); the first three sacral nerves; outlying ganglions near the viscera; and postganglionic fibers. In general, this system innervates the same structures but has a regulatory function opposite that of the sympathetic nervous system. These efferent fibers act to restore stability for quieter activity.

Surgical procedures most frequently performed on the autonomic nervous system by neurosurgeons are discussed here, but surgeons in other disciplines perform some of them.

Sympathectomy. Resection or division of the sympathetic ganglions and nerve fibers of the autonomic nervous system is performed in an attempt to increase peripheral circulation or to decrease the pain of peripheral vascular disease or intractable pain of other organic origin. It may be an emergency procedure to relieve severe vasospasm after arterial embolism or freezing of an extremity. The paravertebral ganglionic chains and/or nerve fibers that innervate the affected area are resected or divided. The procedure may be termed sympathetic ganglionectomy or splanchnicectomy,

but usually the surgical procedure is specified by the location of the ganglions and nerves. (General and vascular surgeons also perform some of the following surgical procedures.)

Upper Cervical Sympathectomy. Upper cervical sympathectomy is done to increase the blood supply in the internal carotid arteries. Through an anterior cervical approach in the neck, the superior cervical ganglion is resected. Ptosis of the eyelid may occur postoperatively because this ganglion innervates eyelid retraction.

Cervicothoracic Sympathectomy. Cervicothoracic sympathectomy may be performed to treat Raynaud phenomenon of the upper extremities by relieving the chronic vasoconstrictive process or to relieve angina pectoris or causalgia. Through a transaxillary-transpleural incision, the stellate ganglion of the middle cervical ganglionic chain is hemisected and the lower half resected along with the second through fifth thoracic nerve ganglions. In select patients, video-assisted thoracoscopy is used to perform sympathectomy to treat Raynaud phenomenon, thoracic outlet syndrome, reflex sympathetic dystrophy, and hyperhidrosis of the upper limbs.

Thoracic Sympathectomy. Thoracic sympathectomy is usually done for relief of the chronic intractable pain of biliary and pancreatic disease. Through a posterior paravertebral incision over the transverse processes of the thoracic vertebrae, the ganglions of the sixth through twelfth thoracic nerves are resected and the splanchnic nerves divided.

Thoracolumbar Sympathectomy. Thoracolumbar sympathectomy is performed for the treatment of essential hypertension. Usually done in two stages, bilateral resection is necessary to reduce blood pressure by altering the vascular tone and denervating the viscera. With the patient prone or in a lateral position, a paravertebral incision parallel to the vertebral column extends from the ninth rib downward and then curves anteriorly toward the iliac crest. The lower half of the thoracic and the first through third lumbar chains with the ganglions and splanchnic nerves are resected.

Lumbar Sympathectomy. Lumbar sympathectomy may be of some value in the treatment of lower extremity vasospastic disease, such as Raynaud phenomenon and Buerger disease; ischemic ulcers as a result of vasospasm of the peripheral vessels; and some types of causalgia. Usually through a flank incision, the lumbar chain and ganglions located in the retroperitoneal space between the vertebral column and the psoas muscle are resected from above the second to below the third ganglions.

Presacral Neurectomy. The hypogastric nerve plexus may be resected for relief of idiopathic intractable dysmenorrhea and pelvic pain.

Vagotomy. Truncal vagotomy is total vagal denervation of all structures below the diaphragm. Selective vagotomy is performed more frequently to denervate a specific branch of the vagal nerve.

Somatic Nervous System

As cranial and spinal nerves extend out from the CNS into plexuses and peripheral nerve branches throughout the body, the somatic nervous system provides involuntary control over sensations and both voluntary and involuntary control over muscles. Loss of sensation and muscular control occurs distal to the site of severed or compressed nerve fibers. Sensation and function will be restored only if regeneration of nerve axons takes place distally from an unobstructed axis cylinder proximal to the site of disruption.

Nerve injuries in the lower extremity tend to be a result of a major impact, such as an automobile accident; upper extremity injuries are more often associated with industrial accidents. Nerve injuries usually are associated with multisystem trauma such as fractures and lacerations. An injury may occur at any point along a peripheral nerve (e.g., from penetrating trauma that severs the nerve or blunt trauma that produces contusions or traction to the nerve). Lower extremity nerves do not recover as rapidly as do upper extremity nerves.

Most peripheral nerve surgery is performed to repair traumatic nerve injury in an extremity. Dissection is also done to remove tumors or relieve pain. Etiologic factors determine the location and length of the skin incision.

Neurorrhaphy. Neurorrhaphy (suturing of a divided nerve) must provide precise approximation of the nerve ends if function is to be restored. Primary repair may be accomplished by suturing the epineurium, or outer sheath. Under magnification of the operating microscope, accurate fascicular alignment and epineural end-to-end suturing of larger nerve bundles constitute the desired technique to enhance regeneration of function. For a successful result, nerves are not repaired under tension. Primary repair soon after injury may be advantageous to align the fascicles.

A tumor, such as a neurofibroma or posttraumatic neuroma, is excised. If the nerve ends can be brought together without tension, they are anastomosed. Silastic membrane may be wrapped around the anastomosis to prevent adhesions with the surrounding tissue.

Neurolysis. Neurolysis (freeing of a nerve from adhesions) relieves pain and restores function. Release of the transverse carpal ligament overriding the median nerve in the wrist affords relief of carpal tunnel syndrome, for example.

Neurotomy, Neurectomy, and Neurexeresis. Neurotomy is division or dissection of nerve fibers. Neurectomy is excision of part of a nerve. Neurexeresis is extraction or avulsion of a nerve. These procedures may be performed to relieve localized peripheral pain.

Bibliography

Alberts MJ et al: Recommendations for the establishment of primary stroke centers, *JAMA* 283(23):3102-3109, 2000.

Bogomolny DL: Functional MRI in the brain tumor patient, *Topic Magnet Res Imag* 15(5):325-335, 2004.

Brettler S: Endovascular coiling for cerebral aneurysms, *AACN Clin Issues* 16(4):515-525, 2005.

Franges EZ: When a headache is really a brain tumor, *Nurse Pract* 31(4):47-51, 2006.

Gerzeny M, Cohen A: Advances in endoscopic neurosurgery, *AORN J* 67(5):957-965, 1998.

Graham CA, Cloughesy TF: Brain tumor treatment: Chemotherapy and other new developments, *Semin Oncol Nurs* 20(4):260-272, 2004.

Phillips J: Neuroscience critical care: The role of the advanced practice nurse in patient safety, *AACN Clin Issues* 16(4):581-592, 2005.

Plowman PN: Stereotactic intracranial radiotherapy has come of age, *J R Coll Physicians Lond* 34(3):273-281, 2000.

Stewart-Amidei C: Managing symptoms and side effects during brain tumor illness, *Exp Rev Neurotherapeutics* 5(6 Suppl):S71-76, 2005.

Suh, JH et al: Update of stereotactic radiosurgery for brain tumors, *Curr Opin Neurol* 17(6):681-686, 2004.

Taillibert S et al: Palliative care in patients with primary brain tumor, *Curr Opin Oncol* 16(6):587-592, 2004.

Youssef AS et al: Transcranial surgery for pituitary adenomas, *Neurosurgery* 57:168-175, 2005.

Chapter 38

Spinal Surgery

CHAPTER OBJECTIVES

After studying this chapter, the learner will be able to:
- Describe the anatomy of the vertebral column and spinal cord.
- Describe to implications of dermatome and myotome distributions.
- Discuss the implication of an individualized plan of care for each type of spinal surgery.
- Differentiate between the types of spinal position devices and operating beds.
- Compare the salient points of spinal surgery that apply to orthopedic and neurologic procedures.

CHAPTER OUTLINE

KEY TERMS AND DEFINITIONS

Ankylosis   Mineralization and solidification of a movable joint.
Approach   Method of incising and accessing the body.
The approach is planned according to the type of procedure and location of the disease or injury. Knowing the approach will help the circulating nurse and scrub person plan the positioning and instrumentation for the surgical procedure.
- **Anterior approach** Entering the body through the front of the neck, chest, or abdomen.
- **Posterior approach** Entering the body through the back of the neck, chest or lower spine.
- **Transoral approach** Entering the body through the mouth to the back of the pharynx.

Decompression   Release of spinal pressure by cutting away segments of the vertebral bone.
Dermatomes   Levels of cutaneous sensory innervation from specific areas of the cord to the peripheral nervous system.
Idiopathic   Unknown or uncertain origin.
Kyphosis   Exaggerated thoracic curvature of the spine.
Lordosis   Exaggerated lumbar curvature of the spine.
Myotomes   Levels of muscle innervation from the spinal cord.
Osteoporosis   Wasting and demineralization of bone.
Paralysis   Decreased ability to move voluntarily.
- **Paraplegia** Injury between the levels of T1 to T8; with injury between the levels T9 to T10, the individual may be able to sit up.
- **Hemiplegia** Injury to one side of the nervous system.
- **Quadriplegia** Injury above the level of T1.

Radiculopathy   Pain that travels up or down a nerve pathway.
Retroperitoneal   Behind the peritoneal cavity without entering the sac.
RSD   Reflex sympathetic dystrophy.
Scoliosis   Lateral curvature of the spine. Can be combined with kyphosis (kyphoscoliosis).
Spondylosis   Bony degeneration of the vertebral column with mineral deposits.
Stagnara wake-up test   The patient is awakened during the surgical procedure and asked to move his or her feet. The patient does not feel pain and is given an amnesic medication.
Stenosis   Narrowing of a passage.
Thenar   The web space between the index finger and the thumb.
Transperitoneal   Through the peritoneal cavity.

HISTORICAL BACKGROUND

Spinal disease was reported in a 4600-year-old document known as the Edwin Smith Papyrus. The papyrus describes 48 case studies with 6 cases specifically related to spinal injury. The descriptions include vertebral subluxation and dislocation, quadriplegia, paraplegia, and cervical spine injury.

The descriptions of the cervical spine injuries gave the ancient practitioners significant clues about the extent of the injury, the ability to recover, and when to understand that recovery was not possible. Many of the clues concerning cord structure and function were not deciphered until 4000 years after they were originally recorded. One description of a cervical injury indicates that the arms and legs did not move or have sensation, but the erectile reflexes were intact. The patient was unknowingly incontinent of urine. This case history describes the spinal reflex arc that remains intact despite the high level of cervical spine trauma.

The practitioner was advised to withhold treatment because recovery was not possible. At this point in history, no distinction was made between the bony vertebrae and the soft tissue of the spinal cord.

Later practitioners, such as Hippocrates (460-375 BC) demonstrated some success with back injury by devising traction tables and ladders for distracting the vertebral column and realigning the bony architecture. Hippocrates noted the spinal reflex arc without understanding its role in bypassing the brain for motor activity. He extended his teachings to include postulating that the kidneys and genitals were somehow connected to the spine. He went so far as to indicate that he thought sperm was produced by the spine.

Galen (AD 130-200) clarified the extent of potential injury and loss of sensation and motor at various levels of the spinal cord. He performed detailed dissection and described the layers of the meninges and the nerve roots. Galen named the most common spinal deformities such as scoliosis, kyphosis, and lordosis. Avicenna (AD 980-1037) added to Galen's work by noting that the brain and cord were separate structures and that the central canal of vertebral column was a protective cage for the spinal cord.

Surgeons and anatomists continued to study the cord and its mysteries by detailed dissection and the use of microscopy. Gerard Blasius (1625-1692), a Dutch anatomist described the "H" pattern of the gray matter and the white covering of the cord in cross section. Benedict Stilling (1810-1879) devised a microtome capable of shaving fine layers of cord in cross section that revealed the ascending and descending tracts and fibers. Bror Rexed (1914-2000), a Swedish anatomy professor, further defined the structure of the gray matter as having 10 layers with clear axonal connections.

Each scientific discovery concerning the spinal cord brings medicine and surgery closer to solving age-old problems associated with paralysis and death related to spinal cord injury. Current work with stem cells has shown promise for cord regeneration and treatment of what was previously thought to be fatal cord damage.

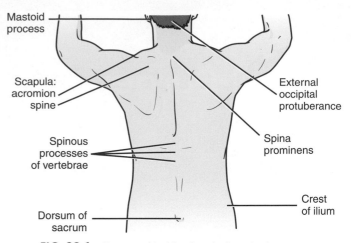

FIG. 38-1   Topographical landmarks for spinal surgery.

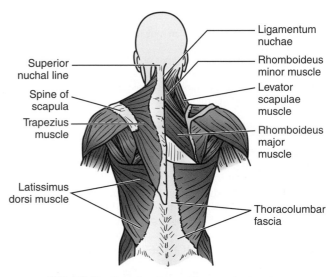

FIG. 38-2   Dorsal surface with muscular borders.

ANATOMY AND PHYSIOLOGY OF THE SPINAL CORD AND VERTEBRAL COLUMN

The vertebral column and spinal cord comprise the posterior aspect of the trunk of the body. The relationship between the bones and nerves is evaluated first from a topographic perspective by assessing the alignment of specific external landmarks (Fig. 38-1). The external dorsal musculature frames the margins of the surgical landmarks used in planning the posterior incision for spinal surgery (Fig. 38-2).

The configuration of the spinal curvature is dependent on chronologic and idiopathic factors. Each age-group, as shown in Figure 38-3, *A*, displays a different set of normal spinal curves based on physiologic development. Abnormal curvatures can be age related but sometimes idiopathic without consideration for age (Fig. 38-3, *B*).

The spinal cord is between 17 and 20 inches (43 to 50 cm) long and passes through a central canal in the vertebral column to the level of the second or third lumbar vertebra (Fig. 38-4). Pairs of spinal nerve roots branch off to each side of the body from 31 segments of the spinal cord as it passes through the vertebrae.

The spinal nerves are as follows:
- Eight pairs cervical
- Twelve pairs thoracic
- Five pairs lumbar
- Five pairs sacral
- One pair coccygeal

The spinal nerves carry sensory and motor impulses between the central nervous system (CNS) and the peripheral nervous system (PNS). The cord is composed of gray matter (cell bodies) on the inside and white matter (nerve fibers) on the outside. This is the exact opposite of the substance of the brain. The ventral nerve roots are the motor axons to the muscles and glands and the dorsal nerve roots are the sensory dendrites (Fig. 38-5). The dorsal root ganglion is easily entrapped by the bony vertebrae and causes pain and disability.

The cephalad portion of the cord begins at the base of the brain at the foramen magnum.

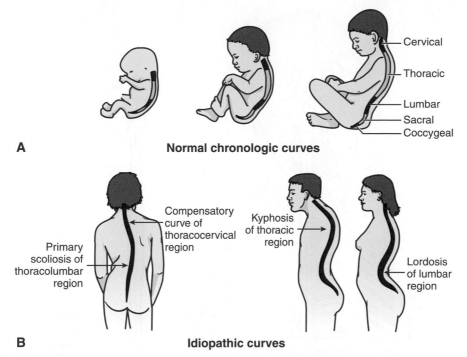

FIG. 38-3   Natural and pathologic spinal curves. **A**, Normal chronologic curves. **B**, Idiopathic curves.

The first thickened area of the spinal cord is at the C7 to T1 junction, forming the brachial plexus. Compromise of the brachial plexus caused by bony impingement of the cervical or upper thoracic vertebrae will result in arm and hand pain and muscular weakness with thenar wasting.

The caudal portion of the spinal cord thickens and ends at L1 to form the conus medullaris before terminating in a fibrous tail known as the cauda equina (horse's tail) (Fig. 38-6). The nerve fibers that extend beyond L2 to L3 form the lumbosacral plexus.

The blood supply to the spinal cord arises from the vertebral artery. The radicular artery of Adamkeiwicz supplies blood to the lower third of the cord. Occlusion of this artery will cause paraplegia. Venous drainage is through the intervertebral vein that drains into the azygos venous system.

The meninges cover the cord to the level of the second or third lumbar vertebra. They terminate in a fibrous band (filum terminale) that extends through the lumbar vertebrae and sacrum and attaches to the coccyx. The dura is not attached or continuous with the central canal of the vertebral column.

Vertebrae

All vertebrae have similar bony characteristics that form a circular canal to house the spinal cord. The structure of a vertebra includes:

- A thick, cylindric body that bears a portion of the weight of the torso.
- Two posterolateral extensions that form the proximal bony vertebral (neural) arch. These extensions form thick pedicles that connect to flatten laminae posteriorly. The laminae connect at the spinous process,

forming a circle. Each pedicle has a notch superiorly and inferiorly to seat the vertebrae above and below.
- A transverse, wing-shaped spinous process that is formed by the connection of the posterior laminae. The central foramen shapes the spinal canal.

The bony structure of the vertebral column extends from the foramen magnum at the base of the skull to the coccyx (Fig. 38-7, *A*). The 33 vertebrae, which provide support for the body, vary in size and shape according to location and are separated by flexible discs over the anterior surface of the body (Fig. 38-7, *B*). Each disc is composed of two parts: an exterior annulus fibrosus and an interior gel referred to as the nucleus pulposus.

The seven cervical vertebrae are in the neck and form the secondary curvature. They are lighter weight with a smaller disc-bearing body.

The top two cervical vertebrae, C1 atlas and C2 axis, have clearly distinct landmarks. The atlas laminae form a circle around the odontoid process of the axis so the head has a wide range of circular and linear motion (Fig. 38-8). The atlas-axis complex has no disc or spinous process and is considered to be strongest vertebra of the cervical portion of the vertebral column.

The 12 thoracic vertebrae articulate posteriorly with the ribs to form a cage around the thoracic organs, forming a primary curvature. The spinous processes are low profile and smaller than the lower vertebrae. The body and discs of the thoracic vertebrae are thinner and are designed to bear minimal weight.

The five lumbar vertebrae are posterior to the retroperitoneal cavity and are designed to carry the heaviest load of the entire vertebral column with the least amount of flexi-

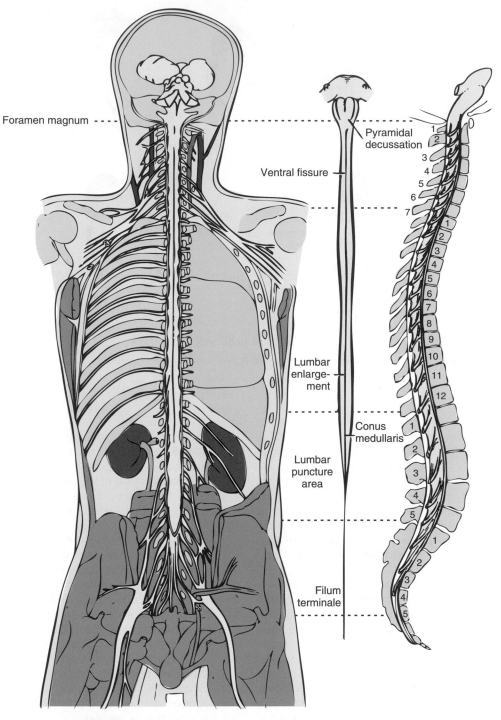

FIG. 38-4   Spinal nerves.
(Modified from Mettler FA: Neuroanatomy, *ed 2, St. Louis, 1948, Mosby.)*

bility. The body and disc of each lumbar vertebra is thick and forms a secondary curvature. Figure 38-9 illustrates the combined lumbar vertebra-disc unit.

The five sacral vertebrae are fused in the adult to form the sacrum and the four fused coccygeal vertebrae form the coccyx (Fig. 38-10). Collectively, these two sets of fused vertebrae form the posterior aspect of the pelvic girdle.

Each vertebra is connected to the other by a series of ligamentous fibers (Fig. 38-11). The vertebral column measures about 28 inches (71 cm) in the average-size adult. The physiologic relationship between the spinal cord, spinal nerves, and the bony vertebral column affects multiple body systems if the curvature is misaligned or some pathology changes the size of a foramen or joint.

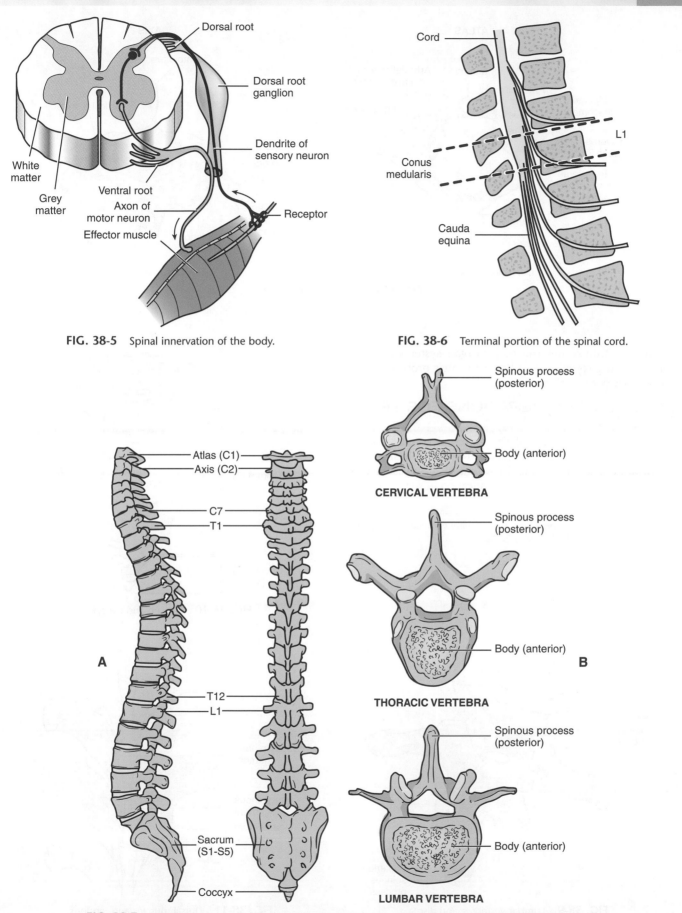

FIG. 38-5   Spinal innervation of the body.

FIG. 38-6   Terminal portion of the spinal cord.

FIG. 38-7   Vertebral column. **A,** Vertebral column: lateral view and posterior view. **B,** Differentiation of vertebrae.

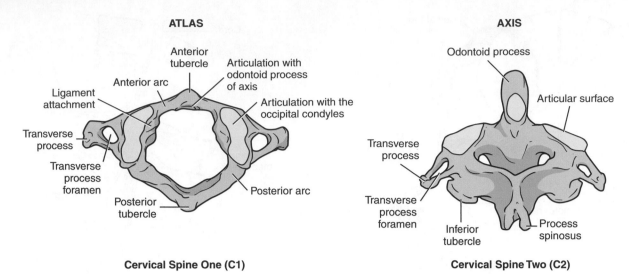

FIG. 38-8   Altas C1 and axis C2.

Figure 38-12 illustrates the major organ systems and the corresponding spinal nerves that can cause problems with physiologic functioning.

SPECIAL CONSIDERATIONS FOR SPINE SURGERY

Because of the proximity of the vertebral column to the spinal cord, both neurosurgeons and orthopedic surgeons perform surgical procedures in this area. Many surgeons have attained subspecialty board certification in spine surgery.[1]

---

[1]Dwyer AP et al: Should there be a subspecialty certification in spine surgery? *Spine* 27(13):1478-1483, 2002.

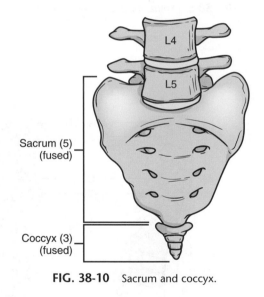

FIG. 38-10   Sacrum and coccyx.

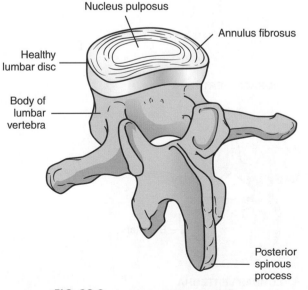

FIG. 38-9   Lumbar vertebrae and disc.

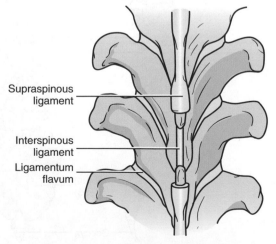

FIG. 38-11   Dorsal muscles and tendons.

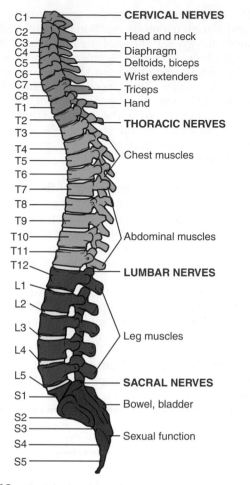

FIG. 38-12 Physiologic relationship between the spinal cord, spinal nerves, and vertebral column.

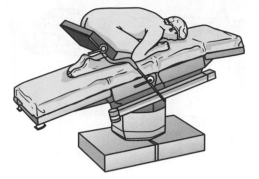

FIG. 38-13 Kneeling-crouching position for spinal surgery.

Both disciplines use power drills, power saws, microscopes, and computer imaging to correct problems in the spinal column; however, many surgeons feel that spine surgery is a specialty unto itself because of the multidisciplinary approaches applied in the correction of spinal problems.

Diagnostics

For diagnosis of spinal conditions, computed tomography (CT) detects abnormal bone. CT and magnetic resonance imaging (MRI) evaluate spinal injuries. MRI and myelography outline soft tissue abnormalities, such as disc degeneration, protrusion, or rupture. Because it is noninvasive and seems as effective, MRI is replacing myelography.

Positioning for Spinal Surgery

Positioning for spinal surgery can require the patient to be placed in either the supine or prone position depending on the type of approach necessary for the planned procedure. Most facilities have specialized operating beds that accommodate the modifications needed for adequate exposure of the surgical site. Some surgical body positions provide distraction of the vertebrae for more direct access to specific regions of the spine.

Considerations for patient positioning include prevention of untoward injury such as pressure areas, pinch points on jointed tables, falls, wrong site surgery, and venous stasis. Positioning a patient in the prone position is a multistep procedure. The patient is given general anesthesia on the transport cart, intubated, and catheterized. A minimum of four people are needed to turn the anesthetized patient into the prone position onto the specialized operating bed.

A few prone positions simulate kneeling or crouching, which means that the patient may be a full lift and body flexion before coming into contact with the surface of the operating bed. Figure 38-13 shows the kneeling-crouching position used by some surgeons for lower spine procedures. This posture constricts the patient's circulation and increases the risk for embolization.[2]

The Jackson table (Fig. 38-14) and the Jackson-Wilson table with the central arch (Fig. 38-15) are used for posterior spinal incisions. Each type of specialty spinal table allows the surgeon to position the patient for optimal vertebral position and exposure of the surgical site.

Instruments Used for Spinal Surgery

Surgical instruments used for spinal surgery for the posterior approach are designed to be used in narrow, deep incisions. The incisions used for surgery of the posterior spine involve paramedian dissection and retraction of several muscle layers. These incisions are very deep and do not always offer a visual advantage to the surgeon and team. The scrub person can prepare for this type of incision by providing medium to large self-retaining retractors in pairs because a matching pair will be used in the cephalad and caudad margins. Some surgeons prefer an angled or jointed Weitlaner or Beckman style.

An assortment of bone debulking rongeurs (Kerrison and Cloward) and curettes with a variety of jaw angles (forward biters, back biters, side biters, up biters, and down biters) are used to remove segments of lamina and spinous process. High-speed drills are sometimes used to reduce bony bulk.

---

[2]Rigamonti A et al: Prone versus knee-chest position for microdiscectomy: A prospective randomized study of intraabdominal pressure and intraoperative bleeding, *Spine* 30(17):1918-1923, 2005.

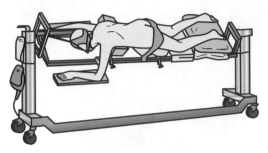

FIG. 38-14   Jackson spinal table.

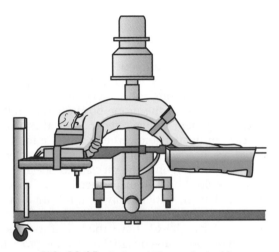

FIG. 38-15   Jackson-Wilson spinal table.

Graspers used include bayonet-style forceps with and without bipolar energy. Sharp dissectors used for soft tissue such as the dura will include #3 and #7 scalpels with several #10, #11, and #15 blades. Blunt dissectors such as Penfields and other periosteal elevators are commonly used. Manual retractors are size-appropriate and angled to provide a clear field of vision for the surgeon. Nerve hooks are used.

Other standard medium and long instruments are used throughout spinal procedures for the posterior and anterior approaches. Keep in mind that any anterior approach will require basic soft tissue sets such as laparotomy instruments and retractors in addition to instruments specific to spinal procedures. Micro instruments are used for microscopic procedures.

Anesthesia Considerations

The anesthesia provider monitors and manipulates the patient's physiology. The patient's airway, breathing, and circulation are under constant surveillance by gross visual exam and by technologic devices. Airway and breathing are compromised by the prone positions used for the posterior spinal approach. The patient's chest excursion is decreased and the intraabdominal pressure is released by allowing the abdominal cavity to rest in a dependent position. The loose abdomen permits the vena cava to remain at a low pressure, preventing excess venous oozing around the vertebral column and cord.

Airway. The patient under general anesthesia who is intubated and placed in a prone position is at high risk for loss of a patent airway. The shape of the trachea and the bifurcation of the bronchi create a complex scenario in which the tip of the endotracheal tube can slip into one bronchus, aerating only one lung. The opposite lung is not adequately ventilated and the level of oxygen saturation decreases. The patient can become hypoxic. The anesthesia provider should remain vigilant about the endotracheal tube position within the trachea and the level of oxygen saturation in the patient's blood.

Intraoperative Neural Monitoring of the Spinal Cord. Some spinal surgeons prefer to monitor sensory and motor activity of the brain and spinal cord during surgery (Fig. 38-16). Intraoperative neural monitoring during the procedure gives the surgeon an early indication of the condition of the cord and spinal nerves as each layer of soft or compact tissue is manipulated.

Dermatomal mapping and Stagnara "wake-up" tests also are reliable techniques for monitoring spinal cord function. In the latter test, the patient must be awake enough to respond to the surgeon's command to move the foot.

Radiologic Use During Spine Surgery. The surgeon usually has a scout radiograph performed. A spinal needle is inserted into the patient's back to the level of the vertebrae targeted for the surgical procedure. The metal needle serves as a marker and confirmation that the procedure is being performed at the correct level of the spine (Fig. 38-17).

Additional radiographs may be taken during the procedure if hardware or appliances are implanted into the bone or surrounding tissue. The follow-up films before closure provide documentation of the spinal procedural level and structural integrity of implants.

Modeling with Scans. Preoperative MRI images can be used to create a 3-D computer model of the affected vertebrae and discs. The computer model allows the surgeon to see the target vertebrae and discs from all directions before incising the skin.[3]

Microscope. The use of the operating microscope was introduced in the late 1960s. Microdiscectomy is a discectomy performed under the operating microscope that is displayed on a video monitor. The video monitor enables the entire team to see the surgical site and anticipate the surgeon's next steps.

Robotic-Assisted Spinal Surgery. Precision tissue manipulation and dissection is made possible by robotic-assisted instrumentation. Some of the systems in use offer the surgeon a greater freedom of hand and wrist motion in close quarters. Some maneuvers made by robotic instrumentation are not possible in the realm of human range of motion. The surgeon's armamentarium is greatly expanded by using robotics for extremely delicate procedures.

[3]Haughton V: Medical imaging of intervertebral disc degeneration, *Spine* 29(23):2751-2756, 2004.

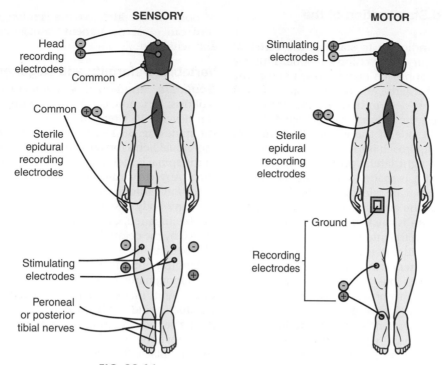

SENSORY

Head recording electrodes

Common

Common

Sterile epidural recording electrodes

Stimulating electrodes

Peroneal or posterior tibial nerves

MOTOR

Stimulating electrodes

Sterile epidural recording electrodes

Ground

Recording electrodes

FIG. 38-16   Intraoperative spinal cord monitoring.

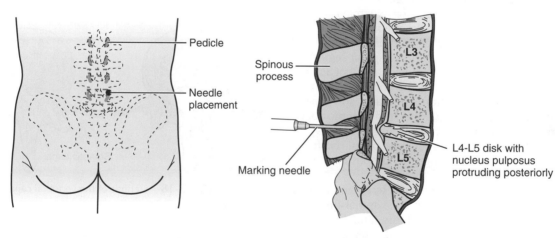

Pedicle

Needle placement

Spinous process

Marking needle

L3

L4

L5

L4-L5 disk with nucleus pulposus protruding posteriorly

FIG. 38-17   Needle localization of surgical level.

Hemostasis. Meticulous hemostasis is necessary in the vertebral and spinal canals. Hematoma formation can create pressure and cause irreparable damage to the nervous system. Compressed cottonoids or patties are used for clearing blood and for applying topical agents such as thrombin. Some surgeons use cotton balls for tamponade pressure after tumor resection. Cotton balls and cottonoids are counted and accounted for in the same manner as other sponges. Topical thrombin can be used for superficial oozing. Thrombin is never injected because it will cause a fatal systemic thrombotic response.

Care is taken to avoid leaving absorbable hemostatic agents in any neural or bony space. Most absorbable agents swell in response to absorption of blood and cause compression in a constricted area. Pressure on the spinal cord or nerves can cause paralysis or other permanent deficit. In 2004, the U.S. Food and Drug Administration (FDA) issued an advisory concerning retained absorbable hemostats in neural spaces.

Bipolar electrosurgery is commonly used to minimize the amount of neural tissue involved with the effects radiofrequency coagulation. Hemostasis for the cut edges of bone can be attained with bone wax or a paste made of powdered antibiotic and saline. Bone wax can act as a mechanical barrier to osteogenesis in some individuals.

Graft Materials and Stabilization of the Vertebrae

Spinal fusion may be indicated to stabilize the vertebral column after spinal injury or excision of bone. Either a posterior or an anterior approach may be used to place the bone grafts. A combined anterior and posterior spinal fusion may be required for severe deformities. The anterior fusion is performed first. Unless the lesion or bone fragment to be removed is on the right side of the vertebral column, an anterior thoracolumbar approach is used through an incision with the patient in the right lateral position (left side up). A retroperitoneal incision is made for an anterior lumbar approach. These approaches are safer on the left side because the surgeon works near the aorta, which is more resistant to inadvertent injury than is the vena cava on the right.

Bone grafts are placed in the intervertebral spaces or along the spinous processes to bridge over or to stabilize the defect. The rib removed for an anterior thoracolumbar approach is used for grafting. Homogeneous cancellous bone from the bone bank may be needed to provide a larger quantity of bone than can be obtained from the rib or an autogenous graft from the crest of the patient's ilium. Cancellous bone rather than cortical bone is usually preferred for spinal fusion. Bone grafts may be used with or without internal fixation devices. The goals of spinal fusion are to achieve stability, rigidity, and correction of deformity. The combined use of internal fixation devices with bone grafts may facilitate postoperative care and early ambulation.

Complex procedures are performed for sublaminar wiring, pedicle screw fixation, and internal vertebral stabilization or fusion. Many spinal implant systems are available. All have the common goal of immobilizing spinal segments; each offers significant biomechanical advantages, but all have potential complications. The surgeon chooses the most appropriate device for the location, approach, and type of deformity and instability. For example, the posterior body and ligamentous structures in the cervical spine may be disrupted by a flexion-compression type of injury. Interspinous wiring and bone grafting provide posterior neck fusion for stability.

In the thoracolumbar spine, pedicular screw and plating systems can be used in conjunction with spinal fusion in treatment of fractures, spondylolisthesis, and idiopathic scoliosis. Cotrel-Dubousset rods, hooks, and screws; the Texas Scottish Rite Hospital (TSRH) system of pedicle screw fixation with rods and cross-links; Luque rods and sublaminar wires; or Wisconsin spinous process wires may be used to provide decompression of spinal nerve roots and vertebral alignment after posterior thoracolumbar spinal fusion. Kaneda, Zielke, Dwyer, or Dunn devices are used when an anterior approach is preferred. Each device has its own set of instrumentation for installation; these are not interchangeable.

PATHOLOGY OF THE VERTEBRAE AND CORD

Disc Degeneration and Rupture

Compression on the Spinal Cord or Nerve Roots. The central canal of the vertebral column can become narrowed, causing compression on the cord (Fig. 38-18). Urgent decompression is necessary if the pressure begins to cause symptoms. Decompression is performed by removing segments of bone at the affected site. Prolonged pressure on the cord can cause permanent damage and loss of function and sensation.

Vertebral Deformity and Degeneration

Scoliosis. An idiopathic lateral curvature of the spine is scoliosis. It is more common in young females, although it can develop in later years with other bony deformities of the spine (Fig. 38-19). The diagnosis is made by having the individual bend forward and observing the linear direction of the spinal bones (Fig. 38-20). The curvature worsens with time. Any curvature of 40% or more requires correction. (Additional information can be found at www.scoliosis.org.)

Many body systems are affected by scoliosis. Digestion can be impaired. Chest excursion and respiratory effort are altered by the deformity that results in the ribcage (Fig. 38-21). The patient has an altered and unsteady gait.

Surgical options include several types of rodding instrumentation, hardware systems, and biografting using allograft or autograft material. Each has a certain amount of failure risk and should not be used in the presence of osteoporosis. After a period of years the graft material may be solid enough to remove the hardware. Most surgeons prefer to leave the rods in place. The surgical approach can be anterior or posterior depending on the type of instrumentation used and the type of correction desired. The most commonly used surgical scoliosis correction systems are as follows:

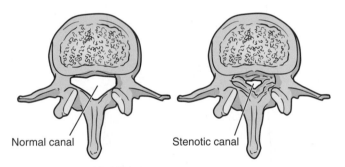

Normal canal   Stenotic canal

FIG. 38-18   Stenosis of the vertebral canal.

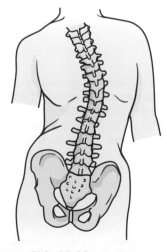

FIG. 38-19   Scoliosis.

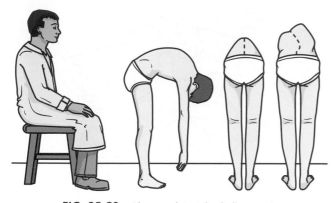

FIG. 38-20   Abnormal vertebral alignment.

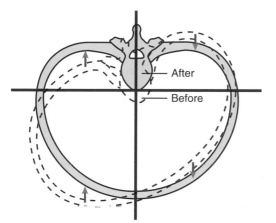

FIG. 38-21   Configuration of rib deformity in scoliosis.

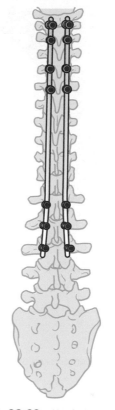

FIG. 38-22   Harrington rods.

1. Harrington rigid metallic rods used for the correction of spinal curvature greater than 60% were introduced in the 1960s. The rods are placed using a posterior approach. The patient is in a body cast for about 6 months postoperatively (Fig. 38-22). The rods can fracture over time because the main fixation is at the ends of the rods.

2. Luque rods are flexible L-shaped bilateral rods wired to the vertebral column to reverse the abnormal angle of the spine by 10%. There is a higher risk of injury because each custom curved segment is wired close to many levels of the spinal nerves. The patient does not need a brace postoperatively.

3. Cotrel-Dubousset features flexible rods with hooks and set screws that use biomechanical principles to reverse the abnormal spinal bends. This system preserves the natural curves of the spine. The system is complex and may require the patient to wear a brace after surgery. This system can be used for kyphoscoliosis.

4. Zelke instrumentation is similar to Cotrel-Dubousset but is used for double curvatures. An anterior approach is commonly used. A body brace is worn postoperatively.

5. TRSH system preserves the natural curves with a series of rods and hooks affixed with nuts and bolts to correct lateral rotation of the vertebrae. These rods can be used for kyphoscoliosis. A brace is not always necessary postoperatively.

6. Isola system is a series of rods and drop-in screws that provides a stable correction of spinal curvature using an anterior transthoracic approach with the patient in a lateral position. Each disc is removed and grafted. Each vertebral body is drilled and has a screw placed for fixation of the rods. These rods can be used for kyphoscoliosis of 40 to degrees and may not require a body brace after surgery. This system can be used for adolescents and adults.

7. Drummond instrumentation uses a Harrington rod on the concave side of the spine and a Luque rod on the convex side. Each vertebra is individually wired. The patient wears a cast or brace postoperatively.

Kyphosis.   Osteoporosis is a degeneration and demineralization of bone that causes compression of the vertebral bodies at regions of spinal curvature (Fig. 38-23). The flattening of the vertebral body causes a loss of height and decreases the accommodation of the movement of the spinal cord and major organ systems (Fig. 38-24). Respiratory effort can be compromised by a decrease in thoracic space. Kyphoplasty is performed percutaneously by the introduction of a catheter and balloon assembly into the collapsed vertebral body (Fig. 38-25, *A*). The balloon is expanded to reproduce the vertebral height, then is removed and replaced by bone cement. The cement hardens to maintain the space created by the kyphoplasty balloon (Fig. 38-25, *B, C*).

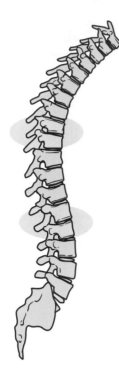

FIG. 38-23   Areas of compression treated with kyphoplasty.

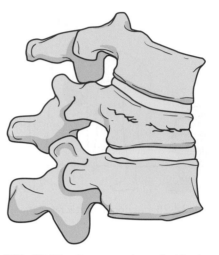

FIG. 38-24   Compressed vertebral body.

Spinal Tumors

Spinal tumors may begin with slowly progressing problems like bladder or bowel weakness and vague symptoms such as back pain and radiculopathy. Thoracic intraspinal tumors represent higher rates of morbidity in the presence of spinal cord atrophy and arachnoid scarring. Diagnostic process is prolonged because the symptoms are not consistent.

Most spinal tumors are readily diagnosed with MRI, and if they metastasize they travel to the bone first. Other cancers such as prostate, lung, and breast metastasize to the vertebrae through hematologic routes and can infiltrate the dura to the cord. About 55% of spinal tumors are metastatic in origin. Symptoms usually are related to spinal cord pressure.

The posterior segment of the vertebral arch is removed to expose the dura over the involved section of the spinal cord. The dura is incised and retracted with sutures. The tumor is excised, and the dura is closed tightly to prevent leakage of cerebrospinal fluid (CSF). Both intrinsic and extrinsic spinal cord tumors can be removed by laser with decreased tissue trauma. The laser is especially useful in areas difficult to reach by dissection, such as the foramen magnum or anterior spinal cord.

Tumors of the spinal area are classified as one of the following types:

1. *Extradural:* outside the dural layer of the meninges. Many of these are benign, such as lipomas, chondromas, granulomas, and abscesses.
2. *Intradural:* under the dural layer of the meninges, not invasive in the spinal cord. These tumors are frequently well circumscribed and slow growing. They arise from the cells of the proximal nerve roots. They can be noted with myelograms.

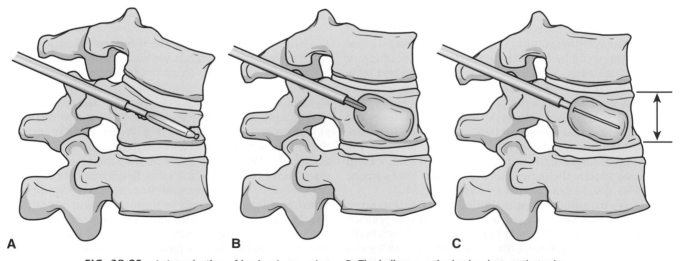

FIG. 38-25   **A,** Introduction of kyphoplasty catheter. **B,** The balloon on the kyphoplasty catheter is expanded. **C,** Bone cement is used to displace the kyphoplasty balloon and maintain vertebral height.

3. *Hemangioblastoma:* vascular tumor in neural tissue. More common in 30- to 40-year-old males 2:1. These tumors can be associated with von Hippel-Lindau disease. More common in the cervical or thoracic areas.

4. *Astrocytoma (glial tumor)* of the spinal cord is rare and is found in 30- to 50-year-old males more than females. MRI reading looks very cystic and thickened. Large segments can be removed with irrigation-aspiration systems like CUSA.
   a. Diffuse fibrous type: harder to remove. Most spinal astrocytomas are this type.
   b. Circumscribed: more clearly defined and have a better prognosis for excision. Less invasive to surrounding tissue.

5. *Intraspinal intramedullary:* slow-growing tumor inside the tissues of the spinal cord. More common in females. These grow more aggressively in children than in adults. Cervical and thoracic areas are the most common primary sites. Sacral tumors tend to metastasize readily to bone.

6. *Ependymoma tumors* arise from the ependymal cells that line the central canal, from the ventriculus terminalis of the conus, and from the filum terminale with cells disseminated by the cerebral spinal fluid. Some are encapsulated with many superficial vessels. Total removal of an encapsulated tumor may eliminate the need for postoperative radiation.
   a. Myxopapillary ependymal tumors arise exclusively in the filum terminale and the conus medullaris and are more common in young males.
   b. Metastasis from areas of the brain

Spinal Trauma

During World War I 80% of spinal cord–injured soldiers died within the first 2 weeks of the wounding. Little was known about special treatment and surgical decompression, so most of the wounded died from complications associated with the spinal cord injury, not the actual damage to the cord. Immobility and infection were leading causes of death. By World War II specialized units were developed in response to scientific understanding of the cord and its function, greatly increasing the survival rate.

Vertebral fractures, with or without dislocation, can cause spinal cord compression that denervates nerve tracts below the injury. Spinal cord injury may also be caused by penetrating or stretching trauma or by damage to blood vessels that supply the cord.

Spinal cord injuries are classified as follows:
- *Complete.* The patient lacks sensation, proprioception (position sense), and voluntary motor function below the level of the spinal cord damage. Lesions above the fifth cervical vertebra (C5) will cause partial to complete diaphragmatic paralysis. Injury in the cervical region will result in quadriplegia (i.e., functional impairment from the neck down). Lumbar cord injuries lead to paraplegia (i.e., excluding paralysis of the upper extremities).
- *Incomplete.* Some sensory, proprioceptive, and motor impulses are present. Loss of function depends on the extent and location of the injury. This is sometimes seen at the lower aspect of the cord below L1 in the region of the cauda equina. Bowel or bladder can be affected without impairing mobility.

Spinal cord edema or hematoma can cause a cord lesion to ascend and worsen the neurologic deficit. Resultant paralysis may be relieved if the surgical procedure to remove bone fragments or to drain a hematoma compressing the spinal cord is done within a very short time after injury. Results are frequently discouraging. Damage to the cord may be too extensive for return of function, or at best, return may be incomplete. Care is taken in moving and positioning the patient to avoid further paralysis. The patient should be logrolled (i.e., turned or lifted without flexing the vertebral column).

A lumbar puncture with pressure readings may be done. If a block in the flow of spinal fluid is present, a laminotomy or laminectomy is done to decompress the spinal cord in a patient with complete paralysis or partial paralysis that is becoming progressively worse. A laminectomy may also be done to remove bone fragments. Internal fixation may be combined with decompression for thoracolumbar fractures.

Temperature control and monitoring of fluid and electrolyte balance are essential to the outcome for the patient with a spinal cord injury. The patient loses thermoregulatory ability after injury and tends to assume the temperature of the environment. Lack of vascular adaptation affects fluid balance. Pulmonary edema and left ventricular failure can occur. Pulmonary embolus also is a potential complication.

Technologic advances in surgical treatment, stabilization, and electrical stimulation have given patients with spinal cord injuries hope for regaining partial or full function.

SURGICAL PROCEDURES OF THE SPINE

Discectomy

Intervertebral disc injuries can happen anywhere along the vertebral column, but usually occur between the lumbar vertebrae and are caused by lifting heavy objects or by twisting the spine. The nucleus pulposus can herniate or rupture through a tear in the annulus fibrosus and posterior ligament (Fig. 38-26). This protrusion, referred to as a herniated disc or ruptured or slipped disc, compresses the spinal nerve roots or spinal cord within the spinal canal against the vertebra. This causes pain along the dermatomes from the lumbar or sacral region to one or both lower legs (Fig. 38-27). Pain may radiate down the sciatic nerve pathway to the leg. During the surgical procedure the herniated nucleus pulposus or ruptured portion of the annulus fibrosus is excised (Fig. 38-28).

Microdiscectomy or percutaneous discectomy may be used to remove a herniated lumbar nucleus pulposus with minimal surgical manipulation. Microdiscectomy permits exposure of the herniated nucleus pulposus through a 1- or 2-inch (2.5- to 5-cm) incision without extensive manipulation of the paraspinal muscles or removal of a large section of lamina. The skin incision is shorter than required for a standard laminectomy; therefore, recovery time is decreased.

Percutaneous Discectomy

Percutaneous lumbar discectomy is an endoscopic procedure to remove a focal bulge–type herniated disc, usually at the level of L4-L5. It is done with the patient under local anesthesia, usually with IV sedation, because the patient must be alert enough to assess radicular pain in the leg.

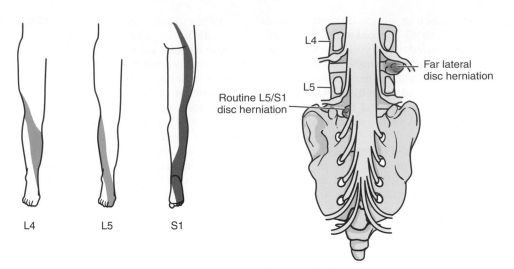

FIG. 38-26   Herniated disc at L5-S1 causes pain along the associated dermatomes.

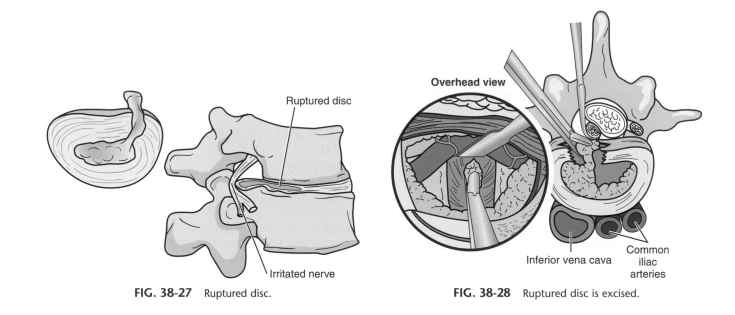

FIG. 38-27   Ruptured disc.

FIG. 38-28   Ruptured disc is excised.

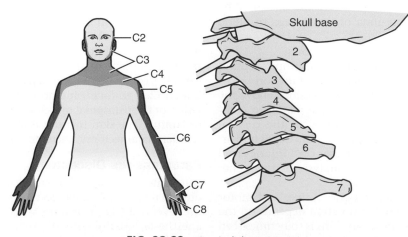

FIG. 38-29   Cervical dermatome.

The patient may be either prone or in a lateral decubitus position. A trocar is inserted through the skin and soft tissue into the disc capsule. Under fluoroscopic control, a cutting probe (Nucleotome) is inserted through the outer cannula. The herniated nucleus pulposus is excised and aspirated to relieve pressure on the spinal nerve root.

Cervical Spine

The cervical dermatome distribution is one of the prime indicators of the location of the injury or pathologic lesion (Fig. 38-29).

Transoral Approach. The patient is positioned supine with the back rest of the operating bed elevated. The head is stabilized in a headrest and the airway is intubated with a nasotracheal tube (Fig. 38-30). The retractors are placed in the pharynx to retract the tongue and the soft palate. The uvula is retracted upward by using a transnasal loop. The teeth are protected by tooth guards or moist sponges (Fig. 38-31). The transpharyngeal incision is made to access the retropharyngeal space. The high cervical spines C1-C2 can be repaired or stabilized.

Anterior Cervical Approach. The anterior cervical spine can be exposed through a transverse skin incision in the neck and dissection through the cleavage plane between the carotid artery and the esophagus (Fig. 38-32). The anterior cervical incision is created along the lateral muscular cleavage line or transversely across the anterior neck (Fig. 38-33). Medium self-retaining retractors are placed in the incision at right angles to provide exposure of the vertebral body while displacing the esophagus and trachea (Fig. 38-34). Care is taken to identify the nerves and vessels. Anterior cervical dissection can cause complications with speech and swallowing postoperatively.

The spinous processes and laminae remain intact when the anterior approach is used. A ruptured intervertebral disc and/or a fracture-dislocation with bone fragments compressing the cervical spinal cord or nerve roots can be completely explored at the level of the vertebral body (Fig. 38-35). Removal of the posterior margins of the vertebral bodies may be indicated to complete the decompression of the nerve root.

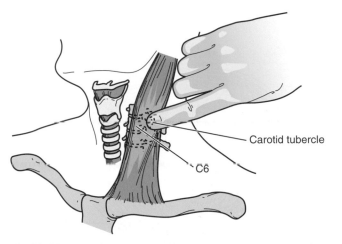

FIG. 38-32 Surgical landmarks for anterior cervical approach for cervical spine surgery.

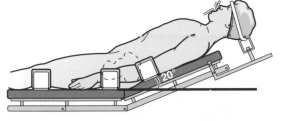

FIG. 38-30 Position for transoral cervical surgery.

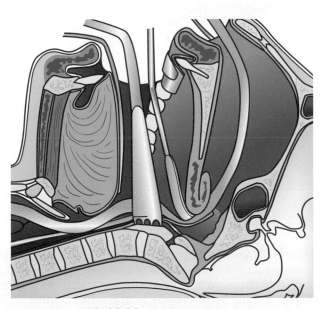

FIG. 38-31 Transoral retractors.

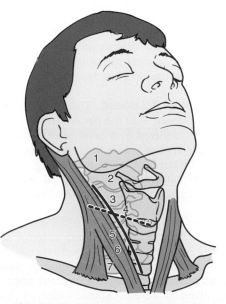

FIG. 38-33 Anterior cervical incisions.

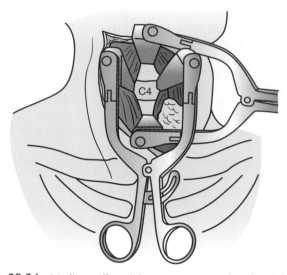

FIG. 38-34   Medium self-retaining retractors are placed at right angles.

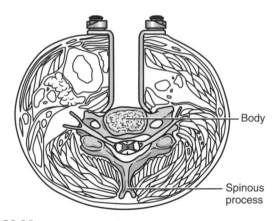

FIG. 38-35   Cross section of retracted tissue at the level of the cervical vertebrae.

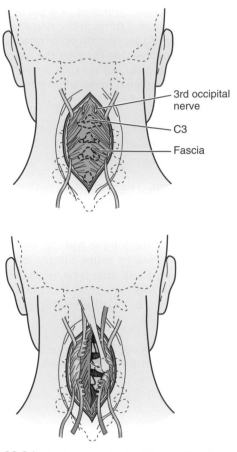

FIG. 38-36   Posterior cervical incision and laminectomy.

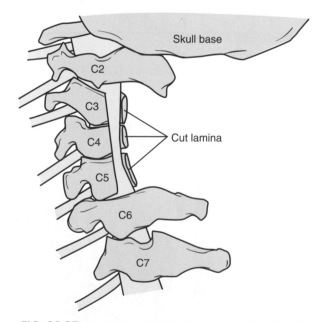

FIG. 38-37   Posterior cervical laminectomy at three levels.

The operating microscope is a valuable adjunct to anterior cervical intervertebral discectomy and for an anterior approach to other cervical spinal lesions. A bone graft may be placed between the vertebral bodies for interbody fusion.

Posterior Cervical Approach. The lower posterior cervical spines can be accessed with the patient in the prone position with the head stabilized in a head-positioning frame. The incision is made vertically over the cervical spinous processes (Fig. 38-36). The laminae are removed (Fig. 38-37) and the remaining cervical spines are stabilized with plates and screws to minimize instability (Fig. 38-38).

Thoracic Spine

Anterior Thoracic Approach. An anterior approach is used for thoracic vertebral disc herniations, spinal cord tumors, or vertebral body fractures. A thoracic surgeon assists with a transthoracic approach. Fractured bone fragments can be stabilized by anterior spinal fusion or placement of posterior rods by costotransversectomy in the thoracic region.

Posterior Thoracic Approach. Posterior thoracic spinal procedures do not involve a full thoracotomy. Positioning is similar to that used for lower posterior spinal procedures and the incision is performed in the same manner as a lumbar incision.

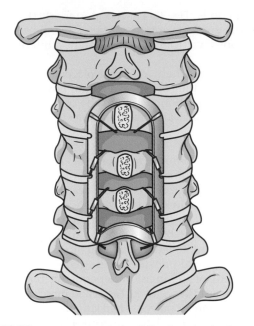

FIG. 38-38   Posterior cervical stabilization after laminectomy.

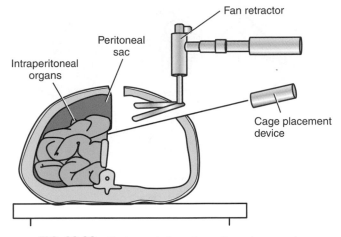

FIG. 38-39   Supine anterior retroperitoneal approach.

Lumbar Spine

Anterior Transperitoneal Lumbar Approach. The anterior transperitoneal approach is performed on a supine patient through an abdominal incision like a laparotomy and enters the peritoneal cavity. Large table-mounted retractors may be used to provide exposure.

Anterior Retroperitoneal Lumbar Approach. The anterior retroperitoneal approach is performed on a patient in a supine or lateral position and involves an incision into the abdomen that is used to dissect the planes behind the peritoneal cavity from the abdominal wall (Fig. 38-39). The peritoneal cavity is displaced laterally and retracted away from the retroperitoneal space.

The retroperitoneal method is used for endoscopic spine surgery and placement of interbody cages for stabilization (Fig. 38-40). The cages are small metallic frames that are packed with bone graft material and inserted between the bodies of the vertebrae. The graft-filled cages can be

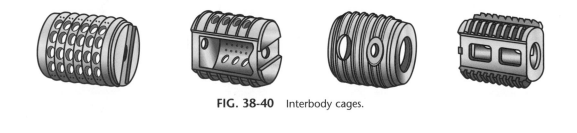

FIG. 38-40   Interbody cages.

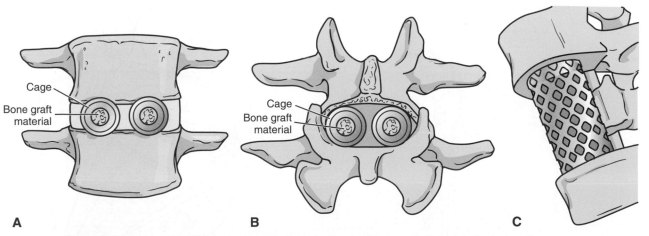

A   **B**   **C**

FIG. 38-41   **A,** Anterior interbody cages. **B,** Posterior interbody cages. **C,** Open interbody cage in anterior placement.

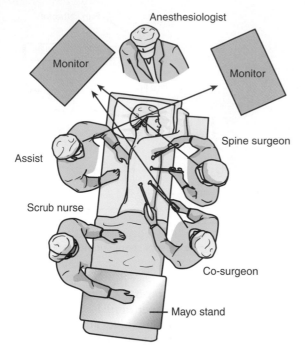

FIG. 38-42   Placement of the team for spinal endoscopy.

placed anteriorly (Fig. 38-41, *A*) or posteriorly (Fig. 38-41, *B*) though the disc space between the vertebral bodies or can be positioned vertically in the anterior interbody space (Fig. 38-41, *C*).

The endoscopic method of cage placement is commonly performed with the patient in a lateral position. The team is strategically positioned around the operating bed so the monitors are in a clear range of vision (Fig. 38-42).

Posterior Lumbar Approach. Removal of the spinous process(es) and lamina from one or more vertebrae is performed to expose an intervertebral or spinal cord lesion. A posterior laminectomy is usually carried out through a vertical midline skin incision with the patient positioned prone position (Fig. 38-43). The patient may be positioned prone on a Jackson table or Wilson or Andrews frame to arch the spine forward, to reduce epidural blood loss by lowering the intraabdominal pressure on the vena cava.

The extent of the incision depends on the number of lumbar laminae to be removed. Fascia and muscles are retracted to expose the spinous processes and laminae. These are sharply debulked and dissected with a rongeur, as necessary, for exposure of the spinal cord dura, spinal nerve roots, or an

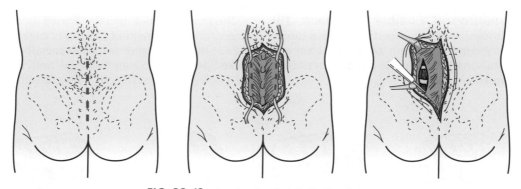

FIG. 38-43   Lumbar incision for laminectomy.

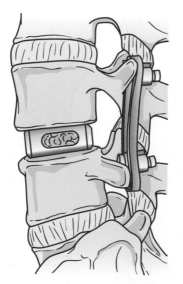

FIG. 38-44   Interbody cage with plates and screws.

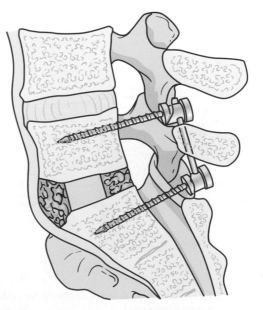

FIG. 38-45   L5-S1 fusion with bone graft and rods with screws.

interlaminar lesion. An intervertebral disc, spinal cord tumor, bone fragments, and extradural or intradural foreign bodies are removed after the laminectomy is completed. Cages can be placed during an open spinal procedure as part of the stabilization after a laminectomy. Figure 38-44 shows an interbody cage packed with bone graft material and stabilization with plates and screws. Figure 38-45 shows an L5-S1 fusion with bone graft for fusion with stabilization with short rods and screws.

Bibliography

Balabhadra R et al: Anterior cervical fusion using dense cancellous allografts and dynamic plating, *Neurosurgery* 56(5):1405-1411, 2004.

Biafora S et al: Arterial injury following percutaneous vertebral augmentation: A case report, *Spine* 31(3):84-87, 2006.

Crosby ET: Airway management in adults after cervical spine trauma, *Anesthesiology* 104(6):1293-1318, 2006.

Gabay M: Absorbable hemostatic agents, *Am J Health Syst Pharm* 63(13):1244-1253, 2006.

Gaines RW: The use of pedicle-screw internal fixation for the treatment of spinal disorders, *J Bone Joint Surg Am* 82(10):1458-1476, 2000.

Goodrich JT: The history of spine surgery in the ancient and medieval worlds, *Neurosurg Focus* 16(1):1-13, 2004.

Grauer J et al: Similarities and differences in the treatment of spine trauma between surgical specialties and location of practice, *Spine* 29(6):685-696, 2004.

Kayanja M et al: The mechanics of polymethylmethacrylate augmentation, *Clin Orthop Relat Res* 443:124-130, 2006.

Ledlie JT: Kyphoplasty treatment of vertebral fractures: 2-year outcomes show sustained benefits, *Spine* 31(1):65-66, 2006.

Nussbaum DA et al: A review of complications associated with vertebroplasty and kyphoplasty as reported to the Food and Drug Administration medical device related web site, *J Vasc Interv Radiol* 15(11):1185-1192, 2004.

Papadopoulos EC et al: Outcome of revision discectomies following recurrent lumbar disc herniation, *Spine* 31(13):1473-1476, 2006.

Rao RD et al: Does anterior plating of the cervical spine predispose to adjacent segment changes? *Spine* 30(24):2788-2792, 2005.

Schizas C et al: Microendoscopic discectomy compared with standard microsurgical discectomy for treatment of uncontained or large contained disc herniations, *Neurosurgery* 57(4 Suppl):357-360, 2005.

Schubert A et al: Anesthesia for minimally invasive cranial and spinal surgery, *J Neurosurg Anesth* 18(1):47-56, 2006.

Theocharopoulos N et al: Fluoroscopically assisted surgical treatments of spinal disorders: Conceptus radiation doses and risk, *Spine* 31(2):239-244, 2006.

Togawa D et al: Histological evaluation of biopsies obtained from vertebral compression fractures: Unsuspected myeloma and osteomalacia, *Spine* 30(7):781-786, 2005.

Voggenreite G: Balloon kyphoplasty is effective in deformity correction of osteoporotic vertebral compression fractures, *Spine* 30(24):2806-2812, 2005.

Winslow CP et al: Dysphonia and dysphagia following the anterior approach to the cervical spine, *Arch Otolaryngol Head Neck Surg* 127(1):51-55, 2001.

Chapter 39

Ophthalmic Surgery

CHAPTER OBJECTIVES

After studying this chapter, the learner will be able to:
- Identify the pertinent anatomy of the eye and surrounding structures.
- Describe the procedures performed on the eye for glaucoma.
- Discuss the advantages and disadvantages of intraocular lens implantation.
- Describe the actions of mydriatic and miotic drugs.

CHAPTER OUTLINE

KEY TERMS AND DEFINITIONS

Aphakic   Without a natural or prosthetic lens.
BSS   Balanced salt solution used for eye irrigation.
Capsulorrhexis   During cataract surgery a continuous circular rent is created in the anterior capsule during to allow removal or phacoemulsification of the nucleus of the opacified lens.
Cataract   Cloudy or yellowed lens of the eye.
Cyclodialysis   Surgical opening between the anterior chamber and the suprachoroidal space to decrease elevated pressure within the eye in glaucoma.
Discission   Cut into soft tissue such as a cataract.
Gonioscopy   Examination of the anterior chamber with a special lens.
Haptic   Tiny flexible prong used to secure a prosthetic intraocular lens.
IOL   Intraocular lens.
Phacoemulsification   Irrigation and aspiration of a cataract using ultrasonic vibrations.
Pneumoretinopexy   Repositioning of a detached retina by use of a gas or air bubble in the vitreous.

SUPPLEMENTAL MATERIAL ON EVOLVE WEBSITE   *evolve*

http://evolve.elsevier.com/BerryKohn
- Content Updates
- Glossary
- Full Set of Perioperative Flash Cards
- Interactive Key Term Flash Cards
- Student Activities
- Tips for the Scrub Person and Circulating Nurse: Strabismus Correction, Vitrectomy
- WebLinks

HISTORICAL BACKGROUND

Disorders of the eye have been well documented throughout history. The word *cataract,* an opacification of the crystalline lens of the eye, is originally derived from a Greek word translated to mean "mist of a waterfall." The cataract has been called by various names throughout history (e.g., pearl of the eye).

Cataract awareness probably extends back at least 3000 years. This belief is supported by the finding of Bronze Age (2000-1000 BC) instruments, such as those used for an ancient couching or reclination treatment. Couching consisted of striking a blow to the front of the eye with a sharp instrument to spontaneously dislocate the opacified lens and push it back into the vitreous cavity. Light then entered the pupil. Couching was performed by the Hindus, Greeks, Romans, and Arabs.

In the early Christian era, Celsus differentiated between incipient (beginning) and mature cataracts. Galen thought the white opacity to be partly in the lens and partly in the aqueous humor in the form of a membrane floating between the lens and the iris. That belief was held, and couching was practiced sporadically until 1745, when Jacques Daviel (1693-1762), a French surgeon, performed the first deliberate lens extraction on a monk from a local monastery. During the first half of the twentieth century, extracapsular cataract extraction was the accepted technique until an intracapsular technique became popular in the mid-1940s.

The first corneal transplant in which a scarred cornea was replaced with a clear donor cornea was performed around 1817. It failed because animal tissue (xenograft) was used instead of human tissue (allograft). The first reported full-thickness graft of full corneal depth to remain clear occurred in 1905. Although attempted in the interval, corneal transplantation did not become an established technique until 1950, when Ramone Castroviejo (1905-1987) developed the procedure. Since then, the technique has been refined to produce a high rate of favorable outcomes. Castroviejo promoted the donation of eyes after death that resulted in the formation of eye banks throughout the world.

In the early eighteenth century, attempts to implant lenses were unsuccessful. The modern era of plastic intraocular lens implantation evolved from an incidental observation. Surgeons in England noted a lack of reactivity to plastic fragments from shattered plane canopies that penetrated the eyes of fighter pilots during World War II. Posterior chamber lenses placed in the 1950s produced disappointing long-term results, mainly because of dislocation. These lenses had to be removed because of inadequate fixation.

The first series of anterior chamber lenses, which were placed in front of the iris, sometimes produced delayed corneal damage. The iris-supported lenses were designed to avoid this complication but are seldom used because of mechanical problems such as dislocation and corneal irritation. Modifications in the design of anterior chamber lenses have reduced complications. Since the 1960s the posterior chamber lens has attained the greatest popularity.

The development of fluorescein angiography by American ophthalmic surgeon Alfred Edward Maumenee, Jr. (1913-1998) demonstrated visualization of the entire retinal vascular tree by the injection of a fluorescing dye and expanded the knowledge of retinal and choroidal physiology and disease. This increased knowledge resulted in improved vision care therapy.

The advent of ophthalmic lasers that provide ablation of pathologic conditions with light energy was a great step forward. In many patients, laser therapy obviates the need for some surgical procedures. Initially used primarily for vascular diseases such as diabetic retinopathy, laser use has expanded to include corneal reshaping and the treatment of glaucoma and secondary membranes. Ophthalmologists pioneered the use of medical lasers and operating microscopes.

ANATOMY AND PHYSIOLOGY OF THE EYE

A thorough understanding of the anatomic structure and physiology of the eye is fundamental to a comprehension of the surgical procedures.

The eyeballs are framed bilaterally by the bony orbits. Each orbit comprises seven separate bones: the maxilla, palatine, frontal, sphenoid, zygoma, ethmoid, and lacrimal bones. Foramina, fissures, and grooves provide stability and access for vessels, nerves, and attachments. Adjacent anatomic structures include the lacrimal apparatus medially, the extraocular muscles and their attachments, and the sinuses.

The globe, or eyeball, is situated within the bony orbit and is surrounded by a padding of fatty tissue. Its position is maintained by extraocular muscles and fascial attachments. The sclera, the white outer tissue layer of the globe, is contiguous with the transparent avascular cornea anteriorly. The conjunctiva is the mucous membrane that lines the inner side of the upper and lower eyelids and the exposed portion of the sclera, except for the cornea (Fig. 39-1).

The eyeball is divided into two segments: anterior and posterior. The anterior segment of the eye includes the cornea, the anterior chamber filled with aqueous fluid (humor), the circular pigmented iris, and the lens. The lens consists of a clear, transparent, gelatinous protein encased in a capsule. It is supported by a series of suspensory ligaments called zonules. The posterior segment, the portion of the eye behind the lens, contains the vitreous fluid (which must be clear for vision), the retina, and the choroid linings, which are the vascular nourishing layers (Fig. 39-2).

Innervation of vision and sensory transmission is derived from the second cranial nerve (optic nerve) (Fig. 39-3). Motor innervation extends from the third cranial nerve (oculomotor nerve) to the rectus muscles. The superior

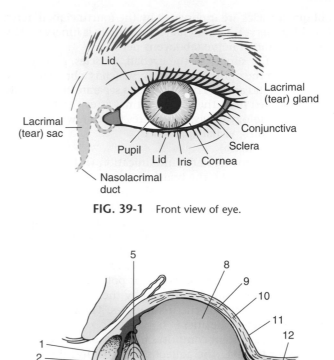

FIG. 39-1 Front view of eye.

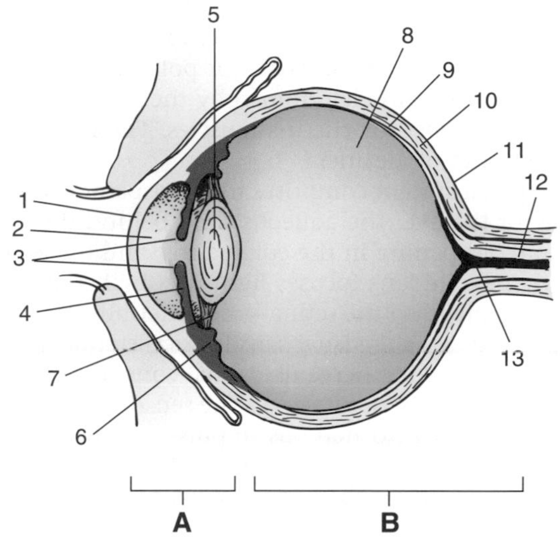

FIG. 39-2 Anatomy of the eye. **A,** Anterior segment. *1,* Cornea; *2,* anterior chamber; *3,* pupil; *4,* iris; *5,* lens; *6,* ciliary body; *7,* zonule. **B,** Posterior segment. *8,* Vitreous body; *9,* retina; *10,* choroid; *11,* sclera; *12,* optic nerve; *13,* central retinal artery.

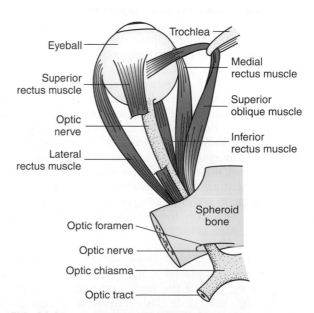

FIG. 39-3 Location of optic nerve in relation to eye muscles.

oblique muscles are innervated by the fourth cranial nerve (trochlear nerve). The lateral rectus muscle is innervated by the sixth cranial nerve (abducens nerve).

The arterial supply of the eyeball, muscles, and eyelids comes from the ophthalmic artery, which is a branch of the internal carotid artery. The retina has a separate blood supply that is derived from the central retinal artery and vein.

The physiology of vision requires the following:

- Functioning visual apparatus
- Source of light
- Intact neurovascular communication with the brain
- Interpretation by the brain of what is seen

The eye resembles a camera with a compound lens system. Light rays emanating from an object in the field of vision are transmitted to the eye, where they traverse the optical system to reach the retina. The retina corresponds to the film of the camera. The area of highest sensitivity for details is called the macula, which is located approximately in the center of the retina at the posterior pole. The intensity of light is automatically determined by the size of the pupil, which is controlled by the iris muscles. The iris functions like the shutter of a camera.

The optical system comprises the transparent cornea, or window of the eye; the aqueous fluid behind the cornea; the pupil, or opening in the colored iris; and the lens. The naturally flexible lens focuses light rays by bending them to form an image on the retina—the innermost layer of the eye that contains the visual sensory nerve endings. These cells are connected to nerve fibers that converge toward the brain to become the optic nerve. The sensory cells translate patterns of light into nervous impulses, which are transmitted to the brain via the optic nerve. The occipital portion of the brain interprets the images of light rays registered on the retina.

OPHTHALMIC SURGICAL PATIENT CARE

Impaired vision may produce prolonged severe stress and alter the patient's self-image. Most patients with impaired vision are older adults. When caring for these patients, the health care provider should reassure them, exercise patience, give directions clearly, anticipate needs, and check their comfort level. Specific patient care considerations include but are not limited to the following:

1. Urinary urgency can be a problem in geriatric patients or in patients receiving diuretic medication. Although the patient should void before coming to the operating room (OR), offer the patient the use of a bedpan or urinal before he or she transfers to the operating bed. Severe urinary urgency can cause increased intraocular pressure (IOP) during the procedure. Strain and gross movement are dangerous and are to be avoided.
2. The surgeon and circulating nurse verify the intended surgical site with the patient and with the office records. After confirmation and to avoid error, some surgeons place an indelible mark on the side of the patient's neck that corresponds to the affected eye.
3. The patient is placed in the supine position on the operating bed so the head and body are aligned. Most ORs use a dedicated ophthalmic operating bed that can be used during the procedure and to transport the patient to the postprocedural recovery area (Fig. 39-4). The top of the head is in line with the edge of the operating bed for accessibility. The head should not be turned greatly in either direction; the head is stabilized in a ring-shaped pillow (donut). The patient's gown is untied at the neck to prevent pressure. Any obstruction to venous circulation can cause undue increased IOP, which can produce a loss of vitreous humor when the eye is opened. To assist venous return from the head, the operating bed is tilted so the patient's head is elevated by 5 to 10 degrees. For long procedures, an egg crate–type or gel pad mattress may be placed on the bed. Additional padding may be needed to position kyphotic or lordotic patients.
4. Skin preparation and draping procedures are performed according to routine. Sterile plastic drapes are often placed over woven textile drapes to contain lint, especially before lens implantation. A patient with a drape over the face is often apprehensive and afraid of suffocating. To help eliminate the feeling of claustrophobia, the drape can be placed over a Mayo stand or clipped to an IV pole to create a tentlike space above the patient's nose and mouth (Fig. 39-5). Oxygen is delivered via nasal prongs or insufflated to the facial area beneath the drape at 6 to 8 L/min.

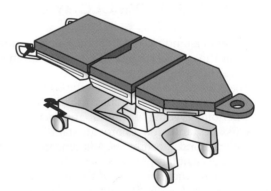

FIG. 39-4   Dedicated ophthalmic bed.

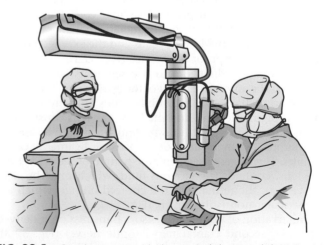

FIG. 39-5   Creating a tent with the surgical drape and the Mayo stand for patient comfort.

An electrosurgical unit (ESU) is not to be used in an oxygen-rich environment because of the increased risk of ignition.

5. A quiet, stimulant-free environment is provided for the awake patient who is receiving a local anesthetic.

6. Because the patient has no defensive blink reflex to protect the retina from light exposure, some surgeons use a sterile, opaque pupillary shield to protect the patient's retina from phototoxic damage caused by prolonged exposure to illumination of the microscope. Some scopes have a sensor near the eyepiece that dims the light source when the surgeon is not looking directly into the scope. The light reverts back to the desired intensity when the surgeon is positioned at the eyepiece.

7. The team should prepare for emergencies by anticipating problems. Fast action can make the difference between a seeing eye and a nonseeing eye postoperatively. The following are potential complications:
   a. A systemic reaction to medications or local anesthetic drugs and cardiac arrest.
   b. A loss of vitreous, which requires the removal of vitreous from the anterior chamber with a vitreotome to prevent prolapse of the wound, severe inflammation, or an updrawn pupil.
   c. An expulsive hemorrhage or an expulsion of ocular contents, which requires a sharp knife (e.g., Beaver blade, Wheeler knife) for fast cutdown into the pars plana area and an 18-gauge needle or cannula attached to a syringe to aspirate blood and reduce pressure in the vitreal compartment in an effort to save the eye and vision (Fig. 39-6).
   d. Instrument failure. Hand aspiration devices should be available for immediate use.

8. A wide variety of fine-size absorbable and nonabsorbable sutures is used. The scrub person follows the manufacturer's recommendations for handling these delicate materials and needles with the appropriate needle holders. Special techniques are used in microsurgery.

9. Hemostasis is attained with bipolar cautery and bipolar eraser pencil. Sponges are spear shaped and consist of precut compressed cellulose on sticks (Fig. 39-7).

10. No foreign material should be introduced into the surgical wound. In intraocular procedures, no portion of any instrument or item intended to enter the eye should be touched by a gloved hand. To remove any debris or impurity, intraocular lenses (IOLs) are soaked and rinsed in balanced salt solution (BSS) and sometimes lubricated with sodium hyaluronate (Healon) before insertion.

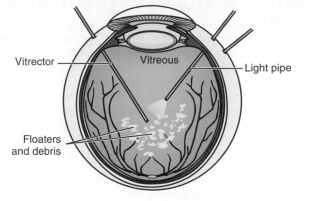

FIG. 39-6   Pars plana vitrectomy for emergency bleeding.

11. Inflammation should be kept as minimal as possible, because even slight inflammation may result in total functional loss. Steroids are often administered locally, subconjunctivally and, sometimes, systemically. The eye may respond violently to the slightest amount of trauma.

12. Antibiotic drops are often instilled topically for 24 hours preoperatively and postoperatively.

13. A sterile eye pad is commonly applied at the conclusion of the surgical procedure. A protective plastic or metal shield may be secured over the eye pad to guard against mechanical injury. Absorbable corneal shields may be used.

14. The patient should not be permitted to participate in the move from the operating bed after intraocular procedures; this prevents a sudden rise in IOP and/or dislocation of the IOL implant.

15. Arm restraints are essential for infants and young children. Restraints are applied to adults only under extreme circumstances, such as disorientation. The use of side rails is standard procedure for all patients undergoing ophthalmic surgery.

An important aspect of postoperative care is informing the patient not to get out of bed alone. A fall or injury to the eye can nullify an otherwise successful surgical procedure. The patient must not do anything to increase IOP (e.g., bend over at the waist, lift heavy objects). Deep breathing postoperatively is encouraged, but coughing is avoided because it could increase IOP and rupture the suture line. The patient should report any postoperative pain, swelling, redness, or discharge. The outcome of ophthalmic procedures includes a cosmetic as well as a functional aspect.

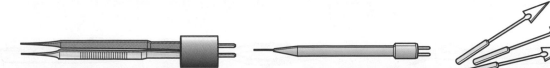

McPherson bipolar ESU forceps   Bipolar ESU eraser pencil   Cellulose spears (absorbent)

FIG. 39-7   Instruments for hemostasis of the eye.

SPECIAL FEATURES OF OPHTHALMIC SURGERY

The patient undergoing ophthalmic surgery faces impairment or loss of vision if the outcome of the surgical intervention is unfavorable. Special features of ophthalmic surgery aim to prevent such a loss. Surgical procedures on the eye are extremely delicate and require precision instrumentation, a steady hand, and quiet surroundings. The operating microscope, all accessory equipment, and microinstruments should be set up and checked before the surgical procedure. The outcome of the procedure depends on the condition of the instruments.

Ophthalmic Instrumentation

The tips of these expensive, fragile microinstruments should be protected and handled with extreme care before, during, and after use. Eye instrumentation is unique to the specialty. With rare exception are any of the following used in any other type of surgery:

- Self-retaining lid retractors and scissors (Fig. 39-8)
- Graspers and manual retractors (Fig. 39-9)
- Enucleation and measuring devices (Fig. 39-10)
- Punctum plug and forceps (Fig. 39-11)
- Corneal trephine (Fig. 39-12)

Operating Microscope

Most ophthalmic surgeons use the operating microscope for intraocular procedures. When the operating microscope is used, the operating bed should be mechanically secure and the patient's head should be stabilized. Inadvertent movement is not tolerated because of the minute surgical field. The headrest should be narrow so it does not obstruct the surgeon's approach to the surgical site from the sides of the vertical column of the microscope. The patient is instructed about the importance of remaining still during the surgical procedure. Otherwise, the patient could easily move out of the field of vision under the microscope or precipitate a complication.

The assistant observes the surgical procedure through an assistant's ocular and irrigates the cornea with BSS to prevent drying (Fig. 39-13). The assistant should bring to the surgeon's attention any potentially unsatisfactory situation that the surgeon cannot observe from his or her position. Some scrub persons are trained to first-assist. The surgeon and the assistants should limit their caffeine intake before the procedure to promote steady hands when using microinstrumentation under the microscope.

Ophthalmic Drugs

Many drugs are critical to the preparation of the eye for the surgical procedure. Orders for patient preparation often contain common abbreviations that identify the eye(s) to receive drops: OD (right eye), OS (left eye), and OU (both eyes); however, the Joint Commission on Accreditation of Healthcare Organizations (JCAHO) has advised that the use of abbreviations can lead to human error and recommends not using them in the interest of patient safety. Before skin preparation, the circulating nurse instills the medications and anesthetic drops as ordered. The following procedures should be observed when instilling eye drops:

1. Wash your hands.
2. Identify the correct medication, eye, and patient.
3. Check for allergy or sensitivity
4. Explain the procedure to the patient
5. Tilt back the patient's head, and tell the patient to look up. While gently pulling down on the lower lid,

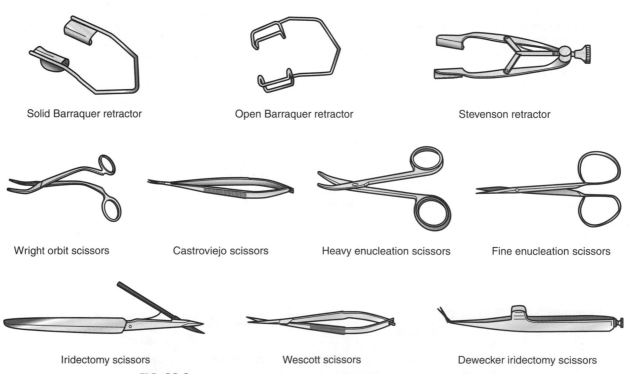

Solid Barraquer retractor   Open Barraquer retractor   Stevenson retractor

Wright orbit scissors   Castroviejo scissors   Heavy enucleation scissors   Fine enucleation scissors

Iridectomy scissors   Wescott scissors   Dewecker iridectomy scissors

FIG. 39-8   Eye instrumentation: self-retaining lid retractors and scissors.

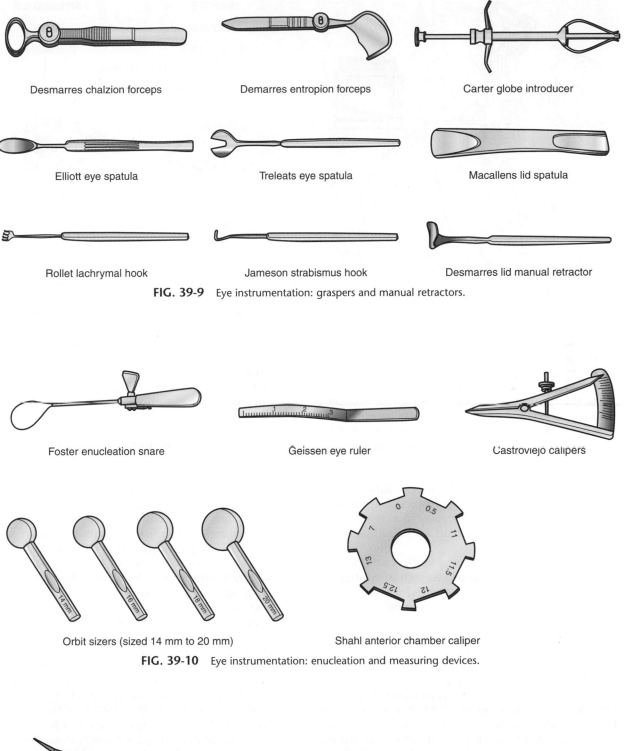

Desmarres chalzion forceps

Demarres entropion forceps

Carter globe introducer

Elliott eye spatula

Treleats eye spatula

Macallens lid spatula

Rollet lachrymal hook

Jameson strabismus hook

Desmarres lid manual retractor

FIG. 39-9 Eye instrumentation: graspers and manual retractors.

Foster enucleation snare

Geissen eye ruler

Castroviejo calipers

Orbit sizers (sized 14 mm to 20 mm)

Shahl anterior chamber caliper

FIG. 39-10 Eye instrumentation: enucleation and measuring devices.

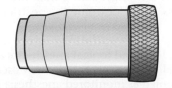

FIG. 39-11 Punctum plug and forceps.

FIG. 39-12 Corneal trephine for tissue cadaver tissue procurement.

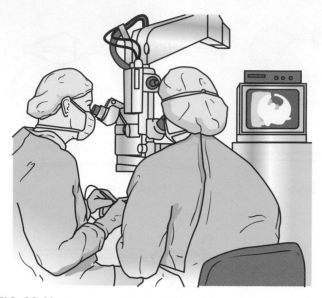

FIG. 39-13   Surgeon and first assistant using a ceiling-mounted microscope.

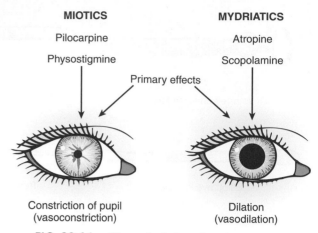

FIG. 39-14   Effects of miotic and mydriatic drugs.

instill the medication in the middle third of the inner aspect of the lower lid. Release the lid while the patient slowly closes the eye to retain the drop; let the patient close the eye between repeated drops. In a struggling child, have a parent tilt the child's head back and close both eyes. Instill the medication at the inner canthus. The drop will roll into the eye as the child opens it.

Some medications, such as atropine, may have a systemic effect. To prevent drainage into the tear duct, nose, and stomach, gently blot excess fluid. In small infants or young children, systemic absorption is avoided by applying finger pressure over the lacrimal sac region (inner canthus) of both eyes simultaneously for 1 minute.

6. Administer only the specified number of drops.
7. Read the label on the vial before each instillation.
8. Each patient should receive a fresh, single-use, disposable vial of medication that is discarded after use.

Mydriatic and Miotic Drugs.
Medications may be given to alter the size of the pupil (Fig. 39-14), including:

- *Mydriatic drops.* 2.5% or 10% phenylephrine (Neo-Synephrine) to dilate the pupil.
- *Mydriatic-cycloplegic drops.* 1% cyclopentolate hydrochloride (Cyclogyl), 1% atropine, and 0.25% scopolamine (Isopto-Hyoscine) to dilate the pupil, paralyze the ciliary body, diminish the reaction to trauma, and prevent anterior synechiae (e.g., adherence of iris to the lens). These drugs are longer acting than phenylephrine.
- *Miotic drops.* 2% pilocarpine to constrict the pupil.

Local and Topical Anesthesia.
Except in children and select patients, local and topical anesthetics are commonly used for ophthalmic surgical procedures. Most surgical procedures are scheduled as monitored anesthesia care (MAC) or attended local. An anesthesia provider monitors the patient and administers oxygen and/or supplements the local anes-

thetic if necessary. Intravenous (IV) midazolam (Versed) and/or fentanyl (Sublimaze) or propofol (Diprivan) is often given to relax the patient. The sedative effects of these agents increase the patient's tolerance to procedures. If a general anesthetic is used, the usual general anesthesia routines are followed.

Local anesthesia consists of the following:

1. Topical instillation of anesthetic drops. The drug used may be 0.5% proparacaine (Ophthaine), 0.5% tetracaine (Pontocaine), or 2% lidocaine (Xylocaine MPF [methylparaben-free]). Most surgeons prefer to use this method in combination with moderate sedation.
2. Local infiltration by injection of the lids and tissue around the eyes with anesthetic medication.
3. Retrobulbar block. An absolutely quiet eye is necessary, especially at high magnifications of the microscope. When general anesthesia is used, some surgeons administer a retrobulbar block for immobility and to lower IOP. A popular solution for this block consists of a mixture of equal parts of 2% or 4% lidocaine and 0.75% bupivacaine 3.75 units/mL for penetration. A 25-gauge × 1½-inch (3.8-cm) needle with a sharp, rounded point (e.g., Atkinson needle) and a 5-mL syringe are used. The surgeon inserts the needle behind the eyeball to anesthetize the globe and paralyze the muscles. The patient is asked to look up and away from the injection site and is told that a slight burning sensation may accompany the injection. Up to 5 mL of solution may be slowly and carefully injected.

Retrobulbar block may be followed by intermittent massage of the eye to soften it, lower IOP, and facilitate surgical manipulation during cataract extraction, especially when insertion of an IOL is being contemplated. Massage is continued until the IOP is lowered to a satisfactory level (e.g., 10 to 12 scale reading on sterile Schiøtz tonometer). Some surgeons apply the Honan balloon pressure device to soften the eyeball after a retrobulbar block (Fig. 39-15). In using this device, a small inflatable balloon is placed directly over the closed eyelid and is secured with a strap around the head. The balloon is inflated to 30 to 40 mm Hg for 5 to 10 minutes to lower intravitreal pressure.

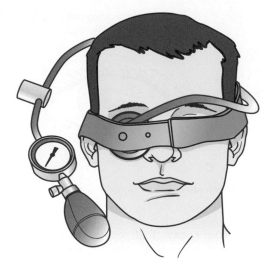

FIG. 39-15 Honan apparatus for softening the eyeball preoperatively.

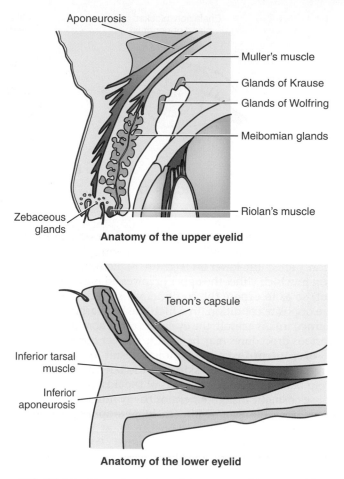

Anatomy of the upper eyelid

Labels: Aponeurosis, Muller's muscle, Glands of Krause, Glands of Wolfring, Meibomian glands, Riolan's muscle, Zebaceous glands

Anatomy of the lower eyelid

Labels: Tenon's capsule, Inferior tarsal muscle, Inferior aponeurosis

FIG. 39-16 Normal anatomy of the upper and lower eyelids.

4. Peribulbar anesthesia. This is an alternative to retrobulbar injection. With this method, injections are made in the soft tissue superior and inferior to the globe rather than behind it. A greater amount of the same anesthetic solution used for retrobulbar injection is used for peribulbar anesthesia. With this procedure, adequate anesthesia is obtained without the risk of retrobulbar hemorrhage.

Ophthalmic Solutions. Extreme and constant care must be used with ophthalmic solutions. Nearly all of these solutions are colorless and may be stored in similar receptacles. These solutions are immediately and individually labeled by the scrub person; the solution is discarded if the identification is missing. Solutions for intraocular use must be separated from all other solutions. Ideally, these solutions should be filtered with micropore filters before injection.

Epinephrine or other sympathomimetics may have side effects when used with some anesthetic agents. Therefore, the surgeon should check with the anesthesia provider before using medications intraoperatively. Medications that may induce vomiting are also avoided. Any straining or gross movement may cause intraocular hemorrhage, a sudden rise in IOP that results in a loss of vitreous, or the expulsion of ocular contents through the wound; all of these conditions can cause blindness.

OCULAR SURGICAL PROCEDURES

For convenience, surgical treatment of the eye can be divided into two main classifications:
1. *Extraocular.* Conditions affecting the exterior surface of the eye, eyelid, or the orbit.
2. *Intraocular.* Conditions pertaining to the interior contents of the eye

Extraocular Procedures

Eyelid. The anatomy of the upper and lower eyelids is described in Figure 39-16.

Excision of Neoplasm of the Eyelid. Tissue may be excised with a knife, an ESU, diathermy, or cryosurgery. An extremely common but benign tumor of the lid is the chalazion—a cystic alteration of one of the oil-secreting meibomian glands in the lid (Fig. 39-17, *A*). The resulting accumulation of oil forms a hard tumor of the lid and requires excision. The excision is usually an office or ambulatory surgical procedure.

Chalazion is differentiated from a stye by the location on the lid. Styes are small infected lash follicles (Fig. 39-17, *B*).

After removal of a malignant lesion of the lid, plastic procedures such as Z-plasty, sliding flaps from adjacent areas, or full- or partial-thickness flaps from the opposing lid are used to close the defect.

Correction of Ptosis. Ptosis, a drooping of the upper lid, may be acquired in adulthood but is more commonly congenital. For the levator aponeurosis procedure, an incision is made on the front surface of the lid to expose the tarsus and the aponeurosis. The tarsus is sutured to the aponeurosis, and the skin incision is closed. For the frontalis suspension procedure, the anterior surface of the upper lid is incised at the crease and two smaller incisions are made above the eyebrow. A graft of fascia or synthetic material is attached to the tarsus and passed through the deep lid tissue and brought out through the eyebrow incisions. The graft material is secured, and the skin incisions are closed.

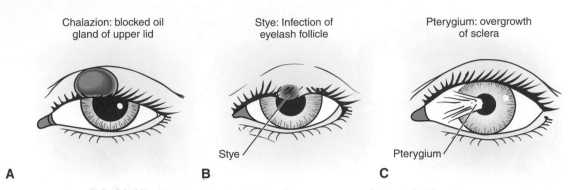

Chalazion: blocked oil
gland of upper lid

Stye: Infection of
eyelash follicle

Pterygium: overgrowth
of sclera

Stye

Pterygium

A   B   C

FIG. 39-17 Common benign lesions of the eye commonly treated with surgery.

Repair of Acquired Malformation of the Eyelid. Conditions such as senile ectropion or entropion most commonly affect the lower lid (Fig. 39-18). Ectropion is a condition in which either the upper or lower lid is everted (turned out) so as to expose the conjunctival surface. Entropion is the opposite condition, in which the lid margin is inverted (turned in). As a result, the eyelashes often abrade the cornea. Various procedures may be used to correct both conditions.

Blepharoplasty. A common result of aging is the stretching of the eyelid skin and the bulging of orbital fat from between the muscle fibers of the lids. Both conditions cause cosmetic disfigurement or baggy lids and, in extreme cases, may obstruct vision. In blepharoplasty, redundant fold(s) of skin and herniated pockets of fat are removed and defects in the muscle layer are repaired. Transconjunctival blepharoplasty is performed by making a small incision into the conjunctiva of the lower lid and removing fat pads. Small bleeders are cauterized with a disposable electrosurgical pencil. Blepharoplasty is commonly performed by plastic surgeons and are described completely in Chapter 40.

Lacrimal Apparatus

Lacrimal Duct Dilation. Lacrimal duct dilation is performed for excessive tearing. A series of probes, graduated in size, are introduced one by one into the duct system to permit freer drainage of tears.

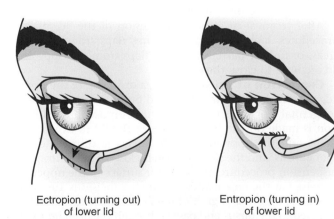

Ectropion (turning out)
of lower lid

Entropion (turning in)
of lower lid

FIG. 39-18 Ectropion and entropion are surgically treated to realign the eyelash line for normal function.

Dacryocystectomy. Extirpation or removal of the lacrimal sac is performed for chronic dacryocystitis. This procedure does not reestablish the tear drainage system.

Dacryocystorhinostomy. Construction of a new opening into the nasal cavity from the lacrimal sac is performed to correct congenital malformation of or trauma to the nasolacrimal duct. A new tear drainage system is constructed.

Extraocular Muscle.
Procedures on the oculomotor muscles, which control eye movement, are performed to correct misalignment that interferes with the ability of the two eyes to remain in simultaneous focus on a viewed object. The surgical procedures correct muscle imbalance by strengthening a weak muscle or by weakening an overactive one. Although commonly performed on children, these muscle procedures may be required in adult patients for the following:

- Untreated childhood strabismus (squint)
- Unsatisfactory result from a childhood surgical procedure
- Trauma to the brainstem or to the orbit with resultant muscle injury or paralysis
- Systemic disease (e.g., thyroid exophthalmos) and muscle paralysis
- Cerebrovascular accident (CVA) with resultant muscle paralysis

Orbit

Decompression. Decompression is the treatment for severe exophthalmos, or a protrusion of the eyeball(s), that does not respond to medical treatment.

Orbital Tumors. Depending on the location of the orbital tumor, exploration may be approached through a lateral wall or the roof of the orbit. This procedure may involve a multidisciplinary team of surgeons.

Surgical Removal of the Eye.
After removal of an eyeball, the patient is fitted with an artificial eye to restore cosmetic appearance. A spherical implant, such as silicone, plastic, tantalum, or hydroxyapatite, may be used to line the orbit and provide support for a prosthetic eye. The eye muscles are sutured to the implant, thereby providing natural movement, allowing the growth of surrounding tissue, and preventing the lower lid from sagging. The type of prosthesis that can be used depends on the procedure used to remove the eyeball.

Enucleation. Enucleation is the complete removal of the eyeball and the severing of its muscular attachments.

The muscle stumps are preserved, with the space between the stumps forming a pocket for the spherical plastic artificial eye. Overlying fasciae and conjunctivae are closed to hold the prosthesis in the socket. The contraction of eye muscles causes the prosthesis to move in the socket, simulating normal eye movements.

Eye prostheses are usually round or oval and can be textured or smooth. Some have pegs upon which the colored iris cap attaches. Others contain a magnet that adheres to the back of the visible colored iris portion. Sizes can be between 12 and 22 mm.

Evisceration. Evisceration removes the contents of the eyeball only; the outer sclera and muscles are left intact for attachment to a prosthesis. This procedure reduces the danger of transmitting an intraocular infection to the orbit and brain. Predisposing factors for evisceration include destruction of the eyeball by injury or disease and absolute glaucoma (hard blind eye).

Exenteration. Exenteration is the removal of the entire eye and orbital contents, including tendon, fatty, and fibrous tissues. This procedure is performed for a malignant tumor of the lids or eyeball that has extended into the orbit. Extensive plastic reconstruction is necessary before an artificial eye can be fitted.

Cornea. Although it consists of resilient tissue, the continually exposed cornea is especially susceptible to injury and infection.

Cauterization. Cauterization with chemicals or heat is sometimes used for a corneal ulceration that does not respond to antibiotics. This is sometimes performed for herpes simplex virus infections of the corneal epithelium. Cauterization may be used in conjunction with topical antiviral agents.

Pterygium. Pterygium is a benign growth of conjunctival tissue over the corneal surface. Although usually slow-growing, pterygia can become fairly aggressive, especially in southern climates. A significant decrease in visual acuity secondary to induced astigmatism and corneal scarring can result from the abnormal growth. A popular surgical technique devised for the eradication of pterygia is the bare sclera method. This method involves excision of the entire pterygium, leaving an area of bare sclera. Beta radiation may be used as an adjunct to surgical treatment (see Fig. 39-17, *C*).

Corneal Transplantation (Keratoplasty). With keratoplasty, a damaged cornea is removed and replaced with a healthy cornea from a human donor (Fig. 39-19). The cornea must be clear to permit light to enter and focus on the retina. Thus this procedure is indicated when scars or opacities on the cornea reduce or destroy vision by preventing the transmission of a clear image. Corneal opacity may result from degenerative changes, scars from chemical burns, perforated corneal ulcers, trauma, or edema after a cataract surgical procedure. In addition, ocular surgery such as phacoemulsification, vitrectomy, and IOL implantation has the potential to damage the corneal endothelium.

Because the cornea is avascular, keratoplasty is the most successful transplantation procedure and has considerably less rejection phenomena than all other tissues except bone. The greatest advance in technique to reduce the rate of rejection and the restriction of activity during convalescence

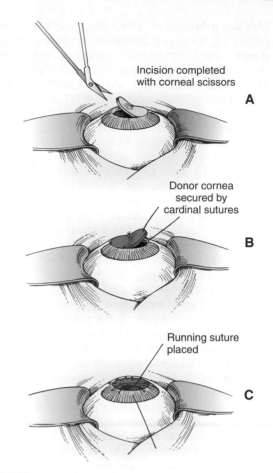

FIG. 39-19 Corneal transplantation (keratoplasty). **A,** Damaged cornea is excised with corneal scissors. **B,** Donor cornea is secured by cardinal sutures. **C,** Continuous suture remains in situ.

has been the use of the operating microscope and microsutures. Continuous 10-0 or 11-0 nylon sutures are left in situ with minimal tissue reaction. Two types of grafts are used:

1. *Full-thickness grafts.* The common type. The entire diameter of the corneal graft (6.5 to 8 mm) is replaced (penetrating keratoplasty).
2. *Partial-thickness or lamellar grafts.* Less popular. Only the top layer of the cornea, not its entire depth, is replaced (lamellar keratoplasty).

An opaque cornea is an optically nonfunctioning one. The goal is to provide recipients with the highest quality corneal tissue. A fresh, healthy cornea cut from the promptly enucleated eye of a relatively young donor within 4 to 6 hours of death is considered the best for transplantation. The cornea should be transplanted to the surface of the recipient eye, which has a healthy retina and optic nerve, as soon as possible to preserve viability and to prevent opacity. The acceptable times for collection of tissue after death and transplantation may vary among eye banks. The National Institutes of Health (NIH) have established the National Eye Institute. (More information is available at www.nei.nih.gov.)

Donor tissue criteria include the following:

1. The consent for enucleation must conform with state laws. A certified eye bank technician may enucleate the eyes.

2. Medical information about the potential donor is evaluated. Some conditions that preclude the use of donor tissue are an unknown cause of death, previous intraocular surgery, Reye syndrome, lymphosarcoma, rabies, and transmissible diseases such as hepatitis, human immunodeficiency virus (HIV), and Creutzfeldt-Jakob disease (CJD). Donor information must be documented on the donor screening form that accompanies the tissue. A copy should be filed at the eye bank.

3. The endothelium, the very sensitive inner single layer of corneal cells, must be kept intact for eventual transparency of the graft. The entire donor globe is removed. Important factors to optimize the success of the transplant include sterile technique, the removal of as much conjunctiva as possible from the donor globe, the avoidance of damage to or contamination of the removed eyes, and the use of appropriate transport containers and preservation methods.

4. The donor's eyes are cooled as soon as possible to prevent deleterious effects. The placement of ice bags over the eyes promptly after death slows the metabolism of corneal cells. In general, the sooner the enucleated eyes are refrigerated, the better the quality of the donor tissue. Enucleated eyes are placed in a controlled environment at the eye bank.

5. The donor's cornea is carefully evaluated for epithelial defects, clarity, the presence of any foreign body, or any evidence of jaundice or infection. Endothelial cell count is a determining factor in estimating the prognosis of the transplant. The higher the count and the more regular the cellular pattern, the better the tissue. Age is not a deterrent if tissue is acceptable for transplantation, but donors younger than 70 years are preferred. The evaluation form must be completed and must accompany the tissue. The transplant surgeon also may receive specular microscopic photographs of the endothelium. Donor tissue preservation methods include the following:

   a. *Preservative medium.* Optisol-GS sterile buffered tissue culture contains the antibiotics gentamicin and streptomycin and allows refrigerated storage for 3 to 7 days. Intermediate-term corneal storage in Chen Medium at 4° C for 2 weeks has rapidly gained popularity without consequence to the tissue. Chen Medium also contains streptomycin and gentamicin, but contains 7% dextran to eliminate the bicarbonate and reduce the amount of sodium chloride required to maintain a high metabolic profile in the corneal tissue. In the OR, the surgeon should inspect the container before using the cornea. If the cornea is cut to size for use, the remaining corneoscleral rim should be placed in a culture medium and sent to the laboratory for culture. The incidence of positive cultures is low. The cornea should not be used and the eye bank should be notified if the medium is turbid or contaminated, such as by a crack in the container.

   b. *Cryopreservation.* Both cryopreserved corneal and scleral tissue can be used for transplantation or for patching purposes. In general, their use is limited to emergency procedures when fresh tissue is not available. Usually this tissue is used less than 6 months after cryopreservation. Precise freezing and defrosting methods are of crucial importance in preventing injury to the endothelium. Corneal metabolism resumes with defrosting; therefore, when the solution is thawed, the team should work rapidly because of the extreme time limitation. The tissue should be placed immediately within its natural anatomic environment to enhance the potential for successful grafting.

Regardless of the storage method, tissue preferably is used as soon as practical after donation. In the OR, adequate preparation, teamwork, and standardized transplantation procedures are imperative. The recipient eye is trephined to receive the donor cornea. A separate sterile donor table is set for the surgeon to use in preparing the donor tissue to the exact measurement needed for the recipient eye. During the procedure, gentamicin, cefazolin, and methylprednisolone are administered under the conjunctiva.

After the surgical procedure, a tissue recipient information form is completed to indicate how the tissue was used. This form is mailed to the eye bank, where it is kept on file. If the tissue is contaminated, the donor number and source can easily be traced. Information on the forms includes recipient medical information; previous keratoplasties; the date, type, and details of the current surgical procedure; and the estimate of success. The patient is instructed to report any symptoms, such as redness, light sensitivity, vision loss, or pain. A patch is worn for 1 to 4 days. Protective eyewear should be worn during the day and a firm patch should be worn for sleeping for several months postoperatively. Sutures can be removed after a few months or may be left in permanently.

Suitable corneal tissue is in limited supply, which places restraints on transplantation. Numerous eye banks in the United States constitute the Eye Bank Association of America, which is tangentially associated with the International Eye Bank. These groups are central clearinghouses for the distribution of accessible tissue. They follow a stringent code of ethics in their functions to inform the public of the need for eye donations, to procure donated eyes, to assist in the optimal use of donor corneas locally, or to arrange for transportation to an area of greater need. Tissue procurement is facilitated by the following:

- Distribution of donor forms from eye banks and organ donation organizations.
- Organ donation consent forms affixed to driver licenses. Family consent is still required before procurement.
- Education of medical and health care personnel to alert them to ask families of deceased patients for donations. Some state laws require a donation request.

Phototherapeutic Keratectomy. In phototherapeutic keratectomy (PTK), scar tissue is removed from the cornea with an excimer laser. This procedure restores vision that has been blocked by scars from an infection, injury, or inherited condition. PTK may obviate the need for a corneal transplant. (More information about excimer lasers can be found at www.excimernet.com.)

Refractive Keratoplasty. Refractive keratoplasty (corneal reshaping) includes a group of surgical procedures designed to alter the shape and refractive power (i.e., focusing power) of the cornea to minimize the optical problems of myopia, aphakia, keratoconus, hyperopia, and astigmatism:

1. Radial keratotomy reduces myopia (nearsightedness) by making multiple small radial incisions in the cornea to approximately 90% of its depth (Fig. 39-20). These incisions allow stretching and flattening of the anterior corneal surface, which corrects the refractive error by reducing corneal curvature and bringing light to a focus closer to or on the retina (Fig. 39-21).

   Radial keratotomy is performed on patients who have occupational requirements for a visual acuity level without the use of glasses or contact lenses, such as certain airline, police, and firefighter positions. The procedure also may be performed for cosmetic reasons. Potential complications include perforations of the cornea, permanent corneal scarring, glaring or variable vision, injury to the lens (causing cataract), and infection. Long-term results are somewhat unpredictable but are improved with microsurgical techniques. This procedure should be limited to patients with healthy eyes. Only low amounts of nearsightedness can be corrected with this procedure.

2. Keratomileusis and keratophakia procedures modify corneal refractivity by using a computerized technique to insert a lathed button of corneal tissue into the cornea. If the patient is the donor (keratomileusis), the anterior lamellae of the cornea are removed, reshaped by cryolathing, and then sutured in place. For keratophakia, the tissue is obtained from another donor and may be preserved. The lenticule is cryolathed during the surgical procedure, inserted intralamellarly into the recipient cornea, and sutured into place.

   Keratomileusis and keratophakia require a highly specialized, experienced team and costly equipment—the computer and the cryolathe for shaping the corneal button. With keratophakia, research is ongoing to develop other materials that may be used in place of human donor tissue. Plastic with a very high water content (similar to continuous-wear contact lens material) has been used.

3. Epikeratophakia is performed to correct extreme refractive errors such as aphakia (absence of lens, which induces extreme hyperopia), myopia, or keratoconus (cone-shaped cornea, which causes extreme astigmatism). The recipient corneal epithelium is removed, and a previously cryolathed and preserved donor button of corneal tissue is sutured onto the corneal surface of the recipient.

4. Corneal sculpting (photorefractive keratectomy [PRK]) is performed to reshape the corneal surface or to remove scars or other surface irregularities. The excimer laser is used to reshape the front corneal contour to correct nearsightedness, farsightedness, and astigmatism. The laser beam removes minute amounts of corneal tissue with each pulse wave without burning through or heating the tissue.

5. Laser-assisted in situ keratomileusis (LASIK) is performed to correct myopia (nearsightedness). A combination of excimer laser and keratome is used to remove layers of the cornea. A small flap is raised in the center of the corneal dome (Fig. 39-22). The laser is used to remove microlayers of tissue. The flap of corneal tissue is replaced without the need for suturing (Fig. 39-23).

6. Intrastromal corneal rings can be placed to elevate the border of the cornea, causing the central portion to recede. This implantable device was approved for use in 1998 and consists of two arc-shaped segments that are implanted in the circumferential stroma of the cornea. It can be removed surgically if vision correction is not satisfactory (Fig. 39-24).

Intraocular Procedures

Iris. Some ophthalmic surgeons subspecialize in anterior segment surgery on the iris, and lens or in posterior segment surgery on the vitreous body, retina, and sclera. Both types of surgery require specialized instrumentation. Most surgeons use the operating microscope for intraocular procedures.

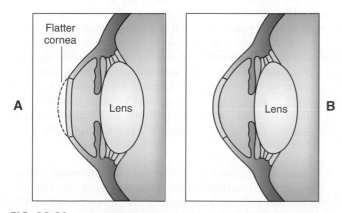

FIG. 39-20 Corneal incisions for visual improvement of myopia. **A,** Radial keratotomy (RK). **B,** Astigmatic keratotomy (AK).

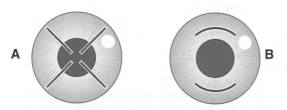

FIG. 39-21 Side view of incised corneas. **A,** Radial keratotomy (RK). **B,** Astigmatic keratotomy (AK).

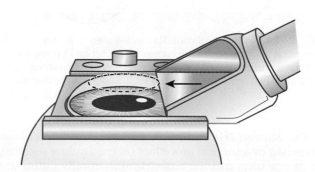

FIG. 39-22 Keratotome used to raise the corneal flap for LASIK surgery.

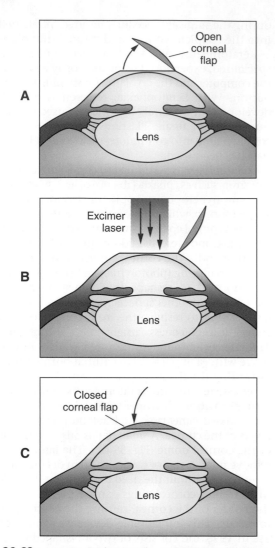

FIG. 39-23   Laser in situ keratomileusis (LASIK). **A,** Top layer of cornea is opened like a flap with keratome. **B,** Excimer laser removes thin layers of exposed corneal surface. **C,** Cornea is replaced.

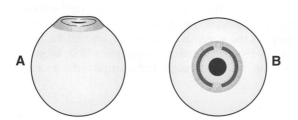

FIG. 39-24   Intrastromal corneal rings are used to form a depression in the center of the cornea for correction of myopia. **A,** Intrastromal corneal ring in place. The center of the cornea flattens. **B,** Two arcs form a circle under the edges of the cornea.

Excision of Iris Prolapse.   Prolapse may follow an eye laceration or a surgical procedure on the anterior segment. Fresh prolapses may be reduced mechanically during the surgical procedure or pharmacologically with drugs. Older prolapses should be excised to avoid an intraocular infection.

Glaucoma.   Glaucoma is a disease characterized by abnormally increased intraocular fluid pressure; it often involves the iris. If uncontrolled, glaucoma progresses to atrophy of the optic nerve, hardening of the eyeball, and blindness. The incidence of glaucoma in people older than 40 years increases with each decade. There is a familial predisposition to the disease.

IOP is estimated in one of three ways:

1. A Schiøtz tonometer records the depth of indentation of the cornea by a plunger of known weight. The degree of indentation is calibrated on the tonometer to correspond to the IOP. The normal numerical value is 10 to 22 mm Hg. The tonometer can be sterilized for use in the OR for preoperative pressure measurement.
2. An applanation tonometer attached to a biomicroscope (slit lamp) records the force required to flatten a specified area of cornea. This method is considered to be the most accurate. The normal value is 10 to 21 mm Hg.
3. An air-puff device measures the force of a reflected amount of air blown against the cornea.

People suspected of having glaucoma undergo additional testing. Tonography continuously measures the rate of aqueous outflow with an electric tonometer. Visual fields detect diminished peripheral vision. Gonioscopy determines the structure of the angle between the iris and the cornea. Two basic types of glaucoma are classified anatomically by the size of this angle: (1) narrow-angle or angle-closure glaucoma, and (2) wide-angle or open-angle glaucoma.

If the angle is narrow, the iris may mechanically obstruct the outflow of aqueous. This will cause the pressure within the eye to rise and will precipitate an attack of acute glaucoma—an emergency situation that is very painful. Surgical intervention, usually a laser iridotomy, affords relief. It is always necessary to widen the angle for this condition and reduce pressure to avoid damage to the optic nerve. Surgical iridectomy occasionally is necessary.

Wide-angle or open-angle glaucoma is the most common type of glaucoma. It is a chronic type, is often of insidious onset, and may cause permanent visual loss before being detected. The obstruction is not mechanical but is a physiologic lack of ability to filter aqueous. Surgical procedures for this type of disease are performed only if medical and laser therapies are unsuccessful. Laser therapy to the trabecular meshwork (trabeculoplasty) offers an alternative to conventional surgical procedures for some glaucoma patients. One of the following surgical procedures may be preferred:

- Iridectomy (excising a sector of iris) or iridotomy (cutting a small opening in the iris) is performed to deflate the mechanical obstruction, thus increasing drainage by permitting the normal outflow of aqueous from the posterior to the anterior chamber. Another use of iridectomy is to create a new optical pupillary opening to improve visual acuity for patients with corneal or lens opacity caused by injury or cataract not associated with glaucoma.
- Filtering-type procedures, of which there are many variations such as trephining and trabeculectomy, create an artificial fistula between the angle of the anterior chamber and the subconjunctival space to bypass the usual blocked outflow channels. Iridectomy is usually performed as part of the procedure to eliminate

blockage of the fistula by the underlying iris. The neodymium:yttrium-aluminum-garnet (Nd:YAG) laser may be used to reopen filtering sites that have scarred closed after previous surgery for glaucoma. The holmium (Ho):YAG laser may be used to create an opening in the sclera (sclerostomy) to promote filtration.

- Cyclodialysis, cyclodiathermy, and cyclocryotherapy are performed to diminish aqueous secretion by the ciliary body. Cyclodialysis involves severing the blood supply of the ciliary body. Cyclodiathermy and cyclocryotherapy use the application of heat or cold, respectively, for the same purpose.

Secondary glaucoma is often a complication of an inflammation such as iritis, which usually responds best to medical treatment. On the other hand, neoplasm, vascular obstruction, trauma, or hemorrhage and other causes of obstruction to aqueous drainage may require surgical intervention. Treatment is directed to the primary cause.

Congenital glaucoma, from an inherent defect in the trabecular meshwork or a systemic disorder, manifests soon after birth.

Cataract.

A cataract is an opacification of the crystalline lens, its capsule, or both. The more or less opaque lens does not transmit clear images to the retina. Symptoms are related to the location and configuration of the opacity. The cause may be a known metabolic or systemic disease, toxic material, radiation, trauma, or genetic factors, or the etiologic factors may be unknown. People are more prone to develop degenerative cataracts with advancing age. Although cataracts often develop in both eyes, each cataract tends to mature at a different rate and only one is removed at a time. Most ophthalmologists perform cataract surgery as an ambulatory surgical procedure.

Cataracts may be classified as one of the following:

- Congenital
- Senile or primary
- Secondary, resulting from local or systemic disease or eye injury

Surgical removal, followed by appropriate optical rehabilitation, is the only treatment. The surgical procedure to be performed is determined by the patient's age and type of cataract. The procedure is selected according to visual requirements, general health, and the potential for rehabilitation. Cataract extraction with implantation of an intraocular lens is the most frequently performed surgical procedure in adults, and the advent of microsurgery has revolutionized this procedure (Fig. 39-25).

Extracapsular Extraction. With extracapsular extraction (ECCE), the lens is delivered through a small incision in the region of the limbus (the junction of the cornea and sclera). The anterior capsule is incised with a cystotome (a miniature hook-shaped knife) or with a capsulorrhexis forceps. The nucleus is delivered by manual expression, or it may be aspirated by phacoemulsification. The remaining cortex is extracted by irrigation-aspiration, sparing the posterior capsule, which is left in place. Automated mechanical irrigation-aspiration devices generally are used. Some surgeons prefer a manual technique using a two-way cannula and syringe. The wound is closed with a few sutures.

ECCE with preservation of the posterior capsule has revolutionized the practice of artificial lens implantation. The implant can be placed at the time of cataract extraction. It resides in the posterior chamber behind the iris and rests on the posterior capsule. The implant is therefore positioned in almost the identical location of the lens it replaces.

The physiologic advantage of ECCE, with or without phacoemulsification and/or lens implant, is protection of the vitreous and retina by the clear posterior lens capsule, which then serves as an anatomic barrier between the posterior and anterior segments of the eye. Occasionally the posterior capsule remains opaque. Nd:YAG laser capsulotomy is performed at a later date to provide an optically clear opening.

The following innovations have enhanced the advantages of ECCE:

1. An operating microscope with coaxial illumination to clearly view the posterior capsule during aspiration.
2. A phacoemulsifier to remove the nucleus through a tiny (3- to 3.5-mm) incision. The smaller wound facilitates healing and causes less distortion of corneal curvatures.
3. An automated irrigation-aspiration system with an electronic sensor to remove all cortex remnants. This minimizes local foreign protein reaction.

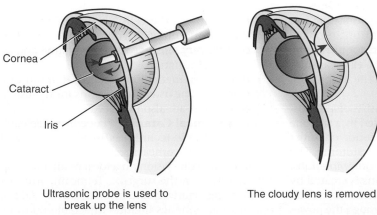

Cornea

Cataract

Iris

| Ultrasonic probe is used to break up the lens | The cloudy lens is removed | An intraocular lens is inserted |

FIG. 39-25 Removing the cloudy lens and placing an intraocular lens in its place.

4. An Nd:YAG laser to atomize posterior capsule opacity. The laser achieves a better result than discission/needling, which requires a second surgical intervention. The laser can be used immediately postoperatively, or the procedure can be delayed. The laser can be used under a drop of local anesthetic without requiring an incision and without causing blood loss.

5. An intraocular foldable lens designed to achieve insertion into the posterior chamber through a small incision.

Intracapsular Extraction. Intracapsular extraction (ICCE) is not commonly used unless the natural lens is displaced. Advance planning is necessary on the rare occasions in which it is performed. The entire lens, intact within its capsule, is delivered through a moderate-size incision made in the region of the limbus. Before delivery, an iridectomy or multiple iridotomies are performed, chiefly to prevent iris prolapse and to preserve communication between the anterior and posterior chambers. Depending on the surgeon's preference, the lens is grasped by a forceps, suction device, or cryoextractor.

A miniaturized, sterile disposable cryoextractor facilitates the removal of fragile or dislocated cataracts. The cryoprobe freezes onto the surface of the cataract, thus obtaining secure adherence. The freezing technique greatly reduces the inadvertent rupture of the capsule during extraction. The scrub person should have a BSS irrigator available for use in case it is necessary to unfreeze an unintentional attachment of the cryoextractor to the iris or cornea. The wound is closed watertight with multiple sutures, commonly 10-0 nylon.

With ICCE, the visual axis is free of remnants that might proliferate or opacify to obstruct vision. The success rate for regaining vision is high, but the popularity of this procedure has waned. Fluorescein angiography has identified a number of patients who developed cystoid macular edema postoperatively, resulting in marked loss of visual acuity. ICCE may also be followed by retinal detachment.

Linear Extraction. Linear extraction is performed in young adults. In this procedure, a small incision is made through the limbus. The anterior capsule is incised, and the major portion of it is excised with a cystotome. The soft cataractous material is irrigated from the anterior chamber.

Phacoemulsification. Although the aspiration technique is commonly used in young people, it was not successful in older adults with senile cataracts until the late 1960s. At that time a sophisticated machine, the phacoemulsifier, was developed to break up (fragment) and remove firm, insoluble lens nuclei. This machine, with components for ultrasonic vibration and irrigation-aspiration, permits extracapsular extraction through a very small incision in the limbus. All functions are controlled by foot pedal.

The handpiece of the phacoemulsifier consists of a disposable, hollow, titanium alloy needle surrounded by a silicone sleeve. The needle is inserted into the anterior chamber after removal of the anterior capsule with a cystotome. The activated needle breaks up the lens with ultrasonic vibrations; the linear motion of the ultrasonic vibrations is created by electrical impulses. This process generates heat. A cooling pump circulates coolant, either fluid or air, through the power cord. While the lens is thus emulsified, a constant flow of BSS irrigating solution through the sleeve prevents heat buildup. The irrigation-aspiration flow is automatically regulated to maintain anterior chamber depth. The aspirator removes the fragments. After the cortex (material surrounding the lens nucleus) is removed by irrigation-aspiration, the posterior capsule may be polished with an instrument to remove any residual cortex. The posterior capsule is left intact unless an opacity remains, in which case it may be incised during the initial surgical procedure or at a future time. The limbal incision is closed with one stitch. Newer methods do not require any suturing.

Appropriate checks should be made before use of the handpiece, and the integrity of the vacuum and irrigating systems must be confirmed. The handpiece should be disassembled for cleaning and sterilization and then reassembled on the sterile field before use. The handpiece can be steam sterilized as a single unit.

In the newer computerized machines, the phacoemulsification and aspiration settings are preset. To avoid error, the scrub person and circulating nurse work closely with the surgeon to monitor the various functions of the machine in use. They should also observe the transparent tubes for the flow of aspirate. Aspirated fluid is contaminated and is discarded postoperatively in the same manner as all blood or body fluid.

Phacoemulsification has certain advantages:
- It dramatically shortens convalescence time. The patient usually returns to full activity in 1 or 2 days.
- It uses a small incision and minimal sutures, which promotes healing.
- It retains the posterior capsule of the lens to preserve a more physiologically normal condition. The occurrence of post–lens extraction edema and retinal detachment is thereby diminished.
- The posterior capsule supports an implanted IOL. Postoperative astigmatism is minimized.

Phacoemulsification also has disadvantages:
- It is not suitable for all patients. Contraindications are corneal disease, a dislocated lens, a shallow anterior chamber, difficult-to-dilate pupils, and completely hard, stonelike cataracts.
- It requires special techniques that, if not thoroughly mastered, may precipitate surgical complications such as temporary or permanent corneal damage (opacification), prolapse of the lens into the vitreous, and vitreous loss.
- It may injure the cells because of the necessary substantial amount of anterior chamber irrigation. Corneal cells are very sensitive to manipulation and can respond by loss of function.
- It requires meticulous technical monitoring of the machine. The usual precautions for the use of electrical equipment are also observed.

Clear Corneal Cataract Procedure. Foldable IOLs and topical anesthetic techniques have been integral with the use of "no stitch" corneal incisions. Patient selection includes the ability to fixate vision on a focal point and cooperate with commands from the surgeon. Tetracaine intraocular drops are used preoperatively and intraoperatively. Additional intraoperative anesthetics include injectable lidocaine without preservatives for infusion into the anterior chamber.

Rehabilitation After Cataract Extraction. Rehabilitation after cataract extraction consists of substitution for the missing part, the lens, so the optical system can function to focus incoming light on the retina. Patients with no optical substitute see only blurred objects of large size. Rehabilitation may be accomplished by spectacles (glasses), contact lenses, or IOL implantation.

Spectacle correction of aphakia, the absence of the lens, provides focusing of light. The spectacle lens is approximately 2 cm in front of the original lens and magnifies images so they are approximately 35% larger than those the patient saw before development and extraction of the cataract. This magnification requires considerable readjustment to judge distances. In addition, peripheral areas are distorted. The spectacle type of replacement is intolerable in patients who have good vision in the unaffected eye because an attempt to fuse the dissimilar images of the two eyes causes double vision.

A contact lens often is used to replace the optical deficiency caused by cataract extraction. This lens rests on the cornea only 2 to 3 mm from the original lens and thus causes only 7% magnification and provides a full, undistorted field of vision. It is difficult for some older adults to handle and care for contact lenses because of a lack of manual dexterity, arthritic hand and finger joints, or visual defects in the opposite eye. For these patients, an implanted IOL is a feasible and popular alternative.

Implantation of Intraocular Lens. IOL implantation is a microsurgical procedure in which an IOL is implanted in almost the identical position of the original lens and therefore does not change the size of the retinal image. Spatial displacement as seen by the aphakic eye and narrowing and distortion of the visual field are eliminated, thereby producing early visual rehabilitation. With spatial displacement, orientation in space is changed—objects are not where they appear to be.

An IOL is intended to remain in situ permanently. The implant is usually inserted through the same incision used to remove the defective, natural lens; this is called primary insertion. Some surgeons prefer to implant the lens at a later time; this is referred to as secondary insertion. The type of IOL used is contingent on the type of cataract extraction the surgeon chooses. Anterior chamber lenses are inserted in conjunction with ICCE or as secondary implants. Posterior chamber lenses are used after ECCE.

The prescription of the implanted lens (refractive power) involves complex preoperative calculations based on the patient's corneal curvature as determined by keratometer readings, anterior chamber depth, and eyeball axial length. Ultrasonography is helpful in making these determinations preoperatively. The information obtained is fed into a computer that automatically calculates the appropriate refractive power of the IOL.

Numerous IOLs of different shapes and sizes are available. Figure 39-26 depicts a common type of implantable lens. The optical portion of a hard lens is made of an inert plastic, polymethyl methacrylate (with or without an ultraviolet blocker), that has been polished to a microscopic smoothness. Flexible and foldable lenses are made of silicone elastomer and acrylic resin.

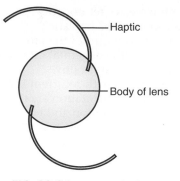

FIG. 39-26 Intraocular lens.

The fixation portion has springlike supports or loops, called haptics, made of plastic (usually polypropylene). Some lenses are secured with polypropylene sutures. Lenses differ in design and method of fixation, and they can be classified according to placement or method of fixation.

Anterior Chamber (Angle Fixation). An anterior chamber lens consists of a band of plastic long enough to traverse the anterior chamber from one angle to the other. The optical portion is centrally located in the anterior chamber, in front of the pupil and iris. The pupil remains mobile because iris adhesions are not required for fixation. Although anterior chamber lenses are sometimes inserted primarily, they are popular lenses for secondary insertion.

Posterior Chamber (Capsular or Ciliary Body Fixation). Posterior chamber lenses are placed behind the iris and pupil, where the patient's own lens used to be. Placement of the IOL in the most normal physiologic position results in stabilization of the iris; less irritation of the uveal tract; a reduced tendency to iritis, secondary glaucoma, and cystoid macular edema; and stabilization of the optics. Posterior lenses permit safe dilation of the pupil if necessary to examine or treat posterior structures of the eye, such as the retina.

With capsular fixation, the lower loop of the haptic is inserted into a pocket of capsule created during extraction of the cataract. The lens does not touch the iris, and the pupil is free to move. With ciliary fixation, the haptics are placed between the iris and the posterior capsule. They rest on the corona (inner rim) of the ciliary body.

Pros and Cons of Intraocular Lens Implantation. The final decision to implant an artificial lens rests with the surgeon, who should exercise good judgment to avoid serious complications.

Indications for implantation are the following:
- Older adult patients with disabling bilateral cataracts and others who cannot adapt to contact lenses
- Patients with occupations having specific visual requirements (e.g., airplane pilots) or a difficult working environment (e.g., ranchers in a dusty area)
- Children with a traumatic cataract, thus preventing amblyopia

Contraindications for implantation are the following:
- Impossibility for follow-up to observe patient for late complications
- Ocular conditions such as poorly controlled glaucoma or previous retinal detachment

- Diabetic proliferative retinopathy
- Poor result in previous implant
- Patient anxiety in regard to the procedure
- Young patients with congenital cataracts
- Endothelial corneal dystrophy
- Cataracts associated with recurrent iritis

Advantages to IOL implantation are the following:
- Superior spatial orientation and binocular vision
- Permanency of device unless complications develop
- Additional option for post-cataract extraction refractive correction
- Unrestricted pupillary dilation if necessary

Complications with IOL implantation are the following:
- Corneal damage or latent edema
- Prolonged inflammation such as iritis or vitritis
- Cystoid macular edema
- Secondary cataract (i.e., opacification of the anterior vitreous) from recurrent iritis
- Corneal opacity (rare with posterior implants)
- Dislocation or malposition of the lens, which can damage the cornea (fortunately rare)

The type of approach used to repair a dislocation depends on the amount of dislocation. With the anterior approach, an anterior vitrectomy is performed to remove the vitreous in front of the lens, followed by removal or repositioning of the lens. With the posterior approach, the vitrector is used to remove the lens and/or vitreous through the pars plana. The IOL can be repositioned or removed.

Retina. Defects in the continuity of the retina can occur after accidental or surgical trauma or as a result of certain degenerative diseases. The dense network of capillary vessels in the retina makes the eyes vulnerable to microvascular disease. Retinopathy is a noninflammatory degenerative disease of the retina.

Retinal changes can occur in patients with diabetes (i.e., diabetic retinopathy). Diabetes can affect every part of the eye, causing lens changes (cataract), palsied extraocular muscles, glaucoma, or corneal problems. A person who has had diabetes for more than 15 years has a significant likelihood of having some form of retinopathy, which generally occurs bilaterally. The severity of retinopathy may differ from one eye to the other. Retinopathy is classified as one of the following:

- *Background or nonproliferative.* With this type of retinopathy, disease is confined to the retinal surface. Bulges or microaneurysms form in retinal capillary walls, eventually permitting leakage and the deposition of exudates. Intraretinal hemorrhages occur and are reabsorbed. Progressive changes in capillary membranes lead to the blockage of capillaries, resulting in retinal ischemia. Deterioration then progresses to the proliferative stage.
- *Proliferative.* In the proliferative stage, new blood vessels emerge from the retina and form in the surrounding tissues in an effort to relieve retinal anoxia (i.e., neovascularization). These fragile vessels may rupture spontaneously, producing hemorrhage into the retina and/or vitreous humor. The eventual result may be partial or complete blindness. Panretinal photocoagulation (PRP) is one method of eliminating abnormal vascularization.

PRP consists of the application of hundreds of laser burns to the peripheral retinal tissue to partially destroy it, thereby reducing the retinal metabolic need for oxygen. After neovascularization has occurred, laser therapy is less effective in delaying or stopping the destructive process. Therefore, early diagnosis and treatment are crucial. In an effort to prevent the formation of new vessels, lasers are used to cauterize minute hypoxic areas of tissue before damage occurs.

Laser light is used for cauterizing bleeding vessels, for diabetic retinopathy, and for other retinopathies such as central serous retinopathy with swelling of the macula, angiomas and hemangiomas, aneurysms, and small tumors. Laser light is absorbed selectively by three pigments in the retina: macular xanthophyll, hemoglobin in the retinal and subretinal blood vessels, and melanin in the retinal pigment epithelium. Laser therapy is not effective in correcting severe retinal damage or detachment.

Repair of Detached Retina. The retina can become separated from its surrounding nourishing layer, the choroid (Fig. 39-27). This detachment may occur in any region of the retina. Primary retinal detachment is characterized by a hole in the retina. Secondary detachment may result when blood, fluid, or a tumor gets behind and displaces the retina; this type of detachment is not necessarily accompanied by a hole. The seepage of vitreous fluid into the potential space between the retina and the choroid causes the retina to become detached, and a serious visual disturbance results. Enucleation is usually indicated for tumor-caused detachment.

Reattachment is effected only by surgical intervention. The retinal defect is sealed off, and often the subretinal fluid is drained. The specific procedure used to achieve retinal reattachment is determined by the type and location of the detachment. All or some of the following procedures may be used in combination:

- *Diathermy.* The traditional procedure involves diathermy coagulation to the area of the sclera overlying the region of the retinal defect. The resultant localized inflammation acts to seal off the break. Coagulation is delivered by a specialized short-wave diathermy unit.

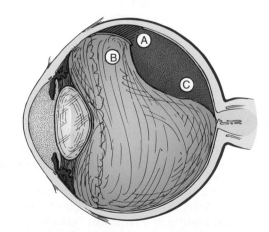

FIG. 39-27 Detached retina. *A,* Retinal break. *B,* Vitreous. *C,* Fluid or blood behind the retina.
(From Glaser BM: Surgical retina. In Ryan SJ et al, eds: Retina, *ed 2, vol 3, St. Louis, 1995, Mosby.)*

- *Cryosurgery.* Some surgeons prefer cryosurgery because of the type of adhesion obtained. The therapeutic applications of cryosurgery are basically similar to those of diathermy, and the tissue reactions superficially resemble each other. Cryosurgery is often used for anterior tears.
- *Scleral buckling.* Internal elevation of the sclera may be increased by the scleral buckling procedure. This technique involves implantation of a wedge of silicone episclerally or intrasclerally. An encircling band of silicone may be used to keep constant external pressure on the buckle. Figure 39-28 depicts the result of this procedure.
- *Intraocular gas tamponade.* Injection of room air or absorbable inert gas into the vitreous cavity can be used to create an intraocular tamponade. Room air absorbs after 5 days. Inert gases such as short-acting sulfahexafluoride (SF_6), intermediate-acting perfluoroethane (C_2F_6), or long-acting perfluorooctane (C_3F_8) are sometimes used to approximate the retina to the choroid (i.e., flatten the retina against the choroid).

With pneumoretinopexy, the patient remains in a seated position for a superior tear or prone for a tear near the macula. This position is maintained for several weeks postoperatively so the gas bubble can successfully rise to close the retinal hole. The position and length of time in that position is determined by the ophthalmologist according to each patient's need. Pneumoretinopexy is less invasive than scleral buckling for securing a retinal detachment (Fig. 39-29).

- *Intraocular fluid tamponade.* Silicone oil has been approved by the U.S. Food and Drug Administration (FDA) for use as a vitreous substitute in securing a retinal detachment that cannot be corrected through conventional surgical intervention. Silicone oil is used for long-term intraocular tamponade. It is removed by the ophthalmologist several months postoperatively. Patients with proliferative vitreoretinopathy with inferior breaks benefit from a blended silicone solution that is heavier than the vitreous. A blend of perfluorohexyloctane and silicone referred to as Densiron has been shown to

effect a repair to the detached lower retina in 90% of patients in clinical trials. The Densiron is removed between 12 and 14 weeks postoperatively.
- *Laser therapy.* Laser therapy can be used to secure the retina, except in severe detachment. A laser is often used to secure small posterior tears. (See the following discussion of laser therapy.)

Glaucoma and infection are potential postoperative complications of retinal reattachment. Glaucoma may be caused by congestion of the uvea by the buckle, increased IOP, or movement of injected gas from the desired site, causing blockage of outflow channels of aqueous humor. Infection is evident by swelling, purulent drainage, and a loss of optical clarity.

Laser Therapy. The laser delivery system uses the binocular microscope of the slit lamp, thus providing stereopsis and greater magnification. The nature of the laser beam permits extremely rapid delivery of radiant energy to produce a sharply defined burn. The small lesion it produces can be placed close to the macula. Exposure can be as brief as $\frac{1}{100}$ second and the treated area as small as 50 mm (less than $\frac{2}{1000}$ inch) in diameter. Because of this short exposure time, immobilization of the eye is unnecessary unless the treated area is close to the macula, the central region of the retina with the clearest visual acuity. Accidental injury of the macula may result in a loss of central vision. Pupillary dilation is essential to avoid macular burn.

The argon laser is effective in treating retinal holes or tears and diabetic retinopathy. The krypton laser can be used to treat lesions closer to the macula and to treat retinal bleeding because of its poor absorption of the yellow pigment of the retina. The krypton spectrum is poorly absorbed by the red pigment of hemoglobin. Therefore, it may be used effectively to treat retinal bleeding in the presence of blood in the vitreous humor. Under these circumstances the argon blue laser is ineffective because of absorption by even a small amount of blood.

Photocoagulation. A retinal hole not surrounded by any detachment may be prophylactically sealed by xenon or laser photocoagulation. These therapeutic modalities, which are usually performed in an ophthalmic treatment area rather than the OR, were the outgrowth of traumatic retinal burns caused by watching an eclipse of the sun.

The xenon arc photocoagulator uses an intense source of multiwavelength light furnished by a xenon tube. The light is optically focused and concentrated into a delivering device that is basically an indirect ophthalmoscope. The latter can be used both to view the area to be treated and to aim the light beam. The light may be directed to any of the pigmented (light-absorbing) layers of the eye, such as the iris or retina. These darker layers readily absorb the white light of the xenon tube.

The optical system of the eye is used in the process of focusing the light beam on the desired area. The power setting and exposure time are completely controlled by the operating ophthalmologist. The pupil of the eye under therapy is dilated to give maximum visibility to the surgeon. The eye is immobilized by local anesthesia to prevent undesired movement, which could result in a burn to an area other than the one desired. Anesthesia also prevents pain from the intensity of the heat. Vitreous shrinkage that possibly leads to an inoperable detachment can be a complication.

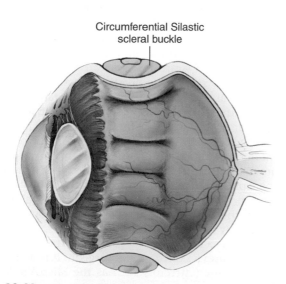

Circumferential Silastic scleral buckle

FIG. 39-28 Compressive effects of scleral buckle. *(From Glaser BM: Surgical retina. In Ryan SJ et al, eds: Retina, ed 2, vol 3, St. Louis, 1995, Mosby.)*

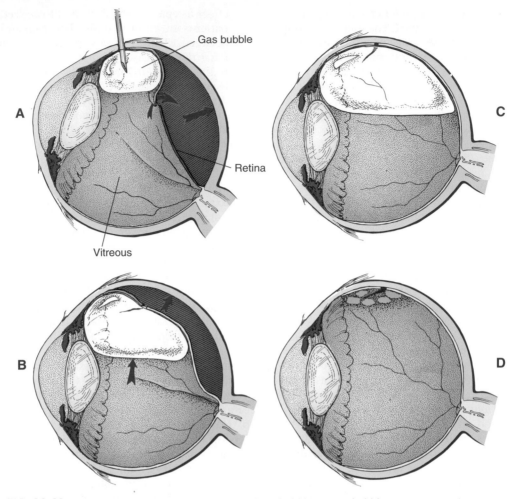

FIG. 39-29   Pneumoretinopexy. **A,** Introduction of gas bubble. **B,** Gas bubble compresses retina.
C, Tamponade formed by gas bubble. **D,** Gas bubble eventually absorbs.
(From Glaser BM: Surgical retina. In Ryan SJ et al, eds: Retina, ed 2, vol 3, St. Louis, 1995, Mosby.)

Vitrectomy. Vitrectomy is the deliberate removal of a portion of the vitreous humor, also called vitreous body, that fills the space between the lens and the retina. Therapeutically it is performed for vitreal opacities, vitreal hemorrhage, and certain types of retinal damage or detachment. In addition to other causes, endophthalmitis (i.e., inflammation of the internal tissues of the eyeball) and the presence of an intraocular foreign body may result in vitreal opacity. In general, the candidates for vitrectomy have substantially impaired vision and complicated conditions preoperatively.

Whereas aqueous fluid is a clear liquid, vitreous is normally a transparent, gelatinous, viscid material containing fibrils. The vitreous helps give shape to the eyeball and serves a refractive function. It permits light rays to pass through it to the retina after the rays have traversed the lens. Diagnostically, the removal of a small amount of vitreous provides a sample for microbiologic study in suspected endophthalmitis. The procedure also provides tissue for biopsy to establish the diagnosis of intraocular tumors.

Alterations in the vitreous can have serious consequences. The loss of vitreous during surgical procedures is a dreaded complication, particularly of cataract extraction.

Subsequent to retinal hemorrhage, which is common in patients with diabetes, bands of scar tissue may opacify the vitreous as well as adhere to the retina near the original bleeding vessel. Traction on the retina by these bands or further cicatrization (scarring) can lead to retinal tears or detachment. A persistent hemorrhage, lasting more than 1 year, is permanent. It will not absorb spontaneously.

For years the vitreous was considered an inaccessible, inoperable area. Research and the advent of microsurgery have changed this belief. A loss of vitreous from the posterior segment during a cataract procedure is relatively innocuous if the anterior segment is cleared of vitreous. Thus no residual strands are present to cause traction effects or to block visual function. In addition, the eye tolerates subtotal vitreal excision in the posterior segment if the vitreous body is proportionately replaced with BSS.

Vitrectomy is a microsurgical procedure that lasts 2 to 3 hours and requires a skilled retinal surgeon. It is performed with a vitreotome (vitrector) such as the MicroVit. These devices, which incorporate a micromotor, terminate in a needlelike tube that contains a cutting mechanism for severing abnormal adhesions and cutting obstructive tissue into small pieces. In addition, the vitreotome has auxiliary connections for the aspiration of vitreous, debris, or blood from the posterior segment.

Vitreous is replaced with BSS via a separate infusion cannula to maintain adequate IOP. A fiberoptic light source or pic is inserted into the vitreous to illuminate the posterior portion of the globe. Various vitrectomy systems are available, but all have cutting, suction, and illumination systems. The machine may have an automatic or hydraulic pole for rapidly regulating the height of the BSS bottle.

The scrub person and circulating nurse should assemble and check equipment before the surgical procedure begins. The vitreotome handpiece is attached to sterile tubing, which is connected to a power console. One person activates the various switches while the other tests the suction vacuum and cutting function. Suction is tested at maximum pressure. The tip is placed in sterile saline and activated until fluid reaches the collection bottle. The pressure is then lowered to the surgeon's preference.

To assess cutting, the switch is activated and the tip is checked visibly and audibly for movement. The infusion catheter is primed with a solution of the surgeon's choice to remove air bubbles that could disturb the view in the posterior segment. The manufacturer's manual should be consulted.

A local anesthetic is administered unless the patient's condition necessitates a general anesthetic. There are two approaches to the vitreous body:

1. Through the posterior segment via the pars plana (i.e., the anterior attachment of the retina). Because the pars plana has no visual function, entry here is relatively atraumatic and poses minimal risk for retinal detachment. The anterior segment remains intact, and IOP is maintained. This approach is used to incise opacified vitreous, old hemorrhage, or bands of scar tissue, thereby giving a clear view of the retina and restoring visual function.
2. Through the anterior segment via incision at the limbus (i.e., junction of the cornea and sclera). A small opening is made, and the tip of the vitrector is introduced. The vitreous is exposed through the pupillary opening. This approach is used to remove vitreous inadvertently displaced into the anterior chamber during cataract removal to avoid postoperative complications. The vitreous volume is replaced with BSS. Anterior vitrectomy also is used to correct retinal traction in retinopathy in premature infants (retrolental fibroplasia).

Vitrectomy is intricate and requires special equipment. The surgeon may request a bipolar cautery with a Charles clip attachment for actively bleeding intraocular vessels. A bipolar pencil or "eraser" may be used intraocularly. A handheld or "sew-on" contact lens placed onto the cornea enhances the view of the posterior chamber. A metal ring is sewn into place at two points around the limbus, encircling the cornea. Viscous material is placed on the cornea, and the lens of choice is placed down in the ring. Occasionally, a lensectomy is performed during vitrectomy to facilitate the view of the posterior segment.

After the removal of vitreous, before wound closure, and with the retina in clear view, the retina is inspected for defects such as holes or vascular abnormalities. If these are found, treatment is applied by means of endocryotherapy, a freezing application delivered by intraocular probe or by a laser delivered by an intraocular device. These maneuvers may be accompanied by the injection of air or inert gas to push the retina into physiologic position.

Postoperatively, patients may experience considerable pain that requires medication, ice packs, and steroid eyedrops for treatment of inflammation. After vitrectomy, patients will experience aphakia if the lens was removed for visualization of the posterior segment, and they will eventually need optical correction such as that needed after cataract extraction. Vitrectomy can significantly improve vision.

Complications of vitrectomy include iatrogenic retinal damage, vitreous hemorrhage, or cataract formation from damage to the lens. A secondary surgical procedure may be required to repair the retina (e.g., a scleral buckling procedure or intraocular tamponade). No present treatment for retinopathy is free of danger. To save vision, some tissue is destroyed or sacrificed.

EYE INJURIES

Various forms and degrees of trauma may occur as a result of injury. All types of injuries require immediate appraisal by an ophthalmologist. A delay in treating even minor injuries may result in a temporary or permanent loss of vision. Complications include hemorrhage, infection, iritis or tears of the iris, retinal tears or detachment, macular edema, and secondary cataract. Treatment may be immediate or secondary if a delay is necessary because of life-threatening injuries. Improved surgical management, such as vitrectomy and microsurgery, has reduced the loss of vision in severely injured eyes. An optimum result is especially crucial in patients with bilateral eye injuries. If possible, patients with eye injuries should be kept in the supine position until seen by an ophthalmologist.

Evaluation of the injury may necessitate sedating or anesthetizing the patient to prevent further damage at examination. Pressure to the eye must be avoided because bone fragments may be displaced or the globe contents emptied.

Injuries may be simple and involve only the external layers, or they may be compound and include the inner structures. They may be nonpenetrating (usually caused by a blunt object) or penetrating (caused by a sharp object). The more structures involved, the more difficult it is to salvage the eye.

Treatment is determined by the type or combination of injuries and aims to do the following:

- Promote healing and prevent anatomic distortion by reparative techniques
- Preserve and/or restore maximum vision
- Control pain by medication
- Prevent infection and inflammation through the administration of antibiotics and steroids

Nonpenetrating Injuries

Burns. Burns may be caused by ultraviolet radiation, such as sunlamps or sunlight, or by an electric flash. These types of burns are basically self-limited and are rarely surgical. A chemical burn constitutes an emergency. The initial treatment consists of flooding the cornea with water. Alkali burns may be further neutralized by prompt irrigation of the epithelium-denuded cornea with ethylenediaminetetraacetic acid (EDTA). This is especially important if discrete particles of alkali are superficially embedded within tissue. EDTA deactivates an enzyme (collagenase) and neutralizes soluble alkali such as sodium hydroxide (lye). Severe burns may be treated with specific amino acids, EDTA, or acetylcysteine (Mucomyst) to inhibit the continued destruction of the cornea by collagenase; however, these burns often progress to corneal opacity and blindness.

Contusions of the Globe. Contusions of the globe may or may not require surgical treatment. If hemorrhage is present, treatment consists of bed rest and antiglaucoma therapy to control IOP. It is not unusual for a secondary hemorrhage to occur on the third or fourth day after injury. If IOP remains high, blood staining of the cornea and damage to the optic nerve may result. It is then sometimes necessary to perform a paracentesis, in which an incision is made into the anterior chamber to drain the blood. If an organized clot is found, judicious irrigation may supplement the incision.

Penetrating Injuries

Lacerations of the globe may occur with or without a retained foreign body and with or without prolapse of the ocular contents. In injuries to the globe, an ophthalmic surgeon should repair both the eye wound and the tissues adjacent to the eye.

With a penetrating injury there is the possibility of an eventual sympathetic ophthalmia—an inflammation of the uninjured eye. Antitetanus therapy should be included in the treatment of these injuries.

Vitrectomy and lensectomy have rendered salvageable some massive injuries that formerly were inoperable. Such injuries include extensive lacerations with cataract formation, vitreous hemorrhage, and retinal damage.

Without a Foreign Body

Eyelid Laceration. Lacerations are repaired according to anatomic principles. Plastic repair involves approximation of the anatomic layers. Penetrating wounds, such as animal bites, are debrided. If the laceration includes the lacrimal canaliculus (duct for the passage of tears), special probes are used to identify the proximal portions for rejoining. Lacerations of the lacrimal canaliculus may be repaired by suturing over one of two types of stents. The Quickert-Dryden tubing consists of a length of flexible silicone with a malleable metal lacrimal probe swaged onto each end. One end of the probe is inserted through the upper lid canaliculus, and the other end is inserted into the lower lid canaliculus. Both ends exit via the tear sac and nasolacrimal canal into the nose. The lacerated canaliculus is then sutured over the tubing, which is removed after healing takes place. Some surgeons prefer the rigid Veirs stainless steel rod, which is inserted into the lacerated canaliculus. A suture swaged to one end permits withdrawal of the rod after healing.

Conjunctival Laceration. Conjunctival laceration is usually debrided and, unless large, is permitted to heal without suturing. If the laceration is large and there is a loss of conjunctival tissue, sutures or rotating flaps of conjunctiva may be necessary for repair.

Corneal and Scleral Lacerations. A small corneal laceration may be covered with a protective soft contact lens to seal it and hold the edges together. A larger wound requires accurate appositional sutures that are best placed using the operating microscope. The microscope is especially useful for irregular, complicated, or multiple tears.

Some irregular corneal lacerations not easily closed by direct suturing may be closed and the leak stopped by the application of cyanoacrylate glue. A soft contact lens is usually placed as a bandage over the freshly glued cornea. A conjunctival flap can be placed to achieve a similar seal, but it is used less frequently. A large laceration may require a penetrating keratoplasty as an emergency procedure to ensure the integrity of the eye.

Adequate exploration, particularly of a scleral wound, is necessary both to determine the extent of injury and to ensure uncovering of the entire wound for repair. In instances of vitreous fluid presentation or loss, it is preferable to remove the fluid from the wound and the anterior chamber with the vitreotome before proceeding with repair. This is performed to prevent undesirable vitreous adhesions from developing postoperatively.

Posterior Rupture of the Globe. Rupture of the globe usually involves the herniation of retinal and uveal tissue into the orbit. Although such injuries are self-healing, the eye is irreparably damaged. This injury usually results in enucleation. Avulsion (tearing) of the optic nerve produces permanent blindness even though the rest of the globe may be intact.

With a Foreign Body

Extraocular injuries are usually not extensive. An intraocular foreign object is removed very gently under sterile conditions to avoid secondary infection and further trauma. A corneal foreign body is removed with a sharp probe (spud), and the surrounding rust ring is removed with a rotating burr. The type, size, and position of other intraocular foreign bodies should be determined accurately before removal. Localization is accomplished by the following:

- Direct vision with an ophthalmoscope
- Computed tomography (CT) scan
- Berman locator, a small but extremely sensitive version of a metal detector, which may indicate the exact location of a ferrous metallic foreign body
- Radiographic study, using a contact lens containing radiopaque landmarks (Sweet's localizer)

Fragments of ferrous metals often can be retrieved by using the attraction of a strong electromagnet. In some cases these foreign bodies can be withdrawn along the path of entry. Nonmagnetic foreign objects present a more serious problem. Often they are secured only by passing a delicate forceps into the globe. Such instrumentation is combined with a partial vitrectomy, thus obtaining satisfactory results.

In summary, traumatic injuries may introduce infection or produce a severe inflammatory reaction to a greater degree than do elective surgical procedures. Proper early treatment is indicated to save vision. Early intervention, before scar formation, may be necessary in some patients.

OPHTHALMIC LASERS

The use of an ophthalmic laser is often a safe alternative to conventional surgery for ablation of a pathologic condition. The color and wavelength of each laser determine which part of the eye it can best treat. Specific wavelengths destroy disease in tissues whose pigments are capable of discriminating absorption of that wavelength. Conversely, the selected wavelength should be only minimally absorbed by the vital adjacent tissues to be preserved. The ophthalmologist controls the power, intensity, and direction of the laser beam. The beam precisely cauterizes tissue and blood vessels, preventing bleeding. Each laser has selective uses:

- *Blue-green argon.* For a retinal detachment, tear, or hole; diabetic retinopathy; macular neovascular lesions; laser trabeculoplasty, to lower IOP and facilitate aqueous outflow in select patients with open-angle glaucoma; iridotomy, in place of iridectomy by incision; and to create a small opening in the iris that allows aqueous to enter the anterior chamber (angle-closure glaucoma). The use of this laser may reduce the threat of endophthalmitis, a serious postoperative complication. Adherence of the iris to laser treatment sites (synechiae) is a complication of laser trabeculoplasty. A portable laser is available for intraoperative use. It permits surgeons to work inside rather than through the eye while the patient is under general anesthesia.
- *Red-yellow krypton.* For blood vessel aberrations of the choroid (common to senile macular disease) in which abnormal vessels damage adjacent nerve tissue; for lesions in the perimacular region (the laser beam passes through cloudy vitreous hemorrhage); and for retinal vascular diseases, such as proliferative diabetic retinopathy and retinal detachment.
- *Invisible pulsed neodymium:yttrium-aluminum-garnet (Nd:YAG).* For preoperative anterior capsulotomy before extracapsular cataract extraction; posterior capsulotomy (discission) after extracapsular cataract extraction to make an opening in an opaque capsule and thus permit light to reach the retina; and lysis or severing of strands of vitreous and/or fibrous bands in the posterior segment that cause cystoid macular edema. Cloudy areas of tissue interfering with vision are painlessly pushed aside, resulting in immediate improvement in sight. Rather than producing the effect by absorption, energy is released almost entirely at the point of focus. Problems in both anterior and posterior parts of the eye are treatable (e.g., with optical iridectomy and photocoagulation of retinal disorders). Unlike with the visible light lasers, the Nd:YAG laser does not require the target tissue to be pigmented for effectiveness.
- *Visible excimer.* Argon-fluoride in the ultraviolet range. Used for shaping the cornea, as in lamellar keratectomy, to correct refractive disorders.
- *Invisible holmium:YAG (Ho:YAG).* For sclerostomy to create an opening in the sclera that promotes filtration for glaucoma. It can also be used for corneal sculpting.

The following are advantages of laser therapy:

- Possibility of infection is minimal. Treatment is noninvasive and sterile, which is an advantage to diabetic and susceptible patients.
- Pain is minimal. Only a topical anesthetic is required unless many retinal areas are treated with a high-energy laser.
- It is performed as an ambulatory procedure.
- The appropriate amount of energy is concentrated in a very small area.
- The light is highly flexible, which seems to do little damage to the clear medium it traverses.
- The laser light is selectively absorbed. Ideally, only desired tissue is affected.
- It is useful in a poor-risk surgical patient or one who has had a previous unsuccessful surgical procedure.

Bibliography

Alio JL et al: Correction of presbyopia by technovision central multifocal LASIK, *J Refract Surg* 22(5):453-460, 2006.

Bourne WM et al: Comparison of Chen Medium and Optisol-GS for human corneal preservation at 4 degrees C: Results of transplantation, *Cornea* 20(7):683-686, 2001.

Hara T, Hara T: Ten-year results of anterior chamber fixation of the posterior chamber intraocular lens, *Arch Ophthalmol* 122(8):1112-1116, 2004.

Kennedy RH et al: Eye banking and screening for Creutzfeldt-Jakob disease, *Arch Ophthalmol* 119(5):721-726, 2001.

Muraine MC et al: Deep lamellar keratoplasty combined with cataract surgery, *Arch Ophthalmol* 120(6):812-815, 2002.

Ray S et al: Management of vitreoretinal complications in eyes with permanent keratoprosthesis, *Arch Ophthalmol* 120(5):559-566, 2002.

Sanchez P et al: Risk factors for infectious disease in corneal transplant screening, *Eye Contact Lens Sci Clin Pract* 32(3):124-127, 2006.

Walker R, Rodgers J: Diabetic retinopathy, *Nurs Stand* 16(45):46-52, 2002.

Chapter 40

Plastic and Reconstructive Surgery

CHAPTER OBJECTIVES

After studying this chapter, the learner will be able to:
- Identify pertinent anatomy of the integumentary system.
- List four primary reasons for plastic surgery.
- Differentiate between autografts, allografts, and xenografts.
- Describe the techniques of skin and tissue grafting.
- Discuss the importance of fluid balance in the burn patient.

CHAPTER OUTLINE

KEY TERMS AND DEFINITIONS

Aesthetic Pleasing form.
Debride Remove dead tissue from wound edges to reveal vital tissue.
Dermatome Instrument for graft procurement. Can be mechanized or freehand knife style.
Dorsal surface The back of the hand.
Eschar Tissue layer that forms over a burn site.
Expander A silicone sac placed beneath the skin and gradually expanded to increase the surface area of the skin to cover a defect.
Flap A multilayer tissue segment used as a surface cover. Can remain attached to a vascularized pedicle or can be a separate segment anastomosed to a new vascular attachment.
FTSG Full thickness skin graft that consists of the epidermis and dermis.
Graft A portion of tissue used as a surface cover. Not vascularized.
Mesher A mechanical device used in the sterile field to cut slits into a skin graft to expand the surface area.
Ptosis Drooping of a part such as an eyelid or breast.
Replant Reattach a severed part. Involves the anastomosis of vessels, nerves, and compact tissue.
STSG Split thickness skin graft that consists of the epidermis and a thin layer of papillary dermis.
"Take" The process of physiologic acceptance and integration of a graft or flap.
Volar surface Palm side of the hand.

HISTORICAL BACKGROUND

Plastic surgery was probably the first form of surgery. Egyptian papyrus scrolls tell of skin grafts and pedicle flaps to replace deficiencies as early as 3500 years ago. Egyptian mummies have been found with artificial ears and noses. In India more than 2000 years ago, the Hindus became skilled in transferring tissue to form noses for those who had lost them as a punishment. Ancient records verify other attempts to improve appearance.

During the fourteenth and sixteenth centuries, restorative procedures for the nose, lips, and ears were performed by Italian surgeons, such as Gasparé Tagliacozzi (1545-1599), who described the creation of a tube graft from the arm to the nose for reconstructive rhinoplasty. In 1872, French orthopedic surgeon Louis Ollier (1830-1900) developed a method for thinly sliced freehand skin grafts that was later modified by German surgeon Karl Thiersch (1822-1895). Thiersch made split-thickness skin grafting popular in 1874. He was a supporter of Lister and introduced aseptic technique during the Franco-Prussian war.

During World Wars I and II the development of military plastic and reconstructive surgery centers led to rapid progress in the rehabilitation of casualties with maxillofacial and hand injuries. Plastic surgeons worked closely with other specialists in treating many types of war injuries. They found that by replacing lost skin with grafts, fractures under these areas healed better and more quickly and parts returned to normal function sooner.

SPECIAL FEATURES OF PLASTIC AND RECONSTRUCTIVE SURGERY

Plastic surgery has been called the "Surgery of Millimeters" because of the critical margin between good and poor cosmetic results. Each millimeter lack or excess of tissue can have a psychological impact on the patient. If the patient thinks his or her appearance has improved, the patient's personality and self-image may improve and others may respond more positively to him or her. The term *plastic* means "to mold or give form."

Plastic surgeons practice their art on virtually any part of the body. They attempt to restore both form (aesthetic appearance) and function. Some plastic surgeons limit their practice to specific areas, such as the head and neck, hand, or breast. The surgeon specifically trained in the art of plastic surgery frequently is a member of a multidisciplinary team to assist with the repair of defects and/or restoration of function. The results depend not only on the skill of the plastic surgeon and the team but also on the age, health status, skin texture, bone structure, extent of the defect, and healing capacity of the patient.

Many plastic and reconstructive surgical procedures are performed on an ambulatory basis; many are performed with the patient under local anesthesia with sedation. The surgeon performs the simplest and safest procedure that will provide a realistic outcome.

Scars are inevitable whenever skin is incised or excised. The incision is made along natural skin lines whenever possible. The plastic surgeon attempts to minimize scar formation by meticulous realignment and approximation of underlying tissues and wound edges. Many plastic procedures involve only the subcuticular tissues and skin. Reconstructive procedures may include manipulation of underlying cartilage, bones, muscles, tendons, nerves, and blood vessels. Replacement tissues or other structural substances come from several sources as follows:

- *Autograft.* Use tissue from self
- *Isograft.* Use tissue from genetically identical person
- *Allograft.* Use tissue from same species
- *Xenograft.* Use tissue from different species
- *Bioengineered graft.* Graft source from combined biologic and synthetic materials
- *Synthetic graft.* Substance from nonbiologic source

Preoperative instruction to patients include to avoid aspirin and not to smoke for at least 2 weeks before an elective surgical procedure. Aspirin and other substances have an anticoagulant action that can affect bleeding, causing hematoma formation. Box 40-1 lists medications and substances that may promote postoperative bleeding. Smoking causes vasoconstrictive ischemia that can affect wound healing, causing tissue necrosis. Photographs are commonly taken preoperatively, intraoperatively, and postoperatively for planning, documentation, and teaching purposes.

General Considerations in Plastic Surgery

1. Pressure points are protected during prolonged procedures. Microvascular plastic and reconstructive surgical procedures may take several hours to complete. The patient should be positioned on a gel pad mattress. Bony prominences should be well padded to prevent tissue necrosis.

BOX 40-1   Medications and Substances That May Promote Postoperative Bleeding

PRODUCTS THAT CONTAIN ASPIRIN (EXAMPLES)
Aleve
Aspergum
Bufferin
Congespirin
Darvon
Ecotrin
Empirin
Excedrin

ANALGESICS THAT HAVE AN ASPIRIN-LIKE EFFECT ON BLEEDING (EXAMPLES)
Dolobid
Norgesic
Oxycodone
Pepto-Bismol
Percodan
Soma
Talwin
Voltaren

MEDICATIONS THAT CONTAIN IBUPROFEN (EXAMPLES)
Advil
Midol
Naprosyn
Nuprin
Postel
Sine-Aid
Toradol

ANTICOAGULANTS (EXAMPLES)
Coumadin
Dicumarol
Heparin
Panwarfin
Periactin

HERBAL SUBSTANCES THAT MAY HAVE AN ANTICOAGULANT EFFECT (EXAMPLES)
Some fish oils
Vitamin E
Ginkgo biloba
Licorice
Garlic
Clove
Ginseng
Ginger
Feverfew
Chamomile
Aloe vera

2. Sterile dye, such as methylene blue, indigo carmine, gentian violet, Bonney's blue, or brilliant green, is often used to outline areas for incision. This can be done with a sterile marking pen or stylus before or after the skin is prepped. Some surgeons will use intravenous fluorescent dye and a black light (Wood's lamp) to confirm vascularity of a flap.

3. Exposure of both sides for comparison is usually required for surgical procedures on the breast, face, ears, and neck. Photography is commonly used preoperatively, intraoperatively, and postoperatively. Equalization of tissue manipulation and excision is matched to preoperative measurements written on a full-size image of the body part undergoing the surgical procedure. Figure 40-1 depicts the areas marked for facial procedures. The nose is measured in comparison to the distance between the zygomatic arches (Fig. 40-2). Contemporary surgeons are using terrain mapping for procedures such as facial allogenous transplants (Fig. 40- 3).

4. Draping often exposes much skin surface, which is unavoidable. A fenestrated sheet frequently cannot be used. The opening does not give adequate exposure, especially for skin grafting. Use towels, self-adhering plastic sheeting, and minor and medium sheets under and around the areas, according to need, to drape as much of the patient as possible. Drapes can be secured with nonpiercing towel clips, skin staples, or sutures.

5. Local anesthesia is used for many surgical procedures on adults. Epinephrine may be added to help localize the agent, prolong the anesthetic action, and provide hemostasis. Care is taken not to use epinephrine in digits, ears, or other areas of terminal blood supply. Short 26- or 30-gauge needles are used for injection.

   a. The surgeon may administer a digital nerve block for procedures of the finger. The patient's hand is placed palm down and a hypodermic needle is inserted through the webspace closest to the affected digit. The surgeon will aspirate to check clearance of all vessels. Then lidocaine 1% or 0.05% without epinephrine 1 mL is injected in the volar space (the region of the palmer surface). As the needle is withdrawn 1 mL is injected at the level of the dorsal space (the region closest to the dorsum of the hand).

6. Nos. 15 and 11 scalpel blades are routinely used to cut small structures. Smaller blades, such as Beaver style, may be used.

7. An electrosurgical unit (ESU) pencil may be used to cut or coagulate during incision. Small, handheld battery-operated units are useful for tiny bleeders. Overuse of the ESU can cause devitalization of tissue and delay healing.

8. Instruments must be small for handling delicate tissues. Iris scissors, mosquito hemostats, fine-tipped tissue forceps, and other small-scale cutting, holding, clamping, and exposing instruments are part of the routine plastic surgery setup. Microinstruments are needed for microsurgical techniques.

9. Nerve stimulation may be used to help identify nerves, especially in craniofacial, neck, and hand reconstruction procedures.

10. Bone, cartilage, or skin grafts may be needed. Grafts and tissues can be used from several different sources for surface and subsurface modifications. Graft materials should not be allowed to dry out. Place in a basin with a few drops of saline. Do not place in a folded moist

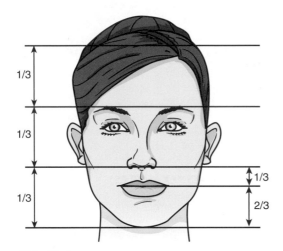

FIG. 40-1 Facial measurement for plastic surgery.

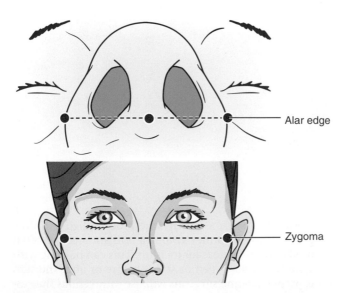

FIG. 40-2 Nasal measurements are planned in relation to the zygoma for plastic surgery.

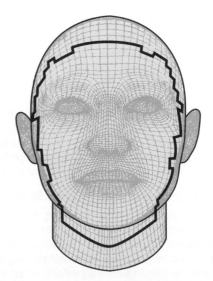

FIG. 40-3 Facial terrain measurements for full face transplant.

sponge because this could be discarded from the field to the sponge bucket by accident.

11. Prosthetic implants may be used in plastic surgery to reconstruct subsurface soft tissue and cartilage defects. They cannot be used unless there is adequate soft tissue coverage. They cannot be used in an infected area.

12. Suture sizes range from 2-0 through 7-0, depending on the location and tissue, with sizes 8-0 through 11-0 sutures for microsurgery. The material used varies according to the personal preference of the surgeon. Synthetic nonabsorbable and absorbable polymers are used more commonly than are natural materials, because they cause less tissue reaction.

13. Atraumatic swaged-on needles of small diameter with sharp cutting edges minimize trauma to superficial tissues. A needle holder with an appropriately fine tip is used with these delicate, curved needles.

14. Skin staples may be used to close skin or to secure skin grafts.

15. Wound closure strips may be used as skin dressings with sutures or to supplement closure with skin staples.

16. Closed-wound suction drainage is frequently used to drain flaps to prevent seroma and hematoma formation.

17. Fine mesh gauze may be used for the contact dressing. This may be impregnated with petrolatum or an oil emulsion, with or without medication, to cover denuded areas. Several types of sterile nonadherent dressings are commercially available. Dry gauze is not used on a denuded area because it adheres and acts as a foreign body, causing granulomas.

18. Pressure dressings may be used after extensive surgical procedures to splint soft tissues and prevent contractures. Even pressure keeps fluid formation in tissues or under a skin graft to a minimum. Commercial compression garments or dressings for various body areas are preferred by some plastic surgeons. Some dressings may be sutured into place. Donor graft sites require bulkier dressings because they have multiple pinpoint bleeders that ooze freely.

19. Stent fixation is a method of obtaining pressure when it is impossible to bandage an area snugly, such as the face or neck. A form-fitting mold may be taped over the nose like a splint. Long suture ends can be tied criss-crossed over a dressing to immobilize it and exert gentle, even pressure.

Tissue may be approximated, supplemented, excised, transferred, or transplanted. Many procedures are done in stages before complete reconstruction and restoration of function are achieved. Tissue flaps and grafts, prosthetic implants, and external prosthetic appliances may be required for functional and cosmetic restoration as a result of ablative surgery or trauma.

Psychologic Support for Patients Undergoing Plastic and Reconstructive Surgery

Physical appearance affects self-image and self-esteem. Patients can develop inferiority complexes and introverted personalities because of congenital or acquired alteration in body structure. The defect may not affect physiologic function but may predispose the person to psychologic crippling if it is not corrected to the individual's satisfaction.

Adults who are dissatisfied with their body image may believe that a change in personal appearance will solve their social, marital, sexual, or business problems. The plastic surgeon assesses the patient's psychologic status, motivations, and expectations before scheduling a surgical procedure. Realistic, attainable outcomes are identified. The patient should be emotionally stable and aware of the potential outcomes. The surgeon should carefully obtain informed consent. Psychologic assessment and preparation are advisable preoperatively and are essential before surgical procedures that may result in disfigurement.

Extensive reconstruction for severe congenital deformities is done in stages, often over months or years. These patients require prolonged psychologic support and encouragement.

Plastic and reconstructive surgery, either therapeutic or cosmetic, evokes emotional responses from the patient, family or significant others, and the entire perioperative team. Anticipation of the final outcome, which can be seen by the patient and others, often creates temporary psychosocial reactions such as depression and isolation. Positive reassurance of progress in improvement of physical appearance and during emotional crises is essential throughout the perioperative period. Perhaps the surgeon-nurse-patient-family relationship is closer when a person undergoes alteration of physical appearance than with other types of surgery.

The patient may be physically healthy but may suffer alterations in self-esteem related to a perception of a defect in appearance. Care must be given in a manner that protects the self-esteem of the patient and respects the family's dignity. This requires communication, understanding, and empathy. Preoperative teaching and discharge planning prepare the patient and the family for postoperative rehabilitation.

Categories of Plastic and Reconstructive Surgery

Four main categories of problems are treated by plastic surgeons:

1. Congenital anomalies, especially in the structure of the face and hands. Other disciplines may surgically treat genitourinary or orthopedic deformities.
2. Aesthetic appearance, especially of the body surface and subsurface, particularly the face and breasts.
3. Benign and malignant neoplasms, especially those leaving large soft tissue defects. Resection of extensive tumors other than those involving the skin or head and neck is not usually within the province of the plastic surgeon initially, but the patient may be referred for reconstructive surgery and rehabilitation. Frequently, reconstructive procedures are done in conjunction with another specialty surgeon at the time of tumor resection.
4. Traumatically acquired disfigurements, especially facial lacerations, hand injuries, and burns. The objective of the plastic surgeon is to restore function, as well as body image.

SKIN AND TISSUE GRAFTING

Denuded areas of the body are resurfaced by transplanting or transferring segments of skin and other tissues from an uninjured area (donor site) to the injured area (recipient site). The plastic surgeon prefers to transfer tissues of compatible color, texture, thickness, and hair-bearing characteristics. Soft tissue autografts are used whenever possible. They are classified as follows according to the source of their vascular supply (which is essential for viability):

- *Free graft.* Tissue is detached from the donor site and transplanted into the recipient site. It derives its vascular supply from the capillary ingrowth from the recipient site. Figure 40-4 depicts regions of the body suitable for autologous graft procurement.
- *Pedicle flap.* Tissue remains attached at one or both ends of the donor site during transfer to the recipient site. The vascular supply is maintained from the vessels preserved in the pedicle of the donor site. Advancement flaps, rotational flaps, rhomboid flaps, and transverse rectus abdominis myocutaneous (TRAM) flaps and latissimus dorsi flaps (Fig. 40-5) are forms of pedicle flaps.
- *Free flap.* Tissue, including its vascular bundle, is detached from the donor site and transferred to the recipient site. Composite free flaps may include muscle, bone, and skin. Microvascular anastomoses between arteries and veins in the flap or autograft and recipient site establish the vascularity necessary for viability (Fig. 40-6).

Deformities caused by loss of soft tissue substance, such as trauma from accidental injury, tumor resection, or radiation therapy, may require a graft to fill in deficiencies and restore contours or to cover tendons and bones. Free grafts, pedicle flaps, and free flaps may be taken from various areas of the body to reconstruct soft tissue defects.

Grafting from one area of the body to another requires a process referred to as "take." The recipient site has to accept the donor tissue for the graft to take or remain as a permanently viable tissue replacement. The skin graft take occurs in three steps. During the first 48 hours, plasma accumulates at the contact area of the graft. This keeps the tissue vitalized before circulation is established. The second phase is the start of capillary ingrowth. And the last step is the anastomosis of vascular channels. If the graft does not take, it sloughs off and necroses.

Skin Graft Knives and Dermatomes

A dermatome is a cutting instrument designed to excise split-thickness skin grafts. The thickness of the graft can be calibrated by adjusting the depth gauge. The width of the graft is determined by the width of the cutting blade. Blades are detachable and disposable, which always ensures a sharp new blade for every patient. The cutting depth should always be reset at zero after changing blades. The length, width, and depth of the graft may be limited by the type of dermatome used and the surface from which the graft is procured (Fig. 40-7).

Freehand Skin Graft Knives and Dermatomes. Freehand knife dermatomes are used when the surface can be stabilized for precision cutting. The depth of the cut is determined by the setting on the blade gauge and adjusted by turning screws on the handle. Most styles have disposable blades. American surgeons Vilray Blair (1871-1955) and James Barrett Brown (1899-1971) developed a freehand knife that was modified by later plastic surgeons. The original style was designed like a straight razor but was later modified to include a roller for more accurate depth measurement (see Fig. 40-7, *C, D*).

Drum-Style Skin Graft Dermatomes. Padgett and Reese dermatomes consist of one half of a metal drum, which is one half of a circle (see Fig. 40-7, *B*). A metal handle through

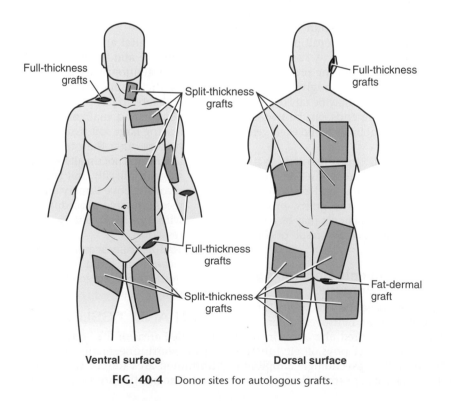

FIG. 40-4   Donor sites for autologous grafts.

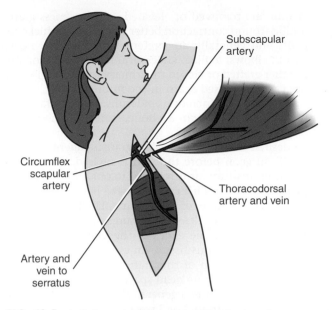

FIG. 40-5   Latissimus dorsi vascularized flap for breast reconstruction.

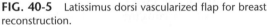
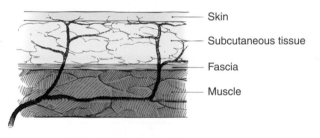

FIG. 40-6   Myocutaneous free flap.

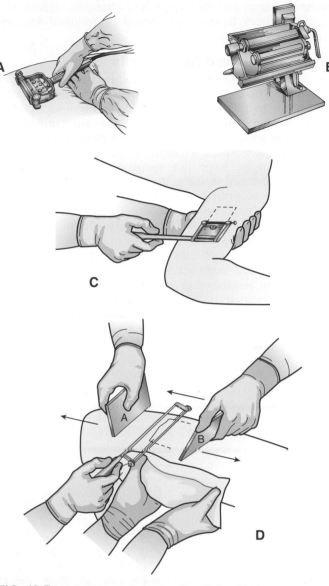

FIG. 40-7   Dermatomes. **A,** Powered oscillating blade–type dermatome with depth gauges on each side of blade. **B,** Drum-type dermatome to manually cut skin graft. **C,** DeSilva freehand skin graft knife. **D,** Assistant provides countertraction for use of a manual Watson skin graft knife.

the center of the drum has an arm on each end. These arms hold the bar that carries the blade. The bar swings around the drum to cut the graft. The size of the graft is limited by the width and length of the drum. An adhesive is placed on both the skin surface and the drum to keep the skin in contact with the drum. The knife blade is moved from side to side as slight tension is exerted on the skin by rotating the drum. The drum-type dermatome is used on flat, open areas, because it is bulky. Its use is limited by the body contour and the amount of suitable skin on the donor site.

Dermatome tape is used with the Reese dermatome. Packaged sterile, the tape has an adhesive coating on each side, covered with a paper backing. The backing is removed on one side and applied to the drum, taking care to line up the edges of the tape and the drum. After the backing paper is removed from the other side of the tape, the drum is placed on the skin, which adheres to it.

When a drum-type dermatome is being handled, the blade carrier is always grasped to prevent its swinging around the drum and seriously injuring the hands. The dermatome is left in the sterile rack when not in use or until the blade is removed.

Powered Skin Graft Dermatomes.   Oscillating blade–type dermatomes may be electric or air powered with compressed

nitrogen or air. The length of the graft is limited only by the donor site. The surgeon checks the adjustable-depth gauge before cutting the graft (see Fig. 40-7, *A*). The oscillating blade, free of vibrations, takes an accurate graft from donor sites that overlie firm structures, such as bone. The oscillating blade–type dermatome generally is not used on the abdominal wall, where underlying support is not firm.

Care is used in handling these precision dermatomes. If the dermatome is electric, the circulator should remove the foot pedal after the graft is taken. If the dermatome is air powered, the scrub person and surgeon should place a thumb under the lever on the handle while preparing the instrument for use. These dermatomes cannot be immersed in water or put in a washer-sterilizer or ultrasonic cleaner. The manufacturer's instructions should be followed for use, care, and sterilization.

Types of Skin and Tissue Grafts

Skin Grafts. The epidermis, including the basal layer of the dermis that generates new skin, is transplanted from a donor site to a recipient site, in which it becomes a part of living tissue in that area. Adherence to healthy underlying tissue and adequate vascularity are necessary for graft take (survival). A fibrin layer forms to bind the graft to the recipient site and to provide nourishment until vascularization is established in the graft. The depth of the graft (Fig. 40-8) varies according to its purpose:

* *Split-thickness graft.* The epidermis and half of the dermis to a depth of 0.010 to 0.035 inch (0.3 to 1 mm) are removed. The donor site heals uneventfully unless it becomes infected. Split-thickness grafts are widely used to cover large denuded areas on the back, trunk, and legs and can be meshed to cover larger areas. The donor site can be reused in 2 to 3 weeks after healing.
* *Full-thickness graft.* The epidermis, dermis, and occasionally subcutaneous fat at a depth greater than 0.035 inch

(1 mm) are removed or elevated. Full-thickness grafts inhibit wound contraction better than do split-thickness grafts and generally are preferred on the face, neck, hands, elbows, axillae, knees, and feet. The donor site is either grafted or closed by primary intention. Donor site cannot be used again in the future.

* *Composite graft.* Includes epidermis, dermis, fat, and other structures such as bone, cartilage, nerve, or tendon.

The desired thickness of a skin graft is determined by the plastic surgeon before the skin is incised. The appropriate cutting instrument is selected to obtain the graft.

Split-Thickness Thiersch Graft. Removed with a freehand skin graft knife or dermatome, Thiersch grafts are used to cover superficial defects. The surgeon may use sutures or skin staples along the edges of the graft to hold it to underlying subcutaneous tissue. An even-pressure dressing is secured over the top of the graft. This prevents movement and helps obliterate dead space in the recipient site. The skin of the donor site regenerates rapidly, and the same area can be used again in 2 or 3 weeks if necessary. If a thin graft is taken and the site remains infection-free, that donor site may be used again sooner.

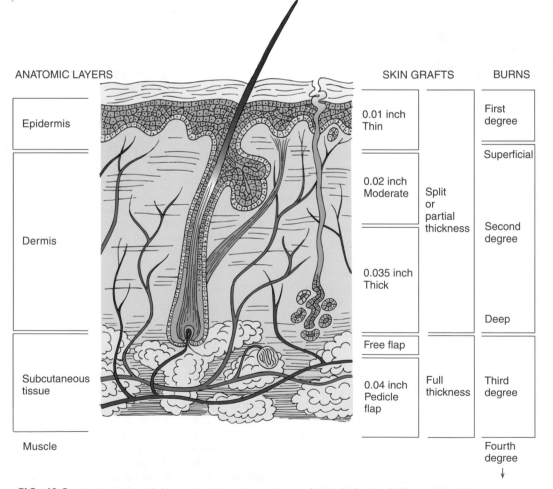

FIG. 40-8   Cross section of skin and subcutaneous tissue, relative thickness of skin grafts, and categorization of burn injury.

Split-Thickness Mesh Graft. A mesh graft makes it possible to obtain a greater area of coverage from a split-thickness skin graft. After removal with a dermatome, the graft is placed on a plastic derma carrier, cut side down. This is a rigid base to keep the graft spread out flat while it is put through a mesh dermatome. This instrument cuts small parallel slits in the graft. When expanded, the slits become diamond-shaped openings (Fig. 40-9). This permits expansion of the graft to cover an area three times as large as the original graft obtained from the donor site. The mesh graft can be placed over the recipient site with slight tension. The increased edge exposures are conducive to rapid epithelialization. The mesh allows serum to escape through the openings. If a mesh dermatome is not available or is not feasible to use, slits can be made with a knife blade in the donor graft to accomplish the same purposes.

Although this method covers a larger area and contours well, much of the wound has to heal by secondary intention, causing scar contracture. The healed area maintains a "cobblestone" appearance.

Full-Thickness Wolfe Graft. Wolfe graft is cut exactly to the size and shape of the recipient site with a skin graft knife. It is sutured into place under normal skin tension. Full-thickness grafts are used on the face, neck, or hands to fill in superficial denuded areas and over joints to prevent contractures. This graft does not become viable readily on granulated surfaces, and the amount that can be transferred is much more limited than with Thiersch graft.

To ensure viability, the donor graft must be held in apposition to healthy tissue in the underlying recipient site. The surgeon tacks the edges of the graft with sutures or staples. The middle portion may be "quilted" (i.e., affixed) with sutures or staples. The graft is covered with an even-pressure dressing.

Free Composite Grafts

A composite graft usually includes skin, subcutaneous tissue and cartilage, bone, or other tissues. The viability of the graft depends on ingrowth of the vascular system from the recipient site.

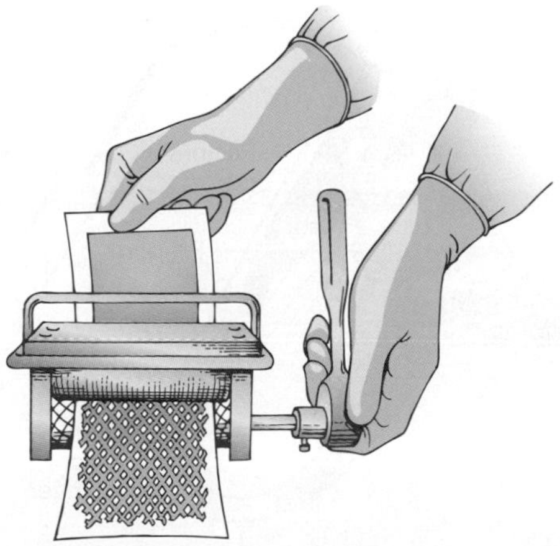

Free Omental Grafts

A free graft of omentum can be used to provide contour in a soft tissue defect in the face or neck, to resurface an area such as the scalp, to provide vascular support for bone and skin grafts around prosthetic materials, and to control wound infection, such as in the chest wall. Omentum will localize inflammation and wall off infection. It will not resorb when grafted. Omentum resected from the peritoneal cavity can be transplanted to an avascular area if sufficient blood vessels are available for microvascular anastomoses to the gastroepiploic artery and vein in the graft. Split-thickness skin grafts cover the omental graft.

Pedicle Flaps

Creation of a pedicle flap may be the procedure of choice to reconstruct deformities of soft tissue loss that will create or that have created an obvious aesthetic or functional disability for the patient. The pedicle, which is the attachment of elevated tissue to the donor site, must contain a vascular bundle to maintain blood supply to the tissue. Pedicle flaps are constructed from several types of tissues and sources of vascular bundles. Nasal reconstruction is commonly done this way (Fig. 40-10).

Flap survival seems to depend on a reduction in vascular resistance or an increase in arterial perfusion pressure, or both. Several techniques are used to monitor circulation in the flap intraoperatively and postoperatively.

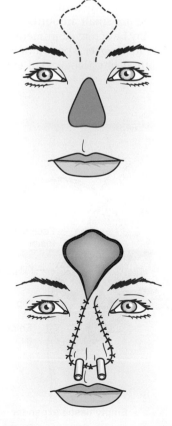

FIG. 40-10 Pedicle flap nose reconstruction.

FIG. 40-9 Split-thickness skin graft being passed through mesh dermatome. Mesh graft expands to obtain greater coverage of recipient graft area.

Arterialized Tissue Flap. A full-thickness skin graft contains a vascular bundle within subcutaneous tissue and skin. Arterialized flaps may contain the following:

- Axial vasculature from axial vessels that supply a fairly definite area of skin and subcutaneous tissue. A direct cutaneous artery flows through the length of the flap.
- Random or local vasculature from a subdermal plexus. Random flaps do not have a specific blood vessel within the flap. These are usually small flaps created around the head or neck.
- Both axial and random vasculature. A deltopectoral flap, for example, has axial vessels from the sternal region and random vessels in the deltoid area.

Depending on the proximity of the recipient site to the donor site, the pedicle flap will be one of the following types:

Rotational Flap. One end of the flap is rotated and sutured to the recipient site to cover a denuded area. The flap tissue is obtained from an area near the recipient site. Arterialized skin pedicle flaps with axial vasculature are rotated in a one-stage procedure. Random rotational pedicle flaps can be used in the face, because vascularity is sufficient in the head and neck.

Cross-Finger Flap. Tissue at the donor site is undermined and rotated to cover a small defect in an adjacent digit.

Tissue Expansion Flap. The surface of the dermal-epidermal layer can be increased by implanting a tissue expansion device subcutaneously, close to the defect (Fig. 40-11). Available in many sizes and shapes, the device has a soft, pliable silicone pouch connected by tubing to a self-sealing inflation reservoir. After insertion under a designated area for creation of the skin flap, the pouch is filled with saline by injecting small amounts into the reservoir. Rapid expansion may be achieved immediately in the head or neck area or gradually over a period of weeks to months in other areas. Natural physiologic skin expansion occurs.

The dermis stretches and thins while the epidermis duplicates itself without changing thickness. Tissue will increase to about 1½ times the width of the device.

The vascular network that develops produces more viable tissue than that of other pedicle flaps. The tissue has similar color, texture, and thickness as the recipient site. The expanded tissue is advanced or transferred to cover the defect, helping to minimize scarring and donor site deformity. Tissue expansion flaps are used for scalp and facial defects, breast reconstruction, and other soft tissue defects. They can be used for closure of large donor site defects.

Myocutaneous Flap. Pedicle myocutaneous flaps allow safe and rapid transfer of tissue over long distances to cover large defects and vital structures. They are used, for example, to close soft tissue defects in the lower extremities, to cover pressure sores on paraplegics, and to reconstruct contour after head and neck resection and mastectomy.

A myocutaneous flap incorporates the muscle with its overlying fascia, subcutaneous tissue, and skin. It receives a vigorous blood supply from the vascular pedicle that supplies the underlying muscle (see Fig. 40-6). It may include a neurovascular bundle with nerve fibers to innervate the muscle in the flap. Usually done as a one-stage procedure, myocutaneous flaps can be created from the following and other muscles:

- Trapezius
- Sternocleidomastoid
- Platysma
- Latissimus dorsi
- Pectoralis major
- Rectus abdominis
- Gracilis
- Gluteus maximus
- Tensor fascia lata
- Biceps or quadriceps femoris

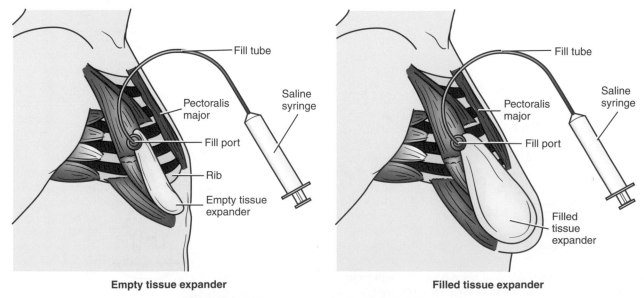

Empty tissue expander   **Filled tissue expander**

FIG. 40-11 Tissue expander under the pectoralis muscle.

Fasciocutaneous Flap. Mobilized fascia, subcutaneous tissue, and skin are transferred as pedicle flaps similarly to the way myocutaneous flaps are transferred. The donor site may need to be covered with a split-thickness graft.

Muscle Flap. A divided section of a muscle with its proximal blood supply intact can be rotated over a soft tissue defect, such as an ulcer on the leg or buttock. A vascularized muscle flap may be covered with a split-thickness skin graft.

Neurosensory Flap. Sensory nerves may remain intact in a flap with other tissues or be restored by microneural anastomosis or by nerve grafting. Preservation of nerves in a vascularized flap becomes important when sensation is critical to function, as in the hand or foot.

Omental Flap. Omentum is mobilized from the peritoneal cavity, without compromise of the vascular pedicle, to cover an infected mediastinal wound or a defect in the chest wall, such as after resection for irradiation necrosis or a neoplasm. The vascularity of donor omentum revascularizes the reconstructed chest wall recipient site. Split-thickness skin grafts, which may be mesh grafts, cover the omental flap. If additional rigidity is needed to restore the chest wall, polypropylene mesh may be sutured inside the ribcage to supplement the strength of the omental flap.

Microsurgical Free-Flap Transfer

Composite free flaps or grafts of tissue are resected and transplanted from one area of the body to another to cover a denuded area, to restore function, or to restore body contour. Microsurgical techniques allow one-stage transfer of tissues. The main artery and vein supplying donor tissues must be anastomosed to vessels in the recipient site under the operating microscope. Often two teams work simultaneously at donor and recipient sites. These are lengthy, tedious procedures, often taking many hours to complete.

Fasciocutaneous Graft. Free grafts of fascia with overlying skin, with or without underlying muscle, may be transferred. For example, temporalis fascia may be transplanted into another area in the face.

Free Muscle Graft. Free island grafts of functional muscle can be resected and transplanted to replace motor function in another area. Although only a small percentage of the graft survives, significant regeneration of muscle occurs. Free muscle, transferred by microvascular techniques and covered with a split-thickness skin graft, promotes healing of infected wounds.

Vascularized Muscle Pedicle Free Flap. In a multistaged procedure, a myocutaneous flap is raised at the donor site and allowed to develop a new, isolated vascular system before free transfer to a recipient site. The vascular system in the muscle underlying the skin flap branches out to supply the skin. At the final stage, the newly vascularized muscle pedicle is dissected free from the donor site. The donor site may need to be covered with a split-thickness graft. Under the operating microscope, arteries and veins in the flap are anastomosed to vessels at the recipient site. Two teams may complete the final stage: one prepares and closes the recipient site and the other frees the flap and closes the donor site. The advantage of this type of flap is that the surgeon can select donor skin that will best provide color, texture, bulk, and contour at the recipient site, such as on the face.

Neurovascular Free Flap. Fascicles of nerves must be anastomosed to restore sensation; in addition, microvascular anastomoses of arteries and veins are needed to maintain viability of the donor tissue. A neurovascular free flap, also known as a sensate flap, may be taken from the scapular region. Many surgeons use the scapular flap because it is easy to dissect, has a long vascular pedicle, and creates a minimal donor site deformity. Other donor sites include the medial and lateral thigh and the lateral aspect of the upper arm.

Free Autologous Bone Graft. Vascularized autografts of bone are superior in strength and are less prone to deossification and structural weakness than are conventional bone grafts. Anastomosis of the vascular bundle with a free rib, for example, may increase the chance of survival of the donor bone graft in a poorly vascularized recipient site (Fig. 40-12).

Composite Myoosteocutaneous Free Flap. A composite flap of skin, muscle, and bone provides soft tissue bulk, internal structural support, and external coverage in one-stage reconstruction of compound defects after head and neck resection. The skin and iliac crest on a vascular pedicle from the deep circumflex artery may be preferred. The scapula and tissue from the upper arm provide an alternative donor site. Or the skin, soft tissue, and latissimus dorsi muscle along with a portion of an underlying rib may be dissected free, preserving the thoracodorsal vessels for anastomosis at the recipient site. Other donor sites include the radial forearm and the fibula with the dorsalis pedis muscle.

Digital Transfer. Microneurovascular techniques are used for replantation of traumatically amputated digits. Less common is the toe-to-thumb transfer, called the free wrap-around neurovascular flap, performed when an amputated thumb cannot be salvaged. Skin from the dorsum of the foot, the great toe (including tendons and bone), and the second toe web space are transferred as a sensate flap to the hand.

After bone fixation and tendon anastomoses, arterial circulation and venous drainage are established under the microscope. Digital nerves are anastomosed to reinnervate sensation and function. Other toes can be similarly transferred for finger reconstruction.

Replantation of Amputated Parts

Replantation may be attempted to salvage a traumatically amputated digit, hand, or entire upper extremity. A severed foot or lower extremity presents more formidable problems because of the functional necessity for weight bearing. The victim of amputation of the scalp, nose, external ear, or penis also is a candidate for replantation. Using microsurgical techniques, replanted parts can survive with varying degrees of effectiveness.

Functional recovery, up to 80% of normal in some patients, may take up to a year or longer because it takes time for nerves to regenerate (approximately 2 inches [5 cm] per

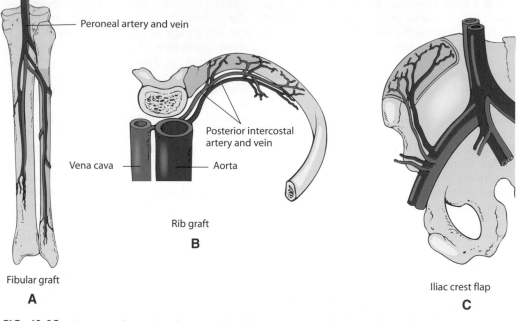

FIG. 40-12   Common donor sites for vascularized bone grafts. **A,** Fibular graft. **B,** Rib graft. **C,** Iliac crest graft.

month). A team of specialists in hand surgery or of plastic surgeons with microvascular skill is vital to success in these arduous procedures.

Correct care and preservation of the severed part for transport with the patient is also vital to success. The amputated part should be placed dry into a plastic bag, which is then sealed and immersed in crushed ice inside an insulated container (e.g., Styrofoam) to retard melting of the ice during travel. The part should not be warmed, frozen, or packed in dry ice. Rapid transport and cooling with ice will buy time.

Initial treatment involves assessment of the total patient. The patient and family should be supported emotionally but not given definitive promises in regard to outcome. The surgeon considers numerous factors when planning for replantation: the need for the part, associated disease and injuries, economic and psychologic factors, and age. Two criteria are of special significance:

1. The replanted part should have potential for being useful.
2. There should be no undue risk to the general safety of the patient if the procedure is performed.

Replantation is more successful in young patients than in older patients. Also, incomplete amputations are more successful because they have intact subcutaneous venous circulation in the skin bridges. Restoration is much more difficult in crush injuries than in sharp, clean amputations. Contraindications to replantation include:

• Prolonged warm ischemia
• Severe bruising or crushing injury
• Multiple fractures or injury at different levels in the same digit
• Associated injuries that preclude the effort

Supportive therapy after injury includes tetanus toxoid, intravenous (IV) antibiotics, fluid replacement therapy, blood products, and judicious administration of anticoagulants.

Preoperative patient preparation is in anticipation of a long procedure. The surgical procedure may take from 4 to 16 hours. The patient is placed on a gel-filled mattress. The head, scapulae, sacrum, and heels are padded. A footboard may be used and antiembolic stockings or sequential compression devices applied. An indwelling Foley catheter is inserted if the procedure will take longer than 2 hours. Most replantations of the hand are done with the patient under moderate sedation and an axillary or supraclavicular block with a long-acting agent, such as bupivacaine (Marcaine) without epinephrine. General anesthesia is used for children and may be needed for adults for a long procedure.

These surgical procedures usually involve a two-team approach: one team prepares the recipient site with the patient's hand and arm positioned on a hand table (Fig. 40-13), and the other prepares the severed or distal part.

In the operating room (OR) the amputated part is cleansed with Ringer's lactate or normal saline. Debridement of crushed tissue is carried out. Vessels are isolated for repair, and vessel patency is ensured. The basic steps of replantation of digits or extremities include (Fig. 40-14):

1. Identify proximal and distal tendons, nerves, and vessels.
2. Shorten bone within an acceptable limit necessary for tension-free repair of blood vessels, nerves, and soft tissues.
3. Stabilize the skeletal structure, such as with internal wire fixation techniques, to maintain joint continuity and fusion in functional position. Small plates and screws may be used.

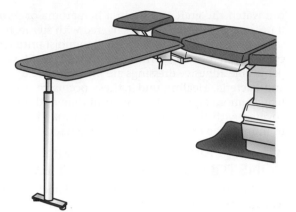

FIG. 40-13   Specialized hand table. The team is seated around the table.

4. Suture tendons and ligaments, both extensors and flexors, appropriately to lessen the junctional scar process that can inhibit motion.
5. Anastomose arteries and nerves. The vessels may be flushed with heparin solution, and systemic anticoagulants may be given. Antispasmodic agents may be needed.
6. Anastomose veins. A general rule is that more veins are anastomosed than are arteries to provide sufficient venous return and thereby minimize edema. Swelling creates pressure that impedes circulation, leading to necrosis. Leech therapy may be indicated to lessen the effects of diminished venous drainage and swelling.[1]

---

[1]www.leechesusa.com for more information.

7. Repair soft tissues and close the skin.
8. Perform a skin graft or tissue flap or transfer if necessary.

Microsurgical techniques are necessary for nerve, artery, and vein repairs of structures that have an external diameter of 1 mm or less.

To avoid constriction, a circumferential bandage is not applied. Instead, a foam bandage is used. The dressing is padded to prevent pressure sores and nerve damage. The original dressing is not changed for 10 days unless indicated.

Postoperative care is extremely important. Dressings must be checked carefully because even slight manipulation can cause great damage. Checking only the tip of the digit for circulation is not adequate. Circulation is verified by cautiously looking into the dressing to check the capillary refill, color, temperature, and drainage. A Doppler and a temperature probe may be used to evaluate arterial circulation. Patients are not permitted to smoke or chew tobacco, because nicotine is a vasoconstrictor. Constriction of vessels may reduce circulation and cause devitalization of tissue.

The many hours expended by the OR team initially to achieve a successful repair of all structures can relieve the patient of subsequent procedures. The objective is to obtain maximal return of function by minimizing permanent disability. Physical and occupational therapies are important in rehabilitation.

General Considerations for All Tissue Autografts

1. Hypothermia is avoided. Room temperature should be increased to 75° to 80° F (24° to 27° C).
2. For long procedures, the patient should be positioned on a gel pad mattress.
3. Skin may be prepped with a colorless antiseptic agent so that the plastic surgeon can see the true skin color and assess the vascularity of the donor graft.

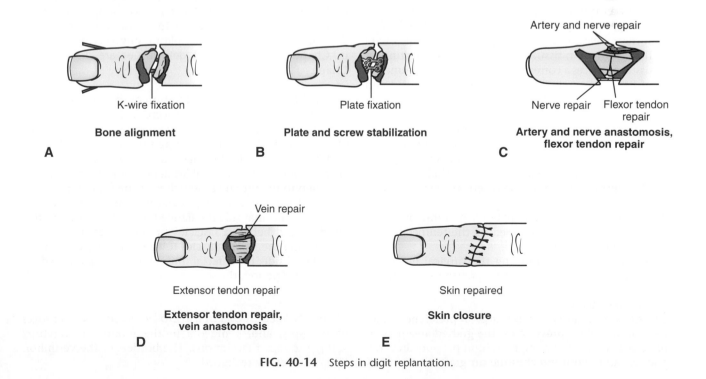

K-wire fixation	Plate fixation	Artery and nerve repair
Bone alignment	**Plate and screw stabilization**	Nerve repair Flexor tendon repair
A	**B**	**Artery and nerve anastomosis, flexor tendon repair** **C**

Vein repair

Extensor tendon repair

Extensor tendon repair, vein anastomosis

D

Skin repaired

Skin closure

E

FIG. 40-14   Steps in digit replantation.

4. Donor and recipient sites are prepped and draped separately but concurrently. Care is taken that cross-contamination does not occur from one site to the other.

5. The recipient site is covered with a sterile drape until the surgeon is ready to apply a free graft or pedicle flap if preparation of the donor site will be the first procedure. If the recipient site must be prepared to receive the donor graft or flap, the donor site is covered.

6. A separate sterile instrument table is prepared for the donor site. This includes appropriate instruments for obtaining the graft or flap and dressings for the donor site. Two surgical teams may work simultaneously.

   Place the dermatome on a separate, small sterile table, never on the recipient instrument table. Handle dermatomes carefully so that the depth gauge is not disturbed. Care is taken to disconnect the power when loading the blades to prevent accidental activation of the device.

7. Grafts are kept moist by placing them in a basin and covering with normal saline. A free flap should be kept in cool saline until the recipient site is prepared. Ice may damage tissues and should be avoided.

8. The operating microscope and appropriate microinstruments must be in readiness for microvascular and neurologic anastomoses.

9. Tissue viability must be ensured. A sterile device may be needed during the surgical procedure to identify major blood vessels underlying a graft. Assessment of the patency of vessels and perfusion of the flap is possible through several types of monitoring.
   a. *Doppler probe.* A Doppler probe is placed on the recipient site preoperatively to obtain baseline measurements for comparison with postoperative measurements. The device has an audible pulsation sound and a digital readout. Ultrasonic Doppler probes also may be used for monitoring arterial vascularity of a part.
   b. *Photoplethysmographic disc.* A disc applied to the flap surface measures reflected light from pulsatile blood flow changes in tissue. A change in blood volume in tissue produces a corresponding change in the amount of light reflected. These changes are amplified and displayed on an oscilloscope.
   c. *Fluorometer.* A fluorescing dye is injected IV, and fluorescence is measured with a fluorometer to evaluate perfusion of the flap. Fluorescein and an ultraviolet Wood's lamp are used to check patency and perfusion. The room is darkened to see fluorescence. A photomultiplier may be used to amplify skin fluorescent emission.
   d. *Thermocouple probe.* The patency of a microvascular anastomosis can be assessed by the temperature in surrounding tissues.

10. Hemostasis is obtained during the surgical procedure with the use of warm saline packs, pressure, or thrombin.

11. An ESU is used very sparingly to prevent the devitalization of tissues.

12. Dressings over grafts vary by surgeon preference. Stent fixation to obtain pressure on the grafted area may be preferred. Some plastic surgeons omit pressure dressings and use an exposure technique on grafts so that they

can watch the graft and drain a hematoma or seroma if necessary. The graft is kept covered with sterile, moist saline gauze dressings to keep the skin moist until revascularization occurs. Synthetic moisture- and vapor-permeable adhesive dressings are impermeable to liquid and bacteria. Healing under these occlusive dressings may be more rapid and less painful than at donor sites covered with fine mesh gauze. A cast may be applied to immobilize extremities for pedicle flaps.

HEAD AND NECK PLASTIC AND RECONSTRUCTIVE PROCEDURES

Some plastic surgeons specialize in head and neck oncology or reconstruction, or both. Others limit their practice to aesthetic, or cosmetic, surgery.

Soft Tissue Reconstruction

Defects in soft tissues of the face or scalp, usually as a result of trauma, may be reconstructed by advancement of tissue expanded from an adjacent area. This technique ensures consistent skin color, texture, and hair-bearing characteristics. Other types of grafts or flaps may be necessary or preferred.

Craniofacial Surgical Procedures

The plastic surgeon usually heads the multidisciplinary team that performs the complex craniofacial procedures discussed in Chapter 41. Many of the concepts developed for these procedures are applied in less-complicated surgical procedures. A variety of extracranial osteotomies, with or without bone grafts, reshape the bony framework of the face and skull. The desired aesthetic and functional results can be obtained only by painstakingly careful planning, dissection, and repositioning.

Maxillofacial and Oral Surgical Procedures

Plastic surgeons reconstruct soft tissue defects around and in the mouth that are caused by trauma or surgical resection. Those maxillofacial procedures involving bony structures that may also be performed by plastic surgeons are discussed in Chapter 41. Congenital deformities are discussed in Chapter 8.

Facial Nerve Grafting. Restoration of the quality of facial expressions in a patient with severe facial nerve paralysis can be accomplished by transfacial nerve grafting. Segments of nerve grafts are brought through tunnels across the lips from the normal side of the face to the paralyzed side. These are anastomosed to the distal facial nerve on the normal side and then to the proximal branches of the injured nerve on the paralyzed side. The overpull of the mouth and lower face toward the normal side is balanced when the nerve graft is anastomosed between fascicles of the intact facial nerve innervating the facial muscles to the same fascicles on the denervated side. If the facial muscle has been paralyzed for a prolonged period, the serratus muscle from the chest wall may be transplanted and innervated by the facial nerve.

Repair of Lacerations of the Lip or Mouth. Wound edges of the lip(s) and/or mucosa in the mouth are carefully sutured to repair lacerations. The borders of the vermilion line are carefully realigned.

Excision of Leukoplakia. Chronic irritation can result in an abnormal whitening of the mucous membrane of the lip and tongue (leukoplakia), a lesion primarily seen in heavy smokers. Sharp dissection or a CO_2 laser is used to resect a precancerous lesion.

Excision of a Lip Tumor. Excision of a lip tumor may be minor, with V-wedge excision, or extensive, depending on the stage of malignancy. Extensive lesions require a flap procedure for reconstruction.

Lip Reconstruction. Lips can be adequately reconstructed by a variety of techniques to restore sensation and motor function after trauma or surgical resection. Lip cancer is the most common type of cancer in the upper respiratory and digestive tracts. Surgical procedures to reconstruct lips may be classified as follows:

- Repair by primary closure of the remaining lip segments.
- Full-thickness cross-lip flaps from the opposite lip.
- Arterialized or myocutaneous flaps from adjacent cheek or nasolabial tissue.
- Distant flaps. Arterialized and innervated myocutaneous flaps from the forehead or deltopectoral region may be used. These require staged procedures. Free microvascular composite grafts are done in one stage.

The ideal repair yields a lip that is not tight and that has a good vermilion border, an adequate sulcus (philtrum), good sensation, and good muscle tone.

Aesthetic Procedures

Procedures are not always performed for aesthetic purposes alone. They may restore function as well as correct a facial deformity or defect.

Blepharoplasty. Redundant skin and/or protruding orbital fat is excised to correct deformities of the upper or lower eyelids of one or both eyes. Blepharochalasis (loss of elasticity of the skin of the eyelids) can occur at any age and usually is of unknown cause. Dermatochalasis primarily involves hypertrophy of the skin of the upper lids. Resection of the excessive redundant skin removes the mechanical visual obstruction caused by these two conditions. Protrusion of intraorbital fat into the lids is the most common eyelid deformity. It is often familial and is sometimes seen in patients as young as 20 years. This fat is removed from the compartments in the upper and/or lower lids to correct the deformity. This may be associated with dermatochalasis. A free graft of cartilage and mucosa from the nasal septum may be necessary to reconstruct lower eyelid defects after excision for tumor. Hypertrophy of the orbicularis muscle appears as a horizontal bulge below the lower lid margin. A skin-muscle flap resection may be performed. A surgical procedure for lifting the eyebrows will secondarily correct a hooding deformity of the upper lids caused by ptosis of the eyebrows.

These procedures are usually performed with the patient under local anesthesia. An upper lid incision is made in a natural skinfold; an incision in the lower lid is just under the eyelash line (Fig. 40-15). If the patient wears dentures, he or she should wear them to the OR because facial contour is distorted without them. The surgeon could remove too much or too little redundant skin.

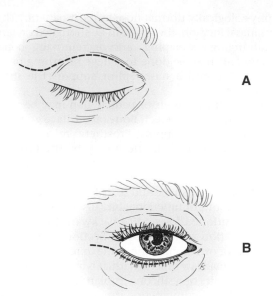

FIG. 40-15 Incisions for blepharoplasty. **A,** Upper eyelid. **B,** Lower eyelid.

Because of the proximity to the eyes, protrusion of periorbital fat may impair vision. Oculoplastic procedures may be performed by an ophthalmologist. Through a conjunctival incision, subconjunctival fat may be removed with a CO_2 laser. An eyelid procedure also may be necessary to protect the eye in a patient with facial nerve paralysis caused by trauma or tumor resection. A gold weight, between 0.05 and 1.2 g, or a spring can be inserted in the upper eyelid with the patient under local anesthesia. This protects the eye by allowing the eyelid to blink.

Otoplasty. Deformities of one or both external ears of an adult are usually the result of burns or traumatic avulsion. A segment of external ear that is partially or completely amputated often can be reattached to the remaining segment and buried beneath a flap of postauricular skin. The area over a completely severed auricular cartilage, which cannot be sutured back in place, is covered with a split-thickness skin graft initially.

Later reconstruction may include insertion of cartilage autograft taken from the patient's ribcage, a cartilage allograft, or a porous polyethylene or silicone prosthetic implant. The porous implant allows vascular and soft tissue ingrowth that reduces the risk of infection and extrusion—potential complications with a silicone implant. The graft or implant is buried beneath a segment of turned-down temporoparietal fascia. Then the area is covered with a split-thickness skin graft from the scalp or a full-thickness graft from the opposite postauricular area.

Rhinoplasty. Reshaping of the nose, although usually performed for cosmetic alteration desired by the patient, may be necessary to correct defects caused by trauma or surgical resection of neoplasms. Subtle changes with limited nasal reduction or augmentation of the nasal tip with the patient's own nasal cartilage can result in an aesthetically attractive and physiologically normal nose in most patients. Through an intranasal incision, the nose can be shortened or narrowed by rearranging, reshaping, and/or removing bone and cartilage. This may be done to relieve breathing problems. Nasal packing and a nasal splint support the structures postoperatively.

A free composite graft or pedicle flap may be necessary to close a large tissue defect. Bone or cartilage grafts may be needed for skeletal support. Prosthetic reconstruction for partial or total loss of the nose may be the procedure of choice.

Mentoplasty. The shape and size of the chin can be altered for aesthetics and/or functional bite disorders. The mandible can be repositioned forward or backward to change alignment in relation to the maxilla. Sections are removed to reduce size, or osteotomies are made to reshape the chin. An abnormally small jaw (micrognathia) is augmented with bone or cartilage grafts or a silicone implant or by advancing the mandible. Lip incompetence (inability to bring the lips together without tension) may be corrected during the same surgical procedure.

Rhytidoplasty. Commonly referred to as a face lift, rhytidoplasty involves extensive dissection from above the ear, both in front of and behind the pinna, downward along the jaw line and upper neck (Fig. 40-16, *A*). The skin is freed from underlying fascia. Wrinkles and folds caused by the normal aging process smooth out as the skin is lifted up and sutured in place. Dissection beneath the platysma muscle, referred to as the submuscular aponeurotic system (SMAS) procedure, minimizes the amount of skin undermined (Fig. 40-16, *B*). The platysma is sutured back to the mastoid (Fig. 40-16, *C*). Redundant skin is trimmed away.

A modified lift can be attained by using Contour Thread, a clear barbed suture under the skin to lift the bilateral fascial planes. Using this suture is considered minimally invasive. No excess tissue is trimmed away. Patients are advised to minimize the stress over the sutured areas for 3 months by wearing a chin strap at night and avoid traction on the tissues of the face. More discussion of Contour Thread is found in Chapter 28 located under synthetic sutures—Barbed Polydioxanone (Quill Suture, Contour Threads). This clear synthetic self-anchoring suture is approved for use by the FDA. It is used for dermal suturing without the need for knotted ends. The surface of the suture has raised barbs that are angled from the center to the ends in both directions.

Frequently other procedures, such as blepharoplasty or rhinoplasty, accompany this surgical procedure. Meticulous hemostasis is essential to prevent hematoma formation, the foremost complication of rhytidoplasty. Hypotensive anesthesia may be used to help reduce this incidence. Closed-wound suction drainage is frequently used with or without a pressure dressing applied after the surgical procedure.

Face Transplant. Surgeons in France and China performed successful partial face transplants in 2006. Full face transplants are in the planning stage at the Cleveland Clinic in Cleveland, Ohio. Traumatic injury to the face can cause massive facial tissue loss for which there is no cosmetic or functional replacement. Microvascular anastomosis has made

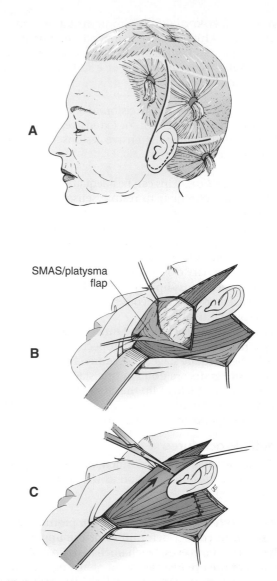

FIG. 40-16   Rhytidoplasty (face lift). **A,** Incision from above ear and in front of and behind pinna. **B,** Dissection beneath and elevation of platysma flap (submuscular aponeurotic system [SMAS] procedure). **C,** Platysma muscle is sutured back to mastoid.

free-flap allogeneic transfer possible, and antirejection drugs offer the promise of long-term take.

Soft Tissue Augmentation. Fat transplantation may be done by mini-liposuction and injection of the patient's own tissue. Fat cells are withdrawn from the lower abdomen, hips, or thighs into a syringe through a hypodermic needle. The fat then is injected into areas around the lips or eyes to smooth wrinkles or into hollow spaces in the cheeks or other facial defects. This procedure may be done in conjunction with a rhytidoplasty. The correction is not permanent, because the fat cells will die.

A purified form of bovine dermal collagen can be injected for the same purposes. A series of injections of small amounts of the collagen are deposited to fill small soft tissue defects or to smooth out wrinkles.

Hair Replacement. Hair follicles can be transplanted from the posterior aspect of the scalp to bald or balding areas. Hundreds of micrografts (4 mm) and minigrafts (4.5 mm) are implanted in staged rows over the entire bald area to change the hairline (Fig. 40-17). A new hairline can be initially established with rotational flaps from other parts of the scalp. This may necessitate tissue expansion. If hair loss is not complete, hair follicle grafts complement and thicken the existing hair. Several transplantation sessions may be necessary to achieve the final result the patient is seeking.

PLASTIC AND RECONSTRUCTIVE PROCEDURES OF OTHER BODY AREAS

Adipose Tissue

Lipectomy is an excision of excessive fat and redundant skin from the upper arms, abdomen, buttocks, thighs, or other body areas.

Liposuction. Localized areas of fat deposits are removed by suction-assisted lipectomy, known as liposuction, to alter body contours. Males and females differ in areas of localized fat deposits (Fig. 40-18). Most surgeons prefer to inject target tissue with 1% lidocaine with 1:100,000 epinephrine in saline to create a tumescent effect to plump up the fat and firm the surface. This solution also reduces blood loss during the surgical procedure. The average adult dosage range for tumescent injection should not exceed 7 mg/kg of lidocaine and in general should not total more than 500 mg.

A blunt, hollow, curved or straight metal cannula (Mercedes cannula) measuring 1.5 to 6 mm with multiple openings in the distal shaft connected to a suction machine is inserted through small skin incisions (Fig. 40-19). The cannula is moved back and forth along the axial plane, parallel to the skin surface, to bluntly dissect and aspirate cores of fat in a honeycomb pattern. This pattern allows for uniform tissue contouring. A laser beam may be used through the cannula to vaporize fat rather than suction it out. The laser diminishes bleeding by coagulating vessels. The patient's hematocrit

level decreases by 1% for each 150 mL of fat removed by conventional liposuction.

Suction-assisted lipectomy may be used in conjunction with conventional abdominoplasty. It is also used to remove fat from the neck and chin, upper arms, breasts, flanks, buttocks, thighs, knees, and ankles. It can be used to defat transfer flaps and to treat some forms of lymphedema and lipomas. The amount of fat removed should not exceed the ability of the overlying skin to contract and may be between 1500 and 2000 mL.

If tumescence is used, 2500 to 3000 mL may be removed without complications. Large fluid volume shifts follow lipectomy, so the inflow and suction contents should be monitored closely. The incisions are sutured and reinforced with wound closure strips, and compression garments are worn for 10 days to 2 weeks postoperatively to control edema and help skin remodeling.

Postoperative discharge planning should include advising the patient that each cannula port site will ooze serosanguineous fluid for a few days. Padding the bed at home is recommended. Removing and donning the compression garment can be difficult because of the tightness required for the synthetic elastic to be effective. The patient can shower with the compression garment on using a liquid antibacterial soap and dry the garment area with a cool hair dryer. If the garment is removed, the reapplication is easier if the patient's body is completely dry and body powder is applied to the skin.

Abdominoplasty. Abdominoplasty includes excising excess, lax abdominal wall skin and adipose tissue and tightening abdominal wall musculature. This is usually a cosmetic procedure referred to as a "tummy tuck." Physical discomfort or the inability to perform personal hygiene because of a large pannus that hangs like an apron over the lower abdomen and genital region may be a functional indication for the procedure. Its purpose is not to make an obese person thin. The most suitable patient is of ideal weight and in good health. Causes of the abdominal wall laxity include pregnancy, marked weight loss, and the aging process.

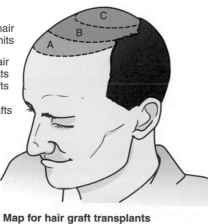

A. 1 hair follicular units

B. 2-3 hair follicular units and linear grafts

C. Linear grafts

Map for hair graft transplants

A

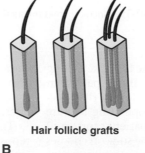

Hair follicle grafts

B

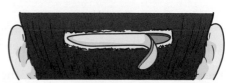

Hair strip graft

C

FIG. 40-17   Hair transplantation.

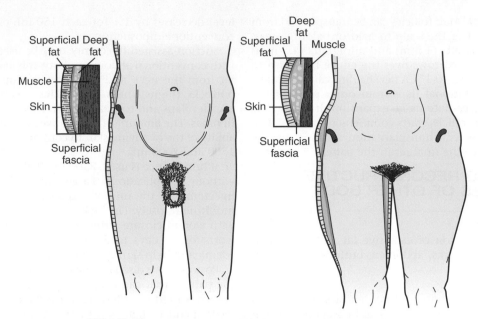

FIG. 40-18   Fat distributions differ between males and females.

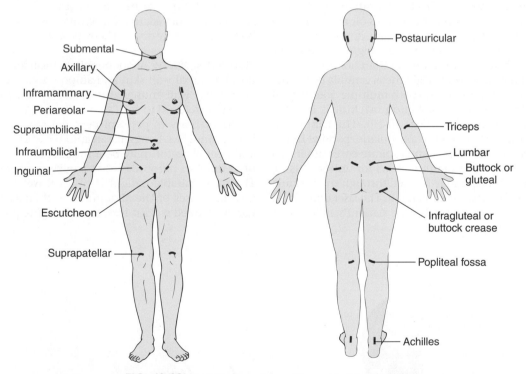

FIG. 40-19   Incision areas for suction-assisted lipectomy.

Preoperatively the primary incision line is marked along a natural skinfold using a marking pen with the patient in a standing position. After the administration of the anesthetic agent, the head and foot of the operating bed are elevated 15 to 20 degrees to anteflex the patient's torso and decrease abdominal tension (Fig. 40-20). The surgeon chooses either a low transverse incision from one anterior superior iliac crest to the other or a combination transverse–secondary vertical incision in a fleur de lis pattern (Fig. 40-21). The typical area of dissection extends subcutaneously to the costal margins and xiphoid process superiorly and to the mid- to lateral axillary lines laterally.

The umbilicus is preserved on a vascularized stalk and repositioned in the abdominal wall after the rectus muscle is tightened (plicated) and excess skin, subcutaneous tissue, and fat are resected. When wound closure is completed,

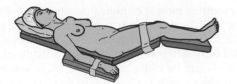

FIG. 40-20   Patient positioning for abdominoplasty.

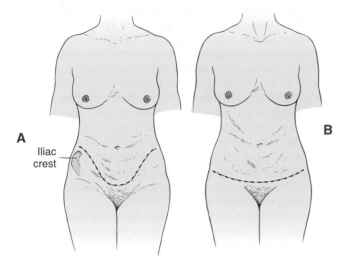

FIG. 40-21   Abdominoplasty incisions. **A,** Medial to iliac crest for patient who desires high "French cut" swimsuit. **B,** In natural abdominal skin crease fold below iliac crest.

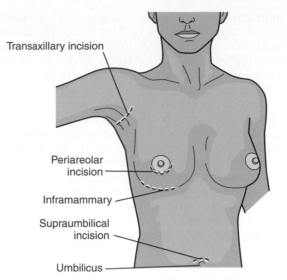

FIG. 40-22   Common incisions for breast implant placement.

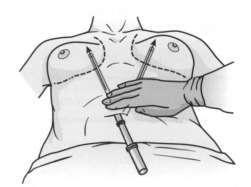

FIG. 40-23   TUBA: Transumbilical breast augmentation.

the abdominal wall should be flat and smooth. Closed suction drainage, a bulky pressure dressing, and an abdominal binder are used to prevent hematoma formation and eliminate dead space.

Postoperatively the patient is restricted to complete bed rest with the head and foot of the bed flexed for 24 hours and then may ambulate progressively.

Breast

Breasts can be enlarged, reduced, or reconstructed. Unilateral augmentation or reduction is sometimes performed to correct asymmetry of the breasts.

Augmentation Mammoplasty. A bilateral mammoplasty usually is performed for aesthetics on a woman who desires larger breasts. Inflatable implants are inserted under breast tissue or the underlying pectoralis muscles and then filled with sterile saline solution through self-sealing valves.

The breast implant can be inserted through a periareolar, transaxillary, inframammary, or supraumbilical endoscopic approach (Figs. 40-22 and 40-23). The periareolar incision, made around the outside border of the lower half of the areola, is the most difficult for insertion of the implant, but it leaves the most inconspicuous scar. The transaxillary incision in the axilla does not scar the breast. The inframammary incision, the most common, is made transversely along the submammary fold. The implant is inserted into a pocket formed between the mammary gland and pectoralis muscle or under the muscle (Fig. 40-24).

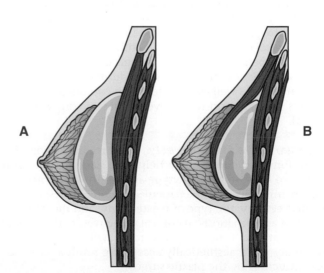

FIG. 40-24   Placement of breast implants. **A,** Placement of implant under the mammary gland and above the pectoralis muscle. **B,** Placement of implant under the pectoralis muscle.

An implant can also be inserted through a supraumbilical endoscopic approach (TUBA). This technique eliminates an incision into the breast. A single incision is made in the superior border of the inner aspect of the umbilicus. An endoscope is tunneled between the fascia and subcutaneous tissue up to the breast.

Subpectoral pockets are dissected to accommodate breast implants. The dissection can be performed bluntly or by saline balloon expansion. The endoscope permits visual placement of a deflated expander between the breast tissue and the pectoralis muscle. The expander is filled with sterile saline solution, through a fill tube, to create a pocket for the implant. After insertion through the endoscope into the pocket, the deflated implant is inflated with sterile saline solution and the fill tube is removed.

Implants are supplied sterile by the manufacturer. The manufacturer's instructions for sterilization of nonsterile implants must be followed. Sterile packages should not be opened by the circulating nurse until the surgeon selects the appropriate-size implants. Silastic sizers are frequently used to make this determination. The implant identification card should be put in the patient's chart and each implant's catalog and lot number recorded.

The woman with breast implants is not excluded from routine screening mammography programs. Additional radiologic images may be taken to visualize all of the breast tissue. Ultrasonography may be performed at the same time to confirm the integrity of the implant. Studies have shown that the risk of rupturing the implant is not increased by compression during mammography if performed according to the American College of Radiology standards.

Capsular contraction, hematoma, infection, and skin necrosis are potential complications after prosthetic implantation for breast augmentation performed either unilaterally or bilaterally. Because of reported incidences of rupture and leakage, with the possibility of the development of autoimmune disease, implants containing silicone gel are not used for breast augmentation or reconstruction unless women are enrolled in a controlled clinical study.

Explantation, or removing a ruptured or leaking silicone implant, frequently is complicated by intracapsular adhesions. Control of bleeding points is critical, to prevent silicone emboli in open blood vessels. This necessitates meticulous capsular dissection and hemostasis during removal of the implant shell, as well as irrigation with copious amounts of sterile saline solution to remove viscous silicone from the wound.

Reconstructive Mammoplasty.
Breast reconstruction after mastectomy psychologically helps the patient cope with an altered body image. The type and timing of reconstruction are influenced by the patient's psychologic response to the mastectomy, the type of mastectomy, and the patient's diagnosis and prognosis. Technical maneuvers of the general surgeon at the time of mastectomy will influence the possibility of an aesthetically acceptable result after breast reconstruction by the plastic surgeon.

To reconstruct breast contour, an implant may be inserted beneath the muscle layers at the time of subcutaneous mastectomy.

After modified radical or radical mastectomy, the wound should be well healed, the scar mature, and the skin well vascularized before implantation. A prosthesis can be implanted only when reliable skin is available to cover it. Skin flaps should be cut as thickly as is consistent with a curative mastectomy. If sufficient skin flaps are not available, the plastic surgeon may use a tissue expander or transfer a pedicle skin flap from the abdomen or back to the chest wall.

Immediate breast reconstruction, or a delay of only a few days, after a modified radical mastectomy can be psychologically advantageous in women who have small lesions and no metastases. A latissimus dorsi myocutaneous flap may be used with an inflatable implant. A vertical or TRAM island flap with the vascular bundle from the superior epigastric vessels can be used without an implant (Fig. 40-25). These flaps can also be used immediately or weeks to months after mastectomy for reconstruction. Aesthetically, the end result is a semblance of a breast in weight and consistency. The goal is fullness rather than projection from the chest. An areola and nipple complex may be constructed in a second-stage surgical procedure. Dermapigmentation (a form of tattooing) may be used to create natural color and shading resembling the nipple-areola complex.

The techniques described may be contraindicated in markedly obese patients and in some patients who do not have a sufficient amount of autogenous tissue for breast reconstruction. Another option is to place a tissue expander under the pectoralis muscle (see Fig. 40-11). When the desired

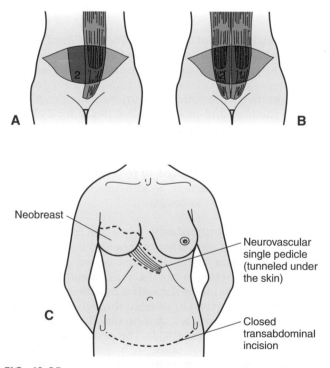

FIG. 40-25 Transverse rectus abdominis myocutaneous (TRAM) flap. **A,** Single TRAM flap with one rectus muscle used for neobreast. **B,** Both rectus muscles can be dissected for neobreasts if bilateral mastectomy is performed. **C,** Closed abdominal incision spans transversely from iliac crest to iliac crest. The neobreast remains attached to the vascular stalk to preserve viability of the breast mound created by the TRAM flap.

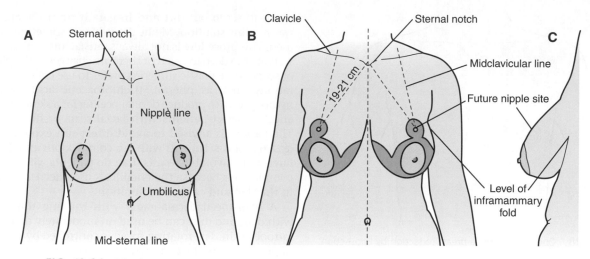

FIG. 40-26   Nipple symmetry measurement. **A,** Measurements are taken from the clavicle to the nipple. The midline is marked from the sternal notch to the umbilicus. **B,** The desired placement of the elevated nipple line is measured in a triangulated line based on the midline sternal notch. The average distance is 19 to 21 cm. **C,** The final measurement is taken laterally from the inframammary fold to the central breast anteriorly.

expansion is achieved, usually slightly larger than the other breast, the expander can be replaced with a permanent prosthesis.

One type of expander/mammary prosthesis has a detachable reservoir and tubing to convert the expander into a permanent prosthesis. If this technique is not an option and the patient does not have adequate tissue in the lower abdomen or back, transfer of a microvascular free flap may be the procedure of choice. The vascular pedicle from a transverse abdominis rectus, superior gluteal, or inferior gluteal myocutaneous free flap may be anastomosed to the axillary or thoracodorsal vessels.

Reduction Mammoplasty. Hyperplasia of the breasts is reduced by resection of skin and glandular tissue. Reduction mammoplasty is usually sought by women for comfort, as well as aesthetic improvement of body image. The nipple-areola complexes are mobilized and transferred intact with the underlying breast tissue, maintaining the blood and nerve supply (Fig. 40-26). The excess skin and glandular tissue may be excised with a scalpel, dermatome blade, or laser (Fig. 40-27). Because breast tissue is very vascular, attention to hemostasis is important. The CO_2 laser offers the advantage of coagulating small blood vessels and sealing lymphatics as tissue is incised. A hemostatic scalpel can be used for the same purposes.

Reduction of the Male Breast. Reduction of the male breast is carried out for gynecomastia, a pathologic condition that consists of bilateral or unilateral enlargement of the male breast. Gynecomastia occurs primarily after 40 years of age or during puberty and is usually related to alterations in the normal hormonal balance. All subareolar fibroglandular tissue is removed, followed by reconstruction of the resultant defect. Some surgeons perform liposuction-assisted procedures to debulk the male breast (Fig. 40-28). If liposuction is used, a compression vest is worn for 4 to 6 weeks postoperatively. Carcinoma can occur in the male breast.

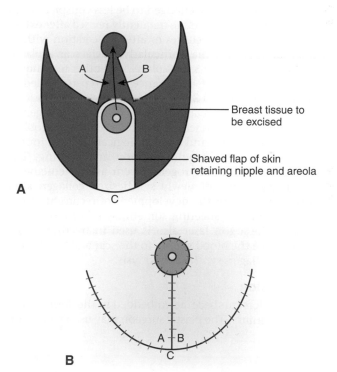

FIG. 40-27   Breast reduction. **A,** A keyhole incision is made in the breasts bilaterally. The tissue is deepithelialized and the nipple is repositioned at the apex of the keyhole. **B,** The nipple is circumferentially sutured in place. The inframammary tissue is approximated vertically, followed by closure of the inframammary fold.

Scars

Scar formation, the body's mechanism for healing wounds, is inevitable whenever skin is incised or injured. The plastic surgeon attempts to make a scar a fine line and as level and

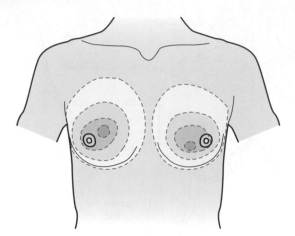

FIG. 40-28 Contours for male breast reduction by liposuction.

smooth as possible at the time of primary wound closure or as a secondary scar revision.

Scar Revision. The plastic surgeon can excise an aesthetically displeasing scar, realign wound edges, and resuture or close them with anticipation of a better cosmetic result. The direction of a scar can be changed to be less conspicuous in the natural skin lines. Scars are frequently revised after extensive reconstructive procedures or after a laceration with or without soft tissue trauma, particularly a facial scar. Z-plasty, W-plasty, M-plasty, lazy-S, Y-V–plasty, and other techniques are used to improve the appearance of a hypertrophied or prominent scar (Fig. 40-29).

Keloid formation, an abnormal deposition of collagen in healing skin wounds, presents a particularly difficult problem for the plastic surgeon and a psychological problem for the patient. Keloids may require excision and grafting. The administration of a lathyrogenic agent and colchicine to inhibit cross-linking of newly synthesized collagen after grafting may prevent the development of recurrent keloid formation. Silicone sheeting sometimes helps reduce the bulkiness. The argon laser also is used in treating keloid scars to reduce the blood supply to the scar and to alter the balance of collagen synthesis and lysis.

Dermabrasion

Dirt and cinders can become embedded in the dermis from a brushburn injury. The plastic surgeon may use a stiff nylon brush to scrub out dirt and irrigate it from the area with warm saline solution. Medical sandpaper sometimes can be used. This procedure is not always satisfactory if many pitted scars are too deep to reach or there are changes in the pigment of scars. Some plastic surgeons prefer to use chemical preparations, such as phenol, trichloroacetic acid, or alpha-hydroxy acid, to produce dermal peeling for a skin-smoothing effect in select patients with facial scars or fine wrinkles. The patient is advised to avoid direct sun exposure for at least 6 months. Patients with fair complexions and thin skin have more favorable results than do patients with dark, oily complexions because the chemicals used decrease melanin in the skin and cause discoloration.

A high-speed dermabrader with rotating tips covered with diamond dust can be used on moderately damaged or tattooed skin. The rotating speed is controlled by regulation of pressure from the compressed nitrogen gas power source. Older dermabraders have narrow bands of waterproof, steam-sterilizable sandpaper mounted on an electric, air-powered, or battery-operated drill. Care is taken by the team to wear appropriate eye protection to shield against splashes and aerosolization of blood and fluids.

Facial resurfacing also can be accomplished with the CO_2 laser. The depth of beam penetration is controlled by the focus of the beam. Full-face laser resurfacing promotes continuity of skin color and texture rather than spot removal of facial scars (Table 40-1).

Skin Cancer

Because overexposure to sunlight is the primary cause of skin cancer, most skin cancers occur on areas of the face, neck, and ears. Basal cell carcinoma, squamous cell carcinoma, and malignant melanoma are the three types of skin cancer. Certain types of nevi are skin lesions that may be precancerous and therefore should be removed. Skin lesions may be removed by the following methods:

- Excision and closure with sutures, grafts, or flaps
- Punch biopsy with closure by second intention
- Cold knife excision for frozen section
- Electrosurgical curettage and electrodesiccation
- Cryosurgery
- Laser surgery
- Radiation therapy

Mohs micrographic surgery is a technique used to excise advanced, recurrent, or poorly defined basal cell or squamous cell carcinomas of the skin with minimal excision of normal

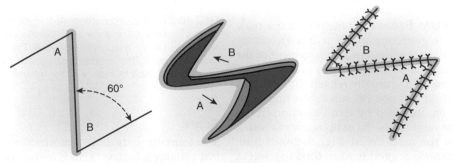

FIG. 40-29 Z-plasty technique of scar revision.

TABLE 40-1	Examples of Lasers Used for Skin Surface Modifications	
Type of Laser	Spectrum of Light	Notes
Argon	Blue-green	Used for treatment of superficial vascular lesions, pigmented areas and some inflammatory lesions; absorbed by hemoglobin
CO_2	Infrared	Has a red aiming beam to make the invisible infrared laser visible; absorbed by water
Tunable dye (Candela)	Yellow	Used to treat port-wine stains and vascular ectasia; very selective vascular destruction; absorbed by pigmented tissues
KTP:YAG	Green	Used to treat tattoos, vascular lesions, and pigmented lesions; good for removal of black, yellow, or blue; works well for dark-skinned patients; articulated arm
Alexandrite	Red	Used to treat tattoos, particularly blue, black, and green; not good for orange or yellow; fiberoptic: flexible arm

From Fortunato NM, McCullough SM: *Plastic and reconstructive surgery,* St. Louis, 1998, Mosby.
CO_2, Carbon dioxide; *KTP:YAG,* potassium titanyl phosphate:yttrium-aluminum-garnet.

tissue. The bulk of the clinically evident tumor is excised initially. Then the lesion is resected by serial tangential excision (i.e., underlying tissue layers are removed with 1- to 3-mm borders). Each layer is numbered and charted for size and location. A map of the corresponding margins of each layer is drawn. The tissue is frozen, cut into sections, and examined microscopically (Fig. 40-30).

The patient may be allowed to leave the OR and wait in a waiting room for the results. The surgeon removes additional layers of tissue or extends dissection until microscopic examination determines that all cancer cells have been removed. A map of the excisional area is created, then the wound is closed. Small wounds may be left open to heal by second intention. Others may be sutured or covered with a rotational myocutaneous flap from an adjacent area. Large denuded areas may require a split- or full-thickness skin graft. If a cartilage graft is needed, cartilage may be transferred from the auricle (pinna) of the ear to the transplant site.

Mohs surgery is not used for excision of malignant melanomas. Primary melanomas are treated according to their anatomic site and level of cutaneous penetration. A wide margin of normal tissue is excised around the melanoma. Skin grafts often are required. Regional lymph node dissection may be indicated to control metastatic disease.

BURNS

Skin and underlying tissues can be destroyed by thermal, chemical, or electrical injury. Burns are open wounds. As in other injuries, initial treatment is aimed at saving the patient's life. Then the treatment is directed toward preserving or restoring to normal, or as near normal as possible, the patient's bodily functions and appearance as rapidly as possible. Depending on the depth, extent, and location of the burn, reconstruction may extend over long periods, from months to years. The patient must be helped to accept the disfigurement; thus rehabilitation from a psychologic standpoint is important. Psychotherapy, as well as surgery and physiotherapy, may be necessary to promote as early a return to normalcy and usefulness as possible.

Classification of Burns

The severity of the injury is determined by the location and the cause of the burn. The Abbreviated Burn Severity Index

(ABSI) is a five-variable scale used to evaluate burn injury severity and the probability of survival. The five variables are sex, age, presence of inhalation injury, presence of full-thickness burn, and percentage of total body surface burned. An ABSI score of 2 to 18 is calculated by the summation of coded values for each variable. Burns are classified by depth and extent as soon after injury as possible. Many burns are a combination of depths. The depth of a burn is classified by the degree of tissue involvement:

- *First-degree superficial burn.* Only the outer layer of the epidermis is involved in a first-degree burn. Superficial erythema, redness of the skin, and tissue destruction occur, but healing takes place rapidly.
- *Second-degree partial-thickness burn.* All epidermis and varying depths of the dermis are destroyed in a second-degree burn. This is usually characterized by blister formation, pain, and a moist, mottled red or pink appearance. Hair follicles and sebaceous glands may be destroyed. Reepithelialization can occur provided that the deepest layer of the epithelium is viable. Superimposed infection can interfere with healing. Thickened scars form after healing of deep second-degree burns.
- *Third-degree full-thickness burn.* The skin, with all of its epithelial structures and subcutaneous tissue, is destroyed in a third-degree burn. This is characterized by a dry, pearly white or charred-appearing surface void of sensation. The destroyed skin forms a parchment-like eschar over the burned area. If removed or left to slough off, eschar leaves a denuded surface that can extend to the fascia. Third-degree burns require skin grafts for healing to occur unless the area is small enough for closure by reepithelialization.
- *Fourth-degree burn.* Sometimes referred to as char burns, fourth-degree burns may damage bones, tendons, muscles, blood vessels, and peripheral nerves. An electrical burn, for example, causes damage much deeper than is apparent on the skin surface. Often, necrotic muscle and bone must be excised.

Estimation of Burn Damage

Two methods are used to estimate the total percentage of body surface burned and the percentage of each degree of burn.

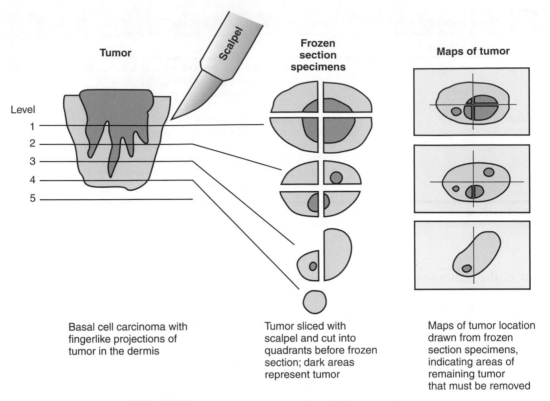

FIG. 40-30   Mohs microscopic excisional tissue mapping.

Lund-Browder Chart.
The percentage sizes of the head and lower extremities differ in infancy, childhood, and adulthood. According to the guidelines of the Lund-Browder chart (Fig. 40-31), the percentage of burn is estimated on the basis of age in addition to the anatomic location of the burn.

Rule of Nines.
The body surface of an adult can be divided into areas equal to multiples of 9% of the total body surface (Fig. 40-32).

Initial Care of the Burn Patient
Patients admitted to the emergency department with obvious burns may have multiple injuries and/or a pretrauma medical history that will complicate treatment. Initial care must include the following measures:

1. *Stop the burning process.* All clothing, jewelry, and metal and synthetic objects in contact with the patient's skin are removed.
2. *Ensure a patent airway.* The respiratory system may be damaged from inhalation of superheated air or toxic gases. Immediate nasotracheal intubation with assisted mechanical ventilation may be necessary. Soft endotracheal tubes are preferred for prolonged intubation. Tracheotomy may be required several days later for prolonged respiratory assistance if the patient cannot be weaned from the ventilator. Bronchoscopy is performed routinely to evaluate the extent of tracheobronchial damage.
3. *Establish IV fluid therapy.* Blood samples are drawn for laboratory analysis and type and crossmatching when a venipuncture or cutdown is performed to establish

an IV route for fluid and nutritional administration. Fluid and electrolyte balance must be restored as quickly as possible. Fluid, electrolytes, and protein are lost through changes in capillary permeability, causing intravascular volume shifts to interstitial tissues. Fluid shifts are directly proportional to the depth and extent of the burn.

Several formulas for determining fluid replacement have been developed to maintain plasma volume during the first 24 hours (Table 40-2). The calculated fluid replacement time begins at the time of injury, not when the patient arrives in the emergency department. A crystalloid solution of Ringer's lactate is infused initially because its hypertonic state decreases fluid loss from the intravascular space. Colloid-containing fluid, fresh frozen plasma, and other nutrients may be infused after the first 24 hours.

4. *Insert an indwelling Foley catheter.* Urine specimens are sent for analysis. Urine is checked for pH and specific gravity at frequent intervals. The hourly output is recorded. Adequate fluid replacement should maintain an output of at least 30 Ll/hr.
5. *Cleanse the wound.* All burns are treated aseptically. A mild cleansing agent, such as povidone-iodine, and warm water or saline solution are used to gently remove debris and loose, devitalized tissue. Copious amounts of water, along with appropriate neutralizing agents, are used to cleanse and irrigate chemical burns. After cleansing, wet sheets under and around the patient must be removed and dry, sterile ones applied. Nonwoven sheets specifically designed for burn care are commercially available.

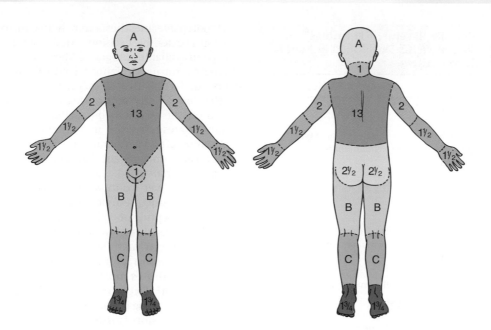

Relative percentage of areas affected by growth	Age in Years					
	0	1	5	10	15	Adult
A— ½ of head	9½	8½	6½	5½	4½	3½
B—½ of one thigh	2¾	3¼	4	4¼	4½	4¾
C—½ of one leg	2½	2½	2¾	3	3¼	3½
Total percent burned			2°⁺		3°⁻	

FIG. 40-31   Lund-Browder chart to determine relative percentage of areas of burns on child's body.

6. *Estimate the percentage and depth of the burn.* Definitive treatment may be completed in the emergency department, or the patient may be transported to an immersion tank for further cleansing and debridement or to the OR for initiation of further therapy as indicated by assessment of the burn. The burned area is covered with sterile or clean linen for transfer of the patient from the emergency department.
7. *Assess the patient's preexisting medical history and other injuries.* The patient may have a chronic illness, such as diabetes or heart disease that must be stabilized as part of the treatment regimen. Withdrawal from alcohol or drugs may cause physiologic disturbances. The patient may have suffered other injuries in the accident causing the burn. Abuse may be suspected, particularly in a child or older person. Appropriate interventions must be taken. The burn may not be the first priority if, for example, the patient has a head injury, ruptured internal organs, or fractures.
8. *Prepare the patient for transport.* The patient may go from the emergency department directly to a burn unit, the OR, or some other care area. The attending physician may initiate therapy before referral to a plastic

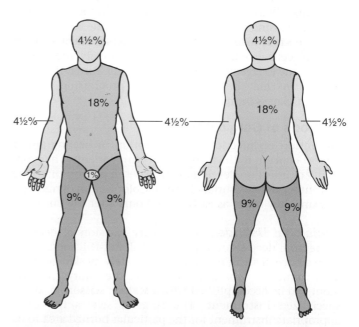

FIG. 40-32   Rule of nines chart to estimate burn injury to an adult.

TABLE 40-2	Fluid Replacement Formulas* for Burn Patients Developed at Major Burn Centers

First 24 Hours	Second 24 Hours
PARKLAND HOSPITAL	
Crystalloid	
4 mL Ringer's lactate/% burn/kg	Dextrose 5% in water
One half during first 8 hours	maintenance
One half during next 16 hours	
Colloid	
None	0.5 mL/% burn/kg
BROOKE ARMY HOSPITAL	
Crystalloid	
2 mL Ringer's lactate/% burn/kg	Dextrose 5% in water
One half during first 8 hours	maintenance
One half during next 16 hours	
Colloid	
None	0.5 mL/% burn/kg
MASSACHUSETTS GENERAL HOSPITAL	
Crystalloid	
1.5 mL Ringer's lactate/% burn/kg	None specified
One half during first 8 hours	
One half during next 16 hours	
Colloid	
0.5 mL/% burn/kg	None specified
None during first 4 hours	
One half during second 4 hours	
One half during next 16 hours	

*Formula is calculated as percent of total body surface (% TBSA) × each kilogram (kg) of body weight × milliliters (mL) of fluid.

surgeon. If available, hyperbaric oxygen (HBO) therapy may be used. HBO produces marked vasoconstriction, decreasing the loss of serum through the burn surface. This may reduce the need for fluid replacement. Oxygen in cells around the burn may positively affect burn tissue to regenerate and begin healing. Partial-thickness burns may be prevented from progressing to full-thickness burns.

Methods of Surgical Treatment

Prevention of infection and promotion of healing are of utmost concern in the treatment of burn patients. The probability of infection developing increases in proportion to the percentage of body surface burned. Colonization of microorganisms may begin as early as 24 hours after the burn.

Excisional Debridement. Primary excision of necrotic tissue from deep second-degree and all full-thickness third-degree burned areas, followed immediately by skin grafting, is performed as soon as possible after the injury. Debridement can be accomplished with a scalpel, scissors, or other specialized instrument. The surgeon selects the most appropriate instrument for the particular burned area to be excised. Layers of burned tissue are removed sequentially until capillary bleeding indicates that tissue is viable.

Hypotensive anesthesia may help control massive blood loss during extensive excisions. Mesh grafts are frequently used to expand available autografts. Micro–skin grafting is another alternative for maximizing a split-thickness autograft. The donor skin is cut with scissors into tiny particles that are placed on the dermal side of an allograft. This dermal surface is placed on the recipient burn site. The skin particles grow together to resurface the area; then the allograft is rejected.

An allograft or xenograft may be applied to temporarily cover an area until regeneration proceeds or sufficient autografts can be harvested. Skin substitutes also are available to temporarily cover wounds, both recipient and donor sites. A composite silicone-nylon membrane with a chemically bonded polypeptide of collagen (Biobrane) will adhere to the wound surface to inhibit infection and control fluid loss. Another artificial material incorporates a layer of bovine hide collagen onto a layer of silicone. These biologic dressings and skin substitutes must be changed periodically.

Tangential Excision. Burned tissue is excised until normal dermal tissue is reached below the depth of the wound. Tangential excision is usually the procedure of choice for deep partial-thickness burns of the dorsum of the hands or on the arms or legs. It is advantageous to minimize contractures. The wound base, containing some viable dermal structures necessary for regeneration, is covered with a split-thickness autograft. Early tangential excision and grafting in one procedure for body surface burns can reduce mortality and septic complications and shorten hospitalization.

Escharectomy. Full-thickness eschar is excised down to the fascia when viable tissues in more superficial layers are not evident, except on the hands, neck, or face. All denuded areas created by excision are covered with a biologic dressing for 3 to 5 days. They are then grafted with full-thickness autografts. Frequently, split-thickness mesh grafts must be used to spread over large areas and allow seepage of serous fluids. These are not placed on the face and neck or over joints. If sufficient skin is not available for autografting, allografts or xenografts continue to be used as biologic dressings for short periods. They are changed every 3 to 5 days.

Other Surgical Procedures. During the course of hospitalization, a burn patient may come to the OR for one or many procedures.

Escharotomy. Shrinkage of eschar may occur and cause a tourniquet effect in circumferential burns of the extremities or thorax. Bilateral incisions through the eschar, not including the fascia, are made to improve circulation to a lower extremity. Multiple incisions on the chest wall relieve respiratory distress. Sites of incisions avoid major peripheral nerves to prevent irreversible neurologic complications.

Fasciotomy. If adequate decompression does not occur after escharotomy, the incision may be extended into underlying fascia. Fascia may need to be incised in the arm if compromised circulation is evident.

Amputation of Digits. Amputation may be necessary to control infection in the extremity and prevent septicemia if escharotomy is unsuccessful.

Debridement. Debridement of underlying tissues helps prevent extension of tissue loss. Nonviable tendons, cartilage, or bone may be excised, such as from the hand, ear, or skull.

Full-Thickness Skin Grafts. With or without tarsorrhaphy, full-thickness skin grafts are used to prevent contracture of the eyelids. The cornea must be protected from exposure.

Split-Thickness Skin Grafts. Autografts are applied to debrided areas as rapidly as possible. The hands and face are the first priority to restore function; joints and flexion creases are second to prevent contractures; and the extremities and trunk are the lowest priority. Skin from donor sites is cut thin if the site will be used again. Mesh grafts are frequently used to cover very large surfaces or irregular areas such as the perineum. Grafts are held in place with staples or sutures and dressings to achieve apposition and immobilization.

Tissue Expansion. If sufficient normal skin is available, a tissue expander may be placed beneath subcutaneous tissue to broaden the width for future use as a local flap to cover an adjacent burned area after excision of scar tissue or for better closure of the donor site.

Myocutaneous Flaps. Myocutaneous flaps, either on a pedicle or by free microvascular transfer, may be used in the reconstruction of burn wounds.

Biologic Dressing Changes. Instead of leaving a biologic dressing in place until rejection, with attendant inflammatory reaction, a biologic dressing is usually replaced every few days until the area is ready for an autograft or skin for an autograft is available. Biologic dressings may be allografts of human skin from a living or cadaver donor, placental or amniotic membranes, or a xenograft of porcine skin. Porcine dressings frequently are applied initially on second-degree burns as a temporary dressing or used in conjunction with extensive excisional therapy. Synthetic skin substitutes may be preferred. A biologic dressing is used for several reasons:

- It helps control infection by covering denuded areas.
- It prevents loss of serum.
- It decreases pain.
- It seems to stimulate the formation of epithelium in dermis under it.
- It promotes growth of granulation tissue.

Dressing Changes. Occlusive dressings, if used, must be changed frequently to control infection harboring under them. An antimicrobial or chemotherapeutic agent may be applied as an integral part of the dressing. The following considerations apply:

1. Silver sulfadiazine (Silvadene) cream applied directly to the burned area makes removal of a dressing less painful and does not disturb the healing process as it is removed. It is an effective topical antimicrobial and produces no metabolic side effects; some patients have developed neutropenia and delayed wound healing after its use.

   Fresh cream is applied after cleansing and debridement. A layer of fine mesh gauze is laid over it (unless the open-exposure method will be used for further healing). Then soft, absorbent material, such as fluffed gauze, and a preformed splint may be used. These are held in place by a cotton elastic bandage. An occlusive dressing may be used to hold a hand, foot, or joint in functional position. Silver sulfadiazine is not used if the patient has a sulfa allergy.

2. Mafenide acetate (Sulfamylon) cream penetrates intact eschar rapidly and is quite successful in reducing bacterial counts to optimal levels for skin grafting. Application directly on the burned area is painful for the patient after cleansing and debridement. It may cause maceration under the dressing. Absorption may result in metabolic acidosis; thus the acid-base balance must be closely monitored. Prolonged use may lead to renal or pulmonary complications.

3. Silver nitrate solution is used infrequently. After cleansing and debridement, multiple-thickness dressings are applied to the area. These are kept saturated with 0.5% silver nitrate solution and changed every 12 hours. For debridement, sterile distilled water is used for irrigation because saline may cause the precipitation of silver salts. It is ineffective in treating established wound infection because it does not penetrate intact eschar. Care is taken to avoid splashing silver nitrate solution onto walls and floors, because staining can occur. If disposable drapes and gowns are not used, stained linen must be laundered separately from other linen.

Serial Biopsy Cultures. Through two linear incisions, a biopsy of tissue, including subcutaneous fat, is excised for culturing. This is done every 2 or 3 days, until the eschar begins to separate, to monitor the colonization of microorganisms in the wound. The results of serial biopsy culture enable the surgeon to make decisions specific to the therapeutic needs of the patient. An antimicrobial or chemotherapeutic topical agent is selected or changed according to these results.

Treatment of Curling's Ulcer. Gastrointestinal complications may occur anytime from the early postinjury period through rehabilitation. Complaints must be carefully evaluated. The patient who develops massive bleeding from a stress ulcer in the stomach and duodenum (Curling's ulcer) must be operated on. Vagotomy with antrectomy is most frequently performed by a general surgeon.

Treatment of Marjolin Ulcer. An ulceration caused by malignant changes (Marjolin ulcer) can develop in the surface area of a burn scar. As long as 20 years after the burn, a prolonged ulceration can lead to squamous cell carcinoma of the skin. The ulcer should be excised.

Environmental Considerations for Burn Patients

1. Environmental control is perhaps the essence of burn therapy. The environment must protect the wound from further injury and microbial invasion. A burn wound is always potentially contaminated until epithelialization occurs. Open exposure of the wound to room air may be the choice of the plastic surgeon for select patients. Regardless of the method of treatment, the following adjuncts are used—if the equipment is available—in the care of burn patients, in addition to strict adherence to all of the principles of aseptic technique.

   a. Reverse isolation technique may be practiced to protect the patient, whose resistance is low, from infection from personnel. Caps, masks, shoe covers, sterile gowns, and sterile gloves are worn by all personnel attending the patient. This may be referred to as protective isolation.

   b. Laminar, or downward unidirectional, airflow away from the wound helps minimize airborne contamination.

c. A plastic isolator protects the patient. Personnel do not directly enter this isolation unit. Patient care is given through clear plastic access walls. The environment around the patient inside the isolator is controlled at 90° F (32° C) and 94% relative humidity to conserve heat loss by evaporation.

2. Patients with extensive burns may be placed on a Stryker frame or a CircOlectric bed specially designed to facilitate handling and turning. They are transported to the OR on these frames or beds. Patients must be turned slowly and gently because they are often hypovolemic after the injury.

3. Hypothermia must be prevented. The patient's thermoregulatory mechanism is altered by the destruction of skin that normally acts as an insulator. Heat loss is the greatest single problem the burn patient faces in the OR.

   a. The room temperature should be increased to between 80° and 90° F (27° and 32° C) with low relative humidity of about 30% to 40%.

   b. The OR must be ready to receive the patient directly from the burn unit. The patient should not wait in a cool holding area or corridor. Concern is for the patient's thermoregulation and potential for infection.

   c. A warm hyperthermia blanket should cover the operating bed. The patient should be exposed as little as possible. Cover with warm blankets.

   d. The patient's temperature should be monitored with a rectal or esophageal probe.

   e. Solutions should be warmed before irrigation or infusion.

   f. Operating during nighttime hours is advantageous for the patient because the normal schedule for oral intake is not interrupted.

4. Hypnosis and biofeedback techniques can reduce potential postanesthetic complications when many surgical procedures are necessary to achieve acceptable functional and aesthetic results after a burn. The OR environment must be quiet to be conducive to hypnotic suggestions given to the patient.

After the initial assessment of a severely burned patient, a prolonged period of treatment begins. A multidisciplinary team must coordinate the treatment plan to achieve the best possible clinical outcome for the patient. As with all plastic surgery patients, both physiologic support and psychosocial support are essential to successful rehabilitation.

Bibliography

Adams DC et al: The running bolster suture for full-thickness skin grafts, *Dermatol Surg* 3(1):92-94, 2004.

Batra RS: Surgical techniques for scar revision, *Skin Therapy* 10(4):4-7, 2005.

Chepeha DB et al: Leech therapy for patients with surgically unsalvageable venous obstruction after revascularized free tissue transfer, *Arch Otolaryngol* 128(8):960-965, 2002.

Dixon P et al: Transumbilical breast augmentation, *AORN J* 72(4):615-625, 2000.

Fortunato NM, McCullough SM: *Plastic and reconstructive surgery*, St. Louis, 1998, Mosby.

Goodman T: *Core curriculum for plastic and reconstructive surgical nursing*, ed 3, Pitman, NJ, 1998, American Society of Plastic and Reconstructive Surgical Nurses.

Gore DC et al: Association of hyperglycemia with increased mortality after severe burn injury, *J Trauma* 51(3):540-544, 2001.

Harcourt D, Rumsey N: Psychological aspects of breast reconstruction: A review of the literature, *J Adv Nurs* 35(4):477-487, 2001.

Homicz MR, Watson D: Review of injectable materials for soft tissue augmentation, *Facial Plastic Surg* 20(1):21-29, 2004.

Mendez-Eastman S: Full-thickness skin grafting: A procedural review, *Plastic Surg Nurs* 24(2):41-47, 2004.

Moran SL et al: TRAM flap breast reconstruction with expanders and implants, *AORN J* 71(2):354-362, 2000.

Moss R et al: Body contouring with ultrasound-assisted lipoplasty, *AORN J* 71(2):370-385, 2000.

Nouri K, Rivas MP: A primer of Mohs micrographic surgery: Common indications, *Skin Med* 3(4):191-196, 2004.

Chapter 41

Otorhinolaryngologic and Head and Neck Surgery

CHAPTER OBJECTIVES

After studying this chapter, the learner will be able to:
- Identify the pertinent anatomy of the ear, nose, and throat.
- Describe the care of the patient having an otorhinolaryngologic procedure.
- List the main types of hearing loss and the treatments.
- Discuss the psychologic effects of head and neck surgery.
- List the precautions of caring for the patient with a tracheostomy.

CHAPTER OUTLINE

KEY TERMS AND DEFINITIONS

Anomaly   Abnormal development.
Cleft   A separation of tissue.
Glossoptosis   Prolapsed tongue.
Gnathia   Jaw structure.
Suture   Joint between skull bones that ossifies with age under normal circumstances.

SUPPLEMENTAL MATERIAL ON EVOLVE WEBSITE   *evolve*

http://evolve.elsevier.com/BerryKohn
- Content Updates
- Glossary
- Full Set of Perioperative Flash Cards
- Interactive Key Term Flash Cards
- Student Activities
- Tips for the Scrub Person and Circulating Nurse: Myringotomy, Tonsillectomy and Adenoidectomy, Radical Neck Dissection
- WebLinks

HISTORICAL BACKGROUND

Recognition of abnormal conditions of the ear, nose, and throat began in early times. Some of the first permanent records are attributed to the Egyptians. Breathing was thought to occur through the ears via the eustachian tubes. Therefore, attempts were made to remedy deafness and ear discharges. The study of anatomy of the ear, nose, and throat antedated the Christian era, leading to the practice of primitive procedures in India.

Hippocrates realized that irregular teeth could cause various mouth and ear disorders. He also recognized otitis media, as well as the fact that congenital deafness was incurable.

GENERAL CONSIDERATIONS IN EAR, NOSE, AND THROAT PROCEDURES

Surgical procedures of the structures of the head and neck region are not within the province of any one surgical specialty. Subspecialists from many disciplines, most notably general surgeons, plastic surgeons, otolaryngologists, and dentists, limit their surgical practice to specific types of problems involving areas of the head and/or neck. Training in these subspecialties is included in specialty postgraduate programs.

Otorhinolaryngology has traditionally been concerned with research and surgical treatment of diseases of the ear *(oto)*, nose *(rhino)*, and throat *(laryngo)*. Advances in scientific knowledge, diagnostic capabilities, and technology have broadened the scope of this field, which has led to subspecialization. General otorhinolaryngologists, commonly called ear, nose, and throat (ENT) surgeons, practice within the total scope of this specialty. Other surgeons confine their practice to one of the subspecialties: otology, facial surgery, or head and neck oncology. The certifying body for this specialty is the American Board of Otolaryngology, Head and Neck Surgery.

Dental and skeletal deformities of alignment and function coexist with aesthetic appearance. These deformities may be congenital, or they may be caused by trauma or disease. They may interfere with breathing, eating, swallowing, speaking, seeing, or hearing. A multidisciplinary team of surgical specialists is often required to reconstruct complex deformities. This team may be all-inclusive with a plastic surgeon, neurosurgeon, oral surgeon, orthodontist or prosthodontist, otolaryngologist, ophthalmologist, and general surgeon; or it may be limited to two or three specialists. The team may also include a radiologist, anesthesia provider, psychiatrist, speech pathologist, and social worker, plus, of course, the patient care staff. A team includes all of the specialties needed for complete preoperative assessment, intraoperative care, and postoperative rehabilitation of the individual patient.

Specific considerations include:
1. Preoperative explanations and postoperative instructions are vital to the outcome. For example, after ear or nasal procedures the patient must avoid blowing the nose, which would force air up the eustachian tube, potentially causing infection; force air through the incision; or dislodge a graft. To sneeze, both the nose and mouth should be open.
2. Communication is a major problem for patients with loss of hearing or voice. Touch is an effective means of conveying concern and letting the patient know he or she is not abandoned. Pencil and paper or a Magic Slate can be useful for the patient to communicate.
3. Care with antiseptic solutions is necessary because they are very painful and irritating if they are allowed to touch a perforated eardrum or get into the eyes. Some solutions, such as chlorhexidine or hexachlorophene, can cause permanent damage. Consult the manufacturer's recommendations before use.
4. The patient may experience anxiety with drapes over the head. Air and oxygen (6 to 8 L/min) administered during the otologic procedure afford relief. Care is taken not to permit the use of cautery in an oxygen-rich environment. Oxygen is combustible.

    Some surgeons prefer a turban-style head drape. Figure 41-1 depicts the method used to create a turban from a drape.

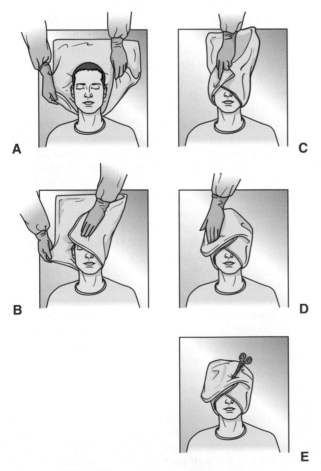

FIG. 41-1 Making a head drape turban.

5. Although a surgical area, such as the oral cavity, is often contaminated, sterile equipment and sterile technique are preferred to avoid introducing blood-borne exogenous microorganisms.
6. Anesthesia is mainly local. Use of local anesthesia minimizes bleeding and postoperative discomfort in addition to affording the surgeon observation of patient response. It allows patient cooperation. The presence of an endotracheal tube during general anesthesia can distort features during the surgical procedure.
    a. A qualified perioperative nurse monitors vital signs and the electrocardiogram (ECG) in the absence of an anesthesia provider. The nurse records the amount of local anesthesia administered and documents the patient's intraoperative responses.
    b. Patients undergoing local anesthesia may wear pajama-type bottoms or underpants to the operating room (OR) in some facilities.
7. Microsurgical otologic and laryngeal procedures, endoscopies, and laser procedures commonly require general anesthesia.
    a. The patient is intubated to maintain the airway and prevent aspiration of blood.
    b. The anesthesia machine may be positioned near the patient's side or feet. The endotracheal tube is taped; all connections must be tight, and tubes must be unkinked. The anesthesia provider usually sits alongside the operating bed (Fig. 41-2).
    c. Eyelid edema caused by facial trauma may expose the conjunctiva. Lubricate with ophthalmic ointment or artificial tears to minimize corneal damage.
8. Various solutions and medications are on the table. Each container should be accurately and clearly labeled for foolproof distinction between, for example, cocaine, lidocaine, and epinephrine.
9. Illumination is provided by the overhead spotlight, the operating microscope, the endoscope, or the surgeon's fiberoptic headlight. Some want the room darkened.
10. Instrumentation is varied to suit the area. It includes very delicate, small endoscopic and microsurgical implements in addition to bone instruments because of the extensive involvement of cartilage and bone in the facial structures and skull. These areas have relatively little soft tissue. Many instruments are angulated to permit insertion without obscuring visualization.
11. Special care with electric appliances is indicated. Electrocoagulation is used to control oozing. Compressed air or nitrogen drills with a foot-pedal control are used on bone, such as the mastoid area. A number of drills for extremely fine work, such as stapes sculpturing, are powered by small electric motors fitted into a handpiece.
12. Various types of fiberoptic endoscopes with appropriate accessories are used. The diameter of aspirating tubes and forceps is small enough to pass through and the length is long enough to extend beyond the end of the scope. The lighting mechanism and all accessories should be checked for working order before the patient is brought to the room.

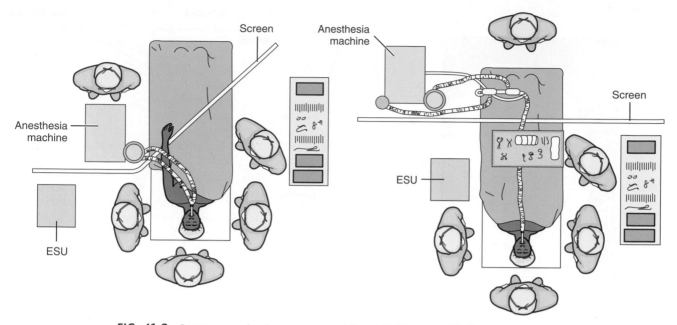

FIG. 41-2   Room setup plan for ear, nose, and throat (ENT) cases. *ESU,* Electrosurgical unit.

13. Cryosurgery may be used to destroy tissue in accessible areas, especially those that bleed profusely if incised.

14. CO_2 lasers are used to vaporize tissue. Argon lasers coagulate tissue by heat generation. Potassium titanyl phosphate (KTP) lasers coagulate to shrink or debulk tissues. Neodymium:yttrium-aluminum-garnet (Nd:YAG) lasers cut and coagulate to minimize bleeding. Appropriate instrumentation and attachments must be available for each type of laser. Laser surgery is usually done in conjunction with the operating microscope or endoscope. All safety precautions are taken to avoid ignition and injury when a laser is used.

15. Microsurgical techniques are used because they facilitate distinction between normal and diseased tissue and allow more accurate dissection.

16. Sponges and compressed patties are relatively small and are a distinct hazard when blood-soaked, because they can occlude an airway. All items used in the OR are counted or accounted for in their entirety at the end of the procedure.

17. One or two drops of blood can obscure a microsurgical field. Hemostatic aids should be ready at all times. Gelfoam pledgets soaked in 1:1000 epinephrine are used frequently. Handle tissue grafts and gelatin sponges with forceps—not the hands.

18. Irrigation equipment and solution at body temperature should be available to remove bone dust, clean burrs, and rinse suction apparatus. Cannulas with very fine suction tips should be irrigated constantly to avoid blockage.

19. Suction should be available at all times and should include several patent cannulas. The degree of suction should be variable. Suction-irrigators are used with sinus endoscopes.

20. Tissue grafts must be kept from drying out before use. A convenient method is to place the graft on a moist cellulose sponge in a sterile, covered Petri dish. Some surgeons intentionally dry a temporalis fascia graft to facilitate handling. This type of graft may also be flattened and thinned in a small press.

21. Many procedures are done with the patient in a slight reverse Trendelenburg's position or with a roll under the shoulders. Some surgeons prefer to have the patient in a modified beach-chair position. This helps anatomic positioning and controls bleeding.

EAR

Anatomy of the Ear

The structures of the outer and inner ear (Fig. 41-3, *A* and *B*) are concerned with two functions:
1. Hearing (i.e., receiving sound, amplifying it, and transmitting it to the brain for interpretation)
2. Maintaining body equilibrium

Anatomically, the ear is divided into three parts: external, middle, and inner.

External Ear. The external, or outer, ear consists of the auricle, or pinna, composed of cartilage except for the lobe; skin; and the external auditory canal. The meatus of the auricle leads, via the ear canal, to the tympanic membrane or eardrum. This membrane separates the external and the middle ear. A color change of the translucent eardrum, visible through a speculum, may be indicative of middle ear disease. The outermost lining of the tympanic membrane is derived from tissue of the ear canal. The inner lining is continuous with the middle ear mucosa. The eardrum protects the middle ear but may be perforated by injury or pressure built up in the middle ear by infection.

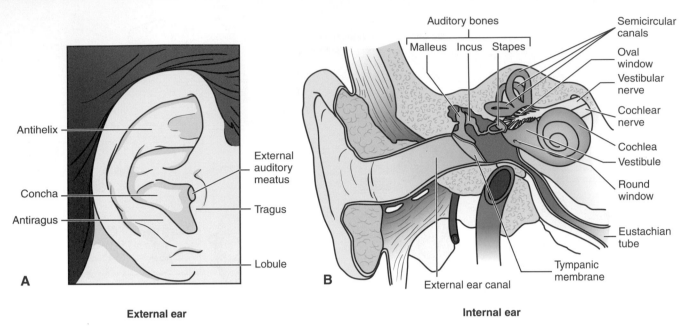

FIG. 41-3   **A,** Anatomy of the outer ear. **B,** Anatomy of the inner ear.

Middle Ear. The middle ear consists of the tympanic cavity, a closed chamber that lies between the tympanic membrane and the inner ear. Within this cavity are the three smallest bones in the body—an ossicular chain comprising the malleus, incus, and stapes. They resemble a hammer, anvil, and stirrups, respectively. The malleus, which is attached to the eardrum, joins the incus, the extremity of which articulates with the stapes, the innermost bone. The footplate of the stapes fits in the oval (vestibular) window, an opening in the wall of the inner ear.

The bones of the ossicular chain must be able to move mechanically to conduct sound from the eardrum to the inner ear. The round (cochlear) window, also between the middle and the inner ear, equalizes pressure that enters through the oval window.

The middle ear opens into the nasopharynx by way of the eustachian tube. Normally closed during swallowing or yawning, the eustachian tube aerates the middle ear cavity. This mechanism is essential for adequate hearing.

Posteriorly the middle ear exits to the mastoid process. This inferior projection of the temporal bone is a honeycomb of air cells lined with mucous membrane. Because the antrum of the mastoid process connects with it, middle ear infection may produce mastoiditis. The middle ear is situated in the tympanic portion of the temporal bone; the inner ear is situated in the petrous portion, which integrates with the base of the skull. The tympanic portion also forms part of the ear canal.

Inner Ear. The end organs of hearing and equilibrium are situated in the inner ear. The two main sections—cochlear and vestibular—have distinct, although coordinated, functions. The cochlea, a bony spiral, relates to hearing. The vestibular labyrinth, which is composed of three semicircular canals, relates to equilibrium. These structures house two separate fluids—endolymph and perilymph—which nourish and protect the hearing receptors. Neuroepithelium of the organ of Corti, the end organ of hearing, holds thousands of minute hair cells, which respond to sound waves that enter the cochlea via the oval window. Neuroepithelium of the vestibular portion also contains hair cells. Rapid head motion produces current in the endolymph that may result in nausea or vertigo. The eighth cranial (vestibulocochlear) nerve governs reflexes to muscles to maintain equilibrium and controls hearing.

Proximal Structures. The middle and the inner ear are adjacent to many important structures. The seventh cranial (facial) nerve is enclosed in a bony canal running through the tympanic cavity and mastoid bone. The meninges of the temporal lobe of the brain are also near the middle ear and the mastoid. Facial paralysis, meningitis, and intracranial infection, such as brain abscess, are potential complications of ear infection.

The major blood vessels are the internal carotid artery and internal jugular vein, as well as the lateral sinus. Thrombosis and infection of the lateral sinus of the dura mater are potentially lethal complications of otitis media, with or without mastoiditis.

Physiology of Hearing

Sound or pressure waves enter the auricle. They pass along the ear canal to the tympanic membrane. The vibration of the waves is transmitted across the middle ear sequentially by the ossicles. Amplification of sound is enhanced to some extent by mechanical action of the ossicles but mainly by aerial ratio. A large volume of sound wave pressure from the tympanic membrane funnels to a small reactive area, the stapedial footplate, intensifying sound. At the footplate of the stapes, sound pressure is transferred to the inner ear via the oval window. The hair cells of the organ of Corti are set in motion by disturbance of the inner ear fluids as sound wave pressure moves from the oval to the round window. Mechanical energy is converted to electrical potential, which is delivered to the brain along the eighth cranial nerve. The brain interprets the impulse (sound) as hearing.

Pathology of Hearing

Hearing affects the quality and quantity of interpersonal interactions. It is a major sense for communicating within one's environment. Loss of hearing therefore affects social relationships. The type of deafness or hearing loss in varying degrees may result from the following:

1. Disease, such as otosclerosis, in which changes in the bony capsule of the labyrinth occur. Otosclerotic bone invades the stapedial footplate, resulting in its fixation and ultimate inability to vibrate in the oval window. Hearing loss is gradual but progressive. This type of deficiency can be surgically corrected when auditory nerve endings are not destroyed.
2. Trauma, such as a perforated eardrum, requiring repair to restore function and aerial ratio.
3. Infection, usually controlled by antibiotics. Although it is more common in children, infection may also occur in adults. It may cause accumulation of fluid in the middle ear. Mastoiditis results from extension of otitis media.
   a. Serous otitis media may result from obstruction of the pharyngeal orifice of the eustachian tube. If blocked, for example, by hypertrophied adenoid tissue, infection, or allergic swelling, the eustachian tube is unable to equalize pressure because air cannot enter the middle ear from the pharynx. The vacuum or negative pressure thus created causes serum to be drawn into the tympanic cavity from blood vessels in the middle ear mucosa. Recurrent otitis media may require drainage of purulent exudate if conservative treatment fails.
   b. Acute otitis media may require drainage of purulent exudate if conservative treatment fails.
   c. Chronic otitis media with or without mastoiditis may follow recurrent otitis media with tympanic membrane perforation. It can produce a chronically draining ear.

Differential Diagnosis. Measurements that compare bone conduction with air conduction are important in differential diagnosis. Bone conduction refers to hearing as transmitted through the skull; air conduction refers to transmission of sound waves from the tympanic membrane to the inner ear via air. Hearing loss caused by a defect in the external or middle ear, referred to as conductive loss, is a mechanical obstruction of air conduction that usually can be helped by surgical intervention. When the decrement is in the inner ear, referred to as perceptive or sensorineural loss, damage to nerve tissue and/or sensory paths to the brain is not benefited by a surgical procedure. Cochlear nerve endings are the main component of sensorineural hearing (Fig. 41-4).

Auditory acuity and function are measured by various tests. The audiogram is one measurement tool. Computer-

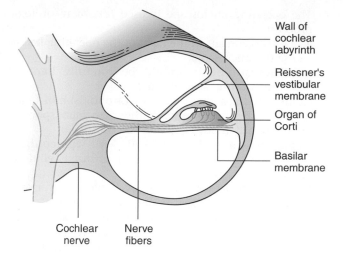

FIG. 41-4 Cross section of cochlear labyrinth with sensory neural mechanism.

averaged tomography is used to measure and analyze electrical impulses, known as auditory brainstem responses, from the brain and cortical auditory pathway. An acoustic reflex latency test of the stapedius reflex provides information about hearing sensitivity. Auditory brainstem evoked potentials assess the patient's hearing threshold.

Surgical Procedures of the Ear

Current techniques, instrumentation, lasers, and the operating microscope have enhanced the capability of otologists.

General Considerations

1. Local anesthesia may be used for a minor procedure on the external ear, but general anesthesia generally is used to avoid patient movement while the surgeon is manipulating delicate structures in the middle or inner ear.
   a. Inhalation anesthesia may be given by facemask for a short procedure, with the anesthesia provider seated at the head of the operating bed.
   b. The anesthesia provider sits alongside the operating bed with the patient facing him or her when the patient is intubated for a major procedure.
   c. Hypotensive anesthesia may be employed to create a bloodless field, especially during microsurgery.
   d. Nitrous oxide diffuses into cavities, causing expansion of the middle ear. This can present a hazard in a grafting procedure, for example; nitrous oxide is discontinued before placement of a graft in the middle ear.
   e. General anesthesia may be supplemented with a local agent in some procedures, often with epinephrine to control bleeding.
2. The patient's head is turned with the affected side up and stabilized in a donut. The dependent pinna should be protected from pressure.
3. Lint-free drapes are preferred. It is mandatory that gloves be free of powder and lint. The formation of a granuloma in the oval window can cause irreversible sensorineural hearing loss.

4. The operating microscope is used for many otologic procedures.
   a. The surgeon sits at the head of the operating bed to use the microscope.
   b. Microinstruments should be carefully handled before, during, and after use.
5. Compressed absorbent patties (cottonoids) moistened with normal saline solution, rather than gauze sponges, are frequently used. They must be counted.
6. Hemostasis may be achieved with epinephrine, absorbable hemostatic sponges or oxidized cellulose, laser, and bone wax.
7. Prosthetic devices should be available in an assortment of types and sizes. Tissue allografts may be used.
8. A nerve stimulator may be used to identify facial, acoustic, cochlear, and/or vestibular nerve branches. Evoked potential audiometry also may be used to monitor the seventh and eighth cranial nerves.
9. Bone instruments, including powered drills, are used for opening the temporal bone.
10. CO_2, Nd:YAG, argon, and KTP lasers are used during otologic procedures to control bleeding, divide nerves, and/or vaporize tissues.
11. Pressure dressings are usually applied. Some surgeons place 1 drop of phenylephrine (Neo-Synephrine) in the ear canal postoperatively.

External Ear Procedures

Removal of a Foreign Body. Removing a foreign body from the outer canal is performed most frequently in children. The object is washed out or removed to prevent purulent infection. A plant seed or vegetable foreign body, such as a pea, is not irrigated, because it may swell in the ear and increase the difficulty of removal. General anesthesia sometimes may be required. Trauma should be minimal during removal of a foreign body to prevent stenosis of the canal or perforation through the eardrum.

Drainage of a Hematoma. Usually a result of injury, a hematoma is drained to avoid infection with subsequent chondritis and deformity of the auricle.

Excision of a Tumor. The extent of the surgical procedure to excise a tumor, either benign or malignant, depends on the size and type of tumor. The skin of the pinna is vulnerable to actinic (chemical) changes caused by radiant energy during exposure to the sun. Basal cell lesions do not metastasize, but squamous cell carcinoma often does. Primary cancer may be excised by a wide or wedge excision with primary closure or a wide excision with a skin graft. If the lesion is extensive, partial or total pinnectomy may be necessary. The area can be skin-grafted and reconstructed cosmetically with a prosthesis. Radical temporal bone resection is indicated if the bone (canal) is involved. Neck dissection may be indicated if nodal metastases are present.

Middle Ear Procedures

Mastoidectomy. Mastoidectomy, the eradication of mastoid air cells, may be indicated to relieve complications of acute or chronic mastoiditis. Mastoidectomy is more commonly performed in conjunction with a reconstructive procedure (see "Tympanomastoid Reconstruction"). A cholesteatoma can form after repeated infections (Fig. 41-5).

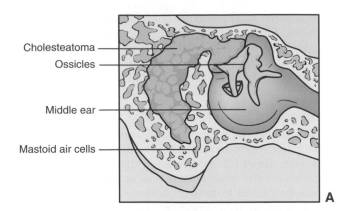

Mastoid air cells and cholesteatoma

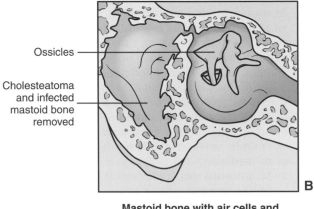

Mastoid bone with air cells and cholesteatoma removed

FIG. 41-5 **A,** Mastoid air cells and cholesteatoma. **B,** Mastoid bone with air cells and cholesteatoma removed.

Simple Mastoidectomy. The mastoid process is opened behind the ear. Air cells are removed by drilling through bone with small burrs, without involving the middle ear or external canal.

Modified Radical Mastoidectomy. Simple mastoidectomy and removal of the posterior wall of the ear canal provide drainage from the mastoid into the canal. The tympanic membrane and middle ear ossicles are preserved.

Radical Mastoidectomy. A radical mastoidectomy is performed for chronic mastoiditis. The middle ear cavity and mastoid antrum are combined into a single cavity for inspection and cleaning. Mastoid air cells are removed. The ossicles and tympanic membrane are partially removed. The stapes and facial nerve are preserved.

Tympanoplasty. Tympanoplasty, as a general term, refers to any procedure performed to repair defects in the eardrum and/or middle ear structures for the purpose of reconstructing sound conduction paths. The degree of hearing improvement after tympanoplasty is related to the degree of damage. Preferably, the ear should be uninfected at the time of the surgical procedure. If not, infected tissue is debrided. As microsurgical procedures, tympanoplasties are classified into five types:

1. Type I (myringoplasty) is closure of a perforation in the tympanic membrane caused by infection or trauma.

The ossicular chain is normal. Autogenous fascia or a vein is used to repair the perforation. A vein graft is taken from the patient's forearm or hand. Fascia, more commonly used as a patch over a perforation, is obtained from the temporalis muscle.

2. Type II is closure of a perforated tympanic membrane with erosion of the malleus. The graft is placed against the incus or remains of the malleus.

3. Type III replaces the tympanic membrane to provide protection for the stapes and round window. The tympanic membrane, malleus, and incus have been destroyed by disease. The stapes is intact and mobile. A homograft of tympanic membrane with attached malleus and incus is placed in contact with the normal stapes, permitting transmission of sound.

4. Type IV is similar to type III except that the head, neck, and crura of the stapes are missing. The mobile footplate may be left exposed with the graft placed around it. The air pocket between the graft and the round window provides sound protection for the round window. To conserve the middle ear hearing mechanism, homograft transplantation of tympanic membrane and ossicles may be used to rebuild the chain.

5. Type V is similar to type IV except that the stapedial footplate is fixed because of otosclerosis (osteospongiosis). A fenestra (small opening) is made in the horizontal semicircular canal. The homograft seals off the middle ear to provide sound protection for the round window.

Reconstruction of the middle ear may be done with a synthetic bioinert material such as high-density polyethylene sponge (Plastipore). Fibrin glue also is used. Partial and total ossicular replacement prostheses have been developed.

Tympanomastoid Reconstruction. Tympanoplasty may be combined with either simple or radical mastoidectomy. The mastoid is drained and cleaned before reconstruction of the eardrum or middle ear ossicles. After incision behind the auricle, the tympanic membrane and tympanic cavity are inspected. The mastoid antrum is entered by drilling through mastoid bone.

Sometimes in chronic otitis media, the mucous membrane of the tympanic cavity is replaced by epithelium from the ear canal as it grows through a perforation in the eardrum. Desquamated skin cells that cannot escape form a ball or cyst, known as a cholesteatoma. If present in the middle ear or mastoid, a cholesteatoma is removed during mastoidectomy and/or tympanoplasty. If left intact, a cholesteatoma can cause permanent hearing loss, balance disturbance, infection, and facial nerve paralysis.

Stapedectomy and Stapedotomy. Conductive hearing loss can result from fixation of the stapes, most often caused by otosclerosis. The surgeon aims to restore vibration from the incus to the mobile oval window membrane to transmit sound. A stapedectomy involves partial or total removal of the stapes. A partial stapedectomy removes only the fixed footplate (Fig. 41-6); a total stapedectomy removes the entire stapes, including the footplate. A stapedotomy (small opening into the footplate) may be the preferred procedure. The opening is made with a handheld perforator, microsurgical power drill, or laser. An argon, CO_2, or KTP laser may be used for this purpose. A low-wattage lasing beam

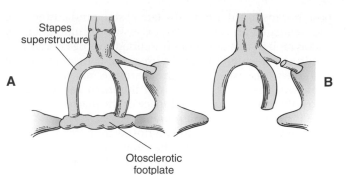

FIG. 41-6   Partial stapedectomy. **A,** Stapes superstructure attached to fixed otosclerotic footplate. **B,** Footplate removed; superstructure remains.

avoids thermal damage to the perilymph and inner ear structures. After partial or total stapedectomy or stapedotomy, the remaining superstructure is used to reconstruct the sound-conducting mechanism.

An incision is made deep in the canal near but not in the eardrum. The eardrum is folded over, giving access to the middle ear. The stapes is disconnected from the incus, fractured by fine microinstruments, and removed. The oval window is sealed by a graft of vein, perichondrium, fascia, fat, or an absorbable hemostatic sponge over the oval window. A prosthesis is inserted and connected to the incus and to the graft, thus restoring sound conduction. Prostheses are made of various inert materials such as polyethylene, stainless steel, or tantalum.

By performing the microsurgical procedure with the patient under local anesthesia, the surgeon can reposition the eardrum and use his or her voice to test whether the patient's hearing is improved. Otosclerosis usually involves both ears, but stapedectomy is performed on only one ear at a time.

Stapes Mobilization. The stapes is manipulated at the footplate to restore normal function. A break through an otosclerotic lesion is achieved by means of transcrural pressure or direct application of chisels and picks to the footplate. A mobile, unaffected portion of a functioning stapes remains. Various techniques are used, with or without the use of prosthetic devices. The advantage of the procedure is that the preserved stapedial footplate provides natural protection for the inner ear. The disadvantage is that frequently a continuing otosclerotic process causes the footplate to become refixed. Therefore stapedectomy is more popular because it produces long-lasting results.

Stapes procedures are performed under direct vision with the operating microscope. The procedures do not disturb the integrity or position of the eardrum.

Removal of Middle Ear Vascular Tumors. The argon laser is absorbed by red pigment. Therefore, it is suited for removal of small vascular tumors in the middle ear, such as glomus tympanicum tumors. The argon laser acts by photocoagulation.

Inner Ear Procedures

Endolymphatic Sac Shunt. The endolymphatic sac is an appendage of the membranous inner ear located in the posterior fossa, anterior to the lateral sinus and posterior to the semicircular canals. An excessive accumulation of endolymph in this sac causes the episodic vertigo (dizziness), tinnitus (ear ringing), and sensorineural hearing loss of Meniere's disease. Through a simple mastoidectomy approach, the sac is opened and the inner ear is drained into either the subarachnoid space or the mastoid. A shunt tube is inserted to maintain drainage.

Labyrinthectomy. In labyrinthectomy the vestibular labyrinth is removed from the inner ear to correct incapacitating vertigo. This results in loss of vestibular function and hearing.

Vestibular Neurectomy. A middle fossa approach to the internal auditory canal for vestibular neurectomy combines otologic and neurosurgical procedures. Through a temporal bone craniotomy incision, dura of the floor of the middle fossa is elevated to expose structures in the superior portion of the internal auditory canal. The superior and inferior vestibular nerves, which control equilibrium, are sectioned to control intractable vertigo. The cochlear nerve, the hearing portion of the eighth cranial nerve, is not damaged, thus preserving hearing. A graft of temporalis muscle is placed over the exposed internal auditory canal to prevent leakage of cerebrospinal fluid.

Removal of an Acoustic Neuroma. Acoustic neuroma resection may be performed by an otologist and/or a neurosurgeon, depending on its location and the extent of neurologic involvement. An acoustic neuroma is a slow-growing, encapsulated, benign tumor of the eighth cranial (acoustic) nerve. It originates in the neural sheath in the internal auditory canal but grows to involve nerve fibers in the posterior fossa. Initially the patient experiences unilateral hearing loss and disturbances, especially tinnitus, and equilibrium problems such as mild vertigo. The syndrome may resemble Meniere's disease or an expanding intracranial tumor. Early differential diagnosis is enhanced by brainstem evoked response audiometry, vertebral angiography, and small-volume air-contrast computed tomography (CT).

A small neuroma, confined to the internal auditory canal, may be resected by the otologist using microsurgical technique through a middle fossa approach to preserve hearing. If a translabyrinthine approach is used to gain access to the internal auditory canal posterior to the inner ear structures, the patient will have total hearing loss after the surgical procedure. Acoustic neuromas extending into the cranial cavity are resected by the neurosurgeon. The CO_2 laser may be used to excise acoustic neuromas through a transmastoid or craniotomy approach. Cerebrospinal fluid leak and meningitis are complications of the craniotomy approach.

For select patients, stereotactic radiosurgery can be performed on an outpatient basis with local anesthesia. Hearing is preserved in 50% of these patients.

Implantation of a Cochlear Prosthesis. Cochlear implants have been used for adults since the 1980s, but it was not until the 1990s that they were used for children. A cochlear implant can restore perception of sound to patients who have profound sensorineural deafness not responsive to external amplification of a hearing aid. They are indicated for use in patients who have intact eighth cranial nerve function and are older than 2 years. The implant is an electronic device that converts sound waves into electrical signals to stimulate cochlear nerve fibers in the absence of functioning hair cells. Several devices are available. All of them have external and internal components (Fig. 41-7). The external part, which is attached behind the ear, has a microphone/transmitter and a speech processor/receiver. The internal part has a receiver/stimulator and electrode/channel(s) that is threaded through the cochlea.

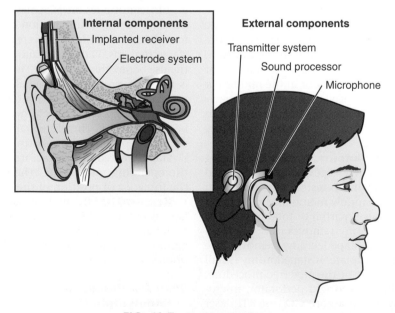

FIG. 41-7 Cochlear implant.

The internal electrode attaches to wires permanently implanted in the cochlea. Through a postauricular incision, a simple mastoidectomy is performed. Under the operating microscope, the facial recess between the posterior canal and the facial nerve is enlarged to expose the chorda tympani nerve and the middle ear. The electrode is securely seated in the mastoid cavity and placed through a recess into the middle ear. It is directed through an opening made in the round window into the scala tympani until it meets resistance. Placement is critical. A plug of fascia from the temporalis muscle is placed around the electrode at the round window to prevent perilymph leakage.

The internal electrode stimulates the auditory nerve to interpret sound. The single-channel model stimulates the nerve randomly so that the patient can discern environmental sounds but not speech. A multichannel electrode enables the patient to distinguish environmental sounds and some speech by differentiating the frequency, volume, and pitch of sound waves. With a single-channel electrode, a ground wire is placed under the temporalis muscle in the mastoid or middle ear. A multichannel electrode does not have a ground wire. The internal receiver is sutured in position over the temporal bone behind the ear. Electromagnetic components and/or a titanium enclosure for the receiver may act as an electrical ground device. Only a bipolar active electrode should be used if electrosurgery is necessary after placement of the receiver.

The external microphone/transmitter component of the implant activates the internal receiver/stimulator. Transmission may be percutaneous or transcutaneous. In the percutaneous model, a direct wire to a receiver implanted behind the ear connects the transmitter. In the transcutaneous model, the transmitter converts electrical energy into magnetic currents that pass through intact skin to the receiver. In both models, sound enters the microphone and is transmitted to a speech processor, worn outside the body, where it is encoded into electrical signals or energy and amplified. The coded signals return to the transmitter and are passed to the internal receiver. The patient can adjust amplification of environmental sounds.

NOSE

Anatomy of the Nose

The supporting structures of the nose consist of two nasal bones and the nasal processes of the maxillary bones superiorly, the lateral cartilages and connective tissue inferiorly, and the septum. The septum, composed of bone posteriorly and cartilage anteriorly, divides the nose into two chambers lined by mucous membrane. The anterior portion, or vestibule, holds the nasal hairs. The external anterior orifices are called nares.

The internal portion of the nose, the nasal cavity (Fig. 41-8) extends to the nasopharynx, the space behind the choanae (funnel-like posterior nasal orifices). The nose communicates with the ear via the eustachian tube. The hard and soft palates divide the nasal and oral cavities. The ethmoid bone separates the nasal and cranial cavities.

The paranasal sinuses are the frontal, maxillary, ethmoid, and sphenoid. Ostia (openings from the sinuses and nasolacrimal ducts) are located in the nasal lateral walls. The ostia provide a drainage system for the sinuses, as well as aerate them. Three turbinate bones (superior, middle, and

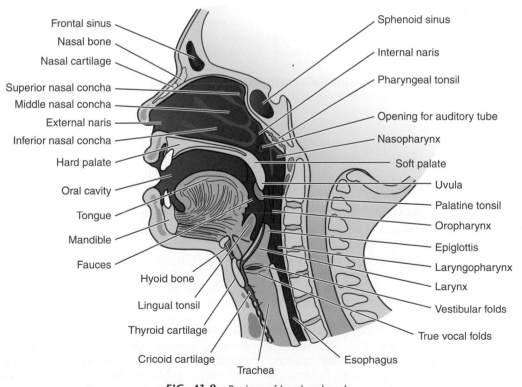

FIG. 41-8   Regions of head and neck.

inferior) are also situated in the lateral walls. These bones are covered with a vascular mucosa. Beneath each turbinate is a corresponding meatus. Tears drain into the nose through the nasolacrimal duct that enters the inferior meatus. Drainage from the paranasal sinuses is passed to the nose through the middle and superior meatus.

External and internal carotid arteries and their branches supply blood to the nasal region. Because of the extensive vascularity, lymphatic supply, and proximity to the brain, infections on or about the face are potentially very dangerous. Microorganisms may readily be carried to or thrombi may form in the cavernous sinus. The sense of smell is derived from the first cranial (olfactory) nerve. The sensory nerve supply of the nasal area is associated with the trigeminal or fifth cranial nerve.

Physiology of the Nose

- It provides filtered air to the respiratory system. Fine cilia in the mucous membranes propel mucus toward the nasopharynx. Air is warmed and moistened as it passes to the trachea and lower respiratory tract.
- It contains the end organs for smell in the olfactory epithelium, which differs from other nasal epithelium. When nasal obstruction blocks off the olfactory epithelium, loss of smell (anosmia) results. The senses of smell and taste are closely related.

Surgical Procedures of the Nose

Nasal procedures are concerned with two factors: adequate ventilation to accessory spaces and adequate drainage from them. Abnormalities in structure, congenital or traumatic, and disease processes hinder function. Corrective procedures are done to relieve obstruction, to ensure drainage, to resect tumors, or to control bleeding (epistaxis).

General Considerations

1. CT and rhinoscopy are often performed preoperatively to diagnose the nature and extent of pathologic conditions, especially in the paranasal sinuses.
2. Many nasal procedures are performed with the patient under local anesthesia with or without intravenous (IV) sedation.
   a. Topical 4% cocaine may be sprayed on the nasal mucosa or applied with soaked, compressed, absorbent patties (cottonoids) or sponges put in the nostrils. Cocaine produces vasoconstriction, as well as anesthesia. The patties should be accounted for at the end of the procedure.
   b. A local agent, often lidocaine hydrochloride, 1% or 2%, is injected into the middle meatus. Epinephrine usually is used for vasoconstriction to control bleeding.
   c. When general anesthesia is indicated, a pack is placed in the pharynx to prevent aspiration of blood after the patient is intubated.
3. Paranasal sinuses and tissues underlying the mucosa are considered sterile. Therefore, instrumentation should be sterile although the nasal cavity is considered a contaminated area because the instrumentation is entering a vascular bed. Venous drainage could easily carry microorganisms to the cavernous sinus, causing an intracranial infection.

4. CO₂, Nd:YAG, and KTP lasers may be used. Endoscopes also are used. All equipment and accessories should be checked for working order.
5. Nasal packing is inserted at the end of most procedures except endoscopic sinus and laser procedures. A mustache dressing may be placed under the nose to act as a drip pad. Postoperatively the patient should be positioned in a head-up position to minimize bleeding. Ice is placed over the nasal bridge for the first 48 hours. The ice should be used in 20-minute intervals only.

Nasal Cavity Procedures. The supporting structures surrounding nasal air passages can be injured or displaced. Acute or chronic disease processes can cause dysfunction or obstruction.

Epistaxis. Most nosebleeds are caused by trauma, usually at Kiesselbach's plexus of arteries and veins (also known as Little's area) in the anterior part of the nasal septum (Fig. 41-9). Dehumidified air may cause changes in the mucosa and splitting of tiny vessels. Bleeding may be spontaneous, as in patients with arteriosclerosis, hypertension, or blood dyscrasia. Epistaxis is usually anterior and unilateral. In people with systemic disease, such as leukemia, or with severe fracture, the bleeding is frequently posterior and more severe. Management involves locating the precise bleeding site and promptly instituting appropriate therapy. Severe hemorrhage places the patient in a precarious condition. Hypovolemia should be corrected preoperatively.

Anterior Pack. Local vasoconstriction and pressure on the side of the nose will control most nosebleeds. Electrocoagulation or silver nitrate is used to provide hemostasis at the bleeding point as needed. When bleeding is from the anterior ethmoid artery, inaccessible to cautery, packing is applied to the area of depression between the septum and the middle turbinate.

Posterior Pack. A posterior pack may be necessary for constant pressure when bleeding is severe in the posterior part of the nose. The pack consists of rolled gauze securely tied to the middle of a length of narrow tape or strong string; commercial packs are available. To control infection and odor, gauze is lubricated with antibiotic ointment before insertion. After a catheter is passed into the mouth via the nose, one end of the tape is tied to the oral end of the catheter. The catheter and attached tape are then drawn back through the mouth and out one nostril, thereby pulling the pack up into the nasopharynx. Thus one end of the tape comes out the nose, the other end out the mouth. These ends are secured to the patient's cheek with adhesive tape. The nasal end is taped to prevent the pack from slipping into the throat; the oral end facilitates removal of the pack. Some oozing may persist in spite of packing. The pack is left in place until bleeding is arrested, usually for at least 48 hours, but prolonged use can lead to otitis media or paranasal sinusitis.

Patients with postnasal packs are often apprehensive and uncomfortable. They must breathe through the mouth. Posterior packs tend to reduce arterial oxygen tension. All patients, especially geriatric patients or those with marginal pulmonary function, should be observed carefully for respiratory problems that may result from the pack dropping into the hypopharynx.

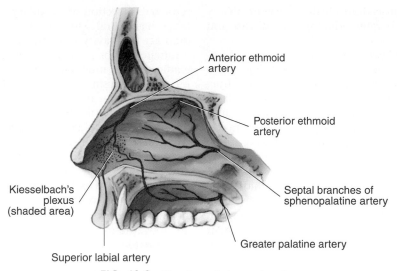

FIG. 41-9 Blood supply to nasal cavity.

Artery Ligation. A microsurgical procedure is performed to control persistent nasal hemorrhage by reducing the blood supply to the posterior portion of the nose. Some surgeons prefer artery ligation to packing, or it may be performed with a pack in place. Through an incision in the oral mucosa, removal of the posterior wall exposes the maxillary sinus for transantral ligation. Terminal branches of the internal maxillary artery, a branch of the external carotid artery, are exposed, identified, and ligated with metallic clips. Electrocoagulation is employed to control intraoperative bleeding, but if bleeding is excessive, creation of a nasoantral window establishes drainage. The replaced posterior mucosal flap is covered with absorbable gelatin sponge, and the incision is closed.

Through an incision along the left side of the nose, ligation of the anterior and posterior ethmoidal arteries is helpful in controlling bleeding in the superior aspect of the nose.

The argon or KTP laser may be used to control severe epistaxis. If a laser is used to control bleeding, nasal packing usually is unnecessary.

Turbinectomy. Chronic engorgement of the middle and/or inferior turbinate causes nasal congestion and rhinorrhea. Rhinitis is frequently an allergic reaction. A KTP laser shrinks turbinates without removing normal mucosa. A CO_2 or Nd:YAG contact laser vaporizes the superficial layer of mucosa without injuring the turbinate or ablating the turbinate. The KTP or CO_2 laser fiber handpiece is directed through a nasal endoscope. Because bleeding is minimal, nasal packing is unnecessary. Electrocoagulation and cryosurgery also have been used to treat soft tissue obstruction and refractory allergic rhinitis.

Nasal Obstruction. Surgical intervention can provide relief for certain types of nasal obstruction. For example, after the mucosa is shrunk with a vasoconstrictor and secretions are suctioned, a foreign body is removed with a forceps. An abscess or hematoma may need to be drained to relieve pressure. Accumulation of pus or blood separates the perichondrium, the connective tissue, from underlying cartilage.

This may cause necrosis of cartilage with resultant deformity. Infection must be eradicated to avoid extension to the brain.

Polypectomy. Polyps (soft, edematous masses) projecting from the nasal or sinus mucosa can obstruct the posterior choanae. Polyps usually are bilateral, but they may be unilateral, single or multiple, and they frequently are infected. In addition to obstructing ventilation, they may obstruct the sense of smell if the olfactory epithelium is blocked. Some polyps may be excised with a wire-loop snare through a nasal speculum or with forceps through an endoscope. Packing is inserted to control bleeding. The KTP laser coagulates the base to debulk large, multiple polyps. The laser fiber can be directed through a straight or angled handpiece. A CO_2 laser can vaporize polyps. The laser is less invasive than other techniques.

Nasal Deformity. Surgical intervention can restore contour and/or improve function after an injury. A deformity in nasal structure also may be corrected to improve cosmetic appearance.

Reduction of a Nasal Fracture. Fracture of the septum or nasal bones often accompanies other trauma to the head. Intranasal manipulation is required to elevate depressed bone or cartilage that may be pushed into the paranasal sinuses. This should be performed as soon as possible to bring the parts into apposition. A delay of 7 to 10 days to permit edema to subside will not affect the outcome. Bleeding from a laceration must be immediately controlled and drained. Intranasal structure compatible with air passage must be preserved.

Septoplasty, Septal Reconstruction, and Submucous Resection. The terms *septoplasty, septal reconstruction,* and *submucous resection* are used interchangeably to describe correction of a deviated nasal septum. Often the result of injury, the condition interferes with breathing and drainage. With the patient under local anesthesia, one side of the septum is incised its entire length. Membranous coverings are detached from cartilage and bone. The deformed part of the septum is removed or straightened and replaced. Bilateral nasal packing is inserted to hold tissues in place and to prevent bleeding. The procedure creates a patent airway and straight septal line, thereby reducing sinus disease and polyp formation.

Rhinoplasty. Rhinoplasty, a procedure to correct deformity of the nose, may be performed by a rhinologist or a plastic surgeon. It is a major procedure involving reconstruction and molding of the bones and cartilages. Septoplasty and rhinoplasty may be performed together; septorhinoplasty restores both function and cosmetic appearance. Local anesthesia and a vasoconstrictor such as 4% cocaine usually are used. Some surgeons prefer to use a nasal spray 30 minutes preoperatively. Both drugs decrease the risk of hypertension during the procedure, which could cause excessive bleeding. The skin is taped postoperatively to maintain the nasal structures in alignment. A rigid shield is applied for protection. This is not removed without a specific order from the surgeon. Temporary ecchymosis from surgical trauma surrounds the eyes postoperatively.

Repair of a Perforated Septum. Perforations occur most often in the anterior cartilage. If bleeding and crusting are severe, the perforation may be covered by rotated mucoperichondrial flaps. Or the mucosa of adjacent intact septum may be denuded and a skin graft applied to cover the perforation. Nasal packing is inserted.

Paranasal Sinus Procedures.

The paranasal sinuses are air-filled spaces in the skull (Fig. 41-10). Because the sinus mucous membrane lining is continuous with the mucous membrane lining of the nose, nasal infection may readily spread to the sinuses. Various procedures provide drainage for patients with chronic sinusitis that may result from allergies or repeated nasopharyngeal infection. Swelling of the nasal mucosa can trap microorganisms within a sinus cavity. Ostial occlusion and abnormalities in the walls of the nasal cavity interfere with breathing, drainage, and smell. Sinus procedures are executed through an external or an intranasal approach or through an endoscope.

Maxillary Sinus Procedure. The maxillary sinuses are located bilaterally between the upper teeth and the eyes.

Caldwell-Luc Procedure (Antrostomy). The maxillary sinus contents are approached through an incision of the oral mucous membrane above the canine teeth. The flap is retracted. A section of maxillary bone is cut out to create a large nasoantral window for aeration and permanent drainage by gravity into the nasal fossa under the inferior turbinate. Polyps and diseased tissue are removed, along with eradication of mucosa. At the completion of the surgical procedure, the sinus is packed with gauze impregnated with antibiotic ointment. One end of the gauze is brought through the window and into the nose. The incision under the upper lip is sutured. The packing is eventually removed through the nose. Antrostomy is usually limited to adults because of unerupted teeth in children. A Caldwell-Luc incision is also used for removal of a tumor in the maxillary sinus.

Ethmoid Sinus Procedures. The ethmoid sinus cells lie bilaterally between the nose and the orbits. The maxillary sinuses are below the ethmoid bones, and the frontal sinuses are above them.

Ethmoidectomy. Diseased tissue is removed from the ethmoid labyrinth, middle turbinate, and meatus. A large cavity is formed to facilitate aeration and drainage. Severe ethmoiditis can cause orbital abscess requiring drainage through an intranasal or external (Lynch) incision that extends from the inner half of the eyebrow down alongside the nose.

Turbinectomy. Removal of portions of the inferior and middle turbinates increases aeration and drainage. The cavity is packed at completion of the surgical procedure.

Frontal Sinus Procedures. The frontal sinuses are situated above the eyes. They are usually approached through the external incision described for ethmoidectomy, or a coronal incision may be made for exposure across the scalp from ear to ear.

Osteoplastic Flap Procedure. The bone covering the frontal sinus is exposed and incised. The contents of the sinus, such as a mucocele (a cyst lined with mucus-secreting glands), are extracted. The lining of the mucocele sac is removed and the cavity packed with fat (from the abdominal wall) to obliterate the sinus with fibrous tissue that fills in the cavity. The incised bone flap is then repositioned, and the incision is sutured.

Killian Procedure. A frontal sinus cavity is reached by removal of the floor or anterior wall of the sinus through an external incision above the eye. A large communication and drainage channel into the nose is formed.

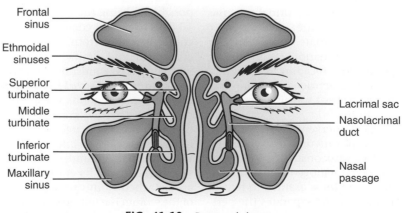

Frontal sinus
Ethmoidal sinuses
Superior turbinate
Middle turbinate
Inferior turbinate
Maxillary sinus
Lacrimal sac
Nasolacrimal duct
Nasal passage

FIG. 41-10 Paranasal sinuses.

Sphenoid Sinus Procedure. The sphenoid sinus is deep—almost in the center of the skull. It may be approached intranasally or via the external ethmoidectomy incision through the eyebrow.

Sphenoidotomy. Sphenoidotomy involves the creation of an opening into the sphenoid sinus for drainage.

Endoscopic Sinus Surgery. Sinuscopes permit direct visualization of the paranasal sinuses and the anatomy of lateral nasal walls. The site of diseased mucosa or obstructive tissue, such as polyps, can be localized for removal, with preservation of some mucosa and restoration of drainage (Fig. 41-11). The mucosa of each sinus has cilia that move air in waveforms. With an endoscopic approach, some ciliary motion may be retained for aeration. The basic principle of endoscopic sinus surgery is that most sinus mucosal disease will resolve if aeration and drainage are reestablished. The extent of the procedure depends on the location of diseased mucosa and the resection necessary to establish drainage. Septal deformities or inferior turbinates causing nasal obstruction may be concurrently corrected (i.e., septoplasty and turbinoplasty). Minor procedures limited to removal of disease from maxillary or ethmoid sinuses usually can be done with topical and local anesthesia. IV sedation or general anesthesia is needed for more extensive procedures, such as ethmoidectomy or sphenoethmoidectomy.

The telescopes of sinuscopes are 2.7 and 4 mm in diameter with 0-, 25- or 30-, 70-, and 120-degree viewing angles. The quartz rod telescope has a solid quartz optical cone in the light post that attaches to a halogen light source. This system provides optimal light transmission through the fiberoptics of the miniaturized scope. An attached suction/irrigation device permits unobstructed viewing. The telescope is inserted intranasally and advanced into the frontal, ethmoid, or sphenoid sinus. It is inserted through a cannula in the canine fossa to reach the maxillary sinus. Many accessory grasping and cutting instruments, including the KTP laser, are used to remove mucosa, lamina, osteum,

and cells. Hemostasis is controlled with epinephrine and cautery or laser. Nasal packing usually is not required.

Functional Procedure. Known as the functional endoscopic sinus surgery (FESS) Messerklinger technique, the surgeon begins at the ethmoid and works anteriorly to the frontal and maxillary sinuses to clear ethmoidal compartments of disease. If a minimal opening of the narrow osteomeatal tract at the anterior ethmoidal sinus will not achieve adequate drainage from other paranasal sinuses, a posterior ethmoidectomy and sphenoidotomy are included in the procedure.

Exenteration. Known as the Wigand procedure, total sphenoethmoidectomy and partial middle turbinate resection are performed, beginning with a sphenoidotomy and working anteriorly to the frontal sinus. This creates a broad opening of the sphenoidal, ethmoidal, frontal, and maxillary sinuses. To avoid the optic nerve, dissection does not extend beyond the lateral wall of the sphenoid. Visual evoked potentials monitor optic nerve function; the eyes are uncovered. The endoscopic procedure may be done bilaterally.

Resection of Tumors. Osteoma, a benign tumor, can arise from bones around the paranasal sinuses. Although rare, primary carcinoma and sarcoma do occur in the frontal, ethmoid, sphenoid, and maxillary sinuses. Most originate in the maxillary sinus. The incidence increases with age. The sinuses are proximal to the orbits, oral cavity, and base of the skull. A tumor in the maxillary sinus may be associated with oral or nasal symptoms, such as loosening of the upper teeth, bleeding from the nose, or asymmetry of the face. A malignant lesion in the ethmoid sinus may be accompanied by displacement of the eye, disturbance of smell, and nasal obstruction. Chronic sinusitis is thought to play an etiologic role because of an associated replacement of respiratory epithelium by stratified squamous cells. Most sinus tumors are squamous cell carcinomas. Often the bony walls are invaded and destroyed by the time symptoms appear, because the tumor tends to extend in all directions. Exploratory surgery by a Caldwell-Luc incision provides the best chance of early diagnosis. Radical craniofacial resection may be indicated.

ORAL CAVITY AND THROAT
Anatomy and Physiology of the Oral Cavity and Throat

The oral cavity is lined with thick mucous membrane. This squamous mucosa connects with the nasopharynx superiorly and the hypopharynx below. The hard palate, part of the maxillary bone, forms the floor of the nasal cavity and the anterior part of the roof of the mouth. The soft palate, a musculomembranous structure posterior to the hard palate, occludes the nasal cavity during speech and swallowing. These functions are aided by the uvula, a small conical appendage (tonguelike structure) that projects from the posterior free margin of the soft palate. It contains the uvular muscle covered by mucous membrane. The tongue, occupying much of the oral cavity, joins the soft palate and pharynx posteriorly by folds of mucous membrane.

The throat refers to space surrounded by the soft palate, the palatoglossal and palatopharyngeal arches, the base of the tongue, and the pharynx. The funnel-shaped pharynx is subdivided into the nasopharynx (above), oropharynx

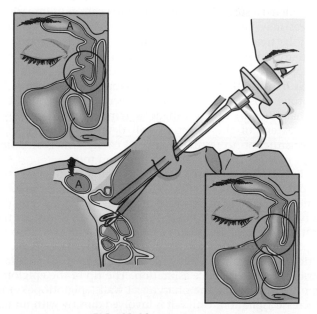

FIG. 41-11 Sinusoscopy.

(middle), and hypopharynx (below). The nasopharynx communicates with the nasal cavity through the posterior choanae. The oropharynx includes the base of the tongue anteriorly, the tonsillar fossae laterally, and the oropharyngeal walls of the throat posteriorly. The hypopharynx leads from the oropharynx to the larynx, trachea, and esophagus. The pharynx, posterior to the larynx and the nasal and oral cavities, consists of constrictor muscles essential to swallowing. The proximity of food and air passages and the joint function of the pharynx in their passage contribute to the hazard of aspiration.

The nasopharynx and oropharynx contain masses of lymphoid tissue. The adenoids (pharyngeal tonsils) hang from the nasopharyngeal roof; the lingual tonsils are in mucosal crypts. The palatine tonsils lie on either side of the oropharynx. These, referred to as the tonsils, are supported in the tonsillar fossae by anterior and posterior pillars. A fibrous capsule adheres to each laterally.

The salivary glands are located in the soft tissue walls of the oral cavity. The six major paired glands are the submandibular, sublingual, and parotid glands. The parotid glands are the largest. The ducts of these major glands, in addition to lesser glands, secrete saliva into the mouth. Saliva functions to moisten and lubricate food to aid in swallowing, to dissolve some substances and enzymatically digest starches, and to facilitate tasting.

Surgical Procedures of the Oral Cavity and Throat

Pathologic conditions may affect the lips, tongue, floor of the mouth, palates, salivary glands, or pharynx. The oral region is one of the most vascular areas of the body. Hemostasis may be achieved with an electrosurgical unit (ESU), hemostatic scalpel, argon beam coagulator, or laser. Lasers are used to vaporize both benign and malignant superficial and subepithelial lesions.

Abnormalities result from congenital malformation, improper occlusion or jaggedness of teeth, and infection, but most commonly they result from trauma and neoplasms. Adequate reconstruction restores the lining, internal structural support, soft tissue, and external coverage. Many of the craniofacial, maxillofacial, and dentofacial procedures previously described in this chapter are performed through intraoral incisions. Plastic surgeons, oral surgeons, laryngologists, or a multidisciplinary team may perform the following procedures through intraoral or extraoral incisions.

Excision of Salivary Gland Tumors. Benign mixed tumors of the salivary glands are more common than are malignant tumors and most frequently are located in a parotid gland. Most tumors can be removed by dissection, and some can be removed by cryosurgery. The incision is of adequate size to expose the entire gland and the facial nerve. A nerve stimulator is used to identify the nerve and its branches. Injury to the nerve results in postoperative facial paralysis.

Parotidectomy. Parotidectomy, excision of a parotid gland, is performed through an incision in the neck below the angle of the mandible and extending upward to one or both sides of the ear (Fig. 41-12). A swelling beneath the skin in the area in front of or below the ear is almost invariably

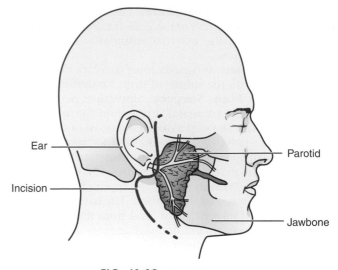

FIG. 41-12 Parotidectomy.

within the substance of the parotid gland. This may be a benign, mixed, or malignant tumor. Benign lesions localized superficially may be excised by superficial subtotal parotidectomy. Lesions deep within the gland, extending under the mandible, frequently displace the soft palate in the oral cavity. Radical neck dissection or hemimandibulectomy may be indicated to remove a highly invasive malignant tumor. For most parotid tumors the facial nerve can be isolated and preserved during total parotidectomy, unless the nerve is inextricably involved by the tumor. If the facial nerve is to be sacrificed, the nerve may be primarily grafted, with the great auricular nerve as a graft, to prevent total facial nerve paralysis.

Excision of Oral Carcinoma. Primary malignant lesions may occur in the lower lip, tongue, or floor of the mouth. Because of the proximity of cervical lymph nodes, metastasis occurs early. A painful, bleeding ulcer is considered a suspicious symptom. Oral cancer in its earliest stages may be asymptomatic and painless. Small tumors may be treated with only irradiation, local excision with primary closure, or vaporization with a laser beam. Larger lesions compel more extensive procedures.

Subtotal Glossectomy or Hemiglossectomy. In subtotal glossectomy or hemiglossectomy, part (subtotal) or half (hemi-) of the tongue is removed (glossectomy). The extent of the resection will determine the type of reconstruction to resurface the oral cavity. Innervated free flaps may be used to maintain bulk and tone.

Total Glossectomy. All of the tongue and often the floor of the mouth are resected. A pectoralis major myocutaneous island flap is more advantageous than are the cervical, pectoral, or forehead flaps also used to restore the intraoral lining. Respiratory embarrassment and chronic aspiration are significant problems after glossectomy. Cricopharyngeal myotomy may be performed to facilitate swallowing and reduce aspiration. The tip of the epiglottis is often sutured to the pharyngeal wall (epiglottopexy) to decrease aspiration. Unless it is involved directly with tumor, the larynx is preserved. Laryngeal suspension, achieved by placing a heavy suture around the mandibular ramus, holds the larynx laterally. Extension into the larynx and cervical metastases are indications for unilateral or bilateral neck dissection, usually with laryngectomy. A tracheotomy is always performed with a total glossectomy to maintain an airway. For postoperative alimentation, a nasogastric tube is inserted before closing the pharynx.

Procedures of the Nasopharynx

Uvulopalatopharyngoplasty. Increasing the air space in the oropharynx corrects obstructive sleep apnea (OSA) caused by anatomic relationships in some patients. OSA can cause oxygen desaturation during apneic episodes that occur during sleep. This can lead to life-threatening pulmonary and systemic hypertension, cardiac dysrhythmias, and neurologic dysfunction if untreated. Upper airway obstruction may be caused by nasal obstruction, a deviated nasal septum, hypertrophied adenoids and/or tonsils, or mandibular retrognathism (overbite), which may be surgically corrected. To diagnose OSA in patients who do not have obvious abnormalities, airway obstruction can be viewed during sleep with fiberoptic nasopharyngoscopy and fluoroscopy. Obstruction of air passage for more than 10 seconds is diagnostic. Oxygen saturation of the blood is 85% in moderate cases and less than 60% in severe obstructive cases. Some of the oropharyngeal muscles may become atonic and collapse inward, and the soft palate may drop down. Patients who have a large, drooping soft palate and at least moderately redundant lateral pharyngeal walls or large tonsils are good candidates for uvulopalatopharyngoplasty. These patients have moderate apnea but do not have severe cardiac dysrhythmias.

The patient is continuously monitored during induction of anesthesia. The surgeon is present and an emergency tracheotomy tray is available in case the patient's airway becomes obstructed.

The full thickness of mucosa is resected from the posterior margin of the soft palate, including the uvula, and most of the anterior tonsillar pillar. The lesser palatine artery is ligated. The tonsils or mucosa of the tonsillar fossae is resected. The remaining posterior tonsillar pillar is sutured to the resected anterior pillar. The palate is closed laterally. The extent of tissue removal varies according to the width and depth of the patient's oropharyngeal space.

Adenoidectomy. Adenoidectomy, the removal of hypertrophied adenoid tissue from the nasopharynx and behind the posterior choanae, may be performed in adults to relieve upper airway obstruction. This is more commonly performed in children, often to prevent recurrent otitis media. Adenoid tissue usually atrophies after adolescence.

The patient is supine. General anesthesia is administered, and the patient is intubated. Adenoids can be resected with an adenotome and curette or vaporized with a CO_2 laser. Bleeding is more easily controlled with the laser. An electrocautery and/or gauze sponges soaked in epinephrine may be used after sharp dissection. Occasionally a posterior nasal pack is needed.

Procedures of the Oropharynx

Tonsillectomy. Chronically infected or hypertrophied tonsils are most frequently removed in childhood (Fig. 41-13).

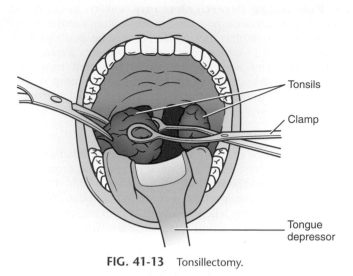

FIG. 41-13 Tonsillectomy.

Even slightly enlarged tonsils can obstruct airflow to the lungs during sleep in an adult. Tonsillectomy may significantly improve symptoms of sleep apnea, with or without uvulopalatopharyngoplasty.

A CO_2, Nd:YAG, argon, or KTP laser may be used to excise tonsils from the tonsillar fossae. The patient is supine. General anesthesia is administered. The endotracheal tube and cuff must be protected, and other laser precautions must be taken around the oral cavity. A smoke evacuator should be available with a CO_2 laser. A handheld laser may be used, or a beam may be directed through the microscope.

Local anesthesia is frequently used for adult tonsillectomy. The patient is in semi-Fowler's or a sitting position on the operating bed or sits in a specially designed chair. The throat is anesthetized with a topical agent and local infiltration. With sharp and blunt dissection, each tonsil is separated from the pillars and capsule and removed from the fossa with a tonsil snare. Attention is given to hemostasis to prevent aspiration; suture ligatures, free ties, and/or absorbable ligating clips may be used. Bleeding can be difficult to control and can occur postoperatively with this technique. Less intraoperative bleeding occurs with laser tonsillectomy.

Incision and Drainage of a Peritonsillar Abscess. Less common since the advent of antibiotics, incision into the anterior tonsillar pillar may be necessary to drain purulent material posterior to the tonsillar capsule after acute tonsillitis.

Resection of a Tonsillar Tumor. A localized squamous cell carcinoma of the tonsil may be resected by dissection or with cryosurgery. An en bloc resection includes the primary tumor and nodes. Metastatic nodes are common. Superior progression of the tumor may reach the supratonsillar fossa, soft and hard palates, and uvula. Inferiorly the tumor may spread to the posterior and lateral walls of the larynx, base of the tongue, and pyriform sinus. Neck dissection may be indicated for regional disease. Surgery may be combined with preoperative or postoperative radiation therapy. The most common complications are fistula formation and delayed healing.

Pharyngeal Diverticulectomy. Diverticulectomy, or removal of sacs or outpouching of lower pharyngeal mucous membrane in which food collects, may be performed in extreme cases in which regurgitation presents a hazard of aspiration. The neck of the sac is dissected from the posterior pharyngeal wall and ligated. The stump of the excised sac is inverted into the pharyngeal wall. Diverticula may be removed endoscopically.

Dental Procedures

Just as the scope of many medical-surgical specialties, such as otolaryngology–head and neck surgery, has broadened, so has dentistry. Likewise, subspecialization within dentistry, through extensive specialized postgraduate education, has given OR practice privileges to dentists who perform surgical procedures in and around the oral cavity. Among these are the following:

- *Oral surgeon.* Oral surgery may be limited to exodontia (extraction of teeth) and minor surgery in the oral cavity. It may also include correction of dentofacial deformities (i.e., oral and maxillofacial surgery). A qualified oral surgeon is competent to complete a history and physical examination and thus determine the patient's ability to undergo the proposed surgical procedure.
- *Orthodontist.* Orthodontics focuses on irregularities of the teeth, malocclusion, and associated facial problems.
- *Prosthodontist.* Prosthodontics is concerned with artificial restoration of intraoral and external facial structures.
- *Periodontist.* Periodontics is the treatment and prevention of disease in the gingiva (gum), underlying soft tissues, and alveoli surrounding the teeth.

Patients with medical problems admitted to the hospital by oral surgeons and all patients admitted for dental care have an admission history, physical examination, and evaluation of their overall medical risk by a physician preoperatively. This physician is responsible for the care of a preexisting condition and any medical problem that arises during hospitalization.

Just as physicians from various specialties function as members of a multidisciplinary team, so do oral surgeons and dentists, each contributing to the dental health of the patient. Frequently they also function as collegial members of the teams involved in craniofacial or maxillofacial surgery. They assist with reconstruction of the face, correction of jaw deformities, and establishment of optimal dental occlusion. For example, the orthodontist may move teeth before a maxillofacial or oral surgeon repositions the jaws to correct malocclusion. Many patients undergo both preoperative and postoperative orthodontia. Prosthodontics may be necessary to replace missing teeth. Prosthodontists also may fit an artificial nose postoperatively after rhinectomy for a tumor or trauma.

Patients seeking dentofacial treatment usually have functional problems. These may include difficulty with mastication (chewing) and deglutition (swallowing), speech problems, abnormal tongue posture, or lip incompetence. A dental surgical procedure is defined as any manipulation, cutting, or removal of oral or perioral tissues and tooth structures where bleeding occurs. Oral surgeons and periodontists perform these procedures.

Periodontics. Diseases that affect the gingiva, bone, and supporting structures such as periodontal ligaments can occur at any age. Periodontal disease is the primary cause of tooth loss in adults older than 35 years. Treatment usually takes place in the periodontist's office. Patients who have medical problems, such as hemophilia or some other blood dyscrasia, severe diabetes, or heart disease, are admitted to the hospital. Periodontal plastic surgery encompasses resective, regenerative, and reconstructive techniques.

Gingivectomy. Portions of the gingiva, mucous membrane, and underlying soft tissue that covers the alveolar process and surrounds the teeth are excised to remove deep pockets of plaque, calculus, and inflamed soft tissue. The CO_2 laser may be used for this procedure.

Mucogingivoplasty. Plastic surgery around the teeth and gums is done primarily to reduce inflammation, prevent accumulation of bacteria, and stop sensitivity. Another indication is to rebuild bone and soft tissue destroyed by disease or trauma. Excessive gum tissue is excised to contour or reshape the gingiva for improved physiologic form or aesthetics. The alveoli may be reconstructed to change their shape and height. Gingival margins may be reshaped for the site of a false tooth or fixed bridge. Gingival grafting or augmentation done before or during orthodontic treatment may reduce the risk of recession of gum tissue from around the roots of teeth. Autogenous mucogingival free grafts from the hard palate or pedicle flaps from adjacent tissues may be used to cover receded alveolar mucosa or an exposed tooth root. Flaps or grafts are used to augment inadequate zones of masticatory gingiva. Gingival onlay grafts are also used to enhance ridges where trauma or extraction has resulted in a reduced ridge, thus correcting an aesthetic defect.

Alveolar Ridge Reconstruction. The alveolar ridge is the bony remains of the alveolar process of the maxilla or mandible that formerly contained the teeth. Some edentulous patients have atrophic maxillae and/or mandibles or bony defects caused by trauma or tumor resection that will not support artificial dentures. The alveolar ridges can be augmented or reconstructed.

Inlay Bone Grafts. Bone grafts are used for augmentation of the maxillae and/or mandible. A prevascularized autogenous rib graft may be transplanted into a maxillary defect; microvascular anastomoses revascularize the graft. Composite grafts of freeze-dried cadaver rib with autogenous particulate cancellous bone and marrow may be preferred in the maxilla. Iliac bone used to augment the mandible calvaria may be harvested from the frontal, parietal, or occipital cranial bones for maxillofacial bone grafts. Calvarial bone undergoes less resorption than rib and iliac bone because of its dense blood supply; graft tissue revascularizes rapidly. Titanium osseointegration fixtures may be used to secure calvarial bone grafts in place.

Dental Implant. Fixtures are implanted into the gingiva and attached to bone to replace or augment lost dentition. Dental implants may replace a single tooth or missing teeth. They are made of biocompatible metals, most commonly titanium, and may be coated with ceramic, carbon, or sapphire. Several types are used:

- *Endosteal implant.* A threaded screw, cylinder, or flat blade is implanted in an alveolus in the maxilla or mandible. The number of implants placed depends on availability of bone and the number of teeth to be replaced. The fixture is covered with soft tissue. By the process of osseointegration, a perimucosal seal and bond develop between the gingiva and the surface of the implant. Some implants have small holes that allow bone to grow through them to secure the implant. After a minimum of 3 (for the mandible) to 6 (for the maxilla) months, a second-stage procedure is performed to connect a solid post to the implanted fixture. This extends slightly above the gingiva. The artificial tooth is attached to this post with tiny screws. Osseointegration provides firm, immobile support and distributes the stress of chewing evenly within the jaw.
- *Subperiosteal implant.* The implant is placed beneath the periosteum directly onto the alveolar bone. This type of implant is used when bone is insufficient to support an endosteal implant.
- *Transosteal implant.* A bone plate with retaining posts, similar to the mandibular staple (see following) is used when the patient has severe mandibular alveolar ridge atrophy.

Mandibular Staple. The staple fastener prosthesis is implanted as an alternative to bone grafting to restore the ability of the mandible to support a denture. The titanium alloy (Tivanium) device has two transosteal pins with a set of fasteners and lock nuts between them on the curved cross-arch connecting plate. The staple is inserted with a drill guide and twist drills specifically designed for it. The staple is evenly seated in the holes drilled in the mandible to the point of contact with the inferior border.

A scratch or bend may weaken the staple and may result in a fracture of the device. A deformed staple will not fit into the drill holes properly. The prosthesis is carefully protected and is handled very little before implantation.

NECK

Anatomy and Physiology of the Neck

The neck connects the head and trunk of the body. It is supported by the cervical vertebrae posteriorly and muscles anteriorly and laterally. The larynx, leading to the trachea, and the proximal end of the esophagus pass within the muscular structure. The vascular, nervous, and lymphatic systems leading to and from the head also pass through the neck. The thyroid and parathyroid glands lie along the trachea on the anterior aspect at the base of the neck.

Larynx. The larynx, situated anteriorly between the hypopharynx superiorly and the trachea inferiorly, consists of three major cartilages supported by ligaments and muscles: the thyroid cartilage, which protects the soft inner structures; the cricoid cartilage directly beneath it; and the paired arytenoid cartilages posterior to the thyroid and joined to the cricoid. The thyroid cartilage is incomplete posteriorly, but the cricoid is a complete ring. The cricothyroid space lies between the thyroid and cricoid cartilages.

The larynx functions as an organ for speech and for closure of the glottis during swallowing to protect the respiratory passage and prevent aspiration. The epiglottis, an elastic cartilage covered with mucous membrane at the root of the tongue in the hypopharynx, covers the superior opening of the larynx during swallowing.

Extrinsic muscles open and close the glottis, the space between the true vocal cords. Intrinsic muscles regulate vocal cord tension. Movement of the paired arytenoid cartilages opens and closes the glottis. Folds of mucous membrane covering muscle line the larynx. The two upper folds are the false cords; the two lower folds are the true vocal cords. The true vocal cords attach to the arytenoid cartilages posteriorly and to the thyroid cartilage anteriorly. The cords are an integral part of phonation. They vibrate to produce sounds by rhythmically moving air particles. Production of vocal sound involves coordination of the musculature of the lips, tongue, soft palate, pharynx, and larynx. The mouth and pharynx are the resonating cavities.

The tenth cranial (vagus) nerve innervates the larynx. Its major branch to the larynx is the recurrent laryngeal nerve (Fig. 41-14). Trauma to the nerve can result in laryngeal paralysis, which is devastating if both nerves are paralyzed.

Trachea. The trachea is a 10- to 11-cm tube composed of rings of cartilage anteriorly and membrane posteriorly. This membrane also forms the anterior wall of the esophagus (the musculomembranous canal between the pharynx and the stomach). The trachea extends from the lower larynx to the carina in the chest, where it bifurcates to form the right and left main bronchi, leading to the lungs.

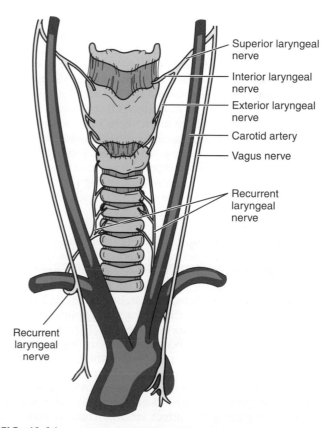

FIG. 41-14 Anatomy of the superior laryngeal and recurrent laryngeal nerves.

Surgical Procedures of the Larynx

Trauma or disease involving laryngeal cartilages, mucous membrane, or the vocal cords can obstruct respiration and/or speech. Surgical procedures are directed toward diagnosis of the cause and elimination of obstruction to maintain the larynx's dual functions in respiration and phonation.

Laryngoscopy. Laryngoscopy is a visual examination of the mucous membrane lining of the larynx and vocal cords with a lighted instrument, with or without the adjunct magnification of the operating microscope. Laryngoscopy is performed for diagnosis, biopsy, and/or treatment of laryngeal lesions, including the following:

- Foreign body, such as a coin, watch battery, or small toy.
- Papilloma of the vocal cords, which prevents accurate cord approximation and a normal voice.
- Laryngeal polyps, with stripping of polypoid mucosa to alleviate recurrence.
- Juvenile papilloma (multiple growths on the larynx, epiglottis, vocal cords, and trachea). These may be treated by cryosurgery or a laser beam in lieu of excision.
- Leukoplakia (a white thickening on the vocal cords, causing hoarseness). The lesion is examined histologically for differentiation from carcinoma.
- Laryngeal web (adherence of the anterior aspects of the vocal cords as a result of removal of mucous membrane or after inflammation). After excision, a metal or plastic plate may be placed between the cords until normal mucous membrane regenerates. The plate is then removed.

Preoperative preparation and endoscopic technique are similar for laryngoscopy, esophagoscopy, and bronchoscopy. General anesthesia usually is used, but local topical anesthesia may be preferred for some patients. The patient is supine with the neck hyperextended and head supported. As after any anesthetization of the throat, postoperative orders include nothing by mouth (NPO) status for a specific number of hours until throat reflexes have returned, to prevent aspiration.

Indirect Laryngoscopy. In indirect laryngoscopy a laryngeal mirror is inserted through the mouth to the base of the tongue. With the patient in a sitting position, light is reflected to the area by the surgeon's headlamp. During this simple diagnostic procedure, a biopsy or polypectomy can be performed.

Direct Laryngoscopy. In direct laryngoscopy a rigid, hollow, tubular laryngoscope is inserted into the larynx for direct visualization. Suction tubes and grasping forceps are maneuvered through the handheld laryngoscope. Fiberoptic light carriers are connected to a light source. Endoscopic principles as discussed in Chapter 32 are applicable.

Suspension Microlaryngoscopy. For microlaryngoscopy the laryngoscope becomes self-retaining by suspension in a special appliance placed over the patient's chest. This gives the surgeon bimanual freedom in use of the operating microscope. The microscope provides binocular vision and magnification in critical inaccessible areas or areas difficult to visualize by direct laryngoscopy. A standard operating microscope with a 400-mm lens is used. Microlaryngeal instruments are added to the basic setup for direct laryngoscopy. Suspension microlaryngoscopy is used for most intralaryngeal procedures.

Laser Microlaryngoscopy. The CO_2 laser was introduced in laryngology by Jako and Strong in 1971. It was initially used for removal of recurrent laryngeal papillomas. Now CO_2 and other lasers are used to remove a variety of benign and malignant lesions in the respiratory tract, particularly in the larynx. For example, the argon laser may be used for treatment of hereditary hemorrhagic telangiectasia (dilated groups of capillaries) in the larynx.

A micromanipulator, used to direct the laser beam, is coupled to the operating microscope. The microscope lens focuses the beam. Reflecting mirrors defocus the beam to reach into otherwise inaccessible areas. Microlaryngeal instruments are used in addition to specific laser instruments. For example, anterior commissure vocal cord retractors with suction attachments are used to clear the smoke of tissue vaporization for visibility.

Laser Safety. The laser is a safe instrument when used around the oral cavity and neck only when safety precautions are taken as follows:

1. The patient's eyelids should be taped shut and covered with moistened sponges to prevent injury from inadvertent reflection of the laser beam from a metal surface.
2. The patient's face should be covered with a moist towel so that only the oral cavity is exposed.
3. The patient's teeth should be protected from the pressure of the laryngoscope and from the laser beam.
4. Only noncombustible anesthetic gases are used. Anesthetic gases can be ignited by the laser. Nitrous oxide should not be used. Oxygen concentration may be decreased to between 21% and 30% during the lasing phase of the procedure.
5. A stainless steel or laminated aluminum and silicone endotracheal tube or a ventilating bronchoscope avoids the danger of ignition. Polyvinyl chloride and latex endotracheal tubes cannot be used because they are heat labile. Red rubber and silicone tubes may be wrapped with reflecting aluminum tape, but the tip is not always sufficiently protected if exposed to the laser beam. Ignition of endotracheal tubes has occurred. Moist gauze or compressed patties, attached to strings, are placed through the suspended laryngoscope to protect the balloon in the cuff of the tube from rupture by stray or reflected laser beams. The balloon should be filled with sterile normal saline solution, which may be tinted with methylene blue dye, so that the balloon will not ignite if ruptured. If a cuff does rupture, immediate replacement of the tube is necessary. A tracheotomy tray should be available for emergency use.
6. Combustible materials, such as sponges and drapes, are kept moist. Water effectively inhibits penetration of laser energy into surrounding tissue and materials.
7. Division of a blood vessel larger than 0.5 mm requires ligation or electrocoagulation.
8. All other precautions for laser surgery are taken.

Laryngeal Injuries. Patients with abnormal laryngeal conditions bear close watching for respiratory distress. The anterior, unprotected location of the larynx predisposes it to trauma, such as a crushing injury. Treatment is concerned primarily with maintenance of the airway, which may be occluded by edema, hematoma, torn mucosa, or cartilaginous fragments.

Cricothyrotomy (emergency incision into the larynx) and/or tracheotomy (incision into the trachea) may be necessary to open the airway or to prevent asphyxia. An intraluminal stent inserted into the larynx superior to the tracheostomy tube and fixed to it for stabilization may be worn for several months until the laryngeal laceration heals and an intralaryngeal airway re-forms. The stent is used to mold the tissues.

Preservation of the voice is also a major concern. Severe laryngeal injury may result in permanent voice impairment. In unilateral vocal cord paralysis, because of muscle atrophy and muscle imbalance, a weak, hoarse ("air-spilling") voice is present. Inadequate glottic closure can be treated by injection of Teflon (Polytef) paste into the affected cord to augment its size and thus help to bring the two cords into apposition. The injected material becomes firm and retains its shape. A functioning cord and marked improvement in voice quality result. This modality is used commonly when the recurrent laryngeal nerve is affected. It is not indicated for acute glottic incompetence. A suspension of Gelfoam powder in saline can be used for temporary augmentation until compensation or the need for permanent augmentation occurs.

Procedures for Carcinoma of the Larynx.
Procedures vary depending on the size and location of the lesion, extent of invasion, and presence of regional or distant metastasis, as well as the patient's age, general condition, and rehabilitative capacity. Classification of malignant lesions by location includes glottic (true cords), supraglottic (above true cords), and infraglottic (below true cords) lesions. In the early stages, cancer of the larynx is one of the most curable of all malignant tumors because of the sparse lymphatic supply in the region of the vocal cords. Radiologic study of the lesion by various methods, such as contrast laryngography, is a valuable adjunct in selecting an appropriate therapeutic modality. Laryngograms can identify mucosal irregularity, vocal cord thickening, or a tumor and can outline the lesion as well as portray functional alteration of laryngeal structures.

Symptoms vary as well. Hoarseness for more than 2 weeks' duration often is a result of cord fixation by a malignant glottic lesion. Dysphagia is suggestive of a tumor at the esophageal opening. Dyspnea from airway obstruction is a late manifestation.

Whenever possible, the surgeon will perform a conservative laryngectomy to retain some natural voice. These procedures yield the same rate of cure of selected cancers as a radical procedure—total laryngectomy—without sacrificing phonation, deglutition, or respiratory function. A neck stoma is usually necessary for breathing.

Laryngofissure with Partial Laryngectomy. Laryngofissure (division of or opening into the larynx) may be necessary to remove a foreign body or tumor. Laryngofissure with partial laryngectomy through an incision in the thyroid cartilage is performed to remove a large tumor confined to one vocal cord. A tracheotomy is performed to maintain the airway. Postoperative hoarseness may diminish as scar tissue forms to replace excised vocal cord.

Supraglottic Laryngectomy. The epiglottis, false cords, and hyoid bone are removed in a supraglottic laryngectomy when a tumor is located in the epiglottis (i.e., is supraglottic). A horizontal incision is made above the true vocal cords, thus preserving voice and a normal airway. Neck dissection may be done simultaneously. A temporary tracheotomy is always part of the procedure because of the danger of aspiration and postoperative edema. With the epiglottis removed, liquids in particular can easily spill into the trachea. A cuffed tracheostomy tube is a necessary precaution postoperatively.

Vertical Hemilaryngectomy. In hemilaryngectomy through a vertical incision, one true cord, false cord, arytenoid, and half of the thyroid cartilage are removed. The epiglottis, cricoid, and opposing cords are preserved. After healing, scar tissue fills in the surgical defect, almost approximating the remaining vocal cord. Thus the patient has a usable although hoarse voice and satisfactory airway and can eat normally. Sometimes a muscle flap is used for glottic reconstruction to improve voice quality. A prophylactic tracheotomy usually is done to protect the airway. Subcutaneous emphysema (i.e., infiltration of air under the skin) is a potential complication.

Total Laryngectomy. A radical procedure, total laryngectomy is performed for advanced lesions involving the larynx and/or hypopharyngeal area, with or without neck dissection. The entire larynx, hyoid bone, cricoid cartilage, two or three tracheal rings, and strap muscles are removed. This resection destroys the connection between the pharynx and the trachea. Pharyngeal walls and the lower trachea are preserved. The pharyngeal opening to the trachea is closed, thus leaving the pharynx open only to the esophagus. The patient breathes and expels bronchial secretions through a permanent stoma at the base of the anterior neck. This is created by suturing the tracheal stump to the skin (tracheostomy). The size of the stoma should be recorded on the patient's record in the event of emergency need for a tube at a later time. In patients with a permanent stoma, resuscitation is always via the stoma.

The nose no longer humidifies the air to the lungs. The sense of smell is also lost, because the nasal olfactory epithelium is not stimulated by inhalation. Acclimatization to air intake through the neck constitutes a major adjustment for the patient.

A nasogastric tube is inserted during the surgical procedure for temporary feeding. Although the patient no longer has a normal voice, normal eating is resumed after healing takes place.

The formation of a salivary fistula is one complication of laryngectomy. Swallowed saliva leaks out through a weakness in the pharyngeal suture line and through the skin. Rupture of the carotid artery, especially in preirradiated patients, is another complication. This may occur if radical neck dissection was performed also, which places the artery in the surgical area.

Rehabilitation should begin preoperatively at the time of diagnosis and include the family. It incorporates input from many professional disciplines, because major disability results from the surgical procedure. In working with a speech pathologist, some patients learn to develop esophageal speech. By intake of a bolus of air into the esophagus and vibration by cricopharyngeal muscles, sound is produced to articulate speech. Patients unable to perfect the technique may use an artificial larynx—an electronic device that includes pitch and volume.

Many patients are unable to acquire usable esophageal speech, with or without the artificial larynx. Some of these patients have undergone surgical procedures to rebuild a functioning glottis or to create a permanent tracheo-esophageal fistula to shunt pulmonary airflow to the pharynx for phonation. Aspiration pneumonia caused by leakage of saliva and food is a major problem after these procedures. Also, pharyngeal constrictor muscle spasms or stenosis may inhibit speech rehabilitation. Voice restoration for these aphonic patients may be enhanced by a valved prosthesis. This is inserted through a tracheoesophageal fistula to allow free flow of air into the esophagus for phonation, to prevent aspiration, and to maintain patency of the fistula. Three types of one-way valve voice prostheses are used:

- The Blom-Singer duckbill prosthesis, so named from the shape of the slit valve, is a silicone tube with retention flanges (collarlike projections). The fistula for the prosthesis is created through an esophagoscope inserted into the cervical esophagus. A needle is introduced to puncture the posterior tracheal wall and anterior esophagus at the superior aspect of the laryngectomy stoma. A rubber catheter stent is inserted through the puncture to maintain patency during healing. When the prosthesis is fitted, the flanges are taped to the peristomal skin. The patient occludes the stoma to produce a voice.
- The Blom-Singer tracheostoma valve and low-pressure prosthesis has a diaphragm that opens during normal respiration and closes in response to expiratory airflow for speech. The circular valve is recessed slightly into the tracheostoma, with the housing fixed to the peristomal skin with a hypoallergenic adhesive. The patient does not manually occlude the stoma during speech.
- The Panje voice prosthesis, commonly known as the voice button, is a biflanged silicone valve inserted into a simple tracheoesophageal stab wound. An insertion guide is used to place the prosthesis through the tracheostoma into the created fistula. The patient occludes the stoma to speak.

Practical help and moral support are offered to the newly laryngectomized patient by others who are members of support groups, such as the International Association of Laryngectomees and the Lost Chord Club. The American Cancer Society is also a resource for assistance.

Laryngeal Transplant.
In January of 1998, Marshall Strome of the Cleveland Clinic Foundation transplanted a larynx and a portion of a trachea into a 40-year-old man whose larynx was crushed in a motor vehicle accident 19 years previously. He was able to speak a few words within 12 hours of the procedure. The full extent of recovery will not be known for years; however, the patient, Timothy Heidler, has since become a motivational speaker and has joined the church choir. Other patients have had the benefit of laryngeal transplants since this successful transplant. The earliest documented attempt to transplant a larynx was in 1969 in Belgium.

Surgical Procedures of the Esophagus

Esophageal disorders may be acquired or congenital. Abnormalities result from trauma, inflammation, neoplasm, or dysgenesis. A gastroenterologist and/or laryngologist may study them.

Esophagoscopy.
Endoscopic direct visualization of the interior of the esophagus is performed to remove foreign bodies; to obtain biopsy, brush cytologic, or secretion specimens for diagnosis; and to examine the esophagus and esophageal orifice of the stomach for organic disease. Inspection is made for diverticula, varices, strictures, lesions, or a hiatal hernia, which may manifest as symptoms of obstruction, regurgitation, or bleeding.

Esophagoscopes are either rigid, hollow metal tubes or the flexible fiberoptic type of scope that reduces discomfort and trauma. Accessory instruments, such as aspiration tubes and biopsy forceps, are similar for all endoscopes. Removal of an obstructing mass, such as a steak bolus in the esophagus, is better accomplished with the rigid metal scope. Various sizes of scopes are available to suit the individual patient's situation.

The patient is positioned with the shoulders even with, or a little over, the edge of the body section of the operating bed. The head section is lowered. An assistant holds the patient's head. The patient is encouraged to relax by breathing deeply if the procedure is done with local topical anesthesia. The head is raised or lowered slowly, at the direction of the endoscopist as the esophagoscope is passed, until the neck is hyperextended. The esophagoscope is passed through the mouth and cricopharyngeal lumen to the cardiac sphincter at the esophagogastric junction. The entire area is carefully scrutinized. The esophagus may be distended by insufflation of air to assist in viewing in the presence of stenosis, or a lumen finder may be necessary. The scrub person introduces tips of aspirating tubes, grasping forceps, bougies, and other long accessories into a rigid esophagoscope for the endoscopist.

Removal of Foreign Bodies.
Removal of foreign bodies from the pharynx and/or esophagus is relatively common. People who wear upper dentures are especially prone to swallowing sharp bones that cannot be felt against the covered palate. Pieces of meat or dental bridgework may lodge or become impacted in the food passage, occluding the airway by pressure. This is an emergency situation necessitating provision of a patent airway by endotracheal intubation or tracheotomy and endoscopic removal of the bolus or foreign object. Acute esophageal obstruction increases salivation, creating the danger of tracheopulmonary aspiration.

Children frequently swallow objects, such as watch batteries, coins, buttons, parts of toys, or safety pins, that may remain in the throat. Metallic objects are visible on roentgenograms, but many others are not.

It is dangerous to attempt to push an object toward the stomach because esophageal perforation can result. Esophagoscopy is the method of choice for removal, although the procedure is often difficult and painstaking. All effort is made to prevent trauma, with resultant mediastinitis.

Dilation of a Stricture. The esophageal lumen can narrow because of the formation of scar tissue resulting from inflammation or a burn at any level. Treatment consists of regular dilation with bougies of graduated sizes. Steroid administration is adjunctive therapy.

When an individual suffers a severe burn, such as from swallowing a caustic material, gastrostomy may be indicated to bypass the esophagus until it heals. Dilation of such strictures uses retrograde fusiform bougies with spindle-shaped shafts that are linked together. They are carried through the gastrostomy, up the esophagus, and out the mouth. The treatment is continued for an extended period.

Dilation of a stricture at the cardioesophageal junction may be necessary in patients with cardiospasm (achalasia). Gross dilation above the stricture, often a result of muscular atrophy, leads to regurgitation. Diagnosis is made by roentgenography, esophagoscopy, or gastroscopy. If dilation is unsuccessful, a myotomy at the esophagogastric junction (Heller procedure) is performed to enlarge the opening into the stomach. Severe, unyielding strictures may necessitate stent placement, resection, or esophageal replacement.

Neoplasms of the Esophagus. Most often malignant, neoplasms of the esophagus are treated by resection, photo-dynamic therapy, or irradiation. Dysphagia or obstruction demands immediate investigation. Surgical procedures fall under the classification of gastrointestinal surgery.

Cervical Esophageal Reconstruction. Restoration of continuity of the alimentary tract is a major challenge after ablative surgery of the neck, particularly after cervical esophagectomy or circumferential pharyngectomy. The location of the primary tumor and its extension and the extent of resection are contributing factors in determining the most satisfactory reconstruction. A pectoralis major myocutaneous flap or a free revascularized intestinal autograft will satisfactorily restore continuity in some situations.

Transposition of the mobilized stomach, jejunum, or colon into the neck may be performed when the entire esophagus is resected. Two teams working simultaneously perform this pull-up procedure. The team of general surgeons performs the abdominal dissection to mobilize the stomach or intestine while the other team resects the primary tumor in the neck. The tumor may arise from the hypopharynx, cervical esophagus, or thyroid gland. Radical neck dissection is carried out for extension into the cervical lymph nodes. Anastomosis of the stomach or intestine to an esophageal remnant may be accomplished with a circular intraluminal stapler if the primary esophageal tumor is above the level of the thoracic inlet. Primary pharyngogastric anastomosis may be required for high transection of the pharynx.

Surgical Procedures of the Trachea
Upper respiratory tract obstruction and ventilatory failure may require surgical intervention when the need for intubation or positive pressure ventilation would be long term or of indefinite duration or when severe laryngeal obstruction is present. The obstruction is bypassed or resected.

Tracheotomy and Tracheostomy. Tracheotomy is an incision into the trachea below the larynx. Tracheostomy is the formation of an opening into the trachea into which

a tube is inserted through which the patient breathes. Performed in any age-group to improve or maintain patency of the airway or relieve obstruction, the opening in the trachea provides easy accessibility for suctioning secretions from the tracheobronchial tree or administering anesthetic to patients with facial trauma or burns. A tracheotomy is commonly a controlled prophylactic procedure but can be an acute emergency. An endotracheal tube may provide temporary airway relief before and during the tracheotomy. Indications for tracheotomy include severe trauma to the hypopharynx or larynx, acute laryngotracheal bronchitis or epiglottitis in infants and children, laryngeal edema, prolonged intubation, or any other condition that obstructs respiration.

Tracheotomy is often done with the patient under local anesthesia. The patient is supine with support under the shoulders to hyperextend the neck. A transverse incision is made, producing a better cosmetic result, or a midline vertical incision is made between the cricoid cartilage and the suprasternal notch. The overlying isthmus of the thyroid gland is retracted or divided, and the exposed third and fourth tracheal rings are incised through a midline vertical incision (Fig. 41-15). Use of the ESU is avoided near the open trachea because the oxygen-rich environment supports combustion.

After tracheal aspiration to remove blood and secretions, a tracheostomy tube is inserted with the obturator in place. Immediately after insertion of the tube, the obturator is removed to open the airway. (This remains with the patient constantly in case of future need.) The outer cannula is fixed in place and the inner cannula can be suctioned or removed for cleaning. The wound is closed with a few sutures, or the superficial edges of the area above the tube may be sutured and the area below left with natural tissue approximation to facilitate drainage. A smooth-edged dressing split

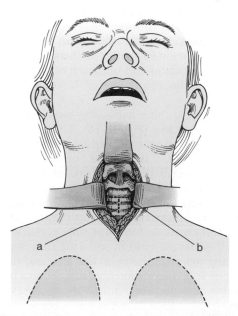

FIG. 41-15 Tracheotomy incisions. Midline vertical incision *(a)* is made between cricoid cartilage and suprasternal notch. Transverse incision *(b)* is used for emergency tracheotomy and cricothyrotomy.

around the tube protects the skin. Commercial tracheostomy dressings are available.

Tapes tied to the ends of the outer cannula are secured around the neck. Proper tension allows insertion of one finger between the tape and skin. If the tapes are tied too tightly, they may compress the jugular vein; if the tapes are tied too loosely, the tube can obtrude with coughing. The tube should not be removed during the first 24 to 48 hours by any person unable to perform a tracheotomy because the tract to the trachea may occlude and not be immediately located.

A sterile tube identical to the one inserted and a tracheotomy set accompany the patient from the OR and constantly remain with him or her until otherwise indicated by the surgeon's order.

A tracheotomy is the creation of an open wound. Although rigid asepsis is not possible, every effort is made to keep contamination to a minimum. Only sterile equipment, with minimal handling, is used to prevent infection. Suctioning through a tracheostomy tube is done as a sterile procedure with a sterile catheter and gloves. Careful suctioning prevents trauma. The catheter is inserted without application of suction, which could injure the tracheal walls and suction out oxygen in the patient with borderline oxygen saturation levels. Suction is applied as the catheter is withdrawn. Sterile solution is run through the catheter after use to clean it and maintain patency. Disposable catheters are recommended; they are used once and discarded.

Some patients who have undergone tracheotomy come to the OR for a change of the tube or other procedure. These patients may require suctioning while waiting in the holding area. Knowledge of and preparation for each patient is a prime responsibility of the circulator. These patients require humidified air, which can be delivered by various devices, to keep secretions liquefied and to prevent drying of tissues. Other needs are constant observation and special communication (e.g., pencil and paper, Magic Slate, picture board). (More information can be found on the Internet at www.bissels.com/trach/htm.)

Tracheostomy Tubes. Although an endotracheal tube may provide ventilation for short-term therapy, a tracheostomy tube is easier to suction and immobilize for extended use. It also reduces the possibility of laryngeal injury and tracheomalacia.

Most tubes have three parts—the outer cannula, inner cannula, and obturator (Fig. 41-16). The inner cannula is periodically removed and cleaned to prevent blockage by crusting of secretions. It is replaced immediately within the outer cannula so that the latter remains free of crusting. The obturator provides a smooth tip during tube insertion to prevent trauma to the tracheal wall. Some plastic tubes do not require an inner cannula because they remain relatively free of crust. If crusts do form, the tube is changed.

Some tubes have a built-in soft cuff that is inflated to eliminate any free space between the tube and the tracheal wall, thus preventing aspiration of drainage down the trachea. Cuffed tubes also facilitate function of any ventilatory apparatus.

A pilot balloon in the inflation line, attached to the outer cannula, indicates cuff inflation or deflation. Proper cuff inflation-deflation is very important. Irritation and pressure

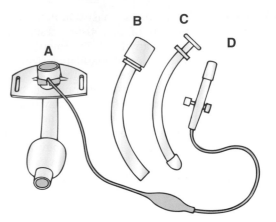

FIG. 41-16 Tracheostomy tube. **A,** Outer cuffed cannula. **B,** Inner cannula. **C,** Obturator. **D,** Pilot balloon in inflation line.

of the cuff against the tracheal wall can cause damage such as ulceration and necrosis of the mucosa, which can lead to infection, tracheobronchial fistula, erosion into the innominate artery, or stenosis from scarring. Precautionary measures include deflation at regular intervals, by the physician's written order, to increase blood flow to the cuff site; use of a low-pressure or controlled-pressure cuff; constant monitoring of intracuff pressure; and minimum inflation to ensure a leak-free system. Overinflation can reduce the tube diameter, as well as cause the cuff to extend over the tip of the tube, thus obstructing ventilation. Or the tracheal wall may herniate over the tube end. Underinflation may cause subcutaneous emphysema. Cuffs also should inflate symmetrically. The amount of air needed for inflation varies with the size of the trachea and the tube. Understandably, less air is needed for larger tubes. Usually 2 to 5 mL of air provides a closed system.

Specific tubes have special variations, such as an opening in the wall opposite the bevel to permit ventilation in case of bevel occlusion. Others have a radiopaque tip that allows radiologic visualization of the tube position. Many have connectors, some of which are a built-in swivel type, permitting lightweight, flexible, easy connection to a ventilating system. These connectors reduce the hazard of accidental disconnection. Still others have a fenestration in the outer cannula, permitting air to flow through the larynx. These tubes are used to allow assessment of spontaneous breathing and coughing in preparation for decannulation in patients no longer requiring mechanical ventilation.

With air passing through the larynx, the patient can speak with the proximal end of the cannula plugged. A so-called speaking tube permits introduction of humidified air and oxygen through a special line, and with upward flow of the gas through the larynx, the patient can speak.

Tracheal Resection. Tracheal obstruction can result from trauma or a tumor, thus occluding the patient's airway. Localized erosion and scarring, causing narrowing of the trachea, can develop from prolonged endotracheal intubation or a tracheotomy. An obstructive or stenotic lesion can be resected and the trachea reconstructed by end-to-end anastomosis. Through a cervical, low-collar skin incision, the upper trachea and subglottis are mobilized. A right posterolateral thoracotomy incision is used for lesions in the distal trachea near the carina, where the trachea bifurcates into the right and left bronchi. A longitudinal incision is made in the stenotic area, and an anode tube (a flexible wire-reinforced endotracheal tube) is inserted into the distal trachea to maintain respiration. The trachea is transected circumferentially above and below the obstructed segment. The laryngeal attachments to the trachea are released, and the suprahyoid muscle is transected. Up to 5 to 6 cm of trachea can be resected and closed by primary anastomosis. The neck is flexed so that the edges of the trachea can be approximated without tension. The neck may be kept flexed during postoperative healing by a heavy suture from the chin to the chest. The patient remains intubated, with the end of the tube located beyond the anastomosis, as a stent, for 1 or 2 days.

Surgical Procedures of the Anterior Neck

Many laryngologists and plastic surgeons, as well as some oral and general surgeons, perform neck dissection when cervical lymph nodes are involved in cancer of the head and neck. A multidisciplinary team, including a thoracic and/or general surgeon, may perform some complex resections and reconstructive procedures.

The patient may be positioned with the neck extended, usually over a thyroid elevator. The arms are secured at the sides of the body and not on armboards, thus preventing distortion of the body contour in the neck region. The operating bed may be tilted into reverse Trendelenburg's position.

Thyroid Procedures. The thyroid gland, located in the anterior aspect of the neck, is composed of two vascular lobes that lie on either side of the trachea and are united by a narrow band, the isthmus (Fig. 41-17). The thyroid hormone controls the rate of body metabolism and may influence physical and mental growth.

Hyperthyroidism (Graves' disease), hypothyroidism, and an enlarged gland (goiter) are the main disorders of the thyroid gland. Drugs, radioactive iodine, and/or surgical resection are used to treat hyperthyroidism. This disease, which is rare in geriatric patients or the very young, affects women more frequently than it does men. Replacement of the thyroid hormone with drug therapy is the specific treatment for hypothyroidism. Oral administration of thyroid extract or iodine may reduce the size of the gland, but surgical excision is frequently necessary to remove benign or malignant tumors.

Thyroid Biopsy. A needle biopsy or an excisional biopsy may be performed to aid in establishing a diagnosis of thyroiditis or differentiating between nodular goiter and carcinoma.

Thyroidectomy. During all thyroidectomy procedures, care is exercised not to damage the laryngeal nerves and parathyroid glands. The patient is positioned supine with the neck hyperextended to provide good exposure of all structures (Fig. 41-18). A transverse collar incision is made in a natural skin crease about 1 inch (2.5 cm) above the clavicle. The cervical fascia is incised vertically in the midline. Throughout the surgical procedure, meticulous hemostasis is maintained. Blood supply arises from the external carotid arteries to the upper poles of the thyroid gland and from the subclavian arteries to the lower poles. The superior laryngeal nerves, which innervate the cricothyroid muscles, and recurrent laryngeal nerves, which innervate the vocal cords, are identified. Trauma to these nerves can result in temporary or permanent laryngeal paralysis. Voice disturbances with hoarseness occur with paralysis of one vocal cord.

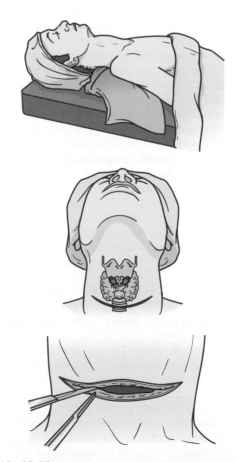

FIG. 41-18 Position and incision for thyroidectomy.

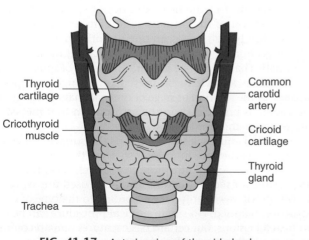

FIG. 41-17 Anterior view of thyroid gland.

Postoperative complications of thyroidectomy include hematoma, edema of the glottis, injury to a recurrent laryngeal nerve, muscle rigidity and spasm (tetany), and acute thyrotoxicosis. A tracheotomy set should remain at the patient's bedside postoperatively for at least 24 hours in the event of respiratory obstruction.

A general surgeon usually performs thyroidectomy. Depending on the pathologic diagnosis, the surgeon chooses the most appropriate procedure for removal of a part of or the entire thyroid gland.

Thyroid Lobectomy. An entire lobe is removed, especially for toxic diffuse goiter, which is usually benign. In case of malignant growth, the lobe and lymph nodes in the neck that drain into the involved area may be dissected.

Subtotal Thyroidectomy. The usual procedure for hyperthyroidism is removal of approximately 5/6 of the thyroid gland. This procedure generally relieves symptoms permanently because the remaining thyroid tissue secretes sufficient hormone for normal function.

Total Thyroidectomy. Excision of both lobes plus the isthmus may be the procedure of choice for palpable disease in both lobes.

Substernal Intrathoracic Thyroidectomy. Invasion of the gland into substernal and intrathoracic regions can cause tracheal obstruction. The sternum may have to be split to remove a large, adherent intrathoracic goiter.

Parathyroid Gland Procedures. The parathyroid glands are small endocrine glands that regulate metabolism of calcium and phosphorus. Four or more glands are located within or are attached to substance of the thyroid gland (two on each side), or they may migrate into the neck or mediastinum. Primary hyperparathyroidism is associated with hypercalcemia, which may be secondary to renal, skeletal, or gastrointestinal disease. A single or multiple glands may be diseased and surgically excised. The incision and exposure are the same as described for thyroidectomy.

Subtotal Parathyroidectomy. A single diseased gland, confirmed by frozen section, is excised. Up to three and a half glands may be removed if all glands appear to be involved, as in diffuse hyperplastic disease. Parathyroid glands are handled by their pedicles to avoid crushing, suturing, or violating the capsule. Inadvertently implanted parathyroid tissue may cause recurrence of disease or persistent or recurrent hypercalcemia. A remnant of normal tissue is left to prevent hypoparathyroidism, which may cause severe tetany. Removed normal tissue may be cryopreserved for autotransplantation in muscle, usually in the forearm, if hypoparathyroidism develops or reoperation is necessary for recurrent or persistent hyperparathyroidism.

Total Parathyroidectomy with Autotransplantation. All parathyroid tissue is removed when all glands are abnormal. First described by William Halsted in 1907, a portion of a gland is immediately transplanted into a vascularized muscle, usually the sternocleidomastoid, which is in the surgical field. Some surgeons prefer to put the transplant in a forearm muscle. This procedure may be done when embedded parathyroid glands are removed in conjunction with a total thyroidectomy. Postoperative supplemental calcium and vitamin D should be considered for treatment of hypoparathyroidism.

Thyroglossal Duct Cystectomy. During fetal development, the thyroid gland descends through the thyroglossal duct from the foramen cecum near the base of the tongue to the neck below the larynx. In adulthood, remnants of this embryonic duct may form a cyst in the anterior midline of the neck. Excision requires removal of the entire cystic sac and a portion of hyoid bone that surrounds the duct.

Cervical and Scalene Lymph Node Biopsy. Biopsy specimens are taken of the cervical and/or scalene nodes for diagnosis of metastatic extension of cancer or tuberculosis into these lymphatic nodes. A thoracic surgeon may perform the procedure.

Neck Dissections

Tumors, benign and malignant, occur in the head and neck regions. Although the origin of many of these neoplasms is technically in the head, the cervical lymph nodes frequently are involved secondarily by metastases from a primary head or neck malignant tumor. Treatment is directed toward definitive management for eradication of the tumor and metastases, with consideration for rehabilitation. In an attempt to eradicate all cancer foci, neck dissection may be performed at a time later than removal of a primary lesion of, for example, the parotid gland or tongue or simultaneously as a one-stage procedure. This composite resection removes the primary tumor and metastatic lesions at the same time en masse. Sometimes metastasis occurs before a primary lesion is discovered.

Various reconstructive techniques provide immediate restoration to improve speech, reestablish oral function, or prevent airway obstruction. Others involve delayed reconstruction. The method of repair depends on the type of defect resulting from excision of the lesion. Preoperatively, the patient's emotional stability is analyzed if the surgical procedure will result in a cosmetic deformity. Reconstruction is planned so that local tissue can be used whenever feasible and normal function is preserved whenever possible. The aim of reconstruction is to restore function and appearance.

Radical Neck Dissection. Malignant tumors of the oral or pharyngeal cavities, cutaneous malignant melanoma, and skin cancer in the head and neck region often require wide resection of the primary lesion and excision of all of the cervical lymph nodes on one or both sides of the neck. This procedure gives the patient with cancer of the cervical lymphatic chain a chance for cure and arrest of spread. When metastasis is known to be present or is highly suspected because of the location or stage of the malignancy, the surgical procedure is predicated on the assumption that metastases are regional and not distant.

The head and neck surgeon plans the surgical procedure with reconstruction in mind, so that the incisions will allow good exposure but provide as much local flap tissue as possible for reconstruction. Incisions used for the tumor resection will necessarily vary according to the type of reconstruction planned. No single surgical procedure can be used to treat all lesions, but certain basic features remain common to all neck dissections (Fig. 41-19).

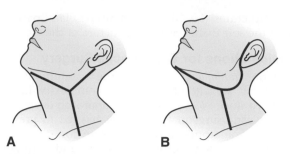

FIG. 41-19 Neck incisions for radical neck dissection. **A,** Block dissection. **B,** Modified Y-incision for block dissection to include radical parotidectomy.

All lymph-bearing tissue from the midline anteriorly to the trapezius muscle posteriorly and from the mandible superiorly to the clavicle inferiorly is removed. All tissue between the deep cervical fascia and the platysma muscle externally is removed except the carotid artery system; the vagus, phrenic, and hypoglossal nerves; and the brachial plexus.

The massive tissue resection (removal en bloc) includes the jugular vein, eleventh cranial (spinal accessory) nerve, sternocleidomastoid muscle, and submandibular salivary gland. Elimination of the motor nerve to the trapezius muscle contributes to muscular atrophy, subsequent shoulder drop on the affected side, and possibly decreased strength in raising the arm.

Various techniques are used to close the large defect in the anterior neck. When the occipital, posterior auricular, facial, and superior thyroid arteries can be preserved, arterialized skin flaps designed to incorporate branches from these vessels can be constructed with the length up to three or four times the width. Otherwise, the length of a flap should not exceed twice the width. A deltopectoral pedicle flap or a pectoralis major myocutaneous free flap may be needed

(Fig. 41-20). An exposed carotid artery is covered. Cervical flaps carrying their own blood supply may be used for this and to restore the oropharyngeal lining intraorally. A pedicle flap of sternocleidomastoid muscle from the clavicle may be an alternative.

The mandible is preserved unless it is involved by direct extension of the tumor into the bone. Access through a mandibular osteotomy or partial mandibulectomy is usually required for effective resection in the posterior oral cavity. Solid bony continuity and realignment of the dental arches are established for functional restoration of speech and chewing. A revascularized free fibular graft, a bone graft from the rib or iliac crest, cancellous bone chips, or a composite graft may be used to stabilize the mandible.

Effective drainage of the wound is important to healing. This is accomplished by use of closed-wound suction drains inserted through stab wounds below the clavicle. Prevention of hematoma protects the viability of the thin skin flaps and facilitates approximation of wound surfaces.

A tracheotomy may be performed to protect the patient from respiratory distress in neck dissection alone. A tracheostomy is always done in a composite radical neck resection.

A feeding gastrostomy tube may be inserted for anticipated extended feeding. This permits suction to avoid aspiration and gastric distention in addition to providing a feeding route. The tube is usually inserted in the OR.

Potential complications of neck dissection are numerous, depending on the tumor itself, irradiation therapy, or necessary sacrifice of vital structures. Intraoperatively, hemorrhage may occur from injury to a major vessel or the thoracic duct. Postoperatively, invasion of overlying skin necrosis into a major vessel wall, such as the carotid artery, can cause an often-fatal blowout of the vessel. Slight previous bleeding may be a forewarning. Balloon occlusion of the carotid artery may be used to prevent hemorrhage.

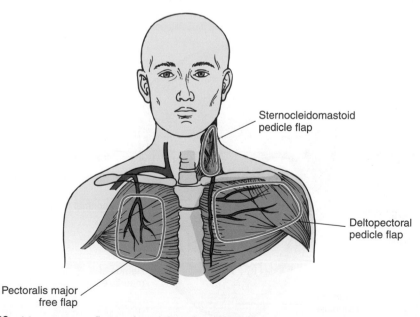

FIG. 41-20 Myocutaneous flap to close defect after radical neck dissection may be deltopectoral pedicle flap, pectoralis major free flap, or sternocleidomastoid pedicle flap.

Although reconstruction begins at the time of primary neck dissection, the patient usually requires considerable postoperative rehabilitation psychologically and staged procedures before cosmetic and functional reconstruction is complete.

FACE AND SKULL
Anatomy and Physiology of the Face

The face is the anterior part of the head, including the forehead, cheeks, nose, lips, and chin, but not the ears. The eyes, situated in the bony orbits, contribute to the features of the face, although they are not technically a part of the face.

The skeletal structure of the face and skull (Fig. 41-21) includes the frontal bone of the forehead. It forms the upper part of the orbits. Divided by sutures (i.e., lines of union between bones), the frontal bone joins the sphenoid and ethmoid, and the paired nasal, lacrimal, maxilla, and zygomatic bones. The posterior orbits are formed by the sphenoid bone, which is shaped like a butterfly with extended wings, and the palatal bones. The medial walls are formed by the ethmoid, lacrimal, and nasal bones and maxilla. The lateral aspect is formed by the zygoma (malar bone), or the cheekbone. The irregularly shaped ethmoid bone also forms the roof and posterior lateral wall of each nasal cavity. The nasal bones form the bridge of the nose between the orbits.

The maxilla (the upper jaw that holds the palate) extends laterally to the zygoma and temporal bone, under the orbit, and along the anterior nasal cavity. The maxillary bones are paired and join in the midline between the nose and the oral cavity. The alveoli that hold the teeth are along the alveolar processes of the maxillae.

The ramus of the mandible (the arch-shaped bone of the lower jaw) articulates with temporal bones at the temporomandibular joints in front of the ears. The alveoli, the tooth-bearing bodies, meet at the alveolar process to form the chin (mental region).

The bony structure of the face is covered with muscles, superficial blood vessels and nerves, epidermis, and dermis.

Other structures (i.e., ducts and sinuses [air spaces]) are also in the soft tissues or bony structure of the face.

Considerations for Craniofacial Surgery

The term *craniofacial* refers to the cranium and face. Craniofacial surgery of increasing complexity has been performed since World War II. The approach developed by French plastic surgeon Paul Tessier has led to previously inaccessible anatomic areas. Exposure for dissection of soft tissues and bone to restore contour and symmetry in practically every type of facial deformity, whether congenital, neoplastic, or traumatic in origin, can be accomplished by a multidisciplinary team of surgeons. This team may include a plastic surgeon, neurosurgeon, anesthesia provider, ophthalmologist, oral surgeon, and otorhinolaryngologist. Some procedures require more than 100 separate maneuvers and may take as long as 14 to 16 hours to complete.

Many of the concepts developed for these very complex procedures are applied in the more common and less complicated procedures to reshape sections of the skull or reconstruct soft tissues. Craniofacial reconstruction should be performed as soon as indicated by the physiologic and psychologic effects of the deformity on the patient, regardless of age. An early surgical procedure not only decreases psychologic trauma but also may prevent craniofacial distortion caused by brain and nerve damage of a disease process or traumatic injury.

Analysis of three-dimensional CT scans and cephalometric tracings accurately superimposed on transparent photographs of the patient preoperatively is essential to determine the extent of the facial deformity and the plan for skeletal rearrangement. The exact size of the defects that will need bone grafts can be determined.

Many procedures involve correction of malocclusion of the mandible at the same time that the orbitocranial skeleton is restructured. Dental models are cut and mounted on an articulator for reference.

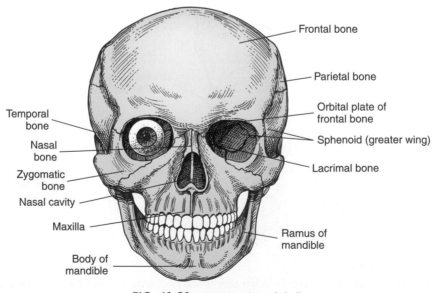

FIG. 41-21 Anterior view of skull.

Hypotensive anesthesia reduces blood loss during these extensive procedures. The patient is continuously monitored throughout the procedure to estimate blood loss. A preoperative tracheotomy may be necessary to maintain an adequate airway postoperatively.

Craniofacial Anomalies

Congenital craniofacial anomalies have a monumental effect on the life and activities of children and their families. These children spend much of their lives in medical and surgical treatment followed by psychosocial therapy. Not only are these children physically deformed in appearance, but they also often have impaired vision, speech, and hearing. In some circumstances the child may be mentally retarded or have other brain injury that results in seizures.

Some of the anomalies are extreme and visually gruesome, but defects that are incompatible with life are complex critical issues to correct in the first few hours or days after birth. The first objective of surgical intervention is to support the child's life functions such as breathing, eating, communicating, and vision. The second objective is to bring the child's form into a more natural appearance. Figure 41-22 depicts the primary areas of the infant's skull that are involved with craniofacial deformity.

The entire therapeutic process is a multidisciplinary effort of many specialized team members. Another issue to consider is that the child may have additional congenital defects of the internal organs or limbs that need to be addressed simultaneously with the head and neck.

Most of the anomalies associated with the head and neck have been categorized by the type of defect and its effect on the development of the face and skull. The main syndromes are as follows:

1. *Craniosynostosis.* Fusion of one or more sutures of the skull. Can be unilateral or bilateral causing facial abnormalities and increased intracranial pressure.
   a. *Scaphocephaly.* Most common type. Closure of the sagittal suture causes an increased anteroposterior length (Fig. 41-23, *A*).
   b. *Plagiocephaly.* Caused by unilateral or unequal coronal synostosis and may involve the lambdoid suture. The face and head are asymmetric (Fig. 41-23, *B*).
   c. *Acrocephaly/oxycephaly/turricephaly.* Caused by fusion of the coronal and frontoethmoidal sutures that increases the vertical axis of the skull referred to as "tower head." Seen in Crouzon disease and Apert syndrome.
   d. *Brachycephaly.* Caused by bicoronal synostosis and sagittal shortening. The head is wide and short. Seen in Crouzon disease (Fig. 41-23, *C*).
   e. *Trigonocephaly.* Least common. Caused by premature closure of the metopic and frontoethmoidal (between the frontal and ethmoid bones) sutures. The skull is triangle shaped with apex on front of forehead with hypotelorism (abnormal decrease in the bony distance between the eyes) (Fig. 41-23, *D*).
2. *Hypertelorism.* A genetic defect that may appear independently, or as a result of a midline facial cleft and/or encephalocele and causes an abnormal increase in the bony distance between the eyes measured between the medial orbital walls. Problems with binocular vision and an absent sense of smell (Fig. 41-24).
3. *Pierre Robin syndrome.* Micrognathia, mandibular hyperplasia, wide cleft palate, glossoptosis (may cause apnea), and feeding difficulties (Fig. 41-25).
4. *Crouzon disease.* Brachycephaly and turricephaly caused by craniosynostosis, midfacial retrusion associated with maxillary hypoplasia, shallow eye orbits to house the globe, optic nerve damage, "bird beak" nose, some mental retardation, and airway difficulty (Fig. 41-26).
5. *Treacher Collins syndrome.* Autosomal dominant defect that causes mandibulofacial dystosis. Caused by lateral facial clefts through the maxilla and malar arches, narrow oropharynx and a high-arched palate with or without a cleft, external ear deformities with or without middle and inner ear defects and conductive hearing loss, lower eyelid deformities, including coloboma (notching of the lower eyelids) and partial to total

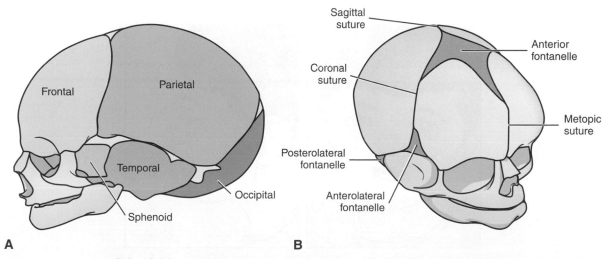

FIG. 41-22   **A,** Bones of the infant skull. **B,** Suture synarthroses of infant skull.

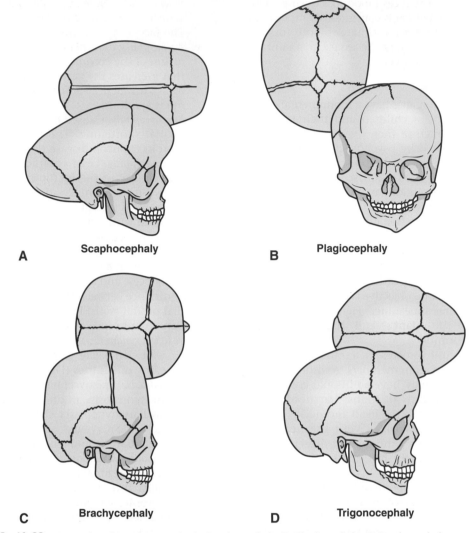

A   **Scaphocephaly**

B   **Plagiocephaly**

C   **Brachycephaly**

D   **Trigonocephaly**

FIG. 41-23   Examples of craniosyostosis: **A**, Scaphocephaly. **B**, Plagiocephaly. **C**, Brachycephaly. **D**, Trigonocephaly.

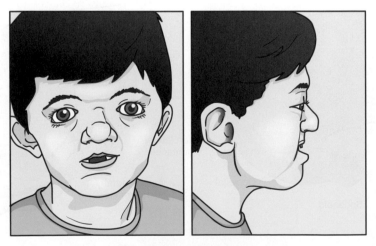

FIG. 41-24   Hypertelorism.

absence of lower lashes, and nasal deformity. May result in esophageal collapse requiring a feeding tube and apnea requiring a tracheostomy (Fig. 41-27).

6. *Craniofacial microsomia.* Caused by the intrauterine interruption of the development of the first and second branchial arches. Also known as oral-mandibular-auricular syndrome. Most common in males. Usually unilateral, but can be bilateral. Can accompany many other defects such as torticollis, craniosynostosis, microtia, facial clefts, absent lung or kidney, cranial nerve abnormality, vertebral malformations, eye malformation, oral feeding problems, and airway collapse.

7. *Apert syndrome.* Also known as acrocephalosyndactyly (autosomal dominant syndrome of anomalies of the extremities, head, and hands). The syndrome is characterized by coronal craniosynostosis, exorbitism, hypertelorism, maxillary hypoplasia, wide, hooked nose, narrow palate with median groove, with or without cleft, bilateral symmetric syndactyly of the hands and/or feet, ankylosis of the elbows, shoulders, and hips. Airway obstruction is secondary to midface hypoplasia necessitating a tracheostomy, and anomalies of the heart, lung, and kidney can be life threatening. Hearing can

be a problem because of malformed eustachian tubes (Fig. 41-28).

8. *Microtia.* Small or absent ears.

Congenital craniofacial deformities are surgically treated by several types of cranial remodeling procedures. Some procedures require the child to wear midface external distraction devices that are tightened daily to cause the face to shift into a forward position. In some conditions the dome of the skull is reshaped by opening the fused sutures and wearing a helmet. Each congenital condition has varying degrees of mental retardation associated with compression of the brain that must be released to minimize the damage.

Craniofacial Procedures

Midface Advancement. The base of the anterior cranial fossae can be exposed through a bifrontal incision to elevate a frontal bone flap. While the neurosurgeon is raising the flap, the plastic surgeon may take donor bone from a rib and/or the iliac crest if autogenous bone grafts will be needed. Harvesting of bone from the calvarium (the upper, dome-like portion of the skull) may be preferred.

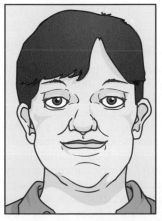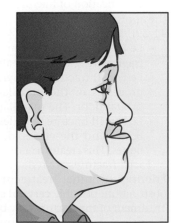

FIG. 41-25 Pierre Robin syndrome.

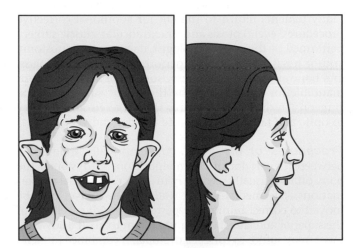

FIG. 41-27 Treacher Collins syndrome.

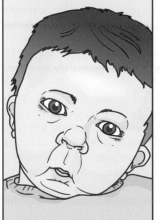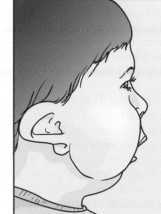

FIG. 41-26 Crouzon disease.

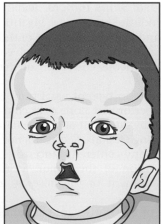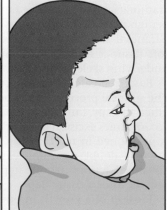

FIG. 41-28 Apert syndrome.

The facial skeleton is separated from the cranial base. The plastic surgeon raises the periorbita, orbital contents, and soft tissue over the dorsum of the nose. The subperiosteum of the anterior maxillae is elevated. Osteotomies are cut in the supraorbital region to mobilize the lateral walls. An anterior maxillary osteotomy, through an infraorbital approach, extends across and below the frontal processes of the maxillae. Osteotomies of the anterior cranial fossae and the medial and lateral orbital walls and floors are completed. The mobilized bones can be functionally advanced in three dimensions as desired. They are then stabilized with a plating system or wired into position.

To maintain stability, bone grafts also are wired into place in the resulting defects. Resorbable plates and fixation are available for use. Demineralized bone blocks, chips, or powder often are preferred to bone grafts to induce osteogenesis. The frontal bone flap is replaced, and the incision is closed.

Mandibular osteotomies may be done before closure to correct alignment of the jaws. Whether this is necessary or not, the mandible is stabilized after closure with intermaxillary wires and suspension wires to the zygomatic arch.

Depending on the deformity, variations of the intracranial and extracranial osteotomies are done to advance, align, or reposition the facial bones and reconstruct soft tissues. Many patients return to the OR for additional corrective procedures: eyelid ptosis and/or extraocular muscle surgery performed by the ophthalmologist; dacryocystorhinostomy and/or nasal reconstruction performed by the rhinologist; and bone augmentation or resection of the maxillae and/or mandible for repositioning by the plastic surgeon or oral surgeon. During all procedures the surgeons avoid injury to optic and facial nerves and to arteries and veins.

Procedures of the Orbit.
An abnormally wide space between (hypertelorism) or malposition of (dystopia) the bony orbits is usually secondary to other craniofacial malformations. The medial orbital walls by themselves may be moved to correct minimal hypertelorism. Advancement of the superior and lateral walls, rather than total orbit advancement, may suffice to correct a dystopia. A combined intracranial and extracranial approach may be necessary to change the angle of the orbits and reposition the medial canthal ligaments of the eyes.

Resection of Nasal or Paranasal Sinus Tumors.
Radical craniofacial resection may be indicated to remove gigantic benign nasal dermoid tumors and malignant tumors of the paranasal sinuses. In a one-stage procedure, all involved soft tissue is excised with simultaneous correction of the underlying skeletal structure.

Basal cell carcinoma is a common type of nasal tumor. The surgical procedure may be performed alone or as combined therapy. Immediate repair by skin graft or pedicle flap accompanies excision of well-defined lesions. Reconstruction is postponed in multicentric (many-centered) cancer or if there is doubt regarding extension of the tumor. More advanced lesions require replacement of the nose by a prosthesis or a tissue flap.

Erosion of a growth in one of the sinuses into an adjacent nasal wall can occlude the air passage. Resection may include partial or total maxillectomy and removal of surrounding tissues. The cavity usually is covered by a skin graft. Unilateral enucleation of the eye may be necessary. A radical surgical procedure for an ethmoid tumor also may involve removal of part of the base of the skull and excision of the maxillary antrum and the palate on the affected side.

In providing maxillofacial prostheses to replace facial structures after various procedures, the prosthodontist works closely with the surgeon and radiation therapist. Splints or stents hold tissue grafts in place, seal cavities from each other, or unite bony segments. A dental prosthesis to close the defect in the upper jaw and an eye prosthesis after enucleation contribute to the patient's rehabilitation after an extensive surgical procedure.

Resection of Craniofacial Tumors and Dysplasia.
Malignant tumors can originate from soft tissues of the face and scalp, the oropharyngeal mucosa, the ear canal, or the lacrimal gland. They can invade the base of the skull. Fibrous dysplasia, a congenital metabolic disturbance that causes an abnormal proliferation of fibrous tissue, can result in asymmetric distortion and expansion of craniofacial bones.

These conditions can collapse the paranasal sinuses; compress the optic nerve or chiasm, causing loss of vision; and cause other functional disabilities. An acute epistaxis (nosebleed) can be life threatening. A combined intracranial and extracranial approach may be used to completely remove the tumor or dysplastic bone. The remaining bony structures may be reshaped or repositioned. Bone grafts and/or prosthetic implants may be used for reconstruction of the forehead, orbits, nose, maxilla, and/or mandible.

Midfacial Fractures.
The facial bones provide a shield for the brain. They also protect the senses of sight, smell, hearing, and taste. Although midfacial fractures and soft tissue injuries are seldom fatal, inadequate treatment can result in disfigurement and sensory impairment. For example, virtually all blindness secondary to trauma is permanent.

Facial fractures should be suspected when the patient complains of pain, malocclusion of the jaws, or diplopia (double vision). Swelling and asymmetry of the face may be obvious. Diagnosis is confirmed by radiograph or a CT scan to identify the bone(s) involved. Rene Le Fort, a French plastic surgeon, pioneered fixation of midface fractures. The Le Fort classification of fractures, which is useful in determining the appropriate method of reduction and stabilization (Fig. 41-29), is as follows:

- Le Fort I fracture is a transverse fracture of the maxilla, fragmenting the upper alveoli and palate.
- Le Fort II fracture is a pyramidal fracture of the frontal processes of the maxillae, the nasal bones, and the orbital floor. The maxillae are freely movable.
- Le Fort III fracture includes zygomas, maxillae, and nasal bones and the ethmoid, sphenoid, and other orbital bones. This creates a craniofacial dysjunction (separation).

Facial fractures are reduced, stabilized, and immobilized. Priorities of initial treatment after injury concern airway obstruction, possible cervical spine injury, and hemorrhage. Treatment of the fracture may be delayed. The surgeon follows the principles of approaching fractures from "inside out, downward up." This means that bony structures are

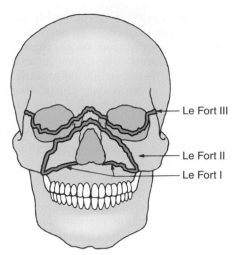

FIG. 41-29 Le Fort facial fractures.

repaired first, then the soft tissues; the mandible or most distal fracture is reduced first before working upward toward the cranium.

The method of bony repair is determined by the complexity of the fracture(s). Intermaxillary fixation combined with interdental wiring, external pin fixation, or rigid internal fixation effect stabilization. Minifacial and midfacial plates, microplates, and mandibular plates may be combined with arch bars or bone grafts.

Reduction of Orbital Fractures. If orbital contents are depressed into the maxillary sinus, surgical exploration through an orbital or a transspinal approach is indicated. The extent of the trauma should indicate the most appropriate surgical management. The injury may involve the rim or the floor of the orbit, or both:

- Fractures of the orbital rim, frequently associated with fractures of the zygoma, are usually detected by the resulting deformity. The fracture is reduced by appropriate means. Fragments are wired into place as necessary.
- A blowout fracture of the orbit may result from a direct blow to the eyeball, which is, in turn, transmitted to the very thin floor of the orbit. A typical fracture is in the medial third of the floor with dislocation of floor fragments into the maxillary sinus. The fracture occasionally may extend into the ethmoid plate. Consequently, orbital contents, which may include the inferior extraocular muscles, are usually herniated into the antrum. This produces limitation of upward gaze and some degree of enophthalmos (recession of the eyeball into the orbit). The herniated orbital contents are reduced from the antrum back into the orbit with special attention to freeing the entrapped muscles. Plastic or silicone sheeting may be used to close the defect in the floor. Or the fragments may be elevated by packing the antrum through a Caldwell-Luc (sinus) approach. The diagnosis may be overlooked unless a laminogram is taken.

Reduction of Nasal Fractures. Fracture of the nasal bones and septum often accompanies other trauma to the head, such as a blowout fracture of the orbit (see above). If the zygoma or maxilla is involved, reduction may be accomplished through a small incision anterior to the ear and

superior to the zygomatic arch. Periosteal elevators are used to raise depressed bone and cartilage fragments. Nasal fractures are splinted with nasal packs and an external splint.

Reduction of Zygomatic Fractures. Dislocations of the zygoma are more common than fractures of the cheek-bone (malar bone). Zygomatic fractures always involve the orbital bones. Those of the zygomatic arch are particularly unstable and require intraosseous or transosseous wire fixation after internal reduction with counterpressure from underneath the arch. Transantral Steinmann pinning may be necessary to maintain reduction of fragments in severely fragmented fractures.

Maxillofacial and Mandibular Procedures. The term *maxillofacial* pertains to the part of face formed by the upper and lower jaws. Most maxillofacial procedures are designed to reconstruct defects in the lips, buccal sulcus, maxilla, alveolar ridge, floor of the mouth, mandible, and/or chin. These defects may be a result of trauma or resection of tumor. Whenever feasible, intraoral incisions are used to minimize facial scarring.

Intermaxillary Fixation of Fractures. After closed or open reduction, fractures of the maxilla and mandible are usually immobilized by interdental wiring if the patient has upper and lower teeth. If the patient is edentulous (without teeth), open reduction and skeletal fixation by circumferential wiring over an intraoral splint or screws and connecting bars may be necessary.

Erich arch bars are shaped along the dental arches. Wires are passed between the teeth to anchor the splints on the upper and lower jaws. Each splint contains a series of small lugs. Tiny rubber bands, placed around opposing lugs, hold the teeth in occlusion. Splints frequently are not used for fixation of these fractures. The teeth may be held in occlusion by wires passed around opposing teeth. After fixation of the mandible or maxilla, wire cutters accompany the patient from the OR and remain at the bedside as long as wires or rubber bands are in place. If the patient experiences respiratory difficulty or vomiting, the wires may have to be cut to prevent aspiration. Fluids may be difficult to swallow.

If microplates can be used for rigid fixation, the interdental wiring may be released after the fixation procedure is completed.

Mandibular Fractures. Some fractures of the mandible can be immobilized by transoral placement of noncompression miniplates. This technique obviates the necessity for interdental wiring. Vitallium, titanium, or stainless steel plates and screws are used for rigid fixation.

Mandibular Reconstruction. Skeletal defects creating loss of mandibular continuity are usually a result of trauma or benign disease. Bone replacement is the most common method of restoring function and contour. The patient's own ilium provides cancellous bone that can be shaped into the configuration of the jaw. A composite graft of a freeze-dried cadaver mandible packed with autogenous cancellous bone chips also can be used. These grafts fill a bony defect but do not provide soft tissue coverage. A vascularized iliac graft is preferable to reconstruct the mandible and a large intraoral defect.

Temporomandibular Joint Syndrome. Persistent pain and dysfunction of the temporomandibular joint (TMJ) can be associated with stress-related bruxism (tensing muscles and grinding teeth), the position of teeth, malocclusion, trauma, arthritis, and other degenerative changes in one or both joints. If TMJ syndrome is unresponsive to conservative treatment, surgical intervention may be indicated.

Arthroscopy. Arthroscopy, usually performed bilaterally, is used to diagnose problems such as scarring or adhesions that do not show up on a CT or magnetic resonance imaging (MRI) scan. Lysis of adhesions, mechanical debridement, and lavage of the TMJ may relieve symptoms. Repositioning or release of the fibrocartilaginous articular disc (meniscus) between the mandibular condyle and the glenoid fossa of the temporal bone may restore function. A 1.7- or 1.9-mm arthroscope with a fiberoptic camera attached is locked into a cannula sheath inserted through an inferolateral puncture wound into the joint capsule. Continuous inflow and outflow of fluid, usually iced Ringer's lactate solution, is necessary to keep the joint distended for visibility and lavage. Therapeutic synovectomy and partial or complete meniscectomy may recontour the joint. A rotary shaver and/or the holmium (Ho):YAG laser may be used. The laser rapidly resects and vaporizes cartilaginous tissue and coagulates bleeding vessels.

Arthroplasty. Open, direct visualization of the disc and condyle may be necessary to correct abnormal relationships. Either a preauricular or postauricular incision may be used to approach the TMJ. The condyle, fossa, and/or articular eminence may be reshaped or resurfaced. A damaged or displaced articular disc can be recontoured and repositioned. It is recontoured with a scalpel or by electrosurgical cutting and then repositioned and sutured in place. If the disc is torn or perforated, it is usually removed. A silicone elastomer implant or titanium alloy prosthesis may be used to reconstruct the joint. The jaw may be immobilized with interdental wiring to stabilize the TMJ during healing.

Orthognathic Surgery. The jaws can be reshaped or repositioned to correct functional bite disorders and/or for aesthetics. Occlusion (closure of teeth) depends on the anteroposterior relationship of the upper and lower jaws. The term *orthognathia*, derived from the Greek words *orthos*, meaning "straight," and *gnathos*, meaning "jaw," relates to treatment of conditions involving malposition of the maxilla or mandible, or both. Malocclusion occurs when teeth do not close together properly. It can cause difficulty in chewing and/or speaking, periodontal disease, and/or TMJ dysfunction. Psychologically debilitating facial deformity and bite disorders of genetic origin or as a result of growth disturbances or trauma include the following:

- *Prognathism.* One or both jaws project forward beyond the normal relationship with the cranial base. If the mandible (lower jaw) protrudes beyond the maxilla (upper jaw), it creates a prominence of chin, concave profile, and underbite. If the maxilla grows beyond the mandible, it creates an overbite.
- *Retrognathism.* One or both jaws are positioned posterior to the normal craniofacial relationship (i.e., behind the frontal plane of the forehead). In reference to the

mandible, the condition is commonly known as a receding chin; this may create an overbite.
- *Apertognathia.* The front teeth do not close because the back teeth come together first, creating an open bite.
- *Micrognathia.* The dental arch, usually of the mandible, is too small to accommodate the teeth. Teeth are pushed out of alignment because they are crowded together.
- *Asymmetry.* A discrepancy in size, shape, or position of the jaws creates an imbalance between the right and left sides of the face.

Preoperative orthodontia may be required to align and level the teeth. The ultimate goal is to achieve functional stability of dentofacial structures with acceptable facial aesthetics. Surgical correction may include extraction of one or more teeth, maxillary and/or mandibular osteotomies with repositioning of bone segments, and/or repositioning of alveoli. Intraorally, bilateral maxillary osteotomies may be performed in conjunction with mandibular osteotomies, or either of these procedures can be done independently to change the shape of the facial contour.

Le Fort Osteotomy. For maxillary deformities, an incision is made in the mucosa of the upper lip. Osteotomies (i.e., bone cuts) are made in the medial and lateral maxillary sinus walls. The vomer is cut just above the floor of the nose. Pterygoid plates are sectioned from the maxilla. The maxilla is movable for reduction, augmentation, or repositioning. The maxilla can be detached from the base of the skull, maintaining vascular supply via the soft palate, and cut into segments to reconstruct the lower face as described for midface advancement. Usually miniplates anchored with screws bridge the osteotomy cuts.

Mandibular Osteotomy. Sagittal split osteotomies through the ramus and vertical osteotomies through the molar region on each side allow backward or forward repositioning of the mandible. If moved posteriorly, bone on the anterior aspect is trimmed for good medullary bone contact. Rigid fixation may be obtained with miniplates or with screws placed percutaneously through stab wounds. The latter are stabilized with an external fixator. If plates and screws are used, intermaxillary fixation as described for fractures may not be necessary.

Postoperative orthodontia may be required to complete closure of spaces around the osteotomies and thus stabilize occlusal function.

Mandibulectomy. Partial or total removal of the lower jaw is performed for extension of a tumor into the bone of the floor of the mouth. It may be performed with glossectomy and radical neck dissection for wide excision. The resultant chin recession is referred to as an Andy Gump deformity. Mandibular replacement combines bone graft and synthetic materials for restoration of speech and appearance. A compound osseocutaneous flap from the iliac crest, with microvascular anastomosis of the deep circumflex iliac artery vascular pedicle, may be transferred for reconstruction. If the patient is dentulous, the relationship of opposing teeth is maintained; if edentulous, the patient wears a denture. Whenever possible, mandible-sparing procedures are done for carcinoma of the tongue.

Bibliography

Akashiba T et al: Relationship between quality of life and mood or depression in patients with severe obstructive sleep apnea syndrome, *Chest* 122(3):861-865, 2002.

Akita S et al: Sleep disturbances detected by a sleep apnea monitor in craniofacial surgical patients, *J Craniofac Surg* 17(1):44-49, 2006.

Baumgartner JE et al: Nonsynostotic scaphocephaly: The so-called sticky sagittal suture, *J Neurosurg* 101(1 Suppl):16-20, 2004.

Bhattacharyya N et al: Efficacy and quality of life impact on adult tonsillectomy, *Arch Otolaryngol* 127(11):1347-1350, 2001.

Fujimori Y et al: Additional distraction osteogenesis after conventional fronto-orbital advancement, *J Craniofac Surg* 16(6):1064-1069, 2005.

Goldstein NA et al: Child behavior and quality of life before and after tonsillectomy, *Arch Otolaryngol* 128(7):770-775, 2002.

Millman RP et al: Simple predictors of uvulopalatopharyngoplasty outcome in the treatment of obstructive sleep apnea, *Chest* 118(4):1025-1030, 2000.

Sannomiya EK et al: Clinical and radiographic presentation and preparation of the prototyping model for pre-surgical planning in Apert's syndrome, *Dentomaxillofac Radiol* 35(2):119-124, 2006.

Sarukawa S et al: Subcranial facial bipartition osteotomy with glabellar reverse V-shaped and temporal approaches instead of the bicoronal approach, *J Craniofac Surg* 17(1):147-151, 2006.

Strome M: Human laryngeal transplantation: Considerations and implications, *Microsurgery* 20(8):372-374, 2000.

Urrego AF et al: The K stitch for hypertelorbitism: Improved soft tissue correction with glabellar width reduction, *J Craniofac Surg* 16(5):855-859, 2005.

Thoracic Surgery

KEY TERMS AND DEFINITIONS

Bougie Long tapered flexible dilator. Some are lighted to be used for transillumination of a tubular anatomic structure such as the esophagus.

Decortication Stripping adhesions from the surface of the pleura.

Fundus Domelike top of stomach near where the esophagus inserts.

Lobectomy Removal of a lobe of the lung.

Mediastinum Cavity within the chest between the pleura that contains the esophagus, trachea, pericardium, and great vessels.

Plication Systematic rows of sutures that stabilize and secure a muscular region such as the diaphragm.

Pleurodesis Introduction of a chemical sclerosing agent into the chest. A powdered antibiotic, talc, or caustic chemical is instilled between the parietal and visceral layers of the pleura to fuse them by creating fibrous adhesions.

Pneumonectomy Removal of a lung.

Poudrage Full-strength powder is placed between pleural tissue layers to create adhesions.

Slurry A loose paste made of fluid and powdered agent used to intentionally create adhesions between two serous surfaces inside a cavity.

Thoracoscopy Rigid endoscopic procedure performed by percutaneous puncture of the thorax.

HISTORICAL BACKGROUND

Interest in the thorax and lungs dates back to ancient times. The brutal practice of dissecting live criminals was documented by Aulus (Aurelius) Cornelius Celsus (AD 3-64), a Roman medical author from the first century. He noted that when the diaphragm, or abdominal transverse septum, was cut, the thorax was widely opened and the person died. Celsus documented the importance of cleanliness in wound care and advocated the use of vinegar for cleansing. His main encyclopedic work, *De re medicina*, consists of eight books on medicine believed to have been written AD 30. These works contained documentation of the four cardinal signs of inflammation, the classic calor (heat), dolor (pain), rubor (redness), and tumor (swelling). In later years, loss of function was added to the list.

Flemish anatomist Andreas Vesalius (1514-1564) used animals to demonstrate to his students the transparent pleura and motion of the lungs beneath it. As exposure was widened and the pleural cavity entered, the lung was seen to collapse. Experimental animals were revived by tracheotomy with a reed pipe used as a tracheostomy tube. The invention of the stethoscope by French physician René Laënnec (1781-1826) facilitated the study of thoracic disease. The 1816 stethoscope was a 12-inch wooden cylinder placed against the patient's chest. It could be disassembled into two parts for storage in his pocket. He kept records of heart and lung sounds to correspond with the findings on autopsy. He gave the sounds names that are currently used in modern medicine, such as bruit, egophony, and rales. Laënnec studied and classified the different stages of tuberculosis and eventually contracted and died from it.

Learning safe access to the pleural cavity and lungs was a difficult step in the development of thoracic surgery. Thoracentesis with a needle and trocar for open drainage of acute empyema was performed in the United States in the mid-nineteenth century. Sporadic attempts at thoracic surgery (e.g., pulmonary resection) in the nineteenth century were accompanied by unacceptable mortality.

In 1913 American surgeon Franz Torek (1861-1938) successfully removed a carcinoma of the esophagus by resecting the ribs. Sucking wounds of the chest created by shell fragments during World War I drew new interest in thoracic problems. In 1920 American surgeon Evarts Ambrose Graham (1883-1957) brought attention to the relationship of the relaxation of vital capacity to the size of an opening in the thorax and in 1923 presented a staged procedure: cautery pneumonotomy and partial excision of the lung. In 1933 he did the first successful pneumonectomy, using exposure by rib resection. Graham noted that most of his cancer patients were cigarette smokers. Graham, a smoker himself, died of lung cancer.

The development of thoracic surgery paralleled advances in diagnostic and surgical endoscopy, endotracheal anesthesia, mechanical ventilation, closed chest drainage systems, and perioperative respiratory care techniques.

Thoracic surgery concerns disorders of the lungs, mediastinum, thoracic esophagus, diaphragm, and chest wall. Surgical intervention is most frequently indicated for neoplasms, traumatic injuries, and vascular disease. Inclusion of vital organs of respiration and circulation within the thoracic cavity mandates special attention to sustaining an oxygenated blood supply to body tissues, especially the brain, during and after the surgical procedure.

ANATOMY AND PHYSIOLOGY OF THE THORAX

An essential balance must be maintained between atmospheric pressure outside the chest and internal pressures within the thoracic cavity to sustain the vital function of respiration. Knowledge of the anatomy and physiology of the chest and thoracic cavity is necessary for an understanding of thoracic surgery.

Thoracic Cavity

The thorax, or chest, is the portion of the trunk between the neck and the abdomen. The thoracic cavity is divided into right and left pleural compartments separated by the mediastinum, which is a separate enclosed space located centrally. Alterations in pressure affecting one side of the thoracic cavity or the mediastinum cause a positional shift of the other compartments.

The bony framework of the thoracic cavity consists of the sternum and costal cartilage anteriorly, 12 pairs of ribs laterally, and 12 thoracic vertebrae posteriorly, all encased within soft tissue. The framework is bounded superiorly by structures of the lower part of the neck and inferiorly by the diaphragm. Eleven external and internal intercostal muscles, which lie between the ribs, have a corresponding artery, vein, and nerve, which require meticulous dissection to avoid inadvertent injury. The arterial blood supply is derived from the internal thoracic artery and the thoracic aorta. Venous drainage is through the mammary veins anteriorly and the azygos and hemiazygos veins posteriorly.

The first seven ribs articulate anteriorly in the midline with the sternum, which is composed of three parts: the manubrium (superiorly), the gladiolus (medially), and the xiphoid process (inferiorly). Ribs one and two articulate with the clavicle and the manubrium. The manubrium and gladiolus join in a projection referred to as the angle of Lewis, a surgical landmark (Fig. 42-1).

Ribs three through seven articulate with the gladiolus (the main sternal body) via the costal cartilage. The eighth,

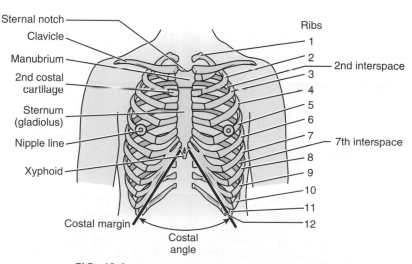

FIG. 42-1 Surgical landmarks of the bony ribcage.

ninth, and tenth ribs are joined anteriorly to the cartilage of the rib above each; the eleventh and twelfth ribs have no anterior fixation. The surgical incisional lines of direction in Figure 42-2 bilaterally overlie the lobes of the lungs on a vertical axis with the sternum (gladiolus) as the thoracic reference point.

The ribs articulate posteriorly with the thoracic vertebrae. The esophagus, trachea, and great vessels leading to and from the neck and arms pass through the small space between the manubrium and the vertebrae. Any structure pushing into this narrow opening (e.g., a mediastinal tumor) may obstruct breathing, venous return from the neck and arms, and swallowing.

Lungs. The lungs lie in the right and left pleural cavities (Fig. 42-3). The main function of these porous, spongy, conical organs is oxygenation of the blood with inspired air and expiration of carbon dioxide. The apex of each extends to the neck; the base rests on the superior surface of the diaphragm.

The right lung, which has three lobes and an oblique fissure and a straighter bronchus, is larger than the left lung, which has two lobes and a more angled bronchus. Blood supply is derived from the two pulmonary arteries and drains into the four pulmonary veins. Lymphatics drain into the bronchopulmonary nodes and into the thoracic duct. Innervation is through the pulmonary plexuses.

The lungs are enveloped by serous membrane, referred to as pleura. The pleura has two layers. The external parietal layer lines the inner surface of the thorax. The inner visceral layer covers the surface of the lung. Small amounts of serous fluid (transudate) are secreted between these layers to allow for smooth interface without friction. Excess inflammation

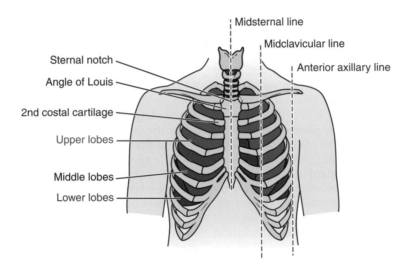

FIG. 42-2 Surgical landmarks: Lines of direction.

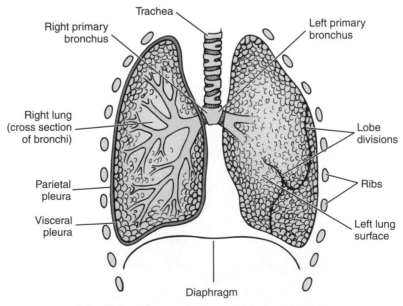

FIG. 42-3 Respiratory system within thoracic cavity.

or fluid accumulation causes pain and impaired respiratory effort. If infected, the transudate becomes exudate containing increased numbers of white blood cells. Severe inflammation causes fibrosis and adhesions of the pleural tissues.

The trachea divides at the carina into two main branches—the bronchi—leading to the right and left lungs. The right lung, with three lobes, is wider and broader than the left lung, because the liver is positioned beneath the diaphragm directly below the base. The left lung has only two lobes and is thinner, longer, and narrower in shape. It shares space in the left side of the chest with the heart, which rests in an area of the left lung referred to as the cardiac notch (Fig. 42-4).

The bronchopulmonary segments within each lung are wedges of tissue separated by veins and thin connective membrane. Although configuration of the segments differs and variations in the bronchi and blood vessels exist between the right and left lungs, it is generally accepted that both lungs normally have 10 bronchopulmonary segments. Although not demarcated by surface fissures, these segments represent zones of distribution of the secondary bronchi and may be excised individually when the segment contains a small lesion, thus preserving the uninvolved portion. Each segmental bronchus subdivides into numerous, increasingly smaller branches that eventually end in terminal bron-

chioles. These fine tubules invested by smooth muscles can constrict to close off the air passage, as in asthma. The terminal bronchioles give rise to respiratory bronchioles from which arise the alveoli. The approximately 300 million alveoli are the functional units wherein oxygenation takes place at the capillary level.

The hilus of the lung, on the mediastinal surface, is the point of entry for the primary bronchus, nerves, and blood vessels. The right primary bronchus is straighter and is a more direct continuation of the trachea. Arterial supply to the lung tissue is derived from the bronchial arteries. Venous drainage is through the bronchial veins, which empty into the azygos system. The pulmonary veins and arteries to and from the heart provide systemic pulmonary circulation. Innervation of the breathing mechanism is by the autonomic nervous system.

Mediastinum. The mediastinum has superior, anterior, middle, and posterior sections, each containing anatomic structures: the thymus lies in the anterior and superior sections, the thoracic aorta lies in the posterior section, the base of the heart and the great vessels lie in the middle, and the esophagus and trachea lie in the superior section. The organs are surrounded and suspended by the loose tissue diffused throughout the mediastinum.

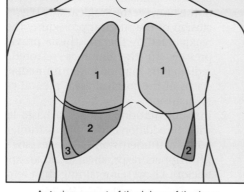

Anterior aspect of the lobes of the lung

Posterior aspect of the lobes of the lung

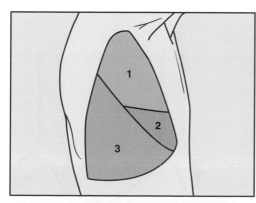

Lateral aspect of the lobes of the right lung

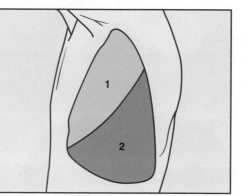

Lateral aspect of the lobes of the left lung

FIG. 42-4 Location of the lobes of the right and left lungs. Patient positioning will be determined for optimal access of the affected lobe(s) or entire lung.

Diaphragm. The diaphragm is a half dome of muscular tissue composed of four embryonic segments (1) dorsal mesentery, (2) septum transversum, (3) two pleuroperitoneal folds, and (4) cervical myotomes that border the inferior aspect of the thoracic cavity. It originates from the six lower ribs on each side, attaches to the xyphoid, and the external and internal arcuate ligaments. Abnormal separation of any of these layers changes the pressure gradient between the peritoneal cavity and the thorax causing a shift of intraabdominal organs cephalad into the chest.

The arterial blood supply arises from the right and left phrenic, intercostal, and internal thoracic arteries. Venous drainage is via the inferior vena cava, the azygos vein on the right and hemiazygos veins on the left. Innervation is from the phrenic nerve that arises from the fourth cervical ramus.

The esophagus, aorta, and vena cava pass from the thorax through the diaphragm into the abdominal cavity. Associated vessels and nerves, such as the vagus nerve follow these three structures through the diaphragm to major organ systems (Fig. 42-5).

Physiology

The size of the thorax varies with the bellows action of the thoracic wall and diaphragm, increasing with inspiration and decreasing with expiration. A partial vacuum between the parietal and visceral pleurae expands the lungs. A negative (subatmospheric) pressure normally within the thorax is essential to life.

Alterations of intrapleural pressure are of major concern, because an uncontrolled opening in the thoracic wall and pressure change can be fatal. Uncontrolled increased positive pressure in one side causes a collapse of the lung on the other side. Referred to as a mediastinal shift, this reaction occurs with entrance of either air or fluid into the pleural cavity, compressing the opposite lung and causing dyspnea. When the mediastinum has moved its limit, it can no longer accommodate a great pressure change; the lung on the affected side collapses. Air in the pleural space between the parietal and visceral pleurae constitutes pneumothorax. Blood in the pleural space constitutes hemothorax.

A mediastinal shift disturbs heart action and circulation. Changes in pressure balance within the thorax reduce vital capacity—the greatest amount of air that can be exchanged in one breath. Many diseases and conditions alter vital capacity (e.g., anesthesia, thoracic tumors, chest trauma).

SPECIAL FEATURES OF THORACIC SURGERY

Entry into the thoracic cavity can be accompanied by pulmonary distress. Team members especially skilled in meeting emergency situations are essential. Patients require close observation and monitoring, because changes may occur rapidly. A pulmonary artery catheter is inserted to monitor pulmonary capillary wedge pressures and arterial blood gases. Equipment for bronchoscopy, esophagoscopy, and mediastinoscopy must be readily available. Other preparations are routinely completed for entry into the chest for intrathoracic procedures:

1. Endotracheal anesthesia permits the lungs to expand and function even when subjected to atmospheric pressure. Administration of anesthesia under controlled positive pressure prevents physiologic imbalance and lung collapse in the presence of controlled pneumothorax. Use of a double-lumen endotracheal tube permits expansion of the unaffected lung and collapse of the lung on the surgical side (Fig. 42-6). At the conclusion of the surgical procedure, the affected lung is reexpanded by the anesthesia provider and negative pressure in the chest is restored. Portable chest radiographs may be taken immediately to assess the status of the surgical area, pleural cavities, and lung reexpansion.

2. Instrumentation includes a basic laparotomy setup with the addition of thoracic instruments. These include bone instruments and a power saw (Fig. 42-7 shows rib strippers/rasps, shears, and an approximator/contractor); a large self-retaining chest retractor/rib spreader (Fig. 42-8); bronchus clamps and lung forceps (Fig. 42-9); and long instruments for work in a deep incision.

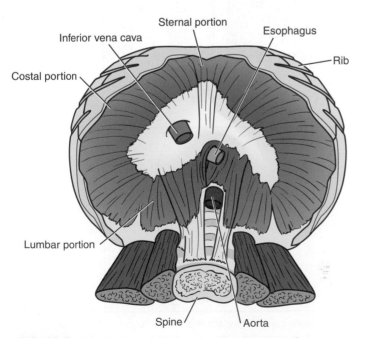

FIG. 42-5 Inferior view of diaphragm with orientation of vena cava, aorta, and esophagus.

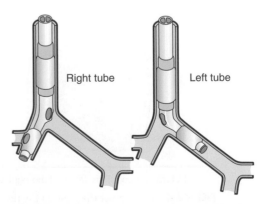

FIG. 42-6 Double-lumen endotracheal tube.

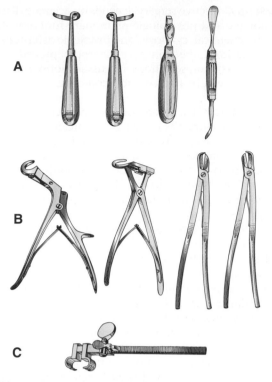

FIG. 42-7   Rib instruments. **A,** Strippers/rasps. **B,** Shears.
C, Approximator/contractor.

Specialty retractors are used to hold lung tissue and displace the bones of the shoulder girdle (Fig. 42-10).

3. A variety of sutures may be used for soft tissues, vessels, and bone. The bronchus usually is closed with staples.

4. Sponges for hemostasis or blunt dissection are placed on long ring-handled forceps. Periosteal bleeding may be controlled by electrocoagulation. Bone wax may be needed to control bone marrow oozing.

5. Blood for transfusion should be available at all times. Hemorrhage is a major threat intraoperatively and postoperatively. Blood may be salvaged for autotransfusion by cell saver and a postoperative drainage salvage reservoir and auto transfusion drain may be used.

6. The surgical field is potentially contaminated by secretions and contact with open air passages when a bronchus is opened and sutured. Used items and instruments are isolated in a discard basin. Maintenance of a dry field is important to prevent aspiration of blood and fluid, which predisposes the patient to postoperative pneumonia.

7. An airtight pleural cavity must be restored and negative pressure maintained for maximum pulmonary function postoperatively. Except after a few specific procedures, a sterile closed water-seal drainage system is essential. Chest tubes are inserted through a stab wound and anchored to the chest wall with suture and tape.

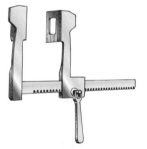

FIG. 42-8   Self-retaining chest retractor/rib spreader.

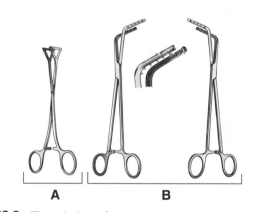

FIG. 42-9   Thoracic tissue forceps. **A,** Bronchus clamps. **B,** Lung forceps.

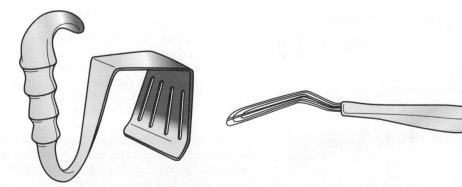

FIG. 42-10   Specialty lung and thoracic retractors.

Two or three tubes are sometimes inserted into the pleural space and connected to separate drainage systems (Fig. 42-11). The tube at the base of the pleural space is usually inserted at the seventh costal interspace, near the anterior axillary line, to evacuate fluid. An upper tube, if indicated, is inserted at the apex through the anterior chest wall at the third costal interspace to evacuate air leaking from the lung. Key points to remember include the following:

a. Connections must be physically tight and securely taped at the time of dressing application. The taped connections should not obscure the observation of drainage.

b. System components must be kept below the level of the patient's body to prevent reentry of air or fluid from the drainage collection system into the pleural cavity.

c. Tubes may be clamped before insertion and connection to the drainage system, depending on the surgeon's preference. Tubes are not routinely clamped at other times unless this is specifically requested by the surgeon.

Access to the Thorax

Surgeon preference and the procedure determine the method of entrance into the thorax. Access may be gained by an anterior, lateral, or posterior approach, or a combination of these. Entrance through the ribcage may be intercostal between the ribs, through the periosteal bed of an unresected rib, or by rib resection. By incising near the top of a rib, the surgeon protects nerves and vessels that lie in the intercostal spaces. An intercostal approach may be used to drain an empyema pocket or mediastinal abscess or to obtain a biopsy specimen of lymph nodes or of a lung.

To enter the thorax via the periosteal bed, the periosteum of the rib is incised and removed from the unresected rib and an incision is made through the bed. For entrance via a rib resection, the periosteum is incised and removed superiorly and inferiorly with a periosteal elevator and the rib is divided. Rib spreaders increase exposure, but if the exposure is still inadequate, the rib above or below the incision also may be resected.

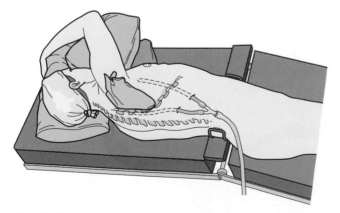

FIG. 42-11 Patient in lateral position with upper and lower chest tubes in place.

Endoscopy. Elective surgery depends on accurate diagnosis by radiologic and physiologic pulmonary function studies and by biochemical, cytologic, and histologic determinations and evaluations. Frequently, endoscopic procedures are performed to obtain secretions and tissue biopsy specimens. Some lesions can be treated endoscopically.

Bronchoscopy. Disorders of the bronchus are most commonly infection, the presence of a foreign body, trauma, or neoplasms. Diagnosis is made by radiologic study and endoscopy. Bronchography (radiologic study of the tracheobronchial tree) is frequently done in conjunction with bronchoscopy. Bronchoscopy (direct visualization of the tracheobronchial tree through a bronchoscope) is done for the following purposes:

• *Diagnosis.* Securing an uncontaminated secretion for culture, obtaining a biopsy specimen, or finding the cause of a cough or hemoptysis

• *Intervention.* Removing a foreign body, excising a small tumor, applying medication, aspirating the bronchi, or providing an airway during performance of a tracheotomy

Foreign bodies in the trachea and bronchi are very serious, requiring a careful history and immediate bronchoscopy with preparation for a potential tracheotomy. Maintaining a safe airway during extraction is a major risk. If the airway is not seriously obstructed, the aspirated foreign body may remain in the bronchus for months without producing symptoms until suppuration develops. Coughing and hemoptysis bring the patient to the physician. Snares and graspers can be used to retrieve foreign bodies.

Bronchoscopes are of two types: a rigid hollow metal tube, and a flexible fiberoptic type. The rigid bronchoscope commonly uses a fiberoptic light carrier attached to a light source to allow visualization of the trachea and primary bronchi. It is the scope of choice for foreign body retrieval and determination of persistent bleeding. It has a side channel incorporated into the length of the instrument and perforations along the sides of the tube to allow oxygenation of bronchi and administration of anesthetic gases if general anesthesia is used.

Aspirating tubes, foreign body or biopsy forceps, and CO_2 laser beams are manipulated through the rigid bronchoscope. Both rigid and flexible fiberoptic bronchoscopes are used for diagnostic and therapeutic procedures.

Flexible bronchoscopy is used frequently for the patient with decreased range of neck motion. Flexible bronchoscopy can be performed via the nasopharynx or orally to the trachea and into the bronchial tree (Fig. 42-12).

Tiny forceps and biopsy brushes can be inserted through the working channel of the flexible fiberoptic bronchoscope to obtain a tissue biopsy specimen. Because the diameter is smaller, the flexible fiberoptic scope reaches into the bronchi of the upper, middle, and lower lobes for examination and/or biopsy. Diagnostic needle aspiration, forceps biopsy, and bronchial brushings and washings are performed in accessible areas. Mediastinal lymph nodes can be aspirated through the flexible bronchoscope. Various types and lengths of aspirating tubes, forceps, and brushes are used to remove tissue and secretions. The neodymium:yttrium-aluminum-garnet (Nd:YAG) or argon laser can be used with either a rigid or a flexible bronchoscope.

If the gag reflex can be controlled, oral rigid bronchoscopy can be performed with the patient under local
anesthesia and intravenous sedation. General anesthesia may
be necessary. The bronchoscope is inserted over the tongue
and through the vocal cords to the trachea. The patient's
head is turned to the right to visualize the left bronchus and
to the left for the right bronchus (Fig. 42-13).

The bronchi may be examined to ascertain the patency
of the tracheobronchial tree or to locate the source of an
obstruction or bleeding. The person who assists the bron-
choscopist introduces tips of instruments into the scope.
Everyone involved with bronchoscopy should wear personal
protective equipment (PPE; gown, gloves, mask, hair cover,
and eye protection) to protect themselves from bronchial
secretions and blood.

Some pulmonary lesions are treated by laser. The CO_2
laser is used for stenosis, granulation tissue, or other obstructive lesions that are not highly vascular. Video-assisted flexible
fiberoptic laser bronchoscopy is more commonly performed
using the Nd:YAG laser. This laser is preferred for vascular
lesions, such as neoplasms, to produce hemostasis as it
cuts. The argon laser is used for photodynamic therapy to
shrink or destroy bronchial tumors. Everyone in the room,
including the patient, is required to wear appropriate eye
protection of the correct optical density for the type of
laser in use.

Airway Stents. Airway obstruction can be relieved by insertion of metal mesh or silicone rubber stents. These may be
straight configuration, T-shaped, or T-Y bifurcation prosthesis

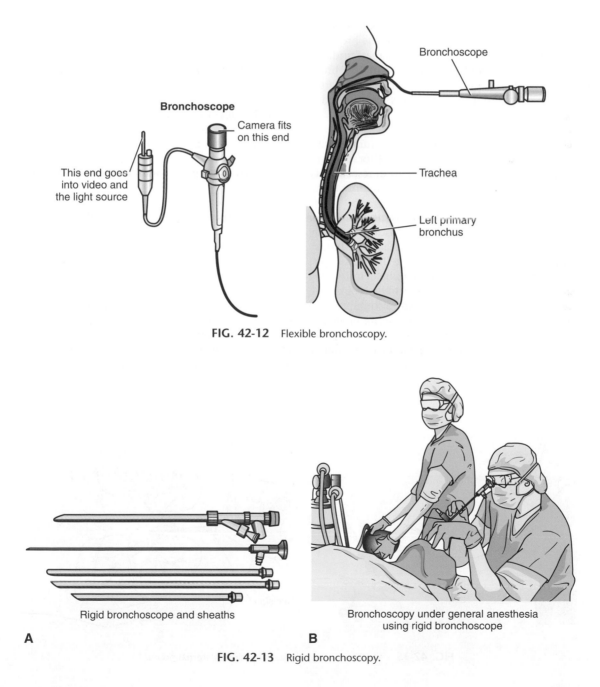

FIG. 42-12 Flexible bronchoscopy.

A Rigid bronchoscope and sheaths

B Bronchoscopy under general anesthesia using rigid bronchoscope

FIG. 42-13 Rigid bronchoscopy.

(Fig. 42-14). Metal stents are permanent and deployed via a rigid bronchoscope over a guidewire. The interstices of the mesh allow for tissue ingrowth providing long-term palliation. Silicone stents are also deployed through a rigid bronchoscope, but are removable.

Positioning is confirmed with radiographs or bronchoscopy. Daily moisture inhalation with a nebulizer is necessary to keep the area moist. Frequent suction may be necessary if the patient cannot clear secretions. Lasers cannot be used in the presence of the stent. It will cause overheating of the tissues, causing uneven pressure and distortion of the lumen of the stent.

The most common reasons for using airway stents are for palliation of obstructing neoplasm, postradiation therapy, after lung transplant, and after fistula repair. Postoperative complications can include stent migration, avulsion, fistula formation, bleeding, and infection.

Ideally, a sterile bronchoscope should be used for each patient. When mucous membranes are intact, the bronchoscope is considered a semicritical item and may undergo high-level disinfection. Thorough cleaning of the bronchoscope and instrumentation is necessary immediately after the procedure. Terminal sterilization is recommended before storage.

Mediastinoscopy.
Mediastinoscopy may immediately follow bronchoscopy. To prevent needless thoracotomy, mediastinoscopy is performed for assessment of resectability in patients with suspected bronchogenic carcinoma and for diagnosis of mediastinal lesions.

Mediastinoscopy uncovers mediastinal lymph nodes for direct visualization and biopsy. Subaortic nodes draining the left lobe of the lung may be out of reach for biopsy with this technique. With the scope, the mediastinoscopist can see down to the carina and about 4 cm distal to it along each bronchus. If more than one biopsy specimen is obtained, each specimen should be placed in a separate container and identified by location. The procedure gives a high percentage of accurate diagnoses and information in staging the extent of a lesion and determining its operability for curative resection. Sometimes a frozen section is done while the patient

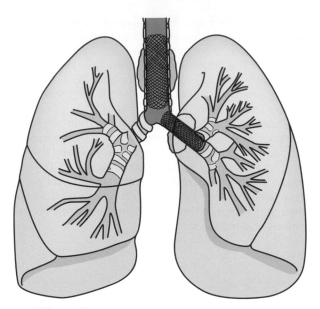

FIG. 42-14   Tracheal and bronchus straight stents.

is in the operating room (OR), with resection performed immediately after a report from the pathologist.

General endotracheal anesthesia is used. The patient is supine with the neck hyperextended and the head turned slightly to the right. A small transverse incision is made in or about 2 cm above the suprasternal notch between the borders of the sternocleidomastoid muscle (Fig. 42-15).

Dissection is carried down to the pretracheal fascia. After blunt dissection, the sterile mediastinoscope is passed behind the suprasternal notch and advanced behind the aortic arch into the superior mediastinum to the level of the carina. Care is exercised because of the proximity of the great vessels to the insertion point of the scope.

Bleeding is controlled by coagulation with an insulated electrosurgical suction tip. Although mediastinoscopy usually is performed without complication, major bleeding may require immediate thoracotomy. A chest radiograph frequently is obtained after mediastinoscopy.

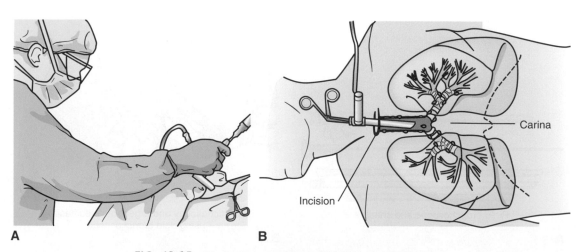

A   **B**

FIG. 42-15   Mediastinoscopy through incision at sternal notch.

Thoracostomy. Closed thoracostomy is performed to establish continuous drainage of fluid from the chest (usually purulent from sepsis or drainage of blood) or to aid in restoring negative pressure in the thoracic cavity. It involves insertion of a tube through an intercostal space via a trocar and cannula.

Thoracoscopy. Thoracoscopy provides visualization of the pleural space, parietal and visceral pleurae, mediastinum, pericardium, and thoracic wall. The need for evaluation of pleural effusion (i.e., the accumulation of fluid, pus, or blood in the pleural space) and the need for obtaining biopsy specimens of pleural or lung tumors are the most common reasons for thoracoscopy.

Definitive treatment of spontaneous pneumothorax (e.g., in patients with cystic fibrosis or in pleural effusion from cancer) using a sclerosing agent for chemical pleurodesis such as a slurry mixture or powder (poudrage) may be performed under thoracoscopic guidance. Materials used for pleurodesis include one or more of the following agents placed through a port:

- Adriamycin
- Bacille Calmette-Guérin
- Bleomycin
- *Corynebacterium parvum*
- Doxycycline
- Doxorubicin
- Fluorouracil
- Iodopovidone
- Nitrogen mustard (alkylating agent)
- Minocycline
- Mitoxantrone
- Quinacrine hydrochloride
- Radioisotopes
- Talc slurry or plain powder
- Tetracycline
- Thiotepa

Fusion of the two pleural layers with a sclerosing agent prevents serous fluid production and accumulation in the chest.

Some of these agents can become systemic, causing side effects such as bone marrow depression. Several types of sclerosing agents such as *C. parvum* work only in the presence of malignancy and are not effective for pneumothorax and normal pleura. Talc can have a residual radiolucent quality that can interfere with chest radiographs.

In patients with empyema and adhesions, a fibrous thickening on the visceral or parietal pleura may restrict pulmonary ventilation. Pulmonary decortication (membrane stripping) removes the restrictive layer or membrane over the lung to reexpand the entrapped lung and fill space remaining after drainage of an empyemic cavity (Fig. 42-16).

Thoracoscopic techniques include video-assisted thoracic surgery for bullous emphysema, pneumonectomy, and debulking of thoracic tumors. Some procedures incorporate aspects of endoscopic and open techniques. An axillary approach to thoracoscopy provides good access to the apex of the lung and satisfactory aesthetic incisional closure. An intercostal incision for thoracoscopy is usually preferred, but in some patients resection of a rib may be necessary to facilitate access to the intrapleural space.

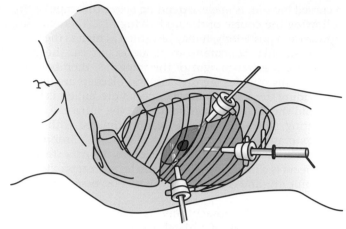

FIG. 42-16 Thoracoscopy for lung biopsy.

A laser can be used to vaporize thickened tissues between the visceral pleura and the lung or between the parietal pleura and the chest wall that impede breathing. Thoracoscopy is used effectively for separation of tissue layers.

General anesthesia is necessary. The patient is in a partial or full lateral thoracotomy position, depending on the preferred access portal sites that the surgeon selects. A small skin incision is made over and carried through the intercostal space of choice. The surgeon incises the parietal pleura to enter the pleural cavity.

After the anesthesia provider deflates the lung, the sterile thoracoscope is inserted into the pleural cavity. When the procedure is completed, the scope is removed and a chest tube is inserted and connected to a sterile closed water-seal drainage system to remove residual air and fluid.

Complications of thoracoscopy include bleeding; injury to thoracic nerves, ducts, or vessels; atelectasis; and respiratory failure. Contraindications to the procedure are a fused lung, inability to tolerate a unilateral deflated lung, and cardiac instability.

Thoracic Incisional Approaches

Factors influencing the location of the thoracic incision include:

- Adequate exposure into the thoracic cavity
- Physiologic intrapleural pressure changes and constant movement of the chest
- Maintenance of integrity of the chest wall and diaphragm
- The condition of the underlying pleura and lung
- The objective of a minimally invasive procedure if possible

Because of its continuity with the neck and abdominal structures, the thoracic cavity may be entered for neck and upper abdominal procedures, as well as for thoracic procedures. Examples include a thoracic aortic aneurysm and pathologic conditions of the esophagus.

Posterolateral Thoracotomy. With the patient in a lateral chest position, a posterolateral incision permits maximum exposure to the lung, esophagus, diaphragm, and descending aorta for exploration of the thoracic cavity. Beginning anteriorly in the submammary fold, about at nipple level, a curved incision is made, extending below the scapular tip, following the course of the underlying ribs. Then curving upward and posteriorly, it may be carried as high as the spine of the scapula. Subcutaneous tissue is incised; the latissimus dorsi, lower margin of the trapezius, rhomboideus, and serratus muscles are divided; and bleeders are ligated. In dividing the serratus muscle, special precaution is taken to avoid the neurovascular bundle on the surface.

During closurehe ribs are reapproximated with a rib approximator/contractor and sutures, the intercostal muscles are sutured, and the incision in the periosteal bed and pleura is closed (Fig. 42-17). Muscles are reapproximated anatomically and sutured; subcutaneous tissue and skin are closed.

Posterolateral thoracotomy is used for pulmonary resections, for repair of a hiatal hernia, and for procedures on the thoracic esophagus or posterior mediastinum.

Anterolateral Thoracotomy. For an anterolateral incision, the patient is supine. Supports are placed under the affected side to tilt the shoulder 20 to 45 degrees for extension of the incision posteriorly. A pad behind the buttocks may rotate the hips slightly.

A submammary incision, immediately below the breast but above the costal margin, extends from the anterior midline to the midaxillary or posterior axillary line. To avoid the axillary apex and a painful scar, the posterior end of the incision is curved downward. Superiorly, access is desired at about the fourth interspace. Further anterior exposure can be gained, if desired, by transecting the sternum and continuing the incision to the contralateral interspace. The pectoralis muscles are divided, the serratus anterior fibers are separated, the intercostal muscles are divided, and the thorax is entered through an intercostal space. When an anterior incision extends to the sternal border, internal mammary arteries and veins are ligated and divided. If the incision is carried far laterally or posteriorly, injury to the long thoracic nerve must be avoided to prevent a winged scapula.

During closure, the sternum is reapproximated with heavy suture, the ribs are approximated with pericostal sutures, and the muscles, subcutaneous tissue, and skin are closed.

Anterolateral thoracotomy is used for resection of a pulmonary cyst or a local lesion or for open lung biopsy.

Thoracoabdominal Incision. With the patient in a lateral position, the thoracoabdominal incision extends from the posterior axillary line to the abdominal midline, paralleling the selected interspace (usually the seventh or eighth). After insertion of a rib spreader, the incision in the intercostal muscles and pleura may be extended posteriorly from within for added exposure. The diaphragm may be divided peripherally. This incision exposes the upper abdomen, retroperitoneal area, and lower aspect of the chest (Fig. 42-18).

In closure, the diaphragm is closed with interrupted sutures. The costal margin is secured by approximating the margins of the divided costal cartilages with suture. Tissue layers are closed in reverse order of incision.

A thoracoabdominal incision is used for repair of a hiatal hernia, for esophagectomy, and in general surgery for resection of retroperitoneal tumors and cardioesophageal lesions.

Median Sternotomy. The patient is supine for a median sternotomy. A vertical incision extends through the midline from the suprasternal notch to the xiphoid process (Fig. 42-19). A power reciprocating saw is used to split the sternum in primary incisions. Reoperative procedures require the use of an oscillating saw to open the sternum. In closure, heavy-gauge stainless steel sutures are used to close the sternum.

A median sternotomy incision is used for simultaneous bilateral pulmonary surgical procedures; for treatment of mediastinal neoplasms or trauma; for pulmonary embolectomy and cardiac and aortic procedures; and for access to the lower cervical and upper thoracic vertebrae. This incision may be preferred for resection of peripheral neoplasms in patients with impaired pulmonary function, particularly in the upper and middle lobes of the lungs.

Partial Sternotomy. When partial sternotomy is used the distal sternum is cut vertically to the level of the manubrium. The patient has a smaller incision and becomes ambulatory sooner postoperatively.

Parasternotomy. Parasternotomy incisions are being used more frequently for minimally invasive cardiac proce-

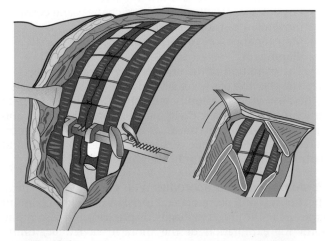

FIG. 42-17   Rib approximation at closure of thoracotomy.

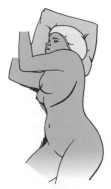

FIG. 42-18   Left thoracoabdominal incision with patient in lateral position.

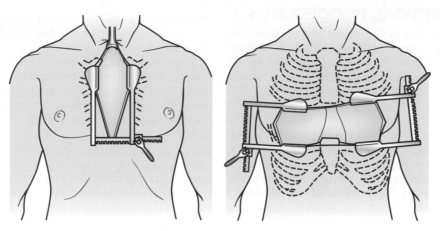

FIG. 42-19   Median sternotomy for lung procedures.

dures. An incision to the left or right of the sternum, without splitting the sternum, allows for visualization of the inner thorax.

Alternative Thoracotomy Incisions. Alternative incisions may be used, such as the following:

- A transaxillary approach for lung biopsy or wedge resection, particularly in the lower lobe; for thoracic sympathectomy or exposure of the second to fifth thoracic ganglia; or for exposure for thoracic outlet syndrome. This vertical incision causes minimal injury to muscles of the chest wall and preserves muscles of the shoulder.
- A supraclavicular (scalene) approach for phrenic nerve section, cervicothoracic sympathectomy, axillary vein thrombosis, or thoracic outlet syndrome. The incision is parallel to the clavicle. The first rib may be resected.
- Cervical mediastinotomy for drainage high in the mediastinum, such as after esophageal perforation.
- Anterior approach for upper dorsal sympathectomy, exposing upper thoracic ganglia.

Lung-Assist Devices

Extracorporeal Membrane Oxygenator. An extracorporeal membrane oxygenator (ECMO) is used as a resuscitative device for adults or children who have potentially reversible respiratory and/or cardiac failure. It also is commonly used to prolong extracorporeal circulation when the patient is in distress after removal from cardiopulmonary bypass. The machine is designed like a cardiopulmonary bypass machine.

ECMO also can be used for a short interim period (several days) to sustain the patient's life while waiting for an organ transplant or after major trauma. Potential complications include bleeding caused by the high-dose anticoagulants required to minimize clotting.

Two methods of extracorporeal membrane oxygenation are the following:

- *Venoarterial bypass.* Cannulation points include the common carotid artery and the internal jugular vein, or the femoral artery and the femoral vein. Venoarterial bypass supports both the heart and lungs by removing deoxygenated venous blood via a vein, removing carbon dioxide, adding oxygen, and returning the oxygenated blood to the body via an artery. The device is used for patients of all ages. It is the method of choice for cardiopulmonary assistance in the preterm neonate, because other appropriately sized assistive devices are unavailable.
- *Venovenous bypass.* The right atrium and the femoral vein are common sites for cannulation. Venovenous bypass supports pulmonary function by oxygenating venous blood and decreasing the circulating venous carbon dioxide level. The advantages are lower mechanical flow rates and decreased risk of arterial emboli. The patient receives ventilatory assistance, which supplements the oxygenation process.

Intravascular Oxygenator. A lung-assist device such as an intravascular oxygenator (IVOX) may be used temporarily to assist the adult patient with respiratory failure or acute respiratory distress syndrome (ARDS). The IVOX allows the patient's damaged lungs to heal. The device is inserted into the common femoral vein and advanced into the vena cava. A chest radiograph is performed to verify placement. It has hundreds of thin-walled hollow fibers made of polypropylene coated with gas-permeable membranes. The gas conduit that exits from the skin has two tubes: one delivers oxygen and the other removes carbon dioxide via diffusion.

The oxygen inlet tube is connected to a pump to produce a flow of oxygen through the lumina of the fibers into venous blood. Carbon dioxide transfers through the outflow membrane, controlled by a vacuum pump. It can provide up to 50% of the patient's gas exchange requirements by bypassing the volume of oxygen to the lungs. By decreasing the airway pressure in the lungs, damaged tissue has a better chance to heal. The IVOX requires minimal anticoagulation and can remain in place for several weeks.

IVOX is less expensive to operate than ECMO and is simpler to operate. It is useful for patients who have had lung transplant and cannot withstand the ventilating pressures associated with oxygenation.

THORACIC SURGICAL PROCEDURES

Pulmonary resection often is the procedure of choice for malignant tumors and benign diseases such as bullous emphysema and tuberculosis. A bronchopleural fistula and pulmonary fibrosis are also among concerns of the thoracic surgeon.

Rib Resection

Rib resection for donor bone procurement requires much of the same instrumentation used for open thoracotomy. A segment of rib is removed (Fig. 42-20). Reconstructive procedures of the ear, mandible, or facial structures commonly employ autologous rib grafts. Equipment and supplies should be immediately available for open thoracotomy or closed chest drainage if hemothorax or pneumothorax should occur.

Mediastinotomy

Anterior mediastinotomy may be indicated when radiographs show hilar or mediastinal nodal involvement inaccessible to mediastinoscopy. With the patient supine and under general anesthesia, an incision is made over the right or left third costal cartilage. The cartilage bed is incised. Extrapleural dissection is carried toward the hilus of the lung, and a biopsy specimen is obtained. If the desired nodes are deep, a mediastinoscope may be inserted through the incision to obtain the biopsy specimen. Alternatively, the pleural space may be entered for a lung biopsy. If this space is entered, closed water-seal chest drainage is required. If it is not entered, the incision is closed in layers without drainage. Mediastinotomy allows assessment of the extent of a lesion or a deformity.

Excision of Lesions. A median sternotomy (i.e., a vertical sternal splitting procedure) may be necessary to resect a cyst or a benign or malignant tumor in the upper anterior mediastinum. Through a posterolateral thoracotomy incision, a tumor may be resected or an abscess drained in the posterior mediastinum.

Correction of a Pectus Deformity. Congenital deformities of the chest wall are usually corrected in childhood. Pectus carinatum (pigeon chest) is forward projection of the sternum, resembling the keel of a boat. Pectus excavatum (funnel chest), which is more common, is caused by elongation of costal cartilages, which pushes the sternum back toward the spine.

Surgical correction of pectus excavatum, sometimes delayed until adolescence or adulthood, is performed to relieve respiratory distress or pressure on the heart from mechanical compression, or for cosmetic improvement. Various techniques may be employed. Usually, with the patient supine and the upper chest slightly hyperextended, costal cartilages are exposed by muscle splitting and/or division through an anterior midline or horizontal inframammary incision. Involved costal cartilages and deformed rib ends are freed from sternal attachments and resected or straightened. The sternum is mobilized and restored to normal position, and its corrected position is maintained by fixation. An alternative method corrects the contour deformity with a silicone prosthesis introduced through an inframammary incision. Dacron patches on the posterior surface stabilize the prosthesis.

Thoracotomy

An incision through the thoracic wall (i.e., thoracotomy) is indicated for drainage of pleural spaces, exploration of the thoracic cavity, or cardiac and pulmonary procedures. Thoracic surgical procedures, exclusive of cardiac procedures, include the following:

Exploratory Thoracotomy. Exploratory thoracotomy is performed as an open procedure to confirm the diagnosis and extent of involvement of bronchogenic carcinoma or other chest disease, such as a mediastinal lesion, when the pathologic process cannot be confirmed by endoscopy. A biopsy specimen is obtained, most often from the lower margin of the upper lobe, for disseminated lung disease. This may be done through an anterior thoracotomy with the patient under local anesthesia. Biopsy specimens are also usually obtained from the mediastinal lymph nodes. Through a posterolateral incision, the lungs and hemithorax are exposed after the ribs are spread and the pleura is opened. Interstitial bleeding and chest trauma are other indications for exploration.

Open thoracotomy may be employed for spontaneous pneumothorax, for large air leaks that prevent reexpansion of the lung, or for persistent leaks and incomplete lung reexpansion. This type of pneumothorax usually occurs from rupture of a bleb on the lung surface. By posterolateral incision through the fourth interspace, an apical bleb may be ligated or the involved segmental area of the lung resected. Abrasion or cauterization of the parietal pleura effects adhesion to the visceral pleura, thereby eliminating future rupture of blebs. Open chest drainage also is used to eliminate an empyemic cavity, which accompanies chronic disease and lung adherence to the chest wall. With this procedure, portions of one or two ribs are removed to aid in the establishment of drainage.

Lung Resection. All or part of a diseased or traumatized lung may be resected (Fig. 42-21). Generally, the indications are neoplasms; emphysematous blebs; and fungal infection, localized residual lung abscess, tuberculosis, and/or bronchiectasis resistant to nonsurgical treatment. Neoplasms are the predominant indication. An anterior intercostal incision with division of costal cartilages above and below the incision may be used for excision of pulmonary nodules or lung biopsy.

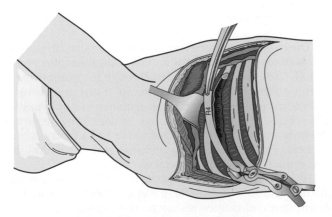

FIG. 42-20   Segmental rib resection.

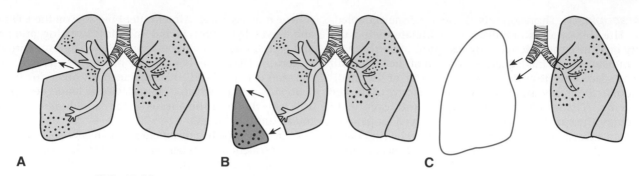

FIG. 42-21 Types of lung resection. **A,** Wedge resection. **B,** Lobectomy. **C,** Pneumonectomy.

A posterolateral incision is commonly employed for lobectomy and pneumonectomy. Endotracheal anesthesia is used. Special precautions in pulmonary resection include meticulous hemostasis and closure of the bronchus, as well as continual attention to cardiopulmonary function preoperatively, intraoperatively, and postoperatively. Particular hazards are hemorrhage, which is difficult to control because of the size and friability of major pulmonary vessels and the proximity of the lungs to the heart; cardiopulmonary insufficiency; and the risk of injury to other intrathoracic structures, such as the vagus, phrenic, and left recurrent nerves and the esophagus. Specific resections include the following.

Segmental Resection. Removal of individual bronchovascular segments of a lobe is preferred when wide excision is not necessary, such as for a pathologic process confined to a segment or for acute hemorrhage. The arteries, veins, and bronchus of the involved segment are ligated and divided. The segment is separated from surrounding lung tissue and removed. The proximal bronchial stump is closed with sutures or staples.

Wedge Resection. Wedge resection is a conservative procedure performed when a lesion is thought to be benign. Along with an adequate margin of normal lung tissue, the diseased peripheral portion of a lobe is removed and the lung tissue is sutured. A stapler may expedite removal and closure. A frozen section is done. If a benign diagnosis is confirmed, the wound is closed in layers and a chest tube is inserted for closed water-seal drainage. If the lesion proves to be malignant, lobectomy or another appropriate procedure may be done. The advantage of wedge resection is its simplicity with minimal blood loss and procedure time.

Lobectomy. One or more lobes of a lung are excised when disease or neoplasm is confined to the lobe. The remaining portion of the lung expands to fill the space formerly occupied by the removed lobe. Through a posterolateral incision, entrance to the chest may be intercostal or by rib resection. The pulmonary pleura is incised and freed from the hilus of the lobe. The arteries and veins to the pulmonary tissue being resected are ligated and divided. The bronchus of the lobe is identified by lung inflation while the bronchus to be resected is clamped.

Suction of blood and secretions from the open bronchus may precede closure of the bronchus by sutures or staples.

A suture line in the bronchus is covered with a flap of parietal pleura to prevent leakage. Dissection is completed, the specimen is removed, and the chest is closed.

Bronchoplastic Reconstruction. Extensive partial pulmonary resection may be followed by bronchoplastic reconstruction to ensure maximum preservation of residual pulmonary tissue. These techniques require successful bronchial anastomoses to retain a patent airway to the bronchioles.

Pneumonectomy. Major indications for excision of an entire lung are malignant neoplasms and extensive unilateral pulmonary disease. The chest wall is opened by a posterolateral incision, the pleura is incised, the lung is exposed, and the pleural cavity is examined. After immobilization of the lung, the hilus is dissected free on all sides. The pulmonary artery and veins are ligated and divided. The bronchus is clamped, divided, and closed with sutures or staples. The bronchus is checked for air leaks by instillation of normal saline solution, and the bronchial stump is covered with surrounding pleura. After wound closure, intrathoracic pressure is measured and residual air aspirated from the hemithorax until the desired pressure is reached. Use of chest drainage is governed by surgeon preference, but usually no chest tube is inserted.

Sacrifice of one lung places the entire responsibility for respiratory and circulatory function on the remaining lung. Potential complications are respiratory insufficiency, cardiac dysrhythmia, and a predisposition for infection because of dead space. The empty hemithorax gradually fills with fluid and eventually consolidates, thus preventing a mediastinal shift. Dehiscence of the bronchial closure may produce a bronchopleural fistula.

Lung Reduction. Lung reduction can be performed for patients who have emphysematous lung disease. In emphysema the lungs have become enlarged because the air sacs are destroyed. By reducing the size of the lungs, efficiency is improved. Minimally invasive techniques have been employed with great success. Clinical trials are in process to validate the efficacy of the techniques.

Patient selection for the procedure is based on the patient's cardiac profile, pulmonary function, and exercise tolerance. Patients with severe disease of the heart or lungs and those who are older than 70 years are usually poor surgical risks for the procedure and are not surgical candidates.

Thoracoplasty. Thoracoplasty is usually done extrapleurally. The chest wall is mobilized to obliterate the pleural cavity or reduce thoracic space by resection of one or more ribs. Indications are inadequate expansion of the lung to fill pleural space after resection, persistent shift of the mediastinum to the empty space after pneumonectomy, or chronic empyema. Tissue fibroses, contracts, and eventually obliterates the space. Thoracoplasty is reserved for patients in whom excessive space in the chest cannot be eliminated satisfactorily by other means to maintain the mediastinum in the midline.

Transplantation of Thoracic Organs. Transplantation of either a single lung or both lungs may be an option for the patient with end-stage pulmonary fibrosis, obstructive lung disease, or cystic fibrosis.

Thymectomy

The thymus gland lies on the pericardium in the anterior mediastinum from its origin in the cervical region around the trachea (Fig. 42-22). The two lobes are separated from the arch of the aorta and great vessels by a layer of fascia. In an adult, the thymus has become smaller and in some cases negligible in size.

Thymectomy is usually performed through a median sternotomy, but the gland may be excised through a transcervical incision. The pericardium, the innominate vein, a portion of the superior vena cava, and a portion of the lung are removed en bloc to resect a thymoma. The phrenic nerve is spared to prevent diaphragmatic paralysis. Thymectomy without en bloc resection may be done to relieve symptoms of myasthenia gravis.

Thoracic Outlet Syndrome

The thoracic outlet is an area bordered by the manubrium anteriorly, the first rib anterolaterally, and the first thoracic vertebra posteriorly. The subclavian artery and vein, the vertebral artery, and the brachial plexus pass through this space (Fig. 42-23). After a neck injury or other postural deformity, changes can occur in the anterior and/or middle scalene muscles, causing intermittent pressure on these vessels and nerves. Symptoms include swelling, sweating, and pain and paresthesia of the upper extremities extending into the fingertips. Diagnosis is made by having the patient raise the arms over the head and simultaneously observing for the Selmonosky triad, which is supraclavicular tenderness, pallor and paresthesia of the affected hand, and weakness of the fourth and fifth digits.

When conservative treatment fails to relieve pain, scalenectomy or scalenotomy is performed. A supraclavicular incision with resection of the first rib or a transaxillary incision is used. In extreme circumstances, bilateral resection of the first rib may be necessary.

CHEST TRAUMA

Trauma to the chest varies in severity and may result in injury to the thoracic wall or intrathoracic organs such as the heart and lungs. If the trauma is severe, the patient is plunged into a critical condition. Rapid initial evaluation of the extent of injury is necessary to preserve life, with priority needs met first. These include resuscitation with relief of airway obstruction, treatment of shock and blood loss, and restoration of normal cardiorespiratory dynamics to the extent possible. Impairment of these dynamics may be caused by various factors such as disturbance of lung expansion or cardiac tamponade.

Trauma is categorized as blunt or penetrating. Blunt trauma usually results from a fall, blow, severe cough, blast, or deceleration injury. The patient may have little overt evidence of chest injury, even though he or she may be bleeding internally from pulmonary contusion. Penetrating wounds are usually caused by a low- or high-velocity missile, such as a knife stab or bullet. Surgical exploration may be required to control bleeding and/or air leak. Open thoracotomy may be performed in the emergency department and the patient brought to the OR with the chest open for further exploration of the wound and for closure.

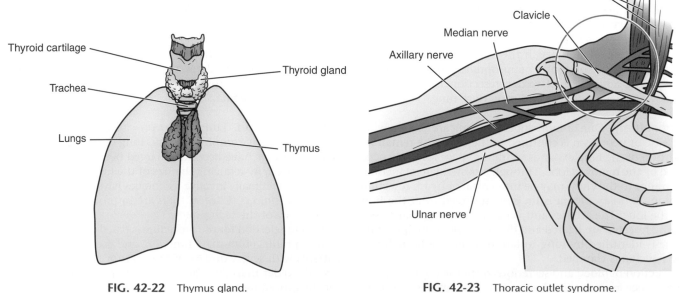

FIG. 42-22 • Thymus gland.

FIG. 42-23 Thoracic outlet syndrome.

Blunt Trauma

Fractured Ribs. Rib fracture is the most common injury to the chest wall, and the fourth to the eighth ribs are the ones mainly involved. Pain may be relieved by an intercostal nerve block. Surgical treatment is usually not required unless sharp edges or displaced bone fragments puncture the pleura or lung. Extensive pneumothorax requires immediate reexpansion of the lungs.

Multiple rib or sternal fractures often produce an unstable chest wall, resulting in flail chest. Normal respiration changes to paradoxic motion of the chest wall. The chest wall collapses on inspiration and expands on expiration. This results in ineffective respiration and coughing. As the chest wall expands, the free-floating sternum is sucked inward, thus impairing ventilation and producing hypoxia. The following measures are used to stabilize the chest wall:

1. Internal stabilization is achieved by controlled mechanical ventilation. An endotracheal tube or tracheostomy tube may be necessary to decrease pulmonary resistance and increase perfusion. Frequent suctioning maintains a clear airway; thus paradoxic motion and dead air space decrease.
2. Surgical stabilization is achieved by inserting pins or wiring fractures together. Fracture of the sternum, scapulae, and clavicles also may be involved in the injury.

Ruptured Organs. Blunt trauma can cause rupture of the diaphragm, aorta, or thoracic tracheobronchial tree, necessitating emergency thoracotomy. Contusions of the lung and pericardium may cause hemorrhage.

Penetrating Wounds

Anatomic visualization of the path of the projectile or instrument producing injury is important. A knife, for example, should not be removed except under the direction of a physician, because it may be penetrating the heart or a major vessel.

Sucking Chest Wound. An open chest wound must be converted to a closed chest wound. Air rushes into an open wound, building up atmospheric positive pressure inside the pleural space. Pneumothorax followed by a mediastinal shift ensues.

Pneumothorax is relieved and further air prevented from entering the chest during respiration by suturing the wound and inserting one or more chest tubes.

Thoracentesis

Air or blood in the pleural cavity may be detected on radiograph and aspirated by a needle and syringe. A chest tube may be inserted into the pleural space percutaneously for closed thoracostomy drainage. If bleeding persists, the chest is opened and vessels are ligated or repaired.

INTRATHORACIC ESOPHAGEAL PROCEDURES

Esophageal disorders may be congenital, or they may be acquired by trauma or disease. Thoracic surgeons may perform esophageal resections for a benign tumor (e.g., leiomyoma) or for relief of obstruction in the thoracic esophagus (e.g., stricture, stenosis, achalasia). Esophageal myotomy with or without fundoplication may relieve obstruction in the lower segment. Resections are performed for malignant tumors. Early detection of esophageal carcinoma increases the rate of cure by surgical resection. Unfortunately, symptoms are not usually apparent in the early stages, so carcinoma of the esophagus generally presents a poor prognosis. Most surgical procedures provide palliation rather than cure. Radical en bloc mediastinectomy may become the procedure of choice, but esophagectomy is more commonly performed.

Esophagectomy

For esophagectomy, the patient is in a lateral position. A posterolateral thoracotomy or thoracoabdominal incision is extended across the chest wall to expose the affected segment of the esophagus (i.e., upper, middle, or lower third). The thoracic cavity is opened, and the mediastinal pleura is incised. The esophagus is dissected away from the aorta and transected above and below the lesion.

For combined thoracoabdominal exposure of a lesion in the lower third of the esophagus, the diaphragm is opened and the stomach mobilized for transection and

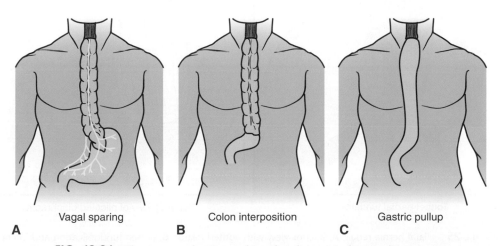

A Vagal sparing	**B** Colon interposition	**C** Gastric pullup

FIG. 42-24 Three approaches to esophageal replacement after esophagectomy.

intrathoracic esophagogastrostomy. In some patients, resection and anastomosis may be performed without thoracotomy by means of a substernal resection to avoid morbidity associated with thoracoabdominal exposure.

High esophageal resection followed by hypopharyngeal reconstruction may be the procedure of choice for tumors in the upper third of the esophagus. Total esophagectomy for tumors in the middle third may be carried out through abdominal and cervical incisions, without thoracotomy. The stomach is mobilized for esophagogastric anastomosis in the neck. Examples of esophageal autologous tissue replacement are depicted in Fig. 42-24.

Repair of a Hiatal Hernia

Repair of herniation of the stomach through the diaphragm may be performed by a general surgeon or by a thoracic surgeon using thoracic routines, such as chest tube insertion with closed water-seal drainage. The surgeon will use a full fundal wrap (Nissen fundoplication) or a partial fundal wrap (Toupet) (Fig. 42-25). Some surgeons will transilluminate the esophagus with a lighted bougie for easier visualization of the structure during open and endoscopic hiatal hernia surgery.

The thoracic approach is preferred in the following situations:

- When exposure from an abdominal approach would be difficult, as with an obese patient

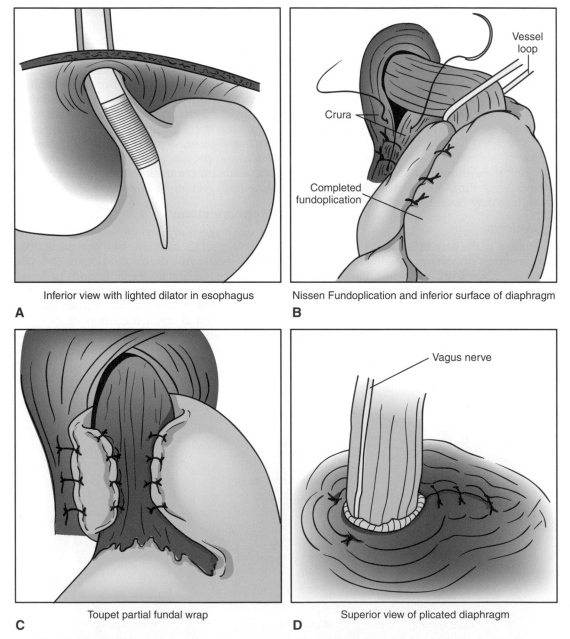

Inferior view with lighted dilator in esophagus

A

Nissen Fundoplication and inferior surface of diaphragm

B

Toupet partial fundal wrap

C

Superior view of plicated diaphragm

D

FIG. 42-25   Hiatal hernia repair. **A,** Inferior view with lighted dilator. **B,** Nissen fundoplication and inferior surface of diaphragm. **C,** Toupet partial fundal wrap. **D,** Superior view of plicated diaphragm.

- When the hernia is incarcerated into the thoracic cavity and would be difficult to reduce through the diaphragm into the abdomen
- When the hernia is recurrent and direct visualization will facilitate the procedure
- When herniation is caused by blunt trauma or a penetrating abdominothoracic wound

Diaphragmatic Pacemaker

Injury to the phrenic nerve can cause full or partial paralysis of the diaphragm. A battery-powered pacing device can be used to stimulate nerve impulses that cause the diaphragm to contract and relax. The device is partially external and partially internal with leads (Fig. 42-26).

COMPLICATIONS OF THORACIC SURGERY

Continuous movement of the chest causes postoperative pain. The patient is likely to breathe shallowly and not adequately raise secretions that accumulate as a result of inhaled anesthetics and sedation. Obstruction in the bronchi from retained secretions can lead to pneumonia and/or atelectasis. The plan of care should include preoperative teaching of breathing techniques to assist the patient in clearing airway secretions.

Development of one pulmonary complication frequently predisposes the patient to development of another. Other potential complications are pneumothorax from an air leak, hemothorax from hemorrhage, and pleural effusion. Empyema and persistent undrained fluid or air pockets can develop in intrathoracic spaces. A bronchopleural fistula may necessitate closure. Pulmonary shunting is also a major complication.

Chylothorax is a potential complication of thoracic surgery. Chylothorax is the leakage of chyle from the thoracic duct of the lymphatic system into the pleural space. This complication may occur in response to trauma or after a surgical procedure in the chest cavity. Surgical repair is performed.

Acute respiratory distress syndrome (ARDS), also known as progressive pulmonary insufficiency or shock lung, may develop in the first 24 to 48 hours after a traumatic injury such as pulmonary contusion or from diffuse or aspiration pneumonia. Beginning with dyspnea, grunting respirations, and tachycardia, signs progress to cyanosis, hypoxemia, and alveolar infiltration. Mortality is high. An IVOX/intravenacaval blood gas exchanger may be used as a temporary booster lung for a patient with ARDS or acute respiratory failure.

Bibliography

Bernier P et al: Video-assisted mini-thoracotomy for thoracic stent-graft implantation: a novel vascular access for endovascular repair, *J Endovasc Ther* 11(2):180-182, 2004.

Chen J et al: Additional minocycline pleurodesis after thoracoscopic surgery for primary spontaneous pneumothorax, *Am J Respir Crit Care Med* 173(5):548-554, 2006.

Cothren C et al: Lung-sparing techniques are associated with improved outcome compared with anatomic resection for severe lung injuries, *J Trauma* 53(3):483-487, 2002.

deSouza A et al: Optimal management of complicated empyema, *Am J Surg* 180(6):507-511, 2000.

Dewey TM, Mack MJ: Lung cancer: surgical approaches and incisions, *Chest Surg Clin North Am* 10(4):803-820, 2000.

Greenberg M et al: The use of fiberoptic bronchoscopy to localize an endobronchial occlusion during repeat thoracotomy, *Internet J Anesthesiol* 9(2): 3, 2005.

Li C, Huang S: Bronchoscopic Nd-YAG laser surgery for tracheobronchial mucoepidermoid carcinoma—A report of two cases, *Int Clin Pract* 58(10):979-982, 2004.

LI LL et al: Quality of life following lung cancer resection: Video-assisted thoracic surgery vs thoracotomy, *Chest* 122(2):584-589, 2002.

Nalaboff KM et al: Endobronchial foreign body extraction: A new interventional approach, *Chest* 120(4):1402-1405, 2001.

Narang S et al: Anesthesia for patients with a mediastinal mass, *Anesthesiol Clin North Am* 19(3):559-579, 2001.

Noppen M et al: Removal of covered self-expandable metallic airway stents in benign disorders: Indications, technique, and outcomes, *Chest* 127(2):482-487, 2005.

Reeves J: Hand you a what? Finding the right instrument when splitting a chest, *Crit Care Nurse* 26(2):S10, 2006.

Stern LE et al: Long-term evaluation of extended thymectomy with anterior mediastinal dissection for myasthenia gravis, *Surgery* 130(4):774-778, 2001.

Theodore N et al: Bilateral thoracoscopic sympathectomy for the treatment of palmar hyperhidrosis in the active duty population, *Military Med* 170(12):1016-1018, 2005.

Wise D et al: Emergency thoracotomy: "How to do it," *Emerg Med J* 22(1):22-24, 2005.

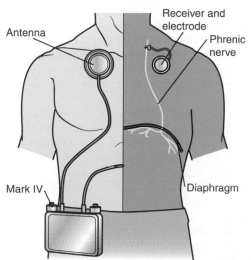

External   Internal

Antenna

Receiver and electrode

Phrenic nerve

Mark IV

Diaphragm

FIG. 42-26   Diaphragmatic pacer for paralyzed diaphragm.

Chapter **43**

Cardiac Surgery

CHAPTER OBJECTIVES

After studying this chapter, the learner will be able to:
- Identify the pertinent anatomy of the heart and great vessels.
- List the types of conduits used for coronary artery bypass grafting.
- Describe the function of a cardiac pacemaker.

CHAPTER OUTLINE

KEY TERMS AND DEFINITIONS

Bicaval Two places on the vena cava.
Conduit Tubular passage for blood.
De-airing Venting air from the heart.
Euvolemia Equilibrium of fluid balance in the body.
Pedunculated Attached by a vascular stalk.
Redo Return to the OR for additional surgery during the postoperative phase. Usually denotes an emergency such as bleeding.

SUPPLEMENTAL MATERIAL ON EVOLVE WEBSITE *evolve*

http://evolve.elsevier.com/BerryKohn
- Content Updates
- Glossary
- Full Set of Perioperative Flash Cards
- Interactive Key Term Flash Cards
- Student Activities
- Tips for the Scrub Person and Circulating Nurse: Coronary Artery Bypass Grafting
- WebLinks

HISTORICAL BACKGROUND

Awareness of the heart transcends the ages. Ancient civilizations revered the heart and considered it the seat of loyalty, bravery, and love. The physiologic properties, such as the heartbeat and its changes under the influence of emotion, gave rise to the importance of the symbolic heart. A warrior in a South American country would remove the beating heart from his enemy in a ritual ceremony and marvel at how it continued to beat. Some cultures performed this rite as part of religious celebration. The mystery associated with the heart and its electrical properties continued through the ages

The circulation of blood was not understood until English physiologist William Harvey (1578-1657) demonstrated that blood makes a complete circuit in the body. Harvey derived knowledge of comparative anatomy from dissections and experiments on the heart chambers, arteries, and veins. Then in 1791 Italian anatomist Luigi Galvani (1737-1798) discovered the fundamentals of electrical stimulation of animal muscle and indirectly discovered how electrical impulses affect the heart.

Cardiopulmonary bypass (CPB) procedures were conceived of as early as 1812. A prototype of the CPB machine was built by Von Frey and Gruber in 1858 and was successful in perfusing a single organ. Development of the CPB machine, which permits safe direct vision for open heart procedures, is credited to John Gibbon, who conceptualized its use for cardiac surgery as early as 1938. In 1953 at Jefferson Medical College in Philadelphia, he performed intracardiac surgery using the first successful pump oxygenator. The procedure to repair an atrial septal defect in an 18-year-old woman was successful.

In 1998 the Cleveland Clinic developed vacuum-assisted venous drainage that decreases the amount of priming solution needed to promote blood flow through the bypass machine from 2.4 L to less than 1 L. This significantly minimizes the risk of postoperative complications such as bleeding, hemodilution, and hemolysis. Cannulas are smaller in diameter and work well in a minimally invasive environment.

Revascularization of an ischemic myocardium to increase blood supply has progressed from abrasion of the epicardium with talcum powder in the 1950s to internal mammary artery implantation and coronary bypass procedures developed in the 1960s. The Cleveland Clinic pioneered advances in coronary artery bypass procedures, starting with F. Mason Sones, who in 1957 developed and refined angiography methods to locate blocked coronary arteries. In 1964 H. Edward Garrett performed the first successful coronary bypass on a human as an emergency procedure in Texas. Rene Favaloro performed the first successful planned coronary artery bypass in 1967 using an autologous interposition saphenous vein graft as a conduit.

The first successful heart transplant by Christiaan Barnard was performed in South Africa in 1967. The advent in 1981 of a combined heart-lung transplant and the implantation of a mechanical artificial heart in 1982 provides hope in the future for patients with end-stage cardiopulmonary disease. Current research is in process concerning the development of an implantable mechanical artificial heart for long-term use.

ANATOMY OF THE HEART AND GREAT VESSELS

Cardiac procedures involve the heart and associated great vessels. To understand diagnostic procedures, hemodynamic monitoring, myocardial preservation techniques, and CPB used in conjunction with cardiac surgery require knowledge of the normal anatomy and physiology of the heart.

The cardiovascular system supplies oxygen and nutrients to body cells and carries waste away from cells by the flow of blood through the system. The heart, blood, and lymph vessels constitute this circulatory system. The heart—the hollow muscular organ located in the thorax—maintains the circulation of blood throughout the body.

HEART

The heart is located in the middle mediastinum slightly left of midline. The heart is a four-chambered muscular "pump" enveloped by a closed, double-layered fibroserous sac—the pericardium. The outer parietal layer forms the sac that contains a small amount of clear serous fluid that lubricates the heart's moving surfaces. The base of the pericardium is attached to the diaphragm; the apex surrounds the great vessels arising from the base of the heart (Figs. 43-1 and 43-2).

The layers of the heart are the epicardium (outer visceral pericardium), myocardium (muscle fibers), and endocardium

(inner membrane lining) (Fig. 43-3). Divided into right and left halves by an oblique longitudinal septum, each half of the heart has two chambers: a thin-walled upper atrium and a thick-walled lower ventricle. The right side of the heart pumps the pulmonary circulation, and the left side of the heart pumps blood into the systemic circulation. The right atrium receives desaturated blood from the inferior and superior venae cavae and the coronary veins. The left atrium receives oxygenated blood from the pulmonary veins. The left ventricle pumps blood into the aorta and the coronary arteries. The heart's rounded apex, formed by the left ventricle, is behind the sixth rib slightly to the left of the sternum. The base is formed by the atria and great vessels.

Valves

Four heart valves promote unobstructed unidirectional blood flow through the chambers (Fig. 43-4). These valves are of two types:
1. *Atrioventricular (AV) valves.* The bases of the cusps (the endocardial leaflets) of these valves attach to the fibrous ring that surrounds their opening between the atrium and ventricle on each side of the heart.
   a. The right tricuspid valve has three cusps, *and lies between the right atrium and ventricle.*
   b. The left mitral valve has two cusps, *and lies between the left atrium and ventricle.*
2. *Semilunar valves.* These valves open to allow blood to flow from the heart chambers into the great vessels.
   a. The pulmonary valve between the right ventricle and the pulmonary trunk has three cusps.
   b. The aortic valve between the left ventricle and the aorta has three cusps.

When the ventricle begins to contract, the AV cusps float up to close the opening, preventing a backflow of blood, as the semilunar valves open. Sequential heart sounds (S_1 and S_2) are heard by stethoscope as the valves open and close.

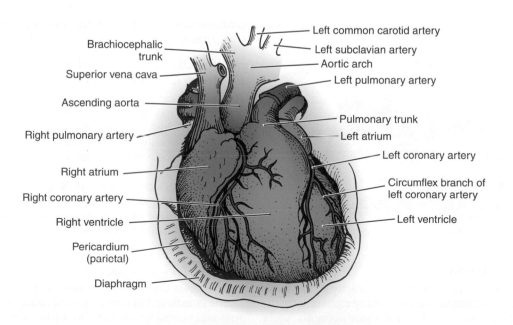

Brachiocephalic trunk
Superior vena cava
Ascending aorta
Right pulmonary artery
Right atrium
Right coronary artery
Right ventricle
Pericardium (parietal)
Diaphragm

Left common carotid artery
Left subclavian artery
Aortic arch
Left pulmonary artery
Pulmonary trunk
Left atrium
Left coronary artery
Circumflex branch of left coronary artery
Left ventricle

FIG. 43-1   Anterior view of heart and great vessels.

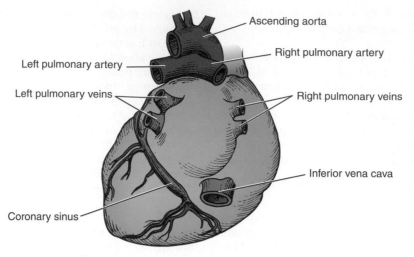

FIG. 43-2   Posterior view of heart and great vessels.

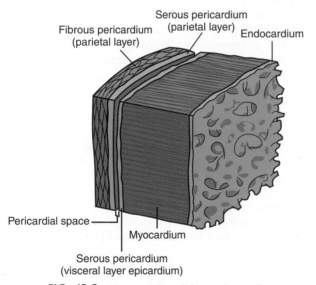

FIG. 43-3   Cross section of the cardiac wall.

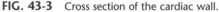
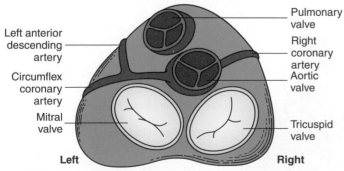

FIG. 43-4   Cardiac valves: superior view with atria removed.

Coronary Circulation

Coronary circulation supplies oxygen directly to the heart muscle and is predominantly anatomically right or left. The coronary arteries arise from the aorta *just above the aortic valve* and, with their branches, supply oxygen and nutrients

to the heart muscle. The coronary arteries fill during the diastolic, or relaxation, phase. The left coronary artery divides shortly after its origin into two main trunks:

1. The anterior descending or interventricular branch courses toward the apex of the heart. Its branches distribute over the anterolateral wall of the left ventricle. Septal branches supply the anterior interventricular septum.
2. The circumflex branch passes posteriorly. Following the AV groove and passing under the left atrial appendage, it meets the right coronary artery at the base of the junction of both ventricles.

The right coronary artery is directed to the right, passing to the posterior aspect of the heart and eventually running between the two ventricles. Its branches supply the posterior interventricular septum. The desaturated coronary blood returns to the venous circulation through the coronary sinus.

The vagus nerve (parasympathetic nervous system) and cardiac branches of the cervical and upper thoracic ganglia (sympathetic nervous system) innervate the heart.

PHYSIOLOGY OF THE HEART
Electrical Conduction System

The conduction system of the heart (Fig. 43-5) permits synchronous contraction of the atria followed by contraction of the ventricles. The right and left sides of the heart function simultaneously but independently. Muscular contractions of the atria and ventricles are controlled by an electrical impulse that originates in the sinoatrial (SA) node. This "pacemaker" is a dense network of specialized Purkinje fibers that begin at the junction of the right atrium and superior vena cava. These fibers become continuous with muscle fibers of the atrium at the node's periphery. The stimulus is passed to the smaller AV node beneath the endocardium in the interatrial septum. A mass of interwoven conductive tissue, this node's specialized fibers are continuous with atrial muscle fibers and the AV bundle of His.

The bundle of His provides conduction relay between the atria and ventricles. Arising from the AV node, the band of conducting tissue passes on both sides of the interven-

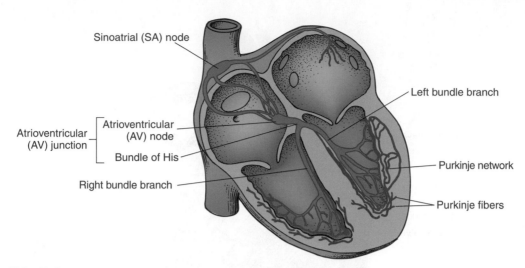

FIG. 43-5 Conducting system within heart. Electrical system is composed of sinoatrial (SA) node; atrioventricular (AV) node and bundle of His at AV junction; left bundle branch; right bundle branch; Purkinje network of Purkinje fibers.

tricular septum, its branches dividing and subdividing to penetrate every area of ventricular muscle and to transmit contraction impulses to the ventricles. Extensions of conductive tissue provide coordinated excitation of myocardium in both atria and ventricles. Each atrial contraction (depolarization) is followed by a period of recharging (repolarization) during which the ventricles contract. Ventricular contraction is followed by a period of recovery while the chambers fill with blood as the atria contract.

Cardiac Cycle

Myocardial contraction is referred to as systole; cardiac relaxation is referred to as diastole. Venous blood from the entire body enters the right atrium via the superior and inferior venae cavae and passes through the tricuspid valve to the right ventricle, from which it is ejected through the pulmonary valve into the pulmonary arterial trunk (Fig. 43-6). Right and left pulmonary arteries originating from the trunk carry the blood to the lungs, where it takes up oxygen and gives off carbon dioxide. Oxygenated blood is transported from the lungs to the left atrium by the pulmonary veins and enters the left ventricle through the mitral valve. Contraction of the left ventricle propels blood through the aortic valve into the aorta, from which it is carried to all parts of the body by arterial branches.

The highest pressure reached during left ventricular systole is the systolic blood pressure. After contraction the ventricle relaxes, during which time systemic intraarterial pressure falls to its lowest level—the diastolic blood pressure. Each contraction of the right ventricle forces blood through the pulmonary valve into the pulmonary arteries to the lungs. In summary, there are two circulations:

1. *Pulmonary.* From the right ventricle to the lungs and back to the left atrium
2. *Systemic.* From the left ventricle to the aorta, to body tissues and organs, and back to the right atrium

SPECIAL FEATURES OF CARDIAC SURGERY

Cardiovascular surgery encompasses the spectrum of clinical pathologic processes associated with congenital anomalies and acquired diseases of the circulatory system. The often complex surgical procedures involving the heart, great vessels, and peripheral blood vessels mandate the need for experienced operating room (OR) teams with special education and training. The goal of cardiovascular surgeons is to restore or preserve adequate cardiac output and circulation of blood to the brain and tissues throughout the body. Technologic advancements in diagnosis, anesthesia, hemodynamic monitoring, extracorporeal circulation, myocardial preservation, prosthetic devices, and transplantation have made possible the correction of many defects and the treatment of cardiovascular diseases.

Cardiac surgery, more than any other surgical specialty, owes its success to teams of experts in chemistry, biology, immunology, biomedical engineering, and electronics, who work cooperatively with courageous surgeons and cardiologists.

Congenital malformations corrected in infancy or early childhood are discussed in Chapter 8. This chapter focuses on surgical procedures performed for acquired heart diseases in adults. The principles of general and thoracic surgery apply to cardiac surgery, but several factors require emphasis:

- Extra minutes are not available, and seconds save lives.
- The team concept is of utmost importance. An experienced team working together can handle emergencies expeditiously.
- Comprehensive physical and psychological preparation of the patient precedes a surgical procedure. Postoperatively the patient is taken to an intensive care unit (ICU). The patient is continuously monitored intraoperatively and postoperatively, including during transport to the ICU.

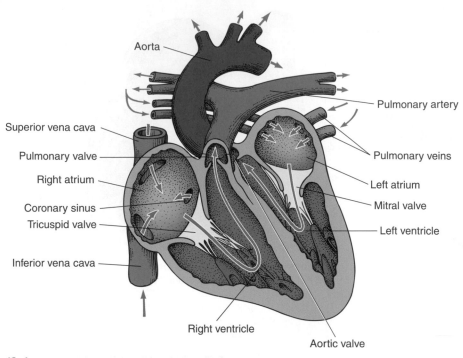

Aorta

Superior vena cava

Pulmonary valve

Right atrium

Coronary sinus

Tricuspid valve

Inferior vena cava

Right ventricle

Aortic valve

Pulmonary artery

Pulmonary veins

Left atrium

Mitral valve

Left ventricle

FIG. 43-6 Circulation of blood through heart. Arrows indicate direction of flow from superior vena cava and inferior vena cava into right atrium, through tricuspid valve into right ventricle, and through pulmonary valve into pulmonary artery. Blood flows from pulmonary veins into left atrium, through mitral valve into left ventricle, and through aortic valve into aorta.

General Considerations

1. The OR for cardiovascular surgery should be equipped with the following:
   a. Cardiac defibrillator, pacemaker, and intraaortic counterpulsation devices.
   b. Cardioplegia (to induce cardiac arrest) and inotropic (to modify cardiac muscle contractility) drugs, including but not limited to the following:
      1) Calcium channel blockers
      2) Dopamine (Intropin)
      3) Dobutamine (Dobutrex)
      4) Epinephrine (Adrenalin)
      5) Intravenous nitroglycerin
      6) Milrinone (Primacor)
   c. Laboratory facilities for blood gas, acid-base balance determinations, potassium, glucose, and hematocrit. Modern analyzers have microprocessors to determine values.
2. The basic thoracic setup is used with the addition of cardiovascular instruments (i.e., various noncrushing vascular and anastomosis clamps, cardiotomy suction tips and sump tubes, and cardiovascular sutures).
3. Prosthetic devices are sterilized by the manufacturer. Care is taken to maintain sterility during placement in the patient. Many types of valves, patches, grafts, and catheters are available. They should be biocompatible, nonthrombogenic, and nonbiodegradable.
   Valves come made of either a bioprosthetic component or metal. Bioprosthetic valves are preserved with glutaraldehyde. They are rinsed in fresh sterile saline

three times to remove the preservative. Some surgeons culture the valve before implantation.
4. Local and/or systemic hypothermia may be used intraoperatively to reduce the body's need for oxygen and to preserve myocardial function. Commercial preparations of sterile slush for local hypothermia are convenient.
5. Intraoperative autotransfusion is often used for blood volume replacement. Blood substitutes such as hetastarch, an albumin substitute for plasma expansion, may be administered. Properly crossmatched blood should be available for transfusion in the event of excessive blood loss. Platelets, stored at room temperature, may be given after CPB to enhance clotting. Often little or no blood is needed for transfusion in many procedures when CPB is used. Also, medications such as aprotinin (Trasylol) may be infused to protect platelet function during CPB.
6. Closed water-seal drainage or suction drainage is used postoperatively to drain the mediastinum and/or pleural space(s) (Fig. 43-7).
7. Many devices are available for cardiac pacing, ventricular support, and treatment of cardiogenic shock. A portable cardiopulmonary support system, external pulsatile pump, and other devices are used. It is critical that these devices be properly sterilized and handled. Read package labels and inserts for the specific manufacturer's instructions. The circulating nurse should affix labels and record serial numbers and identifying data in the patient's chart. In the event of a mechanical failure, this information becomes important. Lot numbers are logged according to facility policy and procedure.

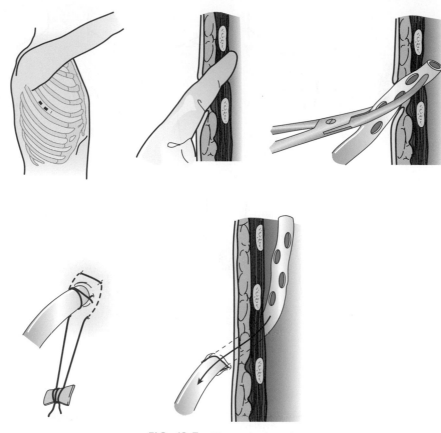

FIG. 43-7   Chest tube insertion.

8. The scrub person should set up a separate table for assembling devices. Check to be certain that all parts are available and functional. A missing component could be catastrophic.

Commonly Used Incisions for Cardiac Surgery

Several different approaches can be used for entering the chest cavity for cardiac surgery (Fig. 43-8).

Median Sternotomy. For median sternotomy the patient is supine. A median sternotomy incision is used for operations of the heart, ascending aorta, and anterior mediastinal structures including the thymus and tumors that lie anterior to the heart.

A vertical incision extends through the midline from the suprasternal notch to approximately 2 inches below the xiphoid process (Fig. 43-9). Retrosternal tissue is dissected. The bony sternum is split (divided) with a powered sternal saw. Caution is used to avoid injury to underlying mediastinal structures, especially if the chest has been opened before. The blade has a safety guard to prevent penetration into the mediastinum.

At closure, heavy-gauge stainless steel wires are placed around or through the sternum, tightly pulled together, and twisted (Fig. 43-10). The ends are buried in the sternum. Other nonabsorbable sutures may be used to provide firm fixation. The linea alba, subcutaneous tissue, and skin are sutured.

Complications are brachial plexus injury from bed-mounted retractors, costochondral separation caused by retraction, infection, nonunion, and keloid formation.

Paramedian Thoracotomy. An incision is made to either the immediate left or right of the sternum for minimally invasive cardiac procedures. A paramedian incision on the left side may also be used to biopsy lymph nodes that reside in the aortopulmonary window that cannot be reached with a mediastinoscope or computed tomography (CT)–guided percutaneous needle. This approach is the Chamberlain procedure.

Transsternal Bilateral Thoracotomy. A bilateral submammary incision is made with the patient supine for transsternal bilateral thoracotomy. In the midline the incision curves superiorly to cross the sternum at the fourth intercostal space level. Lateral extension is to the midaxillary line. The pleural cavity is entered via the interspace after division of the pectoralis muscles. The internal mammary arteries and veins are ligated and divided. The sternum is divided horizontally.

At closure, the sternum is reapproximated securely, the ribs are approximated with pericostal sutures, and the remaining tissue layers are closed.

This incision is referred to as a clamshell and is mostly used for bilateral lung transplants. This incision is less commonly used and causes more discomfort for the patient.

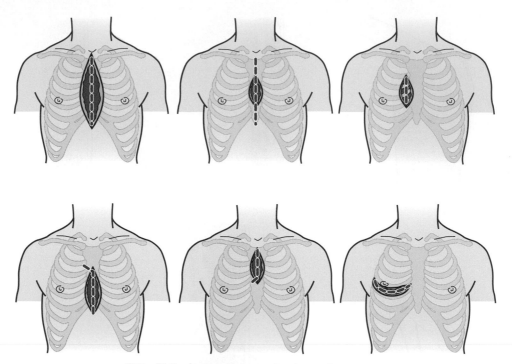

FIG. 43-8   Incisional approaches for cardiac surgery.

Anterolateral or Posterolateral Thoracotomy. Antero-lateral or posterolateral incisions may be preferred for some cardiac procedures such as valve procedures. For some procedures involving the posterior aspect of the heart, the thoracotomy incision is made on the right side (opposite side) of the chest.

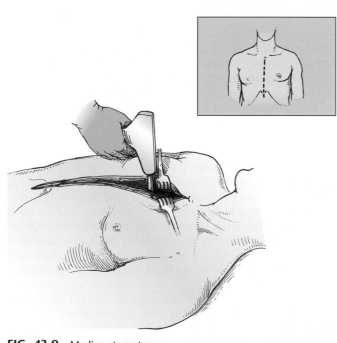

FIG. 43-9   Median sternotomy.
(From Waldhausen JA et al: Surgery of the chest, ed 6, St. Louis, 1996, Mosby.)

Invasive Hemodynamic Monitoring

Although placement of invasive pressure monitoring lines is not their responsibility, perioperative nurses should be aware of the implications of data and the potential for complications, such as thrombus, dysrhythmias, embolus, cardiac arrest, and postoperative infection. For assessment of tissue perfusion, invasive hemodynamic monitoring is used to determine blood pressures in major arteries, veins, and the heart chambers. Indwelling catheter lines are inserted to measure the following:

- Radial and femoral artery pressures.
- Central venous pressure (CVP).
- Pulmonary artery pressure. The Swan-Ganz catheter line determines right atrial, right ventricular, and pulmonary capillary wedge pressures of left ventricular function.

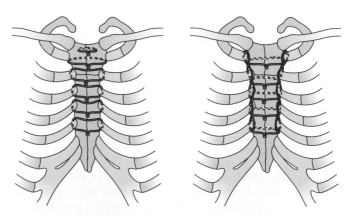

FIG. 43-10   Sternal closure with wire.

It is also used to determine cardiac function as it measures cardiac output, index, oxygen saturation of the central venous system and systemic vascular resistance that, along with pulmonary artery pressures, helps to determine if a patient is hypovolemic, hypervolemic, or euvolemic.

Indwelling intravascular catheters are inserted preoperatively. During a surgical procedure they provide information relative to the effects of anesthetic agents, surgical manipulation of the heart, hypothermia, extracorporeal circulation, induced ischemia, and cardiac arrest. A registered nurse may draw blood samples from the pressure lines at intervals during CPB perfusion for blood gas analysis. Catheter patency is maintained with heparinized flush solutions.

The catheter is flushed with heparinized 5% dextrose in water because inadvertent overload with this solution is less dangerous than is overload with normal saline. Also, an air filter is attached to the end of the pressure tubing as a precaution against fatal air embolism. Every part of the line and filter must be flushed and free of air, or the pressure bag could force a bubble into the left atrium, causing an embolus. In the absence of mitral valve disease, left atrial pressure at the end of atrial diastole, just before the mitral valve opens, indicates left ventricular end-diastolic pressure and therefore left ventricular filling pressure and function.

Postoperatively, hemodynamic monitoring detects dysrhythmias caused by impaired myocardial perfusion, transient reduction in cardiac output with subsequent hypotension, hypovolemia secondary to hemorrhage, and tamponade. Circulating blood volume, pulmonary volume overload leading to pulmonary edema, and reactions to titrated vasopressor drugs also can be identified.

Intraoperative Monitoring

Noninvasive technologies are used intraoperatively to evaluate the effectiveness of some repairs and/or tissue perfusion. These technologies include the following:

- *Transesophageal echocardiography (TEE).* A transesophageal ultrasound probe is used for assessment of graft patency, myocardial perfusion, adequacy of valve replacement, or ventricular function. A Doppler color flow probe also may be useful to quantitatively assess other repairs.
- *Electrophysiologic measurements.* A computerized mapping system is used to identify the focus of dysrhythmias.
- *Near-infrared reflectance spectroscopy.* A device equipped with a sensor is attached to the patient's head. Light transmitted through the skin and skull to the brain is reflected to light detectors in the sensor. Changes in oxygen levels in the brain change light absorption. These changes may alert the anesthesia provider and surgeon to a developing oxygen deficit.

Cardiopulmonary Bypass

CPB is the technique of oxygenating and perfusing blood by means of a mechanical pump-oxygenator system. This apparatus temporarily substitutes for the function of the patient's heart and lungs during cardiac surgery. CPB is used for most intracardiac (open heart) and coronary artery procedures. Venous blood is diverted from the body to the machine for oxygenation (extracorporeal circulation) and is pumped back to the patient (Fig. 43-11).

In preparation for bypass, the patient is systemically heparinized to prevent clot formation within the CPB circuit. Two- or three-stage venous cannulas are inserted into the right atrial appendage and into the inferior vena cava.

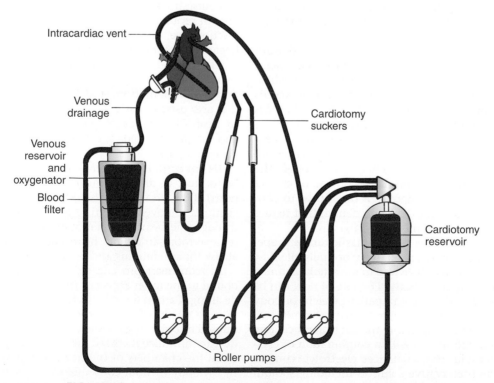

FIG. 43-11   Cardiopulmonary bypass circuit.
(From Waldhausen JA et al: Surgery of the chest, ed 6, St. Louis, 1996, Mosby.)

Venous and arterial cannulation for CPB can be achieved with cannulation of the femoral or subclavian artery and femoral vein. Special arterial cannulas are available for this, and a large-bore chest tube may be used for the femoral venous cannulation.

Bicaval cannulation is done by inserting venous cannulas into the inferior and superior venae cavae. A cannula for return of oxygenated blood to the systemic circulation is placed in the ascending aorta. The femoral or subclavian artery can be used as an alternate site in the presence of an ascending aneurysm, extensive adhesions, or severe calcification of the aorta. Cannulas are connected to the machine by sterile tubing before institution of bypass. During bypass, the lungs are kept deflated and immobilized.

Minimally invasive surgery has given rise to vacuum-assisted venous drainage (VAVD) for the attainment of a bloodless field. This method requires less priming medium for the machine and uses smaller cannulas. VAVD adds negative pressure of 225 to 240 mm Hg to the venous lines for faster decompression of the heart.

The perfusionist who operates the CPB machine must be familiar with its function, care, and operation. The perfusionist may be employed by the cardiac surgeon, a group practice, or the hospital.

Components of a Bypass System

Oxygenator. Oxygen is taken up and carbon dioxide is removed from the blood. The types of oxygenators include the following:

- *Bubble.* Bubbles of oxygen are supplied to the blood by direct blood/gas contact.
- *Membrane.* Oxygen and carbon dioxide diffuse through a permeable Teflon or polyethylene membrane that contains the blood. This method diminishes blood/gas interface. Several types of disposable membrane oxygenators are available.
- *Microporous membrane.* Blood film is separated from ventilating gas by a microporous polypropylene membrane folded like an accordion and operated like a bubble oxygenator. Blood pressure in this oxygenator exceeds gas pressure at all times, thus precluding gas bubbles passing through the microporous membrane.

Heat Exchanger. Incorporated in the circuit, a heat exchanger regulates blood temperature. Water at a thermostatically controlled temperature circulates through the exchanger, which can rapidly produce, control, or correct systemic hypothermia. Hypothermia is often used in conjunction with bypass to reduce oxygen demands of tissues and to protect the myocardium during arrest.

Pump. Rollers turning over sterile plastic tubing propel reheated oxygenated blood in a relatively nonpulsatile flow through a blood filter and bubble trap to the arterial cannula for recirculation through the body. The rate of flow can be varied. It is calculated according to patient weight or body surface area. Reduced flow accompanies hypothermia.

Perfusion. Immediately before the surgical procedure, the machine is primed (filled) with a combination of crystalloid and colloid solutions, a balanced electrolyte component, and a cardiopreservative solution including sodium bicarbonate and heparinized plasma volume expander. Some circuits are heparin coated by the manufacturer.

For a hemodilution technique of priming, the system is filled with fluid that will replace blood diverted to the pump-oxygenator system and is recirculated through the circuit to remove air bubbles. The priming solution should be of sufficient volume and of a suitable hematocrit level so that when mixed with the patient's blood, the resultant buffered plasma will be capable of achieving adequate perfusion and preventing myocardial acidosis. Blood is added as needed to maintain an adequate oxygen-carrying capacity and perfusion rate.

The bypass may be partial or total. In a partial bypass, only a portion of venous return is routed to the pump-oxygenator circuitry; the remaining portion follows the normal systemic circulation. In a total bypass, all venous return is diverted to the machine for total-body perfusion.

Umbilical tapes or Silastic vessel loops are placed around the venae cavae and tightened like a tourniquet to ensure complete drainage and a bloodless field when bicaval drainage is used. The heart is arrested when perfusion tubing is secure.

During perfusion, the patient is monitored intensely (i.e., arterial and venous pressures, body and blood temperatures, blood gases and electrolytes, urinary output, and oxygen consumption). General anesthesia may be maintained by an anesthetic vaporizer that adds vapor to the oxygenating mixture or by intravenous anesthetic.

As the procedure nears completion, the patient is rewarmed to normal body temperature. The cross clamp is removed from the aorta and, as blood fills the heart, the heartbeat is restored. Mechanical ventilation is reestablished, and the patient is gradually weaned from CPB.

After discontinuance of bypass, the cannulas are removed and pursestring sutures around insertion sites are tied. A test dose of protamine sulfate is administered. If the patient is reaction-free, then the full dose is continued until the heparin is completely reversed.

CPB may also be employed in conjunction with deep hypothermia during neurosurgical procedures, in major organ transplantation, and for pulmonary embolectomy. It is also used to assist in the event of ventricular failure, to treat some types of pulmonary dysfunction, and to perfuse an isolated segment of the body for cancer chemotherapy.

De-airing. If an open chamber procedure has been performed, de-airing (venting all the air from inside the heart) of the left ventricle is necessary before the aortic cross-clamp is removed. De-airing is done by placing a needle through the heart and removing the room air. Failure to remove room air from a heart chamber places the patient at risk for air embolus and possible stroke.

In redo heart procedures, the tip of the heart may be bound to the inner aspect of the chest preventing adequate de-airing. Carbon dioxide (CO_2) is used to remedy this situation. CO_2 is heavier than room air and is prophylactically infused into the surgical site continuously during the procedure to minimize the need for de-airing by displacing room air in the chambers of the heart. Residual CO_2 is resorbed by the body without consequence to the patient. De-airing is still performed at the conclusion of the bypass procedure when CO_2 is used.

Myocardial Preservation. A bloodless, motionless field allows direct vision of the heart and its interior for repair of coronary circulation or intracardiac defects. CPB isolates the heart while the body is perfused with oxygenated blood. Cardiac arrest is purposely induced. During bypass, the perfusionist is in control of the patient's body temperature, oxygenation, and preservation of the body and brain. The surgeon assumes responsibility for preservation of the heart. Bypass time is kept to a minimum because injury from myocardial ischemia is time related.

Deliberate arrest may be effected by one or a combination of the following methods:

1. *Aortic cross-clamping.* The aorta is occluded with a vascular clamp proximal to the aortic cannula to block systemic circulation. Ischemic (anoxic) cardiac arrest occurs as the blocked systemic blood within the heart becomes deoxygenated and cardiac metabolic needs are depleted. This technique can be maintained for only a limited period, because myocardial damage and necrosis will occur when the oxygen supply and energy required to maintain the subcellular system are depleted. Cerebrospinal fluid pressure may increase.

2. *Cardioplegia.* Most cardiac surgery is based on the use of cardioplegic solutions used alone or in combination with other techniques discussed. These are preparations of a small amount of potassium in crystalloid, blood, or other solution. Cardioplegia is delivered into the aortic root through the coronary ostia or into the coronary sinus through the right atrium.

• Antegrade infusion: a catheter is placed into the coronary ostia via the ascending aorta above the aortic valve and below the aortic cross clamp (Fig. 43-12). Cardioplegia is infused and flows into the coronary circulation. It is kept out of the left ventricle by a competent aortic valve and systemically by the aortic cross clamp. Between 500 and 1000 mL of solution at 70 mm Hg pressure is initially used. Additional amounts are administered with each anastomosis. Severe coronary disease may cause uneven doses of cardioplegia and interfere with perfusion.

• Retrograde infusion: a catheter is placed into the coronary sinus through the right atrium (Fig. 43-13). Cardioplegia is infused passively at 100 or 200 mL/min and is delivered to the myocardium by first traversing the venous system of the heart and then into the arterial system of the coronary circulation. This method is used during valve surgery and in bypass surgery when proximal lesions of the coronary arteries prohibit adequate antegrade delivery.

Retrograde cardioplegia does not perfuse the right ventricle or the capillary system of the left ventricle as well as antegrade methods. A better continuous flow is attained by placing a venous suction tip near the ostia.

When cardioplegic solution is injected into the coronary artery system, hyperkalemia immediately induces complete electromechanical cardiac arrest. The composition and temperature of the solution and infusion techniques can be determined for each patient's disease process. Some solutions have a calcium antagonist, such as verapamil or nifedipine, to help prevent myocardial ischemia. Some are infused warm; others are infused cold for less myocardial ischemia. Infusion may be continuous or intermittent. In severe proximal coronary disease it may be necessary to give antegrade and retrograde for even distribution of the solution.

Coronary perfusion pressure during administration of the cardioplegic solution may influence regional delivery. When the solution is flushed out of the collateral circulation at the end of the surgical procedure, the heartbeat may resume spontaneously. If not, ventricular fibrillation is treated with countershock.

3. *Hypothermia.* Hypothermia reduces systemic metabolic needs and oxygen requirements. It exerts a protective effect during CPB through a temperature-related decrease of intracellular metabolism, thus allowing tissues to tolerate a prolonged period of decreased perfusion. Hypothermia is an essential component to ischemic myocardial preservation, but because of its calcium-loading effect, cardioplegic arrest precedes initiation of hypothermia.

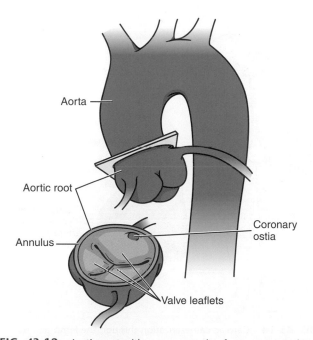

FIG. 43-12 Aortic root with coronary ostia of coronary arteries.

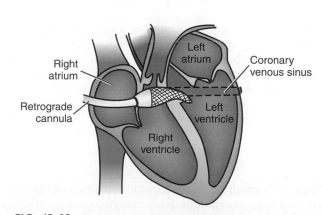

FIG. 43-13 Coronary sinus with retrograde cannula in place.

Local hypothermia can be induced by topical application of iced saline slush around the heart or iced Ringer's lactate solution to the heart externally and/or internally. Cardiac arrest also can be induced by deliberately lowering systemic body temperature moderately to 78.8° to 89.6° F (26° to 32° C) or deeply to below 78.8° F (26° C). This is achieved by a cooling perfusate in the heart-lung machine.

Complications of Cardiopulmonary Bypass. Although excellent results are obtained with most procedures, significant derangements can occur after CPB. These are most obvious in infants or after prolonged surgical procedures in adults. Alterations in clotting may occur as a result of heparinization of blood, mechanical damage to platelets and clotting factors, and direct exposure of blood to oxygen. If trauma or transfusion reaction hemolyzes red blood cells, viscosity in renal tubules may cause tubular necrosis and renal failure.

Inadequate or extended perfusion and oxygenation may promote tissue anoxia and metabolic acidosis. Fluid and electrolyte balance merit close watching, particularly for hypervolemia. When nonblood fluids are used to prime the pump, they may diffuse into interstitial spaces. As this fluid returns to circulation postoperatively, hypervolemia may result. Furthermore, increased levels of aldosterone and antidiuretic hormone induced by the stress of surgery cause retention of sodium and water. Fluids are restricted for 24 hours postoperatively. Cerebral edema and *encephalopathy* at times ensue, for unknown reasons. These developments are generally temporary.

"Post-pump psychosis" consists of visual and auditory hallucinations and paranoid delusions. This often terminates when the patient is transferred from the ICU.

The most severe pulmonary complication of extracorporeal circulation is postperfusion lung syndrome. Its cause is unknown. It is often fatal because of the development of atelectasis, pulmonary edema, and hemorrhage. Metabolic acidosis during bypass may lead to low cardiac output syndrome postoperatively. This occurs most frequently in patients with long histories of cardiac disease.

Diagnostic Procedures

Interference in any part of the circulatory system can jeopardize survival. A surgical procedure is preceded by extensive cardiovascular assessment on the basis of noninvasive and invasive studies that dictate subsequent treatment.

Noninvasive Procedures. Routine examination and electrocardiography are augmented by determination of venous pressure, cardiac output, circulation time, and blood chemistry studies. Chest radiograph reveals the heart's size, position, and outline. Screening or functional capacity testing, such as stress testing, is informative. Pulmonary function tests may detect left ventricular failure. Echocardiography with ultrasonic waves reveals the heart structure and gives information pertinent to congenital heart disease and valvular disease.

Invasive Procedures. Radiographic visualization after injection of a nontoxic radiopaque substance permits study of the heart chambers, great vessels, and coronary circulation.

Radionuclide Imaging. Radionuclide imaging may be used to detect regional reductions in myocardial blood flow and thus help to confirm or deny the diagnosis of myocardial infarction (necrosis of a portion of the myocardium caused by obstruction in a coronary artery). When a patient has "balanced disease," meaning equally blocked throughout all coronary distributions, the radionuclide uptake may be evenly distributed and be questionably interpreted as "normal." The cardiologist will compare all diagnostic findings and determine if cardiac catheterization is the next step to definitive diagnosis despite a "normal" test.

Calcium scoring is also used to determine coronary lesions. This test measures the amount of calcium present in the coronary arteries and is graded to determine the severity of disease.

Angiography. Angiocardiography with intravascular injection of a radiopaque substance permits radiographs of the heart chambers, thoracic vessels, and coronary arteries. Rapid serial radiographs or motion pictures on an enlarged fluoroscopic screen show the heart's outline and the passage of contrast materials in the great vessels. Selective angiocardiography or coronary angiography is done in association with cardiac catheterization to evaluate coronary artery disease and to determine the extent of obstructive disease in the coronary vessels. Aneurysms also may be diagnosed by angiography.

Cardiac Catheterization. Under image intensification fluoroscopy, a sterile catheter is introduced through a cutdown into a brachial vessel in the arm or percutaneously into a femoral vessel in the groin and is passed into the heart or a coronary artery (Fig. 43-14). The procedure permits the following:

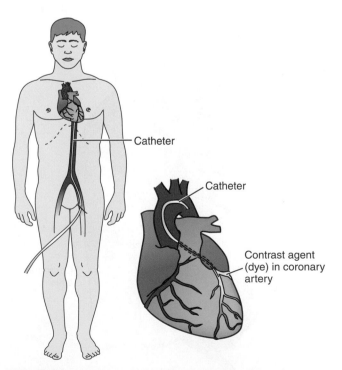

FIG. 43-14   Cardiac catheterization through the femoral artery with the injection contrast agent.

- Evaluation of heart function
- Measurements of intracardiac *and* aortic pressure
- Visualization of the heart chambers
- Calculation of a valve area to determine stenosis

Catheterization is used to diagnose coronary artery disease, valvular heart disease, myocardial disease, or congenital anomalies. It is the ultimate tool for diagnosis of ischemic heart disease.

For study of the coronary arteries, a single catheter is passed and its tip is inserted into the ostia of the arteries for injection of dye and tracing of solution flow. Cinefluorograms record findings. After removal of the catheter, the incision is closed and pressure dressings are applied.

For right-sided heart catheterization, a pulmonary artery catheter is inserted through the vein to obtain pressures in the right atrium and ventricle, pulmonary artery, and pulmonary artery wedge. Measurements of thermodilution, cardiac output, and oxygen saturation also may be obtained. The right internal jugular vein may be cannulated, and a bioptome (a specially designed biopsy forceps) may be advanced to obtain a right endomyocardial biopsy specimen. For left-sided heart catheterization, a catheter is inserted into an artery and advanced through the aortic valve into the left ventricle.

Physiologic monitoring with a multichannel recorder is continuous during the procedure. Potential complications include dysrhythmias, air embolus, thrombosis, and vascular and/or cardiac perforation.

CARDIAC SURGICAL PROCEDURES

The purposes of heart surgery are to correct acquired or congenital anatomic abnormalities, repair or replace defective heart valves, revascularize ischemic myocardium, and improve or assist ventricular function. The hours immediately before the surgical procedure can be a highly stressful period for the patient. Mental stress can cause myocardial ischemia (inadequate blood supply to the heart) without symptoms of chest pain. Therefore, the patient should be monitored from arrival in the OR suite, through induction of anesthesia, and throughout the surgical procedure. Administration of oxygen before induction of anesthesia may be indicated to help reduce stress. Procedures may be performed with or without CPB.

Valvular Heart Disease

Valvular heart disease may arise from a congenital abnormality or can be acquired. Abnormal vibrations or heart murmurs, referred to as S_3 or S_4, may be congenital or the end result of disease such as rheumatic fever or degenerative change. Valves can become thickened and calcified, resulting in loss of valve substance, narrowing of the orifice, and immobility (Fig. 43-15). They then develop insufficiency, fail to close completely, and permit blood leakage or regurgitation. Failure to open completely is caused by stenosis, which impedes blood flow. A defective valve is reconstructed if possible. If the valve is not repairable or if symptoms return after repair, a prosthetic valve is implanted.

Incisional approaches for valve surgery include median sternotomy, anterolateral thoracotomy, and other modifications of lateral thoracotomy. CPB is used for all valve procedures to create and maintain a bloodless field.

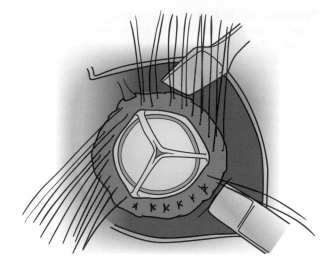

FIG. 43-15 Suturing the annulus of the valve.

Cardioplegia perfusion and administration can be affected by diseased valves. A continual flow of antegrade cardioplegia is given during aortic valve surgery unless the flow obstructs vision. Cannulation of the ostia can cause ostial stenosis. For mitral valve surgery the antegrade flow is interrupted by the mitral valve retractor and requires the aortic root to be de-aired before the procedure can resume.

Restorative Valve Procedures. Restorative and reparative valve surgery is the preferred procedure for most valve diseases. Reconstruction of the patient's own valve may restore normal valve function. Valvuloplasty and annuloplasty are valve-sparing procedures to maintain structural integrity and ventricular function. In valvuloplasty the leaflets are repaired and calcium deposits removed. Some surgeons tuck a Raytec into the ventricle under the valve being repaired. Care is taken to account for this sponge and the particulate during the count performed at closure of the heart.

An annuloplasty ring, either flexible or nonflexible, may be used for support and to provide continuity and permanence of repair. Thromboembolism is less of a threat than it is after valve replacement, thus anticoagulant therapy is not indicated postoperatively.

Valve Replacement. A diseased mitral or aortic valve may be excised and replaced. The surgeon selects the most appropriate procedure and approach—repair versus replacement—and then the type and size of prosthesis to be used.

Several factors are used to determine repair versus replacement of the valve with a mechanical or bioprosthetic valve. These include, but are not limited to, age, life expectancy, body surface area, contraindication to long-term anticoagulation, pathology of the valve, general health and lifestyle of the patient, and comorbidities.

The appropriate valve replacement prosthesis is nontoxic to the patient's system and has an effective valve area to accommodate the patient's body size. Several types of prosthetic heart valves are available. They may be mechanical or biologic.

Mechanical Valves. One type of mechanical valve has discs resembling leaflets of human valves. The discs of some are tilted. The metal ring at the base of the cage may be covered with polyester fabric to facilitate suturing. It also encourages tissue ingrowth, an aid to long-term fixation.

All mechanical valves require long-term anticoagulation with warfarin (Coumadin). Tissue valves may require short-term anticoagulation for 3 to 6 months while endothelialization of the annular ring is being undertaken by the body. Some may elect platelet inhibition with aspirin and platelet inhibitor of choice. However, all tissue valve recipients will require long-term anticoagulation in the presence of atrial dysrhythmias such as atrial fibrillation and atrial flutter.

Biologic Valves. Biologic valves are made from allograft or xenograft (porcine bioprosthesis or bovine pericardial xenograft) donor material. Cryopreserved fresh aortic valve allografts are carefully thawed before use. Glutaraldehyde storage solution is thoroughly rinsed from xenografts with sterile saline before implantation.

Mitral Valve Replacement. Most mitral valve surgery is accomplished through either a medial sternotomy or right thoracotomy. Whichever is used, the pericardium is entered and venous CPB cannulas are placed in the inferior and superior venae cavae. This keeps the surgical site free of blood from the CPB. However, during cardioplegia instillation, blood may inadvertently enter the field. Suction should remain handy.

The atrium is opened and the mitral valve is exposed, inspected, and removed by the circumferential excision and severance of muscular attachments to the ventricular wall. The surgeon usually leaves the annulus, chordae tendineae, and papillary muscles intact. Once the valve has been sized by the surgeon and an appropriate valve placed on the field, interrupted nonabsorbable sutures are then placed all along the annulus in alternating colors. Teflon felt pledgets are commonly used as a buttress under the sutures to prevent the annulus from tearing when the prosthetic valve is seated and the sutures are tied.

Once all sutures have been placed, the valve is lowered into the space formally occupied by the diseased valve, and the sutures are tied (Fig. 43-16). After inspecting the newly implanted valve and ensuring it to be functioning properly, the atrium is closed while blood is allowed to fill the heart displacing the room air. This begins the de-airing process.

Temporary pacing wires may be placed on the epicardium of the right ventricle and atrium. These are brought out through the skin and may be attached to an external pulse generator in the event a bradycardia or other dysrhythmia requiring pacing is encountered during the immediate postoperative course. These are easily removed with gentle traction when deemed appropriate by surgeon.

Aortic Valve Replacement. The surgical procedure for aortic valve replacement is basically the same as that described for mitral valve replacement except that the aortic valve is exposed through a transverse incision in the aorta. The surgical site can be kept free from blood by placing a plastic suction tube into a pulmonary vein and directed backward into the left atrium, across the mitral valve and, finally, into the left ventricle.

Either a mechanical valve or bioprosthesis may be used. Biologic prostheses offer the advantage of a low embolic

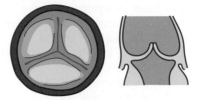
Normal aortic valve

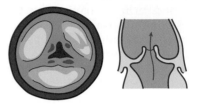
Stenotic aortic valve

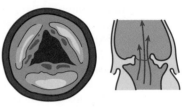
Aortic insufficiency

FIG. 43-16   Aortic valve disease.

rate and obviate the need for prolonged anticoagulation therapy. Cryopreserved fresh aortic valve allograft, from either a donor bank or commercially available allograft, may be preferred. The aortic valve may be replaced with the patient's own pulmonary valve (i.e., an autograft known as the Ross procedure).

Percutaneous Transluminal Balloon Valvuloplasty. An interventional cardiac catheterization procedure, balloon valvuloplasty may be an option to treat valvular stenosis in a high-risk patient who cannot tolerate valve replacement. A catheter with a deflated balloon is inserted under fluoroscopy across a stenosed aortic, pulmonary, tricuspid, or mitral valve. The balloon is repeatedly inflated until the valve is opened.

Coronary Artery Disease

Coronary arteries supplying the myocardium may become stenosed or obstructed, which is referred to as occlusive coronary artery disease or ischemic heart disease. Resultant myocardial ischemia may result in angina or myocardial infarction. Occlusive disease of the coronary arteries characteristically affects vessels in their proximal segments and at the origin of major branches. Significant obstructions can occur in one or all of the coronary arteries simultaneously.

The coronary circulation has four major arteries. The left main coronary artery is the shortest and gives rise to the left anterior descending (LAD) and circumflex (CX) coronary arteries. The right coronary artery (RCA) is the other major coronary artery. The RCA, LAD, and circumflex arteries also can have major branches arising from them. Revascularization to improve blood supply to the myocardium is possible by surgical intervention in selected patients.

Coronary Artery Bypass Graft

For coronary artery bypass grafting (CABG), single or multiple arterial bypasses are done, depending on the number of vessels affected and the degree of obstruction present. The internal mammary (thoracic) artery is the preferred vascular conduit in most patients. Segments of greater saphenous and lesser saphenous veins also are used to bypass coronary artery obstruction. The gastroepiploic, inferior epigastric, and radial arteries also may be used as free grafts. Because the patency rates of cryopreserved saphenous vein and umbilical vein allografts are poor, they are used when no other conduit of choice is available.

The chest is opened by median sternotomy or some other thoracotomy incision for minimal access, and the pericardium is incised. CPB may be used. Most cardiac surgeons wear loupes for magnification while constructing an anastomosis between the graft and the coronary artery. Techniques are influenced by the surgeon's preferred procedure and the extent of grafting.

After the conduit or graft is anastomosed, CPB is discontinued (if used); all incisions are closed and checked for leaks. The pericardium may be left open. The patient is hemodynamically stabilized. The wound is closed in the usual manner for sternotomy with closed water-seal chest drainage.

Off-pump CABG procedures are becoming increasingly popular. The use of a stabilizing retractor assists the surgeon by creating a still area at the site of the distal anastomosis (Fig. 43-17). The use of a carbon dioxide and saline mister-blower helps keep the anastomosis site clear of blood for enhanced vision. Temporary miniature penetrating "bulldog"-style clamps can be inserted into the myocardium and used to occlude the artery by gentle, even compression.

Once the anastomosis is completed, the stabilizer and bulldogs are removed and relocated to the next vessel. The heart is closely monitored for ischemia. CPB is instituted as an emergency measure via the femoral artery and vein if the heart tissue fails to perfuse adequately during the procedure. This approach to coronary artery bypass is especially useful in patients with a calcified ascending aorta where cross-clamping would be contraindicated.

Internal Mammary Artery Conduit. The chest has right and left internal mammary arteries. Because of the potential for a long-term patency rate, at least one internal mammary (IMA) artery can be used as a conduit for myocardial revascularization when the proximal stenosis is greater than 70%. The right internal mammary artery will reach the RCA. The left IMA can be used for revascularization of the LAD but can also reach the diagonal vessel (branch of LAD) and the circumflex. Segments of either right, left, or both internal mammary arteries also are used as free grafts to bypass other diseased coronary arteries.

The IMA may become occluded and threadlike due to what is termed competitive flow when the intact artery senses an equalized flow in minimally occluded vessels. A significant proximal lesion must be present in order for the patient to reap the benefits of the IMA conduit. If the chest is reopened at a later date, care is taken not to transect the IMA.

The left internal mammary artery is dissected up to its origin (termed "taken down") from the subclavian artery, freeing it from the retrosternal aspect of the chest wall (Fig. 43-18). A small amount of tissue is left around the circumference of the artery. After mobilization, the pericardium is notched or opened to minimize tension and distance to the diseased coronary artery. The goal is to prevent tension on the anastomosis, which can cause stenosis or possibly occlusion. Side-to-side or end-to-side anastomosis is performed primarily between the internal mammary artery and the left anterior descending coronary artery, distal to the obstruction (Fig. 43-19).

Saphenous Vein Conduit. The procedure for a saphenous vein bypass graft is expedited by two teams: one harvests the greater and lesser saphenous veins *for use as conduit* while the other opens the chest and prepares for CPB. Methods for saphenous procurement include the open method (Fig. 43-20) and the endoscopic approach (Fig. 43-21). An adequate length of vein is removed to obtain sufficient graft material. The distal end of each vein segment is identified, and the graft is placed in heparinized normal saline solution after it has been harvested. It is handled gently to avoid trauma to the intima. The vein is reversed to permit a normal direction of blood flow through the venous valves into the coronary artery.

The affected coronary artery is opened distal to the obstruction; the proximal end of the saphenous vein is anastomosed end-to-side to the artery, creating the distal anastomosis, thus bypassing the obstruction. Usually a fine 6-0 or 7-0 monofilament nonabsorbable suture is used. The proximal anastomosis is established by creating a small opening in the aorta with a punch and suturing the distal end of the vein to the aperture (Fig. 43- 22).

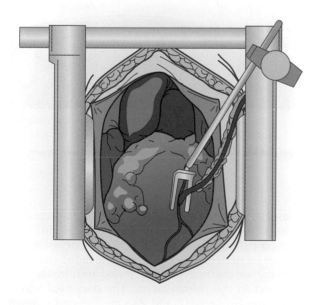

FIG. 43-17 Stabilizing retractor for "off-pump" cardiac procedures.

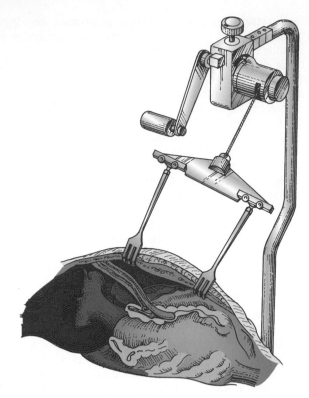

FIG. 43-18   Internal mammary artery procurement using mounted self-retaining retractor.
(Courtesy Rultract, Inc., Cleveland, Ohio.)

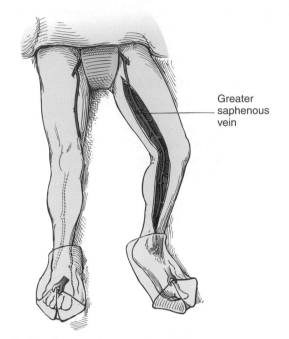

Greater saphenous vein

FIG. 43-20   Open saphenous vein procurement.
(From Waldhausen JA et al: Surgery of the chest, ed 6, St. Louis, 1996, Mosby.)

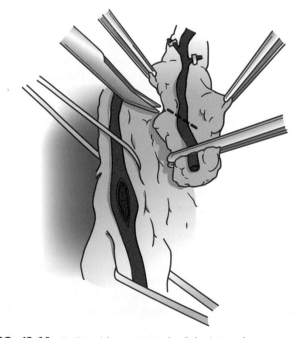

FIG. 43-19   End-to-side anastomosis of the internal mammary artery to a diseased coronary artery.

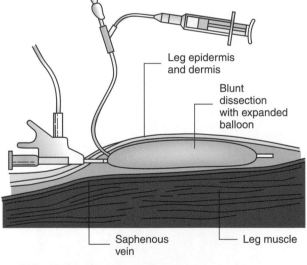

Leg epidermis and dermis

Blunt dissection with expanded balloon

Saphenous vein

Leg muscle

FIG. 43-21   Endoscopic saphenous vein procurement.

Saphenous or other vein or artery bypass grafts are completed before the internal mammary artery is anastomosed to form a vascular conduit. Manipulation of the heart could stress the arterial anastomosis of the IMA (Fig. 43-23).

Radial Artery Conduit.   An arterial conduit is preferred for most patients, because the patency rate remains higher for a longer period. The radial artery can be harvested either via a single incision or endoscopically. The radial artery arises 1 cm distal to the brachial artery and terminates at the distal aspect in the palmar artery. The harvested segment may measure between 12 and 25 cm. The end diameters measure between 3 and 5 mm. The procured segment is usually taken from the patient's nondominant hand.

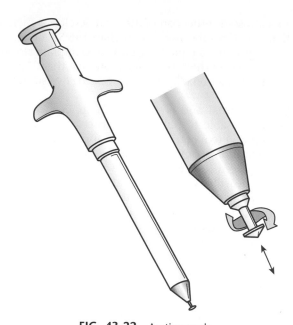

FIG. 43-22 Aortic punch.

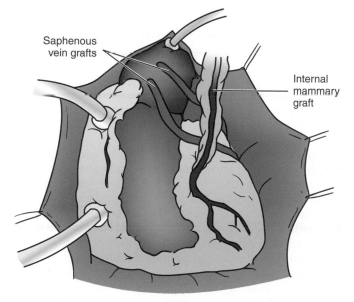

Saphenous
vein grafts

Internal
mammary
graft

FIG. 43-23 Triple conduit bypass. Two saphenous vein grafts with the left internal mammary arterial graft.

In patients undergoing bypass with radial artery conduit harvest, an Allen test or other test deemed appropriate by the surgeon must be undertaken to ensure adequate perfusion of the hand via the ulnar artery.

Though surgical practices vary, a calcium channel blocker is administered preoperatively to avoid vasospasm of the radial artery during procurement. This is usually continued intravenously through postoperative day one when the patient can be switched to an oral form. Many types of calcium channel blockers are available for use (verapamil (Calan), diltiazem [Cardizem], amlodipine [Norvasc]) or combination calcium channel blocker and angiotensin-converting

enzyme (ACE) inhibitor medications may be used (benazepril [Lotrel]).

Coronary Artery Angioplasty. Restoration of perfusion from the left coronary system is possible by direct enlargement of the left main coronary artery lumen in select patients in whom clinical circumstances preclude bypass grafting. A curved incision is made in the lateral aortic wall. Either the posterior or anterior aspect of the left main coronary artery is incised across the stenosis. An autologous onlay pericardial or onlay saphenous vein patch is sutured between the artery and the aortic wall.

Endarterectomy (removal of an organized thrombus and attached endothelium or atherosclerotic fatty plaques from the arterial wall) may be performed in conjunction with left coronary angioplasty or right coronary bypass grafting. Small spatulas, wire loops, miniature abrasive drills, or ultrasonic devices may be used to remove plaque.

Coronary artery angioplasty procedures usually are performed in the cardiac catheterization laboratory (cath lab) or special interventional procedures room in the radiology department. A standby OR team should be available for emergency coronary artery bypass in the event that acute coronary artery obstruction or perforation occurs.

Percutaneous Transluminal Coronary Angioplasty. Percutaneous transluminal coronary angioplasty (PTCA) is performed under fluoroscopy with image intensification. Balloon dilation of the coronary arteries may be the procedure of choice for select patients with significant atherosclerotic narrowing in a major coronary artery (Fig. 43-24). The coronary arteries are approached by either percutaneous femoral artery entry or brachial artery cutdown. A balloon-tipped catheter is passed through a guiding catheter into the area of the coronary artery with atherosclerotic material (plaque). The balloon is inflated by a hydraulic pump to compress plaque against the arterial lining and dilate the arterial wall, thus enlarging the lumen. During the time the balloon is inflated, normal flow of oxygen supplied by the artery to the myocardium is interrupted. Oxygenation distal to the balloon may be maintained with oxygenated perfluorochemical emulsion (Fluosol) flowing through the catheter.

Catheters with ultrasonic devices or tiny drill heads may be used to pulverize atherosclerotic plaque before balloon dilation. Other procedures may be performed as an alternative to or in conjunction with balloon angioplasty.

Laser Angioplasty. An argon laser probe, a neodymium: yttrium-aluminum-garnet (Nd:YAG) optical fiber, or a pulsed excimer laser may be used for laser angioplasty. An integrated system combines direct laser energy and fiberoptics with a balloon angioplasty catheter. The catheter positions the laser fiber, which then vaporizes the plaque or thrombus obstructing the coronary vessels.

Intracoronary Stent. A stent may be inserted to act as a buttress to keep an artery open. The coronary artery to be stented should be at least 3 mm in diameter. The stent, which is permanently implanted at the site of the stenosis, widens the arterial lumen by compressing atherosclerotic plaque against the arterial wall. The stainless steel mesh or springlike coil stent is tightly wrapped around a balloon catheter. As the balloon is inflated, the stent expands. After

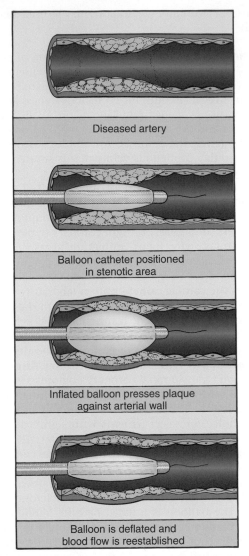

FIG. 43-24   Balloon angioplasty.
(From Canobbio MM: Cardiovascular disorders, *St. Louis, 1990, Mosby.)*

the balloon is deflated and removed, the stent remains in place to provide structural support and keep the artery from collapsing.

Transmyocardial Revascularization (TMR). The myocardium can be revascularized with the creation of a series of channels in an ischemic area of the left ventricle. This procedure is performed through a left thoracotomy incision without the use of CPB. Using a carbon dioxide (CO_2) or holmium (Ho):YAG laser, three to five channels are placed in the distal segment of the left ventricle. Hemostasis is usually established within 45 to 60 seconds. This procedure is used when other conventional therapies cannot be used.

Cardiac Dysrhythmias

Some cardiac rhythm disorders are unresponsive to drug therapy. Normally the electrical cardiac impulse begins at the SA node, thus controlling the rhythm of the heart rate. Fibers from the SA node conduct the impulse through the atria into the AV node and then transmit it along the bundle of His into the ventricles, ending in Purkinje fibers.

Occasionally some other part of the heart develops a rhythmic discharge with a rate more rapid than the SA node. This causes tachycardia (a rapid heartbeat). The impulse also may repeatedly reenter the system, most often at the AV node—bundle of His junction (AV junction), causing overstimulation of the heart.

With epicardial and endocardial mapping techniques, the surgeon is able to pinpoint electrical activity causing dysrhythmia. Preoperatively the mapping procedure is done under fluoroscopy. Electrical impulses from electrode catheters, placed in the heart via a femoral vein, activate sites in the heart to reproduce the abnormal rhythm and to obtain a direct electrocardiogram. Premature cycles, the origin of electrical signals, and accessory pathways can be pinpointed. Intraoperative mapping may be needed to correlate preoperative studies or to identify other sites or pathways masked by antidysrhythmia drugs. The origin and site of a dysrhythmia determine the surgical procedure.

Atrial fibrillation (AF) is one of the most common cardiac dysrhythmias, particularly in patients 50 to 60 years of age. Following cardiac surgery, about 30% of patients will convert to this rhythm. Patients with AF are at very high risk of stroke caused by an embolus, congested heart failure, cardiomyopathy, and death.

Drug therapy commonly includes quinidine, procainamide, sotalol, amiodarone, dofetilide, propafenone, beta blockers, calcium channel blockers, and digoxin. When medical treatments are no longer effective, surgical intervention is necessary. Most patients have left-sided initiating foci near the pulmonary veins, but any of these procedures also can be performed for atrial flutter that is caused by right-sided initiating foci. Ablative treatment near the pulmonary veins causes the risk of pulmonary vein stenosis.

Maze Procedure. The maze procedure, named for the puzzle-like pattern appearance of the incisions introduced by James Cox in 1987, is a cure for AF by interrupting the impulses that cause the dysrhythmias and preserves the contractility of the atria. The procedure requires CPB because both atria are opened and a series of small incisions are made to interrupt the electrical pathways. The scar tissue that forms as a result of the procedure causes the interruption in the pathways. A mitral valvuloplasty is done in conjunction with the maze procedure to improve cardiac performance.

This method has significant success rates for restoring regular sinus rhythm without the use of a pacemaker. Research is being done to develop a minimal access procedure that would not require CPB using saline and epicardially applied bipolar radiofrequency energy. Patients may experience difficulty in increasing their heart rate on exertion and the potential for prolonged conduction, leading to ineffective left atrial contraction.

Maze III Procedure. The maze III incorporates similar techniques to the original maze procedure but requires the removal of both atrial appendages, isolation of the pulmonary veins, and application of cryoablation. Minimally invasive procedures are under development.

Mini Maze Procedure. This uses high radiofrequency ablation. It is similar to the maze III in that it requires isolation of the pulmonary veins altogether or in pairs in conjunction with ablation from the pulmonary veins to the annulus of the mitral valve. This is done without CPB and is highly successful in patients who experience intermittent atrial fibrillation and to a lesser extent in patients with chronic atrial fibrillation.

Radiofrequency Ablation. This treatment of AF involves the use of a surgical probe that creates a series of linear lesions. These lesions encircle the four pulmonary veins and left atrial appendage. The generator supplies temperature-controlled radiofrequency. The surgeon controls the power output.

Cryoablation. This procedure is used to treat the same dysrhythmias as radiofrequency ablation but uses a refrigerant to freeze the affected area to −112° F (−80° C). The maze procedure (maze III) can be modified to incorporate cryoablation that requires less aortic clamp time and decreased chest tube drainage postoperatively. A mitral valve procedure is performed in conjunction if necessary.

Ventricular Aneurysm

Atherosclerotic coronary disease predisposes an individual to myocardial infarction. Ventricular aneurysm (a segmental dilation of the ventricular wall) may develop any time from a few weeks to years after infarction. Predominantly occurring in the left ventricular wall, the aneurysm results from ventricular force on an area of nonfunctioning scar tissue. The thin-walled fibrous aneurysm often contains clots within it. A left ventricular aneurysm usually produces hemodynamic instability manifested by congestive heart failure and ventricular dysrhythmia. The surgeon can excise the aneurysm and reconstruct the ventricle (Fig. 43-25).

The chest is opened by median sternotomy. CPB is established before the adhesion between the aneurysm and pericardium is detached. The ascending aorta is cross-clamped. The aneurysmal sac is opened with a vertical incision, and the area is cleared of thrombus. Fibrotic myocardium is excised circumferentially. Strips of Teflon felt are used as pledgets to prevent tearing of the suture through the ventricle (Fig. 43-26). Before completion of closure, air is removed from the ventricle by suction. The heartbeat is restored, decannulation is performed, and all incisions are closed.

Aneurysmectomy may be done as a single procedure or in conjunction with cardiomyoplasty, valve replacement, coronary artery bypass, or endocardial resection.

Modified Endoventricular Circular Plasty (Dor Procedure). Reconstructive surgery of the transmural anterior ventricular wall with a circular patch plasty was introduced by V. Dor in 1984. This two-layer closure method uses a pursestring suture in the viable inner layer of the myocardium around a scarred aneurysm to minimize the dead area. The dead tissue is excised, and the pursestring is closed to restore the geometry of the ventricle.

Any remaining defect larger than 3 cm can be patched with Dacron. The remaining edges are closed with an interrupted mattress stitch over the outside of the patch with pledgeted nonabsorbable sutures to make it more stable. The result is a more normal left ventricular shape and size.

Atrial Myxoma

Atrial myxoma is a primary cardiac tumor resembling a "cluster of grapes" that usually extends from the endocardium inside the atrium via a pedunculated stalk

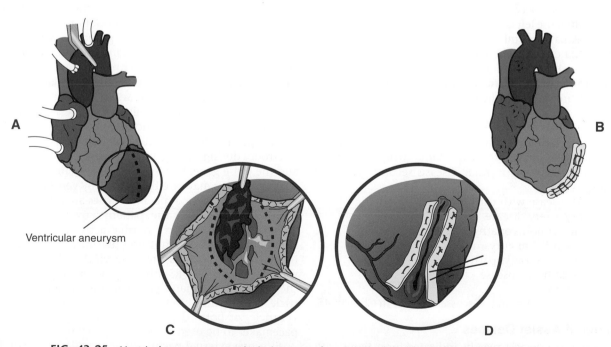

FIG. 43-25 Ventricular aneurysm repair. **A,** Aneurysmal sac is incised. **B,** Clot and excess tissue are removed. The circumscribed area is reinforced with suture. **C,** The edges of the trimmed myocardium are approximated and sutured with felt pledgeted suture bolsters. **D,** The closed myocardium is shown with felt pledgets left in place.

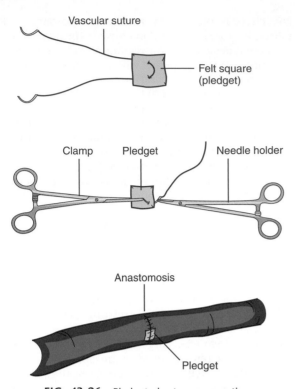

FIG. 43-26   Pledgeted suture preparation.

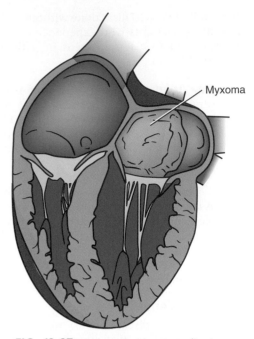

FIG. 43-27   Myxoma: primary cardiac tumor.

(Fig. 43-27). Myxomas are benign and most commonly found in the right atrium but can occur in the left atrium as well as simultaneously in both atria. These benign lesions are dangerous because of their embolic potential and possibility of decreasing the cardiac efficiency. Portions of the myxoma can become dislodged and embolize. If an embolus enters the left atrium, it can lead to a stroke or acute arterial ischemia of a limb or organ.

A myxoma can become enlarged and prolapse into the ventricle, causing incompetence of the tricuspid or mitral valve leading to heart failure. Removal of a myxoma requires CPB. The entire stalk must be removed to prevent regrowth.

Cardiac Transplantation

Cardiac transplantation may be an acceptable option for the patient with limited life expectancy who is incapacitated by end-stage myocardial disease secondary to the following:

- Valvular disease with cardiomyopathy
- Coronary artery disease
- Ischemic cardiomyopathy
- Postmyocardial aneurysm
- Idiopathic cardiomyopathy
- Congenital heart disease
- Cardiac tumor

Cardiac transplantation is discussed further in Chapter 45.

Mechanical Assist Devices

Mechanical assist devices may be indicated for patients with cardiac dysfunction. These devices may be implanted in conjunction with other cardiac surgical procedures or to provide long-term assistance for life-sustaining cardiac function.

Cardiac Pacemaker. The conducting system of the heart may be altered or interrupted at any point by degenerative disease, drugs, or surgical trauma. This may cause syncope, diminished cardiac output, hypotension, dysrhythmias, partial or complete heart block, or sinus bradycardia (sick sinus syndrome). Patients with these conditions may be treated by artificial pacing (i.e., delivery of an electrical impulse by a pacemaker) to correct atrial and ventricular dysrhythmias and to interrupt chronic atrial fibrillation.

A pacemaker consists of a pulse generator, which produces electrical impulses, and leads to carry impulses to stimulating electrodes placed in contact with the heart (Fig. 43-28). A pacing system includes electromyocardial conduction. Lithium batteries supply power for years to the microprocessor of the pulse generator. Platinum alloy or stainless steel electrodes, with leads encased in plastic, may be unipolar or bipolar. With bipolar systems, electric current flows between two electrodes during pacing; it flows between the electrode tip and the pulse generator in unipolar systems.

A pacemaker may be either a standby ventricular demand type or a physiologic type. Both types are intermittent and noncompetitive with the patient's own pacing system. They monitor the heart's normal activity. The impulse to stimulate the heart is not emitted unless the rate of the heartbeat falls below a preset level. Also known as the R wave–inhibited or QRS-inhibited pacemaker, electrodes of the ventricular demand pacemaker are placed in the ventricle. Stimulating electrodes are placed in the atrium or ventricle, or both, depending on the type of physiologic pacemaker to be used.

Effective external pacing for ventricular standstill led to the development of partially implanted electrode leads connected to an external stimulator for long-term pacing for other conditions. Fully implantable pacemaker systems for

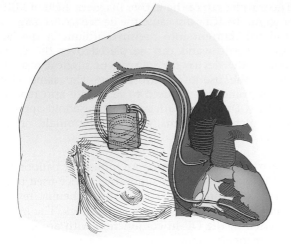

FIG. 43-28   Cardiac pacemaker.
(From Waldhausen JA et al: Surgery of the chest, ed 6, St. Louis, 1996, Mosby.)

long-term use have been available since 1960. An implantable microprocessor generator is hermetically sealed in a metallic container impermeable to body fluids.

Selection of a system depends on the specific pacing requirements of the individual patient. Pacemakers may be temporary or permanent. Endocardial (transvenous) or epicardial (myocardial) electrode leads may be used. Most of these units are programmable to alter pacing function. Temporary pacing is often necessary before and during permanent system implantation. Systemic complete heart block and sinus bradycardia are the most frequent indications for permanent-system implantation. A single-chamber ventricular pacemaker may be implanted. The dual-chamber pacemaker, most commonly in the DDD mode (Table 43-1), senses and synchronously paces both chambers and triggers or inhibits the response to vary the ventricular rate with the atrial rate. Permanent pacing may be initiated by the following devices.

Endocardial Pacemaker.   A transvenous electrode lead is placed in the endocardium and attached to a pulse generator. With the patient under local anesthesia, an incision is made just beneath the clavicle or in the deltopectoral groove, preferably on the side of the chest opposite the patient's dominant hand. The subcutaneous tissue is opened to underlying fascia to create a pocket for the pulse generator.

The lead may be inserted through the cephalic, subclavian, or internal or external jugular vein. Under fluoroscopy, the endocardial electrodes (leads) are advanced via the superior vena cava into the apex of the right ventricle. The leads are attached to the endocardium by one of two ways—passive or active fixation.

In passive fixation, the pacemaking electrode tip has small flexible plastic tines that become attached to the trabeculae of the right ventricle. The endocardium will overgrow these leads, causing a firm attachment.

The electrode used during active fixation has a small threaded tip that is deployed into the endocardium by the surgeon. Atrial leads are directed into the right atrial appendage. The lead is connected to the pulse generator, which in turn is placed into a previously prepared subcutaneous pocket. The incision is primarily closed with or without suction drainage.

Epicardial Electrodes.   With the patient under general anesthesia, epicardial electrodes are placed via a transthoracic approach to the myocardium. For an extrapleural parasternal approach, the pericardium is entered by subperichondral resection of the fifth costal cartilage. Two sew-on or screw-in–type electrodes are implanted 1 cm apart in the myocardium of the right or left ventricle and/or atrium. After the pacing thresholds are measured from an external source, electrode leads are tunneled under the costal margin to the pulse generator implanted in a subcutaneous pocket in the left upper quadrant of the abdominal wall. Water seal chest drainage is necessary only if the pleura were entered.

Precautions with Pacemakers.   Use of an electrosurgical unit (ESU) is usually avoided during placement of a pacemaker or when a surgical procedure is performed on a patient with a pacemaker. Electromagnetic interference may affect the pulse generator, depending on the type of pacemaker. If it is necessary to use the ESU, it should be kept as far away from the pulse generator as possible. The dispersive electrode should be placed on the thigh area, not near the chest.

A pacing system analyzer measures the amount of energy in milliamperes (mA) needed to stimulate the heart. It is used to locate the area of the myocardium where the least

TABLE 43-1	**Identification Code for Cardiac Pacemakers***			
First Letter (Chamber Paced)	Second Letter (Chamber Sensed)	Third Letter (Mode of Response to Sensing of Patient's Heart Rate)	Fourth Letter (Programmable Functions)	Fifth Letter (Tachyarrhythmia Function)
A = Atrium	A = Atrium	I = Inhibited response	P = Programmable rate and output only	N = Normal rate
V = Ventricle	V = Ventricle	T = Triggered response	M = Multiprogrammable	B = Bursts
D = Dual/both chambers	D = Dual/both chambers	D = Dual function/ inhibited and triggered response	C = Communicating noninvasive program	S = Scanning
	O = No sensing	R = Reverse response	O = Nonprogrammable	E = External
		O = No response		

*Sequence of letters describes parameters and functions.

amount of energy will be needed (generally 0.4 to 0.8 mA) and to test functioning of the electrode and pulse generator before placement. Telemetric communication capabilities of some pacemakers allow the surgeon to obtain direct evidence of battery output.

The patient with a pacemaker requires adequate follow-up care. He or she should carry identification containing the serial number, model, rate, manufacturer's name, and date of insertion. The circulating nurse records this information in the patient's chart, along with the time of insertion. Patients with demand or radiofrequency units should be warned to avoid proximity to electromagnetic devices, such as magnetic resonance imaging (MRI) machines, because magnetic interference will stop the pacemaker battery function.

Battery depletion is the most common indication for replacement of the pulse generator. The old generator is removed from the subcutaneous pocket. A new one is connected to the electrode and inserted into the pocket. Occasionally, electrode problems and/or erosion of or infection around the generator require surgical intervention.

Cardioverter-Defibrillator.

The automatic implantable cardioverter-defibrillator (ICD) has the capability of recognizing potential life-threatening episodes of ventricular tachycardia or fibrillation. The system has a pair of sensing electrodes to monitor changes in the heart rate, cycle length, and waveform (Fig. 43-29). After the onset of ventricular tachycardia, two defibrillating electrodes deliver a synchronized shock to terminate it. The electrical conduction pattern of the heart is converted to a more normal pattern. Newer models are capable of pacing, as well as defibrillating. Supplied sterile, the pulse generator of the device is powered by lithium batteries hermetically sealed in a titanium case. The device may be implanted in addition to endocardial resection or other ablation, or instead of a surgical procedure for dysrhythmia. Placement of this device is similar to procedures described for implantation of cardiac pacemakers.

The wavelength of the ESU or magnetic field of MRI can deprogram the ICD and cause the device to discharge aberrant electric current into the myocardium. A specialized electromagnetic wand can be placed over the chest to deactivate the device for subsequent surgical procedures requiring the use of electrosurgery. The same electromagnetic wand can be used to reactivate and reprogram the ICD. ICDs are not affected by household appliances, such as microwave ovens, computer terminals, or television sets.

Intraaortic Balloon Pump.

An intraaortic balloon pump (IABP) is a left ventricular supportive device used to assist a patient with prolonged myocardial ischemia, reversible left ventricular failure, or cardiogenic shock. The IABP can be inserted in the OR in conjunction with an open-heart procedure for circulatory support during weaning from CPB. Because the IABP can be inserted percutaneously via the femoral artery, it can be inserted in an interventional area such as the cardiac cath lab or the ICU when necessary. An IABP reduces left ventricular workload and increases delivery of oxygen to the myocardium, thereby increasing cardiac output and systemic perfusion. An IABP cannot be effective without partial ventricular function.

The cylindrical balloon is inserted into the descending thoracic aorta, just below the left subclavian artery, by way of a femoral artery (Fig. 43-30). The balloon catheter may be inserted percutaneously or by direct vision, or it can be inserted via a prosthetic arterial graft anastomosed end-to-side to the femoral artery. After insertion, the balloon catheter is connected to a pump console.

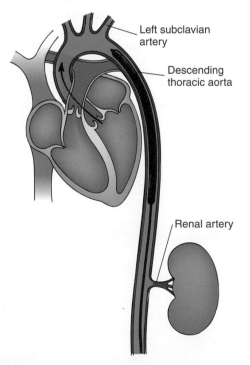

FIG. 43-30 Intraaortic balloon catheter positioned in descending thoracic aorta, above renal artery and below left subclavian artery, via femoral artery.

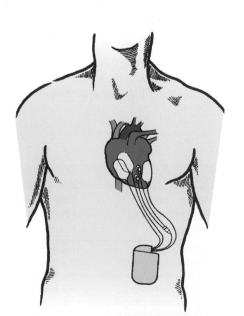

FIG. 43-29 Implantable defibrillator. *(Courtesy Medtronic, Inc., Minneapolis, Minn.)*

The IABP uses principles of counterpulsation. In contrast with systemic arteries, coronary arteries are constricted during systole and fill during diastole. Therefore, inflating the balloon during diastole increases coronary perfusion, aiding contractility and oxygen transport. When the balloon is inflated, the blood volume displaced increases coronary artery pressure. When the balloon deflates during systole, the resistance against which the ventricle pumps is decreased. Balloons vary in size to provide 20, 30, or 40 mL of volume displacement, thus giving a maximum assist without total aortic occlusion. When the balloon is placed and the position is verified by chest radiograph, the complete system is vented of air and filled with either helium or carbon dioxide for balloon inflation, depending on the type of counterpulsator. The ratio of ventricular assist is determined by the individual patient's hemodynamic status.

The pump can be regulated automatically, triggered by an electrocardiogram signal, or operated manually. To prevent potential thrombi, pumping should be continuous. Intraaortic balloons are made of antithrombotic material. The manufacturer's instructions for use should be followed. Pumps are equipped with sensors (e.g., alarm and automatic shut-off) to minimize danger.

Weaning from the IABP is usually gradual, as tolerated by the patient. Lower extremity pulses are checked during and periodically after balloon catheter removal to assess circulation in the foot on the side of the catheter insertion and to check for the presence of clots. Complications associated with an IABP include distal extremity ischemia, thrombus or emboli, gas embolism, arterial or aortic perforation, bleeding, and infection.

Ventricular Assist Device.

A powered ventricular assist device (VAD) can be used to wean patients from CPB when the IABP, drugs, and/or cardiac pacing are ineffective, to support circulation after postinfarction cardiogenic shock or traumatic myocardial contusion, and to provide a temporary bridge for support before transplantation (Fig. 43-31). The VAD has been a significant bridge to transplantation and is useful for cardiac support until a suitable donor is available. The mechanical device maintains systemic and myocardial perfusion while promoting metabolic and hemodynamic recovery of a reversibly damaged myocardium.

The VAD does not depend on cardiac contractility or electrical conduction. It acts as an artificial ventricle. The VAD consists of a flexible polyurethane blood sac, a flexible diaphragm, and a pump assembly enclosed within a rigid polysulfone housing. Inlet and outlet valves maintain unidirectional blood flow. The VAD is attached to the patient via inflow and outflow cannulas. Support can be to the left, right, or both ventricles:

- *Left ventricular assistance (LVA).* Blood is withdrawn from the left atrium into a left ventricular assist device (LVAD) and returned to the ascending aorta. The polyurethane inflow cannula can be inserted into either the left atrium or the left ventricle. The outflow cannula has a segment of woven polyester that is anastomosed end-to-side to the thoracic aorta. The Jarvik 2000 may be the assist device of choice for children and smaller adults who are awaiting a heart transplant.

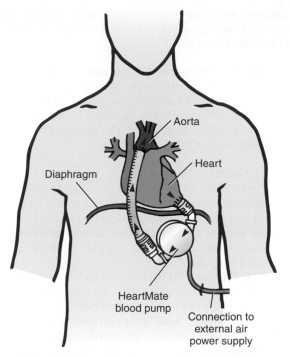

FIG. 43-31   HeartMate ventricular assist device. *(Courtesy Thermo Cardiosystems, Inc., Woburn, Mass.)*

- *Right ventricular assistance (RVA).* Blood is withdrawn from the right atrium into the right ventricular assist device (RVAD) and is returned to the pulmonary artery. The inflow cannula is placed in the right atrium. The outflow cannula is anastomosed end-to-side to the main pulmonary artery.
- *Biventricular assistance (BVA).* Both an LVAD and an RVAD are used to support both ventricles simultaneously.

The cannulas exit the pericardial sac below the costal margin. They are connected to parts of the VAD after removal of all air. Depending on the intended duration of support, the housing is exteriorized or implanted:

- Extracorporeal VAD, used for short-term ventricular assistance, is externally powered pneumatically with compressed air or electrically with centrifugal force. The housing rests on the patient's chest, with the inflow and outflow cannulas passing through the chest wall. The power source is attached to the air-inlet port or pump head. The skin is approximated, or the chest is left open and covered with sterile material sutured to the wound edges. Then the chest is covered with a sterile occlusive dressing. The patient returns to the OR for removal of the device and chest closure or heart transplantation, usually within 10 days.
- Implantable VAD, for long-term use, is an electrically activated pump implanted in the left upper quadrant of the abdomen. The internal battery pack and control unit in the housing are connected to an external battery pack. The cannulas pass through the diaphragm.

The rate of pumping and movement of the diaphragm inside the VAD are programmed by the power console. Another type of LVAD is mounted on a catheter connected to a pump and external motor. The catheter, inserted via the femoral artery or by transthoracic or retroperitoneal approach, draws blood out of the left ventricle and returns it to the descending aorta.

Extracorporeal Membrane Oxygenator. An extracorporeal membrane oxygenator (ECMO) is used as a resuscitative device for patients who have potentially reversible respiratory and/or cardiac failure. It is also commonly used to prolong extracorporeal circulation when the patient is in distress after removal from CPB.

Artificial Heart. Clinical trials are in process to test an artificial heart that can be permanently implanted to maintain circulation in the patient with irreparable myocardial damage or end-stage cardiac disease who does not meet the criteria for cardiac transplantation. A total artificial heart also could be used as temporary support while the patient is awaiting a transplant.

Artificial Heart History. In 1982 William DeVries implanted the first total artificial heart into patient Barney Clark, who lived for 112 days with the device. In 1984 DeVries implanted an artificial heart into a second patient, William Schroeder, who lived 620 days. The Jarvik-7 was an air-driven, double-chambered device that replaced the ventricles. Connector cuffs were sutured to the atria, pulmonary artery, and aorta. These cuffs attached to rims of openings on the device. Power was supplied to the pumping chamber through percutaneous tubes to an external source of compressed air. The patient was essentially tethered to a machine. Many complications, such as emboli, hemorrhage, and infection, were associated with the device.

Recent Advances in Artificial Heart Technology. Abiomed has developed the AbioCor, a fully implantable artificial heart that has been granted permission by the FDA for use in clinical trials on humans since 2001. It is a softball-size self-contained unit with internal rechargeable batteries that can run independently for 30 minutes at a time. The implantable component of the device weighs around 2 pounds and is made of titanium and plastic. There are no external wires; however, an external power pack passes energy through the skin to an internal coil. The external power pack weighs 4 pounds and is recharged every 4 hours. The AbioCor is able to provide complete circulatory support with normal tissue perfusion and no hemolysis, according to current studies. Criteria for use of the AbioCor include biventricular failure without viable treatment alternatives and imminent death within 30 days. The patient's diseased heart is removed with the exception of small atrial attachments (Fig. 43-32).

The first patient to receive the AbioCor implant was Robert Tools, age 59. The implantation was performed in July 2001 at Jewish Hospital in Louisville, Kentucky, by Laman Gray Jr. and Robert Dowling. Mr. Tools lived for 5 months with the device. Ten additional patients have had the device implanted at several heart centers in the United States since, with some success. The second recipient, Tom Christerson, age 71, had the device implanted in September 2001 at the same facility and lived for 512 days with the device. He lived at home and had the opportunity to celebrate his 55th wedding anniversary and the birth of his first great-grandchild.[1]

Investigational studies into a small version of the AbioCor and Penn State Heart will begin in late 2006 or early 2007.

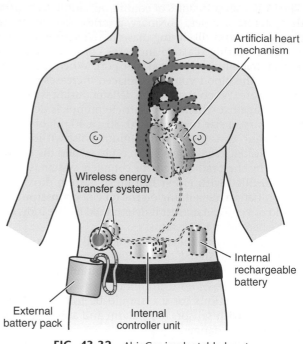

FIG. 43-32 AbioCor implantable heart.

Referred to as AbioCor II, the new unit will be more size appropriate for smaller adults with all components contained within the body.

COMPLICATIONS OF CARDIAC SURGERY

Prevention of complications is a collaborative effort of the surgeon, anesthesiologist, scrub person, and the circulating nurse. The care continuum continues through the patient's stay in ICU and later in the stepdown area. Careful monitoring and management of blood pressure are critical throughout the perioperative care period. Aggressive preoperative evaluation is necessary to screen for patients who are at high risk.

The most common complication of cardiac surgery with or without CBP is stroke. In a patient with atherosclerosis of the coronary arteries the arterial supply of the brain is usually affected. Air embolus is a common complication during valve procedures. Meticulous de-airing of the heart is done by the surgeon before removal of the aortic cross clamp in attempt to prevent air embolus.

Low blood pressure (50 to 60 mm Hg) during bypass can lead to ischemic cerebrovascular accidents of the brain. Hypertensive episodes can lead to hemorrhagic brain insults. Calcium deposits and atheroma that can line the intima of the aorta can embolize during the application and removal of the aortic cross clamp. The surgeon inspects and palpates the aorta to find a section amenable to cross-clamping. There is no guarantee that a plaque will not be dislodged by manipulation or the instrument.

Excessive bleeding can result in cardiogenic shock and alteration of the body's clotting mechanism. Factors that influence clotting include preoperative use of antiplatelet agents, occult liver disease, disruption of an anastomosis due to hypertension or technical malfunction of a suture line, prolonged use of CPB, and ineffective use of protamine for reversal of heparin.

Mediastinal and/or pleural chest tubes are placed to monitor the amount of drainage and, if excessive, may warrant a return to the operating room for exploration or redo.

Postoperative myocardial infarctions (MIs) are infrequent; however, an MI can lead to cardiogenic shock. Postoperative MI can be caused by a kink or acute thrombosis in the newly placed bypass conduit, or air embolus. Acute restrictive pericarditis can obstruct blood flow in a new graft, causing myocardial ischemia.

Organ failure is always a concern with cardiac surgery and CPB. Organ failure can affect any organ system, but is most commonly seen in the kidneys. Low blood pressure caused by an ineffective pump prevents the kidneys from functioning. Acute tubular necrosis (ATN) can result from atherosclerosis of the renal arterial system, leading to kidney failure. Patients with ATN may need hemodialysis for a short time or for life depending on the extent of renal damage. Some patients, who continue to have adequate urine output, may have only a transient rise in their blood urea nitrogen (BUN) and creatinine levels with quick return to normal without the assistance of hemodialysis.

Adult respiratory distress syndrome (ARDS) and other acute respiratory disorders complicate the postoperative outcomes of some patients undergoing cardiac surgery. Preoperative evaluation, especially in smokers, is essential to try to predict and prevent the incidence of postoperative pulmonary disorders.

The bowel and liver are occasionally affected by the surgical experience. Acute liver failure can be first noticed with postoperative bloodwork. A rise in liver function studies (AST, ALT, bilirubin, alkaline phosphatase) can lead to coagulopathies. Bowel that becomes ischemic during bypass can become necrotic in the postoperative course and lead to profound sepsis and death.

Wound infections of the sternum can also lead to horrific sepsis and are managed surgically. The sepsis can result in a prolonged hospital stay or even death. Removing the sternum (sternectomy) is usually a procedure performed by a multidisciplinary team of both cardiac and plastic surgeons. Once the sternum is removed, the plastic surgeon creates a vascularized pedicle flap from the pectoralis muscles or omentum to create a tissue cover for the defect left by the missing sternum. The skin is closed over the flap. The ample blood supply of the muscles and omentum assist with the evacuation of any remaining pathogens and promote wound healing.

Cardiac tamponade occurs when blood and fluids build up around the heart. When blood collects in the pericardium and is not adequately evacuated by the drains, it can collect and begin to compress and compromise the function of the heart. This life-threatening event is first observed when there are increasing right atrial and right ventricular pressures. It is also reflected in a drop of more than 10 mm Hg in systolic blood pressure during the patient's inspiration (pulsus paradoxus). If left untreated cardiac tamponade can lead to hypotension and fatal dysrhythmia.

Electrolyte imbalance in magnesium, potassium, and to a lesser extent, calcium, can lead to serious cardiac dysrhythmias such as sinus bradycardia, supraventricular tachycardia (SVT), ventricular tachycardia (VT), atrial fibrillation, atrial flutter, and ventricular fibrillation (VF). High levels of potassium will cause a fatal dysrhythmia if not medically corrected with medications such as glucose or insulin, furosemide (Lasix), or sodium polystyrene (Kayexalate) or hemodialysis.

Cardiogenic shock may be precipitated by coronary air embolism, pulmonary embolism, myocardial contusion, mechanical venous obstruction, or hypothermia. Precautions are taken intraoperatively to avoid postoperative cardiogenic and/or hemorrhagic shock. Excessive bleeding can result from stress to the clotting mechanism.

Cardiac surgery can be a lifesaving procedure if carefully managed by the entire perioperative team. Attention to sterile technique and patient monitoring is especially critical.

Bibliography

Barassi A: Comparison of three strategies for myocardial protection during coronary artery bypass graft surgery based on markers of cardiac damage, *Clin Biochem* 38(6):504-508, 2005.

Bhat G, Dowling RD: Evaluation of predictors of clinical outcome after partial left ventriculectomy, *Ann Thorac Surg* 72(1):91-95, 2001.

Blaauw Y et al: Treatment of atrial fibrillation, *Heart* 88(4):432-437, 2002.

De Feo, M et al: The risk of stroke following CABG: One possible strategy to reduce it? *Int J Cardiol* 98(2):261-266, 2005.

Dor V: The endovascular circular patch plasty (Dor procedure) in ischemic akinetic dilated ventricles, *Heart Fail Rev* 6(3):187-193, 2001.

Frazier OH et al: Initial clinical experience with the Jarvik 2000 implantable axial-flow left ventricular assist system, *Circulation* 105(24):2855-2860, 2002.

Gavaghan M: Cardiac anatomy and physiology: A review, *AORN J* 67(4):802-822, 1998.

Ghosh S et al: Beating-heart mitral valve surgery in patients with poor left ventricular function. *J Heart Valve Dis* 13(4):622-627, 2004.

Green B: The maze III surgical procedure, *AORN J* 76(1):134-146, 2002.

Imamaki M: A technique for infusion of cardioplegic solution in coronary artery bypass with aortic regurgitation, *J Cardiac Surg* 19(6):539-541, 2004.

Jang GY et al: Recovery of acute myocarditis with biventricular assist device in infant, *Int J Cardiol* 105(3):344-345, 2005.

Jeevanandam V: The quest for permanent ventricular assistance: the role of aortic counterpulsation, *ASAIO J* 50(6):xxxvii-xlii, 2004.

Prassad SM et al: Epicardial ablation on the beating heart: progress towards an off-pump maze procedure, *Heart Surg Forum* 5(2):100-104, 2002.

Ryan WH et al: Mitral valve surgery using the classical "heartport" technique, *J Heart Valve Dis* 14(6):709-714, 2005.

Saad EB, et al: Ablation of atrial fibrillation, *Curr Cardiol Rep* 4(5):379-387, 2002.

Seifert PC: *Cardiac surgery*, St. Louis, 2002, Mosby.

Sorelle R: Cardiovascular news: Totally contained AbioCor artificial heart implanted July 3, 2001, *Circulation* 104(3):9005-9006, 2001.

Zareba KM: The artificial heart—Past, present, and future, *Med Sci Monit* 8(3):72-77, 2002.

Zeltsman D, Acker MA: Surgical management of heart failure, *Annu Rev Med* 53:383-391, 2002.

Chapter 44

Vascular Surgery

CHAPTER OBJECTIVES

After studying this chapter, the learner will be able to:
- Identify the pertinent anatomy of the peripheral vascular system.
- Describe the potential complications associated with peripheral vascular disease.
- Describe the care of the patient with peripheral vascular disease.
- List the differences in aneurysms and their treatment.
- Discuss the vascular access options for hemodialysis.

CHAPTER OUTLINE

KEY TERMS AND DEFINITIONS

Aneurysm   An abnormal outpouching or bulging of an artery.
- **True aneurysm** Progressive dilation of an artery.
- **False aneurysm (pseudoaneurysm)** Injury to all three layers of the arterial wall that permits blood to accumulate in the connective tissue.
- **Dissecting aneurysm** The intima separates from the media. A false passage fills with blood, causing further separation of intima and media.
- **Mycotic aneurysm** Bacterial vegetation embolizes from the valve of the heart to the arteries, where it implants and grows, causing the weakened artery to distend and rupture.

Anticoagulate   Alteration in the cellular activity associated with clotting.

Embolize   Material (i.e., fat, plaque, vegetation, or clot) in a blood vessel becomes bloodborne with the potential for lodging in smaller vascular tributaries.

Iatrogenic   Condition inadvertently caused by the medical or surgical treatment performed by a physician.

Thrombose   Blood within a vascular structure clots and occludes the lumen.

SUPPLEMENTAL MATERIAL ON EVOLVE WEBSITE

evolve

http://evolve.elsevier.com/BerryKohn
- Content Updates
- Glossary
- Full Set of Perioperative Flash Cards
- Interactive Key Term Flash Cards
- Student Activities
- Tips for the Scrub Person and Circulating Nurse: Carotid Endartectomy, Femoral Popliteal Bypass
- WebLinks

HISTORICAL BACKGROUND

For centuries human beings have been plagued with peripheral vascular disease and its complications, such as pain or the loss of an extremity or life. However, little was understood about vascular system disease that causes arterial stenosis or occlusion until the contributions of the Scottish brothers William and John Hunter. Their studies of aneurysm formation, pathology, and treatment provided the foundation for the concepts of modern vascular surgery. William Hunter (1718-1783) was the first to describe an arteriovenous fistula and aneurysm, and John Hunter (1728-1793) performed a successful surgical procedure for a popliteal aneurysm. Others subsequently experimented with vascular anastomoses. Alexis Carrel (1873-1944) received the Nobel Prize in 1912 for his work at the University of Chicago with blood vessel anastomoses, suturing techniques, and animal organ transplantation. The suturing of blood vessels was the vital link necessary for the development of successful vascular surgery.

An endarterectomy to remove a localized vascular occlusion was first performed in 1946. In 1948 the first bypass graft was implanted to treat diffuse vascular disease. In the following decades many surgical procedures have become feasible with the use of improved diagnostic techniques and instrumentation, sutures, synthetic grafts, and microvascular techniques.

In 1983 the American Board of Surgery began a certification program in general vascular surgery. To qualify, candidates must have specialized training and practice in peripheral vascular surgery and be a diplomate of the American Board of Surgery or the American Board of Thoracic Surgery. The Society of Vascular Nursing was founded in 1982. Specialty certification for perioperative vascular nurses was established in 1996.

ANATOMY AND PHYSIOLOGY OF THE VASCULAR SYSTEM

Vessels in the thorax, abdomen, extremities, and extracranial cerebrovascular area constitute the circulatory system (Fig. 44-1). The ascending aorta, which originates from the left ventricle, carries oxygenated blood from the heart to the arteries. The major arteries leading to the head and upper extremities—the brachiocephalic trunk, left common carotid, and subclavian arteries—branch off from the aortic arch in the middle mediastinum above the heart. The thoracic aorta then descends through the posterior mediastinum at the left side of the vertebral column. Passing through the diaphragm, the abdominal aorta descends to the level of the fourth lumbar vertebra, where it bifurcates (i.e., divides) to form the common iliac arteries that lead to the lower extremities. Arteries from the abdominal aorta carry blood to the kidneys and the abdominal and pelvic organs. The femoral artery, which originates from the iliac artery, is the main artery in each leg.

Oxygenated blood flows from the arterial system through the capillary network and returns deoxygenated to the heart via the venous system (Fig. 44-2). The venae cavae enter the right atrium. The superior vena cava, formed by the union of the two brachiocephalic veins, returns deoxygenated

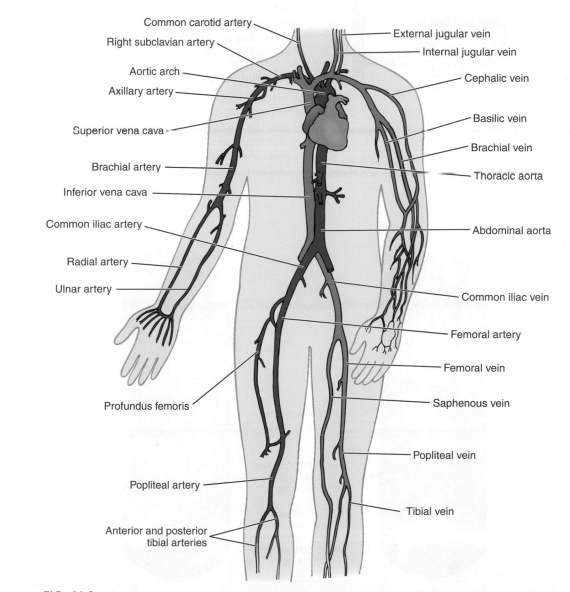

FIG. 44-1   Circulatory system. Arteries (and the heart) are shown as red vessels. Veins are shown as blue vessels.

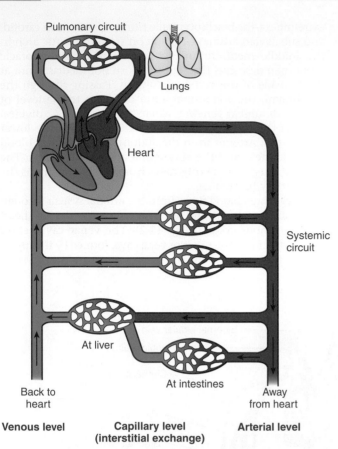

FIG. 44-2   Circulatory system to the capillary level.

venous blood from the head, neck, upper extremities, and chest. The inferior vena cava, which begins at the level of the fifth lumbar vertebra, returns blood from the lower extremities, pelvis, and abdominal organs. There are two exceptions to this oxygenation/deoxygenation pattern:

1. The pulmonary arteries carry deoxygenated blood to the lungs, and the pulmonary veins carry oxygenated blood to the heart.
2. In fetal umbilical circulation, one vein carries oxygenated blood and two arteries carry mixed blood.

Innervation of the arteries and veins is controlled by the efferent vasomotor fibers of the autonomic nervous system. The nerve fibers enter the vessel adventitia (i.e., covering) along the same route as the blood supply. Stimulation of these nerves can cause vasoconstriction that shunts blood to larger organ groups such as the skin or gastrointestinal tract. Some medications cause vasodilation, which relaxes the vessels and slows heart rate to decrease intraluminal pressure.

The vessels are lined with endothelial cells, which when intact do not support platelet aggregation. This property is interrupted when a vessel is injured, and a clot is allowed to form. The endothelial lining also secretes factors that resist clotting, stimulate tissue repair, and synthesize clotting factors.

Arterial Anatomy

Arteries are elastic and constrict in response to hemorrhage. The arterial walls are made up of three layers that are separated by internal and external elastic membranes (Fig. 44-3). The innermost layer is the intima (tunica intima), a single layer of endothelial cells on a thin matrix of hyaluronic acid, collagen, and elastic fibers. The middle layer is the media

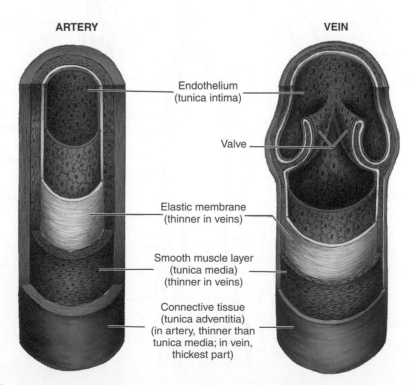

ARTERY   **VEIN**

Endothelium (tunica intima)

Valve

Elastic membrane (thinner in veins)

Smooth muscle layer (tunica media) (thinner in veins)

Connective tissue (tunica adventitia) (in artery, thinner than tunica media; in vein, thickest part)

FIG. 44-3   Cross section of an artery and a vein showing the three layers: tunica intima, tunica media, and tunica adventitia.

(tunica media, or yellow fibrous). It is the thickest of the layers and is composed of a combination of smooth muscle fibers, yellow collagen, and some elastic fibers. The medial layer gives the arterial wall the flexibility and strength to withstand higher internal pressure.

The outermost layer is the adventitia (tunica adventitia, or white fibrous connective tissue). It is the thinnest layer but provides most of the external support for the arterial wall and resistance to overexpansion.

The tissues of the adventitia and the outer third of the media are nourished by a series of capillaries called the vasa vasorum. The rest of the medial layer and the intimal layer are nourished by diffusion from the luminal flow. Terminal arteries, referred to as arterioles, end at the level of the capillary beds in the tissues.

Venous Anatomy

Venous walls are structured in three layers. The innermost layer is the intima and is composed of endothelial cells that produce coagulation factors. The middle layer, or media, is much thinner in the deep venous system and may even be hard to identify microscopically. The superficial veins have a thicker medial layer composed mainly of smooth muscle fibers. This provides some resistance and response to intraluminal pressure changes. The external layer, or the venous adventitia, is composed of loose connective tissue (see Fig. 44-2). Because of lower flow pressure, larger veins have internal semilunar valves to maintain the direction of the blood flow.

The muscular component of the lower extremities provides force during contraction of large muscle groups, which facilitates venous return from the larger peripheral sinusoids. The cerebral veins are an exception; they have no valves. Veins are less elastic than arteries and tend to ooze instead of contracting in response to hemorrhage.

Venous anatomy has three structural components: superficial veins, deep veins, and perforators (also known as communicating veins) (Fig. 44-4). The venous structure and flow of the lower extremities is an example of this system.

At the tissue level, the origin of the venous system at the capillary bed is referred to as venules. The venous drainage of deoxygenated blood from the superficial veins returns through the perforators to the deep veins during muscular contraction. The deoxygenated blood then passes from the deep veins to the inferior vena cava.

Capillary Anatomy

Capillary beds are the vascular nutrition and waste exchange points of the arterial and venous systems. Capillaries are the diameter of a red blood cell and form a network throughout body tissues. Structurally they are a single epithelial cell layer thick, which facilitates the exchange of oxygen and carbon dioxide at the tissue level. They are semipermeable to water and crystalloids but are impermeable to larger molecules such as proteins. Oxygenated blood enters the capillary bed via the arterial system, and deoxygenated blood passively drains into the venous system.

There are no fibrous or muscular layers of the vessels at this level. Lymphatic vessels passively exchange lipids, debris, fluids, proteins, antibodies, and other nutrients at this level in response to skeletal muscle contraction. This fluid is filtered by the lymphatics and is transported through the thoracic duct to the vena cava. The lymphatic vessels are structurally very pliable and have valves to maintain a unidirectional flow.

VASCULAR DISEASE

Vascular diseases that cause occlusion or stenosis are usually acquired diseases. Atherosclerosis is the most common arterial disease. It is a diffuse disease and begins as a disruption of the intima of a large artery. Cholesterol enters the media to stimulate muscle growth, and platelets accumulate around the disruption of the endothelial intima to form plaque or a thrombus. Often this process becomes localized around vessel orifices and branches (i.e., at bifurcations). The disease may produce stenosis (narrowing) and subsequent occlusion or ectasia (dilation) and aneurysm.

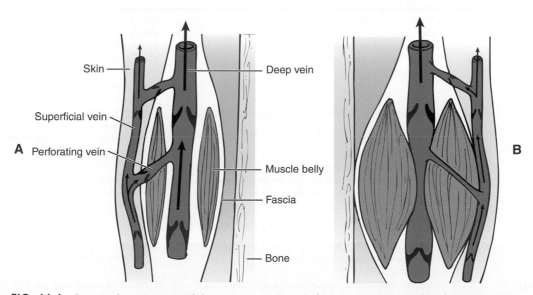

FIG. 44-4 Structural components of deep venous anatomy in lower extremity. **A,** Relaxed state. **B,** With muscle contraction, the perforating veins are squeezed closed.

Atherosclerosis is the principal factor in transient ischemic attacks (TIAs, or "mini strokes"), cerebrovascular accidents (strokes, or "brain attacks"), myocardial infarctions (heart attacks), and aortic stenosis. Risk factors include familial history, a high level of serum cholesterol, smoking, and hypertension (Box 44-1).

Inadequate blood supply causes ischemia in tissues. If left untreated, this can lead to thrombus, embolus, ulceration, necrosis, or gangrene. Venous stasis disease or an obstruction of venous return can cause hemodynamic imbalances. Through vascular surgery, vessels are repaired, reconstructed, or replaced to improve peripheral (systemic) circulation. The most common procedures are performed to revascularize a lower extremity for limb salvage, to repair an aortoiliac aneurysm, and to improve cerebral blood flow through the carotid arteries.

DIAGNOSTIC PROCEDURES

Preoperative assessment of cardiac risk is critically important in planning the care of a patient who requires major vascular surgery. Peripheral arterial and venous diseases are then assessed. Table 44-1 compares the assessment factors of peripheral arterial and venous obstructive diseases in an extremity. Peripheral vascular laboratories, which are similar to cardiac cath labs, have been established in many health care facilities to perform noninvasive and invasive studies before and after surgical intervention.

Noninvasive Procedures

Computed tomography (CT scan) and magnetic resonance imaging (MRI) are noninvasive techniques of choice to confirm a diagnosis of aortic aneurysm, thrombus, or atherosclerotic plaque in arterial walls, especially in the abdominal and carotid circulation. CT scans are good tests to assess the

| BOX 44-1 | Risk Factors for the Development of Peripheral Vascular Disease |

- Advanced age
- Diabetes
- Familial predisposition
- Habitual long periods of standing
- High-fat diet causing high serum cholesterol
- Hypertension
- Obesity
- Repeated pregnancies
- Sedentary lifestyle
- Smoking
- Stress

sizes and stages of vessel occlusions. They can be performed with or without a contrast medium and very quickly in emergency situations. CT scans are somewhat expensive and expose the patient to x-rays.

MRI is useful for evaluating a three-dimensional image of the vessel being studied. This method is contraindicated for patients with stainless steel pacemakers, vena cava filters, or vessel clips, but many patients can benefit from its use. Nonmagnetic materials are not contraindicated. MRI is more expensive than CT scans and takes longer to perform.

Carotid phonoangiography and oculoplethysmography (OPG) are techniques to obtain cerebral blood flow measurements to localize obstructions in the vessels of the head and neck. OPG is contraindicated in patients with intraocular lens implants.

Pulse volume recording (PVR) or photoplethysmography is used to measure systolic pressure in the extremities and digital arterial systems. This test is affected by artifacts and

TABLE 44-1	Comparison of Peripheral Arterial and Venous Obstructive Diseases in an Extremity	
Assessment of Extremity	**Arterial Obstructive Disease**	**Venous Obstructive Disease**
Color	Dusky, blue, gray, mottled, pallor distal to obstruction	Red, purple, brown hemosiderin spots, brawny
Temperature	Cool, cold	Warm, hot
Visual and palpable characteristics	Dry, shiny, flaking skin; vessels not obvious	Moist, peeling skin
	Lack of hair on affected part	Vessels may be tortuous and inflamed
	Thick nails	Thickened tissue
		Hair present on affected part
		Normal nails
Sensation	Numbness, tingling, pain during exercise (intermittent claudication)	Aching, throbbing, tightness, feeling of heaviness; muscles feel fatigued
	Pain at rest in severe disease	Pain decreased by motion or elevation of legs
	Increased pain when exposed to cold	Feels worse at end of day
	Pain can be acute and severe	
Mobility	Painful range of motion; limited flexion and extension caused by avascular necrosis at the tissue level	Painful range of motion; limited flexion and extension caused by congestive edema in joints
	Diminished elasticity	
Size	Not enlarged, average for body build	Swollen, edematous
Integrity of surface layer	Peeling; infarcted; painful, deep, serous, oozing ulcers with defined edges on or between toes	Stasis ulceration; open, draining, shallow ulcers with irregular borders
Pulses	Weak or absent	Present
Condition of digits	Mottled, blackened, fragile, painful; can become gangrenous	Edematous, reddened, painful; can become gangrenous

patient positioning. A diagnosis of deep vein thrombosis (DVT) may be made by phleborheography (PRG), a plethysmographic technique that records the rhythmic changes in venous volume in the legs; these changes are associated with respiration. PRG is not useful for small thrombi or for deep iliac or femoral veins, and the process is time consuming and expensive.

Ultrasonography is a major diagnostic tool for measuring segmental arterial pressures and venous patency in the extremities; it also may be used for abdominal circulation. Doppler color-coded flow imaging and transcranial Doppler imaging are replacing carotid phonoangiography and OPG in the evaluation of carotid circulation. High-resolution, B-mode ultrasound provides real-time images of venous systems in the upper and lower extremities.

Saphenous and cephalic vein mapping accurately measures vein diameter, location, and quality to determine preoperatively if the vein is suitable for use as an arterial conduit in arterial reconstruction. Ultrasound also detects venous thrombosis. With a pulse Doppler blood flow detector, longitudinal and/or transverse cross-sectional scans are obtained and the images are recorded by oscilloscope. A computer-generated print of the image on the screen provides a permanent record of the arteriograph or venograph.

Intraoperative assessment of shunt performance or vessel patency or stenosis, as well as identification of an arteriovenous fistula (AVF), is easily performed with a sterile Doppler probe. An audible signal is transduced and is similar to the sounds transmitted by a Geiger counter (Fig. 44-5).

Invasive Procedures

Selective angiography permits the radiographic study of a particular segment of the vascular system. Aortography visualizes the aorta (Fig. 44-6). Arteriography shows the patency of an artery or a branch of the aorta and its collateral circu-

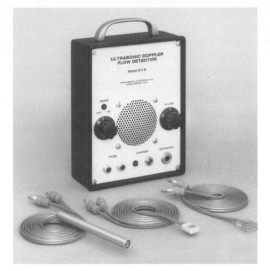

FIG. 44-5 Doppler box and probe.

lation. Phlebography detects DVT, and a venogram visualizes the veins. An angiogram requires the injection of a nontoxic radiopaque substance. The pain associated with injection of intravascular contrast material can be so intense that the procedure may be performed under continuous epidural anesthesia or general anesthesia.

Angioscopy is an endoscopic technique used to visualize the interior of vessels. A small (1.5- to 3-mm) flexible fiberoptic angioscope is coupled to a camera, which allows the view from the angioscope to be seen on a monitor. The lining and structures within the blood vessels are visualized as the scope is advanced within each vessel. For many patients, angioscopy is an alternative preoperative diagnostic tech-

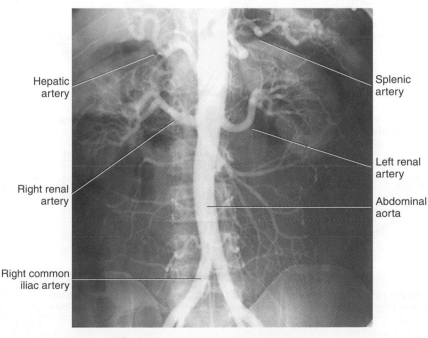

FIG. 44-6 Normal abdominal aortogram.

nique to angiography and may be used to evaluate the effectiveness of therapy intraoperatively. It can reveal retained atherosclerotic plaque or thrombi and suture lines.

Intravascular ultrasonic scanning uses a miniaturized ultrasonic probe at the end of a 5- to 9-French (Fr) catheter. The probe is introduced into the vessel percutaneously. Images of the entire circumference are obtained to determine the thickness of the vessel wall and the distribution of plaque within the wall. This technique may be used both intra-operatively and percutaneously.

SPECIAL FEATURES OF VASCULAR SURGERY

Circulation within the peripheral vascular system affects the brain, internal organs, and extremities. An expanding body of knowledge relating to vascular physiology and the development of the art of vascular surgery has improved the quality of life for many patients with peripheral vascular diseases. Circulatory problems may affect any part of the body, but this discussion focuses on the most common pathologic conditions amenable to vascular procedures performed by vascular surgeons and interventional radiologists. Current surgical trends include open procedures and endovascular techniques.

Vascular injury can occur during invasive diagnostic, monitoring, or therapeutic procedures. Iatrogenic arterial injuries, those resulting from an unexpected outcome of a procedure, can cause loss of function or even death from ischemia, hemorrhage, or embolus. The patient must be carefully observed and monitored for signs of complications during and after vascular procedures. Infection is a devastating postoperative complication that must

be avoided through strict adherence to aseptic and sterile techniques. Other considerations include the following:

- A thorough understanding of the principles of general surgery should be combined with special training in vascular surgical techniques. Speed and accuracy are imperative.
- Local or monitored anesthesia care (MAC) is usually preferred for most conservative interventional procedures. General anesthesia or regional block is used for longer or more extensive procedures.
- Skin preparation is performed very gently. Vascular pathology (i.e. carotid stenosis or aneurysms) should never be rubbed or pressed during the prep because plaque or clots could embolize, causing serious limb or brain damage. Aneurysms could rupture.
- Temperature regulation may be a problem during long procedures or when multiple blood transfusions are given. Warmed fluids can be administered via rapid infusing pumps. Forced-air warming blankets provide a normothermic temperature.
- Meticulous care is exercised during anastomosis of vessels to avoid the danger of postoperative thrombosis and stenosis. To prevent undue trauma to vessels, an assortment of curved and angled scissors, noncrushing vascular clamps, and forceps specifically designed for vascular surgery is included in the instrument setup (Fig. 44-7). Umbilical tape (also called hernia tape) or synthetic vessel loops are used for retraction and vessel control (Fig. 44-8). An operating microscope may be used for anastomosis of vessels. Appropriate instrumentation for microsurgery is made available.

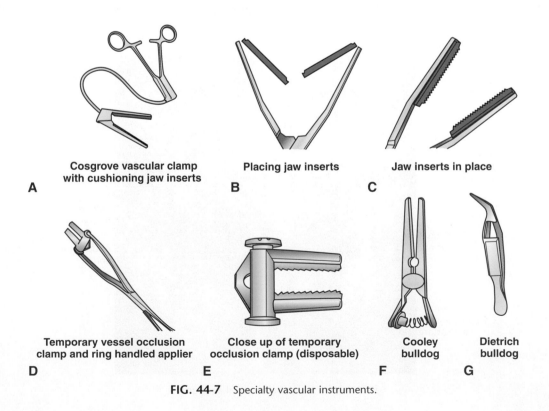

A Cosgrove vascular clamp with cushioning jaw inserts

B Placing jaw inserts

C Jaw inserts in place

D Temporary vessel occlusion clamp and ring handled applier

E Close up of temporary occlusion clamp (disposable)

F Cooley bulldog

G Dietrich bulldog

FIG. 44-7   Specialty vascular instruments.

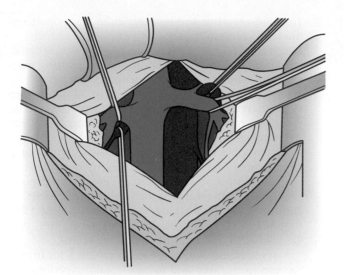

FIG. 44-8 Vessel loops in place for retraction of arteries and venous structures.

Synthetic nonabsorbable suture materials are preferred because they are strong and pass through vessel walls and grafts easily with minimal trauma and tissue reaction. Swaged needles also minimize trauma. A larger swaged suture-to-needle ratio is advantageous to avoid leakage. Holes made in graft materials by the needle are occluded by the larger suture. Double-armed needle sutures are often used for vessel anastomosis.

- Heparinized solution is available for use as an anticoagulant. Preoperatively, heparin (5000 units) may be given subcutaneously for DVT prophylaxis. Intraoperatively, the optimal dose is 70 to 100 units/kg of body weight if given intravenously for immediate systemic effect. Thromboelastography may be used intraoperatively to monitor the effects of heparin administration. Sensitivity to bovine sources of heparin can result in heparin-induced thrombocytopenia (HIT), also known as "white clot" syndrome. Clots composed of fibrin and platelets form after 4 to 15 days of heparin therapy. A severe decrease in the platelet count predisposes the patient to thrombosis and acute arterial occlusion.
- Before closure at the end of the procedure, protamine sulfate, a heparin antagonist, is given to reverse the anticoagulant effect; 1 mg of protamine is given to counteract 100 units of heparin. Protamine is derived from fish semen and testicular tissue and may elicit a sensitivity reaction in patients who are allergic to fish. Patients with type 1 diabetes who take NPH insulin also may be predisposed to a sensitivity reaction to protamine. Some men who have had a vasectomy may exhibit allergic or hypersensitivity reactions.
- Hemostatic agents can be used independently or in combination (Box 44-2). Care is taken not to permit hemostatic materials to be suctioned into the blood-salvage or cell-saving device. These products can be hazardous if permitted to enter the patient's vascular system. Thrombin should be carefully labeled to prevent accidental injection.

BOX 44-2 Hemostatic Agents Used in Vascular Surgery

- *Absorbable gelatin sponge (Gelfoam)* can be used dry or dipped in saline. According to the manufacturer, the patient may have an antigenic reaction when the sponge is soaked in thrombin. The sponge can be applied to the site and removed after 20 seconds or left in the wound; it is absorbed after 4 to 6 weeks. Because it may provide a favorable microbiologic growth medium, it is not used in the presence of infection. It is derived from porcine gelatin and has more of a mechanical than a chemical hemostatic property.
- *Absorbable collagen (Avitene, Hemopad, Helistat),* either in powder, foam, woven, or nonwoven form, induces platelet adhesion and results in the formation of fibrin. It provides both a chemical and a mechanical hemostasis. Because it may provide a favorable microbiologic growth medium, it is not used in the presence of infection. The long-term effects of an in situ collagen hemostat are unknown, but animal studies indicate that it absorbs. It is of bovine origin and can be moistened, but it works better when dry.
- *Oxidized cellulose (Surgicel, Oxycel)* is applied dry over a bleeding site for hemostasis. Although a single layer can be left in the wound and absorbed, it is preferred that a large wad be removed because it may interfere with healing or cause pressure. It chemically destroys thrombin and is not used concurrently with it. Because it may provide a favorable microbiologic growth medium, it is not used in the presence of infection. It has some bactericidal properties against gram-positive and gram-negative microorganisms. The mode of action is mechanical hemostasis when applied to an area of bleeding.
- Fibrin glue is applied by simultaneously placing a combination of cryoprecipitate, bovine thrombin, and/or calcium chloride on the bleeding tissue surface to form a fibrin patch.
- Topical thrombin should be available. Preparations from bovine origin are contraindicated in patients who are sensitive or allergic to these products.

- A vasodilator such as papaverine is used to relax the smooth muscle of the vessel. This prevents endothelial damage during intraluminal irrigation. Vasopressors should be available. Some surgeons use 1% lidocaine.
- Blood is lost by the flushing of clots and debris. Blood loss should be calculated, and blood should be available for replacement if the hematocrit level falls below 26%. During procedures on the great vessels, blood may be salvaged from the thoracic or abdominal cavity for autotransfusion. An autologous blood salvage machine (cell saver) may be used to collect the patient's own blood for autotransfusion. Care is taken not to aspirate hemostatic materials or other debris into the blood suction-salvage device.

Blood should be warmed before transfusion to help prevent inadvertent hypothermia. Consideration is given to the patient who does not want a blood transfusion. Patients undergoing nonemergent procedures should be given the option of donating autologous blood in advance of the procedure.

- For DVT prophylaxis, antiembolic stockings or sequential compression devices should be worn by the patient during and after the surgical procedure in addition to anticoagulant therapy.

• For vascular monitoring, Doppler ultrasound, pulse volume recorder, and/or intravascular imaging techniques are used intraoperatively to monitor hemodynamic changes and to assess blood flow after peripheral vascular reconstruction. A pulmonary artery catheter (Swan-Ganz) is usually inserted to monitor pulmonary artery pressures during and after the procedure.

The most serious immediate postoperative complications are thrombus and hemorrhage. The patient may need to return to the operating room (OR) for immediate correction of these problems. Long-term complications include infection and graft failure by occlusion.

Vascular Grafts

Biologic or synthetic prosthetic vascular grafts are required to bypass a vascular obstruction or to reconstruct vessels. These substitute conduits for blood flow vary in length, diameter, and configuration to meet the requirements of each situation. A graft may be straight or bifurcated into a Y shape. Pieces of biologic or synthetic material may be cut to size for use as patch grafts.

The American National Standards Institute (ANSI) has established requirements for product characteristics and the labeling of textile and nontextile synthetic grafts, vascular allografts, and vascular xenografts. Grafts sterilized in see-through containers or packages permit the surgeon to select the appropriate size after exposure of the surgical site. Manufacturers' instructions for use and handling are strictly followed.

Biologic Vascular Grafts. Autografts, allografts, and xenografts have been used for arterial or venous conduits, but autologous grafts have a higher success rate. Allografts and xenografts have a higher failure rate.

Arterial Conduit. Autologous arteries are procured for coronary artery bypass grafting. The radial, gastroepiploic, or internal mammary arteries are commonly used. Arterial grafts do not thrombose and occlude as readily as do venous grafts.

Venous Conduit. An autologous vein is a suitable graft conduit because it is lined with endothelial cells that inhibit clotting. These cells produce fibrinolytic substances and the plasminogen factor essential to maintain patency. The saphenous vein is commonly used for an autologous arterial bypass or vein graft. If the saphenous vein is not suitable, the basilic or cephalic veins of the arm are sometimes used. A vein graft is used as a conduit in one of three ways:

1. *In situ conduit/bypass.* To revascularize a lower extremity, the saphenous vein is exposed at the proximal and distal aspects but is left in place. The surgeon performs a venotomy at each end of the vein, inserts a valvulotome and/or a disposable valve cutter, and disrupts the internal valves. The occluded artery to be bypassed is ligated distally and proximally and then anastomosed proximally and distally to the saphenous vein. This technique reverses blood flow in the vein and reestablishes the flow of oxygenated blood beyond the level of arterial occlusion. Decreased manipulation and not excising the length of vein minimizes endothelial trauma and preserves antithrombogenic properties.

The vaso vasorum and neurovascular components of the vessel remain intact.

2. *Nonreversed vein graft.* Renal and mesenteric revascularization also can be accomplished by grafting nonreversed segments of the saphenous vein.

3. *Reversed vein graft.* When a segment of saphenous vein is harvested for placement in the arterial system, the vein is reversed from its normal anatomic position so the valves will not obstruct arterial blood flow. Intact valves are used to keep the blood flow unidirectional after anastomosis. Endothelial integrity is maintained by gentle dissection and handling. The surgeon exposes the surgical site while the first assistant, resident, or another surgeon, working at a separate sterile table supplied with fine vascular instruments, ties, and vascular clips, prepares the vein for grafting.

Magnification loupes are worn to check for imperfections in the vein and to tie off leaking perforators. The valves may be cut, especially in small-diameter segments. The vein is flushed with sterile, cold solution (commonly heparinized Plasma-Lyte with papaverine hydrochloride) and immersed in this solution until the recipient site is prepared.

Because the saphenous vein decreases in diameter as it courses distally, a size discrepancy may cause difficulty at the anastomosis attachment sites.

Synthetic Vascular Prostheses. Various forms of synthetic materials are used to construct arterial vascular prostheses. Certain materials are more suitable than others for specific applications. The surgeon selects the most appropriate graft for each patient. Rejection and tissue reaction are minimized if Dacron or Teflon is used.

Knitted Polyester. Knitted polyester (Dacron) grafts are porous enough to allow the ingrowth of fibrous tissue into the interstices. They also are porous enough to allow blood to seep through the material, and therefore they are preclotted before insertion. Preclotting causes the wall of the graft to become impervious to blood by filling the interstices with fibrin. For the preclotting process, the surgeon withdraws blood from the patient at the surgical site before anticoagulation therapy. The scrub person places the blood in a sterile basin containing the graft material. The blood saturates the lumen and all surfaces of the graft. The fabric-fibrin conduit later becomes firmly placed in tissue and provides a hypothrombogenic flow surface.

Filamentous Velour. Knitted velour construction of polyester grafts has uniform porosity for easy preclotting and ensures rapid tissue ingrowth. These types of grafts may be crimped or noncrimped, with velour inside and/or outside. One type, the exoskeleton (EXS) prosthesis, has a spiral polypropylene support fused to the outer surface of noncrimped velour. This graft was developed specifically for use across the knee joint. Another type, in which amikacin is bonded to knitted filamentous velour polyester with a bovine collagen matrix, provides an antibiotic in the prosthetic wall. This type of construction also renders the porous graft impervious to leaks, which eliminates the need for preclotting.

Bonded albumin also reduces porosity and potential thrombosis. Older-style porous grafts required bonding. This was achieved by "baking on" autologous plasma. A porous graft was soaked in the patient's plasma or in allogeneic albumin and was then steam sterilized. This thermal process altered the fibrin and protein elements in plasma.

Woven Polyester. The weave of woven polyester (Dacron) grafts is tight enough to be leakproof, and therefore these grafts do not require preclotting. However, the more inflexible construction limits their use to aortic replacement or for the bypass of large-caliber arteries.

Polytetrafluoroethylene. The microporous wall of polytetrafluoroethylene (PTFE) serves as a lattice framework into which cells grow to become a microthin lining for contact with blood. These prostheses (Gore-Tex, IMPRA) do not require preclotting. Vascular grafts that are constructed of expanded and reinforced PTFE maintain dimensional stability. Configuration may be straight, tapered, or bifurcated. It may be supported by external rings to resist compression.

During the surgical procedure, the inside lumen of the graft may be seeded with the patient's own endothelial cells to sustain patency. The graft may be bonded with an antibiotic before implantation to prevent infection.

Composite Vein Grafts. A composite graft of autogenous vein and synthetic, usually PTFE, may be the surgeon's choice as a substitute for an insufficient length of saphenous vein. The prosthetic graft is anastomosed to a segment of reversed or in situ autogenous vein. The prosthetic graft is cut to match the diameter of the vein.

CONSERVATIVE INTERVENTIONAL TECHNIQUES

Peripheral vascular disease is often managed by a team of collaborating vascular surgeons, cardiologists, and radiologists. Multifaceted care encompasses invasive interventional procedures to treat occlusive disease conservatively. Endovascular procedures are considered minimally invasive conservative management. Vascular instruments and supplies for an open surgical procedure should be immediately available in the event that a vessel is perforated or injured during any of the conservative interventional techniques. A perforation may be closed with sutures; a patch graft, in situ conduit, or synthetic prosthesis may be necessary.

Percutaneous Transluminal Angioplasty

Severe ischemia or incapacitating claudication resulting from localized or segmental stenosis or occlusive disease can be conservatively treated by recanalization to restore the lumen in the obstructed vessel. Atherosclerosis in the iliac, femoral, and popliteal arteries is the most common indication for percutaneous transluminal angioplasty (PTA). Stenosis in the renal arteries also can be treated.

PTA is performed under local anesthesia and fluoroscopy, often in the interventional radiology department by a radiologist, in the angiography or cardiac cath lab by a cardiologist, or in the OR by a surgeon. In the Seldinger technique, the artery is punctured percutaneously with a large-bore needle and a guidewire is introduced. A vessel dilator sheath is advanced over the guidewire into the vessel. The endovascular device is passed through the dilator sheath for the performance of several types of percutaneous procedures. Various techniques are used to dilate a stenotic lesion or to displace or ablate a plaque.

Balloon Angioplasty. A Gruentzig or other type of balloon dilation catheter is passed over the guidewire and positioned across the lesion. Catheters of several diameters with balloons of various widths and lengths are available. Determination of the appropriate balloon size and length is made on the basis of angiogram findings. When the balloon is inflated, atheromatous material is compressed against the arterial wall. It remolds and cracks, splitting the plaque and intima (inner lining) and stretching the media (middle layer) and adventitia (outer layer), thus dilating the lumen of a stenosis or recanalizing an occlusion. The balloon is repeatedly inflated and deflated until the lumen is dilated.

Intraluminal Stent. A prosthetic stent may be placed along the vessel wall to maintain patency after dilation. The Palmaz stent, for example, is a stainless steel mesh tube mounted coaxially on a balloon angioplasty catheter. After the stent is positioned in the artery, the balloon is inflated to expand the stent. The stent remains in place when the balloon is deflated and removed. Stents made of titanium, polypropylene, or other materials either operate in a similar manner or are self-expanding, such as the Gianturco stent (Fig. 44-9).

A specialized method of performing carotid stenting uses a cerebroprotective guidewire and netlike sheath to prevent migration of particulate to the brain (Fig. 44-10). The protective net is positioned before the stent is inserted and deployed.

Laser Angioplasty. With laser angioplasty, a laser fiber is introduced into an occluded artery to destroy plaque or thrombi. The laser usually is used to supplement balloon angioplasty. The procedure may be done percutaneously or as an open surgical procedure via an angioscope. Several different types of laser probes are available. The physician selects the most appropriate probe on the basis of the location and size of the artery and the determination of

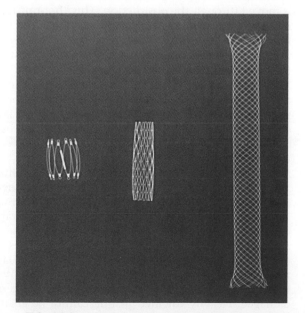

FIG. 44-9 Examples of intraluminal vascular stents.

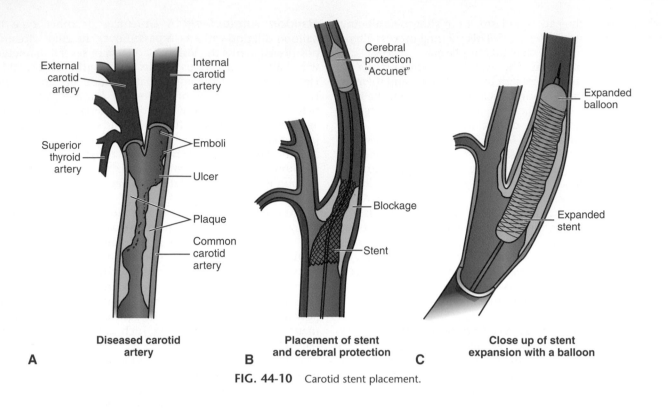

External carotid artery

Internal carotid artery

Superior thyroid artery

Emboli

Ulcer

Plaque

Common carotid artery

Diseased carotid artery

A

Cerebral protection "Accunet"

Blockage

Stent

Placement of stent and cerebral protection

B

Expanded balloon

Expanded stent

Close up of stent expansion with a balloon

C

FIG. 44-10   Carotid stent placement.

the degree of calcification in plaque or other cause of obstruction. The delivery system determines the mechanism of action:

- *Thermal laser.* A thermal laser uses argon or neodymium:yttrium aluminum garnet (Nd:YAG) laser energy to heat the tip of a metal probe at the end of a fiberoptic catheter to a temperature between 392° and 752° F (200° and 400° C). Plaque is vaporized as the tip is moved through the obstruction. This "hot-tip" technique may cause some damage to vessel walls. The laser fiber may be positioned within a balloon to destroy the thrombus selectively or to seal the arterial wall while the vessel is dilated. A temperature between 203° and 230° F (95° and 110° C) in the surrounding tissues dries and disintegrates the thrombus. The combination of pressure from the inflated balloon and diffuse laser energy adheres the loose flaps of arterial tissue back onto the arterial wall; this process is known as arterial welding.
- *Photothermal laser.* A photothermal laser uses contact Nd:YAG laser energy. A sapphire-tipped probe or catheter heats plaque by a photopic effect at the point of contact for vaporization of plaque. This is followed by rapid cooling to prevent damage to the intima.
- *Photochemical laser.* A photochemical laser uses an excimer laser with pulsed energy or a tunable dye laser to destroy plaque with minimal generation of heat. With the athermal action of a "cold laser," the intima is not damaged. Heavily calcified plaque cannot be ablated by an excimer laser.

Intravascular Ultrasonic Energy. An ultrasonic probe on the tip of a catheter can be used to recanalize occluded or stenosed peripheral vessels.

Atherectomy

In an atherectomy, catheter-mounted instruments are used for transluminal removal of atherosclerotic plaque. A high-speed rotating cam, burr, or side cutter is positioned under fluoroscopic guidance. The plaque is pulverized and retrieved to restore the patency of the vessel. These instruments may be used intraoperatively.

Thrombectomy and Embolectomy

For a thrombectomy and embolectomy, a local anesthetic is infiltrated percutaneously. A Fogarty catheter is inserted proximally and advanced into a vessel distally beyond the obstruction. The balloon on the tip is then inflated with heparinized sterile injectable saline. As the catheter is withdrawn, thrombotic or embolic material is removed to restore blood flow to an extremity. This procedure may be performed with fluoroscopy to selectively cannulate vessels. Different types and sizes of catheters and balloons may be used when the blockage is in a native vessel or an artificial graft (Fig. 44-11).

Thrombolytic Therapy

In thrombolytic therapy, streptokinase, urokinase, or tissue-type plasminogen activator (t-PA) may be administered by local bolus infusion into the occluded vessel or directly injected into the thrombus. These drugs activate plasminogen

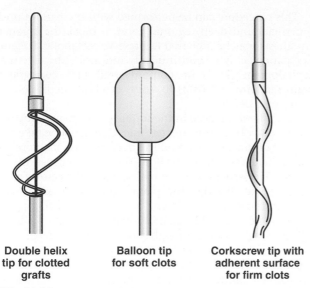

Double helix tip for clotted grafts   **Balloon tip for soft clots**   **Corkscrew tip with adherent surface for firm clots**

FIG. 44-11 Fogarty embolectomy catheter tips in closeup view.

and cause liquefaction of fibrin, thus dissolving the clot or loosening it for removal by balloon catheter. This therapy may be used in conjunction with angioplasty (thrombolysoangioplasty) or infused intraoperatively, especially in tibial vessels, for lower limb salvage.

Streptokinase. Treatment for DVT, pulmonary embolus, or another clotted vessel is facilitated by the use of streptokinase. Streptokinase is derived from a form of betahemolytic streptococci and has an indirect effect that breaks down fibrin. It may not be effective for patients who have antibodies against streptococcus infections. Clots more than 1 week old are not treated with this drug. The maximum effectiveness of this drug is evident within 10 minutes. Reversal of the anticoagulant effect can be accomplished by administering cryoprecipitate or fresh frozen plasma. Some patients will have a sensitivity reaction that can progress to anaphylaxis. Pretreatment with antihistamines and steroids may be indicated.

Urokinase. Urokinase is administered directly into the clot with a catheter in an interventional procedure room equipped with x-ray and fluoroscopy capabilities. Care is taken not to damage the endothelial lining of the vessel. Urokinase causes fewer sensitivity reactions than does strep-

tokinase, but it is expensive to produce. It is derived from fetal kidney cells and urine, and it is reconstituted with sterile water without a bacteriostatic agent.

Tissue-Type Plasminogen Activator. More recent advances in thrombolytic therapy include t-PA, a chemical that occurs naturally as a secretion of the endothelial cell lining of vessels. There is a risk of bleeding when t-PA is used.

VASCULAR SURGICAL PROCEDURES

If conservative therapy is unsuccessful or contraindicated, an open surgical procedure may be indicated.

Arterial Bypass

Occlusive disease or trauma may cause arterial blockage, or arterial injury may indirectly occur near the site of a fracture. The vessel lumen above and below the lesion is usually normal. Vascular reconstruction is performed in an attempt to restore normal circulation. The surgeon selects an appropriate method to bypass the obstruction:

- The involved segment may be excised and the ends anastomosed if they can be approximated without tension.
- If direct anastomosis is impossible, the involved segment is excised, and an autograft or synthetic prosthetic graft is used as a replacement.
- The lesion can be bypassed using the long saphenous vein from one thigh as a vein graft, or a synthetic prosthetic graft may be used. The ends of the graft are anastomosed to the artery proximal and distal to the lesion. The obstructed segment of the artery is not resected.
- The lesion can be bypassed by interposing a prosthetic graft through the subcutaneous tissues between a patent artery and the artery distal to the lesion; this procedure is known as an extra-anatomic bypass. For example, in a femoral-femoral bypass, the graft is placed from the femoral artery of the unaffected leg to the femoral artery of the ischemic leg. In an axillofemoral bypass, the graft is placed from the axillary artery to the femoral artery of the ischemic leg.

Femoropopliteal Bypass. The femoral artery is most prone to obstruction by occlusive vascular disease in a lower extremity. A femoropopliteal bypass, the most commonly performed bypass procedure in an extremity, may be the procedure of choice for severe ischemic disease and limb salvage (Fig. 44-12).

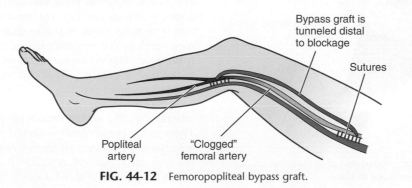

Bypass graft is tunneled distal to blockage

Sutures

Popliteal artery

"Clogged" femoral artery

FIG. 44-12 Femoropopliteal bypass graft.

The patient is placed in the supine position on the operating bed with the thigh of the affected leg slightly abducted and the knee flexed and supported. The entire extremity is prepped and draped to allow adequate exposure. Incisions are made over the femoral and popliteal arteries to expose them and explore the area before bypassing the obstruction in the femoral artery. An autogenous in situ saphenous vein graft, PTFE or noncrimped velour graft, or composite graft may be used. Anastomoses may be visualized with an angioscope. During the surgical procedure, pulsations of the proximal and distal popliteal artery, as well as pulsations in the foot, are checked with a sterile Doppler pulse detector.

Endarterectomy

Atherosclerotic plaque may cause localized stenosis in the major peripheral arteries. An endarterectomy involves the excision of the diseased endothelial lining of the artery and the occluding atheromatous deposits; this leaves a smooth lining (Fig. 44-13). Loosely attached plaque may be removed by dissection in the media with wire-loop strippers, spatulas, and/or catheters. A long-segment endarterectomy may be facilitated in the iliac, femoral, and popliteal arteries with a powered Hall oscillating endarterectomy valvulotome or other high-speed drill to pulverize plaque as described for atherectomy. A saphenous vein or patch graft may be used to close the arteriotomy site. Plaque also can be vaporized from femoral and carotid arteries with a laser. Subsequent inflammation and fibrosis are minimal, and healing is rapid.

Carotid Endarterectomy. One of the most common vascular procedures, a carotid endarterectomy, is performed to prevent a brain attack (stroke) in a patient with severe carotid artery insufficiency. Atherosclerotic plaque at the bifurcation of the common carotid and/or in the internal and external carotid arteries causes localized stenosis or ulceration that impedes cerebral blood flow. Endarterectomy is indicated when this stenosis causes TIAs.

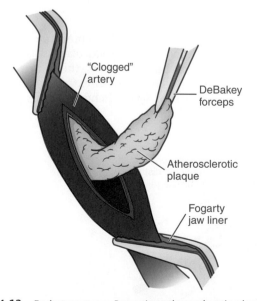

FIG. 44-13 Endarterectomy. Removing atherosclerotic plaque from an artery with Fogarty clamps in place.

This procedure can be performed with the patient under superficial and deep regional cervical block, or a general anesthesia may be preferred to preserve metabolic demands. The patient may be continuously monitored by electroencephalogram (EEG) or computerized EEG topographic brain mapping (CETBM) to assess cerebral circulation and neurologic deficits.

The patient is placed in the supine position, with the head turned away from the affected side. Care must be taken not to place undue extension on the neck because such pressure may occlude vertebral blood flow. The skin is prepped without causing excessive pressure or massage over the carotid artery, which could dislodge the plaque and cause an embolic event in the brain.

In the neck, an oblique incision approximately 4 inches (10 cm) long is carried through subcutaneous tissue, platysma muscle, and the anterior border of the sternocleidomastoid muscle. Retraction of the sternocleidomastoid muscle and jugular vein allows exposure of the common carotid artery and its branches. After systemic heparinization, special vascular instruments are used to clamp above and below the occluded area. In certain instances an intraluminal shunt is inserted in the artery to maintain blood flow to the brain while the plaque is removed. Many surgeons use a shunt routinely; others use an alternative means of cerebral protection, such as deliberate production of mild to moderate hypertension or hypercapnia. Cerebral protection during carotid cross-clamping is a primary concern to prevent serious neurologic complications.

An arteriotomy (incision in an artery) is made in the common carotid artery below the plaque and is extended upward; in the internal and external carotid arteries it begins above the plaque and extends downward. The plaque is dissected free and is removed in its entirety. In addition, most of the underlying media layer is removed. A headlight and magnifying loupes are worn by the surgeon to enhance visibility during dissection and closure of the arteriotomy. To check blood flow, a Doppler pulse detector is used after the artery is closed.

A PTFE or saphenous vein patch graft angioplasty or bypass grafting is occasionally necessary if an adequate lumen cannot be established. Bilateral endarterectomies may be indicated for severe bilateral occlusion, but the surgical procedures are performed at least a week apart.

Aneurysmectomy

An aneurysm is a localized abnormal dilation in an artery that results from the mechanical pressure of blood on a vessel wall that has been weakened by biochemical alterations. There are two types of aneurysms—pseudoaneurysms and true aneurysms. A pseudoaneurysm is usually caused by a break in the integrity of the vessel wall. The pressure from inside the vessel causes all of the layers of the vessel to separate and bulge. This can happen in any artery and requires an open repair.

A true aneurysm does not separate all the layers of the arterial wall. The aneurysmal bulge forms in the media layer. These can take two forms—saccular or fusiform. A fusiform aneurysm is a uniform circumferential dilation. Less common is a saccular aneurysm, a saclike outpouching in the media of the vessel wall (Fig. 44-14).

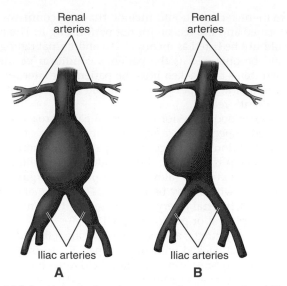

FIG. 44-14 Abdominal aortic aneurysm between renal and iliac arteries. **A,** Fusiform (circumferential) type. **B,** Saccular (saclike) type.

Cystic medial necrosis causes a dissecting aneurysm, usually in the thoracic aorta, in which the media separates from the intima (Fig. 44-15). A dissecting aneurysm can create a false passage for blood the full length of the aorta and cause damage to the vascular attachments of major organs such as the bowel and kidneys. Thoracic dissection requires a thoracotomy and replacement of the diseased portion of the aorta. Figure 44-16 depicts the repaired ascending and descending aorta using synthetic graft material.

Atherosclerosis is the most common cause of an aneurysm, but trauma may also be a factor. The abdominal aorta, thoracic aorta, aortic arch, and popliteal arteries are the vessels most often affected. Diagnostic evaluation combines a physical examination, laboratory findings, and the results of ultra-sonography, CT scan, MRI, and aortography and/or angiography. The location and extent of the lesion determine the operability of the aneurysm and the type of reconstruction. For example, cross-clamping of the descending thoracic aorta to remove an aneurysm will impair blood supply to the spinal cord. Repair in the arch or ascending aorta can impair cerebral and coronary perfusion. Blood flow through the visceral, mesenteric, and renal arteries may be affected by abdominal aortic aneurysmectomy or aortoiliac reconstruction. Vital structures must be protected during aneurysmectomy.

A ruptured aneurysm is a surgical emergency and precludes further evaluation. A transbrachial or transfemoral occluding balloon catheter may be placed in the aorta to prevent an exsanguinating hemorrhage. The surgical procedure is performed immediately.

Open Resection of an Abdominal Aortic Aneurysm.
An abdominal aortic aneurysm (AAA) usually develops between the renal and iliac arteries, although it can occur anywhere along its course. An abdominal aneurysmectomy may be a lifesaving procedure. Serious hazards, including massive hemorrhage, ischemic organs, and injury to ureters and other nearby structures, are associated with the procedure. Renal failure is a potential complication. Modern techniques have greatly reduced elective resection mortality to between 5% and 11%. Ruptured AAA has a mortality of 94%. Survivors of the procedure enjoy the same life expectancy as do other patients with comparable atherosclerotic disease. Early detection is the key. Resection at 4.5 to 5 cm is usually successful.

Constant monitoring of cardiac function with a Swan-Ganz pulmonary artery catheter is used in these high-risk patients. Patients whose condition is unstable may require

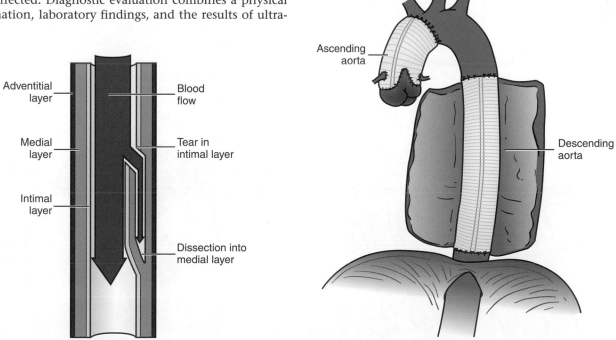

FIG. 44-15 Arterial dissection. The intimal layer tears, and a false passage develops and fills with blood.

FIG. 44-16 Graft examples for thoracic aorta. Thoracic ascending and thoracic descending repairs.

frequent blood gas determinations. Central venous pressure monitoring is a guide for regulating fluid replacement. Blood must be available for transfusion. Autotransfusion may be used if massive hemorrhage is encountered, such as with a ruptured aortic aneurysm. An indwelling Foley catheter is inserted preoperatively, and urinary output is monitored by the anesthesia provider. Mannitol can be infused before aortic cross-clamping to prevent ischemic renal failure. Prolonged cross-clamping can lead to spinal cord or bowel ischemia.

Somatosensory evoked potential (SSEP) monitoring measures primarily dorsal column (sensory) function and minimal anterior cord (motor) function. A time clock should be used to measure the amount of time the aorta is clamped.

Blood flow in the extremities should be checked immediately preoperatively and postoperatively to detect embolic or occlusive problems. Marking the location of the pedal and dorsalis pedis pulses with a marking pen enables rapid location of the appropriate site when they need to be checked intraoperatively. An audible Doppler device generally is used.

With an abdominal aneurysmectomy, a long midline incision from the xiphoid process to the pubis generally is used. The abdomen is thoroughly explored, the small intestinal mesentery is mobilized, and the posterior peritoneum overlying the aorta is incised to expose the aneurysm. A bed-mounted self-retaining abdominal wall retractor and blades helps provide needed exposure (Fig. 44-17).

The small intestine and ascending colon are delivered outside the abdomen to increase exposure and prevent injury. Warm moist tapes, radiopaque towels, plastic sheeting, or a Lahey (bowel) bag may be used to protect these structures. The incisions will extend into the anterior thighs for exploration of the femoral arteries.

Although the situation may be urgent or emergent, care is taken to account for plastic sheeting, towels, and other items used in the abdomen. If counts are aborted because of the patient's condition, documentation in the patient's permanent record should include that the count was not performed and the reason for not performing it. The count should not be listed as incorrect. An abdominal radiograph should be obtained as the patient's condition permits. If known items are packed into the patient for later removal the number and types of items should be documented on the patient's record.

An extended posterior retroperitoneal approach may be preferred, especially in a patient who is obese or has had previous abdominal surgery. The patient is placed in the right lateral position with the left side up. An oblique flank incision is extended along the superior margin of the twelfth rib, which may be resected. The entire abdominal aorta and left renal artery are exposed without needing to enter the pleural or peritoneal cavities.

The kidney, ureter, and peritoneal sac are reflected anteromedially and packed with moist tapes. Exposure is maintained with self-retaining and handheld retractors. If access to the iliac or femoral arteries is required, the patient's hips are rotated to a prone position, and longitudinal incisions are made in the bilateral groins (Fig. 44-18).

Before occlusion of the aorta, blood is withdrawn if needed for preclotting in the graft. Heparin is injected for anticoagulation. Aortic clamps are placed proximal to the aneurysm, and the iliac arteries are clamped distally. The distal aortic stump or iliac arteries may be closed with staples. If the aneurysmal wall is opened, clots and loose intraluminal debris are removed. A tube graft is used if the aneurysm is confined to the aorta. More commonly, a bifurcated graft is sutured in place above the aneurysm and to the common iliac or femoral arteries distally (Fig. 44-19). Branches of other arteries are anastomosed to the graft as necessary, depending on the segment of aorta being replaced. The graft is commonly placed inside the aneurysm (open inclusion method), and the sac is closed over the graft. With the less commonly used closed exclusion method, the graft is placed beside the unopened aneurysm sac.

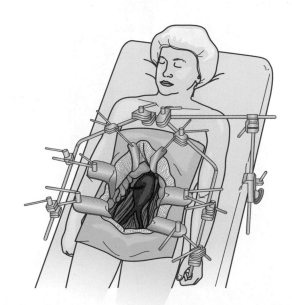

FIG. 44-17 Abdominal aorta exposure for resection.

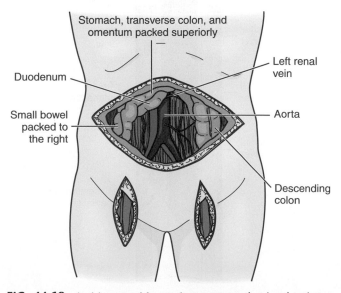

FIG. 44-18 Incisions used for aortic aneurysms that involve the femoral arteries.

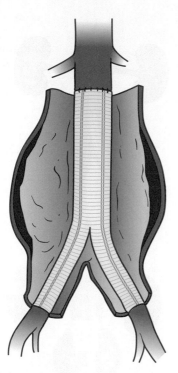

FIG. 44-19 Abdominal aortic graft example. The abdominal aorta and bilateral femoral arteries have been repaired with synthetic graft material.

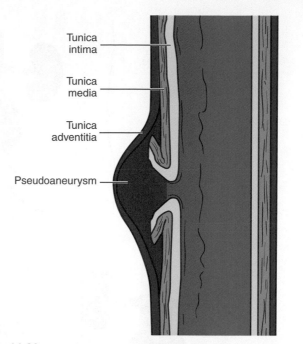

Tunica intima

Tunica media

Tunica adventitia

Pseudoaneurysm

FIG. 44-20 Pseudoaneurysm. The endothelial (tunica intima) and the muscular (tunica media) layers separate, causing a bulge in the outer connective tissue layer of the artery.

Living tissue, either the aneurysm sac or the mesentery, must cover the prosthesis to prevent contact of the prosthesis with the intestines; otherwise a fistula can develop. After the aortic clamps are released, the anastomoses are checked for leakage. The incision is usually closed with nonabsorbable sutures; retention sutures are commonly used for a long midline abdominal incision.

Pseudoaneurysm.

Injury to the arterial layers causes blood to accumulate in the local connective tissue surrounding the vessel, forming an enlarging bulge that can rupture and hemorrhage. Pseudoaneurysm, sometimes referred to as a false aneurysm commonly arises from an iatrogenic source such as arterial intravascular procedure like cardiac catheterization. The most common site is the femoral artery. Pseudoaneurysm differs from true aneurysm because it is caused by an outside source rather than vascular pathology (Fig. 44-20).

Repair of a pseudoaneurysm is performed in the OR and may require the use of a small patch of natural or synthetic graft. Some success has been achieved with localized thrombin injection under ultrasound guidance. Complications include embolization and compression of nerves and tissues in the area.

Endovascular Repair of Abdominal Aortic Aneurysm.

Endovascular AAA repair has the same indications as an open repair. The risk of rupture increases as the diameter of the aneurysm expands, especially if the diameter exceeds 0.5 cm per year. Not all AAAs can be repaired via the endovascular route. Anatomic criteria include having an adequate length of aorta between the renal arteries, the iliac arteries,

and the aneurysmal bulge. The anatomic diameter of the aorta cannot exceed 28 mm, or the graft will not work.

Endovascular grafts can be modular or one piece with limbs that extend into the iliac arteries (Fig. 44-21). The procedure is done by performing bilateral femoral cutdowns and placing guidewires cephalad through the aorta through the femoral artery on the ipsilateral (closest) side.

Aortograms are performed using full-strength contrast medium and a power injector. For a modular aortic stent, the first limb and body of the graft are placed up the guidewire using C-arm guidance and deployed into position. It is pulled caudad into position in the ipsilateral iliac artery and expanded with a balloon filled with half-strength contrast medium to seat the anchors. The second limb is introduced via the contralateral femoral artery and deployed. A unibody design with both limbs attached is positioned in the same manner; however, both distal limbs are seated into the iliac arteries at the same time and expanded.

Advantages of endovascular repair include smaller incisions, less blood loss, and shorter hospital stay. Disadvantages include the possibility of converting to an open method if a complication arises, lack of long-term evaluation of the procedure in humans, endo leak, embolism, and renal artery occlusion.

Standby instrumentation for an open procedure is a must. Blood salvage devices should be used. Doppler and warming devices should be employed as needed throughout the procedure. The team should exercise all precautions for blood and radiation exposure.

Embolectomy

An embolus is a mass of undissolved matter carried by the bloodstream until it lodges in a blood vessel and occludes it. An embolus may be an air bubble, a fat globule, clump

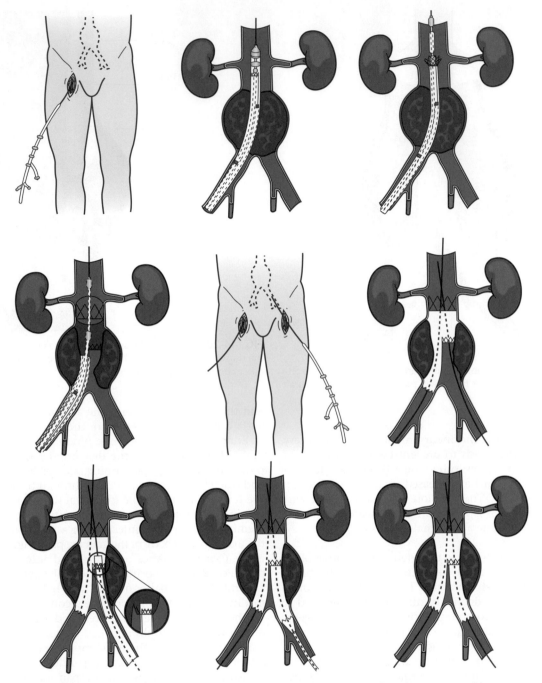

FIG. 44-21   Endovascular repair (ipsilateral and contralateral) of abdominal aortic aneurysm with a modular endograft.

of bacteria, piece of tissue, or foreign body. The occlusion of a blood vessel by an embolus causes various symptoms depending on the size and location of the occluded vessel. The occlusion of a vessel in the brain, lungs, or heart can cause rapid and sudden death.

Surgical intervention is the primary treatment for an embolus unless contraindicated. Select patients may be treated with heparin, vasodilators, and, perhaps, sympathetic blocks. Renal or mesenteric emboli are usually treated by embolectomy or bypass grafting. With an embolectomy, the affected blood vessel is incised and the embolus is removed.

Pulmonary Embolus. The occlusion of a pulmonary artery or one of its branches usually occurs with emboli that originate from veins in the lower extremities or pelvis. Emboli pass up the inferior vena cava to the right side of the heart and are ejected from the right ventricle into the pulmonary artery. A pulmonary embolism may be diagnosed by lung scans, pulmonary angiograms, and phlebograms.

Pulmonary Embolectomy. A massive pulmonary embolism can cause irreversible cardiac arrest or profound refractory hypotension and hypoxemia. If portable cardiopulmonary bypass equipment is available, cannulas can be inserted at the patient's bedside or in the emergency department or intensive care unit. The patient is then transported to the OR. A median sternotomy is performed to establish total cardiopulmonary bypass and to allow access to the pulmonary artery. Pulmonary emboli are removed by manual extraction; by the passage of forceps into both the right and left pulmonary arteries; by the passage of balloon catheters into pulmonary arterial segments; and by squeezing both lungs to force peripheral thrombi through a pulmonary arteriotomy. The incision can be extended for vena caval ligation to prevent recurrent embolization.

Pulmonary Thromboendarterectomy. Chronic pulmonary thromboembolic disease may develop from failure to resolve a massive pulmonary embolus, from repeated embolic episodes, or from a combination of both. The removal of obstructions in the main pulmonary arteries by thromboendarterectomy improves hemodynamics. The procedure is performed with the patient under induced hypothermia and cardiopulmonary bypass; thrombi are removed from the upper, middle, and lower branches of the right pulmonary artery and then from the left pulmonary artery.

Vena Cava Filter. Venous stasis in the deep veins of the lower extremities and pelvis can cause clotting and the potential for embolization via the vena cava through the right atrium to the lungs. Patient conditions that require prophy-

lactic protection from venous embolization are described in Box 44-3. A specialized endovascular filter can be placed via the right jugular or femoral vein under fluoroscopic visualization into the vena cava to prevent emboli from traveling to the lungs (Fig. 44-22). The filter is seated above or below the renal arteries depending on the location of the venous thrombus. The ideal filter should have the following characteristics:
- Low cost
- Lifetime of device is not time limited

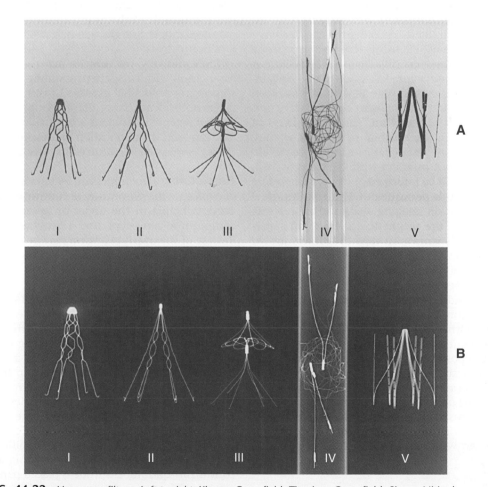

FIG. 44-22 Vena cava filters. *Left to right:* Kimray-Greenfield, Titanium Greenfield, Simon-Nitinol, Gianturco-Bird's Nest, Vena Tech. **A,** Actual filters. **B,** Radiographic images.

- High filtration without flow interruption
- Low access site thrombosis
- Small caliber percutaneous insertion and deployment devices
- Repositioned or removed easily
- Secure fixation to vessel wall
- MRI friendly

Vena cava filters are classified as permanent or temporary. Permanent titanium filters are designed to endothelialize to the vessel wall in as soon as 12 days. A clot that is ensnared in the filter eventually dissolves. The Greenfield filter is a permanent implant that traps and holds clots of 3 mm or larger. If preferred, it can be placed through the femoral vein over a guidewire to the level of L2-3.

The permanent Mobin-Uddin umbrella filter or Greenfield filter is a cone-shaped titanium filter that measures 4.6 cm from apex to base and is ejected and fixed in position below the renal veins and above the point of juncture of the iliac veins. Hooklike prongs anchor the device in the correct orientation to collect clots.

Angiography may be performed during the vena cava filter placement procedure, and the appropriate contrast medium should be readily available. For a high-risk patient, a filter may be placed at the completion of a diagnostic angiogram. A patient with an enlarged, dilated caval lumen 0.3 mm in diameter caused by right heart failure may require placement of a filter in each iliac artery.

The Filcard or Amplatz temporary vena cava filter can be repositioned or removed. Bard has designed the Recovery Filter, which can be removed using the Recovery Cone system for retrieval of the vena cava device.[1] The Gunther Tulip vena cava filter manufactured by Cook allows percutaneous insertion and retrieval from 10 to 14 days after insertion and may be useful for either permanent or temporary prophylaxis against pulmonary embolism. Temporary filters can be placed either through the brachial or femoral arteries. Prolonged placement may result in unsuccessful retrieval.

Titanium filters do not interfere with CT scans or MRI, but the radiologist should be informed of its presence before any imaging procedure is performed. Older stainless steel models cause distortion on imaging scans and are not safe during MRI because of the magnetic qualities and superheating of the metal. Patients with vena cava filters should be instructed to carry wallet cards with the make and model of filter implanted. Following filter placement the patient usually begins anticoagulant therapy.

Complications include lower extremity edema, which may indicate an obstruction in the filter that requires prompt medical attention. Other potential complications include premature deployment of the device or migration. If the device cannot be repositioned by endovascular methods, an open surgical procedure may be performed.

If a vena cava filter cannot be placed, the blood flow within the vena cava may be partially interrupted or plicated with specialized Moretz clips using an open abdominal retroperitoneal approach. This allows blood to return to the right ventricle of the heart without passage of the emboli to the lungs.

[1]www.bardpv.com.

Venous Stasis Disease

When the valves of the veins fail to function normally, increased back pressure of blood causes the veins to become dilated, tortuous, or elongated. These are known as varicose veins. Pain and secondary complications, such as thrombophlebitis and venous stasis ulcers, may follow. It is believed there is a familial tendency toward varicosities caused by incompetent valves, which afflicts both males and females. Habitual long periods of standing, repeated pregnancies, and obesity are other predisposing factors.

A procedure may be performed to bypass a venous obstruction, such as iliac-venous occlusion or femoropopliteal occlusion. Venous valve repair (valvuloplasty) or venous valve transposition may be performed to correct femoral valvular incompetence and severe venous stasis and to salvage the saphenous vein. The perforator or superficial femoral veins may be ligated for severe venous stasis with marked fibrosis and ulcerations. Injection-compression sclerotherapy to treat varicose veins may be preferred to surgical treatment.

Ligation and Stripping of Varicose Veins. For ligation and stripping of varicose veins in a leg, the saphenous vein is excised in toto with the aid of a semiflexible stripping device; this procedure begins at the ankle. Additional incisions are made along the course of the vein to ligate perforator branches as the stripper is moved upward toward the groin. Perforators and branches are occluded with ligating clips and transected. At the groin, an incision is made over the palpated stripper, and the vein is ligated at the saphenofemoral junction.

Preoperatively, the surgeon may mark areas of varicosity for incision with the patient standing at the bedside. Some surgeons use indelible markers During the skin prep, care is taken not to wash away the markings and not to massage areas of potential thrombus accumulation. After closure of the incisions and the application of dressings, the full length of the leg is wrapped in cotton elastic bandages for compression.

Fasciotomy. Decompression by fasciotomy is the treatment of choice for the prevention of compartment syndrome after acute ischemia in the upper or lower extremity. Vascular compromise can occur after a penetrating or crush injury. Release of the overlying fascia may be indicated for clinical evidence of increased pressure, such as pain, edema, pallor, and diminished sensation.

Epidural Spinal Electrical Stimulation. Epidural spinal electrical stimulation (ESES) may be used to improve nutritional blood flow in patients with severe lower limb ischemia. This can lead to the healing of ischemic ulcers. ESES uses a microscope connected to a television camera, television monitor, and video recorder. Intravital capillary microscopy is performed before and after ESES to measure red blood cell velocity in skin capillaries. With the patient in a sitting position, the dorsum of the foot is placed over the microscope. Fluorescein dye is injected intravenously, and the time for perfusion of the capillaries is measured. With the patient under local anesthesia and radiographic control, an epidural electrode is placed parallel to the spinal column. After stimulation of the electrode, perfusion in the foot is tested again.

Vascular Shunts

Normal circulation can be altered to increase or decrease blood flow to a specific organ, either temporarily or permanently. A vascular anastomosis or prosthetic device may be used to establish a route for the diversion of blood flow. For example, vascular isolation of the liver can be achieved with an atrial caval shunt. This shunt permits continuous venous return to the ventricle to sustain cardiac output during the repair of traumatized suprahepatic or retrohepatic vena cava and/or hepatic veins. A straight tube or inflatable balloon catheter may be inserted to establish the shunt.

Portosystemic Shunts. A shunt between the portal and systemic venous systems is definitive treatment for esophageal varices complicated by portal hypertension. This surgical procedure may be only palliative. Many patients have progressive liver disease that eventually leads to liver failure. Shunting does not repair an already damaged liver but can prevent further hemorrhage. Portal hypertension is an increase in portal venous pressure and is caused by the obstruction to intrahepatic blood flow as a result of cirrhosis, hepatitis, or thrombosis. The increased pressure thus produced results in venous dilation that causes varices. The patient also may have ascites. The purpose of the surgical procedure is to reduce portal hypertension and/or portal venous blood flow. The surgeon selects the most appropriate type of shunt to achieve the purpose.

Distal Splenorenal Shunt. Known as the Warren shunt, this procedure involves anastomosis between the splenic vein and the left renal vein. The hilum of the spleen and the tail of the pancreas are exposed through a left subcostal incision. The splenic vein is completely dissected from the pancreas to its bifurcation at the splenic hilum. This technical maneuver preserves portal profusion but eliminates collateral circulation to control bleeding from gastric and esophageal varices by decompression. The splenoportal system must be patent, and there must be adequate distance between the splenic and renal veins for the anastomosis.

An autogenous jugular or external iliac vein graft may be interposed to ensure a tension-free splenorenal anastomosis. A splenectomy may be performed. Other modifications may be made to meet specific patient circumstances.

Mesocaval Shunt. A mesocaval shunt is an option if a splenic vein is too small for a successful splenorenal shunt. A superior mesenteric inferior vena caval shunt is well tolerated by young patients. With a mesocaval shunt, the side of the superior mesenteric vein may be anastomosed to the proximal end of the divided inferior vena cava. An interposition autologous vein or synthetic H-graft may also be used to create a shunt between the inferior vena cava and the superior mesenteric vein.

Portacaval Shunt. A portacaval shunt may be performed with end-to-side or side-to-side anastomosis between the portal vein and inferior vena cava or with an interposition H-graft inserted between the portal vein and inferior vena cava. A ringed PTFE graft may be used, or an autologous graft may be obtained from an internal jugular or saphenous vein. The shunt relieves hypertension by bypassing the obstruction and diverting the return flow of blood to the liver from the portal vein, thus decompressing esophageal varices.

Depending on the type of portosystemic shunt planned by the surgeon, either a subcostal or a transabdominal incision may be used. Two suction setups should be available to evacuate the copious amounts of ascitic fluid that can be anticipated when the peritoneum is opened. Both abdominal and vascular setups are prepared. Pressure within the portal vein is measured with a manometer, via a cannulated branch of the superior mesenteric vein, at the beginning and at the conclusion of the surgical procedure. Because of venous distention and the vascularity of the surgical area, hemorrhage is a major intraoperative hazard. Care is taken to avoid injury to adjacent structures, including the hepatic artery and the common bile duct.

Arteriovenous Shunts and Fistulas. With arteriovenous shunts and fistulas, blood flow from an artery to a vein is established directly and without going through the capillary network. Access to the vascular system through an arteriovenous shunt or fistula is necessary for a patient who is suffering from end-stage renal disease and who is being maintained on long-term chronic hemodialysis.

With the patient under local anesthesia, the endogenous Cimino-Brescia arteriovenous fistula is established internally at the wrist by anastomosis between the radial artery and cephalic vein (Fig. 44-23). This method has the longest functional life of dialysis methods with fewer infections and thrombotic events. This method takes 3 to 4 months to mature before the fistula can be used for dialysis. Creation of a fistula is contraindicated in diabetic patients and patients with peripheral vascular disease.

If the vessels of the wrist and arm are inadequate, a synthetic PTFE graft may be interposed between the artery and vein (Fig. 44-24). A loop fistula may be created with a graft from the brachial artery to the cephalic or basilic vein in the antecubital fossa or from the brachial artery to the axillary vein in the upper arm. A graft access must mature for 3 to 6 weeks before use. The incidence of thrombosis is high.

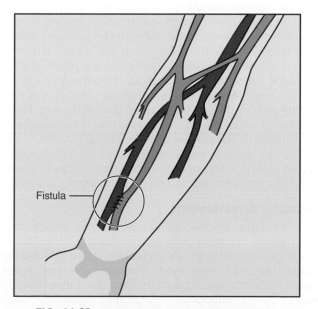

FIG. 44-23   Internal arteriovenous dialysis fistula.

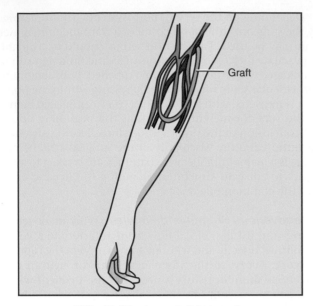

FIG. 44-24 Internal dialysis graft.

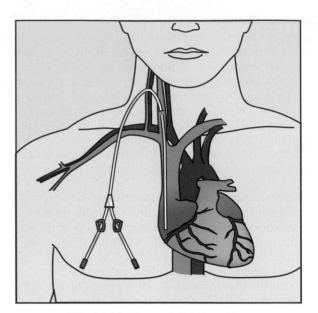

FIG. 44-25 External dialysis catheter.

Enzymatically treated bovine carotid artery xenografts are used occasionally to create arteriovenous shunts or fistulas. Thrombosis and infection are the most common complications. Using a Fogarty balloon catheter, a thrombectomy may reestablish patency. Total explantation of the graft is necessary in the event of a generalized infection.

An external double-lumen dialysis catheter with inflow and outflow tubing that is inserted in the jugular vein to the right atrium can be used for hemodialysis (Fig. 44-25). This type of access is easily inserted and can be used immediately after placement. There is no pain associated with connecting as with percutaneous puncture to access a subcutaneous graft or fistula. Care is taken because these catheters are easily infected and thrombosed. The average usefulness of a catheter is 3 to 6 months. They can be replaced quickly when a problem occurs.

A hemodialysis double–port valve system can be implanted in the anterior chest with two catheters into the right jugular vein to the right atrium (Fig. 44-26). If the right jugular cannot be used, the catheters are passed through the right subclavian vein instead. Placement of the port valves should be planned for patient comfort and tissue stability at 10 or 15 mm below the surface of the skin. Pockets are created under the skin in an area that is not compressed by clothing or shoulder straps of handbags.

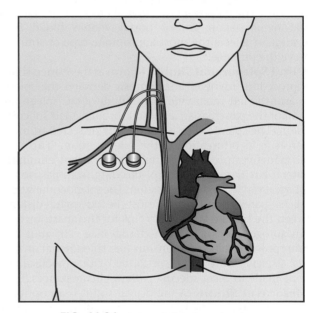

FIG. 44-26 Internal dialysis port system.

The exit valve is place laterally and the return valve is placed medially. Standardized placement helps to prevent errors during cannulation of the valves during dialysis.

Vascular Anastomosis

The operating microscope is needed for microvascular anastomosis of small vessels to revascularize tissue. Patency of the anastomosis depends on factors related to blood flow, coagulation, and vessel spasm. The vessels must be approximated without trapping adventitia in the lumen. Collagen fibers, tissue thromboplastin, and other thrombogenic factors in the adventitia predispose the patient to rapid platelet aggregation that may cause thrombus formation. Interrupted sutures are placed through the full thickness of the vessel wall (i.e., adventitia, media, and intima).

Veins are technically more difficult to anastomose than are arteries, because their walls are thinner and have less substantial muscularis. Anastomoses may be end-to-end or side-to-side. An interpositional vein graft may be needed to add length or to bridge a gap between the ends of either an artery or a vein. A patent artery should pulsate distal to the anastomosis. Although this procedure is used most commonly for tissue transplantation (e.g., vascularized free flaps or replants such as severed digits), the peripheral vascular surgeon may be needed to assist with vascular problems that require microvascular techniques.

Laser-assisted vascular anastomosis, also referred to as vascular tissue welding, fuses medium-size (6 to 8 mm) vessels together to form an anastomosis. The adventitial surface is less thrombogenic than it is after suturing and heals faster with less scar tissue. The argon laser is used for this technique. It may be used to create an arteriovenous shunt at the wrist for hemodialysis, to reattach severed limbs, and to repair damaged vessels.

Limb Salvage

Amputation of a lower extremity may be required for peripheral vascular disease or for lymphedema with lymphangitis. All efforts are made to salvage the limb; amputation is the last resort. Ischemia can cause debilitating pain, skin ulcers, and gangrene, often secondary to smoking or diabetes. Revascularization by the techniques described in this chapter may save the patient from the emotional trauma of amputation. This is a prime objective of the peripheral vascular surgeon.

Bibliography

Allen KB et al: Risk factors for leg wound complications following endoscopic versus traditional saphenous vein harvesting, *Heart Surg Forum* 3(4):325-330, 2000.

Binkert CA et al: Inferior vena cava filter removal after 317-day implantation, *J Vasc Interventional Radiol* 16(3):395-398, 2005.

Chaturvedi S et al: Carotid stent thrombosis: Report of 2 fatal cases, *Stroke* 32(11):2700-2702, 2001.

Dalrymple-Hay MJ et al: Endoscopic vein harvesting with the aid of carbon dioxide insufflation, *Ann Thorac Surg* 71(2):739-741, 2001.

Eggebrecht H et al: Endovascular stent-graft treatment of penetrating aortic ulcer: Results over a median follow-up of 27 months, *Am Heart J* 151(2):530-536, 2006.

Froeschl M et al: Ruptured mycotic pseudoaneurysm of the thoracic aorta, *Cardiovasc Pathol* 15(2):116-118, 2006.

Futterman LG, Lemberg L: A silent killer—Often preventable, *Am J Crit Care* 13(5):431-436, 2004.

Grande WJ et al: Experience with the recovery filter as a retrievable inferior vena cava filter, *J Vasc Interventional Radiol* 16(9):1189-1193, 2005.

Keeling WB et al: Current indications for preoperative inferior vena cava filter insertion in patients undergoing surgery for morbid obesity, *Obesity Surg* 15(7):1009-1012, 2005.

Lewis ME et al: Surgical repair of ruptured thoracic and thoracoabdominal aortic aneurysms, *Br J Surg* 89(4):442-445, 2002.

Mattson MP et al: Folic acid and homocystine in age-related disease, *Ageing Res Rev* 1(1):95-111, 2002.

Medina CR et al: Endovascular treatment of an abdominal aortic pseudoaneurysm as a late complication of inferior vena cava filter placement, *J Vasc Surg* 43(6):1278-1282, 2006.

Michota FA: Venous thromboembolism prophylaxis in medical patients, *Curr Opin Cardiol* 19(6):570-574, 2004.

Middleton WD et al: Diagnosis and treatment of iatrogenic femoral artery pseudoaneurysms, *Ultrasound Quart* 21(1):3-17, 2005.

Roddy SP et al: Composite sequential arterial reconstruction for limb salvage, *J Vasc Surg* 36(2):325-329, 2002.

Salameh JR et al: Carotid endarterectomy in elderly patients: Low complication rate with overnight stay, *Arch Surg* 137(11):1284-1287, 2002.

Singh H et al: Mycotic aneurysm of left anterior descending artery after sirolimus-eluting stent implantation: A case report, *Cathet Cardiovasc Interv* 65(2):282-285, 2005.

Swaminathan TN et al: Numerical analysis of the hemodynamics and embolus capture of a Greenfield vena cava filter, *J Biomech Eng* 128(3):360-370, 2006.

Chapter 45

Organ Procurement and Transplantation

CHAPTER OBJECTIVES

After studying this chapter, the learner will be able to:
- List the criteria for validating brain death.
- Describe the testing performed on tissue before it is suitable for transplantation.
- Discuss the role of the host procurement facility.
- Discuss the psychologic effect of a transplant on the donor and recipient families.

CHAPTER OUTLINE

KEY TERMS AND DEFINITIONS

Apnea   The absence of breathing.
Benching   The sterile process of preparing an organ or tissue for transport to a receiving facility for transplant.
Benching table   A sterile field established away from the primary sterile field for the preparation of an organ or tissue for transplant.
Brain death   No brain function, no reflexes.
Donor   Person who gives an organ or tissue to another person.
Procurement   The process of removing organ(s) from a donor.
Recipient   The person who receives tissue or an organ from another person.
Transplant   The process of taking tissue or an organ from one person and surgically placing it into another person.

HISTORICAL BACKGROUND

The interest in transplantation is many centuries old. Celsus wrote that tissues could survive after grafting from one part of the body to another. Galen attempted to reconstruct facial defects. Centuries later it was observed that full-thickness autografts survived and allografts failed, although the reason for the difference was not understood.

Darwin's theory of evolution and Mendel's laws of heredity shed new light in the nineteenth century, spurring researchers to pursue the study of regenerative capacity in animals. In the early twentieth century, Alexis Carrel and Charles Guthrie performed blood vessel anastomosis, an essential component of organ transplantation. Performing heterotopic heart transplantations in animals, they demonstrated that a heart could be removed, transplanted, and resume beating.

Attempts at kidney transplantation were made in France using animal donors. Although the kidneys made urine, the recipient died within 2 weeks of the procedure. In the 1930s the maintenance of organs in vitro opened the way to organ preservation. The first human-to-human kidney transplant took place in 1933, but the donor and recipient were mismatched blood types. The transplant failed. During the 1940s, expanded information concerning a patient's response to a surgical procedure marked advances in surgical therapy.

Open heart surgery, as well as acquisition of the basic knowledge required for clinical transplantation, evolved in the 1950s. As pioneers in transplantation biology, British immunologist Peter Medawar (1915-1987) and Australian pathologist Sir Frank Macfarlane Burnet (1899-1985) received the Nobel Prize in 1960 for their work on immunologic tolerance of tissue transplantation in animals. Medawar's research identified many factors associated with fetal-maternal immunology.

Many scientific disciplines contribute to and integrate information to aid the progress of clinical transplantation. Foremost among these areas are physiology, genetics, immunology, and pathology. The practical application of clinical transplantation became possible in the 1960s after investigative efforts led to the development of supportive techniques such as cardiopulmonary bypass and immunosuppressive drug therapy.

Kidney transplantation preceded heart transplantation by more than a decade. The first successful kidney transplant was between identical twins in 1954 by Boston surgeon Joseph Murray. Immunosuppression was not used. The first successful heart transplant, performed in 1967 by Christiaan Barnard (1922-2001) in South Africa, expanded the era of clinical organ transplantation. The first human heart recipient lived for 18 days but died from pneumonia as a result of immunosuppressive drugs. American surgeon Thomas Starzl performed the first liver transplant in 1967.

In 1998 the first successful single hand transplant was performed in France by Jean-Michel Dubernard. The patient did not follow through with the prescribed immuno-suppression regimen and subsequently had the hand removed in 2001. Since then, several other countries have trans-planted hands, unilateral and bilateral, with significant success.

In 2000 Malaysian hand surgeon V. Pathmanathan transplanted the arm and hand between infant twin sisters. The donor twin died at birth and her arm was used to replace her sister's deformed arm. No immunosuppression was needed. In 2003, a double hand-forearm transplant was performed in Innsbruck, Austria by Hildegunde Piza. The 41-year-old patient had bilateral amputations caused by a railway accident that left him with 9-cm stumps below the elbow. This was the first limb transplant to involve the entire muscle mass and tendons of the replacement limb. The patient started physiotherapy within 2 weeks of the procedure and had satisfactory small muscle and finger motion within 1 year. Sensory function is improving and is projected to reach an excellent level.

Matt Scott celebrated the seventh anniversary of his single hand transplant at Jewish Hospital in Louisville, Kentucky, in 2006. His transplant is considered to be the first long-term successful cadaver hand transplant. He has enjoyed all of the activities of daily living such as performing multiple two-handed functions and lifting his children. More infor-mation is available at www.handtransplant.com.

Although survival rates vary, most body tissues and organs can be transplanted or grafted. The availability of donor organs remains a problem, although nationwide computerized statistics in 2001 indicate that the number of living related donors exceeds the number of postmortem donors.

TYPES OF TRANSPLANTS

Transplantation is the transfer of an organ or tissue from one person to another or from one body part to another. Concentrated efforts continue in search of compensation for or suitable replacements for deficient tissues and organs. The indication for organ transplantation is irreversible func-tional failure of the organ. The goals of transplantation include changing appearance, restoring function, and/or improving quality of life. (More information is available at www.unos.org and www.organdonor.gov.)

Certain tissues and whole organs can be transplanted and grafted to restore bodily function. The type of transplant selected depends on the purpose of the graft, anatomic function, and availability of the tissue or organ. The types of biologic transplants are listed in Box 45-1.

BOX 45-1   Types of Biologic Transplants

- *Allografts.* Tissue grafted between different or genetically dissimilar individuals of the same species.
- *Autografts.* Tissue grafted in the same person from one part of the body to another. The donor is also the recipient.
- *Bioengineered grafts.* Biologic tissue is combined with synthetic material for implantation.
- *Heterotopic transplant.* Transplant to an anatomically abnormal location in the host. Heterotopic grafts may function normally in the unnatural site.
- *Isografts.* Tissues grafted between genetically identical donor and recipient, as between identical twins.
- *Orthotopic transplant.* Transplant to an anatomically natural recipient site.
- *Xenografts.* Tissues grafted between two dissimilar species; may be used when allograft material is unavailable or a temporary replacement is necessary.

TISSUE TRANSPLANTATION

Some tissues can function normally even after being moved from one area of the body to another or after being obtained from a donor:

- Skin grafts provide a protective surface covering, initially acquiring then eventually losing vascular connection with the host.
- Corneal grafts replace nonfunctioning corneal tissue.
- Bone grafts afford temporary structural supports and a pattern for regrowth of the host's bone; the grafts are then resorbed.
- Ossicles and the tympanic membrane in the ear can be transplanted to restore bone-conduction hearing loss.
- Cartilage restores contour in a defect of cartilaginous facial structures.
- Blood vessel grafts bypass or replace diseased or obstructed segments of vessels.
- Bone marrow restores hematologic and immunologic functions.
- Heart valves replace stenosed or diseased valves.

Tissue transplants can be either autografts or allografts. Xenograft transplants are in the research phases. The American Association of Tissue Banks sets standards for retrieving, processing, storing, and labeling tissues and for donor criteria for allografts (Box 45-2). Tissue for transplantation is procured from suitable cadaver (nonliving) donors, either heartbeating or nonheartbeating, or from a living donor. Table 45-1 details the procurement parameters for tissue allografts. (Additional information is available from the National Institute of Transplantation at www.transplantation.com or the United Network for Organ Sharing at www.unos.org.)

Potential donors are screened to avoid the transmission of infection or disease. Cultures are taken at the time of procurement for microbiologic and serologic testing. Tissue is not transplanted until negative test results are obtained; tissue is discarded if the test result is positive. Living bone donors are tested for human immunodeficiency virus (HIV) immediately after donation and again after 90 days, because seroconversion can be delayed. Recipients also should be tested and should be negative for HIV and hepatitis B virus

BOX 45-2	Donor Selection Criteria for Tissue Allografts

- Negative for viral, bacterial, or fungal infection or disease
- Negative for sexually transmitted disease
- Negative for neurologic disease
- Negative for autoimmune disease
- Negative for metabolic bone disease
- Negative for malignancy or suspected malignant neoplasm
- Negative for disease of unknown origin
- Negative for death of unknown origin
- Negative for use of systemic medication
- Negative for parenteral drug use
- Negative for exposure to toxic substances
- Not ventilator dependent for more than 7 days before brain death
- Not immobile or bedfast for more than 7 days before brain death
- Normothermic 98.6° F (37° C) for more than 7 days before brain death

(HBV). A baseline is essential to establish that the patient was not infected by the act of grafting. Patients with HIV or HBV are not barred from receiving an allograft, but baseline data can help rule out causes for rejection or infection. Incidences of graft failure and superinfection are high in immunocompromised patients with HIV.

Banked tissues are labeled with the donor's name and/or identification number, pertinent medical history, the pathology report of the donor, final culture and serology reports of donors, type and site of donation, date and time of procurement, and method of procurement and preservation.

Bone Marrow Transplantation

Bone marrow transplantation is essentially a tissue transplant. However, because this type of transplantation is fraught with the hazards of rejection, bone marrow is procured and transplanted using a protocol similar to that of organ procurement and transplantation. Bone marrow is transplanted only after conventional treatments have failed to replenish depleted bone marrow cells. The marrow given by infusion

TABLE 45-1	Tissue/Allograft Procurement Parameters		
Age of Donor	Physiologic Status of Donor	Time between Procurement and Grafting	Other Considerations
CORNEA Both sexes: 3 months-80 years	Nonheartbeating cadaver donor	Procured 6-8 hours postmortem at room temperature	Corneas are not perfused tissue. Heartbeating status is unimportant. Tissue may be procured in morgue or setting other than operating room (OR), under sterile conditions.
		Procured 48 hours postmortem if donor has been refrigerated at 39.2° F (4° C)	Corneas are usually used fresh rather than in cryopreserved state.
		Transplanted fresh 7-10 days after procurement	Corneal tissue is not commonly cryopreserved.
		Cryopreserved cornea may be stored for 1 year	
SKIN Both sexes: 14-75 years	Nonheartbeating cadaver donor	Procured 6-8 hours postmortem at room temperature	At least 75% of skin surface should be free of abrasions, scars, or deformities to qualify as donor.
		Procured within 24 hours postmortem if refrigerated at 39.2° F (4° C)	Skin is procured before bone and is taken only from below nipples to knees on ventral surface, and from scapulae to popliteal area on dorsal surface. Tissue is taken to the depth of dermal layer (split thickness). A 70-kg donor can provide 7-8 square feet of skin.
		Cryopreserved skin can be stored for 5 years at −238° F (−150° C)	Newly procured skin is stored at 39.2° F (4° C) in preservation medium for a maximum of 24 hours. Cryopreserved skin is thawed at room temperature not to exceed 59° F (15° C) for use on recipient. Allograft skin is commonly used as a biologic dressing in combination with autograft skin. The recipient autograft is meshed 6:1 and then covered by allograft that has been meshed 2:1. Allograft skin is temporary and is replaced on the recipient every 48-72 hours until natural reepithelialization at the autograft site begins.

TABLE 45-1	Tissue/Allograft Procurement Parameters—cont'd		
Age of Donor	**Physiologic Status of Donor**	**Time between Procurement and Grafting**	**Other Considerations**
ILIAC CREST			
Female: 18-50 years	Nonheartbeating cadaver donor	Procured within 12 hours postmortem at room temperature	Bone is procured after the recovery of any other internal organs and skin. Preferably, bone is procured under sterile conditions; however, it may be procured under clean conditions in a setting such as the morgue and secondarily sterilized by ethylene oxide followed by aeration. Sterile bone can be freeze-dried and stored at room temperature.
Male: 18-70 years		Procured within 24 hours postmortem if refrigerated at 39.2° F (4° C) Cryopreserved bone can be stored for 3 years at –112° F (–80° C)	
JOINTS AND LONG BONE			
Female: 18-50 years	Nonheartbeating cadaver donor	Procured within 12 hours postmortem at room temperature	Bone is procured after the recovery of any other internal organs and skin. Preferably, bone is procured under sterile conditions; however, it may be procured under clean conditions in a setting such as the morgue and secondarily sterilized by ethylene oxide followed by aeration. Sterile bone can be freeze-dried and stored at room temperature.
Male: 18-50 years		Procured within 24 hours postmortem if refrigerated at 39.2° F (4° C) Cryopreserved bone can be stored for 3 years at –112° F (–80° C)	Joints are not used as joints per se but are cut into pieces to fit a defect.
Both sexes: femoral head not age dependent; usually acceptable to age 75	Living nonrelated donor (femoral head or rib)		Living nonrelated donor femoral head can be salvaged during total joint arthroplasty procedure and processed for use as bone plug or ground bone grafting tissue.
HEART VALVES			
Female: 0-40 years Male: 0-35 years	Nonheartbeating cadaver donor	Cryopreserved valves can be used within 1-2 years	Size match is important.

restores hematologic and immunologic functions. Indications for treatment are acute lymphoblastic leukemia, myelogenous leukemia, aplastic anemia, and certain other blood diseases.

Bone marrow transplantation is the only cure for severe combined immunodeficiency disease—a genetic disorder in which a child lacks adequate immune defenses to fight infections. Bone marrow transplants also are given to victims of severe radiation exposure. Contraindications to transplantation are renal or cardiac disease.

With bone marrow transplantation, blood type and human leukocyte antigen (HLA) compatibility are essential. A bone marrow transplant may be one of three types:

1. *Autologous.* The donor is the recipient. Stem cells are collected from the leukemic patient in remission, cryopreserved, and stored to be infused during a subsequent relapse.
2. *Allogeneic.* The donor is HLA-compatible with the recipient. Marrow is harvested for immediate infusion into the recipient.
   a. A syngeneic donor, an identical twin, is preferred.
   b. A genotypically compatible sibling or parent has identical tissue type.
   c. An unrelated allogeneic donor must be HLA-compatible. Graft-versus-host disease (GVHD) is unique to allogeneic bone marrow transplantation.

With GVHD, donor T cells immunologically attach to recipient cells, causing tissue damage at the site of antigen localization.

3. *T cell–depleted marrow.* To prevent GVHD, mature T lymphocytes are removed from donor marrow before infusion into the recipient.

Before transplantation, the recipient is given a high-dose regimen of immunosuppressive chemotherapy to eradicate leukemic, lymphoid, and bone marrow cells, thereby inducing marrow depression. The recipient also receives total body irradiation (TBI) to penetrate the areas resistant to the drugs. During this period of pretransplant preparation, the patient is placed in reverse isolation, preferably in a laminar airflow clean or sterile (germ-free) environment. The patient is closely monitored for the side effects of immunosuppressive chemotherapy and TBI.

After pretransplant protocols have been completed, the donor is hospitalized before the scheduled transplantation. In the operating room (OR), with the patient under general or spinal anesthesia, 500 to 700 mL of bone marrow is aspirated at multiple sites from the iliac crests; the sternum may also be used. The marrow is filtered, heparinized, and placed in sterile containers for infusion. The donor is watched for bleeding and may need blood and fluid replacement.

Marrow is infused into the recipient intravenously or via a Hickman or Broviac catheter over several hours. During this time the patient is constantly attended and closely monitored for adverse reactions. By an unknown process, the marrow migrates into the marrow cavities of the bones. For 10 to 30 days after transplantation, the recipient may receive daily transfusions of lymphocytes, platelets, and granulocytes, preferably taken from the donor, to counteract the predictable side effects of pretransplant immunosuppressive therapy (mainly hemorrhage and infection).

If the marrow is not from an identical twin, blood is irradiated before transfusion to destroy the lymphocytes. Mature blood cells and platelets are unaffected by the irradiation process. Daily marrow aspirations and complete blood counts are performed on the host. The success or failure of transplantation is usually decided after 10 to 20 days, when the new marrow begins to function.

ORGAN TRANSPLANTATION

Organ transplantation can be a lifesaving treatment for some end-stage diseases. Although tissue grafts are commonplace, transplantation of functional, whole, vital organs presents physiologic, philosophic, and ethical dilemmas. A biologically related donor (referred to as a living related donor) makes a supreme sacrifice to become an organ donor; therefore, cadavers are the primary source of organs for transplant. Organ donation is the ultimate gift of life and is given by the donor to the recipient. Transplantation can restore the recipient to near-normal physiologic status.

Kidney transplantation was initially the most successful and principal clinical application of organ transplantation. If a kidney graft fails, the patient may survive by returning to hemodialysis indefinitely before receiving another transplant. This option does not exist for transplants of the heart, liver, pancreas, or the lungs. No practical prolonged artificial support exists for these organs in the event of an allograft failure.

Transplantation of each organ involves unique technical and physiologic problems, but the major barriers and causes of transplant failure are immunologic rejection and infection. Immunodeficiency depends on the amount of immunosuppression the patient receives to prevent rejection. Immunosuppressive agents leave the patient prone to opportunistic infection. Reverse protective isolation may be advisable if the patient develops leukopenia, a decrease in white blood cells. In other aspects of care, transplant recipients are similar to other critical surgical patients with severe chronic illnesses who require measures that minimize the risk of infection.

The American Society of Transplant Surgeons (www.asts.org) and the International Society of Transplantation meet regularly to exchange ideas and information among people of different scientific backgrounds. The aim is to achieve the best possible patient survival rather than merely transplant survival.

The Organ Transplant Registry of the American College of Surgeons, in conjunction with the National Institutes of Health, collects data on transplantation procedures and approves and funds various registries. The Federal Organ Transplantation and Procurement Act of 1983 provided financial grants for the initial development of regional organ procurement centers and a transplant registry. A national taskforce has also been established to analyze medical, legal, ethical, economic, and social issues of concern in organ procurement and transplantation.

Organ banks collect organs and tissues from donors, exchange organs geographically, and register patients in need of a transplant. The register includes information about the patient's blood grouping and tissue typing. Computer lists of patients waiting for donor organs are maintained by the United Network for Organ Sharing (UNOS) and the North American Transplant Coordinator Organization 24-Hour Alert. Regional organ procurement organizations coordinate with these registries to match donated organs with compatible recipients nationwide. The position of the recipient on the waiting list is determined by the severity of the illness.

Other countries have similar mechanisms. For example, the United Kingdom (UK) Transplant Register has membership in the Euro Transplant Register. Organs procured within the UK can be transported by air to another country in Europe, and vice versa, for a histocompatible recipient. The number of patients awaiting transplants exceeds the supply of available donor organs. As a result, many patients die while waiting for a suitable organ to become available.

Many people carry a signed Uniform Donor Card or other identification (e.g., the reverse side of a driver's license) that states that certain or all organs and tissues may be removed for transplantation in the event of death. Such cards or a living will constitutes legal written consent under the Uniform Anatomical Gift Act enacted by all 50 states. Written or telephone consent is still obtained from the family of a potential donor before procurement may commence.

Federal and state laws mandate required-request or routine-inquiry. These laws require that the family of every medically suitable potential donor be asked to consider the donation of organs and tissues. As a result of these laws, organs and tissues are procured in many hospitals and are then transported to organ banks or transplantation centers.

Procurement teams from these centers may go to the community hospital (host facility) to procure organs and tissues.

Time is paramount when critical organs are involved because their value depends on preserving maximum functional viability. The time factor is less urgent with less critical tissue. When a potential donor has been identified, a transplantation coordinator contacts the regional registry and procurement team(s).

Organ Procurement

Immunologic rejection and the shortage of donor organs remain the principal deterrents to transplantation. The goal is selection of a donor-recipient match with adequate histocompatibility to permit an organ to function without complications. Organs and tissues come from two primary sources: cadaver (heartbeating and nonheartbeating) and living related donors (Table 45-2).

Tissue donors may be between newborn and 80 years of age. All donors of vital organs must be free of sepsis or malignant processes, between newborn age and 65 years of age, and have good function of the donor organ(s). Technical aspects of the procurement procedure must ensure the viability of organs throughout the entire period between procurement and transplantation.

Cadaver Donor. Death is confirmed by irreversible cessation of all functions of the brain and brainstem. The criteria for brain death are listed in Table 45-3. To be suitable for organ or tissue donation after death, cadaver donors are classified as either heartbeating or nonheartbeating.

Heartbeating donors are those with confirmed brain death in whom the vital organs can be preserved in vivo. In these donors, brain death usually has resulted from severe neurologic trauma, such as from head or spinal cord injury, hemor-

TABLE 45-2	Organ Procurement Parameters		
Age of Donor	Physiologic Status of Donor	Time Between Procurement and Transplantation	Other Considerations
HEART			
Female: 0-40 years	Heartbeating cadaver donor	3-6 hours, fresh tissue	Heartbeating cadaver donor: total heart and segments of great vessels
Male: 0-35 years	Nonheartbeating cadaver donor	Cryopreserved valves can be used within 1-2 years	Nonheartbeating cadaver donor: heart valves only
			Size match is important
			Donor criteria include no cardiac disease and normal cardiac enzymes
LUNG			
Both sexes: 0-45 years	Heartbeating cadaver donor	1-4 hours	Heartbeating cadaver donor lung(s) may be given en bloc to one recipient The lungs may be separated and/or divided into segments (lobes) for several recipients
	Living related donor		One lobe from living related donor is transplanted into recipient
			Size match is important
			Donor criteria include no evidence of trauma, negative sputum culture, normal chest radiograph
HEART-LUNG EN BLOC			
Both sexes: 0-50 years	Heartbeating cadaver donor	1-4 hours	Heartbeating cadaver donor heart and lungs are transplanted en bloc into recipient
Younger ages preferred			Size match is important
			Donor criteria same as for individual heart or lung donation
LIVER			
Both sexes: 0-45 years	Heartbeating cadaver donor	8-24 hours	Heartbeating cadaver donor liver may be divided into two segments for two separate recipient patients
	Living related donor		Small segment of living related donor's liver is transplanted into recipient
			Size match is important
			Donor criteria include normal liver function, normal liver enzymes and bilirubin, no evidence of trauma

Continued

TABLE 45-2	Organ Procurement Parameters—cont'd		
Age of Donor	**Physiologic Status of Donor**	**Time Between Procurement and Transplantation**	**Other Considerations**
KIDNEY Both sexes: 6 months-60 years	Heartbeating cadaver donor	48-72 hours	Heartbeating and nonheartbeating cadaver donor kidneys are given to two separate recipients
		Ideally, should be transplanted within 12 hours	
	Nonheartbeating cadaver donor in highly selected circumstances	Procured within 45 minutes of cardiac arrest, with immediate in situ cooling	
	Living related donor		One kidney from living related donor is transplanted into recipient Donor criteria include normal renal function, normal serum creatinine, no evidence of trauma
PANCREAS Both sexes: 3 months-60 years	Heartbeating cadaver donor	12-24 hours	Heartbeating cadaver donor pancreas is transplanted as a whole or partial organ for one recipient
	Living related donor		Tail segment of pancreas from living related donor may be transplanted into recipient Donor criteria include normal pancreatic function, normal blood glucose regulation, normal serum amylase, no evidence of diabetes mellitus, no evidence of trauma
KIDNEY-PANCREAS Both sexes: 3 months-60 years	Heartbeating cadaver donor	12-24 hours	Heartbeating cadaver donor kidneys and pancreas are simultaneously transplanted into recipient; Usually performed for diabetic nephropathy Donor criteria are the same as for individual kidney or pancreas donation

TABLE 45-3	Brain Death Criteria
Criteria	**Clinical Assessment**
Irreversible coma not caused by pharmacologic agent, hypothermia, or unknown cause	No response to external stimuli No cerebral brain activity on electroencephalogram (EEG) over a period of 10 minutes EEG activity has no prognostic value for estimation of cerebellar and brainstem activity
Absence of spontaneous movement, decerebrate posturing, and decorticate posturing	Spinal nerve reflexes may be unaffected because these reflexes do not require cortical (brain) activity
Apnea with no spontaneous respiration not influenced by hypothermia or pharmacologic agent	Elevated carbon dioxide in the blood is not a stimulus for breathing No spontaneous respiratory effort for 3 minutes when removed from ventilatory assist device $Paco_2$ greater than 55
No cranial nerve reflexes	Fixed and dilated pupils Pupils are unreactive to light No corneal reflex (no blinking when cornea is touched) No oculocephalic reflex (doll's eyes) No oculovestibular reflex (no response to ice water instilled in ear) No response to pain on face and head (pin prick, supraorbital pressure) No response to upper or lower airway stimulation (no gag or cough reflex when suctioned or stimulated by endotracheal tube)

rhage, or anoxia. Death must occur in a location in which a cardiopulmonary support system is immediately available (i.e., in the emergency department, OR, or other critical care unit).

To be an organ donor, an individual who is brain dead is maintained on mechanical ventilation and/or cardiopulmonary bypass to prevent ischemic damage to the vital organs. Maintenance of a heartbeating donor before and during organ procurement includes the following:

- Systolic blood pressure above 90 mm Hg
- Central venous pressure of 5 to 10 mm Hg
- Hydration with crystalloids and colloids
- Urine output minimum 100 mL/hour (ideally 200 to 300 mL/hour)
- Ventilation with 100% oxygen
- Core body temperature of 98.6° F (37° C)

Nonheartbeating donors are not suitable for the procurement of parenchymal organs. With nonheartbeating donors, cardiopulmonary or ventilatory support was not provided after brain death. As a result, the major organs have suffered thrombosed vascular structures and ischemia. Skin, bone, heart valves, blood vessels, and corneas may be acceptable for procurement from select nonheartbeating donors (see Table 45-1).

Multiple Organ Procurement. The heartbeating donor is brought to the OR and treated with the same respect and care given to any other patient. A sample multiple organ procurement room setup is depicted in Figure 45-1. Organs and tissues are removed under sterile conditions by a procurement team and are preserved and transported to the recipient(s). The procurement team includes two surgeons, two assistants, and a scrub person. A circulating nurse and a scrub person from the host facility assist with the procedure. An anesthesia provider also is necessary to maintain vital functions until the aorta is cross-clamped and cardiopulmonary support is no longer needed. A procurement coordinator from an affiliated organ procurement agency or organ bank usually accompanies the team and assists wherever needed throughout the procurement process. The procurement team brings the necessary supplies for packaging the organ(s) and tissue(s) for transport.

The procurement process includes the following functions:

1. The procurement coordinator facilitates the procurement process by:
   a. Obtaining blood samples and arranging tissue typing to assist the organ bank with the potential placement of procured organs.
   b. Documenting necessary information, making any needed phone calls, and coordinating the host facility personnel with the procurement team.
   c. Assisting the physician with communications with the donor family.
   d. Calling the procurement team.
   e. Assisting the circulating nurse and scrub person with the setup of the procurement room.
   f. The coordinator will bring the necessary cannulas for the organ preservation.
2. The circulating nurse and scrub person assist in the procurement process by:
   a. Gathering sterile supplies that include the following:

1) Laparotomy drape pack and 10 extra medium drapes. Ten or more gowns and gloves will be needed.
2) Nonabsorbable sutures for ligating ties (usually 0, 2-0, 3-0, 4-0 silk) and for closure (usually a size 2 monofilament suture on a large cutting needle) as requested by the surgeon
3) 10 umbilical tapes at least 30 inches long
4) 4 Suction canisters and suction tubings with tips
5) 2 electrosurgical units, 2 dispersive electrodes, and handpieces with long and short blades
6) 12 scalpel blades, No. 10 and No. 15
7) 2 packs bone wax
8) 4 Asepto syringes
9) 20 packs of laparotomy sponges
10) 6 L cold normal saline solution for irrigation
11) Autosuture cart (GIA and TA30) for bowel or pancreas donors

b. Setting up sterile instrumentation that includes the following:
1) Chest tray with sternal saw and self-retaining chest retractor
2) Major abdominal laparotomy tray and large self-retaining abdominal retractor
3) Vascular tray
4) Minor tray for organ preparation table(s) (benching table)
5) Basin set for main table and each benching table

c. Providing nonsterile equipment that includes the following:
1) Two electrosurgical units and dispersive electrodes
2) Suction containers to accommodate at least 24 L of fluid
3) Power source for sternal saw
4) One IV pole for each benching table
5) Warming blanket under the patient
6) Defibrillator
7) Skin preparation solution
8) Isopropyl alcohol (70%) to make slush, or slush machine if available
9) Crushed ice; dry ice is not used for organ preservation
10) Head lights for primary surgeons

d. Medications and blood that will be needed:
1) Heparin 60,000 units
2) Furosemide (Lasix) 20 to 100 mg
3) 2 units of packed red blood cells (typed and crossmatched)

3. The anesthesia provider assists in the procurement process by:
   a. Ventilating the donor with 100% oxygen.
   b. Monitoring electrocardiogram (ECG), blood pressure, urinary output, and fluid and electrolyte balance.
   c. Administering drugs as necessary (e.g., dopamine or dobutamine for vasomotor regulation, muscle relaxants to neutralize spinal reflexes and relax the abdomen, osmotic diuretics for renal function, and heparin for anticoagulation).
   d. Monitoring and replacing blood as appropriate.

e. Monitoring and maintaining core body temperature and initiating cooling: cold fluids, usually Ringer's lactate or Collins' solution with 30,000 units of heparin, are infused intravascularly 10 minutes before the aorta and vena cava are cross-clamped for heart removal.

4. Incisions are made by the procurement surgeon(s) to provide maximum access to organs and tissues:

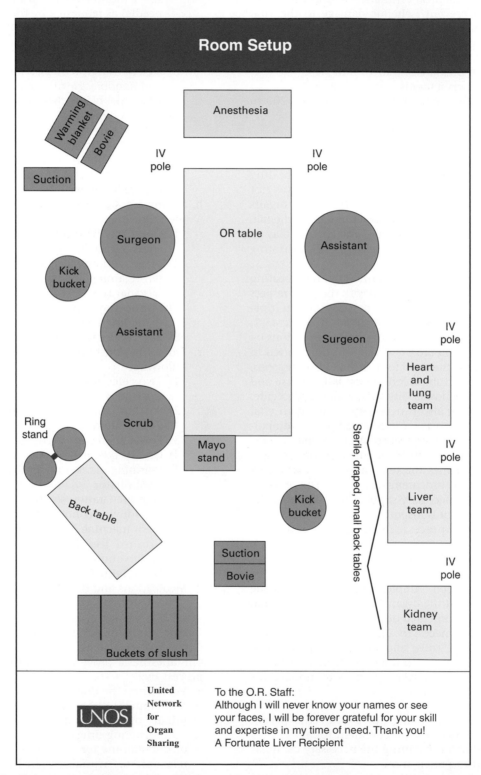

FIG. 45-1   Room setup for multiple organ procurement.
(From Seifert PC: Cardiac surgery: Perioperative patient care, St. Louis, 2002, Mosby. Courtesy of UNOS, United Network for Organ Sharing.)

Procedure: Organ Recovery—Single or Multi-Organ

Skin Prep: Solution varies according to surgeon preference. Prep from clavicle to mid-thigh.

Drapes: Laparotomy drapes are acceptable with a wider area of exposure. Free draping is also acceptable and may be preferred.

Position of Patient: Supine with arms out or tucked, depending on organs to be recovered and surgeon preference. Place warming blanket under patient or use a lower-body Bear Hugger.

Grounding pads, ECG electrodes, and other devices should be placed on the posterior side of the body away from the sterile field.

Suture and Needles Depends upon surgeon preference—<u>examples</u>		Instruments and Equipment Specific tray names will vary according to institution		
Ties:	0, 2-0, 3-0, and 4-0 silk ties* #1 and #4 silk ties*	Basic:	Skin prep tray* Gowns × 5-10* Electrocautery units × 2 Lap tapes* Blades - #10 × 3, #15 × 2, #11 × 2* Suction sets × 2-3 (for large fluid volumes) Suction tips × 2 ea. Yankaur, Poole or octopus Major laparotomy tray	Razors Towels × 5 Grounding pad × 2* Raytec sponges
Suture:	2-0 silk on cutting or taper needle* 4-0 & 5-0 prolene on taper needle* 1 or 2 nylon on cutting needle for closure*			
Other:	Ligaloops/endoloops, umbilical tapes* Vessel paws, bone wax*	Special:	Vascular tray Sternal saw Extra long balfour Vascular stapler (hold) Gallbladder dilators (hold)	Assorted vascular clamps Sternal retractor Mallet GIA, LDS (hold) Large basins × 2-3 (hold)
Hold:	Large and small hemaclips Skin stapler with rotating head			
Dressing:	Sterile 4x4s* Shroud kit*	Extras:	Sterile ice Defibrillator with sterile internal paddles available Headlight available Ice machine available or several bags of unsterile ice IV poles (one for each organ to be recovered)	Slush (or capabilities)**

* Some organ recovery agencies' customized packs will contain these items. Check with your recovery agency to prevent duplication.
** If no slush machine, contact your recovery agency for the formula for making slush. This procedure needs to be initiated at least one hour prior to the recovery case.

Visiting recovery teams may bring additional items, which you may need to autoclave.

FIG. 45-1—cont'd

a. A midline sternal-splitting incision is made from the suprasternal notch to the pubis to remove vital thoracic and abdominal organs (Fig. 45-2). It takes 2 to 3 hours to procure parenchymal organs.
b. Eyeballs are enucleated to procure the corneas. Glass or plastic globes may be put in the sockets to maintain the shape.
c. Skin is taken with a dermatome from flat body surfaces, excluding the upper chest, neck, face, arms, lower legs, and feet (Fig. 45-3). Skin procurement may take 1 to 1½ hours.
d. Skin is excised, and the muscles are separated. Long bones and iliac crests are removed in toto (Fig. 45-4) and are replaced with wooden, fiberglass, or metal dowels to maintain structural integrity. Bone procurement may take 5 to 6 hours to complete.
e. Multiple incisional closures may take 1 to 1½ hours.
5. The sequence of organ removal is coordinated to maintain the viability of the organs. Several small sterile tables should be set up so that organ and tissue packaging for transport can be completed away from the main sterile field. Minor dissection instrumentation may be needed for organ benching
a. Perfused tissues will be taken first.
  1) The kidneys and liver are mobilized and cannulated for in situ cooling.
  2) The aorta is cross-clamped, and the heart is removed first, followed by the liver and then the kidneys, pancreas, and intestines. Mesenteric nodes and the spleen are sampled for tissue typing.
  3) A combined heart-lung procurement may be performed after the other organs have been removed. A bronchoscopy may be necessary for assessment of the lungs. The lungs will be ventilated during the procurement process and a prostaglandin drip will be infused.

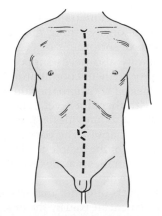

FIG. 45-2 Midline, sternal-splitting incision from suprasternal notch to pubis is made for procurement of thoracic and abdominal organs from heartbeating cadaver donor.

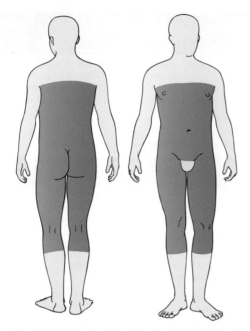

FIG. 45-3 For cadaveric allografts, skin is removed with dermatome from anterior and posterior flat surfaces between midchest and knees.

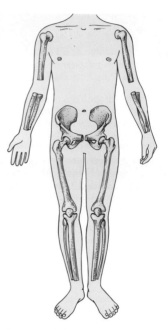

FIG. 45-4 Long bones and iliac crests are procured for bone allografts. Humerus, tibia, and fibula are cut distally. Radius, ulna, and femur are disarticulated at both ends. Pelvis is cut at pubic and sacroiliac joints.

b. Nonperfused tissues are taken last.
   1) Enucleation of the eyes for corneal procurement usually follows retrieval of the parenchymal organs. A certified eye bank technician may do the eye globe procurement.
   2) Skin is then taken, followed by vessels and bone.
6. Closure should be as aesthetic as possible for later viewing at funeral services. Most are done as single-layer closures. Prosthetic bone space-holders are placed. Ice packs are placed over eye sockets and the head of the bed is elevated to minimize fluid accumulation around the eye sockets.
7. The procurement coordinator will provide the necessary paperwork for the surgeons and team to use for documentation.

Additional Considerations in Cadaver Organ Procurement. The procurement coordinator remains at the host facility after the procurement team has departed. The coordinator's role extends into the aftercare given to the donor's body and the psychological support and debriefing of the OR team. After the closure and dressing of all incisional wounds, the donor's body should be bathed and all drainage tubes and IV access lines removed.

The body should be labeled with identification tags and placed on a clean transport cart. The head of the stretcher should be elevated 20 to 30 degrees. Ice packs should be placed over the eye sockets to decrease serous pooling. This will be of benefit to the mortician who prepares the body for viewing. The donor's body is prepared as aesthetically as possible for the benefit of the family and loved ones.

The OR team may experience a sense of sadness and loss. This is normal and to be expected. Death is not a common event in the OR. Although the patient is technically brain dead before arriving in the OR, he or she gives the outward appearance of being sustained on life support as in general anesthesia. After the aorta and vena cava are cross-clamped, ventilatory support is no longer needed and the anesthesia provider turns off the ventilator. The sudden silence can feel overwhelming.

The OR team may need the added support given by the procurement coordinator, who has experienced the same feelings and understands the psychologic impact of each stage of the procurement process. Personnel who specialize in procurement state that they feel the same sense of loss despite years of experience and exposure. An understanding of the outcome is important in the grieving process. Participation in the aftercare of the body helps provide the OR team with a sense of closure and completion of patient care. Some of the same sadness may be shared by the critical care nursing staff members who helped monitor and maintain the donor's vital signs before transfer to the OR. Although the urge to be emotionally strong may exist, it is therapeutic to shed tears of sorrow.

The donor's family also needs support and communication from the procurement coordinator. The coordinator makes himself or herself known to the family and maintains communication with them for several months or longer as needed; he or she also provides referrals for follow-up counseling if the need arises. The coordinator informs the family of the progress of the recipients. In select situations, donor and recipient families may be brought together, thus forming lasting friendships.

The financial aspects of donor maintenance and subsequent organ procurement are paid by the procurement agency and are not the responsibility of the donor's family. Medical bills accumulated before the patient was identified as a potential donor are paid by the donor's family.

Living Related Donor. There are distinct advantages to procuring a kidney, lobe of the liver or lung, tail segment of the pancreas, or marrow from a living related donor. The results are better than are those with nonbiologically related cadaver organs because donor-recipient matches are usually good (identical twin sources are ideal for compatibility). Waiting time is also reduced, and the procedure is planned and performed under controlled circumstances. The ethical concerns include the generalized risk of surgery to the donor.

The use of living donors involves a special protocol:

1. Adult donors, who are preferred over adolescents or children, must be able to give informed consent voluntarily and without coercion. Children are used as donors only for a twin or for a patient with predictable results. If the donor is a minor, court (legal) and parental or guardian consents are required to avoid bias. The donor must fully comprehend the sacrifice; if the physician deems it advisable, a psychiatric examination is included along with intelligence testing.
2. The donor must be in excellent health. The donor's physician confers with him or her and performs the preoperative physical examination to facilitate informed consent. Before a nephrectomy, renal arteriograms are performed to confirm the presence of bilateral kidneys and to identify the renal vasculature.
3. The donor should have no psychiatric complications. Donor reactive depression may follow organ removal if adequate gratitude is not shown by all concerned.

Preservation of Organ Allografts

The successful use of donor tissue depends on rapid organ resection and cooling because the period of ischemia must be kept to a minimum. Long-term preservation of tissue remains a problem; current techniques use a variety of cryoprotective agents. Uncontrolled freezing may produce lethal cell injury. Therefore this technique is used for skin, bone, semen, and blood suspensions but not for whole organs. Hypothermia above freezing at 39.2° F (4° C), with or without the perfusion with cold solutions, reduces general metabolic demands and thereby provides a safety margin. Methods of hypothermia include:

- Simple flush techniques with cold electrolyte solutions and storage by immersion in an electrolyte or flush-out solution in a plastic container that is kept at a hypothermic temperature
- Hypothermic continuous pulsatile perfusion with an oxygenated electrolyte solution

In 1987 potassium-based organ-preservation solutions were developed at the University of Wisconsin by Dr. Folkert Belzer (1930-1995). These solutions are known as UW (ViaSpan) and Belzer MPS solutions, and they extend the preservation time of the liver to 24 hours and of the kidney and pancreas to 72 hours. A total organ perfusion system (TOPS) consists of a machine that pumps an artificial blood substitute through the donor organ during transport. Minicomputers and microsensors regulate pH levels, blood pressure, and nutrient levels. The potential for altering the immunogenicity of an organ and improving its regenerative processes is the focus of research in perfusion techniques. (More information about organ preservation research at the University of Wisconsin is available at sapphire.surgery.wisc.edu/home.htm.)

The organ is placed in a sterile container filled with perfusate. This container is placed in sterile, double-plastic bags and packed in ice. Dry ice is not used. If the organ will be transported to another facility, a Styrofoam ice cooler generally is used as the outer container.

Immunologic Rejection

The body possesses an innate tendency to reject and destroy any foreign material except tissue from an identical twin. Therefore, transplanted cells from donors even slightly dissimilar to the recipient may be rejected.

Organ rejection involves the patient's immunologic system. Both the cellular and the humoral immune systems seem to be involved in the responses to transplanted cells. Activation of the immune system is a response to antigens introduced by the donor graft. An immunologic reaction usually is accompanied by a febrile systemic reaction, local inflammation, and deteriorating function of the graft. A knowledge of antigens, individual-specific and species-specific, and their genetic transmission is important for the avoidance of violent reactions. Many factors influence the strength and rate of a rejection reaction—acquired immunologic tolerance, lymphatic depression, or previous sensitization by blood transfusions, pregnancies, or transplants. Rejection may be reversible with intensive therapy, or it may be progressive and lead to the cessation of transplant function.

Combating Rejection. Attempts must be made to find compatible donors and to minimize rejection. T cells can be spun from donor vertebral marrow and transfused into the recipient to prevent or minimize rejection. This action primes the recipient's system for organ acceptance. The recipient's body can then recognize the transplanted organ as being familiar and thus minimize or prevent rejection.

Preoperative Matching of the Donor to the Recipient. Tissue typing and matching determine the genetic disparity between the donor and the recipient. Histocompatibility implies acceptability by one individual of tissue from another. Histocompatibility tests, although not infallible, assist in donor-recipient selection and result in improved organ survival from both living and cadaver sources. The better the histocompatibility match and degree of genetic similarity between the donor and the recipient, the less serious the rejection.

Histocompatibility testing, or tissue typing, is based on the detection of cell-surface antigens known to affect rejection. Favorable results are expected when few histocompatibility antigens are detected. Preformed antibodies appear to have a harmful effect on graft survival. Histocompatibility testing uses serologic methods that include cell culture techniques and in vitro analysis for the study of cell-to-cell interaction and identification of the mediator of the interaction. Complex assay techniques measure the effects of antibodies and lymphocytes against donor tissue in a culture setup. Cross-matching between the recipient's serum and the donor's peripheral blood target cells is accomplished by multiple serologic reagents or flow cytometry using fluorescent-labeled monoclonal antibodies.

Immunosuppressive Therapy in the Recipient. Specific alterations in immune responses are produced by inactivating or destroying lymphoid cells that are capable of responding to the antigens. The goal is to selectively suppress antigenic reactions to the transplant without impairing the body's defense against pathogenic organisms. To allow the transplant to remain and function, an attempt is made to neutralize or modify the body's protective antigenic mechanisms through the use of various immunosuppressive agents. This barrier can be pierced at least temporarily by creating an increase in transplant tolerance or by paralyzing the recipient's immunologic system. Because the lymphocytes and globulins seem to be mainly responsible for rejection, an attempt is made to vary their synthesis. Antibody formation and immune reaction can be suppressed by certain factors; the protocol for these methods is fairly standard in all transplantation centers.

1. Cyclosporine (Sandimmune), a soil fungus derivative, is a potent immunosuppressant that acts mainly on thymus-derived lymphocytes (T cells), the cells primarily responsible for rejection. This drug reduces rejection, especially in the early or inductive phase, without suppressing the entire immune system. It may be given orally or intravenously. It is always used with low doses of adrenal corticosteroids but usually not with other immunosuppressive agents. Its absorption rate is variable. The toxic effects on the kidneys must be monitored. Verapamil, a calcium channel blocker, may be given to reduce renal toxicity.
2. Immunosuppressive agents, such as FK-506 or 5R-506, may be preferred to cyclosporine to prevent rejection.
3. Monoclonal antilymphocyte globulin, muromonab-CD3 (Orthoclone OKT3), is derived from mouse antibodies and is used for the successful treatment of established allograft rejection without affecting the entire immune system. Monoclonal antibodies have the ability to reverse the initial episode of rejection by binding to specific targeted surface antigens on mature T cells. They suppress only the activity of T cells that cause acute rejection.
4. Polyclonal antilymphocyte globulin, antibodies derived from horse serum, may be used for the induction of immunosuppression or for the reversal of rejection. It usually is given with other immunosuppressive agents.
5. Corticosteroids, such as prednisone, have an antiinflammatory effect that is useful in reversing early rejection reactions. There is an inverse relationship between steroids and lymphocytes. T cells migrate from the circulation to lymphoid tissue.
6. Agents cytostatic or cytotoxic to lymphatic tissue, such as azathioprine (Imuran), suppress the entire immune system and have serious side effects on other systems. They also interfere with DNA synthesis. Extracorporeal perfusion with these drugs and localized radiation to the transplant may be used either separately or concurrently.
7. Heterologous horse or rabbit antithymocyte globulin or antilymphocytic globulin or serum acts against circulating T cells and induces suppressor cells.

The use of immunosuppressive measures is not without complications. Leukopenia and susceptibility to infection are common sequelae. Therapy may not totally abolish rejection by the host but may delay the onset and decrease the incidence of rejection episodes during the crucial first month or two after transplantation.

Pretransplantation Transfusions. Blood transfusions from a living related donor expose the recipient to a limited number of leukocyte antigens and seem to reduce the risk of sensitization to the prospective donor transplant and thereby increase graft survival. Different blood products, including platelets, and pharmacologic conditioning may be part of a pretransplantation transfusion protocol to induce specific immune modification in the recipient. Random preoperative blood transfusions before cadaver organ transplantation may increase the risk of sensitization but may improve allograft survival.

Kidney Transplantation

Kidney transplantation has significantly improved the quality of life for many patients with chronic renal disease. Patients may choose to accept transplantation rather than remain on hemodialysis for the rest of their lives. Indication for transplantation is end-stage renal disease, most often glomerulonephritis, pyelonephritis, polycystic disease, or nephrosclerosis. Recipients may be infants (at least 8 to 12 months with a body weight of 6 to 8 kg) to adults 70 years of age without severe extrarenal disease, malignancy, or active sepsis. Nephrectomy is not performed before transplantation unless the patient has uncontrollable hypertension. Patients with detected presensitization states may need to wait longer for a suitably matched cadaver donor; statistically, these patients have a lower 1-year graft survival rate than do unsensitized patients.

Recipients are carefully prepared preoperatively with kidney dialysis, regulation of fluid and electrolyte intake, pretransplantation transfusions, and control of hypertension. Proper donor-recipient matching is performed.

Donor preparation is equally important. The removal of a kidney is associated with low morbidity, but a living related donor must guard against injuring the remaining kidney for the rest of his or her life. The donor is therefore advised to avoid body-contact sports.

Transplantation Procedure. Unless a cadaver donor organ is used, two adjoining ORs and teams are used for the transplantation procedure. One team procures and preserves the donor kidney, and the other team prepares the recipient site and transplants the kidney.

Donor Nephrectomy. In a living related donor, the kidney is removed through a flank incision (Fig. 45-5). Adequate renal perfusion and urinary output, maintenance of adequate blood pressure and ureteral blood supply, and gentleness in manipulation are extremely important intraoperatively. As soon as the kidney is excised, it is flushed with cold heparinized solution to remove red blood cells. Total ischemia time is usually less than 1 hour. The donor's incision is closed per routine technique.

Recipient Procedure. The iliac fossa is the standard site for transplantation in an adult patient (Fig. 45-6). The hypogastric artery is anastomosed to the renal artery, and the common iliac vein is anastomosed to the renal vein (Fig. 45-7). Reconstruction of the urinary tract is the main technical problem. Ureteroneocystostomy, the implantation of a donor ureter into the bladder, is the preferred technique for urinary drainage. Alternative methods include ureteroureterostomy and ureteropyelostomy.

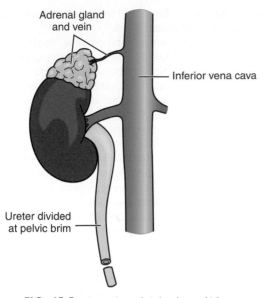

FIG. 45-5   Resection of right donor kidney.

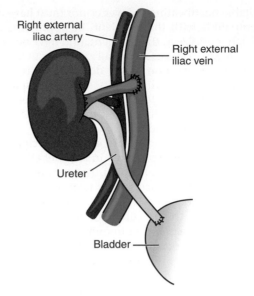

FIG. 45-7   Anastomosis of donor kidney to recipient site.

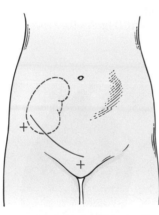

FIG. 45-6   Kidney transplant is placed in the iliac fossa through a lower oblique abdominal incision.

Complications of Renal Transplantation. The complications of renal transplantation may be renal related or extrarenal. The most common renal-related complications include rejection (the dominant cause of graft failure), recurrent nephritis, acute tubular necrosis, and technical failure from genitourinary or vascular problems. Postoperative management is similar to that of other surgical patients, with emphasis on the initial adequacy of renal function, prevention of the hazardous effects of immunosuppressive therapy, and observation for allograft rejection. The following are the possible types of rejection:

- *Hyperacute, caused by presensitization.* Hyperacute rejection is an immediate acute rejection that occurs right after the anastomosis of blood vessels or within 24 hours. It includes thrombosis and extensive destruction of allograft vasculature.
- *Accelerated, caused by presensitization.* With accelerated rejection, the graft may function for up to 5 days, after which there is a rapid loss of renal function. Treatment

for both hyperacute and accelerated rejection is immediate removal of the transplant.

- *Acute.* Acute rejection usually occurs 1 week to 4 months after transplantation and is often reversible unless the immune response is severe. Systemic and local symptoms, as well as reduced urinary output and abnormal laboratory findings, are present.
- *Chronic.* Antibodies developing long after transplantation produce an insidious onset with mild hypertension and diminishing renal function. This type of rejection is not reversible. Acute and chronic rejection may be diagnosed by renal biopsy.

Extrarenal complications are usually caused by immunosuppressive or corticosteroid therapy and include infection (the leading cause of death on a long-term basis), pneumonitis, hepatitis, gastrointestinal bleeding, and psychological problems from a perpetual fear of rejection. Immunosuppressive therapy must be used with caution.

The results of kidney transplantation are gratifying; life can be significantly prolonged. Causes for concern are chronic liver failure and vascular disease (which is a major cause of death in dialysis patients and may occur in a long-term transplant recipient). The incidence of malignant neoplasm in patients surviving renal transplantation more than 1 year exceeds that expected in the general population. (More information about kidney procurement and transplantation is available from the National Kidney Foundation at www.kidney.org.)

Heart Transplantation

Heart transplantation may be performed in select patients with end-stage cardiac disease such as irreversible extensive myocardial failure, widespread atherosclerotic deterioration, or ischemic disease with symptoms at rest. Transplant recipients usually are younger than 55 years and have a life expectancy of less than 1 year. Patients may be following a regimen of dopamine infusion while waiting for a suitable donor.

A suitable heartbeating cadaver donor must have a blood type compatible with the recipient, be approximately the same weight and size as the recipient, and have no evidence of cardiac disease. Donors are usually younger than 40 years.

Optimum preservation of the donor heart is crucial so that it can resume full activity after transplantation. Ischemia time must be less than 6 hours. After removal, the donor heart is rapidly cooled to 39.2° F (4° C) and is transported to the recipient.

The transplantation team prepares the recipient while the donor heart is being procured in another OR or is being transported from another hospital. The recipient is brought to the OR. When the procurement team has inspected the donor heart and deemed it suitable, the transplantation team is notified by the procurement coordinator. After the induction of anesthesia, a pulmonary artery catheter and transesophageal echocardiography (TEE) probe are placed. A median sternotomy is performed.

Most recipients have had previous sternotomies, and adhesions may be present. Careful dissection is necessary to avoid potential embolization from a dilated left ventricle. The myocardium is not manipulated until the aorta is cross-clamped, and the recipient's heart is not mobilized until the donor heart is ready for transplantation. The surgical procedure is similar to routine open heart procedures that use cardiopulmonary bypass. Two surgical modalities are used for cardiac transplantation:

1. *Orthotopic heart transplantation.* The ventricles, atrial appendages, and most of the coronary sinus are excised from the donor heart. The opened atria, aorta, and pulmonary artery of the recipient heart are anastomosed to the donor heart. The sinoatrial nodes of both the donor and the recipient are left intact (Fig. 45-8). Spontaneous nerve regeneration is more likely to occur in younger patients who receive a younger donor organ. Studies have shown that 21% of heart recipients have some sympathetic nerve generation at the ventricular level. The amount of nerve regeneration improves exercise tolerance in the patient.

2. *Heterotopic transplantation.* The donor heart is inserted in an abnormal position in the right side of the chest as an assist device to enhance cardiac function. The recipient's heart is not removed. This less desirable alternative procedure may be indicated when increased pulmonary vascular resistance is a result of left ventricular failure in the recipient's heart. The donor's right atrium is anastomosed to the recipient's right atrium. Anastomoses are completed between the aorta and pulmonary veins of the donor to the left atrium of the recipient (Fig. 45-9).

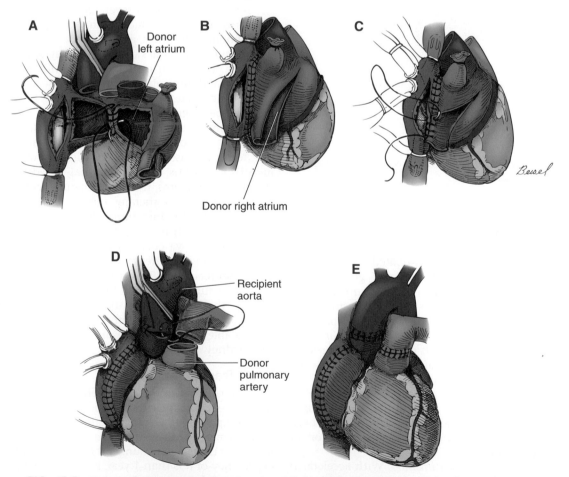

FIG. 45-8   Orthotopic cardiac transplantation. **A** and **B,** Anastomosis of the left atrial wall. **C,** Right atrial anastomosis. **D,** Aortic anastomosis. **E,** The pulmonary artery has been attached.

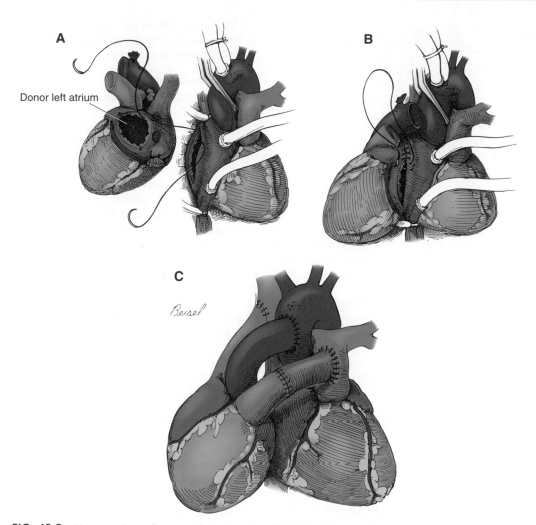

Donor left atrium

FIG. 45-9   Heterotopic cardiac transplantation. **A** and **B,** Left atrial anastomosis. **C,** A remnant of the donor superior vena cava (SVC) is anastomosed to the side of the recipient SVC. The donor ascending aorta and pulmonary artery are anastomosed end-to-side to their respective counterparts. A graft may be interposed between donor and recipient pulmonary arteries to provide additional length.

Most deaths occur in the first 2 postoperative months—the crucial period of immunologic rejection. Electrocardiogram changes such as a drop in voltage, reduced cardiac output, arteritis, myocardial ischemia, and myocardial necrosis occur during rejection. The diagnosis and monitoring of acute rejection may be facilitated by serial transvenous endomyocardial biopsies, which also may confirm the effectiveness of therapy. Under fluoroscopy, a forceps is passed through a catheter into the apex of the right ventricle via the right internal jugular vein and a small sample of myocardium is removed for histologic study.

A major obstacle to long-term survival is the development of obliterative coronary artery disease in the transplanted heart. The rejection process accelerates atherosclerosis. Improvement in survival rates is attributed to early and more accurate diagnosis of rejection and vigorous measures to prevent the atherosclerosis, which is thought to result from immunologic injury to the intima of the coronary vessels. An increase in malignant neoplasms in heart transplant patients has been observed. Patients who have undergone a heart transplant need psychologic support to maintain a will to live and to adjust to problems that may arise at any time.

Combined Heart-Lung Transplantation

The organs of the cardiopulmonary system can be transplanted as a unit. Patients with primary pulmonary hypertension or pulmonary vascular disease secondary to congenital heart disease may be candidates for heart-lung transplantation. Patients with cystic or pulmonary fibrosis and chronic end-stage pulmonary disease also may receive combined transplants. If cardiac function in these patients has not been affected by the disease, their hearts may be used as heartbeating donor cardiac transplants for another patient.

In both the donor and the recipient, the trachea is transected above the carina, and the heart and lungs are removed en bloc. This surgical technique preserves the recipient's phrenic, vagus, and recurrent laryngeal nerves on pedicles, a portion of the right atrium and vena cava, and the aortic arch. A clamshell incision is the approach of choice (Fig. 45-10).

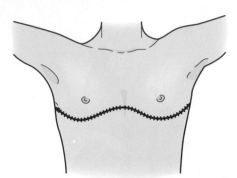

FIG. 45-10 Clamshell incision for double lung transplant.

The donor heart and lungs must fit without compression within the recipient's thoracic cavity. The donor trachea, right atrium, and aorta are anastomosed to corresponding structures in the recipient (Fig. 45-11).

Cyclosporine given both preoperatively and postoperatively enhances healing of the tracheal anastomosis and combats cellular-mediated rejection. Bacterial pneumonia from subclinical bacterial contamination in the donor tracheobronchial tree is the most common cause of morbidity and mortality after heart-lung transplantation.

Lung Transplantation

Transplantation of a single lung, usually the left one, may be performed in a patient with end-stage pulmonary fibrosis who is dependent on oxygen therapy. Both lungs may be replaced sequentially as two single-lung transplants rather than as an en bloc combined heart-lung transplant. Children with bronchopulmonary dysplasia, primary pulmonary hypertension, or congenital hiatal (diaphragmatic) hernia may benefit from a partial lung transplant. A lobe from a living relative may be transplanted instead of a whole lung from a cadaver source.

Optimum preservation of the donor organ is vitally important, and timing is critical. Ischemic time must be less than 4 hours; results improve as ischemic time decreases. Recipient preparation usually occurs simultaneously with donor procurement.

Single-lung transplantation involves bronchus-to-bronchus, pulmonary artery–to–pulmonary artery, and recipient pulmonary veins–to–donor atrial cuff anastomoses. The omentum is wrapped around the bronchus to provide additional blood supply and to support the anastomosis.

Many special problems affect the success of clinical lung transplantation:

- Recipients usually have some degree of pulmonary infection at the time of the surgical procedure. The recipient's remaining lung, if diseased, may be a source of infection.
- Ventilation-perfusion imbalance between the transplanted lung and the remaining lung may result in reduced function of the transplant.
- Imminent rejection is not easily recognized.
- Vascular and fibrotic changes produced by rejection create ischemia and anoxia.
- Healing at the site of bronchial anastomosis is a problem, but less so with cyclosporine and an omental wrap.

- The procedure is technically difficult. The size of the donor lung, hilar structures, and bronchus must approximate those of the recipient.

Liver Transplantation

Hepatic transplantation may be performed in select patients with nonmalignant end-stage liver disease. The ideal recipients are patients with primary liver disease. Successful liver transplantation is performed on infants and children with biliary atresia who develop chronic liver failure or on those with other liver or biliary problems. A preexisting infection in any part of the body is a distinct contraindication because the patient's preoperative status is poor and because the patient lacks the protective proteins normally produced by the liver. Postoperative infection is always a marked danger.

The liver is susceptible to damage from ischemia. However, a donor liver can be preserved for up to 24 hours with the infusion of cold Belzer-MPS solution.

The liver may be separated into two sections and used for two recipients. The left lobe or a left lateral segmental graft may be transplanted into an infant or child; the right side, which is larger, can be transplanted into an adult. For this reduced-size liver transplantation (RSLT) procedure, one team divides the donor organ while another team performs a hepatectomy on the recipient(s).

Successful living related liver transplantation is performed on infants and children with biliary atresia who develop chronic liver failure or on those with other liver or biliary problems. The adult donor gives the left lobe (the smaller lobe) if the recipient is an infant or a child.

Anatomic complexity, friability of tissue, and vascularity of the liver contribute to the technical hazards of liver transplantation (Fig. 45-12). The surgical procedure may take up to 20 hours to complete and requires both extensive dissection as well as ligation of vessels to avoid postoperative hemorrhage. The vena cava must be mobilized. After it is divided, the liver is removed and the donor organ anastomosed to the upper and then the lower vena cava as quickly as possible (Fig. 45-13). During this critical period, venous return from the lower half of the body must be decompressed via a venovenous extracorporeal membrane oxygenation (ECMO) pump from the iliac to the axillary arteries. After anastomoses of the portal vein and hepatic artery, any bleeding must be controlled before reconstruction of the bile duct (Fig. 45-14).

Rejection may be noted by changes in laboratory findings, such as alterations in serum enzyme levels and elevated serum bilirubin. Cellular infiltration of the graft causes impairment of clotting factors, liver cell necrosis, and impaired function. Complications from reconstruction of the biliary tract may lead to graft failure.

Pancreas Transplantation

A variety of techniques have been used in clinical pancreatic transplantation in the treatment of patients with severe diabetes and associated systemic complications. The goal is to provide physiologic islet function to achieve more satisfactory carbohydrate metabolism, to restore normal glucose homeostasis, and to prevent or halt secondary complications associated with diabetes mellitus. The whole

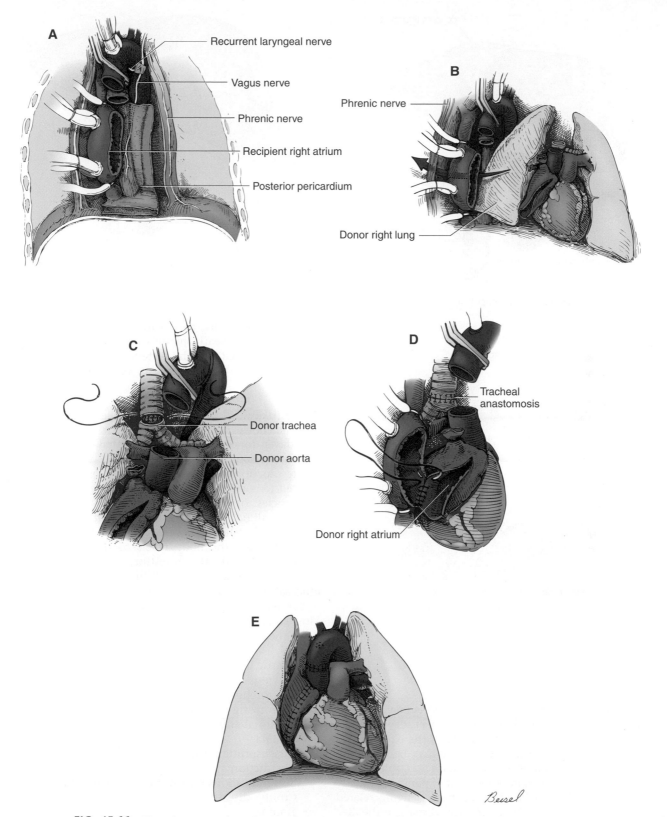

FIG. 45-11   Heart-lung transplantation. **A,** The recipient heart and lungs have been excised, exposing the posterior pericardium. Note the location of the phrenic, vagus, and recurrent laryngeal nerves and the right and left phrenic nerve pedicles. **B,** The recipient heart and lungs are brought onto the field; the right lung is passed beneath the recipient atriocaval remnant and right phrenic nerve to lie in the right pleura; the left lung will be placed beneath the left phrenic nerve and positioned in the left pleural space. **C,** The tracheal anastomosis is performed, followed by the right atrial anastomosis **(D)** and, finally, the aortic anastomosis **(E).**

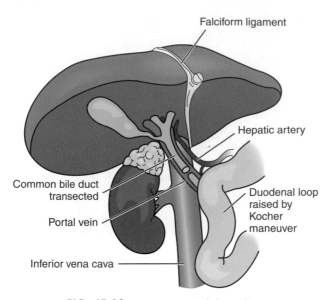

FIG. 45-12   Procurement of donor liver.

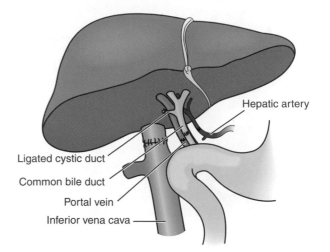

FIG. 45-14   Donor liver in situ after completion of anastomosis.

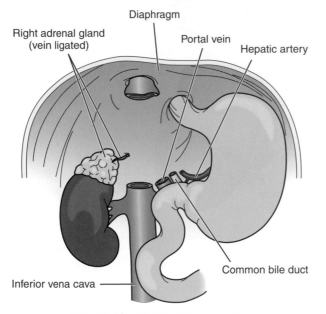

FIG. 45-13   Recipient liver resection.

pancreas, the distal segment, or isolated islets may be transplanted. The whole organ is obtained from a cadaver source. A kidney may be transplanted along with the pancreas.

A composite splanchnic organ graft may be obtained; this type of graft includes the entire pancreas, spleen, and a segment of the duodenum. A segment of pancreas, usually the tail and body, can be obtained from a living related donor and placed into the extraperitoneal space in the iliac fossa. The splenic artery and vein of the donor segment are anastomosed to the external iliac artery and vein of the recipient. Islet cells or beta cells may be isolated for transplantation; beta cells are injected into the liver.

The transplantation procedure must allow exocrine secretions to drain from the pancreatic ducts. This is accomplished most commonly by pancreaticocystostomy for urinary drainage or pancreaticojejunostomy for enteric drainage. Insulin is secreted into the systemic circulation via arterial anastomoses between the donor organ and the recipient vessels.

Small Intestine Transplantation

The small bowel can be procured from a living related donor or cadaver donor. From a living related donor, a minimal segment of 100 to 150 cm of small intestine with a branch of the superior mesenteric artery and vein may be transplanted to correct short-bowel syndrome, genetic enzyme deficiencies, or malabsorption disorders in children. The whole small bowel alone or in combination with the liver and other digestive structures can be used from a cadaver donor. Because the body reacts to the lymphoid tissue transplanted with the intestine, the donor transplant organ may be irradiated to kill the lymph cells but not the mucosal cells.

Survival rates for intestinal transplant are around 50%. Most complications are related to reactions in the lymph tissue, heavy bacterial load of the gut, and technical graft failure.

Pediatric indications for intestinal transplant include:
- Volvulus
- Gastroschisis
- Necrotizing enterocolitis
- Intestinal atresia
- Trauma
- Hirschsprung's disease
- Obstruction

Adult indications for intestinal transplant include:
- Crohn's disease
- Trauma
- Ischemia caused by thrombosis
- Familial polyposis
- Gardner syndrome
- Desmoid tumor
- Radiation enteritis
- Budd-Chiari syndrome

Bibliography

Brown, KA: Liver transplantation, *Curr Opin Gastroenterol* 21(3):331-336, 2005.

Deshpande RR et al: Results of split liver transplantation in children, *Ann Surg* 236(2):248-253, 2002.

Diaz GC et al: Donor health assessment after living-donor liver transplantation, *Ann Surg* 236(1):120-126, 2002.

Fryer JB: Intestinal transplantation: an update, *Curr Opin Gastroenterol* 21(2):162-168, 2005.

Imamura M et al: The first successful DeBakey VAD child implantation as a bridge to transplant, *ASAIO J* 51(5):670-672, 2005.

Jain A et al: Posttransplant lymphoproliferative disorders in liver transplantation: A 20-year experience, *Ann Surg* 236(4):429-436, 2002.

Kamoun M: Mechanisms of chronic allograft dysfunction, *Ther Drug Monitor* 28(1):14-18, 2006.

Machado C: The first organ transplant from a brain-dead donor, Comment in: Neurology, 2006. *Neurology* 64(11):1938-1942, 2005.

Nicholson ML et al: Influence of allograft size to recipient body-weight ratio on the long-term outcome of renal transplantation, *Br J Surg* 87(3):314-319, 2000.

Soin B et al: Xenotransplantation, *Br J Surg* 87(2):138-148, 2000.

Vulchev A et al: Ethical issues in split versus whole liver transplantation, *Am J Transplantation* 4(11):1737-1740, 2004.

Weill D: Donor criteria in lung transplantation: an issue revisited, *Chest* 121(6):2029-2031, 2002.

Index

Ethylene oxide (EO), 225, 302
  sterilization, 315-319
    advantages v. disadvantages of,
      316-317
    aeration time after, 317t, 318-319
    residual products of, 318-319
    types of, sterilizers, 317
    biologic testing of, 319
Eustress, 13
Eutectic mixture of local anesthetics
  (EMLA), 139
Euthanasia, 54-55. *See also* Ethical issues
Evacuation, surgical procedure of, 2t
Evidence
  -based practice, 26, 80
    sacred cows v., 92
  forensic, 119, 122, 123
  sexual assault, 120, 121
Evisceration, 581
Excimer laser, 356-357
Excision
  excisional biopsy, 387, 387f
  surgical procedure of, 2t
Exercise
  aging v., 163
  military preparedness via, 205
Exotoxin, 237, 238
Expander, 848, 866-867
  blood volume, 632-633
Expiration, 533
Explantation
  breast implant, 865-867, 865f
  prosthesis, 389t
Exploration, surgical procedure of, 2t
Exposing instruments, 335-336, 335f, 336f,
  337f, 338f
Exstrophy, bladder, 145-146, 239f
Extracorporeal membrane oxygenator
  (ECMO), 919, 948
Extraction, 2t
  cataract, 150, 826, 841
  extracapsular, 839-840
  intracapsular, 840
  surgical procedure of, 2t
Extravasation, 581
Extubation, 139-140, 420
Exudate, 581
  containing pathogens, 234, 234b
Eyes. *See also* Ophthalmic surgery; Vision
  aging influencing, 167t
  anatomy/physiology of, 827-828, 827f,
    833f
  Bishop eye forceps, 333f
  cornea, 167t, 835-837, 835f, 837f, 973,
    973b
  defense mechanism of, 233
  extraocular procedure, 149-150
  glasses, 269
    leaded, 218
    preoperative removal of, 380
    sideshields for, 259
  glaucoma, 838-839
  goniotomy, 150
  injuries to, 845-846
  lacrimal duct
    dilation, 834
    obstruction, 149
  laser surgery protection for, 360
  lashes, 834, 834f
  -lid, ptosis repair, 149
  muscles of, surgical procedures on,
    149-150
  myringotomy, 150, 150f
  pediatric patient, 150

Eyes (*contd*)
  phototherapeutic keratectomy, 836-837,
    837f
  pupillary distance, 350
  removal of, 834
  stye, 239, 239f, 834, 834f
  visual impairment, 103, 167t

F
Fabric
  dry heat sterilization for, 315
  tensile strength, 581
Face transplant, 850f, 862. *See also*
  Transplant, tissue
  American Association of Oral and
    Maxillofacial Surgeons, 195b
Facemask, 136, 137, 140
FACES Pain Rating Scale, 132-133, 133f
Facilities engineering department, 86-87
Facility-specific policies/procedures,
  20-21
Family
  American Academy of Family Physicians,
    195b
  candidacy for ambulatory surgery
    within, 195
  genetic studies, 389t
  housing/resources of geriatric patient's,
    165
  impact of surgery on, 102, 123
FASA. *See* Federated Ambulatory Surgery
  Association
Fasanella-Servat operation, 149
Fasciculation, 420
Fasciitis, 236f
  necrotizing, 600-601
FDA. *See* Food and Drug Administration
Feces
  containing pathogens, 234, 234b
  fecal-oral disease transmission, 245, 246
  infection transmission via, 236t
Federal Bureau of Prisons, 195b
Federal Medicare Act, 19
Federal Organ Transplantation and
  Procurement Act of 1983, 976
Federated Ambulatory Surgery
  Association (FASA), 193
Female reproductive system, 126, 233,
  695-698, 695f, 696f, 697f, 729f. *See also*
  Gynecologic surgery; Obstetric
  surgery; Pregnancy
  amenorrhea, 694
  amniotic fluid containing pathogens,
    234, 234b
  assisted reproduction, 720-722
  endometrium, 694, 700
  estrogen, 163
  hazards to, 227-228
  hegar uterine dilator, 342f
  hemostatic uterine clamps, 334f
  historical background of, 694-695
  kahn uterine cannula, 334f
  menarche, 694
  menorrhagia, 694
  menstruation, 694
  ova tissue, 389t
  Pap smear, 700
  reproductive sterilization, 53
  sexual assault, 120-121
  sexual intercourse, 167t
  sexually transmitted disease, 240
  Tanner's stages of sexual development,
    694
  transsexual surgery, 757-758

Female reproductive system (*contd*)
  uterine bleeding
    controlling, 552
    diabetes/obesity involving, 107t
  uterine curette, 331, 332f
  uterine sound, 342f
  vaginal infections, 234, 234b, 245, 700
  vaginal procedures, 706-709, 706f, 707f,
    708f, 709f
Femoropopliteal bypass graft, 961-962,
  961f
Fentanyl, 134t, 136, 139, 431t
Ferric subsulfate, 552
Fetus, 126
  cardiovascular defect in, 155-156
  fetal tissue research, 53
  intrauterine fetal surgery, 720, 720f
  vertebral column of, 809
Fever, 233. *See also* Infection;
  Temperature
  toxic shock syndrome causing, 238
Fibrillation, 221
  defibrillator, 219, 619-620, 946, 946f
  ventricular, 618, 619f, 949
Fibrin glue, 573b
File transfer protocol (FTP), 9b
Financial responsibility, 94-96
Fingernails
  acrylic, 196
  operating room hygiene for, 269
Fire safety, 24, 222-224, 222f, 224n, 354.
  See also Burns
  AORN recommended practices, 224,
    224n
  flash fire injury, 24, 214
  National Fire Protection Association, 19,
    214
  oxygen-enriched atmosphere
    requiring, 222-224, 222f
First surgical assistant, 64, 66-78, 68b, 68f,
  75-77, 76f, 77b, 83
  certified nurse midwife-, 77-78
  certified registered nurse-, 75-77, 76f,
    77b
  certified surgical technologist, 10, 33-35,
    33n, 50-52, 52b, 54, 58-59, 65, 65b
  duties of, 69-75, 69f, 70f, 71f, 72f, 73f,
    74f, 75f
  physician assistant, 78
FLACC Behavioral Pain Assessment Scale,
  132, 132n, 132t
Flap, 66, 848, 852-857, 853f, 868, 868f
  arterialized tissue, 856
  myocutaneous, 856, 899, 899f
  pedicle, 855, 855f
Flash/high-speed sterilization, 301,
  310-311, 310t, 311b, 314, 314t
  Association for the Advancement of
    Medical Instrumentation guide to,
    311n
  Association of periOperative Registered
    Nurses on, 311
Floor-mounted microscope, 364-365, 364f
Florae, 231
Fluid specimen, 24, 234, 234b, 259, 388,
  389t, 480-481
Flumazenil, 435
Fluorometer, 860
Fluoroquinolone, 247t
Fluoroscope, 390
Focal length, 350
Focus (microscope), 364
Foley catheter, 140, 680
Follow-up appointment, 196

Mycoplasmal infection, 236, 236t, 239-240, 289, 294t
  mycotic aneurysm, 950
  mycotoxins, 245
Mycosis, 245
Mycotic aneurysm, 950
Mycotoxins, 245
Mydriatics, 832, 832f
Myelography, 393
Myelomeningocele, 154
Myocardial hypertrophy, diabetes/obesity involving, 107t
Myocardial infarction (MI), 936, 949
Myositis, 236f
Myotomes, 807
Myringotomy, intraocular, 121, 150, 150f

N
Nail polish, 196
Naloxone, 140, 435
NANDA-International, 27b
NAON. *See* National Association of Orthopaedic Nurses
Narcan, 140
Narcosis, 420
Narcotics, 199, 421, 434
  reversal, 434-435
Narrative charting, 47
Nasolacrimal duct, congenital obstruction of, 149
Nasopharynx, contamination via, 253
National Association of Orthopaedic Nurses, 59
National Association of Orthopaedic Nurses (NAON), 59
National Board of Surgical Technology and Surgical Assisting (NBSTSA), 57-58, 65
  www.nbstsa.org, 65
National Center for Devices and Radiological Health (NCDRH), 358, 358b
National Commission for Certifying Agencies, 284
National Fire Protection Association (NFPA), 19
  hazard regulation, 214
National Institute for Occupational Safety and Health (NIOSH)
  hazard regulation, 214, 214n
  latex sensitivity, 228-229, 228t
  recommended practices for aseptic technique/safety, 21
National Institute of Health (NIH), 132n
National League for Nursing (NLN), 58-59
National Library of Medicine, 9
National Occupational Research Agenda (NORA)
  chemical hazards, 227
  hazard regulation, 214
NBSTSA. *See* National Board of Surgical Technology and Surgical Assisting
Nd:YAG laser. *See* Neodymium/yttrium/ aluminum/garnet
Near miss, 37
Nebulizer, 140
Neck. *See also* Otorhinolaryngologic surgery
  American Board of Otolaryngology, Head and Neck Surgery, 875
  preparation for surgery of, 520-521
  surgical procedures for, 891-900, 891f, 892f, 895f, 896f, 897f, 899f
  plastic surgery, 860-863, 861f, 862f, 863f

Necrosis, 581
  acute tubular necrosis, 949
  muscular, 106, 106f, 949
  necrotizing fasciitis, 600-601
Needle
  hypodermic, 410, 414, 416f
  interstitial, 113
  loading of, for suturing, 475f, 568f, 569f
  microsurgical, 343f
  needle biopsy, 387
  pediatric, 130f
  percutaneous, biopsy, 387
  radiation therapy interstitial, 113
  spring-loaded, 644
  sterile, 258
  surgical, 566-570, 566n, 567f, 567t, 568f, 569f
  Verres, 142, 643, 644
Negligence, 37, 38. *See also* Legal issues
  accountability v., 18, 37-38, 40-41
  corporate negligence doctrine, 40-41
Neisseria gonorrhoeae, 237t
Neisseria meningitidis, 237t
Nematodes, 246
Neodymium/yttrium/aluminum/garnet (nd:YAG) laser, 357
Neoplasia, 694
Neoplasm, 385
  of eyelid, 833, 834f
  intracranial, 799t
Nephrectomy, 145, 737. *See also* Urologic surgery
Nephrostomy, 145, 737. *See also* Urologic surgery
  percutaneous, 737f
Nerve block, 421, 451. *See also* Anesthesia
Nerve hooks, 344
Neuber, Gustav, 251, 267, 302
Neurologic system, 167t. *See also* Central nervous system; Neurosurgery; Spinal surgery
  diabetes/obesity involving, 107t
Neuromuscular blocker, 139, 435b
Neurosurgery, 787-806. *See also* Central nervous system; Spinal surgery
  adjuncts to visibility, 793
  cranium, 797-805
    arteriovenous malformation, 800f
    Burr holes, 798f
    cerebral artery aneurysm, 801f
    complications of, 804-805
    epilepsy, 803
    extracranial procedures, 803-804
    Hudson brace manual drill, 797f
    injuries, 804, 804f
    intracranial neoplasm, 799t
    stereotactic headframe, 801f
    stereotaxis, 801-802
  diagnostics, 790-791
  hemostasis, 791-793
  historical background of, 787-788
  patient preparation for, 794-796, 794f, 795f, 796f
  pediatric, 152-155, 153f, 154f
  peripheral nerves, 805-806
  prognostics, 791
NFPA. *See* National Fire Protection Association
Nightingale, Florence, 16, 16f, 17b, 58, 302
  environmental theory of, 17b
  Notes on Nursing: What It Is and What It Is Not, 99
NIH. *See* National Institute of Health

NIOSH. *See* National Institute for Occupational Safety and Health
Nitrofurantoin, 247t
Nitroglycerin, 439, 622-623
Nitroimidaxoles, 246, 247t
Nitrous oxide, 139, 430-432, 431t
  -narcotic-relaxant, 139
  occupational health hazards of, 225
Nitze cystoscope, 644, 728
Nitze, Maximilian, 643-644
NLN. *See* National League for Nursing
Noise levels, hospital, 215
Nomenclature, 15
Nonionizing radiation, 213, 219
Nonlipid viruses, 294t
Nonsterile team, 57, 261-262, 262f. *See also* Sterile team
  attire for, 269
  clothing, 269
  members of, 60-63, 61t, 62b
NORA. *See* National Occupational Research Agenda
Norepinephrine, 623, 624
Normovolemic hemodilution technique, 439
North American Association for Ambulatory Urgent Care, 195b
North American Transplant Coordinator Organization 24-Hour Alert, 976
Nose
  anatomy, 883-884, 883f
  nasal secretions containing pathogens, 234, 234b
  nasal speculum, 340f
  obstruction of nasolacrimal duct, 149
  physiology of, 884
  reconstruction, 855, 855f
  surgical procedures for, 884-887, 885f, 886f, 887f
Nosocomial infection, 231
Notes on Nursing: What It Is and What It Is Not (Nightingale), 99
Nothing by mouth (NPO), 196, 373
NPO. *See* Nothing by mouth
Nuclear medicine study, 385
Nurse. *See also* Circulating nurse; Perioperative nurse; Registered nurse; *specific type of care*
  career as, 15
    advanced practice nurse, 82-83
    American Nurses Association, 18, 20, 47-49, 48b, 51-52, 52b, 54, 195b
    American Society of PeriAnesthesia Nurses, 192, 193b
    American Society of Plastic Surgery Nurses, 59
    AORN, 18, 20, 24, 25, 27f, 28, 81, 193, 195b, 206-207, 211n, 311
      recommended practices, 9, 21, 54, 75, 193, 214, 224, 224n, 225n, 304t, 480-481
    Bachelor of Science in Nursing, 82-83
    Canadian Nurses Association, 51
    certified nurse midwife, 77-78
    certified perioperative nurse, 59-61, 60b, 61t, 83
    Cumulative Index to Nursing and Allied Health Literature, 9
    historical roots of, 99
    licensed practical and vocational, 59
    Master of Science in Nursing, 83
    military, 205
    National League for Nursing, 58-59